GYNECOLOGIC CANCER

GYNECOLOGIC CANCER

Controversies in Management

David M. Gershenson, MD
Professor and Chairman
Department of Gynecologic Oncology
The University of Texas M.D. Anderson Cancer Center
Houston, Texas

William P. McGuire, MD
Director
Oncology Service Line and Harry and Jeanette Weinberg
Cancer Institute
Franklin Square Hospital Center
Baltimore, Maryland

Martin Gore, PhD, FRCP
Professor of Cancer Medicine
Director
Rare Cancers Division
The Royal Marsden Hospital
London, United Kingdom

Michael A. Quinn,
MB ChB Glas, MGO Melb, MRCP, FRCOG,
FRANZCOG, CGO
Associate Professor
University of Melbourne
Director of Oncology/Dysplasia
Royal Women's Hospital
Melbourne, Australia

Gillian Thomas, MD
Professor of Radiation, Oncology, Obstetrics and Gynecology
Toronto-Sunnybrook Regional Cancer Center
Toronto, Ontario, Canada

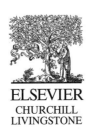

ELSEVIER
CHURCHILL
LIVINGSTONE

ELSEVIER
CHURCHILL
LIVINGSTONE

The Curtis Center
170 S Independence Mall W 300E
Philadelphia, Pennsylvania 19106
or
11830 Westline Industrial Drive
St. Louis, Missouri 63146

GYNECOLOGIC CANCER: Controversies in Management   ISBN 0-443-07142-X
Copyright © 2004 by Elsevier Ltd.

Distributed in the United Kingdom by Churchill Livingstone, Robert Stevenson House, 1-3 Baxter's Place, Leith Walk, Edinburgh EH1 3AF, Scotland, and by associated companies, branches, and representatives throughout the world.

Notice

Gynecology is an ever-changing field. Standard safety precautions must be followed, but as new research and clinical experience broaden our knowledge, changes in treatment and drug therapy may become necessary or appropriate. Readers are advised to check the most current product information provided by the manufacturer of each drug to be administered to verify the recommended dose, the method and duration of administration, and contraindications. It is the responsibility of the licensed prescriber, relying on experience and knowledge of the patient, to determine dosages and the best treatment for each individual patient. Neither the publisher nor the author assumes any liability for any injury and/or damage to persons or property arising from this publication.

The Publisher

Library of Congress Cataloging-in-Publication Data

Gynecologic cancer : controversies in management / [edited by] David M. Gershenson ... [et al.].
   p. ; cm.
  ISBN 0-443-07142-X (alk. paper)
  1. Generative organs, Female--Cancer. I. Gershenson, David M. (David Marc),
  [DNLM: 1. Genital Neoplasms, Female--therapy. WP 145 G9936 2004]
RC280.G5G875 2004
616.99'465--dc22

                                                           2004045146

Acquisitions Editor: Stephanie Donley
Developmental Editor: Alison Nastasi
Project Manager: Peter Faber
Design Coordinator: Gene Harris

Printed in the United States of America.

Last digit is the print number: 9   8   7   6   5   4   3   2   1

This book is dedicated to all those women
with gynecologic cancers who,
in the face of information gaps and therapeutic controversies,
have participated in clinical trials. Their hope, faith, courage,
and the support of their families have taught us
invaluable lessons about the human spirit.

CONTRIBUTORS

David S. Alberts, MD
Regents Professor of Medicine, Pharmacology, and Public Health, University of Arizona School of Medicine; Director, Cancer Prevention and Control, Arizona Cancer Center, Tucson, Arizona
Prevention of Gynecologic Malignancies

Yoland Antill, BMed, FRACP
Research Fellow, Department of Haematology and Medical Oncology, Peter MacCallum Cancer Centre, East Melbourne, Victoria, Australia
Screening and Diagnosis of Ovarian Cancer—High Risk; Management of Complications of Chemotherapy

Grazia Artioli, MD
Fellow, Department of Medical Oncology, University of Chicago Pritzker School of Medicine, Chicago, Illinois
Treatment of Recurrent Endometrial Cancer: Chemotherapy, Hormonal Therapy, and Radiotherapy

Richard E. Ashcroft, MA, PhD
Senior Lecturer in Medical Ethics, Imperial College London, London, United Kingdom
Bioethics

Mark Baekelandt, MD, PhD
Senior Consultant, Department of Gynecologic Oncology, The Norwegian Radium Hospital, Oslo, Norway
Treatment of Recurrent Uterine Sarcomas

Afshin Bahador, MD
Clinical Instructor, Division of Gynecologic Oncology, Department of Obstetrics and Gynecology, University of Southern California Keck School of Medicine, Los Angeles; Section Head, Division of Gynecologic Oncology, City of Hope National Medical Center, Duarte, California
Gynecologic Cancer in Pregnancy

Walter F. Baile, MD
Professor and Chief of Psychiatry, University of Texas M.D. Anderson Cancer Center, Houston, Texas
Death and Dying

Richard R. Barakat, MD
Associate Professor of Obstetrics and Gynecology, Cornell University Weill Medical College; Chief, Gynecology Service, Department of Surgery, Memorial Sloan-Kettering Cancer Center, New York, New York
Prevention of Gynecologic Malignancies

Karen M. Basen-Engquist, PhD, MPH
Associate Professor of Behavioral Science, University of Texas M.D. Anderson Cancer Center, Houston, Texas
Quality of Life in the Gynecologic Cancer Patient

Debra A. Bell, MD
Associate Professor of Pathology, Harvard Medical School; Associate Pathologist, Massachusetts General Hospital, Boston, Massachusetts
Borderline Ovarian Tumors

Doris M. Benbrook, PhD
Associate Professor, Department of Obstetrics and Gynecology, University of Oklahoma College of Medicine, Oklahoma City, Oklahoma
Prevention of Gynecologic Malignancies

Inbar Ben-Shachar, MD
Lecturer, Department of Obstetrics and Gynecology, Hebrew University School of Medicine; Department of Obstetrics and Gynecology, Hadassah Medical Center, Jerusalem, Israel
The Role of Laparoscopy in the Management of Gynecologic Cancers

Ross S. Berkowitz, MD
William H. Baker Professor of Gynecology, Harvard Medical School; Director, Gynecologic Oncology, and Co-Director, New England Trophoblastic Disease Center, Department of Obstetrics and Gynecology, Brigham and Women's Hospital and Dana Farber Cancer Institute, Boston, Massachusetts
Epidemiology, Genetics, and Molecular Biology of Gestational Trophoblastic Disease

Diane C. Bodurka, MD
Associate Professor, Department of Gynecologic Oncology, University of Texas M.D. Anderson Cancer Center, Houston, Texas
Quality of Life in the Gynecologic Cancer Patient

John F. Boggess, MD
Assistant Professor, Division of Gynecologic Oncology, University of North Carolina at Chapel Hill School of Medicine, Chapel Hill, North Carolina
Prevention of Gynecologic Malignancies

Jeffrey Boyd, PhD
Attending Biologist and Member, Department of Surgery and Medicine, Memorial Sloan-Kettering Cancer Center, New York, New York
Hereditary Gynecologic Cancer Syndromes

Mark F. Brady, PhD
Research Associate Professor, Department of Biostatistics, State University of New York at Buffalo, Director of Statistics, GOG Statistical and Data Center, Buffalo, New York
Biostatistics and Clinical Trials

Molly A. Brewer, DVM, MD, MS
Director, Gynecologic Oncology Assistant Professor, Obstetrics and Gynecology, University of Arizona, College of Medicine, Tucson, Arizona
Prevention of Gynecologic Malignancies

Louise A. Brinton, MPH, PhD
Chief, Hormonal and Reproductive Epidemiology Branch, Division of Cancer Epidemiology and Genetics, National Cancer Institute, Rockville, Maryland
Epidemiology of Uterine Cancers;
Prevention of Gynecologic Malignancies

Robert E. Bristow, MD
Associate Professor of Gynecology and Obstetrics, Johns Hopkins University School of Medicine; Director, Kelly Gynecologic Oncology Service, Department of Gynecology and Obstetrics, Johns Hopkins Medical Institutions, Baltimore, Maryland
Management of Advanced Endometrial Cancer;
Management of Complications of Surgery

Robert Brown, MBBS, FRCPA
Associate Lecturer, University of Melbourne Faculty of Medicine; Pathologist, Royal Women's Hospital and Freemasons Hospital, Melbourne, Victoria, Australia
Management of Superficially Invasive Carcinoma of the Cervix

Robert Buckman, MD, PhD
Medical Oncologist and Professor, Department of Medicine, Princess Margaret Hospital, University of Toronto, Toronto, Ontario, Canada; Adjunct Professor, Department of Neuro-Oncology, M.D. Anderson Cancer Center, Houston, Texas
Death and Dying

Henry Burger, MD, FRACP
Honorary Professorial Fellow, Monash University Faculty of Medicine; Emeritus Director, Prince Henry's Institute of Medical Research, Monash Medical Centre, Clayton, Victoria, Australia
Menopause and Hormone Replacement Therapy

Thomas W. Burke, MD
Professor, Gynecologic Oncology, University of Texas M.D. Anderson Cancer Center, Houston, Texas
Advanced-Stage Vulvar Cancer

Higinia R. Cardenes, MD, PhD
Associate Professor of Clinical Radiation Oncology, Department of Radiation Oncology, Indiana University School of Medicine, Indianapolis, Indiana
Treatment of Recurrent Vaginal, Vulvar, and Cervical Cancer

Susan V. Carr, MB, ChB, MFFP, MPhil
Honorary Senior Lecturer, University of Glasgow, Gilmorehill, Glasgow, Scotland, Consultant in Family Planning and Sexual Health, The Sandyford Initiative, Glasgow, Scotland, United Kingdom
Sexuality and Gynecologic Cancer

Jonathan Carter, MD
Associate Professor, Head, Gynaecological Oncology Royal Prince Alfred Hospital; Head, Sydney Gynaecological Oncology Group, Sydney Cancer Centre, Camperdown, Australia
Primary Surgery for Ovarian Cancer

Philip E. Castle, PhD, MPH
Investigator, Hormonal and Reproductive Epidemiology Branch, Division of Cancer Epidemiology and Genetics, National Cancer Institute, NIH, DHHS, Rockville, Maryland
Prevention of Gynecologic Malignancies

Y. M. Chan, MBBS, MRCOG, FHKAM
Honorary Assistant Professor, University of Hong Kong Faculty of Medicine; Medical Officer, Accredited Gynaecological Oncologist, Department of Obstetrics and Gynaecology, Queen Mary Hospital, Hong Kong
Screening, Diagnosis, and Staging of Cervical Cancer

Pui C. (Joan) Cheng, MD
Associate Professor of Gynecologic Oncology and Chief, Section of Gynecologic Oncology and Adjunct Assistant Professor of Medicine, Section of Hematology/Oncology, Tulane University School of Medicine; Chief, Section of Gynecologic Oncology, University Hospital, New Orleans, Louisiana
Gynecologic Cancer in Pregnancy

Cheryl L. Chernicky, MT
Laboratory Supervisor, Department of Obstetrics and Gynecology, University MacDonald Women's Hospital, Cleveland, Ohio
Molecular Biology of Cervical and Vulvar Carcinoma

Christina S. Chu, MD
Assistant Professor, Department of Obstetrics and Gynecology, University of Pennsylvania School of Medicine, Philadelphia, Pennsylvania
Management of Intestinal Obstruction in the Terminal Patient and Management of Ascites

David E. Cohn, MD
Assistant Professor, Division of Gynecologic Oncology, Department of Obstetrics and Gynecology, Ohio State University College of Medicine and Public Health; Attending, Arthur G. James Cancer Hospital and Solove Research Institute, Columbus, Ohio
Vaginal Reconstruction in Pelvic Exenteration

Nicoletta Colombo, MD
Associate Professor of Obstetrics and Gynecology, University of Milan Bicoceni; Director, Gynecologic Oncology Unit, European Institute of Oncology, Milan, Italy
Ovarian Sex Cord–Stromal Tumors

Denise C. Connolly, PhD
Assistant Member, Department of Medical Oncology, Fox Chase Cancer Center, Philadelphia, Pennsylvania
Molecular Biology and Molecular Genetics of Ovarian, Fallopian Tube, and Primary Peritoneal Cancers

Larry J. Copeland, MD
Professor and Chair, Department of Obstetrics and Gynecology, Ohio State University College of Medicine and Public Health; Attending, Arthur G. James Cancer Hospital, Columbus, Ohio
Vaginal Reconstruction in Pelvic Exenteration

Allan Covens, MD
Head, Division of Gynecologic Oncology, University of Toronto, Toronto-Sunnybrook Regional Cancer Center, Toronto, Canada
Fertility and Gynecologic Cancer

Hervé Cure, MD, PhD
Professor of Oncology, Jean-Perrin Anticancer Centre, Clermont-Ferrand and University Hospital, Clermont-Ferrand, France
Dose Intensity in the Treatment of Advanced Epithelial Ovarian Cancer

John Patrick Curtin, MD
Professor and Chair, Department of Obstetrics and Gynecology; Director, Gynecologic Oncology New York University School of Medicine, New York University Medical Center, New York, New York
Early-Stage Cervical Cancer

Dusica Cvetkovic, MS, MD
Postdoctoral Associate, Department of Medical Oncology, Fox Chase Cancer Center, Philadelphia, Pennsylvania
Molecular Biology and Molecular Genetics of Ovarian, Fallopian Tube, and Primary Peritoneal Cancers

Mary Daly, MD, PhD
Director, Cancer Prevention and Control Program, Fox Chase Cancer Center, Division of Population Science, Philadelphia, Pennsylvania
Prevention of Gynecologic Malignancies

Zoreh Davanipour, DVM, PhD
Roswell Park Cancer Center, Cancer Prevention, Epidemiology and Biostatistics, Buffalo, New York
Prevention of Gynecologic Malignancies

Margaret Lorraine Jeune Davy, MBBS, FRANZCOG, FRCOG, CGO
Senior Lecturer, Department of Obstetrics and Gynaecology, University of Adelaide Faculty of Medicine; Director, Gynaecological Oncology, Women's Health Centre, Royal Adelaide Hospital, Adelaide, South Australia, Australia
Primary Fallopian Tube Cancer

Lesa M. Dawson, MD, FRCSC
Assistant Professor, Department of Obstetrics and Gynecology, Memorial University of Newfoundland Faculty of Medicine; Gynecologic Oncologist, Health Sciences Centre, Health Care Corporation of St. John's, St. John's, Newfoundland, Canada
Ovarian Sarcomas

Michael T. Deavers, MD
Associate Professor, Department of Pathology, University of Texas M.D. Anderson Cancer Center, Houston, Texas
Pathology of Vulvar, Vaginal, and Cervical Cancers

Marcela G. del Carmen, MD
Assistant Professor, Harvard Medical School; Attending, Massachusetts General Hospital, Boston, Massachusetts
Management of Complications of Surgery

Susan S. Devesa, MHS, PhD
Chief, Descriptive Studies Section, Biostatistics Branch, Division of Cancer Epidemiology and Genetics, National Cancer Institute, Rockville, Maryland
Epidemiology of Uterine Cancers

Patricia J. Eifel, MD, FACR
Professor and Director of Clinical Research, Department of Radiation Oncology, University of Texas M.D. Anderson Cancer Center, Houston, Texas
Early-Stage Cervical Cancer

Grainne Flannelly, MD, FRCPI, MRCOG
Consultant Obstetritian and Gynaecologist, National Maternity Hospital, Dublin, Ireland
Preinvasive Diseases of the Cervix, Vagina, and Vulva

Gini F. Fleming, MD
Associate Professor of Medicine and Director, Medical Oncology Breast Program, Section of Hematology/Oncology, University of Chicago Hospitals, Chicago, Illinois
Treatment of Recurrent Endometrial Cancer: Chemotherapy, Hormonal Therapy, and Radiotherapy

Jeffrey M. Fowler, MD
Professor and Director, and J.G. Boutselis Chair in Gynecologic Oncology, Ohio State University College of Medicine and Public Health, Division of Gynecologic Oncology, Columbus, Ohio
The Role of Laparoscopy in the Management of Gynecologic Cancers

Eduardo L. Franco, MPH, Dr PH
James McGill Professor of Epidemiology and Oncology and Director, Division of Cancer Epidemiology, McGill University Faculty of Medicine; CIHR Distinguished Scientist, FRSQ Chercheur National, Montreal, Quebec, Canada
Epidemiology of Cervical, Vulvar, and Vaginal Cancers

Francisco A. R. Garcia, MD, MPH
Associate Professor of Obstetrics and Gynecology, University of Arizona School of Medicine, Tucson, Arizona
Prevention of Gynecologic Malignancies

David M. Gershenson, MD
Professor and Chairman, Department of Gynecologic Oncology, The University of Texas M.D. Anderson Cancer Center, Houston, Texas

Giselle B. Ghurani, MD
Fellow in Gynecologic Oncology, University of Miami School of Medicine, Jackson Memorial Medical Center, Department of Obstetrics and Gynecology, Miami, Florida
Urinary Conduits in the Practice of Gynecologic Oncology

Barbara A. Goff, MD
Associate Professor, Gynecologic Oncology, University of Washington, Department of Obstetrics and Gynecology; Gynecologic Oncologist, University of Washington Medical Center, Seattle, Washington
Primary Peritoneal Cancer

Donald P. Goldstein, MD
Professor of Obstetrics, Gynecology, and Reproductive Biology, Harvard Medical School; Director, New England Trophoblastic Disease Center, Brigham and Women's Hospital and Dana Farber Cancer Institute, Boston, Massachusetts
Epidemiology, Genetics, and Molecular Biology of Gestational Trophoblastic Disease

Paul J. Goodfellow, PhD
Professor, Departments of Surgery and Obstetrics and Gynecology, Washington University School of Medicine, St. Louis, Missouri
Molecular Genetics of Endometrial Cancers

Martin Gore, PhD, FRCP
Professor of Cancer Medicine, Director, Rare Cancers Division, The Royal Marsden Hospital, London, United Kingdom

Mark H. Greene, MD
Chief, Clinical Genetics Branch, Division of Cancer Epidemiology and Genetics, National Cancer Institute, Rockville, Maryland
Epidemiology of Ovarian, Fallopian Tube, and Primary Peritoneal Cancers

Benjamin E. Greer, MD
Professor of Obstetrics and Gynecology, University of Washington School of Medicine; Director, Division of Gynecologic Oncology, Department of Obstetrics and Gynecology, University of Washington Medical Center, Seattle, Washington
Management of Complications of Radiotherapy

Kathryn M. Greven, MD
Professor of Radiation Oncology, Wake Forest University Medical School, Winston-Salem, North Carolina
Management of Early-Stage Endometrial Cancer

Perry W. Grigsby, MD
Professor of Radiation Oncology/Nuclear Medicine, Washington University School of Medicine; Staff, Barnes-Jewish Hospital, St. Louis, Missouri
Vaginal Cancer

Jane Groves, BSc, RGN
Specialist Lecturer, University of Central England, Birmingham, and University of Coventry and Warwickshire, Coventry; Macmillan Clinical Nurse Specialist in Gynaecological-Oncology, Good Hope Hospital NHS Trust, West Midlands, United Kingdom
The Gynecologic Cancer Patient and Her Family

Thomas C. Hamilton, PhD
Adjunct Professor, Department of Chemistry, Lehigh University, Bethlehem; Senior Member and Leader of Ovarian Cancer Program, Department of Medical Oncology, Fox Chase Cancer Center, Philadelphia, Pennsylvania
Molecular Biology and Molecular Genetics of Ovarian, Fallopian Tube, and Primary Peritoneal Cancers

Mark G. Hanly, FRCPath (Lond), FCAP
Clinical Associate Professor of Pathology, Director of Anatomical Pathology and Cytopathology Services, Medical College of Georgia, Southeast Georgia Health System Department of Pathology, Brunswick, Georgia
Prevention of Gynecologic Malignancies

Michael R. Hendrickson, MD
Professor of Pathology, Stanford University School of Medicine; Co-Director, Laboratory of Surgical Pathology, Stanford University Medical Center, Stanford, California
Pathology of Uterine Cancers

Lisa M. Hess, MA
Associate Scientific Investigator, Cancer Center Division, College of Medicine, University of Arizona, Tucson, Arizona
Prevention of Gynecologic Malignancies

Jeffrey F. Hines, MD
Instructor, Gynecologic Oncology, Attending Gynecologic Oncologist Department of Obstetrics and Gynecology, Morehouse School of Medicine, Southeastern Gynecologic, LLC, Riverdale, Georgia
Prevention of Gynecologic Malignancies

Michael P. Hopkins, MD
Professor of Obstetrics and Gynecology, Northeast Ohio Universities College of Medicine, Rootstown; Director, Department of Obstetrics and Gynecology, Aultman Health Foundation, Canton, Ohio
Adenocarcinoma of the Cervix

Hedvig Hricak, MD, PhD
Professor of Radiology, Weill Medical College of Cornell University; Chairman, Department of Radiology, Memorial Sloan-Kettering Cancer Center, New York, New York
Imaging of Gynecologic Malignancies

Ian J. Jacobs, MD, MRCOG
Professor of Gynaecological Oncology, St. Bartholomew's Hospital, London, United Kingdom
Screening and Diagnosis of Ovarian Cancer in the General Population

Hilary Jefferies, BSc (Hons), RGN
Specialist Lecturer, University of Central England; Macmillan Clinical Nurse Specialist in Gynaecological Oncology, Birmingham Women's Healthcare NHS Trust, Birmingham, United Kingdom
The Gynecologic Cancer Patient and Her Family

Janne Kaern, MD, PhD
Senior Consultant, Department of Gynecologic Oncology, The Norwegian Radium Hospital, Oslo, Norway
Adjuvant Treatment for Early-Stage Epithelial Ovarian Cancer

Karin Kapp, MD
Associate Professor, Department of Radiotherapy, University of Graz Faculty of Medicine, Graz, Austria
Primary Treatment of Uterine Sarcomas

Joseph Kelaghan, MD, MPH
Program Director, Division of Cancer Prevention, National Cancer Institute, Bethesda, Maryland
Prevention of Gynecologic Malignancies

F. Joseph Kelly, MD
Clinical Assistant Professor, Department of Obstetrics and Gynecology, Division of Gynecologic Oncology, University of South Florida, College of Medicine, Tampa; Gynecologic Oncologist, Lee Cancer Care, Fort Myers, Florida
Perioperative Care

Samir N. Khleif, MD
Naval Hospital Bethesda, National Cancer Institute, Bethesda, Maryland
Biologic Therapy for Gynecologic Malignancies

Wui-Jin Koh, MD
Professor of Radiation Oncology, University of Washington, Department of Radiation Oncology, Seattle, Washington
Locally Advanced Cervical Cancer; Management of Complications of Radiotherapy

Carol Kosary, MA
Mathematical Statistician, Surveillance, Epidemiology, and End Results Program, Surveillance Research Program, Division of Cancer Control and Population Sciences, National Cancer Institute, Bethesda, Maryland
Melanoma of the Female Genital Tract

Joan L. Kramer, MD
Cancer Genetics Fellow, Clinical Genetics Branch, Division of Cancer Epidemiology and Genetics, National Cancer Institute, Rockville, Maryland
Epidemiology of Ovarian, Fallopian Tube, and Primary Peritoneal Cancers

James V. Lacey, Jr, MPH, PhD
Investigator, Hormonal and Reproductive Epidemiology Branch, Division of Cancer Epidemiology and Genetics, National Cancer Institute, Rockville, Maryland
Epidemiology of Uterine Cancers

Rachelle Lanciano, MD
Director, Department of Radiation Oncology, Delaware County Memorial Hospital, Drexel Hill, Pennsylvania
Management of Advanced Endometrial Cancer

Charles Levenback, MD
Professor and Deputy Chairman, Department of Gynecologic Oncology, and Medical Director, Gynecologic Oncology Center, University of Texas M.D. Anderson Cancer Center, Houston, Texas
Lymphatic Mapping of the Female Genital Tract

J. Norelle Lickiss, MD, FRACP, FRCP(Edin)
Clinical Professor (Medicine), University of Sydney Faculty of Medicine, Sydney; Director, Sydney Institute of Palliative Medicine, Royal Prince Alfred Hospital, Camperdown, and Royal Hospital for Women, Sydney, New South Wales, Australia
Pain Control in Patients with Gynecologic Cancer

Harry J. Long, MD
Professor of Oncology, Mayo Clinic College of Medicine; Consultant in Medical Oncology, Mayo Clinic, Rochester, Minnesota
Treatment of Recurrent Vaginal, Vulvar, and Cervical Cancer

Teri A. Longacre, MD
Associate Professor of Pathology, Stanford University School of Medicine; Co-Director of Residency Program, Laboratory of Surgical Pathology, Stanford University Medical Center, Stanford, California
Pathology of Uterine Cancers

M. Patrick Lowe, MD
Fellow in Gynecologic Oncology, University of Southern California Keck School of Medicine, Los Angeles, California
Gynecologic Cancer in Pregnancy

Karen H. Lu, MD
Assistant Professor, Department of Gynecologic Oncology, University of Texas M.D. Anderson Cancer Center, Houston, Texas
Controversies in Endometrial Cancer Screening and Diagnosis; Borderline Ovarian Tumors

Joseph A. Lucci, III, MD
Professor and Director, Division of Gynecologic Oncology, Department of Obstetrics and Gynecology, University of Miami School of Medicine, Sylvester Comprehensive Cancer Center, Miami, Florida
Prevention of Gynecologic Malignancies

David M. Luesley, MA(CANTAB), MD, FRCOG
Professor of Gynaecological Oncology, Birmingham University Faculty of Medicine; Consultant Gynaecological Oncologist, Birmingham Women's Hospital, Birmingham, United Kingdom
Screening, Diagnosis, and Staging of Cervical Cancer

Anais Malpica, MD
Associate Professor, Department of Pathology, University of Texas M.D. Anderson Cancer Center, Houston, Texas
Pathology of Vulvar, Vaginal, and Cervical Cancers

Maurie Markman, MD
Chairman, Department of Hematology/Medical Oncology, Cleveland Clinic Foundation, Cleveland, Ohio
Decision-Making in the Management of Recurrent Epithelial Ovarian Cancer

William P. McGuire, MD
Director, Oncology Service Line and Harry and Jeanette Weinberg Cancer Institute, Franklin Square Hospital Center, Baltimore, Maryland

Michael W. Method, MD, MPH
Vice Chair, Board of Directors/Investigator: Northern Indiana Cancer Research Consortium (NICRC); Director, Oncology Services: Saint Joseph Regional Medical Center, South Bend, Indiana
Prevention of Gynecologic Malignancies

Linda Mileshkin, MBBS, FRACP, MBioeth(Mon)
Fellow, Department of Medicine, University of Melbourne Faculty of Medicine; Consultant Medical Oncologist, Peter MacCallum Cancer Centre, Melbourne, Victoria, Australia
Management of Complications of Chemotherapy

Lori Minasian, MD
Chief, Community Oncology and Prevention Trials Research Group, Division of Cancer Prevention, National Cancer Institute, Bethesda, Maryland
Prevention of Gynecologic Malignancies

Svetlana Mironov, MD
Assistant Professor, Department of Radiology, Weill Medical College of Cornell University; Assistant Attending, Memorial Sloan-Kettering Cancer Center, New York, New York
Imaging of Gynecologic Malignancies

F. J. Montz, MD*
Formerly Professor of Gynecology and Obstetrics, Surgery, and Oncology, Johns Hopkins University School of Medicine, Baltimore, Maryland
Management of Complications of Surgery

Margaret Mooney, MD
Senior Investigator, Surgery Section, Clinical Investigations Branch, Cancer Therapy Evaluation Program, Division of Cancer Treatment and Diagnosis, National Cancer Institute, Bethesda, Maryland
Melanoma of the Female Genital Tract

David H. Moore, MD
Department of Obstetrics and Gynecology, Indiana University Cancer Center, Professor and Chief of Gynecologic Oncology, Indiana University School of Medicine, Indianapolis, Indiana
Treatment of Recurrent Vaginal, Vulvar, and Cervical Cancer

Franco Muggia, MD
Anne Murnick Logan and David H. Logan Professor of Oncology, Departments of Medicine (Cancer Center) and Medicine (Oncology), New York University Cancer Institute, New York, New York
Chemotherapy for Refractory Epithelial Ovarian Cancer

Carolyn Muller, MD, FACOG
Associate Professor of Obstetrics and Gynecology, UT Southwestern Medical Center, Dallas, Texas
Prevention of Gynecologic Malignancies

Arno J. Mundt, MD
Assistant Professor of Radiation and Cellular Oncology and Residency Program Director, University of Chicago Pritzker School of Medicine, Chicago, Illinois
Treatment of Recurrent Endometrial Cancer: Chemotherapy, Hormonal Therapy, and Radiotherapy

*Deceased.

David G. Mutch, MD
Professor, Department of Obstetrics and Gynecology, Washington University School of Medicine; Head, Division of Gynecologic Oncology, Barnes-Jewish Hospital, St. Louis, Missouri
Molecular Genetics of Endometrial Cancers

George L. Mutter, MD
Associate Professor of Pathology, Pathologist, Division of Women's and Perinatal Pathology, Harvard Medical School, Department of Pathology, Brigham and Women's Hospital, Department of Pathology, Boston, Massachusetts
Prevention of Gynecologic Malignancies

Edward S. Newlands, BM, BCh, PhD, FRCP
Professor of Cancer Medicine, Imperial College School of Medicine; Honorary Consultant, Charing Cross Hospital, London, United Kingdom
Management of Gestational Trophoblastic Disease

James L. Nicklin, MBBS, FRANZCOG, CGO
Senior Lecturer (Clinical), Department of Obstetrics and Gynaecology, University of Queensland Faculty of Medicine; Visiting Gynaecologic Oncologist, Wesley Hospital and Royal Women's Hospital, Brisbane, Queensland, Australia
Secondary Surgery for Epithelial Ovarian Cancer

James W. Orr, Jr., MD
Clinical Professor, Department of Obstetrics and Gynecology, University of South Florida College of Medicine, Tampa; Medical Director, Florida Gynecologic Oncology; Medical Director, Lee Cancer Care, Lee Memorial Hospital, Fort Myers, Florida
Perioperative Care

Andrew G. Östör, MD*
Formerly Associate Professor, Department of Obstetrics and Gynecology, University of Melbourne Faculty of Medicine, Melbourne, Victoria, Australia
Pathology of Vulvar, Vaginal, and Cervical Cancers;
* Primary Treatment of Uterine Sarcomas*

Gabriella Parma, MD
Assistant, Gynecologic Oncology Unit, European Institute of Oncology, Milan, Italy
Ovarian Sex Cord–Stromal Tumors

Istvan Pataki, MD
Radiation Oncologist, Department of Radiation Oncology, Delaware County Memorial Hospital, Drexel Hill, Pennsylvania
Management of Advanced Endometrial Cancer

Manuel A. Peñalver, MD
Professor of Obstetrics and Gynecology, University of Miami School of Medicine, Jackson Memorial Medical Center, Department of Obstetrics and Gynecology, Miami, Florida
Urinary Conduits in the Practice of Gynecologic Oncology

Edgar Petru, MD
Associate Professor, Department of Obstetrics and Gynecology, University of Graz Faculty of Medicine, Graz, Austria
Primary Treatment of Uterine Sarcomas

Kelly-Anne Phillips, MBBS, MD
Associate Professor of Medicine, University of Melbourne Faculty of Medicine; Consultant Medical Oncologist, Department of Haematology and Medical Oncology, Peter MacCallum Cancer Centre, East Melbourne, Victoria, Australia
Screening and Diagnosis of Ovarian Cancer—High Risk

Karl C. Podratz, MD, PhD
Professor of Obstetrics and Gynecology, Mayo Clinic, Department of Obstetrics and Gynecology, Rochester, Minnesota
Management of Early-Stage Endometrial Cancer

Michael A. Quinn, MB ChB Glas, MGO Melb, MRCP, FRCOG, FRANZCOG, CGO
Associate Professor, University of Melbourne, Director of Oncology/Dysplasia, Royal Women's Hospital, Melbourne, Australia

Janet S. Rader, MD
Associate Professor, Department of Obstetrics and Gynecology, Division of Gynecologic Oncology, and Department of Genetics, Washington University School of Medicine; Staff, Barnes-Jewish Hospital, St. Louis, Missouri
Prevention of Gynecologic Malignancies

Lois M. Ramondetta, MD
Assistant Professor, Department of Gynecologic Oncology, University of Texas M.D. Anderson Cancer Center, Houston, Texas
Controversies in Endometrial Cancer Screening and Diagnosis

Marcus E. Randall, MD
Chair and William A. Mitchell Professor, Department of Radiation Oncology, Indiana University School of Medicine, Indianapolis, Indiana
Treatment of Recurrent Vaginal, Vulvar,
* and Cervical Cancer*

Nick Reed, MBBS, FRCR, FRCP(Glas)
Honorary Senior Lecturer in Clinical Oncology, University of Glasgow Faculty of Medicine; Consultant Clinical Oncologist, Beatson Oncology Centre, Western Infirmary, Glasgow, Scotland
Treatment of Recurrent Uterine Sarcomas

Danny Rischin, MBBS(Hons), FRACP
Associate Professor, Department of Medicine, University of Melbourne Faculty of Medicine; Head, Solid Tumor Developmental Therapeutics Program, Division of Haematology and Medical Oncology, Peter MacCallum Cancer Centre, Melbourne, Victoria, Australia
Management of Complications of Chemotherapy

*Deceased.

Melissa J. Robbie, MBBS, FRCPA
Honorary Associate, Department of Obstetrics and Gynaecology, University of Melbourne Faculty of Medicine, Parkville; Pathologist, St. Vincent's Hospital/ Mercy Hospital for Women, Melbourne, Victoria, Australia
Pathology of Ovarian, Fallopian Tube, and Primary Peritoneal Cancers

Gustavo Rodriguez, MD
Associate Professor, Department of Obstetrics and Gynecology; Director, Division of Gynecologic Oncology, Feinberg School of Medicine, Northwestern University, Evanston Northwestern Healthcare, Evanston, Illinois
Prevention of Gynecologic Malignancies

Phillip Y. Roland, MD
Director of South Lee County Gynecologic Oncology, Lee Cancer Care, Lee Memorial Hospital, Fort Myers, Florida
Perioperative Care

Lynda D. Roman, MD
Associate Professor of Gynecologic Oncology, University of Southern California Keck School of Medicine, Los Angeles, California
Gynecologic Cancer in Pregnancy

Robert Rome, MBBS, FRCSEd, FRCOG, FRANZCOG, CGO
Senior Fellow, Department of Obstetrics and Gynaecology, University of Melbourne; Associate Director, Oncology and Dysplasia Unit, Royal Women's Hospital, and Gynecologic Oncologist, Freemasons Hospital, Melbourne, Australia
Management of Superficially Invasive Carcinoma of the Cervix

Peter G. Rose, MD
Professor, Division of Gynecologic Oncology, Department of Obstetrics and Gynecology, Case Western Reserve University School of Medicine; Director, Division of Gynecologic Oncology, Cleveland Clinic Medical Center, Cleveland, Ohio
Locally Advanced Cervical Cancer

Stephen C. Rubin, MD
Franklin Payne Professor of Gynecologic Oncology, University of Pennsylvania School of Medicine; Chief, Division of Gynecologic Oncology, University of Pennsylvania Medical Center, Philadelphia, Pennsylvania
Management of Intestinal Obstruction in the Terminal Patient and Management of Ascites

Barnaby Rufford, MBBS, MRCOG
Clinical Research Fellow, St. Bartholomew's Hospital, London, United Kingdom
Screening and Diagnosis of Ovarian Cancer in the General Population

Anthony H. Russell, MD
Associate Professor of Radiation Oncology, Harvard Medical School; Radiation Oncologist, Massachusetts General Hospital, Boston, Massachusetts
Advanced-Stage Vulvar Cancer

Scott Saxman, MD
Associate Professor of Medicine, Uniformed Services University of the Health Sciences F. Edward Hébert School of Medicine; Senior Investigator, Clinical Investigations Branch, Cancer Therapy Evaluation Program, Division of Cancer Treatment and Diagnosis, National Cancer Institute, Bethesda, Maryland
Melanoma of the Female Genital Tract

Peter E. Schwartz, MD
John Slade Ely Professor of Obstetrics and Gynecology and Vice Chairman, Department of Obstetrics and Gynecology, Yale University School of Medicine; Section Chief, Gynecologic Oncology, Yale–New Haven Hospital, New Haven, Connecticut
Hormonal Treatment of Ovarian Cancer

Michael J. Seckl, MBBS, PhD, FRCP
Professor of Molecular Cancer Medicine, Imperial College School of Medicine; Consultant in Cancer Medicine, Department of Medical Oncology, Charing Cross Hospital, London, United Kingdom
Management of Gestational Trophoblastic Disease

Mark E. Sherman, MD
Expert, Hormonal and Reproductive Epidemiology Branch, Division of Cancer Epidemiology and Genetics, National Cancer Institute, Rockville, Maryland
Epidemiology of Uterine Cancers

Michael W. Sill, BS(Chem), PhD(Stat)
Adjunct Instructor; Research Assistant Professor, Biostatistics, Department of Biostatistics, State University of New York at Buffalo; Senior Biostatistician, GOG Statistical and Data Center, Roswell Park Cancer Institute, Buffalo, New York
Biostatistics and Clinical Trials

Steven J. Skates, PhD
Assistant Professor of Medicine (Biostatistics), Harvard Medical School; Assistant Biostatistician, Massachusetts General Hospital, Boston, Massachusetts
Tumor Markers in the Diagnosis and Management of Gynecologic Cancers

Harriet O. Smith, MD
Professor, Department of Obstetrics-Gynecology, University of New Mexico School of Medicine, Albuquerque, New Mexico
Adenocarcinoma of the Cervix

Eugene Sobel, PhD
GOG Statistical and Data Center, Buffalo, New York
Prevention of Gynecologic Malignancies

Gavin C. E. Stuart, MD
Dean, and Professor, Department of Obstetrics and Gynecology, University of British Columbia Faculty of Medicine; Gynecologic Oncologist, British Columbia Cancer Agency, Vancouver, British Columbia, Canada
Ovarian Sarcomas

Charlotte C. Sun, DrPH
Research Instructor, Department of Gynecologic Oncology, University of Texas M.D. Anderson Cancer Center; Adjunct Instructor, University of Texas School of Public Health, Houston, Texas
Quality of Life in the Gynecologic Cancer Patient

Ron E. Swensen, MD
Assistant Professor, Department of Obstetrics and Gynecology, University of Washington School of Medicine; Attending, Division of Gynecologic Oncology, Department of Obstetrics and Gynecology, University of Washington Medical Center, Seattle, Washington
Management of Complications of Radiotherapy

Gillian Thomas, MD
Professor of Radiation, Oncology, Obstetrics and Gynecology, Toronto-Sunnybrook Regional Cancer Center, Toronto, Ontario, Canada

Guillermo Tortolero-Luna, MD, PhD
Associate Professor of Epidemiology, University of Texas School of Public Health; Associate Professor, Department of Gynecologic Oncology, University of Texas M.D. Anderson Cancer Center, Houston, Texas
Epidemiology of Cervical, Vulvar, and Vaginal Cancers

Edward L. Trimble, MD, MPH
Associate Professor, Department of Gynecology and Obstetrics, Johns Hopkins University School of Medicine, Baltimore; Associate Chief (Surgery), Clinical Investigations Branch, Cancer Therapy Evaluation Program, Division of Cancer Treatment and Diagnosis, National Cancer Institute, Bethesda, Maryland
Melanoma of the Female Genital Tract

Claes Tropé, MD, PhD
Professor and Head, Department of Gynecologic Oncology, The Norwegian Radium Hospital, Oslo, Norway
Adjuvant Treatment for Early-Stage Epithelial Ovarian Cancer

Jacobus van der Velden, MD, PhD
Lecturer in Gynecologic Oncology, University of Amsterdam Faculty of Medicine; Staff Specialist in Gynecologic Oncology, Academic Medical Centre, Amsterdam, The Netherlands
Controversies in Early Vulvar Cancer

Paul A. Vasey, MBChB, MSc, MD, FRCP
Reader in Medical Oncology, University of Glasgow Faculty of Medicine; Consultant Cancer Physician, Beatson Oncology Centre, Western Infirmary, Glasgow, Scotland
Primary Chemotherapy for Advanced Epithelial Ovarian Cancer

Jan B. Vermorken, MD, PhD
Professor of Oncology, University Hospital Antwerp; Head, Department of Medical Oncology, University Hospital, Antwerp, Edegem, Belgium
Treatment of Recurrent Uterine Sarcomas

Amanda Vincent, MBBS, BMedSci, PhD, FRACP
Endocrinologist, Menopause Unit and Clinical Nutrition and Metabolism Unit, Department of Endocrinology, Monash Medical Centre, Clayton, Victoria, Australia
Menopause and Hormone Replacement Therapy

Steven E. Waggoner, MD
Associate Professor, Division of Gynecologic Oncology, Case Western Reserve University School of Medicine; Chief, Division of Gynecologic Oncology, University Hospitals of Cleveland, Cleveland, Ohio
Molecular Biology of Cervical and Vulvar Carcinoma

Joan L. Walker, MD
Chief, Section of Gynecologic Oncology, University of Oklahoma School of Medicine; Department of Obstetrics and Gynecology, Section of Gynecologic Oncology, Oklahoma City, Oklahoma
Prevention of Gynecologic Malignancies

Michael J. Wallace, MD
Associate Professor, Interventional Radiology, Department of Diagnostic Radiology, University of Texas M.D. Anderson Cancer Center, Houston, Texas
Interventional Radiology in the Management of Gynecologic Cancers

Bruce Gordon Ward, MBBS, PhD, FRCOG, FRANZCOG, CGO
Mater Medical Centre, South Brisbane, Queensland, Australia
Primary Fallopian Tube Cancer

Michael Wells, BSc(Hons), MD, FRCPath
Professor of Gynaecological Pathology, University of Sheffield Medical School; Honorary Consultant Pathologist, Sheffield Teaching Hospitals, Sheffield, United Kingdom
Hyperplasias of the Endometrium

Haleigh A. Werner, MD
Resident, Department of Radiation Oncology, University of Washington Medical Center, Seattle, Washington
Management of Complications of Radiotherapy

Stephen D. Williams, MD
Professor of Medicine and H.H. Gregg Professor of Oncology, Indiana University School of Medicine; Director, Indiana University Cancer Center, Indianapolis, Indiana
Malignant Ovarian Germ Cell Tumors

Raimund Winter, MD
Professor, University of Graz Faculty of Medicine; Head, Department of Obstetrics and Gynecology, Graz, Austria
Primary Treatment of Uterine Sarcomas

Judith K. Wolf, MD, MS
Associate Professor, Department of Gynecologic Oncology, University of Texas M.D. Anderson Cancer Center, Houston, Texas
Investigational Approaches to the Treatment of Gynecologic Cancers

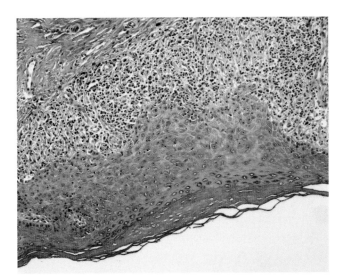

Figure 3–1. Lichen planus, an example of a dermatosis that can be seen in the vulva.

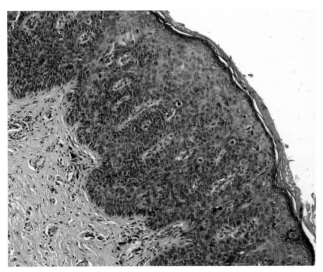

Figure 3–3. Vulvar intraepithelial neoplasia: VIN III, basaloid or undifferentiated type.

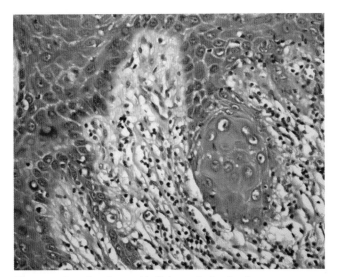

Figure 3–2. Vulvar intraepithelial neoplasia: simplex or differentiated type.

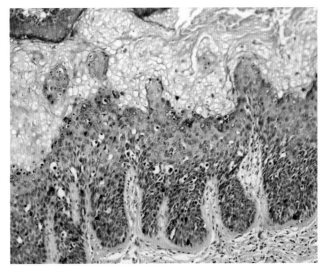

Figure 3–4. Vulvar intraepithelial neoplasia: VIN III, warty or condylomatous type.

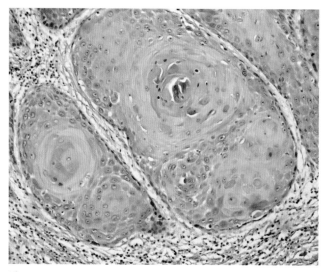

Figure 3–5. Verrucous carcinoma of the vulva. Notice the bulbous pegs and absence of significant atypia.

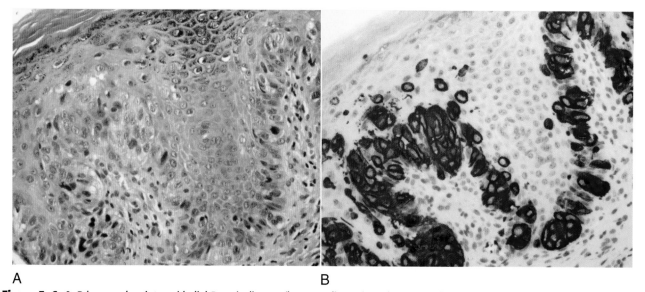

A   B

Figure 3–6. A, Primary vulvar intraepithelial Paget's disease (hematoxylin-eosin stain). **B,** Cytokeratin 7 enhances the neoplastic cells.

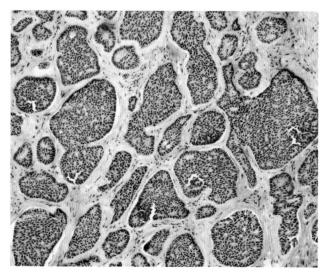

Figure 3–7. Adenoid cystic carcinoma of the Bartholin gland.

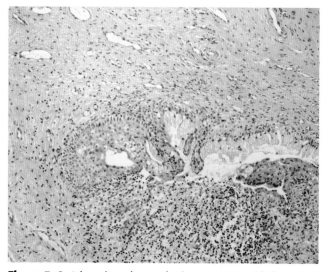

Figure 3–8. Adenosis and metaplastic squamous epithelium.

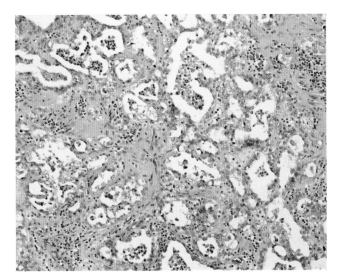

Figure 3–9. Clear cell carcinoma of the vagina.

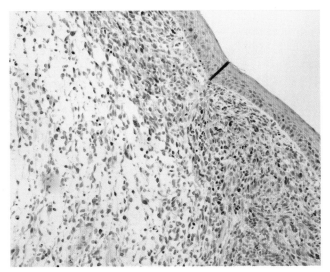

Figure 3–10. Embryonal rhabdomyosarcoma.

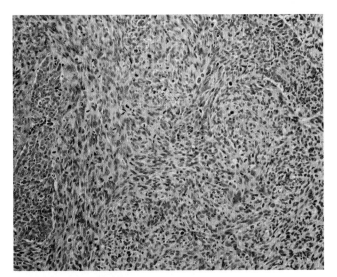

Figure 3–11. Sarcomatoid squamous carcinoma. Islands of typical squamous carcinoma blend into malignant spindle cells.

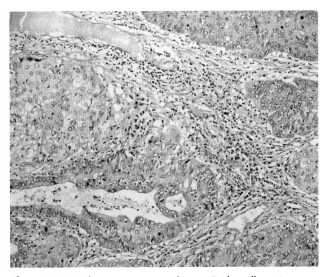

Figure 3–12. Adenosquamous carcinoma. Both malignant squamous and glandular components are present.

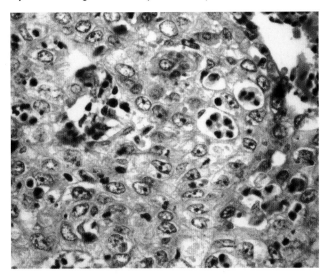

Figure 3–13. Glassy cell carcinoma. The cells have distinct borders, abundant eosinophilic to amphophilic cytoplasm, and large vesicular nuclei with macronucleoli.

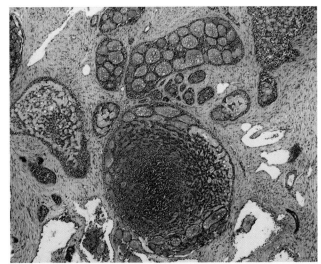

Figure 3–14. Adenoid cystic carcinoma. The tumor has a cribriform pattern with spaces containing mucinous and hyaline material.

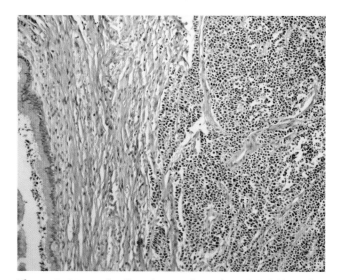

Figure 3-15. Small cell carcinoma. The endocervix is infiltrated by irregular islands and cords of small cells with scant cytoplasm and hyperchromatic nuclei.

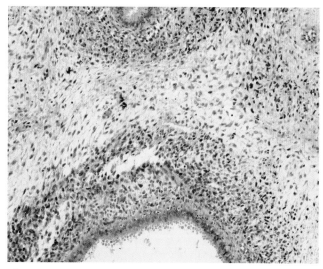

Figure 3-18. Adenosarcoma. The benign glands are surrounded by a hypercellular stromal cuff. Mitotic activity is also present.

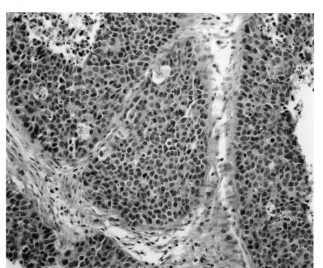

Figure 3-16. Large cell neuroendocrine carcinoma. The tumor cells have moderate amounts of cytoplasm and large nuclei with visible nucleoli. Mitoses and apoptotic figures are frequent.

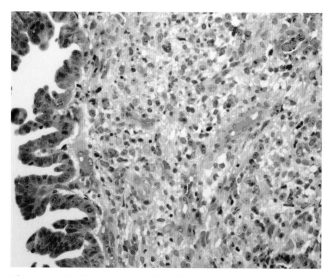

Figure 3-19. Malignant mixed mullerian tumor. Both malignant epithelial (serous carcinoma) and stromal (unclassified sarcoma) components are present.

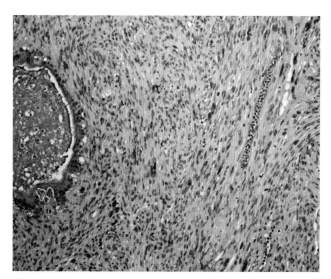

Figure 3-17. Leiomyosarcoma. The tumor has prominent nuclear atypia and mitotic figures.

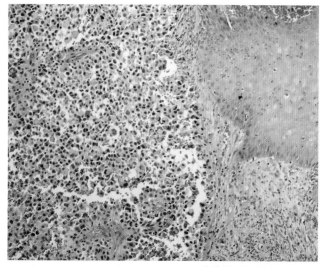

Figure 3-20. Malignant melanoma. The melanoma cells invading the cervical stroma have an epithelioid morphology.

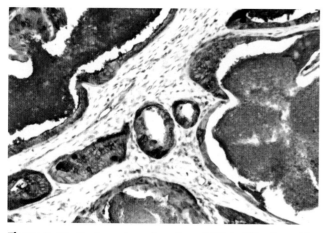

Figure 3–21. Carcinoembryonic antigen (CEA) is diffusely positive in an endocervical adenocarcinoma.

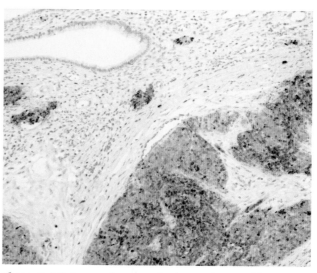

Figure 3–22. Large cell neuroendocrine carcinoma of the cervix diffusely expresses chromogranin.

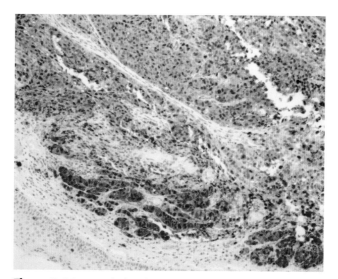

Figure 3–23. A cervical melanoma displays nuclear and cytoplasmic staining for S-100.

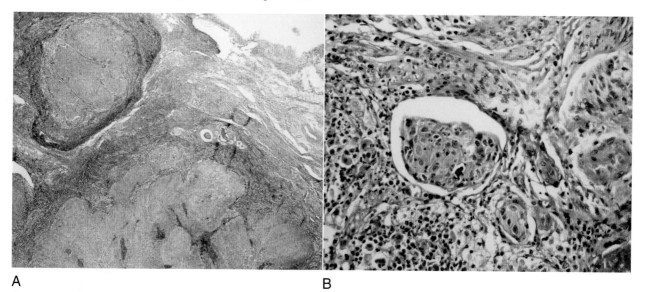

A

B

Figure 3–24. Invasive squamous cell carcinoma of the cervix with deep invasion (**A**) and lymph vascular space invasion (**B**).

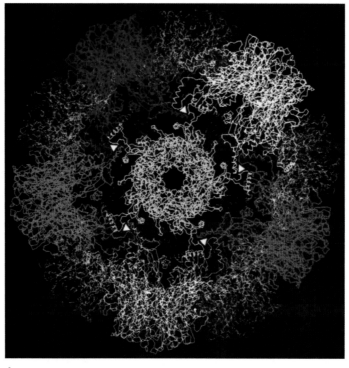

A

Figure 4–3. A, The human papillomavirus (HPV) late protein L1 forms the pentameric assembly unit of the viral capsid shell.

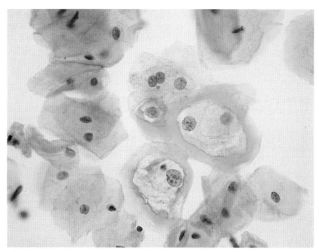

Figure 5-1. Rate of invasive cancer of the cervix after treatment of cervical intraepithelial neoplasia (CIN).

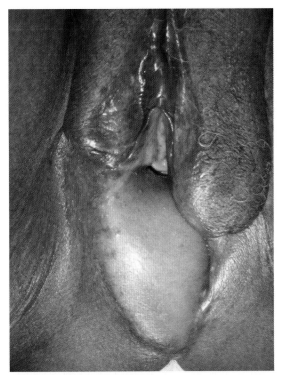

Figure 9–1. Rectus abdominis myocutaneous flap is delivered into the pelvis to construct a neovagina. The patient had developed a recurrence of vaginal carcinoma after primary chemotherapy and radiation therapy, and tumor resection necessitated removal of the posterior and lateral vaginal walls, perineal body, and anorectum.

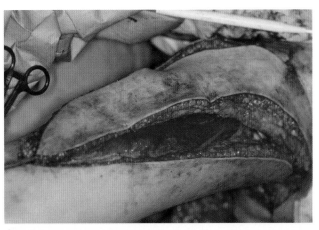

A

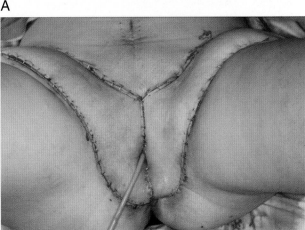

B

Figure 9–2. Tensor fascia lata myocutaneous flap is developed (**A**) and rotated medially (**B**) to cover a large perineal defect after radical vulvectomy and groin node dissection.

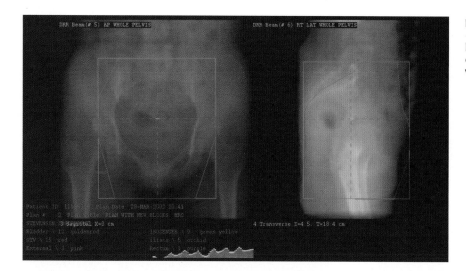

Figure 9–3. A, Pelvic fields (anteroposterior-posteroanterior, right-left laterals) extended inferiorly to cover the entire vagina in a patient with bulky vaginal cuff recurrence.

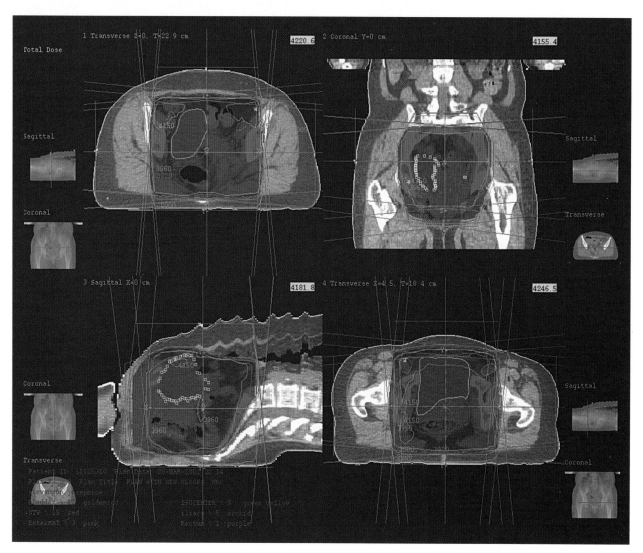

Figure 9–3. cont'd. B, Computed tomography planning, showing isodose "cloud."

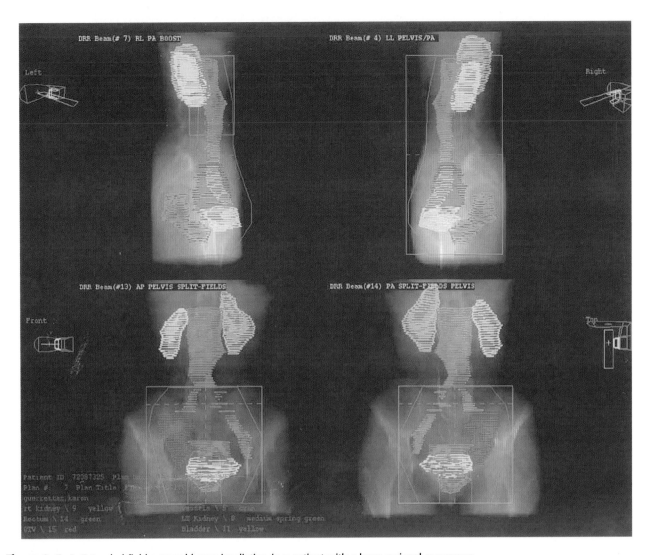

Figure 9–5. A, Extended-field external beam irradiation in a patient with a large regional recurrence.

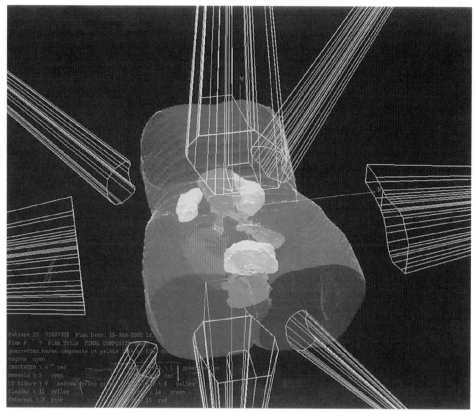

Figure 9–5. cont'd. B, Beam's-eye view of pelvic plus periaortic irradiation followed by boost to the right external iliac recurrence, using three-dimensional conformal therapy.

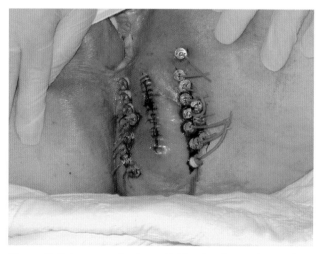

Figure 9–6. Intraoperative interstitial implant in a patient with recurrent vulvar cancer.

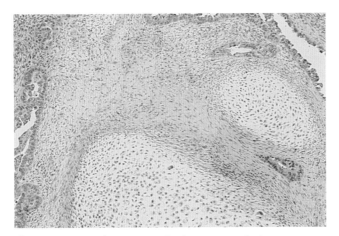

Figure 15–2. Carcinosarcoma. Carcinosarcomas feature an intimate admixture of carcinoma and sarcoma. Note malignant bone and cartilage.

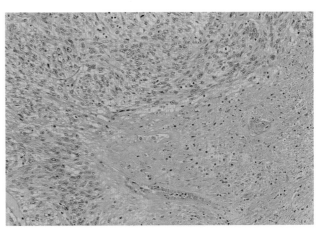

Figure 15–5. Leiomyosarcoma. Coagulative tumor cell necrosis, marked nuclear atypia, and high mitotic index in a typical leiomyosarcoma.

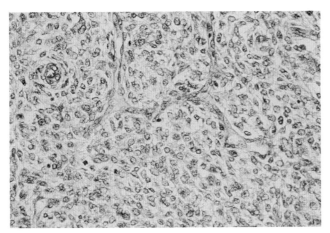

Figure 15–3. Endometrial stromal differentiation. Note individual stromal cells against a background of plexiform vasculature.

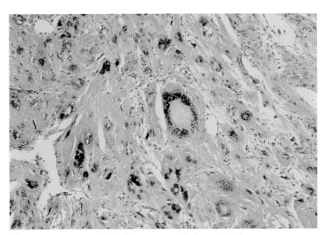

Figure 15–6. Atypical leiomyoma with low risk of recurrence (ALLRR). ALLRR resembles leiomyosarcoma in terms of cytologic atypia, but it lacks both tumor cell necrosis and a high mitotic index (>10 mitotic figures per 10 high-power fields).

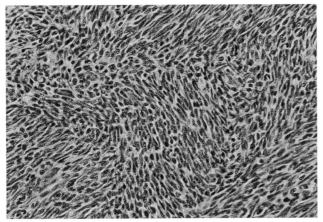

Figure 15–4. Highly cellular leiomyoma. Highly cellular leiomyoma simulates endometrial stromal neoplasms in terms of high cellularity and the inconspicuous cytoplasm of the constituent cells. Thick-walled muscular vessels, desmin positivity, and a fascicular arrangement serve to identify smooth muscle differentiation.

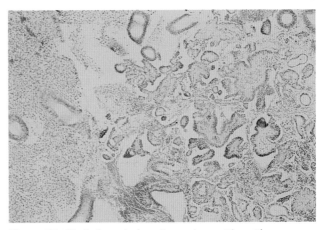

Figure 15–10. Endocervical carcinoma in curettings. The appearance of the carcinoma fragments is distinct from that of the endometrial fragments, suggesting origin from the cervix.

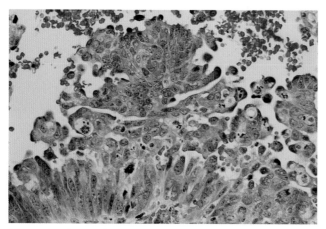

Figure 15–11. Uterine serous carcinoma (USC). USC is usually papillary and features high-grade cytology and easily found (and often abnormal) mitotic figures.

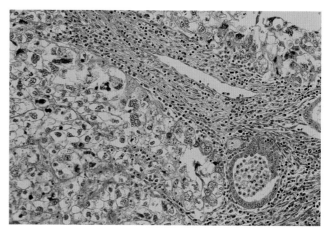

Figure 15–14. Clear cell carcinoma (CCC). CCC has high-grade nuclear features similar to those seen in uterine serous carcinoma. Any architectural pattern may be seen, including papillary structures.

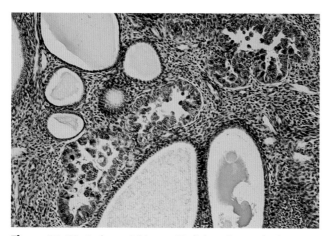

Figure 15–12. Endometrial intraepithelial carcinoma (EIC). EIC typically features focal replacement of benign atrophic endometrial glands by cells with cytologic features identical to those seen in uterine serous carcinoma.

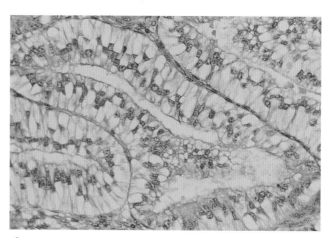

Figure 15–15. Secretory carcinoma. Secretory carcinoma is distinguished from clear cell carcinoma by virtue of its bland cytology and "early secretory" appearance.

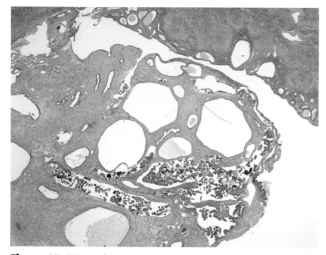

Figure 15–13. Uterine serous carcinoma (USC) in a polyp. Small-volume USC sometimes takes the form of focal involvement of an endometrial polyp.

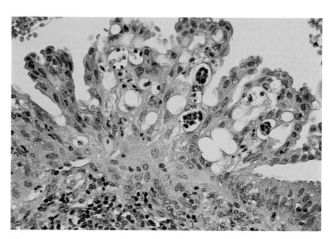

Figure 15–16. Papillary syncytial metaplasia (PSM). PSM features a syncytium of cells with smudged, sometimes hyperchromatic, nuclei. Mitotic figures and prominent nucleoli are absent.

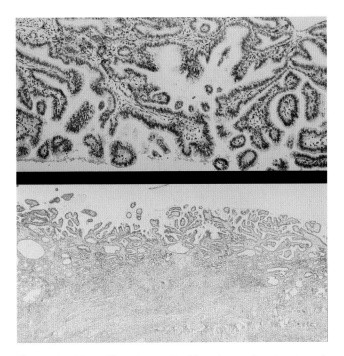

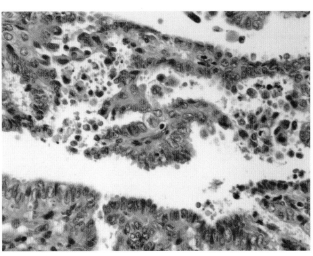

Figure 15–20. Intermediate uterine serous carcinoma (USC)/villoglandular carcinoma (VGC). This case exhibits greater cytologic atypia than the usual VGC and raises management issues.

Figure 15–17. Papillary change. Papillary change denotes stromal cores lined by cytologically bland, nonstratified epithelium.

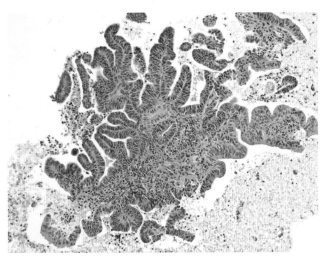

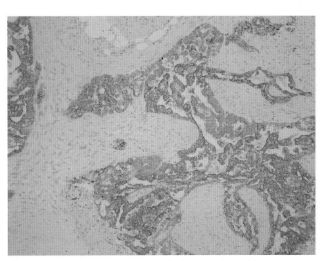

Figure 27–6. This CK7 immunostain is strongly positive, as expected in an ovarian primary tumor (hematoxylin & eosin stain, magnification ×100).

Figure 15–18. Villoglandular hyperplasia. An absence of complex branching and secondary structures distinguishes this pattern from villoglandular carcinoma.

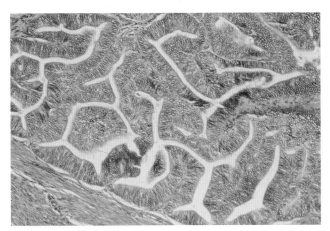

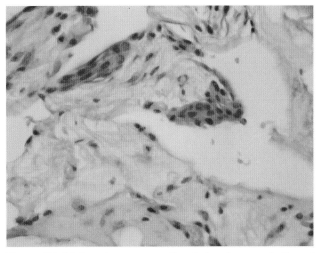

Figure 27–10. Pseudomyxoma peritonei, showing organization of mucin (hematoxylin & eosin stain, magnification ×400).

Figure 15–19. Villoglandular carcinoma (VGC). This case exhibits greater cytologic atypia than the usual VGC and raises management issues.

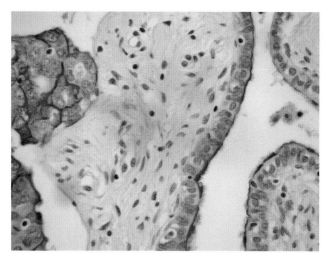

Figure 27–13. The invasive serous tumor on the left shows an immunostaining pattern identical to the normal tubal epithelium on the right (immunoperoxidase to human milk fat globulin, ×400).

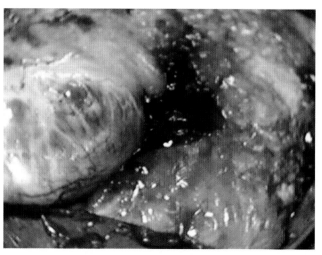

Figure 29–2. Appearance of the gelatinous mucinous ascites typically found with pseudomyxoma peritonei.

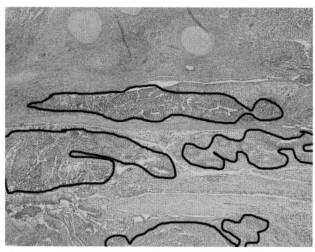

Figure 27–17. The blue areas of primitive neuroepithelium *(outlined)* in this section sum to more than 4 mm², indicating a high-grade immature teratoma (hematoxylin & eosin stain, magnification ×40).

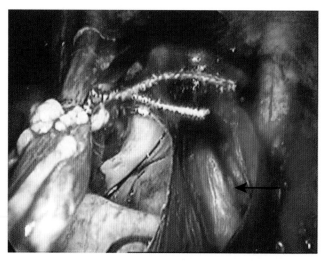

Figure 29–3. Laparoscopic removal of a low-risk ovarian mass. The infundibulopelvic ligament has been tied with extracorporeal knots. The ureter *(arrow)* has been identified and mobilized.

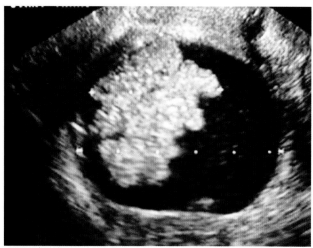

Figure 29–1. Typical transvaginal ultrasound appearance of an early ovarian cancer with prominent internal excrescences or papillations.

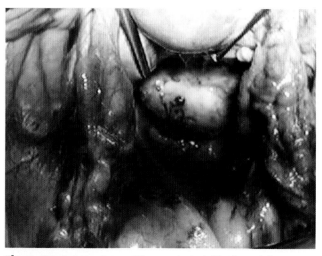

Figure 29–4. Large tumor "drop metastasis" in the cul-de-sac. If such a lesion cannot be shaved off the surface of the rectosigmoid, resection and reanastomosis of the bowel are needed.

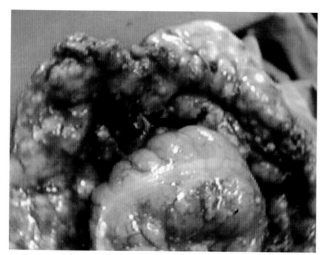

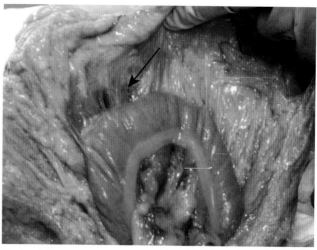

Figure 29–5. The greater omentum is completely replaced by tumor. Usually, an avascular plane can be developed between the tumor-infiltrated omentum and the transverse mesentery. Transverse colectomy is rarely required.

Figure 29–6. The omentum is elevated, showing the underneath side of the transverse colon and the avascular plane to be divided *(arrow)*.

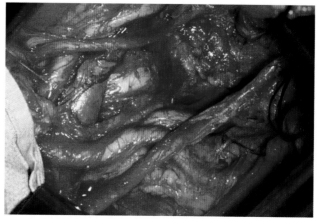

Figure 29–7. Typical appearance of the pelvis after posterior exenteration is performed to clear pelvic disease in a woman with advanced ovarian cancer.

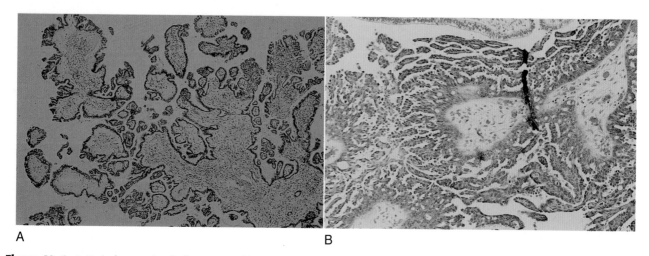

A   B

Figure 40–1. A, Typical serous borderline tumor with irregular, branching papillae. **B,** Serous, borderline tumor with a micropapillary pattern with smooth papillae lined by elongate micropapillae.

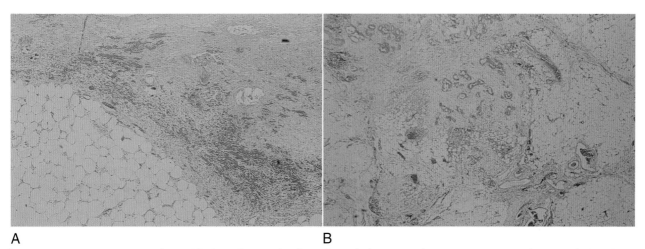

Figure 40–2. A, Noninvasive implant, with sharp demarcation from the underlying normal tissue. **B,** Invasive implant irregularly infiltrates and obliterates the underlying omentum.

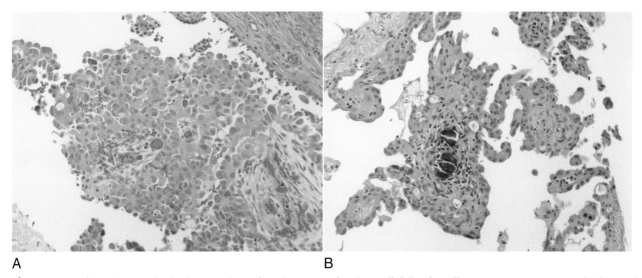

Figure 41–2. Photomicrograph of primary peritoneal carcinoma: **A,** Showing well-defined papillary structures, psammoma bodies, and nuclear crowding. **B,** Showing psammoma bodies.

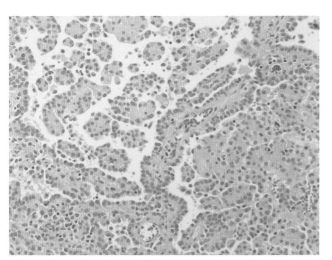

Figure 41–3. Photomicrograph of peritoneal mesothelioma. There are relatively loosely arranged cuboidal cells and poorly defined papillary patterns. The cells have well-spaced nuclei and abundant cytoplasm. There is lack of nuclear crowding.

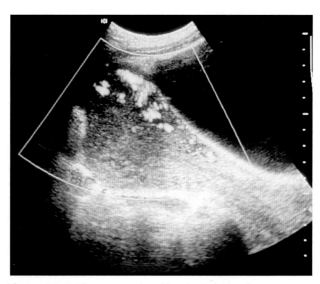

Figure 44–4. Ultrasonography with color Doppler shows persistent gestational trophoblastic disease after removal of a complete hydatidiform mole within the body and wall of the uterus. A typical vesicular or "'snowstorm" appearance of residual molar tissue can be seen within the uterus together with a rich blood supply throughout the endometrium and myometrium. There is no evidence of a fetus.

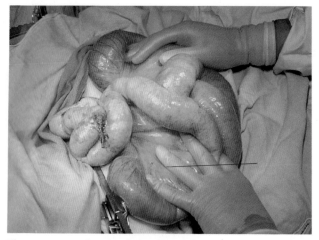

Figure 46–5. Delayed radiation fibrosis of distal small bowel with thickened bowel wall, stenosis of the lumen, and obstruction after pelvic irradiation.

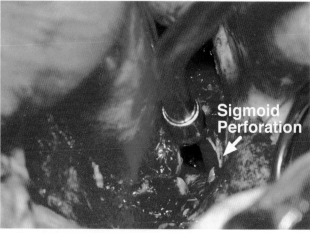

Figure 46–6. Sigmoid perforation with intra-abdominal fecal contamination and abscess after primary irradiation for carcinoma of the cervix in a patient with pelvic inflammatory disease.

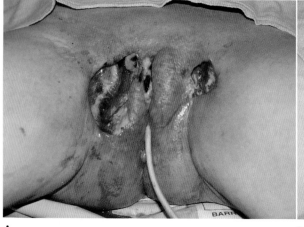

A

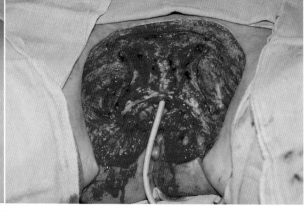

B

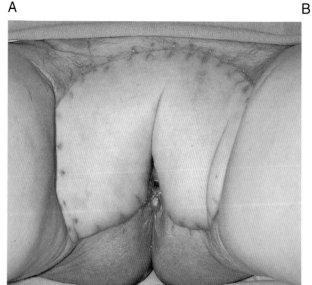

C

Figure 46–9. A, Patient with radiation necrosis of the vulva after primary radiation therapy has secondary infection and osteoradionecrosis, as well as osteomyelitis of the pubis. **B,** Radical vulvectomy and débridement of necrotic tissue with resection of pubis bilaterally back to viable bone of the ischiopubic and ileopubic rami. **C,** After 1 week, pelvic perineal wound reconstruction was performed with a rectus abdominis myocutaneous flap and split-thickness skin graft from the thigh to the abdominal wall.

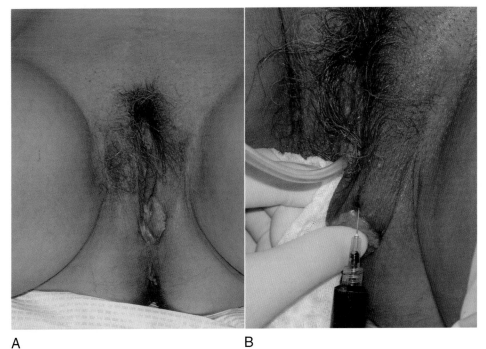

Figure 49–2. A, A 50-year-old patient with a 3-cm squamous carcinoma close to but not involving the midline. **B,** Intradermal peritumoral injection of isosulfan blue. **C,** Isosulfan blue being taken up by cutaneous lymphatic channels. (Courtesy of Dr. Charles Levenback, MD Anderson Cancer Center, Houston, TX.)

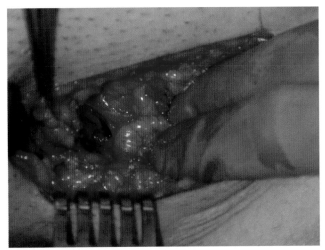

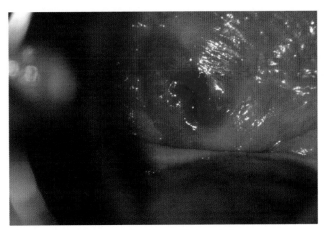

Figure 58–3. Three months after radical trachelectomy.

Figure 49–4. Intraoperative appearance of blue-stained sentinel lymph node. (Courtesy of Dr. Cahrles Levenback, MD Anderson Cancer Center, Houston, TX.)

PREFACE

Discussions regarding a new international textbook in the field of gynecologic oncology originated in January 2000. At the time, editors at Elsevier (formerly Harcourt Health Sciences) in the United Kingdom were interested in publishing a new edition of *Gynecologic Oncology*, edited by the distinguished Australian gynecologist Malcolm Coppleson. After several discussions and meetings, the editors settled on the following characteristics of this new text: It was to be (1) unique among the myriad other textbooks in the discipline, (2) international in its flavor, and (3) comprehensive. Drs. Gershenson and McGuire had made a previous foray into the area of embroilment and dispute with *Ovarian Cancer: Controversies in Management*, published in 1998, and we ultimately made the decision to focus on a much more expansive work on controversies as they relate to gynecologic malignancies, rather than simply duplicating the standard format of many excellent texts already available.

Almost from its inception, we knew that we wanted to populate this book with an international panel of expert contributors. The editors represent four major countries at the forefront of gynecologic oncology patient care, education, and research—Australia, Canada, the United Kingdom, and the United States—and the contributors come from some 12 countries. We also recognized that, because practice patterns vary from one country or region to another, this international flavor would potentially add to the element of controversy within this text. Unlike in the prior textbook on ovarian cancer, however, we are not generally presenting two different viewpoints on each topic but rather attempting to highlight the controversial topics in each area.

The English essayist William Hazlitt stated, "When a thing ceases to be a subject of controversy, it ceases to be a subject of interest." Although controversy can be contentious and destructive, it can also be healthy and illuminating. Striving for the latter approach, we believe that dissection of important controversies in the field will allow both physicians and scientists to identify opportunities and strategies for future research.

We have attempted to provide the reader with not only the usual list of topics included in a textbook on gynecologic cancers but also a menu of topics not commonly covered. Thus, in addition to the sections on each organ site, there are others on complications of cancer treatment, surgical techniques, symptom management, and life during and after cancer treatment. Other miscellaneous topics include investigational approaches to the treatment of gynecologic cancers, hereditary gynecologic cancer syndromes, tumor markers, bioethics, biostatistics and clinical trials, prevention of gynecologic malignancies, gynecologic cancer in pregnancy, melanoma of the female genital tract, interventional radiology, biologic therapy, and imaging of gynecologic malignancies.

We are extremely pleased with the final product and both excited and humbled by the privilege of presenting this new work. We are hopeful that this unique format will stimulate receptivity to various perspectives among physicians worldwide who are caring for women with gynecologic cancers as they meet the challenge to provide excellence in the areas of informed consent, advice, and clinical management.

Finally, we would like to acknowledge and thank the editors at Elsevier—Ms. Stephanie Donley and Ms. Alison Nastasi—for their constant encouragement, and the Elsevier production team and Ms. Marta Abrams at The University of Texas M.D. Anderson Cancer Center for their wonderful assistance in the preparation of this text.

DAVID M. GERSHENSON, MD

WILLIAM P. MCGUIRE, MD

MARTIN GORE, PhD

MICHAEL A. QUINN, MB ChB Glas

GILLIAN THOMAS, MD

Contents

CANCERS OF THE VAGINA, VULVA, AND CERVIX

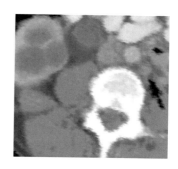

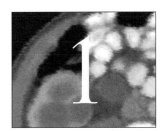

CHAPTER

EPIDEMIOLOGY OF CERVICAL, VULVAR, AND VAGINAL CANCERS

Guillermo Tortolero-Luna and *Eduardo L. Franco*

✦ MAJOR CONTROVERSIES

- What is the role of demographic or socioeconomic factors as determinants of the geographic and racial/ethnic differences in the occurrence of and survival from cervical cancer?
- Has infection with oncogenic human papillomavirus types been established as the necessary causal factor for cervical cancer?
- What is the role of other risk factors for cervical cancer under the necessary causal model of cervical carcinogenesis?
- What is the role of environmental and lifestyle factors in human papillomavirus cervical carcinogenesis?
- Is parity a cofactor for human papillomavirus carcinogenesis or a confounding factor?
- Is use of oral contraceptives a cofactor for human papillomavirus carcinogenesis, or is its association the result of confounding?
- Why is the effect of oral contraceptives different by histologic type and stage?
- Has smoking been established as a cofactor for human papillomavirus–mediated cervical carcinogenesis beyond doubt?
- Are other sexually transmitted infections or inflammation cofactors of interest in human papillomavirus–mediated cervical carcinogenesis?
- What dietary factors have been established as cofactors for human papillomavirus–mediated cervical carcinogenesis?
- What host susceptibility factors influence human papillomavirus–mediated cervical carcinogenesis?
- What is the role of genetic markers of susceptibility to human papillomavirus–mediated cervical carcinogenesis?
- What is the role of human papillomavirus type and concurrent human papillomavirus infection in cervical carcinogenesis?
- What are the roles of human papillomavirus viral load and intratype variation in the risk of persistent human papillomavirus infection and progression to cervical cancer?
- What are some of the unresolved issues that should orient future research on cofactors for cervical cancer?
- What is the role of demographic or socioeconomic factors as determinants of the geographic and racial/ethnic differences in the occurrence of and survival from vulvar cancer?

Continued

- What are the risk factors for vulvar cancer? Is the risk of smoking stronger for vulvar cancer than for cervical cancer?
- What is the role of demographic or socioeconomic factors as determinants of the geographic and racial/ethnic differences in the occurrence of and survival from vaginal cancer?
- Is human papillomavirus infection a necessary cause for vaginal cancer?
- Why is the risk of smoking stronger for vaginal cancer than for cervical cancer?

This chapter presents an overview of the epidemiology of cervical, vulvar, and vaginal cancers. It describes the incidence, mortality, and survival statistics; reviews the current understanding of the role of human papillomavirus (HPV) infection and other cofactors in cervical, vulvar, and vaginal carcinogenesis; and highlights unresolved issues and challenges for future research. The presentation centers on the role of environmental, host, and viral factors in HPV–mediated cervical carcinogenesis. The chapter is organized by the magnitude of the burden on the disease, from cervical cancer to vulvar cancer.

CERVICAL CANCER

Cervical cancer is the second leading malignant neoplasm affecting women worldwide. It continues to be a public health problem particularly in developing countries and among socially disadvantaged populations. Cervical cancer generally affects multiparous women in the early postmenopausal years with enormous social impact, because these women represent the primary source of moral and educational values for their school-age children. Squamous cell carcinomas (SCC) account for 75% to 80% of cases of cervical cancer, whereas adenocarcinomas (ADC) and adenosquamous carcinomas (ASC) account for 10% to 15% of cases.[1] Cervical cancer is preceded by a spectrum of intraepithelial changes classified as cervical intraepithelial neoplasia (CIN), based on the histologic appearance, or squamous intraepithelial lesion (SIL), the terminology favored for cytopathologic diagnosis.[2] This preinvasive phase is asymptomatic, occurs over a long period (10 to 20 years), and is detected by cytologic examination and confirmed by colposcopic-directed biopsy. The incidence of and mortality from cervical cancer declined during the second half of the 20th century, after the introduction of the cytologic screening examination.

Over the last 25 years, HPV infection has gradually taken center stage as the central cause of cervical cancer, owing to the quantity and quality of evidence originating from fundamental and epidemiologic research. More recently, it has been established as the necessary cause for this disease.[3-5] This finding has the potential for expanding the primary and secondary prevention opportunities for cervical cancer. Currently, the greatest promises in these areas lie with immunization against HPV infection and screening using HPV tests,

respectively, as prevention targets to reduce the burden of cervical cancer.

What is the role of demographic or socioeconomic factors as determinants of the geographic and racial/ethnic differences in the occurrence of and survival from cervical cancer?

Cervical cancer is the second most common cancer among women worldwide, preceded only by breast cancer, and accounts for approximately 10% of all cancers in women. It is estimated that approximately 468,000 new cases of cervical cancer and 233,000 deaths from this disease occurred worldwide in the year 2000.[6] In addition, approximately 1,401,000 women were living with cervical cancer in the year 2000 within 5 years of diagnosis.[7] In the United States, cervical cancer is the third most common neoplasm of the female genital tract. In 2003, 12,200 cases of invasive cervical cancer were diagnosed among U.S. women, and approximately 4100 women died from this neoplasm.[8]

Incidence and mortality rates for cervical cancer show a wide geographic variation (Figs. 1-1 and 1-2). Higher incidence and mortality rates are reported in developing countries, where approximately 80% of all cervical cancer cases and deaths occur.[9] Highest rates are reported in Latin America and the Caribbean, sub-Saharan Africa, and South and Southeast Asia, whereas predominantly low rates are reported in most developed countries and in China and western Asia.[6,8,10] In the year 2000, age-adjusted incidence rates ranged from 3.0 per 100,000 women in the Syrian Arab Republic to 94 per 100,000 in Haiti; the age-adjusted mortality rates ranged from 1.3 per 100,000 women in Somalia to 53.5 per 100,000 in Egypt (Table 1-1).[11]

A continuous decline in incidence of and mortality from cervical cancer has been observed in most developed countries during the last 50 years. This decline is mainly attributed to the establishment of organized Papanicolaou (Pap) smear screening programs, to adequate treatment of cervical abnormalities, and possibly to changes in childbearing patterns.[61,12] Meanwhile, in developing countries the rates have continued to increase, have remained stable, or in some instances have decreased slowly. The slower decline in some developing countries that have limited or no screening programs is more likely the result of improvements in socioeconomic conditions in these populations.[9]

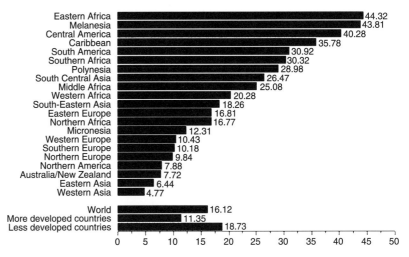

Figure 1–1. Age-adjusted incidence rates for cervical cancer by geographic region: GLOBOCAN, 2000. (From Ferlay J, Bray F, Pisani P, Parkin DM: GLOBOCAN 2000: Cancer Incidence, Mortality and Prevalence Worldwide, Version 1.0. IARC CancerBase No. 5. Lyon, IARC Press, 2001. Available at: http://www-dep.iarc.fr/globocan/globocan.html)

In the mid-1980s, a temporary reverse in the declining trend of incidence and mortality from cervical cancer was documented among women younger than 50 years of age in several developed countries, including England and Wales, the United States, Canada, Finland, Italy, New Zealand, Australia, and Eastern European countries.[1,6,10,13] Similar increases were documented for carcinoma in situ (CIS) of the cervix. In the United States, an increase in incidence rates for CIS was observed in all the Surveillance Epidemiology and End Results (SEER) areas. The increase was first observed among whites in 1985, then among blacks in 1989, and the rates have been higher among whites than blacks.[14] The trend has since reversed, and rates have been declining steadily, once again, since the mid-1990s.[15] This trend, although poorly understood, may be attributed to a birth-cohort effect caused by changes in the prevalence of several risk factors, such as changes in sexual practices, increase in the prevalence of HPV infection, increase in oral contraceptive use, and increased smoking among women born after 1935. However, other factors, such as changes and improvements in coding and registration procedures, increases in screening coverage and hysterectomy rates, decrease in the proportion of cases classified as "uterus not otherwise specified (NOS)," and increase rates of ADC and ASC might have also contributed to this trend.[1,6,10,13] In addition, the increasing trend in CIS is partially attributed to the introduction of the Bethesda classification system, which led to an increased awareness of the importance and complexity of cervical cancer precursors among U.S. physicians.[16]

In the United States, the average annual age-adjusted (2000 U.S. standard population) incidence rate for cervical cancer for the period 1996 to 2000 was 8.7 per 100,000 women.[17] The incidence of cervical cancer increases rapidly with age, reaching a peak at age 45 to 49 years and thereafter leveling off among white women, while continuing to increase among black women (Fig. 1-3). Incidence rates were two times higher among women aged 50 years and older (13.9 per 100,000) than among younger women (6.7 per 100,000).[17] A large racial/ethnic variation in incidence rates is observed in the U.S. population (Fig. 1-4).

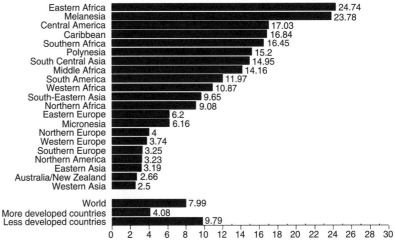

Figure 1–2. Age-adjusted mortality rates for cervical cancer by geographic region: GLOBOCAN, 2000. (From Ferlay J, Bray F, Pisani P, Parkin DM: GLOBOCAN 2000: Cancer Incidence, Mortality and Prevalence Worldwide, Version 1.0. IARC CancerBase No. 5. Lyon, IARC Press, 2001. Available at: http://www-dep.iarc.fr/globocan/globocan.html)

Table 1–1. Highest and Lowest Incidence and Mortality Rates (per 100,000 Women) for Cervical Cancer Worldwide, GLOBOCAN 2000

Incidence		Mortality	
Highest		**Highest**	
Haiti	93.85	Egypt	53.49
Tanzania	61.43	Pakistan	34.17
Zambia	61.08	Kuwait	33.67
Nicaragua	61.08	Tunisia	29.33
Bolivia	58.13	Lebanon	28.93
Malawi	56.16	Malta	26.37
Swaziland	52.16	New Zealand	26.31
Zimbabwe	52.09	China, Hong Kong	26.08
Guinea	51.80	Tajikistan	25.42
Guyana	51.05	Latvia	25.42
Lowest		**Lowest**	
United Arab Emirates	4.57	Rwanda	2.40
Qatar	4.57	Paraguay	2.24
Bahrain	4.57	Congo	2.24
Jordan	4.23	Papua New Guinea	2.21
Finland	4.23	Congo Brazzaville	2.06
Azerbaijan	4.16	Bhutan	1.78
Turkey	3.89	Kenya	1.69
Luxembourg	3.58	Angola	1.50
Iraq	3.27	Uganda	1.32
Syrian Arab Republic	2.99	Somalia	1.27

From Ferlay J, Bray F, Pisani P, Parkin DM. GLOBOCAN 2000: Cancer Incidence, Mortality and Prevalence Worldwide, Version 1.0. IARC CancerBase No. 5. Lyon, IARCPress, 2001: http://www-dep.iarc.fr/globocan/globocan.htm.

Highest incidence rates are reported among Hispanics, followed by blacks and Asian/Pacific Islanders; lower rates are reported among white non-Hispanics and American Indian/Alaskan Natives.[17] Previously, the highest incidence rates in the United States were reported among Vietnamese, Hispanic, Alaskan Native, Korean, and black women; intermediate rates were observed among American Indian, Filipino, and Hawaiian women; and the lowest rates were reported among white non-Hispanic and Japanese women.[18]

The age-adjusted (2000 U.S. standard population) mortality rate from cervical cancer in the United States for the period 1996 to 2000 was 3.0 per 100,000 women.[17] Mortality rates increase with age; however, a steeper increase is observed in blacks, whereas the increase in whites, although steady, is less pronounced (see Fig. 1-3). Mortality rates were more than fourfold higher among women aged 50 years and older (6.9 per 100,000) than among younger women (1.5 per 100,000).[17] Mortality is higher in black women, followed by Hispanics, Asian/Pacific Islanders, American Indian/Alaskan Natives, and white non-Hispanics (see Fig. 1-4).[17]

During the period 1975 to 2000, age-adjusted incidence and mortality rates (2000 U.S. standard population) from cervical cancer declined in both white and black women. Incidence rates declined from 14.8 per 100,000 women in 1975 to 7.6 per 100,000 in 2000; age-adjusted mortality rates declined from 5.6 to 2.8 per 100,000 women during the same period.[17] Although important racial differences have persisted over time, the decline in incidence and mortality has been greater among black women and women aged 50 years and older (Figs. 1-5 and 1-6).[17]

Survival rates vary between developed and developing countries. Higher 5-year relative survival rates for cervical cancer are reported in developed countries such as the United States (71%), Canada (72%), and Europe (59%). Intermediate survival rates are observed among European countries such as England (60%), Denmark (64%), and France (67%).[10] Lower rates are observed in developing countries such as the Philippines (29%) and India (40%).[7,10] In the SEER program the 5-year relative survival rate was higher among women with early-stage cervical cancer (92.2%) than among those with advanced-stage cervical cancer (16.5%).[17] However, only 54% of all cases are diagnosed in a localized stage, and this proportion is lower among black (47%) and older women (39%) (Fig. 1-7). Survival rates are higher among whites (72.9%) than blacks (61.0%) and are inversely related to age (<45 years, 82.4%; 75+ years, 42.3%). After an initial significant improvement in survival rates, they have remained stable during the last 25 years,

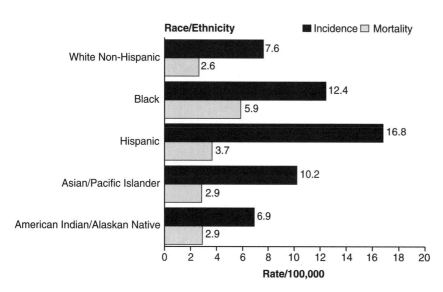

Figure 1–3. Age-specific incidence and mortality rates for cervical cancer—Surveillance Epidemiology and End Results, U.S. 1996–2000. (From Ries LAG, Eisner MP, Kosary CL, et al. (eds): SEER Cancer Statistics Review, 1975–2000. Bethesda, MD, National Cancer Institute, 2003. Available at: http://seer.cancer.gov/csr/1975_2000, 2003.)

Figure 1–4. Age-adjusted incidence and mortality rates for cervical cancer–Surveillance Epidemiology and End Results, U.S. 1996–2000. (From Ries LAG, Eisner MP, Kosary CL, et al. (eds): SEER Cancer Statistics Review, 1975–2000. Bethesda, MD, National Cancer Institute, 2003. Available at: http://seer.cancer.gov/csr/1975_2000, 2003.)

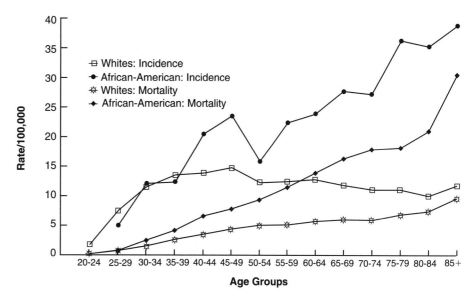

Figure 1–5. Trends in incidence rates for cervical cancer–Surveillance Epidemiology and End Results, U.S. 1975–2000. (From Ries LAG, Eisner MP, Kosary CL, et al. (eds): SEER Cancer Statistics Review, 1975–2000. Bethesda, MD, National Cancer Institute, 2003. Available at: http://seer.cancer.gov/csr/1975_2000, 2003.)

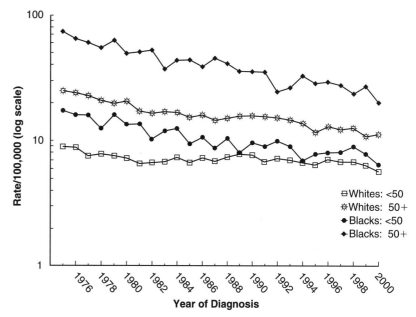

Figure 1–6. Trends in mortality rates for cervical cancer–Surveillance Epidemiology and End Results, U.S. 1975–2000. (From Ries LAG, Eisner MP, Kosary CL, et al. (eds): SEER Cancer Statistics Review, 1975–2000. Bethesda, MD, National Cancer Institute, 2003. Available at: http://seer.cancer.gov/csr/1975_2000, 2003.)

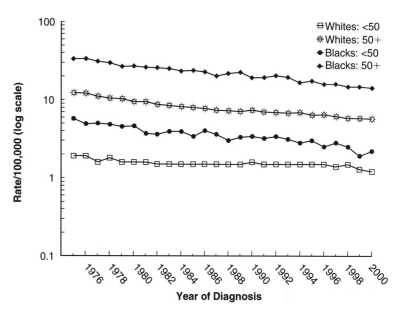

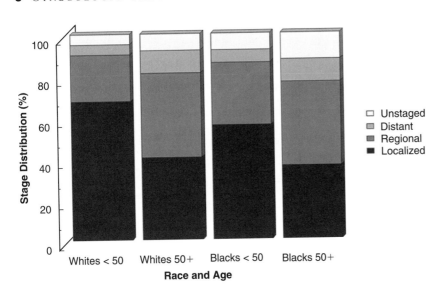

Figure 1–7. Percent distribution of stage of cervical cancer at diagnosis–Surveillance Epidemiology and End Results, U. S. 1992–1999. (From Ries LAG, Eisner MP, Kosary CL, et al. (eds): SEER Cancer Statistics Review, 1975–2000. Bethesda, MD, National Cancer Institute, 2003. Available at: http://seer.cancer.gov/csr/1975_2000, 2003.)

69.1% in 1974–1976 and 71.3% 1992–1999 (Fig. 1-8).[17] This constant trend in survival has been observed in all women except black women younger than 50 years of age, in whom survival rates actually declined 15% during the same period, from 75.2% in 1974–1976 to 64.0 in 1992–1999.[17]

The determinants of these geographic and racial/ethnic differences in incidence, mortality, and survival of cervical cancer, although not well understood, can be partially explained by several indicators of socioeconomic status as well as certain cultural characteristics and language barriers affecting access to adequate screening and medical care.[19] Incidence and mortality rates of cervical cancer increase and survival rates decrease with decreasing social class. In a recent meta-analysis, women of lower socioeconomic status had a 1.6-fold increased risk for CIS and a twofold increased risk for cervical cancer, compared with those of higher status.[20] Socioeconomic status may influence sexual behaviors (both the women's and their partners), increasing the risk of exposure to HPV and other

cofactors. Drain and colleagues[21] found higher incidence rates of cervical cancer in countries with lower health indicators, such as number of physicians per population, percentage of children immunized for measles, infant birthweight, life expectancy of women, female literacy rates, and religion.

In the United States, despite the decrease in incidence and mortality from cervical cancer over the last 25 years, socioeconomic inequalities associated with occurrence of the disease have remained unchanged. Between 1975 and 1999, women living in high-poverty areas in the United States had a 30% higher incidence rate and a 71% higher mortality rate, and the largest burden in these socioeconomically deprived areas was observed among women of minority racial/ethnic groups.[22] In addition, other lifestyle and cultural factors, such as smoking, sexual behaviors, and religion, as well as access to adequate screening, early diagnosis, and treatment, may affect the risk of HPV infection and cervical cancer.[20] To compound these problems, lack of adequate health insurance and other socioeconomic

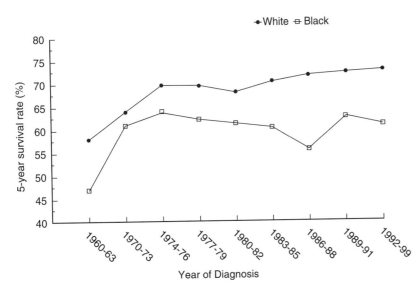

Figure 1–8. Five-year survival rate for cervical cancer by race and year of diagnosis. From Ries LAG, et al: SEER Cancer Statistics Review, 1975–2000. Bethesda, MD, National Cancer Institute, 2003. Available at: http://seer.cancer.gov/csr/1975_2000, 2003.

barriers to medical care further lead to poor clinical outcomes among disadvantaged women. In a recent study, it was demonstrated that socioeconomic status strongly affects cervical cancer survival in the United States but not in Canada, a country that provides universal health care for all its citizens and residents. Disadvantaged patients with cervical cancer in Canada had an almost 50% greater probability of surviving 5 years after diagnosis than their American counterparts.[23]

Has infection with oncogenic human papillomavirus types been established as the necessary causal factor for cervical cancer?

A sexually transmitted etiology for cervical cancer has long been suggested by epidemiologic research. Very early it was hypothesized that cervical cancer was related to sexual activity based on the observations that nuns did not develop cervical cancer and that prostitutes had an increased risk of cervical cancer. Several measures of sexual behavior (e.g., multiple sexual partners, early age at first sexual intercourse, sexual habits of male partners) are consistently associated with an increased risk for cervical neoplasia.[24] Over the years, several sexually transmitted infectious agents have been the focus of research, including herpes simplex virus (HSV), *Chlamydia trachomatis, Trichomonas vaginalis,* cytomegalovirus (CMV), *Neisseria gonorrhoeae,* and *Treponema pallidum.*[24-26] Since the hypothesis of a causal relationship between HPV and cervical neoplasia was first proposed in the mid-1970s,[27] a large body of biologic, clinical, and epidemiologic research has accumulated supporting an etiologic role of some types of HPV in cervical carcinogenesis.[3,4,26,28,29] The association is independent of study population, study design, and HPV detection method.[3,14,28,30-34] More importantly, it meets most of the criteria for causality traditionally used in epidemiologic research, such as strength, consistency, specificity, temporal relationship, biologic gradient, biologic plausibility, coherence, and experimental evidence.[34]

Genital HPV infection is the most commonly diagnosed sexually transmitted infection (STI) in the United States. An estimated 20 million Americans are infected with HPV, and 5.5 million new cases of HPV infection are diagnosed annually in the United States.[35] Approximately 100 HPV types have been described; approximately 40 of them are associated with anogenital disease, and 14 or more are associated with cervical cancer.[36] HPV DNA is detected in more than 90% of cervical cancers (range, 75% to 100%),[4,36,37] in up to 94% of women with preinvasive lesions (cervical SIL), and in up to 46% of women with cytologically normal findings.[3,28,30,38-41] Worldwide, the most common HPV types detected in cervical cancer are HPV-16, -18, -45, -31, -33, -35, -52, and -58; together, they account for 95% of all HPV types in SCCs.[36,37] HPV-16 is by far the most common HPV type detected in cervical precancer and cancer lesions. In a recent meta-analysis, HPV-16 accounted for more than 50%

of all cervical cancer cases, ranging from 45.9% in Asia to 62.6% in North America and Australia.[41] The risk of cervical cancer is higher with specific HPV types (HPV-16, -18, -31, -33, -35, and -45), increasing viral load, and concurrent infection with multiple HPV types.[36,40,42-44] The risk of cervical cancer among HPV-positive women (any type) has been reported to range from 16-fold to 122-fold.[33] Based on a group of studies conducted by the International Agency for Research in Cancer (IARC) between 1997–1998 in seven countries (Brazil, Mali, Morocco, Paraguay, Philippines, Thailand, and Peru), a pooled odds ratio (OR) of 158.2 (95% confidence interval [CI], 113.4 to 220.6) was estimated for the association of HPV with squamous cell cervical cancer.[36] This is among the strongest statistical relations ever identified in cancer epidemiology. In addition, the number of cases of cervical cancer attributed to HPV has been estimated to reach almost 100% if meticulous testing of biopsies and surgical specimens from tumor specimens, including state-of-the-art polymerase chain reaction (PCR) techniques, are used to detect HPV DNA.[4,33]

The association between cervical cancer and HPV infection is unique in cancer epidemiology. Given that it is virtually impossible to identify cervical carcinomas that do not harbor traces of HPV DNA, HPV infection is now considered a necessary causal agent, making alternative, HPV-independent carcinogenic routes implausible at best. In consequence, the magnitude of the association is the largest ever identified in epidemiologic research.[4,36] No other models in cancer causation have identified necessary factors or the magnitude of the associations observed between HPV and cervical cancer.[45] Lung cancer, for example, can occur in the absence of tobacco exposure (active or passive). Similarly, liver cancer may occur in individuals who have never been exposed to the hepatitis B virus.

Despite the causal link between HPV infection and cervical cancer, only a small proportion of HPV infections persist and progress to precancer or cancer, suggesting that HPV infection is a necessary but not a sufficient cause for cervical neoplasia and that other environmental, viral, and host-related factors may also be involved for cervical cancer to occur (Fig. 1-9).

What is the role of other risk factors for cervical cancer under the necessary causal model of cervical carcinogenesis?

The recognition of the causal role of HPV led to new methodologic and statistical challenges[46] and the need to reassess the roles of sexual behaviors and environmental factors previously associated with cervical cancer under this new model of causality. Under the necessary causal model, these factors are considered cofactors instead of independent factors, because their independent effect is observed only in the presence of HPV infection.[26] These factors may influence the acquisition of HPV infection, increase the likelihood of persistent HPV infection (the most critical event in cervical carcinogenesis), or increase the risk of progression from

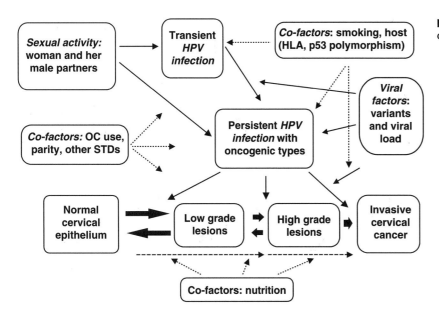

Figure 1–9. A multifactorial model of cervical cancer etiology.

HPV infection to high-grade squamous intraepithelial lesions (HSIL).[47] Environmental factors currently supported by epidemiologic data as potential cofactors in HPV-related cervical carcinogenesis include smoking, high parity, use of oral contraceptives (OC), coinfection with other sexually transmitted agents, and dietary factors.[24,43,47-52] Host-related factors include endogenous hormones, immune response, and genetic susceptibility traits, such as specific human leukocyte antigen (HLA) alleles and haplotypes and polymorphisms in the *TP53* gene.[43,44,52-56] Viral factors include HPV type and variant, viral load, and viral integration.[42,44,57-59]

The reassessment of the role of cofactors in HPV-related cervical carcinogenesis has been conducted using two analytic strategies: adjustment of HPV status by "standard" multivariate modeling using stratified analysis or by logistic regression. However, under the assumption that HPV infection is a necessary cause for cervical cancer to occur, standard epidemiologic approaches to control confounding and assessment of effect modification are not appropriate, and an HPV-positive restricted analysis strategy has been proposed to assess the role of cofactors.[47,60] This approach consists of examining the putative exposure cervical cancer association exclusively among subjects (i.e., cases and controls in a case-control study) whose specimens were positive for HPV DNA of the relevant oncogenic types. By restricting the analysis to HPV-positive subjects, the effect of a given cofactor can be isolated under the assumption that in the absence of HPV the candidate variable would not operate. Unfortunately, this approach is not guaranteed to serve its purpose because of the cross-sectional nature of HPV exposure assessment among women in any control group in a molecular epidemiologic study based on testing at a single time point. Cumulative HPV exposure among disease-free women in such studies cannot be defined; the presence of the virus is merely taken as a proxy of the cumulative cervical exposure to HPV, much like

the situation in case-control studies of the effects of nutrition on cancer that rely on 24-hour recall of dietary items. Because of the transient or intermittent nature of most HPV infections in sexually active women of reproductive age, a single-time-point assessment of the presence of HPV in the cervix carries little predictive value with respect to the overall latency of the relevant cumulative exposure. As a result, many false-negative and false-positive results can be expected in attempting to describe latency-relevant HPV exposure among controls.[45] In consequence, the strategy of restricted analysis described earlier for case-control studies is prone to some degree of misclassification. Ideally, long-term cohort studies with repeated measurements of the virus, lesions, and candidate exposures may provide a more cogent study framework to address the contribution of cofactors. However, such studies are costly and cannot examine associations with invasive cancer. Therefore, the restricted analysis approach used in case-control studies remains the most feasible maneuver to obtain enhanced validity in assessing the role of cofactors, provided its caveats are properly recognized.

The following section provides a brief description of some of the most prominent environmental, host, and viral factors currently being examined as cofactors for HPV-related cervical carcinogenesis.

What is the role of environmental and lifestyle factors in human papillomavirus cervical carcinogenesis?

Is parity a cofactor for human papillomavirus carcinogenesis or a confounding factor? In several case-control studies, high parity or number of live births was found to be consistently associated with cervical cancer and HSIL after controlling for HPV status.[40,61-66] In Denmark, women with two or more pregnancies were found to have a risk of CIS approximately 80% higher than that of nulliparous women.[40] Schiffman and associates[62] observed a threefold increased risk of CIN among women with four or more live births, compared with nulliparous women. A twofold increased risk for CIN III associated with high parity (six or more pregnancies) was observed for Colombian women, but not for Spanish women.[63,67] Herrero and coworkers[61] in Costa Rica observed fivefold and twofold increased risks for invasive cancer among women with 10 or more and 12 or more pregnancies, respectively.

The role of parity among HPV-positive women, using the aforementioned restricted analysis approach, was assessed in a pooled analysis of nine case-control studies conducted by IARC in developing countries[66] and in a review paper of studies reporting on the assessment of cofactors.[47] In the pooled study, a statistically significant association between number of full-term pregnancies and cervical cancer was observed; women with seven or more full-term pregnancies were at 3.8-fold (95% CI, 2.7 to 5.5) increased risk for cervical cancer, and the risk increased with the number of full-term pregnancies (trend, $P < .001$).[66] In addition, early age at first pregnancy was strongly associated with cervical cancer risk. HPV-positive women with a first full-term pregnancy before age 17 years were at 4.4-fold (95% CI, 2.4 to 7.9) increased risk for cervical cancer, compared with HPV-positive nulliparous women, and the risk decreased with increasing age at first full-term pregnancy (trend, $P = .005$).[66] Similar results were observed when the analysis was further restricted to oncogenic HPV types and parous women.[66] This association was also reported in Costa Rica, although the trend was less clear than in the IARC pooled study.[47,50,68] HPV-positive parous women were at 4.6-fold (95% CI, 1.1 to 20.0) higher risk of HSIL and cervical cancer than HPV-positive nulliparous women. The risk was highest among women with four to five pregnancies (OR = 3.5; 95% CI, 1.7 to 7.2) but then seemed to decline with further pregnancies. No association between CIN III/HSIL and parity was reported in other studies in which analysis was restricted to HPV-positive cases and controls.[47,69-71] A stronger association between parity and risk of cervical cancer was evident in the restricted analysis than in the nonrestricted analysis. In the type of analysis not restricted to HPV-positive cases and controls, women with a history of seven or more full-term pregnancies were at a 1.6-fold (95% CI, 1.2 to 2.2) increased risk for cervical cancer, compared with nulliparous women.

Although there is no clear biologic mechanism to support the association between parity and cervical cancer, repeated trauma to the cervix during childbirth and hormonal, immunologic, and nutritional factors have been suggested as mechanisms. The fact that the association persists in HPV-restricted analyses suggests that parity may have a role "downstream" from HPV infection by mediating progression. However, it remains possible that repeated pregnancies have an "upstream" effect as well, because they lead to breaches in the cervical epithelium which could facilitate the establishment and persistence of HPV infection.

Future research is needed to better understand the role of parity as a cofactor for HPV cervical carcinogenesis and to determine the effect of the correlation between parity and other potential cofactors such as smoking and OC use. Similarly, the impact of changes in reproductive patterns on rates of cervical cancer needs to be evaluated, because many developing countries have undergone dramatic reductions in fertility rates in the last two to three decades.

Is oral contraceptive use a cofactor for human papillomavirus carcinogenesis, or is its association the result of confounding? Why is the effect of oral contraceptives different by histologic type and stage? Steroid contraceptive hormones have been hypothesized as a cofactor in HPV-related cervical carcinogenesis. Although results from epidemiologic studies have been inconsistent, most studies have shown an increased risk of cervical cancer.[47,50] However, little is known about the mechanisms by which OCs may increase the risk of acquisition, persistence, and progression of HPV infection to cervical cancer, although recent reviews have provided biologic plausibility to this association.[72,73] In addition, the discovery of hormone receptors in cervical tissue provides further support to the role of OC in cervical carcinogenesis.[72]

Overall, higher risk estimates are reported for CIS and ADC among long-term OC users (5+ years), mostly in cohort studies.[56] Earlier epidemiologic studies showed a weak but consistent, statistically significant association, particularly among long-term OC users.[56,74,75] However, interpretation of these studies is limited by the strong correlation among OC use, sexual behavior (and thus HPV), and patterns of Pap smear screening; by the selection of adequate comparison groups; and by the lack of control for HPV status.[74]

Results from epidemiologic studies in which HPV status was controlled for are conflicting. Most have failed to show an association between HSIL/cervical cancer and various measurements of OC exposure.[28,38,40,56,62,64,67,74,76-78] Long duration of OC use (5+ years) is the exposure measure most consistently found to increase the risk of cervical cancer.[56] In a systematic review, the risk of cervical cancer among studies adjusting for HPV status increased with duration of OC use, from 0.9 (95% CI, 0.7 to 1.1) among users for less than 5 years, to 1.3 (95% CI, 1.0 to 1.7) among users for 5 to 9 years, to 1.7 (95% CI, 1.3 to 2.3) among users for 10+ years. The strongest associations, particularly among current and long-term users, were reported for ADC in situ, followed by invasive ADC.[56,78] Current OC users and OC users for 6+ years were, respectively, at 12.6-fold (95% CI, 2.5 to 64.2) and 6-fold (95% CI, 1.2 to 30.7) increased risks for ADC in situ.[78] Smith and associates[56] also reported an increased risk for ADC. An interaction between OC use and HPV infection has been suggested; however, the evidence is conflicting, is based on small sample sizes, and needs to be interpreted with caution.[62,63,74,76,79]

Similarly, studies restricting analysis to HPV-positive women have shown weak or no association between OC use and HSIL and cervical cancer.[47,50] In the pooled analysis of case-control studies conducted by the IARC, HPV-positive women who had used OC were 42% more likely to develop CIS/cervical cancer than never-users (OR = 1.42; 95% CI, 1.0 to 2.0). This risk was higher for CIS (OR = 2.45; 95% CI, 1.0 to 6.8) than for cervical cancer (OR = 1.29; 95% CI, 0.9 to 1.9).[50] The risks of HSIL and cervical cancer increase with duration of OC use. The increase in risk with duration of OC use has been more consistent across studies than history of use (ever use).[50] Long-term use (5+ years) of OC was associated with a significant increased risk of CIS/cervical cancer (OR = 3.4; 95% CI, 2.1 to 5.5). The risk associated with 5+ years of OC use was higher for cervical cancer (OR = 4.0; 95% CI, 2.0 to 8.0) than for CIS (OR = 2.9; 95% CI, 1.2 to 7.1). Similarly, in Costa Rica, a 3.1-fold (95% CI, 1.1 to 9.1) increased risk for HSIL/cervical cancer was observed among women with two or fewer pregnancies who had used OC for 5+ years.[68] In Manchester, United Kingdom, an increased risk of borderline significance (OR = 1.5; 95% CI, 0.8 to 2.9) was observed for CIN III among OC users for 8+ years.[70] In support of the role of hormonal factors in cervical cancer, a twofold increased risk for ADC and a 1.6-fold increased risk for SCC were reported among obese women (body mass index = 30) after adjustment for HPV status.[80] However, the role of exogenous hormonal factors remains less clear.

The inconsistency of epidemiologic studies on the role of OC use as a cofactor for HPV-related cervical carcinogenesis has been attributed to methodologic differences and control of confounding.[72] In addition, a biologic mechanism to explain the role of OCs as a cofactor for HPV-related cervical carcinogenesis is lacking. Two possible mechanisms have been proposed: increased exposure of the transformation zone to potential carcinogens and increased cell proliferation and transcription. An increased incidence of cervical ectropion among OC users has been reported and would increase the likelihood of exposure of the transformation zone to HPV and other potential carcinogens.[72] However, results from a systematic review of the literature failed to show an association between detection of genital HPV infection and OC use, providing no support to the ectropion hypothesis.[81] The hypothesis of stimulation of cell proliferation and transcription of HPV by estrogens and progesterone has been recently supported.[72,73] Two possible mechanisms have been suggested. One mechanism proposes that steroid hormones increase the expression of HPV E6/E7 oncogenes, promoting degradation of *TP53*, which results in loss of tumor protective activity.[72] The second mechanism suggests that a pathway involving 16α-hydroxiestrone, one of the products of the hydroxylation of estrogens, binds to estrogen receptors, prolonging their proliferative effects, and provides support to the increased risk of cervical cancer observed among long-term OC users.[73] Furthermore, it has been observed that 16α-hydroxylation of estrogens is enhanced in HPV-16 immortalized endocervical cells, suggesting a synergistic effect between high-risk HPV and 16α-hydroxylation.

Further research is needed to identify the biologic mechanism or mechanisms involved in HPV carcinogenesis. These studies need to assess the role of exogenous and endogenous hormonal factors in the bimodal age distribution of HPV infection, as well as the impact of the pattern of use of OC and hormone replacement therapy over time. Epidemiologic studies need to look beyond the confounding effect of sexual activity. Simple adjustment or restriction for HPV status cannot guarantee complete control of confounding because of the problems with this approach (explained earlier). Meticulous adjustment for sexual activity measures in addition to HPV restriction or adjustment may provide a further safeguard by permitting control of the analysis for residual confounding effects remaining due to misclassified HPV status. Adjusting for multiple dimensions of sexual activity may help to minimize the impact of the intrinsic errors that result from assuming that HPV status among control women reflects the complete lifetime exposure that is relevant in terms of its latency to disease onset.

Has smoking been established as a cofactor for human papillomavirus–mediated cervical carcinogenesis beyond doubt? Since the hypothesis of an association between tobacco smoking and cervical cancer was proposed more than 25 years ago, many epidemiologic studies have provided support for this association.[47,82] Most studies have shown a twofold increased risk among smokers and a dose-response relationship with duration and intensity of smoking. This association has been reported in earlier studies before HPV testing, in studies adjusting for HPV status, and in studies restricted to HPV-positive women.[47,82] In most early studies, control of confounding was attained by adjusting for sexual behavior characteristics, particularly the lifetime number of sexual partners and age at first intercourse, as proxy measures for the sexually transmitted pathogen causally linked with the disease. It was suggested that residual confounding, particularly in populations in which cigarette smoking and sexual behavior are highly correlated, were responsible for the observed association.[83] Results from studies controlling for HPV status have been inconsistent. Some studies found a moderate but statistically significant independent effect of smoking on cervical cancer after adjustment for HPV,[28,38,40,61,62,64,76,77,84] whereas others failed to detect an independent effect.[49,67,85-90]

Similar results have been reported in studies restricted to HPV-positive women. The risk of HSIL and cervical cancer among ever-smoker HPV-positive women ranged between 2 and 5, and the risk increased with amount and duration of smoking.[47] Ever-smokers had a twofold increased risk for HSIL/cervical cancer in the pooled analysis of case-control studies conducted by IARC (OR = 2.2; 95% CI, 1.5 to 3.2 for CIS/cervical cancer)[47] and in the nested case-control study conducted in Manchester, UK, for CIN III (OR = 2.2; 95% CI, 1.4 to 3.4).[47,70] The association with current smoking among HPV-positive women was consistent with that observed for ever-smoking. Compared with HPV-positive never-smokers, HPV-positive current smokers were found to be at higher risk for HSIL (OR = 1.9; 95% CI, 1.0 to 3.8) in Denmark[47,69] and for

HSIL/cervical cancer (OR = 2.3; 95% CI, 1.2 to 4.3) in Costa Rica.[47,68] An increased risk for HSIL/cervical cancer was also reported among HPV-positive former smokers, in Denmark (OR = 3.2; 95% CI, 0.9 to 11.4 for HSIL) and in the United States (OR = 2.1; 95% CI, 1.1 to 3.9 for CIS/cervical cancer).[47,69,71] The risk for HSIL/cervical cancer increased with number of cigarette smoked per day and years of smoking in all studies restricted to HPV-positive women[47]; however, only two studies found a significant increasing trend with number of cigarettes per day,[68,70] and only one study found an increasing trend with years of smoking.[70]

The strong epidemiologic evidence for the association between smoking and cervical cancer has been further supported by laboratory and clinical research. Several studies have reported high levels of nicotine and cotinine[91-93] and tobacco-specific N-nitrosamines[94] in cervical mucus of active and passive smokers. In addition, DNA damage in cervical tissue and exfoliated cells of smokers[95-98] and impairment of the local cell-mediated immune response in smokers[93,99] have long been reported. Reduction in the size of cervical lesions was documented among women participating in a smoking cessation intervention,[100] and a higher risk of treatment failure of CIN was reported among smokers after adjustment for HPV status.[101]

More recently, smoking was found to be a predictor of the duration of HPV infection. The median duration of infection was 2.2 months longer among smokers than among never-smokers (10.7 versus 8.5 months).[102] These studies provide biologic plausibility for the association and suggest two possible mechanisms by which tobacco smoking may increase the risk of cervical cancer: as a direct carcinogen and as an immunosuppressor of the host's local immune response, which may indirectly increase the risk of acquisition and persistence of HPV infection and its progression to cervical cancer or the expression of other cofactors.

Despite the consistent evidence in support of the role of smoking as a cofactor in HPV–related cervical carcinogenesis, residual confounding cannot be ruled out, because of the possibility that smoking and duration of smoking may be surrogate measures of HPV exposure (or time since exposure) via sexual activity, and the biologic mechanism by which tobacco smoking might increase the risk of cervical cancer remains unclear.[47] The issue of a residual confounding effect is analogous to the situation described earlier for OC use and requires careful consideration of study design and statistical analysis strategies. In addition, the different effects of smoking on the risks of ADC and SCC, both of them associated with HPV, seems to challenge the understanding of the role of smoking as a cofactor for HPV cervical carcinogenesis.[103]

Are other sexually transmitted infections or inflammation cofactors of interest in human papillomavirus–mediated cervical carcinogenesis?

Over the years, the pursuit of the sexually transmitted etiology of cervical cancer has focused on the role of several STI agents, including HSV, C. trachomatis, T. vaginalis, CMV, N. gonorrhoeae, and T. pallidum.[24,25,76]

After the hypothesis of a causal relationship between HPV and cervical neoplasia was first proposed in the mid-1970s,[27] the attention to other STIs as risk factors for SCC diminished; however, recently there has been an interest in reevaluating the role of STIs, particularly HSV type 2 (HSV-2) and C. trachomatis, as possible HPV cofactors. A possible mechanism whereby STIs could act as HPV cofactors is by inducing local inflammation that facilitates the establishment of HPV infection in the cervical epithelium.

HSV-2 was the focus of intensive study during the 1960s and 1970s. It was proved to be carcinogenic in in vitro and in vivo clinical studies; however, only a fraction of cervical carcinomas contained traces of HSV-2 infection (i.e., viral DNA), suggesting that HSV-2 was not the primary causal factor for cervical cancer.[104]

Several possible mechanisms for the role of HSV-2 in cervical cancer have been proposed. After the possible role of HPV in cervical cancer was suggested, it was hypothesized that HSV-2 and HPV may act synergistically, with HSV-2 initiating mutations and carcinogenesis in HPV-infected cervical cells.[104a] However, the lack of consistency in detecting HSV-2 DNA in cervical cells led researchers to propose a "hit-and-run" mechanism.[105] More recently, in vitro studies have suggested that the Xho-2 subfragment of the HSV-2 genome induces malignant transformation of HPV-immortalized cervical cells.[106] However, Tran-Thanh and colleagues[107] failed to identify HSV-2 Xho-2 or Bgl-IIC DNA.

Serologic studies showed a higher prevalence of HSV-2 antibodies among women with cervical neoplasia than among controls.[24] An increased risk for HSV-2 seropositivity, adjusted for HPV status was also reported in some studies.[77,108,109,109a] However, results continue to be inconclusive.[28,110-114] Lehtinen and associates[114] reported the results from a longitudinal study in the Nordic countries and a meta-analysis of six longitudinal studies. No association between HSV-2 and overall risk of CIS and cervical cancer was observed in the Nordic study (OR = 1.0; 95% CI, 0.6 to 1.7) or in the meta-analysis (OR = 0.9; 95% CI, 0.6 to 1.3).[114]

Contrary to the results obtained from longitudinal studies, results from the pooled analysis of case-control studies conducted by IARC supported a role for HSV-2 as a cofactor of HPV infection in cervical cancer.[65,115] The association was observed after adjusting for HPV status by standard methods and by restricting analysis to HPV-positive cases and controls, and it was higher for ADC (OR = 3.4; 95% CI, 1.5 to 7.7) than for SCC (OR = 2.2; 95% CI, 1.4 to 3.4).[115]

A consistent but modest association between C. trachomatis and cervical cancer that persisted after controlling for HPV status and other potential confounders has been reported.[28,108,109,109a,116-119] However, others failed to show an association with several markers of exposure to C. trachomatis, including antibody determinations,[85,112] culture,[28,108,120] PCR detection,[121] and self-reported history of infection.[77] The risk of cervical cancer among C. trachomatis serologically positive women has been reported to be 1.7 (95% CI, 1.1 to 2.7) after controlling for HPV and smoking status.[116]

The risk was higher with specific *C. trachomatis* serotypes, including serotype G (OR = 6.6; 95% CI, 1.6 to 27.0), serotype I (OR = 3.8; 95% CI, 1.3 to 11.0), and serotype D (OR = 2.7; 95% CI, 1.3 to 5.6).[117] Furthermore, in a IARC multicenter study conducted in Brazil and the Philippines, *C. trachomatis* seropositivity increased by 2.1-fold (95% CI, 1.1 to 4.0) the risk for cervical cancer among HPV-positive women.[119] The association appeared to be more relevant for SCC than ADC. In all, it appears that the lack of consistency in findings across studies suggests that residual confounding due to HPV (because of its sexually transmitted route) may have affected some of the studies finding a positive association with *C. trachomatis*, despite the seemingly careful control for HPV. On the other hand, the effect could be real, the result of a direct inflammatory effect on the cervix (see later discussion). It is obvious that the appropriate testing of this hypothesis will present many challenges for molecular epidemiologists in the future.

Numerous studies have addressed the association between human immunodeficiency virus (HIV) and cervical neoplasia.[25] The Centers for Disease Control and Prevention included invasive cervical cancer in the definition of acquired immunodeficiency syndrome (AIDS)–related conditions in 1992.[122] HIV-positive women have been reported to have higher rates of cervical abnormalities, larger lesions, higher grades of lesions, and higher recurrence rates than HIV-negative women.[123-125] In addition, HIV-positive women have been reported to have higher rates of HPV infection (40% to 95%) and CIN lesions (10% to 36%) than HIV-negative women (23% to 55% and 1% to 12%, respectively).[126-131]

A meta-analysis by Mandelblatt and colleagues[132] concluded that HIV is a cofactor for HPV-related cervical carcinogenesis, and this association seems to vary with the level of immune function. Results from La Ruche and associates[133] in Africa support an interaction between HIV-1 and HPV. Although the biologic mechanism for this interaction is not well understood, it is explained by the effect of HIV infection on the immune system and the existence of a molecular interaction between HIV and HPV.

In summary, understanding of the role of STIs in HPV-related carcinogenesis is limited by the difficulties in investigating the biologic mechanisms involved. STIs may have a direct genotoxic effect or an indirect effect through inflammation. Although HPV infection has not been associated with inflammation, HSV-2 and *C. trachomatis* are associated with cervicitis, which can conceivably lead to breaches in the cervical epithelium, facilitating the establishment of a productive HPV infection that is more likely to persist. The increased cervical permeability that occurs during an STI-induced inflammation may also enhance the role of other carcinogens (e.g., tobacco smoke) or affect the dynamics of antigen processing by Langerhans cells. A somewhat related mechanism, chronic inflammation, may increase the risk of HPV persistence by increasing the production of reactive oxygen species and inhibiting cell-mediated immunity.[52] Taken together, therefore, these pathways support the role of STI-induced inflammation in cervical carcinogenesis.

Alternatively, this association may be spurious and may be a surrogate measure for other high-risk behaviors (i.e., dimensions of sexual activity) associated with an increased risk of exposure to HPV. Although the biologic mechanism for HIV infection as a cofactor for HPV-related carcinogenesis is not completely understood, increasing HIV-associated immunosuppression (levels of CD4-positive lymphocytes lower than $500/mm^3$) is hypothesized to decrease HPV specific immunity, increasing the risk of HPV persistence and progression to preinvasive and invasive cervical lesions.[134]

It is suggested that there is no need for further case-control studies to assess the role of STIs as cofactors for cervical cancer, because this type of study design does not allow the opportunity to rule out the role of STIs as a surrogate measure for other high-risk behaviors associated with an increased risk of exposure to HPV.[52] In other words, no matter how meticulously one conducts an HPV-adjusted or restricted analysis, the possibility of residual confounding always remains. As such, further research using innovative study designs and methods of analysis will be needed to shed light on the complexity of biologic mechanisms for the relation between STIs and inflammation and to corroborate or refute current knowledge. Future longitudinal studies of HPV-positive women, with adequate measures for detection of concurrent STIs, including measures of cervical secretions, will be necessary to determine the role of these STIs as true HPV cofactors or spurious, secondary associations in cervical cancer.[52]

What dietary factors have been established as cofactors for human papillomavirus–related cervical carcinogenesis? Several lines of evidence suggest that dietary factors, particularly vitamin A, carotenoids, vitamin C, vitamin E, and folic acid, may have a protective effect against cervical cancer. The association between vitamin A intake and cervical neoplasia is hypothesized on the basis of the relation of vitamin A to other epithelial tumors, mainly SCCs. The capability of vitamin A to revert metaplastic changes in bronchial epithelium provides a biologic basis for the association with cervical neoplasia.[135] Vitamin C plays a role in the maintenance and protection of the normal epithelium against carcinogens. Folic acid functions as a coenzyme in the metabolism of single-carbon compounds, such as nucleic acid synthesis and amino acid metabolism.[135] Dietary factors may also have a role in cervical immunity and on the progression of HPV infection to cervical neoplasia.[48] It is also hypothesized that subclinical folate deficiency may act as a cofactor in the integration of the HPV genome into host DNA.[136]

However, epidemiologic studies on the association of dietary factors with cervical neoplasia have provided conflicting results.[24,48] Most studies did not support an association between the risk of cervical neoplasia and total vitamin A intake or serum retinol, although the evidence on carotenoids was more consistent with a protective effect on cervical neoplasia.[48] The variability in methods of nutrient measurement, selection of case and comparison groups, and choices of confounding factors controlled in the analyses makes comparison of these studies difficult.[52,137] In addition, the correlation among the various nutrients under study makes interpretation of the results a difficult task. The main limitation in most of the studies is the lack of adjustment for HPV infection.[48,52] In studies with more adequate control of confounding factors, the association between dietary or serum/plasma levels of dietary factors and cervical neoplasia remains inconclusive.[88,95,138-145]

Despite the inconclusive evidence, significant inverse associations with serum β-carotene, lycopene, α-carotene, and tocopherol have been reported with preinvasive and invasive cervical cancer in studies controlling for HPV status.[52] In support of the role of dietary cofactors of HPV in cervical cancer, an inverse association was reported between the risk of HPV persistence and dietary factors, including vegetable intake and plasma levels of cis-lycopene and vitamin B_{12}.[146-148] The role of dietary factors in HPV-mediated cervical carcinogenesis clearly deserves further attention. Because of the complexity of plausible and independent biologic mechanisms, the search for epidemiologic evidence will face many challenges. Regardless of the possible scenarios of interpretation, epidemiologic investigations of the role of diet in cervical cancer will have to contend with appropriately determining HPV exposure while measuring dietary factors using instruments and study designs that minimize measurement error and accommodate latency.

What host susceptibility factors influence human papillomavirus–mediated cervical carcinogenesis?

Most HPV infections are transient; almost 80% of newly diagnosed infections clear within 12 to 18 months after diagnosis, and only a small proportion progress to high-grade lesions or cervical cancer.[31,149-152] Several host and viral factors have been implicated as contributing to the risk of persistence and progression of HPV infection to cervical cancer.[44] The roles of host and viral factors have been the subject of recent literature reviews.[43,44,55,153,154]

The role of the host immune response in the natural history of HPV infection and its progression to cervical neoplasias has been the focus of intensive research over the last decade.[154] Antibody response to HPV infection is considered a key determinant of protective immunity and may play an important role as a marker of past and present infection or as a predictor of HPV-associated cervical neoplasia.[44,153,155] However, the mechanisms of this immune response are not well known. Epidemiologic studies have reported higher seroreactivity to E6 and E7 oncoproteins and to virus-like particles (VLPs) among cervical cancer cases than among controls, ranging between 35% and 59%, and

an increased risk for preinvasive and invasive cervical neoplasia.[156-160]

Seroconversion occurs several months after detection of HPV DNA infection; approximately 60% of women with an incident HPV DNA infection seroconverted within 18 months after detection.[161] No differences in median time to seroconversion were observed with HPV type, although antibody responses to high-risk HPV types have been found to persist longer.[161] These findings are consistent worldwide, and in low and high cancer risk geographic areas.[158,159,162] It is suggested that capsid antibodies may reflect a history of past HPV infection, whereas antibodies to E6 and E7 oncoproteins may be a marker of invasive cervical cancer, with tumor stage and mass determining the magnitude of the response.[160,163] Overall, the antibody response is mainly type-specific and directed against conformational epitopes.[157-159,164,165] Seroreactivity is more likely to be detected among individuals with persistent HPV infection and to increase with number of sexual partners.[159,162,164-166] In addition, HPV-specific serum immunoglobulin A (IgA) and IgG were found to be protective against recurrent HPV infection,[167] and results from a vaccine trial supported the effectiveness of systemic immunization against HPV capsids to prevent persistent infection.[168] As another influence on cervical cancer outcome, seroreactivity to HPV-16 proteins was associated with prognosis of cervical cancer (both disease-free and overall survival).[160,163] HPV-16 VLP IgG antibody–negative cervical cancer patients had a fourfold increased risk of death (95% CI, 1.4 to 11.8), compared with IgG antibody–positive patients after controlling for known prognostic factors including the International Federation of Gynecologists and Obstetricians (FIGO) stage.

There is some evidence indicating that systemic humoral immunity is not necessary for viral clearance.[153] Because HPV transmission and infection are events localized to the genital tract, the mucosal immune response may be more important in determining the outcome of infection than the systemic response.[169] However, few studies have examined local humoral immunity in relation to infection and disease and to epidemiologic and behavioral characteristics. Previous investigations found positive correlations between disease, infection, and local antibody.[159,169-172] These studies observed that a serologic IgA response was associated with infection with oncogenic HPV types, whereas an IgG response was associated with high-grade lesions, suggesting that the former may be a marker of current HPV infection and the latter a marker of cervical neoplasia.[159,169-172] As with the systemic humoral response, a lag of 4 to 12 months between detection of HPV infection and mucosal IgG response was reported, supporting the idea that IgG response might not be a good marker for HPV infection.[161]

There is compelling evidence in the cancer literature, including that of HPV-associated cervical lesions, for a protective role of specific cell-mediated immune responses. Data from epidemiologic studies[154,173] suggest an increased incidence of HPV-associated disease in certain groups of transplant recipients and HIV patients exhibiting immunosuppressed conditions in which cell-mediated immunity, but not the humoral immune function, is affected.[174] Further evidence for the importance of cell-mediated immunity includes (1) infiltration of helper T cells and cytotoxic T lymphocytes in spontaneously regressing warts[175]; (2) depletion of antigen-presenting cells in the cervix of women with cervical neoplasia[176]; and (3) the association of certain HLA haplotypes with cervical cancer risk.[43,177,178] A possible protective role for Th1-type cytokine production, indicative of a strong cell-mediated immunity response, is described in certain chronic parasitic diseases, leprosy, and HIV.[179-181] Furthermore, animal and human research has provided evidence for a protective role of cell-mediated immunity involving Th1-type cytokine production, which could be suppressed by a Th2-type cytokine profile favoring humoral immunity.[182-184]

Nakagawa and associates[173,185] reported that systemic T-cell proliferative responses and cytotoxic T lymphocyte responses to HPV-16 peptides and proteins were detectable in many virgins as well as sexually active women without cervical lesions, but not in those with active disease. Similarly, Tsukui and colleagues[175] reported that the helper T lymphocyte response to HPV antigens, particularly production of interleukin-2 (IL-2), was greater among cytologically normal women than among women with various degrees of progressive cervical neoplasia. The production of Th1 cytokines (IL-2 and interferon-γ), which potentially enhances CMI, was reported to be defective in women with extensive HPV infection, and progression to CIN was associated with a shift from Th1 to Th2 cytokine production.[123,186] Similarly, lymphoproliferative responses to specific HPV E6 and E7 was associated with HPV clearance and regression of CIN.[187,188] In addition, T-cell proliferative responses to HPV-16 E7 peptides was associated with persistence of HPV infection, whereas antigen-specific IL-2 production was associated with both virus clearance and progression of cervical lesions.[183,189]

As with the study of other cofactors, future research on the role of the immune response in HPV-mediated cervical carcinogenesis will require a more in-depth understanding of both systemic and local immune response phenomena at the level of individual HPV types. Understanding the role of the local immune response is of particular importance for vaccine development as a marker of efficacy.

What is the role of genetic markers of susceptibility to human papillomavirus–mediated cervical carcinogenesis? Genetic susceptibility traits, such as specific HLA alleles and haplotypes[43,53] and polymorphisms in the *TP53* gene,[54,55] have been linked to the development of cervical cancer.

HLA genes are involved in antigen presentation to T cells and play a role in the regulation of the cell-mediated Th1 immune response. Certain HLA alleles or haplotypes seem to be involved in susceptibility to HPV infection and cervical neoplasia, probably by

regulating the immune response against HPV infection and ultimately interfering in the establishment of productive persistent infections and cervical lesions.[43] Most research has focused on the study of HLA class II genes rather than HLA class I genes, due primarily to technical factors.[43] A review of the literature by Hildesheim and Wang[43] identified three groups of alleles/haplotypes that have been extensively studied during the last decade. Two of these groups, DQB1*03 alleles (including DQB1*0301, DQB1*0302, and DQB1*0303), and DRB1*1501 and DQB1*0602 alleles, have been associated with an increased risk of disease; whereas, DRB1*13 and DQB1*0603 alleles have been associated with a decreased risk of disease.[43] The most consistent finding is an increased risk of HPV infection and cervical disease in individuals with the DQB1*03 allele.[43,53,179,190-194] This association was observed for preinvasive and invasive disease, and it was consistent in populations worldwide. An increased risk of CIN and cervical cancer was associated with the DRB1*15 allele and the related DRB1*1501-DQB1*0602 haplotype among Hispanic and Swedish patients.[178,195,196] An increased CIN risk among carriers of the haplotype DQA1*0102-DQB1* 0602 in Norwegian[193] and Swedish[196] populations was also documented. Conversely, protective effects have been observed for the DRB1*13 alleles among German, American, and French populations.[191,194,197]

The role of HLA polymorphisms in the acquisition and clearance of HPV infection has been investigated in only a few studies.[53] Testing for HLA-DRB1 and -DQB1 variability, Maciag and colleagues[53] found that the DRB1*0301-DQB1*0201 haplotype was associated with a twofold reduction in risk of HPV infections, regardless of whether they were transient or persistent. The DRB1*1102-DQB1*0301 haplotype was associated with a reduction in risk of persistent infections, whereas DRB1*1601-DQB1*0502 and DRB1*0807-DQB1*0402 were associated with sevenfold and threefold increases in risk of persistence, respectively. Although these results remain to be corroborated, they suggest that much of the HLA class II effects on cervical cancer risk are mediated via their influences on the clearance and maintenance of HPV infection.

Despite the relative consistency of some of the findings in support of a role of HLA in cervical carcinogenesis, several inconsistencies remain. Reasons for these inconsistencies include the high degree of polymorphism of the alleles and methodologic differences such as small sample sizes, variability in control selection, and differences in HLA typing techniques.[194,197] Also of concern is the virtual impossibility for epidemiologic studies to attain enough statistical power and precision to scrutinize the myriad potential associations between individual polymorphisms and specific HPV types, which in theory represent the basic unit for antigen presentation and processing to the immune system. As such, HLA associations will continue to be studied in aggregate form, and by necessity many of the findings emerging from new studies will simply represent chance associations, because of the large number of associations being tested. Such findings are unlikely to be corroborated by future research.

Another host marker of interest is a polymorphism in codon 72 of the *TP53* gene, which codes for two structurally distinct forms of the P53 protein depending on the DNA sequence.[198,199] The association between a homozygous arginine genotype and cervical disease received considerable attention after the demonstration that the arginine form of the P53 protein (P53Arg) was more susceptible than the proline form (P53Pro) to binding and degradation by the HPV-16 and HPV-18 E6 oncoprotein. Individuals with the homozygous arginine form had seven times more susceptibility to HPV-related carcinogenesis than heterozygotes.[200] This finding provided support for a role of cellular genetic factors in HPV-related carcinogenesis. Since then, a large number of clinical and epidemiologic studies have provided inconclusive evidence in support of an increased risk of cervical neoplasia associated with arginine homozygosity in various populations.[54] A meta-analysis by Koushik and colleagues[55] of reports published between 1998 and 2002 identified 45 studies that included a disease-free comparison group and were eligible for inclusion.[55] These studies were conducted in populations worldwide and included preinvasive and invasive cervical lesions, and SCC as well as ADC.[55] Compared with P53Pro homozygosity and P53Arg/Pro heterozygosity combined, P53Arg homozygosity was not associated with an increased risk of cervical neoplasia (OR = 1.1; 95% CI, 0.9 to 1.3). The association was statistically significant for invasive lesions but not for preinvasive lesions, with a small increased risk for SCC (OR = 1.5; 95% CI, 1.2 to 1.9) and ADC (OR = 1.7; 95% CI, 1.0 to 2.7).[55] Reports published after the period of this meta-analysis have continued to be contradictory. Positive associations have been reported between cervical cancer and P53Arg homozygosity in Chile,[201] China,[202] and Mexico,[203] whereas no associations were found in Argentina,[204] central Italy,[205] and Korea.[206]

Several factors may contribute to these inconsistencies, including the possibility of spurious association and the substantial heterogeneity among these studies, particularly the studies of invasive cancer.[55] In the meta-analysis by Koushik and colleagues,[55] the most important factor contributing to between-study heterogeneity was whether or not the genotype frequencies were in Hardy-Weinberg equilibrium. The Hardy-Weinberg law states that "in the situation of random mating (with respect to genotype) and in the absence of mutation, migration, natural selection, or random genetic drift, the amount of genetic variation, represented by the frequency distribution of genotypes, will remain constant from one generation to the next."[55] Studies in which the genotype frequencies significantly deviated from the expected Hardy-Weinberg equilibrium had a greater mean OR than did those studies in which the control group was in equilibrium. However, other methodologic issues related to study design (mostly case-control studies), limited sample sizes, selection of study population, laboratory techniques, and source of DNA may still contribute to these inconsistencies.

Other genetic susceptibility markers for cervical neoplasia of interest that deserve further research include gene products associated with the metabolism of cigarette smoke, such as genetic polymorphisms in cytochrome P450,[207,208] and insulin growth factors (IGFs).[209-211] Future investigations of genetic polymorphism will need close attention to design and methodologic features. These studies should take advantage of special populations or ongoing investigations.[44] Given the relatively low prevalence and heterogeneity of these traits, large sample sizes may be required. Therefore, case-control studies could be the design of choice for such investigations.[55]

What is the role of human papillomavirus type and concurrent human papillomavirus infections in cervical carcinogenesis? There is consistent evidence from cohort studies implicating variability in HPV types in their propensity for persistent infections and in their progression to preinvasive and invasive cervical cancer. A substantially increased risk of preinvasive and invasive cervical cancer exists for women who develop persistent infections with oncogenic HPV types.[28,29,31,32,57,149,212] Moscicki and coworkers[149] observed, among a cohort of 618 HPV-positive adolescents and young women, that those positive for high-oncogenic HPV types had lower regression rates of HPV DNA infection and a 14-fold increased risk (95% CI, 2.5 to 84.5) of developing an HSIL, compared with those positive for low-oncogenic HPV types. Similarly, Ho and colleagues[31,213] observed that infection with high-oncogenic HPV types was a risk factor for persistence of infection. Among Brazilian women, those with high-oncogenic HPV types were 2.6 times more likely to have a persistent infection than women with low-oncogenic types.[214] Furthermore, in the same population, women with a persistent HPV infection with high-oncogenic HPV types had higher incidence rates for any SIL (relative risk [RR] = 10.2; 95% CI, 5.9 to 17.6) and for HSIL (RR = 11.7; 95% CI, 4.1 to 33.3).[212] In addition, median time to progression from atypical squamous cells of undetermined significance (ASCUS) to more severe lesions was shorter, and lesions persisted for longer periods.[215]

The role of concurrent infection with multiple HPV types on the risk of persistence of HPV infection and progression of cervical lesions has been less clear. Higher prevalence of concurrent infection with multiple HPV types was reported among women with mild or moderate cervical abnormalities.[216]

What are the roles of human papillomavirus viral load and intratype variation in the risk of persistent human papillomavirus infection and progression to cervical cancer? In addition to viral type and concurrent multiple infection, viral load and intratypic variation of HPVs have been suggested as risk factors for persistent infection and risk of progression to cervical neoplasia. Viral load has been associated with risk of cervical neoplasia, and it has been suggested as a potential marker of persistent HPV DNA infection.[44,217] However, evidence of its role as a risk factor is still inconclusive, and its value as a prognostic marker of progressive disease is unknown.[44,218] In some studies, a high level of HPV DNA was associated with or predictive of higher-grade lesions,[38,39,42,57,218] although more recent work indicates that high viral loads are more predictive of lower-grade CIN but not of high-grade CIN, suggesting a greater value as a predictor of the initiation of the neoplastic process.[59,217] This finding is consistent with the higher level of viral integration observed in more advanced lesions.[217] Other studies indicate that a high viral load is associated with persistent HPV infections.[219] Studies of Hybrid Capture II technology, using the assay's signal intensity to infer viral load in the specimen, are considered less accurate because they are not normalized by the amount of cellular DNA available for the assay. In addition, they do not provide type-specific information.[59,220,221]

Several factors have been identified that contribute to the inconsistency of results, including differences in measurement methods (e.g., PCR, hybrid capture), use of different cytohistologic classifications, sample quality, and presence of concurrent infection with multiple HPV types.[44]

Testing for molecular variants of HPV provides an extra level of taxonomic detail in ascertaining and monitoring infections that are deemed persistent, decreasing measurement error in epidemiologic studies.[222] Isolates of a given HPV type that have up to 2% nucleotide variation in specific regions of the genome are designated as molecular variants.[223] HPV-16 has been extensively studied, and more than 40 molecular variants have been described.[43,223-226] Sequence analysis of HPV-16, focusing on the noncoding long control region of the viral genome, has led to the identification of five major classes of HPV-16 variants based on geographic relatedness: a European group, two African groups, an Asian group, and an Asian-American group.[225] It seems that particular HPV variants differ in terms of oncogenic potential. In most studies, a higher risk of cervical neoplasia was observed in the presence of non-European variants of HPV-16, compared with European variants.[43,227-229] In a review paper, Hildesheim and Wang[43] reported that infection with non-European variants of HPV-16 was associated with a twofold to ninefold increased risk of HSIL and cervical cancer.[43] This association was consistent in different populations (United States, Latin America, and Japan), was observed in case-control and cohort studies, appeared to be stronger for cervical cancer than for HSIL, and remained after adjustment for age and race.[43,228,229] However, given the correlation between HPV variants, geographic distribution, and race/ethnicity, residual confounding of race/ethnicity as an explanation for the association between non-European and European variants cannot be completely ruled out.[43,228] In a study of Mexican women, the risk of cervical cancer seemed to be more associated with Asian-American variants than with European variants.[230]

Variants involving the coding regions of the HPV genome have also been found to result in varying oncogenic potential.[231] A well-known nucleotide variation is that of position 350 in the E6 gene of HPV-16. In a few studies, the variant with the nucleotide G at 350 was associated with high-grade lesions or progression of CIN[232,233]; however, this has not been observed in other studies.[234-237] Although information on HPV variants of other HPV types is limited, some studies have found an increased risk for cervical neoplasia associated with HPV-18 and HPV-58 non-European variants.[228,238] Furthermore, non-European variants of HPV-16 and HPV-18 have been associated with a higher risk of persistent infection.[228]

Future research on the role of viral factors will need to be expanded to encompass a larger number of HPV types, use of PCR technology, and sequencing of the entire HPV genome to define variants.[44] Despite their adequate size for studying type-specific associations, existing cohort studies that are underway worldwide have only limited statistical capability in examining the natural history of infections at the level of individual variants. Efforts in pooling data and specimens from such studies may prove informative and could enable the exploration of clinically relevant viral polymorphisms that are as yet unsuspected.

What are some of the unresolved issues that should orient future research on cofactors for cervical cancer?

During the last 30 years, laboratory, epidemiologic, and clinical research studies have provided evidence of the roles of certain types of HPV as the necessary causes of cervical cancer.[34] The HPV-cervical cancer model has become a paradigm of progress in cancer research among neoplastic diseases with infectious origins. Research on HPV has progressed at a fast pace since the hypothesis was first proposed in the late 1970s; several primary and secondary prevention strategies have been developed and are undergoing assessment in randomized clinical trials.[12,239,240] Prophylactic and therapeutic trials are under way, and the prevention and treatment of cervical cancer via vaccination against HPV infection is in the foreseeable future.[168,239] Similarly, the value of HPV testing in the screening of cervical cancer and in the triage of women with abnormal cytology is being evaluated.[12,240,241] These strategies have great potential, particularly in high-risk populations in developing countries, where approximately 80% of the cases occur.

Along with fast progress and the potential for prevention of cervical cancer, recognition of the role of HPV infection as a necessary causal agent has led to new methodologic and analytic challenges, the need to reassess the role of previously identified risk factors for cervical cancer, and the need to assess the value of current and new prevention strategies in developed and developing countries.[34,46,242,243]

The understanding of the role of these cofactors is important for the identification of populations or groups of populations at higher risk for persistent HPV infection and progression to cervical neoplasia.

The initial approach to the assessment of confounding and effect modification in HPV-related disease was based on the use of standard epidemiologic multivariate methods by stratified analysis and logistic regression modeling using both HPV-positive and HPV-negative cases and controls. However, after the establishment of HPV as the necessary causal factor for cervical cancer, this approach became inadequate. Under this model of causality, HPV-negative cases cannot conceivably exist and are only the result of misclassification. Additionally, the use of HPV-negative controls is not appropriate because they represent a group of subjects not at risk for cervical cancer. It is suggested that the only possible approach to control for HPV in the assessment of the role of cofactors is by restricting the analysis to HPV-positive subjects only.[46,60] This strategy has already been implemented, taking advantage of several large case-control studies and a prospective-cohort study to reassess the role of several previously established environmental risk factors.[47,65] However, as discussed previously, this strategy is not without pitfalls because of the tenuous assumption that HPV positivity among controls represents their latency-relevant HPV exposure. Any resulting associations from future case-control studies will have to be interpreted cautiously, acknowledging this caveat. Parity, smoking, and OC use are consistently identified as potential cofactors for HPV-related cervical carcinogenesis, and these findings are observed with both analytic strategies.[47,65] ORs for all three factors were slightly higher in the analysis restricted to HPV-positive cases and controls.[47] Despite the less conclusive evidence of the roles of HSV-2 and *C. trachomatis*, restrictive analysis of HPV-positive cases and controls showed a twofold increased risk of cervical cancer associated with these STIs.[65]

The role of dietary factors remains a major challenge for study. The comparison and interpretation of results have been hampered by methodologic limitations inherent to the study of nutritional factors, including data collection methods and generalizability of nutrient databases. Reassessment of the role of nutritional factors using HPV-positive restricted analysis of case-control studies is still pending. In addition to the inconsistent epidemiologic evidence of the role of dietary factors, phase II and phase III chemoprevention trials have failed to support the protective effects of dietary factors in HPV-related carcinogenesis.[47] However, a role in early-stage (as opposed to late) carcinogenesis and several methodologic factors have also been suggested to explain the failure of chemoprevention trials for cervical cancer.[52] In support of the role of dietary factors in the early stages of the carcinogenesis process, several nutrient deficiencies have been associated with the risk of HPV persistence among U.S. Hispanics.[52,147,148,244]

Results from studies of other host cofactors have been less consistent, although in general they tend to support a role in cervical carcinogenesis. To date, most research on host and viral cofactors has been restricted to a small number of HPV types, mainly HPV-16, limiting the interpretation and understanding of the role of these cofactors.[44,51,245] As mentioned earlier, molecular epidemiologic studies have just begun to tap into the complexities of the associations at the level of individual types and variants and to address the natural history on long-term follow-up.

Despite the extraordinary progress in research and the exciting opportunities for primary and secondary prevention of cervical cancer, there is still a need for further, more focused research.[46,245] The role of cofactors in HPV-induced cervical carcinogenesis will continue to be the focus of epidemiologic research in the years to come. Ongoing and future molecular epidemiologic studies will increase understanding of the role of these cofactors and the identification of the biologic mechanisms involved in the carcinogenesis process. This will require the use and development of new molecular tools and novel statistical modeling approaches to understand mechanisms in the natural history of HPV and cervical cancer.

It is suggested that future studies of the role of cofactors should be restricted to HPV-positive subjects; cases in case-control studies should be restricted to high-grade lesions or cervical cancer; and selection of HPV-positivity controls should rely on the use of the most accurate available HPV test or combination tests (e.g., HPV DNA and serologic markers). These studies will need to be large, multicenter, and multidisciplinary to allow for the study of diverse populations in terms of age, race/ethnicity, and geographic distribution. Future studies should ideally be prospective cohort studies with repeated measurements, and they should include a larger number of HPV types and other HPV markers. These studies will require multicenter collaborations to compensate for the low prevalence of some of these markers and the high-degree of polymorphisms of some of the genetic traits of interest. Furthermore, multicenter, multidisciplinary studies will allow better utilization of resources and potentially a reduction in cost.

In addition to the analytic challenges, epidemiologic research faces several study design challenges.[46] New studies will require more accurate definition of HPV exposure, one that takes in consideration the impact of the oncogenicity potential of the types under consideration as a group, the existence of single or multiple infections, the transient or recurrent nature of HPV infection, and the use of other markers of HPV infection (e.g., viral load, integration status, variants), as well as accurate definition of study end points.[46] Cases and controls should be selected based on the research question under study. The impact and interpretation of the HPV-positive restrictive analytic strategy deserves further attention, particularly given that the direction and magnitude of the associations revisited with this approach have remained the same or have been slightly higher estimates than the ones in unrestricted analyses.[47] The role of negative confounding between cofactors and HPV status and the role of selection bias should be addressed in future studies. Another statistical challenge under the HPV-as-necessary-cause model of causality is the estimation of the attributable fraction for the cofactors, given that standard methods to calculate this parameter are not appropriate in the extreme situation in which a cause is deemed necessary.[43,47] In addition, the strong correlations among some cofactors need to be taken into consideration in the analysis and interpretation of results.

Several specific research questions related to the natural history of HPV infection and its progression to cervical cancer have been identified and suggest directions for future research. For the most part, the biologic mechanisms involving these cofactors in HPV-related carcinogenesis are unknown, and proposed hypotheses need further confirmation. Examples of these questions are: What is the meaning of HPV positivity among controls, particularly when measured cross-sectionally? Are HPV-positive controls likely to represent a persistent HPV infection? What is the threshold of duration for a persistent HPV infection beyond which risk of cervical cancer increases? What is the role of exogenous and endogenous hormonal factors in the bimodal age distribution of HPV prevalence observed in some populations? Is the second prevalence peak observed in perimenopausal or postmenopausal women the result of reactivation of latent infection, or does it represent new infections? Does humoral immunity confer long-term type-specific protection against reinfection?

Although preventive strategies were not covered in this chapter, the evaluation of primary and secondary preventive strategies targeted to reduce the risk of acquisition and persistence of HPV infection and the risk of progression to cervical cancer will be the focus of extensive research worldwide. Of paramount importance is the fact that secondary prevention of cervical cancer is gradually shifting from a morphology-based paradigm (i.e., the Pap cytology) to one in which detection of an STI (i.e., HPV infection) becomes the focus. As increasing numbers of otherwise healthy women are told by their physicians that they harbor a sexually transmitted virus that can cause genital cancer, the need for concrete, practical information about HPV will dominate the concerns of health care providers and patients worldwide. Obtaining this information will require specialized research into the transmissibility of HPV, the effectiveness of barrier methods, and the psychological impact of an HPV diagnosis, among other areas. Factors affecting participation in HPV-related clinical research and participation and acceptance of HPV vaccines by adolescent men and women, parents, health care providers, and other groups of society will need to be identified and addressed, in large part by epidemiologic studies.

In addition, future research should explore the role of interpersonal, sociocultural, and social factors. These factors may be important because they influence health behaviors, by which, based on current knowledge, most anogenital HPV infections are transmitted. Social and cultural factors affect health by influencing health behaviors, exposure, and vulnerability to the disease, as well as the access, availability, and quality of health care and health promotion opportunities.[246] Furthermore, interpersonal, sociocultural, and environmental factors explain differences in the prevalence

and incidence of sexually transmitted diseases across societies and subgroups of populations.[247] Such studies would provide valuable information to inform the design, implementation, and evaluation of future primary and secondary preventive strategies, especially in young, socially disadvantaged, and sexually active women from minority populations, in whom cervical cancer continues to be an important health problem and in whom high HPV infection rates are an ever-present problem.

VULVAR CANCER

Vulvar cancer is an uncommon malignant tumor accounting for approximately 9% of all cancers of the female genital tract worldwide.[250] In the United States, the American Cancer Society estimated that in 2003 approximately 4000 women would be diagnosed with vulvar cancer, representing 5% of all cancers of the female genital tract, and 800 women would die from this neoplasm.[8] SCCs constitute the most common histologic type of primary vulvar cancer (90%), followed by melanoma, Bartholin gland carcinoma, basal cell carcinoma, verrucous carcinoma, and Paget's disease.[248] Similar to cervical cancer, invasive vulvar cancer is preceded by a spectrum of intraepithelial changes from mild dysplasia (VIN I), to moderate dysplasia (VIN II), to severe dysplasia (VIN III), to invasive vulvar cancer. The estimated progression rate from VIN to invasive vulvar cancer is approximately 6%, and the risk of progression appears to be higher among older women (40+ years) than among younger women.[248]

What is the role of demographic or socioeconomic factors as determinants of the geographic and racial/ethnic differences in the occurrence of and survival from vulvar cancer?

The geographic pattern of incidence and mortality from vulvar cancer is difficult to describe because of the rarity of the disease and because vulvar cancer is usually grouped with cancers of the vagina, fallopian tubes, and other female genital organs. Higher incidence rates are reported in developing countries such as French Polynesia (4.4 per 100,000), Italy, Argentina, Brazil, and Peru (Table 1-2); lower rates are reported among women in China, Japan, and Korea, and among Asian women in the United States.[249,250] In the United States, the annual age-adjusted (2000 U.S. standard population) incidence rate for vulvar cancer for the period between 1996 and 2000 was 2.2 per 100,000 women.[17] This neoplasm tends to strike older women in their 70s or 80s and is very uncommon in women younger than 35 years of age. The incidence of vulvar cancer increases sharply after age 50 years, and this increasing pattern with age is observed in all racial/ethnic groups. Approximately 66% of cases are diagnosed at 70 years of age or older, whereas only 15% are diagnosed before age 40 years. Mean age at diagnosis of invasive vulvar cancer is between 65 and

Table 1–2. Highest Age-Adjusted Incidence Rates* for Vulvar Cancer Worldwide in 1988–1992

Country	Year	Incidence Rate
French Polinesia	1988-1992	4.4
Italy, Ferrara	1991-1992	3.8
Argentina, Concordia	1990-1994	3.7
Brazil, Porto Alegre	1990-1992	3.6
Italy, Trieste	1989-1992	3.4
Peru, Trujillo	1988-1990	3.4
Canada, Prince Edward Island	1988-1992	3.1
New Zealand, Maori	1988-1992	2.9
U.S., New Orleans: Black	1988-1992	2.7
New Zealand: non-Maori	1988-1992	2.6
Austria, Tyrol	1988-1992	2.6
Canada, Nova Scotia	1988-1992	2.5
Switzerland, Basel	1988-1992	2.5
Canada, Manitoba	1988-1992	2.4
Poland, Lower Silesia	1988-1992	2.4

*Rate per 100,000, age-adjusted to the world standard population.
From Parkin DM, et al: Cancer Incidence in Five Continents VII, IARC, 1997.

70 years; the mean age at diagnosis of noninvasive vulvar neoplasia is about 20 years younger.

During the period 1992–1997, higher age-adjusted (U.S. 1970 standard population) incidence rates were observed among whites (2.3 per 100,000), followed by blacks (1.5), Hispanics (0.8), Asian/Pacific Islanders (0.7) and American Indians/Alaskan Natives (0.5). This racial difference has remained in more recent periods. The age-adjusted (U.S. 2000 standard population) incidence rate during the period 1996–2000 was 2.4 per 100,000 among white women and 1.7 per 100,000 among black women.[17] The diagnosis of vulvar cancer occurs at an earlier age in black women (median, 58 years) than in white women (median, 68 years).[17]

An increasing trend in incidence of vulvar intraepithelial neoplasia (VIN) was reported during the last 25 years or more, whereas the incidence rate of invasive vulvar cancer has remained stable.[251,252] In the United States, the rates for cancer of the vulva increased by an estimated 2.4% annually between 1992 and 1998.[253] Rates are increasing mainly among women younger than 50 years of age, and this trend has been observed in several developed countries, including the United States, Switzerland, Norway, New Zealand, and Austria.[251-256]

Mortality for vulvar cancer is very low; the age-adjusted (2000 U.S. standard population) mortality rate from vulvar cancer in the United States for the period 1996–2000 was 0.5 per 100,000 women.[17] Trends in mortality from vulvar cancer have been less consistent; rates increased from the mid-1970s to the mid-1980s and since then have remained stable.[253] Vulvar cancer is highly curable if detected at early stages. Based on data from nine SEER areas, the overall 5-year relative survival rate for vulvar cancer in the United States for the period 1992–1999 was estimated at 67.9%.[17] Similar 5-year survival rates are reported in Switzerland and Norway.[254,255] Survival decreases with increasing age, stage, grade, inguinal nodes status, and tumor thickness.[255] In addition, poorer survival has been associated with basaloid tumors than with keratinizing tumors; whereas the role of HPV status as a prognostic factor for overall survival and disease-free survival is still inconclusive.[255,257-259]

What are the risk factors for vulvar cancer? Is the risk of smoking stronger for vulvar cancer than for cervical cancer?

The study of the epidemiology of vulvar cancer has been limited primarily because of the rarity of the disease and its etiology remains poorly understood. Most current knowledge on the epidemiology of this neoplasm derives from small clinic-based studies and a few large, population-based, cases-control studies in the United States.[260-262] Results from earlier studies conducted before HPV testing was introduced suggest that vulvar cancer has risk factors similar to those of cervical cancer, including number of sexual partners, smoking, history of STIs, history of abnormal cytologic examination or prior gynecologic cancer, OC use, and dietary factors.[260,263-266] These studies were later extended and reanalyzed after HPV serologic assays became available.

In the early 1990s, three different histologic patterns of vulvar cancer were described—basaloid, warty, and keratinizing—with two distinct etiologic pathways.[267,268] The basaloid and warty patterns together represent a small proportion of all vulvar carcinomas. They are more common in young women, are more frequently found adjacent to VIN, are associated with HPV, and present the same risk factor profile as that of cervical cancer. The keratinizing vulvar carcinomas represent the majority of the vulvar lesions; they occur more often in older women, are not adjacent to VIN, and are not associated with HPV or other risk factors typical of cervical cancer.[267-270] The majority of basaloid or warty tumors (75% to 100%) are HPV DNA positive, whereas only 2% to 23% of the keratinizing carcinomas are HPV positive.[262,267,268,270] Therefore, contrary to cervical cancer, HPV is not considered a necessary cause for vulvar cancer, because it is associated with only a subset of vulvar cancers.[271] After the introduction of the new histologic classification of vulvar cancer, Trimble and colleagues[272] reanalyzed the data from an earlier case-control study[260] and confirmed the two different etiologic patterns of these tumors previously reported. Compared with women with keratinizing tumors, those with basaloid or warty carcinomas were more likely to have had two or more sexual partners (81% versus 43%), to be smokers (94% versus 29%), and to be HPV DNA positive (86% versus 6.3%).

Most epidemiologic studies assessing the role of HPV in vulvar cancer have been limited not only by small sample size but also by their inability to conduct HPV DNA testing in both cases and controls. Most studies of HPV and vulvar cancer have relied on serologic assays for a limited number of HPV types, mainly HPV-16.[262,273-276] Three of these studies included testing for antibodies against HPV-18,[262,275,276] one for HPV-33 antibodies,[275] and one for HPV-6 antibodies.[262] These studies consistently showed that HPV antibody–positive women are at higher risk for vulvar carcinoma compared with HPV antibody–negative women. Stronger associations have been reported for CIS than for invasive vulvar carcinoma, and they have confirmed the different association profiles between HPV and basaloid/warty versus keratinizing carcinomas. Seroreactivity to HPV-16 VLPs was associated with a 5.4-fold increased risk for VIN and a 4.5-fold increased risk for basaloid/warty carcinomas, whereas seroreactivity to HPV-16 E6 or E7 proteins was associated with a 14-fold increased risk for these tumors.[273] An extension of the previous studies by Brinton[277] and Sun[273] and their colleagues, which included 142 cases of preinvasive and invasive vulvar carcinomas and 126 population controls, confirmed a 5.3-fold increased risk (95% CI, 2.5 to 11.1) for all vulvar cancers among HPV-16–seropositive women.[274] Using a small subsample of cases reclassified with the new histologic scheme described earlier, these authors observed a very strong association between HPV-16 seropositivity and VIN (OR = 13.4; 95% CI, 3.9 to 46.5) and a borderline association with basaloid/warty tumors (OR = 3.8; 95% CI, 0.8 to 18.9); no association was observed with keratinizing lesions (OR = 1.6; 95% CI, 0.4 to 7.4).[274] Similarly, Madeleine and coworkers[276] reported that HPV-16 antibody–positive women were at a 3.6-fold increased risk for CIS (95% CI, 2.6 to 4.8) and a 2.8-fold increased risk for invasive cancer (95% CI, 1.7 to 4.7); Carter and associates[262] reported 4.5-fold (95% CI, 3.6 to 6.0) and 3.1-fold (95% CI, 2.0 to 4.9) increased risks, respectively. Furthermore, Bjorge and colleagues,[275] in a nested case-control study conducted in a large population-based cohort in Finland and Norway, found HPV-16 seropositivity to be associated with a 4.5-fold increased risk for vulvar and vaginal invasive cancers combined.

Results on HPV-18 seropositivity have been less consistent.[262,275,276] A twofold increased risk of vulvar carcinoma, both CIS and invasive lesions, was reported among HPV-18–seropositive women by Carter and associates,[262] whereas no effect was reported by Madeleine and coworkers[276] or by Bjorge and colleagues.[275] Of interest, although based on a very small number of subjects, was the 3.3-fold increase risk (95% CI, 0.5 to 23) for vulvar and vaginal cancers combined and the 4.5-fold increased risk (95% CI, 0.5 to 54) for preinvasive vulvar and vaginal cancers combined, found among those women with HPV-33 seropositivity.[275]

Restriction of analysis of the association between HPV-16 seropositivity and vulvar cancer to the HPV DNA–positive stratum seems to have a minimal impact on the estimates of risk[262,276]; however, a stronger association between HPV-16 seropositivity and vulvar carcinoma was reported among HPV-16 DNA-positive women (OR = 4.5) than among HPV-16 DNA-negative women (OR = 2.9).[276]

In addition to HPV, number of lifetime sexual partners, smoking, and HSV-2 seropositivity have been associated with vulvar carcinoma after controlling for HPV serologic status.[274,276] Women with three or more lifetime sexual partners were at a 3.4-fold increased risk for vulvar carcinomas.[274] A 3.2-fold increased risk for vulvar CIS and invasive carcinomas combined,[274] a 1.9-fold increased risk for CIS, and a 1.5-fold increased risk for invasive carcinoma[276] have been reported in association with HSV-2 seropositivity.

Of interest has been the strong association between smoking and the risk of vulvar cancer observed in these studies. A higher risk was observed for current smokers than for ever-smokers, and the association was stronger for CIS than for invasive carcinomas. Current smokers were at a 6.4-fold increased risk for CIS (95% CI, 4.4 to 9.3) and at a 3-fold increased risk for invasive carcinomas (95% CI, 1.7 to 5.3).[276] Restriction of the analysis to HPV-16 DNA–positive subjects only resulted in a 7.1-fold increased risk of vulvar carcinoma among current smokers. Moreover, a possible interaction between HPV-16 seropositivity and smoking has been suggested. Women who were current smokers and HPV-16 seropositive were found to have an 8.5-fold increased risk for vulvar cancer in the study by Hildesheim and associates[274] and an 18.8-fold increased risk in the study by Madeleine and coworkers[276]; the risk was lower among female nonsmokers who were HPV-16 seropositive (2.9-fold and 3.4-fold, respectively), suggesting the role of smoking as a cofactor for vulvar cancer.

In summary, little is known about the epidemiology of vulvar cancer. Epidemiologic studies are difficult to conduct because of the rarity of these lesions. However, existing data are consistent with an association between vulvar cancer and HPV infection, at least for a subset of cases. Data also support the existence of two distinct etiologic pathways for vulvar cancer, one strongly associated with HPV infection (VIN and basaloid/warty carcinomas) and the other not linked to HPV infection (keratinizing carcinomas). Data also suggest smoking and HSV-2 infection as potential cofactors for vulvar neoplasia, as well as a possible interaction between smoking and HPV-16 seropositivity. These salient findings notwithstanding, most epidemiologic studies have been limited in their abilities to study the role of HPV and other risk factors. Studies have relied mostly on serologic assays for HPV testing, because vaginal samples for HPV DNA testing have not been available from control subjects. There is a need for further research to better establish the role of HPV infection and other cofactors in the etiology of vulvar cancer. The magnitude of the association between smoking and vulvar cancer, particularly with CIS, and the possible role of smoking as a cofactor in vulvar cancer deserve future attention, including consideration of the strength of the relation.

Future studies should not combine the two different types of vulvar cancer. Compliance with this distinction will increase the challenge of conducting epidemiologic research of these rare tumors and argues for the need for multicenter efforts. Because of the low incidence of these neoplasms, future epidemiologic research will continue to rely on case-control studies as the most efficient study design for rare conditions. Researchers will need to implement strategies for the collection of cervicovaginal specimens for testing for HPV DNA and other STIs from population-based control subjects, including the use of self-sampling techniques. Many unanswered questions remain about the role of HPV and other environmental, host, and viral factors in vulvar cancer. Studies are needed to address the natural history of the disease, to expand findings to other HPV types, and to further elucidate the roles of smoking and other cofactors in vulvar cancer.

VAGINAL CANCER

Cancer of the vagina is extremely rare. The American Cancer Society estimated that in 2003 approximately 2000 women would be diagnosed with cancer of the vagina and of other nonspecified female genital organs (fewer than 3% of all cancers of the female genital tract), and that 800 women would die from these neoplasms in the United States.[8] SCCs are the most common vaginal malignancy (90%), followed by clear cell ADC and melanoma.[248]

In the United States, the annual age-adjusted (2000 U.S. standard population) incidence rate for vaginal cancer for the period 1996–2000 was 0.7 per 100,000 women.[17] This neoplasm tends to be diagnosed in older women (median age at diagnosis, 69 years); however it seems to be diagnosed at an earlier age in blacks than whites (median, 42 versus 70 years).[17,252,278] The incidence of vaginal cancer increases steadily with age; whereas the incidence of CIS of the vagina reaches a peak between ages 55 and 70 years.

What is the role of demographic or socioeconomic factors as determinants of the geographic and racial/ethnic differences in the occurrence of and survival from vaginal cancer?

During the period 1996–2000, higher incidence and mortality rates were observed among blacks (1.0 and 0.4 per 100,000, respectively) than among whites (0.7 and 0.2 per 100,000, respectively) (Table 1-3).[17] In addition, the diagnosis of vaginal cancer occurs at an earlier age in blacks (median, 42 years) than in whites (median, 70 years), although no differences in survival by race are detected.[17] In analogy to cervical and vulvar cancers, vaginal cancer is preceded by a spectrum of intraepithelial changes from mild dysplasia (VAIN I), to moderate dysplasia (VAIN II), to severe dysplasia (VAIN III), to invasive vaginal cancer.[252] An increasing trend in incidence of vaginal intraepithelial neoplasia (VAIN) was reported during the last 25 years or more, whereas the incidence of invasive vaginal cancer has remained stable.[251,252] Rates of invasive vaginal cancer increase substantially after 65 years of age.[252]

Table 1–3. Age-Adjusted Incidence, Mortality, and 5-year Relative Survival Rates, SEER US 1996–2000

Race	Incidence*	Mortality*	Survival†
Vulvar Cancer			
White	2.4	0.5	76.3
Black	1.7	0.3	67.9
Vaginal Cancer			
White	0.7	0.2	45.9
Black	1.0	0.4	45.4

*Incidence and mortality rates are per 100,000 and age-adjusted to the 2000 US standard population.
†Survival rates are percent.
From Ries et al: SEER Cancer Statistics Review, 1975-2000, Bethesda, MD, National Cancer Institute http://seer.cancer.gov/csr/1975_2000, 2003.

The mortality rate for vaginal cancer is very low; the age-adjusted (2000 U. S. standard population) mortality rate from vaginal cancer in the United States for the period 1996–2000 was 0.4 per 100,000 women.[17] Based on data from nine SEER areas, the overall 5-year relative survival rate for vaginal cancer in the United States for the period 1992–1999 was estimated to be 45%.[17]

Is human papillomavirus infection a necessary cause for vaginal cancer? Why is the risk of smoking stronger for vaginal cancer than for cervical cancer?

It is assumed that vaginal cancer has causal factors similar to those of cervical cancer, including HPV infection.[261] However, this assumption has been based mostly on circumstantial evidence rather than epidemiologic data, primarily because of the rarity of these tumors. Most current knowledge of the epidemiology of vaginal cancer comes from only two large, population-based, case-control studies conducted in the United States.[266,277] In support of the similar etiologic pattern of vaginal and cervical cancers, these two tumors are frequently diagnosed simultaneously.[278,279] Patients are more likely to have a history of other anogenital cancers, particularly cervical cancer,[280] and HPV DNA is found in tissue samples of invasive vaginal carcinoma. HPV seems to play a central role in the causal pathway, because it has been reported in up to 91% of all vaginal cancers.[262,281-282] The prevalence of HPV infection is higher among women with CIS than among those with invasive lesions,[280] and HPV-16 is the most prevalent type, as in cervical cancer.[280,281] HPV-16 antibody–positive women were at a 3.5- to 4.3-fold increased risk for vaginal cancer compared with antibody-negative women.[280,282] A lower but statistically significant risk of vaginal cancer was also observed with seroreactivity to HPV-18 (OR = 2.0; 95% CI, 1.3 to 2.9).[280]

Further supporting the role of HPV infection in vaginal cancer is the finding of a higher prevalence of HPV DNA positivity (98%) among women developing VAIN during follow-up after hysterectomy and radiation treatment for gynecologic cancers, compared with only 13% among women without evidence of these preinvasive lesions.[283]

In addition to HPV infection, other risk factors associated with cervical cancer have also been reported in association with vaginal cancer.[249] A higher risk of vaginal cancer has been observed among women with lower education and income levels.[249,277] Results of the role of sexual behavior have been less conclusive.[249,277] After controlling for HPV serologic status, Daling and colleagues[280] observed a threefold increased risk (95% CI, 1.9 to 4.9) for vaginal cancer among women reporting five or more lifetime sexual partners, and the risk was similar for both CIS and invasive carcinomas.[280] Similarly, an increased risk for vaginal cancer was observed among women who reported having their first sexual intercourse before 17 years of age.[280] HSV-2–seropositive women showed a twofold increased risk of vaginal cancer.[280,282]

Although early studies found a small but not significant association with smoking,[266,277] a more recent report found a twofold (95% CI, 1.4 to 3.1) increased risk of CIS and invasive vaginal carcinomas among current smokers.[280] Smokers of 20 or more cigarettes daily and those smoking for 30 or more years were also at increased risk.[280] The risk was higher for invasive carcinomas than for CIS, and this effect was independent of the measures of smoking exposure used. Of interest is the magnitude of the associations observed between invasive vaginal cancer and the various measures of smoking, which were higher than those observed for cervical cancer: ever-smokers, OR = 3.1; current smokers, OR = 4.6; smokers of 20 or more cigarettes daily, OR = 4.7; and smokers for 30 or more years, OR = 6.7.[280] Hysterectomy was reported to increase the risk of vaginal cancer[277,280,284,285]; however, the association seemed to be observed primarily in women who underwent hysterectomy for benign conditions.[277,280,284]

In summary, little is known about the epidemiology of carcinomas of the vagina. Epidemiologic studies of vaginal cancer have been even more difficult to conduct than those for vulvar cancer, as reflected by the smaller number of published studies. Much like the situation with vulvar cancers, the largest epidemiologic studies have been limited by small sample size and inability to study the role of HPV and other risk factors. Similarly to vulvar cancer, epidemiologic studies have relied mostly on serologic assays for HPV testing. It is possible that the understanding of the epidemiology of vaginal cancer may advance with knowledge gained from the study of cervical cancer and from future preventive strategies targeting cervical cancer, particularly HPV vaccines. However, there is a need for specific research to elucidate the role of HPV and other cofactors in the etiology of this neoplasm and to develop preventive strategies for women at higher risk for the disease. Larger multicenter studies, with collection of adequate vaginal samples for testing for HPV and other STIs, are needed. Finally, the seemingly stronger role of smoking in vaginal cancer than in cervical cancer deserves further research.

References

1. Vizcaino AP, Moreno V, Bosch FX, et al: International trends in incidence of cervical cancer: II. Squamous-cell carcinoma. Int J Cancer 2000;86:429-435.
2. Solomon D, Schiffman M, Tarone R: ASCUS LSIL Triage Study (ALTS) conclusions reaffirmed: Response to a November 2001 commentary. Obstet Gynecol 2002;99:671-674.
3. IARC Working Group: Human Papillomaviruses. (64). IARC Monographs on the Evaluation of Carcinogenic Risks to Human. Lyon, France, International Agency for Research on Cancer, 1995.
4. Walboomers JM, Jacobs MV, Manos MM, et al: Human papillomavirus is a necessary cause of invasive cervical cancer worldwide [comment]. J Pathol 1999;189:12-19.
5. Bosch FX, de SanJose S: Human papillomavirus and cervical cancer: Burden and assessment of causality [review]. J Natl Cancer Inst Monogr 2003;(31):3-13.
6. Parkin DM, Bray FI, Devesa SS: Cancer burden in the year 2000: The global picture. Eur J Cancer 2001;37(Suppl 8):S4-S66.
7. Parkin DM: Global cancer statistics in the year 2000. Lancet 2001;2:533-543.
8. Jemal A, Murray T, Samuels A, et al: Cancer statistics, 2003. CA Cancer J Clin 2003;53:5-26.
9. Sankaranarayanan R, Budukh AM, Rajkumar R: Effective screening programmes for cervical cancer in low- and middle-income developing countries. Bull World Health Organ 2001; 79:954-962.
10. Franco EL, Duarte-Franco E, Ferenczy A: Cervical cancer: Epidemiology, prevention and the role of human papillomavirus infection [comment]. CMAJ 2001;164:1017-1025.
11. Ferlay J, Bray F, Pisani P, Parkin DM: GLOBOCAN 2000: Cancer Incidence, Mortality, and Prevalence Worldwide, Version 1.0. IARC CancerBase No.5. Lyon, France, International Agency for Research on Cancer, 2001.
12. Franco EL: Primary screening of cervical cancer with human papillomavirus tests [review]. J Natl Cancer Inst Monogr 2003; (31):89-96.
13. Beral V, Hermon C, Munoz N, Devesa SS: Cervical cancer. Cancer Surv 1994;19-20:265-285.
14. Franco EL, Ferenczy A: Cervix. In Franco EL, Rohan T (eds): Cancer Precursors: Epidemiology, Detection, and Prevention. New York: Springer-Verlag, 2002.
15. Vizcaino AP, Moreno V, Bosch FX, et al: International trends in the incidence of cervical cancer: I. Adenocarcinoma and adenosquamous cell carcinomas. Int J Cancer 1998;75:536-545.
16. Franco EL, Duarte-Franco E, Rohan TE: Evidence-based policy recommendations on cancer screening and prevention [review]. Cancer Detect Prev 2002;26:350-361.
17. Ries LAG, Eisner MP, Kosary CL, et al: SEER Cancer Statistics Review, 1975-2000. Bethesda, MD, National Cancer Institute, 2003.
18. Miller BA, Kolonel LN, Kolonel LN, et al: Racial/Ethnic Patterns of Cancer in the United States 1988-1992. (NIH Pub. No. 96-4140). Bethesda, MD, National Cancer Institute, 1996.
19. Schiffman MH, Brinton LA, Devessa SS, Fraumeni FM: Cervical cancer. In Schottenfeld D, Fraumeni JF (eds): Cancer Epidemiology and Prevention. New York: Oxford University Press, 1996.
20. Parikh S, Brennan P, Boffetta P: Meta-analysis of social inequality and the risk of cervical cancer. Int J Cancer 2003; 105:687-691.
21. Drain PK, Holmes KK, Hughes JP, Koutsky LA: Determinants of cervical cancer rates in developing countries. Int J Cancer 2002; 100:199-205.
22. Singh GK, Miller BA, Hankey BF, Edwards BK: Area Socioeconomic Variations in U. S. Cancer Incidence, Mortality, Stage, Treatment, and Survival, 1975-1999. NCI Cancer Surveillance Monograph Series, Number 4. (NIH Publication No. 03-5417). Bethesda, MD, National Cancer Institute, 2003.
23. Gorey KM, Holoway EJ, Fehringer G, et al: An international comparison of cancer survival: Toronto, Ontario, and Detroit, Michigan, metropolitan areas. Am J Public Health 1997;87: 1156-1163.
24. Brinton LA: Epidemiology of cervical cancer: Overview. In Muñoz N, Bosch FX, Shah KV, Meheus A (eds): The Epidemiology of Human Papillomavirus and Cervical Cancer. Lyon, France, International Agency for Research on Cancer, 1992, pp. 3-23.

25. Boyle DC, Smith JR: Infection and cervical intraepithelial neoplasia. Int J Gynecol Cancer 1999;9:177-186.

26. Bosch FX, Munoz N: The viral etiology of cervical cancer [review]. Virus Res 2002;89:183-190.

27. zur Hausen H: Human papillomaviruses and their possible role in squamous cell carcinomas [review]. Curr Top Microbiol Immunol 1977;78:1-30.

28. Koutsky LA, Holmes KK, Critchlow CW, et al: A cohort study of the risk of cervical intraepithelial neoplasia grade 2 or 3 in relation to papillomavirus infection. N Engl J Med 1992;327: 1272-1278.

29. Nobbenhuis MA, Walboomers JM, Helmerhorst TJ, et al: Relation of human papillomavirus status to cervical lesions and consequences for cervical-cancer screening: A prospective study. Lancet 1999;354:20-25.

30. Tortolero-Luna G, Mitchell MF, Swan DC, et al: A case-control study of human papillomavirus and cervical squamous intraepithelial lesions (SIL) in Harris County, Texas: Differences among racial/ethnic groups. Cad de Saude Publica 1998;14(Suppl 3): 149-159.

31. Ho GY, Bierman R, Beardsley L, et al: Natural history of cervicovaginal papillomavirus infection in young women. N Engl J Med 1998;338:423-428.

32. Moscicki AB, Hills N, Shiboski S, et al: Risks for incident human papillomavirus infection and low-grade squamous intraepithelial lesion development in young females. JAMA 2001;285:2995-3002.

33. Munoz N: Human papillomavirus and cancer: The epidemiological evidence [review]. J Clin Virol 2000;19:1-5.

34. Bosch FX, Lorincz A, Munoz N, et al: The causal relation between human papillomavirus and cervical cancer [comment] [review]. J Clin Pathol 2002;55:244-265.

35. Koutsky LA: Epidemiology of genital human papillomavirus infection [review]. Am J Med 1997;102:3-8.

36. Munoz N, Bosch FX, de SanJose S, et al: Epidemiologic classification of human papillomavirus types associated with cervical cancer [comment]. N Engl J Med 2003;348:518-527.

37. Bosch FX, Manos MM, Munoz N, et al: Prevalence of human papillomavirus in cervical cancer: A worldwide perspective. International Biological Study on Cervical Cancer (IBSCC) Study Group [see comments]. J Natl Cancer Inst 1995;87:796-802.

38. Morrison EA, Ho GY, Vermund SH, et al: Human papillomavirus infection and other risk factors for cervical neoplasia: A case-control study [comment]. Int J Cancer 1991;49:6-13.

39. Bosch FX, Munoz N, de SanJose S, et al: Human papillomavirus and cervical intraepithelial neoplasia grade III/carcinoma in situ: A case-control study in Spain and Colombia. Cancer Epidemiol Biomarkers Prev 1993;2:415-422.

40. Kjaer SK: Risk factors for cervical neoplasia in Denmark. APMIS Suppl 1998;80:1-41.

41. Clifford GM, Smith JS, Plummer M, et al: Human papillomavirus types in invasive cervical cancer worldwide: A meta-analysis. Br J Cancer 2003;88:63-73.

42. Swan DC, Tucker RA, Tortolero-Luna G, et al: Human papillomavirus (HPV) DNA copy number is dependent on grade of cervical disease and HPV type. J Clin Microbiol 1999;37:1030-1034.

43. Hildesheim A, Wang SS: Host and viral genetics and risk of cervical cancer: A review [review]. Virus Res 2002;89:229-240.

44. Wang SS, Hildesheim A: Viral and host factors in human papillomavirus persistence and progression [review]. J Natl Cancer Inst Monogr 2003;(31):35-40.

45. Franco EL, Rohan TE, Villa LL: Epidemiologic evidence and human papillomavirus infection as a necessary cause of cervical cancer. J Natl Cancer Inst 1999;91:506-511.

46. Wacholder S: Statistical issues in the design and analysis of studies of human papillomavirus and cervical neoplasia [review]. J Natl Cancer Inst Monogr 2003;(31):125-130.

47. Castellsague X, Munoz N: Cofactors in human papillomavirus carcinogenesis: Role of parity, oral contraceptives, and tobacco smoking [review]. J Natl Cancer Inst Monogr 2003;(31):20-28.

48. Potischman N, Brinton LA: Nutrition and cervical neoplasia [review] [erratum appears in Cancer Causes Control 1996;7:402.]. Cancer Causes Control 1996;7:113-126.

49. Ho GY, Kadish AS, Burk RD, et al: HPV 16 and cigarette smoking as risk factors for high-grade cervical intra-epithelial neoplasia. Int J Cancer 1998;78:281-285.

50. Moreno V, Bosch FX, Munoz N, et al: Effect of oral contraceptives on risk of cervical cancer in women with human papillomavirus infection: The IARC multicentric case-control study [comment]. Lancet 2002;359:1085-1092.

51. Schiffman M, Kjaer SK: Natural history of anogenital human papillomavirus infection and neoplasia [review]. J Natl Cancer Inst Monogr 2003;(31):14-19.

52. Castle PE, Giuliano AR: Genital tract infections, cervical inflammation, and antioxidant nutrients: Assessing their roles as human papillomavirus cofactors [review]. J Natl Cancer Inst Monogr 2003;(31):29-34.

53. Maciag PC, Schlecht NF, Souza PS, et al: Major histocompatibility complex class II polymorphisms and risk of cervical cancer and human papillomavirus infection in Brazilian women. Cancer Epidemiol Biomarkers Prev 2000;9:1183-1191.

54. Makni H, Franco EL, Kaiano J, et al: P53 polymorphism in codon 72 and risk of human papillomavirus-induced cervical cancer: Effect of inter-laboratory variation. Int J Cancer 2000;87:528-533.

55. Koushik A, Franco E, Platt RW: P53 codon 72 polymorphism and cervical neoplasia: A review. Cancer Epidemiol Biomarkers Prev (in press).

56. Smith JS, Green J, Berrington DG, et al: Cervical cancer and use of hormonal contraceptives: A systematic review [review] [comment]. Lancet 2003;361:1159-1167.

57. Ylitalo N, Sorensen P, Josefsson AM, et al: Consistent high viral load of human papillomavirus 16 and risk of cervical carcinoma in situ: A nested case-control study [comment]. Lancet 2000; 355:2194-2198.

58. Zerbini M, Venturoli S, Cricca M, et al: Distribution and viral load of type specific HPVs in different cervical lesions as detected by PCR-ELISA. J Clin Pathol 2001;54:377-380.

59. Lorincz AT, Castle PE, Sherman ME, et al: Viral load of human papillomavirus and risk of CIN3 or cervical cancer. Lancet 2002; 360:228-229.

60. Schiffman MH, Castle P: Epidemiologic studies of a necessary causal risk factor: Human papilllomavirus infection and cervical neoplasia. J Natl Cancer Inst 2003;95:E2.

61. Herrero R, Brinton LA, Reeves WC, et al: Risk factors for invasive carcinoma of the uterine cervix in Latin America. Bull Pan Am Health Organ 1990;24:263-283.

62. Schiffman MH, Bauer HM, Hoover RN, et al: Epidemiologic evidence showing that human papillomavirus infection causes most cervical intraepithelial neoplasia [see comments]. J Natl Cancer Inst 1993;85:958-964.

63. Eluf-Neto J: Number of sexual partners and smoking behaviour as risk factors for cervical dysplasia: Comments on the evaluation of interaction [letter; comment]. Int J Epidemiol 1994;23:1101-1104.

64. Yoshikawa H, Nagata C, Noda K, et al: Human papillomavirus infection and other risk factors for cervical intraepithelial neoplasia in Japan. Br J Cancer 1999;80:621-624.

65. Castellsague X, Bosch FX, Munoz N: Environmental co-factors in HPV carcinogenesis [review]. Virus Res 2002;89:191-199.

66. Munoz N, Franceschi S, Bosetti C, et al: Role of parity and human papillomavirus in cervical cancer: The IARC multicentric case-control study [comment]. Lancet 2002;359:1093-1101.

67. Munoz N, Bosch FX, de SanJose S, et al: Risk factors for cervical intraepithelial neoplasia grade III/carcinoma in situ in Spain and Colombia. Cancer Epidemiol Biomarkers Prev 1993;2:423-431.

68. Hildesheim A, Herrero R, Castle PE, et al: HPV co-factors related to the development of cervical cancer: Results from a population-based study in Costa Rica. Br J Cancer 2001;84:1219-1226.

69. Kruger-Kjaer S, Van den Brule AJ, Svare EI, et al: Different risk factor patterns for high-grade and low-grade intraepithelial lesions on the cervix among HPV-positive and HPV-negative young women. Int J Cancer 1998;76:613-619.

70. Deacon JM, Evans CD, Yule R, et al: Sexual behaviour and smoking as determinants of cervical HPV infection and of CIN3 among those infected: A case-control study nested within the Manchester cohort. Br J Cancer 2000;83:1565-1572.

71. Castle PE, Wacholder S, Lorincz AT, et al: A prospective study of high-grade cervical neoplasia risk among human papillomavirus-infected women. J Natl Cancer Inst 2002;94:1406-1414.

72. Moodley M, Moodley J, Chetty R, Herrington CS: The role of steroid contraceptive hormones in the pathogenesis of invasive cervical cancer: A review [review]. Int J Gynecol Cancer 2003;13: 103-110.

73. de Villiers EM: Relationship between steroid hormone contraceptives and HPV, cervical intraepithelial neoplasia and cervical carcinoma [review]. Int J Cancer 2003;103:705-708.

74. Brinton LA: Oral contraceptives and cervical neoplasia. Contraception 1991;43:581-595.

75. Delgado-Rodriguez M, Sillero-Arenas M, Martin-Moreno JM, Galvez-Vargas R: Oral contraceptives and cancer of the cervix uteri: A meta-analysis. Acta Obstet Gynecol Scand 1992;71:368-376.

76. Bosch FX, Munoz N, de SanJose S, et al: Risk factors for cervical cancer in Colombia and Spain. Int J Cancer 1992;52:750-758.

77. Olsen AO, Gjen K, Sauer T, et al: Human papillomavirus and cervical intraepithelial neoplasia grade II-III: A population-based case-control study. Int J Cancer 1995;61:312-315.

78. Lacey JV Jr, Brinton LA, Abbas FM, et al: Oral contraceptives as risk factors for cervical adenocarcinomas and squamous cell carcinomas. Cancer Epidemiol Biomarkers Prev 1999; 8(12): 1079-1085.

79. Negrini BP, Schiffman MH, Kurman RJ, et al: Oral contraceptive use, human papillomavirus infection, and risk of early cytological abnormalities of the cervix. Cancer Res 1990;50: 4670-4675.

80. Lacey JV Jr, Swanson CA, Brinton LA, et al: Obesity as a potential risk factor for adenocarcinomas and squamous cell carcinomas of the uterine cervix. Cancer 2003;98:814-821.

81. Green J, Berrington DG, Smith JS, et al: Human papillomavirus infection and use of oral contraceptives [review]. Br J Cancer 2003;88:1713-1720.

82. Winkelstein W Jr: Cigarette smoking and cancer of the uterine cervix. Banbury Rep 1986;23:329-341.

83. Phillips AN, Smith GD: Cigarette smoking as a potential cause of cervical cancer: Has confounding been controlled? [see comments]. Int J Epidemiol 1994;23:42-49.

84. Parazzini F, Chatenoud L, La Vecchia C, et al: Determinants of risk of invasive cervical cancer in young women. Br J Cancer 1998;77:838-841.

85. Becker TM, Wheeler CM, McGough NS, et al: Cigarette smoking and other risk factors for cervical dysplasia in southwestern Hispanic and non-Hispanic white women. Cancer Epidemiol Biomarkers Prev 1994;3:113-119.

86. Daling JR, Madeleine MM, McKnight B, et al: The relationship of human papillomavirus-related cervical tumors to cigarette smoking, oral contraceptive use, and prior herpes simplex virus type 2 infection. Cancer Epidemiol Biomarkers Prev 1996;5:541-548.

87. Kjaer SK, Engholm G, Dahl C, Bock JE: Case-control study of risk factors for cervical squamous cell neoplasia in Denmark. IV: Role of smoking habits. Eur J Cancer Prev 1996;5:359-365.

88. Kanetsky PA, Gammon MD, Mandelblatt J, et al: Cigarette smoking and cervical dysplasia among non-Hispanic black women. Cancer Detect Prev 1998;22:109-119.

89. Olsen AO, Dillner J, Skrondal A, Magnus P: Combined effect of smoking and human papillomavirus type 16 infection in cervical carcinogenesis. Epidemiology 1998;9:346-349.

90. Roteli-Martins CM, Panetta K, Alves VA, et al: Cigarette smoking and high-risk HPV DNA as predisposing factors for high-grade cervical intraepithelial neoplasia (CIN) in young Brazilian women. Acta Obstet Gynecol Scand 1998;77:678-682.

91. Schiffman MH, Haley NJ, Felton JS, et al: Biochemical epidemiology of cervical neoplasia: Measuring cigarette smoke constituents in the cervix. Cancer Res 1987;47:3886-3888.

92. Hellberg D, Nilsson S, Haley NJ, et al: Smoking and cervical intraepithelial neoplasia: Nicotine and cotinine in serum and cervical mucus in smokers and nonsmokers. Am J Obstet Gynecol 1988;158:910-913.

93. Poppe WA, Peeters R, Daenens P, et al: Tobacco smoking and the uterine cervix: Cotinine in blood, urine and cervical fluid. Gynecol Obstet Invest 1995;39:110-114.

94. Prokopczyk B, Cox JE, Hoffmann D, Waggoner SE: Identification of tobacco-specific carcinogen in the cervical mucus of smokers and nonsmokers. J Natl Cancer Inst 1997;89:868-873.

95. Cuzick J, Singer A, De Stavola BL, Chomet J: Case-control study of risk factors for cervical intraepithelial neoplasia in young women. Eur J Cancer 1990;26:684-690.

96. Phillips DH, She MN: DNA adducts in cervical tissue of smokers and non-smokers. Mutat Res 1994;313:277-284.

97. Simons AM, Mugica van Herckenrode C, Rodriguez JA, et al: Demonstration of smoking-related DNA damage in cervical epithelium and correlation with human papillomavirus type 16, using exfoliated cervical cells. Br J Cancer 1995;71:246-249.

98. Cerqueira EM, Santoro CL, Donozo NF, et al: Genetic damage in exfoliated cells of the uterine cervix: Association and interaction between cigarette smoking and progression to malignant transformation? Acta Cytol 1998;42:639-649.

99. Poppe WA, Ide PS, Drijkoningen MP, et al: Tobacco smoking impairs the local immunosurveillance in the uterine cervix: An immunohistochemical study. Gynecol Obstet Invest 1995; 39:34-38.

100. Szarewski A, Jarvis MJ, Sasieni P, et al: Effect of smoking cessation on cervical lesion size [comment]. Lancet 1996;347:941-943.

101. Acladious NN, Sutton C, Mandal D, et al: Persistent human papillomavirus infection and smoking increase risk of failure of treatment of cervical intraepithelial neoplasia (CIN). Int J Cancer 2002;98:435-439.

102. Giuliano AR, Harris R, Sedjo RL, et al: Incidence, prevalence, and clearance of type-specific human papillomavirus infections: The Young Women's Health Study. J Infect Dis 2002;186:462-469.

103. Lacey JV Jr, Frisch M, Brinton LA, et al: Associations between smoking and adenocarcinomas and squamous cell carcinomas of the uterine cervix (United States). Cancer Causes Control 2001;12:153-161.

104. Franco EL: Viral etiology of cervical cancer: A critique of the evidence [review]. Rev Infect Dis 1991;13:1195-1206.

104a. Zur Hausen H: Human genital cancer: Synergism between two virus infections or synergism between a virus infection and initiating events? Lancet 1982;2:1370-1372.

105. Galloway DA, McDougall JK: The oncogenic potential of herpes simplex viruses: Evidence for a "hit-and-run" mechanism. Nature 1983;302:21-24.

106. Dipaolo JA, Woodworth CD, Coutlee F, et al: Relationship of stable integration of herpes simplex virus-2 Bg/II N subfragment Xho2 to malignant transformation of human papillomavirus-immortalized cervical keratinocytes. Int J Cancer 1998;76:865-871.

107. Tran-Thanh D, Provencher D, Koushik A, et al: Herpes simplex virus type II is not a cofactor to human papillomavirus in cancer of the uterine cervix. Am J Obstet Gynecol 2003;188: 129-134.

108. de SanJose S, Munoz N, Bosch FX, et al: Sexually transmitted agents and cervical neoplasia in Colombia and Spain. Int J Cancer 1994;56:358-363.

109. Dillner J, Lenner P, Lehtinen M, et al: A population-based seroepidemiological study of cervical cancer. Cancer Res 1994; 54:134-141.

109a. Jha PK, Beral V, Peto J et al: Antibodies to human papillomavirus and other genital infectious agents and invasive cervical cancer risk. Lancet 1993;341:1116-1118.

110. Peng HQ, Liu SL, Mann V, et al: Human papillomavirus types 16 and 33, herpes simplex virus type 2 and other risk factors for cervical cancer in Sichuan Province, China. Int J Cancer 1991; 47:711-716.

111. Becker TM, Wheeler CM, McGough NS, et al: Sexually transmitted diseases and other risk factors for cervical dysplasia among southwestern Hispanic and non-Hispanic white women. JAMA 1994;271:1181-1188.

112. Ferrera A, Baay MF, Herbrink P, et al: A sero-epidemiological study of the relationship between sexually transmitted agents and cervical cancer in Honduras. Int J Cancer 1997;73:781-785.

113. Thomas DB, Ray RM, Koetsawang A, et al: Human papillomaviruses and cervical cancer in Bangkok. I: Risk factors for invasive cervical carcinomas with human papillomavirus types 16 and 18 DNA. Am J Epidemiol 2001;153:723-731.

114. Lehtinen M, Koskela P, Jellum E, et al: Herpes simplex virus and risk of cervical cancer: A longitudinal, nested case-control study in the nordic countries. Am J Epidemiol 2002;156: 687-692.

115. Smith JS, Herrero R, Bosetti C, et al: Herpes simplex virus-2 as a human papillomavirus cofactor in the etiology of invasive cervical cancer [comment]. J Natl Cancer Inst 2002;94:1604-1613.

116. Koskela P, Anttila T, Bjorge T, et al: *Chlamydia trachomatis* infection as a risk factor for invasive cervical cancer. Int J Cancer 2000;85:35-39.

117. Anttila T, Saikku P, Koskela P, et al: Serotypes of *Chlamydia trachomatis* and risk for development of cervical squamous cell carcinoma [comment]. JAMA 2001;285:47-51.

118. Wallin KL, Wiklund F, Luostarinen T, et al: A population-based prospective study of *Chlamydia trachomatis* infection and cervical carcinoma. Int J Cancer 2002;101:371-374.

119. Smith JS, Munoz N, Herrero R, et al: Evidence for *Chlamydia trachomatis* as a human papillomavirus cofactor in the etiology of invasive cervical cancer in Brazil and the Philippines. J Infect Dis 2002;185:324-331.

120. Burger MP, Hollema H, Pieters WJ, et al: Epidemiological evidence of cervical intraepithelial neoplasia without the presence of human papillomavirus. Br J Cancer 1996;73:831-836.

121. Claas EC, Melchers WJ, Niesters HG, et al: Infections of the cervix uteri with human papillomavirus and *Chlamydia trachomatis*. J Med Virol 1992;37:54-57.

122. Centers for Disease Control and Prevention: Revised classification system for HIV infection and expanded surveillance definition for AIDS among adolescents and adults. MMWR Morb Mortal Wkly Rep 1993;41:1-15.

123. Lee BN, Follen M, Tortolero-Luna G, et al: Synthesis of IFN-gamma by CD8(+) T cells is preserved in HIV-infected women with HPV-related cervical squamous intraepithelial lesions. Gynecol Oncol 1999;75:379-386.

124. Jay N, Moscicki AB: Human papillomavirus infections in women with HIV disease: Prevalence, risk, and management [review]. AIDS Reader 2000;10:659-668.

125. Conley LJ, Ellerbrock TV, Bush TJ, et al: HIV-1 infection and risk of vulvovaginal and perianal condylomata acuminata and intraepithelial neoplasia: A prospective cohort study [comment]. Lancet 2002;359:108-113.

126. Langley CL, Benga-De E, Critchlow CW, et al: HIV-1, HIV-2, human papillomavirus infection and cervical neoplasia in high-risk African women. AIDS 1996;10:413-417.

127. Maiman M, Fruchter RG, Sedlis A, et al: Prevalence, risk factors, and accuracy of cytologic screening for cervical intraepithelial neoplasia in women with the human immunodeficiency virus. Gynecol Oncol 1998;68:233-239.

128. Massad LS, Riester KA, Anastos KM, et al: Prevalence and predictors of squamous cell abnormalities in Papanicolaou smears from women infected with HIV-1. Women's Interagency HIV Study Group. J Acquir Immune Defic Syndr Hum Retrovirol 1999;21:33-41.

129. Ellerbrock TV, Chiasson MA, Bush TJ, et al: Incidence of cervical squamous intraepithelial lesions in HIV-infected women. JAMA 2000;283:1031-1037.

130. Moscicki AB, Ellenberg JH, Vermund SH, et al: Prevalence of and risks for cervical human papillomavirus infection and squamous intraepithelial lesions in adolescent girls: Impact of infection with human immunodeficiency virus. Arch Pediatr Adolesc Med 2000;154:127-134.

131. Ferenczy A, Coutlee F, Franco E, Hankins C: Human papillomavirus and HIV coinfection and the risk of neoplasias of the lower genital tract: A review of recent developments [review]. CMAJ 2003;169:431-434.

132. Mandelblatt JS, Kanetsky P, Eggert L, Gold K: Is HIV infection a cofactor for cervical squamous cell neoplasia? [comment]. Cancer Epidemiol Biomarkers Prev 1999;8:97-106.

133. La Ruche G, Leroy V, Mensah-Ado I, et al: Short-term follow up of cervical squamous intraepithelial lesions associated with HIV and human papillomavirus infections in Africa. Int J STD AIDS 1999;10:363-368.

134. de SanJose S, Palefsky J: Cervical and anal HPV infections in HIV positive women and men [review]. Virus Res 2002;89:201-211.

135. Schneider A, Shah K: The role of vitamins in the etiology of cervical neoplasia: An epidemiological review [review]. Arch Gynecol Obstet 1989;246:1-13.

136. Butterworth CE Jr, Hatch KD, Soong SJ, et al: Oral folic acid supplementation for cervical dysplasia: A clinical intervention trial. Am J Obstet Gynecol 1992;166:803-809.

137. Giuliano AR: The role of nutrients in the prevention of cervical dysplasia and cancer [review]. Nutrition 2000;16:570-573.

138. Ziegler RG, Brinton LA, Hamman RF, et al: Diet and the risk of invasive cervical cancer among white women in the United States. Am J Epidemiol 1990;132:432-445.

139. Ziegler RG, Jones CJ, Brinton LA, et al: Diet and the risk of in situ cervical cancer among white women in the United States. Cancer Causes Control 1991;2:17-29.

140. Van Eenwyk J, Davis FG, Bowen PE: Dietary and serum carotenoids and cervical intraepithelial neoplasia. Int J Cancer 1991;48:34-38.

141. Van Eenwyk J, Davis FG, Colman N: Folate, vitamin C, and cervical intraepithelial neoplasia [see comments]. Cancer Epidemiol Biomarkers Prev 1992;1:119-124.

142. Liu T, Soong SJ, Wilson NP, et al: A case control study of nutritional factors and cervical dysplasia. Cancer Epidemiol Biomarkers Prev 1993;2:525-530.

143. Batieha AM, Armenian HK, Norkus EP, et al: Serum micronutrients and the subsequent risk of cervical cancer in a population-based nested case-control study. Cancer Epidemiol Biomarkers Prev 1993;2:335-339.

144. Potischman N: Nutritional epidemiology of cervical neoplasia [review]. J Nutr 1993;123(2 Suppl):424-429.

145. Wideroff L, Potischman N, Glass AG, et al: A nested case-control study of dietary factors and the risk of incident cytological abnormalities of the cervix. Nutr Cancer 1998;30:130-136.

146. Sedjo RL, Inserra P, Abrahamsen M, et al: Human papillomavirus persistence and nutrients involved in the methylation pathway among a cohort of young women. Cancer Epidemiol Biomarkers Prev 2002;11:353-359.

147. Sedjo RL, Roe DJ, Abrahamsen M, et al: Vitamin A, carotenoids, and risk of persistent oncogenic human papillomavirus infection. Cancer Epidemiol Biomarkers Prev 2002;11:876-884.

148. Giuliano AR, Siegel EM, Roe D, et al: Dietary intake and risk of persistent human papillomavirus (HPV) infection: The Ludwig-McGill HPV natural history study. J Infect Dis 2003;188:1508-1516.

149. Moscicki AB, Shiboski S, Broering J, et al: The natural history of human papillomavirus infection as measured by repeated DNA testing in adolescent and young women. J Pediatr 1998;132:277-284.

150. Franco EL, Villa LL, Sobrinho JP, et al: Epidemiology of acquisition and clearance of cervical human papillomavirus infection in women from a high-risk area for cervical cancer. J Infect Dis 1999;180:1415-1423.

151. Thomas KK, Hughes JP, Kuypers JM, et al: Concurrent and sequential acquisition of different genital human papillomavirus types. J Infect Dis 2000;182:1097-1102.

152. Liaw KL, Hildesheim A, Burk RD, et al: A prospective study of human papillomavirus (HPV) type 16 DNA detection by polymerase chain reaction and its association with acquisition and persistence of other HPV types. J Infect Dis 2001;183:8-15.

153. Konya J, Dillner J: Immunity to oncogenic human papillomaviruses [review]. Adv Cancer Res 2001;82:205-238.

154. Scott M, Nakagawa M, Moscicki AB: Cell-mediated immune response to human papillomavirus infection [review]. Clin Diagn Lab Immunol 2001;8:209-220.

155. Dillner J, Andersson-Ellstrom A, Hagmar B, Schiller J: High risk genital papillomavirus infections are not spread vertically [review]. Rev Med Virol 1999;9:23-29.

156. de Gruijl TD, Bontkes HJ, Walboomers JM, et al: Immunoglobulin G responses against human papillomavirus type 16 virus-like particles in a prospective nonintervention cohort study of women with cervical intraepithelial neoplasia. J Natl Cancer Inst 1997;89:630-638.

157. Wideroff L, Schiffman M, Haderer P, et al: Seroreactivity to human papillomavirus types 16, 18, 31, and 45 virus-like particles in a case-control study of cervical squamous intraepithelial lesions. J Infect Dis 1999;180:1424-1428.

158. Sun Y, Eluf-Neto J, Bosch FX, et al: Serum antibodies to human papillomavirus 16 proteins in women from Brazil with invasive cervical carcinoma. Cancer Epidemiol Biomarkers Prev 1999;8:935-940.

159. Hagensee ME, Koutsky LA, Lee SK, et al: Detection of cervical antibodies to human papillomavirus type 16 (HPV-16) capsid antigens in relation to detection of HPV-16 DNA and cervical lesions. J Infect Dis 2000;181:1234-1239.

160. Lehtinen M, Pawlita M, Zumbach K, et al: Evaluation of antibody response to human papillomavirus early proteins in

women in whom cervical cancer developed 1 to 20 years later. Am J Obstet Gynecol 2003;188:49-55.

161. Carter JJ, Koutsky LA, Hughes JP, et al: Comparison of human papillomavirus types 16, 18, and 6 capsid antibody responses following incident infection. J Infect Dis 2000;181: 1911-1919.

162. Sukvirach S, Smith JS, Tunsakul S, et al: Population-based human papillomavirus prevalence in Lampang and Songkla, Thailand. J Infect Dis 2003;187:1246-1256.

163. Heim K, Widschwendter A, Pirschner G, et al: Antibodies to human papillomavirus 16 L1 virus-like particles as an independent prognostic marker in cervical cancer. Am J Obstet Gynecol 2002;186:705-711.

164. Matsumoto K, Yasugi T, Oki A, et al: Are smoking and chlamydial infection risk factors for CIN? Different results after adjustment for HPV DNA and antibodies. Br J Cancer 2003; 89:831-833.

165. Viscidi RP, Ahdieh-Grant L, Clayman B, et al: Serum immunoglobulin G response to human papillomavirus type 16 virus-like particles in human immunodeficiency virus (HIV)-positive and risk-matched HIV-negative women. J Infect Dis 2003;187:194-205.

166. Nonnenmacher B, Pintos J, Bozzetti MC, et al: Epidemiologic correlates of antibody response to human papillomavirus among women at low risk of cervical cancer. Int J STD AIDS 2003;14:258-265.

167. Ho GY, Studentsov Y, Hall CB, et al: Risk factors for subsequent cervicovaginal human papillomavirus (HPV) infection and the protective role of antibodies to HPV-16 virus-like particles. J Infect Dis 2002;186:737-742.

168. Koutsky LA, Ault KA, Wheeler CM, et al: A controlled trial of a human papillomavirus type 16 vaccine [comment]. N Engl J Med 2002;347:1645-1651.

169. Tjiong MY, Out TA, ter Schegget J, et al: Epidemiologic and mucosal immunologic aspects of HPV infection and HPV-related cervical neoplasia in the lower female genital tract: A review [review]. Int J Gynecol Cancer 2001;11:9-17.

170. Wang Z, Hansson BG, Forslund O, et al: Cervical mucus antibodies against human papillomavirus type 16, 18, and 33 capsids in relation to presence of viral DNA. J Clin Microbiol 1996;34:3056-3062.

171. Sasagawa T, Rose RC, Azar KK, et al: Mucosal immunoglobulin-A and -G responses to oncogenic human papilloma virus capsids. Int J Cancer 2003;104:328-335.

172. Rocha-Zavaleta L, Pereira-Suarez AL, Yescas G, et al: Mucosal IgG and IgA responses to human papillomavirus type 16 capsid proteins in HPV16-infected women without visible pathology. Viral Immunol 2003;16:159-168.

173. Nakagawa M, Stites DP, Farhat S, et al: T-cell proliferative response to human papillomavirus type 16 peptides: Relationship to cervical intraepithelial neoplasia. Clin Diagn Lab Immunol 1996;3:205-210.

174. Benton C, Shahidullah H, Hunter JAA: Human papillomavirus in the immunosuppressed. Papillomavirus Report 1992;3:23-36.

175. Tsukui T, Hildesheim A, Schiffman MH, et al: Interleukin 2 production in vitro by peripheral lymphocytes in response to human papillomavirus-derived peptides: Correlation with cervical pathology. Cancer Res 1996;56:3967-3974.

176. Iwatsuki K, Tagami H, Takigawa M, Yamada M: Plane warts under spontaneous regression: Immunopathologic study on cellular constituents leading to the inflammatory reaction. Arch Dermatol 1986;122:655-659.

177. Tay SK, Jenkins D, Maddox P, et al: Subpopulations of Langerhans' cells in cervical neoplasia. Br J Obstet Gynaecol 1987;94:10-15.

178. Apple RJ, Erlich HA, Klitz W, et al: HLA DR-DQ associations with cervical carcinoma show papillomavirus-type specificity. Nat Genet 1994;6:157-162.

179. Odunsi K, Terry G, Ho L, et al: Association between HLA DQB1*03 and cervical intra-epithelial neoplasia. Mol Med 1995; 1:161-171.

180. Sher A, Gazzinelli RT, Oswald IP, et al: Role of T-cell derived cytokines in the downregulation of immune responses in parasitic and retroviral infection [review]. Immunol Rev 1992; 127:183-204.

181. Yamamura M, Uyemura K, Deans RJ, et al: Defining protective responses to pathogens: Cytokine profiles in leprosy lesions [erratum appears in Science 1992;255:12]. Science 1991;254: 277-279.

182. Clerici M, Shearer GM: The Th1-Th2 hypothesis of HIV infection: New insights [review]. Immunol Today 1994;15:575-581.

183. de Gruijl TD, Bontkes HJ, Walboomers JM, et al: Immune responses against human papillomavirus (HPV) type 16 virus-like particles in a cohort study of women with cervical intraepithelial neoplasia. I: Differential T-helper and IgG responses in relation to HPV infection and disease outcome. J Gen Virol 1999;80:399-408.

184. de Gruijl TD, Bontkes HJ, van den Muysenberg AJ, et al: Differences in cytokine mRNA profiles between premalignant and malignant lesions of the uterine cervix. Eur J Cancer 1999; 35:490-497.

185. Nakagawa M, Stites DP, Farhat S, et al: Cytotoxic T lymphocyte responses to E6 and E7 proteins of human papillomavirus type 16: Relationship to cervical intraepithelial neoplasia. J Infect Dis 1997;175:927-931.

186. Clerici M, Merola M, Ferrario E, et al: Cytokine production patterns in cervical intraepithelial neoplasia: Association with human papillomavirus infection [see comments]. J Natl Cancer Inst 1997;89:245-250.

187. Kadish AS, Ho GY, Burk RD, et al: Lymphoproliferative responses to human papillomavirus (HPV) type 16 proteins E6 and E7: Outcome of HPV infection and associated neoplasia. J Natl Cancer Inst 1997;89:1285-1293.

188. Kadish AS, Timmins P, Wang Y, et al: Regression of cervical intraepithelial neoplasia and loss of human papillomavirus (HPV) infection is associated with cell-mediated immune responses to an HPV type 16 E7 peptide. Cancer Epidemiol Biomarkers Prev 2002;11:483-488.

189. de Gruijl TD, Bontkes HJ, Walboomers JM, et al: Differential T helper cell responses to human papillomavirus type 16 E7 related to viral clearance or persistence in patients with cervical neoplasia: A longitudinal study. Cancer Res 1998;58: 1700-1706.

190. Odunsi K, Terry G, Ho L, et al: Susceptibility to human papillomavirus-associated cervical intra-epithelial neoplasia is determined by specific HLA DR-DQ alleles. Int J Cancer 1996;67:595-602.

191. Breitburd F, Ramoz N, Salmon J, Orth G: HLA control in the progression of human papillomavirus infections [review]. Semin Cancer Biol 1996;7:359-371.

192. Odunsi KO, Ganesan TS: The roles of the human major histocompatibility complex and human papillomavirus infection in cervical intraepithelial neoplasia and cervical cancer [review]. Clin Oncol (R Coll Radiol) 1997;9:4-13.

193. Helland A, Olsen AO, Gjoen K, et al: An increased risk of cervical intra-epithelial neoplasia grade II-III among human papillomavirus positive patients with the HLA-DQA1*0102-DQB1*0602 haplotype: A population-based case-control study of Norwegian women. Int J Cancer 1998;76:19-24.

194. Hildesheim A, Schiffman M, Scott DR, et al: Human leukocyte antigen class I/II alleles and development of human papillomavirus-related cervical neoplasia: Results from a case-control study conducted in the United States. Cancer Epidemiol Biomarkers Prev 1998;7:1035-1041.

195. Apple RJ, Becker TM, Wheeler CM, Erlich HA: Comparison of human leukocyte antigen DR-DQ disease associations found with cervical dysplasia and invasive cervical carcinoma. J Natl Cancer Inst 1995;87:427-436.

196. Sanjeevi CB, Hjelmstrom P, Hallmans G, et al: Different HLA-DR-DQ haplotypes are associated with cervical intraepithelial neoplasia among human papillomavirus type-16 seropositive and seronegative Swedish women. Int J Cancer 1996;68:409-414.

197. Madeleine MM, Brumback B, Cushing-Haugen KL, et al: Human leukocyte antigen class II and cervical cancer risk: A population-based study. J Infect Dis 2002;186:1565-1574.

198. Harris RW, Forman D, Doll R, et al: Cancer of the cervix uteri and vitamin A. Br J Cancer 1986;53:653-659.

199. Matlashewski GJ, Tuck S, Pim D, et al: Primary structure polymorphism at amino acid residue 72 of human p53. Mol Cell Biol 1987;7:961-963.

200. Storey A, Thomas M, Kalita A, et al: Role of a p53 polymorphism in the development of human papillomavirus-associated cancer [see comments]. Nature 1998;393:229-234.

201. Ojeda JM, Ampuero S, Rojas P: P53 codon 72 polymorphism and risk of cervical cancer. Biol Res 2003;36:279-283.

202. Qie M, Zhang Y, Wu J: Study on the relationship between cervical cancer and p53 codon 72 polymorphism [Chinese]. Hua-Hsi i Ko Ta Hsueh Hsueh Pao 2002;33:274-275.

203. Sifuentes-Alvarez A, Reyes RM: Risk factors for cervico-uterine cancer associated to HPV: p53 codon 72 polymorphism in women attending hospital care [Spanish]. Ginecol Obstet Mex 2003;71:12-15.

204. Abba MC, Villaverde LM, Gomez MA, et al: The p53 codon 72 genotypes in HPV infection and cervical disease. Eur J Obstet Gynecol Reprod Biol 2003;109:63-66.

205. Cenci M, French D, Pisani T, et al: P53 polymorphism at codon 72 is not a risk factor for cervical carcinogenesis in central Italy. Anticancer Res 2003;23:1385-1387.

206. Jee SH, Lee JE, Park JS: Polymorphism of codon 72 of p53 and environmental factors in the development of cervical cancer. Int J Gynaecol Obstet 2003;80:69-70.

207. Goodman MT, McDuffie K, Hernandez B, et al: CYP1A1, GSTM1, and GSTT1 polymorphisms and the risk of cervical squamous intraepithelial lesions in a multiethnic population. Gynecol Oncol 2001;81:263-269.

208. Sierra-Torres CH, Au WW, Arrastia CD, et al: Polymorphisms for chemical metabolizing genes and risk for cervical neoplasia. Environ Mol Mutagen 2003;41:69-76.

209. Mathur SP, Mathur RS, Young RC: Cervical epidermal growth factor-receptor (EGF-R) and serum insulin-like growth factor II (IGF-II) levels are potential markers for cervical cancer. Am J Reprod Immunol 2000;44:222-230.

210. Berger AJ, Baege A, Guillemette T, et al: Insulin-like growth factor-binding protein 3 expression increases during immortalization of cervical keratinocytes by human papillomavirus type 16 E6 and E7 proteins. Am J Pathol 2002;161:603-610.

211. Wu X, Tortolero-Luna G, Zhao H, et al: Serum levels of insulin-like growth factor I and risk of squamous intraepithelial lesions of the cervix. Clin Cancer Res 2003;9:3356-3361.

212. Schlecht NF, Kulaga S, Robitaille J, et al: Persistent human papillomavirus infection as a predictor of cervical intraepithelial neoplasia. JAMA 2001;286:3106-3114.

213. Ho GY, Burk RD, Klein S, et al: Persistent genital human papillomavirus infection as a risk factor for persistent cervical dysplasia [comment]. J Natl Cancer Inst 1995;87:1365-1371.

214. Franco EL: Understanding the epidemiology of genital infection with oncogenic and nononcogenic human papillomaviruses: A promising lead for primary prevention of cervical cancer [comment]. Cancer Epidemiol Biomarkers Prev 1997;6:759-761.

215. Schlecht NF, Platt RW, Duarte-Franco E, et al: Human papillomavirus infection and time to progression and regression of cervical intraepithelial neoplasia. J Natl Cancer Inst 2003;95:1336-1343.

216. Rousseau MC, Villa LL, Costa MC, et al: Occurrence of cervical infection with multiple human papillomavirus types is associated with age and cytologic abnormalities. Sex Transm Dis 2003;30:581-587.

217. Schlecht NF, Trevisan A, Duarte-Franco E, et al: Viral load as a predictor of the risk of cervical intraepithelial neoplasia. Int J Cancer 2003;103:519-524.

218. Josefsson AM, Magnusson PK, Ylitalo N, et al: Viral load of human papilloma virus 16 as a determinant for development of cervical carcinoma in situ: A nested case-control study [comment]. Lancet 2000;355:2189-2193.

219. Brisson J, Bairati I, Morin C, et al: Determinants of persistent detection of human papillomavirus DNA in the uterine cervix. J Infect Dis 1996;173:794-799.

220. Hernandez-Hernandez DM, Ornelas-Bernal L, Guido-Jimenez M, et al: Association between high-risk human papillomavirus DNA load and precursor lesions of cervical cancer in Mexican women. Gynecol Oncol 2003;90:310-317.

221. Dalstein V, Riethmuller D, Pretet JL, et al: Persistence and load of high-risk HPV are predictors for development of high-grade cervical lesions: A longitudinal French cohort study. Int J Cancer 2003;106:396-403.

222. Franco EL, Villa LL, Rahal P, Ruiz A: Molecular variant analysis as an epidemiological tool to study persistence of cervical human papillomavirus infection. J Natl Cancer Inst 1994;86:1558-1559.

223. Bernard HU: Coevolution of papillomaviruses with human populations [review]. Trends Microbiol 1994;2:140-143.

224. Chan SY, Ho L, Ong CK, et al: Molecular variants of human papillomavirus type 16 from four continents suggest ancient pandemic spread of the virus and its coevolution with humankind. J Virol 1992;66:2057-2066.

225. Ho L, Tay SK, Chan SY, Bernard HU: Sequence variants of human papillomavirus type 16 from couples suggest sexual transmission with low infectivity and polyclonality in genital neoplasia. J Infect Dis 1993;168:803-809.

226. Yamada T, Wheeler CM, Halpern AL, et al: Human papillomavirus type 16 variant lineages in United States populations characterized by nucleotide sequence analysis of the E6, L2, and L1 coding segments. J Virol 1995;69:7743-7753.

227. Xi LF, Koutsky LA, Galloway DA, et al: Genomic variation of human papillomavirus type 16 and risk for high grade cervical intraepithelial neoplasia [comment]. J Natl Cancer Inst 1997;89:796-802.

228. Villa LL, Sichero L, Rahal P, et al: Molecular variants of human papillomavirus types 16 and 18 preferentially associated with cervical neoplasia. J Gen Virol 2000;81:2959-2968.

229. Xi LF, Carter JJ, Galloway DA, et al: Acquisition and natural history of human papillomavirus type 16 variant infection among a cohort of female university students. Cancer Epidemiol Biomarkers Prev 2002;11:343-351.

230. Berumen J, Ordonez RM, Lazcano E, et al: Asian-American variants of human papillomavirus 16 and risk for cervical cancer: A case-control study. J Natl Cancer Inst 2001;93:1325-1330.

231. Villa LL: Human papillomaviruses and cervical cancer [review]. Adv Cancer Res 1997;71:321-341.

232. Londesborough P, Ho L, Terry G, et al: Human papillomavirus genotype as a predictor of persistence and development of high-grade lesions in women with minor cervical abnormalities. Int J Cancer 1996;69:364-368.

233. Zehbe I, Voglino G, Delius H, et al: Risk of cervical cancer and geographical variations of human papillomavirus 16 E6 polymorphisms [letter; see comments]. Lancet 1998;352:1441-1442.

234. Bontkes HJ, van Duin M, de Gruijl TD, et al: HPV 16 infection and progression of cervical intra-epithelial neoplasia: Analysis of HLA polymorphism and HPV 16 E6 sequence variants. Int J Cancer 1998;78:166-171.

235. Nindl I, Rindfleisch K, Teller K, et al: Cervical cancer, HPV 16 E6, variant genotypes, and serology [letter; comment]. Lancet 1999;353:152.

236. Hu X, Guo Z, Tianyun P, et al: HPV typing and HPV16 E6-sequence variations in synchronous lesions of cervical squamous-cell carcinoma from Swedish patients. Int J Cancer 1999;83:34-37.

237. Brady CS, Duggan-Keen MF, Davidson JA, et al: Human papillomavirus type 16 E6 variants in cervical carcinoma: Relationship to host genetic factors and clinical parameters. J Gen Virol 1999;80:3233-3240.

238. Chan PK, Chang AR, Cheung JL, et al: Determinants of cervical human papillomavirus infection: Differences between high- and low-oncogenic risk types. J Infect Dis 2002;185:28-35.

239. Lowy DR, Frazer IH: Prophylactic human papillomavirus vaccines [review]. J Natl Cancer Inst Monogr 2003;(31):111-116.

240. Solomon D: Role of triage testing in cervical cancer screening [review]. J Natl Cancer Inst Monogr 2003;(31):97-101.

241. Cuzick J, Sasieni P, Davies P, et al: A systematic review of the role of human papilloma virus (HPV) testing within a cervical screening programme: Summary and conclusions [review]. Br J Cancer 2000;83:561-565.

242. Goldie SJ: Public health policy and cost-effectiveness analysis [review]. J Natl Cancer Inst Monogr 2003;(31):102-110.

243. Miller ABS: Can screening for cervical cancer be improved, especially in developing countries? Int J Cancer 2003;107:337-340.

244. Giuliano AR, Papenfuss M, Nour M, et al: Antioxidant nutrients: Associations with persistent human papillomavirus infection. Cancer Epidemiol Biomarkers Prev 1997;6:917-923.

245. Villa LL, Bernard HU, Kast M, et al: Past, present, and future of HPV research: Highlights from the 19th International Papillomavirus Conference-HPV2001 [review]. Virus Res 2002; 89:163-173.

246. Anderson NB: Solving the puzzle of socioeconomic status and health: The need for integrated, multilevel, interdisciplinary research [review]. Ann N Y Acad Sci 1999;896:302-312.

247. Aral S: Elimination and reintroduction of a sexually transmitted disease: Lessons to be learned? [comment]. Am J Publ Health 1999;89:995-997.

248. Rotmensch J, Yamada SD: Neoplasms of the vulva and vagina. In Kufe DW, Pollock RE, Weichselbaum RR, et al. (eds): Cancer Medicine, 6th ed. Hamilton, Ontario, BC Decker, 2003.

249. Daling JR, Sherman KJ: Cancer of the vulva and vagina. In Schottenfeld D, Schottenfeld D (eds): Cancer Epidemiology and Prevention. New York, Oxford University Press, 1996.

250. Parkin DM, Whelan SL, Ferlay J, et al: Cancer Incidence in Five Continents VII. Lyon, France, IARC, 1997.

251. Sturgeon SR, Brinton LA, Devesa SS, Kurman RJ: In situ and invasive vulvar cancer incidence trends (1973 to 1987). Am J Obstet Gynecol 1992;166:1482-1485.

252. Madeleine MM, Daling JR, Tamini HK: Vulva and vagina. In Franco EL, Rohan TE (eds): Cancer Precursors: Epidemiology, Detection, and Prevention. New York, Springer-Verlag, 2002.

253. Howe HL, Wingo PA, Thun MJ, et al: Annual report to the nation on the status of cancer (1973 through 1998), featuring cancers with recent increasing trends [comment]. J Natl Cancer Inst 2001;93:824-842.

254. Levi F, Randimbison L, La Vecchia C: Descriptive epidemiology of vulvar and vaginal cancers in Vaud, Switzerland, 1974-1994. Ann Oncol 1998;9:1229-1232.

255. Iversen T, Tretli S: Intraepithelial and invasive squamous cell neoplasia of the vulva: Trends in incidence, recurrence, and survival rate in Norway. Obstet Gynecol 1998;91:969-972.

256. Jones RW, Baranyai J, Stables S: Trends in squamous cell carcinoma of the vulva: The influence of vulvar intraepithelial neoplasia. Obstet Gynecol 1997;90:448-452.

257. Ansink AC, Krul MR, De Weger RA, et al: Human papillomavirus, lichen sclerosus, and squamous cell carcinoma of the vulva: Detection and prognostic significance. Gynecol Oncol 1994;52:180-184.

258. Monk BJ, Burger RA, Lin F, et al: Prognostic significance of human papillomavirus DNA in vulvar carcinoma [review]. Obstet Gynecol 1995;85:709-715.

259. Pinto AP, Signorello LB, Crum CP, et al: Squamous cell carcinoma of the vulva in Brazil: Prognostic importance of host and viral variables. Gynecol Oncol 1999;74:61-67.

260. Brinton LA, Nasca PC, Mallin K, et al: Case-control study of cancer of the vulva. Obstet Gynecol 1990;75:859-866.

261. Daling JR, Sherman KJ: Relationship between human papillomavirus infection and tumours of anogenital sites other than the cervix [review]. IARC Scientific Publications 1992; (119):223-241.

262. Carter JJ, Madeleine MM, Shera K, et al: Human papillomavirus 16 and 18 L1 serology compared across anogenital cancer sites. Cancer Res 2001;61:1934-1940.

263. Sherman KJ, Daling JR, Chu J, et al: Multiple primary tumours in women with vulvar neoplasms: A case-control study. Br J Cancer 1988;57:423-427.

264. Sturgeon SR, Ziegler RG, Brinton LA, et al: Diet and the risk of vulvar cancer. Ann Epidemiol 1991;1:427-437.

265. Sherman KJ, Daling JR, Chu J, et al: Genital warts, other sexually transmitted diseases, and vulvar cancer. Epidemiology 1991; 2:257-262.

266. Daling JR, Sherman KJ, Hislop TG, et al: Cigarette smoking and the risk of anogenital cancer. Am J Epidemiol 1992;135:180-189.

267. Crum CP: Carcinoma of the vulva: Epidemiology and pathogenesis [review]. Obstet Gynecol 1992;79:448-454.

268. Kurman RJ, Toki T, Schiffman MH: Basaloid and warty carcinomas of the vulva: Distinctive types of squamous cell carcinoma frequently associated with human papillomaviruses [erratum appears in Am J Surg Pathol 1993;17:536.]. Am J Surg Pathol 1993;17:133-145.

269. Park JS, Jones RW, McLean MR, et al: Possible etiologic heterogeneity of vulvar intraepithelial neoplasia: A correlation of pathologic characteristics with human papillomavirus detection by in situ hybridization and polymerase chain reaction. Cancer 1991;67:1599-1607.

270. Toki T, Kurman RJ, Park JS, et al: Probable nonpapillomavirus etiology of squamous cell carcinoma of the vulva in older women: A clinicopathologic study using in situ hybridization and polymerase chain reaction. Int J Gynecol Pathol 1991;10: 107-125.

271. Gillison ML, Shah KV: Role of mucosal human papillomavirus in nongenital cancers [review]. J Natl Cancer Inst Monogr 2003; (31):57-65.

272. Trimble CL, Hildesheim A, Brinton LA, et al: Heterogeneous etiology of squamous carcinoma of the vulva. Obstet Gynecol 1996;87:59-64.

273. Sun Y, Hildesheim A, Brinton LA, et al: Human papillomavirus-specific serologic response in vulvar neoplasia. Gynecol Oncol 1996;63:200-203.

274. Hildesheim A, Han CL, Brinton LA, et al: Human papillomavirus type 16 and risk of preinvasive and invasive vulvar cancer: Results from a seroepidemiological case-control study [see comments]. Obstet Gynecol 1997;90:748-754.

275. Bjorge T, Dillner J, Anttila T, et al: Prospective seroepidemiological study of role of human papillomavirus in non-cervical anogenital cancers [comment]. BMJ 1997;315:646-649.

276. Madeleine MM, Daling JR, Carter JJ, et al: Cofactors with human papillomavirus in a population-based study of vulvar cancer [erratum appears in J Natl Cancer Inst 1997;89:1896.]. J Natl Cancer Inst 1997;89:1516-1523.

277. Brinton LA, Nasca PC, Mallin K, et al: Case-control study of in situ and invasive carcinoma of the vagina. Gynecol Oncol 1990; 38:49-54.

278. Choo YC, Anderson DG: Neoplasms of the vagina following cervical carcinoma. Gynecol Oncol 1982;14:125-132.

279. Rose PG, Herterick EE, Boutselis JG, et al: Multiple primary gynecologic neoplasms. Am J Obstet Gynecol 1987;157:261-267.

280. Daling JR, Madeleine MM, Schwartz SM, et al: A population-based study of squamous cell vaginal cancer: HPV and cofactors. Gynecol Oncol 2002;84:263-270.

281. Ikenberg H, Runge M, Goppinger A, Pfleiderer A: Human papillomavirus DNA in invasive carcinoma of the vagina. Obstet Gynecol 1990;76:432-438.

282. Hildesheim A, Han C-L, Brinton LA, et al: Sexually transmitted agents and risk of carcinoma of the vagina. Int J Gynecol Cancer 1997;7:251-255.

283. Barzon L, Pizzighella S, Corti L, et al: Vaginal dysplastic lesions in women with hysterectomy and receiving radiotherapy are linked to high-risk human papillomavirus. J Med Virol 2002; 67:401-405.

284. Herman JM, Homesley HD, Dignan MB: Is hysterectomy a risk factor for vaginal cancer? JAMA 1986;256:601-603.

285. Williams WC, Herman JM: Vaginal intraepithelial neoplasia: Methodologic problems in a case-control study. Fam Pract Res J 1990;10:27-35.

CHAPTER

SCREENING, DIAGNOSIS, AND STAGING OF CERVICAL CANCER

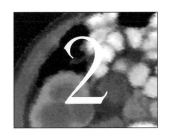

Y. M. Chan   and   David M. Luesley

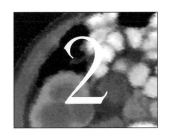

MAJOR CONTROVERSIES

- **What aspect of screening programs is the most important in reducing deaths from cervical cancer?**
- **Is screening in adolescence justifiable?**
- **What is the appropriate age to stop screening?**
- **How can the adverse impact of screening be reduced?**
- **How good is a conventional smear?**
- **Can human papillomavirus testing replace cytologic testing?**
- **Should direct visual inspection be the primary screening method in resource-poor settings?**
- **Does cervicography have a role in screening?**
- **How should human immunodeficiency virus–infected women be screened?**
- **Should smears be taken during pregnancy?**
- **How often does cervical intraepithelial neoplasia become cancer and how long does it take?**
- **What is the best way to treat cervical intraepithelial neoplasia?**
- **Why is staging clinical?**
- **What other investigations have value?**
- **Should staging recognize the importance of lymph node disease?**
- **Does individualized treatment planning improve survival?**
- **Can current imaging technology adequately detect lymph node disease?**

Approximately 500,000 cervical cancers are diagnosed annually worldwide, representing 12% of all cancers diagnosed in women, and about half of those diagnosed will die from their cancer.[1,2] Figure 2-1 shows the global variation in incidence of cervical cancer.

There is convincing evidence that cytologic screening programs are effective in reducing mortality from carcinoma of the cervix.[3-16] Although there are no randomized trials, case-control and cohort studies from a number of developed countries have shown that well-organized cervical screening programs have been effective in reducing cancer incidence and mortality, especially if they have good quality assurance.[17-22]

Potential reductions in disease incidence of 60% to 90% are feasible in the 3 years after screening.[18,20] In the United States, the death rate from cervical cancer has dropped; from being the primary cause of cancer deaths in women, it is now the 12th most common cause.[23]

In contrast, few resource-poor countries have effective cervical screening programs, which explains why the incidence of cervical cancer has not decreased in these countries. In these developing areas of the world, cervical cancer remains the primary cancer killer in women. The failure to establish screening programs in developing countries could be caused by socioeconomic, cultural, or political conditions. With

31

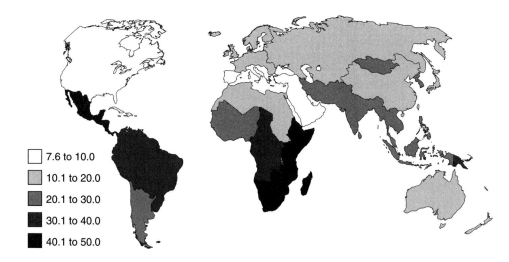

□ 7.6 to 10.0
▨ 10.1 to 20.0
▦ 20.1 to 30.0
▩ 30.1 to 40.0
■ 40.1 to 50.0

Figure 2–1. Global variation in incidence (per 100,000) of cervical cancer. (From Ponten J et al: Strategies for global control of cervical cancer. Int J Cancer 1995;60:2.)

limited and often insufficient resources and poorly developed or nonexistent health care infrastructures, cervical screening may not be perceived as strongly as a health care priority as it is in more affluent nations.

CANCER SCREENING PROGRAMS

An effective screening program should reduce both the incidence of cervical cancer and the mortality from the disease, with minimal adverse impact on the screened population. An organized screening program, as defined by an expert group of the International Union Against Cancer (UICC), should have the following essential elements:[24]

- A defined target population and individuals to be screened
- A defined age at onset and frequency of screening
- Use of personal invitations with given times and places for screening, as well as personal information on the results of screening even for negative cases
- Substantial quality control in taking the smears, making the diagnosis, and evaluating the effects of the program.

The purpose of cytologic screening is to identify those women who have an intraepithelial lesion (cervical intraepithelial neoplasia, or CIN), not those who have cancer. If disease can be detected and treated at this preinvasive stage, outcome should significantly improve. There have been no randomized clinical trials designed specifically to evaluate screening for cervical intraepithelial disease. Such trials are unlikely to be performed, given the established practice and generally accepted health benefit associated with screening. Nevertheless, several important lessons have been learned from the many studies that have been reported.

Types of Programs

What aspect of screening programs is the most important in reducing deaths from cervical cancer?
Cervical screening may be performed either in a structured fashion, to cover all the target population at set intervals, or opportunistically, by performing a test when a woman accesses health care for other reasons. It is now clear that ad hoc or unstructured screening does not necessarily reach the population who really would benefit from regular screening for cervical cancer. Those at high risk for the disease may not be screened, because of the limited accessibility and availability that are associated with opportunistic screening. In addition to being less effective, it is also more costly to perform opportunistic screening than to choose a population-based approach.[24-27] Significant progress in reducing disease burden from cervical cancer has occurred as a result of improved coverage.[19-28]

Age at commencement, interval, and age at discontinuation. Since the introduction of cervical screening programs in developed countries, there has been an ongoing debate with regard to the appropriate age at commencement of screening, the screening interval, and the age at which screening should stop. Table 2-1 shows the variations in cervical screening programs among European countries.[29] Screening programs with varying target age groups and interscreening intervals have been adopted in different populations. As yet, the specifics of the program have not been shown to have a major impact on outcome in terms of cervical cancer deaths. The most important factor appears to be the presence of a program with high coverage of the target population.

The yield in terms of additional treatable cases falls as the screening interval is shortened and as the program is extended to cover people at lower risk. Experience in both Canada and the United Kingdom suggests that there are diminishing returns with increasing frequency of screening in a given cohort of women.[24,30] It probably makes more sense in health-care economic terms to use resources to increase the number of women being screened for the first time than to increase the frequency of screening in women previously screened.

The target age range of a program is a more important determinant of risk reduction than the

Table 2–1. Comparisons of Cervical Screening Programs in European Countries

Country	Year of Initiation	Age Group (yr)	Routine Screening Interval (yr)	Coverage by Organized Screening (%)
Austria	1970	≥20	1	85
Belgium	1994	25-64	3	82.3
Denmark	1967-1990*	23-59	3	90
England	1988	20-64	3-5	84
Finland	1963	30-60	5	89.5
France	1990	25-65	3	22-69
Germany	1971, 1991	≥20	1	46-50
Greece	1991	25-64	2-3	87.8
Ireland	2000	25-60	5	Not available
Italy	1980-1995*	25-64	3	~70
Luxembourg	1962	>15	1	38.9
Netherlands	1996	30-60	5	80
Portugal	1990	20-64	3	51
Spain	1986	25-65	3	41.5
Sweden	Mid-1960s	20-59	3	50-70

*Different counties have different years of initiation of the program.

frequency of screening within the defined age range. The experience of the Nordic countries has shown that a well-organized screening program with a sufficiently wide target age range can be very successful in reducing both the incidence and the mortality of invasive cervical cancer.[19] The importance of good coverage and quality control was also demonstrated by the accelerated decline in mortality in England and Wales after changes were implemented in 1988 (Fig. 2-2).[4,31,32]

Is screening in adolescence justifiable? Women should commence screening after they become sexually active, although how soon after the onset of coital

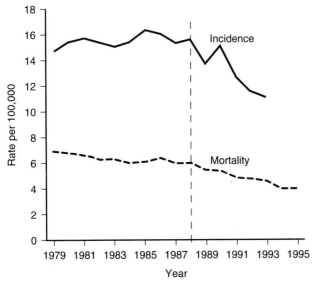

Figure 2–2. Age-standardized incidence and mortality rates of cervical cancer in England from 1979 to 1995 (directly age-standardized using the European standard population). The dashed vertical line represents initiation of computerized call and recall. (From Patnick J: Has screening for cervical cancer been successful? Br J Obstet Gynaecol 1997;104:877.)

activity screening should begin is another matter for debate. Individuals who become sexually active in midadolescence tend to have multiple sexual partners, and they are generally recognized as being at high risk for development of preinvasive and invasive diseases. However, the incidence and mortality rates of cervical cancer among women in their 20s are very low and do not justify screening in adolescence, even if other risk factors for cancer are present. Furthermore, the potential to cause harm from overinvestigation and overtreatment is very real in these young women.[33,34] These factors should be borne in mind when setting the age for commencement of a screening program.

In England and Wales in the mid-1960s, a political decision was made not to pay for Papanicolaou smears in women younger than 35 years of age unless they had had three or more children. During the ensuing decade, the death rate doubled as a result of carcinoma of the cervix in women of that age group. Before 1994, there was an increasing mortality rate among patients age 45 years and younger. The screening program was relaunched in 1988, covering women from 25 to 64 years of age, with quality assurance and computerized call and recall systems. Coverage and quality increased substantially over the next 3 years. Since 1992, 5-year coverage has been greater than 80%. Since 1994, mortality rates even in younger women have dropped, and the trend should continue.[31]

What is the appropriate age to stop screening? At the same time, studies have shown that older women are at increased risk for cervical cancer, with 25% of all cervical cancers and 41% of all deaths from cancer occurring in women older than 65 years of age.[35] The prevalence of abnormal and unsatisfactory cytology findings is also high in this group, about 16 per 1000.[35] Data on screening of older women are conflicting. Some series suggest that screening of women older than 65 years of age is likely to be of benefit, with a 63% improvement in the 5-year mortality rate.[36] However, other series concentrating on well-screened cohorts suggest that a woman who has been regularly screened up until the age of 50 years and has had no abnormal smears is at very low risk and could discontinue screening.[37] The appropriate age to stop screening is still undefined, but as more women enter properly structured programs it is more likely that the age for discontinuation will fall rather than rise.

A working group of the International Agency for Research on Cancer (IARC) used case-control studies to evaluate 10 established screening programs. They showed that protection remains high for 2 years after a negative smear, but thereafter falls with time, and concluded that screening of women age 20 to 64 years every 5 years would protect 84% of them, whereas smears taken every 3 years would protect 91% and annual smears would protect 93%.[28]

Adverse Effects of Screening

Screening policies must consider the balance between benefits and costs. Better health and improved survival come at the cost of the provision of screening, follow-up, and treatment. Human costs include overtreatment, unnecessary follow-up tests and investigations, and worry to those individuals whose positive screening results may not in actuality represent a significant risk. It is important to note that only a proportion of those who test positive have significant pathology. Therefore, in the total population screened, all are exposed to the test, and a proportion have an abnormal test result. Abnormal test results lead to additional intervention and are likely to be associated with some degree of anxiety or disturbance in emotional well-being. Data published over the last three decades clearly indicate that the number of women who have abnormal smears is far in excess of the number who will get cancer, and this cannot be accounted for by intervention alone. The only reasonable conclusion is that only a proportion of "abnormal test results" represent significant disease or situations in which nonintervention might result in cancer. It is this population who are the "health gainers" from screening; the remainder are potential "emotional health losers." As a result, many people suffer some cost to achieve the health gain for the few who benefit. However, the level of technology and understanding of the disease process do not yet allow prediction of which screen-positive individuals will and will not benefit from follow-up tests and treatment. There is considerable activity directed toward using molecular markers of progression to achieve such a selection. These activities remain well within the research arena, although their potential for clinical application is enormous.

How can the adverse impact of screening be reduced? Considerable stress and anxiety can be generated within the screening program, as suggested earlier.[38-42] This is true even in women who eventually receive normal smear reports. Therefore, prescreening counseling is important to avoid undue anxiety if the test should prove to be abnormal. Women should not be lead to believe that an abnormal test result means that cancer is present, a very common misconception. It is also important to explain the limitations of the test so as not to generate unrealistic expectations.

METHOD OF SCREENING

Conventional Cytologic Screening

Pap smears form the basis of conventional cervical screening. The procedure involves scraping the ectocervix (and hopefully the lower portion of the endocervical canal) with an appropriately shaped spatula or brush to collect exfoliated cells. These are then transferred to a glass slide, fixed and stained before examination by a trained technician or cytologist. This is a relatively cheap test and does not require special equipment in the clinics where the samples are collected. The acceptance of the test is good overall, but certain sections of the population, especially older women and members of racial and cultural minority groups,[31] have been slower than others to avail themselves of the test. Screening programs using Pap smears have been shown to be effective in reducing the incidence and mortality rates of cervical cancer.[3-16]

Performance of Conventional Cytology

How good is a conventional smear? The sensitivity of cervical cytology ranges from 30% to 70%, with a specificity of more than 90%.[43-47] Technically, it is incorrect to refer to sensitivity, because sensitivity can be computed only if the whole population sample is subjected to a test regarded as the gold standard. In the case of cytology, this would be histologic assessment of cervical biopsies. Because it is impractical and unrealistic to histologically assess the whole population, a more appropriate description would be "detection rate achieved by cytologic screening." Even in countries where well-organized screening programs achieve high population coverage, there are problems associated with the intrinsic false-negative rate of 30% to 50%. False-negative smears may lead to invasive cancers being missed. In a recent audit, approximately 40% of invasive cancers occurred in women who had been regularly tested.[48] Test failure results from sampling errors, in which the abnormal cells do not get collected or placed on the slide, and reading error, in which a few abnormal cells are not identified among the multitude of normal cells that are also present in a well-taken cervical smear.[49] Cytologic screening is poor at detecting glandular lesions or adenocarcinoma, which account for a growing number and proportion of cervical cancers.[50-53] It should be borne in mind that cervical cytology screening programs do not necessarily depend on one smear in a lifetime. Although an individual test may appear to have an unacceptably high false-negative rate, a series of similar tests spaced throughout a woman's lifetime may have a better performance.

In addition, false-negative smears have medicolegal implications. Cytopathologists may tend to err on the side of caution, leading to an increase in the proportion of smears classified as abnormal. This has the effect of reducing specificity, with the possible consequences of increased anxiety, unnecessary intervention and treatment, and protracted follow-up.

Another major drawback of cervical cytology is its relatively high false-positive rate, which may vary from 5% to 70%, depending on the expertise in interpretation and criteria as to what constitutes a positive test. Even a specificity in excess of 90% means in real terms that 10 women in every 100 screened will receive a false-positive result. Because screening is a population-based activity, this translates into large numbers of women in a given population being given falsely abnormal test results. The performance of the test is, in reality, a combination of factors inherent in the sample itself and the subjective nature of its interpretation. Much time and effort have been directed toward using computers and diagnostic algorithms to minimize this subjectivity, but as yet they have made little impact on clinical practice, and the interpretation of cervical smears is still very much a human activity.

Problems in Classification of Conventional Smears

Although the introduction of and subsequent improvements in the Bethesda system for reporting the results of cervical cytology (Table 2-2)[54] has had a positive impact on the quality and consistency of laboratory performance, the problem of equivocal smears, known as atypical squamous cells of undetermined significance (ASCUS), has been highlighted in a number of studies.[55,56] In one study, even expert cytopathologists could not agree on what constitutes this "grey zone" in cytology,[55] yet such smears account for 60% to 80% of all abnormal smears.[56] More importantly, the majority of those women with histologically confirmed high-grade disease had presented with smears showing ASCUS, or low-grade abnormalities. Only 30% of high-grade disease initially had abnormal smears reported to be high grade.

Liquid-Based Cytology

Sampling and preparation errors have been estimated to be responsible for 70% to 90% of false-negative cervical smears. Because of the collection devices used in taking conventional smears and the subsequent transfer to glass slides, only 20% of the collected cellular population is used.[57-59] Abnormal cells may also be difficult to identify and interpret because of the obscuring effects of air-drying artifact and the presence of

Table 2–2. The 2001 Bethesda System for Reporting Results of Cervical Cytology

Specimen Adequacy
Satisfactory for evaluation (note presence/absence of endocervical/transformation zone component)
Unsatisfactory for evaluation (specify reason)
Specimen rejected/not processed (specify reason)
Specimen processed and examined, but unsatisfactory for evaluation of epithelial abnormality because of (specify reason)

General Categorization (Optional)
Negative for intraepithelial lesion or malignancy
Epithelial cell abnormality
Other

Interpretation/Result
Negative for Intraepithelial Lesion or Malignancy
Organisms
Trichomonas vaginalis
Fungal organisms morphologically consistent with *Candida* species
Shift in flora suggestive of bacterial vaginosis
Bacteria morphologically consistent with *Actinomyces* species
Cellular changes consistent with herpes simplex virus
Other Non-neoplastic Findings (optional to report; list not comprehensive)
Reactive cellular changes associated with
 Inflammation (includes typical repair)
 Radiation
 Intrauterine contraceptive device
Glandular cells status posthysterectomy
Atrophy

Epithelial Cell Abnormalities
Squamous Cell
Atypical squamous cells (ASC)
 Of undermined significance (ASC-US)
 Cannot exclude HSIL (ASC-H)
Low-grade squamous intraepithelial lesion (LSIL)
 Encompassing: human papillomavirus/mild dysplasia/cervical intraepithelial neoplasia (CIN 1)
High-grade squamous intraepithelial lesion (HSIL)
 Encompassing: moderate and severe dysplasia, carcinoma in situ; CIN 2 and CIN 3
 Squamous cell carcinoma
Glandular Cell
Atypical glandular cells (AGC) (specify endocervical, endometrial, or not otherwise specified)
Atypical glandular cells, favor neoplastic (specify endocervical or not otherwise specified)
Endocervical adenocarcinoma in situ (AIS)
 Adenocarcinoma
Other (list not comprehensive)
 Endometrial cells in women ≥40 yr of age

Automated Review and Ancillary Testing (Include as Appropriate)
Educational Notes and Suggestions (Optional)

From Solomon D, Davey D, Kurman R, et al: The 2001 Bethesda System: Terminology for reporting results of cervical cytology. JAMA 2002;287:2116.

blood, mucus, and inflammatory debris. Liquid-based cytology systems aim to overcome these problems.

The cervical samples are taken in the usual manner, and the collection device is rinsed in a vial containing a buffered alcohol liquid preservative. The vial is then transferred to the laboratory, where a slide is prepared from the cells in suspension with a thin, well-distributed layer of cells in a defined area on the slide. Although this method does not use the total cellular population, it does represent a truly random sample of that collected. Furthermore, because the sample is presented to the cytopathologist in a thin, evenly distributed layer, interpretation is less likely to be compromised by obscuring cells, blood, and debris. Studies have shown that this method of slide preparation is associated with an increase in detection of biopsy-proved high-grade cervical disease and a decrease in reports of unsatisfactory smears.[60-66] In one recent meta-analysis, liquid-based cytology was found to be more cost-effective than the Pap smear as a cervical cytologic screening technology.[67]

This technology has already been introduced in the United States and has rapidly become the standard of care. Pilot studies in the United Kingdom are complete, and in Scotland the completed studies have led to a recommendation that liquid-based systems be introduced to replace the conventional Pap smear.

Other advantages of liquid-based technology include the potential to use the remaining fluid for additional tests, including testing for human papillomavirus (HPV). This may be of value in helping management decisions when the result is reported as ASCUS, and indeed this has been recommended since the Bethesda III consensus conference.[54,68,69]

Human Papillomavirus Testing

The causal association between infection with certain HPV types and the development of cervical cancer and its precursor lesions is now beyond doubt.[70-72] Almost all invasive cervical cancers contain high-risk HPV types such as HPV 16, 18, 31, 33, 52, and 58.[73] High-risk HPV is also the most important independent predictor for CIN III. Women infected with high-risk HPV types have relative risks of 40 to 180 for the development of high-grade cervical disease.[74-77] Even higher relative risks (100 to 500) have been reported for persistent HPV infection, which appears to be the key step in cervical carcinogenesis.[78] It is also important to note that only women with abnormal smears and persistence of high-risk HPV in their smears showed progressive CIN disease.[75-80] On the other hand, women without high-risk HPV never showed clinical progression to CIN III.[81,82] Therefore, detection of high-risk HPV identifies individuals who are more likely to develop high-grade CIN or cervical cancer.

Additionally, molecular studies have identified mechanisms by which high-risk HPV types contribute to carcinogenesis.[71,72,83] The World Health Organization and the International Agency for Research on Cancer (IARC) have officially designated HPV types 16 and 18 as carcinogenic agents.

Although a number of different techniques have been used to detect HPV, currently only two are preferred, Hybrid Capture II (HC-II)[84,85] and the polymerase chain reaction (PCR).[86,87] These tests have similar sensitivity and specificity, but PCR is more difficult to use routinely, and particularly in a screening situation. Recent studies using HC-II have consistently documented a high sensitivity (>90%) in the prediction of high-grade CIN or cervical cancer.[56,88-95] Comparative

studies also indicate a higher sensitivity than that achieved by cytology. This could help to identify women with false-negative cytology findings. Specificity is now the major concern, especially in primary screening. False-positive rates of 5% to 20% have been reported.[95]

In developed countries, HPV testing by HC-II has been shown to be practical for managing and triaging women with abnormal smears.[56,88,89,96-99] Those infected with HPV are much more likely to have or to develop high-grade CIN and may benefit from immediate colposcopy. For HPV-negative women, a more conservative follow-up might be indicated.[56,100,101]

The combination of a normal cytology and a negative HPV test carries a negative predictive value of 97% to 100%. The increased reassurance so provided allows safe widening of the screening interval or, for older women, no further screening. This could enable the selection of women who are at risk for high-grade CIN or cancer, allowing a concentration of screening effort in exposed women.

By improving detection of underlying high-grade CIN; reducing the number of repeat smears, colposcopies, biopsies, and unnecessary treatment; and widening the screening interval, the cost-effectiveness of the HPV approach can be demonstrated without diminishing the quality of the service.[56,88,89,96-98] The savings include not only the internal cost but also the emotional cost induced by the close monitoring.

Can human papillomavirus testing replace cytologic testing? One problem with HPV testing is the relatively high prevalence of infection, particularly in young women.[102] Although HPV infection is relatively common, CIN and cervical cancer are not. It is logical to assume that exposure to and infection by HPV, although a prerequisite for the development of cervical cancer, is uncommonly associated with such an outcome. Therefore, the majority of women who test positive for HPV will not develop cancer. A clearer understanding of the final steps in the oncogenic pathway is essential if the full potential of HPV testing is to be realized.

Direct Visual Inspection

Several studies have suggested that direct visual inspection (DVI) of the cervix after the application of 5% acetic acid is almost equivalent to cervical cytology in the detection of cervical carcinoma precursors.[103-108] DVI has several advantages for screening, especially in low-resource settings. It is a low-technology test with minimal infrastructural and equipment requirements. It is not difficult to learn, and nurses or other allied health care workers can be trained to perform the test in a basic primary care clinic. Moreover, it provides an immediate on-site result, allowing for immediate arrangement of follow-up investigations.[103-110]

Should direct visual inspection be the primary screening method in resource-poor settings? Low specificity and low positive predictive values are the major concerns regarding DVI as a screening method, especially if the "screen and treat" policy is to be adopted. Varying definitions used to evaluate performance and the lack of reproducible methods of quality control are the other problems with DVI. The subjective nature of the test, failure to apply sufficient acetic acid for an adequate period, poor visualization of the cervix, and screener fatigue are possible reasons for false-negative results. Nevertheless, DVI may have potential for application in select environments. Studies evaluating the safety, acceptability, and impact of the DVI-based screening program on cancer incidence are currently underway.[109,111]

Cervicography

Cervicography is a technique that attempts to reproduce colposcopy photographically. A photograph of the cervix is taken with a specially designed camera after the application of acetic acid. The camera incorporates a light source and is designed to minimize problems of focus and movement artifact. The procedure can be performed by any trained personnel capable of inserting a speculum and visualizing the cervix.[112] The photographs obtained are sent to an expert for interpretation. Projection of the images onto a screen produces a magnification and resolution similar to those of colposcopy, and interpretation can be performed far more quickly than in a colposcopic examination.

Does cervicography have a role in screening? Studies have shown that cervicography has a significantly better sensitivity than cervical cytology (89% versus 52%), with similar specificity (94% versus 92%).[113] Technically defective cervicograms were reported infrequently (about 5%).[113] However, the role of cervicography in cervical screening has not been determined. The expense of the instrument and the costs of photographic developing make it unlikely to be used for population screening. With improvements in digital imaging and teleconferencing by means of the Internet, increased use of telecervicography has been advocated.

Telecolposcopy

Telecolposcopy is to a certain extent an extension of cervicography, except that the image is recorded in real time and in digital format. In simple terms, a digital video image of a colposcopic assessment is captured. This can be done at a distance from the expert colposcopist, who can either evaluate the image in real time and relay back an opinion or batch-process several examinations. Like any digital image, it can be stored, annotated, manipulated, and transmitted. The technique has obvious applications for teaching and audit, and it may also have a role in the triage of mild cytologic abnormalities. Pilot studies have been conducted,[114,115] and definitive trials are underway.

SPECIAL CIRCUMSTANCES

Human immunodeficiency virus–infected women

In 1993, the Centers for Disease Control and Prevention (CDC) expanded the case definition of acquired immunodeficiency syndrome (AIDS) to include invasive cervical cancer. Cervical cancer is the most common AIDS-related malignancy in women. Once cervical cancer develops in an HIV-infected woman, the disease is more likely to be in an advanced stage, more aggressive, and less responsive to treatment than cervical cancer in a non-HIV-infected woman.[116-121] The recurrence and death rates are higher and the intervals to recurrence and death are shorter in HIV-infected women than in HIV-negative controls.[116-121]

How should human immunodeficiency virus–infected women be screened? The prevalence of CIN is higher among HIV-infected women than in the general population (33% to 41% versus 6%).[122-126] CIN is more difficult to treat in HIV-infected women; in addition, the disease tends to be multifocal, and the chance of persistent or recurrent disease after treatment is higher.[119,127-131] It is estimated that about one of every five HIV-infected women with no evidence of cervical disease initially will develop biopsy-confirmed CIN within 3 years.[132] Moreover, immunosuppression caused by HIV infection may cause a more rapid progression of CIN to carcinoma. These data highlight the need to develop effective cervical cancer prevention programs for HIV-infected women.

Several studies have found that the sensitivity, specificity, and false-negative rates of screening cytology for CIN among HIV-infected women are comparable with those among the general population.[133-136] However, other studies have suggested that cervical screening is not predictive of CIN in HIV-infected women.[137-140] A cytologic diagnosis of ASCUS in HIV-infected women has a 32% risk of associated CIN.[137] A case-control study suggested that cytology findings did not match the biopsy results in 44% of patients and was less severe than the cervical biopsy results in 91% of these mismatches.[139] Cervical cytology also missed 43% of biopsy-proved CIN in this series of HIV-infected women. Moreover, the high prevalence of abnormal cytology findings and CIN and the higher interobserver variation in HIV-infected women limit the usefulness of the Pap smear as a screening tool.

Colposcopically directed punch biopsies are poor predictors of cone or loop excision histology.[141,142] At least 26% and as many as 74% of HIV-infected women with CIN I on punch biopsy may have a significantly worse lesion on cone biopsy despite satisfactory colposcopy findings.[141] Disagreement between punch biopsy and cone histology was evident in 41% of HIV-infected patients in one study.[141] The cone specimen had a higher-grade lesion than was indicated by the punch biopsy in 38% of HIV-infected patients. This is probably a result of the multifocality of the disease.

Despite all these limitations, the cervical smear remains the primary screening method in HIV-infected women. In 1993, the CDC recommended that all HIV-infected women should have cervical screening by Pap smears. If the first smear is normal, the Pap test should be repeated within 6 months to ensure that CIN was not missed on the first smear. If the smear shows ASCUS or any degree of squamous intraepithelial lesions (SIL), the patient should be referred for colposcopy.[143] However, it is unclear whether screening for cervical cancer will improve health outcomes of women infected with HIV.

Invasive cervical cancer currently affects relatively small numbers of HIV-infected women. Most of these women die from opportunistic infections before cervical cancer has a chance to develop. Present data indicate that fewer than 20% of HIV-infected women survive 36 months after the diagnosis of AIDS. However, with improvement in treatment of the disease and increased survival of HIV-infected women, there may yet be an increase in the number of cervical cancers in this group of patients.

Pregnancy

Should smears be taken during pregnancy? In countries without a cervical screening program, pregnancy represents a chance for an opportunistic smear to be taken in the antenatal clinic. Actually, many women start their screening or have smears taken only during pregnancy. In countries with cervical screening programs, the practice of taking opportunistic smears during pregnancy should be avoided.

Cervical smears performed during pregnancy are more prone to sampling errors.[144,145] Contact bleeding is not uncommon at smear taking. The smear taker may perform a less than thorough smear to avoid bleeding from the more vascular cervix. Nevertheless, a properly obtained sample reviewed by an appropriately trained cytologist should represent the true state of the cervix.[146-150] Smears with borderline atypia or low-grade SIL should be repeated in 6 months. Women with smears suggesting high-grade SIL should be referred for colposcopy.

Colposcopy of the pregnant cervix is more complicated than colposcopy of the nonpregnant cervix. Changes in consistency, shape, and vascularity, together with an increased area and rate of squamous metaplasia of the exposed columnar epithelium, can make interpretation of the transformation zone more difficult. Colposcopy, if performed during pregnancy, should be done by someone with adequate experience. Both colposcopically directed biopsy and diathermy loop excision of the cervix can be performed safely during pregnancy.[151-154]

Positive Cervical Screening Results

How often does cervical intraepithelial neoplasia become cancer and how long does it take? It is important to understand the natural history of CIN, because this forms the basis of clinical management of women with abnormal screening results. The continuum model of stepwise progressive changes from mild, to moderate, to severe dysplasia, and to invasive disease as the end result,[155] has been challenged as more has become known with regard to the natural history of the disease.

CIN does not necessarily progress in an orderly fashion to invasive cancer. Minor degrees of CIN may resolve without any form of intervention. Although the transit time from CIN III to invasive cancer is said to be 8, 10, or possibly 20 years, some patients make this transition in a short time. Moreover, a lower-grade CIN lesion can progress directly to invasive cancer. In a review of the literature of almost 14,000 patients monitored for less than 1 year to as long as 20 years, 60% of CIN I lesions regressed, and only 10% progressed to CIN III. In patients with CIN III, one third of the lesions regressed to normal.[156] In a meta-analysis of almost 28,000 patients, progression to cancer was 0.25% with ASCUS, 0.15% with low-grade SIL, and 1.44% with high-grade SIL.[157] Regression to normal occurred in 68% of ASCUS, 47% low-grade SIL, and 35% in high-grade SIL. The problem is the present inability to distinguish between dysplasias that are truly precancerous and those that represent nonspecific proliferations.

Cervical cytology is not a diagnostic tool but a screening test. An abnormal cervical screening test should prompt further investigation, which usually consists of colposcopy and biopsy, with the objective of confirming or excluding invasive cancer or its dysplastic precursors. Most screeners refer women with high-grade abnormalities for colposcopy. For minor abnormalities, the screener is faced with two choices: either to follow up minor abnormalities cytologically, with a risk of missing important abnormalities, or to refer all women with minor cytologic abnormalities for colposcopy, which overwhelms the screening system and increases overtreatment. The choice depends on the referral practice. Referral practices vary based on the availability of resources rather than a sound evidence base. In practice it is difficult to demonstrate any adverse effects of cytologic surveillance compared with colposcopic referral, although the former may be associated with worse long-term compliance.

Treatment of Preinvasive Disease

What is the best way to treat cervical intraepithelial neoplasia? Treatment options include local destructive and excisional techniques. Local destructive techniques should not be used if invasive disease cannot be excluded or if the whole lesion cannot be visualized. This usually necessitates the taking of directed biopsies. Methods of local destruction include

- Electrocoagulation
- CO_2 laser vaporization
- Cold coagulation
- Cryocautery

They are of similar effectiveness, with success rates of between 90% and 98%. There are obvious advantages of excisional methods of management compared with destructive methods, because they allow a much more confident exclusion of early invasive disease, which may be overlooked even by highly trained colposcopists. Excision also combines diagnosis with therapy, obviating the need for an initial assessment plus directed biopsy. Conization is always recommended if colposcopically directed biopsies and endocervical curettage fail to account for significant cytologic abnormalities.

The advent of outpatient loop excision of transformation zone (LEEP or LLETZ) has resulted in the concept of the "see and treat" strategy.[158-161] The specimens containing the whole transformation zone are certainly of better quality than small punch biopsy specimens. Small punch biopsies often underestimate the severity of the lesions, with false-negative rates of 41% to 54% having been reported.[162-165] With LLETZ, early invasive disease can be more reliably excluded. From a patient's perspective, the directed biopsy before planned therapy usually means additional attendance for treatment, if treatment is indicated. However, this approach leads to overtreatment in 10% to 30% of women, with morbidities in a substantial number of women.[33]

DIAGNOSIS

Clinical Symptoms and Signs

Overall, abnormal vaginal bleeding is the most common presenting symptom of cervical cancer. It can manifest in the context of postmenopausal bleeding, irregular menses, or postcoital bleeding. Vaginal discharge is the second most common symptom and is often the herald of advanced disease. Asymptomatic presentation with detection by cervical screening is seen in approximately 10% of cases. Less frequently, other symptoms include pelvic pain or pressure, inguinal or sciatic pain, urinary frequency, and hematuria or oliguria. Symptoms such as these suggest more advanced disease.

With a grossly obvious lesion, a directed punch biopsy or a small excisional biopsy should be performed. Colposcopy may be needed in symptomatic patients who are without a grossly obvious lesion. Colposcopically directed biopsies may establish the diagnosis quite readily, although in the absence of a colposcopically visible lesion, endocervical curettage, endometrial biopsy, or cervical conization may prove expedient. Small directed biopsies are not sufficient for the diagnosis of stage Ia1 and Ia2 lesions because, by definition, the lesion is wholly contained within the biopsy specimen.

Colposcopy should also be considered even if there are grossly obvious cervical lesions, because it is the only reliable method of excluding extension onto the vaginal vault.

STAGING OF DISEASE

Clinical Staging

Why is staging clinical? Cancer of the cervix is usually staged according to the International Federation of Gynecologists and Obstetricians (FIGO) staging system. It is a clinical staging system, and its latest version was released in 1994 (Table 2-3). The justification for persisting with a clinical staging system (as opposed to surgical staging) is that, because the majority of cases will be managed by radiotherapy, clinical staging is necessary if it is to be truly comparative.

Patients should be examined by an experienced gynecologist or clinical oncologist. If the examination is considered unsatisfactory or if there is any discrepancy in the physical findings, the examination

Table 2–3. The 1994 FIGO Staging System for Cervical Carcinoma

Stage 0	Carcinoma in situ, cervical intraepithelial neoplasia grade III	
Stage I	Carcinoma strictly confined to the cervix (extension to the corpus is disregarded)	
	Ia	Invasive carcinoma that can be diagnosed only by microscopy. All macroscopically visible lesions—even with superficial invasion—are allotted to stage Ib carcinomas. Invasion is limited to a measured stromal invasion with a maximal depth of 5.0 mm and a horizontal extension of not more than 7.0 mm. Depth of invasion should be not more than 5.0 mm taken from the base of the epithelium of the original tissue—superficial or glandular. The involvement of vascular spaces—venous or lymphatic—should not change the stage allotment.
		Ia1 Measured stromal invasion of not more than 3.0 mm in depth and extension of not more than 7.0 mm
		Ia2 Measured stromal invasion of greater than 3.0 mm and not more than 5.0 mm with an extension of not more than 7.0 mm
	Ib	Clinically visible lesions limited to the cervix uteri or preclinical cancers greater than Stage Ia
		Ib1 Clinically visible lesions not more than 4.0 cm
		Ib2 Clinically visible lesions greater than 4.0 cm
Stage II	Cervical carcinoma that invades beyond the uterus, but not to the pelvic wall or to the lower third of the vagina	
	IIa	No obvious parametrial involvement
	IIb	Obvious parametrial involvement
Stage III	The carcinoma has extended to the pelvic wall. On rectal examination, there is no cancer-free space between the tumor and the pelvic wall. The tumor involves the lower third of the vagina. All cases with hydronephrosis or nonfunctioning kidney are included, unless they are known to be due to other causes.	
	IIIa	Tumor that involves the lower third of the vagina, with no extension to the pelvic wall
	IIIb	Extension to the pelvic wall and/or hydronephrosis or nonfunctioning kidney
Stage IV	The carcinoma has extended beyond the true pelvis, or biopsy-proved involvement of the mucosa of the bladder or rectum. A bullous edema, as such, does not permit a case to be allotted to stage IV.	
	IVa	Spread of the growth to adjacent organs
	IVb	Spread to distant organs

should be repeated with the patient under general anesthesia. Pretreatment investigations usually include a complete blood count, liver and renal function tests, chest radiography, and intravenous urogram or renal ultrasound. Cystoscopy and sigmoidoscopy may be performed only if clinically indicated. Although staging of cervical cancer is generally clinical, diagnosis and staging of the early invasive lesions relegated to stage I subcategories constitute a special situation in which staging is histologically based. The diagnosis must always derive from histologic evaluation of a cone biopsy, amputated cervix, or hysterectomy specimen. The diagnosis is established only if the surgical margins are free of tumor.

The purpose of staging is to facilitate comparison of results among different institutions or clinical settings. It should be understood that "rules of staging" are intended to specify which subsets of data provide useful and permissible information for classification into staging categories, so that clinical results can be reasonably compared. However, staging should not limit the extent of pretreatment investigations or the subsequent treatment plan. Available information about a tumor, from the standpoint of prognosis, extent of spread, and pathologic and biochemical behavior, is desirable for treatment planning and should not be ignored.

Additional Investigations

What other investigations have value? In practice, computed tomography (CT), magnetic resonance imaging (MRI), and "staging" laparoscopy and laparotomy, are performed in some centers to obtain information useful in treatment planning. However, the results of these studies should not change the clinical stage of the disease.

Unfortunately, the clinical staging process is subjective and provides only approximate estimations for prognostic assessment. This is because wide variations in disease behavior may be included within a single stage or substage.[166,167] Clinical understaging and overstaging are not uncommon when compared with surgical staging. Understaging of up to 20% to 30% in stage Ib, up to 23% in stage IIb, and almost 40% in stage IIIb—and overstaging of about 64% in stage IIIb—have been reported.[168-170] Understaging is usually caused by unrecognized parametrial invasion or lymph node involvement, whereas overstaging occurs when pelvic inflammatory disease or endometriosis (or both) leads to the clinical impression of parametrial involvement.

Should staging recognize the importance of lymph node disease? One of the most obvious criticisms of the current clinical staging system is that it does not take into account the status of the regional lymph nodes. Nodal status is one of the most powerful predictors of outcome in stages I and II disease.[171-175] Furthermore, in surgically managed cases, nodal status becomes known only after primary treatment

has been completed; adverse findings in terms of positive nodes then direct adjuvant radiotherapy. This process not only increases morbidity but a lesser dose of radiation may be prescribed than would be given in a radical radiation setting and thus may be less likely to eradicate nodal disease. For these reasons, some centers are attempting to define nodal status before rather than after the treatment plan is defined.

Surgical Assessment

Cervical carcinoma is generally presumed to spread in an orderly fashion via local and then regional lymphatics.[176] The presence or absence of metastatic disease in the pelvic or para-aortic lymph nodes is an important prognostic factor in cervical cancer, and careful histologic analysis of the lymph nodes is crucial in decision-making for the subsequent therapy. The ability to perform laparoscopic pelvic and para-aortic lymphadenectomy in skilled hands allows for a more comprehensive assessment of the disease without an increased risk of radiation enteric injury should radiation therapy be the chosen primary modality.[177-182] It has been shown that radiation can safely begin within 7 days after surgical staging to avoid treatment delay.[179-182] Significant survival advantage in those patients with debulking of macroscopic nodes before commencement of radiation therapy has also been reported,[183-186] although the therapeutic potential of lymphadenectomy is still somewhat debatable.

Theoretically, surgical staging provides precise documentation of disease extent and thereby allows individualization of therapy. Furthermore, information with regard to the volume and histopathologic variables of the primary lesion may allow for the prediction of risk of local relapse. This knowledge should make possible a more rational and precise approach to treatment planning. In a retrospective review, surgical staging leads to treatment modification in more than 40% of cases.[187,188]

Does individualized treatment planning improve survival? Despite these theoretical advantages, individualization of treatment has not been shown to result in improved outcome, in terms of either reduced morbidity or improved survival. This finding, of course, could be the result of suboptimal treatment, and as yet there are no data available on an individualized treatment approach employing chemoradiation. Of equal importance, many centers do not yet have the laparoscopic expertise to institute a standardized pretreatment nodal assessment program. Surgical staging is not without morbidity, and it may not be practical or feasible in many patients, especially those with very early or very advanced disease. Imaging technology is also advancing rapidly, and it is not inconceivable that MRI, with specific enhancing techniques, might achieve acceptable accuracy levels in the detection of extracervical disease, thus negating the need for endoscopic assessment.

Imaging

Can current imaging technology adequately detect lymph node disease? Lymph node involvement may be evaluated by noninvasive techniques, such as conventional CT or MRI, which provide a sensitivity and specificity of approximately 80% when nodes are greater than 1 cm.[189-192] These values may fall to 24% in cases of lymph nodes with only small metastases. Recent advanced imaging methods, such as positron emission tomography (PET), further improve the prediction of nodal disease.[193-197] Cervical cancers of both squamous and nonsquamous histologies are avid for fluorodeoxyglucose (FDG), and PET-FDG scanning predicts both the presence and the absence of pelvic and para-aortic nodal metastatic disease, with a sensitivity of 91%, a specificity of 100%, a positive predictive value of 100%, and a negative predictive value of 96% in patients with early-stage cervical cancer.[196] In patients with locally advanced disease, PET has a sensitivity of 75%, a specificity of 92%, and a negative predictive value of 92% in detecting para-aortic lymph node metastases.[197] Surgical staging may be avoided in patients with FDG-avid primary tumors and absence of nodal uptake.

Molecular Staging

Despite favorable prognostic features, pelvic recurrence still occurs in about 10% of patients with early-stage cervical cancer. Histologically undetectable or dormant micrometastases in the lymphatic system probably account for disease recurrence after variable disease-free intervals. In a study using cytokeratin 19 transcription as a marker, 50% of patients with early-stage cervical cancer were shown to have occult micrometastases in the lymphatic system.[198] Furthermore, there was a quantitative association between the marker and poor clinicopathologic prognostic features, such as the stage, degree of differentiation, and the presence of lymphovascular invasion.[198]

As with other cancers, there are no methods yet to detect which patients with micrometastases will develop recurrence and how this will affect survival, because not all micrometastases will develop into distant tumors. Evidence from necropsy data and animal models suggests that only a very small fraction of micrometastases continue to grow to form tumors.[199-201] The issue of potential overstaging has been raised. Further studies are definitely needed before these considerations can have clinical application.

Summary

Techniques to screen and treat cervical cancer precursors have had a major impact on the prevention of cervical cancer in developed countries. Now the challenge is to expand this knowledge, in as economic a fashion as possible, to those resource-poor nations where cervical cancer is still a major cause of mortality and morbidity. This will require something more than transference of technology, because such countries are unlikely to be able to support screening as is currently conducted in developed nations.

With regard to established cancer, early and more precise diagnosis appears to be the immediate goal. A better understanding of where the cancer is and how it might behave is an essential prerequisite to a more rational application of multimodality therapies.

REFERENCES

1. Ferlay J, Parkin DM, Pisani P: GLOBOCAN: Cancer Incidence and Mortality Worldwide. IARC Cancer Base 3. Lyons, France, International Agency for Research on Cancer, 1998.
2. Parkin DM, Pisani P, Ferlay J: Estimates of the worldwide incidence of 25 major cancers in 1990. Int J Cancer 1999;80:827-841.
3. Sasieni P, Adams J: Effect of screening on cervical cancer mortality in England and Wales: Analysis of trends with an age period cohort model. BMJ 1999;318:1244-1245.
4. Quinn M, Babb P, Jones J, et al: Effect of screening on incidence of and mortality from cancer of cervix in England: Evaluation based on routinely collected statistics. BMJ 1999;318:904-908.
5. Anttila A, Pukkala E, Soderman B, et al: Effect of organised screening on cervical cancer incidence and mortality in Finland, 1963-1995: Recent increase in cervical cancer incidence. Int J Cancer 1999;83:59-65.
6. Aristizabal N, Cuello C, Correa P, et al: The impact of vaginal cytology on cervical cancer risks in Cali, Colombia. Int J Cancer 1984;34:5-9.
7. Clarke EA, Anderson TW: Does screening by "Pap" smears help prevent cervical cancer? A case-control study. Lancet 1979;2:1-4.
8. Wangsuphachart V, Thomas DB, Koetsawang A, et al: Risk factors for invasive cervical cancer and reduction of risk by "Pap" smears in Thai women. Int J Epidemiol 1987;16:362-366.
9. Zhang ZF, Parkin DM, Yu SZ, et al: Risk factors for cancer of the cervix in a rural Chinese population. Int J Cancer 1989; 43:762-767.
10. Miller AB: Evaluation of the impact of screening for cancer of the cervix. In Hakama M, Miller AB, Day NE (eds): Screening for Cancer of the Uterine Cervix. Lyons, France, International Agency for Research on Cancer, 1986, pp 149-160.
11. Christopherson WM, Lundin FE Jr, Mendez WM, et al: Cervical cancer control: A study of morbidity and mortality trends over a twenty-one-year period. Cancer 1976;38:1357-1366.
12. Boyes DA: The value of a Pap smear program and suggestions for its implementation. Cancer 1981;48(2 Suppl):613-621.
13. Miller AB, Lindsay J, Hill GB: Mortality from cancer of the uterus in Canada and its relationship to screening for cancer of the cervix. Int J Cancer 1976;17:602-612.
14. Johannesson G, Geirsson G, Day N: The effect of mass screening in Iceland, 1965-1974, on the incidence and mortality of cervical carcinoma. Int J Cancer 1978;21:418-425.
15. Geirsson G: Organization of screening in technically advanced countries: Iceland. In Hakama M, Miller AB, Day NE (eds): Screening for Cancer of the Uterine Cervix. Lyons, France, International Agency for Research on Cancer 1986, pp 239-250.
16. Vizcaino AP, Moreno V, Bosch FX, et al: International trends in incidence of cervical cancer. II. Squamous-cell carcinoma. Int J Cancer 2000;86:429-435.
17. Levi F, Lucchini F, Negri E, et al: Cervical cancer mortality in young women in Europe: Patterns and trends. Eur J Cancer 2000;36:2266-2271.
18. IRAC Working Group on Cervical Cancer Screening: Summary chapter. In Hakama M, Miller AB, Day NE (eds): Screening for Cancer of the Uterine Cervix. Lyons, France, International Agency for Research on Cancer, 1986, pp 133-142.
19. Laara E, Day NE, Hakama M: Trends in mortality from cervical cancer in the Nordic countries: Association with organised screening programmes. Lancet 1987;1:1247-1249.
20. IRAC Working Group on Evaluation of Cervical Cancer Screening Programmes: Screening for squamous cervical

cancer: The duration of low risk after negative result of cervical cytology and its implication for screening policies. BMJ 1986;293:659-664.

21. Hakama M, Louhivuori K: A screening programme for cervical cancer that worked. Cancer Surv 1988;7:403-416.

22. Sasieni PD, Cuzick J, Lynch-Farmery E: Estimating the efficacy of screening by auditing smear histories of women with and without cervical cancer. The National Co-ordinating Network for Cervical Screening Working Group. Br J Cancer 1996;73: 1001-1005.

23. Rodu B, Cole P: The fifty-year decline of cancer in America. J Clin Oncol 2001;19:239-241.

24. Hakama M, Chamberlain J, Day NE, et al: Evaluation of screening programmes for gynaecological cancer. Br J Cancer 1985;52: 669-673.

25. Miller AB, Chamberlain J, Day NE, et al: Report on a Workshop of the UICC Project on Evaluation of Screening for Cancer. Int J Cancer 1990;46:761-769.

26. Miller AB: Cervical cancer screening programmes: Managerial guidelines. Geneva: World Health Organization, 1992.

27. Sigurdsson K: The Icelandic and Nordic cervical screening programs: Trends in incidence and mortality rates through 1995. Acta Obstet Gynecol Scand 1999;78:478-485.

28. Ponten J, Adami HO, Bergstrom R, et al: Strategies for global control of cervical cancer. Int J Cancer 1995;60:1-26.

29. Linos A, Riza E: Comparisons of cervical cancer screening programmes in the European Union. Eur J Cancer 2000;36: 2260-2265.

30. Parkin DM, Nguyen-Dinh X, Day NE: The impact of screening on the incidence of cervical cancer in England and Wales. Br J Obstet Gynaecol 1985;92:150-157.

31. Patnick J: Has screening for cervical cancer been successful? Br J Obstet Gynaecol 1997;104:876-878.

32. Gibson L, Spiegelhalter DJ, Camilleri-Ferrante C, et al: Trends in invasive cervical cancer incidence in East Anglia from 1971 to 1993. J Med Screen 1997;4:44-48.

33. Luesley DM, Cullimore J, Redman CW, et al: Loop diathermy excision of the cervical transformation zone in patients with abnormal cervical smears. BMJ 1990;300:1690-1693.

34. Hammond RH, Edmonds DK: Does treatment for cervical intraepithelial neoplasia affect fertility and pregnancy? BMJ 1990;301:1344-1345.

35. Mandelblatt J, Gopaul I, Wistreich M: Gynecological care of elderly women: Another look at Papanicolaou smear testing. JAMA 1986;256:367-371.

36. Fletcher A: Screening for cancer of the cervix in elderly women. Lancet 1990;335:97-99.

37. Fahs MC, Mandelblatt J, Schechter C, et al: Cost effectiveness of cervical cancer screening for the elderly. Ann Intern Med 1992;117:520-527.

38. McDonald TW, Neutens JJ, Fischer LM, et al: Impact of cervical intraepithelial neoplasia diagnosis and treatment on self-esteem and body image. Gynecol Oncol 1989;34:345-349.

39. Marteau TM, Walker P, Giles J, et al: Anxieties in women undergoing colposcopy. Br J Obstet Gynaecol 1990;97:859-861.

40. Barsevick AM, Lauver D: Women's informational needs about colposcopy. Image J Nurs Sch 1990;22:23-26.

41. Bell S, Porter M, Kitchener H, et al: Psychological response to cervical screening. Prev Med 1995;24:610-616.

42. Fylan F: Screening for cervical cancer: A review of women's attitudes, knowledge, and behaviour. Br J Gen Pract 1998;48: 1509-1514.

43. Fahey MT, Irwig L, Macaskill P: Meta-analysis of Pap test accuracy. Am J Epidemiol 1995;141:680-689.

44. Macgregor JE, Campbell MK, Mann EM, et al: Screening for cervical intraepithelial neoplasia in north east Scotland shows fall in incidence and mortality from invasive cancer with concomitant rise in preinvasive disease. BMJ 1994;308:1407-1411.

45. Koss LG: Cytology: Accuracy of diagnosis. Cancer 1989; 64(1 Suppl):249-252.

46. Koss LG: Cervical (Pap) smear: New directions. Cancer 1993; 71(4 Suppl):1406-1412.

47. Reid R, Greenberg MD, Lorincz A, et al: Should cervical cytologic testing be augmented by cervicography or human papillomavirus deoxyribonucleic acid detection? Am J Obstet Gynecol 1991;164:1461-1471.

48. Slater DN, Milner PC, Radley H: Audit of deaths from cervical cancer: Proposal for an essential component of the National Screening Program. J Clin Pathol 1994;47:27-28.

49. Boyes DA, Morrison B, Knox EG, et al: A cohort study of cervical cancer screening in British Columbia. Clin Invest Med 1982; 5:1-29.

50. Liu S, Semenciw R, Probert A, et al: Cervical cancer in Canada: Changing patterns in incidence and mortality. Int J Gynecol Cancer 2001;11:24-31.

51. Vizcaino AP, Moreno V, Bosch FX, et al: International trends in the incidence of cervical cancer. I. Adenocarcinoma and adenosquamous cell carcinomas. Int J Cancer 1998;75:536-545.

52. Sigurdsson K: Quality assurance in cervical cancer screening: The Icelandic experience 1964-1993. Eur J Cancer 1995;31A: 728-734.

53. Mitchell H, Medley G, Gordon I, et al: Cervical cytology reported as negative and risk of adenocarcinoma of the cervix: No strong evidence of benefit. Br J Cancer 1995;71:894-897.

54. Solomon D, Davey D, Kurman R, et al: The Bethesda 2001 Workshop. The 2001 Bethesda System: Terminology for reporting results of cervical cytology. JAMA 2002;287: 2114-2119.

55. Sherman ME, Schiffman MH, Lorincz AT, et al: Toward objective quality assurance in cervical cytopathology: Correlation of cytopathologic diagnoses with detection of high-risk human papillomavirus types. Am J Clin Pathol 1994;102:182-187.

56. Manos MM, Kinney WK, Hurley LB, et al: Identifying women with cervical neoplasia: Using human papillomavirus DNA testing for equivocal Papanicolaou results. JAMA 1999;281: 1605-1610.

57. Joseph MG, Cragg F, Wright VC, et al: Cyto-histological correlates in a colposcopic clinic: A 1-year prospective study. Diagn Cytopathol 1991;7:477-481.

58. Boscha MC, Rietweld-Scheffers PEM, Boon ME: Characteristics of false negative smears in the normal screening population. Acta Cytol 1992;36:711-716.

59. Sherman ME, Kelly D: High-grade squamous intraepithelial lesions and invasive carcinoma following the report of three negative Papanicolaou smears: Screening failures or rapid progression? Mod Pathol 1992;5:337-342.

60. Lee KR, Ashfaq R, Birdsong GG, et al: Comparison of conventional Papanicolaou smears and a fluid-based, thin-layer system for cervical cancer screening. Obstet Gynecol 1997;90: 278-284.

61. Sherman ME, Mendoza M, Lee KR, et al: Performance of liquid-based, thin-layer cervical cytology: Correlation with reference diagnoses and human papillomavirus testing. Mod Pathol 1998;11:837-843.

62. Roberts JM, Gurley AM, Thurloe JK, et al: Evaluation of the ThinPrep Pap test as an adjunct to the conventional Pap smear. Med J Aust 1997;167:466-469.

63. Papillo JL, Zarka MA, St John TL: Evaluation of the ThinPrep Pap test in clinical practice: A seven-month, 16,314-case experience in northern Vermont. Acta Cytol 1998;42:203-208.

64. Bolick DR, Hellman DJ: Laboratory implementation and efficacy assessment of the ThinPrep cervical cancer screening system. Acta Cytol 1998;42:209-213.

65. Linder J, Zahniser D: ThinPrep Papanicolaou testing to reduce false-negative cervical cytology. Arch Pathol Lab Med 1998; 122:139-144.

66. Hutchinson ML, Zahniser DJ, Sherman ME, et al: Utility of liquid-based cytology for cervical carcinoma screening: Results of a population-based study conducted in a region of Costa Rica with a high incidence of cervical carcinoma. Cancer 1999;87: 48-55.

67. Myers ER, McCrory DC, Subramanian S, et al: Setting the target for a better cervical screening test: Characteristics of a cost-effective test for cervical neoplasia screening. Obstet Gynecol 2000;96: 645-652.

68. Wright TC Jr, Cox JT, Massad LS, et al: ASCCP-Sponsored Consensus Conference: 2001 Consensus Guidelines for the management of women with cervical cytological abnormalities. JAMA 2002;287:2120-2129.

69. Stoler MH: New Bethesda terminology and evidence-based management guidelines for cervical cytology findings. JAMA 2002;287:2140-2141.

70. Walboomers JM, Jacobs MV, Manos MM, et al: Human papillomavirus is a necessary cause of invasive cervical cancer worldwide. J Pathol 1999;189:12-19.
71. Giannoudis A, Herrington CS: Human papillomavirus variants and squamous neoplasia of the cervix. J Pathol 2001;193:295-302.
72. Bosch FX, Lorincz A, Munoz N, et al: The causal relation between human papillomavirus and cervical cancer. J Clin Pathol 2002;55:244-265.
73. Bosch FX, Manos MM, Munoz N, et al: Prevalence of human papillomavirus in cervical cancer: A worldwide perspective. International Biological Study on Cervical Cancer (IBSCC) Study Group. J Natl Cancer Inst 1995;87:796-802.
74. Rozendaal L, Walboomers JM, van der Linden JC, et al: PCR-based high-risk HPV test in cervical cancer screening gives objective risk assessment of women with cytomorphologically normal cervical smears. Int J Cancer 1996;68:766-769.
75. Remmink AJ, Walboomers JM, Helmerhorst TJ, et al: The presence of persistent high-risk HPV genotypes in dysplastic cervical lesions is associated with progressive disease: Natural history up to 36 months. Int J Cancer 1995;61:306-311.
76. Ho GY, Burk RD, Klein S, et al: Persistent genital human papillomavirus infection as a risk factor for persistent cervical dysplasia. J Natl Cancer Inst 1995;87:1365-1371.
77. Nobbenhuis MA, Walboomers JM, Helmerhorst TJ, et al: Relation of human papillomavirus status to cervical lesions and consequences for cervical-cancer screening: A prospective study. Lancet 1999;354:20-25.
78. Bosch FX, Rohan T, Schneider A, et al: Papillomavirus research update: Highlights of the Barcelona HPV 2000 International Papillomavirus Conference. J Clin Pathol 2001;54:163-175.
79. Ho GY, Bierman R, Beardsley L, et al: Natural history of cervicovaginal papillomavirus infection in young women. N Engl J Med 1998;338:423-428.
80. Koutsky LA, Holmes KK, Critchlow CW, et al: A cohort study of the risk of cervical intraepithelial neoplasia grade 2 or 3 in relation to papillomavirus infection. N Engl J Med 1992;327:1272-1278.
81. Zielinski GD, Snijders PJ, Rozendaal L, et al: HPV presence precedes abnormal cytology in women developing cervical cancer and signals false negative smears. Br J Cancer 2001;85:398-404.
82. Nobbenhuis MA, Helmerhorst TJ, van den Brule AJ, et al: Cytological regression and clearance of high-risk human papillomavirus in women with an abnormal cervical smear. Lancet 2001;358:1782-1783.
83. zur Hausen H: Papillomaviruses causing cancer: Evasion from host-cell control in early events in carcinogenesis. J Natl Cancer Inst 2000;92:690-698.
84. Schiffman MH, Kiviat NB, Burk RD, et al: Accuracy and interlaboratory reliability of human papillomavirus DNA testing by hybrid capture. J Clin Microbiol 1995;33:545-550.
85. Peyton CL, Schiffman M, Lorincz AT, et al: Comparison of PCR- and hybrid capture-based human papillomavirus detection systems using multiple cervical specimen collection strategies. J Clin Microbiol 1998;36:3248-3254.
86. Sasagawa T, Minemoto Y, Basha W, et al: A new PCR-based assay amplifies the E6-E7 genes of most mucosal human papillomaviruses (HPV). Virus Res 2000;67:127-139.
87. Bernard HU, Chan SY, Manos MM, et al: Identification and assessment of known and novel human papillomaviruses by polymerase chain reaction amplification, restriction fragment length polymorphisms, nucleotide sequence, and phylogenetic algorithms. J Infect Dis 1994;170:1077-1085.
88. Clavel C, Masure M, Bory JP, et al: Hybrid Capture II-based human papillomavirus detection, a sensitive test to detect in routine high-grade cervical lesions: A preliminary study on 1518 women. Br J Cancer 1999;80:1306-1311.
89. Schiffman M, Herrero R, Hildesheim A, et al: HPV DNA testing in cervical cancer screening: Results from women in a high-risk province of Costa Rica. JAMA 2000;283:87-93.
90. Wright TC Jr, Denny L, Kuhn L, et al: HPV DNA testing of self-collected vaginal samples compared with cytologic screening to detect cervical cancer. JAMA 2000;283:81-86.
91. Cuzick J, Sasieni P, Davies P, et al: A systematic review of the role of human papilloma virus (HPV) testing within a cervical screening programme: summary and conclusions. Br J Cancer 2000;83:561-565.
92. Cuzick J, Beverley E, Ho L, et al: HPV testing in primary screening of older women. Br J Cancer 1999;81:554-558.
93. Nindl I, Lorincz A, Mielzynska I, et al: Human papillomavirus detection in cervical intraepithelial neoplasia by the second-generation hybrid capture microplate test, comparing two different cervical specimen collection methods. Clin Diagn Virol 1998;10:49-56.
94. Ferris DG, Wright TC Jr, Litaker MS, et al: Comparison of two tests for detecting carcinogenic HPV in women with Papanicolaou smear reports of ASCUS and LSIL. J Fam Pract 1998;46:136-141.
95. Cuzick J: Human papillomavirus testing for primary cervical cancer screening. JAMA 2000;283:108-109.
96. Cox JT, Lorincz AT, Schiffman MH, et al: Human papillomavirus testing by hybrid capture appears to be useful in triaging women with a cytologic diagnosis of atypical squamous cells of undetermined significance. Am J Obstet Gynecol 1995;172:946-954.
97. Vassilakos P, de Marval F, Munoz M, et al: Human papillomavirus (HPV) DNA assay as an adjunct to liquid-based Pap test in the diagnostic triage of women with an abnormal Pap smear. Int J Gynaecol Obstet 1998;61:45-50.
98. Fait G, Daniel Y, Kupferminc MJ, et al: Does typing of human papillomavirus assist in the triage of women with repeated low-grade, cervical cytologic abnormalities? Gynecol Oncol 1998;70:319-322.
99. Ronnett BM, Manos MM, Ransley JE, et al: Atypical glandular cells of undetermined significance (AGUS): Cytopathologic features, histopathologic results, and human papillomavirus DNA detection. Hum Pathol 1999;30:816-825.
100. Solomon D, Schiffman M, Tarone R; ALTS Study group: Comparison of three management strategies for patients with atypical squamous cells of undetermined significance: Baseline results from a randomized trial. J Natl Cancer Inst 2001;93:293-299.
101. Shlay JC, Dunn T, Byers T, et al: Prediction of cervical intraepithelial neoplasia grade 2-3 using risk assessment and human papillomavirus testing in women with atypia on papanicolaou smears. Obstet Gynecol 2000;96:410-416.
102. Shah, Howley PM: Papillomavirus. In Fields BN, Knipe DM, Howley PM et al. (eds): Virology. Philadelphia, Lippincott-Raven, 1996, pp 2077-2109.
103. Megevand E, Denny L, Dehaeck K, et al: Acetic acid visualization of the cervix: An alternative to cytologic screening. Obstet Gynecol 1996;88:383-386.
104. Sankaranarayanan R, Wesley R, Somanathan T, et al: Visual inspection of the uterine cervix after the application of acetic acid in the detection of cervical carcinoma and its precursors. Cancer 1998;83:2150-2156.
105. Sankaranarayanan R, Shyamalakumary B, Wesley R, et al: Visual inspection with acetic acid in the early detection of cervical cancer and precursors. Int J Cancer 1999;80:161-163.
106. University of Zimbabwe/JHPIEGO Cervical Cancer Project: Visual inspection with acetic acid for cervical-cancer screening: Test qualities in a primary-care setting. Lancet 1999;353:869-873.
107. Denny L, Kuhn L, Pollack A, et al: Evaluation of alternative methods of cervical cancer screening for resource-poor settings. Cancer 2000;89:826-833.
108. Denny L, Kuhn L, Risi L, et al: Two-stage cervical cancer screening: An alternative for resource-poor settings. Am J Obstet Gynecol 2000;183:383-388.
109. Denny L, Kuhn L, Pollack A, et al: Direct visual inspection for cervical cancer screening: An analysis of factors influencing test performance. Cancer 2002;94:1699-1707.
110. Goldie SJ, Kuhn L, Denny L, et al: Policy analysis of cervical cancer screening strategies in low-resource settings: Clinical benefits and cost-effectiveness. JAMA 2001;285:3107-3115.
111. Suba EJ, Raab SS: Cervical cancer screening in developing countries. JAMA 2001;286:3079-3081.
112. Stafl A: Cervicography: A new method for cervical cancer detection. Am J Obstet Gynecol 1981;139:815-825.
113. Kesic VI, Soutter WP, Sulovic V, et al: A comparison of cytology and cervicography in cervical screening. Int J Gynecol Cancer 1993;3:395-398.

114. Ferris DG, Macfee MS, Miller JA, et al: The efficacy of telecolposcopy compared with traditional colposcopy. Obstet Gynecol 2002;99:248-254.

115. Harper DM, Moncur MM, Harper WH, et al: The technical performance and clinical feasibility of telecolposcopy. J Fam Pract 2000;49:623-627.

116. Maiman M, Fruchter RG, Clark M, et al: Cervical cancer as an AIDS-defining illness. Obstet Gynecol 1997;89:76-80.

117. Serraino D, Carrieri P, Pradier C, et al: Risk of invasive cervical cancer among women with, or at risk for, HIV infection. Int J Cancer 1999;82:334-337.

118. Maiman M, Fruchter RG, Serur E, et al: Human immunodeficiency virus infection and cervical neoplasia. Gynecol Oncol 1990;38:377-382.

119. Maiman M, Fruchter RG, Guy L, et al: Human immunodeficiency virus infection and invasive cervical carcinoma. Cancer 1993;71:402-406.

120. Boccalon M, Tirelli U, Sopracordevole F, et al: Intra-epithelial and invasive cervical neoplasia during HIV infection. Eur J Cancer 1996;32A:2212-2217.

121. Fruchter RG, Maiman M, Arrastia CD, et al: Is HIV infection a risk factor for advanced cervical cancer? J Acquir Immune Defic Syndr Hum Retrovirol 1998;18:241-245.

122. Schaafer A, Friedmann W, Mielke M, et al: The increased frequency of cervical dysplasia-neoplasia in women infected with the human immunodeficiency virus is related to the degree of immunosuppression. Am J Obstet Gynecol 1991;164:593-599.

123. Heard I, Jeannel D, Bergeron C, et al: Lack of behavioural risk factors for squamous intraepithelial lesions (SIL) in HIV-infected women. Int J STD AIDS 1997;8:388-392.

124. Maiman M, Fruchter RG, Sedlis A, et al: Prevalence, risk factors, and accuracy of cytologic screening for cervical intraepithelial neoplasia in women with the human immunodeficiency virus. Gynecol Oncol 1998;68:233-239.

125. Massad LS, Riester KA, Anastos KM, et al: Prevalence and predictors of squamous cell abnormalities in Papanicolaou smears from women infected with HIV-1. Women's Interagency HIV Study Group. J Acquir Immune Defic Syndr 1999;21:33-41.

126. Cappiello G, Garbuglia AR, Salvi R, et al: HIV infection increases the risk of squamous intra-epithelial lesions in women with HPV infection: An analysis of HPV genotypes. DIANAIDS Collaborative Study Group. Int J Cancer 1997;72:982-986.

127. Wright TC Jr, Koulos J, Schnoll F, et al: Cervical intraepithelial neoplasia in women infected with the human immunodeficiency virus: Outcome after loop electrosurgical excision. Gynecol Oncol 1994;55:253-258.

128. Holcomb K, Matthews RP, Chapman JE, et al: The efficacy of cervical conization in the treatment of cervical intraepithelial neoplasia in HIV-positive women. Gynecol Oncol 1999;74:428-431.

129. La Ruche G, Leroy V, Mensah-Ado I, et al: Short-term follow-up of cervical squamous intraepithelial lesions associated with HIV and human papillomavirus infections in Africa. Int J STD AIDS 1999;10:363-368.

130. Fruchter RG, Maiman M, Sillman FH, et al: Characteristics of cervical intraepithelial neoplasia in women infected with the human immunodeficiency virus. Am J Obstet Gynecol 1994;171:531-537.

131. Maiman M, Fruchter RG, Serur E, et al: Recurrent cervical intraepithelial neoplasia in human immunodeficiency virus-seropositive women. Obstet Gynecol 1993;82:170-174.

132. Ellerbrock TV, Chiasson MA, Bush TJ, et al: Incidence of cervical squamous intraepithelial lesions in HIV-infected women. JAMA 2000;283:1031-1037.

133. Maiman M, Fruchter RG, Sedlis A, et al: Prevalence, risk factors, and accuracy of cytologic screening for cervical intraepithelial neoplasia in women with the human immunodeficiency virus. Gynecol Oncol 1998;68:233-239.

134. Critchlow CW, Kiviat NB: Old and new issues in cervical cancer control. J Natl Cancer Inst 1999;91:200-201.

135. Spinillo A, Capuzzo E, Tenti P, et al: Adequacy of screening cervical cytology among human immunodeficiency virus-seropositive women. Gynecol Oncol 1998;69:109-113.

136. Wright TC Jr, Ellerbrock TV, Chiasson MA, et al: Cervical intraepithelial neoplasia in women infected with human immunodeficiency virus: Prevalence, risk factors, and validity of Papanicolaou smears. New York Cervical Disease Study. Obstet Gynecol 1994;84:591-597.

137. Holcomb K, Abulafia O, Matthews RP, et al: The significance of ASCUS cytology in HIV-positive women. Gynecol Oncol 1999;75:118-121.

138. Wright TC Jr, Moscarelli RD, Dole P, et al: Significance of mild cytologic atypia in women infected with human immunodeficiency virus. Obstet Gynecol 1996;87:515-519.

139. Del Priore G, Maag T, Bhattacharya M, et al: The value of cervical cytology in HIV-infected women. Gynecol Oncol 1995;56:395-398.

140. La Ruche G, Mensah-Ado I, Bergeron C, et al: Cervical screening in Africa: Discordant diagnosis in a double independent reading. DYSCER-CI Group. J Clin Epidemiol 1999;52:953-958.

141. Del Priore G, Gilmore PR, Maag T, et al: Colposcopic biopsies versus loop electrosurgical excision procedure cone histology in human immunodeficiency virus-positive women. J Reprod Med 1996;41:653-657.

142. Cuthill S, Maiman M, Fruchter RG, et al: Complications after treatment of cervical intraepithelial neoplasia in women infected with the human immunodeficiency virus. J Reprod Med 1995;40:823-828.

143. Centers for Disease Control and Prevention: Sexually transmitted disease guidelines. MMWR Morb Mortal Wkly Rep 1993;42(RR14):90-91.

144. Walker PG: CIN in pregnancy. In Luesley DM, Jordan J, Richart RM (eds): Intraepithelial neoplasia of the lower genital tract. New York, Churchill Livingstone, 1995, pp 221-229.

145. Singer A: Malignancy and premalignancy of the genital tract in pregnancy. In Turnbull A, Chamberlain G (eds): Obstetrics. Edinburgh, Churchill Livingstone, 1989, pp 657-672.

146. Huff BC: Abnormal cervical cytology in pregnancy: A laboratory and clinical dermatologic perspective. J Perinat Neonatal Nurs 2000;14:52-62.

147. Ueki M, Ueda M, Kumagai K, et al: Cervical cytology and conservative management of cervical neoplasias during pregnancy. Int J Gynecol Pathol 1995;14:63-69.

148. Chhieng DC, Elgert P, Cangiarella JF, et al: Significance of AGUS Pap smears in pregnant and postpartum women. Acta Cytol 2001;45:294-299.

149. Kaminski PF, Lyon DS, Sorosky JI, et al: Significance of atypical cervical cytology in pregnancy. Am J Perinatol 1992;9:340-343.

150. Connor JP: Noninvasive cervical cancer complicating pregnancy. Obstet Gynecol Clin North Am 1998;25:331-342.

151. Benedet JL, Selke PA, Nickerson KG: Colposcopic evaluation of abnormal Papanicolaou smears in pregnancy. Am J Obstet Gynecol 1987;157:932-937.

152. Palle C, Bangsboll S, Andreasson B: Cervical intraepithelial neoplasia in pregnancy. Acta Obstet Gynecol Scand 2000;79:306-310.

153. Economos K, Perez Veridiano N, Delke I, et al: Abnormal cervical cytology in pregnancy: A 17-year experience. Obstet Gynecol 1993;81:915-918.

154. Mitsuhashi A, Sekiya S: Loop electrosurgical excision procedure (LEEP) during first trimester of pregnancy. Int J Gynaecol Obstet 2000;71:237-239.

155. Richart RM, Barron BA: A follow-up study of patients with cervical dysplasia. Am J Obstet Gynecol 1969;105:386-393.

156. Ostor AG: Natural history of cervical intraepithelial neoplasia: A critical review. Int J Gynecol Pathol 1993;12:186-192.

157. Melnikow J, Nuovo J, Willan AR, et al: Natural history of cervical squamous intraepithelial lesions: a meta-analysis. Obstet Gynecol 1998;92:727-735.

158. Keijser KG, Kenemans P, van der Zanden PH, et al: Diathermy loop excision in the management of cervical intraepithelial neoplasia: Diagnosis and treatment in one procedure. Am J Obstet Gynecol 1992;166:1281-1287.

159. Bigrigg MA, Codling BW, Pearson P, et al: Colposcopic diagnosis and treatment of cervical dysplasia at a single clinic visit: Experience of low-voltage diathermy loop in 1000 patients. Lancet 1990;336:229-231.

160. Ferenczy A: Management of patients with high grade squamous intraepithelial lesions. Cancer 1995;76(10 Suppl):1928-1933.

161. Holschneider CH, Ghosh K, Montz FJ: See-and-treat in the management of high-grade squamous intraepithelial lesions of the cervix: A resource utilization analysis. Obstet Gynecol 1999;94:377-385.

162. Byrne P, Jordan J, Williams D, et al: Importance of negative result of cervical biopsy directed by colposcopy. BMJ 1988; 296:172.

163. Skehan M, Soutter WP, Lim K, et al: Reliability of colposcopy and directed punch biopsy. Br J Obstet Gynaecol 1990;97: 811-816.

164. Howe D: Colposcopically directed punch biopsy: A potentially misleading investigation. Br J Obstet Gynaecol 1992;99:862.

165. Howe DT, Vincenti AC: Is large loop excision of the transformation zone (LLETZ) more accurate than colposcopically directed punch biopsy in the diagnosis of cervical intraepithelial neoplasia? Br J Obstet Gynaecol 1991;98:588-591.

166. Hacker NF: Clinical and operative staging of cervical cancer. Baillieres Clin Obstet Gynaecol 1988;2:747-759.

167. Heaps JM, Berek JS: Surgical staging of cervical cancer. Clin Obstet Gynecol 1990;33:852-862.

168. Vidaurreta J, Bermudez A, di Paola G, et al: Laparoscopic staging in locally advanced cervical carcinoma: A new possible philosophy? Gynecol Oncol 1999;75:366-371.

169. Lagasse LD, Creasman WT, Shingleton HM, et al: Results and complications of operative staging in cervical cancer: Experience of the Gynecology Oncology Group. Gynecol Oncol 1980;9:90-98.

170. LaPolla JP, Schlaerth JB, Gaddis O, et al: The influence of surgical staging on the evaluation and treatment of patients with cervical carcinoma. Gynecol Oncol 1986;24:194-199.

171. Inoue T, Morita K: The prognostic significance of number of positive nodes in cervical carcinoma stages IB, IIA, and IIB. Cancer 1990;65:1923-1927.

172. Chung CK, Nahhas WA, Stryker JA, et al: Analysis of factors contributing to treatment failures in stages IB and IIA carcinoma of the cervix. Am J Obstet Gynecol 1980;138: 550-556.

173. Chen RJ, Chang DY, Yen ML, et al: Prognostic factors of primary adenocarcinoma of the uterine cervix. Gynecol Oncol 1998;69:157-164.

174. Lai CH, Hong JH, Hsueh S, et al: Preoperative prognostic variables and the impact of postoperative adjuvant therapy on the outcomes of stage IB or II cervical carcinoma patients with or without pelvic lymph node metastases: An analysis of 891 cases. Cancer 1999;85:1537-1546.

175. Ishikawa H, Nakanishi T, Inoue T, et al: Prognostic factors of adenocarcinoma of the uterine cervix. Gynecol Oncol 1999; 73:42-46.

176. Perez CA, Kurman RJ, Stehman FB, et al: Uterine cervix. In Hoskins WJ, Perez CA, Young RC (eds): Principles and Practice of Gynecologic Oncology. Philadelphia, JB Lippincott, 1992, pp 591-662.

177. Dargent DF: Laparoscopic surgery and gynecologic cancer. Curr Opin Obstet Gynecol 1993;5:294-300.

178. Dargent DF: Laparoscopic surgery in gynecologic oncology. Surg Clin North Am 2001;81:949-964.

179. Chu KK, Chang SD, Chen FP, et al: Laparoscopic surgical staging in cervical cancer: Preliminary experience among Chinese. Gynecol Oncol 1997;64:49-53.

180. Childers JM, Hatch K, Surwit EA: The role of laparoscopic lymphadenectomy in the management of cervical carcinoma. Gynecol Oncol 1992;47:38-43.

181. Spirtos NM, Schlaerth JB, Spirtos TW, et al: Laparoscopic bilateral pelvic and paraaortic lymph node sampling: An evolving technique. Am J Obstet Gynecol 1995;173:105-111.

182. Possover M, Krause N, Kuhne-Heid R, et al: Value of laparoscopic evaluation of paraaortic and pelvic lymph nodes for treatment of cervical cancer. Am J Obstet Gynecol 1998;178: 806-810.

183. Cosin JA, Fowler JM, Chen MD, et al: Pretreatment surgical staging of patients with cervical carcinoma: The case for lymph node debulking. Cancer 1998;82:2241-2248.

184. Kinney WK, Hodge DO, Egorshin EV, et al: Surgical treatment of patients with stages IB and IIA carcinoma of the cervix and palpably positive pelvic lymph nodes. Gynecol Oncol 1995; 57:145-149.

185. Fine BA, Hempling RE, Piver MS, et al: Severe radiation morbidity in carcinoma of the cervix: Impact of pretherapy surgical staging and previous surgery. Int J Radiat Oncol Biol Phys 1995;31:717-723.

186. Hacker NF, Wain GV, Nicklin JL: Resection of bulky positive lymph nodes in patients with cervical carcinoma. Int J Gynecol Cancer 1995;5:250-256.

187. Goff BA, Muntz HG, Paley PJ, et al: Impact of surgical staging in women with locally advanced cervical cancer. Gynecol Oncol 1999;74:436-442.

188. Hasenburg A, Salama JK, Van TJ, et al: Evaluation of patients after extraperitoneal lymph node dissection and subsequent radiotherapy for cervical cancer. Gynecol Oncol 2002;84: 321-326.

189. Vercamer R, Janssens J, Usewils R, et al: Computed tomography and lymphography in the presurgical staging of early carcinoma of the uterine cervix. Cancer 1987;60: 1745-1750.

190. van Engelshoven JM, Versteege CW, Ruys JH, et al: Computed tomography in staging untreated patients with cervical cancer. Gynecol Obstet Invest 1984;18:289-295.

191. Whitley NO, Brenner DE, Francis A, et al: Computed tomographic evaluation of carcinoma of the cervix. Radiology 1982; 142:439-446.

192. Togashi K, Nishimura K, Sagoh T, et al: Carcinoma of the cervix: Staging with MR imaging. Radiology 1989;171: 245-251.

193. Grigsby PW, Siegel BA, Dehdashti F: Lymph node staging by positron emission tomography in patients with carcinoma of the cervix. J Clin Oncol 2001;19:3745-3749.

194. Kerr IG, Manji MF, Powe J, et al: Positron emission tomography for the evaluation of metastases in patients with carcinoma of the cervix: A retrospective review. Gynecol Oncol 2001;81: 477-480.

195. Narayan K, Hicks RJ, Jobling T, et al: A comparison of MRI and PET scanning in surgically staged loco-regionally advanced cervical cancer: Potential impact on treatment. Int J Gynecol Cancer 2001;11:263-271.

196. Reinhardt MJ, Ehritt-Braun C, Vogelgesang D, et al: Metastatic lymph nodes in patients with cervical cancer: Detection with MR imaging and FDG PET. Radiology 2001;218:776-782.

197. Rose PG, Adler LP, Rodriguez M, et al: Positron emission tomography for evaluating para-aortic nodal metastasis in locally advanced cervical cancer before surgical staging: A surgicopathologic study. J Clin Oncol 1999;17:41-45.

198. Van Trappen PO, Gyselman VG, Lowe DG, et al: Molecular quantification and mapping of lymph-node micrometastases in cervical cancer. Lancet 2001;357:15-20.

199. Holmgren L, O'Reilly MS, Folkman J: Dormancy of micrometastases: balanced proliferation and apoptosis in the presence of angiogenesis suppression. Nat Med 1995;1:149-153.

200. Luzzi KJ, MacDonald IC, Schmidt EE, et al: Multistep nature of metastatic inefficiency: Dormancy of solitary cells after successful extravasation and limited survival of early micrometastases. Am J Pathol 1998;153:865-873.

201. Cifuentes N, Pickren JW: Metastases from carcinoma of mammary gland: An autopsy study. J Surg Oncol 1979;11: 193-205.

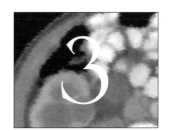

C H A P T E R

PATHOLOGY OF VULVAR, VAGINAL, AND CERVICAL CANCERS

Anais Malpica,   Michael T. Deavers,   and   Andrew G. Ostor

 MAJOR CONTROVERSIES

- **What is the current status of vulvar non-neoplastic epithelial disorders?**
- **Which are the prognostic factors for invasive carcinoma of the vulva?**
- **Is verrucous carcinoma indeed a clinicopathologic entity?**
- **In primary cutaneous vulvar Paget's disease, should the margins be examined by frozen section?**
- **Is the histologic classification of a cervical tumor important for prognosis?**
- **Is immunohistochemical staining helpful in the diagnosis of cervical cancer and for distinguishing among various types of cervical carcinoma?**
- **What are the important histopathologic features for prognosis of cervical cancer?**

VULVAR CANCER

This section presents an updated review of a selected group of disorders of the vulva, including vulvar non-neoplastic epithelial disorders, vulvar intraepithelial neoplasia (VIN), the prognostic factors of invasive carcinoma, verrucous carcinoma, carcinoma of the Bartholin gland, Paget's disease, and atypical melanocytic nevus of the genital region.

What is the current status of vulvar non-neoplastic epithelial disorders?

The current terminology for non-neoplastic epithelial disorders of the vulva was proposed in 1989 by the Nomenclature Committee for the International Society of Gynecological Pathologists.[1] This terminology includes lichen sclerosus, squamous cell hyperplasia (not otherwise specified), and other dermatoses. With

the use of this standardized nomenclature, a plethora of confusing names that had been used in the past, such as vulvar dystrophy, kraurosis, leukoplakia, leukoplakic vulvitis, primary atrophy, sclerotic dermatitis, atrophic vulvitis, and hypertrophic vulvitis, was supposed to disappear. On the other hand, recognition of the clinical and pathologic features of specific dermatoses (e.g., psoriasis, lichen planus, lichen simplex chronicus, spongiotic dermatitis) was considered necessary. At the present time, much work still must be done regarding the abandonment of the above-mentioned obsolete terms and the proper recognition of vulvar dermatoses that are more commonly seen in extragenital sites (Fig. 3-1).

One problem in this area has been the definition of the exact role of lichen sclerosus and squamous hyperplasia in the genesis of invasive squamous cell carcinoma (SCC) of the vulva. Although lichen sclerosus and squamous hyperplasia traditionally have been considered to be of a non-neoplastic nature, more recent studies have found a frequent association between human papillomavirus (HPV)–negative invasive SCC

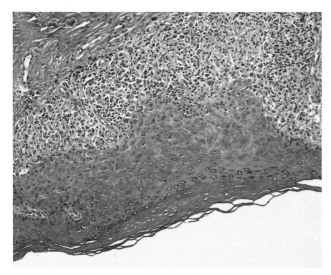

Figure 3–1. Lichen planus, an example of a dermatosis that can be seen in the vulva. See also Color Figures 3-1.

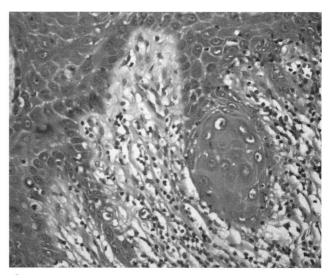

Figure 3–2. Vulvar intraepithelial neoplasia: simplex or differentiated type. See also Color Figure 3-2.

of the vulva in elderly patients and squamous hyperplasia or lichen sclerosus in the adjacent skin.[2-7] Monoclonality and allelic imbalance, which could indicate a neoplastic nature, have been found in some studies of vulvar squamous hyperplasia.[8-10] However, polyclonality and an absence of p53 mutation have also been reported.[11] These controversial results appear to indicate that squamous hyperplasia is unlikely to be a direct precursor of invasive vulvar SCC, but this disorder could be a step in the carcinogenesis sequence in which additional "critical events" must occur.[8]

The association between lichen sclerosus and vulvar invasive SCC has been known for many years. In resected specimens, the incidence of lichen sclerosus in the skin adjacent to invasive SCC has been reported to range from 25% to 61%.[12,13] The exact risk of developing SCC in diagnosed and treated vulvar lichen sclerosus is not known.[14] However, it has been mentioned in the literature that up to 5% of patients with vulvar lichen sclerosus develop carcinoma after long-term follow-up.[15] In one study, it was calculated that women with lichen sclerosus had a relative risk of 246.6% for vulvar carcinoma.[16] As with squamous hyperplasia, some cases of lichen sclerosus have been found to show monoclonality, increased p53 expression, allelic imbalance, and aneuploidy.[8,10,17,18] So far, although the clinicopathologic evidence of an association between lichen sclerosus and vulvar SCC is strong, definitive proof of causation is lacking.[19] As with squamous hyperplasia, it has been proposed that lichen sclerosus could represent a step in the carcinogenesis sequence in which "critical events" must occur.[8,19]

Vulvar intraepithelial neoplasia: a current overview

The VIN nomenclature adopted by the International Society for the Study of Vulvar Disease in 1986[20] and subsequently included in the World Health Organization's classification of female genital tract tumors[21] grades squamous intraepithelial lesions of the vulva according to the level of involvement of the affected epithelium by atypical keratinocytes. In VIN I (mild dysplasia), the lowest third of the epithelium is involved; in VIN II (moderate dysplasia), the lower two thirds of the epithelium is involved; and, in VIN III (severe dysplasia/squamous carcinoma in situ), more than two thirds of the epithelium is involved. This grading system based on the level of epithelial involvement by atypical keratinocytes has also included within the VIN III category a lesion designated as differentiated or simplex VIN III (Fig. 3-2), which is an intraepithelial lesion with the features of a grade 1 SCC confined to the lower portion of the epithelium. The other two types of VIN III, known as basaloid (Fig. 3-3) and warty or condylomatous (Fig. 3-4), indeed show atypical keratinocytes in disarray in more than

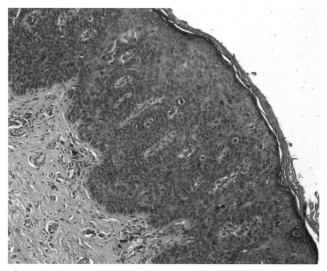

Figure 3–3. Vulvar intraepithelial neoplasia: VIN III, basaloid or undifferentiated type. See also Color Figure 3-3.

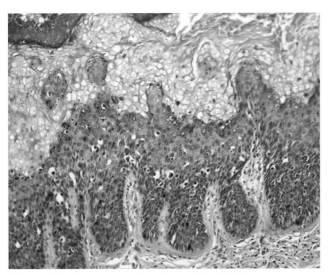

Figure 3–4. Vulvar intraepithelial neoplasia: VIN III, warty or condylomatous type. See also Color Figure 3-4.

two thirds of the epithelium. With the VIN nomenclature, Bowenoid papulosis, Bowenoid dysplasia, Bowen's disease, erythroplakia of Queyrat, simplex carcinoma in situ, and atypia disappear as diagnostic terms.[22,23]

During the last decade it has become increasingly clear that there are two different types of VIN with unique etiologic, pathogenetic, and clinical features.[22] One form, classic VIN, is associated with HPV infection, and the other, differentiated or simplex VIN, is not associated with viral infection. The HPV-associated type of VIN is more common and has been better studied. It occurs predominantly, but not exclusively, in relatively young women, usually in their 30s and 40s. Cigarette smoking has been reported in approximately 60% to 80% of the cases.[22] Condylomata, a history of herpes genitalis, and human immunodeficiency virus (HIV) infection are common in these patients.[22] From the clinical standpoint, classic VIN often produces bulky, whitish, or erythematous plaques. Sometimes it produces pigmented lesions. In more than 40% of the cases, there is multifocal involvement of the vulva. Multicentric intraepithelial or invasive squamous neoplasms of the cervix or vagina have been reported to occur in 18% to 52% of the patients.[22] Classic VIN has been further classified as warty (condylomatous) or basaloid (undifferentiated) by some authors.[24,25] The warty subtype is characterized by a spiked surface, marked cellular pleomorphism, and prominent koilocytes.[24,25] The basaloid subtype has a relatively flat surface and shows replacement of the epithelium by homogeneous small, "undifferentiated" keratinocytes with scanty cytoplasm. Koilocytes may be present but are fewer in number than in the warty subtype.[24,25] The two patterns can coexist in the same lesion, and both subtypes share clinical features and HPV genotypes.[24,25] Because this further classification of the classic VIN adds no significant information from the clinical standpoint, it is not customarily included in pathology reports.

Differentiated or simplex VIN III accounts for 2% to 10% of cases and is typically seen in postmenopausal women.[26,27] Cigarette smoking is seen in approximately 25% of the patients. Multicentric squamous neoplasia involving the cervix and vagina is infrequent, and the vulvar involvement can be multifocal.[26,27] From the clinical standpoint, simplex VIN tend to produce less bulky lesions than does classic VIN. The vulvar lesions usually appear as an ill-defined plaque or as focal, gray-white discoloration with an irregular surface. Histologically, simplex VIN is subtle and can be very difficult to recognize. It can easily be mistaken for acanthosis or squamous hyperplasia.[22] VIN of the simplex type is characterized by a thickened epithelium with a tendency to have elongated and branched rete ridges. Parakeratosis is usually present. There is no significant atypia above the basal or parabasal layers, but large eosinophilic keratinocytes with abnormal vesicular nuclei and prominent intercellular bridges are present mostly in the lower portion of epidermis.[27] Keratin pearls within the rete ridges may be seen. In difficult cases, immunostaining for p53 is helpful. In cases of simplex VIN III, p53 staining of the nuclei of more than 90% of the cells in the lower third of epithelium is seen in two thirds of the cases. In addition, p53-positive cells also extend into higher levels of the epithelium.[27]

The recognition of these two types of VIN, classic and simplex, is important because their behaviors differ significantly. In the classic VIN, the clinical behavior is variable. Local recurrence or persistence has been reported in approximately 7% to 32% of patients who receive surgical treatment ranging from local excision to vulvectomy.[26,28-36] Occult areas of invasive carcinoma have been reported in 6% to 7% of the patients in some studies.[32,36] However, another study showed the presence of occult invasive carcinoma in up to 20% of the patients for whom the resected vulvar skin was submitted in toto.[34] About 3% to 10% of the patients with classic VIN who are treated develop invasive SCC of the vulva later on.[28,29,37] In some patients, VIN III lesions of the classic type that were treated only with biopsy spontaneously regressed.[30,38] At the present time it is not possible to predict the behavior of an individual lesion. Patients at greater risk for progression to invasive SCC appear to be those who are older than 40 years of age or have an immunocompromised status.[22] Young women, especially those with multiple, small, papular, pigmented lesions, may undergo spontaneous regression.[39]

Simplex VIN appears to have a greater potential for progression into invasive SCC than does classic VIN. In one study of VIN III of the simplex type, it was found that 58% of the cases had a prior, synchronous, or subsequent invasive squamous carcinoma.[27]

Which are the prognostic factors for invasive carcinoma of the vulva?

The International Federation of Gynecologists and Obstetricians (FIGO) uses surgical-pathologic staging for vulvar cancer. This staging classification is based on tumor size and adjacent spread, lymph node involvement, and the presence of any distant metastasis.[40] So far, stage is the only significant prognostic factor on multiple regression analysis. Other factors such as tumor diameter, tumor thickness, tumor differentiation, the presence of vascular space invasion, and pattern of tumor growth appear to be prognostic indicators on univariate analysis only.[41]

The application of ancillary techniques such as determination of HPV status, DNA ploidy, morphometric analysis, p53 protein expression, and Ki-67 immunostaining has yielded inconsistent and inconclusive results.[5,41-55] Therefore, none of these techniques is currently being used as a prognostic indicator.

Is verrucous carcinoma indeed a clinicopathologic entity?

Verrucous carcinoma is a highly differentiated, invasive SCC that has a hyperkeratinized, undulating, warty surface; bland cytologic features; and invasion of the underlying stroma as bulbous pegs with a pushing border (Fig. 3-5).[56] The cardinal features that differentiate this type of tumor from a conventional squamous cell carcinoma are the absence of nuclear pleomorphism and the absence of an irregular pattern of infiltration. Giant condyloma of Buschke and Lowenstein is considered to be a synonym for verrucous carcinoma,[56] but the term is confusing and therefore is not recommended.

Verrucous carcinoma accounts for 1% to 2% of all vulvar cancers. This type of tumor is seen primarily in postmenopausal patients. It may invade local structures, has a tendency to recur locally, and has little or no metastatic potential.[56-58] Lymph node metastasis is extremely rare, and its presence should prompt reevaluation of the vulvar tumor for areas of conventional,

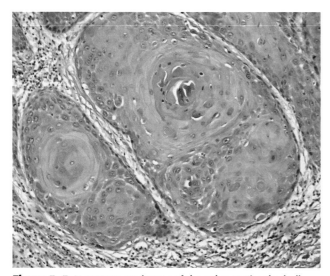

Figure 3–5. Verrucous carcinoma of the vulva. Notice the bulbous pegs and absence of significant atypia. See also Color Figure 3-5.

invasive SCC, which may rarely arise in an otherwise typical verrucous carcinoma (hybrid verrucous carcinoma/invasive SCC).

Verrucous carcinoma has been reported to be associated with HPV, typically HPV-6 or a variant of HPV-6.[59-63] However, a recent study failed to prove this association.[56] Based on current information, it can be stated that verrucous carcinoma does represent a distinct clinicopathologic entity. If the diagnostic features of verrucous carcinoma are seen in a vulvar tumor that has been adequately sampled, local excision without further treatment is still the most adequate therapy.[56]

Vulvar Paget's disease: the proposal of a new classification

Vulvar Paget's disease has most commonly been defined as a carcinoma composed of glandular cells, usually confined to the epithelium, but accompanied by invasive adenocarcinoma in 10% to 20% of the cases.[21]

However, Williamson and Brown[63] presented evidence that vulvar Paget's disease, although it has been considered a single entity,[21] indeed represents a heterogeneous group of epithelial neoplasms. They proposed a new classification, which divides Paget's disease into three major types based on the origin of the neoplastic cells. This new classification is summarized as follows:

Type 1: Primary vulvar cutaneous Paget's disease
Type 2: Paget's disease as a manifestation of an associated adjacent primary, anal, rectal, or other noncutaneous adenocarcinoma
Type 3: Paget's disease as a bladder (urothelial) neoplasia

Type 1 (primary vulvar cutaneous Paget's disease) is further classified as follows. (1) Type 1a Paget's disease (primary vulvar intraepithelial Paget's disease) is characterized by an intraepithelial proliferation of neoplastic glandular cells and could be considered an adenocarcinoma in situ (Fig. 3-6). (2) Type 1b Paget's disease (primary vulvar intraepithelial Paget's disease with invasion) is characterized by the presence of dermal invasion by intraepithelial Paget's cells which can occur in up to 12% of the cases.[64] This type could be considered an intraepithelial neoplasia that became invasive. (3) Type 1c Paget's disease (vulvar Paget's disease presenting as a manifestation of a primary underlying adenocarcinoma of the vulva) is characterized by the additional presence of a primary vulvar adenocarcinoma that is seen in approximately 10% to 20% of the cases.[21] This underlying adenocarcinoma could originate as an adenocarcinoma of the Bartholin gland, a specialized anogenital gland, or other vulvar glandular structures.

Paget's disease as a manifestation of an associated adjacent noncutaneous adenocarcinoma (type 2 Paget's disease) includes Paget's disease associated

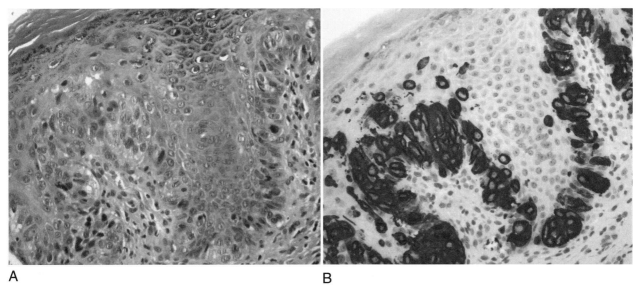

A   B

Figure 3–6. A, Primary vulvar intraepithelial Paget's disease (hematoxylin-eosin stain). **B,** Cytokeratin 7 enhances the neoplastic cells. See also Color Figure 3-6.

with an in situ, invasive rectal, or colonic adenocarcinoma or a cervical adenocarcinoma. Primary perianal Paget's disease with involvement of the vulva is also included in this group.[63]

Paget's disease as a manifestation of bladder (urothelial) neoplasia (type 3 Paget's disease, pagetoid urothelial neoplasia) is a specific type of Paget's disease that characteristically involves the vulvar vestibule, including the periurethral area.

Immunohistochemically, it has been found that primary vulvar Paget's disease (type 1) is immunoreactive for cytokeratin 7 and GCDFP-15 (gross cystic disease fluid protein 15) and, uncommonly, for cytokeratin 20. In contrast, vulvar Paget's disease secondary to anorectal carcinoma is immunoreactive for cytokeratin 20 and consistently negative for GCDFP-15. In cases of vulvar Paget's disease secondary to urothelial carcinoma, the neoplastic cells are positive for cytokeratin 7, cytokeratin 20, and uroplakin III and negative for GCDFP-15.[65]

The differentiation of these three types of vulvar Paget's disease is of utmost importance, because the specific diagnosis has a significant influence on the treatment to be provided.

In primary cutaneous vulvar Paget's disease, should the margins be examined by frozen section?

A careful topographic study by Gunn and Gallager[66] demonstrated that in vulvar Paget's disease the histologically involved area is much greater than the visible lesion. In addition, multicentric foci can occur in grossly normal epithelium.[66] Therefore, even though the frozen section evaluation can render margins free of Paget's disease, there is still a possibility of microscopic residual disease. Frozen section evaluation of grossly normal epithelial margins adjacent to primary

cutaneous vulvar Paget's disease has not been demonstrated either to improve survival or to reduce recurrences.[67-69]

Bartholin gland carcinoma: a tumor with strict diagnostic criteria

For the diagnosis of Bartholin gland carcinoma, the following criteria must be met: (1) the tumor must arise at the site of the gland, (2) it must have a microscopic appearance consistent with Bartholin gland origin, and (3) it must not be metastatic from another site.[21]

The histologic types most commonly seen are adenocarcinomas and SCCs, accounting for 40% of the cases each. Adenoid cystic carcinomas (Fig. 3-7), similar to those occurring in the salivary glands, the

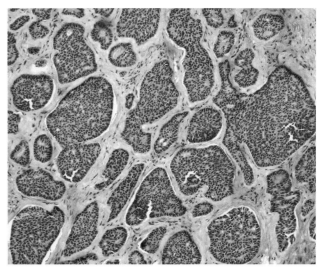

Figure 3–7. Adenoid cystic carcinoma of the Bartholin gland. See also Color Figure 3-7.

upper respiratory tract, and the skin, account for 15% of the cases. Occasionally, adenosquamous carcinomas and transitional cell carcinomas are seen. Each of these account for fewer than 5% of the cases.[21]

Melanocytic lesions of the vulva in young patients: a diagnostic challenge

A known pitfall in pathology is to render an incorrect diagnosis of malignant melanoma on an ill-defined group of melanocytic lesions that occur in the genital area, especially on the vulva of women at the mean age of 23 years. These lesions constitute a distinctive clinicopathologic entity designated atypical melanocytic nevi of the genital type. In a series of 56 such cases, the diagnosis of melanoma was either made or seriously considered in more than one third of the cases.[70]

Atypical melanocytic nevi of the genital type occur in children, adolescents, and women in their 20s. In general, the lesions are asymptomatic and are discovered incidentally during routine clinical examination or self-examination, frequently during pregnancy. Grossly, they can be elevated, in general with a mushroom appearance, or flat. The elevated lesions occur more frequently on the labia majora or the perineum; the flat lesions are usually on the labia minora or periclitoris. Some of the lesions can have black areas and therefore can be clinically worrisome. Unlike dysplastic nevi, atypical melanocytic nevi of the genital type are not typically associated with the presence of dysplastic nevi at other sites.

Histologically, the hallmark of this entity is a proliferation of melanocytes that obscures the dermal-epidermal interface. This proliferation can be continuous or discontinuous with an underlying prominent dermal nevus (seen in up to 50% of the cases). The melanocytic proliferation in the dermal-epidermal interface can be seen in three patterns: nests of melanocytes located immediately beneath the epidermis, intraepidermal nests of poorly cohesive melanocytes, or a continuum of melanocytes crowded across and along the dermal-epidermal interface.[70] Atypia of the melanocytes may be prominent and can raise the possibility of malignant melanoma or dysplastic nevi. The stroma tends to be nondescript.

Dysplastic nevi occur mostly in young women of reproductive age. These lesions are mostly seen in the labia majora and are likely to be associated with dysplastic nevi elsewhere on the skin. Histologically, the nevi can be compound or junctional. The melanocytic nests are within the epidermis, are not numerous, are of variable size, and tend to be in the basal region of the epidermis. Extension of atypical melanocytes into the dermis is not a prominent feature; when it does occur, the cells are arranged as small nests or as single cells. The dermal nests in dysplastic nevi are smaller than the ones seen in atypical melanocytic nevi of the genital area and may or may not show maturation. Another important finding in differentiating these two lesions is the presence of concentric eosinophilic fibroplasia or lamellar fibroplasia in dysplastic nevi.[70]

VAGINAL CANCER

This section reviews the vaginal glandular disorders associated with intrauterine exposure to the diethylstilbestrol, metastatic versus primary carcinomas of the vagina, and vaginal rhabdomyosarcoma.

Vaginal glandular disorders associated with intrauterine exposure to diethylstilbestrol: an update

Diethylstilbestrol (DES), a drug first synthesized in 1938, was administered over a period of three decades to millions of pregnant women throughout the United States and Europe to prevent spontaneous abortion and premature delivery.[71] In 1971, Herbst and colleagues[72] reported a strong association between DES use in pregnancy and the occurrence of vaginal clear cell adenocarcinoma in exposed female offspring. In addition to this finding, it is known that the presence of glandular tissue in the vagina (adenosis) and the metaplastic squamous epithelium associated with adenosis (vaginal epithelial changes) (Fig. 3-8) are also common in DES-exposed females. These changes are seen in up to 34% of these patients.

Adenosis with or without vaginal epithelial changes, more frequently involves the upper third of the vagina and the anterior wall. These changes extend into the middle third of the vagina in 9% and the lower third in 2% of DES-exposed women. Among women with no history of DES exposure, adenosis of the adult type is rare, but when present is similar to the adenosis seen in DES-exposed women.

Two adult (differentiated) forms of adenosis have been described: mucinous, characterized by cells similar to the normal endocervical epithelium, and tuboendometrial, characterized by the presence of cells that resemble endometrial or fallopian tube epithelium. The mucinous type is the more frequently seen; it involves the surface of the vagina and the lamina propria.

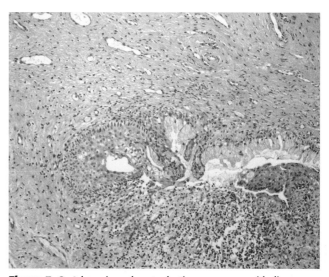

Figure 3–8. Adenosis and metaplastic squamous epithelium. See also Color Figure 3-8.

In contrast, the tuboendometrial type is found in the lamina propria but not on the surface of the vagina.[73] There is also an embryonic (fetal) form of adenosis. This type is the one found in up to 15% of fetuses and stillbirths and sometimes in the vagina of adult women, regardless of the history of DES exposure.[73]

Atypical adenosis characterized by nuclear stratification, nuclear pleomorphism, hyperchromatic nuclei, and prominent nucleoli has been found at the periphery of most clear cell carcinomas.[73]

Clear cell adenocarcinomas of the vagina and cervix are the only tumors associated with DES-exposure. The median age at the time of diagnosis in the DES-exposed U. S. population is 19 years. Clear cell adenocarcinoma develops in approximately 0.014% to 0.14% of exposed girls and women up to the age of 24 years. Approximately 60% of the tumors have been confined to the vagina. In most cases, the tumor involves the upper third and the anterior wall of the vagina. It can range from microscopic size to large. Histologically, this tumor is identical to the clear cell adenocarcinoma of the ovary and endometrium. It is characterized by the presence of clear cells arranged in a combination of architectural patterns including solid, tubulocystic, and papillary (Fig. 3-9). Sometimes there are hobnail cells or flat cells. The latter can appear innocuous, and when this type of epithelium is the only one present in a small sample of tissue, it may be difficult to render a diagnosis of carcinoma.[74]

Carcinoma in the vagina: metastatic tumor must be ruled out

Only 10% to 20% of vaginal malignancies are classified as primary tumors of the vagina.[74] Of the primary vaginal tumors, the most frequently seen is SCC, accounting for 80% of the cases. The criteria to consider a vaginal tumor as primary are strict and include the following: the neoplasm must be located in the vagina without clinical or histologic involvement of the cervix or vulva, and there should not be a history of a previously treated cervical cancer within the 5 years before the detection of the vaginal tumor. Invasive vaginal SCC is a disease of postmenopausal patients with a mean age of 64 years. Most of the tumors involve the upper third and the posterior wall of the vagina.[74]

Adenocarcinomas of the non–clear cell type are rare, and a metastatic origin from the endometrium, endocervix, or intestine should be excluded.

Embryonal rhabdomyosarcoma: the most common vaginal sarcoma

Embryonal rhabdomyosarcoma is the most common vaginal sarcoma. It occurs in children and infants, ranging in age from birth to 41 years (mean age 2 years)[74] This tumor usually arises in the anterior wall of the vagina and appears as papillae, nodules, or polypoid masses with an intact or ulcerated mucosa.[74] Microscopically, the tumor has a loose, myxoid, or edematous stroma. The neoplastic cells have round, oval, or spindle-shaped nuclei and eosinophilic cytoplasm and may show differentiation toward striated muscle cells. Typically, a cambium layer composed of densely packed cells with small hyperchromatic nuclei is located underneath squamous epithelium (Fig. 3-10). Rhabdomyoblasts (strap cells) can be sparse. Their recognition is facilitated by immunohistochemical staining with antibodies against desmin or myoglobin.[74] This tumor has a relatively favorable outcome, with a 90% or greater survival rate.[74]

CERVICAL CANCER

This section presents a review of the various histologic types of malignant tumors of the uterine cervix, the role of immunohistochemical staining in the study of these neoplasms, and the histopathologic features of importance from a prognostic standpoint.

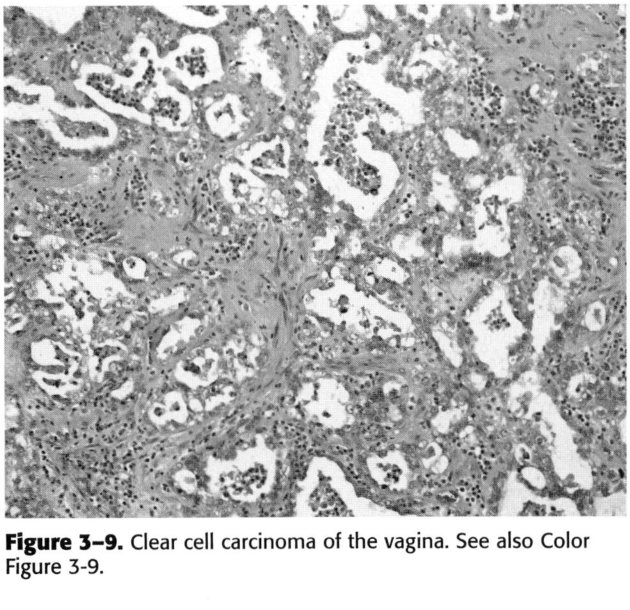

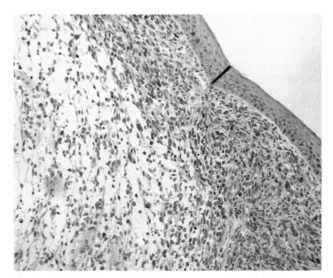

Figure 3–9. Clear cell carcinoma of the vagina. See also Color Figure 3-9.

Figure 3–10. Embryonal rhabdomyosarcoma. See also Color Figure 3-10.

Is the histologic classification of a cervical tumor important for prognosis?

Stage is the single most important prognostic factor in cervical tumors. However, there is a wide variation in survival rates within each stage, and histologic classification accounts for some of these differences. The World Health Organization classification of cervical tumors includes squamous carcinoma, adenocarcinoma, other epithelial tumors, mesenchymal tumors, mixed epithelial and mesenchymal tumors, and other miscellaneous tumors (Table 3-1). SCC, although varying in frequency from one population to another, is the most common cervical tumor and accounts for approximately 75% of all cases. Adenocarcinomas make up approximately 15% of the cases, and other histologic types account for the remainder.[75]

Squamous cell carcinoma. Because SCCs comprise the majority of cervical malignancies, the survival of patients with these tumors is the reference against which others groups are compared. In an analysis of cases from the National Cancer Institute's Surveillance, Epidemiology, and End Results program (SEER), the

Table 3–1. World Health Organization Classification of Cervical Malignancies

Squamous cell carcinoma
  Verrucous
  Warty (condylomatous)
  Papillary
  Lymphoepithelioma-like
Adenocarcinoma
  Mucinous
    Endocervical type
      Adenoma malignum
      Villoglandular
    Intestinal type
      Signet-ring cell
  Endometrioid
  Clear cell
  Serous
  Mesonephric
Adenosquamous carcinoma
Glassy cell carcinoma
Adenoid cystic carcinoma
Adenoid basal carcinoma
Carcinoid tumor
Small cell carcinoma
Large cell neuroendocrine carcinoma
Undifferentiated carcinoma

Leiomyosarcoma
Undifferentiated endocervical sarcoma
Endocervical stromal sarcoma
Embryonal rhabdomyosarcoma
Endometrial stromal sarcoma
Alveolar soft-part sarcoma
Adenosarcoma
Malignant mullerian mixed tumor
Wilms' tumor
Malignant melanoma
Lymphoma and leukemia
Yolk sac tumor
Secondary tumors

5-year survival rates of patients with squamous carcinoma were as follows: stage Ia, 97%; stage Ib, 78.9%; stage IIa, 57.6%; stage IIb, 53.4%; stage III, 33.6%; and stage IV, 13.3%.[75] However, the survival of patients with histologic subtypes of squamous carcinoma may vary. Verrucous carcinoma, a well-differentiated tumor with pushing borders, may present with advanced local disease because of delays in diagnosis, but overall it has a relatively good prognosis.[76] Lymphoepithelioma-like carcinoma, another uncommon variant of SCC, is characterized by a syncytial growth of undifferentiated cells with a prominent lymphoplasmacytic inflammatory infiltrate. These tumors have a greater association with Epstein-Barr virus and a decreased association with HPV-16 and HPV-18 than typical SCC.[77] Although relatively few cases have been reported, these patients appear to have a good prognosis; for example, none of the 15 patients in one study had evidence of metastasis or recurrence.[77] Sarcomatoid SCC is a rare tumor with malignant spindle cells that merge with typical SCC (Fig. 3-11). It has a remarkably poor prognosis, as all of the patients with reported follow-up have died of disease.[78]

Adenocarcinoma. Adenocarcinomas comprise a small portion of all cervical carcinomas, but the incidence of these tumors appears to be increasing.[79] Although there has been considerable controversy regarding the prognosis of adenocarcinoma relative to SCC, many studies have found a worse 5-year survival rate for adenocarcinoma.[80-83] In one study, the 5-year disease-specific survival rate for patients with adenocarcinoma was found to be 72%, compared with 81% for SCC. A second study found the 5-year survival rate for patients with stage I adenocarcinoma to be 53%, compared with 68% for SCC.[81,82] Another large hospital-based study also found significant differences in survival for stages I, II, and III tumors: in stage I disease,

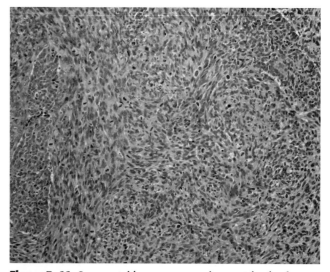

Figure 3–11. Sarcomatoid squamous carcinoma. Islands of typical squamous carcinoma blend into malignant spindle cells. See also Color Figure 3-11.

the 5-year survival rates were 60% for adenocarcinoma and 90% for SCC; in stage II, 47% and 62%; and in stage III, 8% and 36%, respectively.[80] The reason for this difference is unclear, but hypotheses have included delayed detection, an increased rate of distant metastases, and a relative radioresistance of bulky tumors.[81,84]

Some of the subtypes of adenocarcinoma have prognoses that differ from the group as a whole. Villoglandular adenocarcinoma is a well-differentiated tumor that occurs on average in women younger than those with typical adenocarcinoma. In two studies, none of the patients developed recurrent tumor.[85,86] Adenoma malignum (minimal deviation adenocarcinoma) is another well-differentiated adenocarcinoma that is composed of deceptively benign-appearing glands. Although in one recent study only 1 of 6 patients died of disease, an earlier and larger study found a much worse prognosis, with 13 of 22 patients having died of disease.[87,88] Some of the earlier reports of a poor outcome may have been secondary to the advanced stage of the tumors and undertreatment. Clear cell carcinoma of the cervix may arise in association with DES, but it also may arise sporadically. One study of women with clear cell carcinomas who were not exposed to DES did not find the 5-year survival rate to be significantly worse than that for non–clear cell adenocarcinomas.[89] Serous carcinoma of the cervix is histologically similar to papillary serous carcinoma found in the endometrium and ovary. Although the outcome for patients with stage I disease is not significantly different from that of patients with cervical adenocarcinoma overall, advanced-stage tumors have an aggressive behavior.[90] Mesonephric adenocarcinoma is a rare tumor that arises from mesonephric duct remnants in the cervix. Although there have been few reported cases, it appears that stage I mesonephric adenocarcinomas have a better prognosis than adenocarcinomas as a group.[91,92]

Adenosquamous carcinoma. Adenosquamous carcinomas are cervical tumors with a mixture of malignant glandular and squamous components (Fig. 3-12). These tumors are distinct from endometrioid adenocarcinomas with squamous differentiation. They comprise approximately 2% to 3% of cervical cancers and have a worse prognosis than either pure SCC or adenocarcinoma, particularly in advanced-stage disease.[75,93] An analysis of SEER cases found a 5-year survival rate of 54.9% for adenosquamous carcinoma, compared with 67.2% and 67.7% for SCC and adenocarcinoma, respectively.[75] Another, more recent study also found adenosquamous carcinoma to be an independent predictor of poor outcome, especially in patients with advanced-stage disease.[93]

Glassy cell carcinoma. Glassy cell carcinoma is a poorly differentiated variant of adenosquamous carcinoma that comprises approximately 1% of cervical cancers (Fig. 3-13). Two studies have suggested an association with pregnancy,[94,95] and many have reported a poor prognosis for this tumor.[94-98]

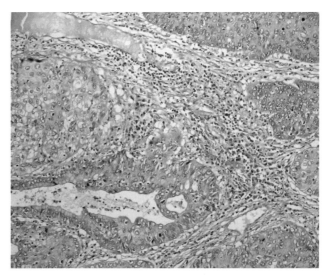

Figure 3–12. Adenosquamous carcinoma. Both malignant squamous and glandular components are present. See also Color Figure 3-12.

Adenoid cystic carcinoma. Adenoid cystic carcinoma is an unusual tumor in the cervix that is histologically similar to adenoid cystic carcinoma of the salivary glands (Fig. 3-14). This tumor has an aggressive behavior, with both frequent lymphatic metastases and hematogeneous spread to the liver, lung, and bones.[99,100] In one study, only 33% of the patients were alive and well at last follow-up; in another, the 3-year survival rate for stage I patients was only 26%.[100,101]

Adenoid basal carcinoma. Adenoid basal carcinoma is a rare tumor with distinctive histologic features. It is characterized by a proliferation of basaloid cells arranged in nests with peripheral palisading. Although they are designated as carcinomas, the behavior of these tumors has been benign, and one group has even suggested changing the name to adenoid basal

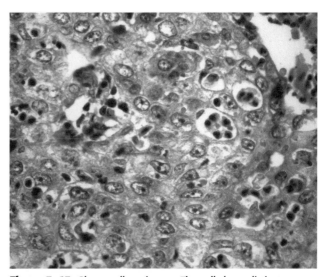

Figure 3–13. Glassy cell carcinoma. The cells have distinct borders, abundant eosinophilic to amphophilic cytoplasm, and large vesicular nuclei with macronucleoli. See also Color Figure 3-13.

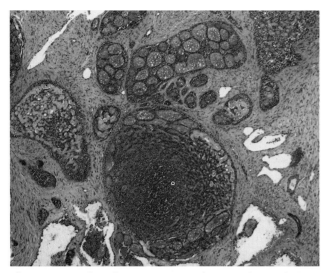

Figure 3–14. Adenoid cystic carcinoma. The tumor has a cribriform pattern with spaces containing mucinous and hyalin material. See also Color Figure 3-14.

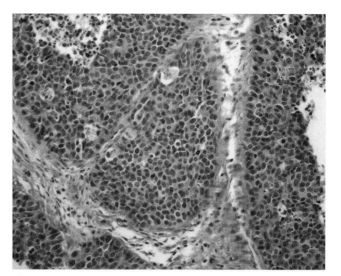

Figure 3–16. Large cell neuroendocrine carcinoma. The tumor cells have moderate amounts of cytoplasm and large nuclei with visible nucleoli. Mitoses and apoptotic figures are frequent. See also Color Figure 3-16.

epithelioma.[102] No patient with typical adenoid basal carcinoma has been reported to have metastases or to have died of disease.[102]

Neuroendocrine carcinoma. The classification of cervical neuroendocrine carcinomas has recently been changed to mirror the nomenclature for pulmonary neuroendocrine tumors.[103] The categories include carcinoid tumor, atypical carcinoid tumor, large cell neuroendocrine carcinoma, and small cell (neuroendocrine) carcinoma. Too few well-documented cases of carcinoid tumor and atypical carcinoid tumor have been reported to draw conclusions about their prognosis. However, small cell carcinoma and large cell neuroendocrine carcinoma are highly aggressive neoplasms.

Small cell carcinomas account for 2% of cervical carcinomas; the overall survival rate is approximately 20%, and the course is relatively short on average, with most patients dying within 2 years after diagnosis (Fig. 3-15).[104,105] Large cell neuroendocrine carcinomas are less common than small cell carcinomas but also have a very poor prognosis (Fig. 3-16). Many patients die shortly after diagnosis, and the overall survival rate is only 20%.[106-108]

Leiomyosarcoma. Although leiomyosarcoma is the most common form of cervical sarcoma, it is a rare tumor and accounts for less than 1% of all cervical malignancies (Fig. 3-17). Similar to leiomyosarcomas of the uterine corpus, cervical leiomyosarcomas have a poor prognosis. Of 12 reported patients

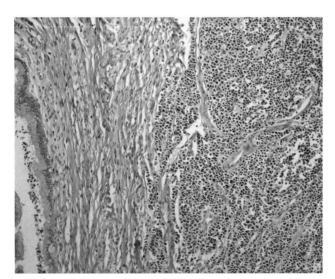

Figure 3–15. Small cell carcinoma. The endocervix is infiltrated by irregular islands and cords of small cells with scant cytoplasm and hyperchromatic nuclei. See also Color Figure 3-15.

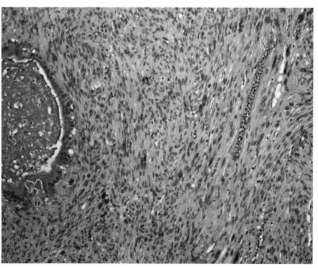

Figure 3–17. Leiomyosarcoma. The tumor has prominent nuclear atypia and mitotic figures. See also Color Figure 3-17.

with available follow-up, only 2 were alive and free of disease.[109,110]

Embryonal rhabdomyosarcoma. Rhabdomyosarcoma is the most common soft tissue sarcoma in children and young adults. Although it is more common in the vagina, embryonal rhabdomyosarcoma may also arise in the cervix. In contrast to leiomyosarcoma, these tumors have a relatively good prognosis, with an overall survival rate of 80%.[111]

Adenosarcoma. Adenosarcoma is a polypoid tumor that contains benign glands and sarcomatous stroma (Fig. 3-18). These tumors are uncommon in the cervix but have a relatively good prognosis. Among reported cases, the disease-free survival rate is 83%.[112]

Malignant mixed mullerian tumor. Malignant mixed mullerian tumors of the cervix are also rare. Like adenosarcomas, they usually manifest as polypoid lesions, but in contrast to adenosarcomas they have both malignant epithelial and stromal components (Fig. 3-19). The majority of these tumors are stage I at presentation, and there is a 42% disease-free survival rate.[113]

Malignant melanoma. Primary cervical melanoma is uncommon, with fewer than 70 cases reported in the literature (Fig. 3-20). Cervical melanomas have an extremely poor prognosis, with a median survival time of 14.5 months. Stage III and IV tumors are uniformly fatal, whereas stages I and II result in 5-year survival rates of 25% and 14%, respectively.[114]

Lymphoma. Cervical involvement by lymphoma is uncommon, with most cases representing secondary spread due to systemic disease. However, low-stage, presumably primary, cases occur and have a good

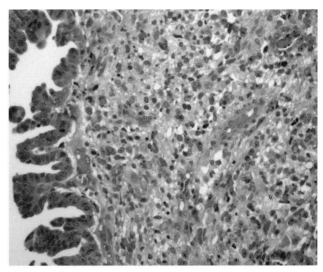

Figure 3–19. Malignant mixed müllerian tumor. Both malignant epithelial (serous carcinoma) and stromal (unclassified sarcoma) components are present. See also Color Figure 3-19.

prognosis. The majority of these cases are diffuse large B-cell lymphomas. The 5-year survival rate is 83%.[115]

Is immunohistochemical staining helpful in the diagnosis of cervical cancer and for distinguishing among various types of cervical carcinoma?

The majority of diagnoses of cervical tumors are established on examination of routine hematoxylin and eosin (H&E) stained slides. However, the morphologic features of the various tumors are not always discrete, and diagnostic difficulties are sometimes encountered in routine H&E stained material. In these instances, immunohistochemistry may be useful.

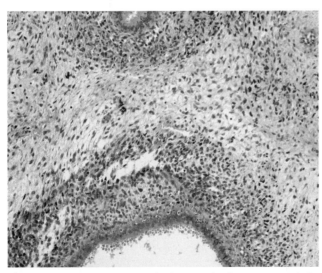

Figure 3–18. Adenosarcoma. The benign glands are surrounded by a hypercellular stromal cuff. Mitotic activity is also present. See also Color Figure 3-18.

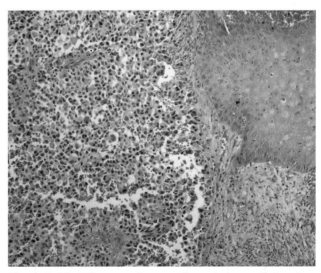

Figure 3–20. Malignant melanoma. The melanoma cells invading the cervical stroma have an epithelioid morphology. See also Color Figure 3-20.

Adenocarcinoma and adenocarcinoma in situ of the cervix may be difficult to differentiate from benign glandular lesions such as microglandular hyperplasia, laminar endocervical glandular hyperplasia, and mesonephric hyperplasia, among others. This problem may arise in small biopsies, and it can be particularly difficult in cases of adenoma malignum. Carcinoembryonic antigen (CEA) is frequently used to help in these instances.[88,116] Cytoplasmic positivity is seen in most cases of endocervical adenocarcinoma and adenocarcinoma in situ, whereas normal endocervical glands are negative (Fig. 3-21). However, the expression of CEA may be only focal in some cases of well-differentiated adenocarcinoma, and because CEA can be positive in squamous mucosa, benign glandular lesions with squamous metaplasia may stain in those areas. Additionally, it has been reported that there can be focal cytoplasmic staining for CEA in endocervical glands with radiation-induced atypia.[117] One study found the addition of Ki-67 and p53 to CEA to be useful in problematic cases.[118] A high Ki-67 proliferation index (>40%), CEA positivity, or both were features of malignant lesions rather than benign mimics in that study, and only malignant neoplasms shared p53 overexpression (>10% of glandular nuclei) and CEA positivity.[118]

Recent studies have shown that p16 is a promising marker for cervical malignant glandular neoplasms. Diffuse strong positivity has been detected in almost all cases of adenocarcinoma and adenocarcinoma in situ tested.[119-121] Benign glandular lesions, in contrast, are negative, weakly positive, or have heterogeneous staining.[120,121] One potential pitfall is that p16 is also expressed in the endometrium.[120]

The distinction between endocervical and endometrial adenocarcinoma is not always obvious based on the histologic examination of tumor present in endometrial biopsy or endocervical curettage specimens, but it is important for determining the appropriate therapy for patients. CEA and vimentin immunohistochemical stains may be useful in addressing this problem. As noted earlier, a majority of endocervical adenocarcinomas are CEA positive (see Fig. 3-21); however, most

endometrial adenocarcinomas are negative for this marker.[122,123] Vimentin, in contrast, is expressed by a majority of endometrial adenocarcinomas but by only a small percentage of endocervical adenocarcinomas.[124,125] Therefore, a CEA-positive/vimentin-negative pattern is supportive of an endocervical origin, whereas a CEA-negative/vimentin-positive pattern favors an endometrial origin.

Given the aggressive behavior of small cell carcinoma and large cell neuroendocrine carcinoma of the cervix and the potential implications for treatment, it is important that these tumors be distinguished from other cervical carcinomas. Although a positive neuroendocrine marker is required for the diagnosis of large cell neuroendocrine carcinoma, it is not a requirement (but can be helpful) for the diagnosis of small cell carcinoma.[103] Chromogranin and synaptophysin are commonly used for this purpose, with synaptophysin being the more sensitive of the two markers (Fig. 3-22).

Mesonephric adenocarcinoma is a rare cervical tumor and can be difficult to identify. Immunohistochemical staining may be useful in distinguishing this variant from other cervical adenocarcinomas. As noted earlier, the majority of endocervical adenocarcinomas are positive for CEA; in contrast, most mesonephric adenocarcinomas are CEA negative.[92] CD10 is another marker that may be useful in making this distinction. Mesonephric adenocarcinomas are generally positive with an apical-luminal pattern, although the staining may be only focal.[126] In contrast, endocervical adenocarcinomas generally are negative for CD10.

Some immunohistochemical characteristics of papillary serous carcinoma of the cervix are worth noting. The majority of endometrial serous carcinomas and ovarian/peritoneal serous carcinomas demonstrate overexpression of p53, usually in a diffuse manner.[127,128] In contrast, most endocervical serous carcinomas are negative for p53.[90] Another difference between

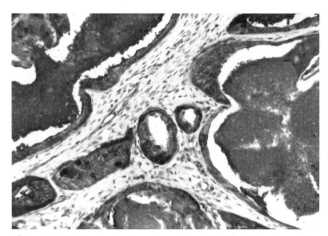

Figure 3–21. Carcinoembryonic antigen (CEA) is diffusely positive in an endocervical adenocarcinoma. See also Color Figure 3-21.

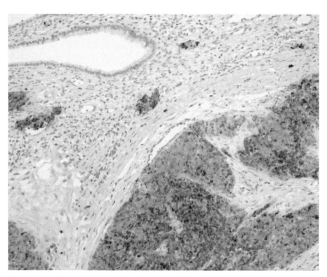

Figure 3–22. Large cell neuroendocrine carcinoma of the cervix diffusely expresses chromogranin. See also Color Figure 3-22.

endocervical and extracervical serous carcinomas is staining for CEA; papillary serous carcinomas of the cervix are frequently CEA positive, whereas noncervical serous carcinomas are negative.[90,129]

Melanomas can be composed of epithelioid cells, spindled cells, or a mixture of the two and therefore may resemble poorly differentiated carcinoma or sarcoma. S-100 and HMB-45 are generally positive in melanomas, whereas cytokeratin stains carcinomas (Fig. 3-23).[130] The markers expressed by a sarcoma depend on the tumor type. Desmin, for example, is found in leiomyosarcomas and rhabdomyosarcomas.

Sarcomatoid squamous carcinomas are highly aggressive cervical tumors that may be confused with malignant mixed mullerian tumors, true sarcomas, or melanomas. Keratin immunohistochemical staining is useful in this differential diagnosis because it is positive in both the epithelioid and the spindle cell components of sarcomatoid squamous carcinoma.[131] However, keratin usually is positive only in the epithelial component of malignant mixed mullerian tumors, and it is absent in malignant melanomas.

What are the important histopathologic features for prognosis of cervical cancer?

Establishing the pathologic stage and the histologic type are important aspects of the histopathologic examination of cervical tumors. However, within each stage for different histologic types, there are other important factors that correlate with survival. These are tumor size, depth of invasion, lymph node metastasis, lymph vascular space invasion, and grade for adenocarcinomas.

The importance of tumor size is indicated by its inclusion in the FIGO staging system for carcinoma of the cervix. In one study, increasing tumor size was correlated with both decreased survival and an increased risk of lymph node metastasis. The 5-year

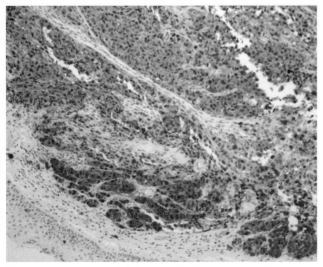

Figure 3–23. A cervical melanoma displays nuclear and cytoplasmic staining for S-100. See also Color Figure 3-23.

disease-free survival rate for patients with tumors 1.0 cm or smaller was 93%; for those with tumors measuring 1.1 to 2.0 cm, it was 76%; for 2.1 to 3.0 cm, 64%; and for greater than 3.0 cm in maximum dimension, 60%.[136] The percentage of patients with lymph node metastases was 3.2% for tumors 1.0 cm or less in maximum dimension and increased to 31.5% for tumors larger than 3.0 cm.[136] Another study found that patients were at greater risk for recurrence and had decreased disease-free survival if they had bulky cervical tumors (>5.0 cm),[132] and yet another study demonstrated that patients with large cervical tumors (>4.0 cm) had twice the frequency of pelvic lymph node metastases and pelvic recurrences as patients with smaller tumors.[133] In the latter study, the patients with larger tumors had a 5-year survival rate of 64.9%, compared with 82.7% for those with smaller tumors.[133] Tumor size is also important in cervical adenocarcinomas, as was demonstrated in two recent studies. In one, the 5-year survival rate for patients with tumors smaller than 3.0 cm was 92%, compared with 76% for patients with larger tumors.[134] In the other study, the 5-year survival rate was 95.3% for patients with tumors up to 3 cm, 63.4% for tumors 3 to 4 cm, and 43.2% for tumors larger than 4 cm.[135]

Another important histopathologic factor included in FIGO staging is depth of tumor invasion. Studies of SCC have found that an increased depth of invasion is associated with an increased risk of lymph node metastasis and decreased progression-free survival (Fig. 3-24A). There were no nodal metastases in one study if the tumors invaded only 3 to 4 mm, and another study found a 4.5% incidence of lymph node metastases with tumors up to 5 mm in depth.[136,137] However, both studies demonstrated a significant increase in the rate of lymph node metastases associated with an increased depth of invasion: 28.9% of cases with invasion greater than 10 mm had lymph node metastases in one of the studies, and 23% of cases with invasion greater than 16 mm had metastases in the other study.[136,137] The depth of invasion was also highly correlated with 5-year disease-free survival in these two studies. In the first study, the rate was 92% for tumors with 5 mm or less invasion and 60% for tumors invading more than 10 mm.[136] The second study was very similar, with 100% disease-free survival for tumors with 3 to 4 mm depth of invasion and 54% progression-free survival for tumors invading more than 10 mm.[137] For adenocarcinomas, increasing depth of invasion is also a significant feature that is associated with recurrent disease.[138,139]

Although lymph node metastasis is not included in FIGO staging, it is an important predictor of tumor behavior. Many studies have found that nodal metastases are highly correlated with overall survival and risk of recurrence. An analysis of FIGO data demonstrated a 5-year survival rate of 89% for patients with negative lymph nodes, compared with 71.8% for those with lymph node metastases.[140] A difference in survival was seen across all stages, and there was also a significant difference in progression-free survival. In addition, the number of lymph nodes involved appears

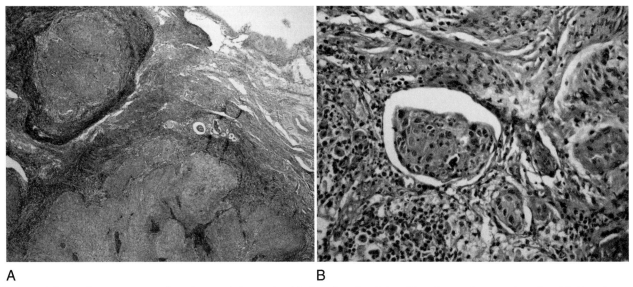

A   B

Figure 3–24. Invasive squamous cell carcinoma of the cervix with deep invasion (**A**) and lymph vascular space invasion (**B**). See also Color Figure 3-24.

to be significant. In one study, the 5-year disease-free survival rate for patients with negative lymph nodes was 77%; for those with one or two positive lymph nodes it was 55%; and for those with more than two lymph nodes involved it was 39%.[136] The significance of lymph node status has also been upheld in studies of cervical adenocarcinoma.[135,139,141] One study found 89.2% overall 5-year survival and 85% disease-free 5-year survival for patients with negative lymph nodes, 61.3% and 51.2% for those with one to two lymph nodes involved, and 13% for those with three or more lymph nodes involved by metastatic carcinoma.[135] Para-aortic lymph node metastases may be more significant than pelvic lymph node metastases, because they are associated with a high rate of recurrences at distant sites, indicative of occult systemic disease.[143]

Lymph vascular space invasion (LVSI) is an important predictor of lymph node metastasis and disease-free survival (see Fig. 3-24B).[137,144,145] In one study, 56.7% of patients with lymph node metastases were found to have LVSI, compared with 21.6% of patients with negative lymph nodes.[144] Patients with LVSI are more likely to experience a recurrence. One study found a 70% increased risk of recurrence in patients with LVSI[146]; this increased risk of recurrence is present even in patients who have negative lymph nodes.[144] Studies of adenocarcinoma have also found LVSI to be significant.[135,139] Patients with LVSI had a 5-year disease-free survival rate of 48.6%, compared with 92.9% for patients without LVSI.[135]

A number of different grading systems have been used for cervical squamous carcinoma, but none appears to be reproducibly effective in predicting prognosis.[137,140] However, tumor grade does appear to influence survival for patients with adenocarcinoma, particularly if nuclear features are included in the grading system.[139,147,148]

REFERENCES

1. Ridley CM, Frankman O, Jones IS, et al: New nomenclature for vulvar disease: International Society for the Study of Vulvar Disease. Hum Pathol 1989;20:495-496.
2. Hording U, Junge J, Daugaard S, et al: Vulvar squamous cell carcinoma and papillomaviruses: Indications for two different etiologies. Gynecol Oncol 1994;52:241-246.
3. Gomez Rueda N, Garcia A, Vighi S, et al: Epithelial alterations adjacent to invasive squamous carcinoma of the vulva. J Reprod Med 1994;39:526-530.
4. Trimble CL, Hildesheim A, Brinton LA, et al: Heterogeneous etiology of squamous carcinoma of the vulva. Obstet Gynecol 1996;87:59-64.
5. Scurry J, Flowers L, Wistuba K, et al: Human papilloma virus, lichen sclerosis and vulvar squamous cell carcinoma. Int J Gynecol Cancer 1998;8:298-306.
6. Rouzier R, Morice P, Haie-Meder C, et al: Prognostic significance of epithelial disorders adjacent to invasive vulvar carcinomas. Gynecol Oncol 2001;81:414-419.
7. Carli P, De Magnis A, Mannone F, et al: Vulvar carcinoma associated with lichen sclerosus: Experience at the Florence, Italy, Vulvar Clinic. J Reprod Med 2003;48:313-318.
8. Pinto AP, Lin MC, Sheets EE, et al: Allelic imbalance in lichen sclerosus, hyperplasia, and intraepithelial neoplasia of the vulva. Gynecol Oncol 2000;77:171-176.
9. Tate JE, Mutter GL, Boynton KA, Crum CP: Monoclonal origin of vulvar intraepithelial neoplasia and some vulvar hyperplasias. Am J Pathol 1997;150:315-322.
10. Lin MC, Mutter GL, Trivijislip P, et al: Patterns of allelic loss (LOH) in vulvar squamous carcinomas and adjacent noninvasive epithelia. Am J Pathol 1998;152:1313-1318.
11. Kim YT, Thomas NF, Kessis TD, et al: P53 mutations and clonality in vulvar carcinomas and squamous hyperplasias: Evidence suggesting that squamous hyperplasias do not serve as direct precursors of human papillomavirus-negative vulvar carcinomas. Hum Pathol 1996;27:389-395.
12. Zaino RJ, Husseinzadeh N, Nahhas W, Mortel R: Epithelial alterations in proximity to invasive squamous carcinoma of the vulva. Int J Gynecol Pathol 1982;1:173-184.
13. Leibowitch M, Neill S, Pelisse M, Moyal-Baracco M: The epithelial changes associated with squamous cell carcinoma of the vulva: A review of the clinical, histological and viral findings in 78 women. Br J Obstet Gynaecol 1990;97:1135-1139.
14. Powell JJ, Wojnarowska F: Lichen sclerosus. Lancet 1999;353:1777-1783.

15. Scurry JP, Vanin K: Vulvar squamous cell carcinoma and lichen sclerosus. Australas J Dermatol 1997;38(Suppl 1):S20-S25.
16. Carli P, Cattaneo A, De Magnis A, et al: Squamous cell carcinoma arising in vulvar lichen sclerosus: A longitudinal cohort study. Eur J Cancer Prev 1995;4:491-495.
17. Carlson JA, Ambros R, Malfetano J, et al: Vulvar lichen sclerosus and squamous cell carcinoma: A cohort, case control, and investigational study with historical perspective. Implications for chronic inflammation and sclerosis in the development of neoplasia. Hum Pathol 1998;29:932-948.
18. Rolfe KJ, Eva LJ, Maclean AB, et al: Cell cycle proteins as molecular markers of malignant change in vulvar lichen sclerosus. Int J Gynecol Cancer 2001;11:113-118.
19. Scurry J: Does lichen sclerosus play a central role in the pathogenesis of human papillomavirus negative vulvar squamous cell carcinoma? The itch-scratch-lichen sclerosus hypothesis. Int J Gynecol Cancer 1999;9:89-97.
20. Wilkinson EJ, Kneale B, Lynch PJ: Report of the ISSVD Terminology Committee. J Reprod Med 1986;31:973-974.
21. Scully RE, Bonfiglio TA, Kurman RJ, et al: Histologic typing of female genital tract tumours. In Scully RE, Poulsen HE, Sobin LH (eds): World Health Organization International Histological Classification of Tumors, 2nd ed. Berlin, Springer-Verlag, 1994.
22. Hart WR: Vulvar intraepithelial neoplasia: Historical aspects and current status. Int J Gynecol Pathol 2001;20:16-30.
23. Kurman RJ, Toki T, Schiffman MH: Basaloid and warty carcinomas of the vulva: Distinctive types of squamous cell carcinoma frequently associated with human papillomaviruses. Am J Surg Pathol 1993;17:133-145.
24. Park JS, Jones RW, McLean MR, et al: Possible etiologic heterogeneity of vulvar intraepithelial neoplasia: A correlation of pathologic characteristics with human papillomavirus detection by in situ hybridization and polymerase chain reaction. Cancer 1991;67:1599-1607.
25. Toki T, Kurman RJ, Park JS, et al: Probable nonpapilloma virus etiology of squamous cell carcinoma of the vulva in older women: A clinicopathologic study using in situ hybridization and polymerase chain reaction. Int J Gynecol Pathol 1991;10:107-125.
26. Abell MR: Intraepithelial carcinomas of epidermis and squamous mucosa of vulva and perineum. Surg Clin North Am 1965;45:1179-1198.
27. Yang B, Hart WR: Vulvar intraepithelial neoplasia of the simplex (differentiated) type: A clinicopathologic study including analysis of HPV and p53 expression. Am J Surg Pathol 2000;24:429-441.
28. Crum CP, Liskow A, Petras P, et al: Vulvar intraepithelial neoplasia (severe atypia and carcinoma in situ): A clinicopathologic analysis of 41 cases. Cancer 1984;54:1429-1434.
29. Buscema J, Woodruff JD, Parmley TH, Genadry R: Carcinoma in situ of the vulva. Obstet Gynecol 1980;55:225-230.
30. Friedrich EG Jr, Wilkinson EJ, Fu YS: Carcinoma in situ of the vulva: A continuing challenge. Am J Obstet Gynecol 1980;136:830-843.
31. Boutselis JG: Intraepithelial carcinoma of the vulva. Am J Obstet Gynecol 1972;113:733-738.
32. Caglar H, Tamer S, Hreshchyshyn MM: Vulvar intraepithelial neoplasia. Obstet Gynecol 1982;60:346-349.
33. Jones RW, McLean MR: Carcinoma in situ of the vulva: A review of 31 treated and five untreated cases. Obstet Gynecol 1986;68:499-503.
34. Chafe W, Richards A, Morgan L, Wilkinson E: Unrecognized invasive carcinoma in vulvar intraepithelial neoplasia (VIN). Gynecol Oncol 1988;31:154-162.
35. Powell LC Jr, Dinh TV, Rajaraman S, et al: Carcinoma in situ of the vulva: A clinicopathologic study of 50 cases. J Reprod Med 1986;31:808-814.
36. Rettenmaier MA, Berman ML, DiSaia PJ: Skinning vulvectomy for the treatment of multifocal vulvar intraepithelial neoplasia. Obstet Gynecol 1986;69:247-250.
37. Jones RW, Rowan DM: Vulvar intraepithelial neoplasia III: A clinical study of the outcome of 113 cases with relation to the later development of invasive vulvar carcinoma. Obstet Gynecol 1994;84:741-745.
38. Bernstein SG, Kovacs BR, Townsend DE, Morrow CP: Vulvar carcinoma in situ. Obstet Gynecol 1983;61:304-307.
39. Jones RW, Rowan DM: Spontaneous regression of vulvar intraepithelial neoplasia 2-3. Obstet Gynecol 2000;96:470-472.
40. Shepherd JH: Cervical and vulvar cancer: Changes in FIGO definitions of staging. Br J Obstet Gynaecol 1996;103:405-406.
41. Lerma E, Matias-Guiu X, Lee SJ, Prat J: Squamous cell carcinoma of the vulva: Study of ploidy, HPV, p53, and pRb. Int J Gynecol Pathol 1999;18:191-197.
42. Ansink AC, Krul MRM, de Weger RA, et al: Human papillomavirus, lichen sclerosus, and squamous cell carcinoma of the vulva: Detection and prognostic significance. Gynecol Oncol 1994;52:180-184.
43. Monk B, Burger R, Lin F, et al: Prognostic significance of human papillomavirus DNA in vulvar carcinoma. Obstet Gynecol 1995;85:709-715.
44. Kaern J, Iversen T, Trope C, et al: Flow cytometric DNA measurements in squamous cell carcinoma of the vulva: An important prognostic method. Int J Gynecol Cancer 1992;2:169-174.
45. Ballouk F, Ambros RA, Malfetano JH, Ross JS: Evaluation of prognostic indicators in squamous carcinoma of the vulva including nuclear DNA content. Mod Pathol 1993;6:371-375.
46. Dolan JR, McCall AR, Gooneratne S, et al: DNA ploidy, proliferation index, grade, and stage as prognostic factors for vulvar squamous cell carcinomas. Gynecol Oncol 1993;48:232-235.
47. Bjerregaard B, Andreasson B, Visfeldt J, Bock JE: The significance of histology and morphometry in predicting lymph node metastases in patients with squamous cell carcinoma of the vulva. Gynecol Oncol 1993;50:323-329.
48. Kohlberger P, Kainz C, Breitenecker G, et al: Prognostic value of immunohistochemically detected p53 expression in vulvar carcinoma. Cancer 1995;76:1786-1789.
49. Scheistroen M, Trope C, Pettersen EO, Nesland JM: P53 protein expression in squamous cell carcinoma of the vulva. Cancer 1999;85:1133-1138.
50. Kagie MJ, Kenter GG, Tollenaar RAEM, et al: P53 protein overexpression, a frequent observation in squamous cell carcinoma of the vulva and in various synchronous vulvar epithelia, has no value as a prognostic parameter. Int J Gynecol Pathol 1996;16:124-130.
51. Emanuels AG, Koudstaal J, Burger MP, Hollema H: In squamous cell carcinoma of the vulva overexpression of p53 is a late event and neither p53 nor mdm2 expression is a useful marker to predict lymph node metastases. Br J Cancer 1999;80:38-43.
52. Hendricks JB, Wilkinson EJ, Kubilis P, et al: Ki-67 expression in vulvar carcinoma. Int J Gynecol Pathol 1994;13:205-210.
53. Hantschmann P, Lampe B, Beysiegel S, Kurzl R: Tumor proliferation in squamous cell carcinoma of the vulva. Int J Gynecol Pathol 2000;19:361-368.
54. Hoffmann G, Casper F, Weikel W, et al: Value of p53, urokinase plasminogen activator, PAI-1 and Ki-67 in vulvar carcinoma. Zentralbl Gynakol 1999;121:473-478.
55. Salmaso R, Zen T, Zannol M, et al: Prognostic value of protein p53 and Ki-67 in invasive vulvar squamous cell carcinoma. Eur J Gynaecol Oncol 2000;21:479-483.
56. Gualco M, Bonin S, Foglia G, et al: Morphologic and biologic studies on ten cases of verrucous carcinoma of the vulva supporting the theory of a discrete clinico-pathologic entity. Int J Gynecol Cancer 2003;13:317-324.
57. Japaze H, Dinh TV, Woodruff JD: Verrucous carcinoma of the vulva: Study of 24 cases. Obstet Gynecol 1982;60:462-466.
58. Gissmann L, de Villiers EM, zur Hausen H: Analysis of human genital warts (condylomata acuminatum) and other genital tumors for HPV type 6 DNA. Int J Cancer 1982;29:143-146.
59. Rando RF, Sedlacek TV, Hunt J, et al: Verrucous carcinoma of the vulva associated with an unusual type 6 human papilloma virus. Obstet Gynecol 1986;67:70-75.
60. Okagaki T: Female genital tumors associated with human papillomavirus infection, and the concept of genital neoplasm papilloma syndrome (GENPS). Pathol Annu 1984;19:31-62.
61. Kondi-Paphitis A, Deligeorgi-Politi H, Liapis A, Plemenou-Frangou M: Human papilloma virus in verrucous carcinoma of the vulva: An immunopathological study of three cases. Eur J Gynaecol Oncol 1998;19:319-320.

62. Van Sickle M, Kaufman RH, Adam E, Adler Storthz K: Detection of human papillomavirus DNA before and after development of invasive vulvar cancer. Obstet Gynecol 1990;76:540-542.

63. Wilkinson EJ: Premalignant and malignant tumors of the vulva. In Kurman RJ, Blaustein A (eds): Blaustein's Pathology of the Female Genital Tract, 5th ed. New York, Springer-Verlag, 2002, pp 99-149.

64. Fanning J, Lambert HC, Hale TM, et al: Paget's disease of the vulva: Prevalence of associated vulvar adenocarcinoma, invasive Paget's disease, and recurrence after surgical excision. Am J Obstet Gynecol 1999;180:24-27.

65. Brown HM, Wilkinson EJ: Uroplakin-III to distinguish primary vulvar Paget disease from Paget disease secondary to urothelial carcinoma. Hum Pathol 2002;33:545-548.

66. Gunn RA, Gallager HS: Vulvar Paget's disease: A topographic study. Cancer 1980;46:590-594.

67. Fishman DA, Chambers SK, Schwartz PE, et al: Extramammary Paget's disease of the vulva. Gynecol Oncol 1995;56:266-270.

68. Crawford D, Nimmo M, Clement PB, et al: Prognostic factors in Paget's disease of the vulva: A study of 21 cases. Int J Gynecol Pathol 1999;18:351-359.

69. Tebes S, Cardosi R, Hoffman M: Paget's disease of the vulva. Am J Obstet Gynecol 2002;187:281-283.

70. Clark WH Jr, Hood AF, Tucker MA, Jampel RM: Atypical melanocytic nevi of the genital type with a discussion of reciprocal parenchymal-stromal interactions in the biology of neoplasia. Hum Pathol 1998;29:S1-S24.

71. Hatch EE, Palmer JR, Titus-Ernstoff L, et al: Cancer risk in women exposed to diethylstilbestrol in utero. JAMA 1998; 280:630-634.

72. Herbst AL, Ulfelder H, Poskanzer DC: Adenocarcinoma of the vagina: Association of maternal stilbestrol therapy with tumor appearance in young women. N Engl J Med 1971;284:878-881.

73. Robboy ST, Anderson MC, Russell P: The vagina. In Robboy SJ, Anderson MC, Russell P (eds): Pathology of the Female Reproductive Tract. London, Churchill Livingstone Harcourt Publishers Limited, 2002, pp 75-104.

74. Zaino RJ, Robby SJ, Kurman RJ: Diseases of the vagina. In: Kurman RJ (ed): Blaustein's Pathology of the Female Genital Tract, 5th ed. New York, Springer-Verlag, 2001, pp 151-206.

75. Kosary CL: FIGO stage, histology, histologic grade, age and race as prognostic factors in determining survival for cancers of the female gynecological system: An analysis of 1973-1987 SEER cases of cancers of the endometrium, cervix, ovary, vulva, and vagina. Semin Surg Oncol 1994;10:31-46.

76. Degefu S, O'Quinn AG, Lacey CG, et al: Verrucous carcinoma of the cervix: A report of two cases and literature review. Gynecol Oncol 1986;25:37-47.

77. Tseng CJ, Pao CC, Tseng LH, et al: Lymphoepithelioma-like carcinoma of the uterine cervix. Cancer 1997;80:91-97.

78. Rodrigues L, Santana I, Cunha T, et al: Sarcomatoid squamous cell carcinoma of the uterine cervix: Case report. Eur J Gynaecol Oncol 2000;21:287-289.

79. Smith HO, Tiffany MF, Qualls CR, Key CR: The rising incidence of adenocarcinoma relative to squamous cell carcinoma of the uterine cervix in the United States: A 24-year population-based study. Gynecol Oncol 2000;78:97-105.

80. Hopkins MP, Morley GW: A comparison of adenocarcinoma and squamous cell carcinoma of the cervix. Obstet Gynecol 1991;77:912-917.

81. Eifel PJ, Burke TW, Morris M, Smith TL: Adenocarcinoma as an independent risk factor for disease recurrence in patients with stage IB cervical carcinoma. Gynecol Oncol 1995;59:38-44.

82. Kleine W, Rau K, Schwoeorer D, Pfleiderer A: Prognosis of the adenocarcinoma of the cervix uteri: A comparative study. Gynecol Oncol 1989;35:145-149.

83. Samlal RAK, van der Velden J, Ten Kate FJW, et al: Surgical pathologic factors that predict recurrence in stage IB and IIA cervical carcinoma patients with negative pelvic lymph nodes. Cancer 1997;80:1234-1240.

84. Lea JS, Sheets EE, Wenham RM, et al: Stage IIB–IVB cervical adenocarcinoma: Prognostic factors and survival. Gynecol Oncol 2002;84:115-119.

85. Jones MW, Silverberg SG, Kurman RJ: Well-differentiated villoglandular adenocarcinoma of the uterine cervix: A clinico-pathological study of 24 cases. Int J Gynecol Pathol 1993;12:1-7.

86. Young RH, Scully RE: Villoglandular papillary adenocarcinoma of the uterine cervix: A clinicopathologic analysis of 13 cases. Cancer 1989;63:1773-1779.

87. Hirai Y, Takeshima N, Haga A, et al: A clinicopathologic study of adenoma malignum of the uterine cervix. Gynecol Oncol 1998;70:219-223.

88. Gilks CB, Young RH, Aguirre P, et al: Adenoma malignum (minimal deviation adenocarcinoma) of the uterine cervix: A clinicopathological and immunohistochemical analysis of 26 cases. Am J Surg Pathol 1989;13:717-729.

89. Reich O, Tamussino K, Lahousen M, et al: Clear cell carcinoma of the uterine cervix: Pathology and prognosis in surgically treated stage IB–IIB disease in women not exposed in utero to diethylstilbestrol. Gynecol Oncol 2000;76:331-335.

90. Zhou C, Gilks CB, Hayes M, Clement PB: Papillary serous carcinoma of the uterine cervix: A clinicopathologic study of 17 cases. Am J Surg Pathol 1998;22:113-120.

91. Clement PB, Young RH, Keh P, et al: Malignant mesonephric neoplasms of the uterine cervix: A report of eight cases, including four with a malignant spindle cell component. Am J Surg Pathol 1995;19:1158-1171.

92. Silver SA, Devouassoux-Shisheboran M, Mezzetti TP, Tavassoli FA: Mesonephric adenocarcinomas of the uterine cervix: A study of 11 cases with immunohistochemical findings. Am J Surg Pathol 2001;25:379-387.

93. Farley JH, Hickey KW, Carlson JW, et al: Adenosquamous histology predicts a poor outcome for patients with advanced-stage, but not early stage, cervical carcinoma. Cancer 2003; 97:2196-2202.

94. Cherry CP, Glucksmann A: Incidence, histology, and response to radiation of mixed carcinomas (adenoacanthomas) of the uterine cervix. Cancer 1956;9:971-979.

95. Seltzer V, Sall S, Castadot MJ, et al: Glassy cell cervical carcinoma. Gynecol Oncol 1979;8:141-151.

96. Talerman A, Alenghat E, Okagaki T: Glassy cell carcinoma of the uterine cervix. APMIS Suppl 1991;23:119-125.

97. Tamimi HK, Elk M, Hesla J, et al: Glassy cell carcinoma of the cervix redefined. Obstet Gynecol 1988;71:837-841.

98. Tsukahara Y, Sakai Y, Ishii J, et al: A clinicopathologic study on glassy cell carcinoma of the cervix. Acta Obstet Gynaecol Jpn 1981;33:699-704.

99. King LA, Talledo OE, Gallup DG, et al: Adenoid cystic carcinoma of the cervix in women under age 40. Gynecol Oncol 1989;32:26-30.

100. Ferry JA, Scully RE: "Adenoid cystic" carcinoma and adenoid basal carcinoma of the uterine cervix: A study of 28 cases. Am J Surg Pathol 1988;12:134-144.

101. Hoskins WJ, Averette HE, Ng ABP, Yon JL: Adenoid cystic carcinoma of the cervix uteri: Report of six cases and review of the literature. Gynecol Oncol 1979;7:371-384.

102. Brainard JA, Hart WR: Adenoid basal epitheliomas of the uterine cervix: A reevaluation of distinctive basaloid lesions classified as adenoid basal carcinoma and adenoid basal hyperplasia. Am J Surg Pathol 1998;22:965-975.

103. Albores-Saavedra J, Gersell D, Gilks CB, et al: Terminology of endocrine tumors of the uterine cervix: Results of a workshop sponsored by the College of American Pathologists and the National Cancer Institute. Arch Pathol Lab Med 1997; 121:34-39.

104. Silva EG, Gershenson D, Sneige N, et al: Small cell carcinoma of the uterine cervix: "Pathology and prognostic factors." Surg Pathol 1989;2:105-115.

105. Gersell DJ, Mazoujian G, Mutch DG, Rudloff MA: Small-cell undifferentiated carcinoma of the cervix: A clinicopathologic, ultrastructural, and immunocytochemical study of 15 cases. Am J Surg Pathol 1988;12:684-698.

106. Gilks CB, Young RH, Gersell DJ, Clement PB: Large cell carcinoma of the uterine cervix: A clinicopathologic study of 12 cases. Am J Surg Pathol 1997;21:905-914.

107. Rhemtula H, Grayson W, van Iddekinge B, Tiltman A: Large-cell neuroendocrine carcinoma of the uterine cervix: A clinicopathological study of five cases. S Afr Med J 2001; 91:525-528.

108. Sato Y, Shimamoto T, Amada S, Hayashi T: Large cell neuroendocrine carcinoma of the uterine cervix: A clinicopathological study of six cases. Int J Gynecol Pathol 2003;22:226-230.

109. Abell MR, Ramirez JA: Sarcomas and carcinosarcomas of the uterine cervix. Cancer 1973;31:1176-1192.

110. Rotmensch J, Rosenshein NB, Woodruff JD: Cervical sarcoma: A review. Obstet Gynecol Serv 1983;38:456-460.

111. Zeisler H, Mayerhofer K, Joura EA, et al: Embryonal rhabdomyosarcoma of the uterine cervix: Case report and review of the literature. Gynecol Oncol 1998;69:78-83.

112. Jones MW, Lefkowitz M: Adenosarcoma of the uterine cervix: A clinicopathological study of 12 cases. Int J Gynecol Pathol 1995;14:223-229.

113. Clement PB, Zubovits JT, Young RH, Scully RE: Malignant mullerian mixed tumors of the uterine cervix: A report of nine cases of a neoplasm with morphology often different from its counterpart in the corpus. Int J Gynecol Pathol 1998;12:211-222.

114. Clark KC, Butz WR, Hapke MR: Primary malignant melanoma of the uterine cervix: Case report with world literature review. Int J Gynecol Pathol 1999;18:265-273.

115. Vang R, Medeiros J, Ha CS, Deavers M: Non-Hodgkin's lymphomas involving the uterus: A clinicopathologic analysis of 26 cases. Mod Pathol 2000;13:19-28.

116. Michael H, Grawe L, Kraus FT: Minimal deviation endocervical adenocarcinoma: Clinical and histologic features, immunohistochemical staining for carcino-embryonic antigen, and differentiation from confusing benign lesions. Int J Gynecol Pathol 1984;3:261-276.

117. Lesack D, Wahab, Gilks CB: Radiation-induced atypia of endocervical epithelium: A histological, immunohistochemical, and cytometric study. Int J Gynecol Pathol 1996;15:242-247.

118. Cina SJ, Richardson MS, Austin RM, et al: Immunohistochemical staining for Ki-67 antigen, carcinoembryonic antigen, and p53 in the differential diagnosis of glandular lesions of the cervix. Mod Pathol 1997;64:242-251.

119. Parker MF, Arroyo GF, Geradts J, et al: Molecular characterization of adenocarcinoma of the cervix. Gynecol Oncol 1997; 64:242-251.

120. Riethdorf L, Riethdorf S, Lee KR, et al: Human papilloma viruses, expression of p16^{INK4A}, and early endocervical glandular neoplasia. Hum Pathol 2002;33:899-904.

121. Negri G, Egarter-Vigl E, Kasal A, et al: P16^{ink4A} is a useful marker for the diagnosis of adenocarcinoma of the cervix uteri and its precursors: An immunohistochemical study with immunocytochemical correlations. Am J Surg Pathol 2003; 27:187-193.

122. Wahlstrom T, Lindgren J, Korhonen M, Seppala M: Distinction between endocervical and endometrial adenocarcinoma with immunoperoxidase staining of carcinoembryonic antigen in routine histological tissue specimens. Lancet 1979;2:1159-1160.

123. Cohen C, Shulman G, Budgeon LR: Endocervical and endometrial adenocarcinoma: An immunoperoxidase and histochemical study. Am J Surg Pathol 1982;6:151-157.

124. Dabbs DJ, Geisinger KR, Norris HT: Intermediate filaments in endometrial and endocervical carcinomas: The diagnostic utility of vimentin patterns. Am J Surg Pathol 1986;10:568-576.

125. Dabbs DJ, Sturtz K, Zaino RJ: The immunohistochemical discrimination of endometrioid adenocarcinomas. Hum Pathol 1996;27:172-177.

126. Ordi J, Romagosa C, Tavassoli FA, et al: CD10 expression in epithelial tissues and tumors of the gynecological tract: A useful marker in the diagnosis of mesonephric, trophoblastic, and clear cell tumors. Am J Surg Pathol 2003;27:178-186.

127. Kounelis S, Kapranos N, Kouri E, et al: Immunohistochemical profile of endometrial adenocarcinoma: A study of 61 cases and review of the literature. Mod Pathol 2000;13:379-388.

128. Goldstein NS, Uzieblo A: WT1 immunoreactivity in uterine papillary serous carcinomas is different from ovarian serous carcinomas. Am J Clin Pathol 2002;117:541-545.

129. Caduff RF, Svoboda-Newman SM, Ferguson AW, et al: Comparison of mutations of Ki-RAS and p53 immunoreactivity in borderline and malignant epithelial ovarian tumors. Am J Surg Pathol 1999;23:323-328.

130. Bacchi CE, Goldfogel GA, Greer BE, Gown AM: Paget's disease and melanoma of the vulva: Use of a panel of monoclonal antibodies to identify cell type and to microscopically define adequacy of surgical margins. Gynecol Oncol 1992;46: 216-221.

131. Steeper TA, Piscioli F, Rosai J: Squamous cell carcinoma with sarcoma-like stroma of the female genital tract: Clinicopathologic study of four cases. Cancer 1983;52:890-898.

132. Werner-Wasik M, Schmid CH, Bornstein L, et al: Prognostic factors for local and distant recurrence in stage I and II cervical carcinoma. Int J Radiat Oncology Biol Phys 1995;32:1309-1317.

133. Horn LC, Fischer U, Bilek K: Histopathological prognostic factors in primary surgically treated cervix carcinoma. Zentralbl Gynakol 2001;123:266-274.

134. Silver DF, Hempling RE, Piver MS, et al: Stage I adenocarcinoma of the cervix: Does lesion size affect treatment options and prognosis? Am J Clin Oncol 1998;21:431-435.

135. Ishikawa H, Nakanishi T, Inoue T, Kuzuya K: Prognostic factors of adenocarcinoma of the uterine cervix. Gynecol Oncol 1999;73:42-46.

136. Sevin BU, Nadji M, Lampe B, et al: Prognostic factors of early stage cervical cancer treated by radical hysterectomy. Cancer 1995;76:1978-1986.

137. Zaino RJ, Ward S, Delgado G, et al: Histopathologic predictors of the behavior of surgically treated stage IB squamous cell carcinoma of the cervix. A Gynecologic Oncology Group study. Cancer 1992;69:1750-1758.

138. Matthews CM, Burke TW, Tornos C, et al: Stage I cervical adenocarcinoma: Prognostic evaluation of surgically treated patients. Gynecol Oncol 1993;49:19-23.

139. Costa MJ, McIlnay KR, Trelford J: Cervical carcinoma with glandular differentiation: Histological evaluation predicts disease recurrence in clinical stage I or II patients. Hum Pathol 1995;26:829-837.

140. Benedet JL, Odicino F, Maisonneuve P, et al: Carcinoma of the cervix uteri. J Epidemiol Biostat 2001;6:5-44.

141. Levêque J, Laurent JF, Burtin F, et al: Prognostic factors of the uterine cervix adenocarcinoma. Eur J Obstet Gynecol Reprod Biol 1998;80:209-214.

142. Sevin BU, Lu Y, Bloch DA, et al: Surgically defined prognostic parameters in patients with early cervical carcinoma. Cancer 1996;78:1438-1446.

143. Lovecchio JL, Averette HE, Donato D, Bell J: 5-Year survival of patients with periaortic nodal metastases in clinical stage IB and IIA cervical carcinoma. Gynecol Oncol 1989;34:43-45.

144. Obermair A, Wanner C, Bilgi S, et al: The influence of vascular space involvement on the prognosis of patients with stage IB cervical carcinoma. Cancer 1998;82:689-696.

145. Roman LD, Felix JC, Muderspach LI, et al: Influence of quantity of lymph-vascular space invasion on the risk of nodal metastases in women with early-stage squamous cancer of the cervix. Gynecol Oncol 1998;68:220-225.

146. Delgado G, Bundy B, Zaino R, et al: Prospective surgical-pathological study of disease-free interval in patients with stage IB squamous cell carcinoma of the cervix: A Gynecologic Oncology Group study. Gynecol Oncol 1990;38:352-357.

147. Berek JS, Hacker NF, Fu YS, et al: Adenocarcinoma of the uterine cervix: Histologic variables associated with lymph node metastasis and survival. Obstet Gynecol 1985;65:46-52.

148. Hopkins MP, Schmidt RW, Roberts JA, Morley GW: The prognosis and treatment of stage I adenocarcinoma of the cervix. Obstet Gynecol 1988;72:915-921.

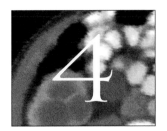

MOLECULAR BIOLOGY OF CERVICAL AND VULVAR CARCINOMA

Steven E. Waggoner   and   Cheryl L. Chernicky

MAJOR CONTROVERSIES

- **How does human papillomavirus infection lead to cervical and vulvar neoplasia?**
- **How does human papillomavirus infection interfere with normal epithelial differentiation?**
- **Besides human papillomavirus infection, what cofactors influence cervical carcinogenesis?**
- **What is the state of vaccine development against human papillomavirus?**
- **What are the common non–human papillomavirus disturbances found in cervical cancers?**
- **What is the molecular biology of vulvar cancer?**
- **What evidence suggests that vulvar cancer may arise from two different pathways?**
- **What disturbances have been identified in tumor suppressor and cell cycle regulatory genes in vulvar cancer?**

Cervical cancer and its precursors remain a significant international health problem. Anogenital infection with certain human papillomaviruses (HPVs) is strongly linked to the development of cervical and, to a lesser extent, vulvar cancer. HPV-derived oncogenes expressed in these malignancies are critical elements in the process of transformation and immortalization, and they are tied to the progression from preinvasive to invasive lesions. Several other cofactors, including behavioral and molecular events, influence the pathogenesis of HPV infection and carcinogenesis. The biologic behavior and response to the treatment of cervical and vulvar cancers may be influenced by HPV- and non-HPV–related alterations found in cervical and vulvar cancers. This chapter reviews the molecular biology of these malignancies and highlights the controversies and challenges in translating our understanding of these molecular mechanisms into future treatments or prevention of these cancers.

Human papillomaviruses

HPVs are DNA tumor viruses that induce proliferative lesions in the mucosal and cutaneous epithelia. HPVs have traditionally been classified as members of the Papovaviridae family, and more than 100 closely related types have been identified. HPV typing is based on genetic sequence rather than serologic reactivity. A new type is defined when DNA sequences in select regions have more than 10% divergence from any of the known HPV types. HPV subtypes or variants have been classified whose genetic sequences differ by less than 10% of known types. Detection of HPV in clinical specimens is normally performed by DNA amplification or DNA/RNA hybrid capture of nucleic acid sequences extracted from target tissues. Most HPVs associated with female anogenital neoplasia are mucotropic, and more than two dozen types have been identified in the genetic material of women with benign, premalignant, and malignant squamous and nonsquamous lesions. Using modern molecular techniques, HPV DNA can be identified in approximately 95% of premalignant and malignant lesions of the cervix. The most common HPV types identified in normal women (in descending order) are types 16, 18, 45, 31, 6, 58, 35, and 33. The most common HPV types in women with cervical cancer in descending order of frequency are types 16, 18, 45, 31, 33, 52, 58, and 35. Other, less commonly identified HPV types have been found in a much higher proportion of women with cervical cancer compared with women without cancer, and they include types 39, 51, 56, 59, 68, 73, and 82. These types should also be considered as oncogenic, even though they are associated with a relatively small percentage of invasive cancers.[1]

The physical state of the HPV genome is strongly associated with the malignant potential of an HPV-infected cell.[2,3] In benign or low-grade lesions, the viral DNAs typically retain their circular construct and exist most often as monomeric plasmids. In most cancers, HPV DNAs are integrated into one or more host chromosomes.[4] This may occur with loss or disruption of one or more of the HPV genes, most commonly *E2*. Sites of integration have been identified near cellular oncogenes, suggesting an interaction between HPV gene products and host factors involved with cellular proliferation and growth regulation in some cases. Most studies show that disruption of host cancer–related genes is not a common event, with integration loci instead distributed widely among the genome.[5,6] Viral integration normally results in loss of infectious virion production, although replication of one or more viral genes becomes linked to all future host DNA replications. The resulting unimpaired HPV oncogene transcription appears to be of greater importance than the function of neighboring host genes.

How does human papillomavirus infection lead to cervical and vulvar neoplasia? The double-stranded DNA of the HPV genome is about 7900 base pairs long. The genome is functionally organized into a region of early (E) genes, whose normal functions are focused on transcription and gene regulation, and late (L) genes, which code for the viral capsid proteins. (Fig. 4-1) A long control region (LCR) separates the E region from the L region. The early region codes for E6, E7, E1, E2, E4, and E5 proteins, and the late region codes for L1 and L2 proteins. The two most important HPV proteins involved in the pathogenesis of anogenital neoplasia are the E6 and E7 proteins. These two transcriptional units encode proteins critical for viral replication. The E6 oncoprotein exerts its main effect by binding to and inactivating the tumor suppressor protein p53 through ubiquitin degradation, which disrupts an inherent cell cycle checkpoint.[7,8] E6 protein also induces cellular telomerase activity.[9] Telomerase synthesizes telomere repeat sequences, which are linked to cell immortalization and are commonly found in transformed cell lines and many cancers.

The E7 oncoprotein binds to and inactivates products of the retinoblastoma gene, *RB1*, which ultimately allows for unchecked cell cycle progression in those cells infected with oncogenic HPV.[10] The E7 protein also interacts with the SMAD complex, which mediates transforming growth factor-β (TGF-β)–induced growth inhibition, a pathway distinct from the RB family of pocket proteins.[11]

On a broader level, HPV E6 and E7 are capable of interacting with chromatin and contribute to the development of genetic instability and subsequent chromosomal aberrations (see "Chromosomal Abnormalities").

Genomic variants of HPV-16 differ in vitro in their abilities to bind to and degrade p53.[12] The variations most commonly identified occur in E6, although E7 mutations also have been identified. Some evidence

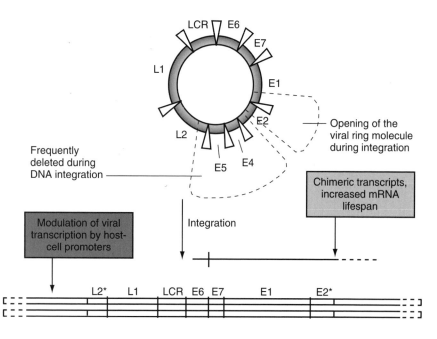

Figure 4–1. The organization of circular HPV DNA and its integration into host-cell DNA. (From zur Hausen H: Papillomaviruses and cancer: From basic studies to clinical application. Nat Rev Cancer 2002; 2:342-350.)

suggests that HPV-16 variants may be more oncogenic than the prototype and carry a higher risk for the development of invasive cervical disease.[13]

E6 and E7 are capable of inducing keratinocyte immortalization in vitro. E6 and E7 protein expression is preserved in almost all invasive cervical cancers studied, and in vitro, antisense nucleotides or monoclonal antibodies directed against E6 or E7 genes result in growth inhibition of HPV-transformed cell lines.[14] These and other purported oncogenic functions of HPV E6 and E7 are summarized in Table 4-1.

E1 proteins are important regulators of HPV DNA replication and appear to be responsible for maintaining viral DNA in its normal closed, circular construct. Mutations of the gene may result in disruption of the viral genome, promoting its integration into the host genome.[15] The E1 and E2 proteins are also involved in the process of cell transformation, further facilitating the immortalization capability of E6 and E7.[16]

The open reading frame of E2 is commonly disrupted during the process of viral integration. Reestablishment of E2 protein production through gene transfer techniques has resulted in repression of HPV E6 and E7 expression, followed by induction of P53 expression in an HPV-18–containing cell line.[17]

E4 encodes a protein that interacts with the cytokeratin network, producing what is called a *koilocyte*.[18,19] The E4 transcript is the most abundant HPV protein in benign warts, but the gene is not highly conserved among the more oncogenic HPV types. E5 encodes a small protein that is often found in the Golgi apparatus and can form complexes with host membrane receptors. Expression of the E5 protein is often lost during viral integration, and although its role in oncogenesis is not well understood, reports suggest a role in activation of the epidermal growth factor receptor.[20,21]

How does human papillomavirus infection interfere with normal epithelial differentiation? Anogenital transmission of HPV normally follows mucosal-to-mucosal contact. Intracellular infection may or may not occur on exposure to HPV and is probably influenced by a number of factors, including HPV type,

Table 4-1. Oncogenic Functions of Human Papillomavirus Early Proteins E6 and E7

Protein	Functions
E6	Interacts with and facilitates degradation of P53
	Targets and abrogates BAK function by promoting its degradation
	Activates telomerase
	Inhibits degradation of SRC family of kinases
	Interacts with chromatin and contributes to genetic instability
E7	Interacts with and degrades retinoblastoma-related proteins
	Stimulates S-phase cyclin A and cyclin E
	Blocks functions of cyclin-dependent kinase inhibitors p21 and p27
	Induces chromosome damage through interactions with centrioles

age at exposure, coexistent cervical infections, host immune function, use of oral contraceptives, and cigarette smoking.

HPV infections are often categorized as productive or proliferative. Productive infections result in the formation of intact, infectious viral particles. Proliferative or nonproductive infections are characterized by viral integration. In each case, the target cell for HPV infection is the basal cell in the anogenital epithelium, with most infections occurring at the squamocolumnar junction of the cervical transformation zone. Most basal cells are committed to squamous cell proliferation through a tightly controlled pathway of differentiation that can be characterized morphologically and molecularly, primarily through expression of different cytokeratins as cells mature throughout the epithelial thickness. Productive HPV gene expression is also tightly linked to epithelial differentiation and normally occurs only in cells that have progressed from the basal layer to the intermediate or suprabasal layers. These cells have lost the capacity for further replication.[22]

Infected basal cells are usually morphologically normal, and the level of HPV gene expression is relatively low. In the suprabasal region, expression of early HPV genes occurs, and with further differentiation, there is induction of all viral genes, including DNA synthesis and transcription of viral capsid proteins.[23] Intact virions are normally present only at the surface or in the most superficial epithelial cells. Morphologically, these infections are recognized as low grade, based mainly on the small risk of progression to cancer if untreated.

Development of high-grade lesions (and ultimately invasive cancer) assumes disruption of the tightly coordinated relationship between epithelial differentiation and viral gene transcription. How this occurs is unknown, but it is probably not caused by a single mechanism. Unregulated expression of E6 or E7 in the basal layer is thought to be a prerequisite for the development of a malignant phenotype. These cells, which retain the capacity to divide, are at risk for additional genotoxic events, many of which may lead to disruption of other pathways tied to cellular replication or apoptosis. Fortunately, the likelihood of transition from a productive, low-risk infection to a proliferative, high-risk infection is quite small.

Besides human papillomavirus infection, what cofactors influence cervical carcinogenesis? The high prevalence of HPV infection in the general population, the long incubation period between HPV infection and cervical cancer, and the observation that most HPV infections and many HPV-associated dysplasias regress without treatment strongly suggest that HPV infection alone is an insufficient cause of invasive cervical cancer.[24,25] Additional cofactors, which may or may not interact directly with HPV, seem to be required before a malignant phenotype arises (Fig. 4-2). Epidemiologic and laboratory evidence suggests interactions between cigarette smoking, use of oral contraceptives, and induced or acquired immune dysfunction as potential cofactors for cervical carcinogenesis. Some studies also

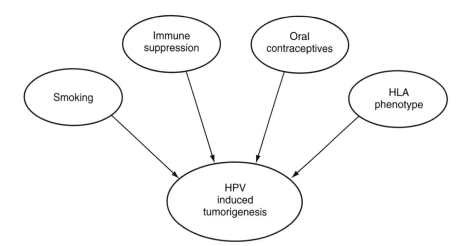

Figure 4–2. Factors other than human papillomavirus (HPV) infection can influence the development of cervical cancer. Smoking causes damage to cervical DNA, which may cooperate with impaired apoptosis in HPV-infected cells. Impaired cellular or humoral immunity inhibits normal host defenses, facilitating persistent HPV infections. Hormones in oral contraceptives can bind to hormone response elements in the HPV genome, upregulating transcription of oncogenic HPV. Polymorphisms in major histocompatibility complex class I and class II genes have been associated with positive and negative risks of cervical neoplasia. A protective effect of human leukocyte antigen (HLA) class II DRB1*13/DBQ1*0603 alleles is the most consistent HLA finding.

point to differences in inherent susceptibility to the development of cervical neoplasia,[26] which may be linked to differences in human leukocyte antigen (HLA) subtypes.

Smoking. An association between cigarette smoking and cervical cancer was suggested as early as 1966, when Naguib and coworkers[27] reported an increased incidence of cervical cancer in smokers compared with nonsmokers. Subsequent epidemiologic studies, including many from outside the United States, have also supported a link between smoking and cervical cancer.[28-31] These studies suggest that smokers have about a fourfold higher risk of developing squamous cell cervical cancer or high-grade dysplasia, even when adjusting for other known risk factors, including HPV infection.

Epidemiologic studies have also been supported by biologic evidence. More than 50 carcinogens are present in tobacco smoke. Tobacco-specific nitrosamines (TSNAs) and polyaromatic hydrocarbons (PAHs) are the two major classes of carcinogens, and they can be found in the tar component of cigarette smoke. The first attempts to produce carcinoma of the cervix in animal models began with the application of crude tar to the genital tract of rats or mice.[32,33] Later, individual chemical carcinogens found in tobacco smoke were tested, including various PAHs such as benzo(a)pyrene. Application of PAHs resulted in a higher incidence of cervical tumors compared with applications of crude tar,[34,35] with more than 70% of treated animals developing invasive cervical tumors and a latency period ranging from 20 to 50 weeks.

Nicotine and its metabolite cotinine can be detected in the cervical mucus of smokers[36] and in concentrations substantially higher than those found in serum. Although neither of these substances is considered carcinogenic, it cannot be assumed these substances have no effect on cervical epithelial cells or HPV.[37]

The TSNA 4-(methylnitrosamino)-1-(3-pyridyl)-1-butanone (NNK) was identified in the cervical mucus of smokers, demonstrating for the first time transportation to the cervix of a chemical carcinogen derived exclusively from tobacco.[38] In vitro, human cervical epithelium is able to metabolize NNK to active intermediates capable of binding to and damaging DNA.[39,40]

Using sensitive analytic techniques, PAHs and their metabolites have also been identified and characterized in human cervical epithelium. In vitro, compared with normal cervical epithelial cells, cells transformed with HPV DNA resist the growth inhibitory effects of benzo(a)pyrene and accumulate higher levels of PAH-derived DNA adducts.[41]

Taken together, these data suggest that exposure of cervical epithelial cells to tobacco carcinogens or other active substances, including nicotine, may cooperate with HPV infections in transformation to a malignant phenotype.

Sex steroids. Evidence has been accumulating that long-term exposure to sex steroids, primarily in the form of oral contraceptive use, is associated with an increased risk of cervical cancer, even when adjusting for HPV status, smoking, and the use of barrier contraceptives. A summary review of this subject, which examined results from 28 studies, reported that increasing duration of oral contraceptive use was associated with an increase in relative risk of cervical cancer from 1.1 (95% CI: 1.1-1.2) for up to 5 years of use to 1.6 (95% CI: 1.4-1.7) for 5 to 9 years and 2.2 (95% CI: 1.9-2.4) for 10 or more years. Results were similar for in situ and invasive cervical cancers and for squamous cell and adenocarcinoma.

The biologic explanations for these epidemiologic associations have not been clearly defined. Sex steroids may influence the risk of cervical cancer by facilitating infection with HPV or affecting the persistence of infection. Sex steroids may alter the squamocolumnar junction or the local immunity of the cervix, either of which could lead to a greater opportunity for oncogenic HPV to transition from a productive infection to a proliferative, oncogenic infection. Nevertheless, some studies do not support the hypothesis that oral contraceptives have a role in facilitation of infection or persistence of HPV.[42,43] A multicenter, case-control study revealed that HPV positivity was not related to oral contraceptive use after controlling for sexual activity and screening history.[44]

There is, however, evidence that suggests a direct influence of sex steroids on HPV gene activity.[45] Steroid hormones can bind to specific glucocorticoid response elements in the HPV genome, and some reports have demonstrated an increase in transcription of oncogenic HPV after exposure to estrogenic substances or progesterone.[46-48] Estrogen and progesterone increase the levels of apoptosis induced by HPV-16 E2 and E7 proteins, an effect that can be blocked by the estrogen receptor antagonist 3-hydroxytamoxifen or the anti-progesterone RU486.[49] In vivo, chronic estrogen exposure has been shown to stimulate the development of squamous cell vaginal and cervical carcinomas in HPV-16 transgenic mice.[50] In another strain of transgenic mice harboring HPV-18 E6 and E7 sequences, exposure to estradiol was associated with an increase in E6 and E7 transcripts and a higher frequency of dysplastic lesions of the lower genital tract compared with a control group of nontransgenic mice.[51]

Immunity and human papillomavirus. The immune response after anogenital exposure to HPV is complex, although much has been learned in the last several years in concert with the quest for an effective HPV vaccine. IgG and IgA antibodies against HPV capsid antigens and, less commonly, E proteins, have been identified in the peripheral blood and cervical secretions of women after infection. Seroconversion typically occurs months after exposure to HPV, and the duration of detectable antibody response varies considerably.[52] Although there does not appear to be significant serologic cross-reactivity between different HPV types, HPV-16 variants seem to have the same seroreactivity. This finding is important given the increasing number of type-specific HPV variants that are being detected in different populations.[53]

However, not all individuals mount an immune response. Immunity may be related to HPV type, whether the exposure is transient or of long duration and an individual's immune competence. The degree of protection against subsequent infection or progression to cancer afforded by the presence of anti-HPV antibodies is not well studied.[54,55] Most infections with HPV are transient. Persistent infections are more common after infection with oncogenic HPV types and high viral loads.[56,57]

It is also likely that host genetic background influences the persistence and perhaps risk of infection with HPV. Humoral, cellular, and innate immune responses may each participate in the susceptibility to infection with HPV and progression to malignancy.[58] Some studies have suggested a role for the major histocompatibility complex (MHC) and risk of developing preinvasive and invasive cervical lesions. The genes for MHC class I (i.e., HLA-A, HLA-B, and HLA-C in humans) and class II (i.e., HLA-DR, HLA-DQ and HLA-DP in humans) molecules are a group of polymorphic genes that encode proteins necessary for the presentation of antigenic peptides to cytotoxic and helper T cells. Polymorphisms in MHC class I and class II genes have been associated with positive and negative risks of cervical neoplasia. A protective effect of HLA class II *DRB1*13/DBQ1*0603* alleles is the most consistent HLA finding in the literature.[59-61]

The association between cervical neoplasia and certain HLA phenotypes has not been consistent. In particular, increased risks of cancer associated with specific HLA gene polymorphisms have often varied with the population studied. In some instances, multiple alleles from different HLA haplotypes appeared necessary before an increased risk of cervical cancer could be demonstrated.[62]

Some of these differences may be explained by geographic variations in HPV-16 E6 polymorphisms. These E6 variants may be associated with differences in oncogenicity and aggressiveness of invasive cancer. There is evidence that HLA phenotypes may recognize the E6 variants with different efficiencies and that the interplay between population-based HLA phenotypes and HPV variants could account for differences in HLA risks described among different populations.[63]

Many HPV proteins are capable of eliciting a lymphoproliferative response. E6- and E7-specific cytotoxic T lymphocytes have been detected in the blood of women with high-grade cervical dysplasia and infiltrating cervical cancers.[64,65] In humans, an impaired immune system, such as after renal transplantation[66] or in association with lupus,[67] is associated with a higher prevalence of HPV infection and a greater tendency for progression to cancer. This relationship is especially true in women infected with HIV. In these women the severity of immune dysfunction correlates with the persistence of HPV infection and the development of cervical cancer has been considered as an indication of progression to acquired immunodeficiency syndrome (AIDS).[68]

One study[69] showed that HPV-16 seropositivity rates did not differ significantly between HIV-positive and HIV-negative women after controlling for other known risk factors. In the HIV-positive cohort studied, the baseline rate of cervical infection with HPV-16 was only 5%, suggesting that the modern use of antiretroviral agents allows for satisfactory control of cervical HPV infection in most cases.

What is the state of vaccine development against human papillomavirus?
Preventative vaccines. Efforts to develop a preventative HPV vaccine have focused on creation of a humoral immune response after exposure to viral capsid proteins, typically the major capsid protein L1. A major advance in vaccine development was the observation that, when expressed in eukaryotic cells, L1 protein self-assembles into particles that closely resemble authentic virons.[70,71] These virus-like particles are noninfectious and contain no oncogenic HPV DNA, and large quantities can be generated using recombinant techniques (Fig. 4-3). Parenteral administration of HPV-16 L1 virus-like particles is well tolerated and reliably induces anti-HPV-16 antibodies.[72]

A multicenter clinical trial enrolling females between the ages of 16 and 23 years demonstrated that an HPV-16 L1 vaccine is able to prevent infection with HPV-16 and the development of HPV-16-associated

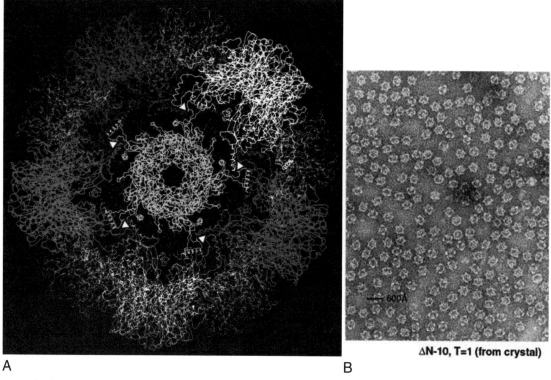

Figure 4–3. A, The human papillomavirus (HPV) late protein L1 forms the pentameric assembly unit of the viral capsid shell. **B,** Recombinant HPV-16 L1 pentamers assemble in vitro into capsid-like structures. These small, virus-like particles are easily obtained from L1 expressed in *Escherichia coli*, which makes them attractive candidate components of papillomavirus vaccines. (From Chen XS, Garcea RL, Goldberg I, et al: Structure of small virus-like particles assembled from the L1 protein of human papillomavirus 16. Mol Cell 2000;5:557-567.) See also Color Figure 4-3A.

cervical dysplasia.[73] By preventing persistent infection with HPV-16, the vaccine may also have the benefit of reducing the risk of sexual transmission of HPV-16 in sexually active individuals.

Because only about 50% of cervical cancers contain HPV-16 DNA sequences, a multivalent vaccine providing immunity against HPV-18 infection and, ideally, against HPV types 31, 33, and 45 could prevent more than 80% of cervical cancers. Many practical issues remain unanswered, including the long-term protection afforded by HPV vaccines, the best time to offer vaccination, and the effectiveness of HPV vaccination in male subjects.[74]

Therapeutic vaccines. Expression of HPV E6 and E7 viral oncoproteins is required for maintaining the growth of cervical cancer cells, a fact that has driven the quest for therapeutic vaccines. The goals of therapeutic vaccination include eliminating or preventing the metastasis of invasive cancer, causing regression of preinvasive lesions or condylomas, and preventing the progression of low-grade lesions to in situ or invasive carcinomas.

E6 and E7 oncoproteins, which are the focus of many therapeutic vaccines, may act as tumor-specific antigens, cooperating with the immune system in animal models of tumor rejection or progression.[75-77] Unfortunately, in humans, the wild-type E7 protein is not a highly effective inducer of a cytotoxic T-cell response. E7 vaccines with enhanced immunogenicity have been developed using a variety of strategies, including creation of L1/E7 chimeric viral-like proteins capable of inducing neutralizing L1 antibodies and E7-specific T cells,[78] the use of dendritic cells pulsed with HPV epitopes,[79] and the use of synthetic E7 gene sequences that yield higher amounts of E7 protein.[80]

Several small trials of vaccination of cervical cancer patients with E6 or E7, or both, proteins or nucleic acid sequences have been completed or are underway. For now, vaccination appears safe and, in some instances, immunogenic. Whether results from these trials will eventually lead to larger studies demonstrating the clinical efficacy of therapeutic vaccines is unknown.[81-83]

What are the common non–human papillomavirus disturbances found in cervical cancers? Cancer is a genetic disease, and the development of a malignant phenotype normally occurs after a series of genetic insults. This may lead to chromosome abnormalities, altered expression of growth factors or their receptors, disturbances in tumor suppressor gene function, or amplification of cellular oncogenes. Aside from the nearly universal expression of HPV E6 and E7 proteins in cervical cancers, additional genetic insults, although common, do not display a particular theme. Observed molecular disturbances in cervical cancers probably reflect a selective growth advantage of clones that have acquired one or more mutations downstream of the transforming properties of HPV E6 and E7. Some of these alterations are related to signaling pathways tied to cell proliferation, differentiation, and perhaps even to metastatic potential and responsiveness to radiation therapy. The next section briefly reviews some of the genetic alterations identified in cervical cancers that are less stringently associated with the direct effects of HPV oncoproteins.

Chromosomal abnormalities. Structural and numeric chromosome abnormalities are commonly identified in cervical cancers and cell lines immortalized with HPV DNA. Derangement in chromosomal integrity appears to be an early event in the pathogenesis of cervical neoplasia, based on studies of premalignant lesions and cultured epithelial cells. Some reports suggest that specific chromosomal disturbances may be linked to progression from preinvasive to invasive carcinoma or transformation from mortal to immortalized phenotypes.[84,85]

The pathogenesis of genetic and chromosomal instabilities in cervical cancer is unknown but is unlikely to arise in response to a common insult. Genetic and chromosomal instabilities have been linked to pathogenic effects of HPV-16 E6 and E7 oncoproteins, with reports suggesting possible interactions of these oncoproteins with mitotic spindles and centromeres.[86]

Chromosomal sites displaying recurrent losses in cervical cancers have included arms 3p, 6p, 11q, 17p, and 18q.[87-89] A number of tumor suppressor genes have been mapped to these chromosome arms, but deletions or alterations in specific genes have not been identified with consistency. Two studies[89,90] have suggested an association between loss of 18q and a poor prognosis, although the mechanism underlying this observation remains unknown.

Signal transduction modulators in cervical cancer. Signal transduction is often used to describe the biochemical interaction between various intracellular (e.g., membrane, cytoplasm) and extracellular compartments of the cell. This process works in a coordinated sequence to regulate the cell cycle, cell-cell interactions, movement, and response to the surrounding microenvironment (Fig. 4-4). Disturbances in signal transduction are frequently observed in human cancers. Translational research in this field has led to the development of new classes of therapeutic agents used to treat cancer.[91] Components of signal transduction that have been most extensively studied in cervical cancer include the epidermal growth factor (EGF) family of cell-surface receptors.

Epidermal growth factor and HER2/NEU receptors. Epidermal growth factor receptor (EGFR) and the related receptor HER2/NEU are transmembrane glycoproteins belonging to the receptor tyrosine kinase family. The ligands for EGFR are EGF and transforming growth factor-α (TGF-α). EGFR is involved in the regulation of several key cellular processes, including cell proliferation, survival, adhesion, migration, and differentiation. Overexpression of the EGFR results in cellular transformation and tumor development in vitro and in vivo. EGFR is expressed in a large proportion of cervical carcinomas but is also found in normal and premalignant lesions.[92] Moderate or strong expression

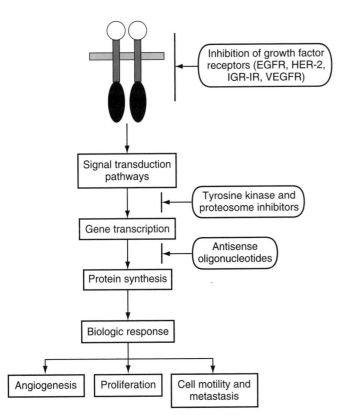

Figure 4–4. Signal transduction works in a coordinated sequence to regulate the cell cycle, cell-cell interactions, movement, and response to the surrounding microenvironment. Strategies aimed at targeting the signaling network are being investigated in women with cervical cancer.

of EGFR is seen more often in malignant cervical lesions.[93] Some,[94,95] but not all,[96] studies have suggested that the expression of EGFR correlates with aggressiveness of cervical carcinoma.

The *HER2/NEU* gene also encodes for a transmembrane glycoprotein with 78% homology to the intracytoplasmic domain of the EGFR. HER2/NEU is a ligandless receptor and exerts its function through formation of heterodimers with other EGFRs.[97] The role of HER2/NEU in cervical cancer is not clear. As is the case with EGFR, some,[98,99] but not all,[100] reports have suggested that amplification of the *HER2/NEU* oncogene is involved in the pathogenesis or biologic behavior of cervical cancer. HER2/NEU protein can be measured in the serum of some patients with cervical cancer. In one report,[101] rising levels of HER2/NEU protein correlated with a more favorable response to therapy compared with patients with decreased or stable levels of HER2/NEU, suggesting that transmembrane portions of HER2/NEU shed during therapy might indicate a more effective destruction of cancer cells.

EGFR and HER2/NEU have become targets for anticancer drug development, and several inhibitors of these receptors are in development or undergoing clinical trials, including the treatment of patients with cervical cancer.

Insulin-like growth factor family and receptors. The insulin-like growth factor (IGF) system comprises a complex network of ligands (IGF-1 and IGF-2), their cognate receptors, IGF-binding proteins (IGFBPs), and IGFBP proteases.[102] Although multiple receptors for the IGFs have been identified, it appears that most of the effects of IGF-1 are mediated through the IGF-1 receptor (IGF-1R), a tyrosine kinase that resembles the insulin receptor. Perturbations in each level of the IGF axis have been implicated in cancer formation and progression in various cell types.[103]

Human cervical cancer cell lines and normal ectocervical epithelial cells express IGF-2 and IGF-1R.[104] The IGF-1R plays key roles in cellular transformation, in maintaining the malignant phenotype, and in cell survival. In vitro, IGF-1R may cooperate with HPV E7-induced transformation and protection from apoptosis.[105] In vitro, downregulation of IGF-1R by antisense RNA can reverse the transformed phenotype of human cervical cancer cells harboring oncogenic HPVs.[106] Tumorigenesis is impaired in nude mice inoculated with cervical cancer cell lines harboring an antisense IGF-1R plasmid. Although there may be a molecular basis for targeting IGF-1R as a potential treatment for cervical cancer, there are no reports of testing this therapeutic approach in humans.

Angiogenesis modulation. Angiogenesis, the formation of new blood vessels from the existing vascular network, is essential for continued tumor growth and metastasis. Tumor vascularity has been reported to be a significant prognostic factor in cervical cancer in some studies.[107,108] Many genes and proteins are involved in angiogenesis, and two—vascular endothelial growth factor (VEGF) and cyclooxygenase-2 (COX-2)—have

been the focus of research in several studies of cervical cancer.

Vascular endothelial growth factor. VEGF is upregulated in response to hypoxia and plays a pivotal role in the development of new blood vessels. VEGF protein and RNA expression have been examined in several studies of cervical cancer. VEGF mRNA was upregulated in cervical cancers compared with normal cervical tissue[109] and was associated with deep stromal invasion and metastasis in another small study.[110]

Some studies have suggested a correlation between VEGF protein expression and prognosis,[95,111] but others have concluded that VEGF protein expression has no prognostic value.[112,113] Because there is no recognized standard for assessing VEGF expression (the extent of tumor staining and the intensity of staining have been used), determining the role of VEGF in the biologic behavior of cervical carcinoma will require much more investigation.[114] Phase II clinical trials using monoclonal antibodies to VEGF are being conducted.

Cyclooxygenase-2 expression. COX-2 is encoded by an early-response gene *(PTGS2)* involved in angiogenesis, and overexpression of COX-2 has been linked to the pathogenesis of several types of cancer. COX-2 expression is induced by many different stimuli, including hypoxia and cytokines. Increased COX-2 expression in cervical cancers has been associated with poor survival and has been linked to resistance of the primary tumor to radiation therapy and neoadjuvant chemotherapy.[115,116] Increased COX-2 expression is also associated with a higher risk of lymph node metastasis,[113] suggesting that the poorer survival seen in women with cervical cancer may not entirely be caused by resistance of the primary cancer to chemoradiation therapy. The potential benefit of COX-2 inhibitors in the treatment of locally advanced cervical cancer is an area of active investigation.

What is the molecular biology of vulvar cancer?

Invasive carcinoma of the vulva is an uncommon disease, accounting for 3% to 5% of cancers of the female genital tract. Most cancers are derived from squamous epithelium, with melanoma, adenocarcinoma, and Paget's disease accounting for most other cell types. The molecular biology of vulvar cancer has not been thoroughly studied, but evidence from many studies suggests that most squamous neoplasias of the vulva evolve along pathways similar to those found in squamous cell cancer of the cervix. Women with vulvar and cervical cancers share many of the same risk factors[117,118] including smoking, a history of genital warts or other sexually transmitted diseases, and immune dysfunction.

What evidence suggests that vulvar cancer may arise from two different pathways? Vulvar cancer can be divided into two broad groups with possible different molecular mechanisms (Fig. 4-5).[119,120] One group is

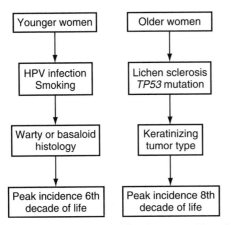

Figure 4–5. Two pathways for the development of invasive vulvar cancer.

characterized by older women (55 to 85 years) who typically develop a keratinizing cancer that is often associated with a prior history of lichen sclerosis or other squamous vulvar dermatoses. These cancers have a high frequency of *TP53* gene mutations, and HPV DNA is often absent, indicating that carcinogenesis may develop through mechanisms distinct from the obligatory relationship between HPV and cervical cancer. In some reports,[121,122] women with HPV-negative tumors or cancers harboring *TP53* point mutations were at increased risk for recurrence and death from vulvar cancer compared with women with HPV-positive tumors or tumors retaining wild-type *TP53*.

The other group of cancers is usually seen in younger women (35 to 65 years old), is often basaloid or warty in appearance, tends to be less invasive, and is associated with a high frequency of detectable oncogenic HPV DNA. Smoking and a history of sexually transmitted diseases are more common in this group of patients.[123,124]

As is the case for cervical cancer, some studies of vulvar cancer have identified disturbances or alterations in cell-cycle regulators, signal transduction modulators, and angiogenesis modulators.

What disturbances have been identified in tumor suppressor and cell cycle regulatory genes in vulvar cancer? *RB1* and *CDKN2A* (formerly designated p16[INK4] and encoding a protein that regulates cyclin D1, an oncoprotein) tumor suppressor genes and the retinoblastoma-related proteins RBL2 (formerly Rb2 or p130) and CDKN1B (formerly KIP1 or P27KIP1) may play important roles in the pathogenesis and progression of vulvar neoplasia. The decrease of expression of these tumor suppressor proteins causes cell proliferation and progression of disease from benign through premalignant to malignant conditions of the vulva.[125,126]

Abnormal cyclin D1 expression is associated with a greater depth of invasion and in combination with loss of RB1 expression may represent an early stage of malignant transformation in vulvar disease.[127] PTEN, which encodes a dual protein and lipid phosphatase, is a tumor suppressor gene located at chromosome 10q23.

This gene affects transcription, translation, and apoptosis and is mutated in a variety of malignancies, including endometrial cancer. *PTEN* mutations are often present in tumor tissue from patients with metastatic disease. *PTEN* mutations were detected in one small study of vulvar carcinomas and were also identified in dysplastic vulvar mucosa, suggesting that *PTEN* mutation may be an early event in vulvar carcinogenesis.[128]

Topoisomerase II is an enzyme that exerts an important role in DNA topology, repair, and replication by breaking and rejoining the DNA double helix. The isoform topoisomerase IIa is a cell cycle–related protein and is expressed in normal and neoplastic cells in the S, G_2, and M phases. Topoisomerase IIa is an applicable proliferation-associated marker in vulvar epithelia and may be a molecular target used to distinguish benign, intraepithelial, and invasive neoplastic epithelial changes.[129]

Signal transduction modulators in vulvar cancer. The two prominent members of the epidermal growth factor receptor family, HER-2/NEU and EGFR, may play a role in vulvar carcinogenesis, although only a few studies have focused on vulvar cancer. In one report, overexpression of HER-2/NEU was associated with lymph node metastasis, suggesting a link between HER-2/NEU and tumor aggressiveness.[130] In another report[131] the A431 vulvar squamous carcinoma cell line was used to demonstrate the efficacy of a murine monoclonal antibody, mAb225, that targets the EGFR. A human/murine chimeric version of this antibody has been produced and shows improved binding and enhanced antitumor activity against human tumor xenografts, with elimination of well-established tumors. This antibody, known as C225, is undergoing evaluation in clinical trials for head and neck cancers, colorectal cancer, and pancreatic cancer.[132]

Angiogenesis modulation in vulvar cancer. Correlations among high VEGF expression, microvessel density, and progression of vulvar cancer have been reported and appear to be associated with worse overall survival.[133,134] In one report, serum concentrations of VEGF were markedly elevated in patients with vulvar cancer compared with healthy female controls and correlated with a significantly shorter disease-free period and a decreased overall survival.[135]

CD44 is a cell adhesion molecule that binds extracellular matrix and is involved in angiogenesis. CD44 isoforms arising from alternative mRNA splicing are implicated in tumor metastases. Patients with vulvar cancer whose tumors express isoform CD44v6 or CD44v3 may have more aggressive cancers.[136,137]

Although information on the molecular biology of vulvar cancer is still emerging, existing studies provide some insight into the interactions among cellular growth, regulatory proteins, angiogenesis factors, and viral oncogenes in the progression of this disease. The significance of these studies, especially as related to biologic behavior and prognosis, is limited by the rarity of the disease and the potential biases inherent in the analysis of archived tissue specimens.

References

1. Munoz N, Bosch FX, de Sanjose S, et al: Epidemiologic classification of HPV types associated with cervical cancer. International Agency for Research on Cancer Multicenter Cervical Cancer Study Group. N Engl J Med 2003;348:518-527.
2. zur Hausen H: Papillomaviruses and cancer: From basic studies to clinical application. Nat Rev Cancer 2002;2:342-350.
3. Choo KB, Pan CC, Han SH: Integration of human papillomavirus type 16 into cellular DNA of cervical carcinoma: Preferential deletion of the E2 gene and invariable retention of the long control region and the E6/E7 open reading frames. Virology 1987;161:259-261.
4. Ziegert C, Wentzensen N, Vinokurova S, et al: A comprehensive analysis of HPV integration loci in anogenital lesions combining transcript and genome-based amplification techniques. Oncogene 2003;22:3977-3984.
5. Tonon SA, Picconi MA, Bos PD, et al: Physical status of the E2 human papilloma virus 16 viral gene in cervical preneoplastic and neoplastic lesions. J Clin Virol 2001;21:129-134.
6. Wentzensen N, Ridder R, Klaes R, et al: Characterization of viral-cellular fusion transcripts in a large series of HPV16 and 18 positive anogenital lesions. Oncogene 2002;21:419-426.
7. Werness BA, Levine AJ, Howley PM: Association of human papillomavirus types 16 and 18 E6 proteins with p53. Science 1990;248:76-79.
8. Scheffner M, Werness BA, Huibregtse JM, et al: The E6 oncoprotein encoded by human papillomavirus types 16 and 18 promotes the degradation of p53. Cell 1990;63:1129-1136.
9. Klingelhutz AJ, Foster SA, McDougall JK: Telomerase activation by the E6 gene product of human papillomavirus type 16. Nature 1996;380:79-82.
10. Chellappan S, Kraus VB, Kroger B, et al: Adenovirus E1A, simian virus 40 tumor antigen, and human papillomavirus E7 protein share the capacity to disrupt the interaction between the transcription factor E2F and the retinoblastoma gene product. Proc Natl Acad Sci U S A 1992;89:4549-4553.
11. Lee DK, Kim BC, Kim IY, et al: The human papilloma virus E7 oncoprotein inhibits transforming growth factor-beta signaling by blocking binding of the Smad complex to its target sequence. J Biol Chem 2002;277:38557-38564.
12. Stoppler MC, Ching K, Stoppler H, et al: Natural variants of the human papillomavirus type 16 E6 protein differ in their abilities to alter keratinocyte differentiation and to induce p53 degradation. J Virol 1996;70:6987-6993.
13. Zehbe I, Wilander E, Delius H, Tommasino M: Human papillomavirus 16 E6 variants are more prevalent in invasive cervical carcinoma than the prototype. Cancer Res 1998;58:829-833.
14. Hu G, Liu W, Hanania EG, et al: Suppression of tumorigenesis by transcription units expressing the antisense E6 and E7 messenger RNA (mRNA) for the transforming proteins of the human papilloma virus and the sense mRNA for the retinoblastoma gene in cervical carcinoma cells. Cancer Gene Ther 1995;2:19-32.
15. Wilson VG, West M, Woytek K, Rangasamy D: Papillomavirus E1 proteins: Form, function, and features. Virus Genes 2002;24:275-290.
16. Romanczuk H, Howley PM: Disruption of either the E1 or the E2 regulatory gene of human papillomavirus type 16 increases viral immortalization capacity. Proc Natl Acad Sci U S A 1992;89:3159-3163.
17. Goodwin EC, DiMaio D: Repression of human papillomavirus oncogenes in HeLa cervical carcinoma cells causes the orderly reactivation of dormant tumor suppressor pathways. Proc Natl Acad Sci U S A 2000;97:12513-12518.
18. Doorbar J, Ely S, Sterling J, et al: Specific interaction between HPV-16 E1-E4 and cytokeratins results in collapse of the epithelial cell intermediate filament network. Nature 1991;352:824-827.
19. Ashmole I, Gallimore PH, Roberts S: Identification of conserved hydrophobic C-terminal residues of the human papillomavirus type 1 E1/E4 protein necessary for E4 oligomerisation in vivo. Virology 1998;240:221-231.
20. Tsai TC, Chen SL: The biochemical and biological functions of human papillomavirus type 16 E5 protein. Arch Virol 2003;148:1445-1453.

21. Fehrmann F, Laimins LA: Human papillomaviruses: Targeting differentiating epithelial cells for malignant transformation. Oncogene 2003;22:5201-5207.
22. Stoler MH: Human papillomaviruses and cervical neoplasia: A model for carcinogenesis. Int J Gynecol Pathol 2000;19:16-28.
23. Demeter LM, Stoler MH, Broker TR, Chow LT: Induction of proliferating cell nuclear antigen in differentiated keratinocytes of human papillomavirus-infected lesions. Hum Pathol 1994;25:343-348.
24. Richardson H, Kelsall G, Tellier P, et al: The natural history of type-specific human papillomavirus infections in female university students. Cancer Epidemiol Biomarkers Prev 2003;12:485-490.
25. Franco EL, Villa LL, Sobrinho JP, et al: Epidemiology of acquisition and clearance of cervical human papillomavirus infection in women from a high-risk area for cervical cancer. J Infect Dis 1999;180:1415-1423.
26. Magnusson PK, Sparen P, Gyllensten UB: Genetic link to cervical tumours. Nature 1999;400:29-30.
27. Naguib SM, Lundin FE Jr, Davis HJ: Relation of various epidemiologic factors to cervical cancer as determined by a screening program. Obstet Gynecol 1966;28:451-459.
28. Winkelstein W: Smoking and cancer of the uterine cervix: Hypothesis. Am J Epidemiol 1977;106:257-259.
29. Slattery ML, Robison LM, Schuman KL, et al: Cigarette smoking and exposure to passive smoke are risk factors for cervical cancer. JAMA 1989;261:1593-1598.
30. Castle PE, Wacholder S, Lorincz AT, et al: A prospective study of high-grade cervical neoplasia risk among human papillomavirus-infected women. J Natl Cancer Inst 2002;94:1406-1414.
31. Hildesheim A, Herrero R, Castle PE, et al: HPV co-factors related to the development of cervical cancer: Results from a population-based study in Costa Rica. Br J Cancer 2001;84:1219-1226.
32. Perry IH, Ginzton LL: The development of tumors in female mice treated with 1:2:5:6 dibenzanthracene and theelin. Am J Cancer 1937;29:680-704.
33. Fusco G: Cancro sperimentale dell'utero e della vagina. Arch Ostet Gynecol 1932;19:15-44, 467-469.
34. Chu EW, Herrold K McD, Wood TA: Cytopathological changes of the uterine cervix of Syrian hamsters after painting with DMBA, benzo(a)pyrene, and tobacco tar. Acta Cytol 1962;6:376-384.
35. Vellios F, Griffin J: The pathogenesis of dimethylbenzanthracene-induced carcinoma of the cervix in rats. Cancer Res 1957;17:364-366.
36. Sasson IM, Haley NJ, Hoffmann D, et al: Cigarette smoking and neoplasia of the uterine cervix: Smoke constituents in cervical mucus. N Engl J Med 1985;312:315-316.
37. Waggoner S, Wang X: Effect of nicotine on proliferation of normal, malignant, and human papillomavirus-transformed human cervical cells. Gynecol Oncol 1994;55:91-95.
38. Prokopczyk B, Cox J, Hu P, et al: Identification of tobacco-specific carcinogens in the cervical mucus of smokers and non-smokers. J Natl Cancer Inst 1997;89:868-873.
39. Prokopczyk B, Trushin N, Leszczynska J, et al: Human cervical tissue metabolizes the tobacco-specific nitrosamine, 4-(methylnitrosamino)-1-(3-pyridyl)-1-butanone, via α-hydroxylation and carbonyl reduction pathways. Carcinogenesis 2001;22:107-114.
40. Melikian AA, Wang X, Waggoner S, et al: Comparative response of normal and of human papillomavirus-16 immortalized human epithelial cervical cells to benzo[a]pyrene. Oncol Rep 1999;6:1371-1376.
41. Smith JS, Green J, Berrington de Gonzalez A, et al: Cervical cancer and use of hormonal contraceptives: A systematic review. Lancet 2003;361:1159-1167.
42. International Agency for Research of Cancer: IARC Monographs on the Evaluation of the Carcinogenic Risk to Humans, vol 72. Hormonal Contraception and Postmenopausal Hormonal Therapy. Lyon, International Agency for Research on Cancer, 1999.
43. Hildesheim A, Schiffman MH, Gravitt PE, et al: Persistence of type-specific human papillomavirus infection among cytologically normal women. J Infect Dis 1994;169:235-240.
44. Moreno V, Bosch FX, Munoz N, et al, for the International Agency for Research on Cancer. Multicentric Cervical Cancer Study Group: Effect of oral contraceptives on risk of cervical

cancer in women with human papillomavirus infection: The IARC multicentric case-control study. Lancet 2002;359:1085-1092.

45. Moodley M, Moodley J, Chetty R, Herrington CS: The role of steroid contraceptive hormones in the pathogenesis of invasive cervical cancer: A review. Int J Gynecol Cancer 2003;13:103-110.

46. de Villiers EM: Relationship between steroid hormone contraceptives and HPV, cervical intraepithelial neoplasia and cervical carcinoma. Int J Cancer 2003;103:705-708.

47. Yuan F, Auborn K, James C: Altered growth and viral gene expression in human papillomavirus type 16-containing cancer cell lines treated with progesterone. Cancer Invest 1999;17:19-29.

48. von Knebel Doeberitz M, Spitkovsky D, Ridder R: Interactions between steroid hormones and viral oncogenes in the pathogenesis of cervical cancer. Verh Dtsch Ges Pathol 1997;81:233-239.

49. Webster K, Taylor A, Gaston K: Oestrogen and progesterone increase the levels of apoptosis induced by the human papillomavirus type 16 E2 and E7 proteins. J Gen Virol 2001;82(Pt 1):201-213.

50. Arbeit JM, Howley PM, Hanahan D: Chronic estrogen-induced cervical and vaginal squamous carcinogenesis in human papillomavirus type 16 transgenic mice. Proc Natl Acad Sci U S A 1996;93:2930-2935.

51. Park JS, Rhyu JW, Kim CJ, et al: Neoplastic change of squamocolumnar junction in uterine cervix and vaginal epithelium by exogenous estrogen in HPV-18 URR E6/E7 transgenic mice. Gynecol Oncol 2003;89:360-368.

52. Onda T, Carter JJ, Koutsky LA, et al: Characterization of IgA response among women with incident HPV 16 infection. Virology 2003;312:213-221.

53. Cheng G, Icenogle JP, Kirnbauer R, Hubbert NL, et al: Divergent human papillomavirus type 16 variants are serologically cross-reactive. J Infect Dis 1995;172:1584-1587.

54. Sun Y, Eluf-Neto J, Bosch FX, et al: Serum antibodies to human papillomavirus 16 proteins in women from Brazil with invasive cervical carcinoma. Cancer Epidemiol Biomarkers Prev 1999;8:935-940.

55. Carter JJ, Koutsky LA, Hughes JP, et al: Comparison of human papillomavirus types 16, 18, and 6 capsid antibody responses following incident infection. J Infect Dis 2000;181:1911-1919.

56. Dalstein V, Riethmuller D, Pretet JL, et al: Persistence and load of high-risk HPV are predictors for development of high-grade cervical lesions: A longitudinal French cohort study. Int J Cancer 2003;106:396-403.

57. Hernandez-Hernandez DM, Ornelas-Bernal L, Guido-Jimenez M, et al: Association between high-risk human papillomavirus DNA load and precursor lesions of cervical cancer in Mexican women. Gynecol Oncol 2003;90:310-317.

58. Wang SS, Hildesheim A: Viral and host factors in human papillomavirus persistence and progression. J Natl Cancer Inst Monogr 2003;31:35-40.

59. Wang SS, Hildesheim A, Gao X, et al: Comprehensive analysis of human leukocyte antigen class I alleles and cervical neoplasia in 3 epidemiologic studies. J Infect Dis 2002;186:598-605.

60. Hildesheim A, Wang SS: Host and viral genetics and risk of cervical cancer: A review. Virus Res 2002;89:229-240.

61. Madeleine MM, Brumback B, Cushing-Haugen KL, et al: Human leukocyte antigen class II and cervical cancer risk: A population-based study. J Infect Dis 2002;186:1565-1574.

62. Glew SS, Duggan-Keen M, Ghosh AK, et al: Lack of association of HLA polymorphisms with human papillomavirus-related cervical cancer. Hum Immunol 1993;37:157-164.

63. Zehbe I, Tachezy R, Mytilineos J, et al: Human papillomavirus 16 E6 polymorphisms in cervical lesions from different European populations and their correlation with human leukocyte antigen class II haplotypes. Int J Cancer 2001;94:711-716.

64. Nimako M, Fiander AN, Wilkinson GW, et al: Human papillomavirus-specific cytotoxic T lymphocytes in patients with cervical intraepithelial neoplasia grade III. Cancer Res 1997;57:4855-4861.

65. Evans EM, Man S, Evans AS, Borysiewicz LK: Infiltration of cervical cancer tissue with human papillomavirus-specific cytotoxic T-lymphocytes. Cancer Res 1997;57:2943-2950.

66. Sillman FH, Sentovich S, Shaffer D: Ano-genital neoplasia in renal transplant patients. Ann Transplant 1997;2:59-66.

67. Dhar JP, Kmak D, Bhan R, et al: Abnormal cervicovaginal cytology in women with lupus: A retrospective cohort study. Gynecol Oncol 2001;82:4-6.

68. Ahdieh L, Munoz A, Vlahov D, et al: Cervical neoplasia and repeated positivity of human papillomavirus infection in human immunodeficiency virus-seropositive and -seronegative women. Am J Epidemiol 2000;151:1148-1157.

69. Viscidi RP, Ahdieh-Grant L, Clayman B, et al: Serum immunoglobulin G response to human papillomavirus type 16 virus-like particles in human immunodeficiency virus (HIV)-positive and risk-matched HIV-negative women. Infect Dis 2003;187:194-205.

70. Kirnbauer R, Booy F, Cheng N, et al: Papillomavirus L1 major capsid protein self-assembles into virus-like particles that are highly immunogenic. Proc Natl Acad Sci U S A 1992;89:12180-12184.

71. Chen XS, Garcea RL, Goldberg I, et al: Structure of small virus-like particles assembled from the L1 protein of human papillomavirus 16. Mol Cell 2000;5:557-567.

72. Harro CD, Pang YY, Roden RB, et al: Safety and immunogenicity trial in adult volunteers of a human papillomavirus 16 L1 virus-like particle vaccine. J Natl Cancer Inst 2001;93:284-292.

73. Koutsky LA, Ault KA, Wheeler CM, et al, for the Proof of Principle Study Investigators: A controlled trial of a human papillomavirus type 16 vaccine. N Engl J Med 2002;347:1645-1651.

74. Goldie SJ, Grima D, Kohli M, et al: A comprehensive natural history model of HPV infection and cervical cancer to estimate the clinical impact of a prophylactic HPV-16/18 vaccine. Int J Cancer 2003;106:896-904.

75. Frazer IH, Leippe DM, Dunn LA, et al: Immunological responses in human papillomavirus 16 E6/E7-transgenic mice to E7 protein correlate with the presence of skin disease. Cancer Res 1995;55:2635-2639.

76. Chen L, Mizuno MT, Singhal MC, et al: Induction of cytotoxic T lymphocytes specific for a syngeneic tumor expressing the E6 oncoprotein of human papillomavirus type 16. J Immunol 1992;148:2617-2621.

77. Chen LP, Thomas EK, Hu SL, et al: Human papillomavirus type 16 nucleoprotein E7 is a tumor rejection antigen. Proc Natl Acad Sci U S A 1991;88:110-114.

78. Jochmus I, Schafer K, Faath S, et al: Chimeric virus-like particles of the human papillomavirus type 16 (HPV 16) as a prophylactic and therapeutic vaccine. Arch Med Res 1999;30:269-274.

79. Ossevoort MA, Feltkamp MC, van Veen KJ, et al: Dendritic cells as carriers for a cytotoxic T-lymphocyte epitope-based peptide vaccine in protection against a human papillomavirus type 16-induced tumor. J Immunother Emphasis Tumor Immunol 1995;18:86-94.

80. Cid-Arregui A, Juarez V, zur Hausen H: A synthetic E7 gene of human papillomavirus type 16 that yields enhanced expression of the protein in mammalian cells and is useful for DNA immunization studies. J Virol 2003;77:4928-4937.

81. Sheets EE, Urban RG, Crum CP, et al: Immunotherapy of human cervical high-grade cervical intraepithelial neoplasia with microparticle-delivered human papillomavirus 16 E7 plasmid DNA. Am J Obstet Gynecol 2003;188:916-926.

82. Steller MA: Cervical cancer vaccines: Progress and prospects. J Soc Gynecol Investig 2002;9:254-264.

83. Galloway DA: Papillomavirus vaccines in clinical trials. Lancet Infect Dis 2003;3:469-475.

84. Heselmeyer K, Schrock E, du Manoir S, et al: Gain of chromosome 3q defines the transition from severe dysplasia to invasive carcinoma of the uterine cervix. Proc Natl Acad Sci U S A 1996;93:479-484.

85. Solinas-Toldo S, Durst M, Lichter P: Specific chromosomal imbalances in human papillomavirus-transfected cells during progression toward immortality. Proc Natl Acad Sci U S A 1997;94:3854-3859.

86. Duensing S, Munger K: The human papillomavirus type 16 E6 and E7 oncoproteins independently induce numerical and structural chromosome instability. Cancer Res 2002;62:7075-7082.

87. Rader JS, Kamarasova T, Huettner PC, et al: Allelotyping of all chromosomal arms in invasive cervical cancer. Oncogene 1996;13:2737-2741.

88. Mullokandov MR, Kholodilov NG, Atkin NB, et al: Genomic alterations in cervical carcinoma: Losses of chromosome heterozygosity and human papilloma virus tumor status. Cancer Res 1996;56:197-205.

89. Harima Y, Sawada S, Nagata K, et al: Chromosome 6p21.2, 18q21.2 and human papilloma virus (HPV) DNA can predict prognosis of cervical cancer after radiotherapy. Int J Cancer 2001;96:286-296.

90. Kersemaekers AM, Kenter GG, Hermans J, et al: Allelic loss and prognosis in carcinoma of the uterine cervix. Int J Cancer 1998;79:411-417.

91. Arteaga C: Targeting HER1/EGFR: A molecular approach to cancer therapy. Semin Oncol 2003;30(Suppl 7):3-14.

92. Lakshmi S, Nair MB, Jayaprakash PG, et al: C-erbB-2 oncoprotein and epidermal growth factor receptor in cervical lesions. Pathobiology 1997;65:163-168.

93. Mathur SP, Mathur RS, Rust PF, Young RC: Human papilloma virus (HPV)-E6/E7 and epidermal growth factor receptor (EGF-R) protein levels in cervical cancer and cervical intraepithelial neoplasia (CIN). Am J Reprod Immunol 2001;46:280-287.

94. Kim YT, Park SW, Kim JW: Correlation between expression of EGFR and the prognosis of patients with cervical carcinoma. Gynecol Oncol 2002;87:84-89.

95. Gaffney DK, Haslam JF, Tsodikov A, et al: Epidermal growth factor receptor (EGFR) and vascular endothelial growth factor (VEGF) negatively affect overall survival in carcinoma of the cervix treated with radiotherapy. Int J Radiat Oncol Biol Phys 2003;56:922-928.

96. Scambia G, Ferrandina G, Distefano M, et al: Epidermal growth factor receptor (EGFR) is not related to the prognosis of cervical cancer. Cancer Lett 1998;123:135-139.

97. Citri A, Skaria KB, Yarden Y: The deaf and the dumb: The biology of ErbB-2 and ErbB-3. Exp Cell Res 2003;284:54-65.

98. Mark HF, Feldman D, Das S, et al: HER-2/neu oncogene amplification in cervical cancer studied by fluorescent in situ hybridization. Genet Test 1999;3:237-242.

99. Nevin J, Laing D, Kaye P, et al: The significance of Erb-b2 immunostaining in cervical cancer. Gynecol Oncol 1999;73:354-358.

100. Ndubisi B, Sanz S, Lu L, et al: The prognostic value of HER-2/neu oncogene in cervical cancer. Ann Clin Lab Sci 1997;27:396-401.

101. Contreras DN, Cobos E, Lox CD: Evaluation of the circulating fraction of the HER-2/neu oncogene in patients with cervical cancer. Eur J Gynaecol Oncol 2002;23:491-495.

102. Yu H, Rohan T: Role of the insulin-like growth factor family in cancer development and progression. J Natl Cancer Inst 2000;92:1472-1489.

103. Grimberg A, Cohen P: Role of insulin-like growth factors and their binding proteins in growth control and carcinogenesis. J Cell Physiol 2000;183:1-9.

104. Steller MA, Delgado CH, Bartels CJ, et al: Overexpression of the insulin-like growth factor-1 receptor and autocrine stimulation in human cervical cancer cells. Cancer Res 1996;56:1761-1765.

105. Steller MA, Zou Z, Schiller JT, Baserga R: Transformation by human papillomavirus 16 E6 and E7: Role of the insulin-like growth factor 1 receptor. Cancer Res 1996;56:5087-5091.

106. Nakamura K, Hongo A, Kodama J, et al: Down-regulation of the insulin-like growth factor I receptor by antisense RNA can reverse the transformed phenotype of human cervical cancer cell lines. Cancer Res 2000;60:760-765.

107. Cooper RA, West CM, Wilks DP, et al: Tumour vascularity is a significant prognostic factor for cervix carcinoma treated with radiotherapy: Independence from tumour radiosensitivity. Br J Cancer 1999;81:354-358.

108. Siracka E, Revesz L, Kovac R, Siracky J: Vascular density in carcinoma of the uterine cervix and its predictive value for radiotherapy. Int J Cancer 1988;41:819-822.

109. Van Trappen PO, Ryan A, Carroll M, et al: A model for co-expression pattern analysis of genes implicated in angiogenesis and tumour cell invasion in cervical cancer. Br J Cancer 2002;87:537-544.

110. Hashimoto I, Kodama J, Seki N, et al: Vascular endothelial growth factor-C expression and its relationship to pelvic lymph node status in invasive cervical cancer. Br J Cancer 2001;85:93-97.

111. Loncaster JA, Cooper RA, Logue JP, et al: Vascular endothelial growth factor (VEGF) expression is a prognostic factor for radiotherapy outcome in advanced carcinoma of the cervix. Br J Cancer 2000;83:620-625.

112. Tjalma W, Weyler J, Weyn B, et al: The association between vascular endothelial growth factor, microvessel density and clinicopathological features in invasive cervical cancer. Eur J Obstet Gynecol Reprod Biol 2000;92:251-257.

113. Kim MH, Seo SS, Song YS, et al: Expression of cyclooxygenase-1 and -2 associated with expression of VEGF in primary cervical cancer and at metastatic lymph nodes. Gynecol Oncol 2003;90:83-90.

114. Lee IJ, Park KR, Lee KK, et al: Prognostic value of vascular endothelial growth factor in stage IB carcinoma of the uterine cervix. Int J Radiat Oncol Biol Phys 2002;54:768-779.

115. Ferrandina G, Lauriola L, Distefano MG, et al: Increased cyclooxygenase-2 expression is associated with chemotherapy resistance and poor survival in cervical cancer patients. J Clin Oncol 2002;20:973-981.

116. Gaffney DK, Holden J, Davis M, et al: Elevated cyclooxygenase-2 expression correlates with diminished survival in carcinoma of the cervix treated with radiotherapy. Int J Radiat Oncol Biol Phys 2001;49:1213-1217.

117. Ferenczy A, Coutlee F, Franco E, Hankins C: Human papillomavirus and HIV coinfection and the risk of neoplasias of the lower genital tract: A review of recent developments. CMAJ 2003;169:431-434.

118. Madeleine MM, Daling JR, Carter JJ, et al: Cofactors with human papillomavirus in a population-based study of vulvar cancer. J Natl Cancer Inst 1997;89:1516-1523.

119. Al-Ghamdi A, Freedman D, Miller D, et al: Vulvar squamous cell carcinoma in young women: A clinicopathologic study of 21 cases. Gynecol Oncol 2002;84:94-101.

120. Hording U, Junge J, Daugaard S, et al: Vulvar squamous cell carcinoma and papillomaviruses: Indications for two different etiologies. Gynecol Oncol 1994;52:241-246.

121. Monk BJ, Burger RA, Lin F, et al: Prognostic significance of human papillomavirus DNA in vulvar carcinoma. Obstet Gynecol 1995;85(Pt 1):709-715.

122. Sliutz G, Schmidt W, Tempfer C, et al: Detection of p53 point mutations in primary human vulvar cancer by PCR and temperature gradient gel electrophoresis. Gynecol Oncol 1997;64:93-98.

123. Rosen C, Malmstrom H: Invasive cancer of the vulva. Gynecol Oncol 1997;65:213-217.

124. Hildesheim A, Han CL, Brinton LA, et al: Human papillomavirus type 16 and risk of preinvasive and invasive vulvar cancer: Results from a seroepidemiological case-control study. Obstet Gynecol 1997;90:748-754.

125. Chan MK, Cheung TH, Chung TK, et al: Expression of p16INK4 and retinoblastoma protein Rb in vulvar lesions of Chinese women. Gynecol Oncol 1998;68:156-161.

126. Zamparelli A, Masciullo V, Bovicelli A, et al: Expression of cell-cycle-associated proteins pRB2/p130 and p27kip in vulvar squamous cell carcinomas. Hum Pathol 2001;32:4-9.

127. Rolfe KJ, Crow JC, Benjamin E, et al: Cyclin D1 and retinoblastoma protein in vulvar cancer and adjacent lesions. Int J Gynecol Cancer 2001;11:381-386.

128. Holway AH, Rieger-Christ KM, Miner WR, et al: Somatic mutation of PTEN in vulvar cancer. Clin Cancer Res 2000;6:3228-3235.

129. Brustmann H, Naude S: Expression of topoisomerase IIalpha, Ki-67, proliferating cell nuclear antigen, p53, and argyrophilic nucleolar organizer regions in vulvar squamous lesions. Gynecol Oncol 2002;86:192-199.

130. Gordinier ME, Steinhoff MM, Hogan JW, et al: S-Phase fraction, p53, and HER-2/neu status as predictors of nodal metastasis in early vulvar cancer. Gynecol Oncol 1997;67:200-202.

131. Mendelsohn J: The epidermal growth factor receptor as a target for cancer therapy. Endocr Relat Cancer 2001;8:3-9.

132. Normanno N, Bianco C, De Luca A, et al: Target-based agents against ErbB receptors and their ligands: A novel approach to cancer treatment. Endocr Relat Cancer 2003;10:1-21.

133. Abulafia O, Triest WE, Sherer DM: Angiogenesis in malignancies of the female genital tract. Gynecol Oncol 1999;72:220-231.
134. Obermair A, Kohlberger P, Bancher-Todesca D, et al: Influence of microvessel density and vascular permeability factor/vascular endothelial growth factor expression on prognosis in vulvar cancer. Gynecol Oncol 1996;63:204-209.
135. Hefler L, Tempfer C, Obermair A, et al: Serum concentrations of vascular endothelial growth factor in vulvar cancer. Clin Cancer Res 1999;5:2806-2809.
136. Rodriguez-Rodriguez L, Sancho-Torres I, Miller Watelet L, et al: Prognostic value of CD44 expression in invasive squamous cell carcinoma of the vulva. Gynecol Oncol 1999;75:34-40.
137. Tempfer C, Sliutz G, Haeusler G, et al: CD44v3 and v6 variant isoform expression correlates with poor prognosis in early-stage vulvar cancer. Br J Cancer 1998;78:1091-1094.

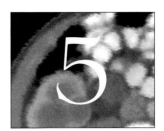

CHAPTER

PREINVASIVE DISEASES OF THE CERVIX, VAGINA, AND VULVA

Grainne Flannelly

 MAJOR CONTROVERSIES

- What is the ideal age range of the population to be screened, and how often should the tests be performed?
- How valid is cervical cytology as a test, and what is the place of new technology in cervical screening programs?
- What screening is recommended for women in high-risk groups?
- Who should be referred for colposcopy?
- Should women with a mildly dysplastic (LoSIL) cervical smear be referred for colposcopy or should the smear be repeated?
- Is mild dysplasia associated with a risk of progression to high-grade disease?
- Which strategy is more efficient?
- Is cytologic surveillance less expensive or associated with less psychological morbidity than immediate colposcopy?
- How should borderline nuclear abnormalities or atypical squamous cells of undetermined significance be managed?
- What is the risk of high-grade cervical intraepithelial neoplasia in women with borderline nuclear abnormalities?
- How should atypical squamous cells of undetermined significance be managed?
- How should cervical intraepithelial neoplasia be treated?
- Who should be treated?
- How should treated women be monitored?
- Are risk factors for recurrence of benefit?
- How long should women be subjected to increased surveillance after treatment?
- What is the role of additional tests in the follow-up period?
- Quality assurance and colposcopy: Who benefits?

This chapter aims to evaluate the screening processes for preinvasive cancer of the cervix, vagina, and vulva and to document current controversies in their management. Each of these areas is dealt with in turn, focusing on their identification, treatment, and follow-up.

MANAGEMENT OF PREINVASIVE DISEASES OF THE CERVIX

Cervical cytology screening programs aim to reduce both the incidence of and mortality from cervical cancer by the detection and effective treatment of preinvasive lesions. In countries where these programs have been well organized, especially in Scandinavia[1,2] and in British Columbia,[3] significant reductions in both mortality and incidence of cervical cancer have resulted. More recently, improvements in the British National Health Service (NHS) Cervical Screening Programme have resulted in a significant reduction in the incidence of invasive cancer of the cervix, from 16 per 100,000 women in 1986 to 9.3 per 100,000 women in 1997. A similar reduction in mortality has resulted, with the rate falling by 7% per year.[4]

Two factors that are of fundamental importance for effective screening of a population are the organization of the program and the validity of the screening test.

Screening programs should be organized in such a way that the target population is adequately identified and "at-risk" individuals in the population are identified and encouraged to avail themselves of screening. There should be adequate facilities for evaluation of smears and for diagnostic confirmation and treatment, with a carefully designed and agreed on referral system and follow-up.[5] Finally, there should be satisfactory quality control in taking the smears, making a diagnosis, providing treatment, and evaluating the effects of the program.

Despite the proved effectiveness of cervical cytology screening, some aspects remain controversial. Considerable differences exist among programs in the definition of the population to be screened and in the frequency with which testing is performed.[6] The place of new technology (including liquid-based cytology) in the screening process, the potential for automated analysis, and the use of human papillomavirus (HPV) testing for selective increased surveillance of high-risk women remain to be determined.[7-10] There has been an increasing focus on quality assurance at all levels of the program, but particularly of colposcopy services, to ensure effective treatment of women with detected cytologic abnormalities, with the goal of preventing invasive cancer and ensuring a prompt return to negative tests.[11-13] Finally, cervical cancer is still a major problem in developing countries where women have access to little or no screening[14-16] and the establishment of relevant and appropriate programs for resource-depleted communities remains a priority for the World Health Organization.[17-20]

Controversies with respect to screening program management

Considerable variation exists between established and proved effective screening programs around the world.[21] The ideal screening program should be acceptable, efficient, and cost-effective[22] and should limit any negative impact on the individual, both physical and psychological.[23] Each individual cervical screening program reflects the expectations of the population as well as its values and resources. In designing protocols, the costs, risks, and side effects of the tests need to be balanced against the expected benefits of early detection and the resultant decrease in disability and lost earnings.

What is the ideal age range of the population to be screened, and how often should the tests be performed?

Age at initiation of screening. Significant variation exists among programs with respect to the age at which cervical screening is started. In most European countries, the starting age is between 20 and 25 years of age. In the Netherlands, cervical screening does not start until the age of 35 years.[24] There is evidence to suggest that teenagers should not undergo cervical screening; the incidence of cervical cancer in teenagers is low,[25] and cervical cytologic screening has not been shown to be effective at reducing the incidence of invasive cancer in women younger than 20 years of age.[26] In addition, the prevalence of transient HPV infection after the commencement of sexual activity is high.[27,28] Cervical screening in this age group may detect prevalent low-grade disease that might have resolved spontaneously if screening were started at a later age.[3] This could result in unnecessary attendances at colposcopy, with the resultant possible negative consequences of increased anxiety and possible overtreatment.

Age at withdrawal from screening. The effectiveness of screening in reducing invasive cancer varies with age; it is greatest in the youngest age groups and least in those older than 70 years.[25] In fact, the reduction in mortality from cervical cancer in women older than 50 years of age is thought by some to be unrelated to the screening process.[29] Biologic factors provide some explanation for this phenomenon, but it is likely that differences in compliance with screening may also be relevant. Women who develop cancer after the age of 55 years are more likely to have deficient screening than younger women.[30] Cervical screening was perceived as essentially a process for younger women and of little relevance to older women in a study of attitudes and perceptions of the screening process in older women who had declined or delayed cervical screening.[31] In addition to compliance, there is evidence that the cervical screening process is less efficient at detecting disease in older women. The detection ratio (number of cancer in situ cases detected per 1000 primary smears) relates both to the sensitivity of the test and to the prevalence of cervical intraepithelial neoplasia (CIN) and has been demonstrated to reach a peak at age 35, decreasing markedly between 35 and 50 years of age, and remaining low thereafter.[32] Selection bias and sampling errors relating to biologic changes in the cervix do not fully explain this phenomenon, and it is likely that a decreasing incidence of CIN after 50 years of age has a contribution to this effect.

In reality, in most screening programs the upper exit age has been assigned arbitrarily, based on the perceived low incidence of CIN in older women.[33] Recent data have questioned the efficacy of screening in women after age 50, with the suggestion that the upper age limit could be reduced to 50 years in well-screened women.[34,35] Early withdrawal of women from the cervical screening program could lead to a substantial reduction of up to 25% in the resources devoted to screening; these resources could then be channeled more effectively into other aspects of health care.[36] However, any such change is likely to increase the overall incidence of cervical cancer unless other steps are taken to compensate.[36] HPV tests may be a useful adjunct, and it has been suggested that an exit screening test combining cervical cytology and HPV testing for high-risk viruses offers the possibility of greater protection for this group of women.[37]

How often should cervical screening tests be performed? The protective effect of cervical screening decreases with the time elapsed since the last smear.[38-41] Attention has focused on the optimal screening interval in an attempt to decrease the incidence of interval cancers. The efficacy of screening according to the screening interval was summarized in a review by the International Agency for Research on Cancer[42]; in the absence of screening, a 20-year-old woman with average risk has a change of about 250 in 10,000 of developing invasive cervical cancer during her lifetime. The percentage reduction in incidence among women age 35 to 64 years is 93.5% with annual screening, 90.8% with screening every 3 years, and 83.6% with screening every 5 years. In a mathematical model, screening at intervals of 3 years retained 97% of the reduction in cervical cancer obtained with annual screening, and this protection was achieved with a significant reduction in cost.[43]

The conclusion is that cervical screening is recommended at least every 3 years from about 20 to 65 years of age.

How valid is cervical cytology as a test, and what is the place of new technology in cervical screening programs? The validity of cervical cytology as a screening tool can be measured by the indices of sensitivity and specificity. Sensitivity is defined as the proportion of persons with a positive test result among those with the disease. Specificity is the proportion of persons with a negative test result among those who are free from the disease. Sensitivity is the best measure of success of screening and indicates the yield. Specificity is the basic measure for disadvantages; poor specificity of the test results in high financial costs and in adverse effects due to false-positive results.

Review of these values for cervical cytology showed an overall sensitivity ranging from 30% to 87% and a specificity of 86% to 99.4%.[8] The sensitivity was slightly lower for mild or moderate dysplasia (78.1%) and slightly higher for severe dysplasia (81.4%) and for invasive carcinoma (82.3%).[44] The relatively poor sensitivity of cervical cytology and resultant false-negative test results has been a cause of concern and traditionally has been compensated for by repeating testing at regular intervals. The incorporation of new technologies into the cervical screening process has been suggested to reduce the incidence of false-negative results, but, because sensitivity and specificity are inversely related, improvement in one of these parameters is associated with a lowering of the other.[45]

Liquid-based cytology. The traditional method for taking a cervical smear involves scraping the cervix and smearing the resultant sample on a glass slide. The interpretation of this test can be difficult due to factors such as air drying of the specimen and the presence of blood and inflammatory exudates that obscure the cells. Liquid-based cytology differs from this conventional technique in that the sample is placed in a liquid that washes the cells, which are then filtered and put on a slide. This procedure has been shown to reduce the percentage of unsatisfactory smears while increasing the detection of high-grade abnormalities.[9,46] This technology has the potential for automated screening[20] and also provides the opportunity for reflex ancillary testing for HPV without the need to take a second test.[47] A possible disadvantage is the increased detection of low-grade abnormalities that may not be clinically relevant, with a consequent increased referral rate for colposcopy. This technology has implications for the cost of screening,[48,49] and its efficacy and cost-effectiveness are currently being studied as part of the NHS Cervical Screening Programme in Great Britain.[50]

Human papillomavirus testing. The epidemiologic pattern of cervical cancer suggests that a sexually transmissible infectious agent might play an important role in the etiology of this disease. It is now widely accepted that HPV is the major infectious agent involved.[51] Specific types, mainly HPV-16 and HPV-18, have been shown to cause the majority of cervical cancers and their high-grade precursor lesions.[51] High-risk HPV DNA can be detected in 99.7% of all invasive cervical cancers.[52] This knowledge has potential applications for prevention and treatment, and clinical trials are currently underway to search for a suitable vaccine.[53] Advances in DNA technology have resulted in the development of commercially available kits that use a hybrid capture technique (HC II); these have been shown to have a 95% sensitivity with a 2.3% positive rate in normal women.[37] The performance of HPV testing in addition to cytology may be a potential adjunct to cervical cytology for primary screening by allowing an increase in screening interval.[54-56] However, the introduction of HPV testing to primary screening is associated with increased cost,[57] and its use for all women has yet to be widely accepted.[58] Selective use of this technology for triaging of women with low-grade cytologic abnormalities for colposcopy[59] or for improving follow-up after treatment[60] may prove a more appropriate application.

Cervical cytology like any screening tool is imperfect. Technological advances may improve the process, but these improvements will incur an increased cost.

What screening is recommended for women in high-risk groups? Within the general population there are defined groups of women who have an increased risk of CIN. Women with renal failure who require dialysis or who undergo renal transplantation have a 5-fold increase in the prevalence of persistence of HPV infection and CIN,[61-63] compared with the general population. These women should have cervical cytology performed at the time of diagnosis, with early referral for colposcopy if there is any abnormality. Women infected with the human immunodeficiency virus (HIV) have an 8-fold increase in the prevalence of CIN.[64] This risk is increased in women with lower CD4 counts.[65] There may be more extensive involvement of the genital tract,[66] and standard treatments for CIN are less effective.[67] Cervical cytology may be relatively insensitive in these women, and current recommendations are for a colposcopic evaluation of the lower genital tract at the time of diagnosis as well as annual cervical cytology testing.[68]

Women with renal failure who need dialysis or transplantation and women with HIV should have a colposcopic assessment at the time of diagnosis, if resources permit, as well as annual cervical cytology screening.

Controversies in Management After an Abnormal Smear

It is only with optimal management after detection of smear abnormalities that the potential of any screening program can be fully realized. The traditional method of assessment was by histologic examination of the tissue obtained by knife cone biopsy.

Colposcopy was introduced in the late 1960s as a diagnostic technique for identifying the probable site of the cytologic abnormality.[69] The ability of colposcopy to discriminate between grades of abnormalities was examined in a meta-analysis of published studies[45]; when the threshold of normal was compared with all cervix abnormalities (atypia, low-grade squamous intraepithelial lesion [SIL], high-grade SIL, cancer), the sensitivity was 96% and the specificity 48%. For the comparison of threshold normal cervix or low-grade SIL with high-grade SIL or cancer, the sensitivity was 85% and the specificity was 69%. Colposcopy is generally an effective means of identifying CIN and obtaining a confirmatory biopsy before treatment.[70] On the other hand, it may result in overtreatment,[71] particularly if combined with diathermy loop excision at the first visit ("see and treat"), and can also cause psychological morbidity.[72-74] Any management policy, therefore, must balance the risks and benefits and should aim to be safe, efficient, and cost-effective. Current controversies in colposcopy relate to referral criteria, methods of treatment and follow-up, and an increased focus on quality assurance and training.

Who should be referred for colposcopy?

Although colposcopy is used worldwide as a secondary event, the threshold for colposcopy referral varies, with colposcopy used as an adjunct to primary screening in some countries. From a public health perspective, this variation in clinical practice relates to the available health care resources as well as the prevalence of disease within a population. Patient expectation, medicolegal considerations, and reimbursement of colposcopists are also factors. There is general agreement that women should be referred for colposcopy after one smear suggesting invasive cancer, because the reported prevalence of cancer in this situation is as high as 56%.[75] Similarly, women with a single smear suggesting glandular neoplasia have reported rates of invasive cancer of 40% to 43%.[76,77] It is generally accepted that women with severe or moderate dysplasia (HiSIL), should be referred for a colposcopic assessment and biopsy. The prevalence rates for CIN grade II/III are 80% to 90% for women with severe dysplasia[78,79] and 74% to 77% for those with moderate dysplasia.[78,80,81] It is with mild changes (LoSIL) and atypical squamous cells of undetermined significance (ASCUS) or borderline nuclear abnormalities (BNA) that the situation is less uniform.

Management of mild dysplasia. Mild dysplasia (LoSIL) is present in 2% to 3% of all cervical smears (Fig. 5-1).[82] The management is controversial because, although many women have trivial changes that regress spontaneously, a significant proportion have CIN III, which will not regress spontaneously and requires treatment.[79,83] Any approach should be effective in reducing the risk of cervical carcinoma and should involve the appropriate use of resources. Two alternative management policies exist. The traditional policy of cytologic surveillance is based on the belief that a majority of these abnormalities will revert to normal over time; referral to colposcopy is reserved for women with persistently abnormal cytologic findings and those who develop severe changes.[84,85] Although retrospective studies of well-organized programs suggest that women who are successfully followed-up do not have an increased risk of cervical cancer if a biopsy is performed when cytologic changes persist,[85] some women lose to surveillance, and these women are definitely at an increased risk of invasive cancer.[85]

The alternative strategy is one of colposcopic assessment after a single cervical smear showing any grade of dysplasia. Advantages of this approach are

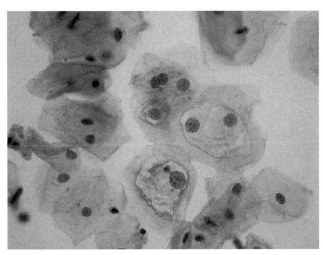

Figure 5-1. Mild dysplasia on a cervical cytology smear. See also Color Figure 5-1.

that it enables a prompt histologic diagnosis and treatment. In addition, it avoids the possibility of incomplete follow-up. Possible adverse effects include both overtreatment and increased anxiety for some women. In 1987, this was the management approach recommended for all women with any dysplasia by the Intercollegiate Working Party on Cervical Cytology Screening.[86] This recommendation has proved to be persuasive; of 210 health districts investigated in a survey carried out by the British Society of Colposcopy and Cervical Pathology (BSCCP), 37% had a policy of immediate colposcopic referral on the basis of a single mildly dysplastic smear.[11] A more recent national guideline suggested referral to colposcopy after a single moderately dysplastic smear but implied that women with mild dysplasia should be referred only if the abnormality persists for 6 months.[87]

The formulation of policy for women with mild dysplasia should not hinge simply on the biology of the disease; psychological and economic considerations also must be taken into account. There may be scope for patient preference if alternative approaches are considered suitable. Furthermore, the high-grade biopsy rate resulting from management of mild dysplasia needs to be considered in each population program.

Should women with a mildly dysplastic (LoSIL) cervical smear be referred for colposcopy or should the smear be repeated? Cytologic surveillance as a management strategy for women with mild dyskaryosis makes sense only if the prevalence of CIN II/III is low and there is clear evidence of significant cytologic regression in most cases over time. Otherwise, significant numbers of women with CIN II/III will have their treatment delayed, others will need to be referred to colposcopy eventually, and a proportion of women with significant disease will be lost to follow-up.

Is mild dysplasia associated with a risk of progression to high-grade disease? Nassiell and colleagues[88] prospectively studied 555 women with mild dysplasia over a period of 12 months, during which time the dysplasia reverted to normal in 62%, persisted in 22%, and progressed to more severe changes in 26%. Fletcher and Soutter[89] observed 666 women who initially had either BNA or mild or moderate dysplasia by cytology over a period of 4.5 years; 24% reverted to a normal cell pattern within that time, and 14% subsequently demonstrated severe dysplasia. In a retrospective study of 1347 women with successful cytologic follow-up after a smear showing mild dysplasia, Robertson[85] reported reversion to negative cytology occurred in 625 (46%) and severe changes in 262 (19%). In the study by Fletcher and Soutter,[89] there was a significant excess incidence of invasive cancer in the 666 women with mild dysplasia managed by cytologic surveillance, compared with the general population. Even reports from well-organized cervical screening programs using a policy of cytologic surveillance have described invasive cancer rates of between 0.6%[85] and 1%,[84] but the authors have concluded that cytologic surveillance is safe provided the woman completes follow-up and that colposcopy is performed if changes persist. However, this view was refuted in a recent reanalysis of previously published studies of cytologic surveillance in such women, which concluded that they clearly had a higher risk of developing invasive cancer despite cytologic follow-up.[90]

Mild dysplasia is associated with a risk of progression to high-grade disease.

Which strategy is more efficient? In a prospective study of 1000 women monitored for up to 2 years after a single mild or moderate dysplastic smear, cytologic surveillance was not found to be an efficient strategy.[91] Among 538 women who presented with a single mildly dysplastic smear, 187 (35%) had CIN III, 101 (19%) had CIN II, 92 (17%) had CIN I, and 158 (29%) had no CIN.[91] Overall, 12% of the women were lost to follow-up, and this figure rose to 25% in the 2-year surveillance group.[91] A single mild smear followed by a nondysplastic smear was associated with a prevalence of CIN III of 25%.[91] Only a minority of the 158 women with mild dysplasia allocated to 2-year surveillance would have fulfilled the criteria for avoiding colposcopic referral.[91] Similar results were reported from another large, prospective randomized controlled trial, which concluded that immediate colposcopy for women with mild dysplasia facilitated earlier diagnosis and treatment of high-grade disease.[92]

Immediate referral for colposcopy represents a more efficient strategy.

Is cytologic surveillance less expensive or associated with less psychological morbidity than immediate colposcopy? A conservative policy is not financially cheaper: an average of six additional smears is required to save each colposcopy referral. Sensitivity analysis shows that the excess cost of a conservative policy increases exponentially as the risk of a subsequent cytologic abnormality exceeds 60%.[93] A cost-effectiveness analysis carried out alongside a randomized clinical trial reported that immediate diagnosis and treatment increased total costs by 50%, but this increased cost was offset by a sharp increase in the number of cases of CIN III detected.[94]

The finding of an abnormal smear and the diagnosis of what is often referred to as "precancer" can be a source of considerable anxiety with particular implications for future fertility, childbearing capacity, and sexual function. Information from patients suggests that the women's anxiety stems from the finding of abnormal cells that are perceived as "cancer cells"[95]; this finding affects her body image, her health status, and her future prospects. Levels of anxiety were measured in two groups of women with mild dysplasia managed by either colposcopy or cytologic surveillance; the former method caused more anxiety. When told that their smear was mildly abnormal, 47% of the immediate-colposcopy group ($n = 182$), compared with 33% of the surveillance group ($n = 163$), thought they had cancer. Although little doubt exists that referral to colposcopy is associated with anxiety, it is clear that women are anxious at the idea of having an abnormal smear that is not being attended to, and a general preference was reported for immediate colposcopy.[96] Some data exist to assert that, in the presence of an abnormal smear, referral for colposcopy is not more stressful than cytologic surveillance.[97] The benefits of immediate colposcopy are early diagnosis, reassurance as to the absence of cancer, prompt treatment, and a return to normal cytology.

Cytologic surveillance is not necessarily a cheaper option, nor is it associated with less psychological morbidity.

How should borderline abnormalities or atypical squamous cells of undetermined significance be managed?
More than 2 million U.S. women receive an equivocal cervical cytologic diagnosis (ASCUS) each year. In Britain, where the British Society for Clinical Cytology (BSCC) terminology is used, the equivalent abnormality is known as BNA. As a result, comparisons of outcomes for these two categories may differ, but the underlying principles for management are the same. Only a minority of women with these findings have high-grade CIN, and in many cases these abnormalities represent a self-limited viral infection with HPV. Strategies for triage to select high-risk women have been explored.

What is the risk of high-grade cervical intraepithelial neoplasia in women with borderline nuclear abnormalities?
Women with koilocytosis were observed over a period of 21 months; only 1.2% had CIN III, and only 16% had any degree of CIN.[98,99] A case-control study of women with follow-up periods ranging from 13 to 106 months after borderline cervical changes demonstrated cytologic progression to CIN III or invasive carcinoma in 22.4%, compared with (0.9%) in a normal control group.[99] The authors concluded that women with BNA have a higher incidence of subsequent high-grade abnormalities, and careful follow-up was advised.

Women with BNA have a higher incidence of subsequent high-grade changes, and careful follow-up is advised.

How should atypical squamous cells of undetermined significance be managed?
The 2001 Bethesda conference split the category of ASCUS into two types: atypical squamous cells HiSIL cannot be ruled out (ASC-H) and atypical squamous cells of undetermined significance (ASC-US).[100] The current consensus guidelines published by the American Society for Colposcopy and Cervical Pathology (ASCCP) recommend immediate colposcopy for women with ASC-H.[101]

The management ASC-US was examined in the ASCUS/LSIL Triage Study (ALTS). This was a multicenter, randomized trial comparing the sensitivity and specificity of three management strategies to detect CIN III: (1) immediate colposcopy, (2) triage to colposcopy based on a combination of HPV results from Hybrid Capture 2 and thin-layer cytology results, and (3) triage based on cytology results alone. The underlying prevalence of histologically confirmed CIN III in women referred with ASCUS was 5.1%. Sensitivity to detect CIN III or greater by testing for HPV DNA was 96.3% (95% confidence interval [CI], 91.6% to 98.8%), with 56.1% of women referred to colposcopy. The sensitivity of a lower cytology triage threshold of ASCUS was 85.3% (95% CI, 78.2% to 90.8%), with 58.6% referred. The authors suggested that testing for high-risk HPV DNA was a viable option in women with ASCUS.[102] The longitudinal results from this study, involving repeated testing, remain to be published, and the optimal management for women with ASCUS smear reports has yet to be determined. In this situation, it has been suggested that consideration of women's triage test preferences should complement overall patient care.[103]

Women with ASC-H should be referred to colposcopy for further investigation. Women with ASCUS have a low prevalence of CIN III. No ideal management strategy exists; the choices available include immediate colposcopy, triage with repeat cytology, and a combination of repeat cytology and HPV testing.

How should cervical intraepithelial neoplasia be treated?
The treatment of any identified precursors of cancer is fundamental to the success of any cervical screening program. This treatment should be effective, safe, and acceptable. It should aim to eradicate all CIN from the cervix and should be tailored to the circumstances of the individual woman.

The treatment of CIN has evolved over the last 30 years away from invasive inpatient procedures, such as hysterectomy and knife cone biopsy, toward simpler outpatient treatments under local anesthesia. Initially, these treatments involved tissue ablation and included radical diathermy,[104] cryotherapy,[105] carbon dioxide laser,[106,107] and cold coagulation.[108-110] The availability of these treatments was of significant benefit to patients in terms of time and money saved, and saved hospital bed space and theater time. These therapies were considered particularly useful for the young patient who had not yet completed her family, because they did not significantly affect subsequent fertility.[110-113]

Strict criteria need to be adhered to when using local ablative treatment. These include a thorough pretreatment assessment (including colposcopy and a colposcopically directed biopsy), an ectocervical lesion that is completely visible, and an absence of colposcopic features of invasive cancer.[114] Concerns regarding the reliability of colposcopically directed biopsies[115,116] and the lack of sensitivity of colposcopy to detect underlying early invasive cancer[117] fueled considerable debate in the early 1990s as to the efficacy and safety of ablative techniques.

Large loop excision of the transformation zone (LLETZ) was introduced in 1988 as a simple outpatient excisional procedure that allows histologic examination of the entire transformation zone, facilitating confirmation of the diagnosis and margins of excision.[118] This treatment is associated with low morbidity,[119] and a single LLETZ procedure does not have an adverse effect on subsequent fertility.[120,121] Its ease of use and the opportunity to treat the patient at the first visit[71,78] led to concerns regarding overtreatment in women with negative histology findings.[122] Despite these concerns, LLETZ has become established as the most widely used method of treatment in the developed world,[11,123] with recommendations that treatment at the first visit be selectively employed by experienced colposcopists who are able to distinguish high-grade from low-grade disease.[122]

The comparative efficacies of the available treatments have been studied.[124,125] The benchmarks of success for any treatment are the rates of invasive cervical cancer after the treatment and the subsequent incidence of recurrent CIN. Conservative outpatient therapy in women with CIN reduces the risk of invasive cancer of the cervix by 95% during the first 8 years after treatment.[126] These risks are illustrated graphically in Figure 5-2. However, even with careful,

long-term follow-up, the risk of invasive cervical cancer among these women is about five times greater than that among the general population of women throughout that period. The effectiveness of alternative surgical treatments for CIN was examined in a Cochrane review of randomized trials, which concluded that no individual type of treatment was superior.[125] Reported nonrandomized series of cryotherapy suggest that single-freeze techniques are associated with a higher risk of persistent disease than a double-freeze technique (6.2% versus 16.3%).[127] Therefore, although LLETZ is the most popular treatment, it is not necessarily a better treatment. Women should be counseled regarding the risk of persistent or recurrent disease and the need for careful and thorough follow-up.

Who should be treated? Women with biopsy-proved CIN II or III should be treated. The natural history of CIN III has demonstrated it to be a true cancer precursor,[128] and, because of the recognized interobserver variation in histologic reporting between grades of CIN,[129] the treatment of CIN II as high-grade disease has been adopted widely. Biopsy-proved adenocarcinoma in situ (ACIS) should be regarded as precancerous[130] and treated by conization[131] or LLETZ,[132] with the aim of obtaining negative excisional margins. The management of biopsy-proved CIN I is controversial, in part because of the lack of reliable data on the natural history of this condition. One study that monitored 566 women for a total of 881 person-years reported resolution of the abnormalities in 306 (54.1%) of the patients, persistent disease in 138 (24.4%), and treatment in 122 (21.5%).[133] Surveillance is a viable option for women with biopsy-proved CIN I if circumstances are favorable in terms of available facilities and patient compliance. Certain safeguards must be applied, with treatment of lesions that persist for 2 years or worsen in grade or size.[134]

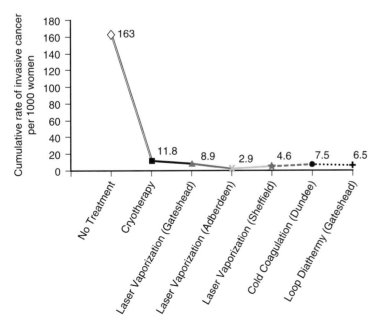

Figure 5-2. Rate of invasive cancer of the cervix after treatment of cervical intraepithelial neoplasia (CIN).

How should treated women be monitored? The increased risk of invasive cancer of the cervix after treatments is more likely to be explained by the progression of inadequately treated persistent disease than by the development of incident CIN. Follow-up protocols involving more intensive screening schedules aim to facilitate the early detection of persistent disease, and all women who have been treated should be so monitored. The effectiveness of any such schedule should be balanced against both the psychological impact of more intensive screening and the health resource implication of monitoring large numbers of treated women. Ideally, schedules should be tailored to the risk of recurrent disease, allowing women who are at low risk to return to routine screening after less intensive surveillance.

Are risk factors for recurrence of benefit? Excisional treatment methods have the advantage that the margins of excision can be determined. Negative margins indicate a lower risk of residual disease, and positive margins a higher risk.[135-140] This is particularly true when the endocervical margins are involved.[138,140] Women who are 40 years of age or older at the time of treatment are also at increased risk.[138,141] Women ages 40 years or older at the time of treatment who have high-grade disease at the margins of excision are a small minority group at particular risk. In one series of 3560 LLETZ treatments, 93 women were in this high risk group, and all of the cancers diagnosed in the follow-up period came from this group.[138] Fertility may not be such an issue for this group of women, and consideration should be given to retreatment and possible hysterectomy rather than conservative follow-up.

How long should women be subjected to increased surveillance after treatment? Most recurrences of CIN are detected in the first 24 months,[137,138,142] but long-term follow-up studies have demonstrated increased risk for at least 10 years after treatment of high-grade CIN.[126] Recent suggestions[126] that women who have had treatment for CIN II/III or ACIS should undergo annual cytology procedures for 10 years before returning to routine screening. Women who have a low risk of recurrence have been identified as those younger than 40 years of age with completely excised, low-grade CIN. The suggestion is that these women should have repeat smears at 6, 12, and 24 months before returning to routine screening.[138]

What is the role of additional tests in the follow-up period? The relative benefit of colposcopy in addition to cytology in the follow-up monitoring of treated women is unproved. Some authors have suggested that it facilitated earlier detection of residual disease,[137,142] but others have not demonstrated an advantage.[143] The difficulty is that women who are potentially at high risk for both residual disease and false-negative cytology results (older women, those with endocervical lesions, and those who have undergone treatment for glandular intraepithelial neoplasia [GIN][131]) are also the women in whom colposcopy is least likely to detect abnormalities.

Women who test positive for HPV DNA after treatment for CIN are at increased risk for recurrent or persistent disease.[60,144] The absence of HPV DNA combined with negative cytology findings at 6 months after treatment has a negative predictive value of 99% and has been suggested as useful in identifying low-risk women.[60] However long-term follow-up data are required to determine the prognostic significance of positive HPV testing in the absence of cytologic or colposcopic evidence of recurrent disease.

Quality Assurance and Colposcopy

In recent years, there has been an increasing focus on the quality of health care services. The four cornerstones of quality assurance are professional performance, use of resources (efficiency), risk management (the risk of harm associated with any intervention), and patient satisfaction with the service.[145] The principal tools for improving the quality of any service are the formulation of evidence-based guidelines and standards of care; the education, accreditation, and continuing professional development of health care providers; and data collection and audit procedures to document any improvement.[146]

Quality assurance and colposcopy: Who benefits? Colposcopy, like any intervention, must be proved to do more good than harm. This is particularly true when the intervention is initiated by the medical population and involves largely a young, asymptomatic group of women. Clearly, the availability of high-quality colposcopy services is of particular relevance to women with an abnormal cervical smear test. There should be access to prompt diagnosis and effective treatment, with adequate information and counseling available at all stages. Quality assurance measures should reduce the risk of significant psychosocial and physical impacts for these women.

Of equal importance are the positive benefits of quality assurance for colposcopists, health authorities, and managers of cervical screening programs. Effective quality assurance measures protect practitioners by the promotion of good clinical practice and the provision of a framework against which to audit local practice. If improvements need to be made, clinical guidelines and standards of care provide clinicians with a negotiating platform to overcome local barriers for change. Health authorities can confirm that accredited colposcopists in accredited colposcopy clinics are providing services with documented evidence of good clinical practice. An additional benefit is the reduction of the risk of medicolegal consequences of adverse outcomes. Finally, the accurate diagnosis and prompt treatment of cancer precursors is fundamental to the effectiveness of screening in reducing the incidence and mortality rates of cervical cancer.

National guidelines should detail evidence based on defined standards of care and good clinical practice.

These data should then allow for both local and national audits. In turn, this should facilitate the establishment of accredited training programs by national and international colposcopy groups. The objectives of any such activities should be:

- To ensure the quality of colposcopic diagnosis and treatment
- To ensure timely access to colposcopy services
- To reduce the psychological impact of colposcopy on women
- To ensure adequate follow-up
- To minimize the risk of incomplete follow-up

Standards of care and clinic administration. It is obvious that colposcopy should be carried out in an appropriate outpatient environment with access to adequate equipment to allow colposcopic assessment, biopsy, and treatment, including access to emergency and resuscitation equipment. There should be clear, written guidelines about the indications for colposcopy, including specific maximum allowable waiting times. In addition, evidence-based written protocols should be available regarding which abnormalities need biopsy and treatment and how any treatment should be performed. These clinics should be provided with adequate medical, nursing, and administrative staffing levels. There is a limit to the number of colposcopy examinations any individual can safely perform in any one session, and it is the responsibility of health care providers to ensure adequate resources to maintain excellent services. The time a woman spends attending the colposcopy is only a fraction of her lifetime screening. Primary care physicians are best placed to provide continuity of care, and there should be a smooth interface between primary care and the colposcopy clinic, to facilitate easy access and prompt communication of both results and management plans. The colposcopy clinic should operate in a closely integrated fashion with the referring cytology and histopathology laboratories.

Indicators of individual performance. Three performance indicators are useful in the assessment of individual practitioners:

- Perceptual ability and documentation of findings
- Rate of biopsy
- Validity of biopsy specimens

Perceptual ability. This performance indicator comprises the ability of an individual to perceive topographic changes on the cervix and to form an opinion as to the probable underlying histology. Because colposcopy is a subjective examination, there can be significant differences in interpretation between observers.[147,148] The most frequent problems in this regard are underestimation of high-grade disease and overestimation of low-grade disease.[45] Attempts to quantify this ability as part of training programs include the standard of 80% accuracy within 1 degree of difference between colposcopy and the underlying

histology (using CIN classification), which has been advocated in both the United States[149] and Canada.[150] The British colposcopy society set the standard based on the functional classification of high-grade and low-grade CIN, with a target accordance of 80%. In addition, it is important that the colposcopist annotate the satisfactory nature of the colposcopic examination as well as the presence or absence of any features of invasion.[87]

Rate of biopsy. In the presence of a satisfactory examination, colposcopically directed punch biopsy becomes the gold standard of diagnosis. This is especially important if an ablative method of treatment is planned. The rate of biopsy has been suggested as a marker of professional performance.[151] The British standards currently indicate that all women with a smear showing moderate or severe dyskaryosis (HiSIL) should have material submitted for histology. If no cervical or vaginal abnormality is obvious, the whole clinical situation should be reevaluated and a LLETZ procedure or conization considered.[152] This is particularly important in the presence of an unsatisfactory colposcopy examination (in which the entire transformation zone is not visible), and it is most common in older women, in whom the transformation zone may revert back up into the endocervical canal.

Women who present with low-grade cytologic abnormalities and who have no abnormalities detected by colposcopy should have a repeat smear performed; if this is normal, it is safe to follow-up cytologically, in either a hospital or a community-based clinic.[133] Women with persistent low-grade cytologic abnormalities should have a biopsy submitted within 2 years.[44]

Validity of biopsy specimens. The colposcopically directed biopsy should be representative of the most severe histologic abnormality of the cervix. The biopsy should be adequate for histologic diagnosis in more than 90% of cases, according to the British (BSCCP, Royal College of Obstetricians and Gynaecologists [RCOG]) guidelines.[153] The positive predictive value of the punch biopsy for CIN II or worse has been advocated as a marker of quality in Italy.[154]

PREINVASIVE DISEASES OF THE VULVA

Definition and Epidemiology

Preinvasive diseases of the vulva are currently designated by the term vulval intraepithelial neoplasia (VIN),[155] as suggested by the International Society for the Study of Vulvovaginal Diseases. This term includes both squamous and nonsquamous lesions. Although some women present with intraepithelial neoplasias of both the cervix and the vulva,[156] significant differences exist between squamous VIN and CIN. VIN is very uncommon, although there is evidence that it is increasing in incidence, particularly among younger women.[155,157,158] The majority of women with VIN are symptomatic, with as many as 79% complaining of pruritus vulvae.[159] However, of symptomatic women who attend a vulvoscopy clinic with suspected VIN, only a minority (4%) will in fact have confirmed VIN.[160]

The true natural history of VIN is difficult to assess, because most of the identified cases of VIN are treated. In a series of 31 cases of VIN, 5 were managed with biopsy alone and all of those progressed to invasive cancer after an interval of between 2 and 10 years.[161] The reported progression rate to invasive cancer after treatment of VIN ranges from 3%[162] to 7%.[163] By contrast, spontaneous regression of histologically proved high-grade VIN has also been reported, particularly in young pregnant women with multifocal disease.[164] To further add to the confusion, many invasive cancers of the vulva occur in association with skin abnormalities other than VIN, such as lichen sclerosis et atrophicus.[165] Paget's disease of the vulva (intraepithelial ACIS) is a rare but clinically important condition that deserves particular attention. Fewer than 1% of gynecologists in the United Kingdom see more than five women with vulvar Paget's disease.[166] Unsuspected microinvasion has been reported in 10% of cases,[167] and 26% of women with Paget's disease of the vulva have another unsuspected carcinoma of the bowel, urogenital tract, or breast.[168]

Diagnosis and Treatment

Colposcopic examination of the vulva is the recommended assessment of women with suspected VIN. The clinical features are neither uniform nor specific. The lesions can be red, white, or pigmented, and the area may appear raised. On palpation, there is commonly a difference in texture, with the abnormal area being coarser, more granular, and less smooth than the normal area. After application of acetic acid, white areas can be identified with variable clarity of the margins.[169] In addition, vascular patterns of punctation and mosaicism can be identified, as in the cervix.[169] Abnormal areas should be biopsied with a Keyes punch biopsy forceps to confirm the diagnosis. Surgical treatment involves wide local excision of the abnormal skin, with at least 5 mm of clear margins. Laser ablation of the area is associated with significant morbidity and an increased incidence of recurrence.[170] Medical treatment with imiquimod has been reported recently in a series of 13 women; complete regression was demonstrated in 8 patients, but 2 of 4 women with apparent partial regression developed invasive cancer.[171] Currently, strategies that use HPV-derived vaccinations are being investigated as treatments for VIN,[172] but the results of such approaches remain to be determined. There is a risk of recurrent intraepithelial and invasive disease after treatment, and long-term follow-up is recommended.

PREINVASIVE DISEASES OF THE VAGINA

Definition and Epidemiology

Vaginal intraepithelial neoplasia (VAIN) is a rare condition that accounts for less than 0.5% of lower genital tract neoplasia.[173] The majority of cases occurs in women who have had a hysterectomy,[174,175] and two thirds of these women have had prior treatment for cervical neoplasia.[174,176] The lesion is located in the upper one third of the vagina in more than 80% of cases.[176] More than half of the cases involve multifocal disease.[174,177] The natural history of this condition was documented in a series of 23 women who were monitored without treatment; persistent disease was noted in 13%, and progression to invasive cancer was noted in 9%.[177]

Diagnosis and Treatment

The colposcopic diagnosis is greatly assisted by the use of aqueous iodine solution, which identifies VAIN as an iodine-negative area. Particular attention is required for the corners of the vaginal vault if the woman has had a hysterectomy. Histologic confirmation should be obtained with a colposcopically directed punch biopsy.

The aim of treatment is to eradicate the VAIN while at the same time preserving sexual function. The anatomy of the vagina and the close proximity of the bladder, bowel, and ureters provide a therapeutic challenge, given that any treatment should reach a depth of at least 1.4 mm.[178] Conservative approaches using ablative techniques have shown variable results. Recurrence rates are high. Reported cure rates are 25% for cryotherapy, 45% for 5-flourouracil therapy, and 69% for laser ablation.[176,179] Surgical excision allows a complete histologic examination of the lesion, including margins, and the diagnosis of occult invasive disease. Surgical excision is recommended as either a primary treatment for high-grade disease or a secondary treatment following failed ablative treatment. Surgical techniques that have been described for this condition include partial vaginectomy via an abdominal[180] or a vaginal[181] approach, wide local excision,[182] and use of a superficial LLETZ procedure.[183] Multifocality is a risk factor for recurrence,[184] and long-term follow-up is required to facilitate detection of any recurrence.

REFERENCES

1. Gustafsson L, Sparen P, Gustafsson M, et al: Efficiency of organised and opportunistic cytological screening for cancer in situ of the cervix. Br J Cancer 1995;72:498-505.
2. Laara E, Day NE, Hakama M: Trends in mortality from cervical cancer in the Nordic countries: Association with organised screening programmes. Lancet 1987;1:1247-1249.
3. Anderson GH, Benedet JL, Le Riche JC, et al: Invasive cancer of the cervix in British Columbia: A review of the demography and screening histories of 437 cases seen from 1985-1988. Obstet Gynecol 1992;80:1-4.
4. Patnick J: Cervical cancer screening in England. Eur J Cancer 2000;36:2205-2208.
5. Hakama M, Louhivuori K: A screening programme for cervical cancer that worked. Cancer Surv 1988;7:403-416.
6. Hakama M, Chamberlain J, Day NE, et al: Evaluation of screening programmes for gynaecological cancer. Br J Cancer 1985; 52: 669-673.
7. Franco E, Syrjanen K, de Wolf C, et al: New developments in cervical cancer screening and prevention. Geneva, Switzerland, June 17-19 1996. Workshop. Cancer Epidemiol Biomarkers Prev 1996;5:853-856.

8. Nanda K, McCrory DC, Myers ER, et al: Accuracy of the Papanicolaou test in screening for and follow-up of cervical cytologic abnormalities: A systematic review. Ann Intern Med 2000;132:810-819.

9. Hutchinson ML, Zahniser DJ, Sherman ME, et al: Utility of liquid-based cytology for cervical carcinoma screening: Results of a population-based study conducted in a region of Costa Rica with a high incidence of cervical carcinoma. Cancer 1999; 87:48-55.

10. Sherman ME, Schiffman MH, Mango LJ, et al: Evaluation of PAPNET testing as an ancillary tool to clarify the status of the "atypical" cervical smear. Mod Pathol 1997;10:564-571.

11. Kitchener HC, Cruickshank ME, Farmery E: The 1993 British Society for Colposcopy and Cervical Pathology/National Coordinating Network United Kingdom Colposcopy Survey: Comparison with 1988 and the response to introduction of guidelines. Br J Obstet Gynaecol 1995;102:549-552.

12. Teale G, Etherington I, Luesley D, Jordan J: An audit of standards and quality in a teaching hospital colposcopy clinic. Br J Obstet Gynaecol 1999;106:83-86.

13. Soutter WP: Criteria for standards of management of women with an abnormal smear. Br J Obstet Gynaecol 1991;98:1069-1072.

14. Kim SJ: Screening and epidemiological trends in cervical cancer. J Obstet Gynaecol Res 1996;22:621-627.

15. Herrero R: Epidemiology of cervical cancer. J Natl Cancer Inst Monogr 1996;21:1-6.

16. Shanta V, Krishnamurthi S, Gajalakshmi CK, et al: Epidemiology of cancer of the cervix: Global and national perspective. J Indian Med Assoc 2000;98:49-52.

17. Cervical cancer control in developing countries: Memorandum from a WHO meeting. Bull World Health Organ 1996;74:345-351.

18. Griffiths M: Screening for cervical cancer in developing countries. BMJ 1992;304:984.

19. Kitchener HC, Symonds P: Detection of cervical intraepithelial neoplasia in developing countries. Lancet 1999;353:856-857.

20. Richart RM: Screening: The next century. Cancer 1995;76: 1919-1927.

21. Chamberlain J: Reasons that some screening programmes fail to control cervical cancer. IARC Sci Publ 1986;76:161-168.

22. Eddy DM: The economics of cancer prevention and detection: Getting more for less. Cancer 1981;47:1200-1209.

23. Nelson JG: Principles and Practice of Screening for Disease. Geneva, World Health Organization, 1968, 2002.

24. Population screening for cervical cancer in The Netherlands: A report by the Evaluation Committee. Int J Epidemiol 1989;18: 775-781.

25. Sasieni P, Adams J: Effect of screening on cervical cancer mortality in England and Wales: Analysis of trends with an age period cohort model. BMJ 1999;318:1244-1245.

26. Wright VC, Riopelle MA: Age at beginning of coitus versus chronologic age as a basis for Papanicolaou smear screening: An analysis of 747 cases of preinvasive disease. Am J Obstet Gynecol 1984;149:824-830.

27. Woodman CB, Collins S, Winter H, et al: Natural history of cervical human papillomavirus infection in young women: A longitudinal cohort study. Lancet 2001;357:1831-1836.

28. Collins S, Mazloomzadeh S, Winter H, et al: High incidence of cervical human papillomavirus infection in women during their first sexual relationship. Br J Obstet Gynaecol 2002;109:96-98.

29. Quinn M, Babb P, Jones J, Allen E: Effect of screening on incidence of and mortality from cancer of cervix in England: Evaluation based on routinely collected statistics. BMJ 1999;318: 904-908.

30. McKenzie CA, Duncan ID: The value of cervical screening in women over 50 years of age: Time for a multicentre audit. Scot Med J 1998;43:19-20.

31. White GE: Older women's attitudes to cervical screening and cervical cancer: A New Zealand experience. J Adv Nurs 1995;21:659-666.

32. Gustafsson L, Sparen P, Gustafsson M, et al: Low efficiency of cytologic screening for cancer in situ of the cervix in older women. Int J Cancer 1995;63:804-809.

33. Royal College of Obstetricians and Gynaecologists: Report of the Intercollegiate Working Party on Cervical Cytology Screening. London: RCOG, 1987.

34. Cruickshank ME: Is cervical screening necessary in older women? Cytopathology 2001;12:351-353.

35. van Wijngaarden WJ, Duncan ID: Upper age limit for cervical screening. BMJ 1993;306:1409-1410.

36. Sherlaw-Johnson C, Gallivan S, Jenkins D: Withdrawing low risk women from cervical screening programmes: Mathematical modelling study. BMJ 1999;318:356-360.

37. Cuzick J, Beverley E, Ho L, et al: HPV testing in primary screening of older women. Br J Cancer 1999;81:554-558.

38. Clarke EA, Hilditch S, Anderson TW: Optimal frequency of screening for cervical cancer: A Toronto case-control study. IARC Sci Publ 1986;76:125-131.

39. Macgregor JE, Campbell MK, Mann EM, Swanson KY: Screening for cervical intraepithelial neoplasia in north east Scotland shows fall in incidence and mortality from invasive cancer with concomitant rise in preinvasive disease. BMJ 1994;308: 1407-1411.

40. Sasieni PD, Cuzick J, Lynch-Farmery E: Estimating the efficacy of screening by auditing smear histories of women with and without cervical cancer. The National Co-ordinating Network for Cervical Screening Working Group. Br J Cancer 1996;73: 1001-1005.

41. Herbert A, Stein K, Bryant TN, et al: Relation between the incidence of invasive cervical cancer and the screening interval: Is a five year interval too long? J Med Screen 1996;3:140-145.

42. Hakama M, Chamberlain J, Day NE, et al: Evaluation of screening programmes for gynaecological cancer. Br J Cancer 1985;52: 669-673.

43. Eddy DM: The frequency of cervical cancer screening: Comparison of a mathematical model with empirical data. Cancer 1987; 60:1117-1122.

44. Soost HJ, Lange HJ, Lehmacher W, Ruffing-Kullmann B: The validation of cervical cytology: Sensitivity, specificity and predictive values. Acta Cytol 1991;35:8-14.

45. Mitchell MF, Schottenfeld D, Tortolero-Luna G, et al: Colposcopy for the diagnosis of squamous intraepithelial lesions: A meta-analysis. Obstet Gynecol 1998;91:626-631.

46. Ferris DG, Heidemann NL, Litaker MS, et al: The efficacy of liquid-based cervical cytology using direct-to-vial sample collection. J Fam Pract 2000;49:1005-1011.

47. Wright TC Jr, Lorincz A, Ferris DG, et al: Reflex human papillomavirus deoxyribonucleic acid testing in women with abnormal Papanicolaou smears. Am J Obstet Gynecol 1998;178: 962-966.

48. Herbert P: Brave new technologies issue: Clever technology looking for a purpose. BMJ 2000;321:51.

49. Austin RM: Implementing liquid-based gynecologic cytology: Balancing marketing, financial, and scientific issues. Cancer 1998;84:193-196.

50. Herbert A, Johnson J: Personal view: Is it reality or an illusion that liquid-based cytology is better than conventional cervical smears? Cytopathology 2001;12:383-389.

51. zur Hausen H: Papillomaviruses in human cancers. Proc Assoc Am Physicians 1999;111:581-587.

52. Walboomers JM, Jacobs MV, Manos MM, et al: Human papillomavirus is a necessary cause of invasive cervical cancer worldwide. J Pathol 1999;189:12-19.

53. zur Hausen H: Papillomaviruses and cancer: From basic studies to clinical application. Nat Rev Cancer 2002;2:342-350.

54. Ratnam S, Franco EL, Ferenczy A: Human papillomavirus testing for primary screening of cervical cancer precursors. Cancer Epidemiol Biomarkers Prev 2000;9:945-951.

55. Schiffman M, Herrero R, Hildesheim A, et al: HPV DNA testing in cervical cancer screening: Results from women in a high-risk province of Costa Rica. JAMA 2000;283:87-93.

56. Wright TC Jr, Denny L, Kuhn L, et al: HPV DNA testing of self-collected vaginal samples compared with cytologic screening to detect cervical cancer. JAMA 2000;283:81-86.

57. Mandelblatt JS, Lawrence WF, Womack SM, et al: Benefits and costs of using HPV testing to screen for cervical cancer. JAMA 2002;287:2372-2381.

58. Duncan I: The case against routine HPV testing in cervical screening. Sex Transm Infect 1998;74:457.

59. Ferris DG, Wright TC Jr, Litaker MS, et al: Triage of women with ASCUS and LSIL on Pap smear reports: Management by repeat Pap smear, HPV DNA testing, or colposcopy? J Fam Pract 1998; 46:125-134.

60. Nobbenhuis MA, Meijer CJ, van den Brule AJ, et al: Addition of high-risk HPV testing improves the current guidelines on

follow-up after treatment for cervical intraepithelial neoplasia. Br J Cancer 2001;84:796-801.

61. Alloub MI, Barr BB, McLaren KM, et al: Human papillomavirus infection and cervical intraepithelial neoplasia in women with renal allografts. BMJ 1989;298:153-156.

62. Fairley CK, Chen S, Tabrizi SN, et al: Prevalence of HPV DNA in cervical specimens in women with renal transplants: A comparison with dialysis-dependent patients and patients with renal impairment. Nephrol Dial Transplant 1994;9:416-420.

63. ter Haar-van Eck SA, Rischen-Vos J, Chadha-Ajwani S, Huikeshoven FJ: The incidence of cervical intraepithelial neoplasia among women with renal transplant in relation to cyclosporine. Br J Obstet Gynaecol 1995;102:58-61.

64. Ellerbrock TV, Chiasson MA, Bush TJ, et al: Incidence of cervical squamous intraepithelial lesions in HIV-infected women. JAMA 2000;283:1031-1037.

65. Fink MJ, Fruchter RG, Maiman M, et al: The adequacy of cytology and colposcopy in diagnosing cervical neoplasia in HIV-seropositive women. Gynecol Oncol 1994;55:133-137.

66. Spitzer M: Lower genital tract intraepithelial neoplasia in HIV-infected women: Guidelines for evaluation and management. Obstet Gynecol Surv 1999;54:131-137.

67. Wright TC Jr, Koulos J, Schnoll F, et al: Cervical intraepithelial neoplasia in women infected with the human immunodeficiency virus: Outcome after loop electrosurgical excision. Gynecol Oncol 1994;55:253-258.

68. Maiman M, Fruchter RG, Sedlis A, et al: Prevalence, risk factors, and accuracy of cytologic screening for cervical intraepithelial neoplasia in women with the human immunodeficiency virus. Gynecol Oncol 1998;68:233-239.

69. Coppleson M: Colposcopic features of papillomaviral infection and premalignancy in the female lower genital tract. Obstet Gynecol Clin North Am 1987;14:471-494.

70. Coppleson M: Current management of lower genital tract preneoplasia. Med J Aust 1991;155:383-388.

71. Luesley DM, Cullimore J, Redman CW, et al: Loop diathermy excision of the cervical transformation zone in patients with abnormal cervical smears. BMJ 1990;300:1690-1693.

72. Marteau TM, Walker P, Giles J, Smail M: Anxieties in women undergoing colposcopy. Br J Obstet Gynaecol 1990;97:859-861.

73. Gath DH, Hallam N, Mynors-Wallis L, et al: Emotional reactions in women attending a UK colposcopy clinic. J Epidemiol Community Health 1995;49:79-83.

74. Freeman-Wang T, Walker P, Linehan J, et al: Anxiety levels in women attending colposcopy clinics for treatment for cervical intraepithelial neoplasia: A randomised trial of written and video information. Br J Obstet Gynaecol 2001;108:482-484.

75. Johnson SJ, Wadehra V: How predictive is a cervical smear suggesting invasive squamous cell carcinoma? Cytopathology 2001;12:144-150.

76. Leeson SC, Inglis TC, Salman WD: A study to determine the underlying reason for abnormal glandular cytology and the formulation of a management protocol. Cytopathology 1997;8:20-26.

77. Cullimore JSJ: The abnormal glandular smear: Cytologic prediction, colposcopic correlation and clinical management. J Obstet Gynaecol 2000;20:403-407.

78. Bigrigg MA, Codling BW, Pearson P, et al: Colposcopic diagnosis and treatment of cervical dysplasia at a single clinic visit: Experience of low-voltage diathermy loop in 1000 patients. Lancet 1990;336:229-231.

79. Soutter WP, Wisdom S, Brough AK, Monaghan JM: Should patients with mild atypia in a cervical smear be referred for colposcopy? Br J Obstet Gynaecol 1986;93:70-74.

80. Anderson DJ, Flannelly GM, Kitchener HC, et al: Mild and moderate dyskaryosis: Can women be selected for colposcopy on the basis of social criteria? BMJ 1992;305:84-87.

81. Soutter WP, Wisdom S, Brough AK, Monaghan JM: Should patients with mild atypia in a cervical smear be referred for colposcopy? Br J Obstet Gynaecol 1986;93:70-74.

82. Bjorge T, Gunbjorud AB, Langmark F, et al: Cervical mass screening in Norway: 510,000 smears a year. Cancer Detect Prev 1994;18:463-470.

83. Walker EM, Dodgson J, Duncan ID: Does mild atypia on a cervical smear warrant further investigation? Lancet 1986;2:672-673.

84. Kirby AJ, Spiegelhalter DJ, Day NE, et al: Conservative treatment of mild/moderate dyskaryosis: Long-term outcome. Lancet 1992;339:828-831.

85. Robertson JJ, Woodend BE, Crozier EH, Hutchinson J: Risk of cervical cancer associated with mild dyskaryosis. BMJ 1988;297:18-21.

86. Royal College of Obstetricians and Gynaecologists: Report of the Intercollegiate Working Party on Cervical Cytology Screening. London: RCOG, 1987.

87. Duncan ID: Guidelines for Clinical Practice and Programme Management. Published by the National Co-ordinating Network, NHS Cervical Screening Programme. Oxford: Oxford Regional Health Authority, 1993.

88. Nasiell K, Roger V, Nasiell M: Behavior of mild cervical dysplasia during long-term follow-up. Obstet Gynecol 1986;67: 665-669.

89. Fletcher A, Soutter WP: Cytological surveillance for mild cervical dyskaryosis. Lancet 1992;340:553.

90. Soutter WP, Fletcher A: Invasive cancer of the cervix in women with mild dyskaryosis followed up cytologically. BMJ 1994;308:1421-1423.

91. Flannelly G, Anderson D, Kitchener HC, et al: Management of women with mild and moderate cervical dyskaryosis. BMJ 1994;308:1399-1403.

92. Shafi MI, Luesley DM, Jordan JA, et al: Randomised trial of immediate versus deferred treatment strategies for the management of minor cervical cytological abnormalities. Br J Obstet Gynaecol 1997;104:590-594.

93. Johnson N, Sutton J, Thornton JG, et al: Decision analysis for best management of mildly dyskaryotic smear. Lancet 1993;342:91-96.

94. Flannelly G, Campbell MK, Meldrum P, et al: Immediate colposcopy or cytological surveillance for women with mild dyskaryosis: A cost effectiveness analysis. J Public Health Med 1997;19:419-423.

95. Lerman C, Miller SM, Scarborough R, et al: Adverse psychologic consequences of positive cytologic cervical screening. Am J Obstet Gynecol 1991;165:658-662.

96. Jones MH, Singer A, Jenkins D: The mildly abnormal cervical smear: Patient anxiety and choice of management. J R Soc Med 1996;89:257-260.

97. Bell S, Porter M, Kitchener H, et al: Psychological response to cervical screening. Prev Med 1995;24:610-616.

98. Dudding N, Sutton J, Lane S: Koilocytosis: An indication for conservative management. Cytopathology 1996;7:32-37.

99. Hirschowitz L, Raffle AE, Mackenzie EF, Hughes AO: Long term follow up of women with borderline cervical smear test results: Effects of age and viral infection on progression to high grade dyskaryosis. BMJ 1992;304:1209-1212.

100. Solomon D, Davey D, Kurman R, et al: The 2001 Bethesda System: Terminology for reporting results of cervical cytology. JAMA 2002;287:2114-2119.

101. Stoler MH: New Bethesda terminology and evidence-based management guidelines for cervical cytology findings. JAMA 2002;287:2140-2141.

102. Solomon D, Schiffman M, Tarone R: Comparison of three management strategies for patients with atypical squamous cells of undetermined significance: Baseline results from a randomized trial. J Natl Cancer Inst 2001;93:293-299.

103. Ferris DG, Kriegel D, Cote L, et al: Women's triage and management preferences for cervical cytologic reports demonstrating atypical squamous cells of undetermined significance and low-grade squamous intraepithelial lesions. Arch Fam Med 1997;6:348-353.

104. Chanen W, Rome RM: Electrocoagulation diathermy for cervical dysplasia and carcinoma in situ: A 15-year survey. Obstet Gynecol 1983;61:673-679.

105. Javaheri G, Balin M, Meltzer RM: Role of cryosurgery in the treatment of intraepithelial neoplasia of the uterine cervix. Obstet Gynecol 1981;58:83-87.

106. Anderson MC: Treatment of cervical intraepithelial neoplasia with the carbon dioxide laser: Report of 543 patients. Obstet Gynecol 1982;59:720-725.

107. Ali SW, Evans AS, Monaghan JM: Results of CO2 laser cylinder vaporization of cervical intraepithelial disease in 1234 patients: An analysis of failures. Br J Obstet Gynaecol 1986;93:75-78.

108. Duncan ID: The Semm cold coagulator in the management of cervical intraepithelial neoplasia. Clin Obstet Gynecol 1983;26:996-1006.

109. Gordon HK, Duncan ID: Effective destruction of cervical intraepithelial neoplasia (CIN) 3 at 100 degrees C using the Semm cold coagulator: 14 years experience. Br J Obstet Gynaecol 1991;98:14-20.

110. Duncan ID: Cold coagulation. Baillieres Clin Obstet Gynaecol 1995;9:145-155.

111. Hollyock VE, Chanen W, Wein R: Cervical function following treatment of intraepithelial neoplasia by electrocoagulation diathermy. Obstet Gynecol 1983;61:79-81.

112. Monaghan JM, Kirkup W, Davis JA, Edington PT: Treatment of cervical intraepithelial neoplasia by colposcopically directed cryosurgery and subsequent pregnancy experience. Br J Obstet Gynaecol 1982;89:387-392.

113. Murdoch JB, Morgan PR, Lopes A, Monaghan JM: The outcome of pregnancy after CO2 laser conisation of the cervix. Br J Obstet Gynaecol 1994;101:277.

114. Creasman WT, Weed JC Jr: Conservative management of cervical intraepithelial neoplasia. Clin Obstet Gynecol 1980;23: 281-291.

115. Buxton EJ, Luesley DM, Shafi MI, Rollason M: Colposcopically directed punch biopsy: A potentially misleading investigation. Br J Obstet Gynaecol 1991;98:1273-1276.

116. Skehan M, Soutter WP, Lim K, et al: Reliability of colposcopy and directed punch biopsy. Br J Obstet Gynaecol 1990;97:811-816.

117. Shafi MI, Finn CB, Blomfield P, et al: Cervical cancer: Need to look and recognise. Lancet 1991;338:388-389.

118. Prendiville W, Cullimore J, Norman S: Large loop excision of the transformation zone (LLETZ): A new method of management for women with cervical intraepithelial neoplasia. Br J Obstet Gynaecol 1989;96:1054-1060.

119. Mor-Yosef S, Lopes A, Pearson S, Monaghan JM: Loop diathermy cone biopsy. Obstet Gynecol 1990;75:884-886.

120. Cruickshank ME, Flannelly G, Campbell DM, Kitchener HC: Fertility and pregnancy outcome following large loop excision of the cervical transformation zone. Br J Obstet Gynaecol 1995;102:467-470.

121. Ferenczy A, Choukroun D, Falcone T, Franco E: The effect of cervical loop electrosurgical excision on subsequent pregnancy outcome: North American experience. Am J Obstet Gynecol 1995;172:1246-1250.

122. Ferris DG, Hainer BL, Pfenninger JL, Zuber TJ: "See and treat" electrosurgical loop excision of the cervical transformation zone. J Fam Pract 1996;42:253-257.

123. Wright TC Jr, Richart RM: Loop excision of the uterine cervix. Curr Opin Obstet Gynecol 1995;7:30-34.

124. Soutter WP: Invasive cancer after treatment of cervical intraepithelial neoplasia. Ann Acad Med Singapore 1998;27:722-724.

125. Martin-Hirsch PL, Paraskevaidis E, Kitchener H: Surgery for cervical intraepithelial neoplasia. Cochrane Database Syst Rev 2000;CD001318.

126. Soutter WP, de Barros LA, Fletcher A, et al: Invasive cervical cancer after conservative therapy for cervical intraepithelial neoplasia. Lancet 1997;349:978-980.

127. Schantz A, Thormann L: Cryosurgery for dysplasia of the uterine ectocervix: A randomized study of the efficacy of the single- and double-freeze techniques. Acta Obstet Gynecol Scand 1984;63:417-420.

128. Mc Indoe WA, Mc Lean MR, Jones RW, Mullins PR: The invasive potential of carcinoma in situ of the cervix. Obstet Gynecol 1984;64:451-458.

129. Robertson AJ, Anderson JM, Beck JS, et al: Observer variability in histopathological reporting of cervical biopsy specimens. J Clin Pathol 1989;42:231-238.

130. Hocking GR, Hayman JA, Ostor AG: Adenocarcinoma in situ of the uterine cervix progressing to invasive adenocarcinoma. Aust N Z J Obstet Gynaecol 1996;36:218-220.

131. Ostor AG, Duncan A, Quinn M, Rome R: Adenocarcinoma in situ of the uterine cervix: An experience with 100 cases. Gynecol Oncol 2000;79:207-210.

132. Houghton SJ, Shafi MI, Rollason TP, Luesley DM: Is loop excision adequate primary management of adenocarcinoma in situ of the cervix? Br J Obstet Gynaecol 1997;104:325-329.

133. Teale GR, Moffitt DD, Mann CH, Luesley DM: Management guidelines for women with normal colposcopy after low grade cervical abnormalities: Population study. BMJ 2000;320: 1693-1696.

134. Shafi MI, Luesley DM: Management of low grade lesions: Follow-up or treat? Baillieres Clin Obstet Gynaecol 1995;9: 121-131.

135. Chang DY, Cheng WF, Torng PL, et al: Prediction of residual neoplasia based on histopathology and margin status of conization specimens. Gynecol Oncol 1996;63:53-56.

136. Dobbs SP, Asmussen T, Nunns D, et al: Does histological incomplete excision of cervical intraepithelial neoplasia following large loop excision of transformation zone increase recurrence rates? A six year cytological follow up. Br J Obstet Gynaecol 2000;107:1298-1301.

137. Flannelly G, Langhan H, Jandial L, et al: A study of treatment failures following large loop excision of the transformation zone for the treatment of cervical intraepithelial neoplasia. Br J Obstet Gynaecol 1997;104:718-722.

138. Flannelly G, Bolger B, Fawzi H, et al: Follow up after LLETZ: Could schedules be modified according to risk of recurrence? Br J Obstet Gynaecol 2001;108:1025-1030.

139. Lopes A, Morgan P, Murdoch J, et al: The case for conservative management of "incomplete excision" of CIN after laser conization. Gynecol Oncol 1993;49:247-249.

140. Murdoch JB, Morgan PR, Lopes A, Monaghan JM: Histological incomplete excision of CIN after large loop excision of the transformation zone (LLETZ) merits careful follow up, not retreatment. Br J Obstet Gynaecol 1992;99:990-993.

141. Paraskevaidis E, Lolis ED, Koliopoulos G, et al: Cervical intraepithelial neoplasia outcomes after large loop excision with clear margins. Obstet Gynecol 2000;95:828-831.

142. Paraskevaidis E, Jandial L, Mann EM, et al: Pattern of treatment failure following laser for cervical intraepithelial neoplasia: Implications for follow-up protocol. Obstet Gynecol 1991;78:80-83.

143. Lopes A, Mor-Yosef S, Pearson S, et al: Is routine colposcopic assessment necessary following laser ablation of cervical intraepithelial neoplasia? Br J Obstet Gynaecol 1990;97:175-177.

144. Paraskevaidis E, Koliopoulos G, Alamanos Y, et al: Human papillomavirus testing and the outcome of treatment for cervical intraepithelial neoplasia. Obstet Gynecol 2001;98: 833-836.

145. Scally G, Donaldson LJ: The NHS's 50th anniversary: Clinical governance and the drive for quality improvement in the new NHS in England. BMJ 1998;317:61-65.

146. Halligan A, Donaldson L: Implementing clinical governance: Turning vision into reality. BMJ 2001;322:1413-1417.

147. Hopman EH, Voorhorst FJ, Kenemans P, et al: Observer agreement on interpreting colposcopic images of CIN. Gynecol Oncol 1995;58:206-209.

148. Hopman EH, Kenemans P, Helmerhorst TJ: Positive predictive rate of colposcopic examination of the cervix uteri: An overview of literature. Obstet Gynecol Surv 1998;53:97-106.

149. Ferris DG, Miller MD: Colposcopic accuracy in a residency training program: Defining competency and proficiency. J Fam Pract 1993;36:515-520.

150. Benedet JL, Anderson GH, Matisic JP, Miller DM: A quality-control program for colposcopic practice. Obstet Gynecol 1991;78:872-875.

151. Cecchini S, Bonardi R, Grazzini G, et al: Training in colposcopy: Experience with a videocolposcopy test. Tumori 1997;83: 650-652.

152. Hellberg D, Nilsson S, Valentin J: Positive cervical smear with subsequent normal colposcopy and histology: Frequency of CIN in a long-term follow-up. Gynecol Oncol 1994;53:148-151.

153. Luesley D: Standards and Quality in Colposcopy. NHSCSP Publication Number 2. NHS publications, NHS cervical screening program, Sheffield 1996.

154. Cecchini S, Iossa A, Grazzini G, et al: Quality control for colposcopy in the Florence screening program for cervical cancer. Tumori 1992;78:291-294.

155. Jones RW: Vulval intraepithelial neoplasia: Current perspectives. Eur J Gynaecol Oncol 2001;22:393-402.

156. Hammond IG, Monaghan JM: Multicentric carcinoma of the female lower genital tract. Br J Obstet Gynaecol 1983;90: 557-561.

157. Basta A, Adamek K, Pitynski K: Intraepithelial neoplasia and early stage vulvar cancer: Epidemiological, clinical and virological observations. Eur J Gynaecol Oncol 1999;20:111-114.

158. Campion MJ, Hacker NF: Vulvar intraepithelial neoplasia and carcinoma. Semin Cutan Med Surg 1998;17:205-212.

159. Sykes P, Smith N, McCormick P, Frizelle FA: High-grade vulval intraepithelial neoplasia (VIN 3): A retrospective analysis of patient characteristics, management, outcome and relationship to squamous cell carcinoma of the vulva 1989-1999. Aust N Z J Obstet Gynaecol 2002;42:69-74.

160. Caschetto S, Caragliano L, Cassaro N, et al: [Screening strategies for vulvar preoplastic and neoplastic lesions]. Minerva Ginecol 2000;52:491-495.

161. Jones RW, McLean MR: Carcinoma in situ of the vulva: A review of 31 treated and five untreated cases. Obstet Gynecol 1986;68:499-503.

162. McNally OM, Mulvany NJ, Pagano R, et al: VIN 3: A clinicopathologic review. Int J Gynecol Cancer 2002;12:490-495.

163. Herod JJ, Shafi MI, Rollason TP, et al: Vulvar intraepithelial neoplasia with superficially invasive carcinoma of the vulva. Br J Obstet Gynaecol 1996;103:453-456.

164. Jones RW, Rowan DM: Spontaneous regression of vulvar intraepithelial neoplasia 2-3. Obstet Gynecol 2000;96:470-472.

165. Crum CP, McLachlin CM, Tate JE, Mutter GL: Pathobiology of vulvar squamous neoplasia. Curr Opin Obstet Gynecol 1997;9:63-69.

166. Tidy JA, Soutter WP, Luesley DM, et al: Management of lichen sclerosus and intraepithelial neoplasia of the vulva in the UK. J R Soc Med 1996;89:699-701.

167. Feuer GA, Shevchuk M, Calanog A: Vulvar Paget's disease: The need to exclude an invasive lesion. Gynecol Oncol 1990;38: 81-89.

168. Preti M, Micheletti L, Ghiringhello B, et al: [Vulvar Paget's disease: Clinico-pathologic review of the literature]. Minerva Ginecol 2000;52:203-211.

169. Coppleson M: Colposcopic features of papillomaviral infection and premalignancy in the female lower genital tract. Dermatol Clin 1991;9:251-266.

170. Shafi MI, Luesley DM, Byrne P, et al: Vulval intraepithelial neoplasia: Management and outcome. Br J Obstet Gynaecol 1989;96:1339-1344.

171. Jayne CJ, Kaufman RH: Treatment of vulvar intraepithelial neoplasia 2/3 with imiquimod. J Reprod Med 2002;47:395-398.

172. Stern PL, Brown M, Stacey SN, et al: Natural HPV immunity and vaccination strategies. J Clin Virol 2000;19:57-66.

173. Cardosi RJ, Bomalaski JJ, Hoffman MS: Diagnosis and management of vulvar and vaginal intraepithelial neoplasia. Obstet Gynecol Clin North Am 2001;28:685-702.

174. Mao CC, Chao KC, Lian YC, Ng HT: Vaginal intraepithelial neoplasia: Diagnosis and management. Zhonghua Yi Xue Za Zhi.(Taipei) 1990;46:35-42.

175. Liu S, Semenciw R, Mao Y: Cervical cancer: The increasing incidence of adenocarcinoma and adenosquamous carcinoma in younger women. CMAJ 2001;164:1151-1152.

176. Rome RM, England PG: Management of vaginal intraepithelial neoplasia: A series of 132 cases with long-term follow-up. Int J Gynecol Cancer 2000;10:382-390.

177. Aho M, Vesterinen E, Meyer B, et al: Natural history of vaginal intraepithelial neoplasia. Cancer 1991;68:195-197.

178. Benedet JL, Wilson PS, Matisic JP: Epidermal thickness measurements in vaginal intraepithelial neoplasia: A basis for optimal CO2 laser vaporization. J Reprod Med 1992;37:809-812.

179. Diakomanolis E, Rodolakis A, Sakellaropoulos G, et al: Conservative management of vaginal intraepithelial neoplasia (VAIN) by laser CO2. Eur J Gynaecol Oncol 1996;17:389-392.

180. Diakomanolis E, Rodolakis A, Boulgaris Z, et al: Treatment of vaginal intraepithelial neoplasia with laser ablation and upper vaginectomy. Gynecol Obstet Invest 2002;54:17-20.

181. Curtis P, Shepherd JH, Lowe DG, Jobling T: The role of partial colpectomy in the management of persistent vaginal neoplasia after primary treatment. Br J Obstet Gynaecol 1992;99:587-589.

182. Cheng D, Ng TY, Ngan HY, Wong LC: Wide local excision (WLE) for vaginal intraepithelial neoplasia (VAIN). Acta Obstet Gynecol Scand 1999;78:648-652.

183. Fanning J, Manahan KJ, McLean SA: Loop electrosurgical excision procedure for partial upper vaginectomy. Am J Obstet Gynecol 1999;181:1382-1385.

184. Dodge JA, Eltabbakh GH, Mount SL, et al: Clinical features and risk of recurrence among patients with vaginal intraepithelial neoplasia. Gynecol Oncol 2001;83:363-369.

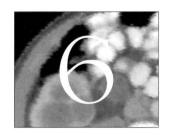

C H A P T E R

CONTROVERSIES IN EARLY VULVAR CANCER

Jacobus van der Velden

 MAJOR CONTROVERSIES

- **What is the definition of early vulvar cancer, and what are the implications for treatment?**
- **What are the questions associated with implementation of the sentinel node technique in vulvar cancer?**
- **What is a unilateral vulvar tumor, and can contralateral groin dissection safely be omitted in these patients?**
- **What should be the extent of the groin dissection?**
- **What should be done when a tumor-free margin of less than 8 mm is found in early vulvar cancer?**
- **Should the goal be margins free from severe dysplasia and lichen sclerosus when early vulvar cancer is surgically treated?**
- **What are the indications for postoperative radiotherapy when positive nodes are found in clinically early vulvar cancer?**

What is the definition of early vulvar cancer, and what are the implications for treatment?

This chapter deals with the problems in staging of vulvar cancer. What must we use when we try to define early vulvar cancer: the clinical TNM staging system or the surgical-pathologic Federation International de Gynecology et Obstetrique (FIGO) staging system? The various systems are discussed with regard to guidance for treatment and prognosis. Two issues are discussed in detail: How must the depth of infiltration in early vulvar cancer be measured? and Is modified treatment for clinically early vulvar cancer sufficient treatment when groin lymph node metastases are also found?

Introduction. Although, in general, a staging system is not meant to be a guideline for treatment but more an instrument for "standardized reporting," many clinicians use the staging system as an aid in deciding how to treat an individual patient. A surgical-pathologic

staging system can never be used in that way, because the information on the extent of the disease becomes available only after the treatment. For that reason, many authors and textbooks still use the old (pre-1988) clinical FIGO staging system to define subgroups such as "early-stage" and "late-stage" vulvar cancer, as the guideline for treatment. However, the only official clinical staging system for vulvar cancer at present is the TNM system (Table 6-1).

In 1988, the FIGO decided to abandon the clinical staging system of squamous cell cancer of the vulva on the basis that the status of the lymph nodes has a major prognostic impact but is not incorporated into this system.

At that time, a surgical-pathologic staging system was introduced in which the presence of metastases in the inguinofemoral nodes resulted in a stage III (unilateral positive nodes) or stage IVA (bilateral positive nodes) designation.[1] Later, in 1994, the FIGO system was again revised based on the recognition of a very early-stage vulvar cancer with a very low risk of lymph node metastases, defined as a tumor with a

Table 6-1. Clinical TNM Staging System for the Vulva

T: Primary Tumor

T1	Tumor confined to vulva, 2 cm in largest diameter
T2	Tumor confined to vulva, >2 cm in diameter
T3	Tumor of any size with spread to urethra and/or vagina and/or perineum and/or anus
T4	Tumor of any size infiltrating the bladder mucosa and/or the rectal mucosa or including the upper part of the urethral mucosa and/or fixed to the bone

N: Regional Lymph Nodes

N0	No nodes palpable
N1	Palpable groin nodes, not enlarged, mobile
N2	Palpable groin nodes, enlarged, firm, mobile (clinically suspect)
N3	Fixed or ulcerated nodes

M: Distant Metastases

M0	No clinical metastases
M1a	Palpable deep pelvic nodes
M1b	Other distant metastases

depth of invasion of less than 1 mm into the stroma and a tumor diameter of less than 2 cm (Table 6-2).[2]

Stage Ia. The depth of invasion is currently defined as the measurement of the tumor from the epithelial-stromal junction of the adjacent most superficial dermal papilla to the deepest point of invasion. Wilkinson originally proposed this definition (Wilkinson method A) and preferred this type of measurement over tumor thickness (method B) or measurement from the deepest rete ridge (method C).[3] This very early vulvar cancer has only a minimal risk of lymph node metastases and was therefore categorized as stage Ia.

One of the reasons to use the Wilkinson A definition is the fact that ulceration or papillomatous tumors either underestimate or overestimate the real infiltration of the tumor into the stroma when tumor thickness is used. However, one of the largest studies to date in

Table 6-2. International Federation of Gynecologists and Obstetricians (FIGO) Staging of Vulvar Carcinoma, 1995 Revision

Stage I	Tumor confined to vulva, 2 cm or less in diameter, no metastases in the groin nodes
Ia	Depth of invasion not exceeding 1 mm (calculated from the nearest dermal papilla)
Ib	All others
Stage II	Tumor confined to the vulva, more than 2 cm in diameter, no metastases in the groin nodes
Stage III	Tumor of any size with adjacent spread to the vagina, urethra, and/or anus; and/or unilateral pathologically confirmed groin lymph node metastases
Stage IV	
IVa	Tumor of any size infiltrating the bladder mucosa and/or rectal mucosa including the upper part of the urethral mucosa, and/or fixed to the bone; and/or pathologically confirmed bilateral groin lymph node metastases
IVb	Distant metastases and/or pathologically confirmed pelvic lymph node metastases

which depth of infiltration was correlated with risk of inguinofemoral lymph node metastases used tumor thickness as definition for depth of infiltration.[4] This makes the scientific basis for use of the definition according to Wilkinson A rather weak.

In the literature on the subject of stage I vulvar carcinomas with tumor infiltration of less than 1 mm, information about important variables, such as how tumor infiltration is measured, treatment, and duration of follow-up, often appears incomplete. When a selection of the literature was made to include only studies in which (1) measurement of tumor infiltration was defined exactly on the basis of method A or B as defined by Wilkinson and (2) the patients all had a groin lymphadenectomy or follow-up of at least 2 years if a groin dissection was not performed, a total of 147 patients were found in seven reports (Table 6-3). It is reassuring to see from Table 6-3 that no positive groin node was seen in the initial operative specimen and no metastasis occurred in the groin when less than 1 mm of invasion was present, regardless of which method was used for calculation of the depth of infiltration. Only a few case reports have been published in which a groin recurrence or positive groin lymph node was found in a patient with a depth of invasion of vulvar carcinoma of less than 1 mm.[4-6] This means that the occurrence of a lymph node metastasis in a patient with a stage IA vulvar carcinoma, regardless of the way in which depth of infiltration is measured (Wilkinson A or B), is very rare. The incidence is too low to justify routine lymphadenectomy in these patients.

If there is still doubt about the reliability of the precise measurement of the depth of infiltration, the sentinel lymph node procedure seems to be a very good alternative for this group of patients with very early vulvar cancer (see Chapter 7).

Clinical stages T1 and T2 with subclinical groin lymph node metastases. One of the major problems when clinical staging is used as the guideline for treatment in vulvar cancer is the fact that subclinical

Table 6-3. Number of Positive Inguinofemoral Lymph Nodes (or Inguinal Recurrences After a Minimum Follow-up Period of 2 Years) in Stage I Superficially Invasive Vulvar Carcinoma, by Infiltration Depth

	0-1 mm		1-2 mm	
Author	N	Positive Nodes, No.	N	Positive Nodes, No. (%)
Method A				
Parker et al[61]	19	0	18	1 (6)
Hacker et al[62]	34	0	19	2 (11)
Hofmann et al[63]	24	0	19	0 (0)
Ross et al[64]	17	0	16	1 (6)
Method B				
Magrina et al[30]	19	0	26	3 (12)
Iversen et al[65]	23	0	12	2 (17)
Struyk et al[66]	11	0	25	2 (8)
Total	147	0	135	11 (8)

Table 6–4. Incidence of Lymph Node Metastases in Relation to Clinical Stage of Disease

Stage	No. Cases	No. Positive Nodes	% Positive Nodes
I	140	15	10.7
II	145	38	26.2
III	137	88	64.2
IV	18	16	88.9

From Berek JS, Hacker NF: Practical Gynecologic Oncology, 3rd ed. Philadelphia, Lippincott Williams & Wilkins, 2000.

inguinofemoral metastases can be present in a considerable number of presumed "early" vulvar cancers.

Iversen showed that 36% of groins that are normal at palpation in patients with all stages of vulvar cancer can harbor metastases.[7] Table 6-4 presents collated data from the literature showing that 10% to 26% of patients with clinically early-stage vulvar cancer have metastases in the groin lymph nodes. This means that clinical staging definitely results in understaging.

Currently, the treatment of choice for early vulvar cancer is a radical local excision of the primary tumor with either a unilateral or a bilateral inguinofemoral lymph node dissection through separate incisions, depending on the site and size of the primary tumor.[8] The issue now is whether modified radical treatment for early vulvar cancer is also a safe treatment for the 10% to 25% of patients with clinically early vulvar cancer but with subclinical lymph node metastases.

A Cochrane overview on the efficacy of this modified treatment in early vulvar cancer concluded that survival was not compromised and morbidity was decreased, compared with historical data in which en bloc resections were used.[9] It was recognized that data from randomized controlled trials were not available. In this review, only the total group of patients with clinically early vulvar cancer was considered; a separate analysis of patients with clinically early vulvar cancer but pathologically late-stage disease was not performed.

Recently, the efficacy of modified treatment in terms of disease-free survival was questioned in several papers.[10-12] De Hullu[10] found that disease-free survival after the triple-incision technique was lower compared with the en bloc technique in patients with early (T1 and T2) vulvar cancer. Overall survival was not compromised. This result can be attributed to the fact that local recurrences can be cured in a large number of cases and do not compromise overall survival, a phenomenon described in earlier studies.[13,14] Of more concern in the study by de Hullu is the relatively higher frequency of regional recurrences (groin and pelvic, also including skin bridge) in the group treated by the triple-incision technique (4%, compared with 9% for the en bloc technique).[10] Regional recurrences are less likely to be cured.[14] As early as 1981, Hacker and colleagues, reporting on the first 100 patients treated by the triple-incision technique, raised concern regarding the efficacy of the modified treatment in patients with positive inguinofemoral lymph nodes.[15] They

found two patients with skin bridge recurrences, and both patients had originally positive nodes. Helm and coworkers, in analyzing patients treated by the triple-incision versus the en bloc technique, stated that "the only group who seemed to fare worse after triple incision surgery were those patients with positive groin nodes."[16] The numbers in the latter study were small, and firm conclusions could not be drawn. In another large series of 100 patients, Grimshaw and coworkers did not see any skin bridge or groin recurrence in patients with positive nodes after the triple-incision technique.[17] However, the corrected survival rate of only 31.2% of patients with positive lymph nodes after modified treatment compares unfavorably with other series, in which survival of 50% or greater is reported.[18]

A similar finding was recently reported by van der Velden and coworkers.[12] They studied the impact of multiple clinical and pathologic variables, including modified treatment, on the recurrence pattern in a subgroup of patients with pathologically late-stage disease on the basis of positive groin nodes. Adjuvant radiation was administered whenever more than one intracapsular tumor metastasis was found, irrespective of the surgical treatment. They found modified treatment to be an independent predictive variable for recurrence-free interval (hazard ratio, 0.52; 95% confidence interval, 0.29 to 0.93). There was an excess of regional recurrences in the group treated by modified treatment. As in de Hullu's study,[10] there was no difference in overall survival.

Summary. Only patients with T1 tumors with a depth of infiltration of less than 1 mm (either measured as tumor thickness or related to the adjacent dermal papilla) can safely be treated without a groin lymph node dissection. This group represents clinically with very early vulvar cancer.

There is a vast body of literature showing that overall survival after modified radical surgery in clinical T1 and T2 vulvar cancer without suspicious groin nodes is not compromised, compared with the en bloc radical vulvectomy as performed in the past. So far there is no evidence for a compromised overall survival rate even when modified treatment is used in clinically early-stage vulvar cancer in the case of subclinical groin metastases, but more data on this subject are definitely needed.

What are the questions associated with implementation of the sentinel node technique in vulvar cancer?

In this section, the role of the sentinel node technique in early vulvar cancer is discussed by means of the following questions:

- Is there already enough evidence to implement this technique?
- Is there a learning curve, and what should be the minimal number of procedures performed before embarking on implementation of this new technique?

- Which technique (blue dye versus technetium) must be used?
- Which patients are suitable candidates for the sentinel node technique?
- Is ultrastaging necessary?

Introduction. Since the first reports on the value of the sentinel lymph node technique in melanoma,[19] this technique has been adopted very rapidly into clinical practice. Currently it is used "routinely" in melanoma and early breast cancer. The introduction of its routine use, however, is not based on thorough clinical trials. No randomized studies in which the new technique was compared with the standard treatment have been reported to date.

Evidence. Levenback and coworkers[20] first reported the use of the sentinel lymph node technique in vulvar cancer in 1994, and since then several reports have been published on its predictive value. Table 6-5 shows a summary of the studies on lymphatic mapping in squamous cell carcinoma of the vulva. The conclusion must be that detection of the sentinel lymph node in vulvar cancer with the use of only a blue dye is unreliable.[20,21] A radioactive tracer, either technetium sulfur colloid or technetium-labeled albumin, is mandatory to get reliable results.

Some advocate a combination of blue dye and technetium to increase the detection rate.[22] There is no evidence from randomized studies for the use of the combined technique, and uncontrolled studies in vulvar cancer in which only technetium was used showed a detection rate of 100% (see Table 6-5).

Learning curve. Both optimal identification of the sentinel node and a low rate of false-negative results are associated with the number of procedures performed by the team involved in the procedure. A study by Cox and colleagues[23] indicated that surgeons need to perform at least 23 procedures to obtain an identification rate of 90% and more than 50 procedures for a rate of 95%. Later, Tafra[24] reviewed the available literature and concluded that at least 20 procedures had to be performed to come to a false-negative rate of less than 5%. Because vulvar cancer is a relatively rare disease and most gynecologic oncologists do not see more than 20 patients per year in total, it is difficult

to get proper experience with this technique. In the Netherlands, an implementation study in vulvar cancer is underway.[10] In this study a minimum of 10 procedures is required before the investigator may start entering patients. The data from Table 6-5 indicate a 100% detection rate with tracer regardless of the number of procedures performed, so it seems reasonable to define experience as, at the least, "performing 10 consecutive procedures with a 100% detection rate."

Candidates for the sentinel procedure. Until more information becomes available, it is clear that only patients with well-defined unifocal tumors, where the injection of the technetium can properly be performed, can undergo the procedure.

Patients with suspicious palpable groin lymph nodes or suspicious lymph nodes detected with other imaging techniques such as ultrasonography or magnetic resonance imaging[25,26] are not good candidates for the sentinel node technique, because there is always the risk that grossly involved lymph nodes may block the lymph flow and subsequently avoid detection with blue dye or technetium, resulting in false-negative scans.[27]

Ultrastaging. The problem of ultrastaging is currently the subject of intense debate. Ultrastaging entails both immunohistochemical staining (IHC) and step-sectioning. To get more reliable insight into possible subclinical metastases, ultrastaging has been proposed by various authors to be used in the sentinel node technique.[22]

No data are available on the prognostic significance of tumor cells found by ultrastaging in lymph nodes of patients with vulvar cancer. Does the presence of tumor cells predict a worse outcome, and, if so, are there strategies to influence this outcome? It has been shown in cervical cancer that patients in whom tumor cells are found in the nodes by various forms of ultrastaging constitute a high-risk group.[28]

One of the major problems, however, is whether this higher risk is caused by more extended regional disease and can be positively influenced by more radical regional node dissection, adjuvant radiation, or adjuvant chemotherapy, or whether it is caused by systemic disease and frequently is not influenced by therapeutic measures. No reliable data are available to

Table 6–5. Overview of the Available Literature on Lymphatic Mapping in Squamous Cell Cancer of the Vulva

Author	N	Tracer	Blue Dye	Sentinel Lymph Node Found (%)	False-Negative Results (No.)
Levenback et al[67]	21	No	Yes	66	0
De Cesare et al[68]	10	Yes	No	100	0
De Cicco et al[69]	15	Yes	No	100	0
de Hullu et al[70]	59	Yes	Yes	100	0
Rodier et al[71]	8	Yes	Yes	100	1
Terada et al[72]	10	Yes	No	100	0
Ansink et al[21]	51	No	Yes	56	2

answer this question. In the aforementioned implementation study, immunohistochemical staining is mandatory, and if the result is positive, a full inguino-femoral lymphadenectomy must be carried out.[10]

Until more data become available, an expert panel on the sentinel node technique in breast cancer recently recommended the following.[22] Each sentinel node should be cut along its longitudinal axis into sections of 1.5- to 2-mm thickness and should be cut at three levels when it is sent in as a frozen section. The rest of the material should be imbedded in paraffin, and for final processing it should be cut in three sections. The panel recommended that IHC should not be used routinely, but only if conventional hematoxylin and eosin–stained slides give rise to suspicion. Several randomized trials are underway to study the clinical meaning of clusters of cells found by IHC. Strong recommendations about the use of IHC can be given only after the results of these studies are known.

Summary. In summary, the sentinel node technique seems to be a promising tool that can lead to further conservation in vulvar cancer surgery. Many questions, such as the role of ultrastaging and the selection of patient groups for this technique, cannot yet be answered and await the results of ongoing trials.

What is a unilateral vulvar tumor, and can contralateral groin dissection safely be omitted in these patients?

In this section, omission of the contralateral groin dissection in unilateral tumors is discussed. What constitutes a unilateral lesion: a marginal distance of greater than 1 cm from an imaginary line drawn from clitoris to anus, or a tumor that does not encroach the midline?

Introduction. The work of Iversen and Aas[29] indicated that the lymph flow from the vulva is predominantly ipsilateral for unilateral lesions, whereas midline lesions drain bilaterally. However, they also showed significant bilateral flow from the anterior labium minus. In agreement with this finding was the observation by Magrina and associates,[30] who found contralateral groin node metastases in 2 of 77 patients with unilateral T1 tumors and negative ipsilateral nodes. Both patients had a unilateral tumor on the labium minus.

Evidence for the safety of an ipsilateral groin node dissection. A collection of retrospective data shows that the risk of contralateral groin metastases in unilateral T1 tumors with negative ipsilateral nodes is indeed very low (Table 6-6). It has to be kept in mind that all of these patients had a bilateral groin dissection. Way[31] showed that doing more sections on blocks of tissue originating from the groin sometimes led to the identification of previously unrecognized micrometastases. This means that evidence for the true safety of omission of the contralateral groin dissection

Table 6–6. Incidence of Positive Contralateral Nodes in Patients with Lateral T1 Squamous Cell Cancer of the Vulva Who Underwent Bilateral Inguinal Node Dissection with Negative Ipsilateral Nodes

Author	Unilateral Lesions, No.	Contralateral Nodes Positive, No. (%)
Wharton et al[73]	25	0 (0)
Parker et al[61]	41	0 (0)
Magrina et al[30]	77	2 (2.6)
Iversen et al[65]	112	0 (0)
Hoffman et al[63]	70	0 (0)
Hacker et al[62]	60	0 (0)
Buscema et al[74]	38	0 (0)
Struyk et al[66]	53	0 (0)
Total	476	2 (0.4)

can come only from cases in which the contralateral groin dissection is actually omitted.

A total of 192 patients with a unilateral T1 tumor treated by an ipsilateral groin dissection only have been described in seven different papers (Table 6-7). The majority of these patients had favorable tumor characteristics, such as invasion of less than 5 mm, absence of vascular space invasion, or well-differentiated tumors. Five patients (2.6%) showed metastases in the undissected contralateral groin. It is important to note that only two out of the five patients in this small series died from their recurrence. In other, larger collated series, a groin recurrence in an undissected groin carries a mortality rate of 90%.[32] Unfortunately the exact locations of the tumors of the five patients are unknown. It would be of interest to know if these tumors were situated at the labia minora, because both imaging studies and retrospective data suggest that tumors on the anterior aspect of the labia minora exhibit contralateral lymph flow.

The fact that the prospective data show less favorable results compared with the retrospective data (2.6% versus 0.4% contralateral groin metastases) and the fact that the patient group from the prospective studies represents a favorable subgroup indicate a possibly greater risk for contralateral groin metastases in the group of patients with unilateral T1 tumors not

Table 6–7. Contralateral Groin Node Metastases in Patients with Lateral T1 Squamous Cell Cancer of the Vulva Who had Omission of the Contralateral Inguinal Node Dissection with Negative Ipsilateral Nodes

Reference	Unilateral Lesions, No.	Contralateral Groin Metastases, No.
Lin et al[42]	14	1
Stehman et al[33]	107	3
Hoffman et al[63]	6	0
Tham et al[75]	7	0
Andrews et al[46]	19	0
Farias-Eisner et al[76]	6	0
Burke et al[40]	33	1
Total	192	5 (2.6%)

selected on the basis of favorable prognostic variables. Still, the risk of dying from a contralateral groin recurrence in small (T1) unilateral vulvar cancers is very low. Therefore, the benefit of omitting a groin dissection on one side seems to outweigh the costs. Frequent follow-up examinations and careful examination of the undissected groin remain mandatory in these patients.

Definition of a unilateral vulvar tumor. In the only prospective study in which contralateral groin dissection was omitted (Gynecologic Oncology Group [GOG] study 74), the definition of a unilateral tumor was "not a midline lesion."[33] Other definitions that are frequently used are "not encroaching the midline" and "greater than 1 cm from the midline."[34] The problem with definitions such as "not a midline lesion" or "not encroaching the midline" is that they are too subjective to be used in clinical practice. The definition of "greater than 1 cm from the midline" seems to be more rational. Heaps and coworkers[35] showed that the risk of local recurrence was 50% when the tumor-free margin was less than 8 mm, whereas substantially fewer recurrences were seen when this margin was greater than 1 cm.

It is not clear from the latter study whether the local recurrences were exactly at the site of the close surgical margins. Still, these data seem to provide sufficient evidence for the safety of using the "greater than 1 cm from the midline" definition for a unilateral lesion. The increasing experience with the sentinel node technique in vulvar cancer will definitely lead to another definition, one that has so far not been used but is more precise and safe: "A tumor is unilateral if no contralateral lymph nodes show tracer activity after a properly performed sentinel node procedure."

Summary. Patients with unilateral vulvar tumors have a very small risk for contralateral lymph node metastases. Omission of the contralateral groin node dissection is therefore acceptable in these cases, providing a safe definition of unilaterality is used. At this time, a unilateral tumor seems to be most safely defined by location greater than 1 cm from the midline. With the introduction of the sentinel lymph node technique, these definitions will soon become redundant.

What should be the extent of the groin dissection?

In this section, the extent of the groin dissection is discussed. Which lymph nodes must be removed from the groin to get optimal tumor control and survival with the least morbidity? In the last decade, controversies have focused on the issue of superficial versus superficial and deep groin node dissection; dissection or nondissection of the fascia lata and cribriform fascia; and whether the saphenous vein should be left intact.

Introduction. The lymphatic drainage from the vulva occurs via two groups of lymph nodes in the groin. Efferent lymphatic channels drain mainly into the superficial (inguinal) lymph node group, situated along the medial half of the inguinal ligament and around the proximal long saphenous vein, particularly where it passes through the cribriform fascia. All of these nodes are located above the fascia lata. A second group of nodes, the deep (femoral) nodes, are situated below the level of the cribriform fascia along the femoral vein. This group consists of only two to four nodes.[36]

Superficial groin node dissection. DiSaia and colleagues (1979) suggested that the deep lymphadenectomy could be omitted to decrease morbidity without compromising survival.[37] This group reported on 50 patients with a vulvar tumor of 2 cm or less in diameter, no clinically suspicious groin nodes, and negative superficial nodes on frozen section in whom the deep groin node dissection had been omitted.[38] No groin recurrences were seen in this group, with follow-up periods longer than 12 months in 84% of the patients. In contrast, a prospective, uncontrolled GOG trial showed that a superficial inguinal node dissection in a very favorable subgroup of T1 patients resulted in a groin recurrence rate of 6%.[33] Later, DiSaia explained their favorable results with the superficial groin node dissection by the fact that frequently the medial part of the cribriform fascia and possibly deep lymph nodes were removed en bloc with the superficial node–containing fat pad.[39] The GOG data are in line with the data of Burke and associates,[40] who found 3 groin recurrences (4%) after a superficial groin dissection with negative nodes in 76 patients. Their somewhat surprising conclusion was that "any degree of groin failure is undesirable but a small percentage of node-negative T1/T2 patients treated with superficial and deep lymphadenectomy also develop groin recurrences."

In large individual series of early-stage or locally advanced vulvar cancer, the risk of groin recurrence after an inguinal and femoral groin dissection with negative nodes was less than 1%.[14,41] Although inguinal dissection with omission of the femoral dissection was introduced to decrease morbidity, even this potential benefit seems unproved. Lin and coworkers[42] showed (in a nonrandomized study) that the frequency of complications related to the groin dissection, such as lymphedema, lymphocysts, wound dehiscence, and infections, did not decrease with omission of the deep groin dissection. They found lymphedema in 2 (13%) of 16 patients after superficial and deep dissection and 5 (17%) of 30 patients after superficial dissection only. The same figures were found for the incidence of lymphocysts. The conclusion must be that a superficial groin dissection, as performed in the GOG study, results in an unacceptable high groin recurrence rate without a certain benefit regarding morbidity. Therefore, it is recommended that both a superficial and a deep groin dissection be performed in every patient for whom a groin dissection is considered. Although it seems that this recommendation is rather straightforward, there is still controversy regarding the extent of this dissection.

What does superficial and deep groin dissection mean? How much lymph node–bearing fat must be removed in a cranial and caudal direction, and in a medial and lateral direction, and what must be the deep margin of dissection? Few clinical data are available to clear this issue, and it must be addressed by combining the scant clinical data with topographical anatomic data. Micheletti and coworkers[43] described a groin node dissection in which the fascia lata and a part of the cribriform fascia over the femoral artery were left intact. This approach was based on their earlier work, in which they found deep groin nodes under the cribriform fascia (e.g., the femoral nodes) only at the medial side of the femoral vein.[36] This method of dissection resulted in a 70% five-year survival rate with optimal groin control.[43] A survey on the technique of groin dissection in the United States was performed by Levenback and coworkers in 1996.[44] Although there was a lot of confusion about the terminology, it was reassuring that most gynecologic oncologists performed a lymph node dissection above the cribriform fascia and medial to the femoral vein, leaving the fascia lata intact as described earlier. A modification of the lateral and medial extent of the groin dissection was presented by Nicklin and associates.[45] In a retrospective study, they analyzed lymphangiograms of patients with vulvar and cervical cancer with the intention of defining the most lateral inguinal node relative to the anterior superior iliac spine. They calculated that by leaving 15% of fatty tissue overlying the lateral part of the inguinal ligament and 20% over the medial part of the inguinal ligament, a 99.8% chance of complete nodal clearance could be achieved. Theoretically, this approach of conserving possible lymph channel–bearing fatty tissue may decrease morbidity, but it needs to be studied prospectively before it can be introduced in clinical practice.

Preservation of the saphenous vein. Another surgical approach that intends to decrease morbidity is preserving the saphenous vein. Preservation of the saphenous vein may be of importance in patients without varicose veins to prevent venous stasis. However, the few papers addressing this issue do not provide evidence of benefit for this group of patients.

Lin and colleagues[42] showed that leg edema occurred in 6 (17%) of 36 patients who had preservation of the long saphenous vein, compared with 5 (13%) of 40 patients in whom this vein was sacrificed. This was confirmed in a study by Hopkins and coworkers,[47] who presented data on 17 patients in whom the saphenous vein was preserved. Paley and associates[48] presented data showing that lymphedema occurred in 36% of patients who had preservation of the saphenous vein, compared with 21% in whom the vessel was removed. These data suggest that sacrificing the saphenous vein does not increase morbidity. Therefore, this vein should be removed en bloc with the lymph node–bearing surrounding fatty tissue.

Sartorius muscle transposition. Other means of reducing morbidity after a groin dissection include the so-called sartorius muscle transposition and covering of the vessels with dura film. The latter method has proved not to be effective in reducing groin morbidity.[49] Sartorius transposition was popularized by vascular surgeons to create a protective barrier against infection after arterial reconstructive surgery. Transposition of the sartorius muscle to cover the inguinal vessels has been widely used to protect the vessels from erosion and even rupture of the artery in case of total wound dehiscence and infection, which were common after en bloc resection. The introduction of the separate incision technique, with a resultant reduction in wound dehiscence and infection, reduced the need for such a transposition. Way[31] reported that five of his patients had vessel rupture, three of whom died, before he started to perform the sartorius transposition, but since he adopted this procedure, no patients had experienced vessel rupture.

Evidence for a negative or positive impact of sartorius muscle transposition procedure on groin infections has not been available until recently. Paley and coworkers[48] reported on the effect of this procedure on wound morbidity after the triple-incision technique. There was an increase in wound breakdown, cellulitis, or both in the patient group in whom the sartorius muscle transposition was omitted, compared with historical controls in whom the procedure had been performed (66% versus 41%). Moreover, in a multivariate analysis, only weight of less than 150 pounds and sartorius transposition were independently associated with a reduction in groin morbidity. Although the sartorius transposition has waned in popularity over the last decade, the aforementioned data may renew interest in the procedure.

Summary. A proper groin node dissection must entail removal of all inguinal lymph node groups situated above the fascia lata as well as the two to four femoral nodes that are located medial to the femoral vein. The fascia lata can be left intact. There is no evidence that preserving the saphenous vein decreases morbidity, whereas there is one study indicating that transposition of the sartorius muscle reduces morbidity in patients after the triple-incision technique.

What should be done when a tumor-free margin of less than 8 mm is found in early vulvar cancer?

Some advocate adjuvant therapy when the tumor-free margin is less than 8 mm, others when it is less than 4 mm. When adjuvant therapy is selected, should it be re-resection or radiotherapy?

Introduction. There is a relationship between the tumor-free margin after resection of a vulvar tumor and the rate of local recurrence. Heaps and coworkers[35] found a vulvar recurrence in 13 of 23 patients who had a tumor-free margin of less than 4.9 mm but in only

8 of 112 patients with a margin greater than 4.8 mm. Recently, de Hullu[10] confirmed these data and also found the frequency of local recurrences to be related to the tumor-free margin. The question is whether the tumor-free margin in itself is an independent prognostic variable for local recurrence. If so, extension of the generally recommended minimal surgical margin of 1 cm to 2 cm or more would probably result in better local control.

Strategies to decrease the local recurrence rate. Although some studies showed no difference in local recurrence rate,[30] others showed that the risk of local recurrence is lower after a radical vulvectomy compared with a modified radical vulvectomy.[10,11] This seems to support the idea of a wider tumor-free surgical margin than the currently recommended 1 cm or more.[8]

There is, however, a major flaw in some of these studies. Although in Heaps' study a logistic model was used to identify the independent prognostic value of a tumor-free margin, only one other variable was tested against a tumor-free margin. A true multivariate analysis, including all prognostic variables, was not performed.[35] In the data published by de Hullu, only a univariate analysis was performed.[10] This implies that the evidence for a tumor-free margin as an independent prognostic variable for local recurrence is not very strong. Extension of the margin of resection from 1 to 2 cm therefore would not necessarily result in a decrease in the local recurrence rate.

Supporting the idea of lowering the number of local recurrences by extending the tumor-free surgical margin is the possibility that recurrences after modified local treatment occur at the original site after a relatively short period. There have been no studies in which the site of the primary vulvar tumor is related to the exact location of the local recurrence, also taking into account the time interval between initial treatment and recurrence. Interesting in this respect are the data published by de Hullu[10] on this time interval. About half of the local recurrences occurred after 2 years. Similar findings were published by Stehman and coworkers,[50] who found a median interval of 3 years. In the series reported by Maggino and associates,[13] 25% of the local recurrences occurred after 4 years. All these data support the concept of new occurrence of local disease in many cases, instead of recurrence of residual disease. These late local recurrences can be cured after secondary surgery in a high percentage of cases. Podratz and coworkers[14] showed that when recurrent disease surfaced 24 months or longer after initial treatment, the subsequent 1- and 5-year survival rates were 84% and 70%, respectively. de Hullu showed that the difference in local recurrence rate between modified radical surgery and radical vulvectomy was significant only after 2 years. Local recurrences occurring after 2 years are more likely to be new tumors. Prevention of these late recurrences is less likely to be influenced by extending the surgical margin from 1 to 2 cm.

These new tumors might even be located far from the original primary tumor. An indication for that is provided by Preti and colleagues,[11] who found that more than 15% of local recurrences on the vulva occur at a site other than that of the primary. The conclusion must be that although a tumor-free margin smaller than 4 to 5 mm constitutes a significant risk factor for recurrence (or re-occurrence), there is no evidence that simply taking a wider margin would be sufficient to prevent local recurrences.

Adjuvant local radiotherapy. What should then be done when a close or positive surgical margin is found in the final pathologic analysis of a resected specimen? In general, when the exact location of the tumor positive margin is known, a re-resection of the area at risk seems logical. There are, however, no data in the literature comparing surgical re-resection with observation in terms of the subsequent risk on local recurrence. Even the study published by Heaps and colleagues[35] does not specify their policy when positive or close surgical margins were found. Some authors currently advocate adjuvant radiation to the primary if a close or positive surgical margin is found. Faul and colleagues[51] treated 62 patients with close or positive surgical margins (less than 8 mm) with either local radiotherapy (n = 31) or observation (n = 31). The adjuvant local radiotherapy group showed a lower incidence of local recurrences (16% versus 58%) and better survival than the observation group. However, the benefit in survival with adjuvant radiotherapy could be accounted for solely by the subgroup of patients who had positive surgical margins. In other words, patients with close surgical margins (greater than 0 but less than 8 mm) did not benefit from adjuvant radiotherapy in terms of overall survival.

Therefore, these data do not support the routine use of adjuvant local radiotherapy in all patients with close surgical margins. However, it can be beneficial for individual patients with positive surgical margins in whom re-resection is not feasible.

Summary. There is firm evidence that patients with close surgical margins are at high risk for local recurrence. Although local re-resection seems most logical from a theoretical point of view, evidence is lacking that it results in a decrease in local recurrence rate. There is not enough evidence to recommend adjuvant local radiotherapy routinely in patients with close surgical margins.

Should the goal be margins free from severe dysplasia and/or lichen sclerosus when early vulvar cancer is surgically treated?

In this chapter, the problem of the treatment of invasive vulvar cancer with adjacent vulvar intraepithelial neoplasia (VIN) or lichen sclerosus vulva (LSV) is discussed. The question is whether associated VIN/LSV increases the risk of local recurrence and, if so, what can be done to lower this risk.

Introduction. One variable that is not often discussed but is, in our experience, important with respect to the risk of local recurrence is the presence of subclinical multifocal disease. Especially in patients with LSV or VIN in whom a local radical excision is performed and LSV or VIN is left in situ, subclinical multifocal disease can be the basis for future local re-occurrences.

Chafe and coworkers[52] in 1988, and later Herod and colleagues,[53] studied the issue of unrecognized invasive carcinoma in patients with VIN. They found subclinical invasive disease in 19% and 16% of patients with VIN. This subclinical disease was very superficial in most of the cases.

Evidence. In both univariate and multivariate analyses, VIN associated with invasive vulvar cancer significantly increased the risk of recurrence ($P < .019$) in a series of 101 patients.[11] However, among the 14 recurrences associated with VIN, 7 were at vulvar, 5 at groin, and 2 at distant sites. Risk assessment was not performed separately for local recurrences. Rouzier and associates[54] correlated multiple histopathologic and clinical variables with survival and local control in 108 patients with vulvar cancer. The group was subdivided into (1) patients with adjacent VIN combined with LSV, (2) those with adjacent undifferentiated VIN, and (3) those with no alterations adjacent to the invasive carcinoma. Adjacent undifferentiated VIN III was a favorable prognostic factor for survival, compared with either no alterations or a combination of VIN and LSV. The combination of VIN and LSV adjacent to the tumor carried the highest risk of local recurrence (35% versus 10% for undifferentiated VIN and 25% for no alterations). Although the literature on this specific subject is scarce, Rouzier's paper supports the theoretical concept of unrecognized invasive disease in VIN or LSV adjacent to the invasive tumor. The consequence must be that adjacent dystrophic lesions should be considered for resection together with the invasive tumor. A superficial resection with margins of 1 cm will suffice, because unrecognized invasive disease within VIN or LSV is early invasive (less than 1 mm of invasion) in most instances.

Summary. Whenever adjacent dystrophy (either VIN or LSV) is present in early vulvar cancer, local eradication must be strongly considered. The decision must also weigh the symptoms and the possible morbidity resulting from the excision.

What are the indications for postoperative radiotherapy when positive nodes are found in clinically early vulvar cancer?

There seems to be no indication for adjuvant radiotherapy when one small, intranodal metastasis is found in the groin nodes. Some also advocate a "wait and see" policy when two or three small, intranodal metastases are found.

Introduction. The status of the lymph nodes and the tumor diameter are the most significant prognostic factors for disease-specific survival in squamous cell cancer of the vulva.[55] Since the original report in 1991, several papers have addressed the issue of the prognostic significance of the pathologic status of the positive lymph nodes. Origoni and colleagues[56] reported on the prognostic value of capsule breakthrough of nodes in patients with vulvar cancer. They found that the presence of capsule breakthrough and a diameter of more than 5 mm of tumor in the nodes predicted a poor outcome. Two other studies dealing with extranodal spread in vulvar cancer presented almost identical results. In the studies of Paladini[57] and van der Velden and coworkers,[58] multivariate analyses indicated that capsule breakthrough was the most significant independent predictor for poor survival.

Paladini also took into account primary tumor parameters, but this did not alter the strong predictive value of extracapsular tumor. Besides extracapsular tumor, the diameter of the tumor in the node[57] or the percentage nodal replacement by tumor[58] also affected survival. Extranodal tumor resulted in poor outcome, even in patients with one positive lymph node, in two of the three studies.[56,58] In the study of Paladini however, extranodal tumor did not result in poor outcome in patients with one positive lymph node.[57] In contrast to the previous studies, extracapsular tumor did not affect survival significantly in the study reported by Burger and colleagues.[59] They analyzed primary tumor parameters and lymph node parameters in regard to their predictive values for survival, using both univariate and multivariate techniques. The 5-year survival rate was not corrected for death due to other causes. Although extranodal tumor did not influence the 5-year survival rate (57% versus 51%), there was a survival difference of 72% versus 58% after 2 years in favor of intracapsular tumor. Because 90% of recurrences in patients with positive nodes occurred within 2 years in this study, the disappearance of the survival difference after 5 years was probably caused by intercurrent deaths rather than deaths due to vulvar cancer. Nevertheless, the crude 5-year survival rate of 51% in patients with extracapsular tumor still compared favorably with the 20% to 30% cancer-related survival rates reported by others.[57,58]

Evidence for efficacy of adjuvant radiotherapy. It is known that there is a greater risk for groin recurrence when patients with positive lymph nodes do not get adjuvant radiotherapy to the pelvis and groin.[18] The greater risk of groin recurrence is predominantly seen in patients with more than two positive nodes.

Burger and colleagues[59] reported only one groin recurrence in 18 patients with positive nodes. They administered groin irradiation after en bloc radical vulvectomy and groin dissection, even if only a single positive node was found. If an extracapsular tumor was present, the dose to the groin was boosted to 60-Gy. The combination of radical vulvectomy with bilateral groin dissection and 60-Gy irradiation apparently results in a very good regional control. In the series by Paladini and associates,[57] who administered radiotherapy only if more than three nodes were positive, 8 of 26 recurrences in patients with positive nodes occurred in the groin. van der Velden, who administered radiotherapy to the groin only if more than two nodes were positive, reported that 12 of 34 recurrences were located in the groin or pelvis.[58] The difference in recurrence rate between the series reported by Burger,[59] in which a very low recurrence rate was found after a high dose of radiotherapy for all patients with positive nodes, and the less favorable results of Paladini[57] and van der Velden[58] supports the efficacy of adjuvant radiotherapy when positive nodes are found.

In contrast to all these data in favor of adjuvant radiotherapy is the report of the National Cancer Data Base (NCDB) on early vulvar cancer published by Creasman and coworkers.[60] The authors concluded that the addition of radiation to the groin in case of positive lymph nodes had no beneficial effect on relative survival. The problem with this retrospective study is selection bias. Patients with one positive node and no adjuvant radiation had a better survival rate than patients who had one positive node and received adjuvant radiation (70% versus 50%, respectively). The selection of patients with one positive node and adjuvant radiotherapy could have been on the basis of other additional poor prognostic factors, such as a single clinically suspicious node or a single node completely replaced by tumor or with capsule breakthrough.

Summary. The majority of results suggests that adjuvant groin radiation is important in obtaining optimal tumor control in the groin. The evidence for the efficacy of adjuvant radiotherapy is strongest in patients with multiple lymph nodes. There are no data to show a beneficial effect of adjuvant groin radiation in patients with one or two intracapsular metastases in a groin lymph node. These patients are well treated with surgery alone.

REFERENCES

1. Creasman WT: New gynecologic cancer staging. Obstet Gynecol 1990;75:287-288.
2. Shepherd JH: Cervical and vulva cancer: Changes in FIGO definitions of staging. Br J Obstet Gynaecol 1996;103:405-406.
3. Wilkinson EJ, Rico MJ: Microinvasive carcinoma of the vulva. Int J Gynecol Pathol 1982;1:29-39.
4. Sedlis A, Homesley H, Bundy BN, et al: Positive groin lymph nodes in superficial squamous cell vulvar cancer. A Gynecologic Oncology Group study. Am J Obstet Gynecol 1987;156:1159-1164.
5. Atamtede F, Hoogerland D: Regional lymph node recurrence following local excision for micro invasive vulvar carcinoma. Gynecol Oncol 1989;34:128-129.
6. Van der Velden J, Kooyman CD, van Lindert ACM, Heintz APM: A stage IA vulvar carcinoma with an inguinal lymph node recurrence after local excision: A case report and literature review. Int J Gynecol Cancer 1992;2:157-159.
7. Iversen T: The value of groin palpation in epidermoid carcinoma of the vulva. Gynecol Oncol 1981;12:291-295.
8. Hacker NF, van der Velden: Conservative management of early vulvar cancer. Cancer 1993;71(4 Suppl):1673-1677.
9. Ansink A, van der Velden: Surgical interventions for early squamous cell carcinoma of the vulva. Cochrane Database Syst Rev 2000;2:CD002036.
10. de Hullu JA: Innovations in treatment of vulvar cancer [thesis]. Groningen, The Netherlands, 2002.
11. Preti M, Ronco G, Ghiringhello B, Micheletti L: Recurrent squamous cell carcinoma of the vulva: Clinicopathologic determinants identifying low risk patients. Cancer 2000;88:1869-1876.
12. van der Velden J, Schilthuis MS, Burger MPM: Enbloc dissection versus triple incision technique in patients with squamous cell cancer of the vulva and positive nodes: The impact on recurrence pattern and survival. Proceedings of the International Gynaecologic Cancer Society. Int J Gynecol Cancer 2002;12:667.
13. Maggino T, Landoni F, Sartori E, et al: Patterns of recurrence in patients with squamous cell carcinoma of the vulva: A multicenter CTF Study. Cancer 2000;89:116-122.
14. Podratz KC, Symmonds RE, Taylor WF: Carcinoma of the vulva: Analysis of treatment failures. Am J Obstet Gynecol 1982;143:340-351.
15. Hacker NF, Leuchter RS, Berek JS, et al: Radical vulvectomy and bilateral inguinal lymphadenectomy through seperate groin incisions. Obstet Gynecol 1981;58:574-579.
16. Helm CW, Hatch K, Austin JM, et al: A matched comparison of single and triple incision techniques for the surgical treatment of carcinoma of the vulva. Gynecol Oncol 1992;46:150-156.
17. Grimshaw RN, Murdoch JB, Monaghan JM: Radical vulvectomy and bilateral inguinal-femoral lymphadenectomy through separate incisions: Experience with 100 cases. Int J Gynecol Cancer 1993;3:18-23.
18. Homesley HD, Bundy BN, Sedlis A, Adcock L: Radiation therapy versus pelvic node resection for carcinoma of the vulva with positive groin nodes. Obstet Gynecol 1986;68:733-740.
19. Morton DL, Lyman GH, Wong JH, et al: Technical details of intraoperative lymphatic mapping for early stage melanoma. Arch Surg 1992;130:392-399.
20. Levenback C, Burke TW, Gershenson DM, et al: Intraoperative lymphatic mapping for vulvar cancer. Obstet Gynecol 1994;84:163-167.
21. Ansink AC, Sie-Go DM, van der Velden J, et al: Identification of sentinel lymph nodes in vulvar carcinoma patients with the aid of a patent blue V injection: A multicenter study. Cancer 1999;86:652-656.
22. Schwartz GF, Giuliano AE, Veronesi U: Proceedings of the consensus conference on the role of sentinel lymph node biopsy in carcinoma of the breast, April 19-22, 2001, Philadelphia. Cancer 2002;94:2542-2551.
23. Cox CE, Bass SS, Boulware D: Implementation of new surgical technology: Outcome for lymphatic mapping of breast carcinoma. Ann Surg Oncol 1999;6:553-561.
24. Tafra L: The learning curve and sentinel node biopsy. Am J Surgery 2001;182:347-350.
25. Moskovic EC, Shepherd JH, Barton DP, et al: The role of high resolution ultrasound with guided cytology of groin lymph nodes in the management of squamous cell carcinoma of the vulva: a pilot study. Br J Obstet Gynaecol 1999;106:863-867.
26. Sohaib SA, Richards PS, Ind T, et al: MR imaging of carcinoma of the vulva. Am J Roentgenol 2002;178:373-377.
27. Fons G, ter Rake B, de Hullu J, et al: False negative sentinel node procedure in a patient with vulva cancer: Proceedings of the International Gynaecologic Cancer Society. Int J Gynecol Cancer 2002;12:658.
28. Van Trappen PO, Gyselman VG, Lowe DG, et al: Molecular quantification of lymph-node micrometastases in cervical cancer. Lancet 2001;357:15-20.
29. Iversen T, Aas M: Lymph drainage from the vulva. Gynecol Oncol 1983;16:179-189.
30. Magrina JF, Webb MJ, Gaffey TA, Symmonds RE: Stage I squamous cell cancer of the vulva. Am J Obstet Gynecol 1979;134:453-459.
31. Way SA: Malignant Disease of the Vulva. Edinburgh, Churchill Livingstone, 1982.
32. Berek JS, Hacker NF: Practical Gynecologic Oncology, 3rd ed. Philadelphia, Lippincott Williams & Wilkins, 2000.
33. Stehman FB, Bundy BN, Dvoretsky PM, Creasman WT: Early stage I carcinoma of the vulva treated with ipsilateral superficial

inguinal lymphadenectomy and modified radical hemivulvectomy: A prospective study of the Gynecologic Oncology Group. Obstet Gynecol 1992;79:490-497.

34. Thomas GM, Dembo AJ, Bryson SC, et al: Changing concepts in the management of vulvar cancer. Gynecol Oncol 1991;42:9-21.

35. Heaps JM, Fu YS, Montz FJ, et al: Surgical pathological variables predictive of local recurrence in squamous cell carcinoma of the vulva. Gynecol Oncol 1990;38:309-314.

36. Borgno G, Micheletti L, Barbero M, et al: Topographic distribution of groin lymph nodes: A study of 50 female cadavers. J Reprod Med 1990;35:1127-1129.

37. DiSaia PJ, Creasman WT, Rich WM: An alternate approach to early cancer of the vulva. Am J Obstet Gynecol 1979;133:825-832.

38. Berman ML, Soper JT, Creasman WT, et al: Conservative surgical management of superficially invasive stage I vulvar carcinoma. Gynecol Oncol 1989;35:352-357.

39. DiSaia PJ: What is the proper extent of an inguinal lymphadenectomy for early vulvar cancer? Gynecol Oncol 1997;64:183-185.

40. Burke TW, Stringer CA, Gershenson DM, et al: Radical wide excision and selective inguinal node dissection for squamous cell carcinoma of the vulva. Gynecol Oncol 1990;38:328-332.

41. Iversen T, Aalders JG, Christensen A, Kolstad P: Squamous cell carcinoma of the vulva: A review of 424 patients, 1956-1974. Gynecol Oncol 1980;9:271-279.

42. Lin JY, DuBeshter B, Angel C, Dvoretsky PM: Morbidity and recurrence with modifications of radical vulvectomy and groin dissection. Gynecol Oncol 1992;47:80-86.

43. Micheletti L, Borgno G, Barbero M, et al: Deep femoral lymphadenectomy with preservation of the facsia lata: Preliminary report on 42 invasive vulvar carcinomas. J Reprod Med 1990; 35:1130-1133.

44. Levenback C, Morris M, Burke TW, et al: Groin dissection practices among gynecologic oncologists treating early vulvar cancer. Gynecol Oncol 1996;62:73-77.

45. Nicklin JL, Hacker NF, Heintze SW, et al: An anatomical study of inguinal lymph node topography and clinical implications for the surgical management of vulval cancer. Int J Gynecol Cancer 1995;5:128-133.

46. Andrews SJ, Williams BT, DePriest PD, et al: Therapeutic implications of lymph nodal spread in lateral T1 and T2 squamous cell carcinoma of the vulva. Gynecol Oncol 1994;55:41-46.

47. Hopkins MP, Reid GC, Vettrano I, Morley GW: Squamous cell carcinoma of the vulva: Prognostic factors influencing survival. Gynecol Oncol 1991;43:113-117.

48. Paley PJ, Johnson PR, Adcock LL, et al: The effect of sartorius transposition on wound morbidity following inguinal-femoral lymphadenectomy. Gynecol Oncol 1997;64:237-241.

49. Finan MA, Fiorica JV, Roberts WS, et al: Artificial dura film for femoral vessel coverage after inguinofemoral lymphadenectomy. Gynecol Oncol 1994;55:333-335.

50. Stehman FB, Bundy BN, Ball H, Clarke-Pearson DL: Sites of failure and times to failure in carcinoma of the vulva treated conservatively: A Gynecologic Oncology Group study. Am J Obstet Gynecol 1996;174:1128-1132.

51. Faul CM, Mirmow D, Huang Q, et al: Adjuvant radiation for vulvar carcinoma: Improved local control. Int J Radiat Oncol Biol Phys 1997;38:381-389.

52. Chafe W, Richards A, Morgan L, Wilkinson E: Unrecognized invasive carcinoma in vulvar intraepithelial neoplasia (VIN). Gynecol Oncol 1988;31:154-165.

53. Herod JJ, Shafi MI, Rollason TP, et al: Vulvar intraepithelial neoplasia with superficially invasive carcinoma of the vulva. Br J Obstet Gynaecol 1996;103:453-456.

54. Rouzier R, Morice P, Haie-Meder C, et al: Prognostic significance of epithelial disorders adjacent to invasive vulvar carcinomas. Gynecol Oncol 2001;81:414-419.

55. Homesley HD, Bundy BN, Sedlis A, et al: Assessment of current International Federation of Gynecology and Obstetrics staging of vulvar carcinoma relative to prognostic factors for survival

(a Gynecologic Oncology Group study). Am J Obstet Gynecol 1991;164:997-1003.

56. Origoni M, Sideri M, Garsia S, et al: Prognostic value of pathological patterns of lymph node positivity in squamous cell carcinoma of the vulva stage III and IVA FIGO. Gynecol Oncol 1992;45:313-316.

57. Paladini D, Cross P, Lopes A, Monaghan JM: Prognostic significance of lymph node variables in squamous cell carcinoma of the vulva. Cancer 1994;74:2491-2496.

58. van der Velden, van Lindert AC, Lammes FB, et al: Extracapsular growth of lymph node metastases in squamous cell carcinoma of the vulva: The impact on recurrence and survival. Cancer 1995;75:2885-2890.

59. Burger MP, Hollema H, Emanuels AG, et al: The importance of the groin node status for the survival of T1 and T2 vulvar carcinoma patients. Gynecol Oncol 1995;57:327-334.

60. Creasman WT, Phillips JL, Menck HR: The National Cancer Data Base report on early stage invasive vulvar carcinoma. The American College of Surgeons Commission on Cancer and the American Cancer Society. Cancer 1997;80:505-513.

61. Parker RT, Duncan I, Rampone J, Creasman WT: Operative management of early invasive epidermoid carcinoma of the vulva. Am J Obstet Gynecol 1975;123:349-355.

62. Hacker NF, Berek JS, Lagasse LD, et al: Individualization of treatment for stage I squamous cell vulvar cancer. Obstet Gynecol 1984;63:155-162.

63. Hofmann JS, Kumar NB, Morley GW: Microinvasive squamous carcinoma of the vulva: Search for a definition. Obstet Gynecol 1983;61:615-618.

64. Ross M, Ehrmann RL: Histologic prognosticators in stage I squamous cell carcinoma of the vulva. Obstet Gynecol 1987; 70:774-784.

65. Iversen T, Abeler V, Aalders JG: Individualized treatment of stage I carcinoma of the vulva. Obstet Gynecol 1981;57: 85-89.

66. Struyk APHB, Bouma J, van Lindert AC: Early stage cancer of the vulva: A pilot investigation on cancer of the vulva in gynecologic oncology centers in the Netherlands. Proceedings of the International Gynaecologic Cancer Society 1989;2:303.

67. Levenback C, Burke TW, Morris M, et al: Potential applications of intraoperative lymphatic mapping in vulvar cancer. Gynecol Oncol 1995;59:216-220.

68. Decesare SL, Fiorica JV, Roberts WS, et al: A pilot study utilizing intraoperative lymphoscintigraphy for identification of the sentinel lymph nodes in vulvar cancer. Gynecol Oncol 1997; 66:425-428.

69. De Cicco C, Sideri M, Bartolomei M, et al: Sentinel node biopsy in early vulvar cancer. Br J Cancer 2000;82:295-299.

70. de Hullu JA, Hollema H, Piers DA, et al: Sentinel lymph node procedure is highly accurate in squamous cell carcinoma of the vulva. J Clin Oncol 2000;18:2811-2816.

71. Rodier JF, Janser JC, Routiot T, et al: Sentinel node biopsy in vulvar malignancies: A preliminary feasibility study. Oncol Rep 1999;6:1249-1252.

72. Terada KY, Shimizu DM, Wong JH: Sentinel node dissection and ultrastaging in squamous cell cancer of the vulva. Gynecol Oncol 2000;76:40-44.

73. Wharton JT, Gallager S, Rutledge FN: Microinvasive carcinoma of the vulva. Am J Obstet Gynecol 1974;118:159-162.

74. Buscema J, Stern J, Woodruff JD: The significance of the histologic alterations adjacent to invasive vulvar carcinoma. Am J Obstet Gynecol 1980;137:902-909.

75. Tham KF, Shepherd JH, Lowe DG, et al: Early vulvar cancer: The place of conservative management. Eur J Surg Oncol 1993; 19:361-367.

76. Farias-Eisner R, Cirisano FD, Grouse D, et al: Conservative and individualized surgery for early squamous carcinoma of the vulva: The treatment of choice for stage I and II (T1-2N0-1M0) disease. Gynecol Oncol 1994;53:55-58.

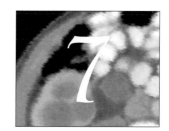

C H A P T E R

ADVANCED-STAGE VULVAR CANCER

Thomas W. Burke and *Anthony H. Russell*

 MAJOR CONTROVERSIES

- **What vulvar lesions should be considered "advanced"?**
- **What treatment approach is most appropriate for the control of locally extensive vulvar disease?**
- **What therapy should follow chemoradiation?**
- **How should gross inguinal lymphadenopathy be managed?**
- **How should occult inguinal node metastases be managed?**

Vulvar cancer is an uncommon malignant lesion. Approximately 90% of these tumors are squamous lesions that arise from the cutaneous surface. The remaining group includes a collection of ultra-rare lesions such as melanoma, adenocarcinoma, sarcomas, Paget's disease, and metastatic lesions from adjacent organs. This section focuses on the management of squamous cancers of the vulva. Even though these tumors arise in an easily visible and palpable site, a significant subset of women choose to ignore symptoms of pruritus, bleeding, and pain and present with advanced local disease. Such cases have become relatively rare as access to health care has improved for most women and the social stigma previously associated with cancers of the lower reproductive tract has dramatically diminished. Many in this group are elderly—sometimes mentally impaired—and are the victims of personal neglect coupled with inappropriate modesty, frank denial, and understandable anxiety. Often they have attempted topical "home" remedies for an extended period. They are sometimes brought in for medical attention when others detect the odor of necrotic tissue, visible evidence of bleeding, or severe pain. An obvious cancer diagnosis can usually be made based on clinical examination revealing a large ulcerated or fungating mass lesion, supplemented by simple punch biopsy (Fig. 7-1).

Squamous tumors of the vulva typically undergo a prolonged local growth phase, with gradual extension to adjacent soft tissue structures. Encroachment on critical midline structures such as the urethra, vagina, anus, or pubic symphysis provides a therapeutic challenge if one tries to balance the desire for curative intent with maintenance of normal function. Careful assessment of the extent of local spread should be the focus of the initial evaluation. Physical examination usually provides the most useful clinical information regarding involvement of perineal soft tissue structures. Cystourethroscopy and proctosigmoidoscopy should be considered for women with large lesions that extend into the deeper anterior or posterior soft tissue spaces. Magnetic resonance imaging can also provide supplemental information about the extent of deep tissue penetration and attachment to periosteum or bone.

A fine superficial network of lymphatic channels courses through the vulvar skin between the vaginal-cutaneous border and the lateral labiocrural folds.[1-3] These lymphatics coalesce superiorly and drain into the superficial group of five to eight inguinal lymph nodes that surround the saphenous venous system. From here, secondary lymphatic channels perforate the cribriform fascia to reach the two or three deep inguinal nodes that lie medial to the femoral vein. Lymphatic flow then proceeds cephalad, beneath the

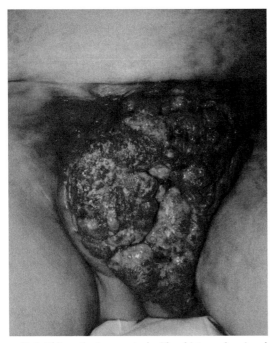

Figure 7–1. This patient presented with a history of perineal pain and bleeding of uncertain duration. Obvious cancer clearly had been present for a significant period and had been ignored by the patient. Biopsy at any site will confirm the diagnosis of squamous cell carcinoma.

Table 7–1. Federation of Gynecologists and Obstetricians (FIGO) Staging of Vulvar Carcinoma

Stage	Clinical Findings
Stage 0	Carcinoma in situ; intraepithelial carcinoma
Stage I	Tumor confined to the vulva or perineum; 2 cm or less in greatest dimension; no nodal metastasis Stage Ia: stromal invasion ≤1.0 mm Stage Ib: stromal invasion >1.0 mm
Stage II	Tumor confined to the vulva or perineum; more than 2 cm in greatest dimension; no nodal metastasis
Stage III	Tumor of any size with adjacent spread to urethra, vagina, or anus; or with unilateral regional lymph node metastasis
Stage IVa	Tumor invades upper urethra, bladder mucosa, rectal mucosa, pelvic bone, or bilateral regional node metastases
Stage IVb	Any distant metastasis, including pelvic lymph nodes

From Creasman WT: New gynecologic cancer staging. Gynecol Oncol 1995;58;157-158.

inguinal ligament, to the pelvic nodal chain. In general, lymphatic flow is unilateral except from midline structures such as the anus and clitoris. Uncommon routes of lymphatic drainage include direct flow to the pelvic nodes from the clitoral area, flow to the deep anorectal nodes from posterior lesions, contralateral flow from a lateral site, and direct flow to the deep inguinal group that bypasses the superficial group. The mechanism of nodal metastasis is thought to be an embolic phenomenon by which malignant cells flow directly to the primary filtering node. Once established within the first-echelon node, metastatic tumor can grow locally to produce clinically evident inguinal adenopathy or spread to adjacent second- and third-echelon nodes.

Distant metastases from vulvar squamous cancer are exceedingly rare. Involvement of para-aortic or scalene nodes is sometimes seen, as is hematogenous dissemination to lung or liver. Such cases are usually refractory to most forms of therapy. Palliative treatment with systemic cytotoxic agents such as cisplatin, irinotecan, 5-fluorouracil (5-FU), or gemcitabine can be offered if the patient desires. This section will not consider management of distant metastatic disease.

What vulvar lesions should be considered "advanced"?

Vulvar cancers are staged according to criteria adopted by the International Federation of Gynecology and Obstetrics (FIGO), as summarized in Table 7-1.[4] A working clinical definition for the term "advanced"

vulvar cancer describes those tumors that cannot be satisfactorily resected by a locally aggressive surgical procedure. In the broad sense, this definition identifies two categories of women with vulvar tumors: those in whom the primary lesion invades functionally important midline structures (T3 or T4 lesions), and those in whom metastases to regional lymph nodes are identified (unilateral or bilateral, occult or gross involvement). Involvement of midline structures is usually readily apparent during examination (Fig. 7-2). It is

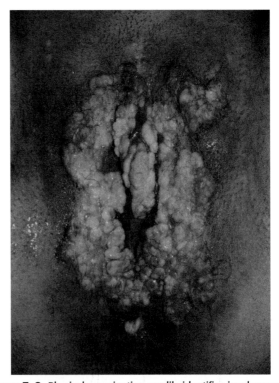

Figure 7–2. Physical examination readily identifies involvement of key midline structures. This extensive central lesion surrounds the urethra and approaches the anal sphincters. Resection with a grossly normal tissue margin would be impossible.

important to consider that primary surgical therapy requires resection of the tumor with a normal tissue margin of 1 to 2 cm to achieve an acceptable rate of local control. Therefore, the examination must include an estimation of the adequacy of achievable resection margins. We have usually required a 2-cm margin for primary resection. However, recent investigation suggests that an uninvolved margin of 1 cm may be adequate.[5-7] The 1-cm fresh tissue margin corresponds to 8 mm of clearance when measured in fixed tissue specimens. These guidelines can be used to assess the adequacy of surgical resection from either frozen-section or final histologic material.

For patients with nodal disease, it is probably useful to further stratify them into those whose nodal disease was discovered during surgical management of presumed "early cancer" and those with clinically evident adenopathy confirmed by fine-needle biopsy during the initial evaluation. The former group should be considered candidates for adjuvant management of potential microscopic residual disease. The latter group needs a management strategy that is capable of eliminating gross regional tumor.

Consequently, three scenarios of advanced vulvar cancer are discussed here: locally extensive cancer without clinically detectable involvement of inguinal lymph nodes, locally extensive cancer with grossly identified nodal spread, and limited local cancer with nodal spread detected after lymph node dissection. In aggregate, this population of patients is challenging to treat, both because of the constraints imposed by age, psychosocial factors, and medical comorbidities, and because it is necessary to coordinate complex multimodality therapy. Contemporary clinical imperatives are to maximize the probability of cancer control with retention of function while minimizing acute and chronic toxicities. These competitive objectives become increasingly divergent as the local-regional extent of cancer advances.

What treatment approach is most appropriate for the control of locally extensive vulvar disease?

The traditional approach to large vulvar tumors was to attempt clearance via ultraradical operation. In many cases, radical vulvectomy with concomitant bilateral groin dissection was combined with pelvic exenteration to resect local and regional disease with a large tissue margin. Long-term survival rates of 25% to 70% were reported for selected series of women whose disease was managed in this way.[8-11] Drawbacks to ultraradical surgical therapy include the operative morbidity of these procedures in elderly women, the high frequency of nodal metastases requiring additional treatment, the loss or alteration of sexual and excretory function, and the development of less radical alternative options. Nevertheless, exenterative procedures remain an option for rare patients whose disease cannot be managed with other modalities or

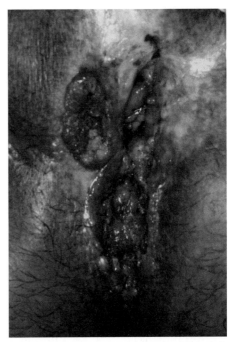

Figure 7–3. This 80-year-old woman developed new ulcerative lesions of the vulva 2 years after radical wide excision of a T2 squamous tumor. External beam irradiation to the groins, lower pelvis, and vulva was given at the time of original diagnosis because of microscopic nodal metastases. Adequate clearance of this recurrence required an exenterative resection.

who develop local pelvic or perineal recurrence after primary treatment (Fig. 7-3).

The use of preoperative external beam irradiation or irradiation given with synchronous chemotherapy (chemoradiation) can substantially reduce the size of many tumors that invade or impinge on functionally important midline structures.[12-30] Frequently, these large lesions can be converted to little or no residual disease that is amenable to limited surgical resection. In fact, the preoperative application of moderate-dose external beam radiotherapy (36 to 54 Gy), followed by planned resection of the tumor bed, has resulted in no residual tumor in a substantial proportion of cases (Table 7-2). Some have supplemented the impact of external beam therapy with interstitial or intracavitary brachytherapy, to apply a higher dose to a discrete tissue volume when surgical resection of residual is anticipated to be inadequate.[31,32]

A growing body of experience is accumulating to support the clinical use of preoperative combined chemoradiation as a strategy to reduce or eliminate bulky vulvar disease (Table 7-3). These findings parallel to those reported in the management of squamous tumors of the cervix, anus, and head and neck sites.[33-39] The Gynecologic Oncology Group (GOG) studied 73 women with stage III or IV squamous vulvar cancers that were judged not to be amenable to resection without exenteration because the disease extended beyond the conventional boundaries of radical vulvectomy.[22] Preoperative chemoradiation, consisting of 47.6 Gy delivered in 1.7-Gy fractions plus two cycles of

Table 7–2. Complete Tumor Clearance after External Beam Irradiation

Reference	Patients (n)	Radiation Dose (Gy)	Pathologic CR No.	Pathologic CR %
Acosta et al.[12] (1978)	14	36-55	5	36
Jafari & Magalotti[16] (1981)	4	30-42	4	100
Hacker et al.[15] (1984)	8	44-54	4	50

CR, complete response.

synchronous cisplatin and 5-FU chemotherapy, converted 69 of 71 women to a resectable status. Ultimately, urinary and fecal continence were conserved in all but 3 patients. This approach provided excellent tumor control with conservation of normal tissue integrity and function for many patients who would otherwise have required exenterative resection to effect tumor clearance. For medically appropriate cases, we favor a similar combined modality approach. External beam doses to the vulva in the range of 45 to 55 Gy are recommended. The regional inguinal and lower pelvic lymph nodes should be incorporated into the treatment volume because of the significant likelihood of small-volume metastasis even in palpably or radiographically normal lymph nodes (Fig. 7-4). Excellent outcomes have been reported with this prophylactic approach.[19,25,40-45] Comparison of nonrandomized case series suggests that chemoradiation may provide better groin control than radiation alone.

Cytotoxic agents employed as components of these combined regimens typically include drugs with effectiveness against squamous lesions and those that are known to potentiate the antitumor effects of ionizing radiation. Many of the regimens reported were adapted from treatment schemes developed for more common squamous cancers. Early series tended to focus on combinations that paired either 5-FU or cisplatin with mitomycin-C or bleomycin. However, since publication of the results of several large trials in women with cancers of the cervix that used either 5-FU plus cisplatin or weekly cisplatin alone, most current regimens employ these agents.[36-39] Although no regimen has demonstrated clearcut clinical superiority, our current preference is to use a prolonged infusion of 5-FU and cisplatin that was originally developed for patients with squamous lesions of the anus.[35]

What therapy should follow chemoradiation?

All women who receive such treatment develop a substantial desquamating response within the treatment field (Fig. 7-5). Although visually impressive, these cutaneous reactions can be managed symptomatically and heal rapidly after completion of the therapy. Some centers then boost the dose to residual tumor or tumor bed with either vaginal brachytherapy or interstitial needle implant.

However, we evaluate the patient for response 3 to 4 weeks after external beam treatment is complete and to plan further surgical therapy. Although several studies have shown that chemoradiation completely eliminates all evidence of cancer, such data have been based on surgical resection of the central tumor bed or sites of suspected residual disease. From a practical standpoint, it is frequently difficult to distinguish between healing vulvar tumor site and residual cancer. We always plan a limited surgical resection, to evaluate the pathologic response and to remove any potential viable cancer, about 6 weeks after chemoradiation. The surgical goal is to remove any abnormal site with a gross normal tissue margin. Presumably, the first phase of therapy has sterilized microscopic extensions and lymphatic emboli within the treatment field, eliminating the requirement for a large tumor-free resection margin.

Groin dissection is not performed, because the inguinal nodes have already been treated during the chemoradiation phase with doses that should control subclinical disease. Significant lower-extremity lymphedema is much more common in women who have been treated with both groin irradiation and groin dissection.[46,47] Consequently, we try to avoid this combination whenever possible.

Table 7–3. Risk of Occult Groin Node Metastasis by Tumor Size

Tumor Diameter (cm)	No Palpable Nodes (Clinical N0)	Palpable/Not Suspicious (Clinical N1)	Total
0-1.0	2/31 (6.4%)	1/5 (20%)	3/36 (8.3%)
1.1-2.0	13/57 (22.8%)	0/17 (0%)	13/74 (17.5%)
2.1-3.0	14/43 (32.5%)	3/11 (27.2%)	17/54 (31.4%)
3.1-5.0	8/28 (28.5%)	3/7 (42.8%)	11/35 (31.4%)
5.0+	3/12 (25%)	1/5 (20%)	4/17 (23.5%)

Adapted from Gonzales-Bosquet J, Kinney WK, Russel AH, et al: Risk of occult inguinofemoral lymph node metastasis from squamous carcinoma of the vulva. Int Rad Oncol Biol Phys 2003;57:419-424.

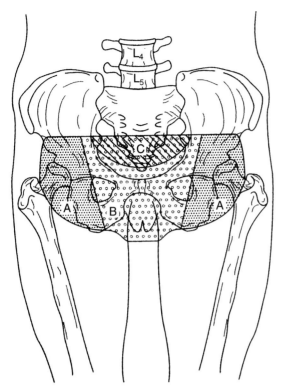

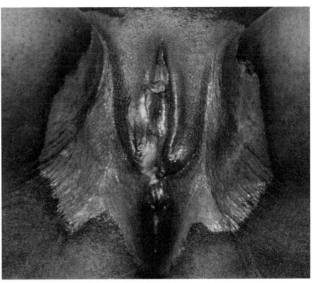

Figure 7–5. Three weeks after completion of chemoradiation using prolonged infusion of 5-fluorouracil and cisplatin, the vulvar skin shows evidence of a widespread desquamation reaction that is healing nicely. A small area of residual ulceration represents a focus of persistent cancer that was removed by limited resection.

Figure 7–4. External beam treatment fields can be designed to provide coverage of the vulva and inguinal and lower pelvic nodes. This strategy is most appropriate for women with high-risk primary disease. Zone A can be treated with mixed photons and electrons or anterior low-energy photons alone, to reduce the dose to the femoral necks. Zone B should be treated with opposed anterior and posterior photons. Zone C may be shielded to reduce the dose to the intestine and urinary bladder. (Reprinted with permission from Russel AH: Radiation therapy for vulvar cancer. In: Eifel PJ, Levenback C (Eds): American Cancer Society Atlas of Clinical Oncology: Cancer of the Female Lower Genital Tract. Philadelphia: BC Decker, 2001, Fig. 14-4, p. 231.)

How should gross inguinal lymphadenopathy be managed?

Clinically palpable inguinal nodal metastases are unusual. Furthermore, clinical evaluation of the superficial groin nodes is notoriously inaccurate. At least 20% of palpably normal nodes contain metastatic cancer, and more than 20% of palpably enlarged nodes are subsequently proven to be histologically negative.[48-55] However, when present, large cancer-containing nodes must be aggressively treated, because the usual doses of external beam therapy are inadequate to control gross disease. Groin failure is debilitating and lethal. If obviously abnormal groin nodes are identified during the initial evaluation, we use fine-needle aspiration to confirm the suspected diagnosis.

Whenever feasible, we attempt to excise or debulk large inguinal node metastases before beginning chemoradiation. This strategy minimizes tumor volume in the groin and allows for better treatment planning by identifying the location and amount of unresectable disease. Hemaclips can be placed to mark the tumor bed or site of residual disease. The depth of

the treatment target can also be determined.[56] Additional boost doses of external beam irradiation can then be added to the standard chemoradiation plan. We do not perform a full lymph node dissection, because doing so would raise the risk of significant post-treatment morbidity in the lower extremity. The surgical goal is to eliminate tumor volume so that subsequent therapy can sterilize small-volume residual or microscopic metastases in adjacent nodes.

Some women present with such extensive nodal involvement (fixed, matted, ulcerated) that any attempt at operative resection is precluded. The GOG treated 46 such women with external beam irradiation and concomitant cisplatin plus 5-FU. Inguinal dissection became technically possible in 37 women, 15 of whom had no histologic evidence of residual nodal cancer.[57] This reversed sequence management plan would appear to offer some opportunity for tumor control in women who would otherwise have incurable disease. Patients who develop groin failure after an attempt at initial control have very limited options and usually are candidates for palliative cytotoxic therapy only.

How should occult inguinal node metastases be managed?

This group includes patients who had initial surgical management of their vulvar cancer that included resection of the primary tumor coupled with some surgical assessment of inguinal lymph nodes. Occult nodal metastasis is a relatively common event in women with vulvar cancer. Although there is some correlation between incidence of nodal metastasis and increasing size of the primary tumor (Table 7-4),[58] a percentage of small tumors will have already

Table 7–4. Results of Chemoradiation for Large Vulvar Cancers

Report	Patients (n)	RT dose (Gy)	Chemotherapy	Response Rate (%)	Alive with NED (%)
Levin et al.[20] (1986)	6	18-60	5-FU/Mito-C	100	67
Thomas et al.[24] (1989)	24	44-60	5-FU/Mito-C	58 (CR only)	78
Carson et al.[27] (1990)	8	45-50	5-FU/Mito-C/CDDP	75 (CR only)	33
Berek et al.[29] (1991)	12	44-54	5-FU/CDDP	92	83
Russell et al.[30] (1992)	25	47-72	5-FU/CDDP	89 (CR = 80)	78
Koh et al.[17] (1993)	20	30-54	5-FU	90 (CR = 50)	49
Scheistroen & Trope[23] (1993)	42	30-45	Bleomycin	67	5
Sebag-Montefiore et al.[28] (1994)	37	—	5-FU/Mito-C	70	—
Eifel et al.[13] (1995)	12	54	5-FU/CDDP	100	49
Lupe et al.[21] (1996)	31	36	5-FU/Mito-C	94	61
Landoni et al.[18] (1996)	58	54	5-FU/Mito-C	80 (CR = 31)	49
Cunningham et al.[26] (1997)	14	50-69	5-FU/CDDP	92 (CR = 62)	29
Moore et al.[22] (1998)	73	47.6	5-FU/CDDP	97 (CR = 48)	55

CDDP, cisplatin; CR, complete response; 5-FU, 5-fluorouracil; Mito-C, mitomycin C; NED, no evidence of disease; RT, external beam radiotherapy.

metastasized to the groin at the time of diagnosis. Some patients in this clinical category have derangements of immune function, including chronic suppression for organ transplantation, chronic steroid therapy, or human immunodeficiency virus (HIV) infection.[59] A variety of approaches for surgical assessment of groin nodes are in common clinical practice, including bilateral superficial and deep groin dissection, unilateral superficial and deep dissection, bilateral or unilateral superficial groin dissection, or lymphatic mapping with a tailored approach to groin dissection.[60-63] In this clinical scenario, the primary disease has typically been adequately excised with clear margins. Occult disease has been identified in one or more nodes in one or both groins. The level of information regarding the extent of nodal involvement may be incomplete.

Patients who fit this profile require careful treatment planning because they have a significant opportunity to obtain long-term survival and cure. Because all obvious cancer has been surgically excised, these women are candidates for truly adjuvant therapy. Data suggest that treatment of occult groin metastases at the time of initial management can provide survival rates approaching 75%.[46,64,65] The desire for aggressive curative therapy must be balanced against the risk of potential complications associated with combined therapy in the groin, including local wound breakdown, chronic lymphangitis, and lymphedema. Although these chronic morbidities are not life-threatening, they are certainly life-altering.

The lack of definitive data has generated multiple areas of minor controversy in this patient subset: Should the vulva be treated along with the groin? Do patients with a single positive node require adjuvant therapy? Should adjuvant therapy be given to both groins if only one contains positive nodes? Should the contralateral groin be treated if one side is positive and the other is undissected? Does the addition of concomitant chemotherapy add any advantage to groin irradiation?

A few clinical trials provide some insights to assist with treatment planning. The GOG conducted a randomized trial in 114 eligible patients that compared pelvic lymphadenectomy with external beam irradiation to the pelvis and groins (but not the tumor bed or vulva) in patients who were found to have inguinal node metastasis.[64] Forty patients had only one positive node. Metastases to pelvic nodes were identified in 15 (28%) of 53 women who had pelvic lymphadenectomy; 9 of these 15 died within 1 year. The overall survival rate at 2 years was 68% for women receiving radiotherapy, compared to 54% for those who had surgical node dissection. Further analysis demonstrated that this survival advantage was limited to women with two or more involved groin nodes (63% for radiotherapy versus 37% for node dissection). The survival difference could be attributed to the markedly reduced incidence of groin failure in irradiated women (5%) compared with those treated surgically (24%). Not surprisingly, the reported incidence of lymphedema was higher in women who received both surgery and radiotherapy. The results of this trial support the routine use of adjuvant postoperative irradiation to both groins and lower pelvis in women with occult metastases to two or more nodes.

Another observation from this study was a 9% incidence of vulvar recurrence noted across both treatment arms. All studies analyzing conservative resection of vulvar tumors report a similar mixture of both new and recurrent tumor within retained vulvar skin.[46,65-68] Undoubtedly, some of these failures might have been prevented by including the vulva within the initial treatment field. However, reliable data to define the magnitude of such a preventive strategy are nonexistent. Clinical experience suggests that isolated recurrences can be curatively resected in about 75% of cases.[69-72] Both treatment strategies have merit. Avoiding initial radiotherapy to the vulva preserves cutaneous and mucosal integrity at the expense of an unknown increase in risk of vulvar failure. From a practical perspective, we use possible predictors of recurrence such as tumor grade, presence of lymph vascular space invasion, and resection margin to select candidates for simultaneous vulvar treatment.[73]

In the absence of comparative data, it is possible to develop a treatment philosophy for groin irradiation in less clearcut settings by evaluating established clinical observations. First, late groin failure is almost always fatal. Second, the presence of nodal spread is the single most important prognostic variable in women with vulvar cancer. Third, the rate of contralateral groin failure is 3% to 9% in women with ipsilateral nodal disease.[46,74] Fourth, radiotherapy to the groins provides a high level of regional tumor control when gross disease in not present. Fifth, groin irradiation has low morbidity when not combined with extensive surgical dissection. Reasonable deductions can then be made to recommend routine adjuvant radiotherapy to both groins and lower pelvic nodes in any woman with a resected nodal metastasis.

The final issue regarding management of resected occult groin metastasis is whether the addition of chemotherapy to planned irradiation is beneficial. There are no available data to assist with this treatment decision. Extrapolation of existing data regarding the effectiveness of chemoradiation in the management of large primary vulvar lesions, cervix cancers, and anorectal tumors tend to suggest that its use in advanced vulvar tumors is desirable. However, against this must be balanced the potential toxicities of combined therapy in elderly women who are recovering from a major operative procedure. Equally important is the potential for combined treatment to result in treatment delay or an incomplete course of radiotherapy. Our current approach is to recommend chemoradiation in medically appropriate candidates, pending the availability of further data.

REFERENCES

1. Iversen T, Aas M: Lymph drainage from the vulva. Gynecol Oncol 1983;16:179-189.
2. Parry-Jones E: Lymphatics of the vulva. J Obstet Gynecol Br Empire 1963;70:751-765.
3. Way S: The anatomy of the lymphatic drainage of the vulva and its influence on the radical operation of carcinoma. Ann R Col Surg Engl 1948;187:3.
4. Creasman WT: New gynecologic cancer staging. Gynecol Oncol 1995;58:157-158.
5. de Hullu JA, Hollema H, Lolkema S, et al: Vulvar carcinoma: The price of less radical surgery. Cancer 2002;95:2331-2338.
6. Faul CM, Mirmow D, Huang Q, et al: Adjuvant radiation for vulvar carcinoma: Improved local control. Int J Radiat Oncol Biol Phys 1997;38:381-389.
7. Heaps JM, Fu YS, Montz FJ, et al: Surgical-pathologic variables predictive of local recurrence in squamous cell carcinoma of the vulva. Gynecol Oncol 1990;38:309-314.
8. Cavanagh D, Shepherd JH: The place of pelvic exenteration in the primary management of advanced carcinoma of the vulva. Gynecol Oncol 1982;13:318-322.
9. Miller B, Morris M, Levenback C, et al: Pelvic exenteration for primary and recurrent vulvar cancer. Gynecol Oncol 1995;58:202-205.
10. Phillips B, Buchsbaum JH, Lifshitz S: Pelvic exenteration for vulvovaginal carcinoma. Am J Obstet Gynecol 1981;141:1038-1044.
11. Thornton WN Jr, Flanagan WL Jr: Pelvic exenteration in the treatment of advanced malignancy of the vulva. Am J Obstet Gynecol 1973;117:774-781.
12. Acosta AA, Given FT, Frazier AB, et al: Preoperative radiation therapy in the management of squamous cell carcinoma of the vulva: Preliminary report. Am J Obstet Gynecol 1978;132:198-206.
13. Eifel PJ, Morris M, Burke TW, et al: Prolonged continuous infusion cisplatinum and 5-fluorouracil with radiation for locally advanced carcinoma of the vulva. Gynecol Oncol 1995;59:51-56.
14. Fairey RN, MacKay PA, Benedet JL, et al: Radiation treatment of carcinoma of the vulva, 1950-1980. Am J Obstet Gynecol 1985;151: 591-597.
15. Hacker NF, Berek JS, Julliard GJF, Lagasse LD: Preoperative radiation therapy for locally advanced vulvar cancer. Cancer 1984;54: 2056-2061.
16. Jafari K, Magalotti M: Radiation therapy in carcinoma of the vulva. Cancer 1981;47:686-691.
17. Koh WJ, Wallace HJ, Greer BE, et al: Combined radiotherapy and chemotherapy in the management of local-regionally advanced vulvar cancer. Int J Radiat Oncol Biol Phys 1993;26: 809-816.
18. Landoni F, Maneo A, Zanetta G, et al: Concurrent preoperative chemotherapy with 5-fluorouracil and mitomycin C and radiotherapy (FUMIR) followed by limited surgery in locally advanced and recurrent vulvar carcinoma. Gynecol Oncol 1996; 61:321-327.
19. Leiserowitz GS, Russel AH, Kinney WK, et al: Prophylactic chemoradiation of inguino-femoral lymph nodes in patients with locally advanced vulvar cancer. Gynecol Oncol 1994;54:112.
20. Levin W, Goldberg G, Altaras M, et al: The use of concomitant chemotherapy and radiotherapy prior to surgery in advanced stage carcinoma of the vulva. Gynecol Oncol 1986;25:20-25.
21. Lupe G, Raspagliesi F, Zucali R, et al: Combined preoperative chemoradiotherapy followed by radical surgery in locally advanced vulvar carcinoma: A pilot study. Cancer 1996;77: 1472-1478.
22. Moore DH, Thomas GM, Montana GS, et al: Preoperative chemoradiation for advanced vulvar cancer: A phase II study of the Gynecologic Oncology Group. Int J Radiat Oncol Biol Phys 1998;42:79-85.
23. Scheistroen M, Trope C: Combined bleomycin and irradiation in preoperative treatment of advanced squamous cell carcinoma of the vulva. Acta Oncol 1993;32:657-661.
24. Thomas G, Dembo A, DePetrillo A, et al: Concurrent radiation and chemotherapy in vulvar carcinoma. Gynecol Oncol 1989; 34:263-267.
25. Whalen SA, Slater JD, Wagner RJ, et al: Concurrent radiation therapy and chemotherapy in the treatment of primary squamous cell cancer of the vulva. Cancer 1995;75:2289-2294.
26. Cunningham MJ, Goyer RP, Gibbons SK, et al: Primary radiation, cisplatin, and 5-fluorouracil for advanced squamous carcinoma of the vulva. Gynecol Oncol 1997;66:258-261.
27. Carson LF, Twiggs LB, Adcock LL, et al: Multimodality therapy for advanced and recurrent vulvar squamous cell carcinoma: A pilot project. J Reprod Med 1990;35:1029-1032.
28. Sebag-Montefiore DJ, McLean C, Arnott SJ, et al: Treatment of advanced carcinoma of the vulva with chemoradiotherapy: Can exentuative surgery be avoided? Int J Gynecol Cancer 1994;4: 150-155.
29. Berek JS, Heaps JM, Fu YS, et al: Concurrent cisplatin and 5-fluorouracil chemotherapy and radiation therapy for advanced-stage squamous carcinoma of the vulva. Gynecol Oncol 1991;42:197-201.
30. Russel AH, Mesic JB, Scudder SA, et al: Synchronous radiation and cytotoxic chemotherapy for locally advanced or recurrent squamous cancer of the vulva. Gynecol Oncol 1992;47:14-20.
31. Carlino G, Parisi S, Montemaggi P, Pastore G: Interstitial radiotherapy with Ir192 in vulvar cancer. Eur J Gynaecol Oncol 1984; 5:183-185.
32. Tod MC: Radium implantation treatment of carcinoma vulva. Br J Radiol 1949;22:508-512.
33. Anal Cancer Trial Working Party, United Kingdom Coordinating Committee on Cancer Research: Epidermoid anal cancer: Results from the UKCCCR randomized trial of radiotherapy alone versus radiotherapy, 5-fluorouracil, and mitomycin. Lancet 1996;348:1049-1054.
34. Bartelink H, Roelofsen F, Eschwege F, et al: Concomitant radiotherapy and chemotherapy is superior to radiotherapy alone in the treatment of locally advanced anal cancer: Results of the European Organization for Research and Treatment of Cancer Radiotherapy and Gastrointestinal Cooperative Groups. J Clin Oncol 1997;15:2040-2049.

35. Rich TA, Ajani JA, Morrison WH, et al: Chemoradiation therapy for anal cancer: Radiation plus continuous infusion of 5-fluorouracil with or without cisplatin. Radiother Oncol 1993;27: 209-215.

36. Morris M, Eifel PJ, Lu J, et al: Pelvic radiation with concurrent chemotherapy compared with pelvic and paraaortic radiation for high-risk cervical cancer. N Engl J Med 1999;340:1137-1143.

37. Keys HM, Bundy BN, Stehman FB, et al: Cisplatin, radiation, and adjuvant hysterectomy for bulky stage IB cervical carcinoma. N Engl J Med 1999;340:1154-1161.

38. Peters WA III, Liu PY, Barrett RJ II, et al: Concurrent chemotherapy and pelvic radiation therapy compared with pelvic radiation therapy alone as adjuvant therapy after radical surgery in high-risk early-stage cancer of the cervix. J Clin Oncol 2000;18: 1606-1613.

39. Rose PG, Bundy BN, Watkins J, et al: Concurrent cisplatin-based chemotherapy and radiotherapy for locally advanced cervical cancer. N Engl J Med 1999;340:1144-1153.

40. Frankendal B, Larsson LG, Westling P: Carcinoma of the vulva: Results of an individualized treatment schedule. Acta Radiol Ther Phys Biol 1973;12:165.

41. Lee WR, McCollough WM, Mendenhal WM, et al: Elective inguinal lymph node irradiation for pelvic carcinomas. Cancer 1993;72:2058.

42. Perez CA, Grigsby PW, Galakatos A, et al: Radiation therapy in management of carcinoma of the vulva with emphasis on conservation therapy. Cancer 1993;71:3703.

43. Petereit DG, Mehta MP, Buchler DA, et al: Inguinofemoral radiation of N0 N1 vulvar cancer may be equivalent to lymphadenectomy if proper radiation technique is used. Int J Radiat Oncol 1993;27:963.

44. Simonsen E, Nordberg UB, Johnsson JE, et al: Radiation therapy and surgery in the treatment of regional lymph nodes in squamous cell carcinoma of the vulva. Acta Radiol Oncol 1984; 23:433.

45. Stehman F, Bundy B, Thomas G, et al: Groin dissection versus groin radiation in carcinoma of the vulva: A Gynecologic Oncology Group Study. Int J Radiat Oncol Biol Phys 1992;24: 389-396.

46. Burke TW, Levenback C, Coleman RC, et al: Surgical therapy of T1 and T2 vulvar carcinoma: Further experience with radical wide excision and selective inguinal lymphadenectomy. Gynecol Oncol 1995;57:215-220.

47. Gould N, Kamelle S, Tillmans T, et al: Predictors of complications after inguinal lymphadenectomy. Gynecol Oncol 2001;82:329.

48. Binder SW, Huang I, Fu YS, et al: Risk factors for the development of lymph node metastasis in vulvar squamous carcinoma. Gynecol Oncol 1990;37:9-16.

49. Curry SL, Wharton JT, Rutledge F:. Positive lymph nodes in vulvar squamous carcinoma. Gynecol Oncol 1980;9:63-67.

50. Goplerud DR, Keettel WC: Carcinoma of the vulva: A review of 156 cases from the University of Iowa Hospitals. Am J Obstet Gynecol 1968;100:550-553.

51. Homesley HD, Bundy BN, Sedlis A, et al: Prognostic factors for groin node metastasis in squamous cell carcinoma of the vulva (a Gynecologic Oncology group study). Gynecol Oncol 1993;49: 279-283.

52. Iversen T, Aalders JG, Christensen A, Kolstad P: Squamous cell carcinoma of the vulva: A review of 424 patients, 1956-1974. Gynecol Oncol 1980;9:271-279.

53. Morley GW: Infiltrative carcinoma of the vulva: Results of surgical treatment. Am J Obstet Gynecol 1976;124:874-888.

54. Morris JM: A formula for selective lymphadenectomy: Its application to cancer of the vulva. Obstet Gynecol 1977;50:152-158.

55. Way S: Carcinoma of the vulva. Am J Obstet Gynecol 1960; 79:692-697.

56. Koh WJ, Chiu M, Stelzer KJ, et al: Femoral vessel depth and the implications for groin node radiation. Int J Radiat Oncol Biol Phys 1993;27:969.

57. Montana GS, Thomas GM, Moore DH, et al: Preoperative chemo-radiation for carcinoma of the vulva with N2/N3 nodes: A Gynecologic Oncology Group study. Int J Radiat Oncol Biol Phys 2000;48:1007-1013.

58. Gonzales-Bosquet J, Kinney WK, Russel AH, et al: Risk of occult inguinofemoral lymph node metastasis from squamous carcinoma of the vulva. Int J Radiat Oncol Biol Phys 2003;57: 419-424.

59. Wright TC, Koulos JP, Liu P, Sun XW: Invasive vulvar carcinoma in two women infected with human immunodeficiency virus. Gynecol Oncol 1996;60:500-503.

60. Ansink AC, Sie-Go DM, van der Velden J, et al: Identification of sentinel lymph nodes in vulvar carcinoma patients with the aid of a patent blue V injection: A multicenter study. Cancer 1999; 86:652-656.

61. de Hullu JA, Doting E, Piers DA, et al: Sentinel lymph node identification with technetium-99m-labeled nanocolloid in squamous cell cancer of the vulva. J Nucl Med 1998;39:1381-1385.

62. Levenback C, Burke TW, Gershenson DM, et al: Intraoperative lymphatic mapping for vulvar cancer. Obstet Gynecol 1994;84:163-167.

63. Terada KY, Coel MN, Ko P, Wong JH: Combined use of intraoperative lymphatic mapping and lymphoscintigraphy in the management of squamous cell cancer of the vulva. Gynecol Oncol 1998;70:65-69.

64. Homesley HD, Bundy BN, Sedlis A, Adcock L: Radiation therapy versus pelvic node resection for carcinoma of the vulva with positive groin nodes. Obstet Gynecol 1986;68:733-740.

65. Berman MD, Soper JT, Creasman WT, et al: Conservative surgical management of superficially invasive stage I vulvar carcinoma. Gynecol Oncol 1989;35:352-357.

66. Farias-Eisner R, Cirisano FD, Grouse D, et al: Conservative and individualized surgery for early squamous carcinoma of the vulva: The treatment of choice for stage I and II (T1-2N0-1M0) disease. Gynecol Oncol 1994;53:55-58.

67. Bryson SCP, Dembo AJ, Colgan TJ, et al: Invasive squamous cell carcinoma of the vulva: Defining low and high risk groups for recurrence. Int J Gynecol Cancer 1991;1:25.

68. Malfetano J, Piver MS, Tsukada Y: Stage III and IV squamous cell carcinoma of the vulva. Gynecol Oncol 1986;23:192-198.

69. Hopkins MP, Reid GC, Morley GW: The surgical management of recurrent squamous cell carcinoma of the vulva. Obstet Gynecol 1990;75:1001-1005.

70. Piura B, Masotina A, Murdoch J, et al: Recurrent squamous cell carcinoma of the vulva: A study of 73 cases. Gynecol Oncol 1993;48:189-195.

71. Podratz KC, Symmonds RE, Taylor WF: Carcinoma of the vulva: Analysis of treatment failures. Am J Obstet Gynecol 1982;143:340-351.

72. Tilmans AS, Sutton GP, Look KY, et al: Recurrent squamous carcinoma of the vulva. Am J Obstet Gynecol 1992;167:1383-1389.

73. Rutledge RN, Mitchel MF, Munsel MF, et al: Prognostic indicators for invasive carcinoma of the vulva. Gynecol Oncol 1991;42:239-244.

74. Stehman FB, Bundy BN, Dvoretsky PM, Creasman T: Early stage I carcinoma of the vulva treated with ipsilateral superficial inguinal lymphadenectomy and modified radical hemivulvectomy: A prospective study of the Gynecologic Oncology Group. Obstet Gynecol 1992;79:490-497.

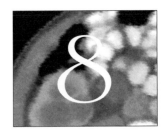

C H A P T E R

Vaginal Cancer

Perry W. Grigsby

 MAJOR CONTROVERSIES

- **What is the appropriate subclassification for stage II disease, and what is the stage assignment for patients with positive groin lymph nodes?**
- **Is the tumor a new vaginal primary or a recurrent lesion?**
- **How should the lymph nodes be evaluated?**
- **What is the role of chemotherapy?**

Vaginal carcinoma is an uncommon malignancy in the United States and worldwide. Vaginal cancers account for approximately 1% to 2% of all female genital neoplasms. The incidence of this tumor appears to be no more than about 1 case in 100,000 women.

Controversial issues pertaining to this uncommon malignancy include its cause and epidemiology, staging and diagnostic evaluation, and therapeutic options. We are in an era of evidence-based medicine in which decisions regarding patient management are often based on the results of prospective, randomized trials. However, there are no prospective, randomized trials for patients with vaginal carcinoma. Our approach to the management of patients with carcinoma of the vagina should logically be based on our best retrospective data and inferences from general principles of cancer management for other tumor sites.

Staging classification

The classification of a tumor as a primary carcinoma of the vagina seems rather straightforward, although some issues need to be addressed. The International Federation of Gynecologists and Obstetricians' (FIGO)[1] definition of carcinoma of the vagina is based on the anatomic location of the tumor and its extensions. According to FIGO, for purposes of tumor staging, the vagina extends from the vulva cephalad to the uterine cervix. Cases should be classified as carcinoma of the vagina when the primary site of growth is in the vagina. Tumor that is present in the vagina but is

shown to be a metastatic lesion from genital or extragenital sites should be classified as metastasis, not carcinoma of the vagina. Lesions that are present on the cervix and vagina are classified as primary cervical cancer. Likewise, lesions that are present on the vulva and in the vagina are classified as primary carcinoma of the vulva. Tumors limited to the urethra should be classified as carcinoma of the urethra.

What is the appropriate subclassification for stage II disease, and what is the stage assignment for patients with positive groin lymph nodes? The current FIGO classification of vaginal carcinoma is shown in Table 8-1. There are two common staging controversies that are not addressed by FIGO. These are the subclassification of stage II disease and the stage assignment of patients with metastases to the groin lymph nodes. The FIGO classification of stage II disease is that the carcinoma has involved the subvaginal tissue but has not extended to the pelvic wall. A proposed modification of the definition of stage II disease by Perez and colleagues[2] assigns stage IIa to tumors with subvaginal infiltration without parametrial involvement and stage IIb to tumors with parametrial infiltration that does not extend to the pelvic wall. Many investigators often use this subclassification of stage II disease. However, investigators have not consistently demonstrated that prognostic significance can be discerned by this subclassification. The stage assignment for patients with metastasis to the groin lymph nodes is not specifically addressed by FIGO. Some investigators assign these patients to stage III,

Table 8–1. FIGO Classification of Vaginal Cancer

Stage	Definition
0	Carcinoma in situ; intraepithelial neoplasia grade III
I	The carcinoma is limited to the vaginal wall.
II	The carcinoma has involved the subvaginal tissue but has not extended to the pelvic wall.
III	The carcinoma has extended to the pelvic wall.
IV	The carcinoma has extended beyond the true pelvis or has involved the mucosa of the bladder or rectum; bullous edema as such does not permit a case to be allotted to stage IV.
IVa	Tumor invades bladder and/or rectal mucosa and/or direct extension beyond the true pelvis.
IVb	Spread to distant organs

From Pecorelli S, Beller U, Heintz AP, et al: FIGO annual report on the results of treatment in gynecological cancer. J Epidemiol Biostat 2000;24:56.

and others assign them to stage IVb. The current American Joint Committee on Cancer (AJCC) assigns patients with T1-T3 tumors with positive inguinal lymph nodes to stage III (Table 8-2). These two controversial staging issues should be resolved to provide consistency in clinical outcome reporting.

Etiology and histology

The frequency distribution of vaginal tumors by histologic type is squamous cell carcinoma in 78%, adenocarcinoma in 4%, endometrioid carcinoma in 1%,

Table 8–2. American Joint Commission on Cancer Staging of Vaginal Cancer

Primary Tumor (T)

TX	Primary tumor cannot be assessed
T0	No evidence of primary tumor
Tis	Carcinoma in situ
T1	Tumor confined to vagina
T2	Tumor invades paravaginal tissues but not to pelvic wall
T3	Tumor extends to pelvic wall
T4	Tumor invades mucosa of the bladder or rectum and/or extends beyond the true pelvis (bullous edema is not sufficient to classify a tumor as T4)

Regional Lymph Nodes (N)

NX	Regional lymph nodes cannot be assessed
N0	No regional lymph node metastasis
N1	Pelvic or inguinal lymph node metastasis

Distant Metastasis (M)

MX	Distant metastasis cannot be assessed
M0	No distant metastasis
M1	Distant metastasis

Stage Grouping

0	Tis	N0	M0
I	T1	N0	M0
II	T2	N0	M0
III	T1-T3	N1	M0
	T3	N0	M0
IVa	T4	Any N	M0
IVb	Any T	Any N	M1

From Greene FL, Page DL, Fleming ID, et al: AJCC Cancer Staging Manual, 6th ed. New York, Springer-Verlag, 2002.

clear cell carcinoma in 3%, melanoma in 4%, and other tumor types in about 10%.[1] Clear cell adenocarcinomas of the vagina are rare and usually occur in patients younger than 30 years who have a history of in utero exposure to diethylstilbestrol (DES). The incidence of this disease was highest for those exposed during the first trimester. DES was used in the 1950s for controlling the symptoms of morning sickness, and its use was discontinued after a few years. The incidence of DES-induced clear cell adenocarcinoma peaked in the 1970s and is rare today.

Metastatic lesions to the vagina are common. All patients with tumors in the vagina should undergo a careful medical history and physical examination to evaluate the possibility of a prior or concurrent cancer. Mazur and associates[3] found that of 269 patients with presumed metastasis to the vagina, 16% were from extragenital sites (most commonly gastrointestinal tract and breast), and 84% were from genital sites. These researchers reported that the most common genital primary tumor sites resulting in metastasis to the vagina were endometrium (78%) and ovary (17%). The lack of a history of cervical cancer with subsequent metastasis to the vagina in their series is interesting in light of the following issue.

Is the tumor a new vaginal primary or a recurrent lesion? A situation that is often encountered clinically but not addressed by FIGO or AJCC and usually only peripherally addressed in the literature is the patient with a questionable history or a documented history of a prior gynecologic malignancy (especially cervical cancer) who presents with a lesion in the vagina. It is often the convention, when reporting results of therapy for patients with vaginal carcinoma, to classify tumors as primary carcinomas of the vagina (in the setting of a prior gynecologic malignancy) if the current vaginal tumor occurred 5 or more years after the initial gynecologic cancer diagnosis and if there is no other clinical evidence of the initial gynecologic lesion. However, this rule is often inconsistently applied, especially in patients with a history of endometrial cancer or cervical cancer.

Patients with a vaginal lesion and a histologic diagnosis of adenocarcinoma consistent with recurrent endometrial cancer fall into two categories: those with a definite history of endometrial cancer and those with a history of a hysterectomy but without sufficient medical records to document a prior endometrial cancer. Regardless of the 5-year rule cited previously, for patients with a proved history of endometrial cancer and a current lesion in the vagina that is adenocarcinoma, the diagnosis that is usually assigned is recurrent endometrial cancer. Patients without a definite diagnosis of a prior endometrial carcinoma but with a histologic diagnosis of adenocarcinoma in a new vaginal lesion are often given the diagnosis of primary vaginal carcinoma.

Paradoxically, patients with a known or questionable history of an in situ or invasive cervical cancer who have undergone a hysterectomy or radiotherapy and present with a squamous cell carcinoma in the vagina are diagnosed as having primary vaginal carcinoma only if the presenting lesion occurs more than 5 years after the initial cancer therapy. In this setting, it is unclear whether the vaginal lesion represents a new carcinoma of the vagina, recurrent cervical cancer, or a human papillomavirus (HPV)–related field effect in these patients. Epidemiologic evidence suggests that squamous cell carcinoma of the vagina has the same risk factors as cervical cancer, including a very strong relationship with HPV infection.[4] Various investigators reporting on vaginal carcinoma have observed that 0% to 60% of patients have undergone a prior hysterectomy and that a cancer diagnosis could be established in up to 35%.[5] Some investigators prefer to exclude all patients with a prior gynecologic malignancy, whereas others include them only if the new lesion occurs more than 5 years after the first diagnosis. The prognosis for patients may be different if there has been a prior cancer diagnosis compared with those without a history of cancer.

Diagnostic Evaluation

Patients with carcinoma of the vagina often present with complaints of vaginal bleeding. A complete medical history should be obtained with emphasis on a history of cancer, radiotherapy, and surgery. A physical examination and a pelvic examination (preferably under anesthesia) should be performed. Biopsies of the primary vaginal lesion and any suspicious areas in the vagina, vulva, and cervix should be obtained. A diagnostic imaging evaluation should be performed to assess lymph node metastasis, distant metastasis, renal status, and the position of the kidneys and ureters. The patterns of lymph node metastasis in patients with vaginal carcinoma are similar to those in patients with cervical carcinoma. For both types of cancer, tumor involvement of the distal one third of the vagina places the patient at a high risk for lymph node metastasis in the inguinal (groin) lymph nodes (as with vulvar and anal carcinomas). Inguinal, pelvic, and para-aortic lymph node regions should be evaluated in patients with vaginal carcinoma.

How should the lymph nodes be evaluated?
Evaluation of the groin lymph nodes should be performed by physical examination and diagnostic imaging. For patients with early-stage vulvar cancer and clinically negative groin lymph nodes, about 20% are found to have histologically positive groin lymph nodes after groin dissection.[6] Patients with vaginal cancer rarely undergo groin lymph node dissection; however, the accuracy of the groin physical examination, particularly for those with advanced disease involving the lower third of vagina, may be similar to that for patients with vulvar cancer. Computed tomography (CT) of the groins, pelvis, and para-aortic region can detect lymph node abnormalities only if the lymph nodes are larger than 1 cm in diameter.

Positron emission tomography (PET) with the glucose analog [^{18}F]fluoro-2-deoxy-D-glucose (FDG) is an imaging method that depends on metabolic, rather than anatomic, alterations to detect disease. The metabolic characteristic that is exploited for oncologic applications of FDG-PET is the increased glycolysis demonstrated by most neoplastic cells. The ability of FDG-PET to detect metastases in normal-sized lymph nodes has been shown to be more sensitive than conventional imaging methods (i.e., CT and magnetic resonance imaging [MRI]). This has been especially true for squamous cell carcinoma of the lung, esophagus, head, neck, and uterine cervix.

We demonstrated that FDG-PET was more sensitive for detecting lymph node metastasis than CT in patients with carcinoma of the uterine cervix.[7] A review of 14 patients with carcinoma of the vagina demonstrated that groin or pelvic lymph node metastasis was present in 43% as detected by FDG-PET compared with only 14% detected by CT (Grigsby, unpublished data, 2002). Because of the increased sensitivity and specificity of FDG-PET compared with CT for cervical cancer,[8] FDG-PET should be considered if available, particularly for patients with advanced carcinoma of the vagina.

Prognostic Factors

The prognosis of patients with vaginal cancer depends on several factors, including features that are similar to the prognostic factors for patients with cervical cancer but are less well documented for patients with vaginal cancer because of the rarity of the disease.

The National Cancer Database of the American College of Surgeons (ACS) has reported that the most significant patient-related prognostic factor is age at diagnosis.[9] The ACS reports that survival was better for younger patients than older patients (90% versus 30%, respectively). This finding has been substantiated by other investigators.[10,11]

Tumor histology can have prognostic significance. Most patients have squamous cell carcinoma or adenocarcinoma, and the survival distinction between patients with these two histologic subtypes is not apparent. There are reports that those with adenocarcinoma have a worse prognosis than those with squamous cell carcinoma.[5] However, others have not verified this finding.[10,12] The poorest survival outcomes are for patients with vaginal melanomas and adults with sarcomas.[9]

Tumor stage, location, and size are three interrelated prognostic factors of major importance. All reports of survival outcome for patients with vaginal carcinoma indicate that tumor stage (as defined by FIGO) is a significant prognostic factor. A summary of 843 reported cases by Piura and colleagues[13] described a 100% 5-year survival rate for patients with stage 0 disease, 64% to 90% for stage I, 31% to 80% for stage II, 0% to 79% for stage III, and 0% to 62% for stage IV. Lesions of the distal vagina have been reported to have a worse prognosis than those in the proximal vagina.[14]

Stage and tumor location are surrogates for tumor size, which may be the most significant prognostic factor if accurately recorded. Tewari and associates[15] reported the results of radiation therapy in 48 patients in whom the tumor size (diameter) ranged from 0.5 to 8 cm (median, 3.2 cm). These investigators reported that survival was significantly better for patients with tumors of less than 3 cm compared with those with tumors larger than 3 cm ($P < .05$). Chyle and colleagues[5] also evaluated tumor size and found that tumor size of larger than 5 cm was associated with a higher local recurrence rate compared with tumors smaller than 5 cm ($P = .003$).

Lymph node metastasis at diagnosis portends a poor prognosis. However, lymph node status as a prognostic factor in patients with vaginal cancer has not been adequately evaluated. The only report of outcome based on lymph node status is by Pingly and colleagues,[16] who found that the 5-year disease-free survivals were 56% for their patients without lymph node involvement and 33% for those with involved lymph nodes.

Intuitively, a physician knows that the radiation dose for a given tumor size is important in controlling the primary tumor. Some reports indicate that local vaginal tumor control is less than desired for patients with advanced-stage disease because of failure to deliver a tumor dose high enough to cure the disease. However, given the limited information that is available, it is impossible to discern from the literature on vaginal carcinoma the appropriate radiation dose for a given tumor size.

The overall treatment time for patients with vaginal cancer has been shown to affect outcome. Lee and associates[17] reported that the pelvic control rate in their patients was 97% if irradiation was completed within 63 days, compared with 54% if treatment was prolonged beyond 63 days ($P = .0003$). Similarly, Pingley and colleagues[16] reported that the disease-free survival rate was reduced from 60% to 30% if the overall treatment time was prolonged.

Treatment

Variables to be considered in the management of patients with vaginal carcinoma include tumor stage, size, and location. Prior treatment with surgery or irradiation should also be considered. Early-stage disease is treated with surgery or irradiation. Advanced-stage disease is treated with irradiation. The use of chemotherapy is discussed in later sections.

Stages 0 and I. Vaginal intraepithelial neoplasia (VAIN) is usually multifocal and commonly occurs in the vaginal apex. VAIN typically occurs in patients with a history of previous treatment for cervical neoplasia. Therapy should be based on the patient's anatomy, the extent of the lesion, and prior treatment. Equivalent results have been reported with wide local excision with or without skin grafting, partial or total vaginectomy with skin grafting, intravaginal use of 5% fluorouracil cream, laser therapy, and intracavitary irradiation.[18-21]

Surgical management of stage I disease consists of a wide local excision or total vaginectomy for lesions less than 0.5 cm thick.[22] Alternatively, intracavitary irradiation can be used to manage these lesions.[20] For lesions that are larger than 0.5 cm or if the tumor histology is adenocarcinoma, total vaginectomy and lymphadenectomy are recommended.[22,23] Irradiation for these more aggressive stage I lesions should include external radiation in addition to brachytherapy.[20,22,24]

Stages II to IVa. Patients with advanced carcinoma of the vagina should be treated with external irradiation and brachytherapy. The external irradiation port is confined to the pelvis, and prophylactic para-aortic irradiation is not routinely administered. Groin irradiation is given when there is groin nodal involvement or given prophylactically when the primary tumor involves the lower one third of the vagina. In a review of 149 patients with vaginal carcinoma who had clinically negative groin lymph nodes and did not receive elective groin irradiation, Perez and colleagues[20] demonstrated that there were no groin failures among 100 patients whose tumors were confined to the upper two thirds of the vagina compared with an 8% groin failure rate if the tumor involved the lower one third of the vagina ($P = .0107$).

External pelvic irradiation and elective groin irradiation should consist of a total of 45.0 to 50.4 Gy given in 1.8-Gy fractions daily. If there is metastatic lymph node involvement of the pelvic or groin lymph nodes, these regions should receive an external irradiation boost dose to 60 to 66 Gy. Adenopathy of greater than 2 cm may be best controlled if excised before the external irradiation.

Brachytherapy is an integral component in the management of patients with vaginal carcinoma. Local control of the primary disease has traditionally been less than adequate. However, with the advent of improved interstitial brachytherapy techniques, local control of the primary tumor has been increasing. Total tumor doses (including external irradiation) ranging from 70 to 85 Gy, depending on tumor size, are sufficient to control the disease in most patients without undue complications.[15,20,25,26]

What is the role of chemotherapy? There are only a few reports of the use of chemotherapy in the management of patients with vaginal cancer. Thigpen and colleagues[27] reported the results of a phase II Gynecologic Oncology Group (GOG) study in which 26 patients with advanced or recurrent carcinoma of the vagina were treated with cisplatin (50 mg/m^2) every 3 weeks. Among 16 patients with squamous cell carcinoma, 1 had a complete response, 5 had stable disease, and 10 patients had disease that progressed. The researchers concluded that there was insignificant activity of cisplatin in advanced or recurrent squamous cell carcinoma of the vagina in the dose and schedule tested. There have been no further GOG studies evaluating the use of chemotherapy in patients with carcinoma of the vagina. Other investigators have reported the use of chemotherapy and concurrent irradiation in the management of advanced-stage disease. Agents that have been used are 5-fluorouracil (5-FU) and mitomycin-C,[11] cisplatin and 5-FU,[28] and cisplatin and epirubicin.[29] However, none of these studies was randomized, and no specific recommendations can be made based on these limited data.

Concurrent cisplatin-based chemotherapy and irradiation is standard therapy for patients with advanced carcinoma of the cervix. Because the cause, histologic features, and natural history of primary vaginal carcinoma are essentially the same as those for invasive carcinoma of the uterine cervix, chemotherapy should be used concurrently with irradiation for patients with advanced-stage carcinoma of the vagina. Because the incidence of vaginal carcinoma is low and the total number of patients developing this disease per year is small, the ability to perform prospective, randomized studies for patients with carcinoma of the vagina is essentially nonexistent. Although no studies exist to support the use of chemotherapy for patients with carcinoma of the vagina, and in reality, none will be performed because of the limited number of available patients, the use of chemotherapy should not be dismissed. This disease is similar in all aspects to invasive carcinoma of the cervix. With the publication of data supporting the use of concurrent cisplatin-based chemotherapy for patients with carcinoma of the uterine cervix,[30-33] it is logical to conclude that concurrent cisplatin-based chemotherapy and irradiation should become standard therapy for patients with advanced-stage invasive carcinoma of the vagina (i.e., stages II, III, and IVa).

Summary

Uniform staging for patients with stage II disease and patients with clinically involved groin lymph nodes should be adopted. The distinction between primary vaginal cancer and recurrent disease in the vagina should be elucidated. The most accurate imaging technology (i.e., CT, MRI, and PET) should be used, when available, to best assess the patient's disease status and therefore more accurately target irradiation. Concurrent chemotherapy and irradiation should become standard therapy for patients with advanced-stage disease.

REFERENCES

1. Beller U, Sideri M, Maisonneuve P, et al: Carcinoma of the vagina. J Epidemiol Biostat 2001;6:141-152.
2. Perez CA, Arneson AN, Galakatos A, Samanth HK: Malignant tumors of the vagina. Cancer 1973;31:36-44.
3. Mazur MT, Hsueh S, Gersell DJ: Metastases to the female genital tract: Analysis of 325 cases. Cancer 1984;53:1978-1984.
4. Daling JR, Madeleine MM, Schwartz SM, et al: A population-based study of squamous cell vaginal cancer: HPV and cofactors. Gynecol Oncol 2002;84:263-270.
5. Chyle V, Zagars GK, Wheeler JA, et al: Definitive radiotherapy for carcinoma of the vagina: Outcome and prognostic factors. Int J Radiat Oncol Biol Phys 1996;35:891-905.
6. Stehman FB, Bundy BN, Thomas G, et al: Groin dissection versus groin radiation in carcinoma of the vulva: A Gynecologic Oncology Group study. Int J Radiat Oncol Biol Phys 1992;24:389-396.
7. Grigsby PW, Siegel BA, Dehdashti F: Lymph node staging by positron emission tomography in patients with carcinoma of the cervix. J Clin Oncol 2001;19:3745-3749.
8. Rose PG, Adler LP, Rodriguez M, et al: Positron emission tomography for evaluating para-aortic nodal metastasis in locally advanced cervical cancer before surgical staging: A surgicopathologic study. J Clin Oncol 1999;17:41-45.
9. Creasman WT, Phillips JL, Menck HR: The national cancer data base report on cancer of the vagina. Cancer 1998;83:1033-1040.
10. Urbanski K, Kojs Z, Reinfuss M, Fabisiak W: Primary invasive vaginal carcinoma treated with radiotherapy: Analysis of prognostic factors. Gynecol Oncol 1996;60:16-21.
11. Kirkbride P, Fyles A, Rawlings GA, et al: Carcinoma of the vagina: Experience at the Princess Margaret Hospital. Gynecol Oncol 1995;56:435-443.
12. Halmstron H, Engquist M: Primary invasive cancer of the vagina. Int J Gynecol Can 1997;7:205-212.
13. Piura B, Rabinovich A, Cohen Y, Glezerman M: Primary squamous cell carcinoma of the vagina: Report of four cases and review of the literature. Eur J Gynaecol Oncol 1998;19:60-63.
14. Ali MM, Huang DT, Goplerud DR, et al: Radiation alone for carcinoma of the vagina: Variation in response related to the location of the primary tumor. Cancer 1996;77:1934-1939.
15. Tewari KS, Cappuccini F, Puthawala AA, et al: Primary invasive carcinoma of the vagina: Treatment with interstitial brachytherapy. Cancer 2001;91:758-770.
16. Pingley S, Shrivastava SK, Sarin R, et al: Primary carcinoma of the vagina: Tata Memorial Hospital experience. Int J Radiat Oncol Biol Phys 2000;46:101-108.
17. Lee WR, Marcus RB, Sombeck MD, et al: Radiotherapy alone for carcinoma of the vagina: The importance of overall treatment time. Int J Radiat Oncol Biol Phys 1994;29:983-988.
18. Wright VC, Chapman W: Intraepithelial neoplasia of the lower female genital tract: Etiology, investigation, and management. Semin Surg Oncol 1992;8:180-190.
19. Krebs HB: Treatment of vaginal intraepithelial neoplasia with laser and topical 5-fluorouracil. Obstet Gynecol 1989;73:657-660.
20. Perez CA, Grigsby PW, Garipagaoglu M, et al: Factors affecting long-term outcome of irradiation in carcinoma of the vagina. Int J Radiat Oncol Biol Phys 1999;44:37-45.
21. Woodman CB, Mould JJ, Jordan JA: Radiotherapy in the management of vaginal intraepithelial neoplasia after hysterectomy. Br J Obstet Gynaecol 1988;95:976-979.
22. Stock RG, Chen ASJ, Seski J: A 30-year experience in the management of primary carcinoma of the vagina: Analysis of prognostic factors and treatment modalities. Gynecol Oncol 1995;56:45-52.
23. Look KY: Organ sparing management for carcinoma of the vulva and vagina. Eur J Gynaecol Ocol 2000;21:439-446.
24. Rubin SC, Young J, Mikuta JJ: Squamous carcinoma of the vagina: Treatment, complications, and long-term follow-up. Gynecol Oncol 1985;20:346-353.
25. Nori D, Dasar N, Albright RM: Gynecologic brachytherapy. I. Proper incorporation of brachytherapy into the current multimodality management of carcinoma of the cervix. Semin Radiat Oncol 2002;12:40-52.
26. Kucera H, Mock U, Knocke TH, et al: Radiotherapy alone for invasive vaginal cancer: Outcome with intracavitary high dose rate brachytherapy versus conventional low dose rate brachytherapy. Acta Obstet Gynecol Scand 2001;80:355-360.
27. Thigpen JT, Blessing JA, Homesley HD, et al: Phase II trial of cisplatin in advanced or recurrent cancer of the vagina: A Gynecologic Oncology Group study. Gynecol Oncol 1986;23:101-104.
28. Grigsby PW, Graham MV, Perez CA, et al: Prospective phase I/II studies of definitive irradiation and chemotherapy for advanced gynecologic malignancies. Am J Clin Oncol 1996;19:1-6.
29. Zanetta G, Lissoni A, Gabriele A, et al: Intense neoadjuvant chemotherapy with cisplatin and epirubicin for advanced or bulky cervical and vaginal adenocarcinoma. Gynecol Oncol 1997;64:431-435.
30. Morris M, Eifel PJ, Lu J, et al: Pelvic radiation with concurrent chemotherapy compared with pelvic and para-aortic radiation

for high-risk cervical cancer. N Engl J Med 1999;340: 1137-1143.

31. Rose PG, Bundy BN, Watkins EB, et al: Concurrent cisplatin-based radiotherapy and chemotherapy for locally advanced cervical cancer. N Engl J Med 1999;340:1144-1153.

32. Keys HM, Bundy BN, Stehman FB, et al: Cisplatin, radiation, and adjuvant hysterectomy compared with radiation and adjuvant hysterectomy for bulky stage IB cervical carcinoma. N Engl J Med 1999;340:1154-1161.

33. Peters WA, Liu PY, Barrett RJ, et al: Concurrent chemotherapy and pelvic radiation therapy compared with pelvic radiation

therapy alone as adjuvant therapy after radical surgery in high-risk early-stage cancer of the cervix. J Clin Oncol 2000;18: 1606-1613.

34. Pecorelli S, Beller U, Heintz AP, et al: FIGO annual report on the results of treatment in gynecological cancer. J Epidemiol Biostat 2000;24:56.

35. Greene FL, Page DL, Fleming ID, et al: AJCC Cancer Staging Manual, 6th ed. New York, Springer-Verlag, 2002.

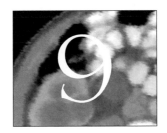

C H A P T E R

TREATMENT OF RECURRENT VAGINAL, VULVAR, AND CERVICAL CANCER

Higinia R. Cardenes,   David H. Moore,   Harry J. Long,   and   Marcus E. Randall

---

MAJOR CONTROVERSIES

- **What patient selection factors are important when considering exenterative surgery for recurrent disease?**
- **Is pelvic exenteration the only surgical option for recurrent cervical or vaginal carcinoma?**
- **What options exist for pelvic reconstruction after radical surgery for recurrent carcinoma of the vagina, vulva, or cervix?**
- **What are the options for urinary diversion in patients undergoing total or anterior pelvic exenteration?**
- **Which patients are candidates for salvage irradiation, and what results can be achieved?**
- **What is the appropriate target volume when treating in-field, central, or regional recurrences after radical surgery?**
- **Which patients are candidates for salvage re-irradiation?**
- **What are the results of combined radiation therapy and chemotherapy in the treatment of recurrent disease?**
- **What are the results of combined surgery and intraoperative radiation therapy in the treatment of recurrent disease?**
- **What options are available for locally recurrent vaginal cancer?**
- **What options are available for locally recurrent vulvar cancer?**
- **What radiotherapeutic options should be considered in the palliative setting?**
- **What is the role of external beam irradiation in patients with recurrent disease in the para-aortic region?**
- **What chemotherapeutic options should be considered for cervical cancer in the palliative setting?**
- **What chemotherapeutic options should be considered for vaginal and vulvar cancer in the palliative setting?**

General Considerations

The patient with recurrent cancer of the female genital tract presents a difficult clinical dilemma. Although optimal therapy has not been defined, local disease is potentially amenable to curative surgery, radiation therapy (RT), or both. Treatment selection factors include primary therapy, extent of the disease at presentation, site of recurrence, local extent of the recurrence, disease-free interval, performance status, and comorbidities.[1-6]

When salvage therapies are contemplated, local recurrence should be biopsy-proven. It is important to evaluate for regional and distant metastases by physical examination and imaging. Generally, patients with pelvic or regional recurrences after definitive surgery alone are managed with external beam radiation therapy (EBRT), often with brachytherapy. Concurrent cisplatin-based chemotherapy may also be recommended. Salvage options for patients with central recurrence after definitive, or adjuvant, RT are limited to radical, usually exenterative, surgery and, in selected patients, re-irradiation using interstitial radiation implants or highly conformal EBRT. Patients with chemotherapy-responsive disease can obtain meaningful palliation in many cases.

Curative-intent retreatment: Surgical considerations

Surgery for recurrent gynecologic cancer was considered futile until the report of Brunschwig[7] in 1948. Better patient selection, anesthesia, operative techniques, and postoperative care have contributed to improved survival and decreased complications and morbidity. Studies have reported mortality from pelvic exenteration of 5% to 8%.[8-10]

What patient selection factors are important when considering exenterative surgery for recurrent disease? Patients determined preoperatively to have significant local extension, involved aortic or pelvic lymph nodes, intraperitoneal disease, or malignant ascites should not undergo laparotomy for attempted pelvic exenteration. The 5-year survival rate for patients with positive pelvic lymph nodes is less than 15% and must be weighed against the mortality of exenterative surgery. Shingleton and colleages[8] subdivided patients into three risk groups using three clinical factors: time from initial therapy to recurrence, size of recurrent tumor, and preoperative pelvic side wall fixation. The highest-risk group included patients with tumors that were larger than 3 cm, fixed to the side wall, and recurred less than 1 year after primary treatment. Within 18 months after exenteration, all these patients died of operative complications or persistent cancer or both.[8] Stanhope and Symmonds[11] reviewed their experience with pelvic exenteration for recurrent disease. When pelvic exenteration was performed for recurrence after RT, the median survival time was

19 months. Despite thorough evaluation, salvage surgery is aborted in more than 25% of cases because of advanced disease found during surgery.[3,12]

Pelvic exenteration results in long-term functional and psychological changes. Ratcliff and associates[13] studied the quality of life in women undergoing pelvic exenteration and reconstruction with a gracilis myocutaneous flap. Twenty one (52%) of 40 patients did not resume sexual activity after surgery, mainly due to self-consciousness about the urostomy or colostomy, vaginal discharge, and vaginal dryness. Surgical refinements such as urinary diversion and pelvic reconstruction and low rectal anastomoses have lessened body image changes. However, Mirhashemi and coworkers[14] found that breakdown or fistula developed after low rectal anastomosis in 50% of patients who had received prior RT. Similarly, Husain and colleagues[15] found that 50% of patients in their series developed anastomotic leaks requiring diverting colostomies.

Is pelvic exenteration the only surgical option for recurrent cervical or vaginal carcinoma? Rutledge and colleagues[16] reviewed 47 patients who underwent conservative surgery for cervical carcinoma recurrent after RT. There were 8 urinary tract fistulas and 7 enteric fistulas, all requiring operative diversion. In a review by Rubin and associates,[17] the 5-year survival rate was 62% among 194 patients with recurrent cervical carcinoma treated with radical hysterectomy. Two patients died of postoperative complications, and the fistula rate was 48%. This suggests that patients with recurrent cervical cancer, initial International Federation of Gynaecologists and Obstetricians (FIGO) stage Ib or IIa, who have recurrent tumors smaller than 2 cm in diameter could be considered for more conservative surgery, although the complication risk is high.

What options exist for pelvic reconstruction after radical surgery for recurrent carcinoma of the vagina, vulva, or cervix? The purposes of vaginal and perineal reconstruction after radical pelvic surgery for recurrent gynecologic cancer are to restore or create vulvovaginal function and to minimize postoperative complications by transferring to the pelvic defect healthy tissue with good blood supply. Many techniques employed for benign disease such as congenital vaginal agenesis—skin grafts, cutaneous flaps, bowel flaps—are not applicable to heavily irradiated patients or for reconstruction of extensive defects after exenterative surgery.

An omental J-flap is created by dividing the omental attachments to the transverse colon, sacrificing either the right or left omental vessels, and unfolding the greater omentum on the preserved vessel. These may be used as interposition flaps for fistula repair and may also be used to form a pelvic "lid" after exenteration, reducing the risk of postoperative small bowel obstruction or fistula. Wheeless[18] described an omental J-flap combined with a split-thickness skin graft to create a functional neovagina. With minor modifications of this technique, the surgeon may use omentum to create a cylinder lined with a split-thickness skin graft and expanded by a soft foam rubber vaginal dilator until healing is complete. Approximately 40% of patients undergoing this operation are able to experience orgasm.[18]

McCraw and colleagues[19] described the gracilis myocutaneous neovagina. Its blood supply arises from the medial circumflex femoral vessels. Rotation of this flap on its neurovascular pedicle preserves muscle innervation, but this usually is not problematic. Burke and associates[20] used gracilis myocutaneous flaps for perineal reconstruction. Most patients underwent this procedure to repair large vulvovaginal defects after surgery for locally recurrent cancer or as part of multimodality treatment of locally advanced disease. Three patients experienced major loss of the cutaneous portion of the flap, but the underlying transposed muscle remained viable. Wound healing was successful in all cases.

In patients with low rectal anastomoses, limited room in the posterior pelvis renders gracilis myocutaneous flap reconstruction more difficult, and neovaginal prolapse can happen. Soper and colleagues[21] noted that the gracilis myocutaneous flap is "bulky," resulting in a lengthy scar along the medial thigh. To circumvent this problem, they used a "short" gracilis myocutaneous flap based on terminal branches of the obturator artery for vulvovaginal reconstruction in 11 patients; 10 of these patients had prior RT, and 9 underwent neovaginal reconstruction after exenteration. No case of vaginal prolapse or donor site infection occurred. Six patients were sexually active after surgery. In a subsequent review,[22] the authors compared 24 patients treated with the use of "short" gracilis myocutaneous flaps versus 22 patients who had undergone reconstruction with "long" flaps and found no difference in major flap loss.[22]

Alternatives to the gracilis myocutaneous flap include the omental J-flap with split-thickness skin grafting[18] and bulbocavernosus myocutaneous flap reconstruction combined with an omental lid. The latter was used by Hatch[23] in eight patients with satisfactory results. With resection of the perineal body and posterior vulva, the bulbocavernosus myocutaneous flap may be unavailable or of insufficient size to form a complete neovagina, and it is, in general, insufficient for the repair of large posterior pelvic defects.

Luo and coworkers[24] reported on the use of an anterolateral thigh fasciocutaneous flap to repair a large vulvar soft-tissue defect in a patient with vulvar melanoma treated with pelvic exenteration. Bilateral gracilis myocutaneous flaps were used for pelvic reconstruction. Only the muscular portions of the flaps survived, but excellent healing at the donor and recipient sites was reported. Long-term function was not described.

A popular myocutaneous flap for pelvic reconstruction is the rectus abdominis flap (Fig. 9-1). Its advantages are easy incorporation into the midline incision and the fact that the long vascular pedicle

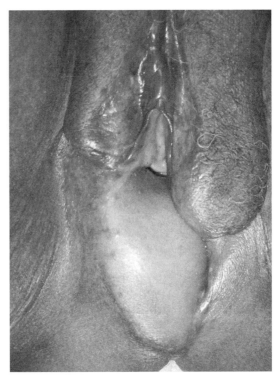

Figure 9–1. Rectus abdominis myocutaneous flap is delivered into the pelvis to construct a neovagina. The patient had developed a recurrence of vaginal carcinoma after primary chemotherapy and radiation therapy, and tumor resection necessitated removal of the posterior and lateral vaginal walls, perineal body, and anorectum. See also Color Figure 9-1.

(inferior epigastric) allows for ample mobilization to virtually anywhere in the groin, vulva, or pelvis. The choice of right or left rectus abdominis myocutaneous flap depends on the presence and location of abdominal incision scars, the integrity of the vascular pedicle, and the presence or necessity of a fecal or urinary tract stoma. An absolute contraindication to its use is a previous Cherney or Maylard incision with division and ligation of the inferior epigastric vessels.

Pursell and associates[25] reviewed their experience with rectus abdominis myocutaneous flaps in 21 patients who underwent pelvic exenteration for recurrent gynecologic cancer and 1 patient who underwent posterior exenteration for recurrent colon cancer. In two patients the flap was used to cover a large perineal defect, and in the remainder it was used to construct a neovagina. Eighteen patients experienced no flap loss. One patient lost one-third of the neovagina, and another patient experienced complete loss. No data were provided regarding sexual function. Others have reported excellent results with the use of this flap for vulvoperineal reconstruction.[26]

Carlson and colleagues[27] used a vertically oriented rectus abdominis myocutaneous flap for vaginal or inguinal reconstruction. Fifteen patients underwent this procedure as part of radical resection for advanced or recurrent gynecologic cancer. One patient experienced wound dehiscence, and three developed necrosis of the cutaneous and subcutaneous portions of the flap. The authors suggested that risk factors for complications with this flap included RT, obesity, and peripheral vascular disease.

Rietjens and coworkers[28] compared two different techniques for vaginal reconstruction—a transverse rectus abdominis musculoperitoneal flap (TRAMP) and an inverted inferior transverse rectus abdominis myocutaneous flap (TRAM)—after radical pelvic surgery or exenteration for recurrent gynecologic or rectal cancer. There was no difference between the groups in terms of prior RT. The vagina became too short or completely closed in the reconstructions with a TRAMP flap but maintained adequate length with the TRAM flap.

In addition to their functional success in pelvic reconstruction, both gracilis and rectus abdominis myocutaneous flaps reduce complications after radical pelvic surgery. Among 45 patients who underwent pelvic exenteration, 16 had vaginal reconstructive surgery with a gracilis myocutaneous flap,[3] Singapore fasciocutaneous flap,[2] or left rectus abdominis myocutaneous flap.[11] The incidence of pelvic abscess was 0%, compared with 27% (6/29) in patients who did versus did not undergo reconstructive surgery ($P = .05$). There were no differences between the two groups with respect to perioperative morbidity or length of hospital stay.[29]

Cardosi and colleagues[30] used a rectus femoris myocutaneous flap for vulvoperineal reconstruction. The patient had undergone tumor resection after previous surgery and RT, leaving a large vulvoperineal defect. Healing was uneventful, the reconstruction was cosmetically acceptable, and the patient's ability to ambulate was not affected.[30]

The tensor fascia lata myocutaneous flap is quite versatile and can be made as large as 25 by 40 cm (Fig. 9-2). Whereas rectus abdominis and gracilis myocutaneous flaps are useful for pelvic reconstruction and neovagina formation, the tensor fascia lata myocutaneous flap is reliable for repair of large inguinal or perineal defects. Chafe and associates[31] achieved excellent results with this flap for vulvar reconstruction after radical vulvectomy.

Inferior gluteal flaps may be used for perineal and vaginal reconstruction. In comparison to rectus abdominis, gracilis, or other myocutaneous flaps, the gluteus perforator-based flap retains the superior blood supply of the myocutaneous flap yet avoids the donor site morbidity associated with muscle transfer or wide cutaneous flaps.[32] This type of flap is used to close large sacral defects, but there is limited experience with it in gynecologic surgery. Loree and colleagues[33] used inferior gluteal flaps in seven patients to reconstruct extensive vulvar, perineal, or vaginal defects. Two patients experienced necrosis at the tip of the flap that required debridement and healing via secondary intention, but no patient experienced complete flap loss.

No method of pelvic reconstruction is superior to all others or applicable to all cases. That many possible options exist should be a source of comfort, not

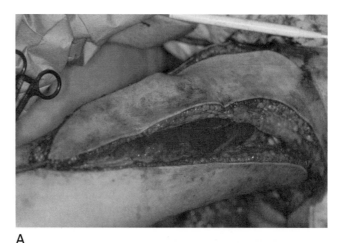

A

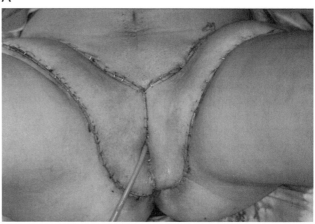

B

Figure 9–2. Tensor fascia lata myocutaneous flap is developed (**A**) and rotated medially (**B**) to cover a large perineal defect after radical vulvectomy and groin node dissection. See also Color Figure 9-2.

consternation, to the pelvic surgeon. An individualized approach to patient care is paramount in the selection of reconstructive procedures.

What are the options for urinary diversion in patients undergoing total or anterior pelvic exenteration?

Urinary diversion is usually required when the urinary tract is involved with recurrent carcinoma or when adequate surgical resection compromises bladder or urethral integrity. Genitourinary tract reconstruction has improved patient survival and quality of life after radical pelvic surgery. Many technical innovations were developed in children with congenital defects or in adults undergoing treatment for bladder carcinoma. Although these same procedures are applicable to patients with gynecologic cancer, equivalent surgical morbidity and mortality should not be expected. Most women with recurrent vaginal or cervical cancer have received prior RT, leading to suboptimal healing and, potentially, postoperative complications. Tunneled ureterointestinal anastomosis, using irradiated ureter and irradiated intestine, may be applicable to the nonirradiated patient but may lead to stricture and urinary obstruction in the patient with recurrent gynecologic malignancy.

Urinary conduits. The ileal conduit, popularized by Bricker,[34] was a revolutionary advance in radical pelvic surgery. Isolation of a segment of ileum as a urinary conduit for ureter implantation substantially reduced the incidence of ascending urinary tract infection and loss of renal function. The major disadvantage is the anastomosis of irradiated small bowel and the implantation of irradiated ureters into irradiated small intestine. The use of sigmoid colon for urinary diversion renders a small bowel anastomosis unnecessary. However, a sigmoid colon urinary conduit may render a low rectal anastomosis more difficult, still requires an anastomosis between irradiated ureters and irradiated bowel, and may result in metabolic derangements such as hyperchloremic acidosis. A transverse colon conduit does not require a small bowel anastomosis. Also, the transverse colon is mobile, and a shorter length of ureter is required to perform the ureterocolonic anastomosis. Use of more proximal, less irradiated ureter plus a nonirradiated colonic segment predictably results in fewer operative complications. Many gynecologic surgeons favor this type of urinary conduit in women who have undergone previous RT.

Few studies have compared methods of conduit urinary diversion. Orr and associates[35] analyzed 115 patients undergoing pelvic exenteration for recurrent gynecologic cancer. Most patients had recurrent cervical carcinoma, and 98% had received RT. Types of urinary diversion were ileal conduit ($n = 97$), transverse colon conduit ($n = 16$), and sigmoid colon conduit ($n = 2$). The rate of urinary fistula associated with ileal conduit urinary diversion was 10%, and all urinary fistulas occurred in patients with an irradiated ileal segment. Stanhope and colleagues[36] reported on 218 patients who underwent urinary diversion, 67% of whom had previously received RT. Ileal conduits ($n = 156$) and sigmoid colon conduits ($n = 62$) were created without stenting the ureterointestinal anastomosis. No difference in conduit complications was seen. The rates of urinary tract fistula (3% versus 5%) and ureteral obstruction (8% versus 11%) were similar for patients with ileal versus sigmoid colon conduits, respectively. Segreti and associates[37] reported on 57 patients who underwent transverse colon conduit urinary diversion. There were no differences in the type or frequency of complications between patients with transverse colon conduits and those with other types of urinary diversion. Hancock and colleagues[38] reported on 212 urinary conduits performed in patients with gynecologic malignancy. Urinary diversion was performed in 154 patients as part of pelvic exenteration for recurrent cancer, in 48 patients because of complications secondary to RT, and in 10 patients for palliation of disease recurrence. Urinary conduits used ileal ($n = 102$) or sigmoid colon ($n = 99$) intestinal segments. There was no difference between the two types of urinary conduit with respect to postoperative complications. The incidence of urinary leak was 3%, equally distributed between the two groups. The authors attributed the low fistula rate to stenting of the ureterointestinal anastomosis and to surgeon judgment in selecting a segment of intestine with minimal RT injury. Stenting is now standard operative technique, regardless of whether a conduit or a continent urinary diversion is performed.

Continent urinary diversion. In 1982, Kock and coworkers[39] reported on the use of a segment of ileum to create a low-pressure continent urinary reservoir that was easy to catheterize and prevented ureteral reflux. Although well suited for urinary diversion in nonirradiated patients, the use of extensive lengths of irradiated ileum is predictably associated with a high rate of postoperative complications.

The Indiana pouch continent urinary reservoir was first described by Rowland and colleagues.[40] Features of this urinary diversion include tunneled ureteral implantations along the tenia of the cecum, the use of the right colon and a short segment of terminal ileum to create a high-capacity pouch, and preservation of the ileocecal valve, which, along with antiperistalsis and tubularization of the terminal ileum, forms an effective continence mechanism. Husain and colleagues[15] reviewed 33 patients who underwent this procedure, 32 of whom had received RT. Two patients experienced early ureteral strictures, successfully managed with temporary percutaneous nephrostomies. Two patients developed late ureteral strictures, which were managed with temporary percutaneous nephrostomy in one patient and with catheter pouch drainage in the other. Five patients experienced nocturnal incontinence. Two patients underwent scar revisions to alleviate stomal stenosis.

The Miami pouch is a modification of the Indiana pouch whereby the length of colon used to create the reservoir is extended to include the entire ascending and proximal transverse colon. The ureters are spatulated and anastomosed without tunneling to the colonic mucosa. Angioli and associates[41] described 77 patients who had undergone Miami pouch continent urinary diversion, 72 of whom had received RT. The perioperative mortality rate was high (12%). Two thirds of the deaths were secondary to sepsis, and all of these patients had undergone at least one reoperation, commonly for abscess or major urinary and/or intestinal leak. Other complications included ureter obstruction, pouch fistula, and anastomotic leak. Ramirez and colleagues[42] reported on 40 patients who underwent Miami pouch continent urinary diversion, mostly as part of pelvic exenteration for recurrent cervical or vaginal carcinoma. All but one had received RT. Postoperative complications related to urinary diversion occurred in 26 patients (65%) and consisted mainly of urinary tract infections or pyelonephritis or both. Six patients underwent surgical intervention to correct complications attributed to the urinary reservoir, including stones, stomal stricture, ureteral anastomotic stricture, and pouch fistula; 90% reported normal conduit function.

The Mainz pouch consists of a reservoir created from the ascending colon, cecum, and two ileal loops. As with the Kock pouch, continence is achieved via intussusception of the distal ileum, and the ureters are implanted into the cecum or ascending colon, using a tunneled, nonrefluxing technique.[43] In a modification of the Mainz pouch described by Leissner and coworkers,[44] approximately 15 to 17 cm of nonirradiated transverse and ascending (or descending) colon is used to construct the pouch reservoir. The colon is detubularized in an antimesenteric fashion, leaving 5 to 6 cm of proximal or distal colon, which is tapered over a Silastic catheter to create the efferent "urethral" segment. A tunneled ureter-colon anastomosis is performed. Among 44 women who underwent this continent urinary diversion, 2 had surgery to correct incontinence problems and 6 required minor procedures to correct stomal stenosis. There was no stenosis or leak of the ureterocolonic anastomosis.

Curative-intent retreatment: Radiotherapeutic considerations

Which patients are candidates for salvage irradiation, and what results can be achieved? Ciatto and associates[45] classified recurrent cervical cancer into three groups according to location: (1) central—confined to the vagina or paravaginal tissues or both, but not extending to the pelvic wall; (2) limited peripheral—tumor limited to one parametrium with extension to the pelvic wall, with or without involvement of the vaginal wall or bone involvement; and (3) massive peripheral—bilateral extension to the pelvic wall, with or without vaginal wall or bone involvement. Patients with central or limited peripheral recurrences are candidates for RT with curative intent.

Retrospective studies have analyzed the outcome of patients with local recurrences of cervical cancer after radical surgery treated with salvage RT and reported survival rates ranging from 30% to 70%. In general, patients with central recurrences have a better outcome than do those with pelvic side wall recurrences.[1,46-48]

What is the appropriate target volume when treating in-field, central, or regional recurrences after radical surgery? Patients who have not received prior RT should receive whole-pelvis EBRT of 40 to 50 Gy to the primary tumor and regional lymphatics. Inguinofemoral lymph node regions should be included in patients who have involvement of the distal third of the vagina or vulvar recurrence (Fig. 9-3).

In patients with vaginal recurrences, the entire vagina should be treated with EBRT or endocavitary brachytherapy to a surface dose of 60 to 65 Gy (Fig. 9-4). Gross tumor volume should receive an additional boost, preferably with an interstitial implant, to bring the total dose to 75 to 85 Gy. The total vaginal mucosal dose from the external and brachytherapy therapy should be limited to 140 Gy in the proximal vagina and 95 Gy in the distal vagina.

Monk and associates[49] advocated EBRT in combination with exploratory laparotomy and "open" interstitial implant for recurrent cancer in the upper vagina after previous hysterectomy. Their rationale was based on the ability to assess the extent of disease more accurately, the possibility of separating bowel and bladder adhesions from the area of the implant, more accurate placement of the needles by direct visualization and palpation of the tumor volume, and the ability to place an omental pedicle graft to separate the bladder and rectum from the implant volume. In 28 patients treated with this technique, the rate of local control was 71%, with 11% experiencing long-term complications. Long-term survival with no evidence of disease was 36%. The authors suggested that high control rates can be achieved in lesions smaller than 6 cm in patients with no previous RT.

Which patients are candidates for salvage re-irradiation? Selected patients who are medically inoperable, technically unresectable, or refuse to undergo exenterative surgery are appropriately considered for re-irradiation to limited volumes. Several techniques are available, and the choice is based on patient- and tumor-related factors and the experience of the radiation oncologist. With EBRT, multiple-beam arrangements using three-dimensional treatment planning are favored. Only limited doses are possible,

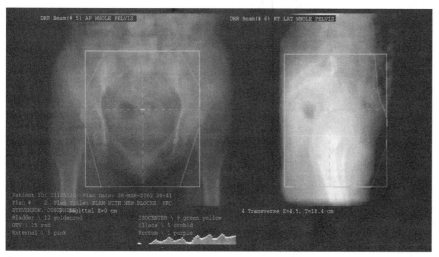

Figure 9–3. A, Pelvic fields (anteroposterior-posteroanterior, right-left laterals) extended inferiorly to cover the entire vagina in a patient with bulky vaginal cuff recurrence.

A

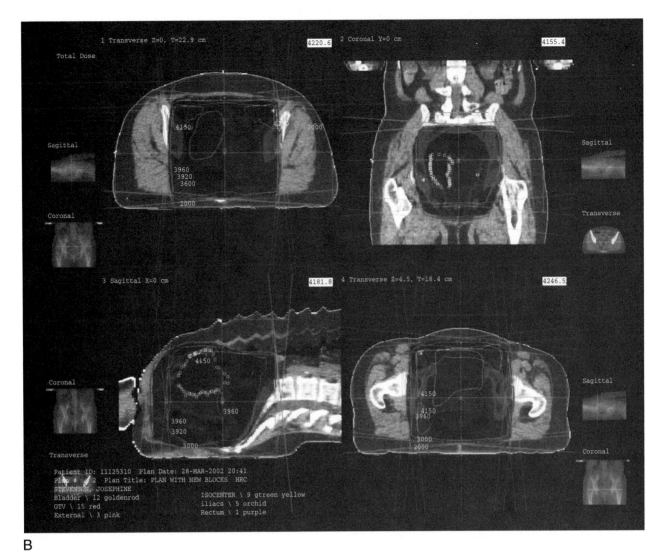

B

Figure 9–3. (cont'd.) **B,** Computed tomography planning, showing isodose "cloud." See also Color Figure 9-3.

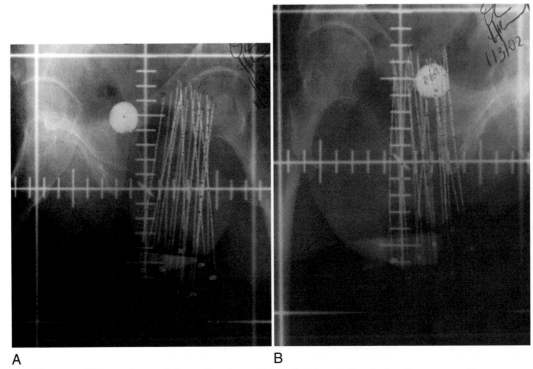

A   B

Figure 9–4. A and **B,** Two oblique orthogonal views of an interstitial implant boost of vaginal cuff recurrence after surgery.

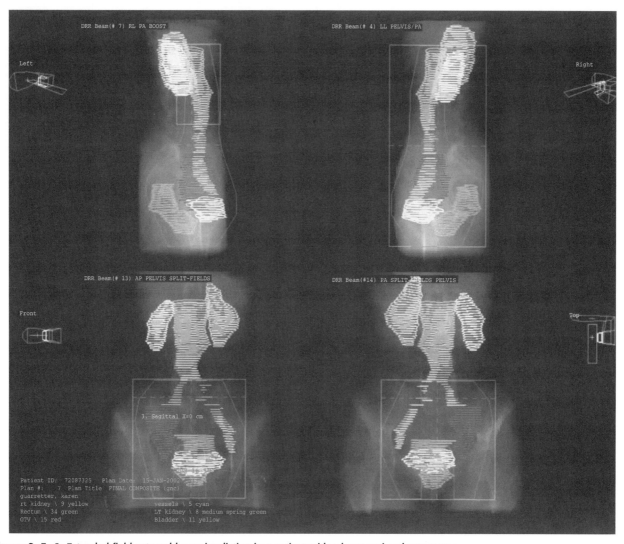

Figure 9–5. A, Extended-field external beam irradiation in a patient with a large regional recurrence.

and a hyperfractionated regimen might be considered in an attempt to decrease late toxicity (Fig. 9-5).

Occasionally, intracavitary or, more commonly, interstitial re-irradiation (IRI) can be used to treat selected patients with clinically definable and localized cervical, vaginal, or vulvar recurrences.[4,50,51] The site and size of the recurrence and the disease-free interval are significant prognostic factors[50,51] (Fig. 9-6). The choice of implant technique (permanent or temporary) and radioisotope is primarily based on tumor volume, geometry, location, patient age and general condition, and suitability for general or regional anesthesia (which is required for temporary iridium 192 implants).

Stereotactic body radiotherapy (SBRT), also known as extracranial stereotactic radioablation (ESR), delivers a small number of high-dose fractions to extracranial targets using a linear accelerator with precise and reproducible target localization. Smaller margins of normal tissue are encompassed, minimizing treatment complications. Blomgren and colleagues[52] reported on 50 patients with 75 tumors in the chest wall and abdomen (the majority pretreated), who received 15 to

45 Gy in one to five fractions at the target periphery. With 6 months of follow-up, 50% had a partial response and 15% had a complete response; after 12 months, these figures were 75% and 30%, respectively. Fifteen patients with 19 extrahepatic abdominal tumors had a mean survival time of 17.7 months, and toxicity was limited.

Curative-intent retreatment: Combined modality considerations

What are the results of combined radiation therapy and chemotherapy in the treatment of recurrent disease? The benefit of concurrent cisplatin-based chemotherapy plus RT in locally advanced cervical cancer has been established in large randomized trials.[53-56] Other phase II and retrospective studies using concurrent RT and 5-fluorouracil chemotherapy[6,57,58] and weekly paclitaxel[59] are encouraging. Given the heterogeneity among patients with recurrent disease, randomized studies are unlikely. However, this combined modality approach may improve locoregional

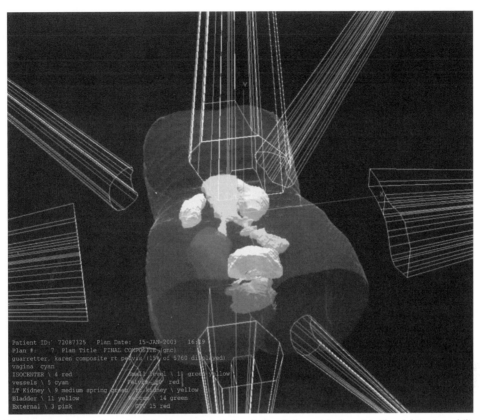

Figure 9–5. (cont'd.) **B,** Beam's-eye view of pelvic plus periaortic irradiation followed by boost to the right external iliac recurrence, using three-dimensional conformal therapy. See also Color Figure 9-5.

control and survival in patients with isolated pelvic recurrences.

What are the results of combined surgery and intraoperative radiation therapy in the treatment of recurrent disease? Patients with microscopically positive or close margins have a dismal prognosis even after exenterative surgery.[60-62] Intraoperative radiation therapy (IORT) allows direct irradiation of a tumor

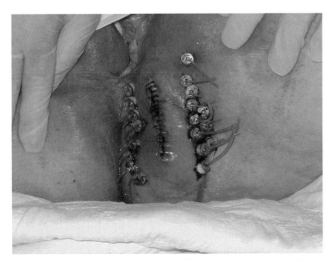

Figure 9–6. Intraoperative interstitial implant in a patient with recurrent vulvar cancer. See also Color Figure 9-6.

bed, potentially sterilizing residual disease after tumor debulking. Advantages of IORT include direct visualization of the target volume and displacement and/or shielding of the surrounding normal tissues. The IORT dose depends on the amount of residual disease, the depth of the target volume, the location in relation to dose-limiting structures (small bowel, plexus, rectum, or bladder), and the prior RT dose.

Limitations in evaluating IORT include small series sizes, limited follow-up, and a wide spectrum of patients with varying amounts of residual disease and initial therapies. Rates of locoregional recurrence and distant metastasis after IORT vary between 20% and 60% and 20% and 58%, respectively. The actuarial survival is poor, with 3- to 5-year survival rates of 8% to 25%.[63-65] Patient selection clearly affects results.

Abe and Shibamoto[66] analyzed prognostic factors after IORT, noting better outcomes in unirradiated patients with central recurrences and in radiated patients after resection of gross recurrence. Grade 3 or higher toxicity is reported in about 35% of patients treated with IORT and commonly includes peripheral nerve injury, gastrointestinal damage (obstruction, perforation, and fistula formation), and ureteral stenosis.

Radical surgical resection with high-dose-rate intraoperative radiation therapy (HDR-IORT) has been reported as salvage therapy in patients with recurrent gynecologic cancer after definitive surgery or RT or both. In one series, patients with complete gross resection had a 3-year local control rate of 83%, compared with 25% for patients with gross residual disease.[67] In the Mayo Clinic series,[68] there was a trend toward reduction of distant metastasis with the addition of chemotherapy, although this did not affect overall survival. As demonstrated in other IORT series, treatment-related late severe complications were frequent (29%).

A combined operative and radiotherapeutic treatment (CORT) procedure was described by Hockel and colleagues[5,69] for recurrent gynecologic malignancies infiltrating the pelvic side wall. The procedure requires surgical exploration demonstrating no intra-abdominal disease, positive contralateral pelvic nodes, or retroperitoneal or bilateral inguinal lymphadenopathy. Gross total tumor resection and a single-plane interstitial implant are performed, encompassing potential microscopic residual disease with a 2-cm margin. Well-vascularized tissue is transposed to the pelvis to reduce the late effects of RT. Pelvic reconstruction is performed, as with exenteration. The tumor bed is irradiated postoperatively, on days 10 through 14, using HDR brachytherapy. In 48 patients, the severe complication rate was 33% at 5 years, and the 5-year survival rate was 44%.

Recurrent vaginal cancer:
General considerations

What options are available for locally recurrent vaginal cancer? In most patients, the primary treatment modality is RT, although surgery is a consideration in some patients with early-stage disease. Patients with recurrent disease after RT have few treatment options. Salvage therapy, when used, has been predominantly exenterative surgery for patients with limited local failures, and palliative RT or chemotherapy, or both, for advanced and metastatic disease. Re-irradiation of small vaginal or pelvic recurrences, using primarily interstitial techniques, has been done with good success.[50,51,70]

Recurrent vulvular cancer:
General considerations

What options are available for locally recurrent vulvar cancer? The most important prognostic factor in recurrent vulvar carcinoma is the site of recurrence. Patients with pelvic recurrences or distant metastases are incurable. Piura and colleagues[71] reported a 5-year survival rate of 35% in 73 women with recurrent carcinoma. Significantly worse outcomes were noted with advanced original disease, positive groin nodes, disease-free interval less than 2 years, or extension beyond the vulva. In multivariate analysis, the site of recurrence was the only significant predictor of survival. Hopkins and associates[72] reviewed 34 patients with recurrent or persistent squamous carcinoma of the vulva. Salvage therapy ws successful in 19 (79%) of 24 patients with negative groin nodes, compared with none of 10 patients

with positive nodes. Tilmans and colleagues[73] reviewed 40 patients with recurrent squamous carcinoma of the vulva. Treatment consisted of surgery or RT or both. No patient with pelvic recurrence or distant metastasis survived. Salvage surgery and RT was successful in 2 of 12 patients with groin recurrences. Of 17 patients with isolated vulvar recurrence, 15 (88%) were alive 2 to 49 months after retreatment.

Palliative-intent retreatment:
Radiotherapeutic considerations

What radiotherapeutic options should be considered in the palliative setting? The Radiation Therapy Oncology Group (RTOG) used 3.7 Gy per fraction twice daily for two consecutive days, at 3- to 6-week intervals, repeated up to three times (maximum tumor dose, 44.4 Gy).[74] Eighty-three (59%) of 142 evaluable patients received three courses of RT, 29 (20%) received two courses, and 29 (20%) received only one course. Among patients completing RT, the response rate was 45%, and 27 patients survived longer than 1 year. The actuarial late complication rate was 5% at 12 months.

In a subsequent phase III study, 136 patients were randomly assigned to rest intervals of either 2 weeks or 4 weeks between the RT courses. There was a trend toward increased acute toxicity in patients with shorter rest periods, but late toxicity and tumor response were not different in the two groups.[75] This schedule offers significant logistic benefits and has been shown to result in good tumor regression and excellent palliation of symptoms.

What is the role of external beam irradiation in patients with recurrent disease in the para-aortic region? Most retroperitoneal recurrences after RT, specifically those infiltrating the pelvic side wall or para-aortic regions, are treated palliatively with systemic or investigational therapy. Grigsby and coworkers[76] reported on 20 patients with recurrent cervical cancer confined to the para-aortic region after definitive RT. The median time between the initial diagnosis and recurrence was 12 months. All patients died within 2 years after recurrence. Patients with disease-free intervals greater than 24 months and those receiving doses greater than 45 Gy had better survival. The poor outcome of these patients reflects the high incidence of both central and distant failures.

Palliative-intent retreatment:
Chemotherapeutic considerations

What chemotherapeutic options should be considered for cervical cancer in the palliative setting? Chemotherapy has been used for the palliative management of advanced or recurrent cervical cancer. In general, the response rates are low and often of short duration. Various factors complicate the use of chemotherapy, including prior surgery and RT, with subsequent limitations in drug delivery and bone marrow reserve. Also, these patients often have compromised renal function that precludes the use of the more active agents.

Single-agent chemotherapy has been the standard treatment for advanced, recurrent, or metastatic squamous cell carcinoma of the uterine cervix. The most active single agents—cisplatin,[77] carboplatin,[78] paclitaxel,[79] and ifosfamide[80]—result in objective regression rates of about 20%, with a median duration of response of about 4 to 6 months. Active single agents can be combined, taking advantage of differences in metabolism, excretion, toxicity, and mechanism of action. In general, most active combinations include a platinum compound and one or more other active single agents. Response rates for combinations are almost double those seen for single agents, but the response duration is short, usually 4 to 5 months, and median survival time is not substantially increased over that seen with single agents. The more drugs included in the combination, the greater the toxicity. Relatively few regimens have been subjected to phase III comparative trials.

Among the most active doublets from phase II trials are combinations of cisplatin with paclitaxel,[81-83] which yield a response rate approaching 50% and a median survival time approximately 4 months longer than that seen with single agents, based on retrospective comparisons. Combinations of ifosfamide plus either cisplatin or carboplatin also demonstrate response rates approaching 50%.[84,85] Newer combinations, including vinorelbine and cisplatin,[86,87] gemcitabine and cisplatin,[88-90] and irinotecan and cisplatin,[91,92] have demonstrated high response rates and are worthy of further evaluation in phase III trials. The triplet of bleomycin, ifosfamide, and cisplatin, as reported by Buxton and associates,[93] was very active, but subsequent trials[94,95] failed to duplicate the high response rate seen. Reports of paclitaxel, ifosfamide, and cisplatin[96] are interesting.

Several[97-103] four-drug combinations have been reported with high overall response rates, but they failed to add substantially to overall survival and were associated with substantial toxicity. These regimens can be given only for short periods because of their toxicity.

Two of the four published phase III trials used single-agent cisplatin as the "standard" regimen. Kumar and coworkers[104] demonstrated a doubling of the response rate with the combination of bleomycin, ifosfamide, and cisplatin, compared with cisplatin as a single agent. This difference was significant but was not associated with a survival advantage. Bloss and associates[95] reported comparable response rates, progression-free survival times, and overall survival times in patients treated with ifosfamide plus cisplatin and with bleomycin, ifosfamide, and cisplatin. In the Gynecologic Oncology Group's randomized trial of cisplatin alone versus cisplatin and ifosfamide versus cisplatin and mitolactol, the combinations produced higher response rates, but there was no improvement in survival, and there was greater toxicity.[105] In the preplatinum era, Sabir and colleagues[106] demonstrated

a significant response advantage with methotrexate plus doxorubicin, compared with weekly low-dose methotrexate alone. No improvement in disease-free survival or overall survival was demonstrated. Edmonson and associates[107] compared bleomycin plus cisplatin with bleomycin followed by the combination of cyclophosphamide, doxorubicin, and cisplatin. This trial also demonstrated a response advantage with the combination, but no survival advantage. Moore and coworkers[108] reported the randomized comparison of single-agent cisplatin versus the combination of paclitaxel plus cisplatin. The combination resulted in a doubling of the response rate (19.4% versus 36.2%) and median progression-free survival time (2.8 versus 4.8 months), but again there was no improvement in survival.

In summary, the available data regarding advanced, recurrent, or metastatic cervical cancer suggest that a number of two-, three-, or four-drug chemotherapy regimens yield response rates approaching 50%. However, time to progression and death are little changed, compared with the results obtained with single-agent cisplatin. Therefore, single-agent cisplatin remains an appropriate therapy for patients with recurrent cervical cancer who do not have a curative-intent option.

What chemotherapeutic options should be considered for vaginal and vulvar cancer in the palliative setting?

Given the rarity of recurrent or metastatic disease in vaginal and vulvar cancer, most chemotherapy reports for treatment are anecdotal or are combined with reports of treatment of advanced or recurrent cervical cancer. In general, regimens that are active in cervical cancer are active in vaginal cancer.

Thigpen and colleagues[109] reported a phase II trial of cisplatin, 50 mg/m^2 every 3 weeks, in 26 patients with advanced or recurrent vaginal cancer. Among the 16 evaluable patients with squamous cell carcinoma, there was 1 complete response (6.2%). Most patients had received prior surgery and RT. Muss and associates[110] reported no responses among 19 evaluable patients who were treated with mitoxantrone, 12 mg/m^2 every 3 weeks. Median survival time of patients with vaginal cancer was 2.7 months. Among other anecdotal reports of responses in trials that included advanced cervical cancer is a report by Long and coworkers[97] in which three patients with advanced vaginal squamous cell carcinoma received treatment with methotrexate, vinblastine, doxorubicin, and cisplatin (MVAC). All patients achieved a complete response of short duration.

At the present time, results of systemic treatment of recurrent or metastatic vaginal and vulvar cancers are largely anecdotal. Although published response rates are low, standard therapy should include cisplatin alone or in conjunction with RT.

References

1. Lanciano R: Radiotherapy for the treatment of locally recurrent cervical cancer. J Natl Cancer Inst Monogr 1996;21:113-115.

2. Rutledge FN, Smith JP, Wharton JT, O'Quinn AG: Pelvic exenteration: Analysis of 296 patients. Am J Obstet Gynecol 1977;129:881-890.

3. Sommers GM, Grigsby PW, Perez CA, et al: Outcome of recurrent cervical carcinoma following definitive irradiation. Gynecol Oncol 1989;35:150-155.

4. Russell AH, Koh WJ, Markette K, et al: Radical re-irradiation for recurrent or second primary carcinoma of the female reproductive tract. Gynecol Oncol 1987;27:226-232.

5. Hockel M, Baussmann E, Mitze M, Knapstein PG: Are pelvic side-wall recurrences of cervical cancer biologically different from central relapses? Cancer 1994;74:648-655.

6. Maneo A, Landoni F, Cormio G, et al: Concurrent carboplatinum/5-fluorouracil and radiotherapy for recurrent cervical carcinoma. Ann Oncol 1999;10:803-807.

7. Brunschwig A: A complete excision of pelvic viscera for advanced carcinoma. Cancer 1948;1:177-183.

8. Shingleton HM, Soong SJ, Gelder MS, et al: Clinical and histopathologic factors predicting recurrence and survival after pelvic exenteration for cancer of the cervix. Obstet Gynecol 1989;73:1027-1034.

9. Roberts WS, Cavanagh D, Bryson SCP, et al: Major morbidity after pelvic exenteration: A seven-year experience. Obstet Gynecol 1987;69:617-621.

10. Soper JT, Berchuck A, Creasman WT, Clarke-Pearson DL: Pelvic exenteration: Factors associated with major surgical morbidity. Gynecol Oncol 1989;35:93-98.

11. Stanhope CR, Symmonds RE: Palliative exenteration: What, when, and why? Am J Obstet Gynecol 1985;152:12-16.

12. Miller B, Morris M, Rutledge F, et al: Aborted exenterative procedures in recurrent cervical cancer. Gynecol Oncol 1993;50:94-99.

13. Ratliff CR, Gershenson DM, Morris M, et al: Sexual adjustment of patients undergoing gracilis myocutaneous flap vaginal reconstruction in conjunction with pelvic exenteration. Cancer 1996;78:2229-2235.

14. Mirhashemi R, Averette HE, Estape R, et al: Low colorectal anastomosis after radical pelvic surgery: A risk factor analysis. Am J Obstet Gynecol 2000;183:1375-1379.

15. Husain A, Curtin J, Brown C, et al: Continent urinary diversion and low-rectal anastomosis in patients undergoing exenterative procedures for recurrent gynecologic malignancies. Gynecol Oncol 2000;78:208-211.

16. Rutledge S, Carey MS, Prichard H, et al: Conservative surgery for recurrent or persistent carcinoma of the cervix following irradiation: Is exenteration always necessary? Gynecol Oncol 1994;52:353-359.

17. Rubin SC, Hoskins WJ, Lewis JL: Radical hysterectomy for recurrent cervical cancer following radiation therapy. Gynecol Oncol 1987;27:316-322.

18. Wheeless CR Jr: Recent advances in surgical reconstruction of the gynecologic cancer patient. Curr Opin Obstet Gynecol 1992;4:91-101.

19. McCraw JB, Massey FM, Shanklin KD, Horton CE: Vaginal reconstruction with gracilis myocutaneous flaps. Plast Reconstr Surg 1976;58:176-183.

20. Burke TW, Morris M, Roh MS, et al: Perineal reconstruction using single gracilis myocutaneous flaps. Gynecol Oncol 1995;57:221-225.

21. Soper JT, Larson D, Hunter VJ, et al: Short gracilis myocutaneous flaps for vulvovaginal reconstruction after radical pelvic surgery. Obstet Gynecol 1989;74:823-827.

22. Soper JT, Rodriguez G, Berchuck A, Clarke-Pearson DL: Long and short gracilis myocutaneous flaps for vulvovaginal reconstruction after radical pelvic surgery: Comparison of flap-specific complications. Gynecol Oncol 1995;56:271-275.

23. Hatch KD: Construction of a neovagina after exenteration using the vulvobulbocavernosus myocutaneous graft. Obstet Gynecol 1984;63:110-114.

24. Luo S, Raffoul W, Piaget F, Egloff DV: Anterolateral thigh fasciocutaneous flap in the difficult perineogenital reconstruction. Plast Reconstr Surg 2000;105:171-173.

25. Pursell SH, Day TG Jr, Tobin GR: Distally based rectus abdominis flap for reconstruction in radical gynecologic procedures. Gynecol Oncol 1990;37:234-238.

26. Zbar AP, Nishikawa H, BeerGabel M: Vertical rectus abdominis myocutaneous transposition flap for total pelvic exenteration in recurrent vulvar carcinoma invading the anus. Tech Coloproctol 2001;5:66.

27. Carlson JW, Carter JR, Saltzman AK, et al: Gynecologic reconstruction with a rectus abdominis myocutaneous flap: An update. Gynecol Oncol 1996;61:364-368.

28. Rietjens M, Maggioni A, Bocciolone L, et al: Vaginal reconstruction after extended radical pelvic surgery for cancer: Comparison of two techniques. Plast Reconstr Surg 2002;109:1592-1597.

29. Jurado M, Bazan A, Elejabeitia J, et al: Primary vaginal and pelvic floor reconstruction at the time of pelvic exenteration: A study of morbidity. Gynecol Oncol 2000;77:293-297.

30. Cardosi RJ, Hoffman MS, Greenwald D: Rectus femoris myocutaneous flap for vulvoperineal reconstruction. Gynecol Oncol 2002;85:188-191.

31. Chafe W, Fowler WC, Walton LA, Currie JL: Radical vulvectomy with use of tensor fascia lata myocutaneous flap. Am J Obstet Gynecol 1983;145:207-213.

32. Judge BA, Garcia-Aguilar J, Landis GH: Modification of the gluteal perforator-based flap for reconstruction of the posterior vagina. Dis Colon Rectum 2000;43:1020-1022.

33. Loree TR, Hempling RE, Eltabbakh GH, et al: The inferior gluteal flap in the difficult vulvar and perineal reconstruction. Gynecol Oncol 1997;66:429-434.

34. Bricker EM: Bladder substitution after pelvic evisceration. Surg Clin North Am 1950;30:1511-1521.

35. Orr JW, Shingleton HM, Hatch KD, et al: Urinary diversion in patients undergoing pelvic exenteration. Am J Obstet Gynecol 1982;142:883-889.

36. Stanhope CR, Symmonds RE, Lee RA, et al: Urinary diversion with use of ileal and sigmoid conduits. Am J Obstet Gynecol 1986;155:288-292.

37. Segreti EM, Morris M, Levenback C, et al: Transverse colon urinary diversion in gynecologic oncology. Gynecol Oncol 1996;63:66-70.

38. Hancock KC, Copeland LJ, Gershenson DM, et al: Urinary conduits in gynecologic oncology. Obstet Gynecol 1986;67:680-684.

39. Kock NG, Nilson AE, Nilson LO, et al: Urinary diversion via a continent ileal reservoir: Clinical results in 12 patients. J Urol 1982;128:469-475.

40. Rowland GR, Mitchell ME, Bihrle R, et al: Indiana continent urinary reservoir. J Urol 1987;137:1136-1139.

41. Angioli R, Estape R, Cantuaria G, et al: Urinary complications of Miami pouch: Trend of conservative management. Am J Obstet Gynecol 1998;179:343-348.

42. Ramirez PT, Modesitt SC, Morris M, et al: Functional outcomes and complications of continent urinary diversions in patients with gynecologic malignancies. Gynecol Oncol 2002;85:285-291.

43. Thuroff JW, Alken P, Riedmiller N, et al: The Mainz pouch (mixed augmentation ileum and cecum) for bladder augmentation and bladder diversion. J Urol 1986;136:17-26.

44. Leissner J, Black P, Fisch M, et al: Colon pouch (Mainz pouch III) for continent urinary diversion after pelvic irradiation. Urology 2000;56:798-802.

45. Ciatto S, Pirtoli L, Cionini L: Radiotherapy for postoperative failures of carcinoma of cervix uteri. Surg Gynecol Obstet 1980;151:621-624.

46. Potter ME, Alvarez RD, Gay FL, et al: Optimal therapy for pelvic recurrence after radical hysterectomy for early-stage cervical cancer. Gynecol Oncol 1990;37:74-77.

47. Ijaz T, Eifel PJ, Burke T, Oswald MJ: Radiation therapy of pelvic recurrence after radical hysterectomy for cervical carcinoma. Gynecol Oncol 1998;70:241-246.

48. Ito H, Shigematsu N, Kawada T, et al: Radiotherapy for centrally recurrent cervical cancer of the vaginal stump following hysterectomy. Gynecol Oncol 1997;67:154-161.

49. Monk BJ, Walker JL, Tewari KS, et al: Open interstitial brachytherapy for the treatment of local-regional recurrences of uterine corpus and cervix cancer after primary surgery. Gynecol Oncol 1994;52:222-228.

50. Randall ME, Evans L, Greven KM, et al: Interstitial re-irradiation for recurrent gynecological malignancies: Results and analysis of prognostic factors. Gynecol Oncol 1993;48:23-31.

51. Wang X, Cai S, Ding Y, Wei K: Treatment of late recurrent vaginal malignancy after initial radiotherapy for carcinoma of the cervix: An analysis of 73 cases. Gynecol Oncol 1998;69:125-129.

52. Blomgren H, Lax I, Goranson H, et al: Radiosurgery of tumors in the body: Clinical experience using a new method. J Radiosurg 1998;1:63-74.

53. Morris M, Eifel PJ, Lu JL, et al: Pelvic radiation with concurrent chemotherapy compared with pelvic and para-aortic radiation for high-risk cervical cancer. N Engl J Med 1999;340:1137-1143.

54. Rose PG, Bundy BN, Watkins EB, et al: Concurrent cisplatin-based chemotherapy and radiotherapy for locally advanced cervical cancer. N Engl J Med 1999;340:1144-1153.

55. Whitney CW, Sause W, Bundy BN, et al: Randomized comparison of fluorouracil plus cisplatin versus hydroxyurea as an adjunct to radiation therapy in stage IIB-IVA carcinoma of the cervix with negative para-aortic lymph nodes: A Gynecologic Oncology Group and Southwest Oncology Group Study. J Clin Oncol 1999;17:1339-1348.

56. Keys HM, Bundy BN, Stehman FB, et al: Cisplatin, radiation and adjuvant hysterectomy compared with radiation and adjuvant hysterectomy for bulky stage IB cervical carcinoma. N Engl J Med 1999;340:1154-1161.

57. Wang CJ, Lai CH, Huang HJ, et al: Recurrent cervical carcinoma after primary radical surgery. Am J Obstet Gynecol 1999; 181:518-524.

58. Thomas GM, Dembo AJ, Black B, et al: Concurrent radiation and chemotherapy for carcinoma of the cervix recurrent after radical surgery. Gynecol Oncol 1987;27:254-263.

59. Cerrotta A, Gardan G, Cavina R, et al: Concurrent radiotherapy and weekly paclitaxel for locally advanced or recurrent squamous cell carcinoma of the uterine cervix: A pilot study with intensification of the dose. Eur J Gynaecol Oncol 2002;23:115-119.

60. Morley GW, Hopkins MP, Lindenauer SM, Roberts JA: Pelvic exenteration, University of Michigan: 100 patients at 5 years. Obstet Gynecol 1989;74:934-943.

61. Shingleton HM, Soong SJ, Gelder MS, et al: Clinical and histopathological factors predicting recurrence and survival after pelvic exenteration for cancer of the cervix. Obstet Gynecol 1989;73:1027-1034.

62. Averette HE, Lichtinger M, Sevin BU, Girtanner RE: Pelvic exenteration: A 15-year experience in a general metropolitan hospital. Am J Obstet Gynecol 1984;150:179-184.

63. Mahe MA, Gerard JP, Dubois JB, et al: Intraoperative radiation therapy in recurrent carcinoma of the uterine cervix: Report of the French Intraoperative Group on 70 patients. Int J Radiat Oncol Biol Phys 1996;34:21-26.

64. Martinez-Monge R, Jurado M, Azinovic I, et al: Preoperative chemoradiation and adjuvant surgery in locally advanced or recurrent cervical carcinoma. Rev Med Univ Navarra, 1997; 41:19-26.

65. Garton GR, Gunderson LL, Webb MJ, et al: Intraoperative radiation therapy in gynecologic cancer: Update of the experience at a single institution. Int J Radiat Oncol Biol Phys 1997;37: 839-843.

66. Abe M, Shibamoto Y: The usefulness of intraoperative radiation therapy in the treatment of pelvic recurrence of cervical cancer. Int J Radiat Oncol Biol Phys 1996;34:513-514.

67. Gemignani ML, Alektiar KM, Leitao M, et al: Radical surgical resection and high-dose intraoperative radiation therapy (HDR-IORT) in patients with gynecologic cancers. Int J Radiat Oncol Biol Phys 2001;50:687-694.

68. Haddock MG, Petersen IA, Webb MJ, et al: IORT for locally advanced gynecological malignancies. Front Radiat Ther Oncol 1997;31:256-259.

69. Hockel M, Schlenger K, Hamm H, et al: Five-year experience with combined operative and radiotherapeutic treatment of recurrent gynecologic tumors infiltrating the pelvic wall. Cancer 1996;77:1918-1933.

70. Gupta AK, Vicini FA, Frazier AJ, et al: Iridium-192 transperineal interstitial brachytherapy for locally advanced or recurrent gynecological malignancies. Int J Radiat Oncol Biol Phys 1999; 43:1055-1060.

71. Piura B, Masotina A, Murdoch J, et al: Recurrent squamous cell carcinoma of the vulva: A study of 73 cases. Gynecol Oncol 1993; 48:189-195.

72. Hopkins MP, Reid GC, Morley GW: The surgical management of recurrent squamous cell carcinoma of the vulva. Obstet Gynecol 1990;75:1001-1005.

73. Tilmans AS, Sutton GP, Look KY, et al: Recurrent squamous carcinoma of the vulva. Am J Obstet Gynecol 1992;167:1383-1389.

74. Spanos WJ, Guse C, Perez CA, et al: Phase II study of multiple daily fractionations in the palliation of advanced pelvic malignancies: Preliminary report of the RTOG 85-02. Int J Radiat Oncol Biol Phys 1989;17:659-662.

75. Spanos WJ, Perez CA, Marcus S, et al: Effect of rest interval on tumor and normal tissue response: A report of Phase III study of accelerated split-course palliative radiation for advanced pelvic malignancies (RTOG 85-02). Int J Radiat Oncol Biol Phys 1993;25:399-403.

76. Grigsby PW, Vest ML, Perez CA: Recurrent carcinoma of the cervix exclusively in the paraaortic nodes following radiation therapy. Int J Radiat Oncol Biol Phys 1993;28:451-455.

77. Bonomi P, Blessing JA, Stehman FB, et al: Randomized trial of three cisplatin dose schedules in squamous-cell carcinoma of the cervix: A Gynecologic Oncology Group study. Journ Clin Oncol 1985;3:1079-1085.

78. Arsenau J, Blessing JA, Stehman FB, McGhee R: A phase II study of carboplatin in advanced squamous cell carcinoma of the cervix: A Gynecologic Oncology Group study. Investigational New Drugs 1986;4:187-191.

79. McGuire WP, Blessing JA, Moore D, et al: Paclitaxel has moderate activity in squamous cervix cancer: A Gynecologic Group study. Journ Clin Oncol 1996;14:792-795.

80. Hannigan EV, Dinh TV, Doherty MG: Ifosfamide with mesna in squamous carcinoma of the cervix: Phase II results in patients with advanced or recurrent disease. Gynecol Oncol 1991;43:123-128.

81. Rose PG, Blessing JA, Gershenson DM, McGehee R: Paclitaxel and cisplatin as first-line therapy in recurrent or advanced squamous cell carcinoma of the cervix: A Gynecologic Oncology Group study. J Clin Oncol 1999;17:2676-2680.

82. Piver MS, Ghamande SA, Eltabbakh GH, O'Neill-Coppola C: First-line chemotherapy with paclitaxel and platinum for advanced and recurrent cancer of the cervix: A phase II study. Gynecol Oncol 1999;75:334-337.

83. Papadimitriou CA, Sarris K, Moulopoulos LA, et al: Phase II trial of paclitaxel and cisplatin in metastatic and recurrent carcinoma of the uterine cervix. J Clin Oncol 1999;17:761-766.

84. Cervellino JC, Araujo CE, Sanchez O, et al: Cisplatin and ifosfamide in patients with advanced squamous cell carcinoma of the uterine cervix: A phase II trial. Acta Oncol 1995;34: 257-259.

85. Kuhnle H, Meerpohl HG, Eiermann W, et al: Phase II study of carboplatin/ifosfamide in untreated advanced cervical cancer. Cancer Chemother Pharmacol 1990;26(Suppl):S33-S35.

86. Pignata S, Silvestro G, Ferrari E, et al: Phase II study of cisplatin and vinorelbine as first-line chemotherapy in patients with carcinoma of the uterine cervix. J Clin Oncol 1999;17:756-760.

87. Coleman RE, Clarke JM, Slevin ML, et al: A phase II study of ifosfamide and cisplatin chemotherapy for metastatic or relapsed carcinoma of the cervix. Cancer Chemother Pharmacol 1990;27:52-54.

88. Duenas-Gonzalez A, Lopez-Graniel C, Gonzalez A, et al: A phase II study of gemcitabine and cisplatin combination as induction chemotherapy for untreated locally advanced cervical carcinoma. Ann Oncol 2001;12:541-547.

89. Duenas-Gonzalez A, Hinojosa-Garcia LM, Lopez-Graniel C, et al: Weekly cisplatin/low-dose gemcitabine combination for advanced and recurrent cervical carcinoma. Am J Clin Oncol 2001;24:201-203.

90. Burnett AF, Roman LD, Garcia AA, et al: A phase II study of gemcitabine and cisplatin in patients with advanced, persistent, or recurrent squamous cell carcinoma of the cervix. Gynecol Oncol 2000;76:63-66.

91. Sugiyama T, Yakushiji M, Noda K, et al: Phase II study of irinotecan and cisplatin as first-line chemotherapy in advanced or recurrent cervical cancer. Oncology 2000;58:31-37.

92. Sugiyama T, Nishida T, Kumagai S, et al: Combination therapy with irinotecan and cisplatin as neoadjuvant chemotherapy in locally advanced cervical cancer. Br J Cancer 1999;81:95-98.

93. Buxton EJ, Meanwell CA, Hilton C, et al: Combination bleomycin, ifosfamide, and cisplatin chemotherapy in cervical cancer. J Nat Cancer Inst 1989;81:359-361.

94. Ramm K, Vergote IB, Kaern J, Trope CG: Bleomycin-ifosfamide-cis-platinum (BIP) in pelvic recurrence of previously irradiated cervical carcinoma: A second look. Gynecol Oncol 1992;46: 203-207.

95. Bloss JD, Blessing JA, Behrens BC, et al: Randomized trial of cisplatin and ifosfamide versus cisplatin, ifosfamide, and bleomycin in advanced squamous cell carcinoma of the uterine cervix: A Gynecologic Oncology Group study. Abstract 49. Gynecol Oncol 2001;80:289.

96. Zanetta G, Fei F, Parma G, et al: Paclitaxel, ifosfamide and cisplatin (TIP) chemotherapy for recurrent or persistent squamous-cell cervical cancer. Ann Oncol 1999;10:1171-1174.

97. Long HJ 3rd, Cross WG, Wieand HS, et al: Phase II trial of methotrexate, vinblastine, doxorubicin, and cisplatin in advanced/recurrent carcinoma of the uterine cervix and vagina. Gynecol Oncol 1995;57:235-239.

98. Papadimitriou CA, Dimopoulos MA, Giannakoulis N, et al: A phase II trial of methotrexate, vinblastine, doxorubicin, and cisplatin in the treatment of metastatic carcinoma of the uterine cervix. Cancer 1997;79:2391-2395.

99. Alberts DS, Martimbeau PW, Surwit EA, Oishi N: Mitomycin-C, bleomycin, vincristine, and cis-platinum in the treatment of advanced, recurrent squamous cell carcinoma of the cervix. Cancer Clinical Trials 1981;4:313-316.

100. Rustin GJ, Newlands ES, Southcott BM, Singer A: Cisplatin, vincristine, methotrexate and bleomycin (POMB) as initial or palliative chemotherapy for carcinoma of the cervix. Br J Obstet Gynaecol 1987;94:1205-1211.

101. Weiner SA, Aristizabal S, Alberts DS, et al: A phase II trial of mitomycin, vincristine, bleomycin, and cisplatin (MOBP) as neoadjuvant therapy in high-risk cervical carcinoma. Gynecol Oncol 1988;30:1-6.

102. Sugimori H, Iwasaka T, Fukuda K, et al: Treatment of advanced cervical cancer by a combination of pepleomycin, vincristine, mitomycin-C, and cisplatin. Gynecol Oncol 1989;34:180-182.

103. Shimizu Y, Akiyama F, Umezawa S, et al: Combination of consecutive low-dose cisplatin with bleomycin, vincristine, and mitomycin for recurrent cervical carcinoma. J Clin Oncol 1998;16:1869-1878.

104. Kumar L, Pokharel YH, Kumar S, et al: Single agent versus combination chemotherapy in recurrent cervical cancer. J Obstet Gynaecol Res 1998;24:401-409.

105. Omura GA, Blessing JA, Vaccarello L, et al: Randomized trial of cisplatin versus cisplatin plus mitolactol versus cisplatin plus ifosfamide in advanced carcinoma of the cervix: A Gynecologic Oncology Group study. J Clin Oncol 1977;15:165-171.

106. Sabir AA, Khoury GG, Joslin CA, Head C: Treatment of recurrent metastatic carcinoma of cervix: A comparison of low dose methotrexate with adriamycin and methotrexate. Clin Oncol (R Coll Radiol) 1989;1:70-74.

107. Edmonson JH, Johnson PS, Wieand HS, et al: Phase II studies of bleomycin, cyclophosphamide, doxorubicin, and cisplatin and bleomycin and cisplatin in advanced cervical carcinoma. Am J Clin Oncol 1988;11:149-151.

108. Moore DH, McQuellon RP, Blessing JA, et al: A randomized phase III study of cisplatin versus cisplatin plus paclitaxel in stage IVB, recurrent or persistent squamous cell carcinoma of the cervix: A Gynecologic Oncology Group study. Abstract 801. Proc ASCO 2001;20:201a.

109. Thigpen JT, Blessing JA, Homesley HD, et al: Phase II trial of cisplatin in advanced or recurrent cancer of the vagina: A Gynecologic Oncology Group study. Gynecol Oncol 1986;23:101-104.

110. Muss HB, Bundy BN, Christopherson WA: Mitoxantrone in the treatment of advanced vulvar and vaginal carcinoma: A Gynecologic Oncology Group study. Am J Clin Oncol 1989;12:142-144.

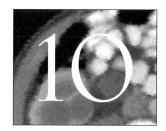

C H A P T E R

MANAGEMENT OF SUPERFICIALLY INVASIVE CARCINOMA OF THE CERVIX*

Robert Rome   and   Robert Brown

 MAJOR CONTROVERSIES

- **What constitutes superficially invasive cancer of the cervix?**
- **Excisional biopsy: loop excision or cold-knife conization?**
- **Which prognostic factors are really important?**
- **Clinical management: what is the value of a conservative approach?**

What constitutes superficially invasive cancer of the cervix?

The introduction of organized screening programs in developed countries has resulted in decreased incidence and mortality from cervical cancer and a noticeable stage shift from more advanced to earlier-stage disease.[1] Small, invasive cancers have become a more frequently encountered clinical problem and are often diagnosed at a younger age in women who wish to retain their childbearing prospects, creating management dilemmas.

The term *microcarcinoma (mikrokarzinöm)* was introduced by Mestwerdt[2] in 1947 to describe small cancers of the cervix that invaded the stroma by less than 5 mm and that had a good prognosis. Since then, there has been considerable controversy and debate about the definition and management of these superficially invasive cancers. There have been numerous attempts by the International Federation of Gynecologists and

Obstetricians (FIGO) and others to develop an acceptable staging system. Terms such as *early stromal invasion, preclinical or occult cancer,* and *microcarcinoma,* which are still descriptively used by some pathologists, have been abandoned in the current FIGO staging system.

The definitions for staging of early cancer of the cervix recommended by the Cancer Committee of FIGO[3] in 1994 (Table 10-1) are more clinically relevant than those hitherto proposed. The current definition pays no regard to lymphovascular space invasion (LVSI), but FIGO urges that its presence or absence be recorded. The FIGO definition also does not use the term *microinvasive cancer.*

The Committee on Nomenclature of the Society of Gynecologic Oncologists (SGO) adopted the following strict definition of microinvasion in 1985. "A microinvasive lesion should be defined as one in which the neoplastic epithelium invades the stroma in one or more places to a depth of 3 mm or less below the basement membrane of the epithelium and in which lymphatic or blood vascular involvement is not demonstrated." The SGO definition pays no heed to the horizontal extent of the tumor.

The purpose of FIGO in defining substage Ia1 and the SGO in defining microinvasive cancer is to indicate small cancers that have an excellent prognosis and that

---

*This chapter is dedicated to the memory of our friend and colleague Professor Andrew Östör, who died in January 2003, in recognition of his contribution to our knowledge of microinvasive cancer of the cervix and particularly its conservative management. This was his life's work, and countless women are the beneficiaries of his legacy.

Table 10–1. FIGO Staging of Early Cervical Cancer: Stage Ia-1b

Stage Ia	Invasive carcinoma that can be diagnosed only by microscopy. All macroscopically visible lesions—even those with superficial invasion—are allotted to stage 1b. Invasion is limited to a measured stromal invasion, with a maximal depth of 5.0 mm and a horizontal extension of not >7.0 mm. Depth of invasion should not be >5.0 mm taken from the base of the epithelium of the original tissue, superficial or glandular. The involvement of vascular spaces—venous or lymphatic—should not change the stage allotment.
Ia1	Measured stromal invasion of not >3.0 mm in depth and extension not >7.0 mm
Ia2	Measured stromal invasion of >3.0 mm and not >5.0 mm with an extension of not >7 mm
Stage Ib	Cancers with a depth of more than 5 mm and/or with a length of more than 7 mm are allocated to stage Ib. The presence (or absence) of capillary-like space involvement should be noted but does not influence stage Ia.

From International Federation of Gynecology and Obstetrics: Staging announcement. FIGO staging of gynecological cancers: Cervical and vulva. Int J Gynecol Cancer 1995;5:319.

may safely be managed by more conservative means. There has also been a growing realization that many cancers in the substage Ia2 category carry a very good prognosis and that many women have been overtreated in the past. Nevertheless, the optimal safe treatment has not been fully defined and remains a contentious subject.

The difficulties with pathologic interpretation of these cancers have been highlighted by several large studies. Sedlis and colleagues[4] reported a Gynecologic Oncology Group (GOG) study of microinvasive carcinoma of the cervix in which 99 (37.4%) of 265 cases were rejected by central pathology review because invasion could not be confirmed and another 18 (6.8%) were rejected because the depth of stromal invasion exceeded 5 mm. Similar high exclusion rates have been reported from the United Kingdom (RCOG) by Morgan and coworkers[5] and by Copeland and associates.[6]

There continues to be controversy surrounding the definition of and the significance of prognostic factors such as LVSI, histologic cell type, and management of these small cancers. In this chapter, we have used the generic term *superficially invasive cancer* to encompass cancers that invade the cervical stroma by no more than 5 mm, just as Mestwerdt did almost 60 years ago.

Diagnosis

Superficially invasive cancers of the cervix do not usually cause symptoms. Most are diagnosed during the investigation and treatment of women with abnormal cervical cytologic results. In the past, the diagnosis was usually made on histologic examination of a cone biopsy, but an increasing proportion is now diagnosed by loop or laser cone biopsy specimens. Occasionally, it is a surprise finding in curettings or a hysterectomy specimen. It is a sine qua non that women who are to undergo hysterectomy for benign reasons should have a current negative Papanicolaou (Pap) smear.

Cytologic features. Occasionally, the possibility of invasive carcinoma is raised on the cytology report, but the reported sensitivity of cytology in predicting superficial invasion varies widely. Ng and associates[7] correctly predicted 27 (87%) of 31 cases based on the presence of nucleoli in tumor cell nuclei. Rome and coworkers[8] found that invasion was predicted cytologically in only 36% of preclinical cancers. Similar experiences have been reported by Andersen and coworkers[9] and Rubio.[10] Pap smears in cases of invasive cervical cancer may also be falsely negative; Rylander[11] reported that 44% of 143 patients diagnosed with invasive cancer had a negative cytologic smear in the preceding 4.5 years, but the exact number that were superficially invasive is unclear.

Because superficially invasive carcinoma in most cases occurs in a background of carcinoma in situ,[12] cytologic smears from these patients typically show features of carcinoma in situ and invasive carcinoma. In superficially invasive squamous tumors,[7,12-14] carcinoma in situ cells show coarse, evenly distributed chromatin and inconspicuous, undifferentiated cytoplasm. With the onset of invasion, nucleoli appear within the nucleus; the chromatin begins to break up, becoming irregular in distribution; and there is clearing of the parachromatin. Accompanying these nuclear changes, the cytoplasm becomes paradoxically more abundant, differentiated, and more squamoid in appearance (Fig. 10-1). A tumor diathesis (i.e., necrotic debris and inflammatory exudate) may be found in 20% of cases.[12] Ng and colleagues[7] found that smears from tumors invading 0.1 to 2.0 mm resembled carcinoma in situ, whereas those invading 3.1 to 5.0 mm looked more like invasive cancer. Most cells derived from early microinvasive cancer were in aggregates and displayed irregular, finely or coarsely granular chromatin, and 10% of cells possessed nucleoli, whereas

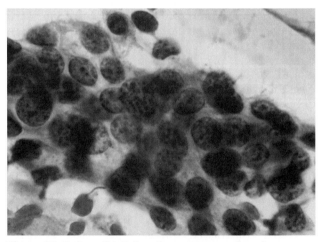

Figure 10–1. Superficially invasive squamous cell carcinoma. This cervical smear shows a syncytial sheet of cells, some with prominent nucleoli and clearing of the parachromatin and others with regular, coarse chromatin indicating high-grade squamous intraepithelial lesions (Papanicolaou stain, magnification × 2400).

carcinoma in situ cells occur as single cells with regular chromatin and lack nucleoli.

The cytologic detection of superficially invasive adenocarcinoma (SIAC) is confounded by the rarity of the lesion and by the array of reactive and proliferative lesions encountered in the cervix.[13-18] In a series of 77 women with SIAC,[19] 71 had previous cervical smears, of which 47 (66%) showed atypical glandular cells that formed pseudosyncytial clusters, crowded cell clusters, acini, cells strips, or isolated cells and showed nuclear hyperchromasia and macronucleoli. Forty of these smears were reviewed,[17] and only 12 displayed additional features suggestive of invasion (i.e., pleomorphic nuclei, coarse and irregular chromatin, karyorrhectic nuclei, and cell detritus).

Histopathology. Invasive carcinomas can be classified according to the world Health Organization (WHO) system.[20] Most superficially invasive cancers of the cervix are squamous cell types (80% to 85%), but an increasing proportion is being recognized as non-squamous types, including adenocarcinomas (15%), adenosquamous carcinomas (3% to 5%), small cell carcinomas, and other rare variants. This trend has been observed in several reports.[21-25]

Clinical decisions are driven by pathologic parameters such as depth of invasion, lymphovascular space involvement, and margin status. Assessment of these features must be based on optimal tissue handled in an optimal way by experienced pathologists.

Superficially invasive squamous cell carcinoma.

Stromal invasion arises predominantly in high-grade squamous intraepithelial lesions of the surface epithelium or from dysplastic squamous epithelium lining endocervical crypts, and only rarely does invasive carcinoma occur beneath normal-appearing epithelium.[12] Before invasion, small foci at the base of the dysplastic epithelium undergo differentiation in which, instead of crowded dysplastic cells with hyperchromatic nuclei and inconspicuous cytoplasm, the cells show abundant eosinophilic, squamoid cytoplasm, and nuclei with prominent nucleoli. From these areas, one or more finger-like projections extend into the stroma—referred to as *early stromal invasion.*[26] These projections penetrate the basement membrane and form cell clusters in the stroma that are usually surrounded by a desmoplastic stromal response accompanied by lymphoplasmacytic inflammation. In early stromal invasion, the stromal invasion is less than 1 mm, and in most instances, it is only a fraction thereof (Fig. 10-2); such cases are virtually all FIGO stage Ia1 cancers.

Several patterns of invasion have been described.[27-29] In the *spray pattern,* finger-like processes or small cell nests invade the stroma separated by uninvolved stroma. This pattern is predominantly seen in superficially invasive tumors and is rarely seen with invasion beyond 3 mm. The *confluent pattern* has fusion of invading processes resulting in anastomosing tongues of tumor with pushing borders and little or no intervening stroma (Fig. 10-3). This pattern is seen in more advanced tumors and may be combined with a spray-type pattern.

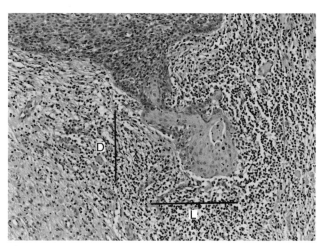

Figure 10–2. Superficially invasive squamous cell carcinoma (early stromal invasion)–FIGO stage Ia1. A tongue of neoplastic cells with cytoplasmic differentiation extends from the base of the surface epithelium, which displays features of high-grade squamous intraepithelial lesions. The depth of invasion (D) is measured from the site of origin of the invasive focus. The horizontal spread (L) is measured across the focus parallel to the surface. If more than one of these foci (i.e., spray pattern) is present, a summation is made of each focus, ignoring intervening stroma. In this case, the depth is 0.2 mm, and the length is 0.25 mm (hematoxylin & eosin, magnification × 200).

In a study of 402 cases of squamous cell carcinoma invading to a depth of 5 mm or less, Takeshima and colleagues[30] found that the confluent pattern was strongly related to the depth of invasion and to the extent of horizontal spread. Sometimes, tumors invade diffusely in small clusters or as bulky, solid growths.

The stromal reaction to invading tumor includes chronic inflammatory cells, edema, and increased vascularity indicative of angiogenesis. These features are useful in detecting invasion. Squamous cell carcinomas may be graded using the modified Broder's system.[20]

A few situations can create diagnostic difficulty in assessing superficially invasive squamous cell

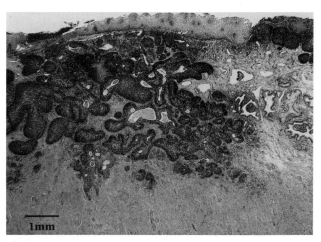

Figure 10–3. Superficially invasive squamous cell carcinoma–FIGO stage Ia2. A more advanced carcinoma with a confluent growth pattern measures 3.0 mm deep and 5.5 mm long. The lymphovascular space invasion at the edge of the tumor does not affect the FIGO staging (hematoxylin & eosin, magnification × 18).

carcinoma (SISCC). Tangential cutting of crypts involved by cervical intraepithelial neoplasia (CIN) may mimic early invasion; these foci have a smooth outline and lack anaplasia, and serial sections reveal confinement to a crypt. Edema and chronic inflammation beneath benign mucosa or CIN may obscure the basement membrane and simulate early invasion. Atypical cells may be entrapped in the stroma along a local anesthetic needle track or by implantation after a biopsy or conization; dysplastic cells are smaller, without the abundant eosinophilic cytoplasm and nucleoli seen in invasive cells. Displacement of dysplastic epithelium along a needle track may simulate LVSI.[31]

Superficially invasive adenocarcinoma. Microinvasive or early adenocarcinoma arises in most cases from adenocarcinoma in situ (ACIS) in the transformation zone. Despite several attempts,[19,32,33] there is no consensus about the definition of SIAC.

A variety of patterns of invasion have been described[32-35] (Figs. 10-4 and 10-5). The Association of Directors of Anatomic and Surgical Pathology[36] have recommended that cervical adenocarcinomas should be graded using architectural and cytologic criteria similar to those used for endometrioid carcinoma in the body of the uterus.

A bewildering array of benign glandular lesions of the endocervix may mimic in situ or invasive adenocarcinoma.[37] ACIS may be confused with endometriosis, inflammatory changes, tuboendometrioid metaplasia, Arias-Stella changes, and the effects of radiation therapy. Invasive adenocarcinoma may be mimicked by tunnel clusters with cytologic atypia,[38] deep nabothian cysts,[39] microglandular hyperplasia,[40,41] mesonephric hyperplasia,[42,43] lobular endocervical glandular hyperplasia,[44] and diffuse laminar endocervical hyperplasia.[45] Benign lesions usually lack

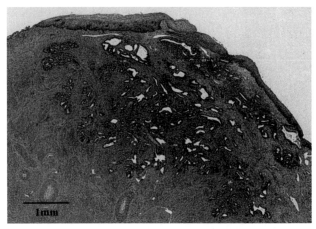

Figure 10–5. Superficially invasive adenocarcinoma—FIGO stage Ia2. A well-differentiated adenocarcinoma shows irregularly shaped glands haphazardly invading cervical stroma deep to the normal endocervical crypts. In this case, the depth is 3.35 mm, and the length is 6 mm (hematoxylin & eosin, magnification × 25).

significant cellular atypia, mitotic activity, or desmoplastic stromal responses, although these features may also be lacking in well-differentiated invasive carcinomas. A variety of immunohistochemical and molecular methods have been advocated to distinguish between reactive or hyperplastic and neoplastic endocervical lesions, but recognition of pseudoneoplastic processes still depends on routine stained slides.[44]

Tumor measurement. The current FIGO staging criteria[3] require measurements of the tumor depth and horizontal spread (length or width). The diagnosis of superficially invasive cancer is best made on conization or hysterectomy specimens. Punch biopsies cannot be properly orientated, and this compromises measurement of depth of invasion.

Tumor *depth and length* should be measured from the histologic slide using a calibrated ocular micrometer. Tumor depth is measured from the basement membrane of the overlying surface epithelium or from the point of origin from an endocervical crypt to the deepest point of invasion. To define the *tumor volume,* a third dimension, the *width,* is required. The most accurate method of determining this requires serial step sectioning through the whole width of the cone using the technique that has been described by Burghardt.[26] It is time consuming and beyond the resources of most service laboratories. Width can also be roughly calculated by taking account of the number of levels or blocks involved (e.g., three blocks that are each 3 mm thick gives a width of 9 mm). Tumor volume is then estimated by multiplying depth, length, and width and is at best a ballpark figure.

In SIAC, the tumor measurements may be more difficult and imprecise because invasion may extend through the basement membrane of the surface epithelium or from anywhere along the crypts; the site of origin cannot be identified in many cases. The use of the deepest normal gland as a marker is helpful but not absolutely reliable because of the infrequent

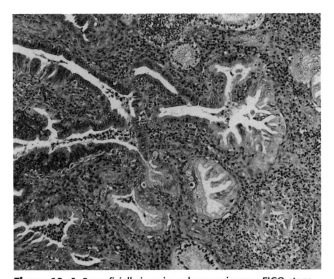

Figure 10–4. Superficially invasive adenocarcinoma—FIGO stage Ia1. Malignant glands with prominent eosinophilic cytoplasm bud from crypts showing adenocarcinoma in situ. A detached invasive focus is surrounded by an inflammatory host response *(bottom right).* In this case, the depth is 2.05 mm, and the length is 4.75 mm (hematoxylin & eosin, magnification × 200).

presence of deep but normal glands that may extend much of the way through the wall. In many cases, depth equates tumor thickness, includes a significant in situ component, and may be a gross overestimate of the depth of invasion.

Multifocality of SISCC has been reported, with frequencies from approximately 12% to 92.5%.[12,46,47] Reich and Pickel[47] identified three patterns of multifocal invasion and suggested criteria for estimating tumor length and width in such cases.

Lymphovascular space involvement. Involvement of vascular spaces by tumor is more common with deeper lesions but may be seen even in tumors less than 1 mm deep.[46] Because it is often not possible to differentiate between lymphatics and blood vessels, a more generic term, LVSI, has been adopted. Shrinkage of fibrous stroma during fixation produces an artefactual clear space around tongues of tumor that resembles vascular space invasion, whereas true LVSI is characterized by an endothelial layer lining the space. Immunohistochemical staining of endothelium using CD31, CD34, or *Ulex europaeus lectin*[48] may be of help, but endothelial cells lining lymphatic spaces may not express endothelial cell markers.[49] Recognition of vascular involvement may be aided by the presence of fibrin thrombi, smooth muscle in the wall of the vessel, and the presence of other vessels in the immediately adjacent stroma.

Specimen processing. The extent of sectioning of excisional biopsies has a major impact on the definitive diagnosis. The wide range of techniques that have been used undoubtedly contributes to the disparate results referred to throughout this chapter and the difficulty in interpreting the literature.

There are no uniform recommendations for the processing of excisional biopsies. Several methods of processing conization specimens are used. *Radial sections* taken from an intact cervix or after opening at the 12-o'clock position produce wedge-shaped blocks that are difficult to section in the vertical plane. Fu[49] estimated that sectioning at a 45-degree angle to the desired vertical plane overestimated the true depth of invasion by 40%. A more widely used method is to take *serial sagittal slices* from one side of the cone to the other. A 15-mm-diameter cone sliced at 2- to 3-mm intervals yields approximately six blocks, which when cut initially at three levels produce 18 slides. Additional levels may be taken if required. The *whole embedding method* advocated by Burghardt[50] and Östör[46] involves bisecting the fixed cone sagittally, embedding the halves in toto and serially step sectioning the block at 200- to 300-µm intervals. This provides 60 to 80 sections and a panoramic view of lesions within the cervix. This method can be duplicated in the other methods by taking levels at 50- to 100-µm intervals when there is cytologic, histologic, or colposcopic suspicion of invasion.

The detection of superficially invasive cancer increases in cold-knife cone biopsies for high-grade squamous intraepithelial lesions (HGSIL) by up to 4% if step serial sections are taken compared with when 10 to 15 sections at 1 per block[51-54] are taken, and the yield increases by 10% if the whole embedding method of Burghardt is used.[26] The detection of LVSI also increases with the extent of sectioning of the specimen. In a series of 30 cases of superficially invasive carcinoma, Roche and Norris[29] found LVSI in 9 (30%) cases in the initial sections and 17 (57%) after an additional 10 levels had been taken. Foci of LVSI may measure 100 to 200 µm (see Fig. 10-3) and may be missed, even by the whole embedding method.

The status of the *surgical margins* of excisional biopsies often has an important influence on management decisions. The margins should be highlighted with one or more ink dyes that will be visible in the sections. The interpretation of margins is easiest in cold-knife conization or hysterectomy specimens because they are usually unfragmented, orientable, and free from thermal artefact.

Lymph nodes. Lymph node dissections contain up to 30 to 50 nodes, all of which should be sectioned. Small lymph nodes are embedded whole, whereas larger nodes are bisected, and both halves are embedded en face. Numerous studies on axillary sentinel lymph nodes in breast cancer have shown that step sectioning, often with immunostaining for cytokeratin, significantly increases the node-positive rate. Sentinel lymph node biopsy for gynecologic malignancies is a recent innovation, and as in axillary sentinel node biopsy for breast cancer, the appropriate handling of the specimen is controversial. If, as in breast cancer and melanoma treatment, sentinel lymph node biopsy proves to effectively predict lymph node status, more detailed examination of these smaller number of nodes would be feasible and would improve the pathologic assessment of lymph node status. It will also introduce the thorny issue of the significance of micrometastatic disease. The absence of pelvic side wall lymph node recurrences in large series of early cervical carcinoma[55] would, however, suggest that micrometastases are not present or are not clinically significant in these early cases.

Colposcopy. Colposcopy has become an integral part of the management of the patient with abnormal cytologic results. The range of colposcopic appearances of early invasive carcinomas has been shown in atlases by Burghardt,[50] Kolstad and Stafl,[56] and Singer and Monaghan.[57]

Several colposcopic features may arouse suspicion of early invasive squamous cell carcinoma. The *vascular pattern* is atypical, with loss of the regular punctate or mosaic pattern that is seen with HGSIL. The vessels lose their regular treelike branching pattern, have various calibers, and have been likened to commas, dots, hairpins, and coils of spaghetti. The intercapillary distance in SISCC is usually variable,[56] and sometimes the vascular pattern is obscured by dense, acetowhite epithelium.

The *area of abnormal epithelium* visible on the ectocervix is usually extensive. This has been observed histologically[58,59] and colposcopically.[60,61] The abnormal transformation zone (TZ) often extends into the endocervical canal and out of colposcopic range, rendering the colposcopic results unsatisfactory in a higher proportion of patients with early invasive cancer than those with HGSIL. Rome and colleagues[8] found that the TZ extended into or was totally confined within the endocervical canal in at least 85% of women with early stromal or occult invasive cancer of the cervix. This led to unsatisfactory colposcopic findings, necessitating an excisional biopsy. This is a reflection of the area of abnormality and the fact that the women with early invasive carcinoma of the cervix are older than those with CIN; postmenopausal women often have retraction of the TZ into the endocervical canal. Benedet and coworkers[62] found lower rates of unsatisfactory colposcopic results of 42% and 28% for microinvasive and occult invasive carcinomas, respectively.

Few researchers have reported the *accuracy of colposcopy* in diagnosing SISCC. Rome and associates[8] correctly predicted 29% (16 of 55) of early stromal invasive cancers with a depth of invasion of less than 1 mm and 50% (36 of 72) clinically occult cancers with a depth of invasion more than 1 mm (up to 7 mm). Murdoch and colleagues[63] also found that colposcopy more accurately predicted invasion when the depth of invasion was more than 1 mm, and similar observations have been made by Benedet and coworkers.[62] The accuracy of colposcopy in SIAC is much less because, just as for ACIS, the colposcopic features of SIAC are not well recognized.[63,68]

Several studies[63-67] have shown that colposcopically unrecognized microinvasive cancer was present in 0.4% to 3% of excisional biopsies done for apparent CIN. These data indicate that many of these superficially invasive cancers are not recognized colposcopically and are surprise findings in excisional biopsies.

In more established, squamous- or glandular-type cancers, the *intercapillary distance* may be increased, and there may be areas of relative avascularity and necrotic exudate due to hypoxia.[56] The *vessels are more fragile*, and there are areas that bleed easily on contact; hence the often reported symptom of post-coital bleeding (PCB). Uecki[69] described *unusual vascular patterns* in early adenocarcinomas, including large vessels that looked like the root of the ginger plant. In these early cancers, the *contour* of the abnormal epithelium is irregular and may assume the appearance of a "miniature mountain range."

Colposcopy facilitates taking a *directed biopsy specimen* from the most abnormal area. If the biopsy shows features of cancer or raises the suspicion of an early invasive cancer, a more definitive excisional biopsy is usually required so that the cancer morphology can be more accurately defined. If the cancer can be seen macroscopically and the biopsy shows frankly invasive cancer the stage is Ib, and definitive treatment can be undertaken without delay.

Excisional biopsy: Loop excision or cold-knife conization?

Largely because of concerns about the possibility of ablating unrecognized invasive cancer,[51] there has been a trend toward excision rather than ablation of CIN. When using an excisional technique, every attempt should be made to excise the entire abnormality and make the procedure both diagnostic and therapeutic. Recent years have also seen a shift from carbon dioxide laser excision to loop electroexcisional procedures (LEEPs) because of the high capital and maintenance costs associated with equipment for the former. The routine use of cold-knife cone biopsy in the treatment of CIN has been abandoned by many because of the associated morbidity, the obstetric sequelae, and the need for general anesthesia. Nevertheless, many authorities believe that cold-knife cone biopsy is still the preferred treatment in some situations.

Loop and laser excision specimens may create diagnostic dilemmas because they may be fragmented, they are often difficult to orientate, and thermal injury may preclude assessment of morphology and excision margins, leading to lamentations from pathologists. Thermal injury may result in coagulative necrosis up to 830 and 750 μm in LEEP and laser conization specimens, respectively.[70] Montz and associates[71] found that, in a series of 25 cases, the tissues were so destroyed as to be inadequate for diagnosis in 4 (16%), and full interpretation of the ectocervical margins was not possible in 8 (32%), and the endocervical margins could not be determined in 12 (44%). Thermal damage to the margin can be minimized by the appropriate blend of cutting and coagulating current.

Uninterpretable or equivocal margins may require a further excisional biopsy, with potentially deleterious impact on fertility and obstetric performance in those for whom conservative management by cone biopsy alone is an option. After excising the specimen, the cervical crater is usually treated with diathermy or laser for hemostasis, and this further destroys epithelium. In the event of invasive cancer extending to the endocervical or stromal margin, this inevitably creates uncertainty about the maximum depth of tumor invasion.

Several studies have compared the efficacy of the various techniques used in the treatment of CIN,[71-73] but there have been no studies comparing the efficacy of the various excisional treatment modalities in superficially invasive cancer. Kennedy and colleagues[67] found 7 (3%) unsuspected invasive malignancies in 237 LEEP specimens, and although they reported the pathologic specimens as "excellent," the endocervical margin was involved in 4 of 6 patients with carcinomas. The higher rate of involved margins is to be expected because of the greater extent of abnormal epithelium associated with superficially invasive cancers.

In view of concerns about specimen quality fragmentation, margin interpretation, and a higher rate of involved margins with LEEP and laser cone biopsies, we prefer a *cold-knife cone biopsy* (i.e., conization) when early invasive cancer is suspected, a high-grade colposcopic abnormality is seen to extend into the endocervical canal, or there is a cytologic high-grade glandular abnormality. Further studies on the relative efficacy of the various excisional treatment modalities for superficially invasive cancers of squamous and glandular histologic types are required, particularly because of the trend toward fertility-sparing surgery.

Which prognostic factors are really important?

Numerous investigators have examined prognostic factors, and the interpretation of published results is confounded, among other reasons, by the changing definitions, variations in the extent of specimen sectioning, lack of central pathology review in multi-institutional studies, and variability of follow-up. In many studies, the horizontal extent was not measured, and some cancers may have exceeded 7 mm and therefore were stage Ib.

The site (e.g., vaginal vault, pelvic side wall, or distant) and nature (e.g., invasive or noninvasive) of recurrences has not always been specified. Some recurrences may have been new tumors or recurrences developing in the vaginal vault[55,75] after a considerable interval and might not have been residual disease or metastases from the original tumor.

Depth of stromal invasion. Depth of the stromal invasion has been the most frequently examined and the most important prognostic factor in cases of superficially invasive cervical cancer. Östör,[28] in an extensive and critical review of the literature, identified 2274 reported cases with stromal invasion less than 1 mm; these are the smaller FIGO stage Ia1 cancers, and many are what pathologists describe as early stromal invasion. Lymph node spread was identified in 3 (1.1%) of 267 patients who had undergone lymph node dissection, and he estimated that in the entire group, 8 (0.4%) suffered invasive recurrence and 2 (<0.1%) died of disease.

In Östör's review, there were also 1324 cases for which the stromal invasion was between 1 and 3 mm, and almost all of these would have fulfilled the FIGO criteria for stage Ia1. Lymph node spread was identified in 7 of 333 patients who had undergone lymph node dissection, but 2 probably had larger cancers. He estimated the risk of lymph node involvement at 1.5%. Twenty-six suffered invasive recurrence, and 9 died, but after excluding cases in which the cancers might have been larger or nonsquamous, the estimated risk of recurrence was 2%, and the risk of death was 0.5%.

The risk of nodal spread becomes clinically relevant when the depth of stromal invasion is between 3 and 5 mm. Table 10-2 shows the details of 1069 patients with squamous cell cancers reported in the literature. The overall rate of lymph node spread was 26 (5.6%) of 467 and ranged from 0% to 13.8%. This range is probably wide because some patients might have had larger

Table 10–2. Lymph Node Involvement, Recurrences, and Deaths in Patients with Squamous Cell Carcinomas and Stromal Invasion of 3 to 5 mm

Study*	No. of Cases	Lymph Node Positive	Recurrent Cancer	Died of Disease
Roche et al.[29] (1975)	21	0/21	Not stated (NS)	NS
Leman et al.[76] (1976)	7	0/7	NS	NS
Iversen et al.[77] (1979)	28	NS	2	1
Sedlis et al.[4] (1979)	21	NS	2	2
Hasumi et al.[78] (1980)	29	4/29	NS	NS
Van Nagell et al.[79] (1983)	32	3/32	3	2
Brémond et al.[80] (1985)	26	0/26	0	0
Creasman et al.[81] (1985)	21	0/NS	1	1
Simon et al.[82] (1986)	26	1/NS	0	0
Maiman et al.[83] (1988)	30	4/30	0	0
Ebeling et al.[84] (1989)	62	NS	3	NS
Kolstad[85] (1989)	187	1/NS	8	3
Schumacher et al.[86] (1989)	16	1/NS	2	1
Tsukamoto et al.[87] (1989)	15	0/NS	1	0
Greer et al.[88] (1990)	5	0/NS	0	0
Burghardt et al.[89] (1991)	16	0/NS	2	2
Chakalova et al.[90] (1991)	10	NS	0	0
Copeland et al.[6] (1992)	59	1/29	2	1
Sevin et al.[91] (1992)	36	2/36	4	4
Jones et al.[92] (1993)	24	0/18	1	0
Östör et al.[55] (1993)	31	0/21	1	1
Buckley et al.[93] (1996)	94	7/94	5	4
Creasman et al.[94] (1998)	188	0/51	0	0
Takeshima et al.[30] (1999)	85	5/73	3	3
Total	**1069**	**26/467** (5.6%)	**38/1012** (3.8%)	**25/950** (2.6%)

*In many of these series, the extent of horizontal spread was not stated. Some may have been FIGO stage Ib1 cancers with spread of more than 7 mm. Some nonsquamous tumors may have been included in some series.

cancers with a horizontal extent of more than 7 mm; because some did not undergo diagnostic cone biopsy before hysterectomy, and there would have been wide variation in the extent of sectioning of the cone biopsies; and because nonsquamous carcinomas might have been included in some series. There were 38 (3.8%) invasive recurrences and 25 (2.6%) deaths.

Horizontal extent, width, and volume. In 1985, the Cancer Committee of FIGO had chosen a horizontal extent of 7 mm as the discriminant between stage Ia2 and Ib cancer and allocated cancers with a length of more than 7 mm to stage Ib.[95] The rationale for this decision probably is based on a case reported in the German literature by Schuller[96] and cited by Burghardt and coworkers.[89] The woman with cervical cancer with stromal invasion of 3 mm and "wide superficial spread" died despite undergoing radical hysterectomy.

Takeshima and associates,[30] in a series of 402 cancers with a depth of invasion of 5 mm or less, noticed that 18% had horizontal spread in excess of 7 mm, thereby making them FIGO stage Ib cancers. They observed that the incidence of lymph node metastases was 2% (2 of 101) in FIGO stages Ia1/Ia2, compared with 7.4% (4 of 54) when the horizontal extent exceeded 7 mm. The recurrence rate was 0.3% (1 of 330) for stage Ia1 or Ia2 disease but 4.2% (3 of 72) when the horizontal extent exceeded 7 mm.

Sevin and colleagues[91] reported a series of 110 patients with stromal invasion of 1 to 5 mm who had undergone pelvic lymph node dissection. Lymph node metastases were found in two patients with stromal invasion of 3 to 5 mm with surface dimensions of 12 and 15 mm, and both had LVSI. Four patients died of recurrent cancer, all of whom had stromal invasion of 3 to 5 mm with surface dimensions ranging from 12 to 22 mm, and three of these patients had LVSI.

Burghardt and Holzer[97] and Lohe and coworkers[98] used tumor volume to define what they called a microcarcinoma. A maximum depth of 5 mm and a maximum length and width of 10 mm (volume of 500 mm³) were the discriminants beyond which tumors were allocated to stage Ib. The largest tumor in their series 97 of 283 microcarcinomas was 420 mm³, and there was LVSI in the surgical specimen. This one patient developed pelvic and distant metastases about 38 months after hysterectomy. The practical problems with volumetric studies in routine laboratory practice have previously been mentioned, but these two studies nevertheless emphasize that tumor volume is probably the most important prognostic factor in early cervical cancer.

Significance of lymphovascular space involvement. The biologic significance of LVSI in superficially invasive cervical cancer has been uncertain, and there has been controversy about whether this finding should influence management. The reported frequency of LVSI in SISCC of the cervix ranges from 8%[12] to 57%.[29] Several large studies have shown that LVSI correlates with the depth of invasion[4,6,29] and with the number of foci of invasion.[29] LVSI may be less common in SIAC,

Table 10-3. Lymphovascular Space Involvement, Lymph Node Metastases, and Recurrence in Tumors with 3 mm or Less Stromal Invasion

LVSI	Pelvic Lymph Node Metastases	Recurrence
Present	4/86 (4.7%)*	6/131 (4.6%)†
Absent	4/757 (0.5%)	10/1556 (0.6%)

*P = .01; risk ratio = 9.18; 95% CI: 1.89-44.61. P value for the difference between lymphovascular space involvement (LVSI) positive and negative status was computed using Fisher's exact test. Data from References 6, 29, 30, 55, 76, 78, 79, 81-83, 91, 99, 100, 101.
†P = .0025; risk ratio = 7.42; 95% CI: 2.36-22.61. P value for the difference between LVSI positive and negative status was computed using Fisher's exact test. Data from References 4, 6, 30, 55, 79, 81-83, 89, 91, 100, 101.

because Östör and associates[32] found it to be present in only 7 (10%) of 77 stage Ia adenocarcinomas.

The accumulated information from the literature indicates that LVSI is an adverse prognostic factor in SISCC and is associated with an increased risk of nodal spread and invasive cancer recurrence. Tables 10-3 and 10-4 show data from studies that examined LVSI, pelvic lymph node involvement, and risk of recurrence for tumors with stromal invasion of 3 mm or less and those with stromal invasion of more than 3 to 5 mm, respectively. Even for tumors with stromal invasion of 3 mm or less, LVSI is associated with a significantly increased risk of pelvic lymph node metastases and recurrence. These data justify the SGO definition of a microinvasive cancer, which excludes such cancers. For the tumors with stromal invasion of more than 3 to 5 mm with LVSI, the increased risk of pelvic lymph node metastases and cancer recurrence is more striking and highly statistically significant. If there is no LVSI, the risk of recurrence is very low (<1%), and this risk seems to be independent of the depth of stromal invasion.

There is a need for more information on LVSI, and it should be documented in each case, as recommended by FIGO. Perhaps further information will come from quantitation of the extent of LVSI as described by Roman and colleagues.[102]

Growth pattern. Fidler and Boyd[103] introduced the term *confluence* in distinguishing occult carcinoma from microinvasive carcinoma, and they found a higher

Table 10-4. Lymphovascular Space Involvement, Lymph Node Metastases, and Recurrence in Tumors with more than 3 to 5 mm Stromal Invasion

LVSI	Pelvic Lymph Node Metastases	Recurrence
Present	13/117 (11.1%)*	16/92 (17.4%)†
Absent	10/295 (3.4%)	3/320 (0.9%)

*P = .006; risk ratio = 8.07; 95% CI: 1.41-9.07. P value for the difference between lymphovascular space involvement (LVSI) positive and negative status was computed using Fisher's exact test. Data from References 6, 29, 30, 55, 76, 78, 79, 81-83, 91, 93, 94.
†P < 10⁻⁸; risk ratio = 22.25; 95% CI: 5.90-57.96. P value for the difference between LVSI positive and negative status was computed using Fisher's exact test. Data from References 4, 6, 30, 55, 79, 81-83, 89, 91, 93, 94.

recurrence rate when there was "invasion by confluent masses of neoplastic cells." Some investigators[6,78,81,87,89] have observed this to be sometimes associated with an adverse outcome. Others[29,30,76,82] have found that a confluent growth pattern does not have prognostic significance. Many of these studies have found the associations between larger tumors, LVSI, and a confluent growth pattern, thereby making its significance as an independent prognostic factor impossible to evaluate. The data appear to support the statement by Roche and Norris[29] that "the confluent pattern is ill defined and vague, its interpretation is highly subjective, and its significance in carcinoma of the cervix invading the stroma to a depth of 5 mm or less is open to question."

Stromal response. It is a characteristic of invasive tumors to have a stromal response. Several investigators[6,55,91,104] have attempted to quantify this and examine it as a prognostic factor in early cervical cancer, but only one[104] has found a lack of stromal response to be an adverse prognostic factor.

Grade. Several studies[55,83,89,105,106] have examined tumor grade as a possible prognostic factor, but there have been no consistent findings in these small tumors.

Histology. There are conflicting opinions about whether SIACs behave similarly to their squamous counterparts. Given their relative infrequency and the variety of histologic subtypes,[20] it is not surprising that these tumors are less well understood.

Several investigators have reported recurrences of SIAC with stromal invasion of 3 to 5 mm. In the largest reported institutional series of 77 stage Ia adenocarcinomas (43 with ≤ 3 mm and 34 with ≥ 3 to 5 mm of stromal invasion), Östör and coworkers[32] reported only one instance of vaginal vault recurrence. This case did not strictly meet the criteria for stage Ia2 disease because the depth of invasion was 3.2 mm, but its horizontal extent was 21 mm, and the estimated volume was 670 mm³. Kaku and associates[107] reported no recurrences in 21 patients with stromal invasion less than 3 mm, but there were two recurrences in 9 patients with stromal invasion of 3 to 5 mm. Schorge and colleagues[108] identified no recurrences in a series of 21 stage Ia1 adenocarcinomas. Covens and coworkers[109] examined tumor volume as a prognostic factor and found no recurrences in 46 patients with tumor volumes less than 600 mm³.

Elliott and associates,[23] however, reported two recurrences in 25 cases of stage Ia1 adenocarcinoma. In one case, the stromal invasion was 1.8 mm, and the tumor recurred in the pelvis; in the second case, stromal invasion was less than 1 mm, and the tumor recurred outside the pelvis. Neither patient had LVSI.

In a population-based study using the SEER database, Webb and colleagues[24] identified 301 stage Ia adenocarcinomas (131 Ia1 and 170 Ia2) managed between 1988 and 1997. There were 140 women who had lymphadenectomy, but there was only one instance (0.7%) of a single positive lymph node. The mean

follow-up period was almost 4 years, and there were no deaths among the 96 women treated by simple hysterectomy.

Smith and coworkers[110] also used the SEER database and added all previously published cases. A total of 1170 cases were identified, including 585 stage Ia1, 358 stage Ia2, and 227 "others" with less defined early disease. Of 531 who underwent lymphadenectomy, 15 (1.28%) had one or more positive nodes; of these, 11 (73.3%) had recurrent disease or died. For stage Ia1 versus Ia2 disease, there were no significant differences in the frequency of positive lymph nodes, disease recurrence, or death. The prognosis for SIAC is good and does not appear to be significantly different from that for SISCC.

A multivariate analysis of prognostic factors was reported by Elliott and associates,[23] who examined age, LVSI status, depth of stromal invasion, histologic cell type, and treatment epoch in 476 cases of FIGO stage 1A cervical cancers treated over a 40-year period. The study failed to predict tumors with a poor prognosis because of the low incidence and small number of recurrences, limiting statistical power.

The problems related to studies of these good-prognosis tumors have been addressed by Copeland[111] in an editorial entitled "Microinvasive Cervical Cancer: The Problem of Studying a Disease with an Excellent Prognosis."

Clinical management: What is the role of a conservative approach?

In general, if the woman is fit, the management of these small tumors should be surgical, with radiotherapy reserved for the unfit, the very elderly, or occasionally used postoperatively if the cancer has been a surprise finding or if nodal spread has been found. Decisions regarding the extent of surgery should take into account multiple factors, including the patient's age, her general health, her wishes regarding fertility, the margins of the excisional biopsy, the risk of residual tumor and local recurrence, the quality of the pathologic examination (particularly the extent of sectioning of the excisional biopsy), tumor morphology, and the risk of nodal spread.

In all cases, the aim of surgery for the primary cancer is to remove all abnormal epithelium with a margin of healthy tissue, and in cases at risk for nodal spread, pelvic lymphadenectomy should be performed. Until recently, this has involved a simple, modified radical or even a radical hysterectomy. Because many women with these superficially invasive cancers are young and wish to preserve their fertility, this approach has been challenged by several studies that examined the place of conservative or fertility-sparing surgery. The surgical margins of the excisional biopsy are very important for decisions about appropriate management of superficially invasive cancers, especially when fertility-sparing surgery is an issue.

For SISCC, there have been several studies[55,76,88,92,112] correlating the surgical margins of the cone biopsy with the incidence of residual CIN or invasive cancer in the subsequent hysterectomy specimen. In these studies, the overall rate of margin involvement was 55% (255 of 463) despite most of the conizations having presumably been performed with curative intent. These data provide further evidence that the area of abnormal epithelium tends to be larger in association with SISCC than with CIN, for which the rate of involved margins is approximately 25% (Rome, unpublished data, 1995). This is an important consideration when SISCC is suspected and cone biopsy may be the definitive treatment. In such cases, abnormal epithelium should be generously excised.

For *negative margins*, the rates of residual CIN in these studies ranged from 0% to 4.2%, but in one,[88] it was as high as 24%. For *positive margins*, the rates of residual disease were much higher and ranged from 39% to 82%. If the apical or stromal margin is positive, there is a small but finite risk that there is a more deeply invasive cancer situated higher in the endocervical canal. Roman and colleagues[112] showed that if the internal margins or the postconization endocervical curettage (ECC) contained dysplasia or carcinoma, the risk of invasion was sufficiently high enough (up to 33%) to warrant repeat conization before definitive treatment. Our experience has been rather different; we found deeper foci of invasion in the hysterectomy specimen after cone biopsy in only 4 (5%) of 77 cases.[8]

For SISCC with stromal invasion of 3 mm or less and no LVSI, the standard treatment has been *simple extrafascial hysterectomy* (i.e., Piver type 1[113]). When the *margins are negative*, there is no LVSI, and the specimen has been adequately sectioned, a *cone biopsy alone* is a safe option, and increasing published data have supported this approach (Table 10-5).[55,85,89,114-117] The caveat is that careful follow-up is essential. In cases managed by cone biopsy alone, *hysterectomy after completion of childbearing* has been advocated by many, but there are few data to support this recommendation. Surveillance is relatively easy, and the recurrence rate is very low, although long-term studies are needed.

When the *endocervical or stromal margins are positive*, further treatment is required because of the very high risk of residual neoplasia. The options include simple extrafascial hysterectomy or repeat cold-knife cone biopsy. Our recommendation is to repeat the cone biopsy if these margins transect invasive cancer (with stromal invasion ≤3 mm) or when these margins transect CIN in cases for which conservation of fertility is desired. When the *ectocervical margins* transect only CIN, a more conservative approach can be taken in patients wishing to conserve fertility. Uninterpretable margins may make decisions very difficult, and optimal specimen quality is essential in these cases.

A special situation applies when the abnormal TZ is very extensive and encroaches onto one or more vaginal fornix. For women wishing to retain their fertility, a cone biopsy with excision of a contiguous vaginal cuff is an option, whereas in cases for which fertility is not an issue, an extended abdominal hysterectomy with excision of a vaginal cuff or an extended vaginal hysterectomy are options. The latter approach is often useful because the vaginal cuff can be defined by using Lugol's iodine at the commencement of surgery, and all iodine negative and abnormal epithelium is excised.

Table 10–5. Reports of Stage Ia Squamous Cell Carcinoma of the Cervix Treated by Cone Biopsy Alone

| Study | Stage | Patients | Recurrence | | Term Pregnancies | Follow-up (Mean) (years) |
			CIN	Invasion		
Kolstad[85] (1989)*	Ia1 Ia2	41	0	4‖	NS	3-17
Burghardt et al.[89] (1991)*	Ia1	93	NS	1¶	NS	NS
	Ia2	18	NS	3**	NS	NS
Morris et al.[114] (1993)*	Ia1 LVSI–	14	1	0	3	0.1-14 (2.2)
Andersen et al.[115] (1993)†	Ia1 LVSI–	31	1	0	NS	NS (3.0)
Östör & Rome[55] (1994)*	Ia1 Ia2	23	0	1††	NS	0-15
Tseng et al.[116] (1997)‡	Ia1 LVSI–	12	1	0	4	6.7
Andersen et al.[117] (1998)†	Ia1 LVSI–	41	1§	0	6	5-12 (6.8)

*Cold-knife cone.
†Combination laser conization.
‡Loop electroexcisional procedure (LEEP).
§Adenocarcinoma in situ.
‖All were local recurrences.
¶Recurrent cervical cancer 12 years after cone biopsy with negative margins.
**Recurrences at 1, 1, and 3 years after cone biopsy; margins were not stated; and one tumor was a clear cell carcinoma cancer.
††Residual cervical cancer manifested 7 years after cone biopsy with an involved apical margin.
LVSI–, no lymphovascular space involvement; NS, not stated.

In cases of nonsquamous neoplasia, the correlation between *negative cone margins* and residual disease is not clear-cut. For ACIS, there is a significantly high incidence of residual disease, with reports ranging from 6% to 40% for negative margins and reports of recurrent disease ranging from 0% to 47%.[118-131] In several instances in these series, there was residual or recurrent invasive adenocarcinoma. Glandular neoplasia may be multifocal, and so-called skip lesions may exist. Östör and coworkers[19] defined skip lesions to be discrete microinvasive adenocarcinomas separated by more than 3 mm in the same lip of the cervix, but they found no instances of skip lesions in a series of 77 cases. Kurian and Al-Nafussi[118] found residual ACIS or SIAC in hysterectomy specimens after loop excisions in 33% of cases, and this correlated with disease involving or within 3 mm of margins.

For SIAC with stromal invasion of 3 mm or less and no LVSI, the standard treatment is simple *extrafascial hysterectomy*. Most of the data on conservative management by *cone biopsy* alone relate to ACIS, and there is a paucity of information on early invasive adenocarcinoma. For stage Ia adenocarcinoma, Östör and associates[32] reported 16 cases (12 with stage Ia1 and 4 with stage Ia2) that were managed conservatively by cone biopsy alone (12 cases) or cone biopsy plus lymphadenectomy (4 cases), and there have been no recurrences. Schorge and colleagues[132] reported 5 cases of stage Ia1 adenocarcinoma (4 cases) or adenosquamous carcinoma (1 case) managed by conization alone. There were no recurrences after a relatively short period of follow-up (6 to 20 months).

These data suggest that selected cases of SIAC can be safely managed conservatively. The margins of excision should be more generous because of the multifocality of the disease and the possibility of skip lesions. For ACIS, Kennedy and coworkers[129] observed that the rate of positive margins was higher in those treated by large loop excision of the TZ than by cold-knife cone biopsy (57.1% and 27.3%, respectively). They concluded that cold-knife cone biopsy was the preferred method of management for patients with ACIS wishing conservative treatment. This conclusion can be extrapolated to cases of SIAC.

There should be a lower threshold for recommending hysterectomy because of the concerns about the high rates of residual ACIS after cones with negative margins in ACIS and the difficulties and limitations of cytology, endocervical curettage, and colposcopy in the follow-up of glandular neoplasms after cone biopsy.[122] The argument for hysterectomy after completion of childbearing is more compelling, but more objective data on surgical margins and the risk of recurrence after treatment by cone biopsy are required.

For SISCC and SIAC invading 3 to 5 mm and with 3 mm or less stromal invasion but with definite LVSI, the standard treatment has been a *modified radical hysterectomy* (i.e., Piver type 2[113]) and *bilateral pelvic lymphadenectomy*, provided the cone biopsy margins are clear of invasive cancer. As long ago as 1948, Willis[133] noticed that small, operable cancers spread by embolization rather than permeation. In superficially invasive cervical cancer, the risk of *parametrial involvement* is known to be miniscule, and several workers[30,55,78,82,83,87,91,98] have assessed the risk. In reports that encompass 1379 patients, there were only two instances of parametrial tumor.[82,87] These data indicate that parametrial excision is unnecessary. The need for excision of a *vaginal cuff* has not yet been adequately addressed in published studies. Studies by Elliott and associates,[23] Östör and Rome,[55] and Yajima and colleagues[134] found a lower incidence of recurrence after an extended or modified radical hysterectomy with excision of the upper vagina than after a simple hysterectomy, despite the fact that many of the patients having a more extended hysterectomy probably had larger cancers. Although more data are needed, it is apparent that the hysterectomy should be extended or modified to include a vaginal cuff but not the parametrium.

In selected cases in which there is a desire to retain fertility, a *cone biopsy combined with a pelvic lymphadenectomy* may be adequate treatment. In such cases, we usually perform the lymphadenectomy *extraperitoneally* as described by Berman and coworkers,[135] whereas others[136] perform it *laparoscopically* in an attempt to decrease morbidity and hospital stay. Another option in stage Ia2 and small stage Ib cancer is *radical trachelectomy and lymphadenectomy*. Interest in this operation was kindled by a report by Dargeant and associates[137] of successful pregnancies after radical trachelectomy for early cervical cancer, and several case series have been reported.[138-140] The lymphadenectomy is often done laparoscopically, and this operation may also include cervical cerclage.

The safety of a conservative fertility-sparing surgery in the management of these superficially invasive cancers with 3 to 5 mm of stromal invasion is yet to be proved, and larger numbers of patients with longer follow-up periods from multi-institutional studies are needed. Studies on *sentinel lymph nodes* in early cervical cancer[141] are relevant and may eventually result in a decrease in the extent and morbidity of pelvic lymph node dissection. Further studies are warranted.

Routine removal of the *ovaries* cannot be justified on the basis of available data. Even in FIGO stage Ib disease, the incidence of ovarian metastases is rare. In the large GOG study,[142] ovarian spread was identified in 4 (0.5%) of 770 patients with squamous carcinoma, 2 (1.7%) of 121 patients with adenocarcinomas, and 0 of 99 patients with adenosquamous or other histologic types. All six patients with ovarian metastases had other evidence of extracervical disease. Kaminski and colleagues[143] found an increase in adnexal neoplasms associated with stage Ib adenocarcinomas, but many of these were benign. Östör and coworkers[32] found no instances of ovarian pathology in 23 cases of SIAC for which adnexectomies were performed.

In women who are medically unfit or whose body habitus precludes such surgery, radiotherapy is the alternative. When a superficially invasive carcinoma with stromal invasion of 3 to 5 mm has been a surprise finding in a hysterectomy specimen, pelvic radiotherapy or pelvic lymphadenectomy should be considered.

Radical parametrectomy such as described by Orr and associates[144] and Chapman and colleagues[145] is not necessary because of the miniscule reported incidence of parametrial involvement.

The *optimal time to perform hysterectomy after cone biopsy* is contentious. An increased risk of febrile morbidity and urinary fistulas in women operated on in 3 weeks after cone biopsy has been reported,[146] but there seems to be no increase in morbidity if surgery is delayed for 6 weeks.[147] Other reports[148,149] have found no correlation between the interval and morbidity and have recommended that surgery should not be delayed because of a recent cone biopsy. However, some cases are unduly vascular in the first few weeks after cone biopsy, and this is unpredictable. This condition most likely results from tissue reaction, inflammation, and possibly infection, and a course of antibiotics in the week or so before surgery is advisable. It seems reasonable to follow the suggestion made by Berek and Hacker[150] and proceed immediately with radical hysterectomy if the surgical margins are involved and there is a significant likelihood of residual cancer but to postpone surgery if the cone margins are clear.

Long-term follow-up after treatment is mandatory to detect residual and recurrent disease and late recurrences. These women seem to be at a lifetime risk for genital tract neoplasia. Even with nonsquamous lesions, disease can recur locally in the vault. The vaginal vault scar itself may be more susceptible to oncogenic influences,[55,75] and in many instances, recurrences are preceded by vaginal intraepithelial neoplasia, which if adequately treated, could prevent the development of invasive cancer.[75] Invasive vaginal recurrence is usually curable, a fact mentioned by Elliott and coworkers,[23] who described five patients with vaginal recurrence who were alive and well 3 to 12 years after treatment of the recurrence.

The overall prognosis for cases of superficially invasive cervical cancer is very good, with a recurrence rate of less than 5% and a death rate of less than 3% for some patients; for those with 3 to 5 mm of stromal invasion and LVSI, the outlook is worse. Multicenter studies using well-defined pathologic criteria, standard treatment protocols, and long-term follow-up may contribute further to our understanding of prognostic factors and optimal treatment. The pathologic diagnosis of these superficially invasive cancers may sometimes be difficult, and close liaison between the pathologist and clinician is important. The use of expert second opinions regarding the pathology and clinical management is encouraged.

REFERENCES

1. Australian Institute of Health and Welfare (AIHW): Cervical Screening in Australia, 1998-1999. AIHW catalogue number CAN 11, cancer series number 16. Canberra, AIHW, 2002.
2. Mestwerdt G: Die Frühdiagnose des Kollumkarzinoms. Zentralbl Gynakol 1947;69:198-202.
3. International Federation of Gynecology and Obstetrics: Staging announcement. FIGO staging of gynecological cancers: Cervical and vulva. Int J Gynecol Cancer 1995;5:319.
4. Sedlis A, Sol S, Tsukada Y, et al: Microinvasive carcinoma of the uterine cervix: A clinicopathologic study. Am J Obstet Gynecol 1979;133:64-74.
5. Morgan PR, Anderson MC, Buckley CH, et al: The Royal College of Obstetricians and Gynaecologists microinvasive carcinoma of the cervix study: Preliminary results. Br J Obstet Gynaecol 1993;100:664-668.
6. Copeland LJ, Silva EG, Gershenson DM, et al: Superficially invasive squamous cell carcinoma of the cervix. Gynecol Oncol 1992;45:307.
7. Ng ABP, Reagan JW, Lindner EA: The cellular manifestations of microinvasive squamous cell carcinoma of the uterine cervix. Acta Cytol 1972;16:5-13.
8. Rome RM, Chanen W, Östör AG: Preclinical cancer of the cervix: Diagnostic pitfalls. Gynecol Oncol 1985;22:302-312.
9. Andersen ES, Nielsen K, Pedersen B: The reliability of preconization diagnostic evaluation in patients with cervical intraepithelial neoplasia and microinvasive carcinoma. Gynecol Oncol 1995;59:143-147.
10. Rubio CA: Cytologic studies in cases with carcinoma in situ and microinvasive carcinoma of the uterine cervix. Acta Pathol Microbiol Scand 1974;82:161-181.
11. Rylander E: Cervical cancer in women belonging to a cytologically screened population. Acta Obstet Gynecol Scand 1976;55:361-366.
12. Ng AB, Reagan JW: Microinvasive carcinoma of the uterine cervix. Am J Clin Pathol 1969;52:511-529.
13. De May RM: Microinvasive squamous cell carcinoma. In De May RM (ed): The Art and Science of Cytopathology. Chicago, ASCP Press, 1996, pp 80-83.
14. Ayer B, Pacey F, Greenberg M: The cytologic diagnosis of adenocarcinoma in situ of the cervix uteri and related lesions. II. Microinvasive adenocarcinoma. Acta Cytol 1988;32:318-324.
15. Nguyen G-K, Jeannot AB: Exfoliative cytology of in situ and microinvasive adenocarcinoma of the cervix. Acta Cytol 1984;28:461-467.
16. Schoolland M, Allpress S, Sterrett GF: Adenocarcinoma of the cervix: Sensitivity of diagnosis by cervical smear and cytologic patterns and pitfalls in 24 cases. Cancer Cytopathol 2002;96:5-13.
17. Mulvany N, Östör A: Microinvasive adenocarcinoma of the cervix: A cytohistopathologic study of 40 cases. Diagn Cytopathol 1997;16:430-436.
18. Kudo R, Sagae S, Hayakawa O, et al: Morphology of adenocarcinoma in situ and microinvasive adenocarcinoma of the uterine cervix: A cytologic and ultrastructural study. Acta Cytol 1991;35:109-116.
19. Östör AG: Early invasive adenocarcinoma of the uterine cervix. Int J Gynecol Pathol 2000;19:29-38.
20. Kurman RJ, Norris HJ, Wilkinson EJ: Tumors of the cervix. In Rosai J, Sobin LH (eds): Tumors of the Cervix, Vagina, and Vulva. Atlas of Tumor Pathology, 3rd series, fascicle 4. Washington, DC, Armed Forces Institute of Pathology, 1992, pp 66-67.
21. Vizcaino AP, Moreno V, Bosch FX, et al: International trends in incidence of cervical cancer II. Squamous-cell carcinoma. Int J Cancer 2000;86:429-435.
22. Vizcaino AP, Moreno V, Bosch FX, et al: International trends in the incidence of cervical cancer I. Adenocarcinoma and adenosquamous cell carcinomas. Int J Cancer 1998;75:536-545.
23. Elliott P, Coppleson M, Russell P, et al: Early invasive (FIGO 1A) carcinoma of the cervix: A clinico-pathologic study of 476 cases. Int J Gynecol Cancer 2000;10:42-52.
24. Webb JC, Key CR, Qualls CR, Smith HO: Population-based study of microinvasive adenocarcinoma of the uterine cervix. Obstet Gynecol 2001;97:701-706.
25. Smith HO, Tiffany MF, Qualls CR, et al: The rising incidence of adenocarcinoma relative to squamous cell carcinoma of the uterine cervix in the United States—A 24 year population based study. Gynecol Oncol 2000;78:97-105.
26. Burghardt E (ed): Early histological diagnosis of cervical cancer: Textbook and atlas. Emanuel A Friedman, trans. Stuttgart, Georg Thieme, 1973, p 259.
27. Fu YS: Pathology of the uterine cervix, vagina, and vulva. In Fu YS (ed): Major Problems in Pathology, vol 21, 2nd ed. London, WB Saunders, 2002, pp 336-341.
28. Östör AG: Pandora's box or Ariadne's thread? Definition and prognostic significance of microinvasion in the uterine

cervix: Squamous lesions. In Rosen PP, Fechner RE (eds): Pathology Annual, part 2. Stamford, Appleton & Lange, 1995, pp 103-136.

29. Roche WD, Norris HJ: Microinvasive carcinoma of the cervix. The significance of lymphatic invasion and confluent patterns of stromal growth. Cancer 1975;36:180-186.

30. Takeshima N, Yanoh K, Tabata T, et al: Assessment of the revised International Federation of Gynecology and Obstetrics staging for early invasive squamous cell cancer. Gynecol Oncol 1999;74: 165-169.

31. McLachlin CM, Devine P, Muto M, Genest DR: Pseudoinvasion of vascular spaces: Report of an artifact caused by cervical lidocaine injection prior to loop diathermy. Hum Pathol 1994;25: 208-211.

32. Östör AG, Rome R, Quinn M: Microinvasive adenocarcinoma of the cervix: A clinicopathologic study of 77 women. Obstet Gynecol 1997;89:88-93.

33. Lee KR, Flynn CE: Early invasive adenocarcinoma of the cervix: A histopathologic analysis of 40 cases with observations concerning histogenesis. Cancer 2000;89:1048-1055.

34. Zaino RJ: Symposium. Part I. Adenocarcinoma in situ, glandular dysplasia, and early invasive adenocarcinoma of the uterine cervix. Int J Gynecol Pathol 2002;21:314-326.

35. Qizilbash AH: In-situ and microinvasive adenocarcinoma of the uterine cervix. A clinical, cytologic and histologic study of 14 cases. Am J Clin Pathol 1975;64:155-170.

36. Association of Directors of Anatomic and Surgical Pathology: Recommendations for the reporting of surgical specimens containing uterine cervical neoplasms. Mod Pathol 2000;13: 1029-1033.

37. Nucci M: Symposium. Part III. Tumor-like glandular lesions of the uterine cervix. Int J Gynecol Pathol 2002;21:347-359.

38. Jones MA, Young RH: Endocervical type A (noncystic) tunnel clusters with cytological atypia: A report of 14 cases. Am J Surg Pathol 1996;20:1312-1318.

39. Clement PB, Young RH: Deep nabothian cysts of the uterine cervix. A possible source of confusion with minimal-deviation adenocarcinoma (adenoma malignum). Int J Gynecol Pathol 1989;8:340-348.

40. Young RH, Scully RE: Atypical forms of microglandular hyperplasia of the cervix simulating carcinoma: A report of five cases and review of the literature. Am J Surg Pathol 1989;13:50-56.

41. Tambouret R, Bell DA, Young RH: Microcystic endocervical adenocarcinomas. A report of eight cases. Am J Surg Pathol 2000; 24:369-374.

42. Ferry JA, Scully RE: Mesonephric remnants, hyperplasia and neoplasia in the uterine cervix: A study of 49 cases. Am J Surg Pathol 1990;14:1100-1111.

43. Seidman JD, Tavassoli FA: Mesonephric hyperplasia of the uterine cervix: A clinicopathologic study of 51 cases. Int J Gynecol Pathol 1995;14:293-299.

44. Nucci MR, Clement PB, Young RH: Lobular endocervical glandular hyperplasia, not otherwise specified: A clinicopathologic analysis of thirteen cases of a distinct pseudoneoplastic lesion and comparison with fourteen cases of adenoma malignum. Am J Surg Pathol 1999;23:886-891.

45. Jones MA, Young RH, Scully RE: Diffuse laminar endocervical glandular hyperplasia: A benign lesion often confused with adenoma malignum (minimal deviation adenocarcinoma). Am J Surg Pathol 1991;15:1123-1129.

46. Östör AG: Studies on 200 cases of early squamous cell carcinoma of the cervix. Int J Gynecol Pathol 1993;12:193-207.

47. Reich O, Pickel H: Multifocal stromal invasion in microinvasive squamous cell carcinoma of the cervix: How to measure and stage these lesions. Int J Gynecol Pathol 2002;21:416-417.

48. Riley CB, Östör AG: Ulex europaeus 1 lectin for demonstration of lymphovascular involvement in microinvasive carcinoma of the cervix. J Histotechnol 1993;16:75-78.

49. Fu YS: Pathology of the uterine cervix, vagina, and vulva. In Major Problems in Pathology, vol 21, 2nd ed. London: WB Saunders, 2002, p 4.

50. Burghardt E: Colposcopy. In Burghardt E, Pickel H, Girardi F (eds): Cervical Pathology: Textbook and Atlas, 3rd ed. Andrew G Östör and Karl Tamussino, trans. Stuttgart, Thieme, 1998, pp 281-284.

51. Anderson MC: Are we vapourising microinvasive lesions? Colposc Gynecol Laser Surg 1987;3:33-36.

52. Boyes DA, Worth AJ, Fidler HK: The results of treatment of 4389 cases of preclinical squamous carcinoma. J Obstet Gynaecol Br Commonw 1970;77:769.

53. Killackey MA, Jones WB, Lewis JL: Diagnostic conization of the cervix: Review of 460 consecutive cases. Obstet Gynecol 1986; 67:766-770.

54. Nichols T, Boyes DA, Fidler HK: Advantages of routine step serial sectioning of cervical cone biopsies. Am J Clin Pathol 1968;49:324-346.

55. Östör AG, Rome R: Microinvasive squamous cell carcinoma of the cervix: A clinicopathologic study of 200 cases with long-term follow-up. Int J Gynecol Cancer 1994;4:257-264.

56. Kolstad P, Stafl A: Atlas of Colposcopy. Baltimore, University Park Press, 1972, pp 95-123.

57. Singer A, Monaghan JM: Lower Genital Tract Precancer—Colposcopy, Pathology and Treatment. Boston, Blackwell Scientific Publications,1994, pp 91-108.

58. Christopherson WM, Parker JE: Microinvasive carcinoma of the uterine cervix. Cancer 1964;17:1123.

59. Tidbury P, Singer A, Jenkins D: CIN3: The role of lesion size in invasion. Br J Obstet Gynaecol 1992;99:583-586.

60. Rome RM, Urcuyo R, Nelson JH: Observations on the surface area of the abnormal transformation zone associated with intraepithelial and early invasive squamous cell lesions of the cervix. Am J Obstet Gynecol 1977;129:565-570.

61. Shafi MI, Finn CB, Luesley DM, et al: Lesion size and histology of atypical cervical transformation zone. Br J Obstet Gynaecol 1991;98:490-492.

62. Benedet JL, Anderson GH, Boyes DA: Colposcopic accuracy in the diagnosis of microinvasive and occult invasive carcinoma of the cervix. Obstet Gynecol 1985;65:557-562.

63. Murdoch JB, Grimshaw RN, Morgan PR, et al: The impact of loop diathermy on management of early invasive cervical cancer. Int J Gynecol Cancer 1992;2:129-133.

64. McIndoe GA, Robson MS, Tidy JA, et al: Laser excision rather than vaporization: The treatment of choice for cervical intraepithelial neoplasia. Obstet Gynecol 1989;74:165-168.

65. Howe DT, Vincenti AC: Is large loop excision of the transformation zone (LLETZ) more accurate than colposcopically directed punch biopsy in the diagnosis of cervical intraepithelial neoplasia? Br J Obstet Gynaecol 1991;98:588-591.

66. Luesley DM, Cullimore J, Redman CWE, et al: Loop diathermy excision of the cervical transformation zone in patients with abnormal cervical smears. Br Med J 1990;300:1690-1693.

67. Kennedy AW, Belinson JL, Wirth S, Taylor J: The role of the loop electrosurgical excision procedure in the diagnosis and management of early invasive cervical cancer. Int J Gynecol Cancer 1995; 5:117-120.

68. Lickrish GM, Colgan TJ, Wright VC: Colposcopy of adenocarcinoma in situ and invasive adenocarcinoma of the cervix. Obstet Gynecol Clin North Am 1993;20:111-122.

69. Ueki M (ed): Cervical Adenocarcinoma—A Colposcopic Atlas. St Louis, Ishiyaku Euro-America, 1985, p 18.

70. Wright TC, Richart RM, Ferenczy A, Koulos J: Comparison of specimens removed by CO_2 laser conization and the loop electrosurgical excision procedure. Obstet Gynecol 1994;79: 147-153.

71. Montz FJ, Holschneider CH, Thompson LD: Large-loop excision of the transformation zone: Effect on the pathologic interpretation of resection margins. Obstet Gynecol 1993;81:976-982.

72. Duggan BD, Felix JC, Muderspach LI, et al: Cold-knife conization versus conization by the loop electroexcision procedure. Am J Obstet Gynecol 1999;180:276-282.

73. Linares AC, Storment J, Rhodes-Morris H, et al: A comparison of three cone biopsy techniques for evaluation and treatment of squamous intraepithelial lesions. J Gynecol Tech 1997;3: 151-156.

74. Mitchell MF, Tortolero-Luna G, Cook E, et al: A randomized clinical trial of cryotherapy, laser vaporization, and loop electrosurgical excision for treatment of squamous intraepithelial lesions of the cervix. Obstet Gynecol 1998;92:737-744.

75. Rome RM, England PG: Management of vaginal intraepithelial neoplasia: A series of 132 cases with long-term follow-up. Int J Gynecol Cancer 2000;10:382-390.

76. Leman MH, Benson WL, Kurman RJ, Park RC: Microinvasive carcinoma of the cervix. Obstet Gynecol 1976;48:571-578.

77. Iversen TR, Abeler V, Kjorstad K: Factors influencing the treatment of patients with stage 1A carcinoma of the cervix. Br J Obstet Gynaecol 1979;86:593-597.

78. Hasumi K, Sakamoto A, Sugano H: Microinvasive carcinoma of the uterine cervix. Cancer 1980;45:928-931.

79. Van Nagell JR, Greenwell N, Powell DF, et al: Microinvasive carcinoma of the cervix. Am J Obstet Gynecol 1983;145:981-989.

80. Brémond A, Frappart L, Migaud C: Étude de 68 carcinomes micro-invasifs du col utérin. J Gynecol Obstet Biol Reprod 1985; 14:1025-1031.

81. Creasman WT, Fetter BF, Clarke-Pearson DL, et al: Management of stage IA carcinoma of the cervix. Am J Obstet Gynecol 1985;153:164-172.

82. Simon NL, Gore H, Shingleton HM, et al: Study of superficially invasive carcinoma of the cervix. Obstet Gynecol 1986;68:19-24.

83. Maiman MA, Fruchter RG, Di Maio TM, Boyce JG: Superficially invasive squamous cell carcinoma of the cervix. Obstet Gynecol 1988;72:399-403.

84. Ebeling K, Bilek K, Johannsmeyer D, et al: Mikroinvasives Karzinom der Cervix Uteri Stadium Ia —Ergebnisse einer multi-zentrischen klinikbezogenen Analyse. Geburtshilfe Frauenheilkd 1989;49:776-781.

85. Kolstad P: Follow-up study of 232 patients with stage Ia1 and 411 patients with stage IA2 squamous cell carcinoma of the cervix (microinvasive carcinoma). Gynecol Oncol 1989;33:265-272.

86. Schumacher von A, Schwarz R: Histopathologische und tumormetrische Untersuchungen am Zervixkarzinom im Stadium 1A. Zentralbl Gynakol 1989;111:516-523.

87. Tsukamoto N, Tunehisa K, Matshukuma K, et al: The problem of stage 1A (FIGO 1985) carcinoma of the uterine cervix. Gynecol Oncol 1989;34:1-6.

88. Greer BE, Figge DC, Tamini HK, et al: Stage Ia2 squamous carcinoma of the cervix: Difficult diagnosis and therapeutic dilemma. Am J Obstet Gynecol 1990;162:1406-1411.

89. Burghardt E, Girardi F, Lahousen M, et al: Microinvasive carcinoma of the uterine cervix (FIGO stage IA). Cancer 1991; 67:1037-1045.

90. Chakalova G, Karagiozov A, Kurlov T: Invasive cervical carcinoma in women up to the age 30. Eur J Gynaecol Oncol 1991; 12:147-151.

91. Sevin BU, Nadji M, Averette HE, et al: Microinvasive carcinoma of the cervix. Cancer 1992;70:2121-2128.

92. Jones WB, Mercer GO, Lewis JL Jr, et al: Early invasive carcinoma of the cervix. Gynecol Oncol 1993:51:26-32.

93. Buckley SL, Tritz DM, van Le L, et al: Lymph node metastases and prognosis in patients with stage 1A2 cervical cancer. Gynecol Oncol 1996;63:4-9.

94. Creasman WT, Zaino RJ, Major FJ, et al: Early invasive carcinoma of the cervix (3 to 5 mm invasion): Risk factors and prognosis. A GOG study. Am J Obstet Gynecol 1998;178:62-65.

95. International Federation of Gynecology and Obstetrics: Staging Announcement: FIGO Cancer Committee. Gynecol Oncol 1986; 25:383-385.

96. Schuller E: Carcinoma colli uteri incipiens. Arch Gynakol 1958; 190:520-548.

97. Burghardt E, Holzer E: Diagnosis and treatment of microinvasive carcinoma of the cervix uteri. Obstet Gynecol 1977;49: 641-653.

98. Lohe KJ, Burghardt E, Hillemanns HG, et al: Early squamous cell carcinoma of the uterine cervix. II. Clinical results of a cooperative study in the management of 419 patients with early stromal invasion and microcarcinoma. Gynecol Oncol 1978;6: 31-50.

99. Averette HE, Nelson JH Jr, Ng ABP, et al: Diagnosis and management of microinvasive (stage Ia) carcinoma of the uterine cervix. Cancer 1976;38:414-425.

100. Seski JC, Abell MR, Morley GW: Microinvasive squamous carcinoma of the cervix. Definition, histologic analysis, late results of treatment. Obstet Gynecol 1977;50:410-414.

101. Bohm JW, Krupp PJ, Lee FYL, Batson HWK: Lymph node metastasis in microinvasive epidermoid cancer of the cervix. Obstet Gynecol 1976;48:65-67.

102. Roman LD, Felix JC, Muderspach LI, et al: Influence of quantity of lymph-vascular space invasion on the risk of nodal metastases in women with early-stage squamous cancer of the cervix. Gynecol Oncol 1998;68:220-225.

103. Fidler HK, Boyd JR: Occult invasive carcinoma cervix. Cancer 1960;13:764-771.

104. Reinthaller A, Tatra G, Breithnecker G, Janisch H: Prognosefaktoren beim Zervixkarzinom der Stadien Ia–IIb nach radikaler Hysterektomie unter besonderer Berücksichtigung der invasiven Stromalreaktion. Geburtshilfe Frauenheilkd 1991; 51:809-813.

105. Larsson G, Alm P, Gulberg B, Grundsell H: Prognostic factors in early invasive carcinoma of the cervix. A clinical, histopathologic and statistical analysis of 343 cases. Am J Obstet Gynecol 1983;146:145-153.

106. La Vecchia C, Franceschi S, Decari A, et al: Invasive cervical cancer in young women. Br J Obstet Gynaecol 1984;91: 1149-1155.

107. Kaku T, Kamura T, Sakai K, et al: Early adenocarcinoma of the uterine cervix. Gynecol Oncol 1997;65:281-285.

108. Schorge JO, Lee KR, Flynn CE, et al: Stage Ia1 cervical adenocarcinoma. Obstet Gynecol 1999;93:219-222.

109. Covens A, Kirby J, Shaw P, et al: Prognostic factors for relapse and pelvic lymph node metastases in early stage I adenocarcinoma of the cervix. Gynecol Oncol 1999;74:423-427.

110. Smith HO, Qualls CR, Romero AA, et al: Is there a difference in survival for 1A1 and 1A2 adenocarcinoma of the uterine cervix? Gynecol Oncol 2002;85:229-241.

111. Copeland LJ: Microinvasive cervical cancer: The problem of studying a disease with an excellent prognosis. Gynecol Oncol 1996;63:1-3.

112. Roman LD, Felix JC, Muderspach LI, et al: Risk of residual invasive disease in women with microinvasive squamous cancer in a conization specimen. Obstet Gynecol 1997;90: 759-764.

113. Piver MS, Rutledge FN, Smith JP: Five classes of extended hysterectomy for women with cervical cancer. Obstet Gynecol 1974;44:265-272.

114. Morris M, Mitchell MF, Silva EG, et al: Cervical conization as definitive therapy for early invasive squamous carcinoma of the cervix. Gynecol Oncol 1993;51:193-196.

115. Andersen ES, Husth M, Joergensen A, Nielsen K: Laser conization for microinvasive carcinoma of the cervix: Short term results. Int J Gynecol Cancer 1993;3:183-185.

116. Tseng CJ, Horng SG, Soong YK, et al: Conservative conization for microinvasive carcinoma of the cervix. Am J Obstet Gynecol 1977;176:1009-1010.

117. Andersen ES, Nielsen K, Pedersen B: Combination laser conization as treatment of microinvasive carcinoma of the uterine cervix. Eur J Gynaecol Oncol 1998;19:352-355.

118. Kurian K, Al-Nafussi A: Relation of cervical glandular intraepithelial neoplasia to microinvasive and invasive adenocarcinoma of the uterine cervix: A study of 121 cases. J Clin Pathol 1999;52:112-117.

119. Hopkins MP, Roberts JA, Schmidt RW: Cervical adenocarcinoma in situ. Obstet Gynecol 1988;71:842-844.

120. Muntz HG, Bell DA, Lage JM, et al: Adenocarcinoma of the uterine cervix. Obstet Gynecol 1992;80:935-939.

121. Im DD, Duska LR, Bosensheim NB: Adequacy of conization margins in adenocarcinoma in situ of the cervix as a predictor of residual disease. Gynecol Oncol 1995;59:179-182.

122. Poynor EA, Barakat RR, Hoskins WJ: Management and follow-up of patients with adenocarcinoma in situ of the uterine cervix. Gynecol Oncol 1995;57:158-164.

123. Widrich T, Kennedy AW, Myers TM, et al: Adenocarcinoma in situ of the uterine cervix: Management and outcome. Gynecol Oncol 1996;61:304-308.

124. Wolf JK, Levenbach C, Malpica A, et al: Adenocarcinoma in situ of the cervix: Significance of cone biopsy margins. Obstet Gynecol 1996;88:82-86.

125. Denehy TR, Gregori CA, Breen JL: Endocervical curettage, cone margins and residual adenocarcinoma in situ of the cervix. Obstet Gynecol 1997;90:1-6.

126. Azodi M, Chambers SK, Rutherford TJ, et al: Adenocarcinoma in situ of the cervix: Management and outcome. Gynecol Oncol 1999;73:348-353.

127. Shin CH, Schorge JO, Lee KR, Sheets EE: Conservative management of adenocarcinoma in situ of the cervix. Gynecol Oncol 2000;79:4-5.

128. Hopkins MP: Adenocarcinoma in situ of the cervix—The margins must be clear. Gynecol Oncol 2000;79:4-5.

129. Kennedy AW, Biscotti CV: Further study of the management of cervical adenocarcinoma in situ. Gynecol Oncol 2002;86: 361-364.

130. Östör AG, Duncan A, Quinn M, Rome R: Adenocarcinoma in situ of the uterine cervix: An experience with 100 cases. Gynecol Oncol 2000;79:207-210.

131. Andersen ES, Neilsen K: Adenocarcinoma in situ of the cervix: A prospective study of conization as definitive treatment. Gynecol Oncol 2002;86:365-369.

132. Schorge JO, Lee KR, Sheets EE: Prospective management of stage 1A(1) cervical adenocarcinoma by conization alone to preserve fertility: A preliminary report. Gynecol Oncol 2000; 78:217-220.

133. Willis RA: Pathology of Tumours. London, Butterworth, 1948, p 167.

134. Yajima A, Noda K: The results of treatment of microinvasive carcinoma (stage 1A) of the uterine cervix by means of simple and extended hysterectomy. Am J Obstet Gynecol 1979;135: 686-688.

135. Berman ML, Lagasse LD, Watiring WG, et al: The operative evaluation of patients with cervical carcinoma by an extraperitoneal approach. Obstet Gynecol 1977;50:658-664.

136. Querleu D, Lebiane E, Castelain B: Laparoscopic pelvic lymphadenectomy in the staging of early carcinoma of the cervix. Am J Obstet Gynecol 1991;164:579-585.

137. Dargent D, Brun JL, Roy M, Remy I: Pregnancies following radical trachelectomy for invasive cervical cancer [abstract]. Gynecol Oncol 1994;52:105.

138. Roy M, Plante M: Pregnancies after radical vaginal trachelectomy for early stage cervical cancer. Am J Obstet Gynecol 1998; 179:1491-1496.

139. Covens A, Shaw P, Murphy J, et al: Is radical trachelectomy a safe alternative to radical hysterectomy for patients with IIA-B carcinoma of the cervix? Cancer 1999;86:2273-2279.

140. Dargeant D, Martin X, Sacchetoni A, Mathevet P: Laparoscopic vaginal radical trachelectomy: A treatment to preserve the fertility of cervical carcinoma patients. Cancer 2000;88:1877-1882.

141. Levenback C, Coleman RL, Burke TW, et al: Lymphatic mapping and sentinel node identification in patients with cervix cancer undergoing radical hysterectomy and pelvic lymphadenectomy. J Clin Oncol 2002;20:688-693.

142. Sutton GP, Bundy BN, Delgado G, et al: Ovarian metastases in stage 1B carcinoma of the cervix: A Gynecologic Oncology Group study. Am J Obstet Gynecol 1992;166:50-53.

143. Kaminsky PF, Norris HJ: Coexistence of ovarian neoplasms and endocervical adenocarcinoma. Obstet Gynecol 1984;64: 553-556.

144. Orr JW Jr, Ball GC, Soong SJ, et al: Surgical treatment of women found to have invasive cervix cancer at the time of total hysterectomy. Obstet Gynecol 1986;68:353-356.

145. Chapman JA, Mannel RS, DiSaia PJ, et al: Surgical treatment of unexpected invasive cervical cancer found at total hysterectomy. Obstet Gynecol 1992;80:931-934.

146. Mikuta JJ, Giuntoli RL, Rubin EL, Mangan CE: The problem of radical hysterectomy. Am J Obstet Gynecol 1977;128:119-125.

147. Samlal RAK, van der Velden J, Schilthuis MS, et al: Influence of diagnostic conization on surgical morbidity and survival in patients undergoing radical hysterectomy for stage IB and IIA cervical carcinoma. Eur J Gynecol Oncol 1997;18:478-481.

148. Orr JW, Shingleton HM, Hatch KD, et al: Correlation of perioperative morbidity and conization to radical hysterectomy interval. Obstet Gynecol 1982;59:726-731.

149. Webb MJ, Symmonds RE: Radical hysterectomy: Influence of recent conization on morbidity and complications. Obstet Gynecol 1979;53:290-293.

150. Berek JS, Hacker NF: Practical Gynecologic Oncology, 3rd ed. Philadelphia, Lippincott Williams & Wilkins, 2000, p 359.

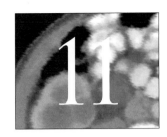

CHAPTER

ADENOCARCINOMA OF THE CERVIX

Michael P. Hopkins and *Harriet O. Smith*

 MAJOR CONTROVERSIES

- Has the incidence of adenocarcinoma increased?
- Is there a precursor lesion of adenocarcinoma in situ?
- Is the etiology of adenocarcinoma in situ the same as for adenocarcinoma?
- What is the optimal management of adenocarcinoma in situ?
- How should early invasive adenocarcinoma be managed?
- Should stage I adenocarcinoma be treated by radical hysterectomy or radiation therapy?
- How should lymph node metastasis in stage I disease be managed?
- How should advanced-stage adenocarcinoma be managed?
- How should recurrent adenocarcinoma of the cervix be managed?
- Do cell type and tumor grade alter survival?
- Can the ovaries by preserved at radical hysterectomy?

Adenocarcinoma of the cervix accounts for approximately 15% to 25% of all cervical malignancies.[1] Unlike squamous cell carcinoma, adenocarcinoma has many histologic variants (Table 11-1) which differ in their predilection for lymph node metastasis and for recurrence. Worldwide, the incidence of adenocarcinoma is increasing, especially among younger women for whom childbearing remains a concern. Nevertheless, because the disease is relatively uncommon, there is no uniformly accepted form of management for adenocarcinoma in situ (AIS) or invasive adenocarcinoma. It is uncertain whether the treatment strategies should be the same as those for squamous cell tumors. This chapter addresses controversies that include the changing trends in incidence of the disease and the cofactors involved; the current management of AIS; early invasive adenocarcinoma; the management of early-stage as opposed to advanced adenocarcinoma; and options for therapy for recurrent adenocarcinoma. Other issues addressed include the role of ovarian conservation in early-stage and advanced disease, its impact on survival, and the effect of histologic subtype on survival.

Has the incidence of adenocarcinoma increased?

Over the past four decades, the overall incidence of all cervical cancers has continued to decline in regions of the world where cytologic screening is routinely practiced. Initially, most institutions and registries reported that the absolute number of adenocarcinoma cases remained constant over time, whereas the proportion of adenocarcinoma relative to squamous cell carcinoma cases increased, and the rise in adenocarcinoma was caused by the decline in all cervical and squamous cell carcinoma incidence rates (Fig. 11-1).[2-7] More recent data, derived from the Surveillance, Epidemiology and End Results (SEER) public-use database, a population-based database of all systematically recorded invasive cancers for about 10% of the population of the United States, indicate that the 5-year average age-adjusted incidence rates for cervical adenocarcinoma increased by 29.1% over 24 years (1973 through 1996).[8] This SEER study, as well as other contemporary reports from population-based registries in Canada, the United Kingdom, and western Europe,

Table 11–1. Modified World Health Organization Histologic Classification of Epithelial Tumors of the Cervix

Squamous Cell Carcinoma	Adenocarcinoma	Other Epithelial Tumors
Microinvasive and invasive	Mucinous	Adenosquamous
Verrucous carcinoma	Endocervical type	Glassy cell carcinoma
Warty carcinoma	Intestinal type	Mucoepidermoid
Papillary squamous cell (transitional)	Signet-ring type	Adenoid cystic
Lymphoepithelioma-like	Endometrioid (with or without squamous metaplasia)	Adenoid basal
	Clear cell adenocarcinoma	Carcinoid-like tumor
	Minimum deviation adenocarcinoma (adenoma malignum)	Small cell carcinoma
	Serous	Undifferentiated carcinoma
	Mesonephric	
	Villoglandular	

Adapted from Wright TC, Ferenczy A, Jurman RJ: Carcinoma and other tumors of the cervix. In Kurman RJ (ed.): Blaustein's Pathology of the Female Genital Tract, 4th ed. New York, Springer-Verlag, 1994, p. 28.

demonstrate that invasive adenocarcinoma cases are increasing, not only in relation to squamous cell carcinoma cases, but also relative to the population at risk.[9-13] More recent data derived from SEER (1973 through 1998, unpublished data; Fig. 11-2) indicate that the age-adjusted incidence rates per 100,000 woman-years for all cervical and squamous cell carcinomas declined by 43.7% (2.07% per year) and 53.3% (2.87% per year), respectively, whereas the rates for adeno-carcinoma and adenosquamous carcinoma increased by 32.4% (1.63% per year) and 32.9% (1.57% per year), respectively.[14] These results mirror those of a Canadian study, which found that adenocarcinoma and adenosquamous carcinoma incidence rates were increasing in younger women,[13] and a recent British study, which reported that the underlying risk of adenocarcinoma was 14 times greater among women born in the early 1960s compared with those born before 1935.[11]

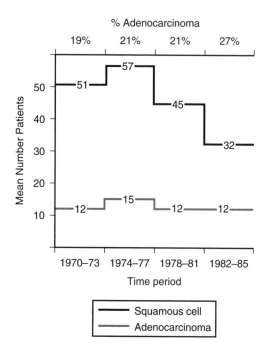

Figure 11–1. Mean number of patients with adenocarcinoma or squamous cell cancer divided by equal 4-year time periods. (From the University of Michigan Medical Center.)

One explanation for these trends is that the methods routinely used today for cytologic screening more effectively identify squamous precursor lesions.[8,10] In the British study previously mentioned, there was a decrease in rates among younger women in the last 2 years of study (1996 and 1997), which supports some protective effect from screening. However, a similar trend was not observed among postmenopausal women, which suggests that screening is less effective in older women, probably because the transformation zone is less accessible.[11] The rise in incidence rates may also be a reflection of changes in sexual practices that began in the 1960s and greater exposure to human papillomavirus (HPV) infection.[11] Population-based registries have reported a decline in the proportion of cervical cancers coded as having unknown histologic classification, and this has been attributed to better recognition of diverse and rare variants by pathologists. Therefore, the increase in adenocarcinoma incidence rates may also be a reflection of improved recognition.[8,12] To address this effect, one registry reviewed all non–squamous cell carcinomas registered between 1966 and 1990 and analyzed trends after reclassification of appropriate cases to adenocarcinoma subtypes. A 3-fold increase in endocervical adenocarcinoma incidence rates among women younger than 35 years, and a 50% decrease among women older than 55 years of age, were found. Additionally, a 3-fold increase in endometrioid adenocarcinoma was found, evenly distributed among all age groups, whereas unfavorable histologies (clear cell, serous, glassy cell, undifferentiated, and not otherwise classified) tended to be found among older women, who also had more advanced-stage disease.[12] Unpublished SEER data similarly indicate no statistically significant changes in the incidence rates of the more rare adenocarcinoma and unclassified subtypes (see Fig. 11-1).

Is there a precursor lesion of adenocarcinoma in situ?

It is unknown whether atypical glandular lesions are precursors to AIS and invasive adenocarcinoma, or whether these findings are merely indicators of significant underlying disease.[15] Studies have indicated

Figure 11–2. Cervical cancer incidence rates. (Unpublished data from the Surveillance, Epidemiology and End Results [SEER] database, 1973-1998.)

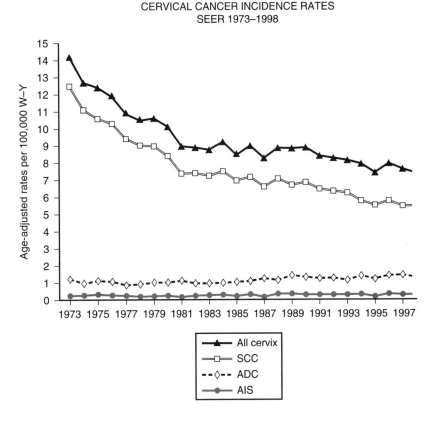

CERVICAL CANCER INCIDENCE RATES
SEER 1973–1998

that 17% to 33% of women with these findings have significant glandular and squamous cell lesions of the cervix or vagina or underlying endometrial carcinoma.[16-21] Although many atypical glandular cells of undetermined significance (AGUS) on cytologic smears merely reflect reparative change, the type known as atypical glandular cells "favor dysplasia" has been associated with underlying intraepithelial neoplasia in 9% to 54% and AIS or invasive cancer in 0% to 8% of cases.[19,21] These observations led to the 2001 Bethesda system modifications that now divide abnormalities less severe than cancer into atypical glandular cells "not otherwise specified" (ACG), atypical glandular cells "favor dysplasia," and AIS.[21] However, because significant underlying disease cannot be excluded on the basis of cytology, the 2001 Consensus Conference on cervical cancer guidelines included colposcopy in the clinical setting of ACG "favor dysplasia," endometrial biopsy for any woman who has atypical endometrial cells or is older than 35 years of age, and excisional biopsy (conization or loop electrosurgical excision procedure [LEEP]) if the colposcopic evaluation is negative. This approach was recommended because AIS and even early adenocarcinoma are often missed at colposcopy.[22]

Most pathologists concur that AIS is an entity distinct from benign glandular changes and invasive adenocarcinoma, although overlapping morphologic features can make this determination difficult.[23-26] As with adenocarcinoma, the number of AIS cases is also increasing. A 12.25% increase in annual incidence rates for AIS (from 10.31 to 14.24 per year per 100,000 women)

was reported in one SEER study.[27] The natural history of AIS is unknown, although there is sound epidemiologic evidence that AIS is a precursor to invasive adenocarcinoma.[23] A population-based analysis of the average ages of women with preinvasive and invasive cervical lesions indicate a 13-year difference among women with AIS compared with adenocarcinoma, and an 18-year difference for squamous cell precursors compared with carcinoma.[27]

Is the etiology of adenocarcinoma in situ the same as for adenocarcinoma?

The etiologies of AIS and invasive adenocarcinoma are unknown. Women with cervical adenocarcinoma also tend to have many characteristics associated with endometrial adenocarcinoma, including obesity and low parity.[28] Depending on the methods used for detection, HPV DNA has been identified in up to 100% of AIS and invasive lesions, and HPV has been implicated as a necessary precursor in recent large-scale epidemiologic studies encompassing women from throughout the world.[29-33] As with squamous cell carcinoma, the most common subtypes associated with malignant tumors are HPV-16 and -18, although most studies demonstrate a preponderance of HPV-18 in adenocarcinomas and HPV-16 in squamous lesions.[29,34-36] Using newer technology, HPV viral DNA has been found in 100% of invasive cancers, supporting the premise that HPV is a necessary prerequisite to cervical cancer including adenocarcinoma.[32]

However, because HPV infections are extremely common and usually transient and the vast majority of infected women do not develop cervical cancer, one or more cofactors are also necessary. A link between cigarette smoking and cervical carcinoma has consistently been found for squamous but not for adenocarcinomatous lesions.[36] More recent data indicate that cigarette smoking is inversely related to cervical adenocarcinoma.[37] Oral contraceptive use has also been implicated as a risk factor for invasive adenocarcinoma in young women (but not in postmenopausal women), and the relative risk appears to increase with duration of use.[38] Long-term use of oral contraceptives and HPV infection also increase the risk of AIS, which provides additional evidence to support AIS as a precursor to invasive adenocarcinoma.[31,38] Of interest, HPV DNA is not usually found in nonmucinous adenocarcinomas including clear cell, squamous, and mesonephric tumors[29]; this fact, along with population-based data demonstrating no change in incidence rates and prevalence in older women with advanced-stage disease, is consistent with differing etiologies for these tumors.[12]

Both AIS and adenocarcinomas have abnormal levels of expression of estrogen receptor and cell cycle–mediated molecules, including cyclin E, p53, p16, p21, and p27.[39] These changes may account for the increased risk associated with contraceptive use,[31,38] as well as noncontraceptive hormone replacement therapy.[40] Although the association between use of oral contraceptives and cervical cancer was initially thought to be specific for adenocarcinoma, long-term use of oral contraceptives in combination with HPV positivity was similarly implicated in squamous cell carcinoma development in a recent study.[41] Another follow-up report of the International Agency for Research on Cancer (IARC) multicenter study identified increased parity as a risk factor for squamous cell carcinoma but not adenocarcinoma.[42]

Together, these results indicate that, although cervical adenocarcinoma and squamous cell carcinoma cell types have many common associations, the cofactors involved are somewhat different. In addition to providing evidence that these lesions are histogenetically related, the association between high-risk HPV subtypes and underlying high-grade squamous dysplasia/AIS also supports a potential role for HPV subtyping to distinguish benign glandular changes from carcinoma precursor lesions, including high-grade squamous dysplasia and AIS.[29,43]

What is the optimal management of adenocarcinoma in situ?

AIS of the cervix was first described in 1953 by Friedell and McKay.[25] Until recently, this entity was seldom reported. Originally, it was strictly defined pathologically as endocervical glands present in the normal location and containing normal epithelium, transitioning into an in situ but malignant-appearing process. In practice, this definition has been expanded to include cases in which the entire gland or glands have been replaced with disease. As long as these changes are within the normal expected location, the lesion is not considered invasive.[1,23-25,44,45] Therefore, AIS constitutes a wide spectrum, ranging from extremely superficial glands, most of which have normal characteristics along with cellular atypia and minimum malignant characteristics, to deep, elongated glands with abundant abnormal cells that extend deep into the endocervical stroma. Using the currently accepted definition, this entire spectrum constitutes AIS. The risks for skip lesions, recurrence, and associated underlying malignancy vary according to the individual features. The management of the individual patient must vary, therefore, based on the extent of disease and on her desire for fertility. The number of microscopic sections sampled at the time of cone biopsy and the amount of endocervical tissue excised may also influence the likelihood of detecting underlying invasive disease.

Until recently, AIS was considered relatively rare. Later reports indicated that there is substantial risk for coincident invasive disease, and for recurrence both of AIS and invasive disease, if management is by conization alone.[46-63] Given the uncertain significance of this pathologic finding, the management of AIS in the individual patient is controversial. Even if conization margins are negative, most reports indicate a substantial risk for residual disease in the hysterectomy specimen.[46,47,50-58] As illustrated in Table 11-2, residual AIS is found in the hysterectomy specimens of up to 25% of

Table 11–2. Residual Disease in Hysterectomy Specimens According to Cone Margin Status and Risk of Recurrence with Observation after Cone Biopsy

Study and Year	Proportion of Negative Margins	Proportion of Positive Margins	Recurrence with Observation
Östör, 2000	2/8	9/12	0/53
Azodi, 1999	5/16	9/16	—
Denehy, 1997	2/7	7/10	—
Wolf, 1996	7/21 (3 invasive)	10/19 (5 invasive)	2/7 (1 invasive)
Poyner, 1995	4/8	3/8	7/15 (2 invasive)
Muntz, 1992	1/12	7/10 (2 invasive)	0/18
Im, 1995	4/9	4/6	0/2
Hopkins, 1988	1/7	4/5	—
TOTAL	27/104 (3 invasive)	64/107 (7 invasive)	7/192 (3 invasive)

cases with negative cone margins. Therefore, most experts recommend at least a standard hysterectomy as treatment.[50-59] If cone margins are positive, the risk of residual disease in hysterectomy specimens may be as high as 80%,[61] and up to 7% of these patients also have invasive disease.[57,58] More worrisome, however, is the approximate 3% incidence of invasive cancer when margins are negative.[57,58,61] This evidence may also be a low estimate, because many registries only record the invasive disease as the final diagnosis. If conization margins are positive, conservative management is not indicated; at a minimum, repeat conization should be performed.[60,61] In one series, 33% of women with positive conization margins were found to have invasive disease in the final hysterectomy specimen.[57]

Although the data are limited with respect to conservative management of cervical carcinoma, at least one large retrospective review cautiously supports fertility-sparing surgery, provided that the conization margins are negative, endocervical sampling has been performed and is also negative, and the patient is committed to close follow-up.[61] The importance of completely excising the endocervical canal by means of a large cylindrical cone has been emphasized.[62] When considering conservative management, most authorities recommend a generous cold knife conization instead of a LEEP procedure,[60] and the endocervical margins must be negative.[45,46,53,58,61] Any attempt at conservative therapy requires extensive patient counseling, because the individual patient may have or may develop recurrent AIS or even invasive adenocarcinoma.[61] With respect to follow-up, frequent surveillance using colposcopy with endocervical sampling is recommended. Compared with squamous cell precursor lesions, colposcopy is a less sensitive instrument for evaluating these patients,[21,22] although the colposcopic appearance of these lesions has been described.[63] Once childbearing is complete, hysterectomy should probably be performed, because the best long-term information available indicates that these women are at substantial risk for recurrence.[55,57,60] In one series, 3 of 21 patients with negative cone margins and 5 of 19 patients with positive margins had invasive disease.[57]

Therefore, if the conization margins are negative and preserving fertility is not a strong consideration, standard simple or abdominal hysterectomy is usually adequate treatment.[44-62] If the conization margins are positive, especially if there is extensive disease and suspicion is high that invasion may be present, modified radical hysterectomy may be justified.[58,63] This approach might also be considered if the cervix is extensively involved with AIS but all of the glands are replaced by malignant-appearing cells.[58,63]

How should early invasive adenocarcinoma be managed?

The current definition for microinvasive squamous cell carcinoma of the cervix was based on the risk of lymph node metastasis coincident with a depth of invasion of less than 3 mm and a breadth of invasion of no more than 7 mm. Additional staging modifications were made to distinguish tumors with 3 to 5 mm of invasion from other stage I disease. For squamous cell carcinoma, extensive literature exists to demonstrate that the risk for lymph node metastasis or recurrence is extremely low (approximately 1%) if the depth of invasion is less than 3 mm and management is by simple hysterectomy or conization.[64,65] Under these circumstances, lymphadenectomy and parametrectomy are no longer advocated.[65] Microinvasive squamous cell disease is considered to be a distinct lesion, and the definition is believed to be readily reproducible among pathologists. Nevertheless, two large prospective studies with centralized pathologic review demonstrated that pathologists disagree in up to 50% of cases.[66,67] In the Gynecologic Oncology Group (GOG) study, 37.4% of cases were rejected from the analysis because of no evidence of invasion and 6.8% because of stromal invasion greater than 5 mm.[65] Nevertheless, it is generally accepted that for squamous cell disease the depth of invasion from the basement membrane can be reproducibly measured. For adenocarcinoma, however, it is intuitively more difficult to measure tumor depth, because many of these lesions arise in glandular crypts distant from the squamocolumnar junction and adjacent basement membrane.[1,23,26] Many pathologists argue that microinvasive adenocarcinoma does not exist; if any invasive component is found, expert pathologists recommend reporting the actual depth of invasion instead of using the term "microinvasion" to describe the findings.[23]

Given these concerns, the management of early invasive adenocarcinoma is necessarily more problematic than that of AIS.[68-82] Until recently, regardless of how superficial the extent of stromal invasion, the mainstay of treatment has been radical hysterectomy and pelvic lymphadenectomy,[68-73] although a few sporadic reports included cases managed by standard hysterectomy or conization, with or without pelvic lymphadenectomy.[68-70,77,79,82,83] In support of radical surgery, the risk of recurrence for AIS and early invasive disease is substantial. Compared with squamous cell lesions, positive lymph nodes in adenocarcinoma substantially reduce the probability of survival,[74,81] and knowledge of lymph node status may identify patients who are likely to benefit from adjuvant radiation therapy and chemotherapy (Fig. 11-3). Many question whether a depth and width of invasion can be reproduced with certainty by pathologists and treating physicians. Recommendations supporting conservative therapy are largely based on review of standard and radical hysterectomy specimens, rather than surveillance of patients after conservative therapy.[76,78-81] The most definitive evidence supporting conservative therapy is Östör's review of the pathology involved, which was followed by a detailed retrospective review of all previously published cases.[76,78]

Additional support for conservative management was obtained with the use of data derived from the SEER database (1983 to 1997).[80,81] When SEER cases

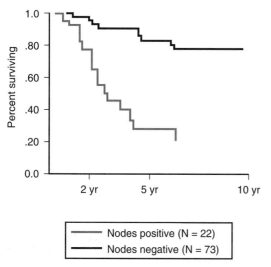

Figure 11–3. Survival in stage I adenocarcinoma of the cervix according to the presence or absence of metastatic disease in the lymph nodes ($P = .001$).

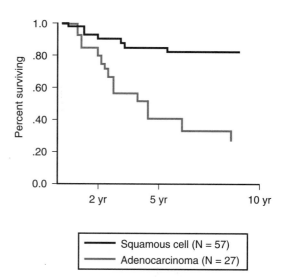

Figure 11–4. Survival by cell type for patients with presumed stage I disease ($P = .001$).

were combined with all previously published reports, a total of 1170 cases were identified (Table 11-3). Overall, the risk for positive lymph nodes was 1.3%, and more than 1% of patients (14/1170) died from the disease.[80,81] These results were similar to those of large series evaluating the risks of recurrence, lymph node positivity, and death for International Federation of Gynecologic Oncologists (FIGO) stages Ia1 and Ia2 squamous carcinoma.[65] Nevertheless, these data must be interpreted with caution. There is no universally accepted definition of "microinvasive" adenocarcinoma agreed on by treating physicians and pathologists. No formal pathology review process exists in SEER, and it is possible that many of these lesions were AIS or precursor lesions. The number of patients who underwent conization before hysterectomy is unknown. The vast majority of all reported cases were managed by standard hysterectomy or radical hysterectomy with or without lymphadenectomy. Therefore, until a formalized review of these cases is completed or prospective data with a centralized pathology review is available, the safest approach in the majority of patients—taking into consideration all of the concerns raised for AIS, in addition to the

presence of early invasive disease—is a standard or modified radical hysterectomy with lymphadenectomy, depending on the lesion's extent. It is important to recognize preoperatively the possibility for more advanced disease in the cervix, to avoid undertreatment. If there is any doubt as to the extent of disease, overtreatment may be preferable. Although the reports are limited, this disease may be more resistant when radiation is added after standard hysterectomy (Figs. 11-4 and 11-5).[82]

The prevalence of this disease is increasing in young women for whom fertility is an important consideration. Under these circumstances, conization with or without pelvic lymphadenectomy has been used. As with AIS, conservative therapy must be individualized. The patient must be informed that she is at substantial risk for recurrent disease, and she must be closely monitored.[84-86] Also, as with AIS, conservative surgery should be considered only after a generous cold knife conization in which the entire transformation zone has been excised with wide negative margins. Even then, the most aggressive approach that includes radical hysterectomy, lymphadenectomy, and radiation therapy does not guarantee cure.[78]

▮ Table 11–3. Summary of All Early Invasive Adenocarcinoma Cases*

Stage	N	No. Undergoing LND	No. with +LND	Recurrence, No. (%)	Death, No. (%)
All Ia1	585	255–276	4	9 (1.54%)	5 (0.85%)
Ia2	358	173	3	7 (1.6%)	4 (1.12%)
Ia1 + Ia2	943	428–449	7	16 (1.70%)	9 (0.95%)
Lesions less well-defined	227	78–87	8	18 (7.93%)	5 (2.20%)
TOTAL	**1170**	**531**	**15**	**34 (2.91%)**	**14 (1.20%)**

LND, lymph node dissection; +LND, one or more positive lymph nodes.
*Type of surgery performed (approximations) = conization (98–99 cases, 8.4%), simple hysterectomy (357–389 cases, 31.9%), radical hysterectomy (460–520 cases, 41.5%), and unknown (149, 12.4%).

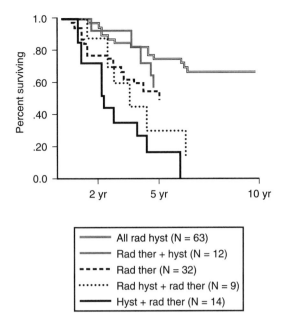

Figure 11–5. Survival by treatment modality for stage I adenocarcinomas of the cervix.

Should stage I adenocarcinoma be treated by radical hysterectomy or radiation therapy?

As with squamous cell carcinoma, treatment options for stages Ib1, Ib2, and IIa adenocarcinomas of the uterine cervix include radical hysterectomy with pelvic and possibly para-aortic lymphadenectomy, radiation therapy, or, in some cases, both.[87-100] Because adenocarcinoma is being diagnosed at earlier stages and the disease is more common in younger women, there are considerable advantages to radical hysterectomy, including preservation of vaginal pliability and ovarian function and the opportunity to avoid potentially adverse effects of pelvic radiation therapy (early and late complications, and the risk of inducing a secondary primary lesion over a normal life span). There are also suggestions that adenocarcinoma may be more radioresistant than squamous cell carcinoma.[94,95] Although there are strong proponents for both approaches, the literature supports a statistically equal probability of survival after either radiation therapy or radical surgery (see Fig. 11-5).[8,87-93] However, larger lesions (2 to 4 cm) may not do as well if managed by primary radiotherapy alone.[93,97,98] If bulky disease is present, the central portion of these tumors may be less sensitive to radiation because of relative cellular hypoxia, and persistent disease is more likely in the hypoxic center of these lesions. These concerns underscore the advantages of radical surgery for patients with stage I adenocarcinoma of the cervix, even when postoperative radiation therapy is likely.[97,98] In one report, the overall survival rate for patients with lesions smaller than 3 cm was 92%, compared with 76% for those with lesions larger than 3 cm. Among surgically treated patients, survival when the lesion size was greater than 3 cm was also significantly

greater (97% versus 77%).[98,100] In general, lymph node metastasis has been found to be a strong predictor of adverse outcome. Although the combination of chemotherapy and radiation therapy for adenocarcinoma is less well understood than that for squamous cell carcinoma, women with stage I cervical cancer who have positive lymph nodes or positive surgical margins have a significantly improved 2-year survival rate (85% versus 62%) if radical surgery is followed by standard radiation therapy and adjuvant chemotherapy.[99]

How should lymph node metastasis in stage I disease be managed?

In several reports, adenocarcinoma not only appears to have a higher predilection for lymph node metastasis than squamous cell cancer[74,81,90,99,100] but also carries an altered prognosis when lymph node metastases are present (see Fig. 11-3). For squamous cell disease, unilateral lymph node metastases reduce the probability of survival from 90% to 60% and, if bilateral pelvic nodes are involved, to between 30% and 40%. As previously mentioned, the likelihood of survival can be improved with the use of postoperative radiation therapy and chemotherapy. For adenocarcinoma, however, the presence of a single positive lymph node has been shown to reduce the survival rate to 30% to 40%, and, if multiple pelvic or para-aortic nodes are involved, the chance of survival may be less than 10%. Nevertheless, there are recent data indicating that survival is not uniformly poor in patients with positive pelvic or para-aortic nodes managed by radiation therapy combined with chemotherapy after radical pelvic surgery.[99,100] These data provide strong support for determining the lymph node status and administering postoperative radiation therapy tailored to the extent of disease. Although the role of adjuvant radiation therapy for adenocarcinoma is uncertain, based on currently available data, all patients found to have positive lymph nodes should receive radiation and adjuvant platin-based chemotherapy.[101-103] Other treatments under investigation in this setting include the use of taxanes as radiation sensitizers.

How should advanced-stage adenocarcinoma be managed?

The prognosis for advanced-stage adenocarcinoma is poor.[5,8] The literature addressing this issue is limited, because more patients with adenocarcinoma appear to present with stage I or stage II disease, rather than with sidewall extension or obvious metastatic spread.[89] Survival of patients with advanced-stage adenocarcinoma have been reported to be poorer than those of patients with squamous cell disease (Fig. 11-6), although population-based data derived from SEER suggest equal survival rates.[8] Differences in survival have been attributed to the large endophytic hypoxic center, which renders these lesions more radioresistant.

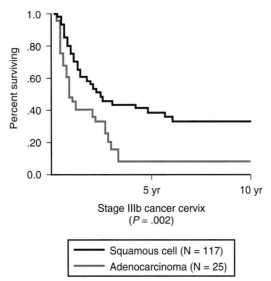

Figure 11–6. Survival for patients with stage III cancer of the cervix according to cell type.

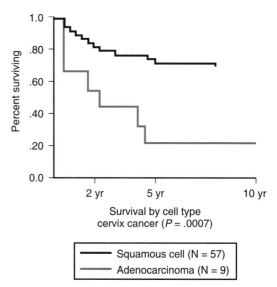

Figure 11–7. Survival for patients with cervical cancer according to cell type after pelvic exenteration.

Although there are few data that specifically address the benefit of adjuvant chemotherapy for advanced-stage adenocarcinoma, most of the available literature supports a survival advantage.[99,101-103] Therefore, therapy currently recommended for advanced-stage adenocarcinoma includes radiation therapy and platin-based chemotherapy. The role of preoperative lymphadenectomy specifically for adenocarcinoma in this setting has not been evaluated. However, data extrapolated from the management of all advanced cervical carcinomas support a role for selective lymph node debulking, and for extended-field radiation in advanced cervical carcinoma. Because these patients may be at greater risk for local recurrence, close surveillance and early recognition of persistent or recurrent disease is warranted.

How should recurrent adenocarcinoma of the cervix be managed?

Unless central recurrence without metastatic disease is found, recurrent adenocarcinoma is uniformly fatal. However, because bulky adenocarcinoma lesions may be less sensitive to radiation therapy, central failures may be amenable to radical pelvic and exenterative surgery. As with squamous cell carcinoma, there are isolated reports of occult metastatic spread, and possible intra-abdominal seeding of the peritoneal cavity has been reported in this clinical setting. Few series have compared survival rates after pelvic exenteration for adenocarcinoma and squamous cell carcinoma. In one report, the survival rate was significantly altered by cell type, but others report that salvage can be successful in a significant portion of these women (Fig. 11-7).[104,105]

Metastatic adenocarcinoma and fixed sidewall disease after radiation therapy carry an extremely poor prognosis. Chemotherapy has been used. As with squamous cell tumors, the responses are brief, but there is no evidence that chemotherapy extends survival. In particular, pelvic recurrences tend to be resistant to chemotherapy. Most available data suggest that adenocarcinoma tumors may be more resistant to chemotherapy than squamous cell tumors, and phase II studies have demonstrated modest responses to most agents, including cisplatin. Patients with advanced disease not amenable to surgery should be offered clinical trial participation.

Do cell type and tumor grade alter survival?

As depicted in Table 11-1, adenocarcinoma of the cervix consists of many subtypes that may differ in biologic aggressiveness.[1,12,106-109] The most common histologic type, endocervical, appears to have the best prognosis, although there are few data that address survival specifically by histologic subtype. A report by Hopkins and colleagues[90] showed no difference in early-stage disease based on cell type (Fig. 11-8).[1,12] In many series, adenocarcinoma subtypes are included in the report of adenocarcinoma. According to the World Health Organization (WHO) classification, adenosquamous carcinomas are classified as "other epithelial tumors," and there are considerable epidemiologic data indicating that adenosquamous carcinoma is more closely linked to squamous cell carcinoma than adenocarcinoma. Although one report indicated that the prognosis for adenosquamous carcinoma was better,[108] most series report poorer survival.[81] The best available data indicate that the incidence rates of rarer lesions (clear cell, serous, papillary serous, undifferentiated, and glassy cell tumors) have not significantly changed, that these lesions tend to affect older women, and that they are associated with more advanced disease.[12] Adenoma malignum, which has been mistaken for benign disease, reportedly has a higher propensity for

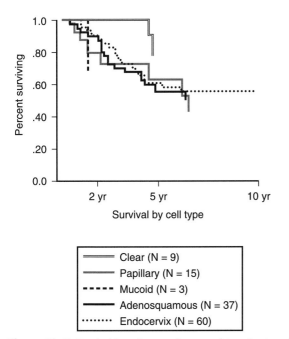

Figure 11-8. Survival by adenocarcinoma subtype in stage I disease (*P* = .65).

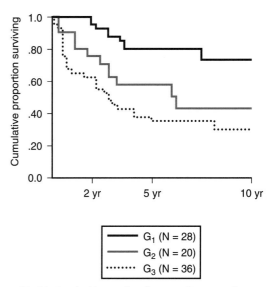

Figure 11-10. Survival by grade, all stages (*P* = .0002).

stage, are at greater risk for lymph node metastasis and have a poorer prognosis (Figs. 11-9 and 11-10).[90]

Can the ovaries be preserved at radical hysterectomy?

Ovarian conservation at the time of radical hysterectomy for adenocarcinoma is controversial, because of isolated reports indicating that it leads to a greater risk for ovarian and intra-abdominal spread.[90,110-115] However, the majority of currently available data

local recurrence and may be less sensitive to radiation therapy.[1] It is also possible that the lower survival rate achieved in women with these tumors is related to the stage at presentation and the degree of tumor differentiation, rather than to the histology per se. In almost all studies, the degree of tumor differentiation alters the prognosis. Patients with poorly differentiated tumors, regardless of the specific cell type identified or the

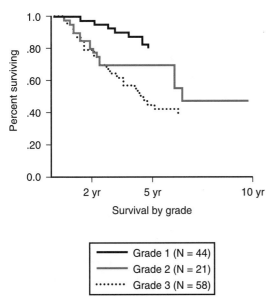

Figure 11-9. Survival by stage I adenocarcinoma of the cervix by tumor differentiation (*P* = .0006).

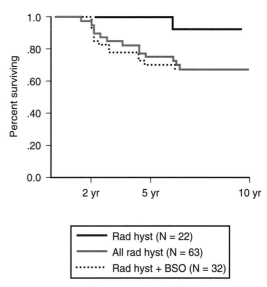

Figure 11-11. Survival by treatment modality for stage I adenocarcinoma of the cervix with or without bilateral salpingo-oophorectomy (BSO).

indicate that ovarian conservation is safe for most patients, and ovarian function may be preserved with careful handling of the ovaries (Fig. 11-11).[90] However, there is a higher risk (2.5%) for ovarian metastasis if deep invasion, parametrial involvement, and lymph node involvement are present. Under these circumstances, careful inspection of the ovaries is necessary if ovarian conservation is to be considered.[110-112]

REFERENCES

1. Wright C, Ferenczy A, Kurman RJ: Carcinoma and other tumors of the cervix. In Kurman RJ (ed): Blaustein's Pathology of the Female Genital Tract, 4th ed. New York, Springer-Verlag, 1994, pp. 279-326.
2. Peters RK, Chao A, Mack TM, et al: Increased frequency of adenocarcinoma of the uterine cervix in young women in Los Angeles County. J Natl Cancer Inst 1986;76:423-428.
3. Schwartz SM, Weiss N: Increased incidence of adenocarcinoma of the cervix in young women in the United States. Am J Epidemiol 1986;124:1045-1047.
4. Anton-Culver H, Bloss JD, Bringman D, et al: Comparison of adenocarcinoma and squamous cell carcinoma of the uterine cervix: A population based epidemiologic study. Am J Obstet Gynecol 1992;186:1507-1514.
5. Hopkins P, Morley GW: A comparison of adenocarcinoma and squamous cell carcinoma of the cervix. Obstet Gynecol 1991;7: 912-917.
6. Nieminen P, Kallio M, Hakama M: The effect of mass screening on incidence and mortality of squamous and adenocarcinoma of cervix uteri. Obstet Gynecol 1995;85:1017-1021.
7. Platz CE, Benda JA: Histology of cancer, incidence and prognosis: SEER population-based data, 1973-1987, female genital tract cancer. Cancer 1995;75:270-294.
8. Smith HO, Tiffany M, Qualls CR, Key CR: The rising incidence of adenocarcinoma relative to squamous cell carcinoma of the uterine cervix in the U.S.: A 24-year population-based study. Gynecol Oncol 2000;78:97-105.
9. Sigurdsson K: The Icelandic and Nordic cervical screening programs: Trends in incidence and mortality rates through 1995. Acta Obstet Gynecol Scand 1999;78:478-485.
10. Hebert A, Singh N, Smith JAE: Adenocarcinoma of the uterine cervix compared with squamous cell carcinoma: A 12-year study in Southampton and South-west Hampshire. Cancer Cytopathol 2001;12:26-36.
11. Saieni P, Adams J: Changing rates of adenocarcinoma and adenosquamous carcinoma of the cervix in England. Lancet 2001;357:1490-1493.
12. Alfsen GC, Thoresen SØ, Kristensen GB, et al: Histopathologic subtyping of cervical adenocarcinoma reveals increasing incidence rates of endometrioid tumors in all age groups: A population based study with review of all nonsquamous cervical carcinomas in Norway from 1966 to 1970, 1976 to 1980, and 1986 to 1990. Cancer 2000;89:1291-1299.
13. Liu S, Semenciw R, Mao Y: Cervical cancer: The increasing incidence of adenocarcinoma and adenosquamous carcinoma in younger women. CMAJ 2001;164:1151-1152.
14. Surveillance, Epidemiology, and End Results (SEER) Stat 4.0. (August 2000 Submission.) Bethesda, MD, U.S. Department of Health and Human Services, Public Health Service, National Institutes of Health, National Cancer Institute, Cancer Statistics Branch, 1999.
15. Goldstein NS, Ahmad E, Hussain M, et al: Endocervical glandular atypia: Does a preneoplastic lesion of adenocarcinoma in situ exist? Am J Clin Pathol 1998;110:200-209.
16. Massad LS, Collins YC, Meyer PM: Biopsy correlates of abnormal cervical cytology classified using the Bethesda system. Gynecol Oncol 2001;82:516-522.
17. Soofer SB, Sidawy MK: Atypical glandular cells of undetermined significance: Clinically significant lesions and means of patient follow-up. Cancer 2000;90:207-214.
18. Chin AB, Bristow RE, Korst LM, et al: The significance of atypical glandular cells on routine cervical cytologic testing in a community-based population. Am J Obstet Gynecol 2000;182: 1278-1282.
19. Chhieng DC, Elgert P, Cohen JM, Cangirella JF: Clinical significance of atypical glandular cells of undetermined significance in postmenopausal women. Cancer 2001;93:1-7.
20. Schoolland M, Allpress S, Sterrett GF: Adenocarcinoma of the cervix: Sensitivity of diagnosis by cervical smear and cytologic patterns and pitfalls in 24 cases. Cancer Cytopathol 2002;96:5-13.
21. Solomon D, Davey D, Kurma R, et al: The 2001 Bethesda System: Terminology for reporting results of cervical cytology. JAMA 2002;287:2114-2119.
22. Wright TC Jr, Cox JT, Massad LS, et al: 2001 Consensus guidelines for the management of women with cervical cytological abnormalities. JAMA 2002;287:2120-2129.
23. Zaino RJ: Glandular lesions of the uterine cervix. Mod Pathol 2000;13:261-274.
24. Jaworski RC: Endocervical glandular dysplasia, adenocarcinoma in situ, and early invasive (microinvasive) adenocarcinoma of the uterine cervix. Semin Diagn Pathol 1990;7:190-204.
25. Friedell GH, McKay DG: Adenocarcinoma in situ of the endocervix. Cancer 1953;6:887-897.
26. Shipman SD, Bristow RE: Adenocarcinoma in situ and early invasive adenocarcinoma of the uterine cervix. Curr Opin Oncol 2001;13:394-398.
27. Plaxe SC, Saltzstein L: Estimation of the duration of the preclinical phase of cervical adenocarcinoma suggests that there is ample opportunity for screening. Gynecol Oncol 1999;75:55-61.
28. Parazzini F, La Vecchia C: Epidemiology of adenocarcinoma of the cervix. Gynecol Oncol 1990;39:40-46.
29. Riethdorf S, Riethdorf L, Milde-Langosh K, et al: Differences in HPV 16- and HPV 19 E6/E7 oncogene expression between in situ and invasive adenocarcinomas of the cervix uteri. Virchows Archiv 2000;437P:491-500.
30. Duggan MA, McGregor SE, Benot JL, et al: The human papillomavirus status of invasive cervical adenocarcinoma: A clinicopathological and outcome analysis. Hum Pathol 1995;2:319-325.
31. Skyldherg BM, Murray E, Lambkin H, et al: Adenocarcinoma of the uterine cervix in Ireland and Sweden: Human papillomavirus infection and biologic alterations. Mod Pathol 1999;12: 675-682.
32. Walboomers JMM, Jacobs MV, Manos MM, et al: Human papillomavirus is a necessary cause of invasive cervical cancer worldwide. J Pathol 1999;189:12-19.
33. Bosch Z, Manos MM, Munoz N, et al: Prevalence of human papillomavirus in cervical cancer: A worldwide perspective. J Natl Cancer Inst 1995;87:796-802.
34. Wallin KL, Wiklund F, Angströam T, et al: Type-specific persistence of human papillomavirus DNA before the development of invasive cervical cancer. N Engl J Med 1999;341:1633-1638.
35. Madeleine MM, Daling JR, Schwartz SM, et al: Human papillomavirus and long-term oral contraceptive use increase the risk of adenocarcinoma in situ of the cervix. Cancer Epidemiol Biol Prevention 2001;10:171-177.
36. Brinton LA, Tashima KT, Leman HF, et al: Epidemiology of cervical cancer by cell type. Cancer Res 1987;47:1706-1711.
37. Lacey JV Jr, Frisch M, Brinton LA, et al: Associations between smoking and adenocarcinomas and squamous cell carcinomas of the uterine cervix (United States). Cancer Cause Control 2001;12:153-161.
38. Ursin G, Peters RK, Henderson BE, et al: Oral contraceptive use and adenocarcinoma of the cervix. Lancet 1994;344: 1380-1394.
39. Lu X, Shiozawa T, Nakayama K, et al: Abnormal expression of sex steroid receptors and cell cycle-related molecules in adenocarcinoma in situ of the uterine cervix. Int J Gynecol Pathol 1999;18:109-114.
40. Lacey JV Jr, Brinton LA, Barnes WA, et al: Use of hormone replacement therapy and adenocarcinomas and squamous cell carcinomas of the uterine cervix. Gynecol Oncol 2000;77:149-154.
41. Moreno V, Bosch FX, Munoz N, et al: Effect of oral contraceptives on risk of cervical cancer in women with human papillomavirus infection: The IARC multicentre case-control study. Lancet 2002;259:1085-1092.
42. Munoz N, Francheschi S, Bosetti C, et al: Role of parity and human papillomavirus in cervical cancer: The IARC multicentre case-control study. Lancet 2002;359:1093-1101.

43. Ronnett BM, Manos MM, Ransley JE, et al: Atypical glandular cells of undetermined significance (AGUS): Cytopathologic features, histopathologic results, and human papillomavirus DNA detection. Hum Pathol 1999;30:816-825.

44. Azodi M, Chambers SK, Rutherford TJ, et al: Adenocarcinoma in situ of the cervix: Management and outcome. Gynecol Oncol 1999;73:348-353.

45. Goldstein NS, Mani A: The status and distance of cone biopsy margins as a predictor of excision adequacy for endocervical adenocarcinoma in situ. Am J Clin Pathol 1998;109:727-732.

46. Denehy TR, Gregor CA, Breen JL: Endocervical curettage, cone margins, and residual adenocarcinoma in situ of the cervix. Obstet Gynecol 1997;90:1-6.

47. Östör AG, Pagano R, Davoren RAM, et al: Adenocarcinoma in situ of the cervix. Int J Gynecol Pathol 1984;3:179-190.

48. Lee KR: Adenocarcinoma in situ with a small cell (endometrioid) pattern in cervical smears. Cancer Cytopathol 1999;87:254-258.

49. Berek JS, Hacker NF, Fu Y-S, et al: Adenocarcinoma of the uterine cervix: Histologic variables associated with lymph node metastasis and survival. Obstet Gynecol 1985;46:46-52.

50. Anderson ES, Arffmann E: Adenocarcinoma in situ of the uterine cervix: A clinico-pathologic study of 36 cases. Gynecol Oncol 1989;35:1-7.

51. Hopkins MP, Roberts JA, Schmidt RW: Cervical adenocarcinoma in situ. Obstet Gynecol 1988;71:842-844.

52. Goldstein NS, Mani A: The status and distance of cone biopsy margins as a predictor of excision adequacy for endocervical adenocarcinoma in situ. Am J Clin Pathol 1998;109:727-732.

53. Etherington IJ, Luesley DM: Adenocarcinoma in situ of the cervix: Controversies in diagnosis and treatment. J Lower Gen Tract Dis 2001;5:94-98.

54. Im DD, Duska LR, Boenshein NB: Adequacy of conization margins in adenocarcinoma in situ of the cervix as a predictor of residual disease. Gynecol Oncol 1995;59:179-182.

55. Poyner A, Barakat RR, Hoskins WJ: Management and follow-up of patients with adenocarcinoma in situ of the uterine cervix. Gynecol Oncol 1995;57:158-164.

56. Muntz HG, Bell DA, Lage JM, et al: Adenocarcinoma in situ of the uterine cervix. Obstet Gynecol 1992;80:935-939.

57. Wolf JK, Levenback C, Maslpica A, et al: Adenocarcinoma in situ of the cervix: Significance of cone biopsy margins. Obstet Gynecol 1996;88:82-86.

58. Hopkins MP: Adenocarcinoma in situ of the cervix: The margins must be clear. Gynecol Oncol 2000;79:4-5.

59. Widrich T, Kennedy AW, Myers TM, et al: Adenocarcinoma in situ of the uterine cervix: Management and outcome. Gynecol Oncol 1996;61:304-308.

60. Lickrish GM, Colgan T, Wright VC: Colposcopy of adenocarcinoma in situ and invasive adenocarcinoma of the cervix. Obstet Gynecol Clin North Am 1993;20:111-122.

61. Krivak TC, Rose GS, McBroom JW, et al: Cervical adenocarcinoma in situ: A systematic review of therapeutic options and predictors of persistent or recurrent disease. Obstet Gynecol Surv 2001;56:567-575.

62. Bertrand M, Lickrish GM, Colgan TJ: The anatomic distribution of cervical adenocarcinoma in situ: Implications for treatment. Am J Obstet Gynecol 1987;157:21-25.

63. Nguyen HN, Averette HE: Special problems in cervical cancer management. Semin Surg Oncol 1999;16:261-266.

64. Elliott P, Cobbleon M, Russell P, et al: Early invasive (FIGO stage IA) carcinoma of the cervix: A clinico-pathologic study of 476 cases. Int J Gynecol Cancer 2000;10:42-52.

65. Benedet JL, Anderson GH: Review: Stage IA carcinoma of the cervix revisited. Obstet Gynecol 1996;87:1052-1059.

66. Creasman T, Zaino RJ, Major FJ, et al: Early invasive carcinoma of the cervix (3 to 5 mm invasion): Risk factors and prognosis. A Gynecologic Oncology Group study. Am J Obstet Gynecol 1998;178:62-65.

67. Morgan PR, Anderson MD, Buckley CH, et al. The Royal College of Obstetricians and Gynaecologists micro-invasive carcinoma of the cervix study: Preliminary results. Br J Obstet Gynaecol 1993;100:664-668.

68. Sachs H, Ikeda J, Brachetti AKJ: Mikroinvasives adenokarzinom and adenocarcinoma in situ der cervix uteri. Med Welt 1975;26:1181-1183.

69. Iversen T, Abeler V, Kjrostad KE: Factors influencing the treatment of patients with stage IA carcinoma of the cervix. Br J Obstet Gynaecol 1979;86:593-597.

70. Qizilbash AH: In situ and microinvasive adenocarcinoma of the uterine cervix: A clinical, cytologic and histologic study of 14 cases. Am J Clin Pathol 1975;64:155-170.

71. Matsukuma K, Tsukamoto N, Kaku T, et al: Early adenocarcinoma of the uterine cervix: Its histologic and immunohistologic study. Gynecol Oncol 1989;35:38-43.

72. Rollason TP, Cullimore J, Bradgate MG: A suggested columnar cell morphological equivalent of squamous carcinoma in situ with early stromal invasion. Int J Gynaecol Pathol 1989;8:230-236.

73. Kaspar HG, Dinh TV, Doherty MG, et al: Clinical implications of tumor volume measurement in stage I adenocarcinoma of the cervix. Obstet Gynecol 1993;81:296-300.

74. Matthews CM, Burke TW, Tornos C, et al: Stage I cervical adenocarcinoma: Prognostic evaluation of surgically treated patients. Gynecol Oncol 1993;49:19-23.

75. Kennedy AW, El Tabakh GH, Biscotti CV, Wirth S: Invasive adenocarcinoma of the cervix following LLETZ (large loop excision of the transformation zone) for adenocarcinoma in situ. Gynecol Oncol 1995;58:274-277.

76. Östör AG, Rome R, Quinn M: Microinvasive adenocarcinoma of the cervix: A clinicopathologic study of 77 women. Obstet Gynecol 1997;89:88-93.

77. Schorge JO, Lee KR, Flynn CE, et al: Stage IA1 cervical adenocarcinoma: Definition and treatment. Obstet Gynecol 1999;93:219-222.

78. Östör AG: Early invasive adenocarcinoma of the uterine cervix. Int J Gynecol Pathol 2000;19:29-38.

79. Kaku T, Kamura T, Kunihiro S, et al: Early adenocarcinoma of the uterine cervix. Gynecol Oncol 1997;65:281-285.

80. Webb JC, Key CR, Qualls CR, Smith HO: Population-based study of microinvasive adenocarcinoma of the uterine cervix. Obstet Gynecol 2001;97:701-706.

81. Smith HO, Qualls CR, Romero AA, et al: Is there a difference in survival for IA_1 and IA_2 adenocarcinoma of the uterine cervix? Gynecol Oncol 2002;85:229-241.

82. Hopkins P, Peters WA, Anderson W, Morley GW: Invasive cervical cancer treated initially by standard hysterectomy. Gynecol Oncol 1990;36:7-12.

83. McHale M, Le TD, Burger RA, et al: Fertility sparing treatment for in situ and early invasive adenocarcinoma of the cervix. Obstet Gynecol 2001;98:726-731.

84. Nagarsheth NP, Maxwell GL, Bentle RC, Rodriguez G: Bilateral pelvic lymph node metastases in a case of FIGO stage IA_1 adenocarcinoma of the cervix. Gynecol Oncol 2000;77:467-470.

85. Zanetta G, Gabriele A, Veccione F, et al: Unusual recurrence of cervical adenosquamous carcinoma after conservative surgery. Gynecol Oncol 2000;76:409-412.

86. Utsugi K, Shimizu Y, Akyama F, Hasmi K: Case report: Is the invasion depth in millimeters valid to determine the prognosis of early invasive cervical adenocarcinoma? A case of recurrent FIGO stage IA_1 cervical adenocarcinoma. Gynecol Oncol 2001;82:205-207.

87. Shingleton HM, Gore H, Bradley DH, Soong S-J: Adenocarcinoma of the cervix: I. Clinical evaluation and pathologic features. Am J Obstet Gynecol 1981;139:799-814.

88. Kilgore LC, Soong S-J, Gore H, et al: Analysis of prognostic features in adenocarcinoma of the cervix. Gynecol Oncol 1988;31:137-148.

89. Eifel PJ, Morris M, Oswald MJ, et al: Adenocarcinoma of the uterine cervix: Prognosis and patterns of failure in 367 cases. Cancer 1990;65:2507-2514.

90. Hopkins P, Schmidt RW, Roberts JA, Morley GW: The prognosis and treatment of stage I adenocarcinoma of the cervix. Obstet Gynecol 1988;72:915-921.

91. Eifel PJ, Burke TW, Delclos L, et al: Early stage I adenocarcinoma of the uterine cervix: Treatment results in patients with tumors ≤ 4 cm in diameter. Gynecol Oncol 1991;41:199-205.

92. Nakano T, Arai T, Morita S, Oka K: Radiation therapy alone for adenocarcinoma of the uterine cervix. Int J Radiation Oncol Biol Phys 1995;32:1331-1336.

93. Eifel PJ, Burke TW, Morris M, Smith TL: Adenocarcinoma as an independent risk factor for disease recurrences in patients with stage IB cervical carcinoma. Gynecol Oncol 1995;59:38-44.

94. West CM, Davidson SE, Burt PA, Hunter RD: The intrinsic radiosensitivity of cervical carcinoma: Correlations with clinical data. Int J Radiat Oncol Biol Phys 1995;31:841-846.

95. Costa MJ, McIlny KR, Trelford J: Cervical carcinoma with glandular differentiation: Histological evaluation predicts disease recurrence in clinical stage I or II patients. Hum Pathol 1995;26:829-837.

96. McLellan R, Dillon MB, Woodruff JD, et al: Long term follow-up of stage I cervical adenocarcinoma treated by radical surgery. Gynecol Oncol 1994;25:253-259.

97. Levêque J, Laurent JF, Burtin F, et al: Prognostic factors of the uterine cervix adenocarcinoma. Eur J Obstet Gynecol 1998; 80:209-214.

98. Silver DF, Hempling RE, Pivers MS, et al: Stage I adenocarcinoma of the cervix: Does lesion size affect treatment options and prognosis? Am J Clin Oncol 1998;21:43-45.

99. Cohn DE, Peters WA III, Muntz HG, et al: Adenocarcinoma of the uterine cervix metastatic to lymph nodes. Am J Obstet Gynecol 1998;18:1131-1137.

100. Irie T, Kigawa J, Minagawa Y, et al: Prognosis and clinico-pathological characteristics of Ib-IIb adenocarcinoma of the uterine cervix in patients who have had radical hysterectomy. Eur J Surg Oncol 2000;26:464-467.

101. Peters WA III, Liu PY, Barrett RJ II, et al: Concurrent chemo-therapy and pelvic radiation therapy compared with pelvic radiation therapy alone as adjuvant therapy after radical surgery in high-risk early-stage cancer of the cervix. Obstet Gynecol Surv 2000;55:491-492.

102. Rose PG, Bundy SN, Watkins EB, et al: Concurrent cisplatin based radiotherapy and chemotherapy for locally advanced cervical cancer. N Engl J Med 1999;340:1144-1153.

103. Morris M, Eifel PJ, Lu J, et al: Pelvic radiation with concurrent chemotherapy compared with pelvic and para-aortic radiation for high-risk cervical cancer. N Engl J Med 1999;340-1137-1143.

104. Crozier M, Morris M, Levenback C, et al: Pelvic exenteration for adenocarcinoma of the uterine cervix. Gynecol Oncol 1995;58:47-48.

105. Morley GW, Hopkins MP, Lindenauer SM, Roberts JA: Pelvic exenteration, University of Michigan: 100 patients at 5 years. Obstet Gynecol 1989;74:934-943.

106. Young RH, Scully R: Villoglandular papillary adenocarcinoma of the uterine cervix: A clinicopathologic analysis of 13 cases. Cancer 1989;63:1773-1779.

107. Jones MW, Silverberg SG, Kurman RJ: Well-differentiated villoglandular adenocarcinoma of the uterine cervix: A clinico-pathological study of 24 cases. Int J Gynecol Pathol 1993; 12:1-7.

108. Chen R-Y, Change D-Y, Yen M-L, et al: Prognostic factors of primary adenocarcinoma of the uterine cervix. Gynecol Oncol 1998;69:157-164.

109. Hopkins MP, Sutton P, Roberts JA: Prognostic features and treatment of endocervical adenocarcinoma of the cervix. Gynecol Oncol 1987;27:69-75.

110. Nguyen L, Brewer CA, DiSaia PJ: Ovarian metastasis of stage IB1 squamous cell cancer of the cervix after radical parametrectomy and oophoropexy. Gynecol Oncol 1998;68: 198-200.

111. Sutton GP, Bundy BN, Delgado G, et al: Ovarian metastases in stage IB carcinoma of the cervix: A Gynecologic Oncology Group study. Am J Obstet Gynecol 1992;166:50-53.

112. Brown JV, Fu YS, Berek JS: Ovarian metastases are rare in stage I adenocarcinoma of the cervix. Obstet Gynecol 1990; 76:623-626.

113. Yamamoto R, Okamoto K, Yukiharu T, et al: A study of risk factors for ovarian metastases in Ib-IIIb cervical carcinoma and analysis of ovarian function after transpositions. Gynecol Oncol 2001;82:312-316.

114. Nakanishi T, Wakai K, Ishikawa H, et al: A comparison of ovarian metastasis between squamous cell carcinoma and adenocarcinoma of the uterine cervix. Gynecol Oncol 2001;82:504-509.

115. Natsuma N, Aoki Y, Kase H, et al: Ovarian metastasis in stage IB and II cervical adenocarcinoma. Gynecol Oncol 1999; 74:255-258.

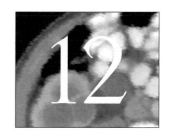

CHAPTER

EARLY-STAGE CERVICAL CANCER

Patricia J. Eifel   and   John Curtin

 MAJOR CONTROVERSIES

- **What is early-stage cervical cancer?**
- **What is the appropriate pretreatment evaluation?**
- **When can patients be treated with fertility-preserving surgery?**
- **Are radical hysterectomy and radiation therapy equally effective treatments for stage Ib-IIa disease?**
- **What are the indications for postoperative radiation therapy?**
- **When should concurrent chemotherapy be added to radiation therapy?**
- **Is there a role for neoadjuvant chemotherapy?**
- **Is there a role for adjuvant hysterectomy?**
- **What factors influence the risks of major complications of treatment?**
- **How does treatment influence sexual function?**

What is early-stage cervical cancer?

Reports of treatment frequently subdivide cervical cancers into "early" and "advanced." However, the designation "early stage" has widely differing meanings in different contexts—all stage I and II cancers, all stage I and IIa cancers, small stage I and IIa (e.g., 4 cm or less) cancers, or stage Ia and Ib1 cancers. Cancers that have spread regionally may or may not be excluded, depending on the intent of the investigator. Most commonly, "early" is meant to refer to cancers that are potentially amenable to curative surgical treatment; however, because the indications for primary surgical treatment are controversial, the types of lesions considered in this group vary considerably.

These different selection criteria have made it difficult to compare experiences and particularly difficult to compare the effectiveness of various treatments. Historically, comparisons have further been complicated by the many changes that have occurred in the International Federation of Gynecology and Obstetrics

(FIGO) definitions of "stage I" disease (Table 12-1).[1-8] In particular, stage Ia or "microinvasive" disease has been inconsistently defined, resulting in a form of stage migration that also influences the composition of cases in the Ib category. The historically vague FIGO definition led clinicians and investigators to accept definitions of microinvasion that ranged from 1 to 5 mm, with or without other limitations on the size or presence of lymphovascular invasion. Eventually, the Society of Gynecologic Oncologists adopted the following definition of stage Ia disease: tumors that invade less than 3 mm without lymphovascular invasion. This definition was widely used in the United States until 1995, when FIGO specified their own somewhat different definition for stage Ia disease (see Table 12-1).[7]

The FIGO staging system roughly groups patients into categories with different average outcomes. However, the stage I and II groups include subsets of patients whose 5-year survival rates range from greater than 90% (e.g., patients with small stage Ib1 tumors and negative lymph nodes) to less than 20%

Table 12–1. Changes in the Definition of Stage I Carcinoma of the Uterine Cervix

1929	League of Nations Health Organization definition of stage I disease: "Cancer strictly confined to the cervix"
	Definition subsequently used by International Federation of Gynecology and Obstetrics
1937	Tumor involving the uterine corpus moved to "stage II"
1950	Tumor involving the uterine corpus moved back to "stage I"
	Preinvasive cancers given a special designation: "stage 0"
1962	New stage Ia category created for tumors designated as having "early stromal invasion"
1972	Stage Ia2 category created for "occult cancer" confined to the cervix
1974	"Occult cancer" given a new designation: "Ib$_{occult}$"
1985	"Ib$_{occult}$" designation eliminated
1995	Current definitions:
	Ia1: Measured invasion of stroma no greater than 3 mm in depth and no wider than 7 mm
	Ia2: Measured invasion of stroma greater than 3 mm but no greater than 5 mm in depth and no wider than 7 mm
	Ib1: Clinical lesions no greater than 4 cm in size
	Ib2: Clinical lesions greater than 4 cm in size

(e.g., patients with bulky endocervical tumors and grossly involved para-aortic lymph nodes). Clinical tumor size and the presence or absence of lymph node metastases are the most powerful determinants of prognosis within stages I and II; these features are commonly used to select treatment and should be (but rarely are) clearly described in reports of outcome.

For the purpose of this chapter, we define early-stage cervical tumors as tumors that are commonly considered to be technically amenable to radical surgical treatment. The discussion focuses on clinical stage I and IIa cancers, although a few clinicians, particularly in certain parts of Europe, advocate surgical treatment even for selected patients with higher-stage disease. Clinicians disagree about the appropriateness of primary surgical treatment for patients with bulky or node-positive stage I-IIa cancers; the arguments for and against such treatment are discussed in the later sections.

What is the appropriate pretreatment evaluation?

A careful pelvic examination, including speculum, bimanual, and rectovaginal examinations, is an important part of clinical staging. However, a separate examination under anesthesia adds little to the initial evaluation of patients with early-stage cervical cancer and is rarely indicated. Cystoscopy and proctoscopy also have a very low yield and are not used in patients with early-stage disease.

For patients who have stage Ia1 cancers without lymphovascular space involvement, the risk of metastatic disease is negligible, and no radiographic staging is necessary. Patients who have more invasive lesions require imaging of the primary tumor site and regional

lymph nodes before definitive treatment is initiated. Several methods can be used to image the pelvis; the selection may vary according to the extent of disease, the anticipated treatment, and the availability and cost of the studies. FIGO limits the studies that can be used to assign a clinical stage to relatively simple studies that are widely available internationally (i.e., plain radiography, intravenous pyelography, barium enema, and bone scan). Today, intravenous pyelography is rarely performed because tomographic imaging modalities that visualize primary and regional disease are also able to detect hydronephrosis caused by tumor.

Findings from the clinical examination and diagnostic imaging about tumor size, parametrial extension, and lymph node involvement correlate with prognosis and are used to select surgery or radiation therapy as the patient's initial treatment. Although clinical evaluation is used to assign a FIGO stage, this method is subjective and frequently inaccurate. The imaging studies permitted for FIGO staging (intravenous pyelography, barium enema, and plain radiography) have a low yield in patients with early-stage disease. However, other imaging studies are useful in selected cases. Although lymphography can detect relatively early metastasis to para-aortic and iliac lymph nodes, it is rarely used today because the special expertise needed to perform and interpret this study is not widely available. Tomographic imaging studies can provide useful information about local and regional areas of involvement, although microscopic involvement cannot be detected and false-positive readings are not uncommon. Tomographic imaging may not be necessary for patients who have small stage Ib1 cancers; however, the risk of parametrial and regional involvement increases and the role of diagnostic imaging becomes more critical with increasing tumor size. Diagnostic imaging methods such as computed tomography (CT) and magnetic resonance imaging (MRI) are clearly superior to clinical examination in determining the presence of enlarged lymph nodes that may harbor metastases. Pelvic examination can be used to estimate tumor size and the presence of gross parametrial extension, but these estimates can also be inaccurate. For example, in a large Austrian study reported by Burghardt and colleagues,[9] 14% of patients with stage Ib disease had histologic evidence of parametrial involvement; interestingly, only 30% of patients with FIGO clinical stage IIb disease who were treated with radical hysterectomy had parametrial involvement, underlining the inaccuracy and possible variability of clinical staging.

For assessment of local disease extent, comparative studies indicate that MRI is superior to CT scanning and in some cases to pelvic examination, particularly in the detection of parametrial invasion, where MRI has an accuracy of 87% to 95%.[10] MRI also has been demonstrated to provide more accurate assessments of tumor diameter and depth of invasion than clinical examination.[11-13] If the clinician only requires information about regional lymph node enlargement and ureteral patency, CT is the most economical study. However, if more detailed images of the primary tumor site are required, MRI is preferred. It is rarely necessary to obtain both studies.

Recently, several studies have suggested that positron emission tomography (PET) may be used to detect regional disease that is missed with CT or MRI. Preliminary studies suggest that PET may be the most useful nonsurgical test for detection of regional metastases.[14,15] Although the high cost and inconsistent reimbursement for PET have limited its use in patients with cervical cancer, further study may lead to an expanded role for PET in the future.

When can patients be treated with fertility-preserving surgery?

Radical hysterectomy and radiation therapy have traditionally been considered the only standard treatments for stage I cervical cancers that invade more than 3 mm. Both treatments result in loss of normal fertility. For patients undergoing radical hysterectomy with preservation of the ovaries, assisted reproduction may be an option. Such patients may be candidates for egg retrieval, in vitro fertilization, and childbirth with the assistance of a gestational surrogate.[16] If radiation therapy is the treatment of choice, patients can consider having eggs retrieved and stored before treatment is begun, although this would delay therapy for at least 4 weeks. Alternatively, the ovaries can be transposed outside the true pelvis before pelvic radiation therapy. When the ovaries are transposed out of the planned radiation field, 50% to 80% of women have continued hormone production and ovulation. Again, a gestational surrogate would be needed to produce a pregnancy.

More recently, several groups have reported the use of radical trachelectomy for early cervical cancers. The goal of this procedure is to resect the primary cancer while maintaining the patient's ability to sustain an intrauterine pregnancy. Radical trachelectomy is usually combined with a laparoscopic pelvic lymph node dissection. Dargent first reported the modern procedure in 1987.[17,18] Since that time, several other institutions have reported their experience with radical trachelectomy.[19-21] There remains some debate as to which patients should be considered for this procedure. In their most recent publication, Dargent and associates[22] stated that candidates should be women who are younger than 40 years of age, want to maintain fertility, and have small, exophytic stage Ia1-IIa cervical carcinomas. Other authors[20] have suggested that the lesions should be smaller than 2 cm and that adenocarcinoma is a relative contraindication. However, two small series reported from the United States[19,21] included a total of 15 patients with adenocarcinomas, none of whom had a disease recurrence. The authors did not describe the histologic types in the 5 patients who required radical hysterectomy or postoperative radiation therapy because of adverse findings.

Patients being considered for radical trachelectomy should be advised that intraoperative or postoperative findings may require that the patient have a full radical hysterectomy or postoperative radiation therapy.

The two most common such findings are positive pelvic lymph nodes and an inability to clear the endocervical margin of cancer. In the series by Schlaerth and coworkers,[19] the two patients in whom the endocervical margin could not be cleared both had lesions greater than 2 cm in diameter. Overall, recurrence rates after radical trachelectomy and pelvic lymphadenectomy have been low and seem to be similar to those reported for similar early lesions treated with radical hysterectomy. Burnett and colleagues[21] summarized the results of four series; there were four recurrences in 152 patients (2.5%) with follow-up time ranging from 23 months to 47 months. Recurrence seems to be correlated with tumor size; in the series by Dargent and associates,[22] the two recurrences occurred in patients with lesions larger than 2 cm.

The goal of radical trachelectomy is a functioning uterus and ovaries. In all series reported, successful pregnancies have been achieved, although the rate of miscarriages and preterm deliveries is high. The increased risk of preterm delivery and its consequences should be included in the preoperative counseling of any patient who is considering radical trachelectomy as an alternative to standard treatment.

Are radical hysterectomy and radiation therapy equally effective treatments for stage Ib-IIa disease?

Radiation therapy and radical hysterectomy are frequently said to be equally effective treatments for patients with early-stage cervical cancer, and reported survival rates of 80% to 90% for patients treated with these two approaches appear to support this contention (Fig. 12-1).[23-42] However, a number of criteria used by clinicians to select patients for one treatment or the other may bias comparisons. Few surgical series include estimates of clinical tumor diameter, but, for those series that do, the results suggest that patients in surgical series may have earlier disease.[23,28,40,41,43] Young women and those who have relatively small, clinically node-negative tumors tend to be preferred for primary surgical treatment. Some surgeons abort hysterectomy procedures if positive lymph nodes are discovered and refer these high-risk patients for radiation therapy. These and other possible selection factors obscure the meaning of uncontrolled comparisons.

There has been only one true randomized trial comparing initial surgery with radiation therapy alone as treatment for early-stage cervical cancer. In that Italian trial, Landoni and colleagues[35] randomly allocated 343 patients with stage Ib or IIa cervical cancer to receive treatment with initial radical hysterectomy and lymphadenectomy or with radiation alone. Patients in the radiation therapy arm were treated with external beam irradiation and low dose-rate intracavitary brachytherapy. Patients in the surgical arm were treated with initial radical type III hysterectomy; patients with parametrial involvement, positive margins, deep stromal invasion, or positive nodes then received

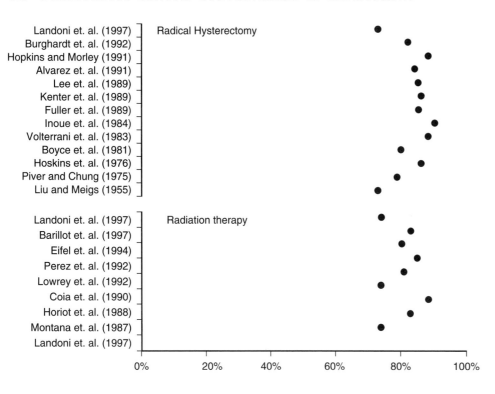

Figure 12–1. Five-year survival rates for patients with stage Ib cervical cancer treated with initial radical hysterectomy or radiation therapy.

postoperative pelvic irradiation. Overall, 62 (54%) of 114 patients with Ib1 and 46 (84%) of 55 patients with Ib2 disease who were randomly assigned to radical hysterectomy received postoperative radiation therapy. The results of the Landoni trial, reported in 1997,[35] demonstrated similar overall survival rates for the two treatments (Fig. 12-2). However, a small subset analysis suggested that initial surgical treatment was superior

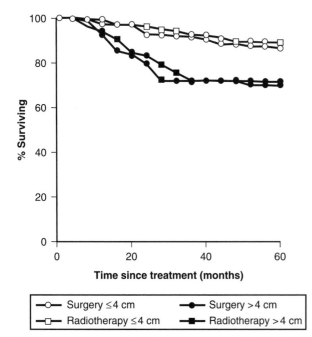

Figure 12–2. Overall survival of patients treated with radiation therapy alone versus initial surgery with or without postoperative radiation therapy according to tumor size. (From Landoni F, Maneo A, Colombo A, et al: Randomised study of radical surgery versus radiotherapy for stage Ib–IIa cervical cancer. Lancet 1997;350:535-540.)

to radiation therapy alone for patients who had adenocarcinomas of the cervix. The overall rate of complications was significantly higher for patients treated with surgery than for those treated with radiation alone. The authors believed that the frequent use of combined-modality treatment in patients treated with initial surgery contributed to the higher complication rate in this group. They concluded that radical hysterectomy was a good treatment for women with small squamous cancers and functioning ovaries, whereas radiation therapy should be considered as primary treatment for older women.

The Landoni trial was completed in 1991 and used treatments that would be considered suboptimal by current standards. The median total dose of radiation delivered to point A (external beam plus low dose-rate irradiation) was 76 Gy, 10 to 15 Gy less than that reported in most U. S. trials. Also, patients with larger tumors treated with radiation and patients requiring postoperative irradiation for positive lymph nodes or positive margins are usually treated with concurrent chemotherapy. Results of prospective trials suggest that treatment with high-dose radiation therapy and concurrent chemotherapy should reduce the recurrence rate after radiation therapy by at least 40%.[44-48] Because no trial has compared high-dose radiation therapy and concurrent chemotherapy with initial surgery, it is difficult to generalize the results of the Landoni trial to current practice.

What are the indications for postoperative radiation therapy?

Although radical hysterectomy is an excellent treatment for patients with early-stage cervical cancer and is frequently sufficient to achieve a cure, some patients who have unexpected intraoperative findings of locally extensive disease may require additional treatment to reduce the risk of local recurrences. Studies have indicated that more than two thirds of the recurrences after radical hysterectomy alone involve the pelvis, suggesting that adjuvant local radiation therapy may be of benefit.[49] Patients with local recurrence also are more likely to experience subsequent distant recurrence than are patients who have their pelvic disease controlled.[50]

Studies have consistently demonstrated a reduced rate of pelvic recurrence after pelvic irradiation in high-risk patients.[51,52] Nevertheless, it has been difficult to demonstrate that radiation therapy improves the overall survival rate in patients with high-risk disease. Several factors may contribute to this problem. Physicians use so many factors to select patients for adjuvant treatment that it is usually impossible in retrospective studies to determine the influence of resulting biases on the outcome of patients receiving treatment. Studies frequently are too small or include too many patients with low-risk tumors to detect or rule out clinically important differences in treatment groups. For these reasons, treatment recommendations have often been based on clinicians' understanding of the risk of recurrence and patterns of disease spread.

Radiation dose is another potential explanation for the lack of a demonstrated survival benefit—the dose of radiation therapy that is usually given after radical hysterectomy may be inadequate. Tumor-bed hypoxia and accelerated repopulation of tumor clonogens probably reduce the ability of radiation therapy to control microscopic residual disease after surgery. Although radiation doses of 55 to 65 Gy routinely are used postoperatively to treat patients with high-risk squamous carcinomas of the head and neck, in the pelvis concern about bowel tolerance often causes clinicians to limit the postoperative radiation dose to 50 Gy or less. This probably contributes to the relatively high pelvic recurrence rates that have been reported in patients whose tumors have high-risk features even when postoperative radiation therapy is given. For example, Peters and associates[44] reported 25 pelvic recurrences in 116 patients who had pelvic radiation therapy (without chemotherapy) after radical hysterectomy for positive lymph nodes, parametria, or margins. Chatani and colleagues[53] reported recurrence rates of 23% for patients with one or two positive lymph nodes and 32% for patients with more than two positive nodes.

Recent Gynecologic Oncology Group (GOG)[52] and Southwest Oncology Group (SWOG)[44] studies have investigated the role of adjuvant treatment in two separate high-risk groups. The SWOG study[44] investigated the role of chemoradiation in patients whose tumors involved the parametrium, surgical margins, or regional lymph nodes. Without radiation therapy, patients who have multiple positive lymph nodes, parametrial involvement, or positive surgical margins have a recurrence risk of 40% or more in retrospective series.[49,51] For patients with these findings, postoperative irradiation is usually recommended to reduce the risk of pelvic recurrence, although the impact of adjuvant

radiation therapy on survival has been difficult to define. In the 1980s, the GOG tried to conduct a randomized trial comparing postoperative pelvic irradiation versus no further treatment after radical hysterectomy in patients with pelvic lymph node involvement. The study had very slow accrual and closed without answering the question. However, in a later trial,[44] the SWOG demonstrated that postoperative treatment with chemoradiation (pelvic radiation plus cisplatin and 5-fluorouracil [5-FU]) resulted in significantly better rates of pelvic disease control and survival than radiation therapy alone in patients with positive lymph nodes, parametria, or margins. These data demonstrate that postoperative chemoradiation is beneficial and suggest that concurrent chemotherapy may be able to compensate for the relatively low dose of radiation that is deliverable in the postoperative setting.

The GOG study[52] suggested that postoperative radiation therapy was beneficial in patients whose tumors had high-risk local features but no histologic evidence of spread beyond the cervix. This randomized trial included 277 patients with negative nodes and local high-risk features. Patients were eligible if they had (1) lymphovascular space invasion with deep stromal invasion, (2) invasion of the middle third and a tumor measuring 2 cm or larger, or (3) superficial invasion and a tumor measuring 5 cm or larger; in addition, all patients with tumors that measured 4 cm or larger were eligible if more than one third of the stroma was involved. Preliminary analysis revealed a significant difference in local recurrence rates—15% in patients who had postoperative radiation therapy versus 28% in those treated with radical hysterectomy alone (Fig. 12-3). Overall, there was a 47% reduction in the risk of recurrence ($P = .008$). In this preliminary analysis, follow-up was too immature for assignment of a significance level to the overall survival comparison, but there were 18 deaths (13%) in the radiation therapy arm versus 30 deaths (21%) in the radical-hysterectomy-only arm (relative mortality rate, 0.64).

Despite this difference, it is apparent that local recurrence continued to be a problem even after postoperative radiation therapy, again suggesting that the dose was insufficient to control disease in a surgically disturbed field. These data suggest several maneuvers that could further decrease the risk of recurrence in patients with high-risk local features. Some clinicians believe that treatment with chemoradiation should be preferred over hysterectomy for patients who are known preoperatively to have high-risk features, particularly patients with bulky tumors. The GOG currently is conducting a trial that compares definitive chemoradiation versus initial radical hysterectomy for patients with stage Ib2 tumors; patients who are treated with initial hysterectomy will receive tailored chemoradiation if their primary tumor has high-risk features or if there is involvement of the surgical margins, parametria, or lymph nodes. Also, the addition of concurrent chemotherapy may further improve the local control rates achieved with postoperative radiation therapy. With further study, it might be possible to identify subgroups of patients with negative lymph nodes and

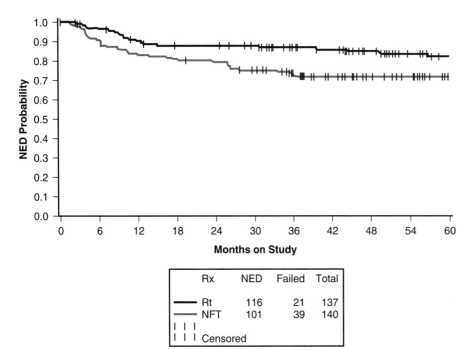

Figure 12–3. Recurrence-free interval for patients who had a radical hysterectomy with findings that indicated an intermediate risk of recurrence. Patients were randomly assigned to receive postoperative pelvic radiation therapy (Rt) or no further treatment (NFT) after hysterectomy. NED, no evidence of disease. (From Sedlis A, Bundy BN, Rotman MZ, et al: A randomized trial of pelvic radiation therapy versus no further therapy in selected patients with stage Ib carcinoma of the cervix after radical hysterectomy and pelvic lymphadenectomy: A Gynecologic Oncology Group Study. Gynecol Oncol 1999;73:177-183.)

Rx	NED	Failed	Total
Rt	116	21	137
NFT	101	39	140

I I I
I I I Censored

local high-risk features who are at particularly high risk for recurrence despite postoperative radiation. Currently, pathologists do not routinely provide detailed information about the extent of tumor-free margins (e.g., measurement of the distance between cancer and the edge of the surgical margins). More detailed information of this type might permit clinicians to more accurately select patients who are at particularly high risk of local recurrence and who might benefit from aggressive adjuvant treatment.

When should concurrent chemotherapy be added to radiation therapy?

In 1999, the results of five randomized studies[44-48] demonstrated the value of concurrent cisplatin-based chemotherapy and radiation therapy for patients with locoregionally advanced cervical cancer. Three of these trials included patients with high-risk stage I and II cervical cancers.

Of the 403 patients included in a trial conducted by the Radiation Therapy Oncology Group (RTOG),[46] 269 had stage I or II disease (the 130 patients with stage I or IIa disease had to have bulky tumors at least 5 cm in diameter or positive pelvic lymph nodes to be eligible). The study was stratified according to stage; those with stage I or II disease who received concurrent chemoradiation including cisplatin and 5-FU had a significantly better survival rate than those treated with radiation alone ($P = .002$).

In another study (Fig. 12-4),[48] the GOG randomly assigned patients with bulky stage Ib squamous carcinomas to receive radiation therapy followed by extrafascial hysterectomy or concurrent cisplatin (40 mg/m^2) or radiation therapy followed by hysterectomy. Although the results of an earlier GOG study

ultimately raised questions about the benefit of adjuvant extrafascial hysterectomy, this later study did demonstrate highly significant improvements in the rates of pathologic complete response and survival in patients treated with chemoradiation.

In a third study,[44] conducted by the SWOG, patients who were treated with initial radical hysterectomy were eligible if they were found to have involved lymph nodes, parametria, or surgical margins; again, patients who were randomly assigned to receive cisplatin and 5-FU concurrently with postoperative pelvic irradiation had better pelvic disease control and survival than did those treated with pelvic irradiation alone (Fig. 12-5). In that study, patients received two cycles of chemotherapy during and two cycles after radiation therapy. The authors noted that patients who completed the entire four cycles of chemotherapy had a better overall survival rate than did those who did not complete the planned treatment. They suggested that this was evidence of a direct effect of systemic chemotherapy on distant micrometastatic disease. However, it is also possible that other features of patients who failed to complete planned treatment were responsible for their poorer outcome. A randomized trial published in 1992 by Tattersall and colleagues[54] failed to show a benefit when adjuvant chemotherapy was given after radical hysterectomy. Also, a large three-arm trial of treatment with initial radiation therapy failed to demonstrate an advantage when adjuvant chemotherapy was added to radiation therapy or chemoradiation.[55] For these reasons, the value of continued chemotherapy after chemoradiation remains uncertain.

These studies strongly suggest that patients who have stage I or IIa cancers that are 5 cm or more in diameter and patients who have pelvic lymph node involvement or positive margins after hysterectomy benefit from concurrent cisplatin-based chemotherapy.

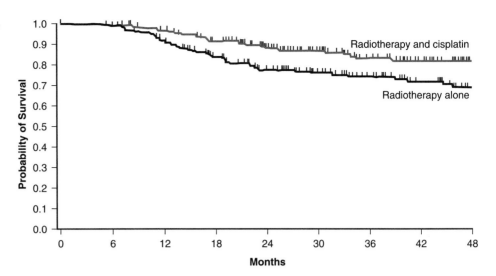

Figure 12–4. Overall survival rates of patients randomly assigned to receive concurrent weekly cisplatin and radiation therapy followed by adjuvant hysterectomy versus radiation therapy and hysterectomy alone. (From Keys HM, Bundy BN, Stehman FB, et al: Cisplatin, radiation, and adjuvant hysterectomy for bulky stage Ib cervical carcinoma. N Engl J Med 1999;340:1154-1161.)

The role of concurrent chemotherapy in patients with low-risk or intermediate-risk stage I or IIa disease is still unclear. The central and pelvic disease recurrence rates for patients who are treated with radiation alone for stage Ib1 cancers (≤4 cm) are approximately 1% and 2%, respectively (Fig. 12-6).[24,28,40] This leaves very little room for improvement with concurrent chemotherapy; radiation therapy alone is probably sufficient for such patients if there is no evidence of lymph node involvement. The role of concurrent chemotherapy in patients who have an intermediate risk of recurrence after hysterectomy is more controversial. In the randomized GOG trial reported by Sedlis and colleagues,[52] postoperative radiation therapy

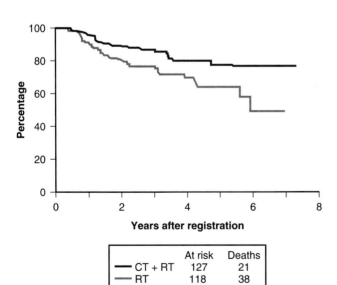

Figure 12–5. Overall survival for patients randomly assigned to receive either posthysterectomy radiation therapy (RT) with concurrent and adjuvant chemotherapy (CT) with cisplatin and 5-fluorouracil (127 patients) or postoperative RT alone (118 patients). (From Peters WA 3rd, Liu PY, Barrett RJ 2nd, et al: Concurrent chemotherapy and pelvic radiation therapy compared with pelvic radiation therapy alone as adjuvant therapy after radical surgery in high-risk early-stage cancer of the cervix. J Clin Oncol 2000;18:1606-1613.)

reduced the risk of pelvic recurrence by about 50% for patients who had an intermediate risk of local recurrence. However, despite this improvement, patients who received pelvic radiation therapy still had a pelvic recurrence rate of 15%, suggesting that more aggressive adjuvant treatment might benefit at least a subset of these patients.

Is there a role for neoadjuvant chemotherapy?

While trials of concurrent chemoradiation were under way, other trials were testing the value of neoadjuvant chemotherapy given before radiation therapy or hysterectomy. These trials frequently documented dramatic responses to chemotherapy, with "downstaging" of lesions. At least seven randomized trials have compared radiation therapy alone versus neoadjuvant chemotherapy followed by radiation therapy in patients with locally advanced lesions. Despite high rates of response to chemotherapy, most of these trials demonstrated no advantage or even poorer survival rates with radiation therapy preceded by chemotherapy, and this approach is no longer favored by most clinicians.[56-62]

More recent studies have evaluated the use of neoadjuvant chemotherapy before radical surgical treatment. One of the largest phase III trials was carried out by Sardi and associates[63] in Argentina. In this trial, 205 patients with stage Ib cervical cancers were randomly assigned to receive surgery alone or surgery after neoadjuvant chemotherapy with vincristine, bleomycin, and cisplatin. All patients received postoperative pelvic irradiation.[63] Response rates and overall survival outcomes were analyzed separately for patients with small stage Ib tumors (<4 cm) and for patients with larger tumors (≥4 cm). For patients with smaller tumors, the rates of overall survival and disease-free survival were similar for the two treatment arms, although patients who received neoadjuvant chemotherapy were less likely to have lymph node metastases detected in their operative specimens. Bulkier tumors were more likely to be resected if the patients had received neoadjuvant chemotherapy (100% versus

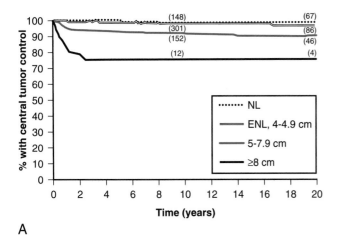

A

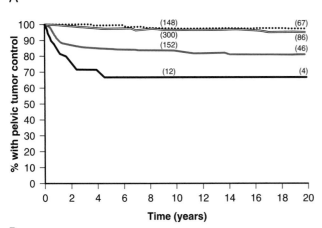

B

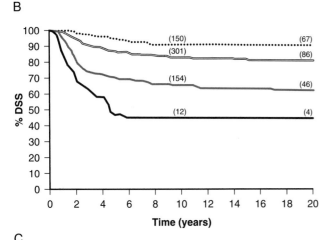

C

Figure 12–6. Rates of central tumor control (**A**), pelvic tumor control (**B**), and disease-specific survival (**C**) for patients grouped according to tumor diameter. The legend refers to all three sets of curves. Numbers in parentheses refer to the number of patients remaining at risk at 5 and 10 years. DSS, disease-specific survival; ENL, enlarged cervix; NL, normal size cervix. (From Eifel PJ, Morris M, Wharton JT, et al: The influence of tumor size and morphology on the outcome of patients with FIGO stage Ib squamous cell carcinoma of the uterine cervix. Int J Radiat Oncol Biol Phys 1994;29:9-16.)

85%). At 7 years, the overall survival rate was significantly better for patients who received neoadjuvant chemotherapy than for control-group patients who had resectable tumors (81% versus 69%) (Fig. 12-7). Another randomized study,[64] which was conducted in

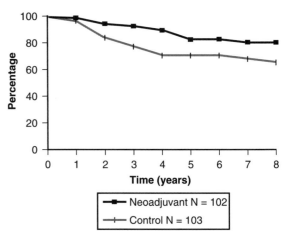

Figure 12-7. Overall survival rates for patients with stage Ib carcinoma of the cervix who were randomly assigned to receive radical hysterectomy followed by pelvic radiation therapy (control) or neoadjuvant chemotherapy followed by hysterectomy and pelvic radiation therapy (neoadjuvant). (From Sardi JE, Giaroli A, Sananes C, et al: Long-term follow-up of the first randomized trial using neoadjuvant chemotherapy in stage Ib squamous carcinoma of the cervix: the final results. Gynecol Oncol 1997;67:61-69.)

patients with locally advanced stage Ib2-III squamous carcinomas, compared radiation therapy alone versus neoadjuvant chemotherapy followed by radical hysterectomy. Thirty-eight patients who had radical surgery with findings of positive lymph nodes or positive surgical resection margins received additional pelvic radiation therapy. For the subset of 174 patients with stage Ib2-IIa disease, overall and progression-free survival rates were significantly better for the patients who received chemotherapy followed by surgery (*P* = .01).[64] The relevance of this trial, which was closed to accrual in 1996, is diminished because it did not include concurrent chemotherapy in the radiation therapy arm. It also has been criticized because of the low dose of radiation (median dose to point A, 70 Gy) and the protracted radiation treatment (more than 10 weeks in 27% of patients). It also should be noted that both of the randomized trials limited eligibility to patients who had squamous lesions; the potential benefit of neoadjuvant chemotherapy for patients with early-stage adenocarcinoma is unknown.

In North America, neoadjuvant chemotherapy has been slow to be accepted. On the basis of the reports of response to neoadjuvant chemotherapy, the GOG sponsored a phase II study of neoadjuvant chemotherapy followed by radical hysterectomy for women with stage Ib2 cancers of the cervix.[65] Encouraging results of this preliminary study led to a randomized trial (GOG 141) that compared treatment with preoperative vincristine and cisplatin followed by radical hysterectomy versus radical hysterectomy alone for patients with "bulky" (>4 cm) stage Ib disease; postoperative chemoradiation therapy was given to patients whose tumors were found to have "high-risk" features. For a variety of reasons, this trial was closed to accrual before accrual was completed. Results have not yet been reported. At this time, there does not appear to be sufficient evidence to support the routine use of neoadjuvant chemotherapy for patients with early-stage cervical cancer.

Is there a role for adjuvant hysterectomy?

The role of adjuvant postirradiation hysterectomy in patients with bulky cervical cancers has sparked controversy for many years. For patients with small tumors, pelvic recurrences are very rare after radiation therapy alone (see Fig. 12-6). Eifel and coworkers[28] reported central and pelvic disease control rates of 99% and 97%, respectively, for tumors that were less than 5 cm in diameter. Even larger (5 to 7 cm) exophytic tumors had a relatively low central recurrence rate of 3%. Similarly, Horiot and associates[31] reported no central recurrences and a pelvic recurrence rate of less than 4% in patients with small stage I tumors. It is difficult to justify the use of adjuvant surgery in such cases because the margin for improvement is so small.

However, for patients with larger tumors, particularly endocervical tumors greater than 5 to 6 cm in diameter, the rate of central recurrence after radiation therapy alone is approximately 10% even when high-dose radiation therapy is delivered without excessive treatment delays. These higher recurrence rates led clinicians to try the strategy of following radiation therapy with a simple extrafascial hysterectomy. In a 1969 retrospective review of the experience at The University of Texas M. D. Anderson Cancer Center, Durrance and colleagues[66] reported a lower rate of pelvic recurrence in women with bulky endocervical tumors (measuring more than 6 cm in diameter) who were treated with radiation followed by extrafascial hysterectomy than in those who were treated with a somewhat higher dose of radiation alone.

After the Durrance report,[66] the popularity of adjunctive hysterectomy increased dramatically. Some clinicians advocated the use of adjuvant hysterectomy in "bulky" tumors that were as small as 3 to 4 cm. However, more recent studies have failed to confirm the value of adjuvant hysterectomy. A reexamination of the M. D. Anderson Cancer Center experience[67] suggested that selection bias could have accounted for much of the difference observed in the Durrance study. Patients who had very large (≥8 cm), poorly responding, or node-positive tumors were more frequently treated with radiation therapy alone, biasing the results. In 1991, the University of Florida compared their institutional experience before and after adoption of adjuvant hysterectomy as standard in patients with bulky (≥6 cm) endocervical tumors.[68] No significant reduction was found in the rate of pelvic recurrences after treatment with combined radiation and adjuvant hysterectomy was adopted as the standard.

Only one prospective randomized trial has attempted to evaluate the benefit of adjuvant hysterectomy. Between October 1984 and November 1991, the GOG entered 282 patients in a study comparing radiation therapy alone with radiation therapy followed by extrafascial hysterectomy; eligible patients had stage Ib squamous carcinomas measuring 4 cm or greater in diameter. Recently publicized results of this trial[69] do not demonstrate any difference in the overall survival

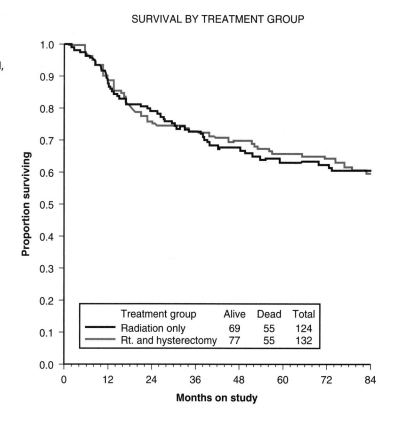

Figure 12–8. Survival rates of patients with stage Ib cervical cancers 4 cm or larger who were randomly assigned to receive either radiation therapy (RT) alone (124 patients) or RT followed by extrafascial hysterectomy (132 patients). (From Keys HM, Bundy BN, Stehman FB, et al: Radiation therapy with and without extrafascial hysterectomy for bulky stage Ib cervical carcinoma: a randomized trial of the Gynecologic Oncology Group. Gynecol Oncol 2003;89:343-353.)

SURVIVAL BY TREATMENT GROUP

Treatment group	Alive	Dead	Total
Radiation only	69	55	124
Rt. and hysterectomy	77	55	132

of patients treated in the two groups (Fig. 12-8). A subset analysis of the results suggests that patients with smaller tumors (4 to 6 cm) may have benefited from adjuvant hysterectomy, whereas those with tumors larger than 6 cm in diameter tended to have a poorer outcome if they were in the adjuvant hysterectomy group; however, the number of patients in each subgroup was very small. As with several other studies performed during this period, the relevance to current practice is limited because the radiation therapy was somewhat protracted (median duration, more than 60 days) and concurrent chemotherapy was not administered.

Complications may be greater with combined therapy, particularly if radical hysterectomy is performed after high-dose radiation therapy.[70,71] O'Quinn and associates[71] reported that, with careful sharp dissection, extrafascial hysterectomy could be performed safely after radiation therapy if the total dose of radiation was reduced by about 15% to 20%; overall complication rates were similar to those after radiation therapy alone, although the rate of fistula formation was increased.[67,72] In another study, Mendenhall and colleagues[68] reported an 18% rate of major complications at 6 years for patients who had adjuvant hysterectomy, compared with 7% for patients treated with radiation therapy alone ($P = .027$).

As outlined earlier, recent studies have demonstrated markedly improved pelvic disease control rates with the addition of concurrent chemotherapy to radiation therapy. Concurrent chemoradiation has increasingly become standard treatment for most patients with bulky stage I-II disease. The very low central recurrence rates achieved with this treatment further reduce the margin for improvement with adjuvant hysterectomy. The GOG has demonstrated[48] that even with combined radiation therapy and hysterectomy, concurrent chemotherapy is required to achieve the best treatment results (see Fig. 12-4). Taken together, these results provide little evidence to justify the routine use of hysterectomy after radiation therapy.

What factors influence the risks of major complications of treatment?

Perioperative complications of radical hysterectomy have become rare with improvements in anesthesia, the use of broad-spectrum antibiotics, and specialized training. Possible late complications of radical hysterectomy include ureteral stricture (usually transient), bladder dysfunction, constipation, wound complications, lymphocyst, and lymphedema. The incidence of postoperative and late complications is related to the type of radical hysterectomy performed and the use of adjuvant radiation therapy. In recent years, surgeons operating on early cervical cancers have increasingly used a modified (class II) radical hysterectomy, which is associated with a lesser risk of serious side effects than the classic class III hysterectomy that was initially described by Meigs.[73] When performing a class II hysterectomy, the surgeon removes the medial half of the cardinal and uterosacral ligaments and ligates the uterine artery at the ureter. Although this procedure has traditionally been limited to patients with FIGO stage Ia disease, recent studies have suggested that it can be used for patients with more invasive early cervical cancers without reducing the chance of cure. Several studies have demonstrated shortened operative times and significantly reduced morbidity with the modified procedure.[74,75] In particular, class II hysterectomy is associated with a lower rate of urologic complications. In a multi-institutional Italian trial in which patients with stage Ib-IIa tumors were randomly assigned to class I or II hysterectomy, Landoni and colleagues[75] reported a 13% rate of urologic complications for patients who had a class II procedure versus 28% with the class III hysterectomy. Photopulos and Zwaag[74] also reported a reduced complication rate with class II hysterectomy, with no fistulas and a mean time to voiding of 16.5 days in 21 patients who had this procedure. The rates of major complications from single institutions vary widely and are difficult to compare because the scoring methods and types of hysterectomy differ or are not specified. Covens and coworkers[76] found that the incidence of major morbidity can differ between surgeons, even within a single facility. They found significantly different rates of perioperative complications (blood loss, operating time, transfusion requirement, and length of hospitalization) between surgeons; the rate of late bladder dysfunction ranged from 0% to 43% for surgeons operating in their facility ($P < .0001$).

Radical surgery is usually contraindicated in patients who have severe heart disease, including unstable angina, congestive heart failure, or a recent history of myocardial infarction; a history of these conditions is an indication for treatment with primary radiation therapy. Radiation therapy is also preferred for patients who have severe pulmonary disease that would increase their risk of complications from anesthesia. On occasion, a patient with an early cervical cancer presents with active thrombotic disease requiring anticoagulation. Although it may be possible to operate on such a patient after placement of a vena cava filter and interruption of anticoagulant therapy, the patient would be better served by the strategy of proceeding directly to radiation therapy. Other conditions that are sometimes considered to be relative contraindications to surgery are obesity and old age. However, single-institution retrospective studies have suggested that patients who are obese and those who are more than 65 years old can, if carefully selected, undergo radical hysterectomy without an increased risk of major complications.[77-80] Selection bias and failure of authors to report the number of patients screened make it difficult to interpret some of these studies. Geisler and Geisler[78] compared 62 women age 65 years or older and a matched cohort of younger women (<50 years of age) who underwent radical hysterectomy for cervical cancer. All of the operations were performed by a single surgeon over an extended period. There were no significant differences in minor or major outcomes; the only notable difference was a longer length of stay after surgery for the older patients. Other studies have examined the impact of obesity on surgical morbidity in patients undergoing radical hysterectomy.[77,79,80] Again, most of these were retrospective studies of carefully selected patients. Cohn and associates[77] found that the procedure was feasible with acceptable morbidity. Other studies have reported longer operating time, an increase in blood loss, and an increase in wound complications with radical hysterectomy in obese women.

The risk of serious complications probably increases if radiation therapy is given after radical hysterectomy. Sedlis and coworkers[52] reported a 7% rate of severe complications (grade 3 or greater) in patients who had radical hysterectomy and postoperative pelvic irradiation, compared with 2.1% for patients who had surgery alone (probability value not stated). Although Landoni and colleagues[35] reported similar overall complication rates for patients who had surgery only versus combined surgery and radiation therapy (24% and 29%, respectively), irradiated patients tended to have more small-bowel obstructions (5% versus 1%) and lymphedema (9% versus 0%). In a review of eight series of patients treated with adjuvant pelvic irradiation, Thomas and Dembo[49] found 39 severe complications in 359 patients (crude incidence, 11%).

The timing and character of late complications differs depending on whether patients have radiation therapy or surgery as their primary treatment. Although the overall rate of major complications after radiation therapy is low, the risk of late complications continues for many years after the treatment. For this reason, complication rates should be calculated actuarially to provide a meaningful understanding of the risk to surviving patients. In a study of 1784 patients treated with primary radiation therapy for stage Ib cervical cancers, Eifel and colleagues[72] reported a 9.3% incidence of major (≥ grade 3) late complications 5 years after radiation therapy. The overall rates of major urinary tract and rectal complications were 2.6% and 2.3%, respectively, at 5 years. Although most rectal complications occurred within the first 2 to 3 years after radiation therapy, there was a protracted risk of developing urinary tract complications (Fig. 12-9). Forty-one patients (1.7%) developed fistulas; the risk of fistula was significantly increased in patients who underwent adjuvant extrafascial hysterectomy or pretreatment laparotomy. The risk of small-bowel obstruction was 3.9% at 5 years and was increased in patients with pretreatment staging laparotomy and thin body habitus. In a more recent review of complications in 3489 patients with stage I-II disease, Eifel and associates[81] reported a strong correlation between major radiation complications and smoking history. Patients who smoked heavily (≥1 pack per day) had a significantly increased risk of urinary tract and gastrointestinal complications; most marked was a more than fivefold increase in the risk of small-bowel obstruction for heavy smokers versus nonsmokers. Other factors that correlated with an increased risk of major complications were thin body habitus, previous or concurrent pelvic infection, pre-radiation therapy staging surgery, and high external radiation dose. Patients who have symptoms or radiographic findings suggestive of tubo-ovarian abscess should not be treated with radiation until the abscess is surgically removed and intravenous antibiotics are administered. Other authors have reported increased complication rates in patients with diabetes mellitus,[82,83] hypertension,[83] inflammatory bowel disease,[84] or young age.[85] Eifel and colleagues[72] did not find a correlation between age and the actuarial incidence of late complications; however, because young women have more years to experience late effects, their lifetime risk is greater than that of older women.

Selection of patients for either primary surgery or primary radiation therapy must include a complete history and physical examination. Some conditions increase the risk of complications after either treatment approach. For example, patients who have severe intestinal adhesions are more likely to have complications from radiation therapy or surgery. In these cases, treatment should be selected by carefully evaluating the risk of complications associated with each treatment. This assessment should include a careful evaluation of the patient's disease extent and an estimate of the likelihood that, if treatment with radical surgery is chosen, high-risk features will be present that necessitate adjuvant radiation therapy. Clinicians must carefully balance the risks and benefits of each treatment in making recommendations for individual patients. However, because radiation-related complications and surgical complications are so different, it is difficult to accurately estimate their relative impact on patients' well-being in the absence of carefully controlled studies that specifically and prospectively address quality of life.

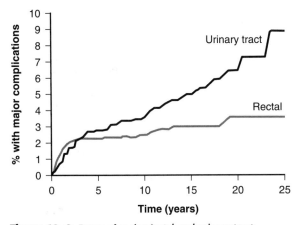

Figure 12–9. Rates of major rectal and urinary tract complications in 1784 patients treated with radiation therapy for stage Ib carcinoma of the cervix. (From Eifel PJ, Levenback C, Wharton JT, et al: Time course and incidence of late complications in patients treated with radiation therapy for FIGO stage Ib carcinoma of the uterine cervix. Int J Radiat Oncol Biol Phys 1995;32:1289-1300.)

How does treatment influence sexual function?

Sexual function is one of many factors that contribute to a patient's overall quality of life. Cervical cancer treatment can affect sexual function in a number of ways, although the impact of treatment on this aspect of women's lives is still poorly understood. Although the risk of sexual dysfunction may be high, there are very few well-designed studies addressing this issue. It is clear, however, that multiple anatomic and psychological factors influence outcome.

Dyspareunia can result from shortening of the vagina due to treatment with radical surgery or radiation therapy. For patients with locally advanced disease, destruction of the paracervical tissues by tumor probably compounds these effects. Diminished estrogen levels after treatment also contribute to vaginal atrophy and dryness. There is a perception that radiation therapy has a greater effect on sexual function than surgical treatment does.[86] However, because treatments are often selected on the basis of patient age and disease extent and because studies of the effects of local treatments rarely correct for these confounding influences, the relative risk of sexual dysfunction from various treatments remains poorly understood. The timing of follow-up evaluations in relation to treatment is also an important influence on measured outcome. The anatomic effects of treatment (particularly radiation therapy) as well as those of aging and hypoestrogenism progress with time.[87,88]

Psychological factors can play an important role in patients' sexual function after treatment. Women with early-stage cervical cancers often are young and of childbearing age. Loss of fertility can have an important impact on their self-image and feelings of sexuality.[89] Concern that the cancer may have been caused by a sexually transmitted virus can influence a patient's attitudes toward sexual relations and her partner. Studies that have focused on determinations of sexual function after either surgery or radiation therapy[88,89] have made clear that sexual function is important to most patients and that the age of the patient at initiation of treatment is not a major factor in outcomes.

Bergmark and coworkers[90] carried out one of the better-designed studies examining the effect of treatment on vaginal function and sexuality among women treated for early-stage cervical cancer. This Swedish study compared patients with stage Ib–IIa disease with a control group of women who did not have a diagnosis of cervical cancer. The control group members were matched with the cancer patients according to age and region of residence, although there were some differences in the age distributions of respondents in the two groups. Anonymous questionnaires about vaginal changes and sexual function were distributed, and the results were analyzed; 77% of the study group and 72% of the controls responded to the survey. Almost 90% of all the treated patients had a surgical procedure; 36% had surgery alone, 22% had surgery plus intracavitary radiation therapy, and 30% had surgery plus external radiation therapy. Only 9% of the women in this study were treated with radiation alone. Sixty-seven percent of the treated patients were taking either systemic or local hormonal therapy, compared with 30% of the control group. Equal percentages of women in the two groups (41%) answered that they had little or no interest in sex in the past 6 months. Compared with control patients, women treated for cervical cancer had higher rates of concern and distress about reduced sexual desire. Cervical cancer patients also reported more problems with short vaginal length (23% versus 3%), insufficient vaginal elasticity (23% versus 4%), and insufficient vaginal lubrication (26% versus 11%). Dyspareunia also was more common among women with cervical cancer. Overall, 26% of cervical cancer patients and 8% of women in the control group reported moderate or much distress due to vaginal changes.

There continues to be an important need for well-designed studies that match comparison groups according to patient age, extent of disease, length of follow-up, and pretreatment sexual function.

REFERENCES

1. International Federation of Gynecology and Obstetrics: Annual report on the results of treatment in carcinoma of the uterus and vagina, vol 14. Stockholm, Kungl. Boktryckeriet P.A. Norstedt & Söner, 1967.
2. International Federation of Gynecology and Obstetrics: Classification and staging of malignant tumors in the female pelvis. Acta Obstet Gynecol Scand 1971;50:1-12.
3. International Federation of Gynecology and Obstetrics: Annual report on the results of treatment in carcinoma of the uterus, vagina, and ovary, vol 15. Stockholm, Kungl. Boktryckeriet P.A. Norstedt & Söner, 1973.
4. International Federation of Gynecology and Obstetrics: Staging announcement: FIGO Cancer Committee. Gynecol Oncol 1986; 25:383-385.
5. International Federation of Gynecology and Obstetrics: Annual report on the results of treatment in gynecological cancer. Int J Gynaecol Obstet 1991;36(Suppl):27-30.
6. International Federation of Gynecology and Obstetrics: Annual report on the results of treatment in gynecological cancer. Stockholm, Radium Hemmet, 1994.
7. International Federation of Gynecology and Obstetrics: Staging announcement: FIGO staging of gynecologic cancers; cervical and vulva. Int J Gynecol Cancer 1995;5:319.
8. League of Nations Health Organization: Inquiry into the results of radiotherapy in cancer of the uterus: Atlas illustrating the division of cancer of the uterine cervix into four stages according to the anatomo-clinical extent of the growth. Stockholm, Kungl. Boktryckeriet P. A. Norstedt & Söner, 1938.
9. Burghardt E, Pickel H, Haas J, et al: Prognostic factors and operative treatment of stages IB to IIB cervical cancer. Am J Obstet Gynecol 1987;156:988-996.
10. McCarthy S, Hricak H: The uterus and vagina. In Higgins C, Hricak H, Helms C (eds): Magnetic resonance imaging of the body. Philadelphia, Lippincott-Raven, 1997, pp. 801-805.
11. Hawnaur JM, Johnson RJ, Buckley CH, et al: Staging, volume estimation and assessment of nodal status in carcinoma of the cervix: Comparison of magnetic resonance imaging with surgical findings. Clin Radiol 1994;49:443-452.
12. Kim SH, Choi BI, Han JK, et al: Preoperative staging of uterine cervical carcinoma: Comparison of CT and MRI in 99 patients. J Comput Assist Tomogr 1993;17:633-640.
13. Wagenaar HC, Trimbos JB, Postema S, et al: Tumor diameter and volume assessed by magnetic resonance imaging in the prediction of outcome for invasive cervical cancer. Gynecol Oncol 2001; 82:474-482.
14. Sugawara Y, Eisbruch A, Kosuda S, et al: Evaluation of FDG PET in patients with cervical cancer. J Nucl Med 1999;40: 1125-1131.
15. Grigsby PW, Siegel BA, Dehdashti F: Lymph node staging by positron emission tomography in patients with carcinoma of the cervix. J Clin Oncol 2001;19:3745-3749.
16. Duska LR, Toth TL, Goodman A: Fertility options for patients with stages IA2 and IB cervical cancer: Presentation of two cases and discussion of technical and ethical issues. Obstet Gynecol 1998;92:656-658.

17. Dargent D: A new future for Schauta's operation through pre-surgical retroperitoneal pelviscopy. Eur J Gynaecol Oncol 1987;8:282-296.

18. Dargent D, Mathevet P: Schauta's vaginal hysterectomy combined with laparoscopic lymphadenectomy. Baillieres Clin Obstet Gynaecol 1995;9:691-705.

19. Schlaerth JB, Spirtos NM, Schlaerth AC: Radical trachelectomy and pelvic lymphadenectomy with uterine preservation in the treatment of cervical cancer. Am J Obstet Gynecol 2003; 188:29-34.

20. Roy M, Plante M: Pregnancies after radical vaginal trachelectomy for early-stage cervical cancer. Am J Obstet Gynecol 1998; 179:1491-1496.

21. Burnett AF, Roman LD, O'Meara AT, et al: Radical vaginal trachelectomy and pelvic lymphadenectomy for preservation of fertility in early cervical carcinoma. Gynecol Oncol 2003;88: 419-423.

22. Dargent D, Martin X, Sacchetoni A, et al: Laparoscopic vaginal radical trachelectomy: A treatment to preserve the fertility of cervical carcinoma patients. Cancer 2000;88:1877-1882.

23. Alvarez RD, Potter ME, Soong SJ, et al: Rationale for using pathologic tumor dimensions and nodal status to subclassify surgically treated stage IB cervical cancer patients. Gynecol Oncol 1991;43:108-112.

24. Barillot I, Horiot JC, Pigneux J, et al: Carcinoma of the intact uterine cervix treated with radiotherapy alone: A French cooperative study. Update and multivariate analysis of prognostics factors. Int J Radiat Oncol Biol Phys 1997;38:969-978.

25. Boyce J, Fruchter R, Nicastri A, et al: Prognostic factors in stage I carcinoma of the cervix. Gynecol Oncol 1981;12:154-165.

26. Burghardt E, Hofmann HMH, Ebner F, et al: Results of surgical treatment of 1028 cervical cancers studied with volumetry. Cancer 1992;70:648-655.

27. Coia L, Won M, Lanciano R, et al: The Patterns of Care Outcome Study for cancer of the uterine cervix: Results of the second national practice survey. Cancer 1990;66:2451-2456.

28. Eifel PJ, Morris M, Wharton JT, et al: The influence of tumor size and morphology on the outcome of patients with FIGO stage IB squamous cell carcinoma of the uterine cervix. Int J Radiat Oncol Biol Phys 1994;29:9-16.

29. Fuller AF, Elliott N, Kosloff C, et al: Determinants of increased risk for recurrence in patients undergoing radical hysterectomy for stage IB and IIA carcinoma of the cervix. Gynecol Oncol 1989; 33:34-39.

30. Hopkins MP, Morley GW: Radical hysterectomy versus radiation therapy for stage IB squamous cell cancer of the cervix. Cancer 1991;68:272-277.

31. Horiot JC, Pigneux J, Pourquier H, et al: Radiotherapy alone in carcinoma of the intact uterine cervix according to G. H. Fletcher guidelines: A French cooperative study of 1383 cases. Int J Radiat Oncol Biol Phys 1988;14:605-611.

32. Hoskins WJ, Ford J, Lutz M, et al: Radical hysterectomy and pelvic lymphadenectomy for the management of early invasive cancer of the cervix. Gynecol Oncol 1976;4:278-290.

33. Inoue T: Prognostic significance of the depth of invasion relating to nodal metastases, parametrial extension, and cell types: A study of 628 cases with stage IB, IIA, and IIB cervical cancer. Cancer 1984;54:3035-3042.

34. Kenter GG, Ansink AC, Heintz APM, et al: Carcinoma of the uterine cervix stage I and IIA: Results of surgical treatment—Complications, recurrence, and survival. Eur J Surg Oncol 1989; 15:55-60.

35. Landoni F, Maneo A, Colombo A, et al: Randomized study of radical surgery versus radiotherapy for stage Ib-IIa cervical cancer. Lancet 1997;350:535-540.

36. Lee Y-N, Wang KL, Lin M-H, et al: Radical hysterectomy with pelvic lymph node dissection for treatment of cervical cancer: A clinical review of 954 cases. Gynecol Oncol 1989;32:135-142.

37. Liu W, Meigs JV: Radical hysterectomy and pelvic lymphadenectomy: A review of 473 cases including 244 for primary invasive carcinoma of the cervix. Am J Obstet Gynecol 1955;69:1-32.

38. Lowrey GC, Mendenhall WM, Million RR: Stage IB or IIA-B carcinoma of the intact uterine cervix treated with irradiation: A multivariate analysis. Int J Radiat Oncol Biol Phys 1992;24: 205-210.

39. Montana GS, Fowler WC, Varia MA, et al: Analysis of results of radiation therapy for stage IB carcinoma of the cervix. Cancer 1987;60:2195-2200.

40. Perez CA, Grigsby PW, Nene SM, et al: Effect of tumor size on the prognosis of carcinoma of the uterine cervix treated with irradiation alone. Cancer 1992;69:2796-2806.

41. Piver MS, Chung WS: Prognostic significance of cervical lesion size and pelvic node metastases in cervical carcinoma. Obstet Gynecol 1975;46:507-510.

42. Volterrani F, Feltre L, Sigurta D, et al: Radiotherapy versus surgery in the treatment of cervix stage Ib cancer. Int J Radiat Oncol Biol Phys 1983;9:1781-1784.

43. Mendenhall WM, Thar TL, Bova FJ, et al: Prognostic and treatment factors affecting pelvic control of stage IB and IIA-B carcinoma of the intact uterine cervix treated with radiation therapy alone. Cancer 1984;53:2649-2654.

44. Peters WA 3rd, Liu PY, Barrett RJ 2nd, et al: Concurrent chemotherapy and pelvic radiation therapy compared with pelvic radiation therapy alone as adjuvant therapy after radical surgery in high-risk early-stage cancer of the cervix. J Clin Oncol 2000;18:1606-1613.

45. Whitney CW, Sause W, Bundy BN, et al: A randomized comparison of fluorouracil plus cisplatin versus hydroxyurea as an adjunct to radiation therapy in stages IIB-IVA carcinoma of the cervix with negative para-aortic lymph nodes: A Gynecologic Oncology Group and Southwest Oncology Group study. J Clin Oncol 1999;17:1339-1348.

46. Morris M, Eifel PJ, Lu J, et al: Pelvic radiation with concurrent chemotherapy compared with pelvic and paraaortic radiation for high-risk cervical cancer. N Engl J Med 1999;340: 1137-1143.

47. Rose PG, Bundy BN, Watkins J, et al: Concurrent cisplatin-based chemotherapy and radiotherapy for locally advanced cervical cancer. N Engl J Med 1999;340:1144-1153.

48. Keys HM, Bundy BN, Stehman FB, et al: Cisplatin, radiation, and adjuvant hysterectomy for bulky stage IB cervical carcinoma. N Engl J Med 1999;340:1154-1161.

49. Thomas GM, Dembo AJ: Is there a role for adjuvant pelvic radiotherapy after radical hysterectomy in early stage cervical cancer? Int J Gynecol Cancer 1991;1:1-8.

50. Stock RG, Chen ASJ, Karasek K: Patterns of spread in node-positive cervical cancer: The relationship between local control and distant metastases. Cancer J Sci Am 1996;2:256-262.

51. Morrow CP: Is pelvic radiation beneficial in the postoperative management of stage Ib squamous cell carcinoma of the cervix with pelvic node metastases treated by radical hysterectomy and pelvic lymphadenectomy? Gynecol Oncol 1980;10: 105-110.

52. Sedlis A, Bundy BN, Rotman MZ, et al: A randomized trial of pelvic radiation therapy versus no further therapy in selected patients with stage IB carcinoma of the cervix after radical hysterectomy and pelvic lymphadenectomy: A Gynecologic Oncology Group study. Gynecol Oncol 1999;73:177-183.

53. Chatani M, Nose T, Masaki N, et al: Adjuvant radiotherapy after radical hysterectomy of cervical cancer: Prognostic factors and complications. Strahlenther Onkol 1998;174:504-509.

54. Tattersall MHN, Ramirez C, Coppleson M: A randomized trial of adjuvant chemotherapy after radical hysterectomy in stage IB-IIA cervical cancer patients with pelvic lymph node metastases. Gynecol Oncol 1992;46:176-181.

55. Lorvidhaya V, Chitapanarux I, Sangruchi S, et al: Concurrent mitomycin C, 5-fluorouracil, and radiotherapy in the treatment of locally advanced carcinoma of the cervix: A randomized trial. Int J Radiat Oncol Biol Phys 2003;55:1226-1232.

56. Chauvergne J, Rohart J, Héron JF, et al: Essai randomisé de chimiothérapie initiale dans 151 carcinomes du col utérin localement étendus (T2b-N1, T3b, MO). Bull Cancer 1990;77:1007-1024.

57. Tattersall MHN, Ramirez C, Coppleson M: A randomized trial comparing platinum-based chemotherapy followed by radiotherapy vs. radiotherapy alone in patients with locally advanced cervical cancer. Int J Gynecol Cancer 1992;2:244-251.

58. Symonds RP, Habeshaw T, Watson ER, et al: Combination chemotherapy prior to radical radiotherapy for stage III and IV carcinoma of the cervix. Clin Radiol 1987;38:273-274.

59. Souhami L, Gil R, Allan S, et al: A randomized trial of chemotherapy followed by pelvic radiation therapy in stage

IIIB carcinoma of the cervix. Int J Radiat Oncol Biol Phys 1991; 9:970-997.

60. Symonds RP, Habeshaw T, Reed NS, et al: The Scottish and Manchester randomized trial of neo-adjuvant chemotherapy for advanced cervical cancer. Eur J Cancer 2000;36:994-1001.

61. Sundfør K, Trope CG, Hogberg T, et al: Radiotherapy and neoadjuvant chemotherapy for cervical carcinoma: A randomized multicenter study of sequential cisplatin and 5-fluorouracil and radiotherapy in advanced cervical carcinoma stage 3B and 4A. Cancer 1996;77:2371-2378.

62. Leborgne F, Leborgne JH, Doldán R, et al: Induction chemotherapy and radiotherapy of advanced cancer of the cervix: A pilot study and phase III randomized trial. Int J Radiat Oncol Biol Phys 1997;37:343-350.

63. Sardi JE, Giaroli A, Sananes C, et al: Long-term follow-up of the first randomized trial using neoadjuvant chemotherapy in stage Ib squamous carcinoma of the cervix: The final results. Gynecol Oncol 1997;67:61-69.

64. Benedetti-Panici P, Greggi S, Colombo A, et al: Neoadjuvant chemotherapy and radical surgery versus exclusive radiotherapy in locally advanced squamous cell cervical cancer: Results from the Italian multicenter randomized study. J Clin Oncol 2002; 20:179-188.

65. Eddy GL, Manetta A, Alvarez RD, et al: Neoadjuvant chemotherapy with vincristine and cisplatin followed by radical hysterectomy and pelvic lymphadenectomy for FIGO stage IB bulky cervical cancer: A Gynecologic Oncology Group pilot study. Gynecol Oncol 1995;57:412-416.

66. Durrance FY, Fletcher GH, Rutledge FN: Analysis of central recurrent disease in stages I and II squamous cell carcinomas of the cervix on intact uterus. AJR Am J Roentgenol 1969;106: 831-838.

67. Thoms WW, Eifel PJ, Smith TL, et al: Bulky endocervical carcinomas: A 23-year experience. Int J Radiat Oncol Biol Phys 1992;23:491-499.

68. Mendenhall WM, McCarty PJ, Morgan LS, et al: Stage IB-IIA-B carcinoma of the intact uterine cervix greater than or equal to 6 cm in diameter: Is adjuvant extrafascial hysterectomy beneficial? Int J Radiat Oncol Biol Phys 1991;21:899-904.

69. Keys HM, Bundy BN, Stehman FB, et al: Radiation therapy with and without extrafascial hysterectomy for bulky stage IB cervical carcinoma: A randomized trial of the Gynecologic Oncology Group. Gynecol Oncol 2003;89:343-353.

70. Rotman M, John MJ, Moon SH, et al: Limitations of adjunctive surgery in carcinoma of the cervix. Int J Radiat Oncol Biol Phys 1979;5:327-332.

71. O'Quinn AG, Fletcher GH, Wharton JT: Guidelines for conservative hysterectomy after irradiation. Gynecol Oncol 1980;9:68-79.

72. Eifel PJ, Levenback C, Wharton JT, et al: Time course and incidence of late complications in patients treated with radiation therapy for FIGO stage IB carcinoma of the uterine cervix. Int J Radiat Oncol Biol Phys 1995;32:1289-1300.

73. Meigs JV: Radical hysterectomy with bilateral dissection of pelvic nodes. In Meigs JV (ed): Surgical treatment of cancer of the cervix. New York, Grune and Stratton, 1954, p. 149.

74. Photopulos GH, Zwaag RV: Class II radical hysterectomy shows less morbidity and good treatment efficacy compared to class III. Gynecol Oncol 1991;40:21-24.

75. Landoni F, Maneo A, Cormio G, et al: Class II versus class III radical hysterectomy in stage IB-IIA cervical cancer: A prospective randomized study. Gynecol Oncol 2001;80:3-12.

76. Covens A, Rosen B, Gibbons A, et al: Differences in the morbidity of radical hysterectomy between gynecological oncologists. Gynecol Oncol 1993;51:39-45.

77. Cohn DE, Swisher EM, Herzog TJ, et al: Radical hysterectomy for cervical cancer in obese women. Obstet Gynecol 2000;96:727-731.

78. Geisler JP, Geisler HE: Radical hysterectomy in the elderly female: A comparison to patients age 50 or younger. Gynecol Oncol 2001;80:258-261.

79. Soisson AP, Soper JT, Berchuck A, et al: Radical hysterectomy in obese women. Obstet Gynecol 1992;80:940-943.

80. Levrant SG, Fruchter RG, Maiman M: Radical hysterectomy for cervical cancer: Morbidity and survival in relation to weight and age. Gynecol Oncol 1992;45:317-322.

81. Eifel PJ, Jhingran A, Bodurka DC, et al: Correlation of smoking history and other patient characteristics with major complications of pelvic radiation therapy for cervical cancer. J Clin Oncol 2002;20:3651-3657.

82. Kucera H, Enzelsberger H, Eppel W, et al: The influence of nicotine abuse and diabetes mellitus on the results of primary irradiation in the treatment of carcinoma of the cervix. Cancer 1987;60:1-4.

83. Potish RA: Importance of predisposing factors in the development of enteric damage. Am J Clin Oncol 1982;5:189-194.

84. Willett CG, Ooi CJ, Zietman AL, et al: Acute and late toxicity of patients with inflammatory bowel disease undergoing irradiation for abdominal and pelvic neoplasms. Int J Radiat Oncol Biol Phys 2000;46:995-998.

85. Perez CA, Breaux S, Bedwinek JM, et al: Radiation therapy alone in the treatment of carcinoma of the uterine cervix. II: Analysis of complications. Cancer 1984;54:235-246.

86. Schover LR, Fife M, Gershenson DM: Sexual dysfunction and treatment for early stage cervical cancer. Cancer 1989;63:204-212.

87. Bruner DW, Lanciano R, Keegan M, et al: Vaginal stenosis and sexual function following intracavitary radiation for the treatment of cervical and endometrial carcinoma. Int J Radiat Oncol Biol Phys 1993;27:825-830.

88. Flay LD, Matthews JH: The effects of radiotherapy and surgery on the sexual function of women treated for cervical cancer. Int J Radiat Oncol Biol Phys 1995;31:399-404.

89. Corney RH, Crowther ME, Everett H, et al: Psychosexual dysfunction in women with gynaecological cancer following radical pelvic surgery. Br J Obstet Gynaecol 1993;100:73-78.

90. Bergmark K, Avall-Lundqvist E, Dickman PW, et al: Vaginal changes and sexuality in women with a history of cervical cancer. N Engl J Med 1999;340:1383-1389.

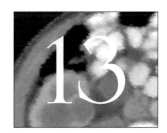

LOCALLY ADVANCED
CERVICAL CANCER

Wui-Jin Koh   and   Peter G. Rose

 MAJOR CONTROVERSIES

- **How should locally advanced cervical cancer be defined?**
- **Is a clinical staging system appropriate?**
- **What is the role of surgical staging?**
- **Have there been improvements in radiation therapy?**
- **Is there a role for routine extended field radiation in this patient population?**
- **Is there a difference between high-dose-rate and low-dose-rate brachytherapy?**
- **Is there a benefit to hyperfractionation?**
- **What is the impact of anemia and tumor hypoxia?**

The publication of five prospective randomized clinical trials in the United States has established the role of concurrent cisplatin-based chemotherapy and radiation for the majority of cervical cancer cases for which radiotherapy is indicated.[1-5] Although the studies had different eligibility criteria, three were specific to patients with locally advanced cervical cancer.[3-5] The dramatic 30% to 50% reduction in the relative risk of death in the five trials prompted a clinical announcement from the National Cancer Institute in February, 1999, which stated that "strong consideration should be given to the incorporation of concurrent cisplatin-based chemotherapy with radiation therapy in women who require radiation therapy for treatment of cervical cancer."[6]

Although this paradigm shift to concurrent chemoradiation represents perhaps the most significant advance in treatment-specific outcome for locally advanced disease over the past 2 decades, there remain areas of ongoing controversy. Issues that require further clarification in the management of locally advanced cervical cancer relate to staging; radiation design and delivery; incorporation of novel

treatment systems; the impact of anemia; optimal combinations of surgery, radiation, and chemotherapy; and post-therapy surveillance recommendations.

How should locally advanced cervical cancer be defined?

The definition of locally advanced cervical cancer is primarily a functional one. It has historically been most useful in determining treatment options or, more specifically, in selecting patients who are not considered candidates for primary surgical management alone. Most practitioners would consider patients with International Federation of Gynaecologists and Obstetricians (FIGO) stage IIb to IVa disease to be included in this category. Either surgery or radiation therapy can be used for the management of stage Ib and IIa cervical cancer, with similar-appearing results. However, significant selection bias exists in determining who is selected for surgery or radiation therapy.[7] Because of controversy regarding the appropriate management of early-stage disease, Landoni and

175

colleagues[8] performed a randomized study of radical surgery versus radiotherapy for stage Ib-IIa cervical cancer. They found no difference in overall or disease-free survival. However, 84% (46/55) of patients with bulky tumors in the surgery group received adjuvant radiation for additional risk factors.

Should patients with Ib2 or IIa disease be uniformly considered candidates for radical hysterectomy, or is there a size threshold beyond which primary surgery would not be advocated? What about the extent of vaginal involvement and adequacy of surgical resection? It has long been recognized that, among tumors limited to the cervix, tumor size is predictive of nodal involvement and survival.[9] Although opinion regarding the appropriate treatment has varied widely, the designation by FIGO of stage Ib1 and Ib2 in 1994 established criteria differentiating the clinical management of smaller versus larger gross cervical tumors limited to the cervix.[10] Finan and colleagues,[11] retrospectively applying the FIGO 1994 definition, reported that patients with stage Ib2 cervical cancer had a significantly higher incidence of nodal metastasis (21% versus 44%) and poorer survival (73% versus 90%) after radical hysterectomy than did patients with stage Ib1, despite the more frequent use of postoperative radiation therapy in the former group (38% versus 72%). Similarly, Trattner and associates[12] found that patients with stage Ib1 cervical cancer had an overall survival rate of 90% at 5 years, compared with 40% for those with stage Ib2 disease. The ideal treatment of stage Ib2 cervical cancer remains controversial, because only limited randomized prospective data are available.

In view of these poor results, a variety of treatment options for this group of patients have been used, including radical hysterectomy followed by radiation or chemoradiation, radiation or chemoradiation followed by routine or selective hysterectomy, neoadjuvant chemotherapy followed by surgery with or without postoperative radiation, and chemoradiation alone. It may be helpful to remember that, for stage Ib2 tumors, two or more modalities for treatment are usually necessary for effective treatment.[13]

The Gynecologic Oncology Group (GOG)[14] has completed a trial comparing radical hysterectomy with or without neoadjuvant chemotherapy. Although the data on progression-free and overall survival are immature, 94% of the patients would warrant postoperative radiation therapy, according to the presence of high or intermediate risk factors found on surgical pathologic analysis. The European Organization of Research and Treatment of Cancer (EORTC) is conducting a randomized trial of neoadjuvant chemotherapy followed by radical surgery versus chemoradiation. The GOG[15,16] is about to initiate a trial comparing radical hysterectomy and tailored radiation therapy versus chemoradiation in stage Ib2 carcinoma of the cervix.

Is a clinical staging system appropriate?

FIGO maintains a clinical staging classification for cervical cancer. This creates a paradox in that assigned FIGO stages, by themselves, may not be well correlated with outcome. In addition to FIGO stage, other clinical factors that are highly significant prognostic factors include lymph node status and tumor size or volume. Furthermore, although it is not mandated by FIGO, contemporary radiation treatment planning for the treatment of cervical cancer in many cases depends heavily on modern imaging technology.

Magnetic resonance imaging (MRI) has been used to assess the extent of cervical stromal, parametrial, and vaginal invasion. The anteroposterior tumor diameter and pelvic lymph node status assessed by MRI are significant prognostic factors in uterine cervical cancer treated with radiation. Compared with computed tomography (CT), MRI is more sensitive in detecting local (i.e., stromal, parametrial, and vaginal) involvement. However, MRI has a similar accuracy to CT for detecting nodal metastases.[17-20] Toita and coworkers[21] reported accurate identification of prognostic factors using MRI to assess local tumor extent and nodal metastasis in 44 patients with cervical cancer treated with radiation therapy.

The American College of Radiology Imaging Network (ACRIN), in conjunction with the GOG,[22] has completed accrual to a prospective study of CT, MRI, and pathologic findings at radical hysterectomy for patients with stage Ib cervical cancer.

Serial MRI examinations before, during, and after radiation therapy have been shown to predict tumor response in cervical cancer.[23] MRI measurement of the tumor regression rate at the midpoint of radiation treatment (45 to 50 Gy) was found to be best for prediction of both local control (fast rate, 84%, versus slow rate, 22%; $P < .0001$) and disease-free survival (63% versus 20%, respectively; $P = .0005$).

Lymphangiography has an increased sensitivity and specificity for nodal metastasis, but its use is uncommon.[24]

Radiologic imaging has provided provocative information predictive of outcome, especially functional imaging.[23,25] This may allow for the selection of patients for less aggressive treatment.[26]

In a retrospective study of GOG data by Stehman and colleagues,[27] the status of the para-aortic lymph nodes at surgical staging was the most significant prognostic factor affecting survival. Among various stages of locally advanced cervical cancer (IIb through IVa), the likelihood of para-aortic nodal metastasis ranges from 19% to 30%. However, in many patients para-aortic nodal metastases are not detected by CT scan. In a prospective study by the GOG, only 34% of patients with para-aortic nodal metastasis were identified by CT.[28] MRI yields a sensitivity very similar to that of CT for para-aortic nodal metastasis.[18-21] Positron emission tomography (PET) is a metabolism-based imaging process that is increasingly used in the effective staging of multiple cancer sites. PET imaging with fluorodeoxyglucose (FDG) has a high avidity for primary cervical tumors, and preliminary experience in cervical cancer has shown improved sensitivity and specificity for the detection of nodal metastases, compared with other imaging modalities (Fig. 13-1). In patients who have undergone surgical staging, the specificity for the positive PET scan in the pelvic nodes

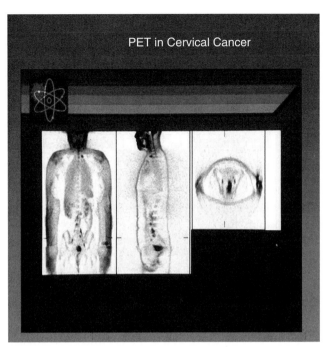

Figure 13–1. Positron emission tomography in cervical cancer. In frontal saggital and cross-sectional views increased radioactivity is seen in the cervix and pelvic, para-aortic and scalene lymph nodes.

has been 90% to 100%. Reinhardt and associates[25] compared the results of MRI and PET for detecting pelvic nodal metastasis in cervical cancer and found that PET had a statistically greater sensitivity (90% versus 64%, $P < .05$).[29]

Among 148 patients with locally advanced cervical cancer who had normal para-aortic nodal anatomy by CT scan or MRI and underwent PET imaging before surgical staging lymphadenectomy, PET had a sensitivity of 78% for detection of para-aortic nodal disease[30-33] (Table 13-1). Park and coworkers[34] correlated cervical cancer nodal tumor size with PET uptake: 67% of nodes larger than 5 mm were detected, as were 80% of nodes larger than 10 mm. The nodal tumors that were missed were most often smaller than 1 cm or microscopic. Grigsby and colleagues[35] performed CT and PET scans on 101 patients before radiation therapy. The survival rate after pelvic radiation therapy for patients with FDG para-aortic nodal uptake (PET+) and normal para-aortic nodal anatomy by CT scanning (CT–) was identical to that for patients who had PET+ and abnormal para-aortic nodal anatomy by CT (CT+) (Fig. 13-2). This finding further confirmed the increased sensitivity of PET for para-aortic nodal

metastasis. Patients who had no suggestion of nodal metastasis on either CT or PET had the best outcome. Although additional studies are needed, it is clear that patients with PET+ nodes have disease in that region. PET may miss small-volume or microscopic nodal metastases.[34] Further studies are needed to determine the sensitivity of PET for detecting small-volume microscopic disease, because patients with this type of metastasis are the population most likely to benefit from the use of extended field radiation therapy with concurrent chemotherapy.

To further evaluate the clinical utility of PET, the GOG is developing a prospective multi-institutional trial of preoperative PET imaging followed by complete pelvic and para-aortic lymphadenectomy in patients with locally advanced disease.

What is the role of surgical staging?

As mentioned previously, the status of the para-aortic nodes in surgical staging is the most significant prognostic factor in survival. In view of the low sensitivity (34%) of CT for para-aortic nodal metastasis, the majority of patients (66%) who have para-aortic nodal metastases are not detected by this modality. Although encouraging data exist for PET, currently Medicare has not approved PET imaging for this use. Furthermore, regardless of improvements in technology, it is apparent that external imaging modalities have a disease volume threshold below which detectability is not feasible. Clearly, there is at present no external imaging modality that allows identification of microscopic tumor deposits. This leaves only surgical staging as an effective method of identifying extrapelvic disease not revealed by CT.

There are two potential benefits to surgical staging. The first is that it permits identification of nodal disease extent, to more accurately guide radiotherapy design and delivery. Numerous authors have reported modification of the radiation field in 18% to 43% of surgically staged patients.[36-38] Another benefit of surgical staging is the ability to debulk grossly positive nodes, some of which are not detected on conventional CT imaging.[39,40] Surgical staging through paramedian retroperitoneal approaches is associated with significantly less radiation morbidity than the transperitoneal approach[41] and does not appear to increase the risk beyond radiation therapy alone. An alternative transverse abdominal retroperitoneal approach was described by Gallup and coworkers.[42] Laparoscopic

Table 13–1. Detection of Para-aortic Nodal Metastasis in Cervical Cancer by Positron Emission Tomography (PET)

Reference, Journal, and Year	N	No. Positive by PET	No. Positive by Pathology	Sensitivity (%)
Rose et al.[30] (J Clin Oncol, 1999)	32	6	8	75
Naranyan et al.[31] (Int J Gynecol Cancer, 2001)	24	4	7	57
Yeh et al.[32] (Oncol Rep, 2002)	42	10	12	83
Lin et al.[33] (Gynecol Oncol, 2003)	50	12	14	86
Total	148	32	41	78

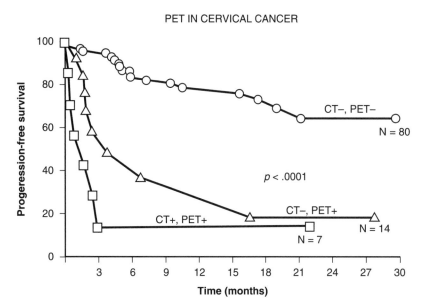

PET IN CERVICAL CANCER

Figure 13-2. Progression-free survival in 101 patients (87 with stage Ib2-IVa) treated with radiation and chemotherapy, based on findings from computed tomography (CT) and positron emission tomography (PET). (From Grigsby PW, Siegel BA, Dehdashti F: Lymph node staging by positron emission tomography in patients with carcinoma of the cervix. J Clin Oncol 2001; 19:3745-3749.)

retroperitoneal approaches have also been studied, with acceptable radiation morbidity.[43] Laparoscopic lymphadenectomy followed by immediate laparotomy demonstrated a false-negative rate of 0% among 12 patients.[44] In a series of 84 patients, nodal metastasis was found in 38.[45] CT scans were available for review in 49 patients, and nodal metastases were surgically detected in 18 of 38 patients with normal CT scans. However, isolated port site recurrences have been identified with this technique.[46]

Retrospective studies have demonstrated that the outcome for patients whose macroscopic nodal disease was resected and that for patients with microscopic nodal disease is similar.[39,40] Patients with macroscopic disease that was resected fared considerably better than those with macroscopic disease that was not resected. Holcolmb and colleagues[34] reported on 274 women with cervical cancer, stages IIb to IVa, treated with primary radiotherapy.[38] Eighty-nine patients who underwent pretreatment staging laparotomy (group 1) were compared with 172 patients who underwent clinical staging (group 2). Para-aortic metastases were detected in 12.3% and intra-abdominal metastases in 4.5% of the patients in group 1. Extended field radiotherapy or systemic chemotherapy or both were given to these patients. The median survival time of patients in group 1 was statistically longer than that of patients in group 2 (29 versus 19 months, P = .01). Multivariate analysis controlling for both stage and age showed that pretreatment staging laparotomy was a significant predictor of survival (P = .03).

Others have argued that the benefits of surgical staging, if any, are minimal.[47] Using a model that employed stage, incidence of para-aortic lymph nodes, and ultimate curability by extended field radiotherapy when para-aortic nodal disease was detected, Petereit and colleagues[48] estimated a potential maximal survival advantage of 6% if routine surgical retroperitoneal node evaluation is performed for all stage and

IIb patients (Fig. 13-3). In a separate study, employing a model of nodal control by radiation and the likelihood of cure by nodal status based on ultimate patterns of failure, Kupets and associates[49] estimated a 1% to 4% maximal improvement in survival for patients who undergo aggressive surgical debulking for nodes 2 cm in diameter or larger (Fig. 13-4). However, this study assumed that patients with failure at distant sites would not have benefited from aggressive pelvic therapy. This assumption is opposed by the Radiation Therapy Oncology Group (RTOG) study of Morris and colleagues,[3] in which patients receiving pelvic radiation therapy and concurrent chemotherapy had not only improved local control but fewer distant recurrences. The former study also failed to evaluate the benefit of extending the radiation field to include para-aortic nodal disease, which would have been expected in 19% to 30% of patients.

An issue that has not been addressed in cervical cancer is the dose of radiotherapy required to control microscopic disease after surgery. It has often been stated that a dose of 45 to 50 Gy is required to control microscopic disease in most cases—however, this is in the surgically undisturbed bed. Postoperative adjuvant pelvic irradiation for high-risk factors after radical hysterectomy, when there is no gross residual disease in the pelvis, leads to only a 50% relative decrease in the pelvic relapse rate.[50-52] Tumor bed hypoxia and accelerated repopulation of any surviving clonogenic cells have been implicated as causes for the decrement in radiation effectiveness.

In head and neck cancer, a randomized trial showed that optimal locoregional control after primary surgery, in patients with completely resected nodal disease, required doses greater than 57 Gy. Among patients with extracapsular nodal extension higher doses (>63 Gy) were required for optimal in-field control.[53] Finally, any putative advantage to surgical staging must be balanced against the delay in radiation therapy as well

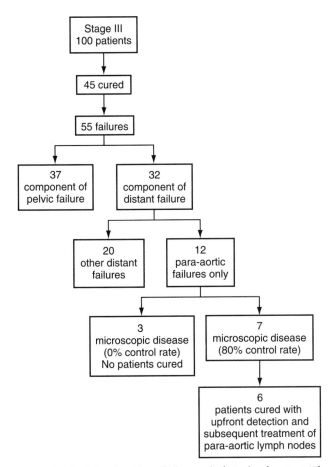

Figure 13–3. Estimate of benefit for surgical staging for stage IIIb cervical cancer. (From Fowler et al. Petereit DG, Hartenbach EM, Thomas GM: Para-aortic lymph node evaluation in cervical cancer: The impact of staging upon treatment decisions and outcome. Int J Gynecol Cancer 1998;8:353–364.)

as the potential for added surgical morbidity. Although the relative benefit of surgical staging can be argued, it must be remembered that cervical cancer affects a younger patient population than any other adult female cancer. Furthermore, extended field radiation with concurrent chemotherapy has been demonstrated to be acceptably tolerable and may be more effective. Finally, because recurrent disease is uniformly fatal, inability to identify and eradicate early metastatic para-aortic disease initially will almost uniformly result in the patient's death.

Have there been improvements in radiation therapy?

CT imaging is already basic to most radiation treatment planning and dosimetry calculation systems. Image fusion will provide better target volume definition. Intensity-modulated radiation therapy (IMRT) represents an exciting new technology in radiotherapy delivery that combines high-resolution imaging, advances in computer treatment software and linear accelerator collimation capabilities, "inverse" planning, and radiation beam flux modulation to produce highly conformal dose distributions that are unachievable with conventional approaches. It has been most widely employed in head and neck and prostate cancers, simultaneously allowing sparing of surrounding normal structures and dose intensification to the tumor target volume. Dosimetric evaluation of its use in gynecologic cancers has shown that IMRT can significantly reduce unwanted radiation exposure to adjacent bowel and bladder while preserving tumor coverage.[54] A pilot clinical experience at the University of Chicago demonstrated significant reduction in acute gastrointestinal toxicity for gynecologic cancer patients undergoing pelvic IMRT, compared with "contemporaneous" historical controls treated with traditional standard techniques.[55] Analysis has also indicated a decrease in chronic gastrointestinal toxicity, as well as acute hematologic suppression, favoring patients treated with IMRT, especially those who also received chemotherapy.[56]

Although there is little doubt that IMRT will gain increasingly widespread clinical application based on its dosimetric superiority over current conventional approaches, questions remain about target definition standardization, intrapatient and interpatient reproducibility, and time-intensive requirements for treatment planning. To implement IMRT for cervical cancer, a paradigm shift in delineation of target volume is required—from historical dependence on bony landmarks to the definition of specific targets based primarily on soft tissue anatomy. However, use of retroperitoneal staging with soft tissue anatomy markers has demonstrated that the traditional bony landmarks do not accurately reflect soft tissue anatomy, owing to significant interpatient variability. The traditional uniformity of pelvic radiation for cervical cancer is modified to direct dose asymmetrically, based on tumor volume distribution. The need for high-resolution imaging, including image fusion technologies, is essential to the accurate definition of target and normal tissue volumes for IMRT.

The need for standardization and target definition in IMRT, especially for clinical trials, has been discussed by the GOG. The radiation oncology committee is seeking to evaluate and establish parameters that are readily and reproducibly applied. An opportunity for "real-time" assessment of individual patient treatment plans lies in "central review," facilitated by electronic submission over the Internet using currently available digital imaging and communication in medicine—radiation therapy (DICOM-RT) data transfer programs.

The role of brachytherapy in cervical cancer is well established. However, historical application of brachytherapy has generally depended on achieving symmetry of insertion relative to the central position of the uterus within the pelvis, thereby creating the classic "pear-shaped" isodose distribution. Although in its infancy, the role of image-guided brachytherapy, in which isodoses are biased toward residual tumor volume, rather than simple central symmetry, should be further assessed.

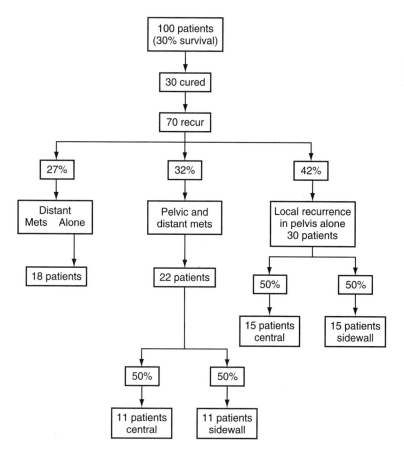

Figure 13–4. Algorithm for cure and recurrence in patients with stage III cervical cancer with positive pelvic lymph nodes. (From Kupets R, Thomas GM, Coverns A: Is there a role for pelvic lymph node debulking in advanced cervical cancer? Gynecol Oncol 2002;87:163-170.)

Is there a role for routine extended field radiation in this patient population?

RTOG 79-20, a randomized trial, demonstrated improved survival for patients with stage IIb and bulky Ib/IIa cervical cancer who received prophylactic para-aortic radiation, compared with pelvic radiation alone. Patients undergoing extended field radiotherapy (which included the para-aortic nodes) had a 10-year overall survival rate of 55%, compared with 44% for those who received treatment to the pelvis only (P = .02).[57] However, a more recent study (RTOG 90-01) showed superiority of concurrent cisplatin/5-FU chemotherapy and pelvic irradiation over the control arm of extended field radiotherapy without chemotherapy, with 5-year overall survival rates of 73% and 58%, respectively (P = .004).[3] Unanswered is the question of whether further therapeutic gain can be achieved by using concurrent chemotherapy and prophylactic para-aortic irradiation in patients with locally advanced cervical cancer. Alternatively, the extension of the para-aortic field may be selectively applied (e.g., in patients with clinically pelvic-confined disease but with multiple pelvic lymph node metastases). The tolerability of concomitant extended field irradiation and cisplatin-based chemotherapy has been reported.[58,59] A randomized trial comparing pelvic versus extended field irradiation in patients with cervical cancer clinically confined to the pelvis (concurrent with weekly cisplatin in both arms) has

been proposed through the GOG but has not been activated at this time.

Underlying the question of prophylactic para-aortic radiation is the assumption that the para-aortic nodes represent the only site of occult extrapelvic disease in some patients, for whom sterilization by radiotherapy would translate to cure (assuming achievable pelvic control). In the absence of routine surgical staging, the incidence of para-aortic nodal metastases is clearly underestimated by routine imaging such as CT or MRI. Because the para-aortic nodes are a "clinically silent site," the rate of failure there as the first site of treatment relapse after pelvic radiation is also undetermined. A GOG surgicopathologic staging study noted positive para-aortic nodes in 21% of stage IIb and 31% of stage III tumors.[28] However, PET imaging demonstrated para-aortic lymphadenopathy in 21% of 101 consecutive patients with cervical cancer cases (stage I through IVa).[35] If PET, or a combination of imaging modalities, can achieve extremely high sensitivity for the detection of small-volume para-aortic metastases and become widely used, the issue of radiation prophylaxis to the para-aortic nodes may become inconsequential. However, currently PET imaging, although more sensitive than CT, has a false-negative rate of 33% for nodal metastasis measuring 0.5 to 1.0 cm.[34]

It is recognized that cervical cancer spreads in a very predictable manner, from the cervix to the pelvic nodes and then to the para-aortic nodes. Furthermore, retrospective reports of para-aortic irradiation have demonstrated improved survival for patients with microscopic versus macroscopic nodal disease (46% versus 21%, respectively).[60,61] This is probably related not only to poorer local control but to the preexisting metastatic disease. Specifically, the use of scalene nodal biopsy in patients with gross para-aortic nodal disease has confirmed malignant scalene nodes in 27%.[62] Although routine scalene nodal biopsy may not be of therapeutic benefit, potential inclusion of these patients into trials of extended field radiation therapy must be recognized as one possible explanation of the potential failure of prophylactic irradiation. Alternatively, because PET imaging has a high sensitivity for macroscopic nodal metastasis but lower sensitivity for microscopic nodal metastasis, prophylactic para-aortic radiation could be used for patients with positive pelvic nodes and negative para-aortic nodes. Patients with no pelvic nodal metastasis could be treated with pelvic radiation alone, because they would at most have microscopic disease in the pelvic nodes.

Is there a difference between high-dose-rate and low-dose-rate brachytherapy?

High-dose-rate brachytherapy has been proposed as an alternative to low-dose-rate brachytherapy for the management of cervical cancer. However, most patients (85% to 88%) are still being treated effectively by low-dose-rate brachytherapy.[63,64] Throughout the world, high-dose-rate brachytherapy has become increasingly popular because it avoids hospitalization, hospital personal exposure to radiation, and prolonged patient immobilization, thereby decreasing the risk of venous thrombosis and its complications. High-dose-rate therapy, as initially used as a substitute for low-dose-rate radiation at identical total doses, was associated with a significant increase in late radiation complications.[65] However, the biologic effective dose of high-dose-rate radiation is greater, and only a fraction (0.54 to 0.6) of the low-dose-rate dose should be applied.[66-68] Greater appreciation for the biologic effective dose has led to lower dose fractions at more frequent intervals, with a lower total dose delivered. Five randomized studies have been performed and demonstrated no difference in outcome, but the studies are flawed.[68-72]

Eifel[73] criticized high-dose-rate therapy because of its narrower therapeutic index, which is more critical for advanced-stage disease, for which the dose must be maximized to effect local control. Petereit and associates[74] from the University of Wisconsin reported a poorer outcome in stage III disease with high-dose-rate therapy, compared with their historical controls. However, this may have been the result of differences in clinical staging by different gynecologic oncologists. Multiple single-institutional experiences suggest general equivalency. Lorvidhaya and Tonusin[75] reported the largest single institutional experience, involving almost 2000 patients from Thailand. In their institution, patients received whole pelvic radiation to a dose of 30 to 50 Gy, with higher pelvic doses for more advanced stages of disease. This was followed by high-dose-rate

therapy at a dose of 6 to 7.5 Gy per application for four to six applications. The investigators reported stage-specific survival and complication rates that were similar to the published experience with low-dose-rate brachytherapy.

GOG and RTOG have accepted the equivalency of high- and low-dose-rate brachytherapy with carefully designed guidelines for use.[76] Both approaches are acceptable if the practitioner is well-trained, careful, and respectful of the potential and limitations of each.

Is there a benefit to hyperfractionation?

Although theoretic benefit does exist with the use of multifractionated irradiation, there is no clinical data to support its benefit in gynecologic cancers. In a phase II study by MacLeod and associates,[77] 61 patients received hyperfractionated radiation therapy for stage IIb to IV cervical cancer. Although 85% completed therapy without treatment breaks, there was one acute treatment-related death. Most concerning was a late toxicity rate of 27%. Additionally, five patients required total hip replacement. Two studies by the GOG used accelerated fractionation with concurrent chemotherapy consisting of either hydroxyurea or cisplatin and 5-FU. These studies, reported by Calkins and coworkers,[78] demonstrated increased morbidity without apparent improvement in cure. In a study by the RTOG of extended field hyperfractionated irradiation with concurrent cisplatin and 5-FU, grade 4 chronic toxicity occurred in 17%.[79] Lastly, the amount of time required for twice-daily fraction therapy is significantly longer; often there is a 6-hour break given between fractions. This converts a 20-minute visit into a 6- to 8-hour session. Compliance with radiation treatment is a major factor for cervical cancer patients. This increased time burden would probably result in significantly less compliance.

Based on the experience in head and neck cancer, there may be a benefit to a concurrent involved-field boost for localized bulky disease/adenopathy.[80]

Hyperthermia

Hyperthermia during concurrent chemotherapy and radiotherapy has been used in locally advanced cervical cancer. van der Zee and colleagues[81] performed a prospective randomized study comparing hyperthermia and standard radiation therapy with radiation therapy alone for locally advanced cervical cancer (stage IIb-IVa). The addition of hyperthermia significantly improved disease-free survival and overall survival at 3 years (51%, versus 27% for radiation alone). The addition of hyperthermia almost doubled the low survival rate of radiation alone. Hyperthermia during concurrent chemotherapy and radiotherapy has been used in locally advanced cervical cancer.[82] Additional studies are needed to determine whether these improvements in survival can be replicated and what improvements over chemoradiation can be achieved.

What is the impact of anemia and tumor hypoxia?

The adverse impact of anemia on outcome after primary radiotherapy for cervical cancer has been well documented in many clinical reviews. The mechanisms underlying this correlation are unclear but may be linked to tumor hypoxia and consequent radioresistance, as well as induction of angiogenesis, increased tumor aggressiveness, and enhanced metastatic potential. A large Canadian multicenter retrospective analysis provided convincing evidence that anemia is an independent negative prognostic factor in cervical cancer.[83] The study found that the average hemoglobin (Hgb) during radiotherapy was more predictive of poor outcome than the pretherapy Hgb was. The adverse impact of anemia during radiotherapy was large, second only to tumor stage in prognostic significance on multivariate analysis. The magnitude of the decrement in survival for anemic compared with nonanemic patients exceeded the expected gain from concurrent chemoradiation strategies. The most provocative suggestion of the Canadian study was that correction of anemia (by transfusion, to a Hgb level of 12 g/dL) abrogated the adverse impact of preexisting anemia.[83] These findings were echoed by another retrospective report from Australia and Austria in which patients received concurrent chemoradiation, although a different threshold Hgb level (11 g/dL) for poor outcome was found.[84] The influence of anemia in masking the potential synergistic benefit of concurrent cisplatin and radiation has even been advanced to explain the negative results of a randomized trial.[85] In evaluating a chemoradiation trial by the GOG, Winter and associates[86] demonstrated that anemia was associated with numerous clinical factors, including nonwhite race, poor performance status, stage III and IV disease, tumor size greater than 4 cm, and protracted radiation (>60 days). Although each of these clinical factors may have adversely affected outcome, a statistical difference in survival was noted for the average weekly nadir hemoglobin levels (AWNH). When separated by clinical stage, patients with AWNH levels of 12 gm/dL survived significantly longer than patients with AWNH levels of 10 gm/dL. However, others have failed to demonstrate a therapeutic benefit to transfusion.[87]

Despite the potential prognostic and therapeutic implications of anemia in cervical cancer, only one small prospective randomized trial directly addressing this issue has been completed, about 3 decades ago. This study indicated improved pelvic control for irradiated patients whose hemoglobin level was corrected by transfusion, but it was hampered by limited patient numbers and lack of stratification.[88] In an attempt to provide definitive answers, the GOG has initiated a prospective multicenter, multinational phase III trial (GOG protocol 0191), in which patients with locally advanced cervical cancer undergoing primary chemoradiation (radiotherapy with concurrent weekly cisplatin at 40 mg/m^2) are randomly assigned to Hgb maintenance at a level of 10 g/dL versus aggressive intervention to raise the Hgb level to 12 g/dL

(by transfusion and erythropoietin). To further elucidate the mechanisms by which anemia may exert its negative effect, correlative translation studies are planned. These include tumor assays of vascular endothelial growth factor (VEGF, a proangiogenic agent), thrombospondin-1 (TSP-1, an angiogenic inhibitor), TP53, CD31 (an endothelial cell surface protein), and carbonic anhydrase IX (CA-IX, a marker for hypoxia). However, this study was closed after an increased incidence of thromo-embolic events were noted with erythropoietin therapy.

Tumor hypoxia, as measured by oxygen electrodes, has been identified in many cervical cancers and is a predictor of poor outcome.[89,90] As noted earlier, there may be a link, but the relationship between anemia and tumor hypoxia remains ambiguous. Regardless of the relationship between these two measures, studies have identified significant modulation of gene expression in hypoxic tumors that may be associated with tumor aggressiveness and progression, including hypoxia inducible factor-1 (HIF-1), TP53, VEGF, platelet-derived endothelial cell growth factor (PDECGF), nitric oxide synthase (NOS), and matrix metalloproteinase (MMP).[91] These provide potential new targets for future therapeutic interventions.

Chemotherapy and Radiation

Choice and schedule. The optimal concurrent chemotherapy regimen is controversial and was debated at the GOG 2003 summer conference. From randomized trials, it can be concluded that cisplatin, either alone or with 5-FU, is superior to hydroxyurea[4,5]; that cisplatin alone is less toxic than cisplatin/5-FU/hydroxyurea[5]; and that cisplatin is superior to 5-FU infusion.[92] Weekly cisplatin meets certain goals as the ideal chemotherapy regimen, including high antitumor activity, acceptable tolerance with concurrent radiation, lower cost, and demonstration of a survival benefit in randomized trials.[92] In a meta-analysis evaluating randomized trials of chemoradiation, a significant improvement in the hazard ratio was seen only for platinum-containing chemotherapy regimens.[93]

Lorvidhaya and colleagues[94] reported on a four-arm, randomized trial comparing radiation; radiation with adjuvant chemotherapy; radiation with concurrent chemotherapy; and radiation with concurrent and adjuvant chemotherapy. The concurrent chemotherapy was mitomycin-C on days 1 and 29 and oral 5-FU on days 1 through 14 and 29 through 42. Adjuvant chemotherapy consisted of three courses of oral 5-FU for 4 weeks, with a 2-week break. The concurrent chemotherapy arm had significantly improved rates of local control and survival. Although other agents, including mitomycin-C and epirubicin, have demonstrated activity with concurrent radiation, their efficacy relative to platinum compounds has not been evaluated. In addition, mitomycin-C was previously abandoned as a radiation sensitizer in North American studies because of a threefold increase in late intestinal complications.[95] Additional agents under study in combination with cisplatin include paclitaxel, topotecan, gemcitabine, and tirapazamine.[96,97] For each of these agents, combination with cisplatin is tolerated and in some cases of metastatic disease is apparently more active. Pattaranutaporn and associates[98] studied the use of pelvic radiation therapy with gemcitabine 300 mg/m^2 weekly, reporting a 90% response rate. A randomized trial comparing weekly cisplatin with weekly cisplatin/gemcitabine before radical hysterectomy demonstrated a higher pathologic response rate in patients treated with the cisplatin/gemcitabine combination.[99]

Biologic agents are also of interest for treatment of locally advanced disease. Cervical cancer frequently expresses the epidermal growth factor receptor EGF-R. The GOG has approved a trial of C-225 and weekly cisplatin as a concurrent radiation sensitizer. The RTOG is currently studying the antiangiogenic effect of the cyclooxygenase-2 (COX-2) inhibitor Celebrex in combination with cisplatin and 5-FU infusion during radiation therapy.

Neoadjuvant strategies. Although neoadjuvant chemotherapy followed by radiation therapy has failed, both in individual studies and in a meta-analysis, to improve the outcome of locally advanced cervical cancer, its role in combination with surgery has not been conclusively determined.[100] Sardi and coworkers[101] performed a randomized trial in which patients with cervical cancer larger than 2 cm were randomly assigned to cisplatin-based neoadjuvant chemotherapy, radical hysterectomy, and radiation therapy versus radical hysterectomy and radiation therapy. The use of neoadjuvant chemotherapy increased tumor resectability and resulted in an improved long-term survival advantage. Conflicting results were reported in a very similarly designed trial by Chang and associates.[102] The largest trial to date was a multicentered Italian trial reported by Benedetti-Panici and colleagues.[103] This trial demonstrated the superiority of neoadjuvant chemotherapy plus radical hysterectomy versus radiation therapy alone. However, the dose of radiation used in the control arm was suboptimal (70 Gy), and radiation-sensitizing cisplatin chemotherapy, the new standard, was not used. To address these issues, the EORTC is conducting a randomized trial of neoadjuvant chemotherapy plus radical hysterectomy versus cisplatin chemoradiation for patients with stage IB$_2$ disease.[15] A meta-analysis by Tierney and colleagues[100] suggests that neoadjuvant chemotherapy plus radical hysterectomy is an acceptable treatment for this disease extent. Whether these findings will hold up against optimal radiation needs to be determined.

No benefit has been shown for neoadjuvant chemotherapy preceding definitive radiotherapy. Indeed, in some trials, despite a high initial response rate and even an appreciable complete response rate to neoadjuvant chemotherapy, a worse survival outcome was noted for radiotherapy after chemotherapy compared with radiation alone.[104,105] Underlying this observation may be the process of accelerated repopulation—a "leaner but meaner" tumor that is reduced in overall size but has an increased number of clonogens within the tumor and a decreased overall potential tumor doubling time. The impact of accelerated repopulation is critical in a modality that is dependent on time and cell kinetics, such as radiation (and also chemotherapy), but perhaps not as important in surgery. In surgery, if the tumor is smaller and more readily resectable, the rate of cell doubling may be inconsequential provided the tumor can be removed in whole. This may explain the difference in outcomes seen with neoadjuvant chemotherapy strategies before radiotherapy versus surgery.

Conclusion

Significant advances in the evaluation and management of locally advanced cervical cancer (stage IIb to IVa) have been achieved in the last decade. Although these improvements are currently in practice in developed countries, they must be applied to the underdeveloped countries to have their greatest impact on survival in this disease.

REFERENCES

1. Peters W III, Liu PY, Barrett RJ II, et al: Concurrent chemotherapy and pelvic radiation therapy compared with pelvic radiation therapy alone as adjuvant therapy after radical surgery in high-risk early-stage cancer of the cervix. J Clin Oncol 2000;18:1606-1613.
2. Keys HM, Bundy BN, Stehman FB, et al: Cisplatin, radiation, and adjuvant hysterectomy compared with radiation and adjuvant hysterectomy for bulky stage IB cervical carcinoma. N Engl J Med 1999;340:1154-1161.
3. Morris M, Eifel PJ, Lu J, et al: Pelvic radiation with concurrent chemotherapy compared with pelvic and para-aortic radiation for high-risk cervical cancer. N Engl J Med 1999;340:1137-1143.
4. Whitney CW, Sause W, Bundy BN, et al: Randomized comparison of fluorouracil plus cisplatin versus hydroxyurea as an adjunct to radiation therapy in stage IIB-IVA carcinoma of the cervix with negative para-aortic lymph nodes: A Gynecologic Oncology Group and Southwest Oncology Group study [comment]. J Clin Oncol 1999;17:1339-1348.
5. Rose PG, Bundy BN, Watkins EB, et al: Concurrent cisplatin-based radiotherapy and chemotherapy for locally advanced cervical cancer. N Engl J Med 1999;340:1144-1153.
6. National Cancer Institute: NCI Clinical Announcement. Bethesda, MD: U. S. Dept. of Health and Human Services, Public Health Service, National Institutes of Health, February 1999.
7. Zola P, Volpe T, Castelli G, et al: Is the published literature a reliable guide for deciding between alternative treatments for patients with early cervical cancer? Int J Radiat Oncol Biol Phys 1989;16:785-797.
8. Landoni F, Maneo A, Colombo A, et al: Randomized study of radical surgery versus radiotherapy for stage IB-IIA cervical cancer. Lancet 1997;350:535-540.
9. Piver MS, Chung WS: Prognostic significance of cervical lesion size and pelvic node metastases in cervical carcinoma. Obstet Gynecol 1975;46:507-510.
10. Creasman WT: New gynecologic cancer staging. Gynecol Oncol 1995;58:157-158.
11. Finan MA, DeCesare S, Fiorica JV, et al: Radical hysterectomy for stage IB1 versus IB2 carcinoma of the cervix: Does the new staging system predict morbidity and survival? [comment]. Gynecol Oncol 1996;62:139-147.
12. Trattner M, Graf AH, Lax S, et al: Prognostic factors in surgically treated stage IB-IIB cervical carcinomas with special emphasis on the importance of tumor volume. Gynecol Oncol 2001;82:11-16.

13. O'Malley D, Rose PG: New recommendations for the treatment of bulky stage I and advanced stage cervical cancer with chemoradiation. Postgrad Obstet Gynecol 2003;23:1-8.

14. GOGO141 (1999, March 26). Treatment of patients with suboptimal ("bulky") stage IB carcinoma of the cervix: a randomized comparison of radical hysterectomy and pelvic and para-aortic lymphadenectomy with or without neoadjuvant vincristine and cisplatin chemotherapy (phase III). www.GOG.fccc.edu/cgibin/protocol/all_protocol_info.pl?protocol_id=GOGO141.

15. EORTC (2002, March 19). Randomized phase III study of neoadjuvant chemotherapy followed by surgery vs. concomitant radiotherapy and chemotherapy in FIGO Ib2 > 4 cm or II B cervical cancer. Retrieved from EORTC on www.eortc.be/protoc/details.asp?protocol=55994.

16. GOGO201 (2002, November 4). Treatment of patients with stage IB2 carcinoma of the cervix: a randomized comparison of radical hysterectomy and tailored chemo-radiation versus primary chemo-radiation. Retrieved from GOG on www.GOG.fccc.edu/cgibin/protocol/all_info.pl?protocol_id=GOGO201.

17. Cobby M, Browning J, Jones A, et al: Magnetic resonance imaging, computed tomography and endosonography in the local staging of carcinoma of the cervix. Br J Radiol 1990;63:673-679.

18. Kim SH, Choi BI, Han JK, et al: Preoperative staging of uterine cervical carcinoma: Comparison of CT and MRI in 99 patients. J Comput Assist Tomogr 1993;17:633-640.

19. Subak LL, Hricak H, Powell CB, et al: Cervical carcinoma: Computed tomography and magnetic resonance imaging for preoperative staging. Obstet Gynecol 1995;86:43-50.

20. Oellinger JJ, Blohmer JU, Michniewicz K, et al: Pre-operative staging of cervical cancer: Comparison of magnetic resonance imaging (MRI) and computed tomography (CT) with histologic results. Zentralbl Gynakol 2000;122:82-91.

21. Toita T, Kakinohana Y, Shinzato S, et al: Tumor diameter/volume and pelvic node status assessed by magnetic resonance imaging (MRI) for uterine cervical cancer treated with irradiation. Int J Radiat Oncol Biol Phys 1999;43:777-782.

22. ACRIN6651/GOGO183 (2002, March 15). ACRIN 6651—Role of radiology in the pretreatment evaluation of invasive cervical cancer. Retrieved from GOG on www.GOG.fccc.edu/cgibin/protocol/all_protocol_info.pl?protocol_id=GOGO183.

23. Mayr NA, Taoka T, Yuh WT, et al: Method and timing of tumor volume measurement for outcome prediction in cervical cancer using magnetic resonance imaging. Int J Radiat Oncol Biol Phys 2002;52:14-22.

24. Eifel PJ, Moughan J, Owen J, et al: Patterns of radiotherapy practice for patients with squamous carcinoma of the uterine cervix: Patterns of care study. Int J Radiat Oncol Biol Phys 1999;43:351-358.

25. Hricak H: MRI: Advance in patient care. J Magn Reson Imaging 2000;12:i.

26. Kodaira T, Fuwa N, Toita T, et al: Comparison of prognostic value of MRI and FIGO stage among patients with cervical carcinoma treated with radiography. Int J Radiat Oncol Biol Phys 2003;56:769-777.

27. Stehman FB, Thomas GM: Prognostic factors in locally advanced carcinoma of the cervix treated with radiation therapy. Semin Oncol 1994;21:25-29.

28. Heller PB, Malateno JH, Bundy BN, et al: Clinical-pathologic study of stage IIB, III, and IVA carcinoma of the cervix: Extended diagnostic evaluation for paraaortic node metastasis. A Gynecologic Oncology Group study. Gynecol Oncol 1990;38:425-430.

29. Reinhardt MJ, Ehritt-Braun C, Vogelgesang D, et al: Metastatic lymph nodes in patients with cervical cancer: Detection with MR imaging and FDG PET. Radiology 2001;218:776-782.

30. Rose PG, Adler LP, Rodriguez M, et al: Positron emission tomography for evaluating para-aortic nodal metastasis in locally advanced cervical cancer before surgical staging: A surgicopathologic study. J Clin Oncol 1999;17:41-45.

31. Narayan K, Hicks RJ, Jobling T, et al: A comparison of MRI and PET scanning in surgically staged loco-regionally advanced cervical cancer: Potential impact on treatment. Int J Gynecol Cancer 2001;11:263-271.

32. Yeh LS, Hung YC, Shen YY, et al: Detecting para-aortic lymph nodal metastasis by positron emission tomography of 18F-fluorodeoxyglucose in advanced cervical cancer with negative magnetic resonance imaging findings. Oncol Rep 2002;9:1289-1292.

33. Lin WC, Hung YC, Yeh LS, et al: Usefulness of (18) F-fluorodeoxyglucose positron emission tomography to detect para-aortic lymph nodal metastasis in advanced cervical cancer with negative computed tomography findings. Gynecol Oncol 2003;89:73-76.

34. Park SY, Roh JW, Park YJ, et al: Positron emission tomography (PET) for evaluating para-aortic and pelvic lymph node metastasis in cervical cancer before surgical staging: A surgicopathologic study. Proc Am Soc Clin Oncol 2003;22:456a.

35. Grigsby PW, Siegel BA, Dehdashti F: Lymph node staging by positron emission tomography in patients with carcinoma of the cervix. J Clin Oncol 2001;19:3745-3749.

36. Goff BA, Muntz HG, Paley PJ, et al: Impact of surgical staging in women with locally advanced cervical cancer. Gynecol Oncol 1999;74:436-442.

37. Odunsi KO, Lele S, Ghamande S, et al: The impact of pre-therapy extraperitoneal surgical staging on the evaluation and treatment of patients with locally advanced cervical cancer. Eur J Gynaecol Oncol 2001;22:325-330.

38. Holcomb K, Abulafia O, Matthews RP, et al: The impact of pre-treatment staging laparotomy on survival in locally advanced cervical carcinoma. Eur J Gynaecol Oncol 1999; 20:90-93.

39. Cosin JA, Fowler JM, Chen MD, et al: Pretreatment surgical staging of patients with cervical carcinoma: The case for lymph node debulking. Cancer 1998;82:2241-2248.

40. Hacker NF, Wain GV, Nicklin JL: Resection of bulky positive lymph nodes in patients with cervical carcinoma. Int J Gynecol Cancer 1995;5:250-256.

41. Weiser EB, Bundy BN, Hoskins WJ, et al: Extraperitoneal versus transperitoneal selective paraaortic lymphadenectomy in the pretreatment surgical staging of advanced cervical carcinoma: A Gynecologic Oncology Group study. Gynecol Oncol 1989;33:283-289.

42. Gallup DG, King LA, Messing MJ, Talledo OE: Paraaortic lymph node sampling by means of an extraperitoneal approach with a supraumbilical transverse "sunrise" incision. Am J Obstet Gynecol 1993;169:307-311.

43. Vasilev SA, McGonigle KF: Extraperitoneal laparoscopic paraaortic lymph node dissection development of a technique. J Laparoendosc Surg 1995;5:85-90.

44. Fowler JM, Carter JR, Carlson JW, et al: Lymph node yield from laparoscopic lymphadenectomy in cervical cancer: A comparative study. Gynecol Oncol 1993;51:187-192.

45. Vidaurreta J, Bermudez A, diPaola G, Sardi J: Laparoscopic staging in locally advanced cervical carcinoma: A new possible philosophy? Gynecol Oncol 1999;75:366-371.

46. Tjalma WA, Winter-Roach BA, Rowlands P, et al: Port-site recurrence following laparoscopic surgery in cervical cancer. Int J Gynecol Cancer 2001;11:409-412.

47. Potter ME, Spencer S, Soon SJ, Hatch KD: The influence of staging laparotomy for cervical cancer on patterns of recurrence and survival. Int J Gynecol Cancer 1993;3:169-174.

48. Petereit DG, Hartenbach EM, Thomas GM: Para-aortic lymph node evaluation in cervical cancer: The impact of staging upon treatment decisions and outcome. Int J Gynecol Cancer 1998;8:353-364.

49. Kupets R, Thomas GM, Coverns A: Is there a role for pelvic lymph node debulking in advanced cervical cancer? Gynecol Oncol 2002;87;163-170.

50. Sedlis A, Bundy BN, Rotman MZ, et al: A randomized trial of pelvic radiation therapy versus no further therapy in selected patients with stage IB carcinoma of the cervix after radical hysterectomy and pelvic lymphadenectomy: A Gynecologic Oncology Group study. Gynecol Oncol 1999;73:177-183.

51. Morrow CP, Bundy BN, Kurman RJ, et al: Relationship between surgical-pathological risk factors and outcome in clinical stage I and II carcinoma of the endometrium: A Gynecologic Oncology Group study. Gynecol Oncol 1991;40:55-65.

52. Koh WJ, Panwala K, Greer B: Adjuvant therapy for high-risk, early stage cervical cancer. Semin Radiat Oncol 2000;10:51-60.

53. Peters LJ, Goepfert H, Ang KK, et al: Evaluation of the dose for postoperative radiation therapy of head and neck cancer: First report of a prospective randomized trial. Int J Radiat Oncol Biol Phys 1993;26:3-11.

54. Portelance L, Chao KS, Grigsby PW, et al: Intensity-modulated radiation therapy (IMRT) reduces small bowel, rectum, and bladder doses in patients with cervical cancer receiving pelvic

and para-aortic irradiation. Int J Radiat Oncol Biol Phys 2001;51:261-266.

55. Mundt AJ, Lujan AE, Rotmensch J, et al: Intensity-modulated whole pelvic radiotherapy in women with gynecologic malignancies. Int J Radiat Oncol Biol Phys 2002;52:1330-1337.

56. Brixey CJ, Roeske JC, Lujan AE, et al: Impact of intensity-modulated radiotherapy on acute hematologic toxicity in women with gynecologic malignancies. Int J Radiat Oncol Biol Phys 2002;54:1388-1396.

57. Rotman M, Pajak TF, Choi K, et al: Prophylactic extended-field irradiation of para-aortic lymph nodes in stages IIB and bulky IB and IIA cervical carcinomas: Ten-year treatment results of RTOG 79-20. JAMA 1995;274:427-428.

58. Varia MA, Bundy BN, Deppe G, et al: Cervical carcinoma metastatic to para-aortic nodes: Extended field radiation therapy with concomitant 5-fluorouracil and cisplatin chemotherapy. A Gynecologic Oncology Group study. Int J Radiat Oncol Biol Phys 1998;42:1015-1023.

59. Malfetano JH, Keys H, Cunningham MJ, et al: Extended field radiation and cisplatin for stage IIB and IIIB cervical carcinoma. Gynecol Oncol 1997;67:203-207.

60. Vigliotti AP, Wen BC, Hussey DH, et al: Extended field radiation for carcinoma of the uterine cervix with positive pariaortic nodes. Int J Radiat Oncol Biol Phys 1992;23:501-509.

61. Stryker JA, Mortel R: Survival following extended field irradiation in carcinoma of the cervix metastatic to para-aortic lymph nodes. Gynecol Oncol 2000;79:399-405.

62. Vasilev SA, Schlaerth JB: Scalene lymph node sampling in cervical carcinoma: A reappraisal. Gynecol Oncol 1990;37:120-124.

63. Eifel PJ, Moughan J, Owen J, et al: Patterns of radiotherapy practice for patients with squamous cell carcinoma of the uterine cervix: Patterns of care study. Int J Radiat Oncol Biol Phys 1999;43:351-358.

64. Nag S, Orton C, Young D, Erickson B: The American brachytherapy society survey of brachytherapy practice for carcinoma of the cervix in the United States. Gynecol Oncol 1999;73:111-118.

65. Souhami L, Seymour R, Roman T: Weekly cisplatin plus external beam radiotherapy and high dose rate brachytherapy in patients with locally advanced carcinoma of the cervix. Int J Radiat Oncol Biol Phys 1993;27:871-878.

66. Orton C, Seyedsadr M, Somnay A: Comparison of high and low-dose rate remote afterloading for cervix cancer and the importance of fractionation. Int J Radiat Oncol Biol Phys 1991;21:1425-1434.

67. Okawa T, Sakata S, Kita-Okawa M, et al: Comparison of HDR versus LDR regiments for intracavitary of cervical cancer: Japanese experience. In Mould RF (Ed.): International Brachytherapy. Veenendaal, The Netherlands: Nucletron, 1992, p. 2013.

68. Patel F, Sharma S, Negi P, et al: Low-dose rate vs. high-dose rate brachytherapy in the treatment of carcinoma of the uterine cervix: A clinical trial. Int J Radiat Oncol Biol Phys 1993;28:335-341.

69. Shigematsu Y, Nishiyama K, Masaki N, et al: Treatment of carcinoma of the uterine cervix by remotely controlled after loading intracavitary radiotherapy with high dose-rate: A comparative study with a low dose-rate system. Int J Radiat Oncol Biol Phys 1983;9:351-356.

70. Teshima T, Inoue T, Ikeda H, et al: High-dose rate and low-dose rate intracavitary therapy for carcinoma of the uterine cervix. Cancer 1993;72:2409-2414.

71. Hareyama M, Sakata K, Oouchi A, et al: High-dose-rate versus low-dose-rate intracavitary therapy for carcinoma of the uterine cervix: A randomized trial. Cancer 2002;94:117-124.

72. Petereit DG, Pearcey R: Literature analysis of high dose rate brachytherapy fractionation schedules in the treatment of cervical cancer: Is there an optimal fractionation schedule? Int J Radiat Oncology Biol Phys 1999;43:359-366.

73. Eifel P: High-dose rate brachytherapy for carcinoma of the cervix: High tech or high risk. Int J Radiat Oncol Biol Phys 1992;24:383-386.

74. Petereit DG, Sarkaria JN, Potter DM, Schink JC: High-dose versus low-dose-rate brachytherapy in the treatment of cervical cancer: Analysis of tumor recurrence. The University of Wisconsin experience. Int J Radiat Oncol Biol Phys 1999;45:1267-1274.

75. Lorvidhaya V, Tonusin A, Changwiwit W, et al: High-dose-rate after loading brachytherapy in carcinoma of the cervix: An experience of 1992 patients. Int J Radiat Oncol Biol Phys 2000;46:1185-1191.

76. Nag S, Abitbol AA, Anderson LL, et al: Consensus guidelines for high dose rate remote brachytherapy in cervical, endometrial, and endobronchial tumors. Clinical Research Committee, American Endocurietherapy Society. Int J Radiat Oncol Biol Phys 1993;27:1241-1244.

77. MacLeod D, Bernshaw D, Leung S, et al: Accelerated hyperfractionated radiotherapy for locally advanced cervix cancer. Int J Radiat Oncol Biol Phys 1999;44:519-524.

78. Calkins AR, Harrison CR, Fowler WC, et al: Hyperfractionated radiation therapy plus chemotherapy in locally advanced cervical cancer: Results of two phase I dose-escalation Gynecologic Oncology Group trials. Gynecol Oncol 1999;75:349-355.

79. Grisby PW, Heydon K, Mutch DG, et al: Long-term follow-up of RTOG 92-10: Cervical cancer with positive para-aortic lymph nodes. Int J Radiat Oncol Biol Phys 2001;51:982-987.

80. Ang KK, Trotti A, Brown BW, et al: Randomized trial addressing risk features and time factors of surgery plus radiotherapy in advanced head-and-neck cancer. Int J Radiat Oncol Biol Phys 2001;51:571-578.

81. Van der Zee J, Gonzalez D, van Rhoon GC: Comparison of radiotherapy alone with radiotherapy plus hyperthermia in locally advanced pelvic tumours: A prospective randomised, multicentre trial. Dutch Deep Hyperthermia Group. Lancet 2000;355:1119-1125.

82. Jones EL, Samulski TV, Dewhirst MW, et al: A pilot phase II trial of concurrent radiotherapy, chemotherapy, and hyperthermia for locally advanced cervical carcinoma. Cancer 2003:98:277-282.

83. Grogan M, Thomas GM, Melamed I, et al: The importance of hemoglobin levels during radiotherapy for carcinoma of the cervix. Cancer 1999;86:1528-1536.

84. Obermair A, Cheuk R, Horwood, et al: Impact of hemoglobin levels before and during concurrent chemoradiotherapy on the response of treatment in patients with cervical cancer. Cancer 2000;92:903-908.

85. Pearcy R, Brundage M, Drouin P, et al: Phase III trial comparing radical radiation therapy with and without cisplatin chemotherapy in patients with advanced squamous cell carcinoma of the cervix. J Clin Oncol 2002;20:966-972.

86. Winter III WE, Maxwell LG, Cunqiao T, et al: The association of hemoglobin with survival in advanced cervical carcinoma patients treated with cisplatin and radiotherapy. Gynecol Oncol 2002;84:479-536.

87. Santin AD, Bellone S, Parrish RS, et al: Influence of allogeneic blood transfusion on clinical outcome during radiotherapy for cancer of the uterine cervix. Gynecol Obstet Invest 2003;56:28-34. Epub 2003 Jul 14.

88. Bush RS: The significance of anemia in clinical radiation therapy. Int J Radiat Oncol Biol Phys 1986;12:2047-2050.

89. Fyles AW, Milosevic M, Pintilie M, Hill RP: Cervix cancer oxygenation measured following external radiation therapy. Int J Radiat Oncol Biol Phys 1998;42:751-753.

90. Hockel M, Vaupel P: Tumor hypoxia: Definitions and current clinical, biologic, and molecular aspects. J Natl Cancer Inst 2001;93:266-276.

91. Dachs GU, Tozer GM: Hypoxia modulated gene expression: Angiogenesis, metastasis and therapeutic exploitation. Eur J Cancer 2000;36(13 Spec No):1649-1660.

92. Lanciano RM: Controversies in cervical and endometrial cancer. Presented at a Gynecologic Oncology Group educational symposium, July 24, 2003, Reno, NV.

93. Green JA, Kirwan JM, Tierney, et al: Survival and recurrence after concomitant chemotherapy and radiotherapy for cancer of the uterine cervix: A systematic review and meta-analysis. Lancet 2002;359:357-358.

94. Lorvidhaya V, Chitapanarux I, Sangruchi S, et al: Concurrent mitomycin C, 5-fluorouracil, and radiotherapy in the treatment of locally advanced carcinoma of the cervix: A randomized trial. Int J Radiat Oncol Biol Phys 2003;55:1226-1232.

95. Rakovitch E, Flyes AW, Pintilie M, Leung PM: Role of mitomycin C in the development of late bowel toxicity following chemoradiation for locally advanced carcinoma of the cervix. Int J Radiat Oncol Biol Phys 1997;38:979-987.

96. Chen MD, Paley PJ, Potish RA, Twiggs LB: Phase I trial of taxol as a radiation sensitizer with cisplatin in advanced cervical cancer. Gynecol Oncol 1997;67:131-136.

97. Craighead PS, Pearcey R, Stuart G: A phase I/II evaluation of tirapazamine administered intravenously concurrent with

cisplatin and radiotherapy in women with locally advanced cervical cancer. Int J Radiat Oncol Biol Phys 2000;48:791-795.

98. Pattaranutaporn P, Thirapakawong C, Chansilpa Y, et al: Study of concurrent gemcitabine and radiotherapy in locally advanced stage IIIB cervical carcinoma [abstract]. Proc Am Soc Clin Oncol 2001;20:390b.

99. Duenas Gonzalez A, Vazquez Govea E, Lopez Graniel CM, et al: Phase II randomized study of cisplatin vs cisplatin/gemcitabine concurrent to radiation in cervical cancer stages IB2-IIB. Proc Am Soc Clin Oncol 2003;22:462a.

100. Tierney JF, Stewart LA, Parmar MK: Can the published data tell us about the effectiveness of neoadjuvant chemotherapy for locally advanced cancer of the uterine cervix? Eur J Cancer 1999;35:406-409.

101. Sardi JE, Giaroli A, Sananes C, et al: Long-term follow-up of the first randomized trial using neoadjuvant chemotherapy in stage IB squamous carcinoma of the cervix: The final results. Gynecol Oncol 1997;671:61-69.

102. Chang TC, Lai CH, Hong JH, et al: Randomized trial of neoadjuvant cisplatin, vincristine, bleomycin, and radial hysterectomy versus radiation therapy for bulky stage IB and IIA cervical cancer. J Clin Oncol 2000;18:1740-1747.

103. Benedetti-Panici P, Greggi S, Colombo A, et al: Neoadjuvant chemotherapy and radical surgery versus exclusive radiotherapy in locally advanced squamous cell cervical cancer: Results from the Italian multicenter randomized study. J Clin Oncol 2002;201:179-188.

104. Souhami L, Gil R, Allan S, et al: A randomized trial of chemotherapy followed by pelvic radiation therapy in stage IIIB carcinoma of the cervix. Int J Radiat Oncol Biol Phys 1991;9:970-997.

105. Tattersall MHN, Larvidhaya V, Vootiprux V, et al: Randomized trial of epirubicin and cisplatin chemotherapy followed by pelvic radiation in locally advanced cervical cancer. J Clin Oncol 1995;13:444-451.

CANCERS OF THE UTERINE CORPUS

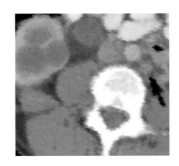

CHAPTER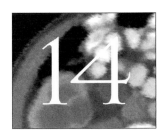

EPIDEMIOLOGY OF UTERINE CORPUS CANCERS

Louise A. Brinton,   James V. Lacey, Jr.,   Susan S. Devesa,   and   Mark E. Sherman

---

 MAJOR CONTROVERSIES

- How much do uterine corpus cancer rates vary geographically and what are the reasons underlying these differences?
- What demographic factors might play a role in the etiology of uterine corpus cancer?
- What factors might explain the observed geographic variation in mortality among whites in the United States?
- Have uterine corpus cancer rates changed over time?
- What factors are associated with survival?
- What factors explain the increased risk of endometrial cancer associated with nulliparity and the decreased risk relating to multiparity?
- What menstrual and reproductive factors other than parity relate to endometrial cancer risk?
- What patterns of oral contraceptive use are most strongly related to decreases in endometrial cancer risk?
- What aspects of exogenous hormone use lead to an increased risk of endometrial cancer?
- Can the adverse effects of estrogens be counteracted by the addition of progestins, and, if so, what is the most effective means by which progestins should be administered?
- What other therapeutic agents affect the risk of endometrial cancer?
- To what extent do body mass and physical activity independently affect risk?
- Which constituents of diet are related to risk?
- Does alcohol consumption affect endometrial cancer risk?
- Does cigarette smoking affect the risk of endometrial cancer, and, if so, what might be the underlying biologic mechanism?
- Do observed relationships with prior medical conditions persist after adjustment for effects of concomitant obesity?
- To what extent do familial factors affect the risk of endometrial cancer?
- Is there a role for environmental factors in the etiology of endometrial cancer?
- How much is known about the natural history of endometrial cancer precursors?
- What is the best system for classifying endometrial cancer precursors?
- What is the epidemiology of endometrial precursors?
- What are the risk factors for endometrial precursors?
- How do endogenous hormones relate to risk?
- Is obesity associated with endometrial cancer independently of endogenous hormones?
- Does the perimenopause represent a crucial period for endometrial cancer?
- What molecular markers might elucidate endometrial carcinogenesis?
- Is there more than one model for endometrial carcinogenesis?

The study of the epidemiology of uterine corpus cancers presents many challenges. Although a large number of factors seem to be strongly predictive of risk (Table 14-1), many of them are highly correlated, requiring a cautious interpretation of causal associations. This issue, along with unclear biologic mechanisms underlying many of the identified risk factors, has led to a number of controversies regarding the epidemiology of the disease. This chapter highlights these controversies and elaborates on additional research that might be useful in increasing the understanding of carcinogenic processes. Information is reviewed relating to the descriptive epidemiology of the disease, known risk factors, and biologic mechanisms mediating these factors.

INCIDENCE, MORTALITY, AND SURVIVAL

According to data from the National Cancer Institute's Surveillance, Epidemiology and End Results (SEER) program,[1,2] an estimated 40,100 cases of cancers of the corpus uteri and cancers of the uterus, not otherwise specified (NOS)—hereafter referred to as uterine corpus cancers—were expected to be diagnosed nationally during 2003. Based on data from 1996 to 1998, the lifetime risk among U. S. women of being diagnosed with uterine corpus cancer is 2.7%, and the lifetime risk of dying from uterine corpus cancer is 0.5%.[1]

Globally, uterine corpus cancer accounted for about 42,000 deaths in 1990,[3] of which 27,500 occurred in developed countries and 14,400 in developing countries.[4] About 6,800 deaths due to this cancer were expected to occur among American women during 2003.[2]

Table 14–1. Risk Factors for Uterine Corpus Cancer

Factors Influencing Risk	Estimated Relative Risk*
Older age	2-3
Residency in North America or Northern Europe	3-18
Higher level of education or income	1.5-2
White race	2
Nulliparity	3
History of infertility	2-3
Menstrual irregularities	1.5
Late age at natural menopause	2-3
Early age at menarche	1.5-2
Long-term use or high dosages of menopausal estrogens	10-20
Long-term use of combination oral contraceptives	0.3-0.5
High cumulative doses of tamoxifen	3-7
Obesity	2-5
Stein-Leventhal disease or estrogen-producing tumor	>5
History of diabetes, hypertension, gallbladder disease, or thyroid disease	1.3-3
Cigarette smoking	0.5

*Relative risks depend on the study and referent group employed.

There is considerable variation in uterine corpus cancer rates, both between and within countries. This has led to questions as to how much of the variation might be explained by reporting differences and the extent to which rates change when individuals migrate from low-incidence to high-incidence areas. Ethnic and racial differences in occurrence have also been noted, raising questions as to probable causes for this variation.

How much do uterine corpus cancer rates vary geographically and what are the reasons underlying these differences?

Internationally, estimated 1990 mortality rates (deaths per 100,000 woman-years, age-adjusted, world standard) varied more than eightfold, from less than 0.4 in China to 4.1 in eastern Europe and the Caribbean and 4.9 in Micronesia/Polynesia.[4] Rates were also low (less than 1) in other parts of Asia and in Africa. Rates in western Europe and North America ranged between 2 and 3 per 100,000. Mortality rates have declined since at least the 1960s in many countries, with narrowing of the international differences.[5]

In contrast to mortality data, which generally exist at the national level because death certificates are legal documents, incidence data from population-based cancer registries are not as widely available. Data from several dozen well-run registries around the world for 1988 to 1992 suggest that incidence rates (age-adjusted, world standard) varied more than threefold.[6] Rates were lowest in parts of China, Japan, India, and Costa Rica (less than 6); intermediate in the Caribbean, Spain, and the United Kingdom; and highest in western Europe, Canada, and North America (Fig. 14-1).[6] The highest rate, 18.4, occurred among U.S. whites. Geographic variation was apparent within many countries, but within-country differences were considerably smaller than those between countries. Rates in urban areas generally exceeded those in neighboring rural areas.[7]

What demographic factors might play a role in the etiology of uterine corpus cancer?

The risk of developing uterine corpus cancer increases rapidly with age during childbearing years (Fig. 14-2). After menopause, rates continue to increase, but at a less rapid pace. Incidence rates for uterine corpus adenocarcinomas are higher among whites than blacks at virtually all ages, with rates twice as high during the perimenopausal years (age 45 to 54). Women of upper socioeconomic status have an elevated risk of uterine corpus cancer.[8,9] It remains unclear the extent to which this relationship is explained by other risk factors correlated with affluence (e.g., over-nutrition, use of estrogen replacement therapy). In contrast to the higher incidence rates among whites,

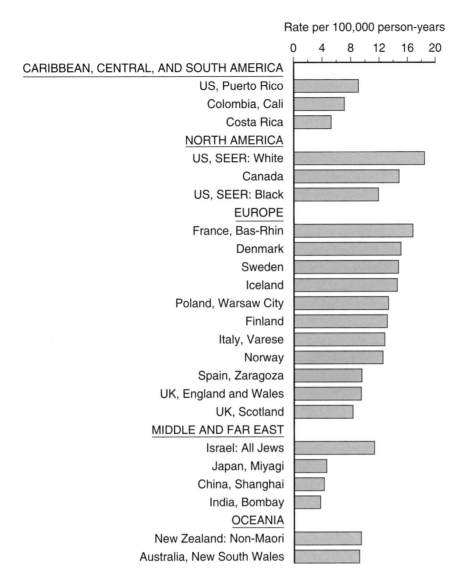

Rate per 100,000 person-years

Figure 14–1. International variation in incidence rates (age-adjusted world standard population) of cancer of the corpus uteri and cancer of the uterus, not otherwise specified (NOS) among women, 1988-1992. (Data from Parkin DM, Whelan SL, Ferlay J, et al: Cancer Incidence in Five Continents, Vol VII. Lyon, IARC Scientific Publishers, 1997.)

mortality rates are higher among blacks over all age groups.

Within the United States between 1988 to 1992, uterine corpus cancer incidence rates were highest among non-Hispanic white and Hawaiian women (Table 14-2).[6] Rates for blacks, Asians, and Hispanics were one half to two thirds those for non-Hispanic whites, and Korean women were at notably low risk. Rates in New Mexico were similar among Hispanic and American Indian women and were lower than among Hispanics in Los Angeles or San Francisco.

The rate of uterine corpus cancer among Chinese women living in Shanghai was only 60% of the rate among Chinese women in Hong Kong or Singapore, whereas the rates among Chinese women in Hawaii and San Francisco were more than twice as high (Table 14-3).[6] Similarly, Japanese women in San Francisco and Hawaii had rates triple those in Japan. Within Israel, women born in Africa or Asia were at considerably reduced risk compared with those born in Israel, Europe, or America.

What factors might explain the observed geographic variation in mortality among whites in the United States?

Considerable geographic variation in uterine corpus cancer mortality rates has been reported within the United States, with notably high rates in parts of the northeast and low rates across the south.[10] Figure 14-3 presents the ranked mortality rates by state economic area for white women during the period 1970 to 1998. The age-adjusted (1970 U.S. standard) rates varied more than threefold, ranging from 1.6 to 5.4 per 100,000 woman-years; the rate was higher than 4 in many areas of the Northeast and Midwest and 3 or lower across the South and mountain states. The regional excess of uterine corpus cancer across the Northeast has been evident for more than four decades.[11] The North-South differences have become more pronounced over time as mortality rates have declined more rapidly in many areas of the south. National data on survival rates among uterine corpus

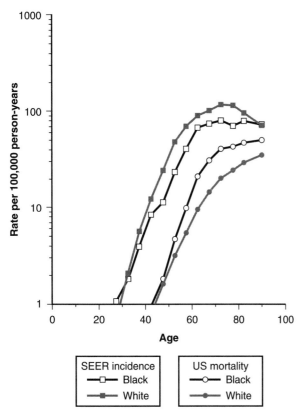

Figure 14–2. Age-specific incidence of cancer of the corpus uteri and cancer of the uterus, not otherwise specified (NOS) in the Surveillance, Epidemiology and End Results (SEER) database and mortality rates among women in the United States, by race, 1990-1998. (Data from Ries LA, Eisner MP, Kosary CL, et al: SEER Cancer Statistics Review, 1973-1998. Bethesda: National Cancer Institute, 2001.

cancer patients are not available, but it is unlikely that geographic variations in survival greatly influence the mortality patterns. Explanations for the geographic patterns are unclear, but they may relate to differences in reproductive behavior, socioeconomic status, and access to medical care, as has been found for breast cancer.[12]

Have uterine corpus cancer rates changed over time?

From the 1950s to the 1990s, age-adjusted uterine corpus cancer mortality rates declined among white and nonwhite women in the United States.[13] During the last two decades of the 20th century, uterine corpus cancer mortality rates continued to decrease, with rates among blacks 60% to 90% higher than those among whites[1] (Fig. 14-4). In 1998, the mortality rates were 5.7 and 3.1 per 100,000 woman-years among blacks and whites, respectively. In contrast, age-adjusted incidence rates consistently have been higher among whites than blacks. Rates peaked during the early 1970s, especially among whites, with the white/black rate ratios exceeding 2; the peaks were related to trends in the use of unopposed estrogens.[14] Rates subsequently declined,

especially among whites during the 1980s, and have been relatively stable since. During the 1990s, incidence was about 40% higher among whites than among blacks.

As shown in Table 14-4, uterine corpus cancer is most commonly diagnosed at localized stages, with recent incidence rates of 17.2 and 8.5 among whites and blacks, respectively. The declines in invasive incidence from 1975-1978 to 1995-1998 were driven by decreases in the rates of localized disease. Rates of localized-stage disease declined at all ages younger than 70 years but increased among older women. Rates of regional-stage disease increased somewhat, and rates of distant disease did not change greatly.

Trends in uterine corpus cancer incidence have varied internationally, including increases in many regions with historically low rates, whereas mortality rates generally have declined.[15]

What factors are associated with survival?

The 5-year relative survival rates among women diagnosed with uterine corpus cancer have not changed greatly since the mid-1970s, with rates consistently higher among whites compared with blacks.[1] Based on more than 14,000 cases diagnosed between 1992 and 1997, 75% of uterine corpus cancers among white women were diagnosed at a localized stage, and 13% at a regional stage (Table 14-5). The stage distribution among black women was not as favorable, with localized and regional stages accounting for 52% and 22% of cases, respectively. The proportion of cases diagnosed at a distant stage was considerably higher among black women than white women—18% versus 8%, respectively. Survival rates varied markedly by stage at diagnosis: 83% or more for women with localized disease versus 28% or less for women with distant spread. The more favorable prognosis among whites compared with blacks persisted for patients within each stage category, perhaps because of differences in extent of disease within stage category, tumor aggressiveness, or aggressiveness or effectiveness of treatment. Some support for true biologic variation by racial ethnicity derives from one analysis that showed moderate racial differences in tumor grade remaining even after control for most recognized risk factors.[16]

RISK FACTORS

The majority of epidemiologic studies have focused on defining the epidemiology of endometrial adenocarcinomas rather than on the rarer cancers, such as sarcomas and synchronous tumors of the endometrium and ovary, whose epidemiology is less clear. A number of risk factors have been identified for endometrial cancer, although in many cases the inter-relationship between factors and the mediating biologic mechanisms are incompletely understood. Most of the controversies center on these two issues.

Table 14–2. Variation in Incidence of Uterine Corpus Cancer* by Racial and Ethnic Group Among U.S. Women (SEER Data, 1988-1992)

	Los Angeles		San Francisco		Hawaii		Connecticut		Seattle		Detroit		Atlanta		New Mexico		Iowa		Utah	
	No.	Rate	No.	Rate	No.	Rate	No.	Rate	No.	Rate	No.	Rate	No.	Rate	No.	Rate	No.	Rate	No.	Rate
Non-Hispanic White†	3326	20.3	1783	19.0	142	15.8	2295	18.9	2233	19.7	2246	19.8	713	15.4	497	16.1	2048	17.9	845	19.2
Hispanic White	617	11.6	155	13.7	—	—	—	—	—	—	—	—	—	—	139	9.7	—	—	—	—
Filipino	74	11.4	49	9.7	52	11.4	—	—	—	—	—	—	—	—	—	—	—	—	—	—
Black	335	11.0	160	12.4	—	—	95	13.7	—	—	362	12.0	163	11.1	—	—	—	—	—	—
Japanese	44	8.1	33	16.5	170	14.6	—	—	—	—	—	—	—	—	—	—	—	—	—	—
Chinese	48	7.3	96	11.9	35	14.3	—	—	—	—	—	—	—	—	—	—	—	—	—	—
Korean	11	2.8	—	—	—	—	—	—	—	—	—	—	—	—	—	—	—	—	—	—
Hawaiian	—	—	—	—	91	20.6	—	—	—	—	—	—	—	—	—	—	—	—	—	—
American Indian	—	—	—	—	—	—	—	—	—	—	—	—	—	—	25	9.6	—	—	—	—

SEER, Surveillance, Epidemiology and End Results program; −, data not available.
*Includes cancers of the corpus uteri and cancers of the uterus, not otherwise specified (NOS); table shows numbers of cases and incidence rates per 100,000 woman-years, age-adjusted using the world standard.
†Includes all whites in Hawaii, Connecticut, Detroit, and Atlanta, and all women in Seattle, Iowa, and Utah.
From Ries LA, Eisner MP, Kosary CL, et al: SEER Cancer Statistics Review, 1973-1998. Bethesda: National Cancer Institute, 2001.

Table 14–3. Variation in Incidence of Uterine Corpus Cancer* by Racial and Ethnic Group and Country of Residence, 1988-1992

Group and Place	No. of Cases	Rate
Chinese		
China, Shanghai	1022	4.3
Singapore: Chinese	366	7.0
Hong Kong	1081	7.3
US, Los Angeles: Chinese	48	7.3
US, San Francisco: Chinese	96	11.9
US, Hawaii: Chinese	35	14.3
Japanese		
Japan, Osaka	1372	4.2
Japan, Miyagi	395	4.6
US, Los Angeles: Japanese	44	8.1
US, Hawaii: Japanese	170	14.7
US, San Francisco: Japanese	33	16.5
Israeli		
Israel: Jews born in Africa or Asia	290	7.9
Israel: Jews born in America or Europe	812	13.4
Israel: Jews born in Israel	209	15.3

*Includes cancers of the corpus uteri and cancers of the uterus, not otherwise specified (NOS); table shows number of cases and incidence rates per 100,000 woman-years, age-adjusted using the world standard.
From Parkin DM, Whelan SL, Ferlay J, et al: Cancer Incidence in Five Continents, Vol. VII. Lyon, IARC Scientific Publishers, 1997.

What factors explain the increased risk of endometrial cancer associated with nulliparity and the decreased risk relating to multiparity?

Nulliparity is a recognized risk factor for endometrial cancer. Most studies demonstrate a twofold to threefold higher risk for nulliparous women compared with parous women.[8,17-19] The association of endometrial cancer with nulliparity has been suggested to reflect prolonged periods of infertility. The hypothesis that infertility is a risk factor for endometrial cancer is supported by studies showing higher risks for married nulliparous women than for unmarried women.[8,9] One study that specifically evaluated infertility as a risk factor for endometrial cancer found a 3.5-fold increased risk for women who reported an inability to get pregnant lasting 3 years or longer.[18] In another study, nulliparous women who sought advice for infertility were at an almost eightfold excess risk compared with nulliparous women without an infertility problem.[17] In a follow-up study from Israel, infertile women were found to have an approximately fourfold increased risk compared with the general population.[20] In that study, women with progesterone deficiencies were at particularly high risk. This finding was noteworthy, given that the means of classifying causes of infertility was based on relatively crude measures. Several ongoing studies that are using well-defined endocrinologic parameters to classify categories of infertility should be even more informative in terms of distinguishing patients who are at high risk for endometrial cancer.

Several biologic alterations linked to infertility have been associated with endometrial cancer risk, including anovulatory menstrual cycles (prolonged exposure to estrogens without sufficient progesterone); high serum levels of androstenedione (i.e., excess androstenedione available for conversion to estrone); and the absence of monthly sloughing of the endometrial lining (residual tissue that may become hyperplastic). Another factor that may be important because of its effect on the amount of free estrogens is the level of serum sex hormone–binding globulin, which has been found to be lower in nulliparous than in parous women.[21]

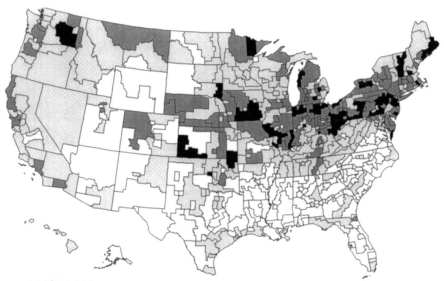

Figure 14–3. Cancer mortality rates among white women for cancer of the corpus uteri and cancer of the uterus, not otherwise specified (NOS), by state economic area (age-adjusted 1970 U.S. population. Updated from http://www3.Cancer.gov/attasplus/), 1970-1998.

US rate = 3.61/100,000
■ 4.26 - 5.37 (highest 10%)
▨ 3.90 - 4.25 (70-89%)
▨ 3.12 - 3.89 (30-69.9%)
□ 2.61 - 3.11 (10-29.9%)
□ 1.62 - 2.60 (lowest 10%)

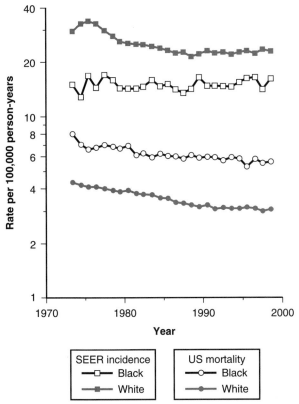

Figure 14–4. Trends in cancer of the corpus uteri and cancer of the uterus, not otherwise specified (NOS) in the Surveillance, Epidemiology and End Results (SEER) (age-adjusted 1970 U.S. population) database and mortality rates incidence among women in the United States by race, 1973-1998. (Data from Ries LA, Eisner MP, Kosary CL, et al: SEER Cancer Statistics Review, 1973-1998. Bethesda: National Cancer Institute, 2001.)

What menstrual and reproductive factors other than parity relate to endometrial cancer risk?

Most studies find that among parous women there is decreasing risk of endometrial cancer with increasing number of births. The age at which a woman has her first liveborn child does not appear to relate to endometrial cancer risk.[8,17,18] However, several recent studies suggest that a last birth occurring late in reproductive life may reduce the risk.[22,23] Although this may reflect unique hormone profiles of women who are able to conceive at older ages, it is also plausible that births at an older age may afford protection by mechanically clearing malignantly transformed cells from the uterine lining. This hypothesis is consistent with observations that the risk of endometrial cancer increases with time since the most recent pregnancy.[22,23] Further support for this hypothesis derives from several studies that have shown reductions in risk among users of intrauterine devices.[24-26] However, it is also possible that these devices may affect risk by causing structural or biochemical changes that alter the sensitivity of the endometrium to circulating hormones.

The relationship of risk to breast-feeding remains controversial. Although a number of studies have failed to show any relationship,[8,9,17] more recent studies suggest that prolonged lactation may offer some protection.[27,28] In one of these investigations, however, the reduced risk did not persist into the age range when endometrial cancer becomes common.[28]

Early age at menarche was found to be related to increased endometrial cancer risk in several studies, although the associations were generally rather weak and trends inconsistent.[8,9,17,18] Several studies found stronger effects of age at menarche among younger women, although this has not been consistently demonstrated.[18] The extent to which these relationships reflect increased exposure to ovarian hormones or other correlates of early menarche (e.g., increased body weight) is unresolved.

Most studies have indicated that the age at menopause is directly related to the risk of developing endometrial cancer.[8] About 70% of all women diagnosed with endometrial cancer are postmenopausal. Most studies support the estimate of MacMahon[29] that there is about a twofold increased risk associated with natural menopause after the age of 52 years, compared with menopause before 49 years of age. Elwood and colleagues[8] hypothesized that the effect of late age at menopause on risk may reflect prolonged exposure of the uterus to estrogen stimulation in the presence of anovulatory (progesterone-deficient) cycles. The interrelationships among menstrual factors, age, and weight are complex, and the biologic mechanisms of these variables operating in the pathogenesis of endometrial cancer are subject to substantial speculation.

Use of oral contraceptives is clearly related to risk (see later discussion), but whether other means of controlling reproduction affect risk remains less clear. As elaborated previously, use of an intrauterine device may be associated with a reduced risk of endometrial cancer. Several studies have suggested that tubal sterilization may result in endogenous hormone alterations. However, a recent study failed to find an association of this procedure with endometrial cancer risk.[30]

What patterns of oral contraceptive use are most strongly related to decreases in endometrial cancer risk?

Users of combination oral contraceptives have been found to experience approximately half the risk for endometrial cancer of nonusers, and long-term users in most studies experience even further reductions in risk.[31-34] Kaufman and associates[34] showed that the reduced risk persisted for at least 5 years after discontinuation, but Weiss and Sayvetz[33] found that the protective effect waned within 3 years. In several studies, the greatest reduction in risk was associated with pills containing high progestin doses, although this finding was not confirmed elsewhere.[32,35] A number of studies have claimed that the protective effect of the pill appears to be greatest among nulliparous women.[18,31] In other studies, the protection has been limited to nonobese women or to those who have not been exposed to noncontraceptive estrogens.[18,33]

Table 14–4. Incidence Trends of Uterine Corpus Cancer* by Race, Stage, and Age (SEER Data, 1975-1978 and 1995-1998)

Population and Type	1975-1978		1995-1998		Change in Rate	
	No. of Cases	Rate	No. of Cases	Rate	Actual	Percent
Whites by Stage						
In situ	970	2.6	245	0.5	−2.1	−79.8
Invasive						
Total	12,194	31.1	11,382	22.9	−8.1	−26.2
Localized	9,821	25.2	8,324	17.2	−8.1	−32.0
Regional	921	2.3	1,612	3.1	0.8	35.4
Distant	677	1.7	831	1.6	−0.1	−3.0
Unstaged	775	1.9	615	1.0	−0.8	−44.8
Blacks by Stage						
In situ	25	0.7	10	0.2	−0.5	−73.5
Invasive						
Total	517	16.2	814	15.7	−0.4	−2.6
Localized	310	9.5	443	8.5	−0.9	−9.9
Regional	73	2.4	179	3.5	1.1	44.2
Distant	74	2.3	124	2.5	0.2	6.5
Unstaged	60	2.0	68	1.2	−0.7	−36.5
Localized Stage among Whites by Age Group (yr)						
30-39	202	4.5	194	2.9	−1.7	−37.0
40-49	758	20.0	818	13.4	−6.6	−33.0
50-59	3,557	90.4	1,960	48.6	−41.8	−46.2
60-69	3,330	112.1	2,214	71.5	−40.7	−36.3
70-79	1,459	75.1	2,185	80.1	5.0	6.7
80+	488	46.6	936	54.8	8.1	17.4

SEER, Surveillance, Epidemiology and End Results program.
*Includes cancers of the corpus uteri and cancers of the uterus, not otherwise specified (NOS); table shows number of cases and incidence rates per 100,000 woman-years, age-adjusted using the 1970 U.S. standard.
From Ries LA, Eisner MP, Kosary CL, et al: SEER Cancer Statistics Review, 1973-1998. Bethesda: National Cancer Institute, 2001.

In contrast to combination oral contraceptives, several studies have shown an increased risk of endometrial cancer among women who had previously used Oracon, a sequential preparation that combined dimethisterone (a weak progestogen) with a large dose of a potent estrogen (ethinyl estradiol).[18,33] The risk associated with the use of other sequential oral contraceptives remains unclear, mainly because these drugs are no longer marketed.

Table 14–5. Distribution of Uterine Corpus Cancer* and 5-Year Relative Survival Rates by Stage at Diagnosis among White and Black Women (SEER Data, 1992-1997)

	White	Black
Cases (N)	14,369	1,019
Stage at Diagnosis (%)		
Total	100	100
Localized	75	52
Regional	13	22
Distant	8	18
Unstaged	4	9
5-Year Relative Survival Rate (%)		
Total	85.8	58.9
Localized	96.9	82.9
Regional	65.1	42.7
Distant	27.7	13.1
Unstaged	47.6	48.9

SEER, Surveillance, Epidemiology and End Results program.
*Includes cancers of the corpus uteri and cancers of the uterus, not otherwise specified (NOS).
From Ries LA, Eisner MP, Kosary CL, et al: SEER Cancer Statistics Review, 1973-1998. Bethesda: National Cancer Institute, 2001.

What aspects of exogenous hormone use lead to an increased risk of endometrial cancer?

Although it is well known that use of estrogen replacement therapy is associated with a 2-fold to 12-fold elevation in risk of endometrial cancer,[36-39] many aspects of the relationship remain less clear. In most investigations, the increased risk did not become apparent until the drugs had been used for at least 2 to 3 years, and longer use of estrogen was generally associated with higher risk.[9,36,37,40] The highest relative risks, reaching 10 to 20, have been observed after 10 years of use, but it is not clear whether there is any additional increase after 15 years. In most studies, cessation of use appears to be associated with a relatively rapid decrease in risk, although a number of studies suggest that elevated risks may continue for some time after discontinuation, possibly for as long as 15 years.[36,37,39,41-43]

All doses of estrogen appear to increase risk, with some evidence that higher doses are associated with greater elevations in risk. Of note is a study showing that even 0.3 mg of unopposed equine estrogen can result in a significant increase in risk.[44] Fewer studies have focused on differences in risk according to cyclic versus continuous regimens of use or whether effects vary with the use of oral synthetic versus conjugated estrogens. However, from the limited data available, it appears that these differences in modes of administration are less important predictors than several other measures of use, notably duration of use and interval since last use.[45] Unresolved is whether use of estrogen patches, creams, or injections can affect risk; given the relationships of risk with even low-dose estrogens, it is plausible that these regimens may confer some increase in risk.

From a number of studies, it appears that estrogen effects are strongest among women who are thin, nondiabetic, or normotensive.[36,41,42,46] These findings suggest that estrogen metabolism differs in these groups of women or that risk is already high enough in obese, hypertensive, or diabetic women that exposure to exogenous estrogens has only a small additional effect.

An interesting observation is that tumors associated with estrogen use generally demonstrate favorable characteristics, including earlier stage at diagnosis, lower grade, and fewer instances of myometrial invasion.[36,47] Estrogen users tend to be younger at diagnosis than patients who have not used estrogen, and the tumors are more frequently accompanied by hyperplasia or adenomyosis.[48,49] These observations may indicate that some advanced endometrial hyperplasias are being diagnosed as endometrial carcinomas; however, several studies and pathologic reviews have shown that the association of estrogen with endometrial cancer persists. Although the estrogen-associated risk is highest for early-stage cancers, the elevated risks also pertain to later-stage disease.[43,47] Therefore, misclassification of endometrial hyperplasias as endometrial cancer probably accounts for only a small portion of the elevation in risk associated with estrogen use.

Can the adverse effects of estrogens be counteracted by the addition of progestins, and, if so, what is the most effective means by which progestins should be administered?

Progesterone has been shown to produce regressive changes in endometrial hyperplasia, a presumed precursor of endometrial cancer. In postmenopausal women with simple hyperplasia, administration of medroxyprogesterone acetate (MPA) in a dose of 10 mg/day for 12 days has been shown to result in conversion of the endometrium to an atrophic or nonhyperplastic pattern.[50,51] This is consistent with the clinical recommendation that combined estrogen-progestin therapy be prescribed for all women with intact uteri. As shown in Table 14-6, studies indicate that the excess risk of endometrial cancer can be significantly reduced if progestins are given for at least 10 days each month.[38,52,53] In several studies, however, subjects who used progestins for fewer than 10 days per month continued to experience some increased risk, with only a slight reduction compared with users of estrogen only.[40,53,54] The sharp contrast between the effects of less than 10 and more than 10 days of progestin use has led to the suggestion that the extent of endometrial sloughing or of "terminal" differentiation at the completion of the progestin phase may play a critical role in determining risk.[40] Although it is now generally accepted that progestins must be administered for at least 10 days each month to provide protection against endometrial cancer risk, it remains questionable whether this regimen is sufficient for complete protection, particularly for long-term users.[55] Few studies have had large numbers of long-term sequential users, and in two studies there was evidence that this pattern of use may result in some persistence of risk.[38,54] Therefore, further studies of long-term users of this regimen are needed.

Table 14–6. Relative Risks of Endometrial Cancer with Use of Sequential or Continuous Progestins Plus Estrogens in Postmenopausal Women

Study and Year	Progestin Days/Cycle	Duration of Use (yr)	Relative Risk	(95% Confidence Interval)
Weiderpass, 1999[53]	<10	>5	2.9	(1.8-4.6)
	Continuous	>5	0.2	(0.1-0.8)
Beresford, 1997[54]	<10	>5	3.7	(1.7-8.2)
	10–21	>5	2.5	(1.1-5.5)
	Continuous	5	1.4	(1.0-1.9)
Pike, 1997[38]	<10	5	1.9	(1.3-2.6)
	≥10	5	1.1	(0.8-1.4)
	Continuous	5	1.1	(0.8-1.4)
Jick, 1993	Not specified	>5	1.3	(0.5-3.4)
Voigt, 1991	<10	>3	2.4	(0.6-9.3)
	≥10	>3	1.1	(0.4-3.6)
Persson, 1989[52]	7–10	3-5	1.2	(0.3-5.5)

Adapted from Archer DF: The effect of the duration of progestin use on the occurrence of endometrial cancer in postmenopausal women. Menopause 2001;8:245-251.

Given the lack of resolution of this issue, there has been increased enthusiasm for prescribing estrogens continuously with progestins. Although Weiderpass and coworkers[53] in Sweden observed a risk considerably below unity for this regimen, Pike and associates,[38] in the United States, found no difference in risk for sequential versus continuous use of progestins. Discrepancies in findings may relate to the use of more potent progestins in Europe.

What other therapeutic agents affect the risk of endometrial cancer?

A number of clinical trials and a population-based case-control study have indicated an increased risk for endometrial cancer among tamoxifen-treated breast cancer patients.[56-59] This is consistent with tamoxifen's estrogenic effects on the endometrium. Elevated risks have been observed primarily among women receiving high cumulative doses of therapy, usually in the range of 15 g or more. One recent study documented a poor prognosis among long-term tamoxifen users who developed endometrial cancer, presumably reflecting less favorable histologies and higher stages of disease at diagnosis.[60] Whether this finding is generalizable to other populations remains unclear.

Increasing use of ovulation induction agents, including clomiphene citrate, has raised concern about potential links with a variety of cancers, including endometrial cancer. Sufficient data are not currently available to determine whether any association exists.[61] One recent report suggested an increased risk of endometrial cancer associated with use of psychotropic medications[62]; additional confirmatory data on this relationship are needed.

To what extent do body mass and physical activity independently affect risk?

Obesity is a well-recognized risk factor for endometrial cancer, with as much as 25% of the disease possibly explained by this factor.[17,63-68] Very heavy women appear to have disproportionately high risks. Brinton and coworkers[17] reported a sevenfold excess risk for women weighing 200 pounds or more, compared with those weighing less than 125 pounds. Although studies have demonstrated significant positive trends of endometrial cancer with both weight and various measures of body mass, including Quetelet's index (weight in kilograms divided by the square of the height in meters), height has not been consistently associated with risk. Obesity appears to affect both premenopausal and postmenopausal endometrial cancer, although possibly through different mechanisms.[9,65,68]

Blitzer and colleagues[69] found a positive association between endometrial cancer and adolescent obesity and hypothesized that long-standing obesity is a more important risk factor than adult weight. However, in several studies that have examined weight both during early adulthood and later in life, contemporary weight and weight gain during adulthood appeared to be most predictive of endometrial cancer risk.[18,66,68,70]

Interest has also focused on determining whether the distribution of body fat predicts endometrial cancer risk. Upper-body fat has been found in several studies to have an effect on endometrial cancer risk independent of body size.[68,71,72] However, other studies have suggested either no effect of body fat distribution or a more crucial role for central obesity.[73-75] Further investigations on this issue are needed, especially studies that consider intervening effects of endogenous hormones.

Several studies have suggested a protective effect of physical activity on endometrial cancer risk that appears independent of relationships with body weight.[63,76-79] However, a number of these studies had internal inconsistencies. For instance, in a recent report,[79] the absence of differences in risk by duration or intensity of physical activity suggested the need for caution before the association is interpreted as causal. A potential relationship is biologically appealing, given that physical activity can result in changes in the menstrual cycle, body fat distribution, and levels of endogenous hormones. The issue therefore deserves attention in future investigations.

Which constituents of diet are related to risk?

Although obesity has been consistently related to endometrial cancer, epidemiologic studies have only recently evaluated the etiologic role of dietary factors. Geographic differences in disease rates (i.e., high rates in Western and low rates in Eastern societies) suggest that nutrition has a role, especially the high content of animal fat in Western diets.[80] Armstrong and Doll[81] demonstrated a strong correlation between a country's total fat intake and endometrial cancer incidence.

Although a number of studies have assessed endometrial cancer risk in relation to consumption of dietary fat, the association remains unclear. A clear assessment of risk depends on careful control for effects of both body size and caloric intake (energy). In the case-control study by Potischman and associates,[82] a relationship with animal fat intake appeared to be relatively independent of other dietary factors. In the case-control study of Goodman and colleagues,[63] some of the effect of fat calories appeared to be explained by body size, although the relationship continued to remain significant. Several other case-control studies, however, failed to confirm a relationship with fat intake.[83,84] In addition, a recent cohort study found just the opposite trend, namely some decrease in risk with relatively high intakes of saturated or animal fat.[64]

More consistent are studies that have shown a possible protective effect of certain nutritional patterns, including reduced risks associated with the consumption of certain micronutrients. For instance, Barbone and associates[83] found no relationship with either animal or vegetable fat intake but found reduced risks related to high intake of certain micronutrients (including carotene and nitrate). In line with this result, a European study found reduced risks among women who reported high intake of fruits and vegetables, specifically those containing high levels of β-carotene.[85] Goodman and colleagues[63] found inverse relationships of risk with consumption of cereals, legumes, vegetables, and fruits, particularly those high in lutein. McCann and coworkers[84] also found evidence for reduced risks among women in the highest quartiles of intake of protein, dietary fiber, phytosterols, vitamin C, folate, α- and β-carotene, lycopene, lutein + zeaxanthin, and vegetables. However, not all studies support relationships with micronutrients, including recently reported results from a large Canadian prospective study.[64]

The quest for protective factors has expanded to include phytoestrogens and consumption of foods high in omega-3 fatty acids, such as fatty fish. Although two studies suggested that consumption of these food items may be beneficial in terms of endometrial cancer risk,[86,87] additional confirmatory studies are needed.

It is clear that further studies are needed to resolve relationships between dietary factors and endometrial cancer risk. These studies should assess the extent to which dietary associations for endometrial cancer are mediated through modifications in hormone metabolism, because both observational and intervention studies have shown higher levels of plasma estrone, estradiol, and prolactin among women who consume a high-fat or omnivorous diet, compared with a low-fat or vegetarian diet.[88-91]

Does alcohol consumption affect endometrial cancer risk?

In a number of studies, regular consumption of alcoholic beverages has been linked to substantial reductions in endometrial cancer risk.[92-95] Several studies noted more pronounced effects among premenopausal or overweight women, suggesting that an attenuation in endogenous estrogen levels may be responsible for the reduced risk.[93,95] However, inconsistent findings from other studies emphasize the need for further evaluation of the relationship between alcohol consumption and endometrial cancer risk.[96-99]

Does cigarette smoking affect the risk of endometrial cancer, and, if so, what might be the underlying biologic mechanism?

A reduced risk of endometrial cancer among smokers has been reported, with current smokers having approximately half the risk of nonsmokers.[92,98,100-105] In a number of studies, the reduced risk associated with smoking was more pronounced in postmenopausal than in premenopausal women.[98,101,103] Several reports found that the reduced risk associated with smoking was most apparent in obese patients.[101,102,104,105] In a recent investigation,[104] smoking also appeared to reduce risks to a greater extent in diabetics and users of postmenopausal hormones, leading to the suggestion that smoking may exert its effects on risk through an antiestrogenic mechanism. In one investigation, cigarette smoking was not related to changes in estradiol levels but did affect serum androstenedione levels,[92] a known source of estrogens in postmenopausal women. A number of issues regarding effects of cigarette smoking on endometrial cancer remain unresolved. Most notably, the extent to which there may be mechanistic differences between premenopausal and postmenopausal women is an intriguing research issue worthy of further pursuit.

Do observed relationships with prior medical conditions persist after adjustment for effects of concomitant obesity?

Numerous clinical reports link polycystic ovary syndrome with an increase in the risk of endometrial cancer, particularly among younger women who present with both conditions.[106-108] However, given that obesity is one of the defining features of this condition, the independence of the two conditions is unclear. In a follow-up study at the Mayo Clinic, women with chronic anovulation were found to be at a threefold increased risk for development of endometrial cancer.[109] Case-control studies have usually had difficulties in obtaining appropriate histories of polycystic ovary syndrome, but several studies have reported increased risks of endometrial cancer among patients who report histories of either hirsutism or acne,[17,110] conditions often associated with hyperandrogenism.

A number of studies have noted a high risk of endometrial cancer among diabetics, but again the issue is whether the association is independent of weight. Two cohort studies[111,112] and a number of case-control studies[17,19,113-115] suggest that the relationship persists when analyses are restricted to nonobese women or are adjusted for the effects of weight. However, in several other studies,[67,116] the effect of diabetes on endometrial cancer risk was apparent only among obese women, suggesting the possible involvement of selected metabolic abnormalities, including hyperinsulinemia. Further research is needed to resolve the association, as well as to elaborate on how specific types of diabetes may be involved.

A variety of other diseases have been suggested as possibly predisposing to endometrial cancer risk, including hypertension, arthritis, thyroid conditions, gallbladder disease, and cholesterolemia. In a number of studies, positive findings may be partially explained by the correlation of the diseases with other factors. Similar to patients with breast cancer, those with previous fractures were found to have a reduced risk of endometrial cancer,[117,118] presumably reflecting the association of lowered bone density with altered endogenous hormone levels.

To what extent do familial factors affect the risk of endometrial cancer?

Several studies have suggested that a family history of endometrial cancer is a risk factor for the disease.[119-122] Data from a family-cancer database in Sweden[120] showed that risk was inversely related to age at diagnosis, with a more than 10-fold excess risk among young (<50 years) daughters of mothers with early-onset diseases. In addition, subjects with a family history of colon cancer were at an increased risk for endometrial cancer, an association that is now well recognized and reflects a role for the dominantly inherited hereditary nonpolyposis colorectal cancer gene.[123] In contrast, studies do not support an etiologic role in endometrial cancer for inherited mutations in either the BRCA1 or the BRCA2 gene.[124] Several investigations have suggested possible disease associations with more common genetic polymorphisms, including the estrogen receptor, methylenetetrahydrofolate reductase (MTHFR), and cytochrome P-450 1A1 (CYP1A1) genes,[125-127] but confirmatory studies are needed.

Is there a role for environmental factors in the etiology of endometrial cancer?

Geographic variations in rates of endometrial cancer, with high rates in certain industrial areas, have led to the suggestion that environmental agents may affect risk. Given the well-recognized influence of hormones on the disease, there has been particular concern about a potential role for certain endocrine disruptors, including dichlorodiphenyltrichloroethane (DDT). Several studies have addressed this issue by comparing levels of DDE (the active metabolite of DDT) in the sera of cases and controls, finding no significant differences.[128,129] Electromagnetic fields have also been of interest, given that they can influence hormone levels. A recent study, however, found no relationship between endometrial cancer risk and use of electric blankets or mattress covers.[130]

The fact that increasing numbers of women are entering the workforce has led to questions about how occupational exposures relate to cancer risk. This issue has only recently begun to be explored with respect to endometrial cancer. In one record linkage study in Finland, endometrial cancer was associated with exposure to animal dander and sedentary work.[98]

▌NATURAL HISTORY AND BIOMARKERS

How much is known about the natural history of endometrial cancer precursors?

The diagnosis of endometrial cancer precursors and carcinoma is usually made on the basis of endometrial biopsy[131] or curettage[132] performed to determine the cause of abnormal vaginal bleeding. Clinical treatment decisions for endometrial lesions depend on lesion severity, patient age, medical history, and patient preferences. Women who are postmenopausal or who have completed childbearing often undergo hysterectomy, whereas younger women who have only mild abnormalities and wish to preserve their fertility increasingly choose conservative management with hormone treatment and repeat sampling.[50,133-135]

The historical acceptance of hysterectomy as first-line therapy[136] may have minimized the impetus for understanding the natural history of endometrial cancer. The existence of multiple different pathologic classification systems, poor diagnostic reproducibility, and the lack of valid population-based screening methods have further compromised the ability to study endometrial cancer precursors. Nonetheless, the realization that many women have undergone unnecessary hysterectomy for highly reversible lesions and the increasing frequency of delayed childbearing have spurred interest in elucidating the natural history of endometrial cancer precursors through multidisciplinary investigations.

Endometrial hyperplasia: A heterogeneous set of pathologic lesions

Most endometrial carcinomas, specifically those histopathologically classified as endometrioid, seem to develop slowly from morphologically defined precursors. Endometrial hyperplasia includes a heterogeneous set of pathologic lesions ranging from immediate endometrial cancer precursors to mild, highly reversible proliferations. Microscopically, these lesions comprise a continuum of morphologic appearances.[137] The earliest lesions consist of slightly crowded and dilated endometrial glands composed of cells with nuclei resembling normal proliferative endometrium; advanced lesions are composed of almost back-to-back glands containing markedly abnormal nuclei, an appearance that closely resembles well-differentiated endometrioid carcinoma.

Most hyperplastic lesions represent innocuous glandular proliferations that regress spontaneously or can be induced to regress with progestins and repeated curettage.[138,139] Occult carcinoma is present in 20% to 45% of women with biopsies diagnosed as endometrial hyperplasia,[140-142] which is usually classified as atypical complex endometrial hyperplasia in the World Health Organization (WHO) classification.

What is the best system for classifying endometrial cancer precursors? Multiple systems have been proposed for classifying endometrial carcinoma precursors.[143] The WHO classification is based largely on a retrospective pathologic review of biopsies and clinical records of 170 women accessioned between 1940 and 1970 at one U. S. reference laboratory.[144] In the WHO system, simple hyperplasia includes dilated glands with mild crowding, and complex hyperplasia consists of more irregularly shaped glands with more severe crowding. These two categories are further subdivided into atypical and non-atypical groups, based on the size and appearance of the nuclei of the glandular cells. In the WHO classification, cytologic atypia is considered to represent the best morphologic predictor of progression to carcinoma.[144] The intraobserver and interobserver reproducibilities of the WHO classification are less than ideal, in part because the criteria for assessing glandular crowding and cytologic atypia are relatively imprecise and morphologic distinctions are somewhat subjective.[145,146]

To improve the diagnostic reproducibility of biopsy interpretation, Bergeron and colleagues[147] proposed a modified WHO classification that collapses atypical hyperplasia and well-differentiated adenocarcinoma into a single category called "endometrioid neoplasia." All other lesions (i.e., non-atypical hyperplasias) are designated simply as "hyperplasia." This classification is predicated on the concept that "endometrial neoplasia" captures all carcinomas or incipient carcinomas (which are treated similarly), rendering further subdivision of the endometrial neoplasia category moot. However, biologic evidence to support this approach is lacking and the cutpoint between endometrial neoplasia and hyperplasia in this system is based on WHO criteria, with the same attendant limitations.

The recent Endometrial Intraepithelial Neoplasia (EIN) system uses morphologic criteria that emerged from retrospective studies using computerized image analysis of endometrial biopsies to identify morphologic features predictive of progression to carcinoma. These features were translated into diagnostic criteria that can be applied with the use of conventional light microscopy: (1) percentage of tissue occupied by glands (i.e., "volume percentage stroma"), (2) heterogeneity in nuclear diameter, and (3) complexity of glandular shape.[148] Microscopically, lesions that measure at least 1 to 2 mm, appear cytologically distinct from surrounding tissue, and display a volume percentage stroma of less than 55% are classified as EIN. Other abnormal proliferative lesions are classified as hyperplasia.

The categories in these three classification systems overlap in complex patterns; which classification best predicts cancer risk and is most reproducible is unclear.[143,149] Although pathologists achieve better interobserver agreement for severe forms of endometrial hyperplasia, diagnoses of milder lesions are less reproducible.[146] Historically, the crucial diagnostic issue for clinical management has been the tendency for general pathologists to misclassify variants of normal endometrium as hyperplastic, leading to excessive treatment. The optimal surrogate end point for endometrial cancer has not been identified, because the risk of progression for endometrial lesions is not well defined. Most studies that have attempted to define those risks have been small and retrospective and have not used statistical methods to account for follow-up time or possible confounders.[144,150-152]

What is the epidemiology of endometrial precursors?
Population-based prevalence estimates and incidence rates for endometrial hyperplasia are difficult to determine because registries usually do not track this diagnosis. One study of 2586 asymptomatic volunteers who were screened for endometrial cancer by direct sampling of the endometrium in combination with a cytologic technique found a similar period prevalence for endometrial hyperplasia and endometrial cancer.[153] In contrast, a summary of 2662 endometrial curettages performed at 11 Dutch hospitals reported 2182 hyperplasias and 480 carcinomas, indicating that invasive cancer is much less common than hyperplasia. However, only 49 of the hyperplasias were classified as atypical, which suggests that the most severe putative precursors are one tenth as common as carcinoma in clinical practice.[154] In short, the scarce data about the reservoir of endometrial cancer and its precursors in populations limit the ability to understand its natural history and accompanying public health issues.

What are the risk factors for endometrial precursors?
Risk factor data for endometrial precursors are rather limited. One comparison of 109 women with hyperplasia and 111 with endometrial cancer reported that unopposed estrogen and obesity were risk factors for both hyperplasia and cancer; however, parity, age at first birth, age at menopause, and body mass were associated only with cancer.[155] A case-control study of 129 women with endometrial hyperplasia without atypia and 258 controls concluded that higher education, obesity, diabetes, and hormone replacement therapy were risk factors for hyperplasia.[156] A retrospective clinical study of 46 cases of endometrial hyperplasia among premenopausal women found that older age, heavier weight, infertility, nulliparity, and family history of colon cancer were associated with increased risk.[157]

Biomarkers of Risk for Endometrial Cancer

How do endogenous hormones relate to risk?
Despite the recognition that endometrial cancer is a hormonally responsive tumor, few studies have assessed its relationships with endogenous hormones. To date, only three large epidemiologic studies have assessed associations with circulating estrogens.[92,158,159] All three studies observed an increased risk of postmenopausal endometrial cancer with increasing levels of estrone after adjustment for other factors, although in one study[158] the association was considerably attenuated after adjustment for body mass. In addition, two studies reported an increased risk with bioavailable (free and albumin-bound) fractions of estradiol and a reduced risk with increasing serum hormone–binding globulin.[158,159] In one investigation,[158] estrogens appeared to be less predictive of premenopausal disease, suggesting that anovulation or progesterone deficiency might be more predictive of risk.

Less well investigated is whether other endogenous hormones are related to endometrial cancer risk. Key and Pike[160] suggested cancer risk is associated with increased cell cycling, which is increased by estrogens and reduced by progesterone. Although progesterone deficiency could therefore be important, no major epidemiologic studies have assessed relationships with progesterone levels. The recognition that the adrenal cortex is the main source of steroid hormones has also led to an interest in adrenal hormones, such as cortisol, androstenedione, dehydroepiandrosterone, and dehydroepiandrosterone sulfate. Two large studies showed positive associations of endometrial cancer risk with serum androstenedione levels.[92,158] In one of these investigations,[158] this association remained after control for estrone levels, leading the investigators to speculate on the importance of aromatase and local conversion of estrone from androstenedione via abnormal endometrial cells.

Other hormone-related biomarkers have only recently been assessed with respect to endometrial cancer, and conclusive relationships are not yet apparent.[159] Of interest, however, are potential relationships with pituitary hormones and insulin-like growth factors.

Is obesity associated with endometrial cancer independently of endogenous hormones? Obesity, which is hypothesized to reflect elevated estrogen levels,[160] seems to represent a key risk factor for both endometrial hyperplasia and carcinoma, but the mechanisms mediating this risk are unclear. One case-control analysis of serum estrogen levels[158] reported that the risk associated with obesity was not entirely mediated by estrogen, especially among premenopausal women.[161] This led to interest in a potential role for insulin levels.[162] However, C peptide levels were found to be unrelated to risk.[163] In another cohort study of postmenopausal women, elevated serum estrogen concentrations appeared to account for the majority of the risk associated with obesity.[159] The relationship of hormones to identified risk factors therefore remains unresolved, supporting the need for further investigations to assess the interrelationships among a variety of risk factors with putative hormone biomarkers.

Does the perimenopause represent a crucial period for endometrial cancer? The "unopposed estrogen" hypothesis, in which exposure to estrogens in the absence of sufficient progestins leads to endometrial proliferation that can develop into endometrial precursors and endometrial cancer, appears to unify the risk and protective factors for endometrial cancer.[164] Key and Pike[160] hypothesized that estrogen levels higher than a certain threshold stimulate endometrial proliferation. In some women, the perimenopause seems to be associated with periodically spiking high levels of unopposed estrogens and anovulatory cycles, which could predispose to cancer development.

What molecular markers might elucidate endometrial carcinogenesis?

Several biomarkers are consistently associated with endometrioid cancer or hyperplasia. Human endometrial tissue expresses two isoforms of the estrogen receptor (ER-α and ER-β) and two isoforms of the progesterone receptor (PRA and PRB), but the role of these receptors in endometrial carcinogenesis is unclear. Expression of both ER and PR isoforms increases in the proliferative phase of the menstrual cycle,[165] but ER-α expression is stronger than that of ER-β near the time of ovulation. In one study, ER-α was detected in 80% of endometrial carcinomas, and ER-β in 36%, with nearly all of the latter showing coexpression of ER-α.[166] Silencing of the PRB gene via promoter methylation has been found in endometrial cancers but not in normal tissue.[167] Endometrial carcinoma may also be associated with a shift toward production of more carcinogenic estrogen metabolites.[168]

Among other markers that have been studied in endometrial tissues, 17β-hydroxysteroid dehydrogenase type 2, which converts estradiol to the less potent estrone, is expressed in secretory endometrium and in a subset of hyperplasias and cancers.[169] Expression of growth factors such as transforming growth factor-β,[170] inflammatory markers such as cyclooxygenase-2,[171] and proliferation and apoptosis markers such as Ki-67 and Bcl-2[172] suggests other markers of potential interest in endometrial carcinogenesis.

The tumor suppressor gene *PTEN* appears to influence several pathways that mediate apoptosis, cell proliferation, and motility.[173] *PTEN* mutations have been identified in up to 83% of endometrial cancers in some case series, as well as in a significant percentage of endometrial hyperplasias. In one report, endometrial samples obtained from about 50% of women with abnormal vaginal bleeding contained small foci of histologically normal glands that showed less of *PTEN* expression.[174] Histologically, normal appearing glands that demonstrated loss of *PTEN* expression may persist for over one year[175] and reflect an early predispositional state for the development of endometrial cancer.[176] If the high prevalence of *PTEN* alterations in non-neoplastic endometrium is confirmed, epidemiologic studies will be needed to determine why most of these foci remain quiescent or regress, whereas a minority expand and develop into precursor lesions.

Microsatellite instability, secondary to inactivating germline mutations in mismatch repair genes (*hMLH1*, *hMSH2*), is characteristic of endometrial cancers that develop in women with hereditary nonpolyposis colorectal carcinoma syndrome.[176] Loss of mismatch repair function of these same enzymes as a consequence of promoter methylation has been found in approximately 20% of sporadically occurring endometrial carcinomas.[177]

Endometrial carcinogenesis: more than one model?

Bokhman[178] first drew attention to the concept that there may be more than one pathway of endometrial carcinogenesis. Based on clinical data, he proposed that about two thirds of endometrial cancers (designated type I) are indolent neoplasms that are related to usual endometrial cancer risk factors that seem to reflect excess estrogen exposure, whereas the remainder (designated type II) are aggressive tumors that seem less related to typical hormonal risk factors mediated. Most endometrioid carcinomas represent the archetype of type I tumors, whereas serous carcinomas seem more characteristic of type II neoplasms.[179] Endometrial hyperplasia is considered to be the precursor of most type I tumors, whereas many type II tumors appear to develop from malignant transformation of atrophic endometrial surface epithelium rather than glandular proliferations. The pathologic lesion that reflects malignant surface change has been referred to by different authors as endometrial intraepithelial carcinoma,[180,181] endometrial carcinoma in situ,[182] and uterine surface carcinoma[183] and may represent the precursor of some invasive type II tumors. The two types display different patterns of molecular markers: *ras* and *PTEN* mutations and mismatch repair defects characterize type I tumors, whereas *TP53* tumor suppressor gene mutations have been found with high frequency in type II tumors.[184,185]

Endometrial carcinogenesis: future directions

The development of a refined model of endometrial carcinogenesis that incorporates genetic alterations, established risk factors, protective exposures, and hormonal imbalances, especially in the setting of anovulation, would enhance the understanding of this disease. The modifiable risk factors, particularly exogenous estrogens and increasing weight, might have crucial effects on distinct lesions at particular points in the spectrum from benign endometrium to invasive carcinoma. Continued efforts to better understand precursor lesions and to clarify the role of potential molecular markers should lead to improved efforts to reduce the population burden of endometrial cancer.

ACKNOWLEDGMENTS: The authors gratefully acknowledge Laure El Ghormli of the National Cancer Institute and John Lahey of IMS, Inc., for data development and figure generation.

REFERENCES

1. Ries LA, Eisner MP, Kosary CL, et al: SEER Cancer Statistics Review, 1973-1998. Bethesda: National Cancer Institute, 2001.
2. Jemal A, Murray T, Samuels A, et al: Cancer statistics, 2003. CA Cancer J Clin 2003;53:5-26.
3. Parkin DM, Pisani P, Ferlay J: Global cancer statistics. CA Cancer J Clin 1999;49:1, 33-64.
4. Pisani P, Parkin DM, Bray F, et al: Estimates of the worldwide mortality from 25 cancers in 1990. Int J Cancer 1999;83:870-873.
5. Mant JWF, Vessey MP: Ovarian and endometrial cancers. Cancer Surv 1994;19:287-307.
6. Parkin DM, Whelan SL, Ferlay J, et al: Cancer Incidence in Five Continents, Vol. VII. Lyon, IARC Scientific Publishers, 1997.
7. Muir C, Waterhouse J, Mack T: Cancer Incidence in Five Continents, Vol. V. Lyon, IARC Scientific Publishers, 1987.
8. Elwood JM, Cole P, Rothman KJ, et al: Epidemiology of endometrial cancer. J Natl Cancer Inst 1977;59:1055-1060.
9. Kelsey JL, LiVolsi VA, Holford TR, et al: A case-control study of cancer of the endometrium. Am J Epidemiol 1982;116:333-342.
10. Devesa SS, Grauman DG, Blot WJ, et al: Atlas of Cancer Mortality in the United States, 1950-1994. Washington, DC, US Government Printing Office, 1999.
11. Pickle LW, Mason TJ, Howard N, et al: Atlas of US cancer mortality among whites, 1950-1980. Washington, DC, US Government Printing Office, 1987.
12. Sturgeon SR, Schairer C, Gail M, et al: Geographic variation in mortality from breast cancer among white women in the United States. J Natl Cancer Inst 1995;87:1846-1852.
13. Devesa SS: Cancers in women. San Diego, Academic Press, 2000.
14. Weiss NS, Szekely DR, Austin DF: Increasing incidence of endometrial cancer in the United States. N Engl J Med 1976; 294:1259-1262.
15. Coleman MP, Esteve J, Damiecki P, et al: Trend in cancer incidence and mortality. Lyon, IARC Scientific Publishers, 1993.
16. Hill HA, Coates RJ, Austin H, et al: Racial differences in tumor grade among women with endometrial cancer. Gynecol Oncol 1995;56:154-163.
17. Brinton LA, Berman ML, Mortel R, et al: Reproductive, menstrual, and medical risk factors for endometrial cancer: Results from a case-control study. Am J Obstet Gynecol 1992;167: 1317-1325.
18. Henderson BE, Casagrande JT, Pike MC, et al: The epidemiology of endometrial cancer in young women. Br J Cancer 1983;47: 749-756.
19. Weiderpass E, Persson I, Adami HO, et al: Body size in different periods of life, diabetes mellitus, hypertension, and risk of postmenopausal endometrial cancer (Sweden). Cancer Causes Control 2000;11:185-192.
20. Modan B, Ron E, Lerner-Geva L, et al: Cancer incidence in a cohort of infertile women. Am J Epidemiol 1998;147:1038-1042.
21. Bernstein L, Pike MC, Ross RK, et al: Estrogen and sex hormone-binding globulin levels in nulliparous and parous women. J Natl Cancer Inst 1985;74:741-745.
22. Albrektsen G, Heuch I, Tretli S, et al: Is the risk of cancer of the corpus uteri reduced by a recent pregnancy? A prospective study of 765, 756 Norwegian women. Int J Cancer 1995;61:485-490.
23. Lambe M, Wuu J, Weiderpass E, et al: Childbearing at older age and endometrial cancer risk (Sweden). Cancer Causes Control 1999;10:43-49.
24. Castellsague X, Thompson WD, Dubrow R: Intra-uterine contraception and the risk of endometrial cancer. Int J Cancer 1993;54: 911-916.
25. Hill DA, Weiss NS, Voigt LF, et al: Endometrial cancer in relation to intra-uterine device use. Int J Cancer 1997;70:278-281.
26. Sturgeon SR, Brinton LA, Berman ML, et al: Intrauterine device use and endometrial cancer risk. Int J Epidemiol 1997;26:496-500.
27. Newcomb PA, Trentham-Dietz A: Breast feeding practices in relation to endometrial cancer risk, USA. Cancer Causes Control 2000;11:663-667.
28. Rosenblatt KA, Thomas DB: Prolonged lactation and endometrial cancer. WHO Collaborative Study of Neoplasia and Steroid Contraceptives. Int J Epidemiol 1995;24:499-503.
29. MacMahon B: Risk factors for endometrial cancer. Gynecol Oncol 1974;2:122-129.
30. Lacey JV Jr, Brinton LA, Mortel R, et al: Tubal sterilization and risk of cancer of the endometrium. Gynecol Oncol 2000;79: 482-484.
31. Combination oral contraceptive use and the risk of endometrial cancer: The Cancer and Steroid Hormone Study of the Centers for Disease Control and the National Institute of Child Health and Human Development. JAMA 1987;257:796-800.
32. Voigt LF, Deng Q, Weiss NS: Recency, duration, and progestin content of oral contraceptives in relation to the incidence of endometrial cancer (Washington, USA). Cancer Causes Control 1994;5:227-233.
33. Weiss NS, Sayvetz TA: Incidence of endometrial cancer in relation to the use of oral contraceptives. N Engl J Med 1980;302: 551-554.
34. Kaufman DW, Shapiro S, Slone D, et al: Decreased risk of endometrial cancer among oral-contraceptive users. N Engl J Med 1980; 303:1045-1047.
35. Rosenblatt KA, Thomas DB: Hormonal content of combined oral contraceptives in relation to the reduced risk of endometrial carcinoma: The WHO Collaborative Study of Neoplasia and Steroid Contraceptives. Int J Cancer 1991;49:870-874.

36. Brinton LA, Hoover RN: Estrogen replacement therapy and endometrial cancer risk: Unresolved issues. The Endometrial Cancer Collaborative Group. Obstet Gynecol 1993;81:265-271.

37. Green PK, Weiss NS, McKnight B, et al: Risk of endometrial cancer following cessation of menopausal hormone use (Washington, United States). Cancer Causes Control 1996;7:575-580.

38. Pike MC, Peters RK, Cozen W, et al: Estrogen-progestin replacement therapy and endometrial cancer. J Natl Cancer Inst 1997;89:1110-1116.

39. Shapiro S, Kelly JP, Rosenberg L, et al: Risk of localized and widespread endometrial cancer in relation to recent and discontinued use of conjugated estrogens. N Engl J Med 1985;313:969-972.

40. Pike MC, Ross RK: Progestins and menopause: epidemiological studies of risks of endometrial and breast cancer. Steroids 2000;65:659-664.

41. Levi F, La Vecchia C, Gulie C, et al: Oestrogen replacement treatment and the risk of endometrial cancer: An assessment of the role of covariates. Eur J Cancer 1993;29A:1445-1449.

42. Mack TM, Pike MC, Henderson BE, et al: Estrogens and endometrial cancer in a retirement community. N Engl J Med 1976;294:1262-1267.

43. Rubin GL, Peterson HB, Lee NC, et al: Estrogen replacement therapy and the risk of endometrial cancer: Remaining controversies. Am J Obstet Gynecol 1990;162:148-154.

44. Cushing KL, Weiss NS, Voigt LF, et al: Risk of endometrial cancer in relation to use of low-dose, unopposed estrogens. Obstet Gynecol 1998;91:35-39.

45. Herrinton LJ, Weiss NS: Postmenopausal unopposed estrogens: Characteristics of use in relation to the risk of endometrial carcinoma. Ann Epidemiol 1993;3:308-318.

46. Jain MG, Rohan TE, Howe GR: Hormone replacement therapy and endometrial cancer in Ontario, Canada. J Clin Epidemiol 2000;53:385-391.

47. Shapiro JA, Weiss NS, Beresford SA, et al: Menopausal hormone use and endometrial cancer, by tumor grade and invasion. Epidemiology 1998;9:99-101.

48. Elwood JM, Boyes DA: Clinical and pathological features and survival of endometrial cancer patients in relation to prior use of estrogens. Gynecol Oncol 1980;10:173-187.

49. Silverberg SG, Mullen D, Faraci JA, et al: Endometrial carcinoma: Clinical-pathologic comparison of cases in postmenopausal women receiving and not receiving exogenous estrogens. Cancer 1980;45:3018-3026.

50. Ferenczy A, Gelfand M: The biologic significance of cytologic atypia in progestogen-treated endometrial hyperplasia. Am J Obstet Gynecol 1989;160:126-131.

51. The Writing Group for the PEPI Trial: Effects of hormone replacement therapy on endometrial histology in postmenopausal women: The Postmenopausal Estrogen/Progestin Interventions (PEPI) Trial. JAMA 1996;275:370-375.

52. Persson I, Adami HO, Bergkvist L, et al: Risk of endometrial cancer after treatment with oestrogens alone or in conjunction with progestogens: Results of a prospective study. BMJ 1989;298:147-151.

53. Weiderpass E, Adami HO, Baron JA, et al: Risk of endometrial cancer following estrogen replacement with and without progestins. J Natl Cancer Inst 1999;91:1131-1137.

54. Beresford SA, Weiss NS, Voigt LF, et al: Risk of endometrial cancer in relation to use of oestrogen combined with cyclic progestagen therapy in postmenopausal women. Lancet 1997;349:458-461.

55. Archer DF: The effect of the duration of progestin use on the occurrence of endometrial cancer in postmenopausal women. Menopause 2001;8:245-251.

56. Andersson M, Storm HH, Mouridsen HT: Incidence of new primary cancers after adjuvant tamoxifen therapy and radiotherapy for early breast cancer. J Natl Cancer Inst 1991;83:1013-1017.

57. Fisher B, Costantino JP, Wickerham DL, et al: Tamoxifen for prevention of breast cancer: Report of the National Surgical Adjuvant Breast and Bowel Project P-1 Study. J Natl Cancer Inst 1998;90:1371-1388.

58. Fornander T, Rutqvist LE, Cedermark B, et al: Adjuvant tamoxifen in early breast cancer: Occurrence of new primary cancers. Lancet 1989;1:117-120.

59. van Leeuwen FE, Benraadt J, Coebergh JW, et al: Risk of endometrial cancer after tamoxifen treatment of breast cancer. Lancet 1994;343:448-452.

60. Bergman L, Beelen JLR, Gallee MPW, et al: Risk and prognosis of endometrial cancer after tamoxifen for breast cancer. Lancet 2000;356:881-887.

61. Benshushan A, Paltiel O, Brzezinski A, et al: Ovulation induction and risk of endometrial cancer: A pilot study. Eur J Obstet Gynecol Reprod Biol 2001;98:53-57.

62. Kato I, Zeleniuch-Jacquotte A, Toniolo PG, et al: Psychotropic medication use and risk of hormone-related cancers: The New York University Women's Health Study. J Public Health Med 2002;22:155-160.

63. Goodman MT, Wilkens LR, Hankin JH, et al: Association of soy and fiber consumption with the risk of endometrial cancer. Am J Epidemiol 1997;146:294-306.

64. Jain MG, Rohan TE, Howe GR, et al: A cohort study of nutritional factors and endometrial cancer. Eur J Epidemiol 2000;16:899-905.

65. La Vecchia C, Parazzini F, Negri E, et al: Anthropometric indicators of endometrial cancer risk. Eur J Cancer 1991;27:487-490.

66. Olson SH, Trevisan M, Marshall JR, et al: Body mass index, weight gain, and risk of endometrial cancer. Nutr Cancer 1995;23:141-149.

67. Shoff SM, Newcomb PA: Diabetes, body size, and risk of endometrial cancer. Am J Epidemiol 1998;148:234-240.

68. Swanson CA, Potischman N, Wilbanks GD, et al: Relation of endometrial cancer risk to past and contemporary body size and body fat distribution. Cancer Epidemiol Biomarkers Prev 1993;2:321-327.

69. Blitzer PH, Blitzer EC, Rimm AA: Association between teen-age obesity and cancer in 56,111 women: All cancers and endometrial carcinoma. Prev Med 1976;5:20-31.

70. Levi F, La Vecchia C, Negri E, et al: Body mass at different ages and subsequent endometrial cancer risk. Int J Cancer 1992;50:567-571.

71. Elliott EA, Matanoski GM, Rosenshein NB, et al: Body fat patterning in women with endometrial cancer. Gynecol Oncol 1990;39:253-258.

72. Schapira DV, Kumar NB, Lyman GH, et al: Upper-body fat distribution and endometrial cancer risk. JAMA 1991;266:1808-1811.

73. Austin H, Austin JM Jr, Partridge EE, et al: Endometrial cancer, obesity, and body fat distribution. Cancer Res 1991;51:568-572.

74. Folsom AR, Kaye SA, Potter JD, et al: Association of incident carcinoma of the endometrium with body weight and fat distribution in older women: Early findings of the Iowa Women's Health Study. Cancer Res 1989;49:6828-6831.

75. Shu XO, Brinton LA, Zheng W, et al: Relation of obesity and body fat distribution to endometrial cancer in Shanghai, China. Cancer Res 1992;52:3865-3870.

76. Shu XO, Hatch MC, Zheng W, et al: Physical activity and risk of endometrial cancer. Epidemiology 1993;4:342-349.

77. Sturgeon SR, Brinton LA, Berman ML, et al: Past and present physical activity and endometrial cancer risk. Br J Cancer 1993;68:584-589.

78. Moradi T, Weiderpass E, Signorello LB, et al: Physical activity and postmenopausal endometrial cancer risk (Sweden). Cancer Causes Control 2000;11:829-837.

79. Littman AJ, Voigt LF, Beresford SA, et al: Recreational physical activity and endometrial cancer risk. Am J Epidemiol 2001;154:924-933.

80. Gusberg SB: Current concepts in cancer: The changing nature of endometrial cancer. N Engl J Med 1980;302:729-731.

81. Armstrong B, Doll R: Environmental factors and cancer incidence and mortality in different countries, with special reference to dietary practices. Int J Cancer 1975;15:617-631.

82. Potischman N, Swanson CA, Brinton LA, et al: Dietary associations in a case-control study of endometrial cancer. Cancer Causes Control 1993;4:239-250.

83. Barbone F, Austin H, Partridge EE: Diet and endometrial cancer: A case-control study. Am J Epidemiol 1993;137:393-403.

84. McCann SE, Freudenheim JL, Marshall JR, et al: Diet in the epidemiology of endometrial cancer in western New York (United States). Cancer Causes Control 2000;11:965-974.

85. Negri E, La Vecchia C, Franceschi S, et al: Intake of selected micronutrients and the risk of endometrial carcinoma. Cancer 1996;77:917-923.

86. Goodman MT, Hankin JH, Wilkens LR, et al: Diet, body size, physical activity, and the risk of endometrial cancer. Cancer Res 1997;57:5077-5085.

87. Terry P, Wolk A, Vainio H, et al: Fatty fish consumption lowers the risk of endometrial cancer: A nationwide case-control study in Sweden. Cancer Epidemiol Biomarkers Prev 2002;11:143-145.

88. Armstrong BK, Brown JB, Clarke HT, et al: Diet and reproductive hormones: A study of vegetarian and nonvegetarian postmenopausal women. J Natl Cancer Inst 1981;67:761-767.

89. Barbosa JC, Shultz TD, Filley SJ, et al: The relationship among adiposity, diet, and hormone concentrations in vegetarian and nonvegetarian postmenopausal women. Am J Clin Nutr 1990;51:798-803.

90. Goldin BR, Adlercreutz H, Gorbach SL, et al: The relationship between estrogen levels and diets of Caucasian American and Oriental immigrant women. Am J Clin Nutr 1986;44:945-953.

91. Prentice R, Thompson D, Clifford C, et al: Dietary fat reduction and plasma estradiol concentration in healthy postmenopausal women: The Women's Health Trial Study Group. J Natl Cancer Inst 1990;82:129-134.

92. Austin H, Drews C, Partridge EE: A case-control study of endometrial cancer in relation to cigarette smoking, serum estrogen levels, and alcohol use. Am J Obstet Gynecol 1993;169:1086-1091.

93. Newcomb PA, Trentham-Dietz A, Storer BE: Alcohol consumption in relation to endometrial cancer risk. Cancer Epidemiol Biomarkers Prev 1997;6:775-778.

94. Swanson CA, Wilbanks GD, Twiggs LB, et al: Moderate alcohol consumption and the risk of endometrial cancer. Epidemiology 1993;4:530-536.

95. Webster LA, Weiss NS: Alcoholic beverage consumption and the risk of endometrial cancer. Cancer and Steroid Hormone Study Group. Int J Epidemiol 1989;18:786-791.

96. Gapstur SM, Potter JD, Sellers TA, et al: Alcohol consumption and postmenopausal endometrial cancer: Results from the Iowa Women's Health Study. Cancer Causes Control 1993;4:323-329.

97. Weiderpass E, Baron JA: Cigarette smoking, alcohol consumption, and endometrial cancer risk: A population-based study in Sweden. Cancer Causes Control 2001;12:239-247.

98. Weiderpass E, Pukkala E, Vasama-Neuvonen K, et al: Occupational exposures and cancers of the endometrium and cervix uteri in Finland. Am J Ind Med 2001;39:572-580.

99. Weir HK, Sloan M, Kreiger N: The relationship between cigarette smoking and the risk of endometrial neoplasms. Int J Epidemiol 1994;23:261-266.

100. Baron JA, Byers T, Greenberg ER, et al: Cigarette smoking in women with cancers of the breast and reproductive organs. J Natl Cancer Inst 1986;77:677-680.

101. Brinton LA, Barrett RJ, Berman ML, et al: Cigarette smoking and the risk of endometrial cancer. Am J Epidemiol 1993;137:281-291.

102. Lawrence C, Tessaro I, Durgerian S, et al: Smoking, body weight, and early-stage endometrial cancer. Cancer 1987;59:1665-1669.

103. Lesko SM, Rosenberg L, Kaufman DW, et al: Cigarette smoking and the risk of endometrial cancer. N Engl J Med 1985;313:593-596.

104. Newcomer LM, Newcomb PA, Trentham-Dietz A, et al: Hormonal risk factors for endometrial cancer: Modification by cigarette smoking (United States). Cancer Causes Control 2001;12:829-835.

105. Parazzini F, La Vecchia C, Negri E, et al: Smoking and risk of endometrial cancer: Results from an Italian case-control study. Gynecol Oncol 1995;56:195-199.

106. Jafari K, Javaheri G, Ruiz G: Endometrial adenocarcinoma and the Stein-Leventhal syndrome. Obstet Gynecol 1978;51:97-100.

107. Wild S, Pierpoint T, Jacobs H, et al: Long-term consequences of polycystic ovary syndrome: Results of a 31 year follow-up study. Hum Fertil (Camb) 2000;3:101-105.

108. Wood GP, Boronow RC: Endometrial adenocarcinoma and the polycystic ovary syndrome. Am J Obstet Gynecol 1976;124:140-142.

109. Coulam CB, Annegers JF, Kranz JS: Chronic anovulation syndrome and associated neoplasia. Obstet Gynecol 1983;61:403-407.

110. Dahlgren E, Friberg LG, Johansson S, et al: Endometrial carcinoma; ovarian dysfunction—A risk factor in young women. Eur J Obstet Gynecol Reprod Biol 1991;41:143-150.

111. Weiderpass E, Gridley G, Persson I, et al: Risk of endometrial and breast cancer in patients with diabetes mellitus. Int J Cancer 1997;71:360-363.

112. Wideroff L, Gridley G, Mellemkjaer L, et al: Cancer incidence in a population-based cohort of patients hospitalized with diabetes mellitus in Denmark. J Natl Cancer Inst 1997;89:1360-1365.

113. Inoue M, Okayama A, Fujita M, et al: A case-control study on risk factors for uterine endometrial cancer in Japan. Jpn J Cancer Res 1994;85:346-350.

114. La Vecchia C, Negri E, Franceschi S, et al: A case-control study of diabetes mellitus and cancer risk. Br J Cancer 1994;70:950-953.

115. Parazzini F, La Vecchia C, Negri E, et al: Diabetes and endometrial cancer: An Italian case-control study. Int J Cancer 1999;81:539-542.

116. Anderson KE, Anderson E, Mink PJ, et al: Diabetes and endometrial cancer in the Iowa women's health study. Cancer Epidemiol Biomarkers Prev 2001;10:611-616.

117. Newcomb PA, Trentham-Dietz A, Egan KM, et al: Fracture history and risk of breast and endometrial cancer. Am J Epidemiol 2001;153:1071-1078.

118. Persson I, Adami HO, McLaughlin JK, et al: Reduced risk of breast and endometrial cancer among women with hip fractures (Sweden). Cancer Causes Control 1994;5:523-528.

119. Gruber SB, Thompson WD: A population-based study of endometrial cancer and familial risk in younger women. Cancer and Steroid Hormone Study Group. Cancer Epidemiol Biomarkers Prev 1996;5:411-417.

120. Hemminki K, Vaittinen P, Dong C: Endometrial cancer in the family-cancer database. Cancer Epidemiol Biomarkers Prev 1999;8:1005-1010.

121. Parslov M, Lidegaard O, Klintorp S, et al: Risk factors among young women with endometrial cancer: A Danish case-control study. Am J Obstet Gynecol 2000;182:23-29.

122. Parazzini F, La Vecchia C, Moroni S, et al: Family history and the risk of endometrial cancer. Int J Cancer 1994;59:460-462.

123. Hemminki K, Li X, Dong C: Second primary cancers after sporadic and familial colorectal cancer. Cancer Epidemiol Biomarkers Prev 2001;10:793-798.

124. Levine DA, Lin O, Barakat RR, et al: Risk of endometrial carcinoma associated with BRCA mutation. Gynecol Oncol 2001;80:395-398.

125. Esteller M, Garcia A, Martinez-Palones JM, et al: Germ line polymorphisms in cytochrome-P450 1A1 (C4887 CYP1A1) and methylenetetrahydrofolate reductase (MTHFR) genes and endometrial cancer susceptibility. Carcinogenesis 1997;18:2307-2311.

126. Esteller M, Garcia A, Martinez-Palones JM, et al: Susceptibility to endometrial cancer: Influence of allelism at p53, glutathione S-transferase (GSTM1 and GSTT1) and cytochrome P-450 (CYP1A1) loci. Br J Cancer 1997;75:1385-1388.

127. Weiderpass E, Persson I, Melhus H, et al: Estrogen receptor alpha gene polymorphisms and endometrial cancer risk. Carcinogenesis 2002;21:623-627.

128. Sturgeon SR, Brock JW, Potischman N, et al: Serum concentrations of organochlorine compounds and endometrial cancer risk (United States). Cancer Causes Control 1998;9:417-424.

129. Weiderpass E, Adami HO, Baron JA, et al: Organochlorines and endometrial cancer risk. Cancer Epidemiol Biomarkers Prev 2000;9:487-493.

130. McElroy JA, Newcomb PA, Trentham-Dietz A, et al: Endometrial cancer incidence in relation to electric blanket use. Am J Epidemiol 2002;156:262-267.

131. Dijkhuizen FP, Mol BW, Brolmann HA, et al: The accuracy of endometrial sampling in the diagnosis of patients with endometrial carcinoma and hyperplasia: A meta-analysis. Cancer 2000;89:1765-1772.

132. Xie X, Lu WG, Ye DF, et al: The value of curettage in diagnosis of endometrial hyperplasia. Gynecol Oncol 2002;84:135-139.

133. Marsden DE, Hacker NF: Optimal management of endometrial hyperplasia. Best Pract Res Clin Obstet Gynaecol 2001;15:393-405.

134. Randall TC, Kurman RJ: Progestin treatment of atypical hyperplasia and well-differentiated carcinoma of the endometrium in women under age 40. Obstet Gynecol 1997;90:434-440.

135. Montz FJ, Bristow RE, Bovicelli A, et al: Intrauterine progesterone treatment of early endometrial cancer. Am J Obstet Gynecol 2002;186:651-657.

136. Kobiashvili H, Charkviani L, Charkviani T: Organ preserving method in the management of atypical endometrial hyperplasia. Eur J Gynaecol Oncol 2001;22:297-299.

137. Huang SJ, Amparo EG, Yao SF: Endometrial hyperplasia: Histologic classification and behavior. Surg Pathol 1988;1: 215-229.

138. Terakawa N, Kigawa J, Taketani Y, et al: The behavior of endometrial hyperplasia: A prospective study. Endometrial Hyperplasia Study Group. J Obstet Gynaecol Res 1997;23: 223-230.

139. Tabata T, Yamawaki T, Yabana T, et al: Natural history of endometrial hyperplasia: Study of 77 patients. Arch Gynecol Obstet 2001;265:85-88.

140. Gucer F, Reich O, Tamussino K, et al: Concomitant endometrial hyperplasia in patients with endometrial carcinoma. Gynecol Oncol 1998;69:64-68.

141. Kaku T, Tsukamoto N, Hachisuga T, et al: Endometrial carcinoma associated with hyperplasia. Gynecol Oncol 1996;60:22-25.

142. Anastasiadis PG, Skaphida PG, Koutlaki NG, et al: Descriptive epidemiology of endometrial hyperplasia in patients with abnormal uterine bleeding. Eur J Gynaecol Oncol 2000;21: 131-134.

143. Zaino RJ: Endometrial hyperplasia: Is it time for a quantum leap to a new classification? Int J Gynecol Pathol 2000;19: 314-321.

144. Kurman RJ, Kaminski PF, Norris HJ: The behavior of endometrial hyperplasia: A long-term study of "untreated" hyperplasia in 170 patients. Cancer 1985;56:403-412.

145. Skov BG, Broholm H, Engel U, et al: Comparison of the reproducibility of the WHO classifications of 1975 and 1994 of endometrial hyperplasia. Int J Gynecol Pathol 1997;16:33-37.

146. Kendall BS, Ronnett BM, Isacson C, et al: Reproducibility of the diagnosis of endometrial hyperplasia, atypical hyperplasia, and well-differentiated carcinoma. Am J Surg Pathol 1998;22: 1012-1019.

147. Bergeron C, Nogales FF, Masseroli M, et al: A multicentric European study testing the reproducibility of the WHO classification of endometrial hyperplasia with a proposal of a simplified working classification for biopsy and curettage specimens. Am J Surg Pathol 1999;23:1102-1108.

148. Mutter GL: Endometrial intraepithelial neoplasia (EIN): Will it bring order to chaos? The Endometrial Collaborative Group. Gynecol Oncol 2000;76:287-290.

149. Baak JP, Orbo A, van Diest PJ, et al: Prospective multicenter evaluation of the morphometric D-score for prediction of the outcome of endometrial hyperplasias. Am J Surg Pathol 2001; 25:930-935.

150. Pettersson B, Adami HO, Lindgren A, et al: Endometrial polyps and hyperplasia as risk factors for endometrial carcinoma: A case-control study of curettage specimens. Acta Obstet Gynecol Scand 1985;64:653-659.

151. Colgan TJ, Norris HJ, Foster W, et al: Predicting the outcome of endometrial hyperplasia by quantitative analysis of nuclear features using a linear discriminant function. Int J Gynecol Pathol 1983;1:347-352.

152. Ortner A, Mikuz G, Jerabek R: Study of prior biopsies of endometrial cancer patients and controls. Cancer Detect Prev 1981;4:475-480.

153. Koss LG, Schreiber K, Oberlander SG, et al: Detection of endometrial carcinoma and hyperplasia in asymptomatic women. Obstet Gynecol 1984;64:1-11.

154. Ausems EW, van der Kamp JK, Baak JP: Nuclear morphometry in the determination of the prognosis of marked atypical endometrial hyperplasia. Int J Gynecol Pathol 1985;4:180-185.

155. Baanders-van Halewyn EA, Blankenstein MA, Thijssen JH, et al: A comparative study of risk factors for hyperplasia and cancer of the endometrium. Eur J Cancer Prev 1996;5:105-112.

156. Ricci E, Moroni S, Parazzini F, et al: Risk factors for endometrial hyperplasia: Results from a case-control study. Int J Gynecol Cancer 2002;12:257-260.

157. Farquhar CM, Lethaby A, Sowter M, et al: An evaluation of risk factors for endometrial hyperplasia in premenopausal women with abnormal menstrual bleeding. Am J Obstet Gynecol 1999;181:525-529.

158. Potischman N, Hoover RN, Brinton LA, et al: Case-control study of endogenous steroid hormones and endometrial cancer. J Natl Cancer Inst 1996;88:1127-1135.

159. Zeleniuch-Jacquotte A, Akhmedkhanov A, Kato I, et al: Postmenopausal endogenous oestrogens and risk of endometrial cancer: Results of a prospective study. Br J Cancer 2001;84: 975-981.

160. Key TJ, Pike MC: The dose-effect relationship between "unopposed" oestrogens and endometrial mitotic rate: Its central role in explaining and predicting endometrial cancer risk. Br J Cancer 1988;57:205-212.

161. Potischman N, Gail MH, Troisi R, et al: Measurement error does not explain the persistence of a body mass index association with endometrial cancer after adjustment for endogenous hormones. Epidemiology 1999;10:76-79.

162. Hale GE, Hughes CL, Cline JM: Endometrial cancer: Hormonal factors, the perimenopausal "window of risk," and isoflavones. J Clin Endocrinol Metab 2002;87:3-15.

163. Troisi R, Potischman N, Hoover RN, et al: Insulin and endometrial cancer. Am J Epidemiol 1997;146:476-482.

164. Akhmedkhanov A, Zeleniuch-Jacquotte A, Toniolo P: Role of exogenous and endogenous hormones in endometrial cancer: Review of the evidence and research perspectives [review]. Ann N Y Acad Sci 2001;943:296-315.

165. Mote PA, Balleine RL, McGowan EM, et al: Colocalization of progesterone receptors A and B by dual immunofluorescent histochemistry in human endometrium during the menstrual cycle. J Clin Endocrinol Metab 1999;84:2963-2971.

166. Utsunomiya H, Suzuki T, Harada N, et al: Analysis of estrogen receptor alpha and beta in endometrial carcinomas: Correlation with ER beta and clinicopathologic findings in 45 cases. Int J Gynecol Pathol 2000;19:335-341.

167. Sasaki M, Dharia A, Oh BR, et al: Progesterone receptor B gene inactivation and CpG hypermethylation in human uterine endometrial cancer. Cancer Res 2001;61:97-102.

168. Newbold RR, Liehr JG: Induction of uterine adenocarcinoma in CD-1 mice by catechol estrogens. Cancer Res 2000;60: 235-237.

169. Utsunomiya H, Suzuki T, Kaneko C, et al: The analyses of 17beta-hydroxysteroid dehydrogenase isozymes in human endometrial hyperplasia and carcinoma. J Clin Endocrinol Metab 2001;86:3436-3443.

170. Parekh TV, Gama P, Wen X, et al: Transforming growth factor beta signaling is disabled early in human endometrial carcinogenesis concomitant with loss of growth inhibition. Cancer Res 2002;62:2778-2790.

171. Cao QJ, Einstein MH, Anderson PS, et al: Expression of COX-2, Ki-67, cyclin D1, and P21 in endometrial endometrioid carcinomas. Int J Gynecol Pathol 2002;21:147-154.

172. Risberg B, Karlsson K, Abeler V, et al: Dissociated expression of Bcl-2 and Ki-67 in endometrial lesions: Diagnostic and histogenetic implications. Int J Gynecol Pathol 2002;21:155-160.

173. Waite KA, Eng C: Protean PTEN: Form and function. Am J Hum Genet 2002;70:829-844.

174. Mutter GL, Lin MC, Fitzgerald JT, et al: Altered PTEN expression as a diagnostic marker for the earliest endometrial precancers. J Natl Cancer Inst 2000;92:924-930.

175. Mutter GL, Ince TA, Baak JP, et al: Molecular identification of latent precancers in histologically normal endometrium. Cancer Res 2001;61:4311-4314.

176. Matias-Guiu X, Catasus L, Bussaglia E, et al: Molecular pathology of endometrial hyperplasia and carcinoma. Hum Pathol 2001;32:569-577.

177. Inoue M: Current molecular aspects of the carcinogenesis of the uterine endometrium. Int J Gynecol Cancer 2001;11:339-348.

178. Bokhman JV: Two pathogenetic types of endometrial carcinoma. Gynecol Oncol 1983;15:10-17.

179. Sherman ME: Theories of endometrial carcinogenesis: A multidisciplinary approach. Mod Pathol 2000;13:295-308.

180. Sherman ME, Bitterman P, Rosenshein NB, et al: Uterine serous carcinoma: A morphologically diverse neoplasm with unifying clinicopathologic features. Am J Surg Pathol 1992;16: 600-610.

181. Ambros RA, Sherman ME, Zahn CM, et al: Endometrial intraepithelial carcinoma: A distinctive lesion specifically associated with tumors displaying serous differentiation. Hum Pathol 1995;26:1260-1267.

182. Spiegel GW: Endometrial carcinoma in situ in postmenopausal women. Am J Surg Pathol 1995;19:417-432.

183. Zheng W, Khurana R, Farahmand S, et al: *p53* immunostaining as a significant adjunct diagnostic method for uterine surface carcinoma: Precursor of uterine papillary serous carcinoma. Am J Surg Pathol 1998;22:1463-1473.

184. Tashiro H, Isacson C, Levine R, et al: *p53* gene mutations are common in uterine serous carcinoma and occur early in their pathogenesis. Am J Pathol 1997;150:177-185.

185. Sherman ME, Bur ME, Kurman RJ: *p53* in endometrial cancer and its putative precursors: evidence for diverse pathways of tumorigenesis. Hum Pathol 1995;26:1268-1274.

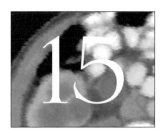

CHAPTER

PATHOLOGY OF UTERINE CANCERS

Michael R. Hendrickson   and   Teri A. Longacre

✦ MAJOR CONTROVERSIES

- Should the traditional "benign-malignant" classification be expanded to reflect different levels of malignancy in the mesenchymal and mixed epithelial/mesenchymal neoplasms of the uterus?
- Is malignant mixed mullerian tumor (carcinosarcoma) really a form of carcinoma (metaplastic carcinoma) rather than a sarcoma? What would be the clinical implications were this true?
- Are there reliable ways of distinguishing the endometrial stromal phenotype from the smooth muscle phenotype, and under what circumstances would this distinction be important?
- What is the difference between "atypical leiomyoma with low risk of recurrence" and a uterine "smooth muscle tumor of uncertain malignant potential" (STUMP)?
- Can endometrial hyperplasia/metaplasia be reliably distinguished from well-differentiated endometrial carcinoma?
- Can the precursor lesions of type I endometrial carcinoma be reliably identified, and can this precursor group be partitioned in a way that reflects increasing levels of risk for development of an endometrial carcinoma?
- Can invasive adenocarcinoma of the cervix be reliably distinguished from invasive adenocarcinoma of the endometrium on endometrial sampling?
- Do coexistent carcinomas of the endometrium and ovary represent synchronous primary tumors or metastases from endometrium to ovary, or from ovary to endometrium?
- Is there a precursor of type II cancers, and how should it be managed?
- How much uterine serous carcinoma (or clear cell carcinoma) in a mixed proliferation is sufficient for a diagnosis of uterine serous carcinoma (or clear cell carcinoma)?
- What is the significance of stage Ia uterine serous carcinoma? Do optimally staged stage Ia uterine serous carcinomas require adjuvant therapy?
- Once a diagnosis of clear cell carcinoma is established, does further diagnostic refinement provide additional prognostic information?
- Does papillary architecture in a nonserous endometrial carcinoma, in and of itself, confer an unfavorable prognosis?

This is a review of selected, managerially relevant problems in malignant and premalignant conditions of the uterine corpus that continue to challenge gynecologic pathologists. Most of these problems have not strongly polarized the gynecologic pathology community and therefore do not lend themselves to a "pros and cons" formulation; however, they represent ongoing areas of active investigation.

UTERINE SARCOMA PROBLEMS

Beyond "Benign" and "Malignant"

Should the traditional "benign-malignant" classification be expanded to reflect different levels of malignancy in the mesenchymal and mixed epithelial/mesenchymal neoplasms of the uterus? One of the major advances in surgical pathology over recent decades has been the gradual abandonment of the traditional "benign-malignant" classification of many differentiated types of neoplasms. As more and more clinicopathologic experience has accrued, the inadequacies of this dichotomous classification for many classes of neoplasms have become apparent; these classifications simply fail to capture the substantial differences in clinical behavior exhibited by the "nonbenign" group. There has been a general trend to retain the benign category (i.e., complete local excision is curative) but to expand the nonbenign group into a number of categories that reflect different patterns of clinically nonbenign behavior. These patterns typically include a consideration of the site of failure (local, regional, or distant); the probability of failure in each of these sites; and the tempo of failure. An example of this trend is the wide acceptance of the ovarian serous neoplasm of low malignant potential (LMP). A useful byproduct of setting out the clinicopathologic characteristics of the particular nonbenign class under consideration is that it replaces the sterile discourse about which of the "nonbenign" categories are "really" malignant with a discussion of the clinicopathologic characteristics of the category and the rational treatment options that follow from the unique behavior of the group.

It is important to emphasize that these clinicopathologic categories (e.g., stage I serous LMP) are not pathologists' hedges; they are well-characterized entities with quite specific behaviors some of which simply resist a comfortable sorting into "benign" or "malignant." To be sure, there are times when it would be clinically irresponsible for a pathologist to be dogmatic about the prognosis of a particular neoplasm (e.g., a particular uterine smooth muscle neoplasm that provides conflicting histopathologic signals). It may be that insufficient experience has been gathered about tumors with this particular constellation of features to know, for example, what the average failure rate is after a particular therapy (e.g., myomectomy). The responsible thing for the pathologist to do in this instance is to hedge and to indicate this situation with a suitable name; the labels used in this circumstance should reflect this very different function (Fig. 15-1). Smooth muscle tumor of uncertain malignant potential (STUMP) is an example of a "hedge" label;

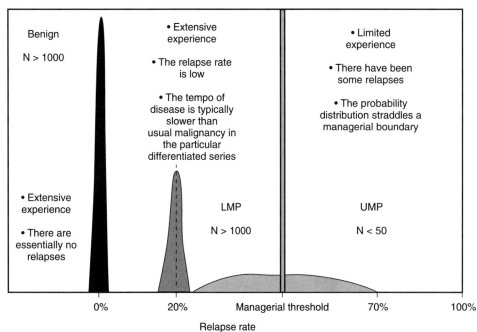

'Benign', 'Low malignant potential' (LMP) and
'Uncertain malignant potential' (UMP) contrasted

Benign
N > 1000

- Extensive
experience

- The relapse rate
is low

- The tempo of
disease is typically
slower than
usual malignancy in
the particular
differentiated series

- Extensive
experience

- There are
essentially no
relapses

LMP
N > 1000

- Limited
experience

- There have been
some relapses

- The probability
distribution straddles a
managerial boundary

UMP
N < 50

0%   20%   Managerial threshold   70%   100%

Relapse rate

Figure 15–1. This diagram makes more explicit the distinction among the clinicopathologic labels, "benign," "low malignant potential" (LMP), and "uncertain malignant potential" (UMP). The subjective probability distribution depicted represents a summary of the informed observer's response to questions of the form, "How probable is it that the *true* relapse rate for LMP (for example) is $(X \pm 0.5)$%?" The value of X is run through all values from 0% to 100%. This assignment usually is based in part on published experience and in part on the expert's personal experience with the entity under consideration. The frequency distribution is centered on the expert's most likely value for the relapse rate (the mean); the width of the curve (the variance) in part reflects the number of cases used for the estimate. The area marked "Managerial Threshold" indicates roughly the range of relapse rates for which a clinically significant difference in therapy and/or prognosis can be obtained.

the circumstances in which it is used are discussed later, in the context of smooth muscle neoplasms.

It is in this spirit that we offer a clinicopathologic classification of uterine mesenchymal and mixed epithelial mesenchymal neoplasms. The histogenetic classification of these neoplasms is relatively complex.[1,2] The primary division is between pure mesenchymal and mixed epithelial/mesenchymal neoplasms. The pure mesenchymal group is further subdivided into those neoplasms that exhibit differentiation normally encountered in the uterus (homologous—i.e., endometrial stromal or smooth muscle), neoplasms exhibiting differentiation not normally present in the uterus (heterologous—e.g., skeletal muscle, cartilage, bone), and neoplasms that are undifferentiated. Of course, the vast majority of neoplasms in this pure mesenchymal group are ordinary leiomyomas. A much smaller percentage of smooth muscle neoplasms are leiomyosarcomas. Most neoplasms exhibiting endometrial stromal differentiation are low-grade sarcomas (endometrial stromal sarcoma); fewer than 10% are benign (stromal nodules). Heterologous differentiation is usually encountered in mixed epithelial/mesenchymal neoplasms, but, rarely, it may be the only differentiated type present; these tumors are almost always malignant.

Any of the malignant mesenchymal patterns of differentiation may be combined with benign or malignant glandular elements to yield, respectively, adenofibroma/adenosarcoma or carcinosarcoma (also known as malignant mixed mullerian tumor). These mixed neoplasms may be further subdivided into homologous or heterologous groups, depending on the phenotype of the mesenchymal component.

These neoplasms exhibit clinical behaviors that range from benign to highly aggressive. Some neoplasms, for example, routinely are diagnosed at high stage, spread locally, disseminate both regionally and distantly, and, over the course of one to several years, characteristically prove fatal. A minority of neoplasms has an intermediate behavior. We distinguish four patterns of clinical behavior exhibited by uterine mesenchymal and mixed epithelial/mesenchymal neoplasms:

Clinical Disease I: *"Benign"*

Local excision is curative

Clinical Disease II: *"Benign, but..."*

Usually clinically benign, but infrequently is diagnosed at high stage or recurs after initial presentation at low stage; indolent clinical course when recurrence recurs; only rarely fatal (e.g., intravenous leiomyomatosis with cardiac involvement)

Clinical Disease III: *"Low Grade Malignancy"*

Sometimes patients present with high-stage disease; recurrence is not unusual; the disease is indolent

Clinical Disease IV: *"Highly Malignant"*

Patients often present with high-stage disease; local, regional and distant failures are typical; rapid evolution is typical

These clinical patterns are correlated with the histogenetic classification of uterine mesenchymal and mixed epithelial/mesenchymal neoplasms in Table 15-1. The classification becomes greatly simplified when this

Table 15–1. Histogenetic Classification of Uterine Neoplasms with Either a Mesenchymal or a Mixed Mesenchymal/Epithelial Phenotype

| Phenotype | Clinical Disease Behavior | | | |
	Type I*	Type II†	Type III‡	Type IV§
Endometrial stromal differentiation	Stromal nodule with or without sex cord elements or glands		Endometrial stromal sarcoma with or without sex cord elements or glands	
Smooth muscle differentiation	Leiomyoma and variants	IVL; atypical leiomyoma with low risk of recurrence; BML; LPD		Leiomyosarcoma: Usual Epithelioid Myxoid
Pure heterologous differentiation	Metaplastic bone or cartilage			Osteosarcoma; chondrosarcoma; liposarcoma; rhabdomyosarcoma; angiosarcoma
Undifferentiated monomorphous spindled cells				Undifferentiated sarcoma
Mixed mullerian differentiation	Adenofibroma; APA	Atypical polypoid adenomyoma of LMP	Adenosarcoma; adenosarcoma with bland sarcomatous overgrowth	Carcinosarcoma (malignant mixed mullerian tumor); adenosarcoma with morphologic malignant stromal overgrowth

*Clinically benign.
†Clinically benign with very few exceptions; if there is dissemination beyond the uterus, the tempo of disease is slow and compatible with long-term survival.
‡Clinically a malignancy of low aggressiveness; local, regional and distant recurrence; slow tempo of disease; fatal in a minority of cases.
§Clinically aggressive malignancy from outset; local, regional, distant spread.
APA, atypical polypoid adenomyoma; BML, benign metastasing leiomyoma; IVL, intravenous leiomyomatosis; LMP, low malignant potential; LPD, leiomyomatosis peritonealis disseminata.

expanded characterization of clinical behavior is used as the organizing principle.

Is Carcinosarcoma Really a Sarcoma?

Is malignant mixed mullerian tumor (carcinosarcoma) really a form of carcinoma (metaplastic carcinoma) rather than a sarcoma? What would be the clinical implications were this true? Neoplasms composed of an intimate admixture of malignant epithelial elements (carcinoma) and malignant mesenchymal elements (sarcoma) arise in a variety of organs (Fig. 15-2). They are most commonly encountered in the female genital tract, particularly the uterine corpus.[1,3,4]

Pathologists have long puzzled over the pathogenesis of these distinctive and easily recognized neoplasms. A number of theories have been proposed to account for this paradoxical mixture of distinct phenotypes that are usually encountered in pure form and are thought to have distinct histogenetic origins.[3] The two most popular theories are the "collision" theory and the "divergence" theory. The first postulates the development of two separate malignancies, which then intermingle to produce a biphasic pattern (i.e., a biclonal origin). The second theory posits a single malignant precursor population that then undergoes clonal evolution in two distinct directions: carcinoma and sarcoma (i.e., a monoclonal origin).

Currently, this is developing into more than a pathologists' discussion of taxonomic niceties; at stake are serious issues relating to therapy. Traditionally, these neoplasms have been grouped with the uterine sarcomas and treated as such. The mounting evidence summarized in the following paragraphs suggests that they are not sarcomas but rather special variant carcinomas—metaplastic carcinomas—and are more appropriately treated with carcinoma therapy. In this view, carcinosarcoma would take its place alongside other high-grade endometrial carcinoma variants such as uterine serous carcinoma (USC) and clear cell carcinoma

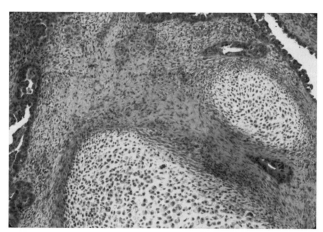

Figure 15–2. Carcinosarcoma. Carcinosarcomas feature an intimate admixture of carcinoma and sarcoma. Note malignant bone and cartilage. See also Color Figure 15-2.

(CCC); indeed, a popular textbook of gynecologic pathology has made this organizational move.[5]

Many terms have been proposed for these distinctive neoplasms, each reflecting a particular investigator's histogenetic bias. In the female genital tract, the most popular terms have been malignant mixed mullerian tumor (MMMT) and carcinosarcoma. For convenience, we will use the label "carcinosarcoma" in the following discussion without committing ourselves to any particular histogenetic account.

In recent years this longstanding histogenetic issue has been attacked anew with the use of modern immunohistochemical and molecular techniques. The metaplastic carcinoma argument rests on three related claims: (1) carcinosarcomas are monoclonal proliferations whose diversity reflects clonal evolution; (2) the originating cell population is epithelial and not mesenchymal; and (3) epidemiologically and clinically, carcinosarcomas are more akin to carcinomas than to pure sarcomas (e.g., leiomyosarcomas). The evidence backing these claims is described in the following paragraphs.

Carcinosarcomas are monoclonal.
Immunohistochemical studies: Immunohistochemical studies have documented the expression of epithelial markers in the sarcomatous components of a large proportion of cases,[6-14] and both epithelial and sarcomatous components have similar P53 profiles.[15,16]

In vitro cell culture studies: Cell lines established from carcinosarcomas have been shown to differentiate into epithelial, mesenchymal, or both biphasic components under various culture conditions.[13,17,18]

Molecular studies: X-chromosomal inactivation assays, P53 mutational analysis, and loss-of-heterozygosity (LOH) studies have all shown the carcinomatous and sarcomatous elements to share common genetic alterations.[19-22] Moreover, identical P53 and K-ras mutations have been demonstrated in both components.[20,23]

Epithelial-to-mesenchymal transition studies: Some investigators have located the histogenesis of carcinosarcoma in the larger framework of epithelial-to-mesenchymal transitions increasingly thought to be typical of the progression of epithelial malignancies.[24]

Carcinosarcomas have an epithelial origin.
Molecular studies: Fujii and colleagues[25] analyzed the loss of specific alleles at 17 chromosomal loci suspected of harboring tumor suppressor genes. They tracked microsatellite markers in multiple, individually microdissected foci of 17 gynecologic carcinosarcomas. By comparing LOH patterns, they deduced the likely temporal order of genetic changes in the evolution of eight individual carcinosarcomas. In no instance was there a progression from pure sarcoma to either carcinoma or carcinosarcoma. Progression from carcinoma to biphasic patterns and then to sarcoma was observed.

Metastases from carcinosarcomas are often composed solely of epithelial elements: The lymph node metastases from carcinosarcomas may consist only of carcinomatous elements, frequently USC.[26]

Clinical profile of carcinosarcoma resembles carcinoma more than sarcoma.

Epidemiologic risk factors: In one large study, carcinosarcomas were shown to have an epidemiologic risk factor profile similar to that of endometrial carcinoma: increased body weight, the use of exogenous estrogen, and nulliparity all were factors that increased the risk of both diseases, whereas oral contraceptive use and current smoking were factors that lowered the risk of both.[27]

Response of carcinosarcomas to carcinoma-type chemotherapy: One study suggested that the response of carcinosarcomas to cisplatin-based chemotherapy resembles that of carcinomas more than sarcomas.[26,28]

The studies described here are scientifically interesting in their own right. However, their managerial relevance will become apparent only as more studies exploring the relative efficacy of carcinoma-type therapy for carcinosarcomas are undertaken.

Stromal Versus Smooth Muscle Phenotype

Are there reliable ways of distinguishing the endometrial stromal phenotype from the smooth muscle phenotype, and under what circumstances would this distinction be important? The distinction between smooth muscle differentiation and endometrial stromal differentiation is of great importance, because the criteria for assessing malignancy differ for the two tumor types. Briefly, for endometrial stromal neoplasms, a diagnosis of malignancy is based not on the intrinsic features of the proliferations but on an assessment of the relationship to the surrounding normal myometrium. In particular, the diagnosis of endometrial stromal sarcoma requires infiltration into the myometrium or intravascular invasion, or both; in the absence of these findings, the stromal proliferation is benign (endometrial stromal nodule). In contrast, the diagnosis of malignancy in the usual smooth muscle neoplasm requires an assessment of the intrinsic histologic features of the neoplasm itself; in particular, the presence and type of necrosis, the degree of cytologic atypia, and the mitotic index. If the margins of a phenotypically ambiguous lesion are pushing, the direction of differentiation makes little difference because cellular leiomyoma and stromal nodules are both clinically benign. On the other hand, although infiltration of myometrium and vascular invasion are criteria of malignancy for endometrial stromal tumors, they may be found in smooth muscle tumors that are clinically benign (e.g., diffuse leiomyomatosis, intravenous leiomyomatosis). In the presence of an irregular myometrial junction or intravascular growth, the pattern of differentiation is crucial.

Smooth muscle differentiation of the usual sort resembles normal myometrium and features fascicles of spindled cells possessing cigar-shaped nuclei and abundant eosinophilic cytoplasm with distinct cell borders (Table 15-2). On the other hand, endometrial stromal differentiation connotes a monomorphous population of blunt, spindled to oblong cells with

Table 15–2. Smooth Muscle (SM) Versus Endometrial Stromal (ES) Differentiation

Technique	ES Cells	Usual SM Cells	Epithelioid SM Cells
Light microscopy—Architecture	Haphazardly arranged cells resembling normal proliferative phase ES cells. Complex plexiform vascular pattern. Hyalin often abundant.	Cells arranged in looping intersecting fascicles. Vascular component not complex. Thick-walled blood vessels are characteristic.	Rounded or polygonal cells with moderate amount of cytoplasm. Neoplasms often exhibit standard SM features focally.
Cytologic features Nuclei Cytoplasm	Blunt, fusiform, uniform, bland Scanty	Elongate, cigar-shaped Moderate amount, typically fibrillar	Round, crumpled Cytoplasm may be totally eosinophilic, clear around the nucleus, clear at the periphery of the cell, or entirely clear. Glycogen (+) in slightly more than half of cases. PAS with diastase (–).
Immunohistochemistry	Normal ES cells: diffusely express CD10 and may express actin and desmin, usually focally; negative for keratin, EMA, and caldesmon. ES sarcoma cells: identical profile, except that the cells in sex cord–like areas can express keratin, EMA, and inhibin.	Uterine SM cells, whether in myometrium or SM neoplasms, almost always express desmin or caldesmon and actin (often all three). May express keratin (usually AE-1) and CD10 (40%-50% of SM tumors contain CD10+ cells). If the cells of a myometrial tumor do not express actin, desmin, or caldesmon, it is probably not of SM type.	Same as spindled SM tumor. A subset, usually composed of clear cells, may express HMB45.*

EMA, epithelial membrane antigen.
*See discussion of perivascular epithelioid cell tumor (PEComa) in Chapter 22.
Data from references 32-42.

scanty cytoplasm and relatively small, uniform nuclei embedded in an abundant reticulin framework. A highly characteristic feature of endometrial stromal differentiation is the delicate arborizing vasculature that sometimes features hyalinization of the arborizing vessels (Fig. 15-3). In other words, the cells forming stromal tumors resemble the cells of the normal proliferative phase endometrium, and only minor deviations from this appearance are allowed.

Confusingly, smooth muscle cells can also come to resemble endometrial stromal cells by losing much of their characteristic eosinophilic, fibrillary cytoplasm and developing closely approximated, round to oblong nuclei of the type more often seen in endometrial stromal cells.[29-31] This pattern has been termed "highly cellular leiomyoma" (Fig. 15-4).[29] A feature that favors smooth muscle differentiation is the presence of thick-walled vessels within the lesion; the vessels in stromal tumors are mainly thin-walled, arching capillaries. A fascicular arrangement of the constituent cells also favors a smooth muscle tumor.

Immunohistochemistry is sometimes (but not always) helpful.[32-42] Caldesmon appears to be a reasonably specific marker for smooth muscle cells, and it is useful in distinguishing cellular leiomyoma from endometrial stromal neoplasms. Endometrial stromal cells are CD10 positive, but so are the cells in one third to one half of smooth muscle neoplasms. We find a panel of desmin, h-caldesmon, and CD10 to be helpful when routine hematoxylin and eosin (H&E) sections are ambiguous as to whether cells of a myometrial lesion are smooth muscle or stromal. Strong desmin or caldesmon staining with weak or absent CD10 favors a smooth muscle tumor, whereas strong CD10 staining with weak or absent desmin and caldesmon staining provides support for endometrial stromal differentiation.

Some cases resist classification for two reasons.[30,43-45] First, all of the cells may share characteristics of both smooth muscle and endometrial stroma. In this respect, they resemble the cells that comprise the normal endometrial-myometrial interface. We might

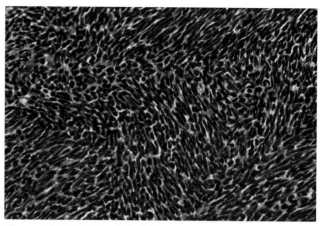

Figure 15–4. Highly cellular leiomyoma. Highly cellular leiomyoma simulates endometrial stromal neoplasms in terms of high cellularity and the inconspicuous cytoplasm of the constituent cells. Thick-walled muscular vessels, desmin positivity, and a fascicular arrangement serve to identify smooth muscle differentiation. See also Color Figure 15-4.

refer to them as stromomyocytes, in analogy to myofibroblasts (cells that simultaneously share characteristics of both myocytes and fibroblasts). The second reason for ambiguity is that some neoplasms are made up of a crazy quilt of zones, each of which exhibits either clearcut endometrial stromal or smooth muscle differentiation. The accumulated literature experience suggests that at least some of these ambiguous neoplasms behave clinically like endometrial stromal sarcoma; for this reason, our practice is to place tumors for which cellular differentiation still remains ambiguous into the endometrial stromal category for purposes of determining therapy and prognosis.

STUMPs versus LMPs

What is the difference between "atypical leiomyoma with low risk of recurrence" and a uterine "smooth muscle tumor of uncertain malignant potential" (STUMP)?
Smooth muscle neoplasms constitute the preponderance of mesenchymal neoplasms encountered in clinical practice. The vast majority are benign and are easily diagnosed; a much smaller group of smooth muscle neoplasms are obviously malignant and are easily identified as leiomyosarcoma. Leiomyomas tend in general to be composed of cytologically bland, mitotically inactive cells, and they typically are non-necrotic, although they may show evidence of recent or remote ischemic damage (so-called degeneration). Leiomyosarcomas, in contrast, are composed of cytologically malignant cells with a high mitotic index and usually are necrotic as a result of rapid tumor growth (Fig. 15-5).

Much effort in the past few decades has been expended on refining microscopic criteria that reliably pick out the clinically benign from the clinically malignant, with the result that the percentage of tumors about which no firm prediction can be made has been

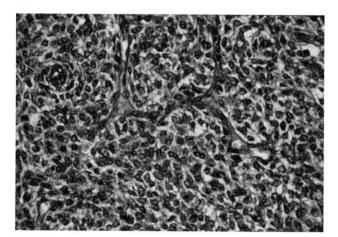

Figure 15–3. Endometrial stromal differentiation. Note individual stromal cells against a background of plexiform vasculature. See also Color Figure 15-3.

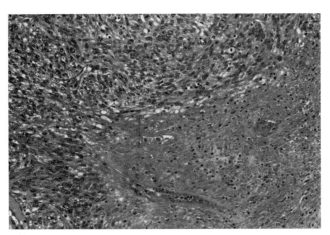

Figure 15–5. Leiomyosarcoma. Coagulative tumor cell necrosis, marked nuclear atypia, and high mitotic index in a typical leiomyosarcoma. See also Color Figure 15-5.

substantially diminished. Our current approach to this differential diagnosis for standard smooth muscle differentiation is set out in Table 15-3.[46] Three features are used to evaluate a uterine smooth muscle neoplasm: (1) the presence or absence of necrosis and its type (hyaline, ischemic necrosis or coagulative tumor cell necrosis), (2) the presence and degree of cytological atypia, and (3) the mitotic index—number of mitotic figures per 10 high-power fields (mf/10 HPF).

When uterine smooth muscle tumors are evaluated using these three criteria, most fall into three groups: benign, malignant, and "atypical leiomyoma with low risk of recurrence" (Fig. 15-6). The last category is a morphologically well-defined group that, in our series, had a failure rate of about 2%, with the tempo

of disease in the one failure being markedly slower than is characteristic of leiomyosarcoma as currently defined. This is an intermediate category, analogous to the LMP surface epithelial tumors of the ovary. It appears in the Clinical Disease II category in Table 15-1. The practical managerial relevance of this group is that when such a smooth muscle neoplasm is encountered in a myomectomy specimen (in a patient who is not unusually risk averse) it is reasonable *not* to perform a completion hysterectomy until childbearing has been completed if close follow-up is feasible.

Applying these criteria to well-preserved, well-sampled tumors permits the classification of the vast majority of smooth muscle neoplasms. In a small minority of cases, the histologic features are still ambiguous and the designation STUMP is warranted. As indicated in Figure 15-1, this term is used in a very different sense than tumor of LMP. In brief, an LMP tumor is a well-defined clinicopathologic category that has a low (but nonzero) failure rate. A STUMP is a tumor whose failure rate is ill defined and which, importantly, straddles some managerially relevant boundary.

We chiefly use the term STUMP when there is ambiguity about one of the evaluated standard features (mitotic index, type of necrosis, degree of atypia), type of smooth muscle differentiation (standard, epithelioid, myxoid) *and* the differential diagnostic possibilities straddle an important managerial boundary. For example, we employ STUMP in a case that combines an absence of necrosis, marked atypia, and a mitotic index that ranges from 5 to 12 depending on how strict the pathologist is in deciding that a hyperchromatic structure is a mitotic figure (or deciding that it is a fragment of a pyknotic nucleus). Here the boundary

Table 15–3. Diagnostic Strategy for Uterine Smooth Muscle Neoplasms*

Mitotic Index (MI), mf/10 HPF	Coagulative Tumor Cell Necrosis	Degree of Cytologic Atypia	Type
Smooth muscle tumors with usual differentiation			
≤20	No	None or no more than mild (i.e., bland cytology)	Leiomyoma (if MI <5) or leiomyoma with increased mitotic figures (if MI ≥5)
>20	No	None or no more than mild (i.e., bland cytology)	Leiomyoma with increased mitotic figures but limited experience
<10	No	Diffuse moderate to severe	Atypical leiomyoma with low risk of recurrence (1/46 failed)
>10	No	Diffuse moderate to severe	Leiomyosarcoma (4/10 failed)
≤10	No	Focal moderate to severe	Leiomyoma with atypia but limited experience
Any	Yes	Any	Leiomyosarcoma (29/39 failed)[†]
Smooth muscle tumor with myxoid stroma			
<5	No	None or mild	Myxoid leiomyoma
Any	No or Yes	Moderate to marked	Myxoid leiomyosarcoma
Smooth muscle tumor with epithelioid differentiation			
<5	No	None or no more than mild	Epithelioid leiomyoma (limited experience)
≥5	No	Any or none	Epithelioid leiomyosarcoma (limited experience)
Any	Yes	Any	Epithelioid leiomyosarcoma (limited experience)

*Based on outcome data from a study of 213 problematic smooth muscle tumors. See text for definitions of morphologic features evaluated.
†Note: Most often there will be significant atypia and/or elevated mitotic counts in leiomyosarcoma in addition to the coagulative tumor cell necrosis; be careful of the case that does not have these additional morphologic features (see text).
From Bell SW, Kempson RL, Hendrickson MR: Problematic uterine smooth muscle neoplasms: A clinicopathologic study of 213 cases. Am J Surg Pathol 1994;18:535-558; Atkins K, Bell SW, Kempson RL, Hendrickson MR: Myxoid smooth muscle neoplasms of the uterus. Mod Pathol 2001;14:132A; and Atkins K, Bell SW, Kempson RL, Hendrickson MR: Epithelioid smooth muscle neoplasms of the uterus. Mod Pathol 2001;14:132A.

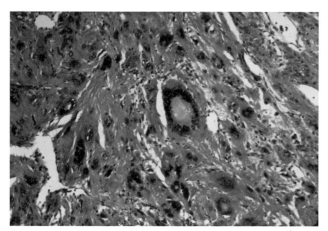

Figure 15–6. Atypical leiomyoma with low risk of recurrence (ALLRR). ALLRR resembles leiomyosarcoma in terms of cytologic atypia, but it lacks both tumor cell necrosis and a high mitotic index (>10 mitotic figures per 10 high-power fields). See also Color Figure 15-6.

straddled separates "atypical leiomyoma with risk of recurrence" and "leiomyosarcoma." In a patient in her reproductive years, this might mean the difference between withholding and performing a hysterectomy.

STUMPs will always be with us; the term gestures toward that ineliminable fringe of cases for which insufficient clinicopathologic information is available to be dogmatic about the potential outcome of patients with this particular constellation of features. They lie in the terra incognita of clinicopathology.

ENDOMETRIAL CARCINOMA PROBLEMS

Our discussion of current controversies in endometrial carcinoma can usefully be organized around a simple two-way classification of these malignancies.

First, carcinomas may be classified in terms of their differentiated histopathologic features (Table 15-4). The endometrium gives rise to a variety of differentiated carcinomas, but more than 80% are glandular neoplasms that resemble the epithelium found in endometrial hyperplasia. Squamous or squamoid ("morular") differentiation is commonly encountered in this endometrioid or usual adenocarcinoma. Other mullerian-differentiated types (e.g., serous, clear cell, mucinous) make up the remainder of endometrial carcinomas, the so-called special variants. These are indicated on the right hand side of Figure 15-7. Endometrial carcinomas may also be grouped with an eye to the hormonal (and associated epidemiologic) background in which they arise: hyperestrogenic settings (type I) or hypoestrogenic settings (type II).[47-51] Patients in the first group (type I) tend to be between 40 and 60 years of age (although carcinoma can develop in younger women, including, in rare instances, those in their 20s). They may have a history of chronic anovulation or estrogen hormone replacement therapy, and the carcinomas are usually well-differentiated, stage I,

Table 15–4. Classification of Endometrial Carcinoma
Endometrioid (usual) carcinoma (includes glandular and villoglandular patterns)
Secretory
Ciliated cell
With squamous differentiation (includes adenoacanthoma and adenosquamous carcinomas—see text)
Special variant carcinomas
Serous
Clear cell
Mucinous
Pure squamous cell
Mixed
Undifferentiated

non-myoinvasive tumors associated with endometrial hyperplasia (found either concurrently or in previous endometrial samplings).[52] Most of the tumors are estrogen receptor (ER) and progesterone receptor (PR) positive and P53 negative and express low levels of the proliferation antigen Ki-67.[48] Patients in this first group have a very favorable prognosis after hysterectomy. In contrast, patients in the second group (type II) tend to be elderly and typically have no history of hyperestrogenism. In these cases, the surrounding non-neoplastic endometrium is almost always atrophic or only weakly estrogen supported, but there may be an in situ component with high-grade cytologic features. The carcinomas that develop in this group of patients are usually of the special variant type with a poor prognosis or are high-grade endometrioid neoplasms that are high stage with deep myoinvasion. They tend to be ER/PR negative, strongly express P53, and show high Ki-67 labeling.[48,53] Not surprisingly, patients with type II cancers are not often cured by hysterectomy.

Combining these two classifications yields three groups around which the topics of this section are discussed: type I endometrioid carcinomas and endometrial hyperplasias; type I special variant carcinomas and endometrial metaplasias; and type II cancers of both types. The great clinical importance of USC warrants discussion of a fourth group, papillary proliferations of the endometrium. Finally, the problem of distinguishing between high-stage uterine carcinoma and synchronous primaries involving extrauterine sites is addressed.

Type I Endometrioid Carcinomas

The majority of patients diagnosed with grade 1 endometrial carcinoma have non-myoinvasive proliferations that are confined to the uterus and are cured by hysterectomy. The same clinical course is seen in patients who harbor less atypical proliferations that, on morphologic grounds, are promising candidates for precursors of type I invasive endometrial carcinoma.

This clinicopathologic fact has frustrated the conventional light microscopic efforts of several generations of

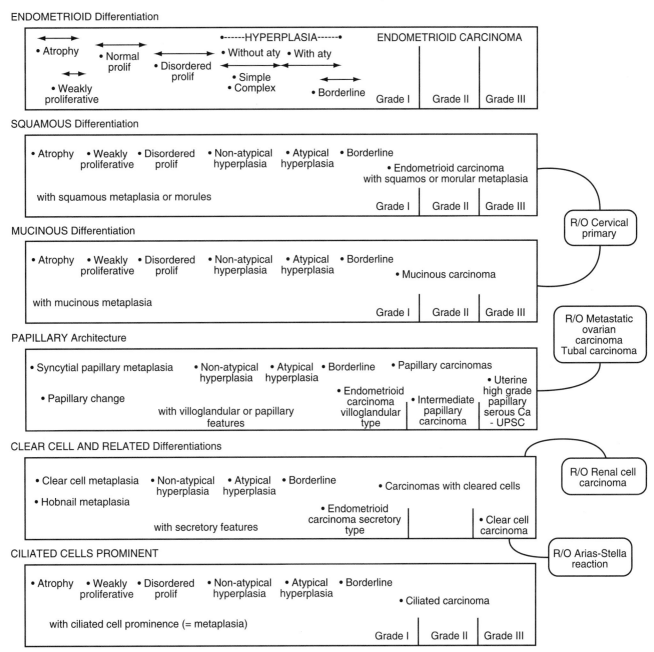

Figure 15–7. The nonsecretory proliferations of the endometrium. The epithelium of nonsecretory endometrial proliferations can have a variety of appearances. Best known is a differential appearance reminiscent of normal proliferative endometrium ("endometrioid"). Alternative differentiated epithelial and architectural patterns are frequently encountered; they include morular, squamous, mucinous, papillary, clear cell, and epithelial with a prominence of ciliated cells. These patterns are often mixed in a single proliferation. They can be further stratified in accordance with their architectural complexity and cytologic atypia. These designations are indicated in the top endometrioid strip and are bracketed by atrophy (left) and grade 3 carcinoma (right). The corresponding designations are indicated in the other strips; they include metaplasia for the benign proliferations and special variant carcinomas for the malignant ones. This diagram can be thought of as a map of endometrial nonsecretory patterns. The histologic pattern is indicated in the vertical direction (y-axis), and the composite degree of architectural complexity and cytologic atypia is indicated in the horizontal direction (x-axis). (From Hendrickson MR, Longacre TA, Kempson RL: The uterine corpus. In Sternberg S, Mills S [eds]: Diagnostic Surgical Pathology, 3rd ed. New York, Raven Press, 1999, p. 2223, Figure 15-9.)

pathologists attempting (1) to arrive at a universally acceptable morphologic definition of well-differentiated endometrial carcinoma and (2) to assess the risk for the development of endometrial carcinoma posed by endometrial proliferations that, morphologically, fall short of clinically malignant proliferations. There is a growing suspicion that the atypical hyperplasia/well-differentiated carcinoma (AH/WDCA) group is, in

principle, resolvable into two groups: a hormonally driven endometrium that is reversible by therapies that interrupt prolonged and sustained estrogen exposure and a morphologically indistinguishable endometrium that may also be hormonally driven but is intrinsically malignant. Recent efforts to deploy morphometry and molecular technology to this task continue to be frustrated by a basic methodologic problem: how does one translate, in a statistically credible fashion, "looks malignant" into "will act malignant"?

Morphologic definition of well-differentiated endometrial carcinoma.

Can endometrial hyperplasia/metaplasia be reliably distinguished from well-differentiated endometrial carcinoma? Determining the point at which endometrial proliferations cease to be hyperplasia/metaplasia and become carcinoma is complicated by a number of factors: (1) a low clinical failure rate (after hysterectomy) over the region of interest; (2) an absence of any dramatic conventional light microscopic change over the region of interest, either in the intrinsic features of the proliferation or in its relation to surrounding normal structures (compare the situation with early invasion in cervical squamous carcinoma); (3) an absence of an abrupt biochemical, cytogenetic, chromosomal, ultrastructural, or immunohistochemical discontinuity over the range of interest (i.e., there is no "gold standard" for malignancy at any other level of examination); and (4) the inability to distinguish between proliferations that at the time of diagnosis have the capacity to invade normal structures from precursor lesions that are not intrinsically malignant but can lead to the development of a proliferation that is malignant.

Elsewhere, we have outlined an argument for using the probability of myoinvasion in the hysterectomy specimen as the outcome variable for studies attempting to distinguish between AH and WDCA.[54] Using myoinvasion as an outcome variable, it becomes apparent that only endometrial proliferations with *extreme* nuclear atypia (specifically, nuclear pleomorphism and prominence of nucleoli) or one of the complex architectural patterns exhibited in the top half of Figure 15-8 (or both) present a low, but significant risk for myometrial invasion.[55]

Most proliferations in this AH/WDCA spectrum are readily placed, with practice, on one side of the line or the other. Problems are created by those cases that straddle the line or represent variations on the AH/WDCA theme that were unanticipated by the criteria. We find the term "borderline lesion" useful in these circumstances. The diagnosis of "borderline" has the advantage of permitting some degree of discretion for the clinician (and the patient) and leaves the clinician's options open: hysterectomy or another sampling, attempted pharmacologic reversal, and resampling. In our opinion, the responsible way of handling this situation is *not* to make a dogmatic pronouncement in the face of what realistically is fairly complete ignorance about the potential of a borderline lesion, but (unpopular as it often is) to pass the uncertainty on to the clinician, who, being in possession of the relevant clinical facts, is in a better position than the pathologist to deal with it in a constructive and informed fashion.[55]

Although the criteria provided here are not particular subjects of controversy, many pathologists continue to make diagnoses of endometrial carcinoma

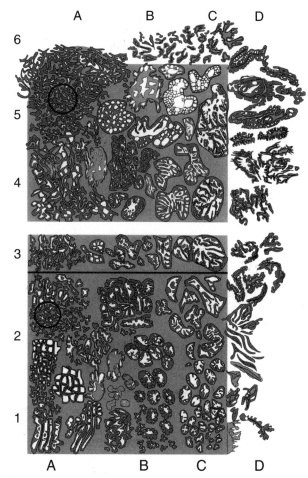

Figure 15–8. Longacre growth chart. Villoglandular carcinoma features architectural complexity in excess of villoglandular hyperplasia but cytologic atypia of at most grade 2. Endometrial proliferations with gland patterns that map to the lower half of the chart are associated with a negligible risk of myometrial invasion and are regarded as benign. These proliferations fall within the range of endometrial hyperplasia/metaplasia and are further designated as atypical when they are associated with cytologic atypia. Occasionally, endometrial proliferations with a low architectural index contain foci with cytologic atypia sufficiently severe to warrant a diagnosis of carcinoma on the basis of cytologic features alone (usually manifested by prominent nucleoli and marked nuclear pleomorphism). In contrast, endometrial proliferations with gland patterns that map to the top half of the chart are associated with myoinvasion with sufficient frequency to warrant a diagnosis of carcinoma regardless of the cytologic features. In unusual cases, endometrial proliferations may feature architectural patterns that are ambiguous in morphologic characteristics, and these patterns are positioned along the borderline zone above the solid line in the lower half of the chart; in these cases, the diagnosis "borderline" is warranted. (From Hendrickson MR, Longacre TA, Kempson RL: The uterine corpus. In Sternberg S, Mills S [eds]: Diagnostic Surgical Pathology, 3rd ed. New York, Raven Press, 1999, p. 2232, Figure 15-29A.)

on the basis of outdated criteria, most of which were unmotivated by independent, evidence-based outcome data. Until clinicians demand such evidence-based criteria for their diagnoses, they will continue to receive diagnoses based on the "It's cancer because I say it's cancer" philosophy, and all efforts at improving the identification of risk lesions and tailoring therapy for such lesions will be subverted.

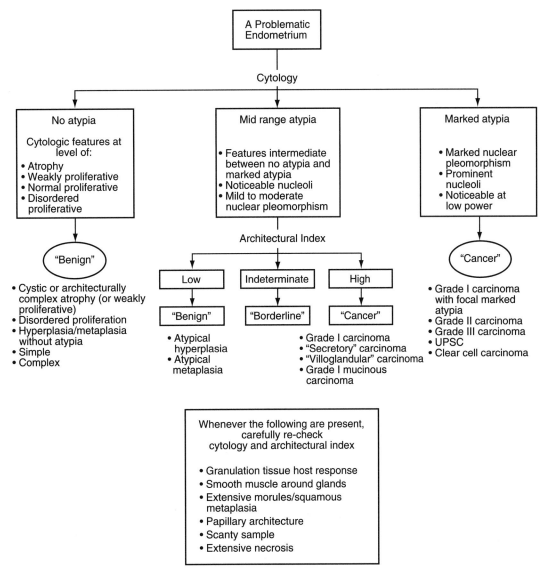

Figure 15–9. An algorithmic approach to problematic uterine sampling. The use of this flow chart requires an adequate sample, an evaluation of the cytologic index (prominence of nucleoli and degree of nuclear pleomorphism), and an evaluation of the architectural index, as indicated in Figure 15-8. (From Hendrickson MR, Longacre TA, Kempson RL: The uterine corpus. In Sternberg S, Mills S [eds]: Diagnostic Surgical Pathology, 3rd ed. New York, Raven Press, 1999, p. 2233, Figure 15-29B.)

In Figure 15-9, we set out an algorithmic approach to the endometrial sampling in cases of suspected carcinoma.

Defining a type I cancer precursor.

Can the precursor lesions of type I endometrial carcinoma be reliably identified, and can this precursor group be partitioned in a way that reflects increasing levels of risk for development of an endometrial carcinoma? There can be little doubt that many of the proliferations subsumed under the heading AH, as it is currently (but variously) defined, constitute an increased risk for the development of endometrial carcinoma as defined previously. However, the magnitude of that risk is currently very much up in the air, and studies that would clarify this issue are beset by formidable methodologic problems. As indicated earlier, pathologists do not routinely use the evidence-based morphologic definition of

well-differentiated endometrial adenocarcinoma. Moreover, the willingness of the surgeon and patient to adopt a wait-and-see attitude given a diagnosis of a possible precancerous lesion is extremely low in the usual age group in which these atypical proliferations develop. For these reasons, the relevant follow-up information needed to clarify this issue is unavailable. In addition, these candidate precursor proliferations are anatomically unstable; they can be reversed by changes in the patient's circulating hormone levels— iatrogenic or endogenous—and the problematic proliferation can be shed spontaneously. It is as though one were attempting to develop a classification of intraepithelial breast lesions in a world where investigators had no universally shared morphologic definition of invasive breast cancer (e.g., the separation of ductal carcinoma in situ and invasive ductal cancer was frequently challenging), where the intraductal lesion changed its appearance with a confusing but unpredictable frequency, and where many of the atypical lesions were treated by bilateral mastectomies.

Despite these methodologic problems, most reports provide evidence that approximately 20% to 30% of women with complex atypical endometrial hyperplasia characterized by glands with marked architectural complexity and crowding, in addition to cytologic atypia, experience progression to a histologic pattern that the investigators deemed morphologic adenocarcinoma. The study published by Kurman and associates[56] demonstrated that no further prognostic insight into risk was provided by grading the degree of atypia.

Substantial attempts have been made in recent years to more specifically identify the endometrial carcinoma precursor using a variety of techniques. Baak and his colleagues have endeavored to identify morphometric criteria for assigning risk levels to hyperplastic endometria. It would appear that, contrary to Kurman and associates,[56] both cytologic and architectural features are required to produce a discriminant function (D-score) that performs adequately.[57-63] Other workers have recruited molecular oncogenetic techniques to the task of identifying precursor lesions, and these have been largely successful in identifying monoclonal endometrial proliferations with specific oncogenetic profiles. Mutter and colleagues[64-68] have translated these molecular observations into conventional light microscopic correlates which roughly correspond to the morphologic features that have traditionally been used to identify those hyperplasias that confer a significant risk for the development of lesions that qualify morphologically as carcinoma. This light microscopic-molecular correlation is encouraging, but the widespread use of expensive technology is impractical, the morphologic correlate of carcinoma used in many of these studies does not appear to be founded on outcome-based criteria, the interobserver agreement using conventional light microscopic stand-ins for the distinction made with these technologies has not been addressed, and, ultimately, the translation of these distinctions into a real-world clinical risk assessment on which treatment recommendations can be based is simply not feasible, based on the data on hand at this time. Conventional light microscopy, with its well-known limitations, continues to be the gold standard for assessing risk.

Type I Special Variant Carcinomas

Special variant carcinomas are important for two reasons: first, the type II special variant carcinomas are of great managerial significance (see later discussion) and, second, the entire group of special variant carcinomas raise anatomic localization issues. A recurring and often difficult problem is distinguishing between an endometrial and an endocervical glandular or papillary primary. Furthermore, several neoplasms (often of identical histologic types) may arise in different components of the mullerian system metachronously or synchronously.

Where is the adenocarcinoma coming from—cervix or endometrium?
Can invasive adenocarcinoma of the cervix be reliably distinguished from invasive adenocarcinoma of the endometrium on endometrial sampling? The distinction between invasive adenocarcinoma of the cervix and that of the endometrium is important, because the surgical and postsurgical approaches to therapy are quite different for carcinomas arising at each of these two sites.[69] A number of strategies are available to approach ambiguous cases (Table 15-5).

To some extent the differentiated type of carcinoma is helpful in assigning primary site; for example, pure squamous carcinomas only very rarely arise in the endometrium. However, all adenocarcinoma subtypes, including endometrioid, can potentially arise from either the uterine corpus or the cervix.

Helpful H&E features that favor an endometrial primary include the finding of an associated endometrioid hyperplasia or metaplasia elsewhere in the endometrium (particularly hybrid mucinous-endometrioid differentiation) and the presence of stromal foam cells. Findings favoring a cervical primary are associated adenocarcinoma in situ involving endocervical glands and a complete dissociation in the endometrial sampling between the appearance of the malignant fragments and the appearance of the associated endometrial fragments. An example is the finding of a dimorphic endometrial sampling consisting of normal secretory endometrium and fragments of adenocarcinoma (Fig. 15-10). The majority of ambiguous cases can be resolved based on these H&E features.[70]

Table 15-5. Distinguishing Endometrial from Endocervical Adenocarcinoma

Technique	Endocervical	Endometrial
Clinical/Radiologic	Dominant mass in cervix	Dominant mass in uterine fundus
Hematoxylin and eosin staining	Cancer-containing fragments differ from endometrial functionalis fragments (dimorphic pattern)	Morphing of malignant fragments with less atypical patterns in other fragments (endometrial hyperplasia/metaplasia)
	ACIS in associated endocervical glands	Stromal foam cells
	Associated squamous CIN	Associated cervical fragments lack ACIS
Immunohistochemistry	CEA positive	CEA negative
	ER and PR negative	ER and PR positive
	Vimentin negative	Vimentin positive
Human papillomavirus in situ	Positive	Negative

ACIS, adenocarcinoma in situ; CEA, carcinoembryonic antigen; CIN, cervical intraepithelial neoplasia; ER, estrogen receptor; PR, progesterone receptor.

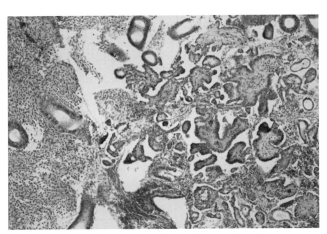

Figure 15–10. Endocervical carcinoma in curettings. The appearance of the carcinoma fragments is distinct from that of the endometrial fragments, suggesting origin from the cervix. See also Color Figure 15-10.

This strategy can be supplemented by localization studies using differential curettage, hysteroscopy, or imaging studies to distinguish primary endometrial from primary endocervical mucinous carcinoma.[71-76]

In persistently ambiguous cases, immunohistochemistry may be helpful. There are no specific immunohistochemical markers that will always distinguish these two possibilities, but a panel of CEA, vimentin, and ER can be useful. Problematic tumors that are CEA positive but negative for ER and vimentin are highly likely to be endocervical in origin, whereas a CEA-negative, ER- and vimentin-positive phenotype strongly favors an endometrial adenocarcinoma.[77-80] Many problematic neoplasms have an intermediate, nonspecific phenotype with this panel, and in these instances human papillomavirus (HPV) in situ hybridization (positive in some cervical primaries) may be an alternative diagnostic strategy.[81]

The problem of synchronous mullerian primary neoplasms.

Do coexistent carcinomas of the endometrium and ovary represent synchronous primary tumors or metastases from endometrium to ovary, or from ovary to endometrium? The coexistence of carcinoma in the endometrium and in the ovary occurs in approximately 10% of patients with "ovarian carcinoma" and slightly more than 5% of patients with "endometrial carcinoma."[82] Whether these tumors represent a primary carcinoma and a metastasis to one site from the other (and hence high-stage neoplasms arising from one of the sites) or are simultaneous primaries (hence both stage I) continues to be a subject of debate, and this problem has significant implications for therapy and prognosis. If both neoplasms are grade 1 and the endometrial neoplasm is not myoinvasive, we think the available published evidence supports the theory that they are simultaneous primaries; under this interpretation, adjuvant therapy is not required.[83-86] However, there are still relatively few outcome data concerning higher-grade or higher-stage simultaneous

tumors, and their treatment is highly variable from one institution to another.

A variety of histologic criteria have been proposed to be of use in determining whether simultaneous cancers represent single or separate tumors, but these have not been independently validated.[84,87] Many of the cancers studied by clonality assays appear to be independent primary tumors, but such studies are limited by small numbers of cases, the inclusion of a high proportion of low-grade cancers, and a variety of methodologic difficulties.[88-90]

A Gynecologic Oncology Group (GOG) study of 74 cases of simultaneous carcinomas reported an excellent prognosis if the tumor was confined to the uterus and ovary, although the risk of recurrence was significantly increased by the presence of histologic grade 2 or 3 tumor within these sites.[82] The presence of pelvic or abdominal metastases was associated with an increased likelihood of recurrence (27.1%, compared with 10% for those tumors confined to the ovary and uterus), but the impact of adjuvant therapy could not be determined due to varying treatment regimens. Although the GOG study constitutes one of the largest prospective series of simultaneous carcinomas with long-term follow-up, its authors cautioned against generalization of their results to other patients with synchronously detected tumors, because the distribution of cell types and histologic grade was somewhat dissimilar from that in earlier retrospective studies.

Type II Carcinomas (both special variant and endometrioid)

All cancers in the type II group are cytologically high grade and clinically aggressive. USC (Fig. 15-11) and CCC, both special variants, dominate this group although these neoplasms may be mixed with high-grade endometrioid components, sometimes possessing cytologically malignant squamous elements. Although the idea is somewhat controversial,

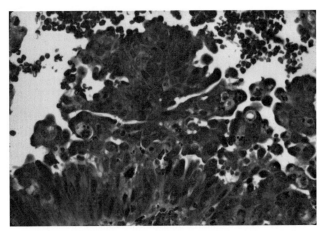

Figure 15–11. Uterine serous carcinoma (USC). USC is usually papillary and features high-grade cytology and easily found (and often abnormal) mitotic figures. See also Color Figure 15-11.

in our opinion there also exists a subgroup of high-grade endometrioid carcinomas, which appear to have a clinicopathologic profile similar to that of USC and CCC, and these are also included in this discussion.

Even though it is now accepted that the type II carcinomas are more clinically aggressive than the type I cancers, several issues have arisen: (1) Is there a precursor lesion for type II cancers? (2) How much USC (or CCC) in a mixed proliferation is sufficient to confer a poor prognosis? (3) Should all type II carcinomas be treated with adjuvant therapy, or is there a subset of low-volume, low-stage type II cancers that can safely be treated without adjuvant therapy?

Type II cancer precursors.
Is there a precursor of type II cancers, and how should it be managed? A precursor lesion for type II cancers has been proposed. As it has been defined, endometrial intraepithelial carcinoma (EIC) is a promising candidate for an in situ lesion.

The initial descriptions of EIC involved USC-like cytologic changes in the endometrium adjacent to USC (Fig. 15-12).[51] Subsequently, such in situ changes were reported in the absence of an endometrial mass, evidence of a thickened endometrium, or myometrial invasion.[91-93] USC-like changes can also be found along the serosa of the uterus and fallopian tubes in conjunction with either in situ USC in the endometrium or an actual tumor mass.

In rare cases, in situ change has been associated with disseminated disease in the absence of invasive uterine cancer.[94] USC confined to endometrial polyps (Fig. 15-13) has also been reported to behave in an aggressive fashion, and this has led to the suggestion that stage Ia type II cancers should be treated aggressively, even if compulsively staged.[95]

In our opinion, despite small studies and case reports suggesting that in situ change may be associated with clinically aggressive disease, the significance of EIC as an isolated finding is still largely undetermined, and

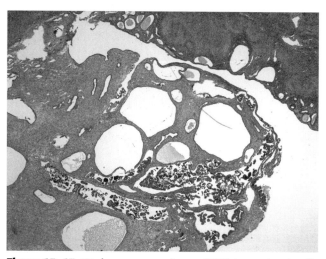

Figure 15–13. Uterine serous carcinoma (USC) in a polyp. Small-volume USC sometimes takes the form of focal involvement of an endometrial polyp. See also Color Figure 15-13.

further studies are warranted to determine the optimum treatment approach.

How much uterine serous carcinoma is needed in a mixed carcinoma to treat it as a uterine serous carcinoma?
How much uterine serous carcinoma (or clear cell carcinoma) in a mixed proliferation is sufficient for a diagnosis of uterine serous carcinoma (or clear cell carcinoma)? The conventional approach to ovarian carcinoma uses a minimum 10% tumor volume of a specific histologic type to warrant a specific diagnostic heading. By convention, many pathologists have used this criterion in endometrial carcinoma. Others, however, believe that, because any percentage of USC (or CCC) is sufficient to confer a poor prognosis in endometrial carcinoma, all cases with any amount of USC or CCC should be diagnosed as such. Only two studies have addressed this issue specifically, and neither found a correlation between percentage of USC and the measured clinical outcomes.[96,97] Although we are of the opinion that the presence of any USC or CCC warrants mention in the diagnostic report, we acknowledge that there are insufficient outcome data regarding the presence of such minimal high-grade cancer, given adequate sampling and staging, to warrant any specific treatment recommendation.

Risk of relapse in surgicopathologically staged Ia uterine serous carcinoma.
What is the significance of stage Ia uterine serous carcinoma? Do optimally staged stage Ia uterine serous carcinomas require adjuvant therapy? The clinical significance and appropriate treatment of USC lacking myometrial invasion, including its putative precursor lesion EIC, is a subject of controversy.[96,98,99] Some USCs pursue an aggressive clinical course even when myometrial invasion is apparently absent or superficial at most (superficial serous carcinoma, or SSC); others may be cured with surgery alone. Because an important feature in assessing prognosis is the

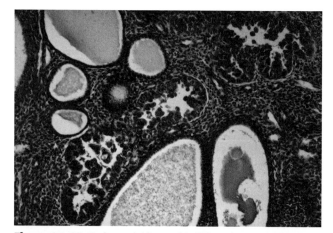

Figure 15–12. Endometrial intraepithelial carcinoma (EIC). EIC typically features focal replacement of benign atrophic endometrial glands by cells with cytologic features identical to those seen in uterine serous carcinoma. See also Color Figure 15-12.

presence or absence of extrauterine disease at presentation, it has been recommended that patients with EIC or SSC undergo meticulous surgical staging at the time of hysterectomy.[99] Because the distinction between EIC and SSC based on the identification of stromal invasion is difficult and these lesions share a unique pattern of clinical behavior, it has been suggested that EIC and SSC measuring 1 cm or less be regarded as "minimal USC."[99] Because there are so few cases with these findings that have been adequately staged and studied, the proposed definitions for EIC and SSC are controversial and require further study.

Grading of clear cell carcinoma.

Once a diagnosis of clear cell carcinoma is established, does further diagnostic refinement provide additional prognostic information? The definition of CCC requires both cytoplasmic clearing (not due to mucin) and high-grade cytologic atypia (Fig. 15-14). At least some cells should have cytoplasmic clearing, but the majority of the neoplastic cells may be eosinophilic. The architecture may be solid, glandular, tubulocystic, or papillary. The cells lining the papillae or glands often are hobnailed. CCC has many mimics. The important elements of the differential diagnosis are indicated in Figure 15-7.

Both USC and CCC are cytologically high-grade neoplasms, and mixtures of the two are relatively common in our experience.[100] There may be discrete areas in the same endometrial sampling with features of the two malignancies, or a "morphed" version of the two may be seen; the latter usually involves papillary structures lined by hobnail cleared cells. This would be an important differential diagnostic problem if the two neoplasms had a clinically significant difference in behavior under current therapy. Because this does not appear to be the case, confusing them is no great diagnostic sin.

Secretory carcinoma is a well-differentiated endometrioid carcinoma with uniform cytoplasmic vacuolization; it specifically lacks the high-grade cytology that defines the CCC (Fig. 15-15). Mucin-containing

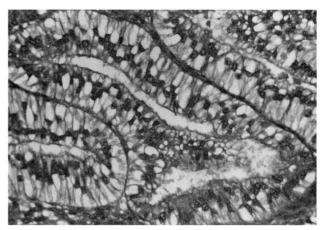

Figure 15–15. Secretory carcinoma. Secretory carcinoma is distinguished from clear cell carcinoma by virtue of its bland cytology and "early secretory" appearance. See also Color Figure 15-15.

cells are cleared, as are glycogen-rich squamoid cells and, occasionally, ciliated cells. The hypersecretory change of Arias-Stella (most commonly seen in pregnancy) may be seen in postmenopausal women taking progestational agents and may mimic CCC.

Although confusing CCC with USC is relatively harmless, confusion with other clear cell proliferations does create mischief. As in studies of CCC of the ovary, nonuniform inclusion criteria in clinicopathologic studies undoubtedly accounts for the substantial differences that exist among series. Those series that report unusually good behavior might involve more lesions at the secretory carcinoma end of the clear cell spectrum, and other series may be more insistent on marked cytologic atypia before a diagnosis of CCC is made.

The question then arises as to whether, with the use of strict criteria (specifically requiring marked cytologic atypia), any additional prognostic information can be extracted by a more fine-grained analysis of the histology. This does not appear to be the case for the architectural pattern, although at least one series reported a correlation between nonsolid architecture and a poor prognosis for stage I CCC.[101-103] Moreover, grading is of little use because the required severe cytologic atypia of a bone fide case ensures a high grade.

Carcinomas Having a Papillary Pattern

Papillary proliferations of the endometrium derive their importance chiefly because of the existence of the highly malignant uterine counterpart of ovarian serous carcinoma—USC. The clinicopathology of USC is well established: high-grade cytology, the characteristic (but not invariable) presence of papillary architecture, frequent presentation at high stage, and the notorious underestimation of surgicopathologic stage by clinical staging.[91,98,100,104-106]

However, not every papillary proliferation in the uterus is malignant, and not all carcinomas with a papillary pattern carry the grave prognosis of USC.[107]

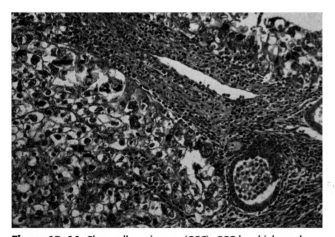

Figure 15–14. Clear cell carcinoma (CCC). CCC has high-grade nuclear features similar to those seen in uterine serous carcinoma. Any architectural pattern may be seen, including papillary structures. See also Color Figure 15-14.

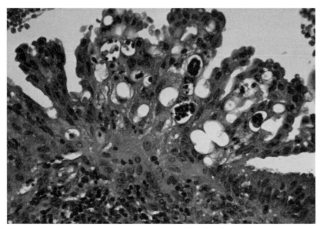

Figure 15–16. Papillary syncytial metaplasia (PSM). PSM features a syncytium of cells with smudged, sometimes hyperchromatic, nuclei. Mitotic figures and prominent nucleoli are absent. See also Color Figure 15-16.

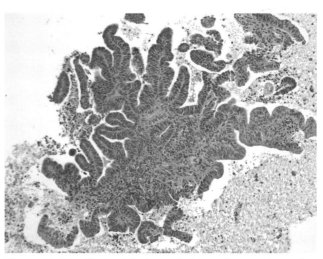

Figure 15–18. Villoglandular hyperplasia. An absence of complex branching and secondary structures distinguishes this pattern from villoglandular carcinoma. See also Color Figure 15-18.

Therefore, it is critical for the pathologist to distinguish among the various papillary neoplastic and non-neoplastic proliferations of the endometrium (Figs. 15-16 through 15-19).

Table 15-6 lists the most important papillary endometrial proliferations, their typical architecture, and the range of allowable cytologic atypia for each. Omitted from the list are those proliferations that may feature papillary architecture but for which the important classifying feature is something else (e.g., cytoplasmic mucin for mucinous carcinoma, prominent cytoplasmic clearing for CCC).

Is villoglandular carcinoma a "bad actor?"

Does papillary architecture in a nonserous endometrial carcinoma, in and of itself, confer an unfavorable prognosis? Well-differentiated endometrial carcinoma quite commonly has a low-power architecture featuring tumor cells supported by a delicate fibrovascular stroma forming papillae with varying degrees of branching (see Fig. 15-8). This pattern, often referred to as villoglandular carcinoma (VGC), may be focal or diffuse, and it often blends imperceptibly into more typical endometrioid carcinoma with the usual glandular pattern.[100,108,109] It is important to note that in both villous and glandular areas, the cytologic features are at most grade 2 or 3. Sometimes small micropapillae are associated with VGC or encountered in other endometrioid carcinomas; the term "endometrioid carcinoma with small nonvillous papillae" has been used for this pattern.[107]

Clinicopathologic studies of VGC have provided conflicting evidence concerning its virulence. Some of the discrepancies are a result of the difficulties in sharply

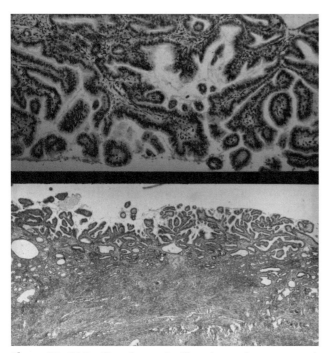

Figure 15–17. Papillary change. Papillary change denotes stromal cores lined by cytologically bland, nonstratified epithelium. See also Color Figure 15-17.

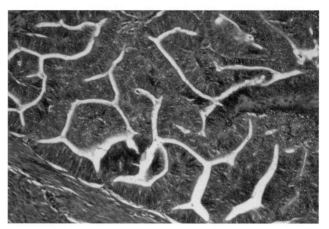

Figure 15–19. Villoglandular carcinoma (VGC). See also Color Figure 15-19.

Table 15–6. Papillary Proliferations of the Endometrium

Anticipated Clinical Behavior	Architecture of Connective Tissue Scaffolding	Cytologic Atypia
Benign		
Papillary syncytial metaplasia	Epithelial stratification with a papillary configuration	Minimal
Papillary change	Three-dimensional papillae	Minimal
Villoglandular hyperplasia	Sheets or folia	Minimal to moderate
Type I carcinomas		
Villoglandular endometrioid carcinoma	Sheets or folia	Moderate to severe
Endometrioid carcinomas with small nonvillous papillae	Epithelial stratification with a papillary configuration	Minimal to moderate
Type II carcinomas		
Uterine (papillary) serous carcinoma	Three-dimensional papillae	Markedly atypical

separating VGC from villoglandular hyperplasia at the benign end of the morphologic spectrum and from USC at the malignant end (see Fig. 15-7).

A consensus is emerging, however, and is perhaps best captured by the results of the GOG study (Protocol 33) of clinical stages I and II endometrial adenocarcinomas. The VGC group in this study, when compared with pure endometrioid carcinoma, tended to be better differentiated but was otherwise statistically indistinguishable from the control group in clinical outcome.[110] Whether VGCs that show a myometrial component have a greater propensity for intravascular growth and lymph node involvement than endometrioid carcinomas of the usual type remains an open question.[109,111]

Currently, VGC is part of the morphologic spectrum of endometrioid carcinoma, and we do not classify it separately or specify it in the diagnosis line. The chief importance of recognizing VGC is for differential diagnostic purposes and to distinguish it from villoglandular hyperplasia on the one hand and

from high-grade papillary carcinoma on the other.[55] Our approach to papillary proliferations of the endometrium is first to assess the cytology and then the architecture. If cytology is grade 3, it is USC; if it is grade 2, then a diagnosis of VGC is warranted, although a small minority of cases remains ambiguous (Fig. 15-20). If grade 1 cytology is present, the distinction lies between villoglandular hyperplasia and grade 1 VGC. This is resolved by an assessment of the proliferation's architecture (see Fig. 15-8): if the papillary pattern lies in the upper part of the figure, we diagnose carcinoma; if in the lower part, a diagnosis of villoglandular hyperplasia is warranted.

REFERENCES

1. Ostor AG, Rollason TP: Mixed tumours of the uterus. In Fox H, Wells M (eds): Haines and Taylor Obstetrical and Gynaecological Pathology, 5th ed. Edinburgh, Churchill Livingstone, 2003, pp. 549-584.
2. Zaloudek C, Hendrickson MR: Mesenchymal tumors of the uterus. In Kurman RJ (ed): Blaustein's Pathology of the Female Genital Tract, 5th ed. New York, Springer-Verlag, 2002, p. 561-605.
3. Wick MR, Swanson PE: Carcinosarcomas: Current perspectives and an historical review of nosological concepts. Semin Diagn Pathol 1993;10:118-127.
4. Colombi RP: Sarcomatoid carcinomas of the female genital tract (malignant mixed mullerian tumors). Semin Diagn Pathol 1993;10:169-175.
5. Zaino RJ: Endometrial hyperplasia and carcinoma. In Fox H, Wells M (eds): Haines and Taylor Obstetrical and Gynaecological Pathology, 5th ed. Edinburgh, Churchill Livingstone, 2003, pp. 443-495.
6. Auerbach H, LiVolsi V, Merino M: Malignant mixed mullerian tumors of the uterus: An immunohistochemical study. Int J Gynecol Pathol 1988;7:123-130.
7. Bitterman P, Chun B, Kurman R: The significance of epithelial differentiation in mixed mesodermal tumors of the uterus: A clinicopathologic and immunohistochemical study. Am J Surg Pathol 1990;14:317-328.
8. Costa MJ, Khan R, Judd R: Carcinoma (malignant mixed mullerian [mesodermal] tumor) of the uterus and ovary: Correlation of clinical, pathologic, and immunohistochemical features in 29 cases. Arch Pathol Lab Med 1991;115:583-590.
9. De Brito P, Orenstein J, Silverberg S: Carcinosarcoma of the female genital tract: Immunohistochemical and ultrastructural analysis of 28 cases. Hum Pathol 1993;24:132-142.

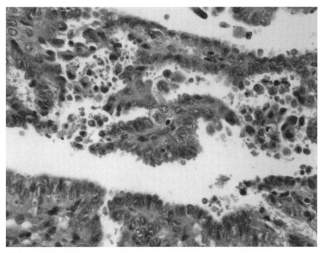

Figure 15–20. Intermediate uterine serous carcinoma (USC)/villoglandular carcinoma (VGC). This case exhibits greater cytologic atypia than the usual VGC and raises management issues. See also Color Figure 15-20.

10. Geisinger K, Dabbs D, Marshall R: Malignant mixed mullerian tumors: An ultrastructural and immunohistochemical analysis with histogenetic considerations. Cancer 1987;59:1781-1790.

11. George E, Manivel JC, Dehner LP, Wick MR: Malignant mixed mullerian tumors: An immunohistochemical study of 47 cases, with histogenetic considerations and clinical correlation. Hum Pathol 1991;22:215-223.

12. Meis J, Lawrence W: The immunohistochemical profile of malignant mixed mullerian tumor: Overlap with endometrial adenocarcinoma [see comments]. Am J Clin Pathol 1990;94:1-7.

13. Gorai I, Yanagibashi T, Taki A, et al: Uterine carcinosarcoma is derived from a single stem cell: An in vitro study. Int J Cancer 1997;72:821-827.

14. Ramadan M, Goudie RB: Epithelial antigens in malignant mixed mullerian tumors of endometrium. J Pathol 1986;148:13-18.

15. Mayall F, Rutty K, Campbell F, Goddard H: P53 immunostaining suggests that uterine carcinosarcomas are monoclonal. Histopathology 1994;24:211-214.

16. Costa MJ, Vogelsan J, Young LJ: P53 gene mutation in female genital tract carcinosarcomas (malignant mixed mullerian tumors): A clinicopathologic study of 74 cases. Mod Pathol 1994; 7:619-627.

17. Gorai I, Doi C, Minaguchi H: Establishment and characterization of carcinosarcoma cell line of the human uterus. Cancer 1993;71:775-786.

18. Emoto M, Iwasaki H, Kikuchi M, Shirakawa K: Characteristics of cloned cells of mixed mullerian tumor of the human uterus: Carcinoma cells showing myogenic differentiation in vitro. Cancer 1993;71:3065-3075.

19. Abeln EC, Smit VT, Wessels JW, et al: Molecular genetic evidence for the conversion hypothesis of the origin of malignant mixed mullerian tumors. J Pathol 1997;183:424-431.

20. Wada H, Enomoto T, Fujita M, et al: Molecular evidence that most but not all carcinosarcomas of the uterus are combination tumors. Cancer Res 1997;57:5379-5385.

21. Torenbeek R, Hermsen MA, Meijer GA, et al: Analysis by comparative genomic hybridization of epithelial and spindle cell components in sarcomatoid carcinoma and carcinosarcoma: Histogenetic aspects. J Pathol 1999;189:338-343.

22. Thompson L, Chang B, Barsky SH: Monoclonal origins of malignant mixed tumors (carcinosarcomas): Evidence for a divergent histogenesis. Am J Surg Pathol 1996;20:277-285.

23. Kounelis S, Jones MW, Papadaki H, et al: Carcinosarcomas (malignant mixed mullerian tumors) of the female genital tract: Comparative molecular analysis of epithelial and mesenchymal components. Hum Pathol 1998;29:82-87.

24. Thiery JP: Epithelial-mesenchymal transitions in tumor progression. Nat Rev Cancer 2002;2:442-454.

25. Fujii H, Yoshida M, Gong ZX, et al: Frequent genetic heterogeneity in the clonal evolution of gynecological carcinosarcoma and its influence on phenotypic diversity. Cancer Res 2000;60:114-120.

26. Silverberg S, Major F, Blessing J, et al: Carcinosarcoma (malignant mixed mesodermal tumor) of the uterus: A Gynecologic Oncology Group pathologic study of 203 cases. Int J Gynecol Pathol 1990;9:1-19.

27. Zelmanowicz A, Hildesheim A, Sherman ME, et al: Evidence for a common etiology for endometrial carcinomas and malignant mixed mullerian tumors. Gynecol Oncol 1998;69:253-257.

28. van Rijswijk RE, Tognon G, Burger CW, et al: The effect of chemotherapy on the different components of advanced carcinosarcomas (malignant mixed mesodermal tumors) of the female genital tract. Int J Gynecol Cancer 1994;4:52-60.

29. Oliva E, Young RH, Clement PB, et al: Cellular benign mesenchymal tumors of the uterus: A comparative morphologic and immunohistochemical analysis of 33 highly cellular leiomyomas and six endometrial stromal nodules, two frequently confused tumors. Am J Surg Pathol 1995;19:757-768.

30. Oliva E, Clement PB, Young RH, Scully RE: Mixed endometrial stromal and smooth muscle tumors of the uterus: A clinicopathologic study of 15 cases. Am J Surg Pathol 1998;22:997-1005.

31. McCluggage WG, Cromie AJ, Bryson C, Traub AI: Uterine endometrial stromal sarcoma with smooth muscle and glandular differentiation. J Clin Pathol 2001;54:481-483.

32. Chu PG, Arber DA, Weiss LM, Chang KL: Utility of CD10 in distinguishing between endometrial stromal sarcoma and uterine smooth muscle tumors: An immunohistochemical comparison of 34 cases. Mod Pathol 2001;14:465-471.

33. Oliva E, Young RH, Amin MB, Clement PB: An immunohistochemical analysis of endometrial stromal and smooth muscle tumors of the uterus: A study of 54 cases emphasizing the importance of using a panel because of overlap in immunoreactivity for individual antibodies. Am J Surg Pathol 2002;26: 403-412.

34. Franquemont D, Frierson H, Mills S: An immunohistochemical study of normal endometrial stroma and endometrial stromal neoplasms: Evidence for smooth muscle differentiation. Am J Surg Path 1991;15:861-870.

35. Fujii S, Konishi I, Katabuchi H, Okamura H: Ultrastructure of smooth muscle tissue in the female reproductive tract: Uterus and oviduct. In Motta PM (ed): Ultrastructure of Smooth Muscle. Kluwer Academic Publishers, 1990, pp. 197-220.

36. Fujii S, Konishi I, Mori T: Smooth muscle differentiation at endometrio-myometrial junction: An ultrastructural study. Virchows Arch A 1989;414:105-112.

37. Baker RJ, Hildebrandt RH, Rouse RV, et al: Inhibin and CD99 (MIC2) expression in uterine stromal neoplasms with sex-cord-like elements. Mod Pathol 1998;11:100A.

38. Rush DS, Tan J, Baergen RN, Soslow RA: h-Caldesmon, a novel smooth muscle-specific antibody, distinguishes between cellular leiomyoma and endometrial stromal sarcoma. Am J Surg Pathol 2001;25:253-258.

39. Nucci MR, O'Connell JT, Huettner PC, et al: h-Caldesmon expression effectively distinguishes endometrial stromal tumors from uterine smooth muscle tumors. Am J Surg Pathol 2001;25:455-463.

40. McCluggage WG, Sumathi VP, Maxwell P: CD10 is a sensitive and diagnostically useful immunohistochemical marker of normal endometrial stroma and of endometrial stromal neoplasms. Histopathology 2001;39:273-278.

41. Watanabe K, Kusakabe T, Hoshi N, et al: h-Caldesmon in leiomyosarcoma and tumors with smooth muscle cell-like differentiation: Its specific expression in the smooth muscle cell tumor. Hum Pathol 1999;30:392-396.

42. Watanabe K, Ogura G, Suzuki T: Leiomyoblastoma of the uterus: An immunohistochemical and electron microscopic study of distinctive tumors with immature smooth muscle cell differentiation mimicking fetal uterine myocytes. Histopathology 2003; 42:379-386.

43. Yilmaz A, Rush DS, Soslow RA: Endometrial stromal sarcomas with unusual histologic features: A report of 24 primary and metastatic tumors emphasizing fibroblastic and smooth muscle differentiation. Am J Surg Pathol 2002;26:1142-1150.

44. Clement PB: The pathology of uterine smooth muscle tumors and mixed endometrial stromal-smooth muscle tumors: A selective review with emphasis on recent advances. Int J Gynecol Pathol 2000;19:39-55.

45. Schammel DP, Silver SA, Tavassoli FA: Combined endometrial stromal/smooth muscle neoplasms of the uterus: A clinicopathological study of 38 cases [abstract]. Mod Pathol 1998;12:124A.

46. Bell SW, Kempson RL, Hendrickson MR: Problematic uterine smooth muscle neoplasms: A clinicopathologic study of 213 cases. Am J Surg Pathol 1994;18:535-558.

47. Bokhman JV: Two pathogenetic types of endometrial carcinoma. Gynecol Oncol 1983;15:10-17.

48. Lax SF, Kurman RJ: A dualistic model for endometrial carcinogenesis based on immunohistochemical and molecular genetic analyses. Verh Dtsch Ges Pathol 1997;81:228-232.

49. Sherman ME, Bur ME, Kurman RJ: P53 in endometrial cancer and its putative precursors: Evidence for diverse pathways of tumorigenesis. Hum Pathol 1995;26:1268-1274.

50. Pere H, Tapper J, Wahlstrom T, et al: Distinct chromosomal imbalances in uterine serous and endometrioid carcinomas. Cancer Res 1998;58:892-895.

51. Sherman ME: Theories of endometrial carcinogenesis: A multidisciplinary approach. Mod Pathol 2000;13:295-308.

52. Lee KR, Scully RE: Complex endometrial hyperplasia and carcinoma in adolescents and young women 15 to 20 years of age: A report of 10 cases. Int J Gynecol Pathol 1989;8:201-213.

53. Fearon ER, Vogelstein B: A genetic model for colorectal tumorigenesis. Cell 1990;61:759-767.

54. Hendrickson MR, Ross J, Kempson RL: Toward the development of morphologic criteria for well-differentiated adenocarcinoma of the endometrium. Am J Surg Pathol 1983;7:819-838.

55. Longacre TA, Chung MH, Jensen DN, Hendrickson MR: Proposed criteria for the diagnosis of well-differentiated endometrial carcinoma: A diagnostic test for myoinvasion. Am J Surg Pathol 1995;19:371-406.

56. Kurman R, Kaminski P, Norris H: The behavior of endometrial hyperplasia: A long-term study of "untreated" hyperplasia in 170 patients. Cancer 1985;56:403-412.

57. Ausems EW, van der Kamp JK, Baak JP: Nuclear morphometry in the determination of the prognosis of marked atypical endometrial hyperplasia. Int J Gynecol Pathol 1985;4:180-185.

58. Baak JP: Further evaluation of the practical applicability of nuclear morphometry for the prediction of the outcome of atypical endometrial hyperplasia. Anal Quant Cytol Histol 1986;8:46-48.

59. Baak JP, Nauta JJ, Wisse-Brekelmans EC, Bezemer PD: Architectural and nuclear morphometrical features together are more important prognosticators in endometrial hyperplasias than nuclear morphometrical features alone. J Pathol 1988;154:335-341.

60. Baak JP, Wisse-Brekelmans EC, Fleege JC, et al: Assessment of the risk on endometrial cancer in hyperplasia, by means of morphological and morphometrical features. Pathol Res Pract 1992;188:856-859.

61. Baak JP, Orbo A, van Diest PJ, et al: Prospective multicenter evaluation of the morphometric D-score for prediction of the outcome of endometrial hyperplasias. Am J Surg Pathol 2001;25:930-935.

62. Baak JP, Kuik DJ, Bezemer PD: The additional prognostic value of morphometric nuclear arrangement and DNA-ploidy to other morphometric and stereologic features in endometrial hyperplasias. Int J Gynecol Cancer 1994;4:289-297.

63. Dunton CJ, Baak JP, Palazzo JP, et al: Use of computerized morphometric analyses of endometrial hyperplasias in the prediction of coexistent cancer. Am J Obstet Gynecol 1996;174:1518-1521.

64. Mutter GL: Endometrial intraepithelial neoplasia (EIN): Will it bring order to chaos? The Endometrial Collaborative Group. Gynecol Oncol 2000;76:287-290.

65. Mutter GL, Baak JP, Crum CP, et al: Endometrial precancer diagnosis by histopathology, clonal analysis, and computerized morphometry. J Pathol 2000;190:462-469.

66. Mutter GL, Chaponot ML, Fletcher JA: A polymerase chain reaction assay for non-random X chromosome inactivation identifies monoclonal endometrial cancers and precancers. Am J Pathol 1995;146:501-508.

67. Nucci MR, Castrillon DH, Bai H, et al: Biomarkers in diagnostic obstetric and gynecologic pathology: A review. Adv Anat Pathol 2003;10:55-68.

68. Mutter GL: Diagnosis of premalignant endometrial disease. J Clin Pathol 2002;55:326-331.

69. Morrow C, Curtin J (eds): Synopsis of Gynecologic Oncology, 5th ed. New York: Churchill Livingstone; 1998.

70. Zaino RJ: The fruits of our labors: Distinguishing endometrial from endocervical adenocarcinoma. Int J Gynecol Pathol 2002;21:1-3.

71. Cacciatore B, Lehtovirta P, Wahlstrom T, Ylostalo P: Preoperative sonographic evaluation of endometrial cancer. Am J Obstet Gynecol 1989;160:133-137.

72. Posniak H, Olson M, Dudiak C, et al: MR imaging of uterine carcinoma: Correlation with clinical and pathologic findings. Radiographics 1990;10:15-27.

73. Hricak H, Lacey C, Schriock E, et al: Gynecologic masses: value of magnetic resonance imaging. Am J Obstet Gynecol 1985;153:31-37.

74. Williams AS, Kost ER, Hermann J, Zahn C: Hysteroscopy in the evaluation and treatment of mucinous adenocarcinoma. Obstet Gynecol 2002;99:509-511.

75. Alfsen GC, Thoresen SO, Kristensen GB, et al: Histopathologic subtyping of cervical adenocarcinoma reveals increasing incidence rates of endometrioid tumors in all age groups: A population based study with review of all nonsquamous cervical carcinomas in Norway from 1966 to 1970, 1976 to 1980, and 1986 to 1990. Cancer 2000;89:1291-1299.

76. Young RH, Clement PB: Endocervical adenocarcinoma and its variants: Their morphology and differential diagnosis. Histopathology 2002;41:185-207.

77. Alkushi A, Irving J, Hsu F, et al: Immunoprofile of cervical and endometrial adenocarcinomas using a tissue microarray. Virchows Arch 2003;442:271-277.

78. McCluggage WG, Sumathi VP, McBride HA, Patterson A: A panel of immunohistochemical stains, including carcinoembryonic antigen, vimentin, and estrogen receptor, aids the distinction between primary endometrial and endocervical adenocarcinomas. Int J Gynecol Pathol 2002;21:11-15.

79. Castrillon DH, Lee KR, Nucci MR: Distinction between endometrial and endocervical adenocarcinoma: An immunohistochemical study. Int J Gynecol Pathol 2002;21:4-10.

80. Kamoi S, AlJuboury MI, Akin MR, Silverberg SG: Immunohistochemical staining in the distinction between primary endometrial and endocervical adenocarcinomas: Another viewpoint. Int J Gynecol Pathol 2002;21:217-223.

81. Staebler A, Sherman ME, Zaino RJ, Ronnett BM: Hormone receptor immunohistochemistry and human papillomavirus in situ hybridization are useful for distinguishing endocervical and endometrial adenocarcinomas. Am J Surg Pathol 2002;26:998-1006.

82. Zaino R, Whitney C, Brady MF, et al: Simultaneously detected endometrial and ovarian carcinomas—A prospective clinicopathologic study of 74 cases: A Gynecologic Oncology Group study. Gynecol Oncol 2001;83:355-362.

83. Choo Y, Naylor B: Multiple primary neoplasms of the ovary and uterus. Int J Gynaecol Obstet 1982;20:327-334.

84. Ulbright T, Roth L: Metastatic and independent cancers of the endometrium and ovary: A clinicopathologic study of 34 cases. Hum Pathol 1985;16:28-34.

85. Montoya F, Martin M, Schneider J, et al: Simultaneous appearance of ovarian and endometrial carcinoma: A therapeutic challenge. Eur J Gynaecol Oncol 1989;10:135-139.

86. Eifel P, Hendrickson M, Ross J, et al: Simultaneous presentation of carcinoma involving the ovary and the uterine corpus. Cancer 1982;50:163-170.

87. Sheu BC, Lin HH, Chen CK, et al: Synchronous primary carcinomas of the endometrium and ovary. Int J Gynaecol Obstet 1995;51:141-146.

88. Fujita M, Enomoto T, Wada H, et al: Application of clonal analysis: Differential diagnosis for synchronous primary ovarian and endometrial cancers and metastatic cancer. Am J Clin Pathol 1996;105:350-359.

89. Emmert-Buck MR, Chuaqui R, Zhuang Z, et al: Molecular analysis of synchronous uterine and ovarian endometrioid tumors. Int J Gynecol Pathol 1997;16:143-148.

90. Lin WM, Forgacs E, Warshal DP, et al: Loss of heterozygosity and mutational analysis of the PTEN/MMAC1 gene in synchronous endometrial and ovarian carcinomas. Clin Cancer Res 1998;4:2577-2583.

91. Sherman ME, Bitterman P, Rosenshein NB, et al: Uterine serous carcinoma: A morphologically diverse neoplasm with unifying clinicopathologic features. Am J Surg Pathol 1992;16:600-610.

92. Ambros RA, Sherman ME, Zahn CM, et al: Endometrial intraepithelial carcinoma: A distinctive lesion specifically associated with tumors displaying serous differentiation. Hum Pathol 1995;26:1260-1267.

93. Spiegel GW: Endometrial carcinoma in situ in postmenopausal women. Am J Surg Pathol 1995;19:417-432.

94. Soslow RA, Pirog E, Isacson C: Endometrial intraepithelial carcinoma with associated peritoneal carcinomatosis. Am J Surg Pathol 2000;24:726-732.

95. Silva E, Jenkins R: Serous carcinoma in endometrial polyps. Mod Pathol 1990;3:120-128.

96. Lim P, Al Kushi A, Gilks B, et al: Early stage uterine papillary serous carcinoma of the endometrium: Effect of adjuvant whole abdominal radiotherapy and pathologic parameters on outcome. Cancer 2001;91:752-757.

97. Carcangiu ML, Chambers JT: Early pathologic stage clear cell carcinoma and uterine papillary serous carcinoma of the endometrium: Comparison of clinicopathologic features and survival. Int J Gynecol Pathol 1995;14:30-38.

98. Gehrig PA, Groben PA, Fowler WC Jr, et al: Noninvasive papillary serous carcinoma of the endometrium. Obstet Gynecol 2001;97:153-157.

99. Wheeler DT, Bell KA, Kurman RJ, Sherman ME: Minimal uterine serous carcinoma: Diagnosis and clinicopathologic correlation. Am J Surg Pathol 2000;24:797-806.

100. Hendrickson MR, Ross J, Eifel P, et al: Uterine papillary serous carcinoma: A highly malignant form of endometrial adenocarcinoma. Am J Surg Pathol 1982;6:93-108.

101. Kanbour-Shakir A, Tobon H: Primary clear cell carcinoma of the endometrium: A clinicopathologist study of 20 cases. Int J Gynecol Pathol 1991;10:67-78.

102. Christopherson W, Alberhasky R, Connelly P: Carcinoma of the endometrium. I. A clinicopathologic study of clear-cell carcinoma and secretory carcinoma. Cancer 1982;49:1511-1523.

103. Abeler V, Kjørstad K: Clear cell carcinoma of the endometrium: A histopathological and clinical study of 97 cases. Gynecol Oncol 1991;40:202-217.

104. Carcangiu ML, Chambers JT: Uterine papillary serous carcinoma: A study on 108 cases with emphasis on the prognostic significance of associated endometrioid carcinoma, absence of invasion, and concomitant ovarian carcinoma. Gynecol Oncol 1992;47:298-305.

105. Cirisano FD Jr, Robboy SJ, Dodge RK, et al: Epidemiologic and surgicopathologic findings of papillary serous and clear cell endometrial cancers when compared to endometrioid carcinoma. Gynecol Oncol 1999;74:385-394.

106. Kupryjanczyk J, Thor AD, Beauchamp R, et al: Ovarian, peritoneal, and endometrial serous carcinoma: Clonal origin of multifocal disease. Mod Pathol 1996;9:166-173.

107. Clement PB, Young RH: Endometrioid carcinoma of the uterine corpus: A review of its pathology with emphasis on recent advances and problematic aspects. Adv Anat Pathol 2002;9:145-184.

108. Chen J, Trost D, Wilkinson E: Endometrial papillary adenocarcinomas: Two clinicopathological types. Int J Gynecol Pathol 1985;4:279-288.

109. Ambros RA, Malfetano JH: Villoglandular adenocarcinoma of the endometrium. Am J Surg Pathol 2000;24:155-156.

110. Zaino RJ, Kurman RJ, Brunetto VL, et al: Villoglandular adenocarcinoma of the endometrium: A clinicopathologic study of 61 cases: A gynecologic oncology group study. Am J Surg Pathol 1998;22:1379-1385.

111. Ambros RA, Ballouk F, Malfetano JH, Ross JS: Significance of papillary (villoglandular) differentiation in endometrioid carcinoma of the uterus. Am J Surg Pathol 1994;18:569-575.

112. Atkins K, Bell S, Kempson RL, Hendrickson MR: Myxoid smooth muscle neoplasms of the uterus. Mod Pathol 2001;14:132A.

113. Atkins K, Bell S, Kempson RL, Hendrickson MR: Epithelioid smooth muscle neoplasms of the uterus. Mod Pathol 2001;14:132A.

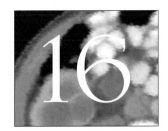

CHAPTER 16

MOLECULAR GENETICS OF ENDOMETRIAL CANCERS

Paul J. Goodfellow and *David G. Mutch*

 MAJOR CONTROVERSIES

- Is inherited endometrial cancer a significant clinical problem?
- How does molecular genetics play into inherited endometrial cancer?
- Are there reliable approaches to identifying patients and families with genetic disease?
- Are family and personal histories of cancers, age of onset, and other diagnostic clues valuable?
- What is the best approach to management of the endometrial cancer patient with inherited disease and her at-risk family members, and how does genetic testing fit into the management plan?
- When should physicians and patients consider genetic testing, and how can they obtain the best test?
- Does endometrial surveillance matter in women who have increased genetic risk for uterine endometrial cancer?
- Where does molecular genetic testing and risk management begin and end, and who is responsible?
- Why is it necessary to understand the genetic basis of endometrial carcinoma?
- Why use molecular markers for endometrial cancer?
- Are there molecular pathologic markers that are useful in the care of women with endometrial cancers?
- When is a marker used in patient care, and are there clinically useful molecular markers for endometrial cancer?

The Meaning and Importance of Inherited Endometrial Cancer

Overview. Inherited cancer susceptibility has been recognized for a large number of malignancies. The Human Genome Project has a heightened awareness of the role that genes play in disease, and it is undeniable that genetics plays a part in the management of several common cancers, including breast and colon carcinomas. These are malignancies for which major (i.e., big effect) genes conferring risk have been identified. A small but significant fraction of patients with breast and colon cancers develop disease because they inherited a mutation in a susceptibility gene.[1] Identifying patients with

genetic disease has ramifications for their management and the management of at-risk family members. It is generally accepted that for patients with inherited breast or colon cancer, more intensive surveillance is of benefit. Early detection of primary cancers and synchronous or metachronous tumors can lead to improved outcomes. There is a growing acceptance that surgical and medical prophylaxis is also of benefit to the patient. The value of more intensive cancer surveillance also applies to the cancer patients' unaffected but at-risk family members.

Inherited endometrial cancer is not well understood. Endometrial carcinoma is a feature of the cancer susceptibility syndrome known as hereditary nonpolyposis

229

colorectal carcinoma (HNPCC), or the so-called Lynch syndrome. Endometrial carcinoma is the second most common malignancy in families that fulfill the clinical diagnostic criteria for HNPCC.[2,3] Some studies have indicated that within HNPCC families, female carriers of the disease-associated mutations have a higher lifetime risk for the development of endometrial cancer than for colorectal cancer.[2] Most studies on familial or inherited forms of endometrial cancer have concentrated on patients with HNPCC or HNPCC-like diseases. Our understanding of inherited endometrial cancer is therefore largely limited to what is seen in colorectal cancer-prone families. Some studies on inherited risk for endometrial cancer have focused on women with early-onset endometrial carcinoma or double primary malignancies (i.e., hallmarks of inherited cancer) but have been limited in their scope.

Is inherited endometrial cancer a significant clinical problem? To answer this question, it is necessary to attempt to define what is meant by inherited endometrial cancer. We know relatively little about familial or inherited forms of uterine cancer. Although endometrial cancer is a key feature of the HNPCC syndrome, which shows clear mendelian-dominant inheritance with high penetrance of the cancer-causing mutation, we do not know if and how often inherited endometrial cancer occurs outside of the HNPCC syndrome (i.e., whether genes other than HNPCC genes can result in inherited endometrial cancer). Futhermore, it is not known whether there are other genes that act alone or in concert to increase risk for endometrial cancer but do not themselves result in simple inheritance patterns. The fact that males are not subject to uterine cancers complicates interpretation of inheritance patterns, much as the largely sex-limited expression of breast cancer susceptibility mutations did in the early investigations of inherited forms of breast cancer. In addition, any female family members who had a hysterectomy for reasons other than uterine cancer provide no information on familial risk, further complicating the interpretation of family histories.

How does molecular genetics play into inherited endometrial cancer? Molecular diagnosis of inherited susceptibility to endometrial cancer is possible in some families, and molecular analysis of endometrial tumors in combination with medical and family history can help identify patients who are at increased risk for genetic disease. Molecular testing is not, however, used in diagnosing endometrial cancer, but rather in assessing risk. When to seek molecular testing is not a straightforward decision. When a patient has a strong family history of cancer, testing is an option that should be considered. More challenging is the patient for whom there is suspicion of inherited cancer susceptibility. A negative gene test does not rule out risk, and there is the danger that both the physician and patient come away with the message that nothing more needs to be done. However, genetic testing with appropriate interpretation of test results can help in

patient management and decision-making. Testing should be seen as the beginning rather than the end of a phase of patient care.

Are there reliable approaches to identifying patients and families with genetic disease? Are family and personal histories of cancers, age of onset, and other diagnostic clues valuable? A family history of cancer is the best indicator of an inherited cancer syndrome but does not necessarily identify all patients with genetic disease. Obtaining a detailed family history is a time-intensive process that cannot be accomplished in most clinics or physician offices. Some practitioners rely on abbreviated family histories that are part of routine physical and history examinations to identify those endometrial cancer patients who are suspicious for inherited cancer susceptibility. Information from what is frequently called a *screening family history* can be used to make decisions about pursuing a more detailed family history or for making a referral to a medical genetics specialist.

After the decision is made that further family history information is required, the patient and her relatives work with a genetic counselor or other suitably trained professional to devise a detailed family history. Typically, a three-generation or deeper pedigree is devised, focusing on identification of all types of cancers in all family members, complete with information on age at onset. Because multiple primary malignancies are a feature of inherited disease, particular attention is given to determining the patterns of synchronous and metachronous malignancies seen in family members. Information on the age at death for family members without cancer is important in the overall assessment of pedigree information and should be sought. In addition to collecting information on malignancies, it is also important to determine whether female family members were diagnosed with endometrial hyperplasia and whether they had a hysterectomy for any reason. Because of the strong association between endometrial and colon cancer risk in HNPCC, information on precancerous colonic lesions should also be obtained. When possible, medical record verification of cancers and precancers should be obtained. The complete family history can then be used to make a clinical diagnosis of inherited cancer susceptibility. Frequently, patients have family histories that suggest increased familial risk for cancer but do not fulfill clinical diagnostic criteria. These women and their families represent a particular challenge for the gynecologic oncologist and genetic specialist because the overall significance of familial risk is difficult to interpret and what it means for the patient and her family members is uncertain.

Early age at diagnosis of endometrial carcinoma and synchronous and metachronous malignancies are features of genetic susceptibility that can be observed in the absence of a family history. Early age at diagnosis or a second malignancy in an endometrial cancer patient are clues that there may be some underlying genetic susceptibility to cancer. Neither of these clinical features, however, is specific to inherited forms of cancer. The mean age of onset of endometrial cancer in the United States is approximately 60 years.[4] Although it might seem logical to consider patients who are diagnosed at age 50 years or younger (i.e., more than a decade earlier than the population mean) as being at increased genetic risk, it is important to bear in mind the potential role of other endometrial cancer risk factors such as obesity and estrogen exposures in those women. Similarly, although multiple primary cancers suggest an underlying genetic susceptibility, the types of cancers and ages at which they developed should be taken into consideration. For example, breast cancer is a common disease, and whether breast cancer is associated with inherited forms of endometrial cancer is a subject of controversy. A late-onset breast cancer in a patient with a previous endometrial cancer may have little connection to inherited cancer susceptibility. Conversely, an endometrial cancer in a patient with a previous breast cancer who received tamoxifen therapy is unlikely to represent a case in which genetic susceptibility accounts for the double primary cancers. On the other hand, colon cancer in an endometrial cancer patient may suggest genetic risk.[5-8] Unlike colon cancer, for which the cardinal features of inherited disease, including ages and patterns of cancers, are well established,[9] endometrial cancer is a malignancy for which a best approach to identifying inherited cases is still to be determined.

Molecular studies can assist in the discovery of inherited forms of endometrial cancer. An analysis of the genes known to be responsible for inherited endometrial cancer (i.e., *MSH2, MLH1, MSH6,* and *PMS2* DNA mismatch repair genes) and discovery of a confirmed pathogenic mutation are the gold standards. Only a small fraction of endometrial cancer patients carry DNA mismatch repair gene mutations, and testing is costly. For patients with strong family histories of cancer consistent with HNPCC, mutation testing should be considered.

Analysis of endometrial tumor DNA to determine if there is a defect in DNA mismatch repair evidenced by microsatellite instability (MSI) may prove useful in identifying cases with DNA repair defects. However, tumor MSI is common in endometrial cancers (approximately 28% have MSI[10]), and in most cases, it is not attributable to inherited mutation in DNA mismatch repair. Most endometrial cancers with MSI have acquired or so-called somatic defects in DNA repair.[11-13] Although no tumor test can accurately point to cases with inherited disease, these tests may yield diagnostic clues.

What is the best approach to management of the endometrial cancer patient with inherited disease and her at-risk family members, and how does genetic testing fit into the management plan? There are several published expert recommendations for the management of women who are at-risk for inherited endometrial cancer. Because the risk for cancer is not limited to the endometrium, the recommendations include approaches to cancer surveillance for other organs. These recommendations evolved from what

was learned from the study of a limited number of families (most with the HNPCC syndrome or HNPCC-like histories). The recommendations and current practices for caring for women with or at-risk for inherited endometrial cancer do not constitute evidence-based medicine. Rather than detailing the recommendations and comparing the different approaches proposed for clinical management of women with or at-risk for endometrial cancer and their at-risk family members, we recommend review of the following information:

American Medical Association web-based continuing medical education (CME) for HNPCC (http://www.ama-assn.org/cmeselec/hnpcc/target/001_cmeinfo/index.html): This reference is for HNPCC in general, with limited emphasis on endometrial carcinoma and other gynecologic pathologies.

American Society for Clinical Oncology:[14] These recommendations represent expert opinion from the gynecologic oncology community and the most relevant recommendations for endometrial cancer concerns.

International Collaborative Group on Hereditary Nonpolyposis Colorectal Cancer (http://www.nfdht.nl): This group offers guidelines for patient management.

Cancer Genetics Consortium recommendations:[15] This publication was among the first to make recommendations for management of women at increased genetic risk for endometrial cancer. It paved the way for studies and specialist consideration of the best approaches.

When should physicians and patients consider genetic testing, and how can they obtain the best test? The rule of thumb should be that when the gynecologic oncologist or other health professional caring for a patient is uncertain, he or she should seek the expert opinion of a clinical geneticist. Patients that fulfill the clinical diagnosis of HNPCC should be offered the option of gene testing (available through a variety of sources). The GeneTests web site (http://www.geneclinics.org), a publicly funded medical genetics information resource developed for physicians and other health care providers, is an excellent resource. Searching this site for endometrial or uterine cancer under the disease category fails to identify a laboratory test. Risk for endometrial cancer and genetic testing are, however, discussed for the HNPCC and PTEN hamartoma tumor syndrome (PHTS). This lack of a searchable test does not mean that testing is not available or is not important. It is simply a reflection of our current lack of understanding of the role that testing might play in the management of endometrial cancer patients.

Does endometrial surveillance matter in women who have increased genetic risk for uterine endometrial cancer? Cancer surveillance is undertaken with the intent to identify and potentially treat malignancies or precancers earlier than would otherwise be possible.

This is predicated on the belief that early treatment will translate to better outcomes. Two interrelated features of endometrial cancer biology make it difficult to determine the benefits of surveillance. One is a general feature of the disease, and the other is specific to inherited forms of endometrial cancer. First, most women with endometrial cancer are symptomatic even with early-stage disease (typically presenting with irregular uterine bleeding), and the overall cure rate is high. By definition, large numbers will be required to see changes from what is generally early detection to even earlier detection. This is compounded by the fact that the overall cancer-free survival for patients with endometrial carcinoma exceeds 80%, and large numbers of patients must be followed to see anything other than a major change in outcome. The second factor that makes it difficult to measure the benefit of endometrial surveillance in women with genetic susceptibility is the modest increase in risk associated with mutation or family history. The overall incidence of HNPCC-associated endometrial cancer is approximately 20% by age 70.[16,17] Although some studies of specific mutations show lifetime risks as high as 40% to 50%,[3,18,19] this may be the case for the minority of genetically susceptible women. A modest increase in risk coupled with the overall early detection and excellent survival makes measurement of the benefit of surveillance difficult. There have been few studies to assess the value of surveillance in genetically susceptible women, and the largest published series suggests that screening may be of little benefit in detecting malignancies.[20] If there is a survival benefit, it may be even more difficult to demonstrate. In the single series published, endometrial cancer-specific survival for patients with HNPCC is indistinguishable from that for women with sporadic disease.[21] That said, there are scant data in the published literature. Several studies are ongoing. The MD Anderson Cancer Center has an active protocol—HNPCC & Endometrial Cancer: Combined Endometrial and Colon Cancer Screening (Protocol #ID01-694)—to assess the feasibility of screening women with HNPCC mutations for both colon and endometrial cancers. Double screening may afford greater benefit than single-organ surveillance. The National Cancer Institute (NCI)–sponsored Gynecologic Oncology Group (GOG) is about to begin a combined surveillance and treatment trial: CPC 0211, Prospective Cohort Study of Gynecologic Cancer Screening and Risk-Reducing Surgery in Women with Hereditary Nonpolyposis Colon Cancer Syndrome (HNPCC). Like the MD Anderson Cancer Center ID01-694 protocol, the GOG trial will prospectively determine the incidence of gynecologic and other cancers in women with HNPCC who elect to participate in intensive surveillance using serial transvaginal ultrasound, endometrial biopsy, and serum CA 125 levels (for women with ovarian tissue at risk) or who elect to undergo risk-reducing surgery. These two studies will include women for whom molecular genetic diagnoses have been made and will provide good indications of the benefits of genetic testing, surveillance, and intervention.

Options for nonsurgical interventions and chemoprevention for genetically at-risk women must be considered. The benefits of these approaches to managing women are even less well understood than surveillance benefits. The MD Anderson Cancer Center is conducting an important trial (HNPCC & Endometrial Cancer: Chemoprevention Using the Oral Contraceptive vs. Depo-Provera, Protocol #ID01-340). For this study, women with a known mutation between the ages of 30 and 50 years are eligible, and funds are available for genetic testing and travel expenses (funded by NCI/DCP, N01-CN-05127).

Where does molecular genetic testing and risk management begin and end, and who is responsible? Molecular genetic testing begins with the cancer patient or an at-risk family member. The gynecologist is frequently responsible for deciding who should be tested, but the decision is shared with the patient. When and how to test has been discussed, as have the current recommendations for management of the patient. These are areas of uncertainty. Even less clear is what to do for family members. Deciding who to consider for testing and how to share family risk data is best handled by a multidisciplinary team that should include oncologists, genetic counselors, and clinical geneticists. The greatest controversy in the genetic management of patients with endometrial cancer and their families is what to do for whom and for how long. There are no simple answers, but it seems safe to say that physician and patient education is needed, as is additional research into the heritability of endometrial and associated cancers and how to prevent, detect, and treat those malignancies.

Patients with molecular diagnoses afford unique opportunities for gaining insights into the causes of tumorigenesis and approaches to treatment. They also represent a population in which cancer-associated morbidity and mortality should be more easily managed than in the general population.

Endometrial Cancer Molecular Markers

Why is it necessary to understand the genetic basis of endometrial carcinoma? Endometrial cancer is the most common gynecologic cancer in the United States. Primary treatment usually consists of exploratory laparotomy, pelvic washings, hysterectomy with bilateral salpingo-oophorectomy, and pelvic and para-aortic lymph node dissection. Subsequent treatment is based on light microscopic assessment of tissues that takes into consideration the histologic differentiation and extent of tumor spread locally and distally. This approach to the evaluation of endometrial cancers and planning for subsequent treatment parallels what is done with many malignancies. However, the surgical staging of endometrial cancers has limitations, and it is generally accepted that better diagnostic and prognostic markers are needed. Elucidating the genetic changes associated with endometrial tumorigenesis holds promise for an improved understanding of endometrial cancer biology and new approaches to the detection and treatment of endometrial cancers and precursor lesions. As noted in the National Cancer Institute's *Report of the Gynecologic Cancers Progress Review Group* (http://prg.nci.nih.gov/gyno/finalreport.html):

> Once cancer has been diagnosed, treatment recommendations are made on the basis of histology and extent of disease...yet response to treatment varies widely among women with the same histologic and clinical features. Many women now run the risk of over-treatment with adjuvant therapy, which can potentially incur unnecessary expense and morbidity. ...molecular and genetic characteristics of tumors should be combined with clinical follow-up data so that molecular markers of risk can be incorporated into the staging system for gynecologic cancers. Molecular and proteomic signatures are needed to supplement or replace the role of histology and extent of disease in treatment decisions, to provide accurate prognostic markers, and as targets for new therapeutic and preventive agents.

Over the past several decades, we have come to understand that cancer is a genetic disease and to accept that the science of cancer genetics is really a study of population genetics. The genetic makeup of the tumor cell determines its behavior, and tumor behavior reflects the variable genetic makeup of the cell populations. Much as common genetic features define a species and differences in the genetic makeup of individuals within the species account for their unique characteristics, there are similarities in the genetic events (i.e., mutations) associated with various cancer types and differences in the genetic makeup of individual tumors and tumor cells. The genetic material and how it is regulated within each normal cell defines what the cell looks like and how it behaves. The cancer phenotype is generally equated with uncontrolled growth that results from a series of mutations. The common genetic alterations that result in the change from normal to cancer cell can be defined for a tumor type, as can the changes unique to a single tumor.

The environment and nongenetic elements play important roles in the many stages of tumor development. The greatest advances in understanding the causes of malignancies have come from our ever-increasing ability to probe the genetic makeup of the cancer cell. Unlike other genetic diseases that result from a single mutation, such as sickle cell disease due to a mutation in the β-globin gene or cystic fibrosis due to mutation in the cystic fibrosis transmembrane conductance regulator, cancers are the results of an accumulation of genetic alterations in genes controlling cell growth, cell death, cell-cell interactions, DNA repair, and a variety of other processes. The best example of genetically defined malignancies can be seen in the work of Vogelstein and colleagues[22,23] on colon cancer. These investigators convincingly demonstrated that the accumulation of a series of mutations is necessary to take normal colon epithelium to premalignant polyps and then on to a frankly malignant tumor.

Three major classes of genes are responsible for the development of cancer: oncogenes, tumor suppressor genes, and DNA repair genes. Oncogenes act as cellular dominants (so-called gain of function effects) and usually promote cell growth. Tumor suppressor genes normally function to negatively regulate cell proliferation, and defects in cancers are recessive (i.e., loss of normal function). Defects in DNA repair and the acquisition of a mutator phenotype appear to be essential for the genotypic and phenotypic progression of cancer.[24]

The cancer cell genome has a signature that defines tumor behavior. We are just beginning to identify and characterize in detail the genetic defects that give rise to malignancies and account for specific tumor features. As technologies improve and our knowledge grows, we should be able to use molecular data to predict the behaviors of cancers much more precisely than is possible using conventional light microscopy. This concept has been demonstrated in a number of malignancies. In colon cancer, loss of DNA mismatch repair, as evidenced by MSI, is associated with improved survival. Response to fluorouracil therapy for stage II or III colon cancers is better in cases in which the tumors have no or limited MSI.[25] This sort of molecular pathologic classification of colon cancers could ultimately be used to make decisions about when to use adjuvant chemotherapy and possibly used in determining what agent is best for a given tumor. In breast cancers, molecular pathologic classification of tumors has been part of clinical management for many years. Hormone receptor status is used in making decisions about what sort of adjuvant therapy will be used.[26-29] *HER2/NEU* oncogene and HER2/NEU protein testing has come to the forefront of breast cancer management.[30]

There are no molecular markers for endometrial cancers in routine clinical use at this time. The NCI-sponsored GOG has recognized the need for better approaches to the management of endometrial cancer and has focused efforts on molecular analysis of tumors. The GOG is about to embark on an ambitious new protocol (GOG-0210) entitled "A Molecular Staging Study of Endometrial Carcinoma." The specimens collected by the GOG in protocol GOG-0210 will be available for a broad range of studies. Endometrial carcinoma lends itself to molecular investigations focused on discovery of diagnostic and prognostic markers. First, there is considerable clinical heterogeneity between and within the various histologic subtypes of endometrial cancer. It is assumed that differences between tumor types and among tumors of the same histologic type are reflections of distinctive molecular fingerprints. Second, there is often a premalignant phase that can be evaluated to search for molecular changes characteristic of the early stages of tumor formation and that are likely to be causally associated with the tumor phenotype. Third, endometrial tissue is easily accessible and usually available for investigation. Preoperative endometrial sampling is routine, the malignancy is clearly definable at the time of surgery in most cases such that tissues can be reliably retrieved for investigations, and tissues in excess of what is required for diagnosis are usually available.

Why use molecular markers for endometrial cancer?

Despite the fact that most endometrial cancer patients are cured with surgery, persistent and recurrent endometrial cancers are significant causes of mortality. The available treatments for recurrent endometrial cancer have limited success. The median survival after recurrence is difficult to determine precisely but has been estimated as being 10 months.[31] The 5-year survival rate for patients who have recurrent disease is only 13%.[32] New and more effective therapies for endometrial carcinoma based on knowledge of the genetic changes that characterize the malignancy, analogous to herceptin therapy for breast cancers, may improve the outcome for women with endometrial cancer.

Adjuvant therapy is a part of the management of women who are at increased risk for recurrent disease. After hysterectomy, irradiation or chemotherapy is used as an attempt to eliminate any remaining tumor cells. In women with early-stage (I and II) endometrial carcinoma, the use and benefits of adjuvant therapy are controversial. Within stage I and II, there are two groups of women with different risks for cancer recurrence based on the available staging methods. Stage Ia patients are at low risk for disease recurrence. Stages Ib, Ic, IIa, and IIb patients are said to be at intermediate risk. For women with intermediate-risk endometrial adenocarcinomas treated with surgery alone, the rate of recurrence is up to 13%.[33] Given the frequency of endometrial cancer, 13% recurrence represents a large number of failures. Pelvic radiation has been the most frequently used adjuvant therapy for women with early-stage endometrial cancer. It is costly and can have serious side effects. The reported complication rates for radiation therapy in endometrial cancer patients have ranged between 4% and 20%.[34-36] In a large, multicenter, randomized trial of adjuvant therapy for stages Ib, Ic, IIa, and IIb endometrioid adenocarcinomas, it was demonstrated that pelvic radiation significantly decreased recurrences but brought about only a small and nonstatistically significant improvement in overall survival.[33] There appears to be a shift away from adjuvant radiation therapy for women with early-stage endometrial cancers because of the uncertainty as to the benefits of treatment. Molecular markers to identify patients who are at very low risk for disease recurrence could help avoid unnecessary adjuvant therapy and, by doing so, lessen the morbidity and expense associated with treating endometrial cancer. Conversely, markers for high-risk disease could be used to target cases for more aggressive treatments at the time of diagnosis. Markers to predict risk of recurrence would directly benefit trials evaluating new treatments.

Are there molecular pathologic markers that are useful in the care of women with endometrial cancers?

The molecular genetics of endometrial cancer have been reviewed elsewhere.[37,38] Epidemiologic and molecular studies have convincingly demonstrated that there are two distinct types of endometrial carcinomas: type I and type II.[39-41] Type I tumors are of the endometrioid histologic subtype; they are usually estrogen related, often low grade and low stage, and tend to occur at a younger age. Type II tumors include papillary serous, clear cell, mucinous, and other histologic variants along with some moderately and poorly differentiated endometrioid carcinomas arising on an atrophic endometrium. Type II cancers generally have a poorer prognosis (typically are higher grade and stage tumors), appear unrelated to estrogenic stimulation, and manifest at a later age.

In this section, we comment on some of the molecular lesions that are seen in endometrial cancers focusing on changes that may have implications in terms of diagnosis or prognosis. It is not surprising that types I and II endometrial cancers have distinctive molecular defects. There have been relatively few molecular markers that are not related to traditional histopathologic variables used in the diagnosis and treatment of endometrial cancer. For convenience, the information has been organized by method of analysis or by individual genes or processes when appropriate.

DNA content: ploidy and cell proliferation. Tumor cell DNA content is a prognostic indicator in many malignancies. Analysis of the DNA content of endometrial cancers has indicated molecular disturbances that might provide more accurate and objective information than standard histologic evaluation.[42-45] In one study, flow cytometric evaluation of the S-phase fraction showed a correlation between S-phase fraction and other proliferation markers in endometrial cancers.[46] The prognostic value of endometrial cancer cell DNA content, however, remains uncertain. Some studies have failed to support the notion that DNA ploidy and S-phase fraction are of prognostic significance or have yielded inconclusive findings.[47,48] Differences in patient populations and methods to measure DNA content could explain why some studies suggest ploidy and S-phase content are prognostic, while others fail to reveal such associations.

TP53 gene. Mutation in the *TP53* tumor suppressor gene is the most commonly observed genetic change found in human cancers.[49] An issue of *Human Mutation*[50] focused on *TP53* and cancer and includes several good reviews on the subject.

TP53 mutation plays a role in most cancers studied, and the prognostic significance for *TP53* aberrations has been demonstrated for many different cancers.[51-57] *TP53* mutation also plays a role in the genesis of endometrial cancers and, in particular, uterine serous carcinomas. Most uterine serous carcinomas have *TP53* mutations.[58-60] The rate of mutation in endometrioid cancers, however, is considerably lower, ranging from 10% to 30%.[61,62] There is also an apparent but less striking association between *TP53* mutation and tumor grade.[63-65]

TP53 mutation status is correlated with a variety of clinicopathologic factors that portend poor outcome.[60] The presence of a *TP53* defect is associated with increased proliferative activity.[65] Increased tumor cell proliferation is a feature of aggressive cancers, which in general correlates well with grade and vice versa.

TP53 mutation status is therefore predictive of tumor aggressiveness.

TP53 mutation status can be determined preoperatively and could be used to identify patients likely to have aggressive disease. Molecular pathologic findings such as *TP53* mutation status could be used in triaging patients to more aggressive therapy. In a study from the Mayo Clinic, endometrial cancers from 134 patients were evaluated for a variety of flow cytometric parameters and molecular markers. The flow cytometric analysis included ploidy, S-phase fraction, and proliferative index. The molecular markers analysis included proliferating cell nuclear antigen, *HER-2/NEU*, and P53. In this cohort, overexpression of P53 (which is equated with mutant *TP53*) clearly defined a subset of patients who were at high risk for disease recurrence and death from their disease.[66] The general indication is that P53 overexpression predicts a more aggressive type of endometrial cancer and could be used as a prognostic tool. Some investigators have failed to demonstrate that P53 overexpression is an independent prognostic indicator but suggest that its use in combination with other markers may prove clinically useful.[67] Additional studies will be required to determine whether P53 analysis could be used in clinical trials or routine care of patients with endometrial cancer.

KRAS2 gene. Mutation in the *KRAS2* member of the *RAS* gene family is seen in 10% to 30% of uterine cancers.[62,64,68-71] Single base changes in codons 12, 13 and 61, seen in all histologic subtypes of endometrial carcinoma, result in a constitutionally activated RAS protein. The frequency of *KRAS2* mutation appears higher in endometrioid adenocarcinomas than in serous carcinomas.[72-74] Mutation appears to be an early event in type I tumors based on the observation that atypical hyperplasia, a precursor to endometrioid carcinoma, frequently harbors *KRAS2* defects.[69,71,75] The relationship between *KRAS2* mutation and clinical and histopathologic features other than histologic subtype is uncertain. Increased RAS activity or *RAS* mutation is correlated with less well-differentiated tumors in some studies but not in others.[76-78] It is unclear whether there is an association between *KRAS2* mutation and outcome.[79,80] The apparently contradictory results may be explained by confounding genetic and environmental factors, coupled with the small sample sizes for many of the molecular studies. However, it seems unlikely that *KRAS2* mutation status is of general prognostic significance. The possibility remains that information on KRAS2 activation could be used in selecting therapies that target the RAS pathway.

Metallothioneins. Metallothioneins represent a family of proteins believed to function in zinc and copper homeostasis in development, zinc metalloprotein metabolism, and detoxification of heavy metals. Metallothioneins are also implicated in the tissue response to stress or injury, providing protection against reactive oxygen species. Normal tissues typically do not express measurable levels of metallothioneins. High-level metallothionein expression is associated with rapidly proliferating tissues and has been described in a wide variety of cancers. Expression appears to correlate with disease progression and poor prognosis in many malignancies including oral squamous, gastrointestinal, and lung cancers.[81,82] For a number of cancers such as bladder, gastrointestinal, and esophageal carcinomas, the association is not clear. In some investigations, there is no apparent relationship between metallothionein expression and outcome, or if there is, it appears to be in subsets of patients receiving specific therapies.[83-90]

In endometrial cancer, metallothionein expression has also been associated with features predictive of outcome.[91,92] Overexpression of metallothioneins was observed in endometrial cancers relative to hyperplasia. It was also positively correlated with grade of tumor and *TP53* mutation status, and there was a trend toward inverse correlation with estrogen receptor (ER) expression.[91] The finding that metallothionein levels are inversely correlated with ER status is not surprising because receptor status is clearly associated with differentiation. There is also a suggestion that metallothionein gene regulation in part may be controlled by hormones. Additional studies are required to determine if metallothionein expression is a marker of aggressiveness in endometrial cancers.

Telomerase. Telomerase activity requires a protein and RNA component. Telomerase levels are low in most normal tissues, with the exception of the germline and activated lymphocytes. Many tumor cell lines, however, express telomerase at high levels. It is believed that telomerase activity is one mechanism by which cells may achieve immortality. Telomerase activity has been correlated with a number of clinicopathologic variables that are known prognostic indicators in many cancers. An issue of *Cancer Letters*, "Telomeres, Telomerase, and The Cancer Cell," includes reviews and commentaries that address the molecular biology of telomerase.[93] Several of the reviews in this issue of *Cancer Letters* deal with the diagnostic, prognostic, and therapeutic implications of telomerase in cancers. There is considerable debate about the prognostic significance of telomerase activity, whether activity in primary tumors mirrors the fraction of proliferating cells, and whether undifferentiated cells automatically upregulate telomerase activity.

The diagnostic, prognostic, and therapeutic potentials of telomerase activity have been evaluated in uterine cancers. Telomerase activity (assessed with the TRAP assay) may prove useful as a diagnostic marker for endometrial carcinoma.[94] Distinguishing between atypical hyperplasia and hyperplasia without atypia by conventional histology is highly observer dependent and challenging for even the most skilled pathologist. Some early studies of telomerase activity in the endometrium suggested that it may not be a good diagnostic marker because normal proliferating cells have measurable and possibly even high activity.[95] As is the case for many malignancies, endometrial cancers and precancerous endometrial lesions frequently express telomerase. Although not every case of atypical endometrial hyperplasia expresses telomerase, telomerase activity may prove very useful as a molecular diagnostic marker.

The prognostic significance of telomerase in endometrial cancers is uncertain. There are contradictory reports on the associations between telomerase activity and conventional prognostic indicators.[96,97] There does seem to be a trend toward associating telomerase activity and tumor aggressiveness with disease-free interval and tumor-related deaths.

Telomerase-based cancer therapy is being explored for many malignancies. Specific inhibition of telomerase is seen as a potential universal cancer therapy and is expected to have fewer side effects than conventional cytotoxic therapies. Research into telomerase inhibition in endometrial cancer lags behind what has been accomplished in other cancer types. There are several reports on changes in telomerase activity in endometrial cancer cells in response to therapy. Yokoyama and colleagues[98] have explored the inhibition of telomerase in endometrial cancer cells. Despite limited research and progress in this area, telomerase-based therapy for endometrial cancers holds particular promise given the generally poor responses to conventional anticancer agents that are seen with most endometrial cancers.

Defective DNA mismatch repair and microsatellite instability. Loss of DNA mismatch repair leads to a molecular phenotype in tumors that is referred to as MSI; MSI reflects a mutator phenotype.[24] Tumors with MSI are believed to have an overall increase in the number of gene mutations attributable to a failure in the DNA mismatch repair apparatus. Approximately 25% of endometrial cancers have defective DNA mismatch repair.[10,13,99-101] MSI is a feature of the tumors (including endometrial carcinomas) that arise in HNPCC patients who have germline defects in a DNA repair gene. Most endometrial cancers with MSI are, however, sporadic. Transcriptional silencing of the *MLH1* gene that is associated with promoter methylation is the most common cause of MSI in endometrial cancers.[11,13,102] MSI in endometrial cancers is more common in type I than in type II tumors.[74,103,104]

Sporadic colon cancers also exhibit MSI. Patients with MSI-positive colon tumors have improved survival.[25,105-108] The prognostic significance of MSI in endometrial cancers is unclear. Some studies suggest a similar association between the presence of MSI and improved outcome,[109] but others show no such relationship.[110,111] The inconsistent findings about the prognostic significance of MSI in endometrial cancers may reflect differences in the patient populations studied, methods used to characterize tumors, and effects of sample size. The well-documented prognostic significance of MSI in specific subsets of colon cancer patients suggests that additional studies of endometrial carcinoma may be warranted.

When is a marker used in patient care, and are there clinically useful molecular markers for endometrial cancer? The discovery of molecular markers for cancer usually relies on retrospective studies. Any new marker that is being considered for clinical use should provide information that is superior to or complements that can be obtained using conventional approaches to the diagnosis and treatment of a malignancy.

There are relatively few molecular markers for endometrial cancers that add clinically valuable information. Most have not been evaluated in prospective trials, and their true value in the management of endometrial cancer patients remains to be determined. There are, however, several interesting candidates. Based on successes in other malignancies, the potential importance of these and other genetic makers is great. A more complete understanding of the genetic basis of uterine cancer development holds promise for the discovery of new diagnostic and prognostic markers. Novel approaches to the prevention, detection, and treatment of endometrial cancer are expected as we begin to elucidate the genetic factors that contribute to the cancer state.

Gynecologists and gynecologic oncologists have important roles in basic and translational endometrial cancer research. This is particularly true in the area of marker discovery. Physicians caring for women with endometrial cancer have a responsibility to help formulate and interpret the results of marker discovery experiments. Moving a molecular marker from the laboratory to the clinic necessitates strong collaboration between researchers and clinicians. Although there may be controversies about which molecular marker is useful in the management of women with endometrial cancer, there is little doubt that molecular genetic studies of endometrial cancers and precursor lesions will lead to advances in patient care.

REFERENCES

1. Frank TS, Critchfield GC: Inherited risk of women's cancers: What's changed for the practicing physician? Clin Obstet Gynecol 2002;45:671-683.
2. Aarnio M, Sankila R, Pukkala E, et al: Cancer risk in mutation carriers of DNA-mismatch-repair genes. Int J Cancer 1999; 81:214-218.
3. Vasen HFA, Wijnen JT, Menko FH, et al: Cancer risk in families with hereditary nonpolyposis colorectal cancer diagnosed by mutation analysis. Gastroenterology 1996;110:1020-1027.
4. Kosary CL, Ries LAG, Miller BA, et al: SEER Cancer Statistics Review, 1973-1992. NIH no. 96-2789. Bethesda, MD, National Institutes of Health, 1995.
5. Brown SR, Finan PJ, Bishop DT: Are relatives of patients with multiple HNPCC spectrum tumours at increased risk of cancer? Gut 1998;43:664-668.
6. Pal T, Flanders T, Mitchell-Lehman M, et al: Genetic implications of double primary cancers of the colorectum and endometrium. J Med Genet 1998;35:978-984.
7. Millar AL, Pal T, Madlensky L, et al: Mismatch repair gene defects contribute to the genetic basis of double primary cancers of the colorectum and endometrium. Hum Mol Genet 1999;9:823-829.
8. Buttin BM, Powell MA, Mutch DG, et al: Increased risk for HNPCC-associated synchronous and metachronous malignancies in patients with MSI-positive endometrial carcinoma lacking *MLH1* promoter methylation. Clin Cancer Res (submitted).
9. Lynch HT, de la Chapelle A: Hereditary colorectal cancer. N Engl J Med 2003;348:919-932.
10. Goodfellow PJ, Buttin BM, Herzog TJ, et al: Prevalence of defective DNA mismatch repair and MSH6 mutation in an unselected series of endometrial cancers. Proc Natl Acad Sci U S A 2003; 100:5908-5913.

11. Esteller M, Levine R, Baylin SB, et al: MLH1 promoter hyper-methylation is associated with the microsatellite instability phenotype in sporadic endometrial carcinomas. Oncogene 1998;16: 2413-2417.

12. Simpkins SB, Whelan A, Babb S, et al: Hypomethylation of the MLH1 promoter region in MSI-positive endometrial carcinomas may be an indicator of inherited cancer susceptibility. Proceed Am Assoc Cancer Res 1999;40:141-142.

13. Gurin CC, Federici MG, Kang L, Boyd J: Causes and consequences of microsatellite instability in endometrial carcinoma. Can Res 1999;59:462-466.

14. Berchuck A, Mutch DG, Karlan BY: The how, when and why of surgical prophylaxis in the high risk patient: Hereditary ovarian and endometrial cancers. J Clin Onc (in press).

15. Burke W, Petersen G, Lynch P, et al: Recommendations for follow-up care of individuals with an inherited predisposition to cancer. I. Hereditary nonpolyposis colon cancer. Cancer Genetics Studies Consortium. JAMA 1997;277:915-919.

16. Watson P, Lynch HT. The tumor spectrum in HNPCC. Anticancer Res 1994;14:1635-1640.

17. Vasen HF, Mecklin JP, Khan PM, Lynch HT: The International Collaborative Group on HNPCC. Anticancer Res 1994;14: 1661-1664.

18. Aarnio M, Mecklin JP, Aaltonen LA, et al: Life-time risk of different cancers in hereditary non-polyposis colorectal cancer (HNPCC) syndrome. Int J Cancer 1995;64:430-433.

19. Vasen HFA, Stormorken A, Menko FH, et al: *MSH*2 mutation carriers are at higher risk of cancer than *MLH*1 mutation carriers: A study of hereditary nonpolyposis colorectal cancer families. J Clin Oncol 2001;19:4074-4080.

20. Dove-Edwin I, Boks D, Goff S, et al: The outcome of endometrial carcinoma surveillance by ultrasound scan in women at risk of hereditary nonpolyposis colorectal carcinoma and familial colorectal carcinoma. Cancer 2002;94:1708-1712.

21. Boks DE, Trujillo AP, Voogd AC, et al: Survival analysis of endometrial carcinoma associated with hereditary nonpolyposis colorectal cancer. Int J Cancer 2002;102:198-200.

22. Fearon ER, Vogelstein B: A genetic model for colorectal tumorigenesis. Cell 1990;61:759-767.

23. Kinzler KW, Vogelstein B: Lessons from hereditary colorectal cancer. Cell 1996;87:159-170.

24. Loeb LA: A mutator phenotype in cancer. Cancer Res 2001;61: 3230-3239.

25. Ribic CM, Sargent DJ, Moore MJ, et al: Tumor microsatellite-instability status as a predictor of benefit from fluorouracil-based adjuvant chemotherapy for colon cancer. N Engl J Med 2003;349: 247-257.

26. Coradini D, Oriana S, Biganzoli E, et al: Relationship between steroid receptors (as continuous variables) and response to adjuvant treatments in postmenopausal women with node-positive breast cancer. Int J Biol Markers 1999;14:60-67.

27. Harvey JM, Clark GM, Osborne K, Allred DC: Estrogen receptor status by immunohistochemistry is superior to the ligand-binding assay for predicting response to adjuvant endocrine therapy in breast cancer. J Clin Oncol 1999;17:1474-1481.

28. Campbell FC, Blamey RW, Elston CW, et al: Quantitative oestradiol receptor values in primary breast cancer and response of metastases to endocrine therapy. Lancet 1981;2:1317-1319.

29. Valavaara R, Tuominen J, Johansson R: Predictive value of tumor estrogen and progesterone receptor levels in postmenopausal women with advanced breast cancer treated with tamoxifen, Cancer 1990;66:2264-2269.

30. Slamon DJ, Leyland-Jones B, Shak S, et al: Use of chemotherapy plus a monoclonal antibody against HER2 for metastatic breast cancer that overexpresses HER2. N Engl J Med 2001;344:783-792.

31. Jereczek-Fossa B, Badzio A, Jassem J: Surgery followed by radiotherapy in endometrial cancer: Analysis of survival and patterns of failure. Int J Gynecol Cancer 1999;9:285-294.

32. Creutzberg CL, van Putten WL, Koper PC, et al: Surgery and postoperative radiotherapy versus surgery alone for patients with stage-1 endometrial carcinoma: Multicentre randomised trial. PORTEC study group: Postoperative radiation therapy in endometrial carcinoma. Lancet 2000;355:1404-11.

33. Roberts J, Brunetto V, Keys H, et al: A phase III randomized study of surgery vs. surgery plus adjunctive radiation therapy in intermediate risk endometrial adenocarcinoma [abstract].

Presented at the 29th Annual Meeting of the Society of Gynecologic Oncologists. February 1998;35:70.

34. MacLeod C, Fowler AR, Ogino I, et al: High-dose-rate brachytherapy in the management of cervical and vaginal intraepithelial neoplasia Int J Radiat Oncol Biol Phys 1998; 40:881-887. Int J Radiat Oncol Biol Phys 1999;43:235-236.

35. Corn BW, Lanciano RM, Greven KM, et al: Impact of improved irradiation technique, age, and lymph node sampling on the severe complication rate of surgically staged endometrial cancer patients: A multivariate analysis. J Clin Oncol 1994;12:510-515.

36. Lewandowski G, Torrisi J, Potkul RK, et al: Hysterectomy with extended surgical staging and radiotherapy versus hysterectomy alone and radiotherapy in stage I endometrial cancer: A comparison of complication rates. Gynecol Oncol 1990;36: 401-404.

37. Hedrick L: The genetic basis of human cancer. In Vogelstein B, Kinzler KW (eds): Endometrial Cancer. New York, McGraw-Hill, 1998, pp 621-629.

38. Goodfellow P: Molecular genetics of uterine malignancies. In Rubin SC, Coukos G (eds): Cancer of the Uterus. New York, Marcel Dekker (in press).

39. Bokhman JV: Two pathogenetic types of endometrial carcinoma. Gynecol Oncol 1983;15:10-17.

40. Deligdisch L, Holinka CF: Endometrial carcinoma: Two diseases? Cancer Detect Prevent 1987;10:237-246.

41. Kurman RJ, Norris HJ: Blaustein's Pathology of the Female Genital Tract. In Kurman RJ (ed): Endometrial Carcinoma, 3 ed. New York, Springer-Verlag, 1987, pp 338-372.

42. Von Minckwitz G, Kuhn W, Kaufmann M, et al: Prognostic importance of DNA-ploidy and S-phase fraction in endometrial cancer. Int J Gynecol Cancer 1994;4:250-256.

43. Zaino RJ, Davis AT, Ohlsson-Wilhelm BM, Brunetto VL: DNA content is an independent prognostic indicator in endometrial adenocarcinoma. A Gynecologic Oncology Group study. Int J Gynecol Pathol 1998;17:312-319.

44. Mangili G, De Marzi P, Vigano R, et al: Identification of high risk patients with endometrial carcinoma. Prognostic assessment of endometrial cancer. Eur J Gynaecol Oncol 2002;23:216-220.

45. Koul A, Bendahl PO, Borg A, et al: TP53 protein expression analysis by luminometric immunoassay in comparison with gene mutation status and prognostic factors in early stage endometrial cancer. Int J Gynecol Cancer 2002;12:362-371.

46. Nordstrom B, Strang P, Bergstrom R, et al: A comparison of proliferation markers and their prognostic value for women with endometrial carcinoma: Ki-67, proliferating cell nuclear antigen, and flow cytometric S-phase fraction. Cancer 1996;78: 1942-1951.

47. Mariani L, Conti L, Antenucci A, et al: Predictive value of cell kinetics in endometrial carcinoma. Anticancer Res 2000;20: 3569-3574.

48. Mariani A, Sebo TJ, Katzmann JA, Keeney GL, et al: Pretreatment assessment of prognostic indicators in endometrial cancer. Am J Obstet Gynecol 2000;182:1535-1544.

49. Koshland DE Jr: Molecule of the year. Science 1993;262:1953.

50. Hum Mutat 2003;21:173-330.

51. Ahrendt SA, Hu Y, Buta M, et al: P53 mutations and survival in stage I non-small-cell lung cancer: Results of a prospective study. J Natl Cancer Inst 2003;95:961-970.

52. Tan DF, Li Q, Rammath N, et al: Prognostic significance of expression of p53 oncoprotein in primary (stage I-IIIa) non-small cell lung cancer. Anticancer Res 2003;23:1665-1672.

53. Rahko E, Blanco G, Soini Y, et al: A mutant TP53 gene status is associated with a poor prognosis and anthracycline-resistance in breast cancer patients. Eur J Cancer 2003;39:447-453.

54. Okuda T, Otsuka J, Sekizawa A, et al: P53 mutations and over-expression affect prognosis of ovarian endometrioid cancer but not clear cell cancer. Gynecol Oncol 2003;88:318-325.

55. Borresen-Dale AL: TP53 and breast cancer. Hum Mutat 2003;21:292-300.

56. Schuijer M, Berns EM: TP53 and ovarian cancer. Hum Mutat 2003;21:285-291.

57. Iacopetta B: TP53 mutation in colorectal cancer. Hum Mutat 2003;21:271-276.

58. Tashiro H, Isacson C, Levine R, et al: P53 gene mutations are common in uterine serous carcinoma and occur early in their pathogenesis. Am J Pathol 1997;150:177-185.

59. Kihana T, Hamada K, Inoue Y, et al: Mutation and allelic loss of the p53 gene in endometrial carcinoma. Cancer 1995; 76:72-78.
60. Kohler MF, Berchuck A, Davidoff AM, et al: Overexpression and mutation of p53 in endometrial carcinoma. Cancer Res 1992;52:1622-1627.
61. Honda T, Kato H, Imamura T, et al: Involvement of p53 gene mutations in human endometrial carcinomas. Int J Cancer 1993;53:963-967.
62. Swisher EM, Peiffer-Schneider S, Mutch DG, et al: Differences in patterns of TP53 and KRAS2 mutations in a large series of endometrial carcinomas with or without microsatellite instability. Cancer 1999;85:119-126.
63. Wachtel SS, Wachtel G, Shulman LP, et al: Identification of p53 mutations in endometrial adenocarcinoma by polymerase chain reaction-single-strand conformation polymorphism. J Soc Gynecol Invest 1994;1:234-237.
64. Enomoto T, Fujita M, Inoue M, et al: Alterations of the p53 tumor suppressor gene and its association with activation of the c-K-ras-2 protooncogene in premalignant and malignant lesions of the human uterine endometrium. Cancer Res 1993;53:1883-1888.
65. Elhafey AS, Papadimitriou JC, El-Hakim MS, et al: Computerized image analysis of p53 and proliferating cell nuclear antigen expression in benign, hyperplastic, and malignant endometrium. Arch Pathol Lab Med 2001;125:872-879.
66. Silverman MB, Roche PC, Kho RM, et al: Molecular and cyto-kinetic pretreatment risk assessment in endometrial carcinoma. Gynecol Oncol 2000;77:1-7.
67. Lundgren C, Auer G, Frankendal B, et al: Nuclear DNA content, proliferative activity, and p53 expression related to clinical and histopathologic features in endometrial carcinoma. Int J Gynecol Cancer 2002;12:110-118.
68. Enomoto T, Inoue M, Perantoni AO, et al: K-ras activation in pre-malignant and malignant epithelial lesions of the human uterus. Cancer Res 1991;51:5308-5314.
69. Duggan BD, Felix JC, Muderspach LI, et al: Early mutational activation of the c-Ki-ras oncogene in endometrial carcinoma. Cancer Res 1994;54:1604-1607.
70. Ignar-Trowbridge D, Risinger JI, Dent GA, et al: Mutations of the Ki-ras oncogene in endometrial carcinoma. Am J Obstet Gynecol 1992;167:227-232.
71. Sasaki H, Nishii H, Takahashi H, et al: Mutation of the Ki-ras protooncogene in human endometrial hyperplasia and carcinoma. Cancer Res 1993;53:1906-1910.
72. Caduff RF, Johnston CM, Frank TS: Mutations of the Ki-ras oncogene carcinoma of the endometrium. Am J Pathol 1995; 146:182-188.
73. Lagarda H, Catasus L, Arguelles R, et al: K-ras mutations in endometrial carcinomas with microsatellite instability. J Pathol 2001;193:193-199.
74. Lax SF, Kendall B, Tashiro H, et al: The frequency of p53, K-ras mutations, and microsatellite instability differs in uterine endometrioid and serous carcinoma: Evidence of distinct molecular genetic pathways. Cancer 2000;88:814-824.
75. Cohn DE, Mutch DG, Herzog TJ, et al: Genotypic and pheno-typic progression in endometrial tumorigenesis: Determining when defects in DNA mismatch repair and KRAS2 occur. Genes Chromosomes Cancer 2001;32:295-301.
76. Long CA, O'Brien TJ, Sanders MM, et al: Ras oncogene is expressed in adenocarcinoma of the endometrium. Am J Obstet Gynecol 1988;159:1512-1516.
77. Scambia G, Catozzi L, Benedetti-Panici P, et al: Expression of ras p21 oncoprotein in normal and neoplastic human endometrium. Gynecol Oncol 1993;50:339-346.
78. Tsuda H, Jiko K, Yajima M, et al: Frequent occurrence of c-Ki-ras gene mutations in well differentiated endometrial adenocarci-noma showing infiltrative local growth with fibrosing stromal response. Int J Gynecol Pathol 1995;14:255-259.
79. Ito K, Watanabe K, Nasim S, et al: K-ras point mutations in endometrial carcinoma: Effect on outcome is dependent on age of patient. Gynecol Oncol 1996;63:238-246.
80. Semczuk A, Berbec H, Kostuch M, et al: K-ras gene point mutations in human endometrial carcinomas: Correlation with clinicopathological features and patients' outcome. J Cancer Res Clin Oncol 1998;124:695-700.

81. Cardoso SV, Barbosa HM, Candellori IM, et al: Prognostic impact of metallothionein on oral squamous cell carcinoma. Virchows Arch 2002;441:174-178.
82. Joseph MG, Banerjee D, Kocha W, et al: Metallothionein expression in patients with small cell carcinoma of the lung: Correlation with other molecular markers and clinical outcome. Cancer 2001;92:836-842.
83. Saga Y, Hashimoto H, Yachiku S, et al: Immunohistochemical expression of metallothionein in human bladder cancer: Correlation with histopathological parameters and patient survival. J Urol 2002;168:2227-2231.
84. Lynn NN, Howe MC, Hale RJ, et al: Overexpression of metal-lothionein predicts resistance of transitional cell carcinoma of bladder to intravesical mitomycin therapy. J Urol 2003;169:721-723.
85. Bahnson RR, Becich M, Ernstoff MS, et al: Absence of immuno-histochemical metallothionein staining in bladder tumor specimens predicts response to neoadjuvant cisplatin, metho-trexate and vinblastine chemotherapy. J Urol 1994;152(Pt 2):2272-2275.
86. Janssen AM, van Duijn W, Kubben FJ, et al: Prognostic signifi-cance of metallothionein in human gastrointestinal cancer. Clin Cancer Res 2002;8:1889-1896.
87. Ofner D, Maier H, Riedmann B, et al: Immunohistochemical metallothionein expression in colorectal adenocarcinoma: Correlation with tumour stage and patient survival. Virchows Arch 1994;425:491-497.
88. Hishikawa Y, Koji T, Dhar DK, et al: Metallothionein expression correlates with metastatic and proliferative potential in squamous cell carcinoma of the oesophagus. Br J Cancer 1999; 81:712-720.
89. Kishi K, Doki Y, Miyata H, et al: Prediction of the response to chemoradiation and prognosis in oesophageal squamous cancer. Br J Surg 2002;89:597-603.
90. Aloia TA, Harpole DH Jr, Reed CE, et al: Tumor marker expres-sion is predictive of survival in patients with esophageal cancer. Ann Thorac Surg 2001;72:859-866.
91. Ioachim EE, Kitsiou E, Carassavoglou C, et al: Immunohisto-chemical localization of metallothionein in endometrial lesions. J Pathol 2000;191:269-273.
92. McCluggage WG, Maxwell P, Hamilton PW, Jasani B: High metallothionein expression is associated with features predictive of aggressive behaviour in endometrial carcinoma. Histo-pathology 1999;34:51-55.
93. Telomeres, Telomerase, and The Cancer Cell [whole issue]. Cancer Lett 2003;194:137-247.
94. Maida Y, Kyo S, Kanaya T, et al: Is the telomerase assay useful for screening of endometrial lesions? Int J Cancer 2002;100:714-718.
95. Bonatz G, Klapper W, Barthe A, et al: Analysis of telomerase expression and proliferative activity in the different layers of cyclic endometrium. Biochem Biophys Res Commun 1998;253:214-221.
96. Ebina Y, Yamada H, Fujino T, et al: Telomerase activity correlates with histopathological factors in uterine endometrial carcinoma. Int J Cancer 1999;84:529-532.
97. Bonatz G, Frahm SO, Klapper W, et al: High telomerase activity is associated with cell cycle deregulation and rapid progression in endometrioid adenocarcinoma of the uterus. Hum Pathol 2001;32:605-614.
98. Yokoyama Y, Wan X, Shinohara A, et al: Hammerhead ribozymes to modulate telomerase activity of endometrial carcinoma cells. Hum Cell 2001;14:223-231.
99. Katabuchi H, van Rees B, Lambers AR, et al: Mutations in DNA mismatch repair genes are not responsible for microsatellite instability in most sporadic endometrial carcinomas. Cancer Res 1995;55:5556-5560.
100. Kowalski LD, Mutch DG, Herzog TJ, et al: Mutational analysis of MLH1 and MSH2 in 25 prospectively acquired RER⁺ endometrial cancers. Genes Chromosomes Cancer 1997;18:219-227.
101. Kobayashi K, Matsushima M, Koi S, et al: Mutational analysis of mismatch repair genes, hMLH1 and hMSH2, in sporadic endometrial carcinomas with microsatellite instability. Jpn J Cancer Res 1996;87:141-145.
102. Simpkins SB, Bocker T, Swisher EM, et al: MLH1 promoter methylation and gene silencing is the primary cause of

microsatellite instability in sporadic endometrial cancers. Hum Mol Genet 1999;8:661-666.

103. Tashiro H, Lax SF, Gaudin PB, et al: Microsatellite instability is uncommon in uterine serous carcinoma. Am J Pathol 1997;150:75-79.

104. Caduff RF, Johnston CM, Svoboda-Newman SM, et al: Clinical and pathological significance of microsatellite instability in sporadic endometrial carcinoma. Am J Pathol 1996;148: 1671-1678.

105. Gryfe R, Kim H, Hsieh ETK, et al: Tumor microsatellite instability and clinical outcome in young patients with colorectal cancer. N Engl J Med 2000;342:69-77.

106. Lothe RA, Peltomäki P, Meling GI, et al: Genomic instability in colorectal cancer: Relationship to clinicopathological variables and family history. Cancer Res 1993;53:5849-5852.

107. Lukish JR, Muro K, DeNobile J, et al: Prognostic significance of DNA replication errors in young patients with colorectal cancer. Ann Surg 1998;227:51-56.

108. Wright CM, Dent OF, Barker M, et al: Prognostic significance of extensive microsatellite instability in sporadic clinicopathological stage C colorectal cancer. Br J Surg 2000;87:1197-1202.

109. Maxwell GL, Risinger JI, Alvarez AA, et al: Favorable survival associated with microsatellite instability in endometrioid endometrial cancers. Obstet Gynecol 2001;97:417-422.

110. Basil JB, Goodfellow PJ, Rader JS, et al: Clinical significance of microsatellite instability in endometrial cancer. Cancer 2000; 89:1758-1764.

111. Peiro G, Diebold J, Lohse P, et al: Microsatellite instability, loss of heterozygosity, and loss of hMLH1 and hMSH2 protein expression in endometrial carcinoma. Hum Pathol 2002;33:347-354.

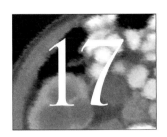

CONTROVERSIES IN ENDOMETRIAL CANCER SCREENING AND DIAGNOSIS

Lois M. Ramondetta and Karen H. Lu

 MAJOR CONTROVERSIES

- Is there a universal screening protocol for low- and high-risk women?
- Are women taking tamoxifen at increased risk for endometrial cancer?
- Is ultrasound examination adequate for screening of women who are taking tamoxifen?
- Should endometrial biopsies be routinely performed on women using tamoxifen?
- Which women are genetically predisposed to endometrial cancer?
- Should women with hereditary nonpolyposis colorectal cancer undergo routine endometrial biopsy?
- What are the risks for obese women?
- What is the value of diagnostic uterine hysteroscopy?
- Do intraperitoneal cancer cells found after hysteroscopy alter prognosis?
- Should patients with endometrial cancer undergo preoperative evaluation with computed tomography or magnetic resonance imaging?
- Can the preoperative serum CA 125 concentration predict lymphatic spread in patients with endometrial cancer?

In 2002, 39,300 women in the United States were diagnosed with endometrial cancer, and 6,600 women died from the disease. This represents an alarming 128% increase in the number of deaths due to endometrial cancer in the United States since 1987. Almost all patients with endometrial cancer (more than 90%) present with postmenopausal bleeding, and, regardless of symptoms, 70% present with stage Ia disease and require no further treatment.[1] Although most patients develop obvious symptoms when the disease is in an early stage, others either are misdiagnosed or are diagnosed when the disease is in a late stage as a result of patient denial, physician oversight, genetic risk, or confusing symptoms, as in the case of a young woman with menometorrhagia.[2,3]

Most authorities do not recommend universal screening for endometrial cancer, and no definitive screening criteria have been established. However, women taking tamoxifen, women with a genetic predisposition to endometrial cancer, and obese women are at increased risk for development of endometrial cancer and may benefit from early-detection strategies. Currently, there are no proved effective screening methods for these high-risk women. Furthermore, the potential benefits of screening high-risk women remain to be determined.

The use of hysteroscopy for diagnosing the disease remains controversial because of the theoretical risks of peritoneal seeding. Although sampling of peritoneal fluid after hysteroscopy suggests that this procedure may lead to positive peritoneal cytology findings, the significance of such a result is unclear.[4-7] The International Federation of Gynecology and Obstetrics (FIGO) staging system suggests that positive cytologic findings significantly worsen the prognosis: patients with positive results are categorized as having stage IIIa disease.[8] However, many have argued that in the absence of other evidence of stage IIIa disease, such as ovarian or serosal metastasis, positive cytology findings should not independently suggest a worse prognosis.[9] Those who argue that positive cytology results alone suggest a worse prognosis are not clear as to how, or even whether, to treat these patients any more aggressively than patients without positive findings. Nonetheless, despite the debated significance of positive cytologic findings in patients with endometrial cancer, the benefits of hysteroscopy in the diagnosis of the disease are not definitive, and its continued use for presymptomatic diagnosis of uterine cancer remains open to question.

Although few disagree that surgical staging is necessary to determine the need for adjuvant treatment, controversy surrounds the use of selective versus complete lymphadenectomy and the possible therapeutic benefits of lymphadenectomy.[10,11] This specific controversy is discussed in Chapter 19. A related issue is the use of preoperative evaluation with magnetic resonance imaging (MRI), computed tomography (CT), or measurement of serum CA 125 levels to reduce extensive and sometimes risky intraoperative staging procedures. The question also arises as to whether preoperative MRI or CT could be avoided if surgical staging findings could help formulate treatment decisions or could even be therapeutic, or furthermore whether thorough surgical staging could be substituted for imaging in all cases.

This chapter focuses on the controversies pertaining to screening for endometrial cancer; the use of hysteroscopy as a diagnostic tool and its effect on staging; and the use of MRI, CT, and CA 125 levels in preoperative evaluation and staging.

Is there a universal screening protocol for low- and high-risk women?

There is no proved indication for universal screening for endometrial cancer. Ninety percent of women presenting with endometrial cancer have postmenopausal bleeding as an early warning sign, and 70% present with disease confined to the uterus. There have been no studies confirming the efficacy of screening for endometrial cancer in the general population.[12,13] In one study, 801 asymptomatic perimenopausal and postmenopausal women underwent endometrial screening biopsies, and only one well-differentiated endometrial cancer was diagnosed.[14] In another study, 597 women with high-risk factors, such as obesity and diabetes, were screened, and only six endometrial cancers were identified.[15] Currently, recommendations for the early detection of endometrial cancer are that

all postmenopausal women with vaginal bleeding should undergo an endometrial biopsy to determine the presence or absence of endometrial cancer. Of all women who present with postmenopausal bleeding, between 4% and 24% have endometrial cancer.[15] In addition, perimenopausal and premenopausal women with irregular bleeding, prolonged menorrhagia, or metrorrhagia should also undergo endometrial biopsy to rule out endometrial cancer.

Are women taking tamoxifen at increased risk for endometrial cancer?

Although screening of the general population for endometrial cancer is not indicated, certain high-risk cohorts, including women who are taking tamoxifen, women with a genetic predisposition to endometrial cancer, and obese women, may benefit from screening. Women using tamoxifen are at an increased risk for development of endometrial cancer.[16-18] In randomized, controlled clinical trials, tamoxifen has been shown to be effective as adjuvant therapy for women with early-stage breast cancer and as a chemopreventive agent in women who are at increased risk for the disease. However, although tamoxifen acts as an antiestrogen in breast tissue, it promotes proliferative activity in the endometrium. Several randomized, prospective clinical trials have reported an increased risk of endometrial cancer in women taking tamoxifen.[16-18] In the National Surgical Adjuvant Breast and Bowel Project (NSABP) B-14 trial, the largest prospective, randomized, placebo-controlled trial of adjuvant tamoxifen in women with early-stage breast cancer in the United States, the rate of endometrial cancer in women who received adjuvant tamoxifen treatment (1.6/1000) was 7.5-fold that in a placebo-treated group (0.2/1000).[16] Because of the unusually low number of endometrial cancers in the placebo group, an additional analysis was performed using a control group of patients with breast cancer from the Surveillance, Epidemiology and End Results (SEER) database. The relative risk of endometrial cancer in women taking tamoxifen in the adjuvant setting was 2.2.[16]

The NSABP P-1 trial was a subsequent large, prospective, randomized placebo-controlled trial testing tamoxifen as a chemopreventive agent in healthy women who were at increased risk for breast cancer. In 1998, the investigators in that trial reported that tamoxifen decreased the incidence of breast cancer but increased the risk of endometrial cancer by 2.53-fold.[19] They added that all of the endometrial cancers were stage I and that no endometrial cancer deaths had occurred by the time of the report. Although women who take tamoxifen are at increased risk for endometrial cancer, this risk is most likely only twofold to threefold. However, given the increase in the number of healthy women who may use tamoxifen as a chemopreventive agent, the question of whether endometrial cancer screening in this cohort is necessary has been raised by both clinicians and patients.

Is ultrasound examination adequate for screening of women who are taking tamoxifen?

The two modalities that have been suggested for monitoring of women who are taking tamoxifen are transvaginal sonography to evaluate the endometrial stripe and endometrial sampling.

Tamoxifen clearly causes thickening of the endometrial stripe, as visualized on transvaginal sonography. However, a number of studies have found a poor correlation between the size of the endometrial stripe and the presence of an endometrial precancerous or cancerous lesion.[20-23] The reason is that cystically dilated glands and subepithelial stromal hypertrophy cause the endometrial stripe to appear thickened on sonography.[21,24] Follow-up biopsies in women whose uterine linings appeared thickened on sonography have shown atrophic endometrium or benign polyps but rarely atypical hyperplasia or cancer.[22,23] In a large prospective study, Gerber and associates[20] used transvaginal sonography to screen 247 postmenopausal women taking adjuvant tamoxifen and 98 control subjects. Of 52 asymptomatic patients with a thickened endometrium, 38 had an atrophic endometrium, 9 had polyps, 4 had hyperplasia, and 1 had endometrial cancer. Of 20 patients who developed abnormal bleeding, 4 had hyperplasia and 2 had cancer. The authors concluded that transvaginal sonography is not indicated for routine screening in asymptomatic women taking tamoxifen but that all women with abnormal bleeding should be evaluated. Although ultrasonography has been suggested for evaluation of the endometrium (especially in patients taking tamoxifen and in those with polyps), we would suggest that histologic evaluation is always needed.

Should endometrial biopsies be routinely performed on women using tamoxifen?

An alternative screening strategy, serial office endometrial sampling, was evaluated by Barakat and associates.[25] Office endometrial sampling provides a histologic specimen to rule out endometrial precancer or cancer, but serial endometrial biopsies may not be acceptable to patients because of the discomfort involved. In addition, cervical stenosis in postmenopausal women limits the usefullness of this technique. Barakat's group used serial endometrial biopsies to evaluate 159 tamoxifen-treated women.[25] Biopsies were obtained at baseline, every 6 months for 2 years, and then yearly for the next 3 years. A total of 635 biopsies were performed, with a median surveillance time of 36 months. Only 1.4% of the endometrial biopsies were abnormal, with one case of complex hyperplasia and no cases of endometrial cancer.

Given the lack of efficacy of the current screening modalities, what should be recommended for women taking tamoxifen? Current consensus opinion recommends endometrial biopsy only for women with abnormal vaginal bleeding.[26] Clearly, women taking tamoxifen should be advised to report to their physician any abnormal bleeding, and in such cases an endometrial biopsy should be performed. In addition, prior to initiating tamoxifen treatment, women should undergo a baseline pelvic examination and Papanicolaou smear. Although the overall risk is small, endometrial cancer remains one of the major concerns of patients who use tamoxifen as a chemopreventive agent. Future studies should focus on identifying those women who are at risk for the development of endometrial cancer while taking tamoxifen.

Which women are genetically predisposed to endometrial cancer?

A second group of women who are at increased risk for endometrial cancer comprises those with an inherited predisposition. Women with hereditary nonpolyposis colorectal cancer (HNPCC), also known as Lynch syndrome, have a 40% to 60% lifetime risk of endometrial cancer, a 60% to 80% lifetime risk of colon cancer, and a 13% risk of ovarian cancer (Fig. 17-1).[27,28] HNPCC results from inheritance of a mutation in one of several mismatch repair genes, including *MLH1*, *MSH2*, *MSH6*, *PMS1*, or *PMS2*. Mutations associated with HNPCC occur most commonly in *MLH1* or *MSH2*. With the availability of commercial genetic testing for *MLH1* and *MSH2*, individuals at high risk can now be identified. Although screening for colon cancer with annual colonoscopy has been shown to improve survival, there are few studies evaluating the benefit of endometrial cancer screening.

Like patients with other inherited cancers, patients with HNPCC-related endometrial cancer are typically

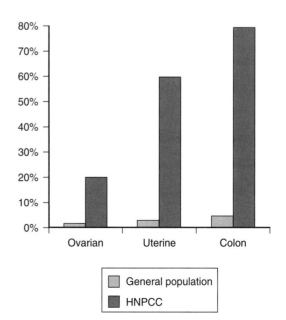

Figure 17–1. Lifetime cancer risks of patients with hereditary nonpolyposis colorectal cancer (HNPCC) compared with the general population.

diagnosed at a younger age than the population as a whole. Several studies have reported that the mean age at diagnosis of endometrial cancer in women with HNPCC is 48 to 51 years.[28-30] Therefore, any proposed screening strategies need to be initiated while women are premenopausal. In 1997, a consensus committee recommended annual endometrial cancer screening in women with HNPCC beginning at age 25 to 35 years.[31] However, the committee did not endorse specific screening methods. Options for screening include transvaginal sonography and office endometrial biopsy. Dove-Edwin and colleagues[32] recently reported on the low efficacy of sonographic screening in women with HNPCC. In 269 women from HNPCC families, no cases of endometrial cancer were detected by abnormal findings during sonographic screening. However, two women in this cohort were diagnosed with endometrial cancer: one presented with postmenopausal bleeding, and one presented with continual menstrual bleeding. Both had stage I disease. Sonographic evaluation of the endometrial stripe in premenopausal high-risk women varies throughout the menstrual period, making it difficult to determine what constitutes normal values of the endometrial stripe. However, transvaginal sonography has the additional benefit of visualization of the ovaries. Future studies will determine whether sonography provides benefit as a screening strategy for women with HNPCC. Clearly, the importance of reporting symptoms of abnormal menstrual or postmenopausal bleeding should be stressed to women with HNPCC.

Should women with hereditary nonpolyposis colorectal cancer undergo routine endometrial biopsy?

Office endometrial biopsy is another option for endometrial screening in women with HNPCC. We currently recommend annual office endometrial biopsy to women who are known mutation carriers, given their substantial risk for endometrial cancer. Future studies to address the efficacy of office endometrial biopsy as a screening tool and concerns about patient tolerability will be important. Finally, women with HNPCC should also be counseled regarding prophylactic hysterectomy and bilateral salpingo-oophorectomy, particularly if prophylactic colectomy is planned.

What are the risks for obese women?

Women who are obese are known to have a substantial risk for development of endometrial cancer, with up to a ninefold increased risk in women who are 50 pounds heavier than their ideal body weight. Although there are currently no recommendations for endometrial cancer screening in obese women, this population should be counseled to report any abnormal vaginal or postmenopausal bleeding. Prompt evaluation by office endometrial biopsy or dilation and curettage (D&C) is warranted.

What is the value of diagnostic uterine hysteroscopy?

Diagnostic hysteroscopy has historically been thought to add sensitivity to the traditional D&C in the diagnosis and evaluation of endometrial cancer.[1] Whether this increased sensitivity is authentic, or whether hysteroscopy could be eliminated as a part of the preoperative workup for endometrial cancer, remains controversial.[33-35]

Historically, the diagnosis and initial staging of endometrial cancer have involved scheduling a fractional D&C and hysteroscopy. More recently, clinicians have begun obtaining office endometrial biopsies, with or without hysteroscopy.[33-35] Certainly, a factor that is more important in the transition from intraoperative to outpatient workup is obtaining the "fractional" portion of the D&C, the endocervical curettage (ECC). The ECC is a necessary step in ruling out endocervical cancer and thus a necessary step in avoiding inappropriate surgical treatment. Theoretically, hysteroscopy allows for a more directed and therefore a more accurate biopsy. False-negative rates of the classic "blind" D&C procedure are 10% to 30%; with the addition of hysteroscopy, the false-negative rate is similarly reported as 20%.[36] On the other hand, endometrial Pipelle biopsies have been shown to have a sensitivity rate for detecting endometrial cancer of 67% but a positive predictive value of 93% and a negative predictive value of 96%.[37] In effect, definitive diagnosis is made only by biopsy; visualization of the endometrium with hysteroscopy, sonography, or even sonohysterography does not significantly add to the histologic diagnosis. This fact supports the discontinuance of hysteroscopy in the diagnostic workup of endometrial cancer (Fig. 17-2).

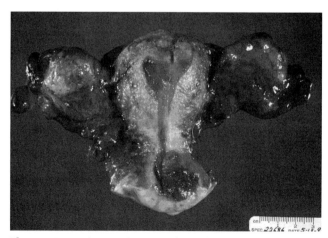

Figure 17–2. Adenocarcinoma of the endocervix. Endocervical curettage is required for diagnosis.

Do intraperitoneal cancer cells found after hysteroscopy alter prognosis?

Another reason to abandon the use of hysteroscopy in the diagnosis of endometrial cancer is that recent reports suggest that dissemination of endometrial cancer cells in patients undergoing hysteroscopy poses a potential serious risk of spreading the cancer within the abdominal cavity.[38-40] Some studies suggest that positive cytology results in the absence of other extraperitoneal findings is a poor prognostic factor. Dissemination occurs either because of distention of the uterine cavity by the pressurized liquid medium with passage of cancer cells via the fallopian tubes or by intravasation and direct penetration of cells into the circulation via injured endometrial vessels. In a parallel observation, the clinical significance of the iatrogenic rupture of an ovarian cystic tumor and potential spread of cancerous cells is still debatable. Similarly, the significance of positive peritoneal washings in a patient with endometrial or ovarian cancer, with or without prior hysteroscopy, is debatable.[41-45] Interestingly, although the FIGO staging system categorizes positive cytology results as a feature of stage IIIa disease, most studies suggest that only in the presence of additional extrauterine disease is this finding ominous.[9] Many oncologists still recommend no additional or adjuvant treatment if positive peritoneal washings are found in the absence of other evidence of extrauterine disease. Kudela and colleagues[40] found that the percentage of positive peritoneal cytologic specimens after hysteroscopy did not differ from the percentage after a D&C. Therefore, hysteroscopy may not have been a significant contributing variable. The more legitimate question pertains to the innate value of the information obtained from hysteroscopy, knowing that histologic diagnosis is still the gold standard. We therefore recommend eliminating hysteroscopy as part of the workup, except in the case of a suspected intraluminal mass or histologic findings suggesting a polypoid structure that might require a directed excision.

Should patients with endometrial cancer undergo preoperative evaluation with computed tomography or magnetic resonance imaging?

Almost 30% of women with grade I endometrial cancer diagnosed by preoperative biopsy need surgical staging by frozen section at the time of hysterectomy.[46-48] Between 20% and 30% of endometrial cancers that are determined to be grade I on histologic analysis of biopsy specimens are either upgraded or found to have unexpected deep invasion at the time of pathologic evaluation.[48] Additional methods to assist in the preoperative identification of patients who need surgical staging would be beneficial for many reasons. First, the preoperative identification of more advanced disease would allow a general obstetrician and gynecologist to arrange for appropriate oncology support or perhaps to refer the patient to a gynecologic oncologist.[11] For example, if biopsy findings suggest low-risk disease and radiologic findings suggest a lack of extrauterine spread, then the surgeon may elect to perform the surgery transvaginally or via a Pfannesteil incision. Second, such knowledge would decrease the risks associated with unnecessary extended lymphadenectomy, especially in a population that so often has several comorbid conditions. MRI or CT of the abdomen and pelvis might decrease the number of unnecessary lymph node dissections and shorten the time in surgery.

Contrast-enhanced MRI of the pelvis has been determined to be better than sonography, CT, or non–contrast-enhanced MRI in determining the depth of myometrial invasion.[49] However, CT and MRI are equivalent in the evaluation of para-aortic and pelvic lymph nodes.[50] Regardless of whether MRI, CT, or another modality such as positron emission tomography (PET) is used, the radiographic information could assist a clinician in planning surgery for patients with contraindications to exploratory laparotomy and extended surgical staging.[51]

However, even with the many advantages of providing the surgeon with all the findings of preoperative images, it is important to acknowledge the limitations of these modalities. First, the false-positive rates for CT and MRI are both 10%, and the false-negative rates range from 8% to 35%. Second, only 10% of metastatic lymph nodes are enlarged, and in patients with endometrial cancer para-aortic lymph nodes may occasionally be positive in the absence of metastatic pelvic lymph nodes. Third, lymph node dissection may be therapeutic, even in the event of microscopic disease, thus suggesting the possibility of undertreatment in some patients with small lymph nodes.

In conclusion, preoperative imaging may be best reserved for patients with high-risk histologic features, elevated liver enzyme concentrations suggestive of liver metastases, elevated CA 125 concentrations, or clinical findings suggestive of cervical involvement.

Can the preoperative serum CA 125 concentration predict lymphatic spread in patients with endometrial cancer?

Although the benefit of a preoperative serum CA 125 measurement is unclear, some have suggested obtaining this value to determine preoperatively the risk of advanced endometrial cancer and lymphatic disease. This recommendation is based on the finding of elevated CA 125 concentrations in patients with lymphatic spread.[52,53] Patients with lymph node metastases were 8.7 times more likely to have a CA 125 level greater than 40 U/mL than were patients without metastases.[52,53] Other studies have shown that a CA 125 level greater than 20 U/mL or grade III histology can correctly identify 75% to 87% of patients requiring lymphandenectomy.[53] Serum CA 125 concentrations greater than 20 U/mL correctly predicted the need for lymphadenopathy in 70% of patients, in contrast to 45% in those with a serum CA 125 greater than 35 U/mL.[54,55]

The use of preoperative testing with imaging and CA 125 measurement for endometrial cancer remains to be determined, but in women whose comorbid conditions suggest increased perioperative risk it may allow reassessment of the situation. Perhaps CA 125 measurements could provide additional valuable information in all cases, but, at the present time, we recommend full surgical staging or selective lymph node sampling based on the projected risk of lymph node metastasis secondary to depth of invasion and histology and encourage new protocols to evaluate the sensitivity of preoperative CA 125 measurement or imaging studies for detecting depth of invasion and lymph node metastasis.

Summary

In conclusion, there is no currently proved benefit to screening of women for endometrial cancer, although high-risk populations have been identified and could be targeted for further research in this area. Additionally, although the preoperative evaluation of patients with diagnosed endometrial cancer using sophisticated imaging techniques and CA 125 measurements may offer additional information, this approach is often inexact and is not precise enough to use in formal treatment planning. Further research is obviously required.

REFERENCES

1. Hawwa ZM, Nahhas WA, Copenhaver EH: Postmenopausal bleeding. Br J Obstet Gynaecol 1970;102:133-136.
2. Burke TW, Tortolero-Luna G, Malpica A, et al: Endometrial hyperplasia and endometrial cancer. Obstet Gynecol Clin North Am 1996;23:411-454.
3. Bokhman JV: Two pathogenic types of endometrial carcinoma. Gynecol Oncol 1983;15:10-17.
4. Bettocchi S, DiVango G, Carmio G, Selvaggi L: Intraabdominal spread of malignant cells following hysteroscopy. Gynecol Oncol 1997;66:165-166.
5. Elit L: Endometrial cancer prevention, detection, management, and followup. Can Fam Physician 2000;46:887-892.
6. Sagawa T, Yamada H, Sakuragi N, Fujimoto S: A comparison between the preoperative and operative findings of peritoneal cytology in patients with endometrial cancer. Asia Oceania J Obstet Gynaecol 1994;29:39-47.
7. Schmitz MJ, Nahhas WA: Hysteroscopy may transport malignant cells into the peritoneal cavity. Eur J Gynaecol Oncol 1994;15:121-124.
8. Mikuta JJ: International Federation of Gynecology and Obstetrics staging of endometrial cancer 1988. Cancer 1993; 71(4 Suppl):1460-1463.
9. Kadar N, Homesley HD, Malfetano JH: Positive peritoneal cytology is an adverse factor in endometrial carcinoma only if there is other evidence of extrauterine disease. Gynecol Oncol 1992;46:145-149.
10. Creasman WT, Morrow CP, Bundy BN, et al: Surgical pathologic spread patterns of endometrial cancer (a GOG study). Cancer 1987;60:2035-2041.
11. Orr JW, Roland PY, Leichter D, Orr PF: Endometrial cancer: Is surgical staging necessary? Curr Opin Oncol 2001;13: 408-412.
12. Eddy D: ACS report on the cancer-related health checkup. CA Cancer J Clin 1980;30:193-240.
13. U. S. Preventive Services Task Force: Guide to Clinical Preventive Services, 2nd ed. Baltimore, Williams & Wilkins, 1996.
14. Archer DF, McIntyre-Seltman K, Wilborn WW, et al: Endometrial morphology in asymptomatic postmenopausal women. Am J Obstet Gynecol 1991;165:317-322.
15. Gerber B, Krause A, Muller H, et al: Ultrasonographic detection of asymptomatic endometrial cancer in postmenopausal patients offers no prognostic advance over symptomatic disease discovered by uterine bleeding. Eur J Cancer 2001;37:67-71.
16. Fornander T, Rutqvist LE, Cedermark B, et al: Adjuvant tamoxifen in early breast cancer: Occurrence of new primary cancers. Lancet 1989;1:117-120.
17. Andersson M, Storm HH, Mouridsen HT: Carcinogenic effects of adjuvant tamoxifen treatment and radiotherapy for early breast cancer. Acta Oncol 1992;31:259-263.
18. Fisher B, Costantino JP, Wickerham DL, et al: Tamoxifen for prevention of breast cancer: Report of the National Surgical Adjuvant Breast and Bowel Project P-1 Study. J Natl Cancer Inst 1998;90:1371-1388.
19. Fisher B, Costantino JP, Redmond CK, et al: Endometrial cancer in tamoxifen-treated breast cancer patients: Findings from the National Surgical Adjuvant Breast and Bowel Project (NSABP) B-14. J Natl Cancer Inst 1994;86:527-537.
20. Gerber B, Krause A, Muller H, et al: Effects of adjuvant tamoxifen on the endometrium in postmenopausal women with breast cancer: A prospective long-term study using transvaginal ultrasound. J Clin Oncol 2000;18:3464-3470.
21. Mourits MJE, Van der Zee AGJ, Willemse PHB, et al: Discrepancy between ultrasonography and hysteroscopy and histology of endometrium in postmenopausal breast cancer patients using tamoxifen. Gynecol Oncol 1999;73:21-26.
22. Cecchini S, Ciatto S, Bonardi R, et al: Screening by ultrasonography for endometrial carcinoma in postmenopausal breast cancer patients under adjuvant tamoxifen. Gynecol Oncol 1996;60:409-411.
23. Cohen I, Rosen DJ, Tepper R, et al: Ultrasonographic evaluation of the endometrium and correlation with endometrial sampling in postmenopausal patients treated with tamoxifen. J Ultrasound Med 1993;12:275-280.
24. Ascher SM, Imaoka I, Lage JM: Tamoxifen-induced uterine abnormalities: The role of imaging. Radiology 2000;214:29-38.
25. Barakat RR, Gilewski TA, Almadrones L, et al: Effect of adjuvant tamoxifen on the endometrium in women with breast cancer: A prospective study using office endometrial biopsy. J Clin Oncol 2000;18:3459-3463.
26. ACOG Committee on Gynecologic Practice: Tamoxifen and endometrial cancer. Washington, DC, ACOG, 1996, p 169.
27. Aarnio M, Sankila R, Pukkala E, et al: Cancer risk in mutation carriers of DNA-mismatch-repair genes. Int J Cancer 1999;81: 214-218.
28. Dunlop MG, Farrington SM, Carothers AD, et al: Cancer risk associated with germline DNA mismatch repair gene mutations. Hum Mol Genet 1997;6:105-110.
29. Watson P, Vasen HF, Mecklin JP, et al: The risk of endometrial cancer in hereditary nonpolyposis colorectal cancer. Am J Med 1994;96:516-520.
30. Vasen HF, Watson P, Mecklin JP, et al: The epidemiology of endometrial cancer in hereditary nonpolyposis colorectal cancer. Anticancer Res 1994;14:1675-1678.
31. Burke W, Petersen G, Lynch P, et al: Recommendations for follow-up care of individuals with an inherited predisposition to cancer. JAMA 1997;277:915-919.
32. Dove-Edwin I, Boks D, Goff S, et al: The outcome of endometrial carcinoma surveillance by ultrasound scan in women at risk of hereditary nonpolyposis colorectal carcinoma and familial colorectal carcinoma. Cancer 2002;94:1708-1712.
33. Gaglione R, Cinque B, Paparatti L, Pistilli E: Hysteroscopy: A milestone in gynecology. Gynaecol Endoscopy 1996;5:19-22.
34. Ian S: Ultrasound, hysteroscopy, and endometrial biopsy in the investigation of endometrial cancer. Best Prac Res Clin Obstet Gynaecol 2001;15:381-391.
35. Obemair A, Geramou M, Gucer F, et al: Impact of hysteroscopy on disease-free survival in clinically stage I endometrial cancer patients. Int J Gynecol Cancer 2000;10:272-275.

36. Zorlu CG, Cobanoglu O, Isik AZ, et al: Accuracy of pipelle endometrial sampling in endometrial carcinoma. Gynecol Obstet Invest 1994;38:272-275.

37. Daniel A, Peters WA: Accuracy of office and operating room curettage in the grading of endometrial carcinoma. Obstet Gynecol 1988;71:612-614.

38. Egarter C, Krestan C, Kurz C: Abdominal dissemination of malignant cells with hysteroscopy. Gynecol Oncol 2000;63: 143-144.

39. Ramono S, Shimoni Y, Muralee D, et al: Retrograde seeding of endometrial carcinoma during hysteroscopy. Gynecol Oncol 1992;44:116-118.

40. Kudela M, Pilka R: Is there a real risk in patients with endometrial carcinoma undergoing diagnostic hysteroscopy (HSC)? Eur J Gynecol Oncol 2001;22:342-344.

41. Creasman WT, Disaia PJ, Blessing J, et al: Prognostic significance of peritoneal cytology in patients with endometrial cancer: Preliminary data concerning therapy with intra-peritoneal radiopharmaceuticals. Am J Obstet Gynecol 1981;144:921-929.

42. Eltabbakh GH, Piver MS, Hempling RE, et al: Excellent long-term survival and absence of vaginal recurrences in 332 patients with low-risk stage 1 adenocarcinoma of the endometrium. Int J Radiat Oncol Biol Phys 1997;38:373-380.

43. Harouny VR, Sutton GP, Clark SA, et al: The importance of peritoneal cytology in endometrial cancer. Gynecol Oncol 1988;72:394-398.

44. Mazurka JL, Krepart GV, Lotoki RJ: Prognostic significance of positive peritoneal cytology in endometrial carcinoma. Am J Obstet Gynecol 1988;158:303-306.

45. Turner DA, Gershenson DM, Atkinson EN, et al: The prognostic significance of peritoneal cytology for stage 1 endometrial cancer. Gynecol Oncol 1989;74:775-780.

46. Kucera E, Kainz C, Reinthaller A, et al: Accuracy of intraoperative frozen-section diagnosis in stage 1 endometrial carcinoma. Gynecol Obstet Invest 2000;49:62-66.

47. Obemair A, Geramou M, Gucer F, et al: Endometrial cancer: Accuracy of the finding of a well-differentiated tumor at dilation and curettage compared with the findings at subsequent hysterectomy. Int J Gynecol Cancer 1999;9:383-386.

48. Zorlu CG, Kuscu E, Ergun Y: Intraoperative evaluation of prognostic factors in stage 1 endometrial cancer by frozen section: How reliable? Acta Obstet Gynecol Scand 1993;72: 382-386.

49. Hricak H, Rubinstein LV, Gherman GM, et al: MR imaging evaluation of endometrial carcinoma: Results of an NCI cooperative study. Radiology 1991;179:829-832.

50. Scheidler J, Hricak H, Yu KK, et al: Radiological evaluation of lymph node metastases in patients with cervical cancer: A meta-analysis. Radiology 1997;278:1096-1101.

51. Kinkel K, Kaji Y, Yu KK, et al: Radiologic staging in patients with endometrial cancer: A meta-analysis. Radiology 1999;212: 711-718.

52. Sood A, Buller R, Burger R, et al: Value of preoperative CA 125 level in the management of uterine cancer and prediction of clinical outcome. Gynecol Oncol 1997;90:441-447.

53. Dotters DJ: Preoperative CA 125 in endometrial cancer: Is it useful? Am J Obstet Gynecol 2000;182:1328-1334.

54. Soper JT, Berchuck A, Olt GJ, et al: Preoperative evaluation of serum CA 125, TAG-72, and CA-15-3 in patients with endometrial carcinoma. Am J Obstet Gynecol 1990;163:1204-1209.

55. Takami M, Sakamoto H, Ohtani K, et al: An evaluation of CA 125 levels in 291 normal postmenopausal and 20 endometrial adenocarcinoma-bearing women before and after surgery. Cancer Lett 1997;121:69-72.

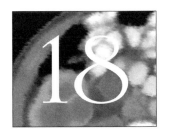

HYPERPLASIAS OF THE ENDOMETRIUM

Michael Wells

MAJOR CONTROVERSIES

- **What is the proper terminology?**
- **What is the reproducibility of diagnosis of endometrial hyperplasia?**
- **What is the role of morphometric analysis in diagnosis?**
- **What is the clonal selection hypothesis of pathogenesis?**
- **What is the distinction between endometrial hyperplasia and adenocarcinoma?**
- **What is the role of hormone replacement therapy in inducing endometrial hyperplasia?**
- **What is optimal management of hyperplasias of the endometrium?**

It has been axiomatic for almost 20 years that there are two types of endometrial adenocarcinoma. The first, of endometrioid type, occurs predominantly in perimenopausal and postmenopausal women, is associated with unopposed estrogen exposure, and arises on the basis of endometrial hyperplasia. The second occurs in elderly women, arises in an atrophic endometrium, and is unassociated with estrogen excess.[1] The paradigm histologic variant for the second type of endometrial adenocarcinoma is high-grade (papillary) serous carcinoma.[2] It has been pointed out, however, that a significant proportion of endometrial carcinomas showing endometrioid differentiation arise from an atrophic, rather than a hyperplastic, endometrium.[3] Endometrioid and serous carcinomas have, in addition to their distinct histologic appearances, distinct molecular profiles (Table 18-1).[2,4] For example, serous carcinoma is characterized by *TP53* mutation and lack of microsatellite instability, whereas endometrioid carcinoma is not. This chapter aims to explain the current understanding of the relationship between endometrial hyperplasia and endometrioid neoplasia of the endometrium and attempts to resolve the controversies associated with endometrial hyperplasias.

Estrogenic stimulation of the endometrium

The normal response of the endometrium to estrogenic stimulation is proliferation that involves both the endometrial glands and stroma, including the stromal vasculature. The appearance of the normal endometrium in the proliferative phase of the normal cycle is well defined and includes epithelial and stromal mitoses, stratification of epithelial cells, and conspicuous blood vessels in the stroma.[5] Although there is some increased tortuosity and convolution of endometrial glands in the late proliferative phase, their walls remain parallel with a consistent amount of intervening stroma. Hyperestrogenic states may have either an endogenous or an exogenous source. The former includes anovulatory cycles, polycystic ovary syndrome, estrogen-secreting tumors (of which granulosa cell tumor is the best example) and obesity (increased peripheral conversion of androgens to estrogen by aromatase in peripheral fat). The most important exogenous source of estrogen is hormone replacement therapy (HRT). To date there is little evidence that environmental estrogens such as phytoestrogens affect the human female genital tract.[6]

Table 18–1. Molecular Profiles of Endometrioid and High-Grade Serous Adenocarcinomas of the Endometrium

Parameter	Endometrioid	Serous
Estrogen/progesterone receptor	+	–
TP53 mutation	–	+
Microsatellite instability	++ (20%-30%)	+ (11%)
PTEN mutation	+ (34%-83%)	–
K-ras mutation	+ (10%-30%)	–
β-catenin mutation	+	–

Unopposed estrogenic stimulation of the endometrium induces hyperplasia, which may be defined as a state of increased cell proliferation, in contrast to hypertrophy, which is the result of an increase in cellular size that leads, in turn, to increased size of an organ (e.g., myocardial hypertrophy in response to systemic hypertension). The changes seen in the perimenopausal endometrium as a consequence of one or more anovulatory cycles may be subtle and are the consequence of unopposed estrogenic stimulation beyond the 14th day of the menstrual cycle. The mild changes that may occur in such circumstances are usually referred to as "disordered proliferation" and include minor variation in glandular size and a little focal glandular crowding.[5] Nevertheless, these changes form a continuum with changes that are regarded as hyperplasia, the distinction between the two being highly subjective. The words used in a histologic report in this situation might take the following form: "The endometrium shows disordered proliferation with mild focal glandular irregularity that is considered to fall short of a diagnosis of endometrial hyperplasia and might reflect the occurrence of one or more anovulatory cycles."

What is the proper terminology?

Over the years, many different and confusing terms have been applied to abnormal proliferations of the endometrium, including adenomatous hyperplasia, cystic hyperplasia, adenoacanthosis, and carcinoma in situ. This history has been extensively reviewed by Zaino.[1] However, for practical purposes, endometrial hyperplasia is usually considered in three main categories: simple, complex, and atypical. *Simple hyperplasia* may be thought of as the physiologic response of the endometrial glands and stroma to unopposed estrogenic stimulation; together with "disordered proliferation," it forms part of the spectrum of this endometrial response. It is questionable whether simple hyperplasia per se is ever the harbinger of neoplastic transformation of the endometrium. Simple hyperplasia is a diffuse abnormality of the endometrium characterized by variability in gland size with a normal gland/stroma ratio (Fig. 18-1). Many of the glands assume a cystic appearance, which may be apparent macroscopically.

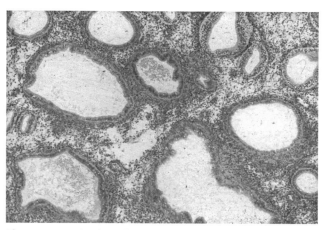

Figure 18–1. Simple endometrial hyperplasia. (From Wells M: Female genital tract. In Underwood JCE [ed]: General and Systematic Pathology, 3rd ed. New York, Churchill Livingstone, 2000, pp 495-519.)

Complex hyperplasia is characterized by architectural irregularity of the glands with an increased gland/stroma ratio in the absence of cytologic atypia (Figs. 18-2 through 18-4); it is also associated with a low risk of transformation to adenocarcinoma. *Atypical hyperplasia,* also referred to as complex atypical hyperplasia, is characterized by an increased gland/stroma ratio and architectural irregularity of the glands, with neoplastic cytologic atypia (epithelial dysplasia) (Fig. 18-5); it is considered to have a 23% to 30% risk of progression to carcinoma.[7]

I have considerable difficulty with the entity of so-called simple atypical hyperplasia and have never made this diagnosis. It is recommended that the use of this nebulous term be abandoned. Conventionally, cytologic atypia is regarded as the most important criterion in distinguishing simple and complex hyperplasias from the lesion that can be regarded as a true precancer with a risk of malignant transformation. The use of the term *atypia* in this context refers to those

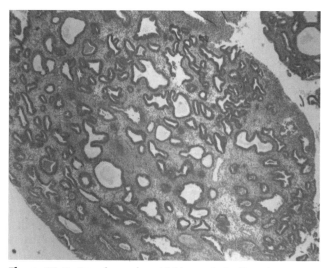

Figure 18–2. Complex endometrial hyperplasia. Note the architectural irregularity of the endometrial glands at low power.

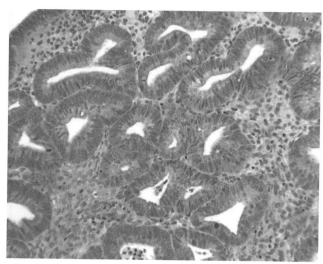

Figure 18–3. Complex hyperplasia. Note the glandular crowding.

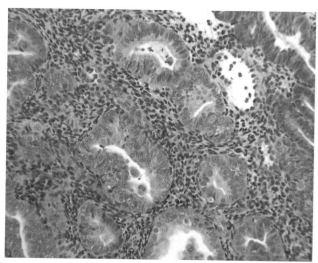

Figure 18–5. Complex atypical hyperplasia (atypical hyperplasia or endometrial intraepithelial neoplasia). Architectural irregularity is associated with a variable degree of cytologic atypia.

cytologic features that histopathologists equate with epithelial malignancy but that may also occur in the absence of invasion, such as variations in the size and shape of nuclei (nuclear pleomorphism), loss of regular stratification of nuclei within the epithelium, prominent nucleoli, and irregularity of nuclear chromatin (see Fig. 18-5). Mitoses are a feature of the normal proliferative endometrial epithelium, so their significance in endometrial hyperplasia is difficult to assess, although there may be abnormal mitotic figures.

Endometrial Intraepithelial Neoplasia

If atypical hyperplasia of the endometrium is a true precancer, then it is probably more appropriate to think of it as an endometrial intraepithelial neoplasia (EIN),[8] not to be confused with the recently defined

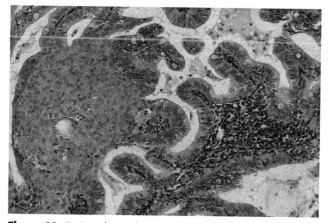

Figure 18–4. Complex endometrial hyperplasia associated with focal squamous metaplasia (squamous morule). (From Wells M: Female genital tract. In Underwood JCE [ed]: General and Systematic Pathology, 3rd ed. New York, Churchill Livingstone, 2000, pp 495-519.)

precursor of high-grade serous carcinoma that has been termed "endometrial intraepithelial carcinoma (EIC)." The latter shows intense p53 protein expression, reflecting *TP53* mutation[2,9]; although it is unquestionably a precancer, it is not regarded as part of the morphologic spectrum of endometrial hyperplasia and therefore is not referred to again in this chapter. There is clearly potential for terminologic confusion, but it should be remembered that, logically, endometrioid neoplasia of the endometrium encompasses EIN and endometrioid endometrial adenocarcinoma, whereas intraendometrial neoplasia encompasses EIN and intraendometrial adenocarcinoma, because an endometrial adenocarcinoma may show invasion of the endometrial stroma in the absence of myometrial invasion. It has been suggested that the term *hyperplasia* be reserved for the categories of simple and complex hyperplasias, which have negligible risk of neoplastic transformation.[10] However, it should be remembered that even the two broad groups of hyperplasia and EIN are not mutually exclusive and may coexist in an individual endometrium (Table 18-2).

What is the reproducibility of diagnosis of endometrial hyperplasia?

The kappa scores for the reproducibility of a diagnosis of cytologic atypia, although better than those for simple versus complex hyperplasia or atypical hyperplasia versus carcinoma, remain sufficiently low as to result in significant interobserver variation in the classification of endometrial hyperplasia.[10] The recognition of significant neoplastic cellular atypia in the endometrial epithelium presents difficulties. The assessment of neoplastic endometrial epithelial atypia in this context is associated with the same difficulties as the histologic diagnoses of glandular intraepithelial neoplasia or glandular dysplasia and adenocarcinoma

Table 18–2. Reconciliation of the Terminology of Endometrial Hyperplasia with the Concept of Endometrial Intraepithelial Neoplasia

Former Classification	Simple hyperplasia	Complex hyperplasia	Atypical hyperplasia
New Classification	Hyperplasia		Endometrial intraepithelial neoplasia (EIN)
			Low grade High grade

in situ in any glandular epithelium (e.g., gastric, colonic, endocervical). It is preferable to use a two-tier classification of low- and high-grade atypias or EIN (see Table 18-2), although it must be conceded that the recognition of such low-grade lesions in the endometrium is particularly difficult and there is little in the literature to guide one in the subtleties of interpreting such lesions.

Despite the problems of interobserver and intraobserver variation in the classification of endometrial "hyperplasia," it is likely that the categories of simple, complex, and atypical hyperplasia will persist for the foreseeable future. Because of the inherent difficulties of interobserver and intraobserver variations, it has been suggested that atypical hyperplasia and well-differentiated adenocarcinoma should also be condensed into a category of *endometrioid neoplasia,* and simple and complex hyperplasia should be combined in the category of *hyperplasia,* along the lines discussed earlier.[10] Combining atypical hyperplasia (EIN and well-differentiated endometrioid adenocarcinoma) into a single category of endometrioid neoplasia is probably a step too far for most pathologists and clinicians, although combining simple and complex hyperplasia into a single category of hyperplasia has much to commend it.

Endometrial Hyperplasia With Superimposed Secretory Changes

It is usual to diagnose endometrial hyperplasia in a proliferative endometrium. Sometimes, however, it may be apparent that secretory changes are superimposed on what is interpreted histologically as a preexisting hyperplasia. Such changes may be induced by endogenous progestogen if, for example, a series of anovulatory cycles is followed by ovulation and secretory transformation (to a greater or lesser extent) of the endometrium. Alternatively, exogenous progestogen may also be responsible if, for example, progestogens are prescribed before an endometrial biopsy or curettage is performed. The histopathologist may also be requested to assess an endometrial biopsy specimen from a patient who is being treated conservatively by exogenous progestogen after a diagnosis of atypical hyperplasia. This problem is usually encountered in the context of the polycystic ovary syndrome (Fig. 18-6). The assessment of such endometria may be difficult, and it should be remembered that the luteal phase of the normal menstrual cycle is associated with considerable tortuosity of glands.

Endometrial hyperplasia versus metaplasia

The endometrium is subject to a wide range of benign metaplastic changes, familiarity with which is crucial if an erroneous diagnosis of endometrial hyperplasia or neoplasia is to be avoided.[1,5] The most common types of metaplasia include squamous (see Fig. 18-4), papillary syncytial, ciliated cell (tubal), mucinous, clear cell, and eosinophilic (oxyphilic). Such changes may be seen in the presence of an endometritis or an intrauterine contraceptive device but also commonly occur in association with endometrial hyperplasia. It is important for the histopathologist not to exaggerate the presence of architectural or, more importantly, cytologic atypia in the presence of such metaplastic changes. Papillary syncytial change (for it may be a reactive rather than metaplastic phenomenon) may give rise to particularly alarming changes when seen in endometrial biopsy or curettage material, because it may be associated with pyknotic nuclei. Characteristically, there is an associated polymorphonuclear leukocyte infiltrate (Fig. 18-7).

What is the role of morphometric analysis in diagnosis?

The value of morphometry has been the identification by quantitative analysis of a subset of objectively measured morphometric parameters that predict the subsequent development of endometrial adenocarcinoma from a preexisting "hyperplasia." Image analysis on hematoxylin- and eosin-stained sections has allowed

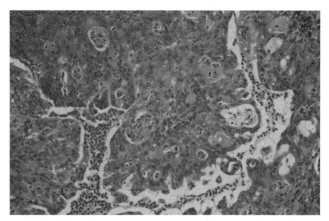

Figure 18–6. Papillary syncytial metaplasia superimposed on atypical hyperplasia (endometrial intraepithelial neoplasia). Such alarming changes may lead to an erroneous diagnosis of adenocarcinoma or even papillary serous carcinoma.

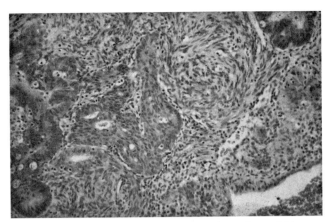

Figure 18-7. Endometrial stromal invasion by endometrioid adenocarcinoma. This is no longer "endometrial intraepithelial neoplasia," but it is still "intraendometrial neoplasia."

the analyses of various architectural and cytologic features. Baak and his colleagues showed that computerized morphometric analysis in association with histologic interpretation is the most reproducible and precise means of identifying EIN.[11-14] Importantly, these workers showed that architectural features in addition to cytologic atypia are useful in the diagnosis of EIN. They demonstrated that glandular crowding in EIN displaces stroma to a point at which the stromal volume is less than about half of the total tissue volume (stroma + epithelium + gland lumen)—in other words, the "volume percentage stroma" is less than 55%. This parameter and other features have been weighted in a predictive formula to yield a so-called D score, which, when applied to endometrial biopsy or curettage material, predicts the likelihood of there being coexisting carcinoma or progression to carcinoma. This finding has been validated by prospective outcome-based and clonal correlation studies.[14]

Experimental evidence has shown that endometrial precancer lesions are monoclonal neoplastic proliferations and that, in those individual cases in which comparison with an adjacent invasive lesion is possible, they bear a sufficiently similar genetic profile to the invasive lesion to indicate a direct neoplastic progression from the preinvasive to the invasive lesion.[14-16] In these preinvasive lesions (EIN), there is a strong correlation between the D score and monoclonality, which Baak and Mutter equated with "precancer."[14-16] The data and arguments for applying these criteria can be found on a web site: www.endometrium.org.

The data of Baak, Mutter, and colleagues[14-16] support the notion that, in contrast to EIN, the term "endometrial hyperplasia" should be reserved for those appearances seen in anovulatory endometrium or in endometrium with prolonged estrogen exposure, which range from proliferative endometrium with cysts (persistent proliferative endometrium) to bulkier endometrium with dilated, contorted glands (previously designated complex hyperplasia). These endometria are polyclonal and do not exhibit microsatellite

instability. Moreover, evidence suggests that patients with true endometrial hyperplasia revert to a normal endometrial pattern after continuous combined hormone therapy.[17,18]

There are two controversial aspects to Baak and Mutter's work. The first is the fact that they equate monoclonality with "precancer." Although neoplastic lesions are invariably monoclonal, this does not necessarily mean that all monoclonal lesions are neoplastic. For example, endometriotic foci have now been shown to be invariably monoclonal.[19,20] Although endometriosis unquestionably has neoplastic potential it would, in my opinion, be quite inappropriate to regard endometriosis per se as a precancer. Endometriosis may show dysplasia or intraepithelial neoplasia of its epithelium, and the evidence suggests that this lesion is a precancer,[21,22] but monoclonality is not confined to this lesion. The second issue is that as many as 44% of cases diagnosed as "complex nonatypical hyperplasias" by conventional histology and even 5% of "simple nonatypical hyperplasias" were shown to be monoclonal on X chromosome and microsatellite analysis and therefore were regarded as endometrial precancers or EIN (see further discussion at www.endometrium.org). In each case, computerized morphometry predicted monoclonality correctly.[14] Therefore, although on the whole there is a good correlation between the morphometric D score and conventional histologic interpretation, there are some cases that would be regarded as endometrial precancers by morphometric and monoclonality criteria but do not show cytologic atypia on conventional morphology. Because cytologic atypia has been regarded hitherto as the main criterion for the diagnosis of endometrial precancer and indeed as a mandate (except in certain rare circumstances) for hysterectomy, the general body of gynecologic pathologists still has some difficulty reconciling these two modes of assessment. Therefore, there is not invariably a close correlation between EIN using the widely accepted conventional (predominantly cytologic) criteria for diagnosing atypical hyperplasia and the morphometric criteria for diagnosing EIN, although the importance of recognizing cytologic atypia in the individual case has recently been acknowledged.[23]

What is the clonal selection hypothesis of pathogenesis?

The most common genetic abnormalities identified in endometrioid adenocarcinoma and its precursors are microsatellite instability (MSI)[24-26] and mutations of the so-called phosphatase and tensin homolog deleted on chromosome 10 gene (PTEN).[23] PTEN is a tumor suppressor gene located on chromosome 10q23.3. It is inactivated either by loss of heterozygosity or by mutation in up to 83% of endometrial adenocarcinomas, and this appears to be an early event. In contrast to the situation that pertains with TP53, in which mutation is associated with increased p53 protein expression, aberration of PTEN is associated with loss of immunohistochemical reactivity for the protein product; such PTEN-negative or "null" glands may be identified in apparently normal proliferative endometrium.[23] A hypothesis has been formulated that there is clonal selection of such abnormal epithelium in response to continuing oncogenic influences, including estrogen, with the ultimate development of endometrioid adenocarcinoma. Because the finding of null glands is quite common and endometrioid adenocarcinoma is relatively uncommon, the implication is that inherent protective mechanisms must cope with these aberrant clones in most cases. Further basic research is required in this area.

What is the distinction between endometrial hyperplasia and endometrial adenocarcinoma?

Much has been written by surgical pathologists on the distinction between atypical hyperplasia and endometrioid adenocarcinoma.[1] Stromal invasion is characterized by stromal fibrosis (see Fig. 18-7) and necrosis, polymorphonuclear leukocyte infiltration of the stroma, and a cribriform growth pattern of neoplastic glandular epithelium. The distinction between high-grade EIN and an invasive lesion may be difficult. From the practical point of view, the recognition of both lesions as neoplastic is the important factor; the real distinction of clinical importance is that between intraendometrial neoplasia (whether EIN or intraendometrial adenocarcinoma) and myoinvasive endometrial adenocarcinoma. With rare exceptions, endometrioid neoplasia, whether intraendometrial or with myometrial invasion, is an indication for hysterectomy. Approximately 40% of hysterectomy specimens removed for "atypical hyperplasia" show endometrial adenocarcinoma, and a significant proportion also show myometrial invasion.[27]

What is the role of hormone replacement therapy in inducing endometrial hyperplasia?

Postmenopausal women represent the major group of patients taking HRT. By virtue of their age, they have a background prevalence (albeit low) of endometrial precancer and cancer that must be taken into account when assessing the risks of HRT. In a study of 801 asymptomatic women, Archer and associates[28] found a prevalence of 5.2% for endometrial hyperplasia and 0.6% for atypical hyperplasia, with one case of endometrial carcinoma. Korhonen and coworkers[29] evaluated endometrial biopsy specimens from 2964 perimenopausal and postmenopausal women who were candidates for HRT and found 68.7% of these to be atrophic, 23.5% proliferative, 0.5% secretory, and 0.6% hyperplastic; 0.07% showed adenocarcinoma, and 6.6% had insufficient tissue for classification. The authors concluded, because of the low yield of endometrial carcinoma, that biopsy is unnecessary before HRT is started in asymptomatic women.

Unopposed estrogen therapy. An association between endogenous hyperestrogenism and endometrial hyperplasia was documented in the 1940s and 1950s, before the introduction of exogenous estrogen therapy. The association between exogenous estrogen therapy and endometrial carcinoma was documented in the 1970s and has repeatedly been confirmed since.[30-34] The reported risk ratio for endometrial carcinoma in women taking unopposed estrogen has varied from 2.3 to 10. The risk increases with increasing daily dose and duration of therapy, and it persists for many years after estrogen therapy has been stopped. The risks of estrogen-related endometrial carcinoma are greater in lean than in overweight women. This implies that exogenous estrogens have an additive (rather than a multiplicative) effect on endometrial carcinogenesis. It also suggests the existence of an upper risk threshold or of some limiting factor (e.g., sex hormone receptors) that impedes the continued efficacy of the combined estrogenic stimulus of obesity and exogenous estrogen beyond a certain level. Data further suggest that the risk of endometrial carcinoma is reduced among women who have used oral contraceptives. It may be that oral contraceptive use renders the endometrium less susceptible to hormonal carcinogenesis.

Studies have repeatedly shown the association between unopposed estrogen therapy and endometrial hyperplasia, and some have shown an association between the dose of estrogen and the prevalence of hyperplasia. The Postmenopausal Estrogen/Progestin Intervention (PEPI) Trial was a large, prospective, randomized, double-blind study which found that women assigned to estrogen alone (0.625 mg conjugated equine estrogen) were significantly more likely to develop simple (27.7%), complex (22.7%), or atypical hyperplasia (11.7%) than those given placebo (simple, 0.8%; complex, 0.8%; atypical, 0%; $P < .001$). This study demonstrated the necessity for baseline and annual endometrial biopsy samples when a high dose of unopposed estrogen such as this is used.[35]

Sequential hormone replacement therapy. It is well established that the addition of a progestogen to an HRT regimen substantially reduces the risk of endometrial carcinoma.[36] Although some studies reported no significant differences in the incidence of endometrial carcinoma among women taking combined HRT compared with women not taking HRT, more recent studies have suggested that the cyclic addition of progestogen to HRT does not completely eliminate the risk. Beresford and colleagues[37] found that the relative risk of endometrial carcinoma in women using a sequential combined regimen of estrogen and at least 10 days of progestogen was 1.3 (95% confidence interval [CI], 0.8 to 2.2) and that this relative risk increased to 2.5 (CI, 1.1 to 5.5) with 5 or more years of use, compared with an odds ratio of 1.0 for women who had never used hormones. This study also showed that fewer than 10 days of progestogen per cycle yielded a relative risk of 3.1 (CI, 1.17 to 5.7), which rose to 3.7 (CI, 1.7 to 8.2) with 5 or more years of use. Weiderpass and associates[38] found that women receiving a sequential combined regimen of estrogen and fewer than 16 days of progestogen per cycle for 5 years or longer had a relative risk for carcinoma of 1.6, compared with controls. Pike and coworkers[39] found no significant increase in the risk for carcinoma among women receiving combined versus sequential HRT, the latter with 10 or more days of progestogen per cycle; however, in women taking sequential HRT with fewer than 10 days progestogen per cycle, an increased risk for carcinoma was found that was of similar magnitude as that for women taking unopposed estrogen.

The PEPI trial found that women taking sequential HRT showed a tendency to develop hyperplasia (simple, 3.4%; complex, 1.7%; atypical, 0%), but the numbers were small and the differences between regimens were not statistically significant. The PEPI trial also reported that of 36 women who developed estrogen-induced hyperplasia during the trial, 34 reverted to normal on discontinuation of the estrogen and introduction of progestogen.[35] In a 1-year prospective, double-blind, randomized, multicenter study of 1724 postmenopausal women, those treated with various combinations of conjugated estrogen and medroxyprogesterone acetate developed endometrial hyperplasia in no more than 1% of cases, compared with 20% among women taking conjugated estrogen only.[40] None of the patients receiving higher medroxyprogesterone dosages developed hyperplasia.

In a multicenter study in the United Kingdom, endometrial biopsy data were generated for women treated with sequential HRT for a mean duration of 2.5 years (range, 1 to 6 years). Complex hyperplasia was found in 5.4% and atypical hyperplasia in 0.7% of the patients. It is possible that these figures, which are higher than those reported previously, reflect the duration of the study, which had a longer mean duration of therapy than previous studies. There were no cases of endometrial carcinoma. Most (76.8%) of the biopsies showing hyperplasia were taken during the progestogen phase of the treatment cycle; 17.8% were taken during treatment with estrogen alone. There were no significant differences in prevalence of hyperplasia between regimens containing 10 versus 12 days of progestogen. Hyperplasia was found to be significantly more prevalent with regimens containing levonorgestrel than with those containing norethisterone acetate (7.3% versus 4.2%, respectively). Hyperplasia was also more prevalent with lower doses of progestogen than with higher-dose therapy. These results suggest that the risk of endometrial hyperplasia may be increased in women treated with sequential HRT containing lower doses of progestogen.[17,18,41]

Broadly similar results were observed in another study, which compared a long-cycle (3-month) sequential HRT regimen with a monthly cycle regimen, progestogen being given for 10 days in each cycle. There was a higher incidence of hyperplasia in the long-cycle group, as well as one case each of atypical hyperplasia and carcinoma. In addition, the long-cycle group had a more irregular bleeding pattern, and, correspondingly, a higher dropout rate.[42]

Continuous combined hormone replacement therapy. Endometrial carcinoma has been reported only rarely in women taking continuous combined HRT regimens. In most cases, however, the women had a history of unopposed estrogen or sequential HRT use with less than 10 days of progestogen, or they had risk factors such as a family history of endometrial carcinoma. As discussed previously, the largest study to date reporting endometrial histology in postmenopausal women taking continuous combined HRT showed no cases of endometrial hyperplasia or malignancy, with an atrophic endometrium being induced in more than two thirds of women during a 9-month treatment period. All of the women who had complex hyperplasia while taking sequential HRT and completed the study reverted to nonhyperplastic endometrial patterns afterward.[17,18]

During the 3 years of the PEPI trial, there were no recorded cases of complex hyperplasia in women treated with continuous combined HRT, compared with 1.7% of 118 women treated with sequential HRT and 0.8% of 119 women treated with placebo.[35] These findings were confirmed by another study that showed no cases of hyperplasia after 2 years of continuous combined hormone replacement therapy.[43]

What is the optimal management of hyperplasias of the endometrium?

Although it is appreciated that atypical hyperplasia is more recalcitrant to exogenous progestogen therapy,[44] at present there is, apart from the recognition of atypical hyperplasia (EIN), no morphologic or other means of predicting which subset of precancers will respond to high-dose progestogen therapy. As a result, the decision whether to treat EIN hormonally or surgically is still largely a clinical one. Hyperplastic glands and stroma typically contain high concentrations of both estrogen and progesterone receptors,[1] but I know of no study that has specifically addressed the correlation between hormone receptor expression of endometrial epithelium and stroma and response to progestogen in atypical hyperplasia (EIN).

Atypical hyperplasia or intraendometrial adenocarcinoma (intraendometrial neoplasia) is, in most circumstances, an appropriate indication for hysterectomy. One exception is the occurrence of these lesions in young women (sometimes in their 20s) with polycystic ovary syndrome. Assessment by modern imaging techniques can give a very reliable indication as to whether myometrial invasion is present. If not, there is a strong case for conservative management with exogenous progestogen, which can be administered by means of an intrauterine device.[45]

Difficulties of interpretation may be encountered when a deliberate decision is made to treat endometrial hyperplasia or EIN by progestogen with repeat endometrial biopsy or curettage. Again, this is usually done in the context of the polycystic ovary syndrome in young women in their 20s or early 30s who have been investigated for infertility. In such circumstances,

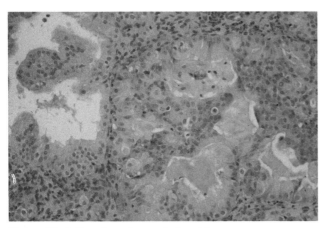

Figure 18–8. Secretory changes induced by exogenous progestogen superimposed on atypical hyperplasia (endometrial intraepithelial neoplasia). This is the endometrium of a young woman with polycystic ovary syndrome.

the histopathologic opinion is crucial to the decision as to whether to continue with conservative treatment or to advise the patient that hysterectomy would be appropriate (Fig. 18-8).

Outpatient endometrial biopsy seems to be an effective means of sampling the endometrium and identifying endometrial hyperplasia in the majority of patients.[46-48] However, awareness of the artefactual changes induced by such procedures is necessary to ensure that hyperplasia is not overdiagnosed.

Conclusions

1. Unopposed estrogenic stimulation of the endometrium is responsible for endometrial hyperplasia. However, the environmental and host factors that determine the development of estrogen-driven neoplasia over and above estrogen-driven hyperplasia remain unanswered.
2. Two categories of endometrial lesion are proposed: endometrial hyperplasia and endometrial neoplasia, the latter divided into intraepithelial and invasive neoplasia (the term "invasive" referring to endometrial stromal invasion). True endometrial hyperplasia very rarely progresses to neoplasia and may be treated hormonally, whereas the lesion formerly designated "atypical hyperplasia" is now regarded as EIN, a condition that is neoplastic from its outset and carries a significant risk of progression to invasive neoplasia.
3. Apart from exceptional circumstances, a diagnosis of atypical hyperplasia (EIN or noninvasive intraendometrial neoplasia) is an indication for hysterectomy. In select patients, there may be a case for conservative management by progestogen treatment and repeat endometrial biopsy. At present, there is no means of predicting which patients with a diagnosis of EIN are likely to respond to such treatment.

4. EIN or endometrial precancer may be identified using morphometric analysis based on a combination of architectural and morphologic features in which the volume percentage stroma is an important parameter. Such lesions show monoclonality, but the recognition of cytologic atypia remains important in assessment of the individual case.
5. The histologic distinction between high-grade EIN (atypical hyperplasia or complex atypical hyperplasia) and an invasive lesion remains problematic. Pragmatically, however, the important distinction is that between intraendometrial neoplasia (either intraepithelial or associated with invasion of the endometrial stroma) and myoinvasive endometrial adenocarcinoma.
6. Abnormalities of *PTEN* are the most common genetic abnormalities in endometrioid endometrial neoplasia and are associated with loss of PTEN protein expression. On immunohistochemical evaluation, the normal endometrium may also show PTEN-negative glands. These glands, though histologically normal, may be the harbinger of endometrial neoplasia arising by a process of clonal expansion. Further confirmatory work is required in this area.
7. Epithelial metaplasia of the endometrium or superimposed secretory changes are sources of diagnostic confusion for the histopathologist interpreting endometrial biopsy or curettage material.
8. Sequential hormone replacement therapy is associated with a slightly increased risk of endometrial hyperplasia. It is questionable whether there is a true increase in the incidence of EIN over and above the background prevalence seen in a population of untreated postmenopausal women.
9. Continuous combined hormone replacement therapy is not associated with an increased risk of endometrial hyperplasia, and complex endometrial hyperplasia may revert to normal histology with such therapy.
10. Endometrial hyperplasia can be diagnosed effectively in outpatient biopsy samples.

REFERENCES

1. Zaino RJ: Endometrial hyperplasia and carcinoma. In Fox H, Wells M (eds): Haines and Taylor Obstetrical and Gynaecological Pathology, 5th ed. New York, Churchill Livingstone, 2003, pp 443-495.
2. Feeley KM, Wells M: Advances in endometrial pathology. In Lowe DG, Underwood JCE (eds): Recent Advances in Histopathology, Vol. 19. New York, Churchill Livingstone, 2001, pp 17-34.
3. Sividris E, Fox H, Buckley CH: Endometrial carcinoma: Two or three entities? Int J Gynecol Cancer 1998;8:183-188.
4. Matias-Guiu X, Catasus L, Garcia A, et al: Molecular pathology of endometrial hyperplasia and carcinoma. Hum Pathol 2001;32: 569-577.
5. Buckley CH: Normal endometrium and non-proliferative conditions of the endometrium. In Fox H, Wells M (eds): Haines and Taylor Obstetrical and Gynaecological Pathology, 5th ed. New York, Churchill Livingstone, 2003, pp 391-441.
6. Burton JL, Wells M: The effect of phytoestrogens on the female genital tract. J Clin Pathol 2002;55:401-407.

7. Kurman R, Kaminski P, Norris H: The behaviour of endometrial hyperplasia: A long term study of "untreated" hyperplasia in 170 patients. Cancer 1985;56:403-412.

8. Mutter GL, and the Endometrial Collaborative Group: Endometrial Intraepithelial Neoplasia (EIN): Will it bring order to chaos? Gynecol Oncol 2000;76:287-290.

9. Ambros RA, Sherman ME, Zahn CM, et al: Endometrial intraepithelial carcinoma: A distinctive lesion specifically associated with tumours displaying serous differentiation. Hum Pathol 1995;26:1260-1267.

10. Bergeron C, Nogales FF, Masseroli M, et al: A multicentric European study testing the reproducibility of the WHO classification of endometrial hyperplasia with a proposal of a simplified working classification for biopsy and curettage specimens. Am J Surg Pathol 1999;23:1102-1108.

11. Baak JPA, Nauta J, Wisse-Brekelmans E, Bezemer P: Architectural and nuclear morphometrical features together are more important prognosticators in endometrial hyperplasias than nuclear morphometrical features alone. J Pathol 1988;154:335-341.

12. Baak JPA: The role of computerized and cytometric feature analysis in endometrial hyperplasia and cancer prognosis. J Cell Biochem 1995;59(Suppl 23):137-146.

13. Dunton C, Baak J, Palazzo J, et al: Use of computerized morphometric analyses of endometrial hyperplasias in the prediction of coexistent cancer. Am J Obstet Gynecol 1996;174:1518-1521.

14. Mutter GL, Baak JPA, Crum CP, et al: Endometrial precancer diagnosis by histopathology, clonal analysis and computerized morphometry. J Pathol 2000;190:462-469.

15. Jovanovic AS, Boynton KA, Mutter GL: Uteri of women with endometrial carcinoma contain a histopathological spectrum of monoclonal putative precancers, some with microsatellite instability. Cancer Res 1996;56:1917-1921.

16. Mutter GL, Boynton KA, Faquin WC, et al: Allelotype mapping of unstable microsatellites establishes direct lineage continuity between endometrial precancers and cancer. Cancer Res 1996;56:4483-4486.

17. Sturdee DW, Ulrich LG, Barlow DH, et al: The endometrial response to sequential and continuous combined oestrogen-progestogen replacement therapy. Br J Obstet Gynaecol 2000;107:1392-1400.

18. Wells M, Sturdee DW, Barlow DH, et al, for the UK Continuous Combined HRT Study Investigators: Effect on endometrium of long term treatment with continuous combined oestrogen-progestogen replacement therapy: Follow up study. BMJ 2002;325:239-242. Full text available at: http://bmj.com/cgi/content/full/325/7358/239. (See also Archer DF: Continuous combined hormone replacement therapy and endometrial hyperplasia [editorial]. BMJ 2002;325:231-232.)

19. Jimbo H, Hitomi Y, Yoshikawa H, et al: Evidence for monoclonal expansion of epithelial cells in ovarian endometrial (sic) cysts. Am J Pathol 1997;150:1173-1178.

20. Tamura M, Fukaya T, Murakami T, et al: Analysis of clonality in human endometriotic cysts based on evaluation of X chromosome inactivation in archival formalin-fixed, paraffin embedded tissue. Lab Invest 1998;78:213-218.

21. Fukunaga M, Nomura K, Ishikawa E, Ushigome S: Ovarian atypical endometriosis: Its close association with malignant epithelial tumours. Histopathology 1997;30:249-255.

22. Ogawa S, Kaku T, Amada S, et al: Ovarian endometriosis associated with ovarian carcinoma: A clinicopathological and immunohistochemical study. Gynecol Oncol 2000;77:298-304.

23. Mutter GL: Diagnosis of premalignant endometrial disease. J Clin Pathol 2002;55:326-331.

24. Levine RL, Cargile CB, Blazes MS, et al: PTEN mutations and microsatellite instability in complex atypical hyperplasia: A precursor lesion to uterine endometrioid carcinoma. Cancer Res 1998;58:3254-3258.

25. Maxwell GL, Risinger JI, Gumbs C, et al: Mutation of the PTEN tumor suppressor gene in endometrial hyperplasias. Cancer Res 1998;58:2500-2503.

26. Esteller M, Catasus L, Matias-Guiu X, et al: hMLH1 Promoter hypermethylation is an early event in human endometrial tumorigenesis. Am J Pathol 1999;155:1767-1772.

27. Janicek M, Rosenshein N: Invasive endometrial cancer in uteri resected for atypical endometrial hyperplasia. Gynecol Oncol 1994;52:373-378.

28. Archer DF, McIntyre-Seltman K, Wilborn WW, et al: Endometrial morphology in asymptomatic postmenopausal women. Am J Obstet Gynecol 1991;165:317-322.

29. Korhonen MO, Symons JP, Hyde BM, et al: Histologic classification and pathologic findings for endometrial biopsy specimens obtained from 2964 perimenopausal and postmenopausal women undergoing treatment for continuous hormones as replacement therapy (CHART2 Study). Am J Obstet Gynecol 1997;176:377-380.

30. Beral V, Banks E, Reeves G, Appleby P: Use of HRT and the subsequent risk of cancer. J Epidemiol Biostat 1999;4:191-210.

31. Rubin GL, Peterson HB, Lee NC, et al: Estrogen replacement therapy and the risk of endometrial cancer: Remaining controversies. Am J Obstet Gynecol 1990;162:148-154.

32. Brinton LA, Hoover RN, and the Endometrial Cancer Collaborative Group: Estrogen replacement therapy and endometrial cancer risk: Unresolved issues. Obstet Gynecol 1993;81:265-271.

33. Grady D, Gebrestsadik T, Kerlikowske K, et al: Hormone replacement therapy and endometrial cancer risk: A meta-analysis. Obstet Gynecol 1995;85:304-313.

34. Levi F, La Vecchia C, Gulie C, et al: Oestrogen replacement treatment and the risk of endometrial cancer: An assessment of the role of covariates. Eur J Cancer 1993;29A:1445-1449.

35. The Writing Group for the PEPI Trial 1996: Effects of hormone replacement therapy on endometrial histology in postmenopausal women. The Postmenopausal Estrogen/Progestin Interventions (PEPI) Trial. JAMA 1996;275:370-375.

36. Voight LF, Weiss NS, Chu J, et al: Progestagen supplementation of exogenous oestrogens and risk of endometrial cancer. Lancet 1991;338:274-277.

37. Beresford SAA, Weiss NS, Voight LF, McKnight B: Risk of endometrial cancer in relation to oestrogen combined with cyclic progestagen therapy in postmenopausal women. Lancet 1997;349:458-461.

38. Weiderpass E, Adami HO, Baron JA, et al: Risk of endometrial cancer following estrogen replacement with and without progestins. J Natl Cancer Inst 1999;91:1131-1137.

39. Pike MC, Peters RK, Cozen W, et al: Estrogen-progestin replacement therapy and endometrial cancer. J Natl Cancer Inst 1997;89:1110-1116.

40. Woodruff JD, Pickar JH, for the Menopause Study Group: Incidence of endometrial hyperplasia in postmenopausal women taking conjugated estrogens (Premarin) with medroxyprogesterone acetate or conjugated estrogens alone. Am J Obstet Gynecol 1994;170:1213-1223.

41. Sturdee DW, Barlow DH, Ulrich LG, et al: Is the timing of withdrawal bleeding a guide to endometrial safety during sequential oestrogen-progestogen replacement therapy? Lancet 1994;344:979-982.

42. Bjarnason K, Cerin A, Lindgren R, Weber T: Adverse endometrial effects during long cycle hormone replacement therapy. Scandinavian Long Cycle Study Group. Maturitas 1999;32:161-170.

43. Nand SL, Webster MA, Baber R, O'Conner V, for the Ogen/Provera Study Group: Bleeding pattern and endometrial changes during continuous combined hormone replacement therapy. Obstet Gynecol 1998;91:678-684.

44. Ferenczy A, Gelfand M: The biologic significance of cytologic atypia in progestogen-treated endometrial hyperplasia. Am J Obstet Gynecol 1989;160:126-131.

45. Montz FJ, Bristow RE, Bovicelli A, et al: Intrauterine progesterone treatment of early endometrial cancer. Am J Obstet Gynecol 2002;186:651-657.

46. Fothergill DJ, Brown VA, Hill AS: Histological sampling of the endometrium: Comparison between formal curettage and the Pipelle sampler. Br J Obstet Gynaecol 1992;99:779-780.

47. Batool T, Reginald PW, Hughes JH: Outpatient Pipelle endometrial biopsy in the investigation of post-menopausal bleeding. Br J Obstet Gynaecol 1994;101:545-546.

48. Piegsa K, Calder A, Davis JA, et al: Endometrial status in postmenopausal women on long-term continuous combined hormone replacement therapy (Kliofem): A comparative study of endometrial biopsy, outpatient hysteroscopy and transvaginal ultrasound. Eur J Obstet Gynecol Reprod Biol 1997;72:175-180.

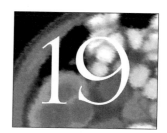

C H A P T E R

MANAGEMENT OF EARLY-STAGE ENDOMETRIAL CANCER

Kathryn M. Greven   and   Karl C. Podratz

 ## MAJOR CONTROVERSIES

- **What is the optimal surgical management of early-stage corpus cancer?**
- **What is the role of adjuvant radiation?**
- **What is the optimal type of adjuvant radiation?**
- **What is the role of adjuvant chemotherapy?**
- **What is the role of hormone replacement therapy?**

Over the last two decades, substantial progress has been made in the understanding of prognostic factors for survival and patterns of disease recurrence for patients diagnosed with endometrial cancer. Adjuvant treatment has evolved from preoperative radiation therapy (RT) for all patients to postoperative RT for selected patients, as determined by patient- and disease-related prognostic factors. However, several controversies still exist in the management of endometrial cancer. Surgical staging has contributed to the knowledge of disease dissemination, but the role of lymphadenectomy is unclear: Should lymphadenectomy be considered therapeutic or merely prognostic? Does the performance of a lymphadenectomy alter patterns of failure and hence the recommendations for adjuvant treatment? Questions also persist regarding the application of adjuvant RT: Which patients need no adjuvant therapy? Which patients can be adequately treated with vaginal brachytherapy alone, or is pelvic RT beneficial for certain patients? Does cytotoxic chemotherapy add to the disease control of high-risk patients? Finally, can patients who survive a diagnosis of endometrial cancer be offered hormone replacement therapy that may improve quality of life?

Etiology and Epidemiology

Endometrial cancer is the most common malignancy of the female reproductive tract. It is exceeded annually in overall frequency only by breast, colon, and lung cancers. During 2002, an estimated 39,300 new cases of endometrial cancer were diagnosed in the United States, and 6600 deaths from this disease occurred.[1] Since 1991, more deaths have occurred annually from endometrial cancer in the United States than from cancer of the cervix. The death rate from endometrial cancer has remained relatively stable over the past two decades even though endometrial carcinoma invariably declares itself early in its natural history and is usually clinically manifested as stage I disease. These sobering statistics suggest the need for reassessment of diagnostic, staging, and therapeutic approaches in the overall management of this neoplasm. The successful treatment of endometrial cancer and a decrease in the death rate may involve the implementation of more definitive treatment algorithms, predicated on an enhanced understanding of the epidemiology, etiology, and biology of epithelial carcinoma of the uterine corpus.

The association of unopposed estrogens, nulliparity, or irregular menses (or combinations of these) with endometrial cancer has been recognized for several decades. More recently, the administration of tamoxifen for the treatment of breast cancer has also been correlated with an increased risk of developing endometrial cancer. Although sources of unopposed estrogens include the administration of estrogen and the presence of a gonadal stromal tumor, the most cogent contemporary demographic characteristic associated with corpus cancer is obesity and polycystic ovary syndrome, specifically in women younger than 40 years of age. These physiologic conditions are associated with elevated serum estrone and estradiol concentrations, reflecting increased levels and peripheral conversion of androstenedione and testosterone.[2] Compounding these increased levels of circulating serum estrogens is the androgen-induced decreased concentration of serum hormone-binding globulin, which further enhances the bioavailability of the steroid hormones associated with endometrial cancer. Multiple studies have demonstrated an association between tamoxifen and endometrial cancer, and the National Surgical Adjuvant Breast and Bowel Project projected a 7.5 relative risk of developing endometrial cancer for women with breast cancer treated with tamoxifen.[3] However, the benefits derived in reduction in breast cancer relapses and life-years saved from tamoxifen ingestion dwarfs the mortality attributed to tamoxifen-induced corpus cancer. The clinicopathologic characteristics of patients with tamoxifen-associated endometrial cancer are similar to those seen in women with a history of unopposed estrogen. The incorporation of progestins in hormone replacement regimens, the liberal use of oral contraceptive agents, and the increased frequency of smoking among women during the past three decades have presumably contributed to the limited increases in the number of cases of endometrial cancer diagnosed annually over the past 15 years.

In 1983, Bokhman[4] described two distinct "pathogenetic types" of endometrial carcinomas. Type I was characterized as a well- to moderately well-differentiated, superficially invasive lesion with a favorable prognosis that was associated with obesity, hyperlipidemia, irregular bleeding of extended duration, estrogenic colpocytology, and hyperplastic endometrium. By contrast, type II lesions were poorly differentiated and deeply invasive carcinomas with a poor prognosis. The associated clinical symptoms were of short duration, with phenotypic characteristics and histologic features suggesting an independence of estrogen. Type I (endometrioid) consists predominantly of the endometrioid histologic subtype (>80%), whereas type II (nonendometrioid) includes papillary serous, clear cell, and undifferentiated subtypes. In a review of the Mayo series, nonendometrioid histology constituted 13% of the sampled cohort and occurred in an older patient population.[5] Clinicopathologic features were divergent. Patients with nonendometrioid histology demonstrated advanced disease: 62% had stage III/IV disease, 73% had poorly differentiated tumors,

44% had myometrial invasion to the serosa, and the 5-year survival rate was 33%, compared with 7%, 11%, 3%, and 92%, respectively, for patients with endometrioid histology.

Assessment of the two dominant histologic subtypes also suggests discrete characteristic precursor lesions. Early-stage endometrioid carcinomas usually occur within proliferative or hyperplastic endometrium (frequently with atypia) and seldom are associated with carcinoma in situ.[6,7] These observations suggest a continuum from normal endometrium through hyperplastic changes to endometrial carcinoma, which in turn implies the potential for reversibility. In fact, several investigators have demonstrated spontaneous or progestin-induced regression of these precursor lesions.[8,9] In addition, reports have documented progestin-induced regressions of well-differentiated endometrioid carcinomas in women younger than 40 years of age who elected to preserve fertility.[10-12] By contrast, serous papillary carcinomas appear to arise within a background of atrophic endometrium, frequently with accompanying carcinoma in situ.[6,7] These observations infer the occurrence of an aberrant molecular event or series of events originating in a single cell and leading to malignant transformation.

The continued integration of clinical and molecular characteristics will facilitate understanding of the etiology of endometrial cancer and provide the potential for target-based therapeutic options. In an analysis of more than 300 patients, Mariani and colleagues[13] observed a significant ($P < .01$) diminution in ligand binding to estrogen receptors (ER) and progesterone receptors (PR) in tumor samples with either grade 3 histology or nonendometrioid subtypes. Alterations in receptor expression, receptor assembly and activation, response element recognition, or receptor degradation are among the potential explanations for loss of hormone binding. Although mutations in the ER appear to be infrequent, recent evidence suggests that promoter site hypermethylation might account in part for the loss of ER.[14] Likewise, differential expression of the PR-α (PRA) and PR-β (PRB) has been reported.[15,16] Considering that PRA appears to downregulate ER action and PRB is the primary activator of progesterone-responsive genes, the loss of either might theoretically result in an unopposed estrogen effect. Clinically, reduced levels of ligand interaction with the ER, PR, or both in endometrial carcinoma samples significantly ($P < .01$) correlates with post-treatment relapses and death from disease.[13]

Alterations in the expression of oncogenes, tumor suppressor genes, and mismatch repair genes have been correlated with clinical outcomes and presumably are involved in the transformation process. The *PTEN* tumor suppressor gene, possessing growth-inhibitory functions, appears to be differentially expressed in endometrial cancers. *PTEN* mutations are infrequently observed in nonendometrioid carcinomas but are relatively common in the endometrioid subtype.[17,18] Although they failed to detect *PTEN* mutations in normal endometrium, Mutter and associates[18] identified mutations in 55% of precursor lesions and in 87% of endometrioid carcinomas. These observations suggest that *PTEN* mutations may play an early role in carcinogenesis and potentially may be predictive of disease progression. Likewise, *KRAS2* mutations have been identified in both complex atypical hyperplasia (CAH) and invasive carcinoma.[19] Furthermore, hypermethylation of the human mut-L homologue 1 (hMLH1) promoter, resulting in silencing of transcription of the corresponding DNA mismatch repair gene, is usually seen in endometrial carcinomas with microsatellite instability and, to a lesser degree, in the precursor CAH lesions.[20,21] By contrast, *TP53* mutations and expression are predominantly associated with high-grade lesions and nonendometrioid subtypes and unfavorable outcomes.[22-24] Exemplary of the potential clinical usefullness of such molecular markers was the report of Silverman and coworkers,[25] in which the pretreatment (dilatation and curettage) overexpression of TP53 and an S-phase fraction of 9% or greater predicted advanced disease and poor outcome. If only one or neither of the markers was abnormal, the 10-year cancer-related survival rate was 90%, compared with 32% if both were abnormal.

Diagnostic Evaluation

The majority of women who are diagnosed with endometrial cancer present with postmenopausal bleeding. For these women, endometrial aspiration biopsy is simple and cost-effective, with greater than 90% accuracy. If the biopsy is negative but the symptoms suggest endometrial cancer, hysteroscopy or dilatation and curettage may be performed. Physical examination must include evaluation of peripheral nodal areas, including the supraclavicular fossa and inguinal regions. Examination of the abdomen should assess hepatomegaly or abnormal masses. Pelvic examination should include inspection of the suburethral area, vaginal mucosa, cervix, and uterine adnexa, as well as assessment of the size of the uterus.

Chest radiography and routine laboratory tests that reflect the complete blood cell count and serum chemistries are usually performed preoperatively.

Although imaging of the abdomen and pelvis is feasible with computed tomography, magnetic resonance imaging, or ultrasound, inclusion of these procedures is not usually justified in a routine workup because of their limited specificity and sensitivity and the associated expense.

Prognostic Factors

Clinical and pathologic stages or extent of disease correlate with the incidence and patterns of disease recurrence for patients with endometrial cancer.[26,27] Histologic grade, depth of myometrial penetration, pathologic subtype, age, lymphovascular penetration, and nodal involvement have all demonstrated prognostic value in predicting recurrence.[28] Various other

Table 19–1. International Federation of Gynecology and Obstetrics (FIGO) Clinical Staging System for Endometrial Cancer, 1971

Stage	Description
I	Carcinoma confined to uterine corpus
Ia	*Sounds ≤8 cm
Ib	*Sounds >8 cm
II	Carcinoma involving the uterine corpus and cervix

*Length of uterine canal.

tumor-related factors have also been recognized as prognostic, including ploidy and proliferative activity.[29] The presence of hormone receptors for progesterone is associated with more favorable outcome.[30] The difficulty with interpreting these prognostic factors is that they are all interrelated, and separating their individual contributions to the patient's outcome is difficult.

The previous clinical staging system (Table 19-1) did not take these characteristics into account.[31] The current staging system recognizes depth of myometrial penetration, histologic grade, and extent of disease as prognostic.[32] The current staging system (Table 19-2) also divides patients with extrauterine disease in a somewhat arbitrary fashion.[32] A prospective surgical staging study (Gynecologic Oncology Group [GOG] Protocol 33) demonstrated that patients with metastasis to pelvic nodes have a better prognosis than those with involved para-aortic nodes.[28] Yet such patients are all categorized as having stage IIIc disease. Patients with serosal involvement, positive peritoneal cytology, or adnexal metastasis (or some combination of these features) are all classified as having stage IIIa disease. However, patients with only one extrauterine site of involvement have a much better prognosis than do patients with multiple sites.[33] Patients who have extrauterine disease with a low-grade histology or involvement of peritoneal cytology alone may have a very favorable outcome.[33] Therefore, recommendations for adjuvant therapy based on the current staging system may be invalid. It is also clear that other factors not taken into account by the current staging system, such as lymphovascular space invasion, older age, and pathologic subtype, as well as unknown variables, contribute to the risk of recurrence.[34]

Table 19–2. International Federation of Gynecology and Obstetrics (FIGO) Staging System for Endometrial Cancer, 1988

Stage	Description
I	Carcinoma confined to the corpus uteri
Ia	Tumor limited to endometrium
Ib	Invasion to less than one half of the myometrium
Ic	Invasion to greater than one half of the myometrium
II	Carcinoma that involves the corpus and the cervix but has not extended outside the uterus
IIa	Endocervical glandular involvement only
IIb	Cervical stromal invasion

What is the optimal surgical management of early stage corpus cancer?

Standard surgical treatment for endometrial cancer includes a total abdominal hysterectomy and bilateral salpingo-oophorectomy. The peritoneum should be carefully examined for the presence of any tumor deposits, and the periaortic or pelvic areas should be examined to detect enlarged lymph nodes. Complete surgical staging includes peritoneal washings with cytologic examination and selective lymph node dissection. Vaginal hysterectomy has been reported to produce an acceptable outcome if an abdominal hysterectomy is precluded because of body habitus or medical condition.[35]

Dr. Karl Podratz's argument in support of routine lymphadenectomy. The progress in managing early-stage endometrial cancer has at best been limited, reflecting traditions (or standard of care), surgical skills, turf issues, and ill-conceived clinical trials. The standard of care in presumed localized disease has routinely included hysterectomy, removal of adnexal structures, and adjuvant RT based on uterine pathologic risk factors. Treatment failures and the accompanying compromised longevity in presumed early-stage corpus cancer are the result of failure to recognize sites of extrauterine dissemination at the time of primary surgical treatment. Furthermore, the adjuvant therapy used has been that dictated by traditional treatment preferences rather than target-based therapy as determined by patterns of failure. Hence, a paradigm shift in the management of early endometrial cancer is needed, with subsequent management predicated on evolving target-based treatment algorithms.

The controversy regarding the role of adjuvant RT in patients with stage I disease is directly linked to the thoroughness of surgical staging. Three prospective studies addressing the value of postoperative pelvic RT observed improved regional control in suboptimally staged patients but failed to demonstrate a significant impact on overall survival.[36-38] Furthermore, evidence is evolving to suggest that pelvic EBRT no longer has an adjuvant role in the management of stage I endometrial cancer after definitive surgical staging. Hence, the management controversy appears to focus on the role of lymphadenectomy in the surgical treatment of early-stage endometrial cancer.

Since the adoption of the current staging system, which is based on pathologic findings, significant management controversy has focused on the role of lymphadenectomy in the surgical treatment of early-stage endometrial cancer. Historically, the assessment of the retroperitoneum at the time of hysterectomy has varied from omission to formal node dissection, as determined by physician biases, surgical skills, or patient characteristics. Assuming that the objectives of lymphadenectomy are diagnostic, prognostic, and therapeutic, the indications for and extent of the pelvic and para-aortic systematic node dissection should be based on the potential for occult lymphatic involvement as predicated by uterine pathology. Therefore, it is reasonable to believe that a subset of patients with low-risk lesions can safely forego node dissection but that patients with moderate- or high-risk lesions can derive diagnostic and therapeutic benefits from definitive staging, including complete lymphadenectomy. Differentiation of these low-risk patients from patients with a higher risk of nodal involvement has been accomplished in various ways. One institutional review determined that when the primary tumor diameter (PTD) (≤2 cm versus >2 cm) was used to discriminate between the traditional low-risk stage Ia or Ib lesion and grade 1 or 2 endometrioid carcinomas, a defined subset of patients was identified that would not benefit from formal node dissection.[39] Of 292 patients with low-risk endometrioid disease, 123 presented with lesions less than or equal to 2 cm. Only three of this group had a recurrence (all in the vagina, and all were salvaged), and no cancer-related deaths were reported. In comparison, patients whose lesions exceeded 2 cm in the greatest dimension had an 8% positive node frequency, an 8% recurrence rate (the majority at distant sites), and 6% cancer-related deaths. Patients in the more favorable subset were almost equally divided between hysterectomy only or hysterectomy plus lymphadenectomy, and both groups experienced a 5-year survival rate of 100%. The subset of low-risk patients (PTD ≤2 cm) accounted for 20% of the overall population and 25% of stage I patients. Based on GOG 33, 10% of clinical stage I patients harbor nodal metastases.[28] However, if the subset of low-risk patients is taken into account (25%), nodal involvement in the remaining 75% would approximate one in every seven women. This would seem to justify inclusion of a lymphadenectomy in the management of early endometrial cancer to search for occult disease.

The extent of the lymphadenectomy in staging of corpus carcinomas—selective node sampling versus formal lymphadenectomy—continues to be debated. Uterine epithelial carcinoma is the only gynecologic malignancy for which node sampling is practiced when assessment of regional lymph nodes is desirable. The literature strongly suggests that the number of identified nodal metastases increases as the extent of sampling expands. Likewise, the number of retroperitoneal failures decreases and survival increases as the number of node-bearing sites sampled increases. Kilgore and associates[40] compared outcomes in patients with four or more sites sampled and patients with no sampling and reported that the more extended dissection yielded survival advantages for the entire population ($P < .001$), for high-risk patients ($P < .001$), and for high-risk patients treated with adjuvant RT ($P = .01$). Furthermore, based on statistical modeling, to ensure an 80% probability of detecting a single positive node if 5% of the nodes are positive, approximately half of the regional lymph nodes would need to be sampled. Hence, to ensure optimal diagnostic potential, formal lymphadenectomies should be encouraged.

In addition to the diagnostic indications, the accumulating literature strongly suggests that formal pelvic and para-aortic lymph node dissection offers potential therapeutic value or, at a minimum, affords

Table 19–3. Recurrence after Formal Lymphadenectomy in Patients with Uterine-confined Endometrial Cancer with Deep Myometrial Penetration (Stage Ic) or Grade 3 Histology not Receiving Pelvic External Beam Radiotherapy

Reference	N	Mean No. of Nodes	Postoperative Brachytherapy	Mean Follow-up (Mo.)	No. of Recurrences
Fanning[41]	66	—*	+	52	2
Orr et al[42]	115	24	+	39	6
Chadha et al[43]	38	7	+	30†	3
Ng et al[44]	77	32	+	45	11
Horowitz et al[46]	117	12	+	65†	11
Straughn et al[45]	128	11	–	30	8‡
Total	541				41§

*Complete pelvic and para-aortic lymphadenectomy; number of nodes not stated.
†Median follow-up.
‡All except one salvaged with radiotherapy.
§Includes 27 distant (5.0% of total), 12 vagina (2.2%), 3 pelvis (0.6%).

the opportunity for modifications in adjuvant therapy. Several institutions have reported outcomes among patients with moderate- or high-risk node-negative stage I endometrial cancer managed with formal lymphadenectomy but without adjuvant external beam radiotherapy (EBRT).[41-46] Vaginal brachytherapy only was administered in five of the six studies, as illustrated in Table 19-3. Collectively, 541 patients with reasonable surveillance intervals experienced an 8% recurrence rate, and 75% of the failures occurred at distant sites. Only 15 failures occurred in the pelvis; 11 were vaginal failures, and all except 1 were salvaged with subsequent RT. These data suggest minimal value for adjuvant whole pelvic RT in patients with completely staged early endometrial cancer. In a retrospective assessment of predictors of lymphatic failure, Mariani and coworkers[47] identified only two risk factors for pelvic side wall failure: cervical stromal invasion and nodal metastases. In the absence of these risk factors, no pelvic side wall failures were observed among 292 patients, compared with a 5-year failure rate of 26% if either or both of these factors were detected at the time of definitive staging. These studies strongly suggest that postoperative adjuvant therapy in patients who have undergone definitive staging (including a formal pelvic and para-aortic node dissection) should focus primarily on the vagina and distant sites.

In summary, the contemporary literature supports the concept of target-based management of neoplasms, as does the evolving database for early endometrial cancer. Because of the low risk of occult extrauterine spread, lymphadenectomy is not indicated for patients with grade 1 or 2 endometrioid carcinomas whose primary tumor is 2 cm or less in diameter and invades only the inner half of the myometrium. After hysterectomy, these pathologic risk factors can readily be assessed by frozen section analysis. However, a complete pelvic and para-aortic node dissection should be encouraged for all other early-stage lesions. The merits of performing a systematic lymphadenectomy are diagnostic, prognostic, and therapeutic. Furthermore, documentation of node-negative stage I disease

eliminates the requirement of EBRT and the associated additional cost, treatment time, and morbidity risk. A target-based treatment algorithm for early-stage endometrial cancer consistent with the current literature is illustrated in Figure 19-1.

Dr. Kathryn Greven's argument against routine lymphadenectomy. There is no doubt that surgical staging of endometrial cancer is more accurate than clinical staging. The GOG enrolled 895 patients with assessable clinical stage I or occult stage II cancer in a surgical staging protocol that was open from 1977 through 1983. Analysis of the data on the first 621 patients demonstrated that 22% had disease outside the uterus, including lymph node metastasis, involvement of the uterine adnexa, intraperitoneal metastasis, or malignant cells in the peritoneal washings.[48] In an update of this protocol, Morrow and colleagues[28] reported that only 48 (5.4%) of the 895 patients had aortic node involvement. Of these 48 patients, 47 had either grossly positive pelvic nodes, grossly positive adnexal metastasis, or deep myometrial penetration, any of which would obviate the need for a para-aortic node dissection. Only 18 patients (2%) had positive pelvic nodes in the absence of other findings. This small number of patients with tumor involving isolated pelvic nodes would not seem compelling enough for physicians to perform a lymph node dissection on most patients with early-stage endometrial cancer.

There is little information to suggest that node dissection alters patterns of recurrence. Morrow and colleagues[28] reported that 55% of total failures occurred in the pelvis in patients who had lymph node dissection without pelvic RT, and 30% of failures occurred in those who had pelvic node dissection as well as pelvic RT. Similarly, Kilgore and associates[40] noted that rates for treatment failure in the pelvis did not differ between patients who had lymphadenectomy and those who did not.

For staging lymphadenectomy to be beneficial, therapeutic alternatives based on the results of such a procedure need to be available. Several institutions

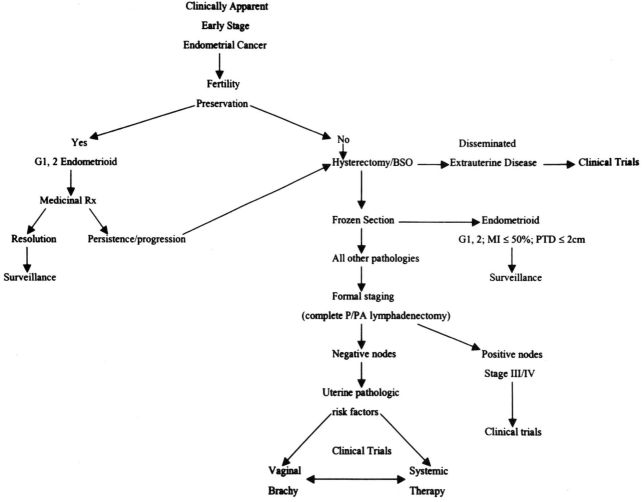

Figure 19–1. Treatment algorithm for early-stage endometrial cancer. BSO, bilateral salpingo-oophorectomy; G, grade; MI, myometrial invasion; P/PA, pelvic/para-aortic; PTD, primary tumor diameter.

have published their experiences with adjuvant vaginal brachytherapy after negative staging lymphadenectomy. These reports indicate that there are some high-risk patients who can be selected for this treatment and have favorable outcomes.[41-45] There are no randomized data to support this observation. In fact, the only randomized data, from patients with early-stage endometrial cancer who were treated with hysterectomy as well as lymphadenectomy, demonstrated that without adjuvant RT there was a 13% pelvic or vaginal recurrence rate that was significantly reduced with the addition of pelvic RT.[36] Also, there are so few patients in certain subgroups that it is not known whether older patients, patients with lymphovascular space invasion, those with cervical stroma invasion, and those with both high grade and deep myometrial penetration can be approached in this way.

Several investigators have established that lymphadenectomy increases the risk of complications, particularly if it is combined with external RT. More blood transfusions, longer hospitalizations, lymphedema, gastrointestinal injury, and the development of lymphocysts have been reported. Morrow and

colleagues[28] reported a 19% rate of surgical complications in the GOG protocol that included many institutions and surgeons. Fanning[41] documented a 6% incidence of serious complications in his group of patients. Mohan and associates[49] documented a 13% rate of significant morbidity after complete surgical staging and vaginal brachytherapy

There is no consensus regarding what type of lymph node evaluation should be performed. Kilgore and colleagues[40] advocated biopsy sampling of "multiple" nodes even though the actual number of nodes sampled ranged from 1 to 55. Fanning[41] did not report the number of nodes recovered, because the "number of lymph nodes counted correlates directly with the pathologist performing the gross and microscopic examinations." Chuang and associates,[50] from MD Anderson Cancer Center, suggested that a selective lymphadenectomy in which nine sites were assessed accurately predicted the lymph node status. The GOG described the required procedure for GOG 33 as follows: "The fat pad over the major vessels beginning at the bifurcation extending to the proximity of the renal vessels was removed in toto. In the pelvis, the retroperitoneal spaces were opened and the lymph bearing tissues over the external and common iliac vessels were removed as well as the lymph bearing tissue in the obturator fossa above the obturator nerve."[48] The reality is that most patients are not operated on by gynecologic oncologists. In the American Cancer Society database,[51] a gynecologic oncologist operated on only 32% of women with endometrial cancer, with an additional 11% having a gynecologic oncologist as an assistant. Only 24% of women operated on by a surgeon other than a gynecologic oncologist had a nodal dissection as part of the staging procedure. Also, there is little consensus among specialists, with only 54% of gynecologic oncologists performing a routine lymphadenectomy. Finally, obesity and comorbid conditions prohibit lymph node dissection in many patients.

Kilgore and associates[40] argued that lymphadenectomy has a therapeutic benefit. Their institutional experience included patients treated between 1969 and 1990. Patient outcomes were primarily analyzed by whether lymphadenectomy was performed; histologic grade, patient age, and depth of myometrial penetration were not analyzed for their influences on patient outcome. Subgroup analysis of 62 patients who had uterine-confined tumors of grade 3 or with deep myometrial invasion demonstrated that patients with multiple pelvic nodes sampled had significantly better survival rates than patients with no nodes sampled; the 5-year survival rates were 85% and 28%, respectively. The latter rate for patients with high-risk uterineconfined disease is lower than for any similar group of patients reported in the literature. Obviously, selection factors must have been important in determining which patients were treated with pelvic node sampling. Yet, this report has been used to support the premise that lymphadenectomy yields a therapeutic benefit for these patients. Another report analyzed patients treated between 1970 and 1979.[52] Similar survival rates were noted among the 245 women who were treated with total abdominal hysterectomy and bilateral salpingo-oophorectomy, compared with 100 women who did not have lymphadenectomy. The authors concluded that lymphadenectomy was prognostic but not therapeutic. In an attempt to resolve this debate concerning the efficacy of lymphadenectomy,

the Medical Research Council began a randomized trial in 1998 in which women were randomly assigned to lymphadenectomy with hysterectomy or to hysterectomy alone. It is hoped that the results of this trial will clarify some of the confusion.

Patterns of Recurrence

A common site of disease recurrence for patients with endometrial cancer is in the pelvis. Many of these pelvic recurrences are in the vagina. Established dictum has been that 50% of the recurrences in the pelvis are in the vagina and the others occur elsewhere in the pelvis. Several published reports provide information on patterns of failure for patients with uterine-confined disease after treatment with surgery alone. Elliott and associates[53] reported a vaginal recurrence risk of 15% for patients not receiving adjuvant RT who had myometrial invasion greater than one third and grade 3 histology. Other pelvic recurrences were not documented. In a randomized GOG study in which all patients were treated with initial total hysterectomy and node dissection, Roberts and coworkers[36] reported 19 pelvic or vaginal recurrences among 202 patients not receiving RT. Most of these patients had low histologic grades and shallow depths of myometrial penetration. Creutzburg and colleagues[38] reported that 14% of patients with no adjuvant treatment after hysterectomy without node dissection had recurrences in the pelvis. However, a high-risk subgroup was identified—those older than 60 years of age with stage Ic and grade 1 or 2 histology, or any age with stage Ib, grade 3 histology—who had a pelvic recurrence rate of at least 19%. Several retrospective studies have been less specific as to the site of disease recurrence (Table 19-4).[54,55]

Some patients with uterine-confined disease are at increased risk for distant metastatic disease spread. These patients are likely to be older, and have high-grade histology, lymphovascular space invasion, deep myometrial penetration, or aggressive histologic subtype (Table 19-5).[22,37,55-60] Mariani and colleagues[61] analyzed 229 patients with stage I (node-negative) endometrial cancer by regression analysis and identified myometrial invasion as the only independent

Table 19-4. Patterns of Disease Recurrence for Patients with Uterine-confined Endometrial Cancer

Reference	Irradiation	Risk Factors	Recurrence (%)		
			Vagina	Pelvis	Total
Elliot et al[53]	None	MI >1/3, G 3	15	NA	NA
Roberts et al[36]	None	Any	9.5	NA	
Carey et al[55]	Inadequate	MI >1/3, G 2 or 3	NA	15	30
Creutzberg et al[38]	None	Ic, G 1 or 2	10	3	13
		Ib, G 2 or 3			
Creutzberg et al[54]	None	Ic, G 1 or 2, age >60 yr	19	NA	
		Ib, G 3			

G, histologic grade; Ib and Ic, pathologic stage; MI, myometrial penetration; NA, not available.

Table 19–5. Incidence of Distant Metastatic Disease for Patients with Uterine-confined Endometrial Cancer

Reference	N	Risk Factors	Distant Recurrence (%)
Aalders et al[37]	44	MI >1/2, G 3	18
Konski et al[57]	12	MI >1/2, G 3	25
Carey et al[55]	129	MI >1/2, II, G 3	14
Greven et al[58]	119	I, G 3	25
Lanciano et al[59]	168	II	19
Mayr et al[60]	23	I/II, G 3	26
Morrow et al[28]	60	MI >1/3, G 2/3	15

G, histologic grade; I and II, pathologic stage; MI, myometrial penetration.

predictor of distant failure. Only 2% of patients with less than 66% myometrial invasion had distant failures, compared with 29% of those with myometrial invasion greater than 66%, suggesting that patients in the latter group would be candidates for clinical trials of adjuvant systemic therapy. Such patients may benefit from the addition of a systemic agent to their adjuvant therapy. This is the rationale for the ongoing Radiation Therapy Oncology Group (RTOG) treatment protocol 9905, which randomly assigns high-risk patients with uterine-confined disease to pelvic RT or pelvic RT with cisplatin followed by cisplatin and paclitaxel.[62]

Most patients with high-grade histology, cervical involvement, or deep myometrial penetration (or some combination of these features) have been treated with adjuvant RT. Because of the incidence of distant metastasis, there has been great interest in the use of systemic therapy for these patients. A report from Mundt and colleagues[63] of patients treated with only chemotherapy and no RT demonstrated a substantial risk of pelvic recurrence. The group of patients who was more likely to have recurrence in the pelvis were those patients treated with chemotherapy alone for stage I or II tumors.

What is the optimal type of adjuvant radiation?

Options for adjuvant radiation therapy. Adjuvant RT can be delivered using EBRT directed to the pelvis, vaginal brachytherapy (colpostats or cylinder), or a combination of both. Treatment can also be directed to the whole abdomen or to an extended field that includes the pelvis and para-aortic region. The goal of pelvic treatment with RT is to treat the pelvic lymph node regions that are at risk of containing microscopic disease as well as the central pelvic region that includes the upper vagina.

When EBRT is given, typical field arrangements usually include a four-field approach. A contrast agent is frequently used to visualize the small intestine. Prone positioning, bladder distention, and the use of a false tabletop have all been reported to decrease the volume of the small bowel within the pelvis. The dose

of radiation is 45 to 50 Gy to the pelvic region given with standard fractionation. It is not known whether field size may be decreased for patients who have had lymph node sampling. However, it is believed that the midpelvis should not be blocked.

If vaginal brachytherapy is the desired treatment modality, colpostats or cylinders can be used to treat the vaginal mucosa. Low-dose-rate (LDR) or high-dose-rate (HDR) techniques have been used. Prescribed doses vary and should be based on dose rate, treatment volume, additional EBRT, and radiation tolerance of normal structures, particularly the bladder and rectum. If brachytherapy is used without EBRT, a dose that has been commonly used for LDR treatment is 60 Gy to the vaginal surface with dose rates of 80 to 120 cGy/hour. Consensus guidelines for HDR treatment have been published.[64] A commonly employed HDR schedule is 700 cGy to 0.5 cm from the cylinder surface, given in three sessions for a total dose of 2100 cGy. In general, it is believed that treatment of the entire length of the vaginal mucosa is unnecessary and may result in excess morbidity from vaginal dysfunction or rectal morbidity due to an increased volume of normal tissue receiving RT. Treatment of the top 5 cm of the vagina should be adequate.

Although some oncologists advocate the combination of vaginal brachytherapy and pelvic RT for select patients, several reports have failed to document an improved outcome with this approach (Table 19-6).[65,66] In general it is not necessary to use both modalities, because the pelvic recurrence rate after either pelvic RT alone or brachytherapy alone has ranged from 0% to 4.5%.[36,53,67] However, it is important to realize that patients treated with both EBRT and brachytherapy tend to have worse prognostic factors, which may have placed them at increased risk of recurrence. It is not possible to ascertain whether patients with advanced stage, close margins, poor histologic subtype, or lymphovascular space invasion may benefit from the addition of a brachytherapy boost to the vaginal apex.

Morbidity of adjuvant radiation. Certainly adjuvant RT can result in a risk of morbidity for patients. Complications are related to treatment volume, daily fractionation, total dose, patient-related variables, treatment techniques, and type of surgical treatment.[68,69] EBRT results in severe chronic sequelae in 5% to 15% of patients. The most significant effects are obstruction of the small bowel, fistula formation, proctitis, chronic diarrhea, vaginal stenosis, and insufficiency fractures of the bone. Several reports have documented that the addition of a lymphadenectomy is an independent factor associated with increased serious morbidity.[68,70,71] Other factors include poor radiation technique with high total dose or the use of only one irradiation field per day as well as prior surgical treatment and older age of the patient. A recently published trial that randomly assigned patients to pelvic RT (46 Gy in 23 fractions) or no further therapy documented actuarial rates of complications at 5 years of 26% and 4%, respectively (Fig. 19-2).[54] Serious sequelae were noted to be 3% and 0%, respectively, at 5 years. The four-field

Table 19–6. Five-year Pelvic Recurrence Rates for Patients Treated with External Beam Radiotherapy (EBRT) Alone or with EBRT plus Brachytherapy for Stage I Endometrial Cancer

Reference	Treatment	N	Pelvic Recurrence (%)
Irwin et al[66]	EBRT	97	5
	EBRT + brachytherapy	217	8
Greven et al[65]	EBRT	173	4
	EBRT + brachytherapy	97	7

box technique was associated with a lower risk of late complications, suggesting that optimization of radiation technique lowers the risk of complications. Notably, these patients had not undergone lymphadenectomy, which might have been anticipated to increase the risk of serious morbidity.

Vaginal brachytherapy alone should have a very low risk of serious long-term sequelae. Greven[69] and

Aalders[37] and their colleagues reported 0% and 0.7% incidence of serious complications, respectively, for patients who had postoperative LDR intracavitary therapy alone. Complications from HDR intracavitary treatment are related to dose and technique.[72] Grade 1 and 2 complications have been observed in the vagina, bladder, and rectum for 25%, 5.5%, and 3% of patients, respectively.[72] Serious complications are rare.[73]

Figure 19–2. Incidence of morbidity after adjuvant pelvic irradiation (RT) or no further therapy. **A,** Grade 1-4 complications and **B,** Grade 2-4 complications. (From Creutzberg CL, van Putten WL, Koper PC, et al: The morbidity of treatment for patients with stage I endometrial cancer: Results from a randomized trial. Int J Radiat Oncol Biol Phys 2001;51:1246-1255.)

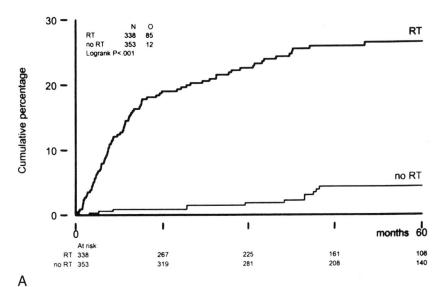

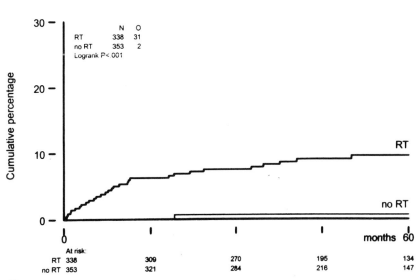

Complications are usually caused by rectal injury or vaginal stenosis and are probably related to the total dose. It is important to be aware of the location of the point of prescription as well as the dose to the rectum and bladder. Isodose curves and calculation of points at the apex of the cylinder, for example, help to decrease the risk of inadvertent overdosage of the vagina.[64]

What is the role of adjuvant radiation?

Outcomes with adjuvant radiation. Patients with favorable prognostic features of low histologic grade and shallow depth of myometrial penetration are unlikely to have metastatic disease found in the lymph nodes. Creasman and associates[48] documented that none of 44 patients with grade 1 histology had positive pelvic or para-aortic nodes, and only 3% of patients with inner or middle third myometrial invasion were found to have positive nodes. These patients have excellent outcomes with vaginal brachytherapy alone, whether or not a staging lymphadenectomy has been performed.[28,42,49,74,75] In fact, low recurrence rates have been documented with no adjuvant RT after hysterectomy.[53,55,76]

EBRT has been shown to decrease the incidence of pelvic recurrences but with no improvement in survival. Several investigators have reported pelvic recurrence rates ranging from 0% to 4.5% for patients with either deeply invasive or high-grade histologic lesions after adjuvant pelvic RT.[34,55,67] Three prospectively randomized trials documented decreased pelvic recurrences with adjuvant pelvic RT. Aalders and associates[37] demonstrated that pelvic recurrence was decreased from 15% to 5% for patients with deep myometrial penetration by the addition of pelvic RT. Roberts and coworkers[36] (GOG 99) reported 19 pelvic recurrences in 202 patients not receiving RT, compared with 1 recurrence in 188 patients receiving pelvic RT. Creutzburg and colleagues[38] reported that 14% of patients had recurrence in the pelvis with no adjuvant treatment after hysterectomy, compared with 4% of those who received pelvic RT (Fig. 19-3).[38] The majority of the patients in each of these trials had shallow depth of penetration, or grade 1 or 2 histology, or both. It is possible that there are subgroups of patients with poor prognostic factors who may demonstrate an improved survival rate in addition to improved pelvic control with adjuvant RT.

Historically, patients with indicators of poor prognosis have typically received RT to the pelvis whether or not the nodes were involved. However, there are a few recent retrospective reports in which patients with uterine-confined disease who had poor prognostic indicators (e.g., high-grade histology, deep myometrial penetration) but negative lymph nodes demonstrated excellent outcomes after treatment with vaginal brachytherapy alone (see Table 19-3).[41-46] These reports indicated that, with proper patient selection, vaginal brachytherapy may be adequate after staging lymphadenectomy and total abdominal hysterectomy.

The only prospective trial comparing vaginal brachytherapy with pelvic RT for such patients

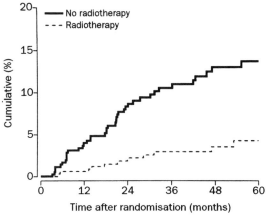

Figure 19–3. Incidence of pelvic recurrences after adjuvant pelvic irradiation or no further therapy. (From Creutzberg CL, van Putten WL, Koper PC, et al: Surgery and postoperative radiotherapy versus surgery alone for patients with stage-1 endometrial carcinoma: Multicentre randomised trial. PORTEC study group. Post Operative Radiation Therapy in Endometrial Carcinoma. Lancet 2000;355:1404-1411.)

suggested an improvement with the addition of EBRT.[37] However, the patients in that randomized trial had not undergone staging lymphadenectomy. Until prospective trials indicate that vaginal brachytherapy and pelvic RT result in equivalent outcomes, this should not be assumed. Certainly, the sequelae after pelvic RT are more serious and more frequent than after vaginal brachytherapy. Patients who are believed to have increased risk of sequelae after pelvic RT because of multiple prior abdominal surgeries, diabetes, hypertension, collagen vascular disease, or other reasons may have an improved therapeutic ratio with adjuvant vaginal brachytherapy.

The National Comprehensive Cancer Network (NCCN) has published guidelines for the treatment of patients with endometrial cancer.[77] Table 19-7 includes the author's proposed guidelines for treatment of patients.

Radiation Alone for Patients With Inoperable Endometrial Cancer

Treatment of endometrial cancer with RT alone is generally reserved for those patients in whom surgery would be considered a high risk. Because endometrial cancer is more prevalent in the population of older adults, many patients have numerous medical problems. Radiation has been used to cure patients with early disease and to achieve palliation in patients with advanced local disease.

The efficacy of primary RT for endometrial carcinoma was demonstrated in the results of several studies that documented 5-year disease-specific survival rates of 60% to 88% for patients with stage I disease and 64%

Table 19–7. Adjuvant Treatment Recommendations for Patients with Endometrial Cancer

Stage	Grade 1	Grade 2	Grade 3
Ia	Observe	Observe	Pelvis RT or vaginal IC
Ib	Observe	Observe or vaginal IC	Pelvis RT
Ic	Pelvis RT or vaginal IC	Pelvis RT*	Pelvis RT*
IIa, MI <50%	Vaginal IC	Vaginal IC	Pelvis RT ± vaginal IC*
IIa, MI >50%	Pelvis RT or vaginal IC	Pelvis RT ± vaginal IC	Pelvis RT ± vaginal IC*
IIb, MI <50%	Pelvis RT ± vaginal IC	Pelvis RT ± vaginal IC	Pelvis RT ± vaginal IC*
IIb, MI >50%	Pelvis RT ± vaginal IC	Pelvis RT ± vaginal IC	Pelvis RT ± vaginal IC*

*Consider chemotherapy/RT protocol. Any patient with lymphovascular space invasion should be considered for pelvic RT. Choices should be made based on balancing the chance of morbidity for each individual patient and the chance of recurrence. Patients who have had full lymphadenectomy have an increased risk of subsequent complications.
IC, intracavitary brachytherapy; MI, muscle invasion; RT, radiation therapy.

to 88% for patients with stage II disease (Table 19-8).[78-82] Pelvic control was documented to range from 86% to 100% for patients with stage Ia disease and from 69% to 88% for patients with stage Ib disease.[75,78] Outcomes for these patients vary because of the clinical assessment of the extent of disease, which has been demonstrated to have inaccuracies compared with pathologic staging. Prognostic factors include better outcomes for patients with stage Ia (compared with Ib) disease, younger patients, patients with well-differentiated tumors (compared with poorly differentiated tumors), and minimal cervical involvement.

Treatment generally includes brachytherapy with or without EBRT. Inferior disease outcome has been reported for patients treated with EBRT alone. Brachytherapy may be administered with LDR therapy including either Heyman or Simon capsules combined with vaginal colpostats or with Fletcher-Suit afterloading tandem and vaginal colpostats. In addition, recent reports with comparable outcomes support the use of HDR applicators for the treatment of endometrial cancer.

Curative treatment doses have included mean total intrauterine exposures ranging from 3500 to 5000 mg/hour. Estimated LDR doses to point A range from 40 Gy to as high as 80 Gy. Patients with histologic grade 3 disease, larger uterine volume, or cervical involvement usually receive EBRT in addition to intracavitary treatment. EBRT doses of 20 to 45 Gy are prescribed. A midline block inserted after 20 Gy may be used to protect the rectum and bladder so that more effective brachytherapy doses can be given. Total doses to point A using EBRT and LDR brachytherapy are usually 85 to 90 Gy. Institutional experiences with HDR brachytherapy have used variable techniques. The American Brachytherapy Society has published treatment guidelines.[64] If HDR therapy is used alone, a suggested fractionation scheme is five fractions of 7.3 Gy per fraction prescribed at 2 cm from the midpoint of intrauterine sources. After EBRT to the pelvis of 45 Gy, two to four fractions ranging from 8.5 Gy to 5.2 Gy prescribed to 2 cm from the midpoint of the intrauterine sources should be acceptable. If treatment planning based on computed tomography, magnetic resonance imaging, or ultrasonography is available, it may be individualized based on the thickness of the uterine wall and fundus.

Treatment is usually well tolerated. The probability of serious complications involving the small bowel, bladder, and rectum was reported to be 5.3% in one series of patients treated predominantly with intracavitary treatment.[78] The complication rate was generally higher in patients who received EBRT in addition to intracavitary treatment.[80]

In conclusion, RT should be considered for any patient with uterine-confined endometrial cancer who

Table 19–8. Definitive Treatment with Radiation Alone for Endometrial Carcinoma

Reference	No. Patients	Treatment	5-Yr DFS Stage Ia/Ib (%)
Clinical stage I			
Knocke et al[78]	235	HDR	85/73*
Nguyen and Petereit[79]	36	HDR	88†
Chao et al[80]	101	LDR ± EBRT	80/84
Kupelian et al[81]	120	LDR	87*
Rouanet et al[82]	108	LDR + EBRT	67/60
Clinical stage II			
Knocke et al[78]	37	HDR ± EBRT	68
Kupelian et al[81]	17	LDR ± EBRT	88*
Rouanet et al[82]	11	LDR + EBRT	64

*Disease-specific survival.
†3-Year DFS.
DFS, disease-free survival rate; EBRT, external beam radiation therapy; HDR high-dose-rate brachytherapy; LDR, low-dose-rate brachytherapy.

is not able to undergo hysterectomy. Pelvic control rates and disease-free survival rates demonstrate that patients can be effectively treated with RT that includes brachytherapy.

What is the role of adjuvant chemotherapy?

Systemic recurrences have been documented in all subgroups of patients with endometrial cancer. Patients with uterine-confined disease who are at the highest risk of distant metastases have deep myometrial invasion, unfavorable histology, lymphovascular involvement, cervix invasion, or high histologic grade. Table 19-5 indicates the frequency of distant relapses in published reports.

Phase II chemotherapy trials in women with advanced or recurrent endometrial cancer have identified doxorubicin, cisplatin, and carboplatin as active agents with response rates of 30% to 35%.[83-85] A trial by the GOG suggested a similar level of activity for paclitaxel. Objective responses were reported in 10 (36%) of 28 evaluable patients treated at a dose of 250 mg/m[3].[86]

There are few institutional or single-armed published reports of the use of cytotoxic agents as adjuvant treatment of endometrial cancer. O'Brien and Killackey[87] treated 26 women with poor-prognosis endometrial cancer with cisplatin, doxorubicin, and cyclophosphamide every 4 weeks for four courses. Pelvic RT was given after administration of systemic chemotherapy. Toxic effects were considered acceptable, but there was no significant difference in disease-free survival for these patients compared with a group of "matched" patients most of whom received adjuvant RT of the pelvis (58% versus 49%).

Burke and associates[88] reported results for 62 patients who had adjuvant treatment with cisplatin and doxorubicin and cyclophosphamide given every 4 weeks for six courses. Thirty-nine patients had preoperative brachytherapy placement. The 3-year survival rate was 82% for the 33 patients without extrauterine disease and 46% for the 29 patients with extrauterine disease.

A phase II trial was completed by the RTOG that included 46 patients treated with a combination of cisplatin and pelvic RT followed by cisplatin and paclitaxel.[89] Toxicity was found to be acceptable.

Currently, two phase III trials designed to test the efficacy of chemotherapy are accruing patients. RTOG 9905 was opened in 2000. This trial randomly assigns women with high-risk uterine-confined disease to pelvic RT alone or pelvic RT with chemotherapy that includes cisplatin and paclitaxel. Accrual has been very slow, because uterine-confined high-risk disease is uncommon. The Nordic Society for Gynecologic Oncology is conducting a trial that randomly assigns women with uterine-confined disease to pelvic RT or pelvic RT followed or preceded by four cycles of cyclophosphamide (Cytoxan) and doxorubicin or epirubicin. Despite the lack of evidence for the efficacy of chemotherapy in this situation, more oncologists are treating women with systemic chemotherapy. Data from this trial or from trials that include patients with more advanced disease may provide information regarding the efficacy of systemic therapy in these patients.

Follow-Up and Quality of Life

What is the role of hormone replacement therapy?

For several decades, the association of endometrial cancer with sources of unopposed estrogens, including obesity, hormone-producing ovarian neoplasms, polycystic ovary syndrome, and estrogen replacement therapy (HRT) has been recognized. These observations were extrapolated and the administration of estrogen to patients diagnosed with endometrial cancer was declared an absolute contraindication. However, an enhanced understanding of the natural history, the clinicopathologic risk factors, and the biology of this disease have provided reasons to challenge the practice of denying estrogen to certain subsets of patients who might benefit from HRT.[90-93] With the possible exception of the stimulation and neoplastic transformation of ectopic endometriosis with estrogens after hysterectomy for endometrial cancer, the post-treatment detection of recurrent endometrioid carcinoma reflects the presence of occult extrauterine spread at the time of primary therapy. Therefore, patients with disease localized to the uterus at the time of surgery are reasonable candidates for HRT. It follows that patients with occult extrauterine disease are at substantial risk for relapse, which may be facilitated by exogenous estrogens in patients with estrogen-induced tumors. Hence, the overriding challenge is the identification, with an acceptable negative predictive value for postoperative recurrence, of those patients who can safely receive HRT. The remaining early-stage patients form two subsets consisting of patients at risk of harboring occult disease that is either estrogen dependent or estrogen independent. The efficacy of administering estrogens to these two subgroups must await clinical trials. Theoretically, the patients at risk for occult estrogen-dependent carcinomas would best be treated with estrogen and progestins, considering the documented potential reversibility of well-differentiated carcinomas.[10-12] With regard to estrogen-independent endometrial carcinomas, the majority are poorly differentiated or nonendometrioid (or both) and are generally estrogen receptor–negative.[13] These observations imply that exogenous estrogens would not alter the natural history of these cancers, but confirmation must await prospective clinical trials addressing these specific subgroups.

Several retrospective studies have assessed outcomes of patients receiving estrogen replacement therapy after definitive management of their endometrial cancers.[90-93] Collectively, these data fail to demonstrate an increased failure rate or a negative impact on survival with estrogen administration. However, inferences that estrogen supplementation was linked to more favorable survival results could readily be accounted for in the apparent differences in age, clinicopathologic risk factors, or receptor status.[90,92,93]

Recently, the GOG initiated a randomized, double-blind trial (GOG 137) assessing the effect of estrogen replacement therapy in women with stages I and II endometrial adenocarcinoma. Of importance to subsequent study analyses, Lee and associates[91] reported that only a single recurrence was detected among 62 low-risk (stages Ia and Ib, grade 1 and 2), non–estrogen-treated patients, and no failures occurred in a similar group of 44 low-risk estrogen-treated patients. These results strongly suggest that women with grade 1 or 2 endometrioid carcinoma with less than 50% myometrial penetration are prime candidates for HRT. Assessing a single institution's referral practice, Mariani and colleagues[39] reported that 47% of all patients whose endometrial cancer was managed surgically presented with stage Ia or Ib and grade 1 or 2 endometrioid cancers. Of these 292 low-risk patients, 123 had a primary tumor diameter of 2 cm or less, and only 3 experienced a recurrence. All of the recurrences were in the vagina, and all were salvaged, with no cancer-related deaths. However, of the 169 patients with a tumor diameter greater than 2 cm, 8% experienced recurrence, 6.5% had recurrence at a distant site, and 6% died of their disease. Myometrial invasion of more than 50% has been reported to be the only independent predictor for hematogenous dissemination[67] and a primary determinant for distant recurrence in stage Ic patients.[94] Therefore, caution must be exercised when interpreting the results of future studies, including GOG 137, and should include appropriate subgroup analyses. The most cogent subgroups in which to analyze the effects of HRT on outcomes will include stage Ib, grade 1 and 2 endometrioid cancer with a tumor diameter greater than 2 cm and all stage Ic, all grade 3, and all non-endometrioid lesions. The assessment of estrogen and progesterone receptor status will likewise be of paramount importance for providing subsequent treatment recommendations, including the potential value of adding progestins.

Summary

The goal of treatment for patients with endometrial cancer should be achieving the best outcome with the least amount of treatment. The current difficulty is defining which patients do not need adjuvant RT, which patients could be adequately treated with vaginal RT, and which patients could benefit from the addition of pelvic RT. The role of lymphadenectomy remains to be defined. Because some patients have a risk of distant metastasis, the role of systemic therapy needs to be further defined. Only 50% of isolated vaginal or pelvic recurrences can be salvaged with RT.[95] Patients who have recurrence with a shorter disease-free interval after surgery are at higher risk for distant metastatic disease and death.[96] If local recurrence is the source of distant dissemination, certainly prevention of recurrence would be beneficial. A similar paradigm has been used to explain the more favorable survival rates of breast cancer patients who were treated with postoperative RT to prevent locoregional recurrence.[97]

Additional research is needed to understand biologic indices that may contribute improved methods of identifying high-risk groups of patients. These indices include nuclear proliferation, oncogene expression, and ploidy. Better prognostic subgrouping is needed. Results from currently accruing trials are eagerly anticipated. Development of trials exploring the efficacy of vaginal brachytherapy is encouraged. Because of the relatively good prognosis for patients with this disease, multiple institutions are needed to provide sufficient numbers of patients to determine the potential effects of any intervention.

REFERENCES

1. Jemal A, Thomas A, Murray T, Thun M: Cancer Statistics, 2002. CA Cancer J Clin 2002;52:23-47.
2. Sherman ME, Sturgeon S, Brinton LA, et al: Risk factors and hormone levels in patients with serous and endometrioid uterine carcinomas. Mod Pathol 1997;10:963-968.
3. Fisher B, Costantino JP, Redmund CK, et al: Endometrial cancer in tamoxifen-treated breast cancer patients: Findings from the National Surgical Adjuvant Breast and Bowel Project (NSABP) B-14. J Natl Cancer Inst 1994;86:527.
4. Bokhman JV: Two pathogenetic types of endometrial carcinoma. Gynecol Oncol 1983;15:10-17.
5. Wilson TO, Podratz KC, Gaffey TA, et al: Evaluation of unfavorable histologic subtypes in endometrial adenocarcinoma. Am J Obstet Gynecol 1990;162:418-423.
6. Ambros RA, Sherman ME, Zahn CM, et al: Endometrial intraepithelial carcinoma: A distinctive lesion specifically associated with tumors displaying serous differentiation. Hum Pathol 1995;26:1260-1267.
7. Spiegel GW: Endometrial carcinoma in situ in postmenopausal women. Am J Surg Pathol 1995;19:417-432.
8. Kurman RJ, Kaminski PE, Norris HJ: The behavior of endometrial hyperplasia: A long-term study of "untreated" hyperplasia in 170 patients. Cancer 1985;56:403-412.
9. Ferenczy A, Gelfand M: The biologic significance of cytologic atypia in progesterone-treated endometrial hyperplasia. Am J Obstet Gynecol 1989;160:126-131.
10. Kim YB, Holschneider CH, Ghosh K, et al: Progestin alone as primary treatment of endometrial carcinoma in premenopausal women. Cancer 1997;79:320-327.
11. Randall TC, Kurman RJ: Progestin treatment of atypical hyperplasia and well-differentiated carcinoma of the endometrium in women under age 40. Obstet Gynecol 1997;90:434-440.
12. Kahu T, Yoshikawa H, Tsuda H, et al: Conservative therapy for adenocarcinoma and atypical endometrial hyperplasia of the endometrium in young women: Central pathologic review and treatment outcome. Cancer Lett 2001;167:39-48.
13. Mariani A, Sebo TJ, Webb MJ, et al: Molecular and histopathologic predictors of distant failure in endometrial cancer. Cancer Detect Prev 2003;27:434-441.
14. Sasaki M, Kotcherguina L, Dharia A, et al: Cytosine-phosphoguanine methylation of estrogen receptors in endometrial cancer. Cancer Res 2001;61:3262-3266.
15. Leslie KK, Kumar NS, Richer J, et al: Differential expression of the A and B isoforms of progesterone receptor in human endometrial cancer cells: Only progesterone receptor B is induced by estrogen and associated with strong transcriptional activation. Ann N Y Acad Sci 1997;828:17-26.
16. Kumar NS, Richer J, Owen G, et al: Selective down-regulation of progesterone receptor isoform B in poorly differentiated human endometrial cancer cells: Implications for unopposed estrogen action. Cancer Res 1998;58:1860-1865.
17. Risinger JI, Hayes K, Maxwell GL, et al: PTEN mutation in endometrial cancers is associated with favorable clinical and pathologic characteristics. Clin Cancer Res 1998;4:3005-3010.

18. Mutter GL, Lin MC, Fitgerald JT, et al: Altered PTEN expression as a diagnostic marker for the earliest endometrial precancers. J Natl Cancer Inst 2000;92:924-930.

19. Mutter GL, Wada H, Faquin WC, Enomoto T: K-ras mutations appear in the premalignant phase of both microsatellite stable and unstable endometrial carcinogenesis. Mol Pathol 1999;52:257-262.

20. Esteller M, Levine R, Baylin SB, et al: MLH1 promoter hypermethylation is associated with the microsatellite instability phenotype in sporadic endometrial carcinomas. Oncogene 1998;17:2413-2417.

21. Esteller M, Catasus L, Matias-Guiu X, et al: hMLH1 promoter hypermethylation is an early event in human endometrial tumorigenesis. Am J Pathol 1999;155:1767-1772.

22. Hamel NW, Sebo TJ, Wilson TO, et al: Prognostic value of p53 and proliferating cell nuclear antigen expression in endometrial carcinoma. Gynecol Oncol 1996;62:192-198.

23. Tashiro H, Isacson C, Levine R, et al: P53 mutations are common in uterine serous carcinoma and occur early in their prognosis. Am J Pathol 1997;150:177-185.

24. Soslow RA, Shen PU, Chung MH, Isacson C: Distinctive p53 and mdm2 immunohistochemical expression profiles suggest different pathways in poorly differentiated endometrial carcinoma. Int J Gynecol Pathol 1998;17:129-134.

25. Silverman MB, Roche PC, Kho RM, et al: Molecular and cytokinetic pretreatment risk assessment in endometrial carcinoma. Gynecol Oncol 2000;77:1-7.

26. Ayhan A, Yarali H, Urman B, et al: Comparison of clinical and surgical-pathologic staging in patients with endometrial carcinoma. J Surg Oncol 1990;43:33-35.

27. Wolfson AH, Sightler SE, Markoe AM, et al: The prognostic significance of surgical staging for carcinoma of the endometrium. Gynecol Oncol 1992;45:142-146.

28. Morrow CP, Bundy BN, Kurman RJ, et al: Relationship between surgical-pathological risk factors and outcome in clinical stage I and II carcinoma of the endometrium: Gynecologic Oncology Group Study. Gynecol Oncol 1991;40:55-65.

29. van Dam PA, Watson JV, Lowe DG, et al: Flow cytometric DNA analysis in gynecological oncology. Int J Gynecol Cancer 1992;2:57-62.

30. Kleine W, Maier T, Geyer H, et al: Estrogen and progesterone receptors in endometrial cancer and their prognostic relevance. Gynecol Oncol 1990;38:59-65.

31. International Federation of Gynecology and Obstetrics: Classification and staging of malignant tumors in the female pelvis. Int J Gynaecol Obstet 1971;9:172.

32. International Federation of Gynecology and Obstetrics: Corpus cancer staging. Int J Gynaecol Obstet 1989;28:190.

33. Greven KM, Lanciano RM, Corn B, et al: Pathologic stage III endometrial carcinoma: Prognostic factors and patterns of recurrence. Cancer 1993;71:3697-3702.

34. Greven KM, Corn B, Case D, et al: Which prognostic factors influence the outcome of patients with surgically staged endometrial cancer treated with adjuvant radiation? Int J Radiat Oncol Biol Phys 1997;39:413-418.

35. Chan JK, Lin YG, Monk BJ, et al: Vaginal hysterectomy as primary treatment of endometrial cancer in medically compromised women. Obstet Gynecol 2001;97(5 Pt 1):707-711.

36. Roberts JA, Brunetto VL, Keys HM, et al: A phase III randomized study of surgery vs. surgery plus adjunctive radiation therapy in intermediate risk endometrial adenocarcinoma (GOG 99) [abstract]. Proc Soc Gynecol Oncol 1998;29:70.

37. Aalders J, Abeler V, Kolstad P, et al: Postoperative external irradiation and prognostic parameters in stage I endometrial carcinoma: Clinical and histologic study of 540 patients. Obstet Gynecol 1980;56:419-427.

38. Creutzberg CL, van Putten WL, Koper PC, et al: Surgery and postoperative radiotherapy versus surgery alone for patients with stage-1 endometrial carcinoma: Multicentre randomised trial. PORTEC Study Group. Post Operative Radiation Therapy in Endometrial Carcinoma. Lancet 2000;355:1404-1411.

39. Mariani A, Webb MJ, Keeney GL, et al: Low-risk corpus cancer: Is lymphadenectomy or radiotherapy necessary? Am J Obstet Gynecol 2000;186:1506-1519.

40. Kilgore LC, Partridge EE, Alvarez RD, et al: Adenocarcinoma of the endometrium: Survival comparisons of patients with and without pelvic node sampling. Gynecol Oncol 1995;56:29-33.

41. Fanning J: Long-term survival of intermediate risk endometrial cancer (stage IG3, IC, II) treated with full lymphadenectomy and brachytherapy without teletherapy. Gynecol Oncol 2001;82:371-374.

42. Orr JW, Holimon JL, Orr PF: Stage I corpus cancer: Is teletherapy necessary? Am J Obstet Gynecol 1997;176:777-788.

43. Chadha M, Nanavati P, Liu P, et al: Patterns of failure in endometrial carcinoma stage IB grade 3 and IC patients treated with postoperative vaginal vault brachytherapy. Gynecol Oncol 1999;75:103-107.

44. Ng TN, Perrin LC, Nicklin JL, et al: Local recurrence in high-risk node-negative stage I endometrial carcinoma treated with postoperative vaginal vault brachytherapy. Gynecol Oncol 2000;79:490-494.

45. Straughn JM, Huh WK, Kelly FJ, et al: Conservative management of stage I endometrial carcinoma after surgical staging. Gynecol Oncol 2002;84:194-200.

46. Horowitz NS, Peters WA 3rd, Smith MR, et al: Adjuvant high dose rate vaginal brachytherapy as treatment of stage I and II endometrial carcinoma. Obstet Gynecol 2002;99:235-240.

47. Mariani A, Webb, MJ, Keeney GL, et al: Predictors of lymphatic failure in endometrial cancer. Gynecol Oncol 2002;84:437-442.

48. Creasman WT, Morrow CP, Bundy BN, et al: Surgical pathologic spread patterns of endometrial cancer: A Gynecologic Oncology Group Study. Cancer 1987;60:2035-2041.

49. Mohan DS, Samuels MA, Selim MA, et al: Long-term outcomes of therapeutic pelvic lymphadenectomy for stage I endometrial adenocarcinoma. Gynecol Oncol 1998;70:165-171.

50. Chuang L, Burke TW, Tornos C, et al: Staging laparotomy for endometrial carcinoma: Assessment of retroperitoneal lymph nodes. Gynecol Oncol 1995;58:189.

51. Partridge EE, Shingleton HM, Menck HR: The National Cancer Data Base report on endometrial cancer. J Surg Oncol 1996;61:111-123.

52. Candiani GB, Belloni C, Maggi R, et al: Evaluation of different surgical approaches in the treatment of endometrial cancer at FIGO stage I. Gyn Oncol 1990;37:6-8.

53. Elliott P, Green D, Coates A, et al: The efficacy of postoperative vaginal irradiation in preventing vaginal recurrence in endometrial cancer. Int J Gynecol Cancer 1984;4:84-93.

54. Creutzberg CL, van Putten WL, Koper PC, et al: The morbidity of treatment for patients with stage I endometrial cancer: results from a randomized trial. Int J Radiat Oncol Biol Phys 2001;51:1246-1255.

55. Carey MS, O'Connell GJ, Johanson CR, et al: Good outcome associated with a standardized treatment protocol using selective postoperative radiation in patients with clinical stage I adenocarcinoma of the endometrium. Gynecol Oncol 1995;57:138-144.

56. Descamps P, Calais G, Moire C, et al: Predictors of distant recurrence in clinical stage I or II endometrial carcinoma treated by combination surgical and radiation therapy. Gynecol Oncol 1997;64:54-58.

57. Konski A, Domenico D, Tyrkus M, et al: Prognostic characteristics of surgical stage I endometrial adenocarcinoma. Int J Radiat Oncol Biol Phys 1996;35:935-940.

58. Greven KM, Randall ME, Fanning J, et al: Patterns of failure in patients with stage I, grade 3 carcinoma of the endometrium. Int J Radiat Oncol Biol Phys 1990;19:529-534.

59. Lanciano RM, Curran WJ Jr, Greven KM, et al: Influence of grade, histologic subtype, and timing of radiotherapy on outcome among patients with stage II carcinoma of the Endometrium. Gynecol Oncol 1990;39:368-373.

60. Mayr NA, Wen B-C, Benda JA, et al: Postoperative radiation therapy in clinical stage I endometrial cancer: Corpus, cervical, and lower uterine segment involvement-patterns of failure. Radiology 1995;196:323-328.

61. Mariani A, Webb MJ, Keeney GL, et al: Hematogenous dissemination in corpus cancer. Gynecol Oncol 2001;80:233-238.

62. Phase III Randomized Study of Adjuvant Radiotherapy with or without Cisplatin and Paclitaxel After Total Abdominal Hysterectomy and Bilateral Salpingo-oophorectomy in Patients

with Stage I or II Endometrial Cancer (RTOG 9905). Current information retrieved from http://www.cancer.gov/Clinical Trials/ on December 13, 2003.

63. Mundt AJ, McBride R, Rotmensch J, et al: Significant pelvic recurrence in high-risk pathologic stage I-IV endometrial carcinoma patients after adjuvant chemotherapy alone: Implications for adjuvant radiation therapy. Int J Radiat Oncol Biol Phys 2001; 50:1145-1153.

64. Nag S, Erickson B, Parikh S, et al: The American Brachytherapy Society recommendations for high-dose-rate brachytherapy for carcinoma of the endometrium. Int J Radiat Oncol Biol Phys 2000;48:779-790.

65. Greven KM, D'Agostino RB, Lanciano RM, et al: Is there a role for a brachytherapy vaginal cuff boost in the adjuvant management of patients with uterine-confined endometrial cancer? Int J Radiat Oncol Biol Phys 1998;42:101-104.

66. Irwin C, Levin W, Fyles A, et al: The role of adjuvant radiotherapy in carcinoma of the endometrium-results in 550 patients with pathologic stage I disease. Gynecol Oncol 1998;70:247-254.

67. Kucera H, Vavra N, Weghaupt K: Benefit of external irradiation in pathologic stage I endometrial carcinoma: A prospective clinical trial of 605 patients who received postoperative vaginal irradiation and additional pelvic irradiation in the presence of unfavorable prognostic factors. Gynecol Oncol 1990;38:99-104.

68. Corn BW, Lanciano R, Greven K, et al: The impact of improved irradiation technique, age, and lymph node sampling on the severe complication rate of surgically staged endometrial cancer patients: A multivariate analysis. J Clin Oncol 1994;12:510-515.

69. Greven KM, Lanciano RM, Herbert SH, et al: Analysis of complications in patients with endometrial carcinoma receiving adjuvant irradiation. Int J Radiat Oncol Biol Phys 1991;21:919-923.

70. Lewandowski G, Torrisi J, Potkul RK, et al: Hysterectomy with extended surgical staging and radiotherapy versus hysterectomy alone and radiotherapy in stage I endometrial cancer: A comparison of complication rates. Gynecol Oncol 1990;36:401-404.

71. Potish RA, Dusenbery KE: Enteric morbidity of postoperative pelvic external beam and brachytherapy for uterine cancer. Int Radiat Oncol Biol Phys 1990;18:1005-1010.

72. Onsrud M, Strickert T, Marthinsen AB: Late reactions after postoperative high-dose-rate intravaginal brachytherapy for endometrial cancer: A comparison of standardized and individualized target volumes. Int J Radiat Oncol Biol Phys 2001;49:749-755.

73. Anderson JM, Stea B, Hallum AV, et al: High-dose-rate postoperative vaginal cuff irradiation alone for stage IB and IC endometrial cancer. Int J Radiat Oncol Biol Phys 2000;46:417-425.

74. Eltabbakh GH, Piver MS, Hempling RE, et al: Excellent long-term survival and absence of vaginal recurrences in 332 patients with low-risk stage I endometrial adenocarcinoma treated with hysterectomy and vaginal brachytherapy without formal staging lymph node sampling: Report of a prospective trial. Int J Radiat Oncol Biol Phys 1997;38:373-380.

75. Petereit DG, Tannehill SP, Grosen EA, et al: Outpatient vaginal cuff brachytherapy for endometrial cancer. Int J Gynecol Cancer 1999;9:456-462.

76. Larson D, Broste SK, Krawisz BR: Surgery without radiotherapy for primary treatment of endometrial cancer. Obstet Gynecol 1998;91:355-359.

77. National Comprehensive Cancer Network practice guidelines for endometrial carcinoma. Oncology 1999;13:45-67.

78. Knocke TH, Kucera H, Weidinger B, et al: Primary treatment of endometrial carcinoma with high-dose-rate brachytherapy: results of 12 years of experience with 280 patients. Int J Radiat Oncol Biol Phys 1997;37:359-365.

79. Nguyen TV, Petereit DG: High-dose-rate brachytherapy for medically inoperable stage I endometrial cancer. Gynecol Oncol 1998;71:196-203.

80. Chao CK, Grigsby PW, Perez CA, et al: Medically inoperable stage I endometrial carcinoma: A few dilemmas in radiotherapeutic management. Int J Radiat Oncol Biol Phys 1996;34:27-31.

81. Kupelian PA, Eifel PJ, Tornos C, et al: Treatment of endometrial carcinoma with radiation therapy alone [review]. Int J Radiat Oncol Biol Phys 1993;27:817-824.

82. Rouanet P, Dubois JB, Gely S, Pourquier H: Exclusive radiation therapy in endometrial carcinoma. Int J Radiat Oncol Biol Phys 1993;26:223-228.

83. Thigpen JT, Buchsbaum HJ, Mangan C, Blessing JA: Phase II trial of adriamycin in the treatment of advanced or recurrent endometrial carcinoma: A Gynecologic Oncology Group study. Cancer Treat Rep 1979;63:21-27.

84. Thigpen JT, Blessing JA, Beecham J, et al: Phase II trial of cisplatin as first-line chemotherapy in patients with advanced or recurrent uterine sarcomas: A Gynecologic Oncology Group study. J Clin Oncol 1991;9:1962-1966.

85. Long HJ, Pfeifle DM, Wieand HS, et al: Phase II evaluation of carboplatin in advanced endometrial carcinoma. J Natl Cancer Inst 1988;80:276-278.

86. Ball HG, Blessing JA, Lentz SS, Mutch DG: A phase II trial of paclitaxel in patients with advanced or recurrent adenocarcinoma of the endometrium: A Gynecologic Oncology Group study. Gynecol Oncol 1996;62:278-281.

87. O'Brien, Killackey M: Adjuvant therapy in "high risk" endometrial adenocarcinoma. Proc ASCO 1994;13:249.

88. Burke TW, Gershenson DM, Morris M, et al: Postoperative adjuvant cisplatin, doxorubicin, and cyclophosphamide (PAC) chemotherapy in women with high-risk endometrial carcinoma. Gynecol Oncol 1994;55:47-50.

89. Greven KM, Winter K, Underhill K, et al: Preliminary analysis of RTOG 9708: Adjuvant postoperative irradiation combined with cisplatin/taxol chemotherapy following surgery for patients with high-risk endometrial cancer. Int J Radiat Oncol Biol Phys 2004, (in press).

90. Creasman WT, Henderson D, Hirshaw W, Clarke-Pearson DL: Estrogen replacement therapy in the patient treated for endometrial cancer. Obstet Gynecol 1986;67:326-330.

91. Lee RB, Burke TW, Park RC: Estrogen replacement therapy following treatment for stage I endometrial carcinoma. Gynecol Oncol 1990;36:189-191.

92. Chapman JA, DiSaia PJ, Osann K, et al: Estrogen replacement in surgical stage I and II endometrial cancer survivors. Am J Obstet Gynecol 1996;175:1195-1200.

93. Suriano KA, McHale M, McLaren CE, et al: Estrogen replacement therapy in endometrial cancer patients: A matched control study. Obstet Gynecol 2001;97:555-560.

94. Mariani A, Webb MJ, Keeney GL, et al: Surgical stage I endometrial cancer: Predictors of distant failure and death. Gynecol Oncol 2002;87:274-280.

95. Sears JD, Greven KM, Hoen HM, et al: Prognostic factors and treatment outcome for patients with locally recurrent endometrial cancer. Cancer 1994;74:1303-1308.

96. Corn B, Lanciano R, D'Agostino R, et al: The relationship of local and distant failure from endometrial cancer: Defining a clinical paradigm. Gyn Onc 1997;66:411-416.

97. Overgaard M, Hansen PS, Overgaard J, et al: Postoperative radiotherapy in high-risk premenopausal women with breast cancer who receive adjuvant chemotherapy. Danish Breast Cancer Cooperative Group 82b Trial. N Engl J Med 1997;337:949-955.

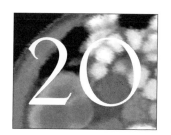

MANAGEMENT OF ADVANCED STAGE ENDOMETRIAL CANCER

Istvan Pataki, Rachelle Lanciano, and Robert E. Bristow

 MAJOR CONTROVERSIES

- **What is the appropriate surgical management of a malignant adnexal neoplasm discovered at the time of surgery for endometrial cancer?**
- **What is the appropriate adjuvant therapy for endometrial cancer with isolated adnexal metastasis?**
- **What is the appropriate adjuvant therapy for synchronous cancers of the endometrium and ovary?**
- **What is the appropriate management of endometrial cancer with positive nodes?**
- **What is the appropriate management of endometrial cancer with positive cytology?**
- **What is the optimal management of stage IVa endometrial cancer?**
- **What is the optimal management of stage IVb endometrial cancer?**
- **What is the optimal management of advanced (stage III/IV) uterine papillary serous carcinoma?**

Endometrial corpus cancer is the fourth most common malignancy among United States women and the eighth most common cause of cancer-related death.[1] The American Cancer Society estimated that 39,300 new cases of uterine corpus cancer would be diagnosed during 2002.[1] Of these, 22% (or approximately 8600 women) would have regional or distant spread of disease. Patients with advanced disease account for the majority of tumor-related deaths and present a significant challenge for clinicians. The therapeutic armamentarium for metastatic endometrial cancer includes surgery, radiation therapy, chemotherapy, hormone therapy, and combinations of these modalities; however, effective management strategies have yet to be precisely defined. This chapter focuses on the more problematic management issues for patients with

International Federation of Gynecology and Obstetrics (FIGO) stage III and IV endometrial cancer.

STAGE III ENDOMETRIAL CANCER

According to FIGO statistics, 13.2% of patients with endometrial cancer submitted to surgical staging are found to have stage III disease.[2] Criteria for Stage III disease include any of the following: surgicopathologic confirmation of tumor spread to the uterine serosa, adnexae, vagina, parametria, pelvic or para-aortic (PA) lymph nodes or positive cytology in peritoneal fluid.[2] For patients who are unable to undergo surgical staging, the FIGO 1971 clinical staging system is invoked, in which stage III reflects extrauterine spread of disease that is clinically confined to the true pelvis.[2]

What is the appropriate surgical management of a malignant adnexal neoplasm discovered at the time of surgery for endometrial cancer?

In the setting of endometrial cancer, a coexistent adnexal mass may represent a metastatic (metachronous) lesion from the endometrial primary, a second (synchronous or dual) primary cancer of the ovary, or a benign condition such as an inflammatory mass. Between 5% and 10% of patients undergoing surgical staging for endometrial cancer are found to have a malignant adnexal neoplasm.[3-6] A critical issue facing the surgeon in such circumstances is determining the extent of the staging procedure. Specifically, surgical staging for endometrial cancer consists of peritoneal cytologic washings and sampling of the retroperitoneal pelvic and PA lymph nodes. In contrast, patients with ovarian cancer are routinely submitted to extended surgical staging, with omentectomy, appendectomy, and peritoneal biopsies in addition to cytologic washings and retroperitoneal lymph node sampling.

At the time of surgical exploration, initial attention should be directed toward removing the adnexal mass and obtaining a frozen-section diagnosis. On completion of the hysterectomy, the uterus should be submitted for immediate intraoperative pathologic inspection. Clearly, discordance between endometrial and ovarian histology implies the presence of two separate primary neoplasms, and extended surgical staging is indicated. Distinguishing between synchronous and metachronous disease is more problematic if the same histologic findings are present in both endometrium and ovary. The most commonly observed concordant histologic subtype is endometrioid. In such instances, intraoperative pathologic evaluation for the presence of deep myometrial invasion, lymphovascular invasion, small (<5 cm) or bilateral ovarian tumors, and a multinodular pattern of ovarian growth may be predictive of ovarian metastasis from an endometrial primary tumor.[7] Some authors have recommended that, if frozen-section findings are consistent with metastatic endometrial cancer, then only retroperitoneal lymph node sampling (as in the endometrial cancer staging protocol) should be performed.[8] On the other hand, 45% to 86% of patients with synchronous (dual) primary endometrial and ovarian lesions have endometrioid histology in both sites.[4,9,10] One could argue, therefore, that the extended staging procedure should still be performed in such circumstances, because differentiation between an endometrial lesion metastatic to the ovary and a synchronous primary ovarian cancer may be possible only on permanent-section pathologic analysis. An additional point of consideration is that adnexal involvement by endometrial cancer can be a marker for other sites of extrauterine spread, with retroperitoneal lymph node metastasis present in 15% to 32%

of such cases.[3,5,6] Perhaps more importantly, as many as 35% of patients with ovarian metastases in fact have upper abdominal disease (FIGO stage IVb) that might go undetected by the standard endometrial cancer staging procedure.[5]

In summary, patients who are found to have malignant adnexal disease at the time of endometrial cancer surgery should, in most circumstances, undergo extended surgical staging, as for ovarian cancer. Even if the endometrial and ovarian histologic tumor types are concordant, the additional information provided by extended staging is useful for both diagnostic purposes and treatment planning and adds little in the way of morbidity to the staging procedure normally performed for an isolated primary endometrial cancer.

What is the appropriate adjuvant therapy for endometrial cancer with isolated adnexal metastasis?

The diagnosis of isolated adnexal metastasis from a primary endometrial cancer can be challenging, particularly if the histologic subtypes are concordant. Molecular analyses of multiple polymorphic DNA markers, patterns of X-chromosome inactivation, mutations in the *PTEN*, *TP53*, or K-*ras* genes, human papilloma virus detection, and allelic loss on chromosome 17q have been used in an attempt to define the lineage relationships between synchronous neoplasms of the endometrium and ovary.[11-15] However, these investigational techniques are time-consuming and labor intensive, and they require additional confirmation of their utility in contemporary clinical practice. In most cases, therefore, the diagnosis of metachronous endometrial and ovarian malignancies is based on the final pathologic analysis. In 1985, Ulbright and Roth[7] empirically proposed major and minor criteria for characterizing ovarian metastasis from a primary endometrial cancer. These criteria included (1) a multinodular ovarian tumor pattern (major criteria), or (2) two or more of the following minor criteria: small (<5 cm) ovary or ovaries, bilateral ovarian involvement, deep myometrial invasion (greater than one-third), vascular invasion, and tubal lumen involvement. Despite little independent verification of their validity, these criteria form the basis for current pathologic diagnostic standards.

The weight of available data suggests that adnexal metastasis from endometrial cancer, as an isolated finding, is associated with a favorable prognosis. In the series of Mackillop and Pringle,[16] the 5-year survival rate for patients with isolated adnexal involvement was 82.3%, which was statistically significantly superior to the 27.7% rate for patients with other sites of intrapelvic spread. Sixty-seven percent of these patients were treated with adjuvant pelvic radiation (PRT) postoperatively. Connell and associates[5] reported a 5-year DFS of 71% for patients with endometrial cancer and isolated adnexal metastasis. Adjuvant therapy for this group consisted of PRT in 75% of cases, chemotherapy in 33%, and hormone therapy in 16%. Among those patients whose retroperitoneal lymph nodes were sampled (and presumably negative), the 5-year DFS was 82%. On multivariate analysis, adnexal involvement was not independently predictive of survival. Similar findings were reported by Mariani and coworkers,[17] who found that adnexal involvement was not an independent prognostic factor for disease-free or overall survival among patients with stage IIIa endometrial cancer. In their series, adjuvant radiation therapy was administered to 84% of patients, and the 5-year survival rate associated with isolated adnexal metastasis was 89%.

Although isolated adnexal involvement by endometrial cancer portends a favorable prognosis, interpretation of the efficacy of adjuvant therapy is complicated by heterogeneous patient populations and postoperative treatment protocols. Whole abdominopelvic radiation therapy has been reported to be highly efficacious in reducing the risk of disease recurrence.[18] Conversely, Takeshima and associates[6] observed a 5-year DFS of 72% for 15 patients with endometrial cancer and isolated ovarian metastasis treated with surgery alone. In the majority of reported series, some form of adjuvant therapy, usually whole pelvic irradiation, was administered. This management strategy has been associated with excellent long-term survival rates (71% to 89%) and probably should be considered the standard of care for patients with the more common endometrioid tumor histology, provided all other staging biopsies are negative. There are insufficient data to reach any definitive conclusion regarding the role of chemotherapy or whole abdominal radiation therapy (WAR) in this setting.

What is the appropriate adjuvant therapy for synchronous cancers of the endometrium and ovary?

The coexistence of cancer of the ovary occurs in approximately 5% of patients with endometrial cancer.[4] The published literature on this phenomenon consists largely of single-institution clinicopathologic studies employing variable histologic criteria. This limitation notwithstanding, it appears that patients with synchronous (dual) primary cancers of the endometrium and ovary have a surprisingly good long-term prognosis.

In one of the earliest reports, Eifel and colleagues[19] observed only a single recurrence among 16 patients with synchronous endometrial and ovarian malignancies of endometrioid histology and identical histologic grade. Ten of these patients received postoperative radiation therapy. Zaino and coworkers[9] reported a long-term survival rate of 71% for 24 patients with synchronous endometrial and ovarian malignancies; deep myometrial invasion and higher histologic tumor grade were associated with a worse prognosis. Eighty-two percent of these patients received postoperative radiation therapy, 45% chemotherapy, and 27% hormone therapy. Investigators from the University of California at Los Angeles reported a

median survival time of 76 months and a long-term survival rate of 55% for 11 patients with simultaneous endometrial and ovarian malignancies, 4 of whom had at least stage II ovarian cancer.[10] Five patients were treated with postoperative chemotherapy, and five received PRT. Pearl and colleagues[20] reported on 16 patients with synchronous dual primary stage I cancers of the endometrium and ovary; 88% of these patients had endometrioid histology in both sites, and 94% had concordant tumor grades. Adjuvant chemotherapy or radiation therapy was administered to 70% of the patients. There were no disease-related deaths, with follow-up ranging from 3 to 144 months. Zaino and associates,[4] reporting for the Gynecologic Oncology Group (GOG), analyzed 74 cases of synchronous endometrial and ovarian cancers in the largest comprehensive study to date. Endometrioid histology was present in both the endometrium and the ovary in 86% of cases, and tumor grade was concordant in 69% of all tumors. Microscopic tumor spread (extragenital) to the pelvis or abdomen was documented in 31% of patients. The presence of extragenital metastasis and higher tumor grade predicted a higher risk of tumor recurrence. For the entire group, the estimated 5-year survival rate was 86%. Because it was not a primary outcome variable, the details of adjuvant therapy were not reported.

It is difficult to determine to what extent the selection of adjuvant therapy contributes to the favorable long-term outcome of patients with synchronous endometrial and ovarian cancers. Consequently, adjuvant treatment for these patients should be based on the "worst-case scenario" for each disease site (Table 20-1). Both endometrial and ovarian cancers can be categorized as having low or high risk for recurrence and disease-related death based on histopathologic and staging criteria. High-risk characteristics for endometrial cancer include deep myometrial invasion, high tumor grade or atypical histologic subtype, lymph/vascular space invasion, extension to cervix or parametria, and nodal involvement. Adjuvant therapy decisions should be based on the collective severity of

Table 20–1. Adjuvant Therapy Recommendations for Patients with Synchronous (Dual) Primary Cancers of the Endometrium and Ovary

Group	Endometrial Cancer	Ovarian Cancer	Adjuvant Therapy
1	Low risk	Low risk	None
2	High risk*	Low risk	TVD radiation†
3	Low risk	High risk‡	Chemotherapy§
4	High risk*	High risk‡	Chemotherapy§ + TVD radiation†

*High-risk endometrial cancer characteristics: deep myometrial invasion, high tumor grade or atypical histologic subtype, lymph/vascular space invasion, extension to cervix or parametria, nodal involvement.
†TVD radiation: tumor volume–directed radiation therapy; may include vaginal apex brachytherapy, whole pelvic irradiation, and/or extended-field irradiation.
‡High-risk ovarian cancer characteristics: FIGO surgical stage Ic or higher, or tumor with grade 3 histology.
§Platinum plus paclitaxel–based combination chemotherapy.

these features. Endometrial cancer patients meeting high-risk criteria (group 2 in Table 20-1) should receive tumor volume–directed radiation therapy, which may consist of vaginal apex brachytherapy, whole pelvic external beam irradiation, or extended-field irradiation (EFRT). Ovarian cancer patients with FIGO stage Ic or more advanced disease, or grade 3 histology, or both, are considered to be at high risk for recurrence and should receive adjuvant platinum/paclitaxel-based combination chemotherapy (group 3 in Table 20-1). Rarely, patients may have high-risk features in both anatomic sites (group 4 in Table 20-1). In such circumstances, both adjuvant chemotherapy and tumor volume–directed radiation therapy should be administered. The microvascular injury associated with external beam radiation treatment may, at least theoretically, compromise subsequent end-organ delivery of cytotoxic drugs. Therefore, adjuvant chemotherapy should probably be administered before irradiation.

What is the appropriate adjuvant therapy for endometrial cancer with positive nodes?

Endometrial cancer with positive lymph nodes is found in about 10% of all patients with a diagnosis of endometrial cancer. In the FIGO pathologic staging system of 1988, these patients are designated as having stage IIIc disease. The GOG reported a large multi-institutional surgical staging study that examined patterns of involvement in 621 patients with clinical stage I and occult stage II disease.[21] This study identified 6% of patients with positive pelvic adenopathy, 3% with both pelvic and PA adenopathy, and 2% with positive PA adenopathy only. This distribution correlates with the known lymphatic drainage of the uterus.

Adverse factors such as grade, depth of invasion into the myometrium, cervical or adnexal involvement, lymphovascular invasion, and histology (e.g., uterine papillary serous carcinoma [UPSC], clear cell [CC] cancer) determine the risk of lymph node involvement, as demonstrated by GOG Protocol 33.[3] The frequency of PA nodal involvement when pelvic nodes are found to be positive is 40% to 50%.[3,22] The 5-year disease-free survival rate (DFS) is significantly worse in patients with positive PA nodes, compared with those without such involvement (35% versus 85%).[21] Within the node-positive group, increasing histologic grade and UPSC/CC histology predict for worse DFS.[23]

The role of surgical lymphadenectomy in endometrial cancer is not well defined. Data by Kilgore and colleagues[24] suggest a therapeutic benefit even for patients with no clinical evidence of lymphadenopathy. A cohort of 205 patients with clinical stage I or II endometrial cancer and pelvic node sampling had better survival that did 208 similar patients without such sampling. Only a limited number of patients were actually found to have positive pelvic nodes, which could not account for the survival benefit seen. This suggests that microscopic disease may be missed

on pathologic examination, but its removal may confer a benefit.[24] If grossly enlarged lymph nodes are encountered, recent data suggest that resection of these nodes is therapeutically beneficial.[22,25,26] Corn and associates[26] described the outcome of patients who underwent total abdominal hysterectomy and bilateral salpingo-oophorectomy (TAH/BSO) plus resection of grossly enlarged PA nodes, followed by pelvic and PA radiation therapy. These results were compared with those of patients who had TAH/BSO and the same radiation therapy, but without resection of grossly enlarged nodes. There was a significant reduction in PA failure rate, from 39% to 13%, when grossly involved PA lymph nodes were resected. The overall 5-year DFS was 46% in the entire group of patients with positive PA nodes. DFS was not analyzed according to presence or absence of PA failure.[26] Mariani and colleagues[25] also confirmed the therapeutic value of PA lymphadenectomy in a report from the Mayo Clinic. Fifty-one patients had positive nodes (pelvic or PA). The 5-year overall survival rate was 77% in patients who underwent PA lymphadenectomy and 42% in those who did not. Other pathologic or treatment factors were not statistically significant for predicting survival, and morbidity was not increased by the addition of PA lymphadenectomy in these patients.[25] Based on all of these data, it is recommended that grossly enlarged lymph nodes be resected when it is safe to do so.

The standard postoperative treatment for stage IIIc disease includes adjuvant radiotherapy. The optimal volume of radiotherapy remains undefined. Possible options are PRT, EFRT, and WAR, all with or without vaginal brachytherapy boost.

Patients who have histologically confirmed positive PA nodes continue to have suboptimal outcomes. Patterns of failure can be pelvic, abdominal, or distant, but they depend on the type of treatment administered, as reported by a number of retrospective series.[21,26-29] Standard treatment for patients with documented PA nodal involvement is EFRT (Table 20-2), or possibly WAR (Table 20-3) after surgical debulking. This was illustrated in a report by Hicks and colleagues,[28] who analyzed 19 patients with documented PA nodal involvement. Patients were treated postoperatively in a nonrandomized fashion with PRT plus progestins, or with EFRT. The median pelvic dose was 5040 cGy, and the median PA dose was 4500 cGy. The 5-year DFS was 27% for the EFRT group, and there were no survivors in the PRT group at 5 years. As seen in Table 20-2, other authors also report 5-year DFS rates in the range of 30% to 40% for patients treated with EFRT.

Patients who have positive pelvic nodes only may be divided into two groups: those with negative PA nodes after nodal sampling and those with unsampled PA nodes. The latter group is known to have a 40% to 50% chance of PA node involvement.[3,21,22,30] A number of authors have reported on adjuvant PRT in patients with positive pelvic nodes, with variable assessment of the PA nodes (Table 20-4).[21,23,27,30-32] Schorge and associates[27] analyzed 20 patients with confirmed pelvic lymph node involvement who had

Table 20–2. Outcome for Endometrial Cancer Patients with Para-Aortic Metastases

Study and Ref. No.	No. of Patients	Type of RT	Failure Pattern (% of Total Population)	Outcome (5-yr DFS)
Morrow et al.[21]	48	37 EFRT 11 no RT	RT: 81% (18% of them in EFRT field) No RT: 56%	36% for whole group
Hicks et al.[28]	19	8 PRT 11 EFRT	PRT: 63% lung, 37% abdominal EFRT: 64% lung, 0% abdominal	PRT: 0% EFRT: 27%
Schorge et al.[27]	15	5 PRT 2 EFRT 8 chemotherapy or observation	RT: 57% (25% of them pelvic) No RT: 50% (50% of them pelvic)	(5-yr OS for 35 stage IIIc patients: 52%)
Corn et al.[26]	26	EFRT (6 preoperative)	(37% pelvic, 39% distant, 27% in para-aortic nodes, 0% only in abdomen)*	40% (5-yr OS: 46%)
Rose et al.[29]	26	17 EFRT 8 PRT 1 Postoperative death	EFRT: 6% pelvic, 29% distant PRT: not stated	EFRT: 65% CSS (median survival: 27 mo) PRT: 12% CSS (median survival: 14.5 mo)

CSS, cause-specific survival; DFS, disease-free survival rate; EFRT, extended-field radiotherapy; OS, overall survival; PRT, pelvic radiotherapy; RT, radiotherapy.
*Percentage of all failures.

either pathologically negative or unsampled PA nodes. Thirteen patients had PRT, with four recurrences (two extrapelvic and two pelvic). The remaining seven patients did not receive any radiotherapy; five of them had recurrences, all extrapelvic. The 5-year DFS was only 55% for the whole group. Morrow and collecgues[21] reported a 5-year DFS rate of 72% (13/18) for patients with positive pelvic lymph nodes and pathologically negative PA nodes treated with PRT. Patterns of failure for this group were not reported. Nelson and coworkers[13] reported on 17 patients with positive pelvic nodes but pathologically negative PA nodes. Thirteen patients received PRT, and four received

WAR. Two patients had failure in the PA nodes, and two others distantly. The authors suggested consideration of EFRT for these surgically staged patients. Because sampling alone may underestimate the true incidence of positive PA nodes, EFRT is a reasonable option for these patients, as well as for those patients with unsampled PA nodes.[30,31]

Given the patterns of relapse for patients without adjuvant radiotherapy, vaginal brachytherapy is a possible consideration for node-positive patients. This was suggested by the results of GOG 94, a phase II study of WAR without vaginal brachytherapy for stage III/IV endometrioid or any-stage UPSC or CC

Table 20–3. Outcome with Whole Abdominal Radiotherapy for High-Risk Endometrial Cancer Patients

Study and Ref. No.	No. of Patients	Stage	Failure Pattern (% of Total Population)	Outcome
Greer & Hamberger[41]	27	63% stage III; 37% stage IV	Not stated	5-yr CSS: 86% stage III, 70% stage IV
Potish[45]	49	Stage I–III	First site: 5 abdominal, 1 distant, 3 abdominal and distant, 2 pelvic, 1 unknown	5-year DFS: 63%
Smith et al.[48]	48	46% stage III/IV EAC; 54% stage I–IV UPSC/CC	EAC: 18%, all distant UPSC/CC: 42% (4 pelvic, 1 abdominal, 6 distant)	3-yr DFS: 79% for EAC, 47% for UPSC/CC
Small et al.[50]	30	47% UPSC; 37% IIIa; 26% IIIc	10% Pelvic, 7% upper abdominal, 7% para-aortic nodes, 10% distant	5-yr DFS: 77%
Stewart et al.[49]	119	18% stage IIIc; 37% UPSC/CC	38% Abdominal/pelvic (first site)	5-yr CSS: 75% for EAC, 57% for UPSC/CC
Axelrod et al.[33]	165	47% of EAC and 53% UPSC/CC (60% of EAC and 46% of UPSC/CC stage IIIc)	Not stated	3-yr OS: 31% for EAC, 33% for UPSC/CC

CC, clear cell carcinoma; CSS, cause-specific survival; DFS, disease-free survival; EAC, endometrioid adenocarcinoma; OS, overall survival; UPSC, uterine papillary serous carcinoma.

Table 20–4. Outcome for Patients with Positive Pelvic Lymph Nodes (PA Nodes Negative or Unknown)

Author	No. of Patients	PA Pathologic Status	Type of RT	Failure Pattern (% of Population)	Outcome
Morrow et al.[21]	18	All negative	PRT: 16 RT: 2	PRT: 25% (25% of them pelvic) No RT: 50% (100% of them pelvic)	5-yr DFS: 75%
Schorge et al.[27]	20	Not stated	PRT: 13 RT: 7	PRT: 15% extrapelvic, 15% pelvic	5-yr OS: 52% for 35 stage IIIc patients
Nelson et al.[31]	17	All negative	EFRT: 13 WAR: 4	0% abdominal/pelvic, 12% in PA nodes, 12% distant	5-yr DFS: 81%
Mundt et al.[30]	30	26/30 Negative	EFRT: 10 PRT: 20	23% pelvic overall, 0% abdominal, 20% PA (all in PRT group)	5-yr DFS: 34% 5-yr CSS: 56%
Lurain et al.[32]	20	(65% had pathologic node assessment)	PRT	Not stated	5-yr DFS: 55%

CSS, cause-specific survival; DFS, disease-free survival; EFRT, extended-field radiotherapy; OS, overall survival; PA, para-aortic; PRT, pelvic radiotherapy; RT, radiotherapy; WAR, whole abdominal radiotherapy.

disease (see later discussion); a 4.2% vaginal failure rate was noted overall.[33] However, there are some data to suggest that the pelvic control rate does not increase with this additional treatment.[23]

Standard PRT typically uses a four-field approach. Conventional field borders are at the top of the fifth lumbar vertebra (L5) superiorly, the bottom of the obturator foramina inferiorly, and 2 cm beyond the widest point of the inlet of the true bony pelvis. For the lateral fields, the anterior border is usually the symphysis pubis, and the posterior border is through the S2-S3 interspace. For EFRT, an anteroposterior-posteroanterior beam arrangement is often used for the PA portion of the fields, to spare the kidneys. The superior border is typically at the T12-L1 or T11-T12 interspace. Computed tomography–based treatment planning can help to avoid normal structures and can ensure adequate coverage of the nodal regions at risk.

The role of WAR for node-positive patients has been controversial. The rationale for this approach was based on patterns of failure suggesting that, in addition to the pelvis, the upper abdomen is a common site of failure after surgical resection for high-risk endometrial cancer with positive nodes.[34-38] Of note, the entity of UPSC was not established in many of these older series. This aggressive histologic subtype is known to have a higher than usual rate of relapse in the upper abdomen, possibly skewing the earlier series.[37,39] In general, although patterns of recurrence do include abdominal sites, these are less often found to be isolated or first sites of recurrence, decreasing the rationale for WAR.[26,40] A number of phase II single-institution studies examining the outcome for these patients after WAR have been reported (see Table 20-3).[41-50]

A recent update of the combined experience from the Mayo Clinic and Beaumont Hospital[49] analyzed 119 patients treated with WAR after TAH/BSO; 37% had UPSC or CC histology. Lymph node sampling was performed for 85% of these 119 patients, and 18% were found to have positive nodes. Patterns of failures by first site were reported. Of a total of 37 failures, combined abdominal/pelvic recurrences were seen in 14 patients, although abdomen-only failures were not reported separately. Vaginal failures were seen in 6 patients, for a total of 20 failures in the treated volume. Distant failures were seen in 17 patients. One third of the patients with endometrioid histology had failure in the lung, in contrast to only 8% of those with UPSC/CC histologies. Twelve percent of patients developed grade 3 or 4 chronic gastrointestinal toxicity, and 2% developed grade 3 chronic renal toxicity. Ten percent experienced bowel obstruction requiring surgical intervention.[49] Interpretation of this and other studies of WAR is hampered by their heterogeneous inclusion criteria and treatments and their retrospective nature. Based on these series that show superior DFS and overall survival rates compared with historical controls, the GOG conducted two trials examining the value of WAR in node-positive and other high-risk patients.

The first trial (GOG 94),[33] the results of which have been presented only in abstract form, was a phase II trial of WAR for surgically staged III/IV maximally debulked (<2 cm) endometrial adenocarcinomas or any-stage UPSC/CC cancer. The total dose to the abdomen was 30 Gy, with a fraction size of 1.5 Gy/day. No liver blocks were used, and posterior kidney blocks were used throughout treatment. A boost to 45 Gy was delivered to the PA region if the PA nodes were positive, and the pelvis received 50 Gy. For all 165 patients treated, the progression-free survival rate was 31% for endometrioid and 33% for UPSC/CC histologies. A similar pattern of relapse was also noted between these two groups, although specific details on the patterns of failure were not provided. The incidence of severe and life-threatening toxicities after surgery was 7.2%, with postoperative cardiovascular events most common (6%); for WAR, the incidence was 32%, with 12.5% bone marrow toxicity, 17.7% acute and chronic gastrointestinal events, and 1.8% hepatic toxicity.[33]

Based on this study, GOG 122 was launched for a similar group of patients. This was a phase III, randomized study comparing combination doxorubicin and cisplatin chemotherapy versus WAR. Accrual was completed in February 2000, and results are pending. The mature results of GOG 122 will provide additional information regarding the efficacy of WAR versus chemotherapy and patterns of failure with each approach after surgery. There are still further questions that this study will not answer, such as the optimal radiotherapy volume, the benefit of concurrent chemoradiation compared with radiotherapy alone, and the appropriate sequencing of adjuvant treatment. Given the high rate of distant failures, as well as the failure rate within the WAR field, exploration of other strategies (e.g., addition of systemic chemotherapy to appropriate radiation) seems worthwhile.

Chemotherapy has been studied as an adjunct to surgery for high-risk endometrial cancer with or without radiation. Aoki and colleagues[51] reported on 61 patients with stage III disease treated with surgery followed by adjuvant cisplatin (70 mg/m²), doxorubicin (40 mg/m²), and cyclophosphamide (500 mg/m²) given every 4 weeks for five cycles. The actuarial 5-year DFS was 78.6%, with the median time to failure being 18 months. Multivariate analysis revealed myometrial invasion (greater than one-half) and lymphovascular invasion to be significantly associated with a decrease in DFS. A low-risk group was defined as those patients with no or only one of these two risk factors, and a high-risk group as those with two or more risk factors. The 5-year DFS was 100% for the low-risk group and 59% for the high-risk group. For high-risk patients with positive lymph nodes, the predominant pattern of failure was locoregional (37.5%); distant failure was less common (12.5%). For high-risk patients with negative nodes, the predominant pattern was abdominal and distant (35.7%). The toxicity of chemotherapy included grade 3/4 neutropenia in 49% but no septic deaths. Dose reduction was necessary in 19.7% of the patients.[51]

Mundt and associates[52] studied 43 patients with high-risk stage I–IV endometrial cancer treated with cisplatin/doxorubicin-based chemotherapy regimens for four to six cycles after surgery. The predominant pattern of failure was pelvic, with 38% vaginal and 26% nonvaginal pelvic failures. Vaginal failures correlated with cervical invasion and adnexal metastases, whereas nonvaginal pelvic failures correlated with deep myometrial invasion and lymph node involvement.[52] These studies of adjuvant chemotherapy alone confirm that the predominant site of failure in the absence of radiotherapy is the pelvis, demonstrating the need for adjuvant radiotherapy.

Concurrent chemoradiation has been studied as an adjuvant treatment that addresses the high rate of pelvic failures described with chemotherapy alone. Frigerio and colleagues[53] reported a feasibility trial of weekly paclitaxel during 50.4 Gy of PRT. After

radiation, three additional courses of paclitaxel were administered; toxicity was mild. To further explore concurrent chemoradiation, the Radiation Therapy Oncology Group (RTOG) completed a phase II trial[54] consisting of TAH/BSO, postoperative PRT with vaginal brachytherapy, and concurrent cisplatin given on days 1 and 28 of radiation therapy. Patients then received four additional cycles of cisplatin and paclitaxel. Eligible patients included those with grade 2 or 3 endometrial adenocarcinoma with either myometrial invasion greater than one-half, stromal invasion of the cervix, or pelvis-confined extrauterine disease. Preliminary results showed locoregional and distant recurrences in 2% and 5% of patients, respectively, at 12 months. Acute toxicity was acceptable, with hematologic toxicity predominant. Grade 3 and 4 long-term complications were seen in 14% and 2% of the patients, respectively.[54] This adjuvant approach is currently being tested against PRT alone in an important phase III study of the RTOG (Protocol 99-05) and the GOG (Protocol 194) for stage I/II endometrial cancer with high-risk features. This trial will shed light on the additional contribution of concurrent chemotherapy in the setting of high-risk endometrial cancer.

The current GOG trial (GOG 184) was designed to evaluate the best chemotherapeutic regimen to be combined with postoperative tumor volume–directed radiation in the treatment of advanced endometrial cancer. Treatment included pelvic irradiation (50.4 Gy), with or without irradiation of the PA nodes (43.5 Gy) depending on PA nodal status, and with or without vaginal brachytherapy depending on cervical involvement. Patients were then randomly assigned to receive doxorubicin and cisplatin, either with or without paclitaxel, every 3 weeks for six courses after the radiotherapy. It is hoped that this ongoing study will clarify the most effective postradiation chemotherapeutic regimen for endometrial cancer and assess the toxicity and quality of life for patients in the setting of aggressive chemotherapy.

At this point, no randomized study has conclusively demonstrated any additional benefit of adjuvant chemotherapy for node-positive or other high-risk patients. Clinical trial participation should be encouraged for such patients. Outside of such trials, given the observed patterns of failure, adjuvant chemotherapy in the context of appropriate radiotherapy could be considered, especially if more effective systemic agents are developed in the future.

What is the appropriate adjuvant therapy for endometrial cancer with isolated peritoneal cytology?

Malignant peritoneal cytology is discovered in only about 10% of patients with clinical stage I or occult stage II endometrial cancer who have undergone surgical staging. In only half of these patients with positive cytology is it an isolated finding.[3] An early study of surgical-pathologic staging for clinical stage I/II endometrial cancer (GOG Protocol 33) revealed a significant decrease in the 5-year survival rate, from 85% to 56%, when peritoneal cytology was positive. Among patients without metastases (PA and pelvic lymph nodes, adnexal metastases, and gross extrauterine disease), positive cytology still remained a significant negative prognostic factor for recurrence-free interval, with a relative risk of 2.4.[21,55]

Positive peritoneal cytology is associated with other known prognostic factors, such as deep myometrial invasion and high grade. Milosevic and coworkers[56] pooled 17 prospective and retrospective studies for stage I endometrial cancer to determine the clinical significance of malignant peritoneal cytology. Malignant cytology was found in 8%, 12%, and 16% of patients with grade 1, 2, and 3 disease, respectively, and in 8% and 17%, respectively, of those with superficial and deep myometrial invasion. A strong association was noted between malignant cytology and disease recurrence, although the associated adverse prognostic factors (e.g., grade 3, deep myometrial invasion) were believed to dominate the clinical course of the disease. Kadar and colleagues[57] confirmed the negative prognostic effect of peritoneal cytology—but only in association with spread to the adnexae, peritoneum, or lymph nodes, and not if disease was otherwise confined to the uterus. They also found a strong association between positive washings and other high-risk features of the endometrial cancer, such as high grade, lymphovascular invasion, and involvement of adnexae, lymph nodes, or peritoneum.[57]

More recent studies shed further light on the effect of positive peritoneal cytology on DFS and patterns of failure. Takeshima and associates[58] performed a clinical-cytopathologic study on 534 patients surgically staged. There was no effect on survival for patients with disease limited to the uterus, grade 1, and depth of myometrial invasion less than one-half (n = 250), regardless of whether the cytology was positive or negative (5-year DFS, 98% versus 100%). For patients with disease limited to the uterus, grade 2 or 3, or depth of myometrial invasion greater than one-half (n = 211), the 5-year DFS decreased from 91% to 77% if cytology results were positive. Positive cytology affected patients with extrauterine disease as well, with a 5-year DFS of 43% if cytology was positive, compared with 72% if negative. The effects of lymphovascular invasion and nonendometrioid histology were not evaluated in this study.

Mariani and colleagues[17] reviewed the Mayo Clinic experience for stage IIIa endometrial cancer and stratified patients by positive cytology only (IIIa1) versus uterine serosa or adnexae involvement (IIIa2). For the 37 patients with positive cytology only (IIIa1), histologic grade 3, nonendometrioid histologic subtype, and lymphovascular invasion significantly predicted a poor prognosis with extra-abdominal sites of failure. Of the 22 patients with stage IIIa1 disease and endometrioid histologic subtype but no lymphovascular invasion, none had a recurrence (77% received WAR or phosphorus 32 irradiation). By contrast, of the 15 stage IIIa1 patients with either nonendometrioid histologic subtype or lymphovascular invasion, 60% had

recurrence, and 78% of the recurrences were outside the abdomen (80% received WAR or ^{32}P). Patients with uterine serosal involvement in this series (n = 6) had a 100% relapse rate in extra-abdominal sites, whereas those with adnexal involvement (n = 8) had a rate of only 25%. Ashman and associates[59] confirmed the poor prognosis associated with solitary serosal involvement (n = 15), reporting a 5-year DFS of 41.5%, with 86% of failures in extraabdominal sites.

The current data support the negative prognostic significance of positive cytology for both uterine-confined and extrauterine endometrial cancer. For uterine-confined disease, risk factors such as grade 2/3, lymphovascular invasion, deep myometrial invasion, and nonendometrioid histology influence the prognosis of patients with positive cytology. Therefore, only patients with grade 1 endometrioid histology, myometrial invasion less than one-half without lymphovascular invasion, and uterine-confined disease have unaffected survival when peritoneal cytology is positive.

Therapy directed at patients with positive peritoneal cytology who are at high risk for recurrence must include strategies to address distant (extra-abdominal) as well as abdominal/pelvic failure patterns, including systemic and tumor volume–directed radiation therapies. Systemic therapy can include progestational agents or chemotherapy. Piver and coworkers[60] reviewed a prospective trial of patients with endometrial carcinoma, confined to the uterus except for malignant peritoneal cytology, treated with 1 year of progesterone (Megace, 160 mg/day) and tumor volume–directed radiation therapy (vaginal versus pelvic radiation). Eighty percent of patients underwent second-look laparoscopy, and 95% were free of disease with negative cytology. The remaining two patients with persistent malignant cytology received an additional year of progesterone and had negative cytology results at third-look laparoscopy. In this study, 89% of patients had grade 1/2 histology, 66% had myometrial invasion less than one-half, 98% had endometrioid histology, 80% had estrogen receptor–positive disease, and 90% had progesterone receptor–positive disease. No patient had developed recurrent endometrial cancer, with a median follow-up of 63 months. Of interest, Hirai and colleagues[61] monitored 34 patients with positive cytology by repeat cytologic analysis via a peritoneal catheter placed intraabdominally when the abdomen was closed at 7 and 14 days after following surgery. Only one patient (3%) had persistence of positive peritoneal cytology at day 14. A GOG trial[62] of advanced/recurrent endometrial cancer treated with medroxy progesterone acetate (200 mg/day) revealed response rates of 37% for progesterone receptor–positive and 8% for progesterone receptor–negative cancer. Therefore, for patients whose cancer is confined to the uterus except for positive peritoneal cytology and who have receptor-positive disease associated with low-risk pathologic features, adjuvant progestational agents with or without tumor-directed radiotherapy is acceptable adjuvant treatment.

The use of chemotherapy and the field definitions of volume-directed irradiation have been previously reviewed. Treatment for patients with positive cytology and high-risk pathologic features needs to be individualized. Radiotherapeutic options include volume-directed therapy that can include WAR, pelvic irradiation (with or without PA nodes), or vaginal brachytherapy alone, depending on the expected locoregional patterns of failure. Systemic options include chemotherapy versus progestational agents, depending on the level of risk and receptor status. Because there is no standard treatment for patients with positive peritoneal cytology, clinical research trials such as those described earlier and other ongoing trials should be considered.

STAGE IV ENDOMETRIAL CANCER

According to FIGO criteria, stage IVa endometrial cancer represents locally advanced disease with invasion of the bladder or rectal mucosa. Patients with any peritoneal implants or distant metastasis (including positive inguinal lymph nodes) meet criteria for stage IVb disease.[2] Stage IV endometrial cancer accounts for just 3% to 13% of all cases, yet it is responsible for 23% of cancer-related deaths in the first year after diagnosis.[2,63-65] The 5-year survival rate for patients with stage IV endometrial cancer ranges from 10% to 25%.[64,65]

What is the optimal management of stage IVa endometrial cancer?

Stage IVa disease is defined by the FIGO staging system as tumor invasion of the bladder or rectal mucosa. Fewer than 5% of all patient with endometrial cancer present with this stage. Overall outcome for these patients is poor. The major controversy in this group of patients centers on the role of surgical intervention, specifically the role of cytoreductive surgery, which may include exenteration. The treatment approach needs to be customized to the extent of disease. Most studies group and evaluate these patients together with those who have stage IVb disease and suggest that maximum cytoreductive surgery is of benefit.[66-69] Chi and colleagues[69] reported on 55 patients with stage IV disease, of whom six were categorized as stage IVa. This and other studies are reviewed later. Postoperative treatment for these patients typically consists of volume-directed radiation therapy, systemic chemotherapy, or both.

What is the optimal management of stage IVb endometrial cancer?

The poor prognosis associated with stage IV disease results, at least in part, from the limited efficacy of radiation therapy, chemotherapy, and hormone therapy against large-volume tumors. With this in mind, attention has been directed toward the role of cytoreductive surgery for advanced metastatic endometrial cancer, the objective being to initiate adjuvant therapy with only minimal residual disease.

Greer and Hamberger[41] reported on 31 patients with intraperitoneal metastases of stage III or IV endometrial cancer treated with postoperative WAR. Ten patients with stage IV disease were left with residual disease of 2 cm or less and had a 5-year survival rate of 70%. There were no 5-year survivors among patients with residual disease measuring greater than 2 cm. Although this study included patients with both stage III and stage IV disease, was of limited size, and did not state the precise extent of initial or residual disease, it was one of the earliest to suggest that adjuvant therapy for advanced endometrial cancer is more successful in the setting of small-volume residual disease.

More recent studies have demonstrated that the prognosis for patients with stage IV endometrial cancer, without an attempt at surgical intervention, is extremely poor. In 1994, Goff and coworkers[66] reported their experience with 47 patients with stage IV endometrial cancer. Twenty-nine patients underwent cytoreductive surgery leaving no "bulky" residual disease, although the specific diameter of tumor residuum was not directly stated. In this study, the group of patients submitted to cytoreductive surgery had a significantly longer median survival time (19 mo) than did the 18 patients who did not undergo primary surgical exploration because of presumed unresectable disease (8 mo). These data clearly demonstrate the prognostic value of cytoreductive surgery leaving "nonbulky" residual disease. McMeekin and coworkers[67] recently reported similar results among 51 patients with stage IV endometrial cancer. The median survival time for patients undergoing surgery (72% of whom had <2 cm residual disease) was 17 months, compared with 6 months if primary surgery was not undertaken. Collectively, these reports indicate that initial surgery has therapeutic as well as diagnostic value; however, the varying surgical selection criteria used in these studies precludes an accurate assessment of true survival benefit.

Two large series have specifically evaluated the survival impact of cytoreductive surgery for stage IV endometrial cancer. Chi and colleagues[69] from the Memorial Sloan-Kettering Cancer Center reported on 55 patients with stage IV endometrial cancer treated with primary surgery. Overall survival was highly correlated with the amount of cytoreductive surgery performed. Forty-four percent of patients were left with optimal (≤2 cm) residual disease and had a median survival time of 31 months. This was a significant advantage compared with patients who underwent cytoreduction but were left with suboptimal (>2 cm) residual disease (12 months) or with patients who had unresectable carcinomatosis (3 months). Furthermore, the authors found no statistically significant difference in survival between those patients with small-volume metastatic disease (≤2 cm) before cytoreduction and those with initially large-volume disease (>2 cm) who

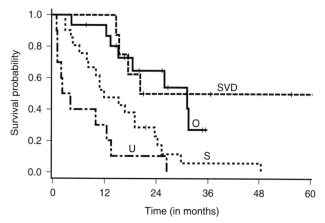

Figure 20–1. Survival of patients with stage IV endometrial carcinoma based on the extent of tumor cytoreduction. SVD, optimally cytoreduced with initial small-volume metastatic disease; O, optimally cytoreduced with initial large-volume metastatic disease; S, suboptimally cytoreduced; U, unresectable. (From Chi DS, Welshinger M, Venkatraman ES, Barakat RR: The role of surgical cytoreduction in stage IV endometrial carcinoma. Gynecol Oncol 1997;67:56-60.)

achieved cytoreduction to an optimal residual volume (Fig. 20-1). These data suggest that surgery may at least partly counterbalance the prognostic influence of tumor biology, if initial tumor size is taken as a marker of biologic aggressiveness. Investigators from the Johns Hopkins Hospital recently reported their experience with 65 patients undergoing primary surgery for stage IVb endometrial cancer.[68] Optimal surgery, defined as residual tumor nodule of 1 cm or less, was achieved in 55.4% of patients and was the strongest predictor of overall survival. Patients undergoing optimal cytoreduction had a median survival time of 34.3 months, compared with 11.0 months for those patients left with residual disease greater than 1 cm (Fig. 20-2). In this study, patients who were left with

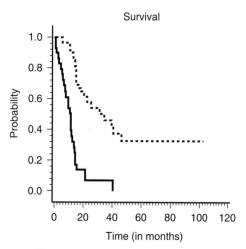

Figure 20–2. Overall survival of patients with stage IVb endometrial carcinoma by residual disease status: *dashed line,* residual disease of 1 cm or less (*n* = 36); *solid line,* residual disease greater than 1 cm (*n* = 29). (From Bristow RE, Zerbe MJ, Rosenshein NB, et al: Stage IVB endometrial carcinoma: The role of cytoreductive surgery and determinants of survival. Gynecol Oncol 2000;78:85-91.)

only microscopic residual disease survived significantly longer (median, 40.6 months) than either patients with optimal but visible residual disease or patients undergoing suboptimal surgery. In summary, the available data suggest that optimal cytoreductive surgery can be accomplished in a significant proportion (44% to 72%) of patients with stage IV endometrial cancer and is consistently associated with improved survival (Table 20-5).

The optimal adjuvant therapy after maximal cytoreductive surgery for stage IVb endometrial cancer has yet to be determined. Postoperative whole abdominopelvic irradiation has been reported to be reasonably efficacious for patients with residual tumor measuring less than 2 cm in maximal diameter.[41,43] However, advanced metastatic endometrial cancer carries a significant risk of distant failure, and adjuvant systemic chemotherapy offers the possible advantage of also treating occult extraperitoneal disease. The most active agents appear to be doxorubicin, cisplatin, and paclitaxel. The combination of doxorubicin and cisplatin has produced overall response rates ranging from 45% to 63%, whereas single-agent doxorubicin therapy is associated with a measurable response in 19% to 27% of patients with advanced or recurrent disease.[70,71] Single-agent paclitaxel has also demonstrated significant activity, with an overall response rate of 36% among chemotherapy-naïve patients with advanced endometrial cancer.[72] Fleming and colleagues,[73] reporting for the GOG, described an overall response rate of 46% for patients with measurable advanced endometrial cancer treated with the combination of cisplatin, doxorubicin, and paclitaxel. Theoretically, the sequential administration of both tumor volume–directed radiation therapy and systemic chemotherapy might provide optimal control of intraperitoneal disease and also reduce the risk of distant failure.[68] The GOG is currently evaluating the efficacy and safety of this combined-modality adjuvant treatment approach for patients with advanced endometrial cancer (Protocol 184). Adjuvant hormone therapy may be a therapeutic alternative for those patients who are considered poor candidates for systemic chemotherapy or irradiation. Among patients with advanced or recurrent endometrial cancer with grade 1 tumor histology or high (≥50 fmol/mg) progesterone receptor content, oral medroxyprogesterone acetate (MPA) is associated with an overall response rate of 37%.[62] Only 8% of cancers with grade 3 tumor histology or low progesterone receptor content respond to such therapy, however.[62]

What is the optimal management of advanced (stage III/IV) uterine papillary serous carcinoma?

The first collected series describing UPSC as a unique histopathologic variant of endometrial cancer were reported independently by Lauchlan[74] and by Hendrickson and associates[39] in the early 1980s. Histologically, these tumors, in comparison with the

Table 20–5. Compiled Studies of Surgery for Stage IV Endometrial Cancer

Study (Ref. No.)	N	Surgical Status	Median Survival Time (mo)	Significance
Goff et al.[66]	29	"No bulky residual"	18	P < .01
	18	No surgery	8	
McMeekin et al.[67]	44	Surgery (72% <2 cm)	17	P = .06
	7	No surgery	6	
Chi et al.[69]	24	≤2 cm	31	P < .01
	21	>2 cm	12	
	10	Unresectable	3	
Bristow et al.[68]	36	≤1 cm	34	P < .01
	29	>1 cm	11	

more common endometrioid adenocarcinomas of the endometrium, more closely resemble serous carcinoma of the ovary and have a distinctly different clinical behavior. Specifically, UPSC has been characterized by an unusual propensity for retroperitoneal, intraperitoneal, and upper abdominal spread.[74-81]

A particularly troublesome feature of UPSC has been the inability to predict extrauterine extension of disease based on the primary tumor pathology.[81-83] This observation has led many authors to advocate routine extended surgical staging, as for ovarian carcinoma, if UPSC pathology is suspected. Those studies that describe patients undergoing omentectomy and peritoneal biopsy in addition to TAH/BSO, peritoneal cytology, and lymph node sampling consistently demonstrate extracorporeal extension of UPSC in 69% to 87% of cases.[80,81,83-85] According to these reports, lymph node metastasis is present in approximately 40% of these cases, and tumor spread to the omentum is discovered in approximately 20% of cases submitted to a rigorous surgicopathologic evaluation.[80-82,86] Geisler and coworkers[81] reported the surgicopathologic findings in 65 cases of UPSC. Twenty-five percent (12 of 48) of patients without grossly evident upper abdominal disease had microscopic abdominal metastases that would not have been detected by the standard endometrial cancer staging operation. Furthermore, 24% of patients with negative lymph nodes had microscopic disease detected in the omentum or abdominal peritoneum. Consequently, extended surgical staging is recommended for all cases in which UPSC pathology is suspected.

Depending on the extent of initial exploration and surgicopathologic sampling, stage IV disease is discovered in 18% to 48% of patients with UPSC.[48,75,76,81,82,86-88] The long-term prognosis in this setting is extremely poor, as evidenced by the reported 5-year survival rates of 0% to 5%.[76,89,90] Recent data indicate, however, that an intensive surgical approach can have a meaningful impact on the clinical course of disease. Investigators from the Johns Hopkins Hospital and the Massachusetts General Hospital reported a combined series of 31 patients with stage IV UPSC submitted to an aggressive attempt at primary cytoreductive surgery.[85] Reflecting the overall poor prognosis of this disease, the median overall survival time for all patients was just 14.4 months, and the 5-year survival rate was 3.9%. Optimal cytoreduction, defined as

residual disease of 1 cm or less in maximal diameter, was achieved in 51.6% of patients and was the most significant predictor of survival outcome. Patients undergoing optimal surgery had a median survival time of 26.2 months, compared with 9.6 months for patients left with suboptimal residual disease. At 24 months, 57.1% of patients with optimal cytoreduction were still alive, compared with 6.7% of patients with large-volume residual disease. Further stratification according to residual tumor burden revealed that patients with only microscopic residual tumor had a significantly longer median survival time (30.4 months) compared with either patients with 0.1 to 1.0 cm residual disease (20.5 months) or patients with suboptimal residual disease (9.6 months) (Fig. 20-3). These data suggest that, as for endometrial cancer in general, a maximal surgical effort is warranted for patients with advanced metastatic UPSC.

Adjuvant treatment strategies for patients with metastatic UPSC continue to evolve. Whole pelvic radiation therapy has been shown to significantly reduce the pelvic relapse rate among patients with stage III disease; however, this group also has a significant risk

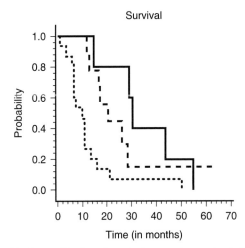

Figure 20–3. Stratification of survival curves by maximal diameter of residual disease (P = .004): *solid line,* microscopic residual (n = 6); *dashed line,* residual disease 0.1 to 1.0 cm (n = 10); *dotted line,* greater than 1 cm residual disease (n = 15). (From Bristow RE, Duska LR, Montz FJ: The role of cytoreductive surgery in the management of stage IV uterine papillary serous carcinoma. Gynecol Oncol 2001;81:92-99.)

of abdominal and extraabdominal failure.[88,90,91] WAR (with pelvic and PA boost) has been used in the adjuvant setting, with long-term survival rates ranging from 50% to 69%.[45,48,91] However, recurrences in extraabdominal sites (liver, lung, supraclavicular lymph node) are frequently observed in patients with advanced-stage UPSC treated with postoperative radiation therapy alone.[91] In an attempt to reduce this risk, systemic chemotherapy has been administered in the adjuvant setting, with mixed results. Early studies used cyclophosphamide, doxorubicin, and cisplatin and yielded objective response rates of 18% to 25% for patients with measurable disease.[89,92] More recently, several groups of investigators have reported favorable results wit therapy based on platinum and paclitaxel.[93-96] Zanotti and coworkers[93] observed objective responses in 89% of patients treated for residual disease after initial surgery and in 64% of patients treated for recurrent UPSC. Using single-agent paclitaxel, Ramondetta and colleagues[96] reported an objective response rate of 77% for patients with advanced or recurrent UPSC.

These data provide a conceptual basis for generating specific treatment strategies based on the surgico-pathologic distribution of metastatic UPSC. Despite a poor long-term prognosis, patients with upper abdominal metastases (stage IVb disease) may derive a significant survival benefit from adjuvant treatment with systemic chemotherapy. Of the available agents, the combination of platinum and paclitaxel has thus far demonstrated the greatest activity and should probably be considered the current standard of care in this setting. Locoregional (stage III) UPSC carries a significant risk of both local and distant relapse. Consequently, these patients may be most appropriately treated with the combined use of sequential platinum- and paclitaxel-based combination chemotherapy and tumor volume–directed irradiation. Contemporary series employing such an approach have reported 5-year survival rates ranging from 31% to 69% for patients with stage III UPSC.[48,84,90] Clearly, additional clinical studies are warranted to better define the most efficacious adjuvant treatment strategies for patients with advanced-stage UPSC.

REFERENCES

1. Jemal A, Thomas A, Murray T, Thun M: Cancer Statistics, 2002. CA Cancer J Clin 2002;52:23-47.
2. Creasman W, Odicino F, Maisonneuve P, et al: Carcinoma of the corpus uteri. In Pecorrelli S, Creasman WT, Pettersson F, et al. (eds): International Federation of Gynecology and Obstetrics Annual Report on the Results of Treatment in Gynecologic Cancer. J Epidemiol Biostat 1998;3:35-62.
3. Creasman WT, Morrow CP, Bundy BN, et al: Surgicopathologic spread patterns of endometrial cancer: A Gynecologic Oncology Group study. Cancer 1987;60:2035-2041.
4. Zaino R, Whitney C, Brady MF, et al: Simultaneously detected endometrial and ovarian carcinomas: A prospective clinicopathologic study of 74 cases. A Gynecologic Oncology Group Study. Gynecol Oncol 2001;83:355-362.
5. Connell PP, Rotmensch J, Waggoner S, Mundt AJ: The significance of adnexal involvement in endometrial carcinoma. Gynecol Oncol 1999;74:74-79.
6. Takeshima N, Hirai Y, Yano K, et al: Ovarian metastasis in endometrial carcinoma. Gynecol Oncol 1998;70:183-187.
7. Ulbright TM, Roth LM: Metastatic and independent cancers of the endometrium and ovary: A clinicopathologic study of 34 cases. Hum Pathol 1985;16:28-34.
8. Chi DS, Barakat RR: Surgical management of advanced or recurrent endometrial cancer. Surg Clin North Am 2001;81:885-898.
9. Zaino RJ, Unger ER, Whitney C: Synchronous carcinomas of the uterine corpus and ovary. Gynecol Oncol 1984;19:329-335.
10. Eisner RF, Nieberg RK, Berek JS: Synchronous primary neoplasms of the female reproductive tract. Gynecol Oncol 1989;33:335-339.
11. Shenson DL, Gallion HH, Powell DE, Pieretti M: Loss of heterozygosity and genomic instability in synchronous endometrioid tumors of the ovary and endometrium. Cancer 1995;76:650-657.
12. Emmert-Buck MR, Chuaqui R, Zhuang Z, et al: Molecular analysis of synchronous uterine and ovarian endometrioid tumors. Int J Gynecol Pathol 1997;16:143-148.
13. Fujita M, Enomoto T, Wada H, et al: Application of clonal analysis: Differential diagnosis for synchronous primary ovarian and endometrial cancers and metastatic cancer. Am J Clin Pathol 1996;105:350-359.
14. Caduff RF, Svoboda-Newman SM, Bartos RE, et al: Comparative analysis of histologic homologues of endometrial and ovarian carcinoma. Am J Surg Pathol 1998;22:319-326.
15. Lin WM, Forgacs E, Warshal DP, et al: Loss of heterozygosity and mutational analysis of the PTEN/MMAC1 gene in synchronous endometrial and ovarian carcinomas. Clin Cancer Res 1998;4:2577-2583.
16. Mackillop WJ, Pringle JF: Stage III endometrial carcinoma: A review of 90 cases. Cancer 1985;56:2519-2523.
17. Mariani A, Webb MJ, Keeney GL, et al: Assessment of prognostic factors in stage IIIA endometrial cancer. Gynecol Oncol 2002;86:38-44.
18. Potish RA, Twiggs LB, Adcock LL, Prem KA: Role of whole abdominal radiation therapy in the management of endometrial cancer: Prognostic importance of factors indicating peritoneal metastases. Gynecol Oncol 1985;21:80-86.
19. Eifel P, Hendrickson M, Ross J, et al: Simultaneous presentation of carcinoma involving the ovary and the uterine corpus. Cancer 1982;50:163-170.
20. Pearl ML, Johnston CM, Frank TS, Roberts JA: Synchronous dual primary ovarian and endometrial carcinomas. Int J Gynecol Obstet 1993;43:305-312.
21. Morrow P, Bundy BN, Kurman RJ, et al: Relation between surgical-pathological risk factors and outcome in clinical stage I and II carcinoma of the endometrium: A Gynecological Oncology Group study. Gynecol Oncol 1991;40:55-65.
22. McMeekin DS, Lashbrook D, Gold M, et al: Analysis of FIGO stage IIIc endometrial cancer patients. Gynecol Oncol 2001;81:273-278.
23. Greven KM, Lanciano RM, Corn B, et al: Pathologic stage III endometrial carcinoma: Prognostic factors and patterns of recurrence. Cancer 1993;71:3697-3702.
24. Kilgore LC, Partridge EE, Alvarez RD, et al: Adenocarcinoma of the endometrium: Survival comparisons of patients with and without pelvic node sampling. Gynecol Oncol 1995;56:29-33.
25. Mariani A, Webb MJ, Galli L, Podratz KC: Potential therapeutic role of para-aortic lymphadenectomy in node-positive endometrial cancer. Gynecol Oncol 2000;76:348-356.
26. Corn BW, Lanciano RM, Greven KM, et al: Endometrial cancer with para-aortic adenopathy: Patterns of failure and opportunities for cure. Int J Radiat Oncol Biol Phys 1992;24:223-227.
27. Schorge JO, Molpus KL, Goodman A, et al: The effect of post-surgical therapy on stage III endometrial carcinoma. Gynecol Oncol 1996;63:34-39.
28. Hicks ML, Piver MS, Puretz JL, et al: Survival in patients with paraaortic lymph node metastases from endometrial adenocarcinoma clinically limited to the uterus. Int J Radiat Oncol Biol Phys 1993;26:607-611.
29. Rose PG, Cha SD, Tak WK, et al: Radiation therapy for surgically proven para-aortic node metastasis in endometrial carcinoma. Int J Radiat Oncol Biol Phys 1992;24:229-233.
30. Mundt AJ, Murphy KT, Rotmensch J, et al: Surgery and post-operative radiation therapy in FIGO Stage IIIC endometrial carcinoma. Int J Radiat Oncol Biol Phys 2001;50:1154-1160.

31. Nelson G, Randall M, Sutton G, et al: FIGO stage IIIC endometrial carcinoma with metastases confined to pelvic lymph nodes: Analysis of treatment outcomes, prognostic variables, and failure patterns following adjuvant radiation therapy. Gynecol Oncol. 1999;75:211-214.

32. Lurain JR, Rice BL, Rademaker AW, et al: Prognostic factors associated with recurrence in clinical stage I adenocarcinoma of the endometrium. Obstet Gynecol 1991;78:63-69.

33. Axelrod J, Bundy B, Roy T, et al: Advanced endometrial carcinoma (EC) treated with whole abdominal irradiation (WAI): A Gynecologic Oncology Group (GOG) study. Proceedings of the Society of Gynecologic Oncologists, No. 99, 1995.

34. Aalders JG, Abeler V, Kolstad P: Clinical (stage III) as compared to subclinical intrapelvic extrauterine tumor spread in endometrial carcinoma: A clinical and histopathological study of 175 patients. Gynecol Oncol 1984;17:64-74.

35. Bedwinek J, Galakatas A, Camel M, et al: Stage I grade III adenocarcinoma of the endometrium treated with surgery and irradiation: Sites of failure and correlation of failure rate with irradiation technique. Cancer 1984;54:40-47.

36. Bruckman JE, Bloomer WD, Marck A, et al: Stage III adenocarcinoma of the endometrium: Two prognostic groups. Gynecol Oncol 1980;9:12-17.

37. Eifel PJ, Ross J, Hendrickson M, et al: Adenocarcinoma of the endometrium: Analysis of 256 cases with disease limited to the uterine corpus: Treatment comparisons. Cancer 1983;52:1026-1031.

38. Genest P, Drouin P, Girard A, Gerig L: Stage III carcinoma of the endometrium: A review of 41 cases. Gynecol Oncol 1987;26:77-86.

39. Hendrickson M, Ross J, Eifel P, et al: Uterine papillary serous carcinoma: A highly malignant form of endometrial carcinoma. Am J Surg Pathol 1982;6:93-108.

40. McMeekin DS, Lashbrook D, Gold M, et al: Nodal distribution and its significance in FIGO stage IIIc endometrial cancer. Gynecol Oncol 2001;82:375-379.

41. Greer BE, Hamberger AD: Treatment of intraperitoneal metastatic adenocarcinoma of the endometrium by the whole-abdomen moving strip technique and pelvic boost irradiation. Gynecol Oncol 1983;16:365-373.

42. Loeffler JS, Rosen EM, Niloff JM, et al: Whole abdominal irradiation for tumors of the uterine corpus. Cancer 1988;61:1332-1335.

43. Martinez A, Podratz K, Schray M, Malkasian G: Results of whole abdominopelvic irradiation with nodal boost for patients with endometrial cancer at high risk of failure in the peritoneal cavity. Hematol Oncol Clin North Am 1988;2:431-446.

44. Gibbons S, Martinez A, Schray M, et al: Adjuvant whole abdominopelvic irradiation for high risk endometrial carcinoma. Int J Radiat Oncol Biol Phys 1991;21:1019-1025.

45. Potish RA: Abdominal radiotherapy for cancer of the uterine cervix and endometrium. Int J Radiat Oncol Biol Phys 1989;16:1453-1458.

46. Frank AH, Tseng PC, Haffty BG, et al: Adjuvant whole-abdominal radiation therapy in uterine papillary serous carcinoma. Cancer 1991;68:1516-1519.

47. Grice J, Ek M, Greer B, et al: Uterine papillary serous carcinoma: Evaluation of long-term survival in surgically staged patients. Gynecol Oncol 1998;69:69-73.

48. Smith RS, Kapp DS, Chen Q, Teng NN: Treatment of high-risk uterine cancer with whole abdominopelvic radiation therapy. Int J Radiat Oncol Biol Phys 2000;48:767-778.

49. Stewart K, Martinez A, Weiner S, et al: Ten-year outcome including patterns of failure and toxicity for adjuvant whole abdominopelvic irradiation in high-risk and poor histologic feature patients with endometrial carcinoma. Int J Radiat Oncol Biol Phys 2002;54:527-535.

50. Small W Jr, Mahadevan A, Roland P, et al: Whole-abdominal radiation in endometrial carcinoma: An analysis of toxicity, patterns of recurrence, and survival. Cancer J 2000;6:394-400.

51. Aoki J, Kase H, Watanabe M, et al: Stage III endometrial cancer: Analysis of prognostic factors and failure patterns after adjuvant chemotherapy. Gynecol Oncol 2001;83:1-5.

52. Mundt AJ, McBride R, Rotmensch J, et al: Significant pelvic recurrence in high-risk pathologic stage I-IV endometrial carcinoma patients after adjuvant chemotherapy alone: Implications for adjuvant radiation therapy. Int J Radiat Oncol Biol Phys 2001;50:1145-1153.

53. Frigerio L, Mangili G, Aletti G, et al: Concomitant radiotherapy and paclitaxel for high-risk endometrial cancer: First feasibility study. Gynecol Oncol 2001;81:53-57.

54. Greven K, Winter K, Underhill K, et al: Preliminary analysis of RTOG 9708: Adjuvant postoperative irradiation combined with cisplatin/Taxol chemotherapy following surgery for patients with high-risk endometrial cancer. Int J Radiat Oncol Biol Phys 51:3, 55.

55. Zaino RJ, Kurman RJ, Diana KL, Morrow CP: Pathologic models to predict outcome for women with endometrial adenocarcinoma. Cancer 1996;77:1115-1121.

56. Milosevic MF, Dembo AJ, Thomas GM: The clinical significance of malignant peritoneal cytology in stage I endometrial carcinoma. Int J Gynecol Cancer 1992;2:225-235.

57. Kadar N, Homesley HD, Malfetano JH: Positive peritoneal cytology is an adverse factor in endometrial carcinoma only if there is other evidence of extrauterine disease. Gynecol Oncol 1992;46:145-149.

58. Takeshima N, Nishida H, Tabata T, et al: Positive peritoneal cytology in endometrial dancer: Enhancement of other prognostic indicators. Gynecol Oncol 2001;82:470-473.

59. Ashman JB, Connell PP, Yamada D, et al: Outcome of endometrial carcinoma patients with involvement of the uterine serosa. Gynecol Oncol 2001;82:338-343.

60. Piver MS, Recio FO, Baker TR, Hempling RE: A prospective trial of progesterone therapy for malignant peritoneal cytology in patients with endometrial carcinoma. Gynecol Oncol 1992;47:373-376.

61. Hirai Y, Takeshima N, Kato T, Hasumi K: Malignant potential of positive peritoneal cytology in endometrial cancer. Obstet Gynecol 2001;97:725-728.

62. Thigpen JT, Brady MF, Alvarez RD, et al: Oral medroxyprogesterone acetate in the treatment of advanced or recurrent endometrial cancer: A dose-response study by the Gynecologic Oncology Group. J Clin Oncol 1999;17:1736-1744.

63. Wolfson AH, Sightler SE, Markoe AM, et al: The prognostic significance of surgical staging for carcinoma of the endometrium. Gynecol Oncol 1992;45:142-146.

64. Vardi JR, Tadros GH, Anselmo MT, Rafla SD: The value of exploratory laparotomy in patients with endometrial carcinoma according to the new International Federation of Gynecology and Obstetrics staging. Obstet Gynecol 1992;80:204-208.

65. Pliskow S, Penalver M, Averette HE: Stage III and stage IV endometrial carcinoma: A review of 41 cases. Gynecol Oncol 1990;38:210-215.

66. Goff BA, Goodman A, Muntz HG, et al: Surgical stage IV endometrial carcinoma: A study of 47 cases. Gynecol Oncol 1994;52:237-240.

67. McMeekin DS, Garcia M, Gold M, et al: Stage IV endometrial cancer: Survival, recurrence, and role of surgery. American Society of Clinical Oncology 2001 Annual Meeting, abstract 821.

68. Bristow RE, Zerbe MJ, Rosenshein NB, et al: Stage IVB endometrial carcinoma: The role of cytoreductive surgery and determinants of survival. Gynecol Oncol 2000;78:85-91.

69. Chi DS, Welshinger M, Venkatraman ES, Barakat RR: The role of surgical cytoreduction in stage IV endometrial carcinoma. Gynecol Oncol 1997;67:56-60.

70. Thigpen T, Blessing J, Homesley H, et al: Phase III trial of doxorubicin +/− cisplatin in advanced or recurrent endometrial carcinoma: A Gynecologic Oncology Group (GOG) study [abstract 830]. Proc Am Soc Clin Oncol 1993;12:261.

71. Aapro M, Bolis G, Chevallier B, et al: An EORTC-GCCG randomized phase II trial of doxorubicin (dox) versus doxcisplatin (CDDP) in endometrial carcinoma [abstract 885]. Proc Am Soc Clin Oncol 1994;13:275.

72. Ball HG, Blessing JA, Lentz SS, et al: A phase II trial of paclitaxel in patients with advanced or recurrent adenocarcinoma of the endometrium: A Gynecologic Oncology Group study. Gynecol Oncol 1996;62:278-281.

73. Fleming GF, Fowler JM, Waggoner SE, et al: Phase I trial of escalating doses of paclitaxel combined with fixed doses of cisplatin and doxorubicin in advanced endometrial cancer and other gynecologic malignancies: A Gynecologic Oncology Group study. J Clin Oncol 2001;19:1021-1029.

74. Lauchlan SC: Tubal (serous) carcinoma of the endometrium. Arch Pathol Lab Med 1981;105:615-618.

75. Chambers JT, Merino M, Kohorn EI, et al: Uterine papillary serous carcinoma. Obstet Gynecol 1987;69:109-113.

76. Carcangiu ML, Chambers JT: Uterine papillary serous carcinoma: A study of 108 cases with emphasis on the prognostic significance of associated endometrioid carcinoma, absence of invasion, and concomitant ovarian carcinoma. Gynecol Oncol 1992;47:298-305.

77. Jeffrey JF, Krepart GV, Lotocki RJ: Papillary serous adenocarcinoma of the endometrium. Obstet Gynecol 1986;67:670-674.

78. Matthews RP, Hutchinson-Colas J, Maiman M, et al: Papillary serous and clear cell type lead to poor prognosis of endometrial carcinoma in black women. Gynecol Oncol 1997;65:206-212.

79. Christopherson WM, Alberhasky RC, Connelly PJ: Carcinoma of the endometrium II: Papillary adenocarcinoma: A clinical pathologic study of 46 cases. Am J Clin Pathol 1982;77:534-540.

80. Goff BA, Kato D, Schmidt RA, et al: Uterine papillary serous carcinoma: Patterns of metastatic spread. Gynecol Oncol 1994;54:264-268.

81. Geisler JP, Geisler HE, Melton ME, Wiemann MC: What staging surgery should be performed on patients with uterine papillary serous carcinoma? Gynecol Oncol 1999;74:465-467.

82. Gitsch G, Friedlander ML, Wain G, Hacker NF: Uterine papillary serous carcinoma: A clinical study. Cancer 1995;75:2239-2243.

83. O'Hanlan KA, Levine PA, Harbatkin D, et al: Virulence of papillary endometrial carcinoma. Gynecol Oncol 1990;37:12-19.

84. Bristow RE, Asrari F, Trimble EL, Montz FJ: Extended surgical staging for uterine papillary serous carcinoma: Survival outcome of locoregional (stage I-III) disease. Gynecol Oncol 2001;81:279-286.

85. Bristow RE, Duska LR, Montz FJ: The role of cytoreductive surgery in the management of stage IV uterine papillary serous carcinoma. Gynecol Oncol 2001;81:92-99.

86. Tay EH, Ward BG: The treatment of uterine papillary serous carcinoma (UPSC): Are we doing the right thing? Int J Gynecol Cancer 1999;9:463-469.

87. Kato DT, Ferry JA, Goodman A, et al: Uterine papillary serous carcinoma (UPSC): A clinicopathologic study of 30 cases. Gynecol Oncol 1995;59:384-389.

88. Ward BG, Wright RG, Free K: Papillary carcinomas of the endometrium. Gynecol Oncol 1990;39:347-351.

89. Nicklin JL, Copeland LJ: Endometrial papillary serous carcinoma: Patterns of spread and treatment. Clin Obstet Gynecol 1996;39:686-695.

90. Craighead PS, Sait K, Stuart GC, et al: Management of aggressive histologic variants of endometrial carcinoma at the Tom Baker Cancer Centre between 1984 and 1994. Gynecol Oncol 2000;77:248-253.

91. Mallipeddi P, Kapp DS, Teng NNH: Long-term survival with adjuvant whole abdominopelvic irradiation for uterine papillary serous carcinoma. Cancer 1993;71:3076-3081.

92. Levenback C, Burke TW, Silva E, et al: Uterine papillary serous carcinoma (UPSC) treated with cisplatin, doxorubicin, and cyclophosphamide (PAC). Gynecol Oncol 1992;46:317-321.

93. Zanotti KM, Belinson JL, Kennedy AW, et al: The use of paclitaxel and platinum-based chemotherapy in uterine papillary serous carcinoma. Gynecol Oncol 1999;74:272-277.

94. Resnik E, Taxy JB: Neoadjuvant chemotherapy in uterine papillary serous carcinoma. Gynecol Oncol 1996;62:123-127.

95. Le TD, Yamada SD, Rutgers JL, DiSaia PJ: Complete response of a stage IV uterine papillary serous carcinoma to neoadjuvant chemotherapy with Taxol and carboplatin. Gynecol Oncol 1999;73:461-463.

96. Ramondetta L, Burke TW, Levenback C, et al: Treatment of uterine papillary serous carcinoma with paclitaxel. Gynecol Oncol 2001;82:156-161.

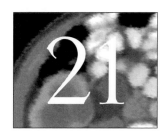

TREATMENT OF RECURRENT ENDOMETRIAL CANCER: CHEMOTHERAPY, HORMONAL THERAPY, AND RADIOTHERAPY

Arno J. Mundt, Grazia Artioli, and Gini F. Fleming

 MAJOR CONTROVERSIES

- **Is salvage radiation therapy effective in patients with endometrial cancer who have relapse after surgery alone?**
- **Does surgery have a role in recurrent endometrial cancer?**
- **Should hormone therapy always be tried before the institution of cytotoxic chemotherapy?**
- **Does paclitaxel/doxorubicin/cisplatin represent standard therapy?**
- **What are the future directions for treatment of recurrent endometrial cancer?**

Endometrial carcinoma is usually diagnosed at an early stage, and it is often perceived as a relatively benign cancer. Only 5% of women have stage IV disease at the time of diagnosis.[1] However, more than 15% of women with endometrial cancer will die from the disease.[2] The most common sites of recurrence are the vaginal vault, pelvis, abdomen, para-aortic nodes, and lung.[3] Once the disease recurs or metastasizes, the prognosis is poor; median survival in Gynecologic Oncology Group (GOG) trials of women treated with either hormonal therapy or chemotherapy has usually been about 1 year or less.[4,5] The serum CA 125 concentration is frequently elevated in women with recurrent disease. When elevated, it may be a useful adjunct in monitoring the response to systemic therapy.[6,7]

RADIATION THERAPY

Is salvage radiation therapy effective in endometrial cancer patients who have relapse after surgery alone?

Approximately half of those patients with endometrial carcinoma who experience relapse after surgery alone have recurrence in the pelvis, including 50% in the vaginal vault.[8,9] Women with an isolated pelvic relapse represent a favorable subset of patients with recurrent disease. Meigs[10] initially reported on the benefit of salvage radiation therapy (RT) in 1929. Today, most women with recurrent disease limited to the pelvis undergo RT, with curative intent.

Table 21–1. Salvage Radiation Therapy in Locally Recurrent Endometrial Carcinoma

Author	Year	N	5-Year Local Control (%)	5-Year Survival (%)
Pirtoli et al[16]	1980	48	Not stated	53*
Greven and Olds[15]	1987	18	44‡	33§
Curran et al[13]	1988	47	48	31
Kuten et al[12]	1989	51	35†	18
Hoekstra et al[20]	1993	26	84*	44
Morgan et al[17]	1993	34¶	60	68
Sears et al[14]	1994	45	54	44
Hart et al[19]	1998	26	65	53
Jereczek-Fossa et al[11]	2000	73	48*	25
Wylie et al[18]	2000	58	65	53

*Crude result.
†Locoregional control.
‡3-Year minimum follow-up.
§No evidence of disease (3-10 year follow-up).
¶All patients had isolated vaginal recurrences.

Table 21-1 summarizes the largest published series of salvage RT in patients with recurrent endometrial carcinoma. Five-year survival rates vary considerably in these reports, ranging from 18% to 68%.[11-20] The best outcomes are seen in women with isolated vaginal recurrences,[12,13,16,18] a long recurrence-free interval,[14,17] low-grade disease,[13,19] adenocarcinoma histology,[18,19] and no prior RT.[17] Local control is achieved in 35% to 84% of patients,[11-20] with the majority of series reporting rates between 40% and 60%.[11,13-15,17,19] One of the most important factors associated with local control is tumor size.[15,18,20] Wylie and colleagues[18] reported 5-year local control rates of 80% and 54% in tumors of 2 cm or less and tumors greater than 2 cm, respectively ($P = .02$). In a review of 26 patients with local recurrence, Hoekstra and associates[20] noted locoregional relapse in 6% of tumors of 4 cm or less, compared with 33% of tumors greater than 4 cm.

The optimal RT approach in these patients involves a combination of pelvic RT and either interstitial or intracavitary brachytherapy. However, small-volume tumors may be treated with vaginal brachytherapy alone, especially if the lesion has been excised. Interstitial brachytherapy has been shown to be useful in patients with a suburethral recurrence.[21] High radiation doses (70 to 85 Gy) are required in all patients with local recurrence. Lower doses are associated with poorer tumor control.[13,17] Overall, treatment is well tolerated, with severe complications seen in 3% to 12% of patients, primarily related to the gastrointestinal tract.[11,12,17,20] Unsurprisingly, patients with a history of prior RT are at high risk for severe sequelae.[12]

Although salvage RT is successful in many women with locally recurrent disease, particularly those with small-volume lesions, it is not successful in approximately half of patients with local recurrence after surgery. These results strongly support the need for close follow-up in all patients with endometrial carcinoma who are treated with surgery alone in order to diagnose local recurrences when they are still curable. A more prudent policy is to treat patients who have high-risk features (deep myometrial invasion, cervical involvement, high-grade tumors) at initial diagnosis, given the known benefits of adjuvant RT.[22,23] Technologic advances in RT, including intensity-modulated whole pelvic RT[22,23] and high dose rate (HDR) brachytherapy,[24] allow adjuvant RT to be delivered with fewer side effects than in the past. Attention needs to be devoted to exploring the use of concomitant chemoradiotherapy approaches in patients with bulky disease recurrences.

SURGERY

Does surgery have a role in recurrent endometrial cancer?

Although adjuvant RT reduces the risk of pelvic recurrence after surgery,[25,26] a subset of patients still develops a local relapse. A potentially curative approach to such patients is salvage surgery. Since the initial report by Brunschwig in 1948,[27] several investigators have reported the outcome of locally recurrent endometrial carcinoma treated with salvage surgery.[27-30] In the largest series to date, Barakat and colleagues[29] reviewed the 50-year experience of pelvic exenteration in recurrent endometrial carcinoma at the Memorial Sloan Kettering Cancer Center. Of the 44 women treated, 34 (77%) had undergone prior RT. The majority of patients underwent either total or anterior exenteration. Overall, the 3-year survival rate was 35%, with 20% of patients surviving for 5 years or longer. However, major complications were noted in 80% of patients, including fistulae, sepsis, wound dehiscence, and pulmonary emboli. Morris and coworkers[27] reported a 5-year disease-free survival rate of 45% in 20 patients treated between 1955 and 1988 at the MD Anderson Cancer Center. All patients had a history of prior adjuvant RT. Consistent with the Memorial Sloan Kettering experience, major complications were common, occurring in 60% of patients.

These results suggest that, although salvage surgery is successful in a subset of women with locally recurrent disease after surgery and RT, it is associated with a high risk of serious sequelae. It is imperative to carefully inform patients of the risks and benefits of this approach. Moreover, only women who are likely to benefit should be considered. Ideal candidates are patients with small-volume, central recurrences who are without evidence of extrapelvic metastases or sidewall extension. At surgery, care must be taken to assess for possible metastases in the abdomen, pelvis, and regional lymph nodes. If abdominopelvic metastases, involved lymph nodes, or extension to the sidewall are found, surgery should be aborted. In select patients with residual disease after surgery, some centers advocate the use of intraoperative RT (IORT).[31,32] Unsurprisingly, the best control rates after IORT are seen in patients with microscopic residual disease.[31]

HORMONE THERAPY

Should hormone therapy always be tried before the institution of cytotoxic chemotherapy?

Endometrial cancers frequently express both estrogen (ER) and progesterone (PR) receptors, and high levels of PR expression have been shown to correlate inversely with stage and grade, as well as being a favorable independent prognostic indicator in some series of early-stage disease.[33-37]

Progestins. Kelly and Baker[38] initially described the activity of progestins in the treatment of advanced endometrial cancer in the *New England Journal of Medicine* in 1961. Six of their 21 patients treated with varying doses of progestins responded to therapy. More recent trials, using stricter response criteria, show response rates in the range of 15% to 25%. Older trials used injectable agents, such as hydroxyprogesterone caproate (HPC, Delalutin), but bioavailability and response rates for intramuscularly injected and oral agents were shown to be similar,[39,40] and more recent trials have used oral medroxyprogesterone acetate (MPA, Provera) or megestrol acetate (MGA, Megace). In general, as can be seen in Table 21-2, higher doses of progestins have not produced response rates superior to those seen with standard doses.[4] Appropriate oral doses are 160 mg/day of MGA or 200 mg/day of MPA.

Tamoxifen and other selective estrogen receptor modulators. Tamoxifen, although it increases the rate of endometrial cancer when used as therapy for breast cancer,[41] can inhibit the growth of endometrial cancer xenografts in athymic mice.[42] It has also been tested in a number of small trials for the treatment of recurrent endometrial cancer, and a 1991 review of eight older studies noted a pooled response rate of 22%.[43] This is probably an overestimate of what would be seen in unselected patients with current evaluation and response criteria; a recently reported GOG trial noted a response rate of only 10% in patients with no prior systemic therapy.[44] Response in that study was inversely correlated with grade; 3 (23%) of 13 grade 1 tumors responded, as did 3 (14%) of 21 grade 2 tumors, and 1 (3%) of 24 grade 3 tumors. An earlier GOG trial in women with recurrence after chemotherapy, progestins, or both, reported no responses at all.[45] Other selective estrogen receptor modulators (SERMS) may also have modest activity against endometrial cancer. A preliminary report on a trial using arzoxifene noted confirmed responses in 7 (22%) of 32 patients, as well as two unconfirmed responses, in a group of women selected for potential endocrine sensitivity (ER- or PR-positive tumors or grade 1 or 2 tumors of endometrioid histology).[46] A second trial rated a response rate of 31%, also in patients selected for potential hormone sensitivity.[46a]

Administration of tamoxifen has been reported to increase expression of the PR in both benign endometrial tissues[47] and endometrial carcinomas.[48,49] This observation has generated trials of combination and sequential therapies with progestins and tamoxifen, but there is no clear evidence that this strategy is superior to therapy with progestins alone. One small Eastern Cooperative Oncology Group (ECOG) randomized phase II trial noted a response rate of 19% with the combination of tamoxifen and MGA, compared with 20% for MGA alone.[50] The GOG recently reported a 27% response rate from a phase II trial of alternating 3-week courses of MGA and tamoxifen.[51]

Other hormonal agents. Gonadotropin-releasing hormone (GnRH) agonists have been tested in a number of small trials. Because most patients with endometrial cancer have undergone bilateral oophorectomy, any effect of these agents could not involve modulation of ovarian hormone production. However, endometrial cancer cells are known to express GnRH receptors,[52,53] and both agonists and antagonists to GnRH can have antiproliferative effects in vitro,[54,55] although these effects are not seen in all studies.[56,57] One of four small published trials showed a 28% response rate,[58] and the others reported 0%, 8% and 11% response rates, respectively.[59,60,60a] Evidence of activity for this group of agents must be considered unconfirmed.

Estrogens in postmenopausal or oophorectomized women result primarily from the conversion of adrenal androgens to estrogens in peripheral adipose tissues by the enzyme aromatase. Significant amounts of aromatase are also found in the stroma of endometrial cancer.[61] There is one case report of a partial response of a progestin-refractory endometrial stromal sarcoma to letrozole.[62] Aromatase inhibitors have been tested in a limited fashion in endometrial carcinoma. The GOG noted only 2 responses (9%) in a trial of anastrazole in 23 patients, 4 of whom had received prior progestin therapy. Fourteen of the patients in that trial had grade 3 histology, nine had grade 2, and none had grade 1. Both of the responders had grade 2 tumors.[63] A preliminary report of a National Cancer Institute of Canada trial evaluating letrozole noted two partial responses among the first 10 evaluable patients.[64]

Table 21–2. Select Trials of Hormone Therapy

Author	Year	Agent	Dose	N	Response Rate (%)	Median Overall Survival Time (mo)	Comments
Progestins							
Reifenstein[108]	1971	HPC	≥1.0 g/wk	314	30	13.6	
Thigpen et al[109]	1986	MPA	150 mg/day	331	18	10.5	
Lentz et al[76]	1996	MGA	800 mg/day	54	24	7.6	
Thigpen et al[4]	1999	MPA	200 mg/day vs 1000 mg/day	145 154	25 15	11.1 7.0	Randomized trial
SERMs							
Slavik et al[45]	1984	TAM	20-40 mg/day	19	0	—	Patients resistant to progestins and/or chemotherapy
Klijn et al[46]	2000	Arzoxifene	20 mg/day	32	22	—	Preliminary result; patients selected for potential hormone sensitivity
McMeekin et al[46a]	2003	Arzoxifene	20 mg/day	31	—	—	Patients selected for potential hormone sensitivity
Thigpen et al[44]	2001	TAM	40 mg/day	68	10	8.8	No prior progestins
Progestins and Tamoxifen							
Fiorica et al[51]	2000	MGA + TAM	MGA 160 mg/day × 3 wk, followed by TAM 40 mg/day × 3 wk	61	27	14	Alternating drugs 56 patients evaluable for response
Panda et al[50]	2001	MGA vs TAM + MGA	MGA 160 mg/day vs TAM 20 mg/day + MGA 160 mg/day	20 42	20 19	12.6 8.6	Randomized phase II trial Both agents taken simultaneously in combination arm
GnRH Agonists							
Jeyarajah et al[58]	1995	Leuprolide	3.75-7.5 mg	32	28	—	Half of patients had prior progestins; one received goserelin instead of leuprolide
Covens et al[59]	1997	Leuprolide	7.5 mg q 28d	25	0	6	Some patients with prior progestins
Lhomme et al[60]	1998	Triptorelin	3.75 mg q 28d	28	8.7	7.2	Two patients with prior progestins, four with prior chemotherapy
Asbury et al[60a]	2002	Goserelin	3.6 mg q 28d	40	11	7.3	
Aromatase Inhibitors							
Rose et al[63]	2000	Anastrozole	1 mg/day	23	9	6	No grade I tumors treated
Sidhu et al[64]	2001	Letrozole	2.5 mg/day	10	20	—	Preliminary report
Ardrogens							
Covens et al[64a]	2003	Danazol	400 mg/day	25	0	14.4	4 patients with elevation in liver enzymes

GnRH, gonadotropin-releasing hormone; HPC, hydroxyl progesterone caproate; MGA, megestrol acetate; MPA, medroxyprogesterone acetate; SERMs, selective estrogen receptor modulators; TAM, tamoxifen.

Other hormonal agents have not yet been shown to have activity in endometrial carcinoma. A trial of danazol showed hepatic txicity in four patients but no responders among twenty-five subjects.[64a] Caution should be used in concluding that an agent is inactive based on small trials of hormonal therapy, because in unselected groups of patients the number who is potentially sensitive might, by chance, be quite small.

Predictive factors for response to hormonal therapy. Factors that have been found to predict for response to progestins and, to a limited extent, to other hormonal therapy, include well-differentiated tumors, long interval between diagnosis and tumor recurrence, and high levels of ERs and PRs, with receptor levels being an independent predictive factor.[65] Attempts have been made to standardize definitions of ER and PR positivity so that patients with endometrial cancer could be selected for hormonal therapy in a manner similar to breast cancer patients.[66,67] A summary of the older literature reported a response rate of 86% in PR-positive patients and only 7% in PR-negative patients.[68] More recent results also suggest a predictive power for receptor status, but they note more modest response rates in PR-positive tumors. For example, the GOG obtained a combined response rate of 37% in PR-positive patients, compared with 7% in PR-negative patients, in their randomized trial of high-versus low-dose MPA. In that trial, receptor status was evaluated locally and was available for only 132 of 299 patients. Grade was also predictive; the response rate was 37% for grade 1 tumors, 23% for grade 2 tumors, and only 9% for grade 3 tumors. A previous GOG trial used MPA at 150 mg/day in 331 patients, with an 18% overall response rate. In the subset of 51 women with measurable disease and known hormone receptor status, response occurred in 4 (40%) of 10 PR-positive patients and in 5 (12%) of 41 PR-negative patients.[4,43]

Hormone receptor measurements. Although most published data suggest that receptor status is predictive of response to hormone therapy, it is not routinely used to select which patients with endometrial cancer might benefit from treatment, because of a number of concerns: some patients defined as "receptor negative" by various cutoff criteria nonetheless respond to hormones; there can be intratumoral variation of receptor status[37]; there can be heterogeneity between the hormone receptor status of the primary tumor and that of metastases; and results at different metastatic sites can be discordant.[69,70] One recent small study using immunohistochemical methods found that in 20 of 30 cases the metastatic tumor maintained the general ER/PR pattern of the primary, but 33% (6/18) of PR-positive primaries had PR-negative metastases.[70] Biopsy of the metastatic disease site for prediction of hormone responsiveness is not always clinically practical. Interestingly, some of the early work in breast cancer suggested similar high rates of discordance between receptor status of primary and metastatic tumors. One series reported that 6 of 9 ER-positive patients developed ER-negative metastases and 4 of 5

PR-positive primary tumors developed PR-negative metastases.[71] In primary breast cancer, positive receptor status does not guarantee response of metastatic disease to hormones, although negative receptor status makes such a response very unlikely.

In older reports, PR was assayed by the biochemical DCC (dextran-charcoal-coated) assay, and there were concerns about contamination with normal adjacent endometrial tissue, which would result in false-positive findings.[72,73] This is not an issue with immunohistochemical assays, but other concerns arise. There are two isoforms of the PR receptor, PRA and PRB, and both of these proteins are expressed in hormone-dependent cancers. There is evidence that a large proportion of tumors expresses a predominance of one or the other isoform. PR-specific antibodies may fail to detect PRB in formalin-fixed, wax-embedded tissue despite their ability to do so by immunoblot analysis.[74] This is of particular concern in the treatment of endometrial cancer, because some recent work suggests that progesterone acts principally through PRB receptors to inhibit cancer cell invasiveness.[75]

Should progestins be used as a first-line therapy in endometrial cancer patients with recurrent disease? Progestins cause weight gain and an increase in thrombotic complications, which are not insignificant issues in a population already predisposed to obesity. However, they are generally less toxic than chemotherapy and can produce durable responses. For example, in the GOG trial of high-dose MGA,[76] overall median survival was only 7.6 months, but the median response duration was 8.9 months, with 4 of 13 responses lasting longer than 18 months and 3 of those still ongoing at the time of publication. Nonetheless, the overall response rate to hormonal therapy in is low. A GOG trial in which unselected patients with advanced or recurrent disease were randomly assigned either to alternating MGA/tamoxifen or to combination chemotherapy was closed because of poor accrual despite the fact that patients assigned to hormonal therapy were crossed over to chemotherapy at the time of progression. It is probable that this reflects discouragement with response rates to hormonal therapy in unselected patients.

Patients with disease that does not require active palliation (e.g., asymptomatic lung metastases) and whose tumors are grade 1 or 2 or are PR positive should consider a trial of hormonal therapy before chemotherapy. Those who respond to an initial trial of hormonal therapy and subsequently relapse should consider a second-line hormonal agent. Poorly differentiated, clear cell, and papillary serous endometrial tumors rarely demonstrate ER or PR expression[77,78] and should generally be treated with chemotherapy initially. This represents a large proportion of women with metastatic disease; about 40% to 50% of patients entered on recent randomized GOG trials for recurrent disease had grade 3 tumors.[79] Patients whose tumors are not hormonally responsive and who are symptomatic because of estrogen deprivation can be considered for palliative estrogen replacement while they undergo other therapies. However, like women receiving anticancer hormonal therapy, they may be at increased risk for deep venous thromboses.

CHEMOTHERAPY

Does paclitaxel/doxorubicin/cisplatin represent standard therapy?

A variety of cytotoxic agents are active in the initial therapy of recurrent endometrial cancer. However, chemotherapy may be toxic in this group of patients, who often are elderly, have frequently received RT to the pelvis, and may have multiple medical comorbidities, including obesity, hypertension, and diabetes. A GOG chemotherapy trial published in 1994 noted that patients entered on the study had a median age of 65 years (range 36 to 90 years), and 68% had prior pelvic RT.[79] However, better supportive care measures have made it possible to use more intensive chemotherapy in this patient population, and newer combination chemotherapy regimens are showing improved response rates.

Results of single-agent trials of commercially available agents in chemotherapy-naïve patients are summarized in Table 21-3, and results in women with previous cytotoxic therapy are summarized in Table 21-4. Only paclitaxel is consistently active in both groups.[80-85] Anthracyclines regularly produce response rates of 20% to 30% as first-line therapy, but, as is the case in ovarian cancer, they appear to have less activity in pretreated patients.[86,87] Alkylating agents, particularly ifosfamide, likewise appear to have activity only in patients without prior chemotherapy.[88] Moreover, ifosfamide, like vincristine and hexamethylmelamine, has been associated with considerable toxicity in this patient population.[68,89,90] An overview of six pre-1975 studies (comprising fewer than 10 patients each) testing 5-fluorouracil noted an overall response rate of 20%[91]; it is possible that response rates would be lower if modern criteria were applied. Most of the patients in the one reported trial of liposomal doxorubicin had prior anthracycline therapy.[92] This drug has less hematologic toxicity than does unencapsulated doxorubicin, and it does not cause alopecia; if meaningful activity can be demonstrated, it may be a useful agent for treatment in a relatively frail group of patients. A GOG trial of liposomal doxorubicin as first-line therapy is ongoing, and several groups are investigating combinations containing liposomal doxorubicin. Trials of thalidomide, topotecan, and oxaliplatin are completed or ongoing.

Table 21–3. Single-Agent Trials in Patients with Endometrial Cancer and no Prior Chemotherapy

Author	Year	Agent	Dose	No. Evaluable	Response Rate (%)
Anthracyclines					
Horten et al[87]	1978	Doxorubicin	50 mg/m²	21	19
Thigpen et al[86]	1979	Doxorubicin	60 mg/m²	43	37
Calero et al[110]	1991	Epirubicin	80 mg/m²	27	26
Taxanes					
Ball et al[80]	1996	Paclitaxel	250 mg/m²/24 hr + G-CSF	28	35.7
Platinum					
Trope et al[111]	1980	Cisplatin	50 mg/m²	11	36
Seski et al[90]	1981	Cisplatin	50-100 mg/m²	26	42
Edmonson et al[112]	1986	Cisplatin	60 mg/m²	14	21
Thigpen et al[84]	1989	Cisplatin	50 mg/m²	49	20
Green et al[85]	1990	Carboplatin	400 mg/m²	23	30
Burke et al[83]	1993	Carboplatin	360 mg/m²	33	33
Alkylating Agents					
Horton et al[87]	1978	Cyclophosphamide	666 mg/m²	19	0
Seski et al[90]	1981	HMM	8 mg/kg/day	20	30
Thigpen et al[113]	1988	HMM	280 mg/m²/day × 14 days	34	9
Barton et al[114]	1989	Ifosfamide	5 g/m²/24 hr	16	12.5
Sutton et al[89]	1996	Ifosfamide	1.2 g/m²/day × 5 days	33	24
Pawinski et al[88]*	1999	Ifosfamide	5 g/m²/24 hr	16	25
		Cyclophosphamide	1200 mg/m²/24 hr	14	14
Vinca Alkaloids					
Thigpen et al[68]	1987	Vinblastine	1.5 mg/m²/day × 5 days	34	12
Broun et al[115]	1993	Vincristine	1.4 mg/m²	33	18
Other					
Omura et al[116]	1978	Methyl-CCNU	150 mg/m² q 6 wk	5	40
Moss et al[117]	1990	Methotrexate	40 mg/m²/wk	33	6
Muss et al[123]	1991	Teriposide (UM 20)	100 mg/wk	5	20
Wadler et al[130]	2003	Topotecan	0.8-1.5 m/m²/day × 5	40	20

CCNU, N-(2-chloroethyl)-N′-cycohexyl-N-nitrosourea; G-CSF, granulocyte colony-stimulating factor; HMM, hexamethylmelamine.
*Randomized phase II trial.

Table 21–4. Single-Agent Trials in Endometrial Cancer Patients with Prior Chemotherapy

Author	Year	Agent	Dose	No. Evaluable	Response Rate (%)
Anthracyclines					
Horton et al[87]	1978	Doxorubicin	50 mg/m^2	9	0
Hilgers et al[118]	1985	Mitoxantrone	10-12 mg/m^2	15	0
Muggia et al[92]	2002	Pegylated liposomal doxorubicin	50 mg/m^2	42	9.5
Taxanes					
Lissoni et al[81]	1996	Paclitaxel	175 mg/m^2/3 hr	19	37
Woo et al[82]	1996	Paclitaxel	170 mg/m^2/3 hr	7	43
Platinum					
Deppe et al[119]	1980	Cisplatin	3 mg/kg	13	31
Thigpen et al[120]	1984	Cisplatin	50 mg/m^2	25	4
Alkylating Agents					
Horton et al[87]	1978	Cyclophosphamide	666 mg/m^2	6	0
Sutton et al[121]	1992	Ifosfamide	1.2 g/m^2/day × 5 days	23	8.6
Pawinski et al[88]*	1999	Ifosfamide	5 g/m^2/24 hr	16	0
		Cyclophosphamide	1200 mg/m^2/24 hr	15	0
Epidophyllotoxins					
Slayton et al[122]	1982	IV etoposide (VP-10)	100 mg/m^2 on days 1, 3, 5	29	3
Muss et al[123]	1991	Teniposide (VM26)	100 mg/m^2/wk	17	6
Rose et al[124]	1996	PO etoposide (VP-16)	50 mg/m^2/day × 21 days	21	0
Other					
Jackson et al[125]	1986	Vincristine	0.25-0.5 mg/m^2 CIV† × 5 days	5	0
von Hoff et al[126]	1991	Fludarabine	18 mg/m^2/day × 5 days	19	0
Moore et al[127]	1999	Actinomycin D	2 mg/m^2	25	12
Miller et al[131]	2002	Topotecan	0.5-1.5 mg/m^2/day × 5	22	9

*Randomized phase II trial.
†Continuous intravenous infusion.

Combination chemotherapy. A large number of combination chemotherapy or chemoendocrine regimens for endometrial cancer have been tested in patients with recurrent disease in small single-institution series.[93] It is difficult to conclude from such reports that any particular regimen is to be preferred. Earlier reports suggested that patients with papillary serous carcinoma were more resistant to cytotoxic chemotherapy.[94,95] However, recent trials suggest that response rates for serous cancers are not different from those for other histologic subtypes of endometrial carcinomas.[96]

One combination that garnered interest was MVAC (methotrexate, vinblastine, doxorubicin, and cisplatin), with a reported response rate of 67% and a median overall survival time of 9.9 months in 30 patients.[97] However, the regimen was toxic and included two drugs of uncertain activity. Taxane/platinum doublets have been of considerable interest recently; response rates of 50% to 75% and median survival times of up to 17.6 months have been reported in a number of small studies.[96,98-100] A response rate of 73% was noted for the triplet of cisplatin, epirubicin, and paclitaxel, but that trial included some patients with stages IIb and III disease.[101]

Randomized trials. Although there have been numerous trials of chemohormonal therapy, only one very small randomized phase II trial comparing chemotherapy

with chemohormonal therapy has been reported[128] (Table 21-5). Although the response rate was higher in the combination arm, overall survival was not superior, and the usual practice remains to use hormones and chemotherapy in sequence, rather than in combination. Table 21-5 shows results of the more recent randomized trials of first-line chemotherapy for recurrent or metastatic endometrial carcinoma. A comparison of doxorubicin with doxorubicin plus cyclophosphamide showed no significant difference in unadjusted response rates or median survival times between the two arms.[79] Two subsequent trials compared single-agent doxorubicin with the combination of cisplatin and doxorubicin.[102,103] The response rate for the combination was significantly higher in both trials, and overall survival with the combination was higher in the European Organization of Research and Treatment of Cancer (EORTC) Gynaecological Cancer Cooperative Group (GCCG) trial, although not in the GOG trial.

Most recently, a preliminary report of the phase III GOG trial testing the three-drug TAP regimen, which combines 3-hour paclitaxel/doxorubicin/cisplatin with granulocyte colony-stimulating factor (G-CSF), against the doublet of doxorubicin/paclitaxel noted an improvement in both response rate and overall survival with the three-drug combination.[104] The upcoming GOG trial will compare the TAP regimen with the carboplatin/paclitaxel doublet, which, as noted,

Table 21–5. Randomized Chemotherapy Trials (First-Line)

Author	Year	Regimen	No. Evaluable	RR (%)	Median OS (mo)	Comments
Ayoub et al[128]	1988	CAF*	20	15	12.4	OS difference not significant
		CAF* + MPA/TAM†	23	43	13.6	
Aapro et al[103]	2003	Dox 60 mg/m²	87	17	7	
		Dox 60 mg/m² + Cis 50 mg/m²	90	43	9	
Thigpen et al[102]	1993	Dox 60 mg/m²	122	27	9.2	
		Dox 60 mg/m² + Cis 50 mg/m²	101	45	9.0	
Thigpen et al[79]	1994	Dox 60 mg/m²	132	22	6.7	No significant difference in unadjusted RR or OS
		Dox 60 mg/m² + Ctx 500 mg/m²	144	30	7.3	
Gallion[5]	2002	Dox 60 mg/m² + Cis 60 mg/m² (6 AM)	169	46	11.2	
		Dox 60 mg/m² + Cis 60 mg/m² (6 PM)	173	49	13.2	
Fleming et al[129]	2000	Dox 60 mg/m² + Cis 50 mg/m²	157	40	12.4	
		Dox 50 mg/m² + Tax 150 mg/m²/ 24 hr + G-CSF	158	44	13.6	
Fleming et al[104]	2002	Dox 60 mg/m² + Cis 50 mg/m²	132	34	12.1	Significant difference in RR and OS
		Dox 45 mg/m² + Cis 50 mg/m² + Tax 160 mg/m² + G-CSF	134	57	15.3	
Ongoing GOG Trial		Tax/Carboplatin Dox 45 mg/m² + Cis 50 mg/m² + Tax 160 mg/m² + G-CSF				

Cis, cisplatin; Ctx, cyclophosphamide; Dox, doxorubicin; GOG, Gynecologic Oncology Group; G-CSF, granulocyte colony-stimulating factor; OS, overall survival; RR, response rate; Tax, paclitaxel.
*CAF = Dox 30 mg/m² on day 1, plus Ctx 400 mg/m² on days 1 and 8, plus 5-fluorouracil 400 mg/m² on days 1 and 8.
†MPA/TAM = Medroxyprogesterone acetate 200 mg/day × 3 wk, alternating with tamoxifen 20 mg/day × 3 wk.

has shown promising activity in a number of phase II trials.

Agents used in women with ovarian cancer often are active in women with endometrial cancer as well; however, as exemplified by the inactivity of oral etoposide as a second-line therapy for endometrial carcinoma, the response profiles for the two tumor types are not necessarily identical. Prior pelvic RT and advanced age make patients with endometrial cancer more susceptible to hematologic toxicity, and most GOG trials give women who have had prior pelvic RT or, who are older than 65 years of age, automatic up-front dose reductions; physicians using regimens for the first time in this patient group should note carefully what dose adjustments were used. It is not clear that there currently exists a standard first-line chemotherapy regimen for women with recurrent endometrial cancer. However, the addition of a taxane to platinum/anthracycline chemotherapy has produced a survival advantage, with a median overall survival time superior to that reported in any other recent randomized trial in this group of patients. The upcoming GOG trial will answer the question of whether the anthracycline is an important addition to a taxane/platinum combination.

What are the future directions for treatment of recurrent endometrial cancer?

Because recurrent endometrial cancer is a relatively unusual cause of cancer death, drug development for this tumor type often lags behind that for more common cancers. Liposomal doxorubicin has well-documented activity in other gynecologic tumor types; if results of ongoing trials suggest meaningful activity against endometrial cancer, it will be a welcome addition to the list of active agents. Gemcitabine has not yet been tested but is a logical candidate for evaluation in this disease.

As is the case with other metastatic solid tumors, different combinations of currently available cytotoxic agents seem unlikely to make a major impact on the course of recurrent endometrial cancer, and alternative approaches need to be explored. About 20% of advanced or recurrent endometrial cancers stain 3+ for the oncoprotein HER2/NEU using the Herceptest immunohistochemical assay,[104] and a GOG phase II trial of trastuzumab (anti-HER2 monoclonal antibody) in women with HER2-overexpressing endometrial cancer for whom chemotherapy has failed is ongoing. Vaccine and adoptive immunotherapy approaches that are being developed for HER2-overexpressing breast cancer may be applicable to HER2-overexpressing endometrial cancer as well. Likewise, 60% to 90% of endometrial carcinomas have been reported to overexpress epidermal growth factor receptor (EGFR, HER1), and may therefore be candidates for regimens incorporating EGFR-targeting monoclonal antibodies or small-molecule tyrosine kinase inhibitors.[105-107] Trials of erlotinib (OSI-774, Tarceva) and gefitinib (ZD 1839, Iressa) in patients with carcinoma of the endometrium are currently ongoing. Enrollment of patients in clinical trials testing new approaches should remain a priority.

REFERENCES

1. Pettersson F, Creaseman WT, Shepherd JH: Annual Report on the Results of Treatment in Gynecologic Cancer. Stockholm, International Federation of Gynecology and Obstetrics, 1995, p 22.
2. Jemal A, Thomas A, Murray T, et al: Cancer Statistics, 2002. CA Cancer J Clin 2002;52:23-47.
3. Cirisano FD Jr, Robboy SJ, Dodge RK, et al: The outcome of stage I-II clinically and surgically staged papillary serous and clear cell endometrial cancers when compared with endometrioid carcinoma. Gynecol Oncol 2000;77:55-65.
4. Thigpen JT, Brady MF, Alvarez RD, et al: Oral medroxyprogesterone acetate in the treatment of advanced or recurrent endometrial carcinoma: A dose-response study by the Gynecologic Oncology Group. J Clin Oncol 1999;17:1736-1744.
5. Gallion HH, Brunetto VK, Lentz SS, et al: Standard timed doxorubicin plus cisplatin versus circadian-timed doxorubicin plus cisplatin in patients with FIGO stage III/IV or recurrent endometrial carcinoma. A Gynecologic Oncology Group Study. Society of Gynecologic Oncologists 2002;84:487.
6. Abramovich D, Markman M, Kennedy A, et al: Serum CA-125 as a marker of disease activity in uterine papillary serous carcinoma. J Cancer Res Clin Oncol 1999;125:697-698.
7. Cherchi PL, Dessole S, Ruiu GA, et al: The value of serum CA 125 and association CA 125/CA 19-9 in endometrial carcinoma. Eur J Gynaecol Oncol 1999;20:315-317.
8. Ingersoll FM: Vaginal recurrence of carcinoma of the corpus: Management and prevention. Am J Surg 1971;121:473-477.
9. Aadlers JG, Abeler V, Kolstad P: Recurrent adenocarcinoma of the endometrium: A clinical and histopathological study of 379 patients. Gynecol Oncol 1984;17:85.
10. Meigs JV: Adenocarcinoma of fundus of uterus: Reporting concerning vaginal metastases of this tumor. N Engl J Med 1929;201:155-160.
11. Jereczek-Fossa B, Badzio A, Jassem J: Recurrent endometrial cancer after surgery alone: Results of salvage radiotherapy. Int J Radiat Oncol Biol Phys 2000;48:405-413.
12. Kuten A, Grigsby PW, Perez CA, et al: Results of radiotherapy in recurrent endometrial carcinoma: A retrospective analysis of 51 patients. Int J Radiat Oncol Biol Phys 1989;17:29-34.
13. Curran WJ Jr, Whittington R, Peters AJ, et al: Vaginal recurrences of endometrial carcinoma: The prognostic value of staging by a primary vaginal carcinoma system. Int J Radiat Oncol Biol Phys 1988;15:803-808.
14. Sears JD, Greven KM, Hoen HM, et al: Prognostic factors and treatment outcome for patients with locally recurrent endometrial cancer. Cancer 1994;74:1303-1308.
15. Greven K, Olds W: Isolated vaginal recurrences of endometrial adenocarcinoma and their management. Cancer 1987;60:419-421.
16. Pirtoli L, Ciatto S, Cionni L, et al: Salvage with radiotherapy of postsurgical relapses of endometrial cancer. Tumori 1980;66:475-480.
17. Morgan JD 3rd, Reddy S, Sarin P, et al: Isolated vaginal recurrences of endometrial carcinoma. Radiology 1993;189:609-613.
18. Wylie J, Irwin C, Pintilie M, et al: Results of radical radiotherapy for recurrent endometrial cancer. Gynecol Oncol 2000;77:66-72.
19. Hart KB, Han I, Shamsa F, et al: Radiation therapy for endometrial cancer in patients treated for postoperative recurrence. Int J Radiat Oncol Biol Phys 1998;41:7-11.
20. Hoekstra CJ, Koper PC, van Putten WL: Recurrent endometrial adenocarcinoma after surgery alone: Prognostic factors and treatment. Radiother Oncol 1993;27:164-166.
21. Greven KM: Interstitial radiation for recurrent cervix or endometrial cancer in the suburethral region. Int J Radiat Oncol Biol Phys 1998;48:831-834.
22. Roeske JC, Lujan A, Rotmensch J, et al: Intensity-modulated whole pelvic radiation therapy in patients with gynecologic malignancies. Int J Radiat Oncol Biol Phys 2000;48:1613-1621.
23. Mundt AJ, Lujan AE, Rotmensch J, et al: Intensity-modulated whole pelvic radiotherapy in women with gynecologic malignancies. Int J Radiat Oncol Biol Phys 2002;52:1330-1337.
24. Alektiar KM, McKee A, Venkatraman E, et al: Intravaginal high-dose-rate brachytherapy for stage IB (FIGO grade 1, 2) endometrial cancer. Int J Radiat Oncol Biol Phys 2002;53:707-713.
25. Creutzberg CL, van Putten WL, Koper PC, et al: Surgery and postoperative radiotherapy versus surgery alone for patients with stage-1 endometrial carcinoma: Multicentre randomised trial. PORTEC Study Group. Post Operative Radiation Therapy in Endometrial Carcinoma. Lancet 2000;355:1404-1411.
26. Aadlers J, Abeler V, Kolstad P: Postoperative external irradiation and prognostic parameters in stage I endometrial carcinoma: Clinical and histopathologic study of 540 patients. Obstet Gynecol 1980;56:419-426.
27. Brunschwig A: Complete excision of pelvic viscera for advanced carcinoma: A one stage abdominoperineal operation with end colostomy and bilateral ureteral implantation into the colon above the colostomy. Cancer 1948;1:177-182.
28. Barber HRK, Brunschwig A: Treatment and results of recurrent cancer of corpus uteri in patients receiving anterior and total pelvic exenteration. Cancer 1968;22:949-954.
29. Barakat RR, Goldman NA, Patel DA, et al: Pelvic exenteration for recurrent endometrial cancer. Gynecol Oncol 1999;75:99-103.
30. Morris M, Alvarez RD, Kinney WK, et al: Treatment of recurrent adenocarcinoma of the endometrium with pelvic exenteration. Gynecol Oncol 1996;60:288-291.
31. Garton GR, Gunderson LL, Webb MJ, et al: Intraoperative radiation therapy in gynecologic cancer: Update of the experience at a single institution. Int J Radiat Oncol Biol Phys 1997;37:839-843.
32. Del Carmen MG, McIntyre JF, Fuller AF, et al: Intraoperative radiation therapy in the treatment of pelvic gynecologic malignancies: A review of fifteen cases. Gynecol Oncol 2000;79:457-462.
33. Kadar N, Malfetano JH, Homesley HD: Steroid receptor concentrations in endometrial carcinoma: Effect on survival in surgically staged patients. Gynecol Oncol 1993;50:281-286.
34. Iwai K, Fukuda K, Hachisuga T, et al: Prognostic significance of progesterone receptor immunohistochemistry for lymph node metastases in endometrial carcinoma. Gynecol Oncol 1999;72:351-359.
35. Fukuda K, Mori M, Uchiyama M, et al: Prognostic significance of progesterone receptor immunohistochemistry in endometrial carcinoma. Gynecol Oncol 1998;69:220-225.
36. Nyholm HC, Christensen IJ, Nielsen AL: Progesterone receptor levels independently predict survival in endometrial adenocarcinoma. Gynecol Oncol 1995;59:347-351.
37. Castagnetta L, Lo Casto M, Mercadante T, et al: Intra-tumoural variation of oestrogen receptor status in endometrial cancer. Br J Cancer 1983;47:261-267.
38. Kelley R, Baker W: Progestational agents in the treatment of carcinoma of the endometrium. N Engl J Med 1961;264:216-222.
39. Sall S, DiSaia P, Morrow CP, et al: A comparison of medroxyprogesterone serum concentrations by the oral or intramuscular route in patients with persistent or recurrent endometrial carcinoma. Am J Obstet Gynecol 1979;135:647-650.
40. Kauppila A: Progestin therapy of endometrial, breast and ovarian carcinoma: A review of clinical observations. Acta Obstet Gynecol Scand 1984;63:441-450.
41. Early Breast Cancer Trialists' Collaborative Group: Tamoxifen for early breast cancer: An overview of the randomized trials. Lancet 1998;351:1451-1447.

42. Dardes RC, Bentrem D, O'Regan RM, et al: Effects of the new selective estrogen receptor modulator LY353381.HCl (Arzoxifene) on human endometrial cancer growth in athymic mice. Clin Cancer Res 2001;7:4149-4155.

43. Moore TD, Phillips PH, Nerenstone SR, et al: Systemic treatment of advanced and recurrent endometrial carcinoma: Current status and future directions. J Clin Oncol 1991;9:1071-1088.

44. Thigpen T, Brady MF, Homesley HD, et al: Tamoxifen in the treatment of advanced or recurrent endometrial carcinoma: A Gynecologic Oncology Group study. J Clin Oncol 2001;19:364-367.

45. Slavik M, Petty WM, Blessing JA, et al: Phase II clinical study of tamoxifen in advanced endometrial adenocarcinoma: A Gynecologic Oncology Group study. Cancer Treat Rep 1984;68:809-811.

46. Klijn J, den Hoed Kliniek D: Multicentre phase II study of the selective estrogen receptor modulator (SERM) LY353381 in advanced or recurrent endometrial cancer: Objective responses in progestagen sensitive patients (pts). Proc Am Soc Clin Oncol 2000;19:386a.

46a. McMeekin DS, Gorden A, Fowler J, et al: A phase II trial of arzexifene, a selective estrogen response modulater, in patients with recurrent or advanced endometrial cancer. Gynecol Oncol 2003;90:64-89.

47. Elkas J, Armstrong A, Pohl J, et al: Modulation of endometrial steroid receptors and growth regulatory genes by tamoxifen. Obstet Gynecol 2000;95:697-703.

48. Carlson JA Jr, Allegra JC, Day TG Jr, et al: Tamoxifen and endometrial carcinoma: Alterations in estrogen and progesterone receptors in untreated patients and combination hormonal therapy in advanced neoplasia. Am J Obstet Gynecol 1984;149:149-153.

49. Mortel R, Levy C, Wolff JP, et al: Female sex steroid receptors in postmenopausal endometrial carcinoma and biochemical response to an antiestrogen. Cancer Res 1981;41:1140-1147.

50. Pandya KJ, Yeap BY, Weiner LM, et al: Megestrol and tamoxifen in patients with advanced endometrial cancer: An Eastern Cooperative Oncology Group Study (E4882). Am J Clin Oncol 2001;24:43-46.

51. Fiorica J, Brunetto V, Hanjani P, et al: A phase II study (GOG 153) of recurrent and advanced endometrial carcinoma treated with alternating courses of megestrol acetate and tamoxifen citrate. Proc ASCO 2000;19:379a.

52. Imai A, Ohno T, Iida K, et al: Presence of gonadotropin-releasing hormone receptor and its messenger ribonucleic acid in endometrial carcinoma and endometrium. Gynecol Oncol 1994;55:144-148.

53. Srkalovic G, Wittliff JL, Schally AV: Detection and partial characterization of receptors for (D-Trp6)- luteinizing hormone-releasing hormone and epidermal growth factor in human endometrial carcinoma. Cancer Res 1990;50:1841-1846.

54. Sica G, Schinzari G, Angelucci C, et al: Direct effects of GnRH agonists in human hormone-sensitive endometrial cells. Mol Cell Endocrinol 2001;176:121-128.

55. Grundker C, Gunthert AR, Westphalen S, et al: Biology of the gonadotropin-releasing hormone system in gynecological cancers. Eur J Endocrinol 2002;146:1-14.

56. Kleinman D, Douvdevani A, Schally AV, et al: Direct growth inhibition of human endometrial cancer cells by the gonadotropin-releasing hormone antagonist SB-75: Role of apoptosis. Am J Obstet Gynecol 1994;170:96-102.

57. Bax CMR, Chatzaki E, Gallagher CJ: Investigation of mechanisms responsible for the successful treatment of endometrial cancer with GnRH analogs. In Filicori M, Flamigini C (eds): Treatment with GnRH Analogs: Controversies and Perspectives. Park Ridge, NJ, Parthenon, 1996, pp 173-180.

58. Jeyarajah AR, Gallagher CJ, Blake PR, et al: Long-term follow-up of gonadotrophin-releasing hormone analog treatment for recurrent endometrial cancer. Gynecol Oncol 1996;63:47-52.

59. Covens A, Thomas G, Shaw P, et al: A phase II study of leuprolide in advanced/recurrent endometrial cancer. Gynecol Oncol 1997;64:126-129.

60. Lhomme C, Vennin P, Callet N, et al: A multicenter phase II study with triptorelin (sustained-release LHRH agonist) in advanced or recurrent endometrial carcinoma: A French Anticancer Federation study. Gynecol Oncol 1999;75:187-193.

60a. Asbury RF, Bruncho VL, Lee RB, et al: Goserelin acetate as treatment for recurrent endometrial carinoma: A gynecologic oncology group study. Am J Clin Oncol 2002;25:557-560.

61. Watanabe K, Sasano H, Harada N, et al: Aromatase in human endometrial carcinoma and hyperplasia: Immunohistochemical, in situ hybridization, and biochemical studies. Am J Pathol 1995;146:491-500.

62. Maluf FC, Sabbatini P, Schwartz L, et al: Endometrial stromal sarcoma: Objective response to letrozole. Gynecol Oncol 2001;82:384-388.

63. Rose PG, Brunetto VL, VanLe L, et al: A phase II trial of anastrozole in advanced recurrent or persistent endometrial carcinoma: A Gynecologic Oncology Group study. Gynecol Oncol 2000;78:212-216.

64. Sidhu K, Fyles A, Eisenhauer E, et al: Phase II study of the aromatase inhibitor letrozole in endometrial carcinoma—NCIC CTG IND 126. Proc ASCO 2001;20:192b.

64a. Covens A, Brunetlo VL, Markman M, et al: Phase II trial of danazol in advanced recurrent, or persistent endometrial cancer; A gynecologic oncology group study. Gyn Oncol 2003;89:470-474.

65. Creasman WT: Prognostic significance of hormone receptors in endometrial cancer. Cancer 1993;71:1467-1470.

66. Nyholm HC, Nielsen AL, Lyndrup J, et al: Estrogen and progesterone receptors in endometrial carcinoma: Comparison of immunohistochemical and biochemical analysis. Int J Gynecol Pathol 1993;12:246-252.

67. Ravn V, Havsteen H, Thorpe SM: Immunohistochemical evaluation of estrogen and progesterone receptors in paraffin-embedded, formalin-fixed endometrial tissues: Comparison with enzyme immunoassay and immunohistochemical analysis of frozen tissue. Mod Pathol 1998;11:709-715.

68. Thigpen JT, Kronmal R, Vogel S, et al: A phase II trial of vinblastine in patients with advanced or recurrent endometrial carcinoma: A Southwest Oncology Group Study. Am J Clin Oncol 1987;10:429-431.

69. Runowicz CD, Nuchtern LM, Braunstein JD, et al: Heterogeneity in hormone receptor status in primary and metastatic endometrial cancer. Gynecol Oncol 1990;38:437-441.

70. Niemann TH, Maymind M, Fowler JM, et al: Expression of estrogen receptor and progesterone receptor in advanced stage endometrial cancer. Gynecol Oncol 1999;72:467.

71. Holdaway IM, Bowditch JV: Variation in receptor status between primary and metastatic breast cancer. Cancer 1983;52:479-485.

72. Mortel R, Zaino R, Satyaswaroop PG: Heterogeneity and progesterone-receptor distribution in endometrial adenocarcinoma. Cancer 1984;53:113-116.

73. Zaino RJ, Clarke CL, Mortel R, et al: Heterogeneity of progesterone receptor distribution in human endometrial adenocarcinoma. Cancer Res 1988;48:1889-1895.

74. Mote PA, Johnston JF, Manninen T, et al: Detection of progesterone receptor forms A and B by immunohistochemical analysis. J Clin Pathol 2001;54:624-630.

75. Dai D, Wolf DM, Litman ES, et al: Progesterone inhibits human endometrial cancer cell growth and invasiveness: Down-regulation of cellular adhesion molecules through progesterone B receptors. Cancer Res 2002;62:881-886.

76. Lentz SS, Brady MF, Major FJ, et al: High-dose megestrol acetate in advanced or recurrent endometrial carcinoma: A Gynecologic Oncology Group Study. J Clin Oncol 1996;14:357-361.

77. Carcangiu ML, Chambers JT: Uterine papillary serous carcinoma: A study of 108 cases with emphasis on the prognostic significance of associated endometrioid carcinoma, absence of invasion and comcomitant ovarian carcinoma. Gynecol Oncol 1992;47:298-303.

78. Umpierre SA, Burke TW, Tornos C, et al: Immunocytochemical analysis of uterine papillary serous carcinomas for estrogen and progesterone receptors. Int J Gynecol Pathol 1994;13:127-130.

79. Thigpen JT, Blessing JA, DiSaia PJ, et al: A randomized comparison of doxorubicin alone versus doxorubicin plus cyclophosphamide in the management of advanced or recurrent endometrial carcinoma: A Gynecologic Oncology Group study. J Clin Oncol 1994;12:1408-1414.

80. Ball HG, Blessing JA, Lentz SS, et al: A phase II trial of paclitaxel in patients with advanced and recurrent adenocarcinoma of the endometrium: A Gynecologic Oncology Group study. Gynecol Oncol 1996;62:278-281.

81. Lissoni A, Zanetta G, Losa G, et al: Phase II study of paclitaxel as salvage treatment in advanced endometrial cancer. Ann Oncol 1996;7:861-863.

82. Woo HL, Swenerton KD, Hoskins PJ: Taxol is active in platinum-resistant endometrial adenocarcinoma. Am J Clin Oncol 1996;19:290-291.

83. Burke TW, Munkarah A, Kavanagh JJ, et al: Treatment of advanced or recurrent endometrial carcinoma with single-agent carboplatin. Gynecol Oncol 1993;51:397-400.

84. Thigpen JT, Blessing JA, Homesley H, et al: Phase II trial of cisplatin as first-line chemotherapy in patients with advanced or recurrent endometrial carcinoma: A Gynecologic Oncology Group Study. Gynecol Oncol 1989;33:68-70.

85. Green JB 3rd, Green S, Alberts DS, et al: Carboplatin therapy in advanced endometrial cancer. Obstet Gynecol 1990;75:696-700.

86. Thigpen JT, Buchsbaum HJ, Mangan C, et al: Phase II trial of adriamycin in the treatment of advanced or recurrent endometrial carcinoma: A Gynecologic Oncology Group study. Cancer Treat Rep 1979;63:21-27.

87. Horton J, Begg CB, Arseneault J, et al: Comparison of adriamycin with cyclophosphamide in patients with advanced endometrial cancer. Cancer Treat Rep 1978;62:159-161.

88. Pawinski A, Tumolo S, Hoesel G, et al: Cyclophosphamide or ifosfamide in patients with advanced and/or recurrent endometrial carcinoma: A randomized phase II study of the EORTC Gynecological Cancer Cooperative Group. Eur J Obstet Gynecol Reprod Biol 1999;86:179-183.

89. Sutton GP, Blessing JA, DeMars LR, et al: A phase II Gynecologic Oncology Group trial of ifosfamide and mesna in advanced or recurrent adenocarcinoma of the endometrium. Gynecol Oncol 1996;63:25-27.

90. Seski JC, Edwards CL, Copeland LJ, et al: Hexamethylmelamine chemotherapy for disseminated endometrial cancer. Obstet Gynecol 1981;58:361-363.

91. Carbone PP, Carter SK: Endometrial cancer: approach to development of effective chemotherapy. Gynecol Oncol 1974;2:348-353.

92. Muggia FM, Blessing JA, Sorosky J, et al: Phase II trial of the pegylated liposomal doxorubicin in previously treated metastatic endometrial cancer: A Gynecologic Oncology Group study. J Clin Oncol 2002;20:2360-2364.

93. Barakat RR, Grigsby PW, Sabbatini P, et al: Corpus: Epithelial Tumors. Philadelphia, Lippincott Williams & Wilkins, 2000, pp 919-959.

94. Price FV, Chambers SK, Carcangiu ML, et al: Intravenous cisplatin, doxorubicin, and cyclophosphamide in the treatment of uterine papillary serous carcinoma (UPSC). Gynecol Oncol 1993;51:383-389.

95. Levenback C, Burke TW, Silva E, et al: Uterine papillary serous carcinoma (UPSC) treated with cisplatin, doxorubicin, and cyclophosphamide (PAC). Gynecol Oncol 1992;46:317-321.

96. Hoskins PJ, Swenerton KD, Pike JA, et al: Paclitaxel and carboplatin, alone or with irradiation, in advanced or recurrent endometrial cancer: A phase II study. J Clin Oncol 2001;19:4048-4053.

97. Long HJ 3rd, Langdon RM Jr, Cha SS, et al: Phase II trial of methotrexate, vinblastine, doxorubicin, and cisplatin in advanced/recurrent endometrial carcinoma. Gynecol Oncol 1995;58:240-243.

98. Zanotti KM, Belinson JL, Kennedy AW, et al: The use of paclitaxel and platinum-based chemotherapy in uterine papillary serous carcinoma. Gynecol Oncol 1999;74:272-277.

99. Price FV, Edwards RP, Kelley JL, et al: A trial of outpatient paclitaxel and carboplatin for advanced recurrent, and histologic high-risk endometrial carcinoma: Preliminary report. Semin Oncol 1997;24:S15-78-S15-82.

100. Dimopoulos MA, Papadimitriou CA, Georgoulias V, et al: Paclitaxel and cisplatin in advanced or recurrent carcinoma of the endometrium: Long-term results of a phase II multicenter study. Gynecol Oncol 2000;78:52-57.

101. Lissoni A, Gabriele A, Gorga G, et al: Cisplatin-, epirubicin- and paclitaxel-containing chemotherapy in uterine adenocarcinoma. Ann Oncol 1997;8:969-972.

102. Thigpen T, Blessing J, Homesley H, et al: Phase III trial of doxorubicin +/- cisplatin in advanced or recurrent endometrial carcinoma: A Gynecologic Oncology Group (GOG) Study. Proc Am Soc Clini Oncol 1993;12:261.

103. Aapro MS, VanWiljk FH, Bolis G, et al: Doxorubicin versus doxorubicin and cisplatin in endometrial carcinoma: Randomised study (55872). EORTC gynecological cancer group. Am Oncol 2003;14:441-48.

104. Fleming GF, Brunetto VL, Mundt AJ, et al: Randomized trial of doxorubicin (DOX) plus cisplatin (CIS) versus DOX plus CIS plus paclitaxel (TAX) in patients with advanced or recurrent endometrial carcinoma: A Gynecologic Oncology Group (GOG) study. Proc Am Soc Clin Oncol 2002;21:202a.

105. Miturski R, Semczuk A, Postawski K, et al: Epidermal growth factor receptor immunostaining and epidermal growth factor receptor-tyrosine kinase activity in proliferative and neoplastic human endometrium. Tumour Biol 2000;21:358-366.

106. Nagai N, Oshita T, Fujii T, et al: Prospective analysis of DNA ploidy, proliferative index and epidermal growth factor receptor as prognostic factors for pretreated uterine cancer. Oncol Rep 2000;7:551-559.

107. Athanassiadou P, Petrakakou E, Liossi A, et al: Prognostic significance of p53, bcl-2 and EGFR in carcinoma of the endometrium. Acta Cytol 1999;43:1039-1044.

108. Reifenstein EC Jr: Hydroxyprogesterone caproate therapy in advanced endometrial cancer. Cancer 1971;27:485-502.

109. Thigpen T, Blessing J, Disaia P: Oral medroxyprogesterone acetate in advanced or recurrent endometrial carcinoma: Results of therapy and correlation with estrogen and progesterone receptor levels. The Gynecologic Oncology Group experience. In Baulieu EE. Iacobelli S, McGuire WL (eds): Endocrinology and Malignancy: Proceedings of the First International Congress on Cancer and Hormones. Park Ridge, NJ, Parthenon, 1986, pp 446-454.

110. Calero F, Asins-Codoner E, Jimeno J, et al: Epirubicin in advanced endometrial adenocarcinoma: A phase II study of the Grupo Ginecologico Espanol para el Tratamiento Oncologico (GGETO). Eur J Cancer 1991;27:864-866.

111. Trope C, Grundsell H, Johnsson JE, et al: A phase II study of Cis-platinum for recurrent corpus cancer. Eur J Cancer 1980;16:1025-1026.

112. Edmonson JH, Krook JE, Hilton JF, et al: Randomized phase II studies of cisplatin and a combination of cyclophosphamide-doxorubicin-cisplatin (CAP) in patients with progestin-refractory advanced endometrial carcinoma. Gynecol Oncol 1987;28:20-24.

113. Thigpen JT, Blessing JA, Ball H, et al: Hexamethylmelamine as first-line chemotherapy in the treatment of advanced or recurrent carcinoma of the endometrium: A phase II trial of the Gynecologic Oncology Group. Gynecol Oncol 1988;31:435-438.

114. Barton C, Buxton EJ, Blackledge G, et al: A phase II study of ifosfamide in endometrial cancer. Cancer Chemother Pharmacol 1990;26:S4-S6.

115. Broun GO, Blessing JA, Eddy GL, et al: A phase II trial of vincristine in advanced or recurrent endometrial carcinoma: A Gynecologic Oncology Group Study. Am J Clin Oncol 1993;16:18-21.

116. Omura GA, Shingleton HM, Creasman WT, et al: Chemotherapy of gynecologic cancer with nitrosoureas: A randomized trial of CCNU and methyl-CCNU in cancers of the cervix, corpus, vagina, and vulva. Cancer Treat Rep 1978;62:833-835.

117. Muss HB, Blessing JA, Hatch KD, et al: Methotrexate in advanced endometrial carcinoma: A phase II trial of the Gynecologic Oncology Group. Am J Clin Oncol 1990;13:61-63.

118. Hilgers RD, Von Hoff DD, Stephens RL, et al: Mitoxantrone in adenocarcinoma of the endometrium: A Southwest Oncology Group Study. Cancer Treat Rep 1985;69:1329-1330.

119. Deppe G, Cohen CJ, Bruckner HW: Treatment of advanced endometrial adenocarcinoma with cis-dichlorodiammine platinum (II) after intensive prior therapy. Gynecol Oncol 1980;10:51-55.

120. Thigpen JT, Blessing JA, Lagasse LD, et al: Phase II trial of cisplatin as second-line chemotherapy in patients with advanced or recurrent endometrial carcinoma: A Gynecologic Oncology Group study. Am J Clin Oncol 1984;7:253-256.

121. Sutton GP, Blessing JA, Manetta A, et al: Gynecologic oncology group studies with ifosfamide. Semin Oncol 1992;19:31-35.

122. Slayton RE, Blessing JA, Delgado G: Phase II trial of etoposide in the management of advanced or recurrent endometrial

carcinoma: A Gynecologic Oncology Group Study. Cancer Treat Rep 1982;66:1669-1671.

123. Muss HB, Bundy BN, Adcock L: Teniposide (VM-26) in patients with advanced endometrial carcinoma: A phase II trial of the Gynecologic Oncology Group. Am J Clin Oncol 1991;14:36-37.

124. Rose PG, Blessing JA, Lewandowski GS, et al: A phase II trial of prolonged oral etoposide (VP-16) as second-line therapy for advanced and recurrent endometrial carcinoma: A Gynecologic Oncology Group study. Gynecol Oncol 1996;63:101-104.

125. Jackson DV Jr, Jobson VW, Homesley HD, et al: Vincristine infusion in refractory gynecologic malignancies. Gynecol Oncol 1986;25:212-216.

126. von Hoff DD, Green S, Alberts DS, et al: Phase II study of fludarabine phosphate (NSC-312887) in patients with advanced endometrial cancer. Am J Clin Oncol 1991;14:193-194.

127. Moore DH, Blessing JA, Dunton C, et al: Dactinomycin in the treatment of recurrent or persistent endometrial carcinoma: A Phase II study of the Gynecologic Oncology Group. Gynecol Oncol 1999;75:473-475.

128. Ayoub J, Audet-Lapointe P, Methot Y, et al: Efficacy of sequential cyclical hormonal therapy in endometrial cancer and its correlation with steroid hormone receptor status. Gynecol Oncol 1988;31:327-337.

129. Fleming GF, Brunetto VL, Bentley R, et al: Randomized trial of doxorubicin (DOX) plus cisplain (CIS) versus DOX plus paclitaxel (TAX) plus granulocyte colony-stimulating factor (G-CSF) in patients with advanced or recurrent endometrial cancer: A report on Gynecologic Oncology Group (GOG) Protocol no. 163. Proc Am Soc Clin Oncol 2000;19:379a.

130. Wadler S, Levy DF, Lincoln ST, et al: Topotecan is an active agent in the first-line treatment of metastatic or recurrent endometrial carcinoma: Eastern cooperative oncology group study (E3E93). J Clin Oncol 2003;21:2100-2114.

131. Miller DS, Blessinf JA, Lentz SS, et al: A phase II trial of topotecan in patients with advanced, persistent, or recurrent endometrial carcinoma: A gynecologic oncology group study. Gynecol Oncol 2002;87:247-251.

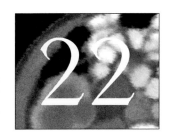

PRIMARY TREATMENT OF UTERINE SARCOMAS

Raimund Winter, Andrew Östör, Karin Kapp, and Edgar Petru

 MAJOR CONTROVERSIES

- **What is the classification of uterine sarcomas?**
- **What is the role of lymphadenectomy in surgical treatment?**
- **What is the role of adjuvant radiation therapy in stage I/II disease?**
- **What is the role of adjuvant chemotherapy in the treatment of uterine sarcomas?**

PATHOLOGY OF UTERINE SARCOMAS

Sarcomas (from the Greek, *sarcos*, "flesh") are malignant tumors of mesenchymal tissues. They may be pure or mixed. The word "mixed" in this context means that the sarcoma contains epithelial elements which may be benign or malignant. Tumors in this category are malignant either by virtue of their histologic features and cell types or by virtue of their growth pattern. The World Health Organization (WHO) classification is detailed in (Table 22-1).[1]

Sarcomas are uncommon, accounting for only about 3% of all uterine malignancies.

Little is known of their pathogenesis. Occasionally tumors have followed pelvic irradiation[2] and are associated with Tamoxifen,[3,4] estrogen therapy or the polycystic ovary syndrome.[5] The usual risk factors for endometrial carcinoma (e.g., unopposed estrogen therapy, diabetes, hypertension) are not thought to apply to sarcomas, although a limited relationship has been claimed for carcinosarcomas by some. Malignant transformation of leiomyomas is extremely rare. Consistent genetic alterations have not been identified.

With the exception of sarcoma botryoides, sarcomas occur in middle-aged or postmenopausal women.[6,7] They are more common in blacks.[8,9]

Sarcomas by virtue of their histologic features and cell types

Leiomyosarcoma. Leiomyosarcomas are malignant tumors of smooth muscle cells. They are typically solitary intramural masses, usually not associated with leiomyomas. They average 8 cm in diameter and have an appearance resembling fish flesh. In contrast to leiomyomas, leiomyosarcomas are soft, do not project above the surrounding myometrium, are poorly circumscribed and often display foci of necrosis and hemorrhage. Rarely, they may be found incidentally in hysterectomy specimens. The usual leiomyosarcoma is composed of fascicles of spindle-shaped cells with abundant eosinophilic cytoplasm, which may contain longitudinal fibrils. The nuclei are pleomorphic, fusiform or cigar-shaped, and hyperchromatic with coarse chromatin and prominent nucleoli. Multinucleated tumor giant cells are common. The margin is usually infiltrating, and vascular invasion is seen in up to 25% of cases. The mitotic rate usually exceeds 10 mitotic figures (mf) per 10 high-power fields (HPF) in the most cellular areas (HPF is defined as that seen by the 40× objective). Some of the mitoses may be abnormal. Tumor cell necrosis (as opposed to the infarct-like type) is typically prominent. Occasionally, however,

Table 22–1. Modified World Health Organization Classification of Mesenchymal and Mixed Tumors of the Uterus

Smooth muscle tumors
   Leiomyoma
      Mitotically active leiomyoma
      Cellular leiomyoma
      Hemorrhagic cellular leiomyoma
      Atypical leiomyoma
      Epithelioid leiomyoma
      Myxoid leiomyoma
      Vascular leiomyoma
      Lipoleiomyoma
Smooth muscle tumor of uncertain malignant potential
Leiomyosarcoma
   Epithelioid leiomyosarcoma
   Myxoid leiomyosarcoma
Other smooth muscle tumors
   Metastasizing leiomyoma
   Intravenous leiomyomatosis
   Disseminated peritoneal leiomyomatosis
Endometrial stromal tumors
   Stromal nodule
   Endometrial stromal sarcoma
Mixed endometrial stromal-smooth muscle tumors
Adenomatoid tumor
Other mesenchymal tumors (benign and malignant)
   Homologous
   Heterologous
Mixed epithelial-mesenchymal tumors
   Benign
      Adenofibroma
      Adenomyoma
      Atypical polypoid adenomyoma
   Malignant
      Adenosarcoma
         Homologous or heterologous
      Carcinosarcoma (mixed mullerian tumor)
         Homologous or heterologous
Undifferentiated
Miscellaneous tumors
   Sex cord–like tumors
   Neuroectodermal tumors
   Lymphoma
   Other

histologically bland-looking tumors declare themselves by distant spread. Presumably, at least some pulmonary nodules from "benign metastasizing leiomyomas" originate from such neoplasms. Variants include the epithelioid and myxoid types. Although rare, these subtypes are important because their histologically bland appearance belies their malignant behavior.

Two rare subtypes, the epithelioid leiomyoma and the so-called smooth muscle tumor of uncertain malignant potential (STUMP), pose clinical problems because of their unpredictable prognosis. The former include leiomyoblastoma, and clear cell leiomyoma. Although most of these are benign, the behavior of epithelioid tumors with two or more of the following features is not established: large size (>6 cm), mitosis count between 2 and 4 mf/10 HPF, significant cytologic atypia, and tumor cell necrosis. The term STUMP is reserved for those neoplasms about which clinicopathologic information is scant, the degree of smooth

muscle differentiation is uncertain, and the microscopic criteria of malignancy are borderline.

Endometrial stromal sarcoma. Endometrial stromal sarcomas are sarcomas composed of cells that resemble normal proliferative-phase endometrial stromal cells but invade the myometrium, often its vascular channels, and occasionally extend into extrauterine vessels. They are multinodular, worm-like lesions that grow in the myometrium, sometimes protruding from the cut ends of blood vessels. They are densely cellular tumors composed of uniform small, round or oval nuclei with scanty cytoplasm. The mitotic rate is usually brisk. Nuclear atypia is mild. A fine network of small arterioles is characteristic. Vascular invasion occurs in approximately 30% of cases and accounts for the former term, "endolymphatic stromal myosis." The sole criterion separating this lesion from the benign stromal nodule is the infiltrating margin of the former.[10-12] For this reason, making the distinction between the two in curettage specimens can be difficult or impossible.

Endometrial stromal sarcomas have traditionally been divided into low-grade and high-grade types. However, more recently it was emphasized that high-grade endometrial sarcoma is so pleomorphic as to bear no resemblance to endometrial stromal cells, and that claiming such a pedigree is no longer tenable.[13] Consequently, the current WHO classification recommends that this term be dropped and replaced by "high-grade endometrial sarcoma" (alternate designations are "poorly differentiated endometrial sarcoma" and "undifferentiated uterine sarcoma").[1]

Mixed endometrial stromal and smooth muscle tumors. Mixed endometrial stromal and smooth muscle tumors are arbitrarily defined as having at least 30% of each component. The word "mixed" in this context refers to a mixture of two mesenchymal elements. Only 15 cases of these rare neoplasms have been fully reported,[14] with another 38 cases reported in abstract form.[15] The terminology used in these reports has varied. In the abstract studies, 22 tumors were designated as "stromal–smooth muscle nodules" and 16 as "low-grade sarcomas." In the other series, the tumors were reported as "endometrial stromal nodules" or "endometrial stromal sarcomas with smooth muscle differentiation" (depending on the margin) with the "mixed" appellation given in parentheses. The mean age at presentation was 38 years (range, 20 to 68 years), with similar symptomatology to that of leiomyomas. In the series of 15 cases, the only tumor with an infiltrating margin recurred as a pure endometrial stromal sarcoma, although the follow-up for the group was short. In the abstract reports, all of the stromal smooth muscle nodules were benign, whereas three of the low-grade sarcomas had extrauterine spread at presentation, recurrences, or both. The recurrent tumors were purely smooth muscle, purely stromal, or a mixture.

Sarcoma botryoides (embryonal rhabdomyosarcoma or botryoid rhabdomyosarcoma). Sarcoma botryoides is a malignant tumor composed of cells with small, round to oval to spindle-shaped nuclei, some of which show differentiation toward striated muscle cells. These tumors occur almost exclusively in infants younger than 2 years of age. Grossly, they are smooth-surfaced, slippery, grape-like lesions that project from the cervix into the vagina, where they are more common (*botrys*, Greek: "bunch of grapes"). Typically, small cells with small, dark, round nuclei are condensed just under the epithelium, making up the celebrated "cambium layer" (*cambium*, Greek: "mantle"). The deeper part of the tumor is edematous. The rhabdomyoblasts are scattered throughout the various layers and often are racquet- or tadpole-shaped with abundant pink cytoplasm containing cross-striations. Rhabdoid differentiation may be enhanced by immunoperoxidase staining. These tumors must be distinguished from benign fibroepithelial polyps with bizarre stromal cells, by the lack of a cambium layer, presence of striated muscle cells and mitoses, and characteristic low-power appearances of the latter.[16-18] Whether sarcoma botryoides is a histologically distinct entity or a site-specific variant of embryonal rhabdomyosarcoma remains debatable, and biologic studies have not yielded a molecular distinction.[19] Rare examples of sarcoma botryoides have been reported in young women; they usually contain cartilage and carry a good prognosis.[20]

Mixed Epithelial/Mesenchymal Tumors

Adenosarcoma. Adenosarcomas are tumor composed of malignant mesenchymal and benign epithelial elements. Grossly, they are superficial polypoid growths that project into and fill the cervix or uterine cavity. Myometrial invasion occurs in about 20% of cases. The cut surface is solid and cystic. Microscopically, these tumors resemble cystosarcoma phylloides of the breast (*phylloid*, Greek: "leaf"), with the broad, leaf-like projections and cysts lined by benign epithelium which usually resembles normal proliferative endometrium. Less commonly the epithelium is mucin-secreting columnar endocervical or squamous in type. The stromal component is endometrial or fibrous, or both. Classically, the stroma is condensed under the surface to form a mantle around the cysts, the so-called cambium layer. Differentiation of this tumor from the benign adenofibroma is difficult and controversial because its cellularity varies from place to place; it is based mainly on the mitotic rate, the cut-off being 2 mf/10 HPF.[21] Nevertheless, adenofibromas placed in the category by the criteria described may recur locally, especially if incompletely excised.[22] Adenosarcomas are indolent tumors with a tendency for late local recurrence in about 20% of cases. They metastasize rarely.

Carcinosarcoma. Carcinosarcomas are tumors composed of mesenchymal and epithelial components, both of which are malignant. Their notoriety as the most malignant of sarcomas has been challenged, precedence now being given to leiomyosarcoma.[7,23] Grossly, they are polypoid growths with necrotic surfaces. The cut surface is variegated, with areas of necrosis, cystic

change, and hemorrhage. A gritty sensation may indicate the presence of cartilage or bone, or both. Although myometrial invasion is the rule, the tumor is rarely confined to a polyp. The stromal component may be homologous (composed of tissues native to the uterus) or heterologous (composed of tissues foreign to the uterus). The homologous components include, in order of frequency, primitive embryonic tissue, nonspecific sarcoma, endometrial stromal sarcoma, or leiomyosarcoma. In some cases, the sarcoma is nonspecific. Heterologous components are most commonly rhabdomyosarcoma, followed by chondrosarcoma, osteosarcoma, and, rarely, liposarcoma. The epithelial element is usually unclassifiable adenocarcinoma or, less commonly, other types of endometrioid adenocarcinoma. Occasionally, squamous carcinoma is also seen.

Carcinosarcomas have traditionally been classified as sarcomas. Their histogenesis, however, has always been contentious, with both monoclonal and biphasic origins having been postulated. More importantly, a number of authorities now believe that carcinosarcomas are metaplastic carcinomas and that it is the epithelial element that "drives" the tumor. In the textbook, *Blaustein's Pathology of the Female Genital Tract*, carcinosarcomas are listed as a variant of endometrial adenocarcinoma.[24] This is of more than just academic interest, because the therapy is different. In particular, the question arises whether the treatment of carcinosarcomas should include routine pelvic lymph node dissection. The arguments advanced for the adenocarcinomatous nature of carcinosarcomas include the following: (1) The two components are of monoclonal origin, as supported by a small number of molecular studies. (2) The mesenchymal elements often express epithelial markers, such as cytokeratins and epithelial membrane antigen. (3) Carcinosarcomas share some of the predisposing factors of endometrioid adenocarcinomas. (4) Carci-nosarcomas are said to respond better to cisplatin-based chemotherapy used for treatment of adenocarcinoma.[25] (5) Pelvic and para-aortic metastases are not uncommon. (6) Metastases are claimed to be pure adenocarcinoma most commonly, rather than sarcoma or a mixture of the two.

The opposing views are set out in *Haines and Taylor's Obstetrical and Gynaecological Pathology*[26]: (1) Some, but not all, of the molecular studies support a monoclonal pathogenesis. (2) Mixed tumors, such as adenosarcomas, do exist, and it is hard to imagine how a sarcoma could derive from benign epithelium. (3) Immunoperoxidase staining is often confusing because pure leiomyosarcomas may express epithelial markers such as cytokeratins and, conversely, poorly differentiated carcinoma may express vimentin, a mesenchymal marker. Furthermore, mesenchymal markers are not as well studied or as distinctive as those of epithelium. Thus the distinction between carcinoma and sarcoma becomes blurred, and in fact there is no single, unequivocal criterion to distinguish between them. (4) The putative shared risk factors are based on a single study of only 29 women, in which the authors concluded that "confirmation of these findings in larger studies is needed."[27] (5) The prognosis of carcinosarcomas is significantly worse than that of grade 3 endometrioid, serous, or clear cell adenocarcinomas. In addition, the presence of this type of tumor is an independent predictor of survival after other factors such as stage, depth of myoinvasion, and vascular involvement are taken into account.[28] (6) The pons asinorum is the nature of metastases, the literature on which is conflicting. A point that has been overlooked is that metastases may vary in their composition in different organs in the same patient. In the new WHO classification, carcinosarcomas are classified under sarcomas.[1]

Smooth muscle proliferations with unusual growth patterns. These tumors include dissecting leiomyoma, intravenous leiomyomatosis, benign metastasizing leiomyoma, parasitic leiomyoma, and disseminated peritoneal leiomyomatosis. These lesions are histologically bland but have a propensity for local spread, recurrence, and distal metastases. A detailed discussion of these rare neoplasms is beyond the scope of this chapter.

Perivascular epithelioid cell tumor (PEComa). The perivascular epithelial cell tumor, or PEComa, is the latest introduction in the galaxy of uterine sarcomas. Whether it is a true clinicopathologic entity remains to be seen. Only a few cases have been reported. Initially described in the lung,[29] the PEComas were called "sugar tumors" because biochemical analysis of tumor tissue revealed a high content of carbohydrates. Grossly, the tumors form intramural uterine masses. Microscopically, they are composed of cells that resemble epithelioid smooth muscle cells but are positive for HMB45, a melanoma marker. Their putative origin is the mythical perivascular epithelioid cell,[30] the presence of which has not been proved in normal tissues. Only 3 of the 12 uterine examples behaved in a malignant fashion, although follow-up was short.[31]

In summary, a number of controversies regarding the histogenesis, classification, and behavior of uterine sarcomas remain. As a group, sarcomas provide a variety of microscopic appearances, which continuously widen the eyes of the most jaded pathologists and clinicians who deal with them (a quote modified from Kraus[32]).

Clinical Features

Three main types of uterine sarcomas are of clinical relevance: leiomyosarcoma, endometrial stroma sarcoma, and mixed mullerian tumors (MMT).

Leiomyosarcoma. Leiomyosarcomas account for about 30% of all uterine sarcomas.[8] The peak incidence is at 50 years of age. The incidence in women undergoing hysterectomy for presumed fibroids is 0.2% for women age 31 to 40 years, 0.9% for 41 to 50 years, 1.4% for 51 to 60 years, and 1.7% for age 61 to 81 years.[33]

Symptoms are nonspecific and include abnormal vaginal bleeding, vaginal discharge, lower abdominal mass, or lower abdominal discomfort. Pulmonary metastases are frequent in patients with advanced disease and can cause respiratory symptoms.[34]

The diagnosis of leiomyosarcoma is usually made histopathologically in a uterus removed for suspected fibroids. Cervical cytology and curettage usually do not reveal the presence of an underlying leiomyosarcoma. Although it was long thought that rapidly growing fibroids were suspicious for sarcoma, Parker and colleagues[35] found only one leiomyosarcoma among 371 such patients. New technologies such as transvaginal color and pulsed Doppler sonography[36] and positron emission tomography with F-fluorodeoxyglucose[37] may improve the preoperative evaluation of patients with uterine tumors.

Endometrial stromal sarcoma. Endometrial stromal sarcomas account for about 15% of uterine sarcomas. The peak incidence of low-grade tumors is before menopause, but the peak incidence of undifferentiated lesions is after menopause. Presenting symptoms are typically menometrorrhagia, postmenopausal bleeding, or lower abdominal discomfort.

Endometrial stromal sarcoma may arise from the stroma of the endometrium or from foci of adenomyosis. The condition is rarely diagnosed at curettage. As with leiomyosarcoma, the preoperative indication is typically uterine fibroids and the diagnosis of endometrial stromal sarcoma is made in the hysterectomy specimen of a uterus removed for presumed uterine fibroids. High-grade or undifferentiated lesions, however, are more likely to be diagnosed with curettage. Early stages are confined to the uterus. In advanced disease, the disease breaks through the uterine wall and spreads via the broad ligament, the parametria, and the adnexa. The disease can spread in the abdomen or to the lungs. Imaging modalities may improve the preoperative diagnosis of endometrial stromal sarcoma.[36,37]

Mixed mullerian tumors. MMTs (the WHO preferred term is carcinosarcoma) account for 40% to 50% of uterine sarcomas and usually occur in postmenopausal women. The mean age of patients with adenosarcoma is 58 years, and that of patients with carcinosarcoma between 60 and 70 years. In one study,[27] carcinosarcoma, like endometrial carcinoma, was associated with nulliparity and obesity.

Clinical symptoms are vaginal bleeding, abdominal or pelvic discomfort, a pelvic mass, and vaginal discharge. Because these tumors grow exophytically, about 40% of patients have tumor in the cervical canal. The diagnosis is made by histopathology of the curettage material.

Prognostic Factors

Uterine sarcomas are generally associated with a poor prognosis. However, these tumors are rare, and the resulting small numbers of patients in individual series make it difficult to analyze prognostic factors in detail.

Leiomyosarcoma. For leiomyosarcoma, tumor stage is the most important prognostic factor.[6,38-43] The prognosis of leiomyosarcoma is considered worse than that of MMT.[23] The mitotic index may have value as a prognostic factor. In a number of studies, the mitotic index was the only statistically significant prognostic factor.[6,7,44,45] In contrast, Evans and associates[46] did not find the mitotic index to be a prognostic factor. Tumor size appears to be a prognostic factor in patients with stage I disease.[42,44] In some studies, premenopausal women have done better than their postmenopausal counterparts.[6,39,43,44,47,48] In other studies, age was not significantly associated with prognosis.[49,50]

Endometrial stromal sarcoma. As with leiomyosarcoma, the stage of the disease is the most important prognostic factor for endometrial stromal sarcoma.[46,51] In a univariate analysis of patients with stage I disease, prolonged overall survival was associated with minor myometrial invasion and a low mitotic index.[52]

Mixed mullerian tumors. The prognosis of patients with MMT is poor. The most important prognostic factor is the surgical stage of the disease, extrauterine spread, and depth of invasion.[11,14,33,53-61] Lymphovascular space involvement is significantly associated with metastases. In a multivariate analysis of 46 patients Nordal and coworkers[2] found extrauterine spread, age, and the percentage of the serous or clear cell component to be significant prognostic factors, whereas mitotic index, vascular invasion, and DNA ploidy were not. Tumor size was a significant prognostic factor in the univariate but not the multivariate analysis. These results may be influenced by the limited number of patients in the series.[2] Marth and colleagues[62] found parity to be an independent prognostic factor, but this was not confirmed by others.[2] In a Gynecologic Oncology Group (GOG) study[7] based on 301 cases of MMT, 167 were classified as homologous and 134 as heterologous. In the univariate analysis, adnexal involvement, lymph node metastases, tumor size, lymphovascular space involvement, histologic grade, cell type, age, positive peritoneal cytology, and depth of invasion had a significant impact on the progression-free interval. In the multivariate analysis, adnexal involvement, node metastases, histologic cell type (heterologous versus homologous), and grade were significant prognostic factors.

Staging. There is no official staging system for uterine sarcomas. These tumors are staged according to the International Federation of Gynecology and Obstetrics (FIGO) system for carcinoma of the corpus uteri.

SURGICAL TREATMENT

There are no randomized studies to guide the surgical treatment of patients with uterine sarcomas. Also, the diagnosis frequently is made only after surgery is completed. If the diagnosis is known, surgery is planned according to the stage of the tumor and the status of the lymph nodes.

Hysterectomy is the cornerstone of treatment for patients with malignancies of the uterus, although preservation of the uterus may be considered for young patients with an incidental diagnosis of low-grade leiomyosarcoma. There are no data to indicate whether a radical hysterectomy decreases the rate of local recurrence.

Surgical staging includes determining the status of the lymph nodes. Sampling procedures may underestimate the incidence of node involvement, compared with systematic removal of the node-bearing tissue. If only enlarged nodes are removed, micrometastases will be missed. In an analysis of patients undergoing systematic lymphadenectomy for endometrial carcinoma, Girardi and associates[63] found that 37% of node metastases in patients with endometrial cancer were smaller than 2 mm. The fact that large tumor deposits, particularly in the para-aortic region, probably cannot be treated effectively by chemotherapy or radiation therapy is an argument for the surgical removal of bulky lymph nodes.

Leiomyosarcoma

Leiomyosarcomas arise in the myometrium and spread through the lymphatic vessels to the regional lymph nodes and the peritoneal cavity. However, in the GOG study,[7] only 3.5% of patients with stage I or II disease who underwent node sampling as part of surgical staging had positive lymph nodes, and only 3.4% had adnexal involvement. Chen[64] described a 15% rate of node involvement in stage I/II disease. In a series of 15 women with surgical staging, Goff and colleagues[34] found node involvement only in patients with peritoneal spread. In contrast, in advanced disease the rate of node involvement is as high as 44%.[34,65,66] Leibsohn and associates[33] reported a 50% rate of node involvement in patients with tumors measuring 6 to 10 cm. Because tumor size is associated with survival, it appears useful to incorporate it into the planning of treatment.

Premenopausal women who are operated on for uterine fibroids frequently desire preservation of the uterus. In stage I/II, premenopausal women appear to have a better prognosis than their postmenopausal counterparts. The ovaries are seldom involved,[7] and leaving the adnexa in situ does not appear to increase the risk of recurrence.[44,67-69] In contrast, Abu-Rustum and coworkers[70] described spontaneous regression of a pulmonary metastasis after salpingo-oophorectomy.

Hysterectomy and bilateral salpingo-oophorectomy are indicated in postmenopausal women. If the diagnosis of sarcoma is known, peritoneal cytology and omentectomy are advisable to evaluate intraperitoneal spread. Intraoperative frozen section analysis appears to be of limited value in patients with leiomyosarcoma.[71] If the diagnosis of leiomyosarcoma is made after vaginal hysterectomy (e.g., in a patient with a presumed myoma in statu nascendi), radiotherapy can be considered (see later discussion), particularly if morcellation was required when the uterus was removed. In patients with advanced disease, debulking surgery appears warranted, with the intention of prolonging quality of life for as long as possible. Isolated pulmonary metastases can be considered for resection. Survival rates of 43% at 5 years have been reported.[72]

The role of lymphadenectomy in patients with leiomyosarcoma appears to be limited, because a high proportion of patients with negative lymph nodes develop recurrence anyway.[34] In contrast, Morrow[73] recommended node sampling, particularly in the para-aortic region.

One of us (R.W.) considers surgical staging adequate only if it includes an assessment of the lymph nodes. It appears justified to omit lymph node dissection in patients with low-grade leiomyosarcoma, in premenopausal women, and in those with a tumor diameter of less than 5 cm. In contrast, nodes should be removed in postmenopausal women with high-grade tumors larger than 5 cm. Because primary surgery is frequently performed without knowledge of the nature of the tumor, these latter patients should be referred to a tertiary referral center and considered for a formal staging procedure. An alternate view should also be considered. Like endometrial cancer, uterine sarcomas initially spread in the pelvis. Both Covens and associates[74] and DiSaia and colleagues[75] found para-aortic node involvement only in patients with positive pelvic nodes. Accordingly, lymphadenectomy should begin in the pelvis, not in the para-aortic region. No patient with positive nodes survived longer than 2 years.[74]

Recommendations for the surgical treatment of leiomyosarcoma are shown in Figure 22-1.

Endometrial Stroma Sarcoma

The difficulties in the diagnosis of endometrial stromal sarcoma resemble those of leiomyosarcoma. Polypoid tumors filling the uterine cavity and extending into the cervical canal can be diagnosed with curettage or biopsy. In a small series of five patients with stage I and two with stage III disease, Goff and coworkers[34] found no metastases. In the series reported by Covens and associates,[74] all three women with low-grade endometrial stromal sarcoma survived for 5 years, whereas three of four women with high-grade lesions died within 2 years. Chang and colleagues[12] questioned the validity of conventional classification of stage I endometrial stromal sarcoma into low-grade and high-grade tumors. In a retrospective analysis that did not supply information on tumor stage, Salazar[76] reported that four of six patients developed recurrence irrespective of adjuvant treatment.

Because very few data are available on the incidence of lymph node involvement in patients with endometrial stromal sarcoma, it is difficult to say whether lymphadenectomy is appropriate for these patients. Surgery should be guided by the general principles of surgery for uterine sarcomas. Recommendations are shown in Figure 22-2.

Mixed Mullerian Tumors

Adenosarcoma. Adenosarcomas have a better prognosis than carcinosarcomas, because most patients are diagnosed with stage I disease.[21,77] Pelvic lymph node metastases are likely if the sarcomatous component makes up more than 25% of the tumor.[78,79] Between 25% and 40% of patients develop a recurrence, most commonly in the vagina or pelvis.[78,79] Recurrences are usually composed primarily of the sarcomatous component.[54,80] The risk of recurrence increases with the proportion of the sarcomatous component, deep myometrial invasion, and spread beyond the uterus.

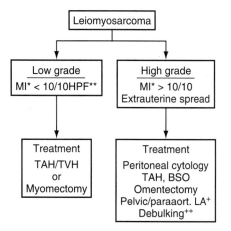

* MI = mitotic index; ** HPF = high power field by 40X objective;
+ Paraaortic lymphadenectomy if pelvic nodes are positive;
++ in advanced stages taking into consideration medical condition and quality of life

Figure 22–1. Algorithm for surgical treatment of leiomyosarcoma. BSO, bilateral salpingo-oophorectomy; HPF, high-power field by 40× objective; LA, lymphadenectomy; MI, mitotic index; TAH, total abdominal hysterectomy; TVH, total vaginal hysterectomy.

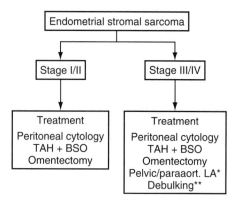

* Paraaortic lymphadenectomy if pelvic nodes are positive;
** taking into consideration medical condition and quality of life

Figure 22–2. Algorithm for surgical treatment of endometrial stromal sarcoma. BSO, bilateral salpingo-oophorectomy; LA, lymphadenectomy; TAH, total abdominal hysterectomy.

Figure 22–3. Algorithm for surgical treatment of mixed epithelial/mesenchymal tumors. BSO, bilateral salpingo-oophorectomy; LA, lymphadenectomy; LVSI, lymphovascular space involvement; RAH, radical abdominal hysterectomy; TAH, total abdominal hysterectomy.

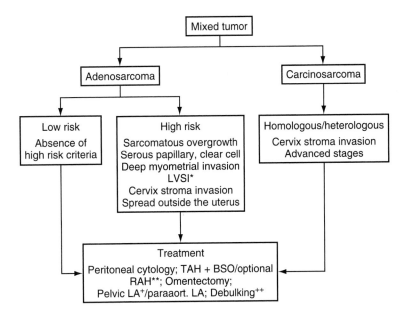

* LVSI = lymph vascular space involvement; ** RAH = radical abdominal hysterectomy;
⁺ paraaortic lymphadenectomy if pelvic nodes are positive; ⁺⁺ taking into consideration medical condition and quality of life

In patients without these risk factors, surgical treatment consists of hysterectomy, bilateral salpingo-oophorectomy, and omentectomy. Radical hysterectomy may be considered in patients with risk factors, extension to the cervical stroma, or parametrial tissue. Para-aortic lymphadenectomy should be considered for patients with positive pelvic nodes. Peritoneal washings and omentectomy are part of surgical staging. Debulking may provide palliation for women with advanced disease. Recommendations are shown in Figure 22-3.

Carcinosarcoma. Carcinosarcomas spread rapidly to the pelvic and para-aortic lymph nodes, the vagina, the adnexa, and peritoneal surfaces. Patients with advanced disease frequently have tumor in the upper abdomen and in the lungs. Metastases may originate from the carcinomatous or the sarcomatous component of the primary tumor. Metastases with both components have been reported.[81] In the GOG study of 301 cases (167 homologous, 134 heterologous), up to 20% of patients with clinical stage I/II disease had lymph node metastases,[7] and 20% had to be reclassified as stage III/IV. The rate of pelvic node involvement was twice that of para-aortic node involvement (15% versus 7.8%), and 5% of the patients had both pelvic and para-aortic node involvement. Morrow[73] reported on a patient who had para-aortic metastases but negative pelvic nodes. The rate of node involvement in patients with clinical stage I/II papillary-serous or clear cell tumors was 30%. Node involvement was found in 68% of patients with spread to the adnexa, compared with 11% of those without adnexal involvement. For both heterologous and homologous stage I/II carcinosarcoma, the rate of adnexal involvement was 12%, positive peritoneal cytology was 22%, cervical involvement was 26%, and extension to the outer half of the myometrium was 38%. Eighty percent of tumors measured between 2 and 10 cm, 50% of tumors were poorly differentiated, and 85% of homologous and 79% of heterologous carcinosarcomas had a mitotic index greater than 16 mf/10 HPF.

The distinction between homologous and heterologous tumors is not relevant for surgical treatment. Because the diagnosis is usually known before surgery, these patients should be operated on by a gynecologic oncologist. Spread beyond the uterus can frequently be assessed by preoperative imaging studies. Radical hysterectomy with bilateral salpingo-oophorectomy may be considered for patients with spread to the cervix or parametrial tissues. For tumors limited to the uterus, total hysterectomy with salpingo-oophorectomy appears sufficient. Covens and associates[74] found no difference in survival for patients with stage I disease treated with regular hysterectomy versus radical hysterectomy. Lymphadenectomy appears to be warranted because of the rate of node involvement in these patients; it should be begun in the pelvis and extended cephalad only if those nodes are positive. Omentectomy and peritoneal washings are part of surgical staging.

The prognosis of patients with spread beyond the uterus is guarded, but surgery should not compromise quality of life in these patients. Recommendations are shown in Figure 22-3.

ADJUVANT TREATMENT

Radiotherapy in the Treatment of Uterine Sarcomas

The role of adjuvant radiotherapy in the management of uterine sarcomas has never been tested in a randomized trial and is still controversial. The data provided in the literature, all of which were retrieved retrospectively, are based on small patient numbers, precluding a definitive conclusion on the efficacy of radiotherapy. In addition, comparisons between individual reports are hampered by differences in patient selection, treatment techniques (i.e., pelvic radiotherapy, brachytherapy, or a combination of both), and the radiation doses delivered. Details of the radiation doses are lacking in most reports. The reasons for employing irradiation are often not stated, suggesting that the decision for referral may be guided by institutional or physician preference.

Postoperative radiotherapy. The results of the majority of reports of the value of adjuvant radiotherapy suggest that adjuvant irradiation increases the rate of pelvic control without affecting survival.

Salazar and colleagues,[76] who analyzed patterns of failure according to treatment modality, found that pelvic control was markedly increased in 31 patients who received postoperative pelvic irradiation 33 patients who were treated with surgery alone. Overall outcome was not affected, because almost 50% of overall failures occurred both in the pelvis and at distant sites, and 47% occurred at sites beyond the pelvis. In a series on 87 patients, Sorbe and coworkers[82] reported significantly fewer pelvic failures among women who received adjuvant radiotherapy ($n = 18$) versus additive radiotherapy ($n = 44$). Although the difference in survival was not significant, there was a trend toward improved survival for patients in the combined modality group. In a large survey on 209 patients, 49% of whom received adjuvant pelvic radiotherapy, George and colleagues[83] found that, although 2-year survival rates according to stage were similar for both groups, the 2-year recurrence rate was lower in patients treated with postoperative radiotherapy.

The fact that distant spread is a major component of failure in uterine sarcomas prompted the Gynecological Oncology Group (GOG) to investigate the value of adjuvant chemotherapy in stage I and II disease in a prospective randomized trial.[84] This trial, in which postoperative irradiation was optional, failed to demonstrate a significant difference in recurrence rate, progression-free interval, or survival. Hornback and associates[85] compared the outcome of 60 women who received adjuvant radiotherapy in this trial with that of 97 women who had surgery alone and found that only 23% of irradiated patients failed in the pelvis, compared with 54% of the nonirradiated group. No difference in progression-free interval was observed. A significant decrease in local recurrence ($P < .01$) was also reported by Covens and colleagues,[74] with no failures among 15 patients who underwent radiotherapy, compared with a 41% failure rate among 22 patients treated with surgery only. With regard to the overall rate of treatment failures, Jereczek and coworkers[86] found that 7 (50%) of 14 patients who received adjuvant radiotherapy had recurrence, only one of which was in the pelvis, as opposed to 12 (70.5%) of 17 nonirradiated patients, with 9 failing locoregionally.

No impact of postoperative radiotherapy on outcome was reported by Tinkler and coworkers.[87] Although approximately half of the 82 patients in their series (50% of whom presented with stage I disease) received pelvic radiotherapy, no differences in local control or survival were observed. Fifty-one of 54 patients who relapsed had evidence of distant spread. Other researchers[88] found that recurrences were decreased in patients with endometrial stromal sarcoma only. However, among the 64 patients with stage I disease (which included 28% leiomyosarcoma, 28% MMT, and 16% endometrial stromal sarcoma), only 16 had received postoperative radiotherapy. Chauveinc and colleagues[89] noted improved pelvic control in all irradiated patients regardless of the histologic type. According to multivariate analysis, however, best results were obtained in patients with endometrial stromal sarcoma. A similar pattern of response was observed by Echt and associates.[90]

In contrast to the studies cited earlier, improved overall survival, disease-free interval, and local recurrence–free interval were reported by Ferrer and colleagues[91] who analyzed a cohort of 103 patients, of whom 52% received pelvic irradiation, with more than half of those also receiving brachytherapy. Actuarial survival at 5 years was 73% with adjuvant radiotherapy and 37% without it. The 5-year disease-free interval increased from 33% to 53%, and the 5-year locoregional recurrence–free interval from 36% to 76%. A survival benefit was shown in a previous study,[92] in which 17 of 76 patients who underwent radiotherapy had improved overall survival ($P = .045$) and relapse-free interval ($P = .005$), whereas no improvement in outcome was observed in 19 patients who received adjuvant chemotherapy. Knocke and colleagues[93] also reported a survival benefit, which appeared to be based on improved pelvic control, for the two subgroups of patients with disease, those confined to the uterus and those patients with endometrial stromal sarcoma.

Few studies have reported separate control rates for the classic types of uterine sarcomas. Retrospective reviews of patients with MMT have shown controversial results. Nielsen and colleagues,[94] in a clinicopathologic analysis of 60 patients with MMT, could demonstrate neither a significant survival advantage for surgery plus irradiation, or for surgery plus chemo-therapy, compared with surgery alone after stratification according to stage nor a difference in pelvic recurrence-free survival. Only a trend toward a decreased rate of pelvic recurrences in patients receiving whole pelvic radiotherapy for stage I/II disease was observed by Chi and associates.[96] This is in contrast to findings by Gerszten and coworkers,[96] who demonstrated that the addition of radiotherapy significantly reduced the local recurrence rate from 55% to 3%, which translated into an improvement in distant failure rates and consequently in survival for patients with stage I/II tumors. Excellent results were also obtained by Manolitsas and colleagues[97] in a pilot study of combined adjuvant chemotherapy and radiotherapy in patients with stage I/II disease. Patients who completed the standard protocol had a significantly better survival ($P = .02$) than patients who did not receive the recommended treatment, with survival rates of 95% and 47%, respectively.

Only one report exists on the role of radiotherapy in patients with leiomyosarcoma.[6] Of 126 patients analyzed, 71.4% presented with stage I/II tumors. Approximately 30% of patients received adjuvant radiotherapy. None of the irradiated patients had failure in the pelvis, as opposed to 14.3% in the surgery-only group. Twenty-three patients with stage I/II developed distant metastases. Only 5 of the irradiated patients failed distantly, compared with 18 of the surgery-only group. Reports on the potential benefit of radiotherapy in endometrial stromal sarcoma[52,98] must be considered anecdotal. Although the reported data on survival and locoregional control appear better than those reported for MMT or leiomyosarcoma, no conclusion can be reached on the effect of adjuvant radiotherapy.

Preoperative radiotherapy. Although preoperative radiotherapy was used in the past[99] and was shown to reduce the incidence of local failure, the rationale for such an approach must be questioned. Only surgery with careful exploration of pelvic and abdominal spread provides the data based on which adjuvant or additive therapeutic modalities can be selected.

Primary radiotherapy. Primary radiotherapy is reserved for patients who are unable to undergo surgery for medical or technical reasons. The belief that uterine sarcomas are "radioresistant" should be modified to "less radiosensitive," because radiotherapy in the adjuvant setting has proved its efficacy in mesenchymal tumors at other sites. Although radiotherapy is clearly inadequate primary treatment for uterine sarcomas, it should nevertheless be consid-ered to delay locoregional progression or to palliate side effects caused by growth into adjacent structures. The same holds for postoperative recurrences in the pelvis or vagina and for distant metastases at sites that can be treated with adequate doses to achieve relief of symptoms.

In conclusion, the role of radiation therapy has not been properly defined because reliable data are still lacking. Although there appears to be a benefit of adjuvant radiotherapy in patients with disease confined to the uterus in terms of improved locoregional control, the subsets of patients who benefit from locoregional treatment are yet to be defined. Only prospective, randomized, multicenter trials with stratification according to the major histologic variants and prognostic factors (e.g. stage, depth of infiltration, lymph node status, grade, menopausal status) can provide these long-needed answers.

Chemotherapy in the Treatment of Uterine Sarcomas

Leiomyosarcoma

Adjuvant chemotherapy. The prognosis of patients with uterine sarcomas is generally poor, with 5-year survival rates of about 50% to 60% in stage I and about 15% in stage II-IV disease. In this context, adjuvant therapeutic interventions are of particular interest. High recurrence rates and a propensity to develop distant metastases make these tumors potential candidates for systemic therapy.

There has been only one randomized study comparing adjuvant doxorubicin with observation in 156 patients after surgery for stage I-II uterine sarcoma. Eight courses of doxorubicin were administered at 60 mg/m[2] every 3 weeks.[98] Overall, there seemed to be a trend toward improved reduced recurrence rates and improved survival in the chemotherapy group (Table 22-2). However, the subgroup analysis of the patients with stage I disease did not reveal any benefit of chemotherapy in this population. In conclusion, there is no clear justification for the use of adjuvant chemotherapy in uterine sarcoma.[100,101]

Palliative chemotherapy. Tables 22-3 and 22-4 list the key efficacy and toxicity data of various single-agent and combination chemotherapy studies in uterine sarcomas, with special emphasis given to leiomyosarcomas. Studies are ranked according to remission rate. In general, the numbers of patients treated within these studies were small and rarely exceeded 30 patients.[102-106] Ifosfamide appeared to be the most active chemotherapeutic agent in advanced leiomyosarcoma.[103,104,107] Combinations with anthracyclines seemed to be modestly more active but significantly more toxic, especially myelotoxic.[103,108]

Table 22–2. Recurrence Rates and Median Survival Time after Adjuvant Chemotherapy with Doxorubicin in Stage I/II Uterine Sarcoma According to Histology

	Recurrence Rate (%)	
Histology	Doxorubicin (n = 75)	Untreated Controls (n = 81)
Leiomyosarcoma	44	61
Homologous carcinosarcoma (MMT)	40	52
Heterologous MMT	37	50
Other histologic subtypes	50	44
Median survival time	73.7 mo	55.0 mo

MMT, mixed mullerian tumor.
From Omura G, Blessing J, Major F, et al: A randomized clinical trial of adjuvant Adriamycin in uterine sarcomas: A Gynecologic Oncology Group study. J Clin Oncol 1985;3:1240-1245.

Table 22–3. Palliative Single-Agent Chemotherapy in Uterine Sarcomas, with Particular Reference to Leiomyosarcomas

Chemotherapy Regimen	No. of Patients	Response	Complete Response	Median Progression-Free Survival Time (mo)	Median Survival Time (mo)	Remarks	Reference
Epirubicin	20	7/20 (35%) 4/13 (31%)*	4/20 (20%) 2/13 (15%)*	—	—	Epirubicin 120 mg/m² q 3 wk; no life-threatening toxicity	Lissoni et al.[119] (1997)
Ifosfamide	35	6/35 (17%)*	0/35 (0)*	—	6.0	11% grade 3-4 neutropenia; 3% grade 4 neurotoxicity; GOG study	Sutton et al.[104] (1992)
Cisplatin	96	1/33 (3%)*	0/33 (0)*	—	7.8	Cisplatin 50 mg/m² q 3 wk as first-line chemotherapy; no life-threatening toxicity; GOG study	Thigpen et al.[106] (1991)
Doxorubicin	39	1/17 (6%)*	0/17 (0)*	—	8.1	—	Hannigan et al.[115] (1983)
Paclitaxel	34	3/34 (9%)*	3/34 (9%)*	—	—	33% grade 3-4 neutropenia; GOG study	Sutton et al.[105] (1999)
Cisplatin	20	1/20 (5%)*	0/20 (0)*	—	—	Cisplatin 50 mg/m² q 3 wk as second-line chemotherapy; GOG study	Thigpen et al.[123] (1986)

*Results for leiomyosarcomas.
GOG, Gynecologic Oncology Group.

Cisplatin alone has only modest activity. Reported experience is scant with paclitaxel and docetaxel. Taxanes may play a role in the design of future studies to improve treatment results. Monotherapy with liposomal doxorubicin, etoposide, or topotecan has only shown marginal activity in phase II studies. Two current phase II GOG studies are investigating the use of dacarbazine, mitomycin C, doxorubicin, and cisplatin (GOG 0131) as well as docetaxel and gemcitabine (GOG 0087) in advanced leiomyosarcoma. Another phase II study is evaluating the efficacy of temozolomide and thalidomide in metastatic or advanced leiomyosarcoma (NCI-G02-2060).

Lung metastases seem to respond more favorably to chemotherapy than do lesions of the liver or the vagina.[109]

Endometrial Stromal Sarcoma

Adjuvant chemotherapy. There are only anecdotal studies on the use of adjuvant chemotherapy in stage I-II endometrial stromal sarcoma. Either doxorubicin or vincristine was used with actinomycin D and cyclophosphamide.[110]

Palliative chemotherapy. Little data exists on chemotherapy in this rare disease. In one GOG-study is listed, in which response rates of 33% were observed in 22 patients treated with ifosfamide.[108]

Palliative hormonal therapy. Endometrial stromal sarcoma is generally rich in estrogen and progesterone receptors. Remissions after gestagens, in particular megestrol acetate, have been reported. In recent years, gonadotropin-releasing hormone analog[111] and aromatase inhibitors[112] have been used.

Carcinosarcoma (mixed mesodermal sarcoma, malignant mullerian tumor)

Adjuvant chemotherapy. In a GOG study, after a minimum follow-up of 2 years, ifosfamide and cisplatin resulted in a progression-free survival rate of 63% and an overall survival rate of 74%.[113] This treatment was associated with grade 3 or 4 neutropenia as well as grade 3 or 4 thrombocytopenia in 63% and 26% of patients, respectively.

In another study, 38 patients with stage I-II MMT received cisplatin and epirubicin in addition to radiotherapy. After complete surgical staging, multimodality therapy resulted in an overall survival rate of 74%. The survival rate was 95% among patients who completed treatment according to the multimodality protocol.[97]

In conclusion, adjuvant treatment results including chemotherapy seem promising but not convincing in this type of uterine tumor.

Palliative chemotherapy. MMTs are usually more sensitive to chemotherapy than leiomyosarcomas.

Table 22–4. Palliative Combination Chemotherapy in Uterine Sarcomas, with Particular Reference to Leiomyosarcomas

Chemotherapy Regimen	No. of Patients	Response	Complete Response	Median Progression-Free Survival Time (mo)	Median Survival Time (mo)	Remarks	Reference
Ifosfamide + doxorubicin	30	16/26 (62%) 10/17 (55%)*	4/26 (15%) —*	12	—	Ifosfamide 2-2.4 mg/m²/day on days 1-5; doxorubicin 20-30mg/m²/day on days 1-3 q 3 wk; G-CSF for 10 days; 63% febrile episodes; 40% grade 2-3 mucositis	Leyvraz et al.[103] (1998)
Cisplatin + ifosfamide + epirubicin	27	15/27 (56%) 4/10 (40%)*	6/27 (22%) 0/10 (0)*	—	15.9	37% grade 3-4 leukopenia; 19% grade 3 thrombocytopenia	Shimizu[117] (2000)
Docetaxel + gemcitabine	18	8/18 (44%)*	3/18 (17%)*	—	—	25% grade 3-4 granulocytopenia; 25% grade 3-4 thrombocytopenia; 5% neutropenic fever	Hensley et al.[118] (2001)
Ifosfamide + doxorubicin	34	10/33 (30%)*	1/34 (3%)*	—	—	Ifosfamide 5 g/m²/day; doxorubicin 50 mg/m²/day q 3 wk; 49% grade 3-4 granulocytopenia; 1 death from sepsis and 1 from cardiotoxicitiy	Sutton et al.[108] (1996)
Doxorubicin + dacarbazine doxorubicin	240	6/20 (30%)* 7/28 (25%)*	NR** NR**	— —	— —	44% grade 3-4 leukopenia; 14% grade 3-4 thrombocytopenia; GOG study	Omura et al.[109] (1983)
Cyclophosphamide + vincristine + doxorubicin + dacarbazine	30	7/30 (23%)	1/30 (3%)	—	—	—	Piver and Rose[120] (1988)
Cisplatin + dacarbazine	19	4/19 (21%)	3/19 (16%)	—	—		
Vincristine + dactinomycin + cyclophosphamide	11	2/11 (18%)	0/11 (0)	—	—		
Doxorubicin + cyclophosphamide	132	3/23 (13%)*	0/23 (0)*	11.0	5.0	No life-threatening Toxicity; GOG study	Muss et al.[121] (1985)
or Doxorubicin Dacarbazine + etoposide + hydroxyurea	39	7/39 (18%)*	2/39 (5%)*	—	—	No life-threatening Toxicity; GOG study	Currie et al.[102] (1996)
Ifosfamide + doxorubicin	11	1/11 (9%)*	1/11 (9%)*	—	—	—	Hawkins et al.[122] (1990)
Ifosfamide	10	1/10 (10%)*	0/10 (0)*	—	—		

*Results for leiomyosarcomas.
G-CSF, granulocyte colony-stimulating factor; GOG, Gynecologic Oncology Group.
**NR, Not reported.

Table 22–5. Palliative Chemotherapy in Endometrial Stromal Sarcoma

Chemotherapy Regimen	No. of Patients	Response	Complete Response	Median Progression-Free Survival Time (mo)	Median Survival Time (mo)	Remarks	Reference
Ifosfamide	22	7/21 (33%)	3/21 (14%)	—	—	Ifosfamide 1.2-1.5 mg/m² /day on days 1-5 q 3 wk; 19% grade 3-4 neutropenia; GOG study	Sutton et al.[107] (1996)

GOG, Gynecologic Oncology Group.

Tables 22-6 and 22-7 list the response, survival, and toxicity data of various single-agent and combination chemotherapy studies ranked according to activity. Similarly to leiomyosarcomas, the numbers of patients treated in these studies have been small, thus precluding definite conclusions. Again, ifosfamide plays a significant role in the treatment of advanced disease. However, treatment with this agent may also be associated with significant toxicity, especially when it is used in combinations. One randomized study compared the combination of cisplatin and ifosfamide alone. Although the response rate was higher in the combination arm (see Table 22-7), no clearcut advantage for combination therapy could be identified.[114]

Cisplatin and doxorubicin are moderately active in MMTs.[106,115] In a GOG study, oral trimetrexate demonstrated insignificant activity only.[116] One current randomized phase III GOG study (GOG 161) is

Table 22–6. Palliative Single-Agent Chemotherapy in Carcinosarcoma of the Uterus (Mixed Mesodermal Sarcoma; Malignant Mullerian Tumor)

Chemotherapy Regimen	No. of Patients	Response	Complete Response	Median Progression-Free Survival Time (mo)	Median Survival Time (mo)	Remarks	Reference
Cisplatin	18	5/12 (42%)	1/12 (8%)	4.5	—	Cisplatin 75-100 mg/m² q 4 wk	Gershenson et al.[124] 1987
Ifosfamide	29	9/28 (32%)	5/28 (18%)	—	—	Ifosfamide 1.2-1.5 mg/m² /day on days 1-5 q 4 wk; GOG study; grade 3-4 neurotoxicity in 2 patients, 1 of whom died from toxicity	Sutton et al.[125] (1989)
Cisplatin	63	12/63 (19%)	5/63 (8%)	—	—	Cisplatin 50 mg/m² q 3 wk as first-line chemotherapy; GOG study	Thigpen et al.[106] (1991)
Cisplatin	34	5/28 (18%)	2/28 (7%)	—	—	Cisplatin 50 mg/m² q 3 wk as second-line chemotherapy; GOG study	Thigpen et al.[126] (1986)
Doxorubicin	19	3/19 (16%)	0/19 (0)	—	5.7	—	Hannigan et al.[115] (1983)
Doxorubicin	15	0/9 (0)	0/9 (0)	—	11.3	Doxorubicin 50-90 mg/m² q 4 wk; 2 septic deaths; cardiotoxicity in 2 patients	Gershenson et al.[128] (1987)

GOG, Gynecologic Oncology Group.

Table 22–7. Palliative Combination Chemotherapy in Carcinosarcoma of the Uterus (Mixed Mesodermal Sarcoma; Malignant Mullerian Tumor)

Chemotherapy Regimen	No. of Patients	Response	Complete Response	Median Progression-Free Survival Time (mo)	Median Survival Time (mo)	Remarks	Reference
Cisplatin + ifosfamide	224	54%	—	—	—	Randomized GOG study; neutropenia grade 3-4 in 60% and 36%, respectively; grade 3-4 CNS toxicity in 14% and 18%, respectively	Sutton et al.[114] (1998)
Ifosfamide		36%	—	—	—		
Doxorubicin + dacarbazine	72	7/31 (23%)	—	—	—	—	Omura et al.[109] (1983)
Doxorubicin		4/41 (10%)	—	—	—		
Doxorubicin + cyclophosphamide or Doxorubicin	20	5/20 (25%)	2/20 (10%)	—	—	No life-threatening toxicity; GOG study	Muss[121] et al. (1985)
Dacarbazine + hydroxyurea + etoposide	33	5/32 (15%)	2/32 (6%)	—	—	4-day regimen; no therapy-related deaths; GOG study	Currie et al.[127] (1996)

CNS, central nervous system; GOG, Gynecologic Oncology Group.

investigating the addition of paclitaxel to ifosfamide in MMT of the uterus. A phase II study is currently evaluating the efficacy of thalidomide in this disease.

In conclusion, ifosfamide, although significantly toxic, seems to be the most active agent in the palliative treatment of MMT.

REFERENCES

1 Tavassoli FA, Devilee P (eds.): Pathology and Genetics of Tumours of the Breast and Female Genital Organs. Lyon, IARC Press 2003, p. 218.
2. Nordal RR, Kristensen GB, Stenwig AE, et al: An evaluation of prognostic factors in uterine carcinosarcoma. Gynecol Oncol 1997;3;316-321.
3. McCluggage WG, Abdulkader M, Price JH, et al: Uterine carcinosarcomas in patients receiving tamoxifen: A report of 19 cases. Int J Gynecol Cancer 2000;10:280-284.
4. Treilleux T, Mignotte H, Clement-Chassagne C, et al: Tamoxifen and malignant epithelial-nonepithelial tumors of the endometrium: report of six cases and review of the literature. Eur Surg Oncol 1999;25:477-482.
5. Chumas JC, Mann WJ, Tseng L: Malignant mixed mullerian tumor of the endometrium in a young woman with polycystic ovaries. Cancer 1983;52:1478-1481.
6. Gaducci A, Landoni F, Sartori E, et al: Uterine leiomyosarcoma: Analysis of treatment failures and survival. Gynecol Oncol 1996; 62:25-32.
7. Major FJ, Blessing JA, Silverberg SG, et al: Prognostic factors in early-stage uterine sarcoma: A Gynaecologic Oncology Group study. Cancer 1993;71:1702-1709.
8. Harlow BL, Weiss NS, Lofton S: The epidemiology of sarcomas of the uterus. J Natl Cancer Inst 1986;76:399-402.
9. Madison T, Schottenfeld D, Baker V: Cancer of the corpus uteri in white and black women in Michigan, 1985-1994: An analysis in trends in incidence and mortality and their relation to histologic subtype and stage. Cancer 1998;83:1546-1554.
10. Norris HJ, Taylor HB: Mesenchymal tumors of the uterus. I. A clinical and pathological study of 53 endometrial stromal tumors. Cancer 1966;19:755-766.
11. Tavassoli FA, Norris HJ: Mesenchymal tumors of the uterus VII: A clinicopathologic study of 60 endometrial stroma nodules. Histopathology 1981;5:1-10.
12. Chang KL, Crabtree GS, Lim-Tan SK, et al: Primary uterine endometrial stroma neoplasms: A clinicopathologic study of 117 cases. Am J Surg Pathol 1990;14:415-438.
13. Evans HL: Endometrial stroma sarcoma and poorly differentiated endometrial sarcoma. Cancer 1982;50:2170-2182.
14. Oliva E, Clement PB, Young RH, Scully RE: Mixed endometrial stroma and smooth muscle tumors of the uterus: A clinicopathologic study of 15 cases. Am J Surg Pathol 1998;22:997-1005.
15. Schammel DP, Silver SA, Tavassoli FA: Combined endometrial stromal/smooth muscle neoplasms of the uterus: Clinicopathologic study of 38 cases. Mod Pathol 1999;12:124A.
16. Norris HT, Taylor HB: Polyps of the vagina: A benign lesion resembling sarcoma botryoides. Cancer 1966;19:227-232.
17. Nucci MR, Young RH, Fletcher CD: Cellular pseudosarcomatous fibroepithelial stromal polyps of the lower female genital tract: An underrecognized lesion often misdiagnosed as sarcoma. Am J Surg Pathol 2000;24:231-240.
18. Östör AG, Fortune DW, Riley CB: Fibroepithelial polyps with atypical stromal cells (pseudosarcoma botryoides) of the vulva and vagina: A report of 13 cases. Int J Gynecol Pathol 1988;7:351-360.
19. Parham DM: Pathologic classification of rhabdomyosarcomas and correlations with molecular studies. Mod Pathol 2001;14: 506-514.
20. Daya DA, Scully RE: Sarcoma botryoides of the uterine cervix in young women: A clinicopathological study of 13 cases. Gynecol Oncol 1988;29:290-304.
21. Clement PB, Scully RE: Müllerian adenosarcoma of the uterus: A clinicopathologic analysis of 100 cases with a review of the literature. Hum Pathol 1990;21:363-381.
22. Östör AG, Fortune DW: Benign and low grade variants of mixed mullerian tumor of the uterus. Histopathology 1980;4:369-382.
23. Olah KS, Dunn JA, Gee H: Leiomyosarcomas have a poorer prognosis than mixed mesodermal tumors when adjusting

for known prognostic factors: The result of a retrospective study of 423 cases of uterine sarcoma. Br J Obstet Gynaecol 1992;99: 590-594.

24. Ronnett BM, Zaino RJ, Elenson LH, Kurman RJ: Endometrial carcinoma. In Kurman RJ (ed): Blaustein's Pathology of the Female Genital Tract, 5th ed. New York, Springer-Verlag, 2002, pp. 538-541.

25. Van Rijswijk REN, Tognon G, Burger CW, et al: The effect of chemotherapy on the differential components of advanced carcinosarcomas (malignant mixed mesedermal tumors) of the female genital tract. Int J Gynecol Cancer 1994;4:52-60.

26. Östör AG, Roccason TP: Mixed tumors of the uterus. In Fox H, Wells M (eds): Haines and Taylor Obstetrical and Gynaecological Pathology, 5th ed. Edinburgh, Elsevier Science, 2002.

27. Zelmanowicz A, Hildesheim A, Sherman ME, et al: Evidence for a common etiology for endometrial carcinomas and malignant mixed mullerian tumors. Gynecol Oncol 1998;69: 253-257.

28. George E, Lillemoe TJ, Twiggs LB, Perrone T: Malignant mixed mullerian tumor versus high-grade endometrial carcinoma and aggressive variants of endometrial carcinoma: A comparative analysis of survival. Int J Gynecol Pathol 1995;14:39-44.

29. Liebow AA, Castleman B: Benign clear cell ("sugar") tumors of the lung. Yale J Biol Med 1971;43:213-222.

30. Pea M, Martignoni G, Zamboni G, Bonetti F: Perivascular epithelioid cell. Am J Surg Pathol 1996;20:1149-1155.

31. Vang R, Kempson RL: Perivascular epithelioid cell tumor ("PEComa") of the uterus: A subset of HMB-45-positive epithelioid mesenchymal neoplasms with an uncertain relationship to pure smooth muscle tumors. Am J Surg Pathol 2002; 26:1-13.

32. Kraus FT. Gynecologic Pathology. St Louis, CV Mosby, 1967.

33. Leibsohn S, d'Ablaing G, Mishell DR, Schlaerth JB: Leiomyosarcoma in a series of hysterectomies performed for presumed uterine leiomyomas. Am J Obstet Gynecol 1990;162: 968-976.

34. Goff BA, Rice LW, Fleischhacker D, et al: Uterine leiomyosarcoma and endometrial stroma sarcoma: Lymph node metastases and sites of recurrence. Gynecol Oncol 1993;50:105-109.

35. Parker WH, Fu YS, Berek JS: Uterine sarcoma in patients operated on for presumed leiomyoma and rapidly growing leiomyoma. Obstet Gynecol 1994;83:414-418.

36. Kurjak A, Kupesic S, Shalan H, et al: Uterine sarcoma: A report of 10 cases studied by transvaginal color and pulsed Doppler sonography. Gynecol Oncol 1995;59:342-346.

37. Umesaki N, Tanaka T, Miyama M, et al: Positron emission tomography with F-fluorodeoxyglucose of uterine sarcoma: A comparison with magnetic resonance imaging and power Doppler imaging. Gynecol Oncol 2001;80:372-377.

38. Blom R, Guerrieri C, Stal O, et al: Leiomyosarcoma of the uterus: A clinicopathologic, DNA flow cytometric, p53, and mdm-2 analysis of 49 cases. Gynecol Oncol 1998;68:54-61.

39. Kahanpaa KV, Wahlstrom T, Grohn P, et al: Sarcomas of the uterus: A clinicopathologic study of 119 patients. Obstet Gynecol 1986;67:417-424.

40. Marchese MJ, Liskow AS, Crum CP, et al: Uterine sarcomas: A clinicopathologic study, 1965-1981. Gynecol Oncol 1984;18: 299-312.

41. Nola M, Babic D, Ilic J, et al: Prognostic parameters for survival of patients with malignant mesenchymal tumors of the uterus. Cancer 1996;78:2543-2550.

42. Nordal RR, Kristensen GB, Kaern J, et al: The prognostic significance of stage, tumor size, cellular atypia and DAN ploidy in uterine leiomyosarcoma. Acta Oncol 1995;34:797-802.

43. Wolfson AH, Wolfson DJ, Sittler SY, et al: A multivariate analysis of clinicopathologic factors for predicting outcome in uterine sarcomas. Gynecol Oncol 1994;52:56-62.

44. Larson B, Silfversward C, Nilsson B, Petterson F: Prognostic factors in uterine leiomyosarcoma: A clinicopathologic study of 143 cases. The /?Radiumhemmet series, 1936-1981. Acta Oncol 1990;29:185-191.

45. Pautier P, Genestie C, Rey A, et al: Analysis of clinicopathologic prognostic factors for 157 uterine sarcomas and evaluation of a grading score validated for soft tissue sarcoma. Cancer 2000;88: 1425-1431.

46. Evans HL, Chawla SP, Simpson C, Finn KP: Smooth muscle neoplasms of the uterus other than ordinary leiomyoma: A study of 46 cases, with emphasis on diagnostic criteria and prognostic factors. Cancer 1988;62:2239-2247.

47. Mayerhofer K, Obermair A, Windbichler G, et al: Leiomyosarcoma of the uterus: A clinicopathologic multicenter study of 71 cases. Gynecol Oncol 1999;74:196-201.

48. Vardi JR, Tovell HMM: Leiomyosarcoma of the uterus: A clinicopathologic study. Obstet Gynecol 1980;56:428-434.

49. Barter JF, Smith EB, Szap CA, et al: Leiomyosarcoma of the uterus: Clinicopathologic study of 21 cases. Gynecol Oncol 1985; 21:220-227.

50. Hart WR, Billman JK Jr: A reassessment of uterine neoplasms originally diagnosed as leiomyosarcomas. Cancer 1978;41: 1902-1910.

51. El-Naggar AK, Abdul-Karim FW, Silva EG, et al: Uterine stromal neoplasms: A clinicopathologic and DNA flow cytometric correlation. Hum Pathol 1991;22:897-903.

52. Bodner K, Bodner-Adler B, Obermair A, et al: Prognostic parameters in endometrial stroma sarcoma: A clinicopathologic study in 31 patients. Gynecol Oncol 2001;81:160-165.

53. Bekkers RL, Willemsen WN, Schijf CP, et al: Leiomyomatosis peritonealis disseminata: Does malignant transformation occur? A literature review. Gynecol Oncol 1999;75:158-163.

54. Blom R, Guerrieri C: Adenosarcoma of the uterus: A clinicopathologic, DNA flow cytometric, p53 and mdm-2 analysis of 11 cases. Int J Gynecol Cancer 1999;9:37-43.

55. Eddy GL, Mazur MT: Endolymphatic stromal myosis associated with tamoxifen use. Gynecol Oncol 1997;64:262-264.

56. Fukunaga M, Ishihara A, Ushigome S: Extrauterine low-grade endometrial stromal sarcoma: Report of three cases. Pathol Int 198;48:297-302.

57. Ordi J, Stamatakos MD, Tavassoli FA: Pure pleomorphic rhabdomyosarcomas of the uterus. Int J Gynecol Pathol 1997;16:369-377.

58. Quade BJ, Pinto AP, Howard DR, et al: Frequent loss of heterozygosity of chromosome 10 in uterine leiomyosarcoma in contrast to leiomyoma. Am J Pathol 1999;154:945-950.

59. Roth E, Taylor HB: Heterologic cartilage in the uterus. Obstet Gynecol 1966;27:838-844.

60. Tietze L, Guenther K, Hoerbe A, et al: Benign metastasizing leiomyoma: A cytogenetically balanced but clonal disease. Hum Pathol 2000;31:126-128.

61. Tsushima K, Stanhope CR, Gaffey TA, Lieber MM: Uterine leiomyosarcomas and benign smooth muscle tumors: Usefulness of nuclear DNA patterns studied by flow cytometry. Mayo Clin Proc 1988;63:248-255.

62. Marth C, Windbichler G, Petru E, et al: Parity as an independent prognostic factor in malignant mixed mesodermal tumors of the endometrium. Gynecol Oncol 1997;64:121-125.

63. Girardi F, Petru E, Heydarfadai M, et al: Pelvic lymphadenectomy in surgical treatment of endometrial cancer. Gynecol Oncol 1993;49;177-180.

64. Chen SS: Propensity of retroperitoneal lymph node metastasis in patients with stage I sarcoma of the uterus. Gynecol Oncol 1989;32;215-218.

65. Fleming WP, Peters WA, Kumar NB, Morley GW: Autopsy findings in patients with uterine sarcoma. Gynecol Oncol 1984;19: 168-172.

66. Rose PG, Piver MS, Tsukada Y, Lau T: Patterns of metastasis in uterine sarcoma: An autopsy study. Cancer 1989;63: 935-938.

67. Berchuck A, Rubin SC, Hoskins WJ, et al: Treatment of uterine leiomyosarcoma. Obstet Gynecol 1988;71:845-850.

68. Gard GB, Mulvany NJ, Quinn MA: Management of uterine leiomyosarcoma in Australia. Aust N Z J Obstet Gynaecol 1999; 39:93-98.

69. Van Dinh T, Woodruff JD: Leimyosarcoma of the uterus. Am J Obstet Gynecol 1982;144:817-823.

70. Abu-Rustum NR, Curtin JP, Burt M, Jones WB: Regression of uterine low-grade smooth muscle tumors metastatic to the lung after oophorectomy. Obstet Gynecol 1997;89:850-852.

71. Schwartz LB, Diamond MP, Schwartz PE: Leiomyosarcomas: clinical presentation. Am J Obstet Gynecol 1993;168; 180-183.

72. Levenback C, Rubin SC, McCormack PM, et al: Resection of pulmonary metastases from uterine sarcomas. Gynecol Oncol 1992;45;202-205.

73. Morrow CP: Leiomyosarcoma. In Morrow CP, Curtin JP (eds): Gynecologic Cancer Surgery. New York, 1996, pp. 613-616.

74. Covens AL, Nisker JA, Chapman WB, Allen HH: Uterine sarcoma: An analysis of 74 cases. Am J Obstet Gynecol 1987; 156:370-374.

75. Di Saia PhJ, Morrow CP, Boronow R, et al: Endometrial sarcoma: Lymphatic spread pattern. Am J Obstet Gynecol 1978;130:104-105.

76. Salazar OM, Bonfiglio TA, Patten SF, et al: Uterine sarcomas: Analysis of failures with special emphasis on the use of adjuvant radiation therapy. Cancer 1978;42:1161-1170.

77. Swisher EM, Gown AM, Skelly M, et al: The expression of epidermal growth factor receptor, HER-2/Neu, p53 and Ki-67 antigen in uterine malignant mixed mesodermal tumors and adenosarcoma. Gynecol Oncol 1996;60:81-88.

78. Kaku T, Silverberg SG, Major FJ, et al: Adenosarcoma of the uterus: A Gynecologic Oncology Group clinicopathologic study of 31 cases. Int J Gynecol Pathol 1992;11:75-88.

79. Seidman JD, Wasserman CS, Aye LM, et al: Cluster of uterine mullerian adenosarcoma in the Washington, DC metropolitan area with high incidence of sarcomatous overgrowth. Am J Surg Pathol 1999;23:809-814.

80. Gollard R, Kosty M, Bordin G, et al: Two unusual presentations of müllerian adenosarcoma: Case reports, literature review, and treatment considerations. Gynecol Oncol 1995;59:412-422.

81. George E, Manivel JC, Dehner LP, Wick MR: Malignant mixed müllerian tumors: An immunochemical study of 47 cases, with histogenetic consideration and clinical correlation. Hum Pathol 1991;22:215-223.

82. Sorbe B: Radiotherapy and/or chemotherapy as adjuvant treatment of uterine sarcomas. Gynecol Oncol 1985;20:281-289.

83. George M, Pejovic MH, Kramar A, and Gynecologic Cooperating Group of French Oncology Centers: Uterine sarcomas: Prognostic factors and treatment modalities—Study on 209 patients. Gynecol Oncol 1986;24:58-67.

84. Omura G, Blessing J, Major F, et al: A randomized clinical trial of adjuvant Adriamycin in uterine sarcomas: A Gynecologic Oncology Group study. J Clin Oncol 1985;3:1240-1245.

85. Hornback NB, Omura G, Major FJ: Observations on the use of adjuvant radiation therapy in patients with stage I and II uterine sarcoma. Int J Radiat Oncol Biol Phys 1986;12:2127-2130.

86. Jereczek B, Jassem J, Kobierska A: Sarcoma of the uterus: A clinical study of 42 pts. Arch Gynecol Obstet 1996;258:171-180.

87. Tinkler SD, Cowie VJ: Uterine sarcomas: A review of the Edinburgh experience from 1974 to 1992. Br J Radiol 1993;66: 998-1001.

88. Rose PG, Boutselis JG, Sachs L: Adjuvant therapy for stage I uterine sarcoma. Am J Obstet Gynecol 1987;156:660-662.

89. Chauveinc L, Deniaud E, Plancher C, et al: Uterine sarcomas— The Curie Institut experience: Prognosis factors and adjuvant treatments. Gynecol Oncol 1999;72:232-237.

90. Echt G, Jepson J, Steel J, et al: Treatment of uterine sarcomas. Cancer 1990;66:35-39.

91. Ferrer F, Sabater S, Farrus B, et al: Impact of radiotherapy on local control and survival in uterine sarcomas: A retrospective study from the Group Oncologic Catala-Occita. Int J Radiat Oncol Biol Phys 1999;44:47-52.

92. Moskovic E, Macsweeney E, Law M, Price A: Survival, patterns of spread and prognostic factors in uterine sarcoma: A study of 76 patients. Br J Radiol 1993;66:1009-1015.

93. Knocke TH, Kucera H, Dörfler D, et al: Results of postoperative radiotherapy in the treatment of sarcoma of the corpus uteri. Cancer 1989;83:1972-1979.

94. Nielsen SN, Podratz KC, Scheithauer BW, O'Brien PC: Clinicopathologic analysis of uterine malignant mixed müllerian tumors. Gynecol Oncol 1989;34:372-378.

95. Chi DS, Mychalczak B, Saigo PE, et al: The role of whole-pelvic irradiation in the treatment of early-stage uterine carcinosarcoma. Gynecol Oncol 1997;65:493-498.

96. Gerszten K, Faul C, Kounelis S, et al: The impact of adjuvant radiotherapy on carcinosarcoma of the uterus. Gynecol Oncol 1998;68:8-13.

97. Manolitsas TP, Wain GV, Williams KE, et al: Multimodality therapy for patients with clinical stage I and II malignant mixed müllerian tumors of the uterus. Cancer 2001;91:1437-1443.

98. Weitmann HD, Kucera H, Knocke TH, Pötter R: Surgery and adjuvant radiation therapy of endometrial stromal sarcoma. Wien Klin Wochenschr 2002;114:1-2.

99. Perez CA, Askin F, Baglan RJ, et al: Effects of irradiation on mixed müllerian tumors of the uterus. Cancer 1979;43:1274-1284.

100. Nordal RR, Thoresen SO: Uterine sarcomas in Norway 1956-1992: Incidence, survival and mortality. Eur J Cancer 1997;33:907-911.

101. Peters WA III, Rivkin SE, Smith MR, Tesh DE: Cisplatin and Adriamycin combination chemotherapy for uterine stromal sarcomas and mixed mesodermal tumors. Gynecol Oncol 1989;34:323-327.

102. Currie J, Blessing J, Muss H, et al: Combination chemotherapy with hydroxyurea, dacarbazine, and etoposide in the treatment of uterine leiomyosarcoma: A Gynecologic Oncology Group study. Gynecol Oncol 1996;61:27-30.

103. Leyvraz S, Bacchi M, Lissoni A, et al: High response rate with the combination of high-dose ifosfamide and doxorubicin for the treatment of advanced gynecologic sarcomas. Proc ASCO 1998;17:354a.

104. Sutton G, Blessing J, Barrett R, McGehee R: Phase II trial of ifosfamide and mesna in leiomyosarcoma of the uterus: A Gynecologic Oncology Group study. Am J Obstet Gynecol 1992;166:556-559.

105. Sutton G, Blessing J, Ball H: Phase II trial of paclitaxel in leiomyosarcoma of the uterus: A Gynecologic Oncology Group study. Gynecol Oncol 1999;74:346-349.

106. Thigpen T, Blessing J, Beecham J, et al: Phase II trial of cisplatin as first-line chemotherapy in patients with advanced or recurrent uterine sarcomas: A Gynecologic Oncology Group study. J Clin Oncol 1991;9:1962-1966.

107. Sutton G, Blessing J, Park R, et al: Ifosfamide treatment of recurrent or metastatic endometrial stromal sarcomas previously unexposed to chemotherapy: A study of the Gynecologic Oncology Group. Obstet Gynecol 1996;87:747-750.

108. Sutton G, Blessing J, Malfetano J: Ifosfamide and doxorubicin in the treatment advanced leiomyosarcomas of the uterus: A Gynecologic Oncology Group study. Gynecol Oncol 1996;62: 226-229.

109. Omura G, Major F, Blessing J, et al: A randomized study of Adriamycin with or without dimethyl triazenoimidazole carboxamide in advanced uterine sarcomas. Cancer 1983;52: 626-632.

110. Berchuck A, Rubin S, Hoskins W, et al: Treatment of endometrial stromal tumors. Gynecol Oncol 1990;36:60-65.

111. Mesia A, Demopoulos R: Effects of leuprolide acetate on low-grade endometrial stromal sarcoma. Am J Obstet Gynecol 2000;182:1140-1141.

112. Maluf F, Sabbatini P, Schwartz L, et al: Endometrial stromal sarcoma: Objective response to letrozole. Gynecol Oncol 2001; 82:384-388.

113. Sutton G, Blessing J, Carson L, et al: Adjuvant ifosfamide, mesna, and cisplatin in patients with completely resected stage I or II carcinosarcoma of the uterus: A study of the Gynecologic Oncology Group. Proc ASCO 1997;16:362a.

114. Sutton G, Brunetto V, Kilgore L, et al: A phase III trial of ifosfamide alone or in combination with cisplatin in the treatment of advanced, persistent, or recurrent carcinosarcoma of the uterus: A Gynecologic Oncology Group Study. Gynecol Oncol 1998;68:137-141.

115. Hannigan E, Freedman R, Elder K, Rutledge F: Treatment of advanced uterine sarcoma with Adriamycin. Gynecol Oncol 1983;16:101-104.

116. Fowler J, Blessing J, Burger R, Malfetano J: Phase II evaluation of oral trimetrexate in mixed mesodermal tumors of the uterus: A Gynecologic Oncology Group Study. Gynecol Oncol 2002; 85:311-314.

117. Shimizu Y: Combination of consecutive low-dose cisplatin with ifosfamide and epirubicin for sarcoma uteri. Proc ASCO 2000; 19:391a.

118. Hensley M, Venkatrama E, Maki R, Spriggs D: Docetaxel plus gemcitabine is active in leiomyosarcoma: Results of a phase II trial. Proc ASCO 2001;20:353a.

119. Lissoni A, Cormio G, Colombo N, et al: High-dose epirubicin in patients with advanced or recurrent uterine sarcoma. Int J Gynecol Cancer 1997;7:241-244.
120. Piver S, Rose P: Advanced uterine sarcoma: Response to chemotherapy. Eur J Gynaecol Oncol 1988;9:124-129.
121. Muss H, Bundy B, DiSaia P, et al: Treatment of recurrent or advanced uterine sarcoma. Cancer 1985;55:1648-1653.
122. Hawkins R, Wiltshaw E, Mansi J: Ifosfamide with and without adriamycin in advanced uterine leiomyosarcoma. Cancer Chemother Pharmacol 1990;26(Suppl):26-29.
123. Thigpen T, Blessing J, Wilbanks G: Cisplatin as second-line chemotherapy in the treatment of advanced or recurrent leiomyosarcoma of the uterus: A phase II trial of the Gynecologic Oncology Group. Am J Clin Oncol 1986;9:18-20.
124. Gershenson D, Kavanagh J, Copeland L, et al: Cisplatin therapy for disseminated mixed mesodermal sarcoma of the uterus. J Clin Oncol 1987;5:618-621.
125. Sutton G, Blessing J, Rosenshein N, et al: Phase II trial of ifosfamide and mesna in mixed mesodermal tumors of the uterus. Am J Obstet 1989;161:309-312.
126. Thigpen T, Blessing J, Orr J, DiSaia P: Phase II trial of cisplatin in the treatment of patients with advanced or recurrent mixed mesodermal sarcomas of the uterus: A Gynecologic Oncology Group study. Cancer Treat Rep 1986;70:271-274.
127. Currie J, Blessing J, McGhee R, et al: Phase II trial of hydroxyurea, dacarbazine, and etoposide in mixed mesodermal tumors of the uterus: A Gynecologic Oncology Group study. Gynecol Oncol 1996;61:94-96.
128. Gershenson D, Kavanagh J, Copeland L, et al: High-dose doxorubicin infusion therapy for disseminated mixed mesodermal sarcoma of the uterus. Cancer 1987;59:1264-1267.

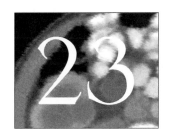

TREATMENT OF RECURRENT UTERINE SARCOMAS

Nick Reed,   Mark Baekelandt,   and   Jan B. Vermorken

 MAJOR CONTROVERSIES

- **What are the major patterns of spread and post-treatment follow-up?**
- **What are the options for treatment of recurrent uterine sarcomas?**
- **What are the potential new modalities for treatment of recurrent uterine sarcoma?**

What are the major patterns of spread and post-treatment follow-up?

Uterine sarcomas continue to provide a major challenge to treatment, both for management of the primary presentation and for relapse. These rare tumors represent a diverse group that have been lumped together because of their common origin in the gynecologic tract, making interpretation of data on prognosis and treatment difficult. It is now recognized that the various types behave as clinically distinct cancers, with significant differences in patterns of spread. Whereas carcinosarcomas (CS) have a pattern of spread characterized by local extension and regional lymph node metastases (Table 23-1), similar to endometrial adenocarcinomas, endometrial stromal sarcomas (ESS) more typically have locoregional extension into the parametrium, broad ligament, and adnexal structures. In contrast, leiomyosarcomas (LMS) are far more likely to spread directly to the lungs.[1] Recent molecular evidence, backed by some clinical evidence, has suggested strong similarities between CS and carcinomas of the endometrium, and even evidence for a common etiology.[2-4] In a study on lymph node involvement in LMS and ESS, none of the women without extrauterine disease had any lymph node metastases detected, but nevertheless 40% of them later experienced a distant failure.[5] In 84% of cases, the lung was involved as a site of recurrence. This pattern of relapse is consistent with hematogenous spread. In an autopsy study on 73 patients with a mixture of all types of uterine sarcomas, the presence of pulmonary metastases was not associated with retroperitoneal lymph node metastasis or intraperitoneal disease.[6] There is also a considerable divergence of these tumor types in time to relapse. LMS are much more likely to metastasize early, whereas ESS have been known to relapse up to 20 years after primary presentation. This has important bearing on the method and duration of follow-up care.

It therefore is evident that three separate protocols for management of these patients after primary treatment should be developed. Optimally, follow-up monitoring is done in a multidisciplinary clinic, where they may be seen by a specialist (gynecologic, medical, or radiation oncologist) and where, in the event of a problem, immediate cross-referral is available. Furthermore, given the relative rarity of these tumors (although they seem to become increasingly more common), management arguably should be centralized, whenever feasible, to the regional gynecologic cancer service. Local agreement should be obtained as to the frequency of follow-up and the type and frequency of investigations to be carried out. Again, because of the rarity of these cancers, local or regional cooperative groups should produce their own standardized protocols that adhere to national or, better still, international agreements on recommended follow-up procedures. Follow-up care for these patients is important, because even low-stage uterine sarcomas have high recurrence rates, and certainly for ESS this may be a very late phenomenon. A number of patients will have recurrence with

Table 23–1. Frequency of Lymph Node Metastases in Uterine Sarcoma (%)

Nodes	Carcinosarcoma	Leiomyosarcoma
Pelvic	15–20	3–5
Para-aortic	7	Not available

After Major FJ, Blessing JA, Silverberg SG, et al: Prognostic factors in early-stage uterine sarcoma: A Gynecologic Oncology Group study. Cancer 1993;71: 1702-1709.

limited disease in the pelvis, in the abdomen, or retroperitoneally; detection of these relapses is important, because these patients still may be candidates for radical surgery.

The main method of follow-up is clinical examination. In addition, blood investigations, including complete blood count, routine biochemical profile, and specific markers, as well as imaging investigations, may be used. New tumor markers are likely to become available in the near future. Because most patients with pelvic relapse have symptoms, clinical history taking and physical examination, including a gynecologic examination, are important. However, patients with more distant metastases, particularly in the lung, may not be symptomatic. The use of routine assessment of the complete blood count and biochemical profile is questionable in the asymptomatic patient. A regular chest radiograph is probably more important in view of the development of occult or silent lung metastases. The use of more sophisticated imaging procedures such as ultrasonography, computed tomography, and magnetic resonance imaging (or even positron emission tomography) depends on the local availability of these modalities and may be influenced by economic factors. If possible, local relapse should be confirmed by cytologic or histologic means, although in the future the use of tumor markers may become more reliable.

What are the options for treatment of recurrent uterine sarcomas?

Surgery, radiation therapy, chemotherapy, and hormone therapy may all play relevant roles in the management of relapsed disease, although for some patients the use of best supportive care and early intervention by palliative care physicians may be appropriate. For some patients, the time frame of the relapse may be so fast that no effective treatment can be offered. However, it is recommended that review of the pathology be carried out, and that the use of molecular markers (which may give information about estrogen or progesterone receptor status) and central review by a multidisciplinary team should be the first priority. Ideally, all of these patients should be registered in a Rare Tumor Registry, as has been proposed and developed by the Gynecological Cancer Intergroup (GCIG). Registration will additionally provide information about the availability of any current studies or trials and research protocols.

Surgery. Surgery is the standard of care for those patients with a relapse that is localized or limited to a single or a few well-circumscribed lesions within the pelvis, abdominal cavity, or retroperitoneum. As for other (recurrent) soft tissue sarcomas, the intention should be curative: complete resection with tumor-free margins.[7,8] Palliative surgery should be considered on the basis of the individual patient's symptoms, with the aim of improving quality of life.

Surgery may also be considered for patients with localized, isolated metastases in the lung or liver. Several studies have shown that patients with histologically verified pulmonary metastases from uterine sarcoma, who have no extrathoracic tumor and in whom disease is anticipated to be resectable, can obtain impressive long-term survival rates.[9,10] Levenback and colleagues[9] showed that patients with unilateral disease had a significantly better survival than patients with bilateral metastases. Perhaps counterintuitively, disease-free interval before surgery was not a prognostic factor in any of the studies. Similarly, wedge resection of liver metastases should be considered for patients with anticipated good prognosis and performance status. In combination with such procedures, the use of chemotherapy before or after surgery (or both) should be discussed with a multidisciplinary team, the importance of which is emphasized once more in the frame of treatment planning for patients with recurrent uterine sarcoma.

Radiation therapy. The role of radiotherapy in these patients is mainly for symptom control. Patients may present with vaginal bleeding, discharge, or pain. If there is localized disease at the vaginal vault or in the pelvis, it can be treated effectively by a short course of radiotherapy. For patients with very extensive disease, short courses of treatment, giving either 20 Gy in four or five fractions or 30 to 35 Gy in ten fractions to relatively small volumes, can be very effective. For patients with a better performance status and anticipated longer survival, palliative doses of 40 to 45 Gy may be considered.

Radiotherapy also may have a valuable role in the treatment of bone metastases or lung metastases causing hemoptysis, situations in which a short palliative course of treatment can relieve symptoms. Similarly, if brain metastases occur and life expectancy is thought to exceed 2 to 3 months, a course of cranial irradiation can lead to good local tumor control and allow patients to be weaned off steroids. Radiotherapy can also be considered for patients who develop para-aortic lymph node metastases causing pressure effects. Finally, there is a small number of patients who has truly localized relapse and is not considered for any form of surgical intervention. In these cases, high-dose radiation is justifiable, with the patients usually being treated in the same manner as if primary radiation were being given. Whole pelvic radiation to a dose of 40 to 50 Gy over 4 to 5 weeks would usually be considered, with either an external boost or vaginal brachytherapy.

Hormone therapy. Estrogen receptors (ER) and progesterone receptors (PR) are detected in about 30% to 55% of uterine sarcomas.[11,12] Most studies show that ESS have a higher ER and PR content than LMS. The presence of ER and PR makes hormone treatment justifiable, although there is little standardized information with regard to its efficacy. Several anecdotal reports have described responses to hormone therapy (progestational agents and tamoxifen).[11-14] A recent report described an objective response of 9 months' duration, in a patient with an ER-rich ESS, to the third-generation aromatase inhibitor, letrozole.[15] A phase II trial of letrozole in patients with recurrent ESS is under consideration in Europe (European Organization of Research and Treatment of Cancer [EORTC]). Thus far, the data are too scarce to make any firm recommendations regarding the appropriate use of hormone therapy in patients with recurrent uterine sarcomas.

Chemotherapy. The high overall recurrence rate of sarcomas, even in low-stage disease, together with their propensity to recur at distant sites, underscores the need for effective systemic therapy. However, the rarity of the disease has made it difficult to develop clinical studies with sufficient power. Also, there is no evidence that chemotherapy for metastatic uterine sarcomas is likely to be curative. Its use is only palliative, but good palliation may be achieved with careful patient selection. Chemotherapy should also be considered in combination with surgery, radiation therapy, or both. It is especially with the use of chemotherapy that one must differentiate among the tumor subtypes. The differences in patterns of spread were discussed previously. In addition, most LMS and high-grade CS metastasize within 12 to 18 months, whereas lower-grade CS and ESS may behave in a much more indolent manner. Furthermore, there are significant differences in sensitivity to the chemotherapy agents, with certain drugs having considerable activity in one tumor type and virtually no activity in another. Therefore, in future clinical studies, the efficacy of therapies for the different histologic types should be studied in separate patient populations. The reported activities of different single agents and combination regimens in various types of uterine sarcomas are given in Tables 23-2 and 23-3.

Another intriguing point particularly applies to CS, in which metastases frequently contain epithelial components only.[16] This fact leads many to question whether CS are truly sarcomatous tumors or whether they are metaplastic epithelial carcinomas. It may help explain the differential response rates, particularly to platinum drugs, and it also reinforces the importance of central pathologic review of these uncommon tumors, so that the correct treatment can be offered at the outset.

Carcinosarcoma. Dealing first with CS, it is apparent that they are chemosensitive tumors. However, many of the patients who do achieve a response have remissions lasting no more than 6 to 12 months, although occasionally a patient has a significantly longer

Table 23–2. Single-Agent Activity in Various Types of Uterine Sarcomas

Agent	Response Rate (%)	Histologic Type	Study and Ref. No.
Doxorubicin	16	Any	Omura et al[17]
Doxorubicin	19	Any	Muss et al[25]
Cisplatin	19	CS	Thigpen et al[20]
Cisplatin	3	LMS	Thigpen et al[20]
Ifosfamide	32	CS	Sutton et al[22]
Ifosfamide	17	LMS	Sutton et al[31]
Ifosfamide	33	ESS	Sutton et al[28]
Paclitaxel	9	LMS	Sutton et al[30]
Paclitaxel	8	LMS	Gallup et al[42]
Topotecan	11	LMS	Miller et al[43]

CS, carcinosarcoma; ESS, endometrial stromal sarcoma; LMS, leiomyosarcoma.

remission. From the literature, it is apparent that several classes of drugs emerge as having greater activity. One must be careful in looking at the older reports, which frequently lumped all uterine sarcomas together; it is only more recently that distinctions have been made among the subtypes. Doxorubicin, cisplatin, ifosfamide, and dacarbazine have single-agent activity in CS. Response rates for single-agent therapy range from 0% to 10% for doxorubicin[17,18] to 18% to 42% for cisplatin[19-21]; for ifosfamide, a single-agent response rate of 32% has been reported.[22] Today, however, these drugs generally are not used as single agents, and it is therefore not surprising that combination chemotherapy results in an improvement in the response rates at the expense of increased toxicity. In the EORTC phase II trial 55923, a 56% overall response rate was observed in 32 assessable patients with CS who were treated with a combination of cisplatin, doxorubicin, and ifosfamide.[23] This trial confirmed the chemosensitivity of CS to platinum-based chemotherapy, but the authors emphasized that the myelotoxicity and nephrotoxicity associated with this regimen gave it an unfavorable toxicity profile.

Thus far, only a single phase III trial has been conducted on CS as a separate entity.[24] In this GOG trial, 194 evaluable patients with advanced, recurrent, or persistent CS were treated with ifosfamide with or without cisplatin. Response rates (36% versus 54%) and progression-free survival times slightly favored the combination treatment, but there was no significant difference in overall survival (RR = .80; P = .071), and the combination produced significantly more toxicity. The other two published randomized trials on combination chemotherapy in uterine sarcoma have included mixtures of the different histologic types.[17,25] Although these studies showed no differences in survival for the combination chemotherapy regimens compared with the single-agent arms, they were heavily underpowered for each histologic type. As a result, no conclusions can be drawn with regard to the value of combination chemotherapy in the treatment of advanced or recurrent uterine sarcomas.

Of the newer chemotherapy drugs, paclitaxel is probably the one that is most active. Single-agent

Table 23–3. Response Rates for Various Combination Regimens in Uterine Sarcoma

Combination	Response Rate (%)	Histologic Type	Study and Ref. No.
Vincristine/actinomycin D/cyclophosphamide	26	Any	Hannigan et al[44]
Doxorubicin/dacarbazine	24	Any	Omura et al[17]
Doxorubicin/cyclophosphamide	19	Any	Muss et al[25]
Cyclophosphamide/doxorubicin/cisplatin	76	CS	Willemse et al[45]
Cisplatin/doxorubicin/dacarbazine	33	CS	Baker et al[46]
Pegylated liposomal doxorubicin/paclitaxel	19	CS	Campos et al[47]
Doxorubicin/ifosfamide + granulocyte colony-stimulating factor (G-CSF)	77	CS	Leyvraz et al[33]
Topotecan/paclitaxel	29	CS	Fuller et al[48]
Cisplatin/ifosfamide	54	CS	Sutton et al[24]
Cisplatin/doxorubicin/ifosfamide	54	CS	van Rijswijk et al[23]
Doxorubicin/ifosfamide	30	LMS	Sutton et al[32]
Doxorubicin/ifosfamide	55	LMS	Leyvraz et al[33]
Mitomycin/doxorubicin/cisplatin	23	LMS	Edmonson et al[34]
Docetaxel/gemcitabine	53	LMS	Hensley et al[35]

CS, carcinosarcoma; ESS, endometrial stromal sarcoma; LMS, leiomyosarcoma.

activity of 18% was reported in a group of patients who had undergone prior treatment and had had no responses to other drugs.[26] The current GOG Protocol 161 is looking at the combination of paclitaxel and ifosfamide, compared with ifosfamide alone. However, as might have been expected, there is also interesting evidence of activity of paclitaxel and carboplatin in doses used in the treatment of epithelial ovarian cancer. A recent report by Duska and coworkers[27] showed a 55% complete response rate, with an additional 17% of patients achieving a partial response, yielding a total response rate of 72% in 26 patients with ovarian CS who received paclitaxel and platinum chemotherapy as first-line treatment. This study also showed an interesting median survival time of 27 months. The TEC combination (paclitaxel/epirubicin/carboplatin) is being examined in a phase II study by the Nordic Society for Gynecologic Oncology (NSGO).

A word of caution must be introduced with regard to the use of ifosfamide in patients who have either poor performance status or have bulky pelvic disease. These patients are more likely to have problems with ifosfamide toxicity, making this an area in which specialist teams who are used to administering this drug should be involved. This again reinforces the view that these cases should be managed by multidisciplinary teams, and not by the oncologist who only occasionally sees a patient with a relapsed uterine CS. Given the difficulties in administering ifosfamide, many clinicians prefer to avoid use of this drug. In addition, ifosfamide administration generally requires inpatient admission and rescue therapy with mesna. Regimens based on carboplatin and paclitaxel (with or without an anthracycline) that can be given in an outpatient setting clearly have significant pharmacoeconomic advantages and are more convenient for the patient. Therefore, although ifosfamide may be a very active drug in this setting, schedules based on carboplatin and paclitaxel are likely to be more frequently used.

Given the rarity of these tumors, one must conclude by recommending that these patients should, whenever possible, be entered into clinical trials, because this is the only way in which knowledge of the management of this disease can be advanced. Because a number of patients with uterine sarcoma have a history of pelvic irradiation, modification of the clinical trial design in this area should also be considered, to permit patients with previous malignancy (in remission for longer than 5 years) to be entered into studies. For those situations in which the patient is reluctant or ineligible to enter into a clinical trial, the previously mentioned carboplatin- and paclitaxel-based schedules or the cisplatin/ifosfamide/doxorubicin (PIA) regimen is recommended. Patients who are deemed ineligible for combination chemotherapy can be treated with single-agent carboplatin or cisplatin.

Endometrial stromal sarcoma. Because this is the rarest of the three major gynecologic sarcomas, there is proportionally less evidence available. However, much of the data suggest kinship with the CS subtype and by and large indicate activity for the same drugs: cisplatin, carboplatin, doxorubicin, ifosfamide, and paclitaxel. Again, the recommendation must be that patients should be entered into clinical trials whenever possible. One of the few clinical trials that specifically looked at ESS was a single-agent phase II study with ifosfamide, reported by Sutton and colleagues,[28] which showed a 33.3% response rate. Berchuck and associates[29] reported a 50% response rate to doxorubicin alone or in combination in 10 patients with recurrent ESS. In summary, with regard to the use of cytotoxic chemotherapy, the recommendations for CS would also be advised for ESS.

Leiomyosarcoma. LMS are clearly the most aggressive of these tumors, and a relapse rate of up to 70% within 2 years has been reported. It has also been shown that the incidence of para-aortic lymph node metastases at presentation is significantly lower than for CS. Because these tumors are much more likely to metastasize by hematogenous spread, lung and liver metastases are more likely to be seen.

The response rates to the agents tested in LMS are clearly different from those for CS. Thigpen and colleagues[20] observed a response rate of only 3% to cisplatin in a series of 33 patients with LMS. Similarly, Sutton and coworkers[30] reported a 9.1% response rate to paclitaxel in 33 patients with LMS. In contrast, a 25% response rate was observed with doxorubicin in a study by Omura and associates,[17] and a 17% response rate for ifosfamide was reported by Sutton's group.[31] The combination of doxorubicin and ifosfamide has produced promising results, with response rates varying from 30% to 55%.[32,33]

Because of preliminary observations favoring the use of mitomycin, doxorubicin, and cisplatin (MAP) chemotherapy in LMS, the Gynecologic Oncology Group (GOG) looked at this combination, specifically in LMS.[34] Only moderate activity was demonstrated, with 9% of patients achieving a complete response and 14% having a partial response, for an overall response rate of 23%. More exciting results were published by Hensley and coworkers,[35] who tested the combination of gemcitabine and docetaxel in a group of patients who had been heavily pretreated. Among their 34 patients, 3 achieved complete responses and 15 partial responses, for an overall response rate of 53%; almost half of these patients were pretreated with either doxorubicin or doxorubicin and ifosfamide. The toxicity of the regimen was reported to be very acceptable. The high response rates were surprising, given the fact that these two drugs administered as single agents have relatively low activities, and the authors offered several interesting possible explanations for this apparent synergism. This is clearly an active and potentially very interesting combination, and it may allow the development of new schedules. Again, patients should be preferentially entered into clinical trials, so as to improve our knowledge and understanding of the behavior of this disease and the efficacy of treatment.

The novel marine compound, ecteinascidin (ET-743), has shown interesting activity in soft tissue sarcomas[36,37] and seems to be of particular interest in regard to LMS of the uterine tract. A pooled analysis of pivotal phase II trials in soft tissue sarcomas demonstrated response rates for LMS in general and for uterine LMS in particular approaching 20% (data on file, PharmaMar). A randomized phase III trial comparing ecteinascidin with ifosfamide is to be launched by the EORTC Gynecologic Cancer Group.

What are the potential new modalities for treatment of recurrent uterine sarcoma?

Although single cytotoxic agents and several combinations have demonstrated some activity, they have thus far failed to show a clear impact on the survival of patients with uterine sarcomas. Most likely, future advances in sarcoma treatment will depend on increased insight into the molecular genetics of the disease (or diseases). Molecular markers will allow better determinations of prognosis and better stratification of patients in clinical trials. Microarray-based expression assays may reveal clinically relevant expression patterns, which in turn could lead to novel therapeutic targets (e.g., signal transduction, apoptosis). Significant progress has been made in genome-wide expression profiling of soft tissue tumors, including demonstration of strikingly distinct gene expression patterns in synovial sarcomas, gastrointestinal stromal tumors (GISTs), neural tumors, and a subset of LMS, possibly leading to a new and improved classification of these tumors.[38]

An example of this evolution is the use of imatinib (STI571, Gleevec) in GIST. C-Kit, a tyrosine kinase, is frequently mutated and constitutively activated in GIST. In two recent reports, high rates of objective responses and disease stabilization were reported with imatinib, a specific inhibitor of c-Kit tyrosine kinase in patients with unresectable or metastatic GIST.[39,40] In a study of 38 mesenchymal tumors of the uterus and ovary, however, only 1 of 24 uterine sarcomas (CS, ESS, and LMS) expressed c-Kit, and in fewer than 5% of the cells.[41] It therefore seems unlikely that patients with uterine sarcomas will benefit from therapy with tyrosine kinase inhibitors such as STI571.

Conclusions

1. Given the rarity of the different types of uterine sarcomas, information on the optimal management of advanced and recurrent disease is insufficient. Therefore, physicians should be motivated to include these patients in clinical trials.
2. Given the differences in sensitivity to treatment among the various subtypes of uterine sarcomas, future trials must be histology-specific.
3. Pathology expertise in interpreting these tumors is critical, and access to central review is advised in the absence of local expertise.
4. Follow-up of patients with uterine sarcoma is important; meaningful second-line treatments are available, and long disease-free periods can be obtained in selected patients.
5. Surgery has an important role in the treatment of localized and limited relapses of uterine sarcoma and of isolated lung or liver metastases.
6. The main role of radiotherapy is for the palliation of symptoms of recurrent disease.
7. Different single agents have substantial activity in different types of uterine sarcoma: cisplatin and ifosfamide in CS and ESS, and doxorubicin in LMS.
8. Although they have demonstrated higher response rates, the few reported trials of combination chemotherapy have failed to show a convincing survival benefit in favor of the combinations. In general, however, these trials have been underpowered. Cooperative groups should make an effort to develop sufficiently large trials that have the power to answer clinically relevant questions.

9. Significant advances are awaited from the molecular profiling of these diseases. The ability of microarray-based techniques to study the expression of thousands of genes simultaneously opens the possibility of a different, more clinically relevant classification of sarcomas, as well as identification of new targets for therapy.

10. The Rare Tumor Registry being developed by the GCIG, which includes a web site containing expert guidelines and recommendations for clinical studies, can act as an invaluable educational tool and should be available beginning in 2004.

REFERENCES

1. Major FJ, Blessing JA, Silverberg SG, et al: Prognostic factors in early-stage uterine sarcoma: A Gynecologic Oncology Group study. Cancer 1993;71:1702-1709.

2. Amant F: Etiopathogenesis of uterine sarcomas: A study on genetic, hormonal and ethnic factors (dissertation). Leuven, Belgium, Leuven University Press, 2002.

3. Gorai I, Yanagibashi T, Taki A, et al: Uterine carcinosarcoma is derived from a single stem cell: An in vitro study. Int J Cancer 1997;72:821-827.

4. Reed NS, Mangioni C, Malmstrøm H, et al: First results of a randomized trial comparing radiotherapy versus observation postoperatively in patients with uterine sarcomas: An EORTC-GCG study [abstract]. Int J Gynecol Cancer 2003;13(Suppl 1):4.

5. Goff BA, Rice LW, Fleishhacker D, et al: Uterine leiomyosarcoma and endometrial stromal sarcoma: Lymph node metastases and sites of recurrence. Gynecol Oncol 1993;50:105-109.

6. Rose PG, Piver MS, Tsukada Y, Lau T: Patterns of metastasis in uterine sarcoma: An autopsy study. Cancer 1989;63:935-938.

7. Wang Y, Zhu W, Shen Z, et al: Treatment of locally recurrent soft tissue sarcomas of the retroperitoneum: Report of 30 cases. J Surg Oncol 1994;56:213-216.

8. Lewis JJ, Leung D, Woodruff JM, Brennan MF: Retroperitoneal soft-tissue sarcoma: Analysis of 500 patients treated and followed at a single institution. Ann Surg 1998;3:355-365.

9. Levenback C, Rubin SC, McCormack PM, et al: Resection of pulmonary metastases from uterine sarcomas. Gynecol Oncol 1992;45:202-205.

10. Mountain CF, McMurtrey MJ, Hermes KE: Surgery for pulmonary metastasis: A 20-year experience. Ann Thorac Surg 1984;38:323-330.

11. Wade K, Quinn MA, Hammond I, et al: Uterine sarcoma: Steroid receptors and response to hormonal therapy. Gynecol Oncol 1990;39:364-367.

12. Sutton GP, Stehman F, Michael H, et al: Estrogen and progesterone receptors in uterine sarcomas. Obstet Gynecol 1986;68:709-714.

13. Piver MS, Rutledge FN, Copeland L, et al: Uterine endolymphatic stromal myosis: A collaborative study. Obstet Gynecol 1984;64:173-178.

14. Gynecological Group, Clinical Oncological Society of Australia: Tamoxifen in the treatment of advanced and recurrent uterine sarcomas: Results of a phase II study. Cancer Treat Rep 1988;6:811.

15. Maluf FC, Sabbatini P, Schwartz L, et al: Endometrial stromal sarcoma: Objective response to letrozole. Gynecol Oncol 2001;82:384-388.

16. Van Rijswijk REN, Tognon G, Burger CW, et al: The effect of chemotherapy on the different components of advanced carcinosarcomas (malignant mixed mesodermal tumors) of the female genital tract. Int J Gynecol Cancer 1994;4:52-60.

17. Omura GA, Major FJ, Blessing JA, et al: A randomized study of adriamycin with and without dimethyl triazenoimidazole carboxamide in advanced uterine sarcomas. Cancer 1983;52:626-632.

18. Gershenson DM, Kavanagh JJ, Copeland LJ, et al: High-dose doxorubicin infusion therapy for disseminated mixed mesodermal sarcoma of the uterus. Cancer 1987;59:1264-1267.

19. Thigpen JT, Blessing JA, Orr JW, DiSaia PJ: Phase II trial of cisplatin in the treatment of patients with advanced or recurrent mixed mesodermal sarcoma of the uterus: A Gynecologic Oncology Group study. Cancer Treat Rep 1986;70:271-274.

20. Thigpen JT, Blessing JA, Beecham J, et al: Phase II trial of cisplatin as first-line chemotherapy in patients with advanced or recurrent uterine sarcomas: A Gynecologic Oncology Group study. J Clin Oncol 1991;9:1962-1966.

21. Gershenson DM, Kavanagh JJ, Copeland LJ, et al: Cisplatin therapy for disseminated mixed mesodermal sarcoma of the uterus. J Clin Oncol 1987;5:618-621.

22. Sutton GP, Blessing JA, Rosenshein N, et al: Phase II trial of ifosfamide and mesna in mixed mesodermal tumors of the uterus: A Gynecologic Oncology Group study. Am J Obstet Gynecol 1989;161:309-312.

23. van Rijswijk REN, Vermorken JB, Reed N, et al: Cisplatin, doxorubicin and ifosfamide in carcinosarcoma of the female genital tract: A phase II study of the European Organization for Research and Treatment of Cancer Gynecological Cancer Group (EORTC 55923). Eur J Cancer 2003;39:481-487.

24. Sutton G, Brunetto VL, Kilgore L, et al: A phase III trial of ifosfamide with or without cisplatin in carcinosarcoma of the uterus: A Gynecologic Oncology Group study. Gynecol Oncol 2000;79:147-153.

25. Muss HB, Bundy B, DiSaia PJ, et al: Treatment of recurrent or advanced uterine sarcoma: A randomized trial of doxorubicin versus doxorubicin and cyclophosphamide. A phase II trial of the Gynecologic Oncology Group. Cancer 1985;55:1648-1653.

26. Curtin JP, Blessing JA, Soper JT, DeGeest K: Paclitaxel in the treatment of carcinosarcoma of the uterus: A Gynecologic Oncology Group study. Gynecol Oncol 2001;83:268-270.

27. Duska LR, Garrett A, Eltabbakh GH, et al: Paclitaxel and platinum chemotherapy for malignant mullerian tumors of the ovary. Gynecol Oncol 2002;85:459-463.

28. Sutton G, Blessing JA, Park R, et al: Ifosfamide treatment of recurrent or metastatic endometrial stromal sarcomas previously unexposed to chemotherapy: A study of the Gynecologic Oncology Group. Obstet Gynecol 1996;87:747-750.

29. Berchuck A, Rubin SC, Hoskins WJ, et al: Treatment of endometrial stromal tumors. Gynecol Oncol 1990;36:60-65.

30. Sutton G, Blessing JA, Ball H: Phase II trial of paclitaxel in leiomyosarcoma of the uterus: A Gynecologic Oncology Group study. Gynecol Oncol 1999;74:346-349.

31. Sutton GP, Blessing JA, Barrett RJ, McGehee R: Phase II trial of ifosfamide and mesna in leiomyosarcoma of the uterus: A Gynecologic Oncology Group study. Am J Obstet Gynecol 1992;166:556-559.

32. Sutton GP, Blessing JA, Malfetano JH: Ifosfamide and doxorubicin in the treatment of advanced leiomyosarcomas of the uterus: A Gynecologic Oncology Group study. Gynecol Oncol 1996;62:226-229.

33. Leyvraz S, Bacchi M, Lissoni A, et al: High response rate with the combination of high-dose ifosfamide and doxorubicin for the treatment of advanced gynecologic sarcomas [abstract]. Proc Am Soc Clin Oncol 1998;17:354a.

34. Edmonson JH, Blessing JA, Cosin JA, et al: Phase II study of mitomycin, doxorubicin, and cisplatin in the treatment of advanced uterine leiomyosarcoma: A Gynecologic Oncology Group study. Gynecol Oncol 2002;85:507-510.

35. Hensley ML, Maki R, Venkatraman E, et al: Gemcitabine and docetaxel in patients with unresectable leiomyosarcoma: Results of a phase II trial. J Clin Oncol 2002;12:2824-2331.

36. Demetri GD: ET-743: The US experience in sarcomas of soft tissues. Anticancer Drugs 2002;13(Suppl 1):7-9.

37. Brain EGC: Safety and efficacy of ET-743: The French experience. Anticancer Drugs 2002;13(Suppl 1):11-14.

38. Nielsen TO, West RB, Linn SC, et al: Molecular characterisation of soft tissue tumors: A gene expression study. Lancet 2002;359:1301-1307.

39. von Mehren M, Blanke C, Joensuu H, et al: High incidence of durable responses induced by imatinib mesylate (Gleevec) in patients with unresectable and metastatic gastrointestinal stromal tumors (GISTs) [abstract]. Proc Am Soc Clin Oncol 2002;21:403a.

40. Judson IR, Verweij J, van Oosterom A, et al: Imatinib (Gleevec) an active agent for gastrointestinal stromal tumors (GIST), but not for other soft tissue sarcoma (STS) subtypes not

characterized for KIT and PDGF-R expression: Results of EORTC phase II studies [abstract]. Proc Am Soc Clin Oncol 2002;21:403a.

41. Klein WM, Kurman RJ: Lack of expression of c-kit protein (CD117) in mesenchymal tumors of the uterus and ovary. Int J Gynecol Pathol 2003;22:181-184.

42. Gallup DG, Blessing JA, Andersen W, Morgan MA: Evaluation of paclitaxel in previously treated leiomyosarcoma of the uterus: A Gynecologic Oncology Group study. Gynecol Oncol 2003; 89:48-51.

43. Miller DS, Blessing JA, Kilgore LC, et al: Phase II trial of topotecan in patients with advanced, persistent or recurrent uterine leiomyosarcomas: A Gynecologic Oncology Group study. Am J Clin Oncol 2000;23:355-357.

44. Hannigan EV, Elder KW, Rutledge FN: Treatment of advanced uterine sarcoma with vincristine, actinomycin D and cyclophosphamide. Gynecol Oncol 1983;15:224-229.

45. Willemse PHB, Bouma J, Hollema H: Cisplatin in gynecologic carcinosarcoma [letter]. J Clin Oncol 1992;10:1365.

46. Baker T, Piver MS, Caglar H, Piedmonte M: Prospective trial of cisplatin, adriamycin and dacarbazine in metastatic mixed mesodermal sarcomas of the uterus and ovary. Am J Clin Oncol 1991;14:246-250.

47. Campos S, Penson RT, Matulonis UA, et al: A phase 2 and pharmacokinetic/dynamic study of Doxil and weekly paclitaxel chemotherapy for recurrent mullerian tumors [abstract]. Proc Am Soc Clin Oncol 2000;19:410a.

48. Fuller AF, Penson RT, Supko JG, et al: A phase I/II and pharmacokinetic study of 96-hour infusional topotecan and paclitaxel chemotherapy for recurrent mullerian sarcomas [abstract]. Proc Am Soc Clin Oncol 2000;19:392a.

Cancers of the Ovary, Fallopian Tube, and Peritoneum

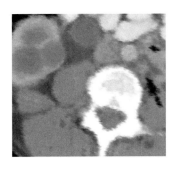

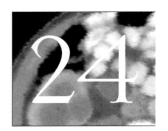

EPIDEMIOLOGY OF OVARIAN, FALLOPIAN TUBE, AND PRIMARY PERITONEAL CANCERS

Joan L. Kramer   and   Mark H. Greene

✦ MAJOR CONTROVERSIES

- What are the epidemiologic characteristics of ovarian cancer?
- What are the possible mechanisms of ovarian carcinogenesis?
- What factors are known to modify the risk of ovarian cancer in humans?
- How does parity affect the risk of ovarian cancer?
- What is the effect of oral contraceptives on ovarian cancer risk?
- Does age at menarche influence the risk of ovarian cancer?
- Is there a relationship between lactation and ovarian cancer risk?
- What are the effects of age at menopause and gynecologic surgery?
- Is there an association of menopausal hormone therapy with ovarian cancer?
- Is infertility a risk factor for ovarian cancer?
- Does exposure to psychotropic medications affect the risk of ovarian cancer?
- Do certain analgesic medications reduce the risk of ovarian cancer?
- Is talc exposure an ovarian cancer risk factor?
- To what extent does family history contribute to the risk of ovarian cancer?
- Which genetic syndromes are associated with ovarian cancer?
- What are the epidemiologic characteristics of primary carcinoma of the fallopian tube?
- What are the epidemiologic characteristics of extraovarian primary peritoneal cancer?

Few aspects of gynecologic cancer are as fraught with controversy as are the issues related to the etiology of ovarian cancer. The past decade has seen a series of major advances in understanding the pathobiology of this clinically challenging malignancy, but much remains uncertain. This chapter reviews the highlights of ovarian cancer epidemiology and etiology, focusing on issues that are likely to be of interest to the practicing gynecology clinician.

What are the epidemiologic characteristics of ovarian cancer?

Although the vast majority of malignant ovarian tumors are epithelial in origin, cancers also can derive from the other cell types that are present in the ovary: tumors that develop from ovarian germ cells are classified as dysgerminomas and teratomas; tumors derived from follicular cells are designated sex cord–stromal

Table 24–1. Cumulative Probability (%) of Developing or Dying of Invasive Ovarian Cancer from Birth to the End of the Age Interval Specified

Age (yr)	All Women Developing	All Women Dying	White Women Developing	White Women Dying	Black Women Developing	Black Women Dying
0-9	<0.01	<0.01	<0.01	<0.01	<0.01	<0.01
10-19	0.01	<0.01	0.01	<0.01	<0.01	<0.01
20-29	0.05	<0.01	0.05	<0.01	0.04	<0.01
30-39	0.12	0.01	0.13	0.01	0.08	0.01
40-49	0.29	0.06	0.30	0.06	0.19	0.05
50-59	0.60	0.19	0.63	0.20	0.36	0.14
60-69	1.00	0.42	1.06	0.45	0.63	0.31
70-79	1.41	0.73	1.51	0.79	0.91	0.53
80-89	1.67	0.98	1.77	1.06	1.06	0.65
90+	1.72	1.04	1.83	1.13	1.10	0.69

From Feuer EJ, Wun LM: DEVCAN: Probability of Developing or Dying of Cancer Software, Version 4.2. Bethesda, MD: National Cancer Institute, 2002.

tumors, most often granulosa cell tumors; and stromal elements of the ovary may give rise to sarcomas (e.g., fibrosarcoma). However, these malignancies are quite rare and, consequently, the incidence of epithelial ovarian cancer is generally approximated by the incidence of ovarian cancer as a whole.

In the United States, ovarian cancer accounts for 4% of newly diagnosed cancers in women, with 25,400 new cases expected during 2003; 14,300 deaths are expected to result from ovarian cancer in 2003, representing 5% of all female cancer deaths. The cumulative probabilities of developing, or dying from, ovarian cancer among U.S. women are 1.4% and 0.7%, repectively, by age 80 (Table 24-1). Although ovarian cancer is rare in women younger than 40 years of age, the incidence rises with increasing age and peaks in the fifth decade, after which the rate plateaus.[1] Because the majority of women who develop ovarian cancer eventually die of the disease, mortality rates vary with incidence rates (Table 24-2). Ovarian cancer incidence rates vary among different populations. Rates are highest among Caucasian women in Europe and the United States, with lower rates in women from Central and South America.[2] Latina women living in the United States have rates approaching those of white women from other ethnic groups. Asian women generally have lower rates, although these rates increase among individuals of Japanese or Chinese descent living in the United States.[3] The incidence of ovarian cancer is generally lower among black women in the United States than among white women (Tables 24-2 and 24-3).[4]

Epithelial ovarian neoplasms are commonly separated into "invasive" and "borderline" categories. The borderline tumors are also referred to as tumors of "low malignant potential," because of their lower histologic grade and more favorable disease prognostic characteristics. Approximately 20% of all ovarian neoplasms are borderline tumors.[5-7] Invasive ovarian cancers are further subclassified by histologic subtype. Serous histology is most frequently seen, accounting for 56% of ovarian cancers in a contemporary Canadian series.[8] Mucinous tumors are the second most frequent, at 18%, followed by endometrioid cancers (16%) and clear cell tumors (6%). Some consider the clear cell and endometrioid subtypes to have similar histogenetic origins, and at times these are grouped together. "Other, unclassified" and mixed epithelial tumors accounted for 3% of the total in the Canadian series. Incidence rates for the serous and endometrial subtypes

Table 24–2. Surveillance, Epidemiology, and End Results (SEER) Race-Specific, Age-Adjusted Incidence Rates for Invasive Ovarian Cancer (11 Registries, 1992–1999)*

Age (yr)	All Races	White	Black	American Indian/Alaska Native	Asian or Pacific Islander	Hispanic
All	17.1	18.1	12.2	8.7	12.6	13.2
0-19	0.8	0.8	0.6	0.7	1.1	0.9
20-29	4.0	4.1	3.2	1.1	4.2	4.4
30-39	7.8	8.2	4.4	3.7	8.0	5.8
40-49	17.6	18.6	11.8	9.9	15.6	13.7
50-59	32.6	34.7	20.8	16.8	27.7	24.6
60-69	46.7	50.3	33.7	16.5	30.0	37.4
70-79	58.6	62.2	48.9	30.2	31.1	42.7
80+	57.7	60.2	45.7	42.4	30.7	42.7

*Rates are expressed as cases per 100,000 women per year, age-adjusted to the U.S. population from the 2000 census.
From Ries L, Eisner M, Kosary C, et al: SEER Registries: SEER Cancer Statistics Review, 1973-1999. Bethesda, MD: National Cancer Institute, 2002.

Table 24–3. Surveillance, Epidemiology, and End Results (SEER) Race-Specific, Age-Adjusted Mortality Rates for Invasive Ovarian Cancer (Total United States, 1990–1999)*

Age (yr)	All Races	White	Black	American Indian/Alaska Native	Asian or Pacific Islander	Hispanic
All ages	9.2	9.5	7.8	4.9	4.7	5.7
0-19	0.0	0.0	0.0	0.0	0.0	0.0
20-29	0.2	0.2	0.3	0.4	0.2	0.3
30-39	1.1	1.1	1.1	0.9	0.9	0.9
40-49	4.8	5.0	3.7	3.3	3.9	3.2
50-59	14.3	14.9	10.8	7.3	9.6	9.2
60-69	28.9	29.9	24.5	15.9	14.3	17.2
70-79	45.8	47.0	40.5	21.9	18.1	26.8
80+	55.1	56.1	48.3	29.4	23.5	34.9

*Rates are expressed as cases per 100,000 women per year, age-adjusted to the U. S. population from the 2000 census.
From Ries L, Eisner M, Kosary C, et al: SEER Registries: SEER Cancer Statistics Review, 1973-1999. Bethesda, MD: National Cancer Institute, 2002.

peaks between the ages of 70 and 74 years; there is a slightly later peak for mucinous tumors, and a *much* earlier peak (ages 55 to 59 years) for clear cell tumors[9] (Table 24-4).

What are the possible mechanisms of ovarian carcinogenesis?

Incessant ovulation hypothesis. The "incessant ovulation" hypothesis of ovarian carcinogenesis, originally put forth in 1972 by Fathalla, postulated that the disruption and cellular injury in the ovarian epithelium that occurs with each ovulation requires time to heal appropriately and that, without an adequate rest period, the repair can become disordered, leading to neoplastic transformation.[10] Furthermore, each injury and repair cycle is thought to stochastically increase the opportunity for erroneous DNA repair. It has been postulated that some ovarian cancer risk modifiers, such as pregnancy and oral contraceptive (OC) use, reduce the "ovulation age" by providing a respite from ovulation, diminishing the need for repair to the ovarian surface epithelium, and thereby reducing the risk of ovarian cancer.[11,12]

Table 24–4. Histology-Specific, Age-Standardized Incidence Rates for Invasive Ovarian Cancer (Canadian Cancer Registry, 1991–1993)

Histologic Subtype	Rate*
All types, combined	13.71
Serous	4.61
Mucinous	1.72
Endometrioid	1.28
Clear cell	0.60
Other epithelial	3.57
Carcinoma not otherwise specified	1.29

*Age-standardized incidence rate per 100,000 women per year.
From Zhang J, Ugnat AM, Clarke K, Mao Y: Ovarian cancer histology-specific incidence trends in Canada 1969-1993: Age-period-cohort analyses. Br J Cancer 1999;81:152-158.

Ovulation is also linked to the formation of clefts and inclusion cysts, which are lined with ovarian epithelium and are found within the ovarian stroma. Ovarian cancer appears to arise from surface epithelium that is trapped within the ovarian stroma, rather than from the ovarian surface itself. Some authors propose that these inclusion cysts represent preneoplastic lesions, and that it is the proliferation and subsequent transformation of the ovarian epithelium lining these cysts that leads to cancer.[13] This theory is based on observations that the ovarian surface epithelium lining the clefts and inclusion cysts develops metaplastic changes with time. Rather than the normal squamous or cuboidal morphology, these cells take on a more columnar shape. They then become positive for markers found in ovarian neoplasia, such as CA 125 and E-cadherin. The cells lining these cysts have also been noted to develop histologic dysplasia and other morphologic signs of neoplastic progression.[14,15]

Gonadotropin hypothesis. The "gonadotropin hypothesis" derives support from both animal models and epidemiologic data. Pituitary hormones are required for ovarian tumor development in various rodent models. In these models, conditions that are characterized by a decrease in peripheral circulating estrogens, and a consequent increase in pituitary gonadotropin secretion, are associated with an increase in ovarian tumor development. Ovaries exposed to the chemical carcinogen dimethylbenzanthrene (DMBA) will develop tumors after they are transplanted into oophorectomized mice, but not if those mice have had their pituitaries removed.[16] Irradiated (hormonally inactivated) ovaries transplanted into rodent hosts with intact ovaries remain tumor free, but they often develop tumors if transplanted into oophorectomized hosts.[17]

Even in the absence of an external carcinogen, the incidence of ovarian cancer in rodents is markedly increased if both ovaries are implanted into the spleen.[18] The ovarian hormone secretions from intrasplenic ovaries enter the portal circulation and are then metabolized by the liver before entering the systemic circulation. The resulting decrease in peripheral circulating estrogens triggers an increase in pituitary gonadotropin secretion. Under these conditions, the risk of malignant transformation within the intrasplenic ovaries is increased.[18] If circulating estrogen levels are maintained (through administration of supplemental estrogen or the retention of an ovary in its original, native position), these tumors do not develop, presumably because the estrogen suppresses gonadotropin secretion. Additional support for the gonadotropin hypothesis is found in the observation that exogenous gonadotropins speed the development of tumors in intrasplenic ovaries.[18]

Cramer and Welch[19] theorized that increased levels of gonadotropins are not directly mutagenic to the ovarian epithelium; rather, the elevated levels of gonadotropins induce ovarian secretion of estrogen, which then acts locally (in a paracrine manner) to induce proliferation and subsequent transformation of ovarian epithelium. The circulating hormones alter gonadotropin secretion, which in turn influences ovarian hormone secretion. Therefore, the reduction in ovarian cancer risk seen in parous women and subsequent to the use of OCs could be explained by the decreases in gonadotropin secretion that characterize these two states.

Androgen hypothesis. In 1998, Risch[20] put forth the hypothesis that androgens have an important role in the pathogenesis of ovarian cancer. This theory is based on evidence that ovarian epithelial cells contain androgen receptors and therefore should be capable of responding to androgenic signals.[21,22] The ovarian epithelium is exposed to androgenic steroids from both ovarian and adrenal sources, including androstenedione, dehydroepiandrosterone, and testosterone.[23] In vitro studies indicate that androgens can stimulate growth of normal ovarian epithelial cells in tissue culture,[24] as well as the growth of ovarian cancer cell lines.[25] Androgens have also been found to stimulate proliferation of ovarian epithelium in guinea pigs, leading to the formation of cysts, papillomas, and adenomas.[26]

Some epidemiologic data also support this hypothesis. For example, a population-based case-control study found higher levels of androgens (androstenedione and dehydroepiandrosterone) in women who subsequently developed ovarian cancer than in matched controls.[27] Polycystic ovary syndrome, which is characterized in part by increased levels of androgens, was associated with an increased risk of ovarian cancer in a large cohort study,[28] although data from another study failed to find such an association.[29] According to this hypothesis, the reduction in ovarian cancer risk that is associated with the use of OCs would be expected based on suppression of androgen levels.[30]

Progesterone hypothesis. In contrast to the risk-enhancing effect of androgens, Risch[20] found evidence of a *protective* role for progesterone in relation to ovarian cancer risk. Beginning with the observation that normal ovarian epithelium contains progesterone receptors,[22] Risch found support for this hypothesis in both animal and epidemiologic studies. For example,

the domestic laying hen (*Gallus domesticus*), which is known to spontaneously develop epithelial ovarian cancer, has proved to be a useful animal model.[31] One study found the 3-year incidence of ovarian cancer in hens older than 2 years of age to be 24%.[32] Because inhibition of ovulation by feed restriction decreases but does not eliminate ovarian cancer risk in this model, strategies to alter risk independent of their effects on ovulation can be studied. In the anovulatory bird, the risk of ovarian cancer decreases further with the administration of a combination OC preparation, and it decreases even further if the birds are given progestin alone.[33] These results imply that the estrogenic component of combination OCs may blunt the protective effect associated with progestin administration.

Molecular studies performed in macaque monkeys provide additional support for this hypothesis. In this animal model, progesterone induces, and estrogen inhibits, apoptosis of ovarian epithelial cells. If estrogen and a progestin are given together, the combination produces an intermediate result.[34]

These animal data are consistent with observations that suggest an increased risk of ovarian cancer among postmenopausal women taking estrogen alone, which is somewhat tempered by the coadministration of progesterone.[35] Other epidemiologic data support a protective role for progesterone. Pregnancy, which is accompanied by markedly increased levels of progesterone, is associated with a decrease in ovarian cancer risk. Combination OCs contain progestational agents, and their administration is also linked with decreased risk of ovarian cancer.[36] Progestin-only OCs, which only partially (or incompletely) suppress ovulation, are nonetheless associated with decreased risk of ovarian cancer.[37] However, the use of depot medroxyprogesterone acetate, a long-acting progestational contraceptive, had no demonstrated effect on the risk of ovarian cancer in the one study that examined this relationship.[38]

What factors are known to modify the risk of ovarian cancer in humans?

How does parity affect the risk of ovarian cancer?

The protective effect of parity on ovarian cancer risk is well documented, with supporting evidence seen in both case-control and prospective cohort studies. For example, a pooled analysis of three European hospital-based case/hospital-based control studies found that parous women were at reduced risk of ovarian cancer compared with nulliparous women, with a relative risk (RR) of 0.7 (95% confidence interval [CI], 0.6 to 0.8).[39] In this analysis, women reporting four or more term pregnancies had a 40% reduction in risk when compared with nulliparous women.

Subsequently, a collaborative analysis of multiple U.S. case-control studies was published.[40] The Collaborative Ovarian Cancer Group combined data at the individual subject level from 12 studies, which involved a total of 2197 ovarian cancer cases and 8893 controls. Six of the studies had hospital-based controls, and the remainder used various population-based methods for ascertaining controls. For population studies, parous women had a marked decrease in the risk of ovarian cancer, with an odds ratio (OR) of 0.5 (95% CI, 0.4 to 0.6). Although data from the studies with hospital-based controls yielded evidence of a more modest protective effect, with a pooled OR of 0.8 (95% CI, 0.6 to 0.9), this discrepancy was largely accounted for by differences in parity between the study populations. The fitted OR per full-term pregnancy was similar across the different study populations, with an OR of 0.81 per pregnancy for population studies, compared with 0.87 for hospital studies. Therefore, each additional pregnancy reduced the risk of ovarian cancer by 13% to 19%. Risk also decreased with increasing parity in both study populations. Population-based data indicated that the greatest protection was associated with the first full-term pregnancy.

The association of parity with a decreased risk of ovarian cancer has also been confirmed in prospective cohort studies. Analysis of data from the Nurses' Health Study, for example, revealed that parous women overall had a 45% reduction in risk when compared with nulliparous women. In addition, the benefit seen increased with increasing parity, so that (in one model) each birth was associated, incrementally, with a 16% reduction in ovarian cancer risk.[41] It is unclear, at present, whether the effects of gravidity and parity are independent or are simply two different measures of the same basic association.

What is the effect of oral contraceptives on ovarian cancer risk? The effect of OCs on ovarian cancer risk has also been extensively evaluated in both case-control and cohort studies. Case-control studies have estimated risk reductions ranging from 30% to 60% for ever-users versus never-users.[40,42] A meta-analysis found that risk decreased with increasing duration of OC use. One year of OC administration was associated with an 11% reduction in risk, whereas 5 or more years' exposure decreased the risk by 50%,[43] an estimate that was confirmed in a subsequent study.[44]

Multiple cohort studies have also confirmed the ovarian cancer risk reduction associated with OC use.[35,45] In the Oxford Family Planning Association study, for example, the risk of ovarian cancer was decreased by 60% among those who had ever used OCs, with a significant trend for decreasing risk with increasing duration of use.[45]

Does age at menarche influence the risk of ovarian cancer? Although the previously cited pooled analysis of 12 U.S. case-control studies demonstrated a weak trend of decreasing ovarian cancer risk associated with increasing age at menarche, this finding was not confirmed in other case-control[42,46] or cohort studies.[41] Therefore, age at menarche cannot be considered an established risk factor for ovarian cancer, based on currently available data.

Is there a relationship between lactation and ovarian cancer risk? A modest protective effect for breast-feeding was demonstrated in population-based case-control studies. A 19% risk-reduction was seen among parous women who breast-fed, and the association persisted after adjustment for parity.[40] A larger protective effect of breast-feeding was seen in an Italian case-control study, with risk decreased by 50% among those who breast-fed for at least 12 months. This association persisted after adjustment for covariates (95% CI, 0.4 to 0.8).[42] Although a crude risk reduction of 29% with lactation was seen in an Australian case-control study, this effect failed to reach significance when adjusted for parity.[47] It is likely that breast-feeding is associated with, at best, a modest decrease in risk of ovarian cancer, although the data on this subject are sparse.

What are the effects of age at menopause and gynecologic surgery? Although a few European case-control studies found a modest increase in ovarian cancer risk with increasing age at "natural"(i.e., non-surgical) menopause,[46,48] other case-control studies found no evidence for such an effect.[40,42] Two large cohort studies[35,41] also found no relationship between age at menopause and risk of ovarian cancer. A meta-analysis combining data from six population-based case-control studies showed a weak association, which was not statistically significant (hazard ratio [HR], 1.1; 95% CI, 1.0 to 1.2).[49]

However, hysterectomy without complete oophorectomy has been associated with an estimated ovarian cancer risk reduction of 33% to 36% in various studies.[40,50,51] In addition, data from both cohort and case-control studies indicate a significant effect of tubal ligation (with retention of the ovaries) on ovarian cancer incidence and mortality. In the Nurses' Health Study, the incidence of ovarian cancer was found to decrease by 67% after tubal ligation.[51] Another study, using ovarian cancer *mortality* as the end point, found a significant protective effect after tubal ligation, with mortality decreasing by one third.[52]

Case-control studies estimate a more modest reduction in risk associated with tubal ligation. A cancer center–based case-control study showed a 48% risk reduction,[53] whereas a large Australian case-control study estimated the reduction in risk to be 39%.[50] A smaller World Health Organization study showed a 28% decreased risk, which failed to reach statistical significance.[54]

The mechanism for the decrease in risk associated with either of these gynecologic surgeries is not clear. Some have argued that the risk reduction seen is actually an artifact resulting from screening of the ovaries for cancer during these elective procedures. If this were true, however, one would expect diminishing benefit with increasing time since the surgery, and this is not seen. Others have asserted that both hysterectomy and tubal ligation decrease the access of talc (or other putative environmental carcinogens) to the ovary. The relative risk associated with perineal talc use has been estimated to be 1.3, with a minority of women reporting talc exposure. Therefore, the magnitude of the benefit that is seen with tubal ligation and hysterectomy is greater than what could be accounted for simply by removal of the putative talc-related risk alone.

Still others have postulated that these procedures may lead to a decrease in ovarian function and ovulation, perhaps through an alteration in ovarian circulation. Although the major blood supply to the ovaries is left intact as a result of these procedures, and there is no evidence that tubal ligation is associated with decreased levels of circulating ovarian hormones, there are no data on hormone levels in the microenvironment of the ovary after these surgeries. In addition, most studies of ovarian function after tubal ligation have limited follow-up to the first 12 months after the procedure, so little is known of long-term hormonal effects. In one report,[65] the decrease in breast cancer mortality associated with tubal sterilization argues for an alteration in ovarian steroidogenesis after the procedure; a second study failed to confirm this observation.[56]

Is there an association of menopausal hormone therapy with ovarian cancer? The effect of menopausal hormone therapy (MHT, also called estrogen replacement therapy or hormone replacement therapy) on ovarian cancer risk has been debated. Findings from various case-control studies have been contradictory, with some studies supporting an increased risk of ovarian cancer with MHT[39,48] and others finding no significant association.[40,57] An early meta-analysis suggested that the association between MHT and ovarian cancer was statistically significant,[58] but a later meta-analysis argued to the contrary.[59]

Prospective cohort studies have helped to clarify this situation. Analysis of a cohort of 211,581 women selected from the original cohort of the American Cancer Society Cancer Prevention Study II found that ever-users of MHT had an RR for ovarian cancer death of 1.2 (95% CI, 1.1 to 1.4), compared with never-users. Risk increased with increasing duration of estrogen use, such that those who used estrogen for greater than 10 years had 2.2 times the risk of death from ovarian cancer than those who never took MHT (95% CI, 1.5 to 3.2).[36]

In addition, data from the follow-up study of the participants in the Breast Cancer Detection Demonstration Project showed that in those who had ever taken MHT (in the form of estrogen given without a progestin) had an ovarian cancer RR of 1.6 (95% CI, 1.2 to 2.0). Risk also increased with increasing duration of use, such that those who took estrogen for 20 years or longer had a risk more than three times greater than that of never-users (RR, 3.2). The addition of progesterone to the hormone regimen appeared to modulate the risk downward. The group of women who had a progestin added after initial treatment with estrogen alone showed only a trend toward increased risk, with an RR of 1.5 (95% CI, 0.9 to 2.4). Among those women who took *only* the combination of estrogen and progestin, there were but 18 ovarian cancer deaths (in 42,400 person-years of follow-up), and no significant alteration of risk was demonstrated.[35]

Therefore, the weight of the more recent evidence, derived from the methodologically superior prospective cohort study design, suggests that MHT, particularly estrogen alone, is associated with a modest but significant increase in the risk of ovarian cancer. Although these data suggest that the combination of estrogen and progesterone may be safer than estrogen treatment alone in regard to ovarian cancer risk, long-term administration of this combination regimen is no longer considered appropriate in the routine health maintenance of postmenopausal women. A large randomized, controlled trial of a combination of oral estrogen with progesterone (versus placebo) was halted early because of an excess of adverse events (e.g., breast cancer, stroke, pulmonary embolus, coronary heart disease) in those taking the active drug.[60] For this reason, a new study of the effects of long-term combination MHT on ovarian cancer risk can no longer be contemplated, and all further data on this issue will have to come from follow-up of previously defined cohorts.

Is infertility a risk factor for ovarian cancer? There are conflicting reports regarding the effect of infertility on ovarian cancer risk. Women with fertility problems often differ from those without such problems in terms of other established ovarian cancer risk factors, such as parity or OC use. This issue is further complicated by the need to separate the biologic effects of infertility alone from the effects of the medications used to treat this condition. Initial case reports of ovarian cancer associated with ovulation induction prompted concern, because the medications used to stimulate ovulation act by increasing gonadotropin levels. Both the incessant ovulation hypothesis and the gonadotropin hypothesis predict that the use of these medications can lead to increased risk of ovarian cancer.

The oral agent clomiphene citrate, for example, produces an increase in pituitary gonadotropin secretion, which in turn stimulates ovulation.[61] Gonadotropin therapy, consisting of various formulations of follicle-stimulating hormone (FSH), or FSH and luteinizing hormone (LH), is given by injection to stimulate ovulation. If it is the trauma of ovulation alone that leads to an increased risk of ovarian cancer, one might expect an increased incidence of ovarian cancer among those women who responded to treatment with multiple ovulations, particularly those who used the medications for multiple cycles. If, instead, it is elevated levels of gonadotropins that increase then risk, then women who have been treated with any of these medications could be at increased risk.

The initial case reports were followed by the publication of case-control data indicating that infertile women who used fertility drugs had an elevated risk of ovarian cancer when compared with women without a diagnosis of infertility.[40] Women who had not used fertility medications showed no alteration in risk. In 1994, a study of a cohort of infertile women was published. Among the 3837 women studied, there were 11 cases of ovarian cancer, compared with the 4.4 cases that were expected. Of those 11 cases, 4 were invasive epithelial cancers, 5 were epithelial ovarian tumors of borderline malignancy, and the remaining 2 were granulosa cell tumors. More than half of the women in the cohort had been treated with clomiphene, but fewer than 4% had received gonadotropin therapy. Although any use of ovulatory stimulants was associated with an increased risk of ovarian cancer, this increase was most dramatic among those women who had used clomiphene for more than 12 cycles, with an RR of 11 (95% CI, 1.5 to 81.3).[62]

Other studies attempted to clarify the effects of infertility medications on ovarian cancer risk by examining women who were referred for infertility treatment. An Australian study[63] of women who had been referred to a clinic specializing in in vitro fertilization found no evidence of an increased incidence of ovarian cancer in the entire cohort. Additionally, both those who had received fertility medication and those who had not had similar risks.

A meta-analysis[64] of eight case-control studies found that fertility drug use in *nulligravid women* was associated with an elevated risk of *borderline tumors*, but the risk of invasive ovarian cancer was not elevated. Nulligravid women who had attempted to become pregnant for more than 5 years had a 2.7-fold increased risk of ovarian cancer, compared with those who tried to conceive for less than 1 year. Among those who were nulliparous but who had been pregnant, fertility drug use was not associated with increased risk.

Effects of parity and other reproductive risk factors also make interpretation of the effect of infertility on the risk of ovarian cancer difficult to isolate. For example, in one case-control study, a higher proportion of cases than controls reported a history of infertility, giving a crude OR of 1.5, but cases were also more likely to be nulliparous and less likely to have taken OCs. In addition, only 43% of cases and 52% of controls knew their fertility status. After adjustment for these important covariates, the increased risk associated with long-term infertility was no longer significant. A subgroup analysis indicated that nulliparous women who reported infertility but had not been treated for it had a risk of ovarian cancer that was 2.5 times that of nulliparous women who did not report infertility.[65] In contrast, difficulty becoming pregnant was reported by 14% of women in one cohort study, with 17% of those nulligravid. The incidence of death from ovarian cancer was not increased in the infertile women.

An Israeli study[66] that was suggestive of an increased incidence of ovarian cancer in a cohort of infertile women observed only 12 cases among 2496 study subjects; the result was not statistically significant (standardized incidence ratio [SIR], 1.6; 95% CI, 0.8 to 2.9). The authors of the study noted that the observed difference in ovarian cancer incidence could be explained if half the cohort were nulliparous. In addition, there was no significant difference in incidence of ovarian cancer between those women who were treated with ovulatory stimulants and those who were not.

In summary, there is little convincing evidence that infertility itself increases the risk of ovarian cancer. Among women treated with ovulatory stimulants, there is evidence of an increased incidence of ovarian tumors of borderline malignancy, but thus far the evidence does not support an increased risk of invasive epithelial ovarian cancer.

Does exposure to psychotropic medications affect the risk of ovarian cancer? Psychotropic medications, such as amphetamines, sedatives, barbiturates, anticonvulsants, antidepressants, and antipsychotics, have been inconsistently associated with an increased risk of ovarian cancer. A case-control study from New England found that use of any of these medications for at least 6 months was associated with increased ovarian cancer risk, with an RR of 1.6 (95% CI, 1.1 to 2.3). This association was largely limited to medications that act through dopaminergic or GABAergic mechanisms, as opposed to serotoninergic medications.[67] However, another case-control study failed to corroborate this association.[68]

Data from a large cohort study did suggest a modest increase in the risk of ovarian cancer with the use of any psychotropic medication, as reported at the time of the baseline questionnaire (RR, 1.5). However, these results failed to reach statistical significance because of the small number of incident cases (47); the resulting 95% CIs were quite wide, 0.7 to 3.2.[69]

Do certain analgesic medications reduce the risk of ovarian cancer? The effect of analgesics such as acetaminophen, aspirin, and other nonsteroidal anti-inflammatory drugs (NSAIDs) on ovarian cancer risk remains controversial. Case-control studies have provided conflicting evidence of a protective effect for acetaminophen. One study examined the relationship between continuous use of "analgesic medications" (defined as intake of aspirin, acetaminophen, or ibuprofen at least weekly, for 6 months or longer) and ovarian cancer risk. The analysis revealed no significant effect of either aspirin or ibuprofen consumption on ovarian cancer risk but did suggest a significant protective effect for the use of acetaminophen, with an adjusted OR of 0.5 (95% CI, 0.3 to 0.9).[70] Experimental studies in rodents demonstrating uterine and ovarian atrophy at high doses of acetaminophen, and decreased ovarian-cyst formation at lower doses, suggested a biologic basis for this observation.[71] Another case-control study found a similar risk reduction with acetaminophen use, with an OR of 0.6 (95% CI, 0.3 to 0.9).[72] However, two other case-control studies found little evidence of a relationship between acetaminophen intake and ovarian cancer risk.[73,74] The reason for these conflicting results is not clear.

Data from various cohort studies are also contradictory. One study suggested a 45% decrease in the risk of ovarian cancer death with daily acetaminophen use, but the finding failed to reach statistical significance.[75] Two other cohort studies found no evidence of a relationship between acetaminophen intake and ovarian cancer risk.[76,77]

Some of these same studies also analyzed the effect of aspirin use on risk and found no significant association.[70,72,73,76] A 40% to 50% risk reduction associated with intake of NSAIDs was seen in some studies,[73,76] but others found no such relationship.[70,74]

In summary, there are insufficient data in support of a protective effect of acetaminophen or NSAIDs to recommend the clinical use of these agents to reduce the risk of ovarian cancer. Further studies are needed to clarify this association, which, if real, would have significant clinical implications.

Is talc exposure an ovarian cancer risk factor? A number of case-control studies have found that application of talc to the perineum is associated with an increase in the risk of ovarian cancer. A meta-analysis of case-control studies found a modest increase in ovarian cancer incidence among women who reported exposure to talc (adjusted RR, 1.3; 95% CI, 1.1 to 1.5).[78] Similar increases in ovarian cancer risk, ranging from 1.3 to 1.5, were found in three additional case-control studies published after the meta-analysis.[47,79,80] Subsequently, Ness and colleagues[81] reported case-control data indicating an increased risk of ovarian cancer associated with conditions potentially related to ovarian inflammation, including talc use.

An association between the use of talc and an increased risk of ovarian cancer was not supported by analysis of the Nurses' Health Study, which collected prospective data from a cohort of more than 78,000 women. Although 40% of the cohort reported ever using talc, fewer than 15% reported ever using talc on a daily basis. Ever-use of perineal talc did not increase the risk of ovarian cancer (RR, 1.1; 95% CI, 0.9 to 1.4), and the risk was not increased with daily use. Theorizing that women who had undergone a tubal ligation or hysterectomy could be considered to be relatively protected from ovarian exposure to talc, the analysis was repeated excluding those women, but the association between talc exposure and ovarian cancer risk remained null (RR, 0.97; 95% CI, 0.7-1.3).[82]

Reports that the National Toxicology Program intended to review talc for possible listing in the 10th edition of the *Report on Carcinogens* triggered much debate. The International Agency for Research in Cancer (IARC) had previously designated talc containing asbestiform fibers as a human carcinogen but had indicated that the evidence regarding cosmetic (nonasbestiform) talc was insufficient.[83] The IARC also asserted that there was inadequate evidence for carcinogenicity to animals from any type of talc.[83] The National Toxicology Program indicated that studies published subsequent to the IARC review provided sufficient further evidence that talc is carcinogenic to humans to merit a listing in the 10th edition of the *Report on Carcinogens*. These studies suggested an association between exposure to talc in occupational settings and cancer risk in humans, as well as an association between use of talcum powder and cancer risk. However, at this time, the National Toxicology Program has deferred action on this listing and has indicated a need to establish a clear definition of the agent or agents in talc that are involved in human exposure.[84]

Overall, the aggregate data related to talc exposure are most reasonably interpreted as suggesting that the risk, if present, is small.

To what extent does family history contribute to the risk of ovarian cancer?
Family history of ovarian cancer. A family history of ovarian cancer has long been recognized as a risk factor for developing the disease, but estimates of the magnitude of this risk have varied. An Australian case-control study[47] demonstrated that ovarian cancer risk was significantly increased among women who had a first-degree relative with a history of ovarian cancer (RR, 3.9; 95% CI, 1.6 to 9.7); the RR increased to 4.8 when corrected for parity. In a pooled analysis of seven case-control studies, 4% of ovarian cancer patients had a history of ovarian cancer in first-degree relatives. This family history was associated with a substantial increase in ovarian cancer risk, compared with no such family history (RR, 5.4; 95% CI, 3.5 to 8.4).[44] A study of a cohort of first-degree relatives of ovarian cancer patients showed no increased risk of cancer, all sites combined, but did document an increased the incidence of ovarian cancer (SIR, 2.8; 95% CI, 1.8 to 4.2). The risk seemed higher if the affected relative was a sister (SIR, 3.7; 95% CI, 2.3 to 5.7) rather than a mother (SIR, 0.6; 95% CI, 0.0 to 3.1).[85]

Analyzing all previously published ovarian cancer case-control and cohort studies, a meta-analysis from 1998 found a pooled RR of 3.1 (95% CI, 2.6 to 3.7) for first-degree relatives of ovarian cancer cases. A gradient in risk was observed among specific classes of first-degree relatives: mothers of ovarian cancer patients were at least risk (RR, 1.1; 95% CI, 0.8 to 1.6), sisters were at higher risk (RR, 3.8; 95% CI, 2.9 to 5.1), and daughters appeared to have the highest risk (RR, 6.0; 95% CI, 3.0 to 11.9). In addition, risk increased with increasing number of affected family members. With one first-degree relative affected, the cumulative risk of developing ovarian cancer by 75 years of age was estimated to be 4.0%; with two affected relatives, the risk increased to 14%. For reference purposes, the analogous figure for women with no family history was less than 1%.[86]

Several attempts have been made to explore the question of whether the ovarian cancer risk factors identified from epidemiologic studies of unselected women with ovarian cancer behave in a similar fashion among ovarian cancer patients who have a positive family history of the disease. A cohort study examined the association of parity and ovarian cancer risk in individuals stratified by family history and found that nulliparous women with a family history were at higher risk of ovarian cancer than parous women with a family history of the disease, the same pattern previously observed in general population studies.[87] A population-based case-control study found that the risk of ovarian cancer was decreased by 50% in women with a family history of the disease who had used OCs for at least 4 years, again paralleling the general population data.[88] A large Italian case-control study suggested that women with both the standard risk factors and a family history were at greater risk than those with one, the other, or neither.[48] These analyses did not take into account the presence or absence of germline mutations in the ovarian cancer susceptibility genes.

Which genetic syndromes are associated with ovarian cancer?

BRCA1 and BRCA2. Between 5% and 10% of ovarian cancers are considered hereditary in origin, the result of germline mutations in cancer predisposition genes. Most of these cancers are part of the syndrome known as hereditary breast and ovarian cancer (HBOC) and can be attributed to germline mutations in the genes *BRCA1* or *BRCA2*. Both *BRCA* genes follow an autosomal dominant mode of inheritance and fit a tumor suppressor model of action. *BRCA1* is a large gene found on the long arm of chromosome 17.[89] The lifetime risk of ovarian cancer for women carrying a mutated form of *BRCA1* has been estimated at 40% to 60%,[90-92] with a lifetime risk of breast cancer approaching 90% in some families.[92,93] Female carriers of *BRCA1* mutations also have a risk of fallopian tube carcinoma estimated at 50 to 120 times that of the general population,[90,94] as well as a marked increase in the risk of primary peritoneal cancer (RR, 45).[90]

Study of HBOC kindreds with no evidence of linkage to the *BRCA1* gene led to the discovery of a second predisposition locus on chromosome 13, designated *BRCA2*.[95] Like *BRCA1*, *BRCA2* is a large gene with multiple documented disease-associated mutations scattered across its span. A region within exon 11 of *BRCA2* has been designated the "ovarian cancer cluster region," because mutations within this area are more likely to be statistically associated with ovarian cancer. The lifetime risk of ovarian cancer for female carriers of *BRCA2* mutations is lower than that reported for *BRCA1*, having been estimated at 16% to 27%.[92] Ovarian cancer in *BRCA2* mutation carriers tends to occur at a later age than in those with *BRCA1* mutations (57.5 versus 51.2 years).

Estimates of penetrance of the *BRCA* genes vary according to the population studied. Initial estimates were based on cancer incidence in the families used for linkage analysis and gene-finding, which were selected because of the occurrence of multiple cases of breast and ovarian cancer in multiple generations. In contrast, significantly lower penetrance estimates are found in studies that target populations that are more similar to the general population.

HNPCC. Ovarian cancer is also part of the spectrum of cancers seen in the hereditary nonpolyposis colorectal cancer syndrome (HNPCC). HNPCC is an autosomal dominant disorder that is associated with defects in the genes responsible for DNA mismatch repair. Although HNPCC is most characteristically associated with early-onset colon cancers, it is also characterized by increased risks of a number of extracolonic malignancies, including cancers of the endometrium and ovary, as well as cancers of the stomach, small bowel, and upper urinary tract. The cumulative risk of ovarian cancer by age 70 years among persons with mutations in one of the mismatch repair genes is approximately 12%,[96] compared with the general population risk of 1.4%. Although these risks are not as dramatically elevated as those associated with *BRCA1/2*, they are still 8 to 9 times higher than the expected risks among women in the general population.

Other familial cancer syndromes. The *Carney complex,* a syndrome clinically manifested by primary pigmented nodular adrenal disease, cardiac and skin myxomas, blue nevi, and endocrine disorders, has been associated with ovarian tumors, including both adenomas and adenocarcinomas.[97] *Peutz-Jeghers syndrome,* characterized by pigmented lesions on the lips, gastrointestinal hamartomatous polyps, and mutations in the *STK11* gene, is associated with an incidence of carcinoma estimated at 20% to 50%. Although gastrointestinal cancers are the most common malignancy associated with this syndrome, affected females may develop ovarian neoplasms. Tumors arise from the ovarian surface epithelium or from ovarian stromal cells, and they include the sex cord tumor with annular tubules, Sertoli cell tumors of the ovary, and mucinous epithelial ovarian cancers.[97] Ovarian carcinoids have been reported in association with the *multiple endocrine neoplasia type 1* syndrome. This syndrome is more characteristically associated with parathyroid adenomas and secretory tumors of the pancreas or gastrointestinal tract.[97] Juvenile granulosa cell tumors of the ovary have been associated with *Ollier's disease* enchondromatosis) in several case reports.[98] The *nevoid basal cell carcinoma syndrome,* which has been linked to the gene *PTCH,* is associated with an increased incidence of ovarian fibromas.[99] Further details regarding the hereditary ovarian cancer syndromes are presented in Chapter 62.

What are the epidemiologic characteristics of primary carcinoma of the fallopian tube?

Primary carcinoma of the fallopian tube is extremely rare, with an annual incidence estimated at 3.6 per 1,000,000 women per year in the United States.[100] The incidence of fallopian tube cancer increases with advancing age, with little risk before age 25 years; the incidence peaks between 60 and 64 years of age. In 20% of cases, cancer of the fallopian tube is diagnosed simultaneously with a cancer of another site.[100] Because the diagnosis of primary carcinoma of the fallopian tube is made so infrequently, it is often grouped together with ovarian neoplasms in statistical databases. In a population-based dataset, women with fallopian tube carcinoma had better survival, stage for stage, than did women with epithelial ovarian cancer.[101] Although a number of investigators have published case series of patients with fallopian tube carcinoma in which the clinicopathologic characteristics of this cancer are summarized,[102-104] to date no systematic studies designed to assess risk factors have been published.

There has been a resurgence of interest in this rare cancer with the realization that carriers of mutations in the *BRCA* genes are at increased risk of primary carcinoma of the fallopian tube. Case reports have linked fallopian tube carcinoma with germline mutations in both *BRCA1*[105,106] and *BRCA2*.[107] A Canadian study[108] found that 7 women from a population-based series of 45 cases of fallopian tube cancer were carriers of BRCA mutations. In some cases, investigators have demonstrated loss of heterozygosity at the wild-type BRCA1 allele in these tumors, evidence supporting an etiologic link between the BRCA mutation and the development of the fallopian tube malignancy.[106] In addition, two studies have demonstrated a dramatically increased risk for this disease among BRCA1 carriers, with estimated RRs between 48 and 120.[90,94]

The most pragmatic consequence of recognizing that the fallopian tube is one of the organs at risk for malignant transformation in women with germline mutations in BRCA1 or BRCA2 is the need to consciously include the fallopian tube when performing risk-reducing bilateral oophorectomy. It would be imprudent at best to leave some or all of the fallopian tube behind when attempting a surgical procedure that has cancer risk reduction as its primary goal. Optimal surgical technique assumes even greater importance now that most of these procedures are done laparoscopically. Special attention must be paid to avoid leaving a remnant of ovarian tissue at the distal end of the utero-ovarian ligament, and the proximal end of the fallopian tube should be transected as close to the uterine cornua as possible.

A new, and currently unresolved, issue that has been raised in this context centers on acknowledging that, in the absence of a hysterectomy, the interstitial (intramural) segment of the fallopian tube is inevitably left in situ when a bilateral salpingo-oophorectomy is performed. This portion of the fallopian tube, which resides within the muscular wall of the uterus, is very short, and part of its mucosa consists of endometrial rather than fallopian tube tissue, but theoretically there is still a concern that this fragment of retained fallopian tube carries the potential for malignant transformation. To date, there are no reports in the literature of carcinoma arising in the interstitial portion of the fallopian tube. In fact, the majority of these carcinomas occur at the distal, fimbriated end of the tube. Nonetheless, this concern has led some investigators to suggest that risk-reducing surgery in this context should include a hysterectomy.[105]

Currently, the data required to permit a fully informed decision about this choice are lacking; consequently, hysterectomy has not become a standard part of the risk-reducing surgical procedure. The increased morbidity associated with adding a hysterectomy to laparoscopic salpingo-oophorectomy must be factored into this decision as well. On the other hand, the use of MHT or tamoxifen as a breast cancer prevention strategy is considerably simplified in the absence of a uterus. If a recent preliminary report[94] suggesting a significant excess risk of endometrial cancer in BRCA1 mutation carriers is confirmed, then the pendulum will undoubtedly swing toward including a hysterectomy. For the moment, it seems most appropriate to suggest that elective hysterectomy should at least be considered at the time risk-reducing salpingo-oophorectomy is discussed with a patient who is genetically at risk, and that this decision should be made on a case-by-case basis.

What are the epidemiologic characteristics of extraovarian primary peritoneal cancer?

Extraovarian primary peritoneal carcinoma (PPC), which is characterized by widely disseminated malignancy along the peritoneal surfaces with little or no involvement of the ovary, is also known as serous surface papillary carcinoma, papillary serous carcinoma of the peritoneum, or extraovarian peritoneal serous papillary carcinoma. Although PPC more commonly occurs in women with intact ovaries, it has also been diagnosed in women years after oophorectomy for benign conditions.[109] PPC has long been recognized as a distinctive clinical entity, but it was not until the 1990s that a formal definition was developed. The Gynecologic Oncology Group (GOG) limits the diagnosis of PPC to cases in which (1) both ovaries are physiologically normal in size or enlarged by a benign process; (2) the involvement in the extraovarian sites is greater than the involvement on the surface of either ovary; (3) ovarian involvement, if present, either (a) is confined to the ovarian surface epithelium with no evidence of cortical invasion, (b) involves ovarian surface epithelium and underlying cortical stroma but with any given tumor size less than 5×5 mm, or (c) includes tumor less than 5×5 mm within the ovarian substance with or without associated surface disease; and (4) the histology is serous mullerian.[110] Therefore, by definition, PPC is histologically indistinguishable from serous ovarian carcinoma. Some investigators have proposed broadening this definition to include other histologic types, such as endometrioid, clear cell, and mucoid.[111] Because there is no separate staging system for PPC, it is usually staged using the system for ovarian carcinoma, with most cases classified as stage III or IV.

Studies of loss of heterozygosity at various gene loci within tumor tissue have provided evidence that some PPCs are multifocal in origin.[112] A multifocal origin appears to be more common in carriers of BRCA1 mutations[113] than in women with wild-type BRCA1. PPC is similar to ovarian carcinoma in terms of frequency of aneuploidy and overexpression of TP53 protein, but a higher proportion of PPCs overexpress HER-2/neu.[114]

The clinical presentation of PPC often mimics that of advanced ovarian carcinoma. In one series of 199 women with presumed ovarian cancer, 29 cases (15%) were found on laparotomy to fit the criteria for extraovarian PPC.[115] In another series, 25 of 96 patients with a preoperative diagnosis of stage III or IV ovarian adenocarcinoma were found after surgical staging to have PPC.[116]

There are few descriptive epidemiologic data available concerning PPC. A study comparing 50 women with PPC with 503 women classified as having primary ovarian carcinoma found that the former group was significantly older than the latter (mean, 64 versus 55 years). PPC was also associated with a later age at menarche (13.3 versus 12.8 years). Differences in parity between these two groups of patients did not reach statistical significance, nor were there significant differences with regard to other ovarian cancer risk modifiers, such as OC use and family history.[117]

The association between PPC and a family history of ovarian cancer has been documented most convincingly in HBOC families. In 1982, investigators reported "intra-abdominal carcinomatosis" in 3 of 28 high-risk women who had previously undergone prophylactic oophorectomy.[118] Since then, additional cases of PPC have been documented in women with strong family histories of ovarian cancer who had their ovaries removed to decrease their risk of cancer.[119] These observations have raised questions regarding the effectiveness of oophorectomy as a risk-reducing strategy, because some women developed an ovarian cancer–like illness despite having the surgery. In one series of 324 women with strong family histories of ovarian cancer who underwent risk-reducing oophorectomy, PPC subsequently developed in 6 women.[119] The *BRCA* mutation status of these persons was not known, nor were quantitative estimates of PPC risk provided for this case series.

Molecular studies of tumor samples have linked PPC to *BRCA1*,[120] and germline mutations in *BRCA1* were found in 11% of women with PPC in one small series.[121] A larger, population-based Israeli series demonstrated that the prevalence of the Ashkenazi founder *BRCA* mutations was similar in women with PPC (28%) and in women with stage III or IV ovarian cancer (30%), regardless of family history.[122] These rates contrast with an estimated 2% carrier rate in the general Ashkenazi population. Recent data indicate that the risk of PPC is dramatically increased among carriers of *BRCA1* mutations, with an RR of 44.6 (95% CI, 24.9 to 80.2), based on 13 cases from 699 families reported to the Breast Cancer Linkage Consortium.[94]

The development of PPC after prophylactic oophorectomy in high-risk women is viewed by many as a failure of this surgical procedure to prevent ovarian cancer. Certainly, women contemplating surgical removal of their ovaries as a means to reduce the incidence of ovarian cancer need to be made aware that a modest risk of PPC will persist after surgery. However, the assertion that surgery reduces the risk of ovarian cancer by only about 50%[123] clearly represented a misinterpretation of the data cited as the basis for that estimate.[124] This error has inappropriately discouraged some high-risk patients and their health care providers concerning the potential benefit of risk-reducing surgery.

In fact, removal of the ovaries in carriers of *BRCA* mutations is associated with major reductions in both breast and BRCA-associated gynecologic cancers. In a retrospective study[125] of women with known deleterious *BRCA* mutations, 251 women who had undergone bilateral prophylactic oophorectomy were matched to 292 control women who had both ovaries intact. After excluding the 6 cases of ovarian cancer (stage I) found incidentally at the time of risk-reducing surgery, the women who underwent oophorectomy had a 96% reduction in ovarian cancer risk (HR, 0.04; 95% CI, 0.01 to 0.16). In addition, the risk of breast cancer was significantly decreased in the oophorectomy group (HR, 0.5; 95% CI, 0.3 to 0.8). The magnitude of risk reduction is impressive, even taking into account the inherent bias of the retrospective study design. In a small prospective study[126] of oophorectomy versus surveillance in *BRCA* mutation carriers with a mean follow-up time of 24.2 months, investigators found 1 case of PPC among 98 women who underwent oophorectomy, compared with 4 cases of ovarian cancer plus 1 case of PPC among the 72 women who chose surveillance. The incidence of breast cancer was also reduced in the oophorectomy group, with 3 cases diagnosed, compared with 8 cases in the surveillance group. Analyzing both breast and gynecologic cancers together, risk was reduced by 75% by oophorectomy (HR, 0.2; 95% CI, 0.1 to 0.7). Therefore, salpingo-oophorectomy is best viewed as a means to reduce (but not completely eliminate) the risk of cancer among women at increased genetic risk.

Summary

The major story regarding ovarian cancer etiology over the past 15 years is the discovery of *BRCA1/2* and the mismatch repair genes as the basis of several important genetic syndromes that underlie inherited susceptibility to ovarian cancer. These molecular advances are now being leveraged into an improved understanding of the biology of the sporadic counterpart of this disease. Such insight may translate into novel targeted therapeutic strategies.

These discoveries have also spawned a series of as yet unresolved clinical challenges regarding optimal management in genetically susceptible women, including questions about the behavior of conventional ovarian cancer risk factors in the high-risk context; the nature, timing, morbidity, and benefits associated with risk-reducing surgery; and the role of chemoprevention-based intervention strategies. The recognition of parity as a proven risk factor, and of OCs and gynecologic surgery as conferring major protection against ovarian cancer, has led to major advances in our understanding of the pathogenesis of ovarian cancer, even though the mechanism by which surgery reduces risk remains elusive.

The relationship between infertility and the risk of ovarian cancer, and that between talc exposure and ovarian cancer, remain controversial despite decades of research. Although much has been learned, there is still much work ahead in the struggle to bring this difficult disease under control. The recognition that estrogen appears to be an ovarian cancer risk factor and that progestins represent a promising risk-reducing option is shaping the direction of chemoprevention research for this cancer.

REFERENCES

1. Jemal A, Murray T, Samuels A, et al: Cancer statistics, 2003. CA Cancer J Clin 2003;53:5-26.
2. Ferlay J, Bray F, Pisani P, Parkin D: GLOBOCAN 2000: Cancer incidence, mortality and prevalence worldwide, Version 1.0. IARC Cancer Base No. 5. Lyon, IARC Press, 2001.

3. Herrinton LJ, Stanford JL, Schwartz SM, Weiss NS: Ovarian cancer incidence among Asian migrants to the United States and their descendants. J Natl Cancer Inst 1994;86:1336-1339.

4. Ries L, Eisner M, Kosary C, et al: SEER cancer statistics review, 1973-1999. Bethsda, MD: National Cancer Institute, 2002.

5. Katsube Y, Berg JW, Silverberg SG: Epidemiologic pathology of ovarian tumors: A histopathologic review of primary ovarian neoplasms diagnosed in the Denver Standard Metropolitan Statistical Area, 1 July-31 December 1969 and 1 July-31 December 1979. Int J Gynecol Pathol 1982;1:3-16.

6. Modugno F, Ness RB, Wheeler JE: Reproductive risk factors for epithelial ovarian cancer according to histologic type and invasiveness. Ann Epidemiol 2001;11:568-574.

7. Zanetta G, Rota S, Chiari S, et al: Behavior of borderline tumors with particular interest to persistence, recurrence, and progression to invasive carcinoma: A prospective study. J Clin Oncol 2001;19:2658-2664.

8. Risch HA, Marrett LD, Jain M, Howe GR: Differences in risk factors for epithelial ovarian cancer by histologic type: Results of a case-control study. Am J Epidemiol 1996;144:363-372.

9. Zhang J, Ugnat AM, Clarke K, Mao Y: Ovarian cancer histology—Specific incidence trends in Canada 1969-1993: Age-period-cohort analyses. Br J Cancer 1999;81:152-158.

10. Fathalla MF: Factors in the causation and incidence of ovarian cancer. Obstet Gynecol Surv 1972;27:751-768.

11. Casagrande JT, Louie EW, Pike MC, et al: "Incessant ovulation" and ovarian cancer. Lancet 1979;2:170-173.

12. Henderson BE, Ross RK, Pike MC, Casagrande JT: Endogenous hormones as a major factor in human cancer. Cancer Res 1982;42:3232-3239.

13. Feeley KM, Wells M: Precursor lesions of ovarian epithelial malignancy. Histopathology 2001;38:87-95.

14. Tresserra F, Grases PJ, Labastida R, Ubeda A: Histological features of the contralateral ovary in patients with unilateral ovarian cancer: A case control study. Gynecol Oncol 1998;71:437-441.

15. Auersperg N, Wong AS, Choi KC, et al: Ovarian surface epithelium: Biology, endocrinology, and pathology. Endocr Rev 2001;22:255-288.

16. Krarup T: 9:10-Dimethyl-1:2-benzantracene induced ovarian tumours in mice. Acta Pathol Microbiol Scand 1967;70:241-248.

17. Kaplan H: Influence of ovarian function on incidence of radiation-induced ovarian tumors in mice. J Natl Cancer Inst 1950;11:125-132.

18. Capen CC, Beamer WG, Tennent BJ, Stitzel KA: Mechanisms of hormone-mediated carcinogenesis of the ovary in mice. Mutat Res 1995;333:143-151.

19. Cramer DW, Welch WR: Determinants of ovarian cancer risk: II. Inferences regarding pathogenesis. J Natl Cancer Inst 1983;71:717-721.

20. Risch HA: Hormonal etiology of epithelial ovarian cancer, with a hypothesis concerning the role of androgens and progesterone. J Natl Cancer Inst 1998;90:1774-1786.

21. Galli MC, De Giovanni C, Nicoletti G, et al: The occurrence of multiple steroid hormone receptors in disease-free and neoplastic human ovary. Cancer 1981;47:1297-1302.

22. al Timimi A, Buckley CH, Fox H: An immunohistochemical study of the incidence and significance of sex steroid hormone binding sites in normal and neoplastic human ovarian tissue. Int J Gynecol Pathol 1985;4:24-41.

23. Burger HG: Androgen production in women. Fertil Steril 2002;77(Suppl 4):3-5.

24. Edmondson RJ, Monaghan JM, Davies BR: The human ovarian surface epithelium is an androgen responsive tissue. Br J Cancer 2002;86:879-885.

25. Ahonen MH, Zhuang YH, Aine R, et al: Androgen receptor and vitamin D receptor in human ovarian cancer: Growth stimulation and inhibition by ligands. Int J Cancer 2000;86:40-46.

26. Silva EG, Tornos C, Fritsche HA Jr, et al: The induction of benign epithelial neoplasms of the ovaries of guinea pigs by testosterone stimulation: A potential animal model. Mod Pathol 1997;10:879-883.

27. Helzlsouer KJ, Alberg AJ, Gordon GB, et al: Serum gonadotropins and steroid hormones and the development of ovarian cancer. JAMA 1995;274:1926-1930.

28. Schildkraut JM, Schwingl PJ, Bastos E, et al: Epithelial ovarian cancer risk among women with polycystic ovary syndrome. Obstet Gynecol 1996;88:554-559.

29. Pierpoint T, McKeigue PM, Isaacs AJ, et al: Mortality of women with polycystic ovary syndrome at long-term follow-up. J Clin Epidemiol 1998;51:581-586.

30. Murphy A, Cropp CS, Smith BS, et al: Effect of low-dose oral contraceptive on gonadotropins, androgens, and sex hormone binding globulin in nonhirsute women. Fertil Steril 1990;53:35-39.

31. Fredrickson TN: Ovarian tumors of the hen. Environ Health Perspect 1987;73:35-51.

32. Papasolomontos PA, Appleby EC, Mayor OY: Pathological findings in condemned chickens: A survey of 1,000 carcasses. Vet Rec 1969;84:459-464.

33. Rodriguez GC, Carver D, Anderson K, et al: Evaluation of ovarian cancer preventive agents in the chicken [abstract 140]. Gynecol Oncol 2001;80:316.

34. Rodriguez GC, Walmer DK, Cline M, et al: Effect of progestin on the ovarian epithelium of macaques: Cancer prevention through apoptosis? J Soc Gynecol Investig 1998;5:271-276.

35. Lacey JVJ, Mink PJ, Lubin JH, et al: Menopausal hormone replacement therapy and risk of ovarian cancer. JAMA 2002;288:334-341.

36. Rodriguez C, Patel AV, Calle EE, et al: Estrogen replacement therapy and ovarian cancer mortality in a large prospective study of US women. JAMA 2001;285:1460-1465.

37. Rosenberg L, Palmer JR, Zauber AG, et al: A case-control study of oral contraceptive use and invasive epithelial ovarian cancer. Am J Epidemiol 1994;139:654-661.

38. Depot-medroxyprogesterone acetate (DMPA) and risk of epithelial ovarian cancer: The WHO Collaborative Study of Neoplasia and Steroid Contraceptives. Int J Cancer 1991;49:191-195.

39. Negri E, Franceschi S, Tzonou A, et al: Pooled analysis of 3 European case-control studies: I. Reproductive factors and risk of epithelial ovarian cancer. Int J Cancer 1991;49:50-56.

40. Whittemore AS, Harris R, Itnyre J: Characteristics relating to ovarian cancer risk: Collaborative analysis of 12 US case-control studies. II. Invasive epithelial ovarian cancers in white women. Collaborative Ovarian Cancer Group. Am J Epidemiol 1992;136:1184-1203.

41. Hankinson SE, Colditz GA, Hunter DJ, et al: A prospective study of reproductive factors and risk of epithelial ovarian cancer. Cancer 1995;76:284-290.

42. Greggi S, Parazzini F, Paratore MP, et al: Risk factors for ovarian cancer in central Italy. Gynecol Oncol 2000;79:50-54.

43. Hankinson SE, Colditz GA, Hunter DJ, et al: A quantitative assessment of oral contraceptive use and risk of ovarian cancer. Obstet Gynecol 1992;80:708-714.

44. Hartge P, Whittemore AS, Itnyre J, et al: Rates and risks of ovarian cancer in subgroups of white women in the United States. The Collaborative Ovarian Cancer Group. Obstet Gynecol 1994;84:760-764.

45. Vessey MP, Painter R: Endometrial and ovarian cancer and oral contraceptives: Findings in a large cohort study. Br J Cancer 1995;71:1340-1342.

46. Franceschi S, Parazzini F, Negri E, et al: Pooled analysis of 3 European case-control studies of epithelial ovarian cancer: III. Oral contraceptive use. Int J Cancer 1991;49:61-65.

47. Purdie D, Green A, Bain C, et al: Reproductive and other factors and risk of epithelial ovarian cancer: An Australian case-control study. Survey of Women's Health Study Group. Int J Cancer 1995;62:678-684.

48. Tavani A, Ricci E, La Vecchia C, et al: Influence of menstrual and reproductive factors on ovarian cancer risk in women with and without family history of breast or ovarian cancer. Int J Epidemiol 2000;29:799-802.

49. Schildkraut JM, Cooper GS, Halabi S, et al: Age at natural menopause and the risk of epithelial ovarian cancer. Obstet Gynecol 2001;98:85-90.

50. Green A, Purdie D, Bain C, et al: Tubal sterilization, hysterectomy and decreased risk of ovarian cancer. Survey of Women's Health Study Group. Int J Cancer 1997;71:948-951.

51. Hankinson SE, Hunter DJ, Colditz GA, et al: Tubal ligation, hysterectomy, and risk of ovarian cancer: A prospective study [see comments.]. JAMA 1993;270:2813-2818.

52. Miracle-McMahill HL, Calle EE, Kosinski AS, et al: Tubal ligation and fatal ovarian cancer in a large prospective cohort study. Am J Epidemiol 1997;145:349-357.

53. Cornelison TL, Natarajan N, Piver MS, Mettlin CJ: Tubal ligation and the risk of ovarian carcinoma. Cancer Detect Prev 1997;21:1-6.

54. Rosenblatt KA, Thomas DB: Reduced risk of ovarian cancer in women with a tubal ligation or hysterectomy. The World Health Organization Collaborative Study of Neoplasia and Steroid Contraceptives. Cancer Epidemiol Biomarkers Prev 1996;5:933-935.

55. Calle EE, Rodriguez C, Walker KA, et al: Tubal sterilization and risk of breast cancer mortality in US women. Cancer Causes Control 2001;12:127-135.

56. Brinton LA, Gammon MD, Coates RJ, Hoover RN: Tubal ligation and risk of breast cancer. Br J Cancer 2000;82:1600-1604.

57. Hempling RE, Wong C, Piver MS, et al: Hormone replacement therapy as a risk factor for epithelial ovarian cancer: Results of a case-control study. Obstet Gynecol 1997;89:1012-1016.

58. Garg PP, Kerlikowske K, Subak L, Grady D: Hormone replacement therapy and the risk of epithelial ovarian carcinoma: A meta-analysis. Obstet Gynecol 1998;92:472-479.

59. Coughlin SS, Giustozzi A, Smith SJ, Lee NC: A meta-analysis of estrogen replacement therapy and risk of epithelial ovarian cancer. J Clin Epidemiol 2000;53:367-375.

60. Rossouw JE, Anderson GL, Prentice RL, et al: Risks and benefits of estrogen plus progestin in healthy postmenopausal women: Principal results from the Women's Health Initiative randomized controlled trial. JAMA 2002;288:321-333.

61. Archer DF, Hofmann G, Brzyski R, et al: Effects of clomiphene citrate on episodic luteinizing hormone secretion throughout the menstrual cycle. Am J Obstet Gynecol 1989;161:581-589, discussion.

62. Rossing MA, Daling JR, Weiss NS, et al: Ovarian tumors in a cohort of infertile women. N Engl J Med 1994;331:771-776.

63. Venn A, Watson L, Bruinsma F, et al: Risk of cancer after use of fertility drugs with in-vitro fertilization. Lancet 1999;354:1586-1590.

64. Ness RB, Cramer DW, Goodman MT, et al: Infertility, fertility drugs, and ovarian cancer: A pooled analysis of case-control studies. Am J Epidemiol 2001;155:217-224.

65. Mosgaard BJ, Lidegaard O, Kjaer SK, et al: Infertility, fertility drugs, and invasive ovarian cancer: A case-control study. Fertil Steril 1997;67:1005-1012.

66. Modan B, Ron E, Lerner-Geva L, et al: Cancer incidence in a cohort of infertile women. Am J Epidemiol 1998;147:1038-1042.

67. Harlow BL, Cramer DW, Baron JA, et al: Psychotropic medication use and risk of epithelial ovarian cancer. Cancer Epidemiol Biomarkers Prev 1998;7:697-702.

68. Coogan-PF, Rosenberg L, Palmer JR, et al: Risk of ovarian cancer according to use of antidepressants, phenothiazines, and benzodiazepines (United States). Cancer Causes Control 2000;11:839-845.

69. Kato I, Zeleniuch-Jacquotte A, Toniolo PG, et al: Psychotropic medication use and risk of hormone-related cancers: The New York University Women's Health Study. J Public Health Med 2000;22:155-160.

70. Cramer DW, Harlow BL, Titus-Ernstoff L, et al: Over-the-counter analgesics and risk of ovarian cancer. Lancet 1998;351:104-107.

71. National Toxicology Program: Toxicology and carcinogenesis studies of acetaminophen (CAS no 103-9-2) in F344/N rats and B6C3F1 mice (feed studies). NIH publication no 93-2849. Tehnical Report Series no. 394. Research Triangle Park, NC: National Institutes of Health, 1993.

72. Moysich KB, Mettlin C, Piver MS, et al: Regular use of analgesic drugs and ovarian cancer risk. Cancer Epidemiol Biomarkers Prev 2001;10:903-906.

73. Rosenberg L, Palmer JR, Rao RS, et al: A case-control study of analgesic use and ovarian cancer. Cancer Epidemiol Biomarkers Prev 2000;9:933-937.

74. Meier CR, Schmitz S, Jick H: Association between acetaminophen or non-steroidal antiinflammatory drugs and risk of developing ovarian, breast, or colon cancer. Pharmacotherapy 2002;22:303-309.

75. Rodriguez C, Henley SJ, Calle EE, Thun MJ: Paracetamol and risk of ovarian cancer mortality in a prospective study of women in the USA. Lancet 1998;352:1354-1355.

76. Fairfield KM, Hunter DJ, Fuchs CS, et al: Aspirin, other NSAIDs, and ovarian cancer risk (United States). Cancer Causes Control 2002;13:535-542.

77. Friis S, Nielsen GL, Mellemkjaer L, et al: Cancer risk in persons receiving prescriptions for Paracetamol: A Danish cohort study. Int J Cancer 2002;97:96-101.

78. Gross AJ, Berg PH: A meta-analytical approach examining the potential relationship between talc exposure and ovarian cancer. J Exp Anal Environ Epidemiol 1995;5:181-195.

79. Cook LS, Kamb ML, Weiss NS: Perineal powder exposure and the risk of ovarian cancer. Am J Epidemiol 1997;145:459-465.

80. Chang S, Risch HA: Perineal talc exposure and risk of ovarian carcinoma. Cancer 1997;79:2396-2401.

81. Ness RB, Grisso JA, Cottreau C, et al: Factors related to inflammation of the ovarian epithelium and risk of ovarian cancer. Epidemiology 2000;11:111-117.

82. Gertig DM, Hunter DJ, Cramer DW, et al: Prospective study of talc use and ovarian cancer. J Natl Cancer Inst 2000;92:249-252.

83. Overall Evaluations of Carcinogenicity: An Updating of IARC Monographs Volumes 1 to 42 [Suppl 7]. IARC Monographs on the Evaluation of the Carcinogenic Risks to Humans. Lyon: IARC Press, 1987, p 349.

84. National Toxicology Program 10th Report on Carcinogens: Status of Talc Nomination. Available at http://ntp-server. niehs. gov/NewHomeRoc/Talcstatus.html. Accessed 10/10/2002.

85. Auranen A, Pukkala E, Makinen J, et al: Cancer incidence in the first-degree relatives of ovarian cancer patients. Br J Cancer 1996;74:280-284.

86. Stratton JF, Pharoah P, Smith SK, et al: A systematic review and meta-analysis of family history and risk of ovarian cancer. Br J Obstet Gynaecol 1998;105:493-499.

87. Vachon CM, Mink PJ, Janney CA, et al: Association of parity and ovarian cancer risk by family history of breast or ovarian cancer in a population-based study of postmenopausal women. Epidemiology 2002;13:66-71.

88. Walker GR, Schlesselman JJ, Ness RB: Family history of cancer, oral contraceptive use, and ovarian cancer risk. Am J Obstet Gynecol 2002;186:8-14.

89. Hall JM, Lee MK, Newman B, et al: Linkage of early-onset familial breast cancer to chromosome 17q21. Science 1990;250:1684-1689.

90. Brose MS, Rebbeck TR, Calzone KA, et al: Cancer risk estimates for BRCA1 mutation carriers identified in a risk evaluation program. J Natl Cancer Inst 2002;94:1365-1372.

91. Easton DF, Ford D, Bishop DT: Breast and ovarian cancer incidence in BRCA1-mutation carriers. Breast Cancer Linkage Consortium. Am J Hum Genet 1995;56:265-271.

92. Ford D, Easton DF, Stratton M, et al: Genetic heterogeneity and penetrance analysis of the BRCA1 and BRCA2 genes in breast cancer families. The Breast Cancer Linkage Consortium. Am J Hum Genet 1998;62:676-689.

93. Ford D, Easton DF, Bishop DT, et al: Risks of cancer in BRCA1-mutation carriers. Breast Cancer Linkage Consortium. Lancet 1994;343:692-695.

94. Thompson D, Easton DF: Cancer incidence in BRCA1 mutation carriers. J Natl Cancer Inst 2002;94:1358-1365.

95. Wooster R, Neuhausen SL, Mangion J, et al: Localization of a breast cancer susceptibility gene, BRCA2, to chromosome 13q12-13. Science 1994;265:2088-2090.

96. Aarnio M, Sankila R, Pukkala E, et al: Cancer risk in mutation carriers of DNA-mismatch-repair genes. Int J Cancer 1999;81:214-218.

97. Papageorgiou T, Stratakis CA: Ovarian tumors associated with multiple endocrine neoplasias and related syndromes (Carney complex, Peutz-Jeghers syndrome, von Hippel-Lindau disease, Cowden's disease). Int J Gynecol Cancer 2002;12:337-347.

98. Gell JS, Stannard MW, Ramnani DM, Bradshaw KD: Juvenile granulosa cell tumor in a 13-year-old girl with enchondromatosis (Ollier's disease): A case report. J Pediatr Adolesc Gynecol 1998;11:147-150.

99. Evans DG, Ladusans EJ, Rimmer S, et al: Complications of the naevoid basal cell carcinoma syndrome: Results of a population based study. J Med Genet 1993;30:460-464.

100. Rosenblatt KA, Weiss NS, Schwartz SM: Incidence of malignant fallopian tube tumors. Gynecol Oncol 1989;35:236-239.

101. Kosary C, Trimble EL: Treatment and survival for women with fallopian tube carcinoma: A population-based study. Gynecol Oncol 2002;86:190-191.

102. Rosen AC, Klein M, Hafner E, et al: Management and prognosis of primary fallopian tube carcinoma. Austrian Cooperative Study Group for Fallopian Tube Carcinoma. Gynecol Obstet Invest 1999;47:45-51.

103. Alvarado-Cabrero I, Young RH, Vamvakas EC, Scully RE: Carcinoma of the fallopian tube: A clinicopathological study of 105 cases with observations on staging and prognostic factors. Gynecol Oncol 1999;72:367-379.

104. Baekelandt M, Jorunn N, Kristensen GB, et al: Carcinoma of the fallopian tube. Cancer 2000;89:2076-2084.

105. Paley PJ, Swisher EM, Garcia RL, et al: Occult cancer of the fallopian tube in BRCA-1 germline mutation carriers at prophylactic oophorectomy: A case for recommending hysterectomy at surgical prophylaxis. Gynecol Oncol 2001;80:176-180.

106. Zweemer RP, van Diest PJ, Verheijen RH, et al: Molecular evidence linking primary cancer of the fallopian tube to BRCA1 germline mutations [see comments.]. Gynecol Oncol 2000;76:45-50.

107. Rose PG, Shrigley R, Wiesner GL: Germline BRCA2 mutation in a patient with fallopian tube carcinoma: A case report. Gynecol Oncol 2000;77:319-320.

108. Aziz S, Kuperstein G, Rosen B, et al: A genetic epidemiological study of carcinoma of the fallopian tube. Gynecol Oncol 2001; 80:341-345.

109. Weber AM, Hewett WJ, Gajewski WH, Curry SL: Serous carcinoma of the peritoneum after oophorectomy. Obstet Gynecol 1992;80:558-560.

110. Bloss JD, Liao SY, Buller RE, et al: Extra-ovarian peritoneal serous papillary carcinoma: A case-control retrospective comparison to papillary adenocarcinoma of the ovary. Gynecol Oncol 1993;50:347-351.

111. Chu CS, Menzin AW, Leonard DG, et al: Primary peritoneal carcinoma: A review of the literature. Obstet Gynecol Surv 1999;54:323-335.

112. Muto MG, Welch WR, Mok SC, et al: Evidence for a multifocal origin of papillary serous carcinoma of the peritoneum. Cancer Res 1995;55:490-492.

113. Schorge JO, Muto MG, Welch WR, et al: Molecular evidence for multifocal papillary serous carcinoma of the peritoneum in patients with germline BRCA1 mutations. J Natl Cancer Inst 1998;90:841-845.

114. Kowalski LD, Kanbour AI, Price FV, et al: A case-matched molecular comparison of extraovarian versus primary ovarian adenocarcinoma. Cancer 1997;79:1587-1594.

115. Killackey MA, Davis AR: Papillary serous carcinoma of the peritoneal surface: Matched-case comparison with papillary serous ovarian carcinoma. Gynecol Oncol 1993;51:171-174.

116. Ben Baruch G, Sivan E, Moran O, et al: Primary peritoneal serous papillary carcinoma: A study of 25 cases and comparison with stage III-IV ovarian papillary serous carcinoma. Gynecol Oncol 1996;60:393-396.

117. Eltabbakh GH, Piver MS, Natarajan N, Mettlin CJ: Epidemiologic differences between women with extra-ovarian primary peritoneal carcinoma and women with epithelial ovarian cancer. Obstet Gynecol 1998;91:254-259.

118. Tobacman JK, Greene MH, Tucker MA, et al: Intra-abdominal carcinomatosis after prophylactic oophorectomy in ovarian-cancer-prone families. Lancet 1982;2:795-797.

119. Piver MS, Jishi MF, Tsukada Y, Nava G: Primary peritoneal carcinoma after prophylactic oophorectomy in women with a family history of ovarian cancer: A report of the Gilda Radner Familial Ovarian Cancer Registry. Cancer 1993;71: 2751-2755.

120. Bandera CA, Muto MG, Welch WR, et al: Genetic imbalance on chromosome 17 in papillary serous carcinoma of the peritoneum. Oncogene 1998;16:3455-3459.

121. Bandera CA, Muto MG, Schorge JO, et al: BRCA1 gene mutations in women with papillary serous carcinoma of the peritoneum. Obstet Gynecol 1998;92:596-600.

122. Menczer J, Chetrit A, Barda G, et al: Frequency of BRCA mutations in primary peritoneal carcinoma in Israeli Jewish women. Gynecol Oncol 2003;88:58-61.

123. Schrag D, Kuntz KM, Garber JE, Weeks JC: Decision analysis: Effects of prophylactic mastectomy and oophorectomy on life expectancy among women with BRCA1 or BRCA2 mutations. N Engl J Med 1997;336:1465-1471.

124. Struewing JP, Watson P, Easton DF, et al: Prophylactic oophorectomy in inherited breast/ovarian cancer families. J Natl Cancer Inst Monogr 1995;17:33-35.

125. Rebbeck TR, Lynch HT, Neuhausen SL, et al: Prophylactic oophorectomy in carriers of BRCA1 or BRCA2 mutations. N Engl J Med 2002;346:1616-1622.

126. Kauff ND, Satagopan JM, Robson ME, et al: Risk-reducing salpingo-oophorectomy in women with a BRCA1 or BRCA2 mutation. N Engl J Med 2002;346:1609-1615.

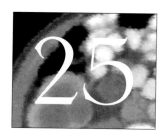

SCREENING AND DIAGNOSIS OF OVARIAN CANCER—HIGH RISK

Yoland Antill   and   Kelly-Anne Phillips

MAJOR CONTROVERSIES

- **What constitutes high risk?**
- **What is the most appropriate screening method?**
- **What is the most appropriate screening interval?**
- **What is the most appropriate age at which to commence screening?**
- **Is screening the best way to manage risk, and what are the alternatives?**
- **What are the future directions for the development of screening tools?**

What constitutes high risk?

The population cumulative lifetime risk for epithelial ovarian cancer in Western women is about 1%.[1] However, subgroups of women who are at much higher risk for the disease can be identified. No strong environmental risk factors for ovarian cancer have been identified. Risk rises with increasing age, particularly after 40 years of age, but after this factor is controlled, the most important risk factors are family history[1] and the presence of a germline mutation in a gene that can predispose to ovarian cancer. The two major familial cancer syndromes associated with a substantially increased risk for epithelial ovarian cancer are the hereditary breast/ovarian cancer syndrome and hereditary nonpolyposis colorectal cancer syndrome (Table 25-1) (HNPCC).

BRCA1 and BRCA2. Two genes have been identified that are associated with the hereditary breast/ovarian cancer syndrome.[2,3] Germline mutations in these genes, *BRCA1* and *BRCA2*, predispose women mainly to breast cancer but also to ovarian cancer and, to a lesser extent, carcinoma of the fallopian tube and primary peritoneal cancer (Fig. 25-1). For female carriers

of a mutation in *BRCA1 or BRCA2*, the risk of developing ovarian cancer by 70 years of age has been estimated to be between 15% and 66%[4-7]; the risk for *BRCA2* mutation carriers on average is less than for *BRCA1* mutation carriers.[5]

In the general population, it has been estimated that fewer than 0.2% of individuals carry a germline mutation in *BRCA1* or *BRCA2*.[8] However, in some ethnic populations there is a high prevalence of mutations in *BRCA1* and *BRCA2* due to founder effects. Founder effects occur when a population expands after having been small in number and geographically or reproductively isolated. In individuals of Ashkenazi Jewish descent, there are three founder mutations (185delAG and 5382insC in *BRCA1* and 6174delT in *BRCA2*), which are present in approximately 2% of the population overall.[9] Therefore, a higher proportion of ovarian cancer cases among Jewish women are caused by underlying mutations in these genes. For a woman with ovarian cancer in the general population, the chance of carrying a mutation in *BRCA1* or *BRCA2* is between 5% and 11%, whereas for a Jewish woman with ovarian cancer, the chance of having an underlying mutation is much higher, between 30% and 60%.[10-12]

Table 25–1. Genes Associated With Hereditary Ovarian Cancer

Syndrome	Gene	Type of Ovarian Cancer	Lifetime Risk (%)	Other Cancers Associated with the Syndrome
Breast/ovarian syndrome	BRCA1 BRCA2	Epithelial ovarian cancer	10–60	Breast, fallopian tube, primary peritoneal cancer, others
Hereditary nonpolyposis colorectal cancer (HNPCC)	MLH1 MSH2 MSH6 PMS1 PMS2	Epithelial ovarian cancer	10	Colon, rectal, endometrial, gastric, small bowel, urinary tract

Although the age at onset of ovarian cancer is lower in women with a germline mutation in BRCA1 than for women in the general population, BRCA1 and BRCA2 mutations do not seem to be responsible for very-early-onset ovarian cancer. In a population-based British study of 101 women with invasive epithelial ovarian cancer diagnosed before 30 years of age, no germline mutations in BRCA1 or BRCA2 were identified.[13] Other studies have demonstrated that ovarian cancers are rarely diagnosed before the age of 40 years in BRCA1 or BRCA2 mutation carriers.[14,15] However, in general, BRCA1-associated ovarian cancers occur at an earlier age than either BRCA2-associated or nonhereditary ovarian cancers. Conversely, the average age at diagnosis of ovarian cancer in a BRCA2 mutation carrier is similar to that in women with nonhereditary ovarian cancer.[10,14,15] In a Canadian population-based study of ovarian cancer, the average age at diagnosis

was 51.2 years for BRCA1 mutation carriers, 57.5 years for BRCA2 mutation carriers, and 57.8 years for women in whom no mutation was identified.[15] Women diagnosed before the age of 40 years were less likely to have a mutation in BRCA1 or BRCA2 than women diagnosed in any other age group.

The Gilda Radner Familial Ovarian Cancer Registry in New York State contains data on more than 1616 families with "familial ovarian cancer" (defined as two or more affected first- or second-degree relatives with epithelial ovarian cancer).[16] In a recent review of the first 1000 families enrolled, the age at onset of ovarian cancer was significantly younger (53.5 years) than for women in the general population (60.8 years). On average, a decrease in age at diagnosis of ovarian cancer was seen in successive generations. In 131 families whose family history was complete for three generations, all with at least three members affected by ovarian cancer, the mean age at diagnosis for daughters was 43.3 years; for mothers, 55.0 years; and for grandmothers, 60.77 years. In a study of consecutive cases of ovarian cancer in Jewish women presenting to Memorial Sloan-Kettering Cancer Center, the age at diagnosis was younger (56 years) in women with BRCA1 or BRCA2 mutations than for women without a mutation (63 years).[14] Women with a BRCA1 mutation had a mean age at diagnosis 8 years earlier than that of women with a BRCA2 mutation (54 versus 62 years). No cancers were found in mutation carriers before the age of 30 years, and, among the six cancers that were diagnosed between the ages of 30 and 40 years, four were in BRCA1 mutation carriers and two were in noncarriers. Similarly, in another hospital-based study of 208 Jewish women with ovarian cancer, the mean age at diagnosis for the 57 BRCA1 mutation carriers was lower than that for the 29 BRCA2 mutation carriers (50.8 versus 62.1 years).[10]

The ovarian cancer risk for BRCA1 and BRCA2 mutation carriers appears to be influenced by both genetic and environmental modifying factors. The site of gene mutation in BRCA1 or BRCA2 may be important for determining the absolute level of risk. Several studies have reported that mutations towards the 3' end of BRCA1 result in a reduced risk for ovarian cancer compared with mutations in other areas of the BRCA1 gene,[17-19] although other studies have found no such effect.[15,20] A lower risk for breast cancer and a higher risk for ovarian cancer has been seen for

FAMILY HISTORY REPRESENTATIVE OF
BREAST/OVARIAN SYNDROME

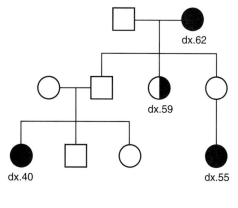

■ Breast cancer

□ Ovarian cancer

Figure 25–1. Several features of the hereditary breast and ovarian cancer syndrome are demonstrated by this pedigree. Women within such families are at high risk for both ovarian cancer and breast cancer, unless they can be documented not to carry the specific gene mutation that is present in other family members with cancer. Bilateral breast cancer or multiple primary tumors may also be seen. Although breast cancer is uncommon in men even in these high-risk families, men can carry the causative gene mutation and transmit it to their daughters.

individuals who carry a mutation in the middle third of the *BRCA2* gene (the so-called ovarian cancer cluster region), compared with those with mutations at other sites in *BRCA2*.[15,21,22] Several studies have suggested that polymorphisms (changes in DNA sequence that have no or little effect on protein function and therefore are not pathogenic) present in other genes may further modify the penetrance (the likelihood that an individual will develop cancer if she has inherited a germline mutation) of *BRCA1* and *BRCA2* for ovarian cancer, but further studies are required to confirm their relevance.[23-25] Retrospective studies of the potential protective effect of the oral contraceptive pill on ovarian cancer risk have had conflicting results.[25,26] A single retrospective study suggested that tubal ligation in *BRCA1* mutation carriers may result in a substantial reduction in their risk for ovarian cancer.[28]

Mismatch repair genes. The HNPCC syndrome is characterized by substantially increased lifetime risks for colorectal cancer but also for some types of noncolonic tumors, including epithelial ovarian cancer (Fig. 25-2). The two genes that are most frequently mutated in the germline in HNPCC carriers are *MLH1* and *MSH2*, although germline mutations in other mismatch repair genes can also be responsible.[29] The cumulative lifetime risk for ovarian cancer for female carriers may be as high as 10%, but such women are also at substantially increased risk for the development of endometrial cancer, with the cumulative lifetime risk estimated at between 40% and 60%.[30,31] In fact, for female mutation carriers, the risk of gynecologic malignancy is higher than their estimated lifetime risk for colorectal cancer.[31]

FAMILY HISTORY REPRESENTATIVE OF HNPCC

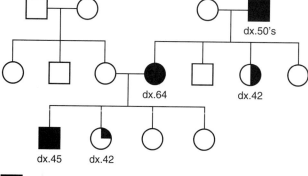

■ Colorectal cancer

◨ Ovarian cancer

◪ Endometrial

Figure 25–2. This pedigree demonstrates several features typical of a family with hereditary nonpolyposis colorectal cancer syndrome (HNPCC). The most common cancers associated with this syndrome are endometrial and colorectal cancers. This family also illustrates the fact that the gene mutation can be expressed in both sexes and inherited from either parent. An autosomal dominant pattern of inheritance should also be noted.

Retrospective data on 80 ovarian cancer patients collected by the International Collaborative Group on HNPCC, showed that the mean age at diagnosis was relatively young at 42.7 years.[32] Similarly, in a review of 120 families entered on the HNPCC register from a single Australian center, the mean age of diagnosis of ovarian cancer was 48.3 years (range, 29 to 74 years).[33] In contrast to ovarian cancer occurring in nonmutation carriers, in the International Collaborative Group dataset, most tumors were well or moderately differentiated and 85% were FIGO stage I or II at diagnosis.[32] However, the retrospective nature of these data and the fact that ascertainment was via HNPCC families rather than population based may have biased the data toward tumors with better prognosis.

What is the most appropriate screening method?

Cancer screening. Screening is the application of a relatively simple and inexpensive test to a well population with the aim of distinguishing those who have a disease from those who do not.[34] In order for screening to be both useful and cost-effective, several determinants should be met.

1. The disease must have a preclinical phase during which the screening test can be used for diagnosis.[34] The majority of women with ovarian cancer do not present until late in the course of their disease,[35,36] most likely because of the lack of symptoms associated with early-stage disease. Unlike cervical cancer, for example, there is no known distinct precancerous phase, and the interval between early- and late-stage disease is poorly defined in both nonhereditary and hereditary ovarian cancer. It may be possible to identify a "molecular preclinical phase," based on the report of Jazaeri and colleagues,[37] who analyzed ovarian cancers with the use of microarray techniques. They were able to demonstrate that ovarian cancers occurring in the setting of a germline BRCA1 mutation had a different molecular profile from those occurring in the setting of a BRCA2 germline mutation. Interestingly, the subgroup of serous papillary cancers, which were not caused by germline mutations in BRCA1 or BRCA2, could be broadly divided into two groups on the basis of their gene expression profiles. Despite the absence of germline mutation, they did in fact have either "*BRCA1*-like" or "*BRCA2*-like" molecular profiles. These data, if confirmed, suggest that there are common molecular steps in the pathogenesis of ovarian cancers, and further knowledge of the specifics of the early molecular changes may assist the development of a molecular screening test.

2. If the disease is discovered during the preclinical phase, there must be available therapy that significantly alters the outcome when compared with treatment for the same disease once it becomes symptomatic.[34] Survival for women with stage I or II ovarian cancer is far better than for those with more

advanced disease,[38] suggesting that early diagnosis could improve survival in women with ovarian cancer. However, the natural history of ovarian cancer for both mutation carriers and noncarriers remains unclear. It is not known, for example, whether ovarian cancer progresses in an orderly manner through stages I to IV, as does the adenoma-carcinoma sequence of colonic cancer, or whether it effectively arises as an advanced-stage cancer.

Furthermore, there is controversy regarding whether the prognosis of equivalent stages of ovarian cancer differs between mutation carriers and noncarriers. It is a potentially important issue when one considers the rationale for screening high-risk women. For example, if the prognosis for treated hereditary ovarian cancer were better, stage for stage, than that for treated nonhereditary ovarian cancer, there would be increased justification for screening of high-risk women, because treatment of early-stage disease in mutation carriers would be more effective than in noncarriers.

There are conflicting data regarding the prognosis for women with ovarian cancer and a known *BRCA1* or *BRCA2* gene mutation, compared with women who have nonhereditary ovarian cancer. Rubin and associates[39] showed in a retrospective study that women with advanced ovarian cancer resulting from a germline *BRCA1* mutation had a significantly longer median survival time (77 months) than did matched controls with no family history suggestive of a hereditary cancer syndrome (29 months). Similarly, Ben David and colleagues[40] reported on 896 ovarian cancer cases from the National Israeli Study of Ovarian Cancer. Germline mutations in *BRCA1* or *BRCA2* were found in 26.1% of cases. There was a significant difference in median survival time favoring mutation carriers (51.2 versus 33.1 months). Three similar but smaller studies showed comparable results.[41-43] Conversely, at least three studies did not show a survival advantage for women whose ovarian cancers occurred in the setting of a germline mutation.[44-46] These data are difficult to interpret because of methodologic issues.[47] Even less is known about the outcomes for women with mutations in mismatch repair genes who develop ovarian cancer.

3. In order for the screening tool to be cost-effective, the disease must have a high prevalence in the population to be screened.[34] This represents the most important argument for screening of high-risk women, because the prior probability of disease being present is substantially higher in this subgroup of the population, as evidenced by the increased lifetime risks outlined earlier.

4. The test should be simple to perform and should be acceptable to technician and patient alike.[34] To date, screening tests used for ovarian cancer have been found to be acceptable to women in the general population.[48,49] Women at high risk may have greater cancer-related anxiety and therefore may be more willing to undergo screening in an attempt to reduce their cancer risk.[50] Conversely, some studies

have shown that high-risk women with overwhelming anxiety are less likely to adhere to surveillance guidelines.[51] Women who underwent surgical procedures for false-positive screening results were found to have increased levels of anxiety and generalized distress up to 1 year after their surgery.[52] However, another study found that false-positive screening results were associated with an increase in anxiety that resolved after a short time without ongoing adverse effects.[53,54]

5. Ideally the test should have both high sensitivity and specificity. Often however, one is sacrificed in order to improve the other. In high-risk women, any screening test is likely to have a higher specificity than in the general population, because of the higher incidence of the disease. Nevertheless, it is important for any screening test to have very high specificity, because the majority of women with positive test results go on to have surgical exploration. It would not be acceptable for a large number of women to undergo surgical intervention in order to find one carcinoma. The screening tests currently available for ovarian cancer include serum CA 125 measurement and imaging by ovarian ultrasonography.

Serum CA 125. The CA 125 antigen is derived from the coelomic epithelium. Overexpression of the antigen occurs in several malignant and benign conditions, and this limits the effectiveness of serum CA 125 measurement as a screening test for ovarian cancer. Conditions that cause peritoneal or mesothelial changes can result in an increase in serum CA 125 levels. Physiologic rises are seen at the time of menstruation, during the first trimester of pregnancy, and after delivery.[55] Benign conditions such as endometriosis, uterine fibroids, infection, and postoperative inflammation are well recognized to result in elevated serum CA 125 concentrations.

Bast and coworkers[56] demonstrated that elevations in serum CA 125 were seen more frequently in women with ovarian carcinoma (82%) than in women from the general population (1%), women with benign disease (6%), or women with nongynecologic cancers (28.5%). The same group retrospectively analyzed CA 125 levels in stored serum from a woman who subsequently developed ovarian cancer. They noted that the patient's CA 125 levels had started to increase a year before her clinical diagnosis.[57] It was then postulated that serum CA 125 might be a suitable screening test to detect early ovarian cancer in asymptomatic women.

Large population studies have been carried out to determine whether serum CA 125 can be used in isolation for early detection of ovarian cancer in the general population.[58-60] Zurawski and colleagues[58] conducted a retrospective case-control study of 39,300 women who had donated blood samples to a Swedish serum bank. Compared with matched controls, significant differences in serum CA 125 concentrations were documented from samples taken up to 24 months before a subject's diagnosis of ovarian cancer. These results prompted two prospective studies. Einhorn and associates[59] performed a longitudinal study of a cohort of 175 women, selected from a large population of apparently healthy women, who were found to have CA 125 levels higher than 30 U/mL. Serial CA 125 measurement, pelvic examinations, and transabdominal ultrasound studies were performed at regular intervals. Six ovarian cancers were diagnosed during the period of follow-up, two each in stages Ia, IIb, and IIIc. Helzlsouer and coworkers[60] analyzed CA 125 in serum collected over a 12-year period from more than over 11,000 women older than 18 years of age. Ovarian cancer was diagnosed in 37 women, and the sensitivity of the serum CA 125 level for ovarian cancer within 3 years of diagnosis was 57%. Both clinically and economically, neither of these studies demonstrated that serum CA 125 measurements would be useful as a screening test for ovarian cancer in the general population.

To try to improve the sensitivity of serum CA 125 as a screening test for ovarian cancer, Skates and colleagues[61] developed the Risk of Ovarian Cancer Algorithm (ROCA), which uses serial CA 125 measurements rather than a single reading. The algorithm is based on the observations that serum CA 125 levels correlate with tumor volume and that tumor growth is exponential in the early phase of disease. It was developed using the CA 125II assay (a newer, high-affinity antibody that has a 50% reduction in assay variability) on stored samples in the postmenopausal subset of the Swedish population used in the study of Einhorn's group. The probability that a woman has ovarian cancer is calculated by means of a mathematical model that includes the absolute level of CA 125 as well as the rate of rise over time. This algorithm has a very high specificity of 99.7%, with a sensitivity of 83%, and therefore has a much higher positive predictive value (16%), compared with that seen in previous screening studies using single-point estimations of CA 125. The relevance of this algorithm to premenopausal women and to women who are at substantially increased risk for ovarian cancer is the subject of ongoing studies.

Ultrasonography. Transabdominal ultrasonography was originally used to look for structural abnormalities and volume of the postmenopausal ovary.[62] It was found to be more reliable than clinical examination at detecting ovarian enlargement.[63] To enable optimal visualization of the ovaries through the bladder, women are required to have a full bladder. Obesity and distortion of the pelvic anatomy reduce the rate at which the ovaries can be detected. Transvaginal ultrasound imaging has now superseded transabdominal ultrasonography as the method of visualizing the ovaries. It is less influenced by body morphology, does not require a full bladder, and, on average, takes 5 to 10 minutes to complete. Initial studies established that transvaginal ultrasonography was effective for determining abnormal ovarian morphology and volume and was well tolerated.[64,65]

To further improve the sensitivity of ovarian ultrasound imaging for cancer screening, Bourne and coworkers[66] introduced the use of color flow Doppler imaging to detect intraovarian vascular change together with measurement of impedance to blood flow.

The technique is based on the theory that rapidly growing tumors are likely to have significant blood vessel growth before stromal growth and that the Doppler imaging technique will detect the physiologic changes associated with blood vessels before morphologic changes occur in the ovary. Their research suggested that the presence of an invasive cancer is less likely in the absence of intratumoral neovascularization and a high pulsatility index. However, later studies showed that low impedance flow can also be seen in benign tumors and even in normal ovaries at the time of ovulation; although malignant lesions tended to have higher rates of blood flow and lower resistance indices, no specific cutoff values have yet been determined.[36,67]

Studies of transvaginal ultrasound imaging as a sole modality in women at potentially increased risk for ovarian cancer have been disappointing to date. In a first phase screening study of 1601 self-referred, asymptomatic women who had a first- or second-degree relative affected by ovarian cancer, Bourne and colleagues[68] reported that 61 of the women had abnormal transvaginal ultrasound findings, but only 7 of them were found to have a primary ovarian cancer at laparotomy. Five of these cancers were stage Ia (including three borderline rather than malignant tumors), one was stage IIa, and one was a stage III carcinoma. Since the screening, five interval cancers have also been diagnosed, including three ovarian cancers (24 to 44 months after last screening examination) and two primary peritoneal cancers (2 and 8 months after last screen).

Multimodality studies in women at high risk. Use of a single modality (i.e., serum CA 125 measurement or ultrasound imaging) for ovarian cancer screening appears to be inadequate, but it has been postulated that a combination of the two techniques might increase the predictive value of ovarian cancer screening. Jacobs and colleagues[48] conducted a large study of postmenopausal women, who were at average risk for ovarian cancer, to assess the screening efficacy of the combination of serum CA 125 with ultrasonography. Women initially had a serum CA 125 measurement. Levels greater than 30 U/mL were considered abnormal, and those women with high levels were recalled for a transabdominal ultrasound study. Those with a normal ultrasound result had the CA 125 measurement repeated every 3 months; those with abnormal results were referred to gynecologists or general practitioners for further management. All women were administered an annual follow-up questionnaire. A total of 22,000 women were enrolled on the study, of whom 340 were investigated for increased CA 125 levels. Forty-one ultrasound studies were thought to be abnormal, and those women were referred for further investigations. Nineteen cases of ovarian cancer were diagnosed, 11 of which were detected as a result of both an elevated CA 125 concentration and abnormal transabdominal ultrasound findings. In addition to the 21,951 apparently true-negative results, there were 8 false-negative and 30 false-positive results. At 2 years, the specificity was 99.9% and the sensitivity 78.6%.

The same group of women was then asked to participate in a randomized trial to determine the impact of 3 years of annual screening by the same two-step process.[35] A total of 10,977 women were randomly assigned to the control arm, and the remaining 10,958 women received ongoing annual screening. A total of 468 women from the screened group had an elevated CA 125 concentration warranting further investigation with transvaginal ultrasound imaging. Of these, 29 underwent surgical exploration, which revealed 6 cases of ovarian cancer and 23 cases of benign findings only. In the next 7 years after the screening period, a further 10 women in the screening arm were diagnosed with ovarian cancer, as were 20 women from the control arm. Although the study was not powered to look at differences in mortality, the median survival time after diagnosis for women from the screened group was longer than that for women from the control group (72.9 versus 41.8 months).

A number of studies investigating the effect of multimodality ovarian screening in women at increased risk for ovarian cancer have been reported and are summarized in Table 25-2. Self-referred women older than 25 years of age who had at least one first-degree relative or two second-degree relatives with ovarian cancer were enrolled in a prospective study to evaluate ovarian cancer screening with the use of transvaginal ultrasonography with color flow Doppler and CA 125 measurements.[69] A CA 125 level greater than 35 U/mL was considered abnormal and prompted a repeat test 2 to 3 months later. A progressive rise in CA 125 concentration in excess of 95 U/mL, or a doubling of the level over 3 months, was considered abnormal and warranted further investigations using imaging techniques. All women, regardless of CA 125 level, were examined by transvaginal ultrasonography with color flow Doppler to determine the volume, morphology, pulsatility index, and resistive index. For premenopausal women, this procedure was scheduled during the follicular phase of the menstrual cycle. All abnormal scans were repeated 8 to 12 weeks later, with surgical referrals for those women who had persistent abnormalities or a mass that was increasing in size. The mean age of the group was 41 years, and only 15% were postmenopausal. Only 23% had more than one relative with ovarian cancer, so the majority of participants had a moderate rather than a high lifetime risk for ovarian cancer. No cases of ovarian cancer were detected among the 386 women enrolled over a 2-year period. The problems reported with these methods of screening parallel those of other high-risk and general population studies. CA 125 levels were abnormal in about 10% of the subjects (42 in total, 41 of whom were premenopausal), but in most cases (84%) the level had normalized by the time of the second repeat study. Of eight women with persistently elevated CA 125 levels (three of whom also had abnormal transvaginal ultrasound results), five went on to have surgical investigation, the results of which were all benign. Ten other women who underwent surgical investigation for persistent abnormalities on transvaginal ultrasound with normal CA 125 levels also had benign findings

at operation. Although ultrasound was highly accurate in estimating the size and morphology of ovarian masses, only 57% of postmenopausal and 87% of premenopausal ovaries could be identified. CA 125 levels were strongly influenced by menopausal status, phase of the menstrual cycle, and oral contraceptive use.

Belinson and coworkers[70] reported the findings of the first 2 years of The Cleveland Clinic Foundation Familial Ovarian Cancer Registry, which was established in 1991. Eligible women were older than 25 years of age and had at least one first-degree relative or two second-degree relatives with ovarian cancer, or one first-degree relative with breast cancer and one second-degree relative with ovarian cancer. Of note, it is not clear from the published report whether these affected relatives were from the same side of the family. If not, many of the individuals included in this study may have been at moderate rather than high risk for ovarian cancer. A CA 125 level and transvaginal ultrasound study with color flow Doppler were done at the initial visit. Follow-up recommendations were made based on the risk assessment derived from examination of the family history and investigation findings; these were not documented in the published paper. Of 137 women enrolled in the program, most were premenopausal, with a mean age of 43 years, and only 40 had more than one relative with ovarian cancer. The initial CA 125 level was elevated in five patients, all of whom were premenopausal. Only one cancer was diagnosed in a woman, with an abnormal transvaginal ultrasound and an elevated CA 125 concentration of 45 U/mL. Operative findings revealed a stage IIIb ovarian carcinoma. The total cost of the tests to find one carcinoma was $68,848. Although the registry is ongoing, the implementation of screening has become limited to those who are from high-risk families and older than 35 years of age.

The first reported prospective study, of a group of 845 moderate- and high-risk women who participated in an ovarian and breast cancer screening program, were reported by Dørum and colleagues.[71] The women were divided into one of three groups for follow-up: those with a history of breast cancer ($n = 49$), those with a history of ovarian cancer ($n = 42$), and unaffected women ($n = 754$). The mean age of unaffected women was 41.3 years. Women underwent annual breast and pelvic examination, CA 125 measurement, cervical smear, transvaginal ultrasonography, and mammography with or without breast ultrasonography from the age of 25 years or 10 years earlier than the youngest affected woman in the family. Women with multicystic cysts, thick septa, excrescences, or irregular patterns and variety of the sonolucency of the tumors were identified as having a greater malignant potential and underwent surgery. Women with simple ovarian cysts less than 2 cm in diameter had a repeat transvaginal ultrasound study 2 to 3 months later and then underwent laparoscopy if the cyst persisted or had increased in size. For women with a CA 125 level higher than 35 U/mL, the blood test was repeated 2 to 3 months later, and if they were persistently elevated laparoscopy

Table 25–2. Ovarian Cancer Screening: Familial Studies

Author	Muto et al.[69]	Belinson et al.[70]	Dørum et al.[71]	Karlan et al.[36,72]	Scheuer et al.[75]
Study population	Age >25 yr; ≥1 FDR or ≥2 SDR with OC; Self-referred or referred by primary care provider	Age >25 yr; ≥1 FDR with OC (expanded after 2 yr to include 2 SDR with OC or 1 SDR with OC and 1 FDR with BC); Self-referred or physician-referred	≥FDR or SDR (if via male relative) with OC and/or ≥FDR or ≥SDR (if via male relative) with BC ≤60 yr and/or ≥SDR (if via male relative) with OC and BC ≤60 yr; Self-referred or referred by local hospital or doctor	>35 yr; ≥1 FDR with BC, CRC, OC, or endometrial cancer; ≥1 SDR with OC; or personal history of BC; Living in Los Angeles area; Self-referred or physician-referred	Known *BRCA1* or *BRCA2* mutation; Identified via genetic program at Memorial Sloan-Kettering Cancer Center
N	384	137	803	1261	62‡
Mutations	Not assessed in any patient	Not assessed in any patient	Not assessed in any patient	*BRCA1:* 3/4; *BRCA2:* 0/4*	*BRCA1:* 156/233; *BRCA2:* 77/233
Personal history of BC	None reported	None reported	49	18†	143
Screening method	Single : CA125 and TVUS	Baseline CA125 and TVUS, with follow-up based on results	Yearly CA 125 and TVUS	CA 125 and TVUS: 1991–1995, every other year; 1995 and later, annually	Pelvic examination every 6–12 months, TVUS monthly, and CA 125 monthly
No. abnormal tests	CA 125: 42; TVUS: 89	CA 125: 5; TVUS: 7	Not assessed in any patient	CA 125: 68†; TVUS: 52†	Either CA 125 or TVUS: 22/62
No. operations for benign disease	28	0	Not stated	Not stated	5
No. cancers diagnosed	0	Stage IIIb OC: 1	Borderline tumors: 4; Stage I OC:1; Stage II OC: 1; Stage III OC: 10	Stage I OC: 3; PPC: 7	Stage I or II OC: 4; PPC: 1

BC, breast cancer; CRC, colorectal cancer; FDR, first-degree relative; OC, ovarian cancer; PPC, primary peritoneal carcinoma; SDR, second-degree relative; TVUS, transvaginal ultrasonography.
*Mutation testing carried out only in women diagnosed with BRCA-related gynecologic cancer.
†Missing data.
‡Includes women eligible for both breast cancer and ovarian cancer surveillance.

was performed. Women with a previous personal history of estrogen receptor–positive breast cancer were eligible for the study and after the initial round of screening were considered for therapeutic oophorectomy. Of the 16 ovarian cancers diagnosed, 4 were borderline tumors, 1 was stage I carcinoma, 1 was a stage II adenocarcinoma, and 10 were stage III carcinomas. Therefore, although this approach resulted in the detection of ovarian tumors, most of these were either advanced-stage malignancies or early-stage borderline tumors, for which early detection is unlikely to substantially affect mortality.

The Gilda Radner Ovarian Cancer Detection Program was established in July 1991 for women who are considered to be at increased risk for development of ovarian cancer on the basis of their family history. Eligible women are older than 35 years of age and have a family history of at least one first-degree relative with breast cancer, colon cancer, ovarian cancer, or other gynecologic cancer, or a second-degree relative with ovarian cancer.[72] Participants were screened for ovarian cancer with the use of second-yearly transvaginal ultrasound and measurement of serum CA 125 (together with analysis of other blood and urine specimens for other biomarkers) until 1995, when the protocol was amended to annual screening. The initial results of this follow-up study and a subsequent update have been published.[73,74] A total of 1261 participants have been screened 6082 times. Three stage I ovarian carcinomas and seven primary peritoneal carcinomas have been diagnosed.[73] In four cases, abnormal ultrasound findings triggered surgical exploration. Three of these women had early-stage disease; however, it is important to note that two of the three were borderline tumors, one with serous and one with mucinous pathology. All three of these women had normal serum CA 125 levels. New, marked elevations in CA 125 concentration resulted in surgical intervention in a further two cases. Despite normal transvaginal ultrasound results, both patients had stage III peritoneal carcinoma with extensive and bulky abdominal disease but only miliary superficial ovarian involvement. The remainder had both normal or stable transvaginal ultrasound findings and CA 125 results at the visit before diagnosis (two of these only six months before diagnosis). The incidence of ovarian cancer in this study, 0.81%, was similar to that reported by Bourne and colleagues,[68] 0.69% in a similarly designed study.

Liede and associates[74] recently reported data concerning the subgroup of 290 healthy Jewish women enrolled in the program. Genetic testing was performed in 213 of these women for the three Jewish founder mutations (185delAG in BRCA1, 5382insC in BRCA1, and 6174delT in BRCA2), and 33 founder mutations were detected (27, 4, and 2 cases, respectively). Eight BRCA-related gynecologic malignancies (two cases of ovarian cancer, one fallopian tube cancer, and five primary peritoneal cancers) were diagnosed during the first 10 years of screening of the 290 Jewish women in the cohort. All but one of these women carried a germline mutation. Only two of the eight were diagnosed with early-stage disease (one stage Ic and one stage IIc), and

the rest had advanced disease at the time of diagnosis. Five of the women ultimately diagnosed with malignancy had had normal screening results 6 months before diagnosis. There is no comment in either this report[74] or that of Karlan's group[73] in 1999 regarding the number of patients that underwent surgical investigation for benign conditions or the rate of complications from screening or subsequent investigations.

Prospective follow-up data were recently published for women who were found to have a mutation in BRCA1 or BRCA2 between May 1995 and October 2000 at the Memorial Sloan-Kettering Cancer Center. Scheuer and colleagues[75] reported outcomes of women who elected to undergo prophylactic surgery compared with those who elected to undergo screening for both breast and BRCA-related gynecologic cancers. Mutation carriers who elected to undergo ovarian cancer screening rather than prophylactic oophorectomy were advised to undergo six-monthly or annual gynecologic examinations and six-monthly transvaginal ultrasound studies together with serum CA 125 determinations. Breast surveillance recommendations were also made but will not be discussed here. At a mean follow-up time of only 17 months (range, 2.3 to 40.2 months), 4 of the 89 women who elected ovarian cancer screening had been diagnosed with ovarian cancer and 1 with primary peritoneal cancer. All tumors were stage I or II at the time of surgery. Abnormal ultrasound findings prompted four of these surgical explorations, whereas elevated CA 125 concentrations were noted in two. At the time of publication, no interval cancers had been diagnosed. In addition, five women underwent surgical exploration and were found to have benign conditions, and 12 women had resolution of abnormal findings at subsequent screenings and did not undergo surgical intervention. The authors reported that the combination of CA 125 measurement and transvaginal ultrasonography in this study had a specificity of 90.9% and sensitivity of 71%.

In the studies outlined here, it was disappointing that a large percentage of the tumors detected as the result of abnormal test findings were already at an advanced stage, despite the use of combined modality screening.[68,70,71,73] Furthermore, there was a high rate of false-positive scans,[70,71,73] resulting in unnecessary surgical exploration.

When assessing the research to date in this area, the reader must be aware of several points. There was significant heterogeneity among the populations studied. The eligibility criteria for each study varied, making comparisons difficult. Most patients recruited to these studies did not meet criteria indicating a high risk for the development of ovarian carcinoma; the majority would be considered to be at moderate risk at most. The intervals between scheduled tests and procedures after an abnormal screening test also varied. Because of this diversity among the studies published to date, it is difficult to form a consensus opinion with regard to the most appropriate screening regimen for high-risk women. American and European consensus panels have therefore been cautious in their recommendations for ovarian cancer screening in high-risk women.

Nevertheless, although the application of current ovarian cancer screening modalities in the general population is not economically justified, in high-risk populations the same tests are thought to have a potentially higher predictive value (because of the higher disease prevalence) and are recommended.[76,77]

What is the most appropriate screening interval?

The screening interval is an area of considerable controversy, although various groups have developed recommendations. In 1994, the National Institutes of Health (NIH) consensus development panel recommended annual screening with a rectovaginal pelvic examination, serum CA 125 measurement, and transvaginal ultrasonography for women with a hereditary ovarian cancer syndrome (with an assumption of autosomal dominant inheritance pattern).[76] The authors commented that these recommendations were promulgated despite a lack of data to support a reduction in mortality with these screening investigations. The Cancer Genetics Studies Consortium later recommended the use of transvaginal ultrasonography and serum CA 125 measurements at 6- or 12-month intervals but maintained that the optimal screening interval is not yet known.[78] The French National Ad Hoc Committee's recommendations were for twice-yearly pelvic examinations and annual transvaginal ultrasonography with color flow Doppler. The committee also recommended that in premenopausal women the ultrasound study should be performed during the follicular phase of the menstrual cycle.[77]

Most relevant studies have been published shortly after the commencement of screening of participants. The Gilda Radner Familial Ovarian Cancer Registry, one of the longest-running surveillance programs, moved from second-yearly to annual screening in 1995.[73] This decision was based on the Registry's experience and that of Bourne and Campbell's group,[68] in which the detection of late-stage disease after a previously normal screening result was of concern. They recommended that screening should be done at least more often than every 2 years.[36] In the most recently published study,[75] and the one that has been most promising in terms of the proportion of early-stage carcinomas detected, the screening interval was 6 months. This screening regimen was adapted from the Cancer Genetics Studies Consortium recommendations.[78]

Consideration needs to be given to the psychological effects that screening may have on high-risk women, with particular reference to the likelihood of their having at least one, and possibly several, false-positive screening result during their lifetime. Wardle and colleagues[54] evaluated the psychological impact of true-negative and false-positive results in a high-risk group of women participating in an ultrasound screening program. A questionnaire was used to assess the psychological state of participants, their coping style, and their anxiety about the risk of cancer before and after the initial screening procedure, after subsequent screening tests for abnormalities found on the initial ultrasound study, and again after surgery (for persistent abnormalities). Of 302 women, 69 had abnormalities detected at the first round of screening; 64 of these women had a second scan, with 20 going on to have surgical investigation. No ovarian cancers were detected at surgery. Women who had a normal scan result at baseline had significantly reduced psychological distress and worries about cancer after than before the test. Women recalled for testing who had "information-seeking" coping styles and those women who were referred for surgical evaluation had the highest levels of distress. At follow-up assessment, anxiety levels in women with negative findings at surgery were found to have returned to baseline. Early data from an ongoing prospective study of women with *BRCA1* or *BRCA2* mutations undergoing surveillance for breast and ovarian cancer also suggested that anxiety may be exacerbated by false-positive test results.[51] Some research has also indicated that increased levels of anxiety may interfere with adherence to screening recommendations.[51]

What is the most appropriate age at which to commence screening?

The recommendations for screening (annual rectovaginal pelvic examinations, serum CA 125 measurements, and transvaginal ultrasound studies) from the NIH consensus panel[76] currently apply to women who are at high risk for ovarian cancer, from age 25 to 35 years, regardless of whether the patient is known to have a gene mutation or indeed what type of mutation. Since these recommendations were published, important new information regarding the likely age at onset of ovarian cancers in mutation carriers has come to light. As discussed previously, women with a *BRCA1* mutation are more likely to develop ovarian cancer 5 to 10 years earlier than women in the general population, but for women with a *BRCA2* mutation the age at onset is more in keeping with that of women with a negative family history. Ovarian cancer before the age of 40 years is rare even among *BRCA1* mutation carriers, so many now consider that screening for ovarian cancer should commence in *BRCA1* carriers at about the age of 35 years and in *BRCA2* carriers at about 40 to 45 years of age. Although the risk of ovarian cancer in women from families with HNPCC is less than that in those with *BRCA1* or *BRCA2* mutations, the age at onset is even earlier than in the former group. Additionally, the relatively high risk for early-onset endometrial cancer in such individuals means that most investigators recommend commencement of gynecologic surveillance at age 25 to 30 years.[32]

Is screening the best way to manage risk, and what are the alternatives?

Prophylactic oophorectomy. Recent data confirm that prophylactic oophorectomy in women who carry a mutation in *BRCA1* or *BRCA2* reduces the risk for both

BRCA-associated gynecologic cancer and breast cancer.[79-81] In a retrospective, multi-institutional study, Rebbeck and associates[80] showed a 96% reduction in risk for BRCA-associated gynecologic cancer among 259 mutation carriers who had undergone bilateral prophylactic oophorectomy, compared with 292 matched mutation carriers who had not undergone this procedure; similarly, there was a 53% reduction in breast cancer risk. The mean age at bilateral prophylactic oophorectomy was 42 years. In a prospective single-institution study, researchers at Memorial Sloan-Kettering Cancer Center showed that, with a mean follow-up of only 24.2 months, there was a 75% reduction in the risk for BRCA-associated gynecologic cancer or breast cancer among 98 mutation carriers who underwent salpingo-oophorectomy, compared with 72 mutation carriers who chose cancer screening.[79] A recent population-based case control study from Israel has shown similar results to these two clinic-based studies.[81] In that study there was a 71% reduction in ovarian and related cancers in BRCA mutation carriers who had undergone bilateral oophorectomy (Table 25-3).[76]

A key controversy related to prophylactic oophorectomy in high-risk women has been the question of their residual risk for primary peritoneal cancer after surgery. Based on the most recent data,[16,79,80,82] this risk appears to be small and does not negate the efficacy of prophylactic oophorectomy in reducing overall cancer risk.

Another controversy relates to the timing of prophylactic oophorectomy in such women. For carriers of a BRCA1 or BRCA2 mutation, the risk of very-early-onset ovarian cancer is low. Therefore, prophylactic surgery can probably be safely postponed until childbearing is complete. For carriers of a BRCA1 mutation, prophylactic surgery might be best considered at 35 to 40 years of age. For BRCA2 mutation carriers, it may be reasonable to postpone prophylactic oophorectomy until age 45 to 50 years, because of the generally later onset of these tumors. For those with no documented mutation, the optimal age for prophylactic oophorectomy should be guided by the family history, with particular reference to the earliest age at which ovarian cancers have occurred in that family.

Prophylactic surgery in women who carry a mutation in BRCA1 or BRCA2 should include removal of the fallopian tubes. Carcinoma of the fallopian tube is part of the clinical spectrum of BRCA-associated gynecologic cancer,[83,84] and the additional morbidity resulting from removal of the tubes at the time of prophylactic oophorectomy is minimal. Such prophylactic surgery can be done laparoscopically in most cases.[85]

More controversial is the issue of whether such women should also undergo hysterectomy. Hysterectomy at the time of prophylactic oophorectomy has been recommended by some because it eliminates the risk of endometrial cancer should the woman wish to use tamoxifen as a breast cancer chemopreventive agent.[86] A perhaps more important issue relates to the use of hormone replacement therapy after prophylactic oophorectomy. This is often recommended to prevent acute menopausal symptoms such as hot flushes and vaginal dryness, but it has also been thought that such an approach might prevent the long-term complications of early menopause, including osteoporosis and coronary heart disease. If the uterus is left in situ, then combined oral hormone replacement therapy with both an estrogen and a progestin is recommended, because unopposed estrogen increases the risk for endometrial cancer.[87] However, evidence from the general population is mounting that combined oral hormone replacement therapy substantially increases breast cancer risk compared with estrogen-only replacement therapy. Also, the risk for coronary heart disease, stroke, and pulmonary emboli is substantially elevated in women who take combined oral hormone replacement therapy.[88] Hysterectomy at the time of prophylactic oophorectomy in high-risk women would eliminate the need to use replacement oral progestins (to decrease the endometrial cancer risk associated with unopposed estrogen). Other approaches (e.g., direct endometrial progestin) to optimize the risk/benefit ratio for the various cancer-related and non–cancer-related adverse outcomes, while leaving the uterus in situ, require further study.[89]

Oral contraceptives. Oral contraceptive use is associated with a marked reduction in ovarian cancer risk in the general population.[90] In a retrospective case-control study in which the subjects were members of hereditary breast/ovarian syndrome families, any past use of the oral contraceptive pill was shown to reduce the ovarian cancer risk for BRCA1 and BRCA2 carriers by about 50%, with decreasing risk seen for increasing duration of use.[26] Conversely, in a population-based case-control study of Jewish women in Israel, ovarian cancer risk was not reduced in BRCA1 or BRCA2 carriers who had used the oral contraceptive pill (see Table 25-3).[27] The discrepant results of these two studies may be explained by differences in their

▮ **Table 25–3.** Ovarian Cancer Risk Reduction Strategies for *BRCA1* and *BRCA2* Mutation Carriers		
Strategy	Risk Reduction (%)	Study and Ref. No.
Prophylactic salpingo-oophorectomy	71–96	Rebbeck et al.,[80] Rutter et al.[81]
Oral contraceptive pill	0–50	Narod et al.,[26] Modan et al.[27]
Tubal ligation	63*	Narod et al.[28]

*Protective effect seen only in *BRCA1* mutation carriers.

design, but further studies are required to determine the impact of oral contraceptive use on ovarian cancer risk in high-risk women. Any potential benefit of oral contraceptives in terms of reduction in ovarian cancer risk for high-risk women must be weighed against the potential for increased breast cancer risk, especially in *BRCA1* or *BRCA2* carriers, in whom the baseline risk for breast cancer is already very high. The available evidence suggests that oral contraceptives do increase the risk for breast cancer in mutation carriers.[91-93]

Tubal ligation. Tubal ligation has been associated with a reduction in the risk for ovarian cancer in the general population in a number of studies.[94-96] In a retrospective case-control study, Narod and colleagues[28] demonstrated a lower ovarian cancer risk for *BRCA1* mutation carriers who had had tubal ligation, compared with those who had not (see Table 25-3). After adjustment for possible confounding factors such as oral contraceptive use, parity, history of breast cancer, and ethnic group, the odds ratio was 0.39. In the same study, no protective effect of tubal ligation was seen for *BRCA2* mutation carriers. However, the sample size of *BRCA2* carriers was small, so an important effect may have been missed. The findings from another recently published study are also consistent with a reduced risk for ovarian cancer in mutation carriers who undergo tubal ligation.[81] Given these data, one option for *BRCA* mutation carriers might be to undertake tubal ligation after childbearing is complete and to delay prophylactic oophorectomy (if desired) until age 35 to 40 years in *BRCA1* carriers, and age 45 to 50 years in *BRCA2* carriers.

What are the future directions for the development of screening tools?

Clearly, current screening methods are less than optimal for use in high-risk populations. The capacity to detect early-stage disease has not been well demonstrated, and the number of interventions for ultimately benign disease is too high. The need for newer, sensitive and specific biomarkers for ovarian cancer is evident. A number of potential tumor markers, including lysophosphatidic acid (LPA), are currently being investigated. LPA, originally purified from the ascitic fluid of a patient with known ovarian cancer, is thought to play a role in the stimulation of cancer cell growth.[97] Researchers have found significantly higher serum levels in women who have ovarian cancer, compared with those who have benign conditions and other types of cancer. One study showed increased levels of LPA in 9 of 10 patients with stage I epithelial ovarian cancer and in all 24 patients with stages II, III, or IV disease.[97] Other substances of interest include galactosyltransferase, inhibin proaC immunoreactive forms, and CA 72-4.[98]

With rapid progression in the field of gene technology, screening for ovarian cancer may dramatically change in the coming years. Current and future research in genomics, transcriptional profiling, and proteomics will allow detailed investigation of DNA, RNA, and protein levels in tumors, serum, and other substances. It is hoped that this will translate into the identification of novel biomarkers for cancer that in turn may be used either alone or with other existing tests for cancer screening in at-risk populations.

Proteomics is a new, cost-effective technology using substances such as serum, plasma, urine, and ascites to detect low-molecular-weight molecules in a high-throughput, nonbiased approach.[99] Linked with highly sophisticated bioinformatics, a number of "protein signatures" can be established that differentiate one condition from another. Using serum from patients with ovarian cancer, Petricoin and coworkers[100] were able to establish five discriminating proteomic patterns for ovarian cancer. These were then used to try to distinguish women with or without ovarian cancer in a group of 116 women from high-risk ovarian families, 50 of whom had a known cancer. The test was able to correctly identify all 50 women with ovarian cancer, including the 18 women with stage I carcinomas. Of the 66 women without cancer, 63 were identified as not having cancer, giving a sensitivity of 100% (95% confidence interval [CI], 93 to 100) and a specificity of 94% (CI, 84% to 99%). The positive predictive value of this test in this study was 94% (CI, 84% to 99%). Trials to confirm these results in both high- and low-risk groups are currently underway at the National Cancer Institute.

Microarray analysis is a process that allows assessment of the level of expression of thousands of genes in many tumors concurrently. With the use of this technique in ovarian cancer cell lines, Mok and associates[101] were able to detect an increase in prostasin along with other proteins in cancerous cells compared with normal ovarian epithelial cell lines. Other researchers had determined that, like CA 125, prostasin is more often associated with late-stage disease and with serous subtypes rather than early-stage or mucinous cancers. They found that a combination of prostasin and CA 125 measurements improved the sensitivity and specificity of the screening test in a group of 37 patients and 100 controls. A number of other potential tumor markers have been identified with the use of microarray technology.[99] Although the search continues for suitable markers, it is thought that combinations of these will be able to be used for the early detection of ovarian cancer.

The screening of high-risk women for ovarian cancer is an important yet challenging issue. Several groups have developed and published screening recommendations despite the absence of good evidence of benefit for any approach. Much further research is needed, and, whenever possible, high-risk women who require ovarian cancer screening should be entered onto high-quality clinical trials.

REFERENCES

1. Edmondson RJ, Monaghan JM: The epidemiology of ovarian cancer. Int J Gynecol Cancer 2001;11:423-429.

2. Miki Y, Swenson J, Shattuck-Eidens D, et al: A strong candidate for the breast and ovarian cancer susceptibility gene *BRCA1*. Science 1994;266:66-71.

3. Wooster R, Bignell G, Lancaster J, et al: Identification of the breast cancer susceptibility gene BRCA2. Nature 1995;378: 789-792.

4. Struewing JP, Hartge P, Wacholder S, et al: The risk of cancer associated with specific mutations of BRCA1 and BRCA2 among Ashkenazi Jews. N Engl J Med 1997;336:1401-1408.

5. Ford D, Easton DF, Stratton M, et al: Genetic heterogeneity and penetrance analysis of the BRCA1 and BRCA2 genes in breast cancer families. The Breast Cancer Linkage Consortium Am J Hum Genet 1998;62:676-689.

6. Antoniou AC, Gayther SA, Stratton JF, et al: Risk models for familial ovarian and breast cancer. Genet Epidemiol 2000;18: 173-190.

7. Anglian Breast Cancer Study Group: Prevalence and penetrance of BRCA1 and BRCA2 mutations in a population-based series of breast cancer cases. Br J Cancer 2000;83:1301-1308.

8. Ford D, Easton DF, Peto J: Estimates of the gene frequency of BRCA1 and its contribution to breast and ovarian cancer incidence. Am J Hum Genet 1995;57:1457-1462.

9. Roa BB, Boyd AA, Volcik K, Richards CS: Ashkenazi Jewish population frequencies for common mutations in BRCA1 and BRCA2. Nat Genet 1996;14:185-187.

10. Moslehi R, Chu W, Karlan B, et al: BRCA1 and BRCA2 mutation analysis of 208 Ashkenazi Jewish women with ovarian cancer. Am J Hum Genet 2000;66:1259-1272.

11. Abeliovich D, Kaduri L, Lerer I, et al: The founder mutations 185delAG and 5382insC in BRCA1 and 6174delT in BRCA2 appear in 60% of ovarian cancer and 30% of early-onset breast cancer patients among Ashkenazi women. Am J Hum Genet 1997;60:505-514.

12. Hirsh-Yechezkel G, Chetrit A, Lubin F, et al: Population attributes affecting the prevalence of BRCA mutation carriers in epithelial ovarian cancer cases in Israel. Gynecol Oncol 2003; 89:494-498.

13. Stratton JF, Thompson D, Bobrow L, et al: The genetic epidemiology of early-onset epithelial ovarian cancer: A population-based study. Am J Hum Genet 1999;65:1725-1732.

14. Boyd J, Sonoda Y, Federici MG, et al: Clinicopathologic features of BRCA-linked and sporadic ovarian cancer. JAMA 2000;283: 2260-2265.

15. Risch HA, McLaughlin JR, Cole DE, et al: Prevalence and penetrance of germline BRCA1 and BRCA2 mutations in a population series of 649 women with ovarian cancer. Am J Hum Genet 2001;68:700-710.

16. Piver MS, Jishi MF, Tsukada Y, Nava G: Primary peritoneal carcinoma after prophylactic oophorectomy in women with a family history of ovarian cancer: A report of the Gilda Radner Familial Ovarian Cancer Registry. Cancer 1993;71: 2751-2755.

17. Gayther SA, Warren W, Mazoyer S, et al: Germline mutations of the BRCA1 gene in breast and ovarian cancer families provide evidence for a genotype-phenotype correlation. Nat Genet 1995; 11:428-433.

18. Friedman LS, Ostermeyer EA, Szabo CI, et al: Confirmation of BRCA1 by analysis of germline mutations linked to breast and ovarian cancer in ten families. Nat Genet 1994;8:399-404.

19. Shattuck-Eidens D, McClure M, Simard J, et al: A collaborative survey of 80 mutations in the BRCA1 breast and ovarian cancer susceptibility gene: Implications for presymptomatic testing and screening. JAMA 1995;273:535-541.

20. Thompson D, Easton D, Breast Cancer Linkage Consortium: Variation in BRCA1 cancer risks by mutation position. Cancer Epidemiol Biomarkers Prev 2002;11:329-336.

21. Gayther SA, Mangion J, Russell P, et al: Variation of risks of breast and ovarian cancer associated with different germline mutations of the BRCA2 gene. Nat Genet 1997;15:103-105.

22. Thompson D, Easton D, Breast Cancer Linkage Consortium: Variation in cancer risks, by mutation position, in BRCA2 mutation carriers. Am J Hum Genet 2001;68:410-419.

23. Wang WW, Spurdle AB, Kolachana P, et al: A single nucleotide polymorphism in the 5¢ untranslated region of RAD51 and risk of cancer among BRCA1/2 mutation carriers. Cancer Epidemiol Biomarkers Prev 2001;10:955-960.

24. Phelan CM, Rebbeck TR, Weber BL, et al: Ovarian cancer risk in BRCA1 carriers is modified by the HRAS1 variable number of tandem repeat (VNTR) locus. Nat Genet 1996;12: 309-311.

25. Levine DA, Boyd J: The androgen receptor and genetic susceptibility to ovarian cancer: Results from a case series. Cancer Res 2001;61:908-911.

26. Narod SA, Risch H, Moslehi R, et al: Oral contraceptives and the risk of hereditary ovarian cancer. N Engl J Med 1998;339: 424-428.

27. Modan B, Hartge P, Hirsh-Yechezkel G, et al: Parity, oral contraceptives and the risk of ovarian cancer among carriers and non-carriers of a BRCA1 or BRCA2 mutation. N Engl J Med 2001;345:235-240.

28. Narod SA, Sun P, Ghadirian P, et al: Tubal ligation and risk of ovarian cancer in carriers of BRCA1 or BRCA2 mutations: A case-control study. Lancet 2001;357:1467-1470.

29. Peltomaki P, Vasen HF: Mutations predisposing to hereditary nonpolyposis colorectal cancer: Database and results of a collaborative study. The International Collaborative Group on Hereditary Nonpolyposis Colorectal Cancer. Gastroenterology 1997;113:1146-1158.

30. Dunlop MG, Farrington SM, Carothers AD, et al: Cancer risk associated with germline DNA mismatch repair gene mutations. Hum Mol Genet 1997;6:105-110.

31. Aarnio M, Sankila R, Pukkala E, et al: Cancer risk in mutation carriers of DNA mismatch repair genes. Int J Cancer 1999;81: 214-218.

32. Watson P, Bützow R, Lynch HT, et al: The clinical features of ovarian cancer in hereditary nonpolyposis colorectal cancer. Gynecol Oncol 2001;82:223-228.

33. Brown GJ, St John DJ, Macrae FA, Aittomaki K: Cancer risk in young women at risk of hereditary nonpolyposis colorectal cancer: Implications for gynecologic surveillance. Gynecol Oncol 2001;80:346-349.

34. Hulka BS: Cancer screening: Degrees of proof and practical application. Cancer 1988;62(8 Suppl):1776-1780.

35. Jacobs IJ, Skates SJ, MacDonald N, et al: Screening for ovarian cancer: A pilot randomised controlled trial. Lancet 1999;353: 1207-1210.

36. Karlan B, Platt LD: The current status of ultrasound and color Doppler imaging in screening for ovarian cancer. Gynecol Oncol 1994;55:S28-S33.

37. Jazaeri AA, Yee CJ, Sotiriou C, et al: Gene expression profiles of BRCA-1 linked and BRCA-2 linked, and sporadic ovarian cancers. J Nat Cancer Inst 2002;94:990-1000.

38. International Federation of Gynecology and Obstetrics: Annual report on the results of treatment in gynaecological cancer. Int J Gynecol Obstet 1989;28:189-190.

39. Rubin SC, Benjamin I, Behbakht K, et al: Clinical and pathological features of ovarian cancer in women with germline mutations of BRCA1. N Engl J Med 1996;335:1413-1416.

40. Ben David Y, Chetrit A, Hirch-Yechezkel G, et al: Effect of BRCA mutation on the length of survival in epithelial tumours. J Clin Oncol 2002;20:463-466.

41. Aida H, Takakuwa M, Nagata H, et al: Clinical features of ovarian cancer in Japanese women with germline mutations of BRCA1. Clinical Cancer Res 1998;4:235-240.

42. Berchuck A, Heron KA, Carney MA, et al: Frequency of germline and somatic BRCA1 mutations in ovarian cancer. Clin Cancer Res 1998;4:2433-2437.

43. Cass I, Baldwin RC, Varkey T, et al: Improved survival in women with BRCA-associated ovarian carcinoma cancer. 2003; 97:2187-2189.

44. Pharoah PDP, Easton DF, Stockton DL, et al: Survival in familial, BRCA1 associated and BRCA2 associated epithelial ovarian cancer. Cancer Res 1999;59:868-871.

45. Johannsson Ó, Ranstam J, Borg A, Olsson H: Survival of BRCA1 breast and ovarian cancer patients: A population-based study from Southern Sweden. J Clin Oncol 1998;16: 397-404.

46. Wojciechowska-Lacka A, Markowsha J, Skasko E, et al: Frequent disease progression and early recurrence in patients with familial ovarian cancer primarily treated with paclitaxel and cisor carboplatin (preliminary report). Eur J Gynaecol Oncol 2003; 24:21-24.

47. Phillips KA, Andrulis IL, Goodwin PJ: Breast carcinomas arising in carriers in mutations in BRCA1 or BRCA2: Are they prognostically different? J Clin Oncol 1999;17:3653-3663.

48. Jacobs I, Prys Dadis A, et al: Prevalence screening for ovarian cancer in postmenopausal women by CA 125 measurement and ultrasonography. BMJ 1993;306:1030-1033.

49. Zurawski VR, Knapp RC, Einhorn N, et al: An initial analysis of preoperative CA 125 levels in patients with early stage ovarian carcinoma. Gynecol Oncol 1988;30:7-14.

50. Schwartz M, Lerman C, Daly M, et al: Utilization of ovarian cancer screening by women at increased risk. Cancer Epidemiol Biomarkers Prev 1995;4:269-273.

51. Hensley ML, Castiel M, Robson ME: Screening for ovarian cancer: What we know, what we need to know. Prim Care Cancer 2001;20:1601-1607.

52. Wardle FJ, Collins W, Pernet AL, et al: Psychological impact of screening for familial ovarian cancer. J Nat Cancer Inst 1994; 85:653-657.

53. Pernet AJ, Wardle J, Bourne TH, et al: A qualitative evaluation of the experience of surgery after false positive results in screening for familial ovarian cancer. Psychooncology 1992;1:217-233.

54. Wardle FJ, Pernet A, Collins W, Bourne TH: False positive results in ovarian cancer screening: One year follow-up of psychological status. Health Psychol 1993;10:33-40.

55. Verheijen RHM, von Mengorff-Pouilly S, van Kamp GJ, Kenemans P: CA 125: Fundamental and clinical aspects. Cancer Biol 1999;9:117-124.

56. Bast RC, Klug TL, St John E, et al: A radioimmunoassay using a monoclonal antibody to monitor the course of epithelial ovarian cancer. N Engl J Med 1983;309:883-887.

57. Bast RC, Siegal F, Runowicz C, et al: Elevation of serum CA 125 prior to diagnosis of an epithelial ovarian carcinoma. Gynecol Oncol 1985;22:115-120.

58. Zurawski VR, Orjaseter H, Andersen A, Jellum E: Elevated serum CA125 levels prior to diagnosis of ovarian neoplasia: Relevance for early detection of ovarian cancer. Int J Cancer 1988;42:677-680.

59. Einhorn N, Sjövall K, Knapp R, et al: Prospective evaluation of serum CA 125 levels for early detection of ovarian cancer. Obstet Gynecol 1992;80:14-18.

60. Helzlsouer KJ, Bush TL, Alberg AJ, et al: Prospective study of serum CA 125 levels as markers of ovarian cancer. JAMA 1993; 269:1123-1126.

61. Skates SJ, Feng-Ji X, Yin-Hua Y, et al: Toward an optimal algorithm for ovarian cancer screening with longitudinal tumour markers. Cancer 1995;76:S2004-S2010.

62. Campbell S, Goessens L, Goswamy R, Whitehead M: Realtime ultrasonography for determination of ovarian morphology and volume. Lancet 1982;20:425-426.

63. Granberg S, Wiklan M: A comparison between ultrasound and gynaecological examination for detection of enlarged ovaries in a group of women at risk for ovarian cancer. J Ultrasound Med 1988;7:59-64.

64. Higgins RV, van Nagell JR, Donaldson ES, et al: Transvaginal sonography as a screening method for ovarian cancer. Gynecol Oncol 1989;34:402-406.

65. Van Nagell JR, Higgins RV, Donaldson ES, et al: Transvaginal sonography as a screening method for ovarian cancer: A report of the first 1000 cases screened. Cancer 1990;65:573-577.

66. Bourne T, Campbell S, Steer C, et al: Transvaginal color flow imaging: A possible new screening technique for ovarian cancer. BMJ 1989;299:1367-1370.

67. Taylor KJW, Schwartz PE: Cancer screening in a high risk population: A clinical trial. Ultrasound Med Biol 2001;27:461-466.

68. Bourne T, Campbell S, Reynolds KM, et al: Screening for early familial ovarian cancer with transvaginal ultrasonography and color blood flow imaging. BMJ 1993;306:1025-1029.

69. Muto MG, Cramer DW, Brown DL, et al: Screening for ovarian cancer: The preliminary experience of a familial ovarian cancer centre. Gynecol Oncol 1993;51:12-20.

70. Belinson JL, Okin C, Casey G, et al: The familial ovarian cancer registry: Progress report. Cleve Clin J Med 1995;62:129-134.

71. Dørum A, Kristensen GB, Abler VM, et al: Early detection of familial ovarian cancer. Eur J Cancer 1996;32A:1645-1651.

72. Karlan BY, Raffel LJ, Crvenkovic G, et al: A multidisciplinary approach to the early detection of ovarian carcinoma: Rationale,

73. Karlan BY, Baldwin RL, Lopez-Luevanos E, et al: Peritoneal serous papillary carcinoma, a phenotypic variant of familial ovarian cancer: Implications for ovarian cancer screening. Am J Obstet Gynecol 1999;180:917-928.

74. Liede A, Karlan BY, Baldwin RL, et al: Cancer incidence in a population of Jewish women at risk of ovarian cancer. J Clin Oncol 2002;20:1570-1577.

75. Scheuer L, Kauff N, Robson M, et al: Outcome of preventative surgery and screening for breast and ovarian cancer in BRCA mutation carriers. J Clin Oncol 2002;20:1260-1268.

76. National Institute of Health Consensus Development Panel on Ovarian Cancer: Ovarian Cancer: Screening, treatment, and follow-up. JAMA 1995;273:491-497.

77. Eisinger F, Alby N, Bremond A, et al: Recommendations for medical management of hereditary breast and ovarian cancer: The French National Ad Hoc Committee. Ann Oncol 1998;9:939-950.

78. Burke W, Daly M, Garber J, et al: Recommendations for follow up care of individuals with an inherited predisposition to cancer. II. BRCA1 and BRCA2. Cancer Genetics Study Consortium. JAMA 1997;277:997-1003.

79. Kauff ND, Satagopan JM, Robson ME, et al: Risk-reducing salpingo-oophorectomy in women with a BRCA1 or BRCA2 mutation. N Engl J Med 2002;346:1609-1615.

80. Rebbeck TR, Lynch HT, Neuhausen SL, et al: Prophylactic oophorectomy in carriers of BRCA1 or BRCA2 mutations. N Engl J Med 2002;346:1616-1622.

81. Rutter JL, Wacholer S, Chetrit A, et al: Gynecologic surgeries and risk of ovarian cancer in women with BRCA, and BRCA2 Ashkenazi founder mutations: an Israel population-based case control study. J Natl Cancer Inst 2003;95:107-108.

82. Struewing JP, Watson P, Easton DF, et al: Prophylactic oophorectomy in inherited breast/ovarian cancer families. J Natl Cancer Inst Monogr 1995;17:33-36.

83. Agoff SN, Mendelin JE, Grieco VS, Garcia RL: Unexpected gynecologic neoplasms in patients with proven or suspected BRCA-1 or -2 mutations: Implications for gross examination, cytology, and clinical follow-up. Am J Surg Pathol 2002;26: 171-178.

84. Aziz S, Kuperstein G, Rosen B, et al: A genetic epidemiological study of carcinoma of the fallopian tube. Gynecol Oncol 2001;80: 341-345.

85. Russell JB: Laparoscopic oophorectomy. Curr Opin Obstet Gynecol 1995;7:295-298.

86. Fisher B, Costantino JP, Wickerham DL, et al: Tamoxifen for prevention of breast cancer: Report of the National Surgical Adjuvant Breast and Bowel Project P-1 Study. J Natl Cancer Inst 1998;90:1371-1388.

87. Weiderpass E, Adami HO, Baron JA, et al: Risk of endometrial cancer following estrogen replacement with and without progestins. J Nat Cancer Inst 1999;91:1131-1137.

88. Writing Group for the Women's Health Initiative Investigators: Risks and benefits of estrogen plus progestin in healthy postmenopausal women: Principal results from the Women's Health Initiative randomized controlled trial. JAMA 2002;288: 321-333.

89. Pike MC, Ross RK: Progestins and menopause: Epidemiological studies of risks of endometrial and breast cancer. Steroids 2000; 65:659-664.

90. Vessey MP, Painter R: Endometrial and ovarian cancer and oral contraceptives: Findings in a large cohort study. Br J Cancer 1995;71:1340-1342.

91. Ursin G, Henderson BE, Haile RW, et al: Does oral contraceptive use increase the risk of breast cancer in women with BRCA1/ BRCA2 mutations more than in other women? Cancer Res 1997;7:3678-3681.

92. Grabrick DM, Hartmann LC, Cerhan JR, et al: Risk of breast cancer with oral contraceptive use in women with a family history of breast cancer. JAMA 2000;284:1791-1798.

93. Narod SA, Dube MP, Klijn J, et al: Oral contraceptives and the risk of breast cancer in BRCA, and BRCA2 mutation carriers. J Natl Cancer Inst 2002;94:1773-1779.

94. Hankinson SE, Hunter DJ, Colditz GA, et al: Tubal ligation, hysterectomy and the risk of ovarian cancer. J Am Med Assoc 1993;270:2813-2818.

95. Whittemore AS, Harris R, Itnyre J: Characteristics relating to ovarian cancer risk: Collaborative analysis of 12 US case-control studies. II: Invasive epithelial ovarian cancers in white women. Am J Epidemiol 1992;136:1184-1203.
96. Rosenblatt KA, Thomas DB, and the WHO Collaborative Study of Neoplasia and Steroid Contraceptives: Reduced risk of ovarian cancer in women with tubal ligation or hysterectomy. Cancer Epidemiol Biomarkers Prevent 1996;5:933-935.
97. Xu Y, Shen Z, Wiper DW, et al: Lysophosphatidic acid as a potential biomarker for ovarian and other gynecologic cancers. JAMA 1998;280:719-723.
98. Menon U, Jacobs IJ: Recent developments in ovarian cancer screening. Curr Opin Obstet Gynecol 2000;12:39-42.
99. Mills G, Bast R, Srivastava S: Future for ovarian cancer screening: Novel markers from emerging technologies of transcriptional profiling and proteomics [editorial]. J Natl Cancer Inst 2001;93:1437-1439.
100. Petricoin EF, Ardekani AM, Hitt BA, et al: Use of proteomic patterns in serum to identify ovarian cancer. Lancet 2002; 359:572-577.
101. Mok SC, Chao J, Skates S, et al: Prostasin, a potential serum marker for ovarian cancer: Identification through microarray technology. J Natl Cancer Inst 2001;93:1458-1464.

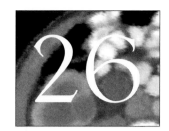

CHAPTER

SCREENING AND DIAGNOSIS OF OVARIAN CANCER IN THE GENERAL POPULATION

Barnaby Rufford and Ian J. Jacobs

 MAJOR CONTROVERSIES

- **Is ovarian cancer a disease that is amenable to a screening program?**
- **Who should be screened?**
- **What screening tests should be used, and what are they looking for?**
- **How should these screening tests be used?**
- **What is the optimal screening interval?**
- **Can ovarian cancer screening reduce mortality from ovarian cancer?**
- **Can we prevent ovarian cancer?**
- **What should we aim for in the future?**

Ovarian cancer is the most common gynecologic malignancy and the fourth most common cause of death from cancer in the developed world. Only cancers of the breast, colon, and lung cause more deaths. It also carries the worst prognosis of the gynecologic cancers, with an overall 5-year survival rate of 30%. A key factor contributing to this poor prognosis is the late presentation of the cancer, which is related to the ovaries' position within the peritoneal cavity, resulting in minimal local irritation or interference with vital structures until ovarian enlargement is considerable or metastasis occurs. Seventy percent of women are diagnosed with stage III or IV disease, with 5-year survival rates of 15% to 20% and less than 5%, respectively.[1] Despite an increase in understanding of the molecular events underlying malignancy and advances in surgery and chemotherapy, there has only been a slight improvement in the overall prognosis of ovarian cancer during the past 30 years. Women whose cancer is diagnosed at an early stage do have a significantly improved prognosis, with a survival rate of more than 80% for stage I disease and more than 90% for those diagnosed with stage Ia disease.[2] A potential way to improve outcome may be to detect the condition at an early stage, when the prognosis remains relatively good, with the use of a screening program. This chapter reviews eight major issues related to the introduction of an ovarian cancer screening program in the general population.

Is ovarian cancer a disease that is amenable to a screening program?

The World Health Organization (WHO) has established a set of principles to guide the development of a screening program. If a screening program is likely to be successful, the disease should fulfill most of the criteria:

- *The condition should pose an important health problem.* Ovarian cancer is the most common gynecologic malignancy in the developed world, with an estimated 23,000 new cases per year in the United States, and carries a poor prognosis, with a 5-year survival of approximately 30%.

- *The natural history or progression of the disease should be well understood.* Retrospective serum analysis shows evidence of increased CA 125 levels years before ovarian cancer is discovered by symptoms or ultrasound.[3] This suggests a disease process that follows a path from preclinical disease gradually to advanced metastatic disease. Despite advances in the understanding of ovarian carcinogenesis, there is no known precursor lesion. There are no data on how long ovarian cancer takes to progress from early to advanced disease. Although some have hypothesized that early-stage ovarian cancer may represent a different disease process from advanced disease and never progress, there is no evidence to support this.

- *There should be a recognizable early stage of the disease.* Although there is not a recognized premalignant condition, the existence and good prognosis of stage I disease is well documented.

- *Treatment of the disease at an early stage should be of more benefit than if treatment is delayed.* The 5-year survival rate for stage Ia disease is greater than 90%, compared with 15% to 20% for stage III and 5% for stage IV disease.

- *There must be a suitable test.* The CA 125 tumor marker and ultrasound have been shown to detect preclinical ovarian cancer in a substantial proportion of cases.

- *The test should be acceptable to the population.* Transvaginal ultrasound scanning and CA 125 blood tests have been demonstrated to be acceptable tests in large, prospective trials.

- *There should be adequate facilities for the diagnosis and treatment of abnormalities detected.* CA 125 assays and ultrasound are widely available, as are the facilities for surgical and medical treatment of ovarian cancer. Earlier diagnosis may result in a reduction in the burden on existing facilities.

- *For diseases of insidious onset, screening should be repeated at regular intervals determined by the natural history of the disease.* There is no doubt that ovarian cancer screening needs to be an ongoing program. However, the lack of knowledge about rate of disease progression means that the optimal screening interval has yet to be determined.

- *The chance of physical or psychological harm to those screened should be less than the chance of benefit.* The benefit in terms of ovarian cancer mortality is not yet clear, but current screening strategies achieve a high specificity and positive predictive value. Studies have also indicated that there are no long-term psychological sequelae from false positive results.

- *The costs of screening should be balanced against the benefit it provides.* A computer model estimated a cost of less than $100,000 per year of life saved, which compares favorably with many medical interventions.[4]

The WHO criteria for a screening program appear to be largely fulfilled, although some areas of controversy remain. Some of these areas are discussed in the following sections.

Who should be screened?

Although screening women at known high lifetime risk for developing ovarian cancer is likely to result in the highest positive predictive value, approximately 90% of ovarian cancers occur in women who do not fall in this high-risk group. To make a significant impact on overall mortality, a screening strategy needs to be aimed at the general population. The median age for developing ovarian cancer is 59 years, and less than 15% of ovarian cancers occur in women younger than 50 years of age. It would therefore seem reasonable to start screening the general population at 50 years of age. Many of the ovarian malignancies that occur in younger women are nonepithelial cancers and are therefore not amenable to screening with CA 125 determinations. Screening premenopausal women has a higher false-positive rate than screening postmenopausal women because of physiologic and benign premenopausal conditions that are associated with increased levels of CA 125 and ultrasound abnormalities. Law and colleagues[5] used national statistics to determine the number of years of life lost through deaths from a particular cancer at each age. They concluded that screening would be most effective (i.e., associated with the largest number of years of life saved per person screened) if done 5 years before the loss of life peaked. The peak age range for ovarian cancer was 55 to 59 years, and the researchers' argument provides further justification for using 50 years as the cutoff for general population screening. It would seem reasonable to direct one screening program at the high-risk population and a second program at the general population of women 50 years of age or older. It may also be possible to identify subgroups of risk within this general population. This may involve targeted screening of those with the vague symptoms that are often reported by women with ovarian cancer (even those with stage I disease), significantly before their eventual clinical diagnosis,[6] or by selection based on risk factors such as menopausal status, years of oral contraceptive use, and parity. It may also be possible to look for low penetrance genetic predispositions (e.g., single-nucleotide polymorphisms) to identify women with moderately increased susceptibility to ovarian cancer by virtue of their genetic profile.

What screening tests should be used, and what are they looking for?

A central principle of cancer screening is detection of a preinvasive or early invasive cancer, thereby reducing disease mortality and the morbidity of treatment.[7,8] Many solid cancers have a preinvasive or intraepithelial phase. The cervical cancer model illustrates this well. About 30% of high-grade intraepithelial lesions of the cervix may progress to invasive disease if left untreated.[9] Other cancers associated with detectable premalignant conditions include those of the esophagus, large bowel, endometrium, and vulva.

The hallmark of these preinvasive lesions is the presence of an intraepithelial lesion with the histologic features of cancer but the absence of destructive stromal invasion. Borderline ovarian tumors, otherwise called ovarian neoplasms of low malignant potential or ovarian intraepithelial neoplasms, fulfill the histologic criteria of preinvasive lesions. However, there is no convincing evidence that borderline tumors are precursors of invasive ovarian cancers. Although they can occasionally be multifocal at presentation in a manner suggestive of metastatic disease, studies have shown that although most metastatic invasive ovarian cancers are clonal in nature, metastatic multifocal borderline tumors are frequently not from the same clone.[10] Borderline and invasive ovarian cancers do not share similar genetic events. The tumor suppressor gene *TP53* is mutated in ovarian cancers in up to 75% of cases, but it is rarely mutated in borderline tumors. *KRAS* mutations occur relatively frequently in borderline tumors and uncommonly in ovarian cancers, with the exception of mucinous cystadenocarcinomas.[11-14] Borderline tumors are rarely aneuploid, whereas cancer is typically so.[15] Although borderline tumors resemble intraepithelial neoplastic lesions, there is no convincing evidence that they are the precursor lesions for most ovarian cancers.

The other lesion that has been considered as a possible precursor lesion for ovarian cancer is the benign ovarian neoplasm. If a large proportion of ovarian cancers arose in this way, removal of benign cysts in a screening program would affect future ovarian cancer incidence. Crayford and coworkers[16] analyzed data from a cohort of 5479 self-referred, asymptomatic women who participated in ovarian cancer screening trials and who had been followed up for an average of 15 years. Two hundred two women had bilateral salpingo-oophorectomies as a result of findings on ultrasound screening. The removal of persistent ovarian cysts was not associated with a decrease in the proportion of expected deaths from ovarian cancer. The main limitations of this study were the use of ovarian cancer mortality rather than incidence as the end point, the absence of a control group, and the fact that 59% of the lesions removed were physiologic or simple cysts rather than benign neoplasms. Hartge and associates[17] assessed whether asymptomatic complex ovarian cysts detected on ultrasonography in postmenopausal women were precursors to ovarian cancer. In 20,000 postmenopausal women enrolled in an ongoing randomized cancer screening trial, they compared the risk factor profile of women with complex, benign ovarian cysts with the established risk factors for ovarian cancer. These women did not share the same risk factor profile as women with ovarian cancer, suggesting that most complex, benign ovarian cysts and other clinically suspicious abnormalities detected on ultrasonography

were not immediate precursors of ovarian cancer. A true precursor lesion for ovarian cancer has yet to be identified, limiting the goal of screening to detection of asymptomatic, preclinical, low-volume disease.

The ovaries are not easily accessible. Although vaginal examination is important in assessing symptomatic women, it lacks the sensitivity and specificity required for a first-line screening test in asymptomatic women. In one study, only 30% of women who had ovarian masses on transvaginal ultrasound had an abnormal pelvic examination.[18]

Visualization or direct sampling to detect malignant disease or, perhaps in the future, a premalignant condition is being investigated in preliminary studies using office laparoscopy and cytologic examination of brush samples from the ovarian surface in screening high-risk populations. The possibility of using optical methods such as optical spectroscopy is also being investigated. The main options for screening involve serum tumor markers and ultrasound scanning.

Of the ovarian tumor markers, the most extensively studied is CA 125. It is an antigenic determinant on a high-molecular-weight glycoprotein recognized by the mouse monoclonal antibody, OC125, developed using an ovarian cancer cell line as an immunogen. CA 125 was first discovered in 1981.[19] Levels are raised in 50% of stage I and 90% of stage II ovarian tumors.[20] CA 125 levels may also be raised in a range of other physiologic and pathologic conditions that may be gynecologic or nongynecologic, benign or malignant (Table 26-1). This causes particular problems in screening the high-risk

Table 26–1. Examples of Conditions Found in Association with Increased CA 125 Levels

Gynecologic Conditions
Endometriosis
Fibroids
Hemorrhagic ovarian cysts
Menstruation
Acute pelvic inflammatory disease
Pregnancy (first trimester)

Gastrointestinal and Hepatic Conditions
Acute pancreatitis
Colitis
Chronic active hepatitis
Cirrhosis
Diverticulitis

Miscellaneous Conditions
Pericarditis
Polyarteritis nodosa
Renal disease
Sjögren's syndrome
Systemic lupus erythematosus

Malignancies
Bladder
Breast
Endometrium
Lung
Liver
Non-Hodgkin's lymphoma
Ovary
Pancreas

population, because many of these women are premenopausal, and the CA 125 level may fluctuate with the menstrual cycle or may be elevated by conditions such as endometriosis. The specificity of CA 125 as a screening tool can be improved using serial determinations over time.[21] An algorithm has been developed in postmenopausal women from the general population that determines the risk of ovarian cancer based on CA 125 profile with time.[22] This is based on the observation that women with ovarian cancer have increasing levels of CA 125, even if below 30 U/mL, whereas women without ovarian cancer have static or decreasing levels even if they remain above 30 U/mL. The risk of ovarian cancer (ROC) calculation for interpretation of serum CA 125 levels is based on the behavior of serial CA 125 levels among volunteers in the initial multimodal ovarian cancer screening trials.[22-27] The ROC for an individual is calculated using a computer algorithm based on Bayes theorem that compares an individual's serial CA 125 levels to the pattern in known cases and controls. The closer the CA 125 profile to the CA 125 behavior of known cases of ovarian cancer, the greater the risk of ovarian cancer. The final result is presented as the individual's estimated risk of having ovarian cancer. A ROC of 2% implies a risk of 1 in 50.[28] Compared with a single cutoff value, this approach has decreased false-positive results while increasing sensitivity because women with normal but rising levels are identified. The greater the rate of rise in CA 125 levels, the greater is the risk of ovarian cancer.

The latest in a series of tumor markers that have been assessed is plasma lysophosphatidic acid (LPA), a bioactive phospholipid with mitogenic and growth factor–like activities that may have a potential role in ovarian cancer diagnosis and screening.[29] Its sensitivity is reported to be 100% in advanced disease and 90% in stage I disease, with an overall specificity for ovarian cancer of 90%. In a series of stage I and II cancers in which CA 125 and LPA levels were assessed, LPA was elevated in more than 90%, whereas CA 125 was elevated in only 50%.[30]

An exciting possibility involves detecting ovarian cancer using bioinformatics to identify proteomic patterns in serum that distinguish neoplastic from non-neoplastic disease. Petricoin and colleagues[31] reported that a proteomic pattern completely discriminated symptomatic patients with a malignant pelvic mass from a control group. In their set, the proteomic pattern achieved a sensitivity of 100%, a specificity of 95%, and a positive predictive value of 94%. This approach may have great potential, but because it has not been assessed in preclinical samples from asymptomatic women with ovarian cancer, its value in screening is unclear.

Ultrasound has been studied as a screening test for ovarian cancer for more than 2 decades. Transabdominal scanning lacked specificity, and in the key early study involving 5540 women, 50 underwent surgical investigation for each case of ovarian malignancy detected.[32] Specificity has improved with the introduction of transvaginal scanning and the use of morphologic scoring systems for interpreting scans.[33] This scoring

system was used in a Kentucky ovarian cancer screening trial using transvaginal sonography, and it reduced the number of women undergoing surgical investigation to 10 for each case of malignancy detected.[34] Some investigators have used color flow Doppler imaging to assess vasculature and blood flow characteristics in ovarian masses. Malignant masses have increased blood flow during diastole, helping to distinguish them from benign ones.[35,36] Bourne and coworkers[37] reported the results of screening 1601 women with a positive family history of ovarian cancer who underwent transvaginal ultrasound examination with color flow Doppler imaging. Sixty-one (3.8%) women were referred for surgery as a result of positive scan findings. Six primary ovarian cancers were detected; five were stage I. However, because of the subjective nature of Doppler imaging, it has failed to make the anticipated impact on reducing false-positive results in other screening trials. In the largely premenopausal group of women who undergo familial ovarian cancer screening, the increased incidence of benign and physiologic ovarian lesions create problems with false-positive rates similar to those seen with CA 125 testing.

How should these screening tests be used?

There are three main strategies for using screening tests:

1. An ultrasound approach based on primary screening with transvaginal ultrasound is used, with repeat testing after a fixed interval if an abnormality is detected.
2. Multimodal screening incorporates primary screening using a serum marker, usually CA 125, with repeat assessment of the marker and transvaginal ultrasound as a second-line test. CA 125 results are interpreted using the ROC algorithm previously discussed.
3. A combined approach uses serum CA 125 and transvaginal ultrasound scanning as first-line tests to maximize the detection rate, and its use is usually limited to screening the high-risk population.

The optimal screening strategy has yet to be established and will depend on the target population. Results from the large, prospective studies of screening for ovarian cancer in the general population suggest that sequential multimodal screening has superior specificity and positive predictive value compared with strategies based on transvaginal ultrasound alone. However, ultrasound as a first-line test may offer slightly greater sensitivity for early-stage disease. An ultrasound-based strategy may have a greater impact on ovarian cancer mortality, albeit at a higher price in terms of surgical intervention for false-positive results.[38]

What is the optimal screening interval?

An important way to influence the sensitivity, specificity, and cost-effectiveness of a screening program is to vary the screening interval. It may be appropriate to have a fixed screening interval or to alter the interval according to a woman's level of risk. Frequent screening is likely to be chosen if a disease progresses rapidly, if there is significant variation in disease progression between individual women, and if it is justified for the cost. Most trials have empirically chosen annual screening. If the screening interval is too short, it will lead to higher false-positive rates with resultant higher cost and morbidity. If, however, the screening interval is too long, we may miss the opportunity of detecting women with early-stage disease. Based on a model of CA 125 data from screening trials, Skates and associates[3] estimated the CA 125-positive preclinical phase of the disease in the general population to be about 1.9 years. Jacobs and colleagues[24] reached a similar estimate of 1.4 years based on the

expected versus observed cases at a prevalence screen. This suggests that annual screening is a reasonable interval. Studies are under way to determine the optimal screening intervals for patients at high risk.

Can ovarian cancer screening reduce mortality from ovarian cancer?

Over the past decade, large, prospective population studies with long-term follow-up in the United Kingdom, United States, and Japan have provided very encouraging results regarding the performance of the established screening tests and strategies for the general population. Most studies, however, have had single-arm and nonrandomized designs (Tables 26-2 and 26-3).

Table 26–2. Prospective Studies of Ovarian Cancer Screening Using Ultrasound Strategy in the General Population

Study	Main Features	Screening Strategy	No. Screened	No. of Invasive EOCs Detected*	No. of Positive Screens	No. of Positive Screens per Cancer Detected
USS-Only Approach						
USS (Level 1 Screen), then repeat USS (Level II Screen)						
Pavlik et al.[100] (2000); DePriest et al.[101] (1997); van Nagell et al.[102] (1995)	Age ≥50 yr and postmenopausal or ≥30 yr with family history	TVS, annual screens, mean of four screens per woman	14,469	11 (6) (5 stage I)	180	16.3
Sato S et al.[103] (2000)	Part of general screening program, retrospective	TVS	51,550	22 (17 stage I)	324	14.7
Hayashi et al.[104] (1999)	Age ≥50 yr	TVS	23,451	3 (3)	258	†
Tabor et al.[105] (1994)	Age 46-65 yr	TVS	435	0	9	—
Campbell et al.[106] (1989)	Age ≥45 yr (mean, 53 yr) or with family history (4%)	TAS, three screens at 18-mo intervals	5479	2 (3) (2 stage I)	326	163
Millo et al.[107] (1989)	Age ≥45 yr or postmenopausal (mean, 54 yr)	US (not specified)	500	0	11	—
Goswamy et al.[108] (1983)	Age 39-78 yr, postmenopausal	TAS	1084	1 (1 stage I)		
USS and CDI (Level I Screen)						
Kurjak et al.[109] (1994)	Age 40-71 yr (mean, 45 yr)	TVS and CDI	5013	4 (4 stage I)	38	9.5
Vuento et al.[110] (1995)	Age 56-61 yr (mean, 59 yr)	TVS and CDI	1364	(1)	5	—
USS (Level I) and Other Test (Level II Screen)						
Parkes et al.[111] (1994)	Age 50-64 yr	TVS, then CDI if TVS positive	2953	1 (1 stage I)	15‡	15
Holbert et al.[112] (1994)	Age 30-89 yr, postmenopausal	TVS, then CA 125 if TVS positive	478	1 (1 stage I)	33§	33
Schincaglia et al.[113] (1994)	Age 50-69 yr	TAS, then aspiration or biopsy	3541	2 (0 stage I)	98	9.5

*The number of borderline or granulosa tumors detected is shown within parentheses on the first line of the entry; the number of stage I tumors is shown in parentheses on the second line.

†Only 95 women consented to surgery, and there are no follow-up details on the remaining women.

‡Eighty-six women had abnormal ultrasound scan results before CDI.

§Only 11 of these women underwent surgery.

CDI, color flow Doppler imaging; EOC, epithelial ovarian cancer; TAS, transabdominal ultrasound; TVS, transvaginal ultrasound, USS, ultrasound scanning.

Table 26–3. Prospective Studies of Ovarian Cancer Screening Using CA 125 as the Primary Test in the General Population

Study	Main Features	Screening Strategy	No. of Screened	No. of Invasive EOCs Detected*	No. of Positive Screens	No. of Operations per Cancer Detected
CA 125 Only						
Einhorn et al.[21] (1992)	Age ≥40 yr	Serum CA 125	5,550	6 (2 stage I)	175†	29†
CA 125 (Level I Screen), then Ultrasound (Level II Screen)						
Jacobs et al.[23-25] (1988, 1993, 1996)	Age ≥45 yr (median, 56 yr), postmenopausal	Serum CA 125, TAS if CA 125↑	22,000	11 (4 stage I)	41	3.7
Jacobs et al.[26] (1999)	Age ≥45 yr (median, 56 yr), postmenopausal	RCT, serum CA 125, TAS/TVS if CA 125↑, three screens	10,958	6 (3 stage I)	29	4.8
Grover et al.[114] (1995)	Age ≥40 yr (median, 51 yr) or with family history (3%)	Serum CA 125, TAS/TVS if CA 125↑	2,550	1 (0 stage I)	16	16
Adonakis et al.[115] (1996)	Age ≥45 yr (mean, 58 yr)	Serum CA 125, TVS if CA 125↑	2,000	1 (1) (1 stage I)	15	15
Total				19 (1)	101	5.3

*The number of borderline or granulosa tumors detected is shown within parentheses on the first line of the entry; the number of stage I tumors is shown in parentheses on the second line.
†Not all of these women underwent surgical investigation because the study design involved intensive surveillance rather than surgical intervention.
EOC, epithelial ovarian cancers; RCT, randomized, controlled trial; TAS, transabdominal ultrasound; TVS, transvaginal ultrasound.

The only randomized, controlled trial reported was that of Jacobs and colleagues.[26] This pilot randomized, controlled trial assessed multimodal screening with sequential CA 125 determinations and ultrasonography. Participants were all U.K. residents, postmenopausal, and 45 years old or older. Exclusion criteria were a history of bilateral oophorectomy or ovarian cancer. The 22,000 women who had previously taken part in an ovarian cancer prevalence screen were randomized to two groups: a screened group and a control group. Screening involved primary screening with CA 125 measurement and ultrasonography for all women with a CA 125 measurement above 30 U/mL. Ovarian volume was assessed on ultrasonography, and women with abnormal ultrasound findings were referred for surgical investigation. Of 29 women referred for surgical investigation, 6 had an index cancer (defined as invasive primary epithelial cancers of the ovary and fallopian tube and excluded borderline ovarian cancers). Of the 23 patients with false-positive results, 14 had benign ovarian tumors, 4 had fibroids, 2 had adenocarcinoma of unknown origin, and 3 had no abnormality. The positive predictive value of screening was 20.7%, and there was no surgical mortality or serious morbidity. Another 10 women in the screening group developed an index cancer during the follow-up of 8 years. Twenty women developed an index cancer in the control group. Survival time from randomization for the 16 women who had an index cancer in the screened group was significantly longer than that of the 20 women in the control group (P = .0112). The median survival time of women with index cancers in the screened group was 72.9 months, compared with

41.8 months for women with index cancers in the control group (Fig. 26-1). The study was not designed to have the power to show a difference in mortality, but it was the first randomized, controlled trial of ovarian cancer screening and did show a significant survival difference. It showed acceptable patient compliance and positive predictive value.

The results from this pilot study formed the basis for a larger, randomized controlled study in the United Kingdom. The United Kingdom Trial of Ovarian Cancer Screening (UKCTOCS), commenced in 2001. The study aims to recruit 200,000 women and randomize them in a 1:1:2 ratio into ultrasound screening, multimodal screening, and control groups. The primary end point of the trial is ovarian cancer mortality. Secondary end

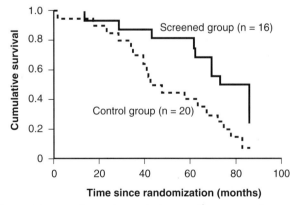

Figure 26–1. Kaplan-Meier survival curves for women who developed index cancers in the screening and control groups.

points include the physical morbidity associated with ovarian cancer screening, the resource implications of screening and the resulting interventions, the feasibility of population screening for ovarian cancer as reflected by uptake of invitations and compliance rates with annual screening, and a comparison of the performance of two screening strategies for ovarian cancer. A final objective is to establish a unique serum bank for future assessment of novel tumor markers. Women are being recruited over 3 years from 13 regional collaborating centers. They are invited to participate from the age and sex registers of the health authorities related to the collaborating centers. Inclusion criteria are as follows:

- Age 50 to 74 years: A minimum age of 50 years was chosen because ovarian cancer is relatively uncommon before this age; a maximum of 74 years was chosen because over this age all-cause mortality during 7 years of follow-up is likely to be high and confound interpretation of the end point of ovarian cancer mortality.
- Postmenopausal status: Status is determined by more than 2 months of amenorrhea after a natural menopause or hysterectomy or more than 12 months of hormone replacement therapy commenced for menopausal symptoms. Postmenopausal status is required because the frequency of benign and physiologic conditions associated with an increased CA 125 level and ultrasound abnormalities decreases after the menopause, and consequently, the false-positive rate is lower than in premenopausal women.

Exclusion criteria are as follows:

- Women with a history of bilateral oophorectomy are excluded.
- Women with currently active nonovarian malignancy are excluded. Women with a history of cancer are eligible if they have no known persistent or recurrent disease and have not received treatment for more than 12 months. This does not include pre-malignant disease or breast cancer treatment with estrogen receptor antagonists. This exclusion is required to minimize false-positive CA 125 results due to previously diagnosed malignancies.
- Women with a history of ovarian malignancy are excluded.
- Women at significantly increased risk of ovarian cancer as suggested by their family history (Table 26-4) are excluded because of the ethical difficulties in potentially randomizing high-risk women to a control group. These women are eligible for the United Kingdom Familial Ovarian Cancer Screening Study (UKFOCSS), which is a nonrandomized study.
- Women participating in other ovarian cancer screening trials are excluded.

Women in the eligible age group are identified on the health authority registers and are mailed letters inviting them to join the study. Those who accept are invited to a recruitment visit, where the study is explained, eligibility confirmed, consent obtained, and blood taken. They are asked to complete a quality of life

Table 26–4. Definition of Individuals at High Risk for Ovarian Cancer

The individual is a first-degree relative (i.e., mother, sister, daughter) of an affected member of a high-risk family, defined by the following criteria:

1. The family contains two or more individuals with ovarian cancer who are first-degree relatives.
2. The family contains one individual with ovarian cancer and one individual with breast cancer diagnosed before 50 years of age; individuals are first-degree relatives.
3. The family contains one individual with ovarian cancer and two individuals with breast cancer diagnosed before 60 years of age; individuals are first-degree relatives.
4. The family contains an affected individual with a mutation of one of the known ovarian cancer predisposing genes.
5. The family contains three individuals with colorectal cancer, with at least one case diagnosed before 50 years of age, as well as one case of ovarian cancer; all are first-degree relatives.
6. Criteria 1, 2, and 3 can be modified when paternal transmission is occurring. Families in which affected relatives are related by second degree through an unaffected intervening male relative who has an affected sister are eligible.

questionnaire. They are then randomized to the control group or a screening group by computer allocation:

Control arm (50% of women): These women's general practitioners are asked to keep on file the letter explaining their participation and to refer women with a suspected ovarian cancer to the gynecologic oncologist at their regional center. This is done to ensure similar care for women in the control and study groups.

Ultrasound arm (25% of women): These women are assessed using transvaginal ultrasound or by transabdominal ultrasound scanning if the former approach is not possible or acceptable. Ovarian size and morphology are documented. Women with normal scans or scans showing only a simple ovarian cyst of less than 5 cm in diameter and 60 cc in volume are routinely followed up with annual screening. After unsatisfactory results, scans are repeated in 6 to 8 weeks. Women who have an ovarian abnormality have another scan in 6 to 8 weeks, and if this abnormality is confirmed, they are referred to a gynecologic oncologist.

Multimodal arm (25% of women): These women undergo venipuncture for CA 125 assay and calculation of the ROC algorithm. Those with normal results have repeat venipuncture on an annual basis. Women with an intermediate ROC result have repeat venipuncture in 12 weeks, and the ROC is recalculated. Those with an elevated ROC value have another CA 125 test and an ultrasound scan in 6 to 8 weeks. Those with abnormalities on ultrasound are referred to a gynecologic oncologist; if the scan is normal, the ROC is recalculated. A small group of women with markedly elevated ROC values based on CA 125 determinations proceed to surgery even if the ultrasound findings are normal.

Women referred to a gynecologic oncologist from the screening arms are considered for surgery.

According to investigation findings, this may involve laparoscopic bilateral salpingo-oophorectomy or a laparotomy. Based on these findings, a decision may be made to manage some women conservatively.

Follow-up of all women includes asking them to complete a questionnaire at 3, 5, and 7 years after randomization. Women participating in the study are also tagged on the health service registry, so the study is aware of any new cases of cancer or deaths from cancer in the study population.

In addition to the UKCTOCS study, ovarian cancer screening is part of the large National Cancer Institute–sponsored Prostate, Lung, Colorectal, and Ovarian (PLCO) Cancer Screening Trial. This two-arm, randomized trial incorporates ultrasound, CA 125, and pelvic examination and aims to involve 74,000 women between 55 and 74 years old. There are 10 screening centers nationwide with balanced randomization to intervention and control arms. For ovarian cancer screening, women have a CA 125 determination at entry and annually for 5 years, and they have a transvaginal ultrasound scan at entry and annually for 3 years. Participants will be followed up for at least 13 years from recruitment.[39,40]

These studies should give a definitive answer about whether ovarian cancer screening reduces mortality at the end of this decade.

Can we prevent ovarian cancer?

The potential benefits of a reduction in mortality by detecting ovarian cancer at the preclinical stage by screening have been discussed, as have the limitations of having to screen for preclinical disease as opposed to premalignant disease. However, the greatest reduction in mortality may be achieved by preventing disease from occurring in the first instance. Strategies that may be used to prevent ovarian cancer are discussed in the following sections.

Lifestyle. Lifestyle and environmental factors have a major impact on the incidence of cancer. Although there is no single risk factor for ovarian cancer as there is, for example, with cigarette smoking and carcinoma of the lung, there are a number of factors that influence the incidence of ovarian cancer.

Exercise. Whether there is any relationship between levels of physical activity and ovarian cancer is widely debated. A case-control study found that leisure-time physical activity was associated with a reduced incidence of epithelial ovarian cancer.[41] Women who reported high levels of physical activity had a relative risk of developing ovarian cancer of 0.73 (0.56-0.94) compared with those who reported low levels, after adjustment for age, parity, oral contraceptive pill use, tubal ligation, and body mass index. However, diet and other lifestyle variables were not controlled for, and the level of physical activity may be a marker for a healthy lifestyle. This trend was supported in an Italian study that found a corresponding reduction in risk of ovarian cancer with increased physical activity across all age groups.[42] However, an evaluation of the Nurses' Health Study cohort found no inverse association between recreational physical activity and ovarian cancer risk, and although not statistically significant, it raised the possibility of a modest increase in ovarian cancer risk with frequent vigorous activity.[43] The Iowa Women's Health Study found an increased relative risk (RR = 2.1) for women with a high level of exercise compared with those with a low level. A positive association was also found with an increased waist-to-hip ratio.[44] There is no definitely established link between exercise levels and ovarian cancer incidence.

Diet. There is only limited evidence linking diet and the risk of ovarian cancer. An Italian case-control study found an association between a greater consumption of red meat and an increased risk of developing ovarian cancer (OR = 1.53), but a decreased risk was found with the consumption of fish (OR = 0.51) or vegetables (OR = 0.47 [raw], 0.65 [cooked]).[45] Data from the Iowa Women's Health Study found a statistically significant decreased risk of ovarian cancer with increased consumption of green, leafy vegetables and suggested an increased risk with increased consumption of eggs, cholesterol, and lactose.[46] This appears to corroborate earlier data,[47] and it has been hypothesized that the divergent fat consumption between northern and southern Europe could explain the difference in ovarian cancer mortality.[48,49] However, other evidence points to no association between fat and ovarian cancer.[50,51] Some studies have found milk consumption to be protective against ovarian cancer,[52,53] and others have found a relationship between increased consumption of some carotenoids and decreased ovarian cancer risk,[54,55] but further studies have not confirmed this.[56] There is insufficient evidence to substantiate a definite link between diet and ovarian cancer.

Parity. The relationship between increasing parity and reducing risk of epithelial ovarian cancer is well documented. A collaborative analysis of 12 U.S. case-control studies found a decreasing risk of ovarian cancer with increasing parity.[57] Parous women had a lower risk than nulliparous women (OR = 0.76, 95% CI: 0.63-0.93 in hospital studies; OR = 0.47, 95% CI: 0.40-0.56 in population studies). Risk decreased with increasing parity among the parous women. Each additional pregnancy after the first conferred the same risk reduction of about 14%, which is smaller than the 40% risk reduction associated with the first term pregnancy. Failed pregnancies also appeared to be protective, although less so than term pregnancies. No association was found with age at first pregnancy in this study.

Another large, epidemiologic analysis agreed with the protective effects of increasing parity. Women with five or more births had a relative risk of ovarian cancer of 0.4 compared with nulliparous women. Each pregnancy conferred a risk reduction of about 20%.[58] This study found a significant protective effect of increasing age at first pregnancy, with women having their first child at 35 years or older having a relative risk of 0.61(95% CI: 0.44-0.81) compared with those who first gave birth before the age of 20 years. Other studies agreed with this finding.[59,60] Increasing age at last birth has also been identified as a protective factor.[60] Several other studies have confirmed the protective effects of pregnancy.[60-63] It has been suggested by some studies that the more recent a pregnancy, the greater the protective effect it has (i.e., the protective effect of pregnancy may reduce over time).[59,60] However, other studies have failed to confirm this finding.[64]

The protective effect of pregnancy also appears to extend to carriers of gene mutations. One study interviewed and successfully completed mutation analysis for 840 Jewish women with ovarian cancer and 751 controls. The investigators showed a statistically significant reduction in ovarian cancer risk with each live birth in carriers of BRAC1/2 mutations and in noncarriers.[65]

Breast-feeding. Breast-feeding appears to reduce ovarian cancer risk. An Italian study found an odds ratio of 0.5 (95% CI: 0.3-0.7) for women who had breast-fed for longer than 12 months compared with women who had never breast-fed.[66] Breast-feeding for a shorter period was also protective (OR = 0.6, 95% CI: 0.5-0.9). Whittemore and colleagues,[57] in their collaborative analysis of 12 U.S. case-control studies, found a significant reduction in ovarian cancer risk with breast-feeding that reduced further with increasing duration but was most effective in the first 6 months after delivery than the subsequent period. Other studies have found a similar risk reduction.[57,67-69]

Fertility. The first study to suggest an association between fertility treatment and an increased risk of ovarian cancer was the collaborative analysis of 12 case-control studies. It found an odds ratio of 2.8 (95% CI: 1.3-6.1) for women who had ever used fertility drugs compared with those with no history of infertility. The risk was highest among nulliparous women, with an odds ratio of 27.0 (95% CI: 2.3-315.6). However this study did not provide adequate controls for confounding and protective factors. The link between fertility drugs and an increased risk of ovarian cancer has been supported by other studies,[70,71] but still other studies have not supported this link.[72-75] The relationship between ovarian stimulation and ovarian cancer remains uncertain. A strong link seems unlikely, but it remains possible that fertility drugs cause a modest increase in risk.

Hormone replacement therapy. Epidemiologic studies looking for an association between hormone replacement therapy (HRT) and ovarian cancer have yielded conflicting results, with positive and negative associations being reported. However, the temporal association between HRT use and ovarian cancer risk has frequently been overlooked, with most studies looking at current and recent use, and it is possible that there is a significant delay between HRT use and any effect on risk. Oral contraceptive pill use and pregnancy most often occur in the third and fourth decades of life,

whereas their protective effects are seen on average 2 to 3 decades later. A study by Lacey and coworkers[76] found a positive association with use only during the 2 years before diagnosis, and the large Cancer Prevention Study II[77] found a positive association only with more than 10 years of use and with use within 15 years of death. It is possible that HRT use stimulates the growth of preexisting, undiagnosed ovarian cancers, rather than increasing the risk of malignant transformation. On the basis of these studies, there does not appear to be a compelling case for an association between HRT and ovarian cancer.

Surgery.
Tubal ligation. The beneficial effects of tubal ligation on reducing the risk of ovarian cancer have been demonstrated in a number of studies. Statistically significant reductions in ovarian cancer were observed in the collaborative analysis of 12 U.S. case-control studies (OR = 0.59, 95% CI: 0.38-0.53 for the hospital-based data).[57] There was no association with age at surgery or time since surgery. Other studies have supported these data.[78-82] This benefit extends to carriers of the BRCA1 mutation.[83]

Hysterectomy. Simple hysterectomy with ovarian preservation appears to reduce ovarian cancer risk. Analyzing the data of 12 case-control studies, Whittemore and associates[57] found a significantly reduced risk in hospital-based studies but not in population-based studies. Significant risk reductions were also found in other studies,[62,78-81] although one study did not find a significant reduction in risk.[84]

Possible mechanisms that have been hypothesized for these reductions in risk include local alterations in blood flow, increasing anovulation, and the reduction in carcinogens reaching the ovary through the lower genital tract.

Prophylactic oophorectomy. Those at increased risk of ovarian cancer because of their family history may elect to have their ovaries removed to eliminate or at least reduce their risk of developing the disease. This is not a realistic option in the general population, except in selected cases as part of a surgical procedure being undertaken for another reason. It seems reasonable to assume that prophylactic oophorectomy would result in the elimination of—or at least a considerable reduction in—the risk of subsequent ovarian cancer. There is good evidence supporting this, with prophylactic oophorectomy in BRCA1 and BRCA2 gene carriers being shown to significantly reduce the risk of ovarian cancer, celomic epithelial cancer, and breast cancer.[85-87]

Chemoprevention.
Oral contraceptive pill. It is well established that the combined oral contraceptive pill protects against epithelial ovarian cancer. The largest study reported, the Cancer and Steroid Hormone Study (CASH), showed that oral contraceptive use, even for a few months, reduced the risk by 40% for women between the ages of 20 and 54 years (RR= 0.6). The effect probably takes

from 5 to 10 years to become apparent, but it persists long after the use of oral contraceptives ends. protection exists regardless of the formulation of combined oral contraceptive used. The effect is greater among those who have used the contraceptive pill for a longer duration, with a relative risk of 0.2 for users of oral contraceptives for more than 10 years.[67] Numerous other studies have found similar reduction in risk of ovarian cancer in oral contraceptive pill users.[57,69,88,89]

Most of the studies that have shown this risk reduction were based on women who have used the older, higher-dose, 50-μg estrogen preparations. The benefits are independent of the dose of estrogen or progestin.[90] This protective effect extends to carriers of mutations in the BRCA1/2 gene.[91]

The mechanism by which the oral contraceptive pill reduces the risk of ovarian cancer is the subject of debate. There are several theories about the

Table 26–5. Oral Contraceptives and Ovarian Cancer Risk

Study	Study Type	Cases	Controls	Relative Risk Overall	Comments
Chiaffarino et al.[63] (2001)	C-C	1031	2411	0.5	Figure for ≥5 years
Modan et al.[65] (2001)	C-C	832	2257		5.8% (1.5-10) per year for nonmutation carriers but no risk reduction in mutation carriers at 0.2% (−4.9-5.0)
Greggi et al.[66] (2000)	C-C	440	868	0.4 (0.3-0.6)	Low-risk population
Ness et al.[90] (2000)	C-C	767	1367	0.6 (0.5-0.8)	Protection unaffected by estrogen or progesterone dose
Beard et al.[116] (2000)	C-C	103	103		
Beral[117] (1999)	Coh	55	Cohort 46,000	0.6 (0.3-1.0) $P < .05$	Royal College of General Practitioners' Oral Contraception Study
Narod et al.[91] (1998)	C-C	207	161	0.5 (0.3-0.8)	Cases all mutation carriers
Hankinson et al.[118] (1995)	Coh	260	Cohort 121,700		Nurses' Health Study
Vessey et al.[119] (1995)	Coh	42	Cohort 15,292	0.4 (0.2-0.8)	Oxford Family Planning Study
Purdie et al.[120] (1995)	C-C	824	860		
Risch et al.[62] (1994)	C-C	450	564	0.52 (0.39-0.71)	Benefit with and without hysterectomy
Rosenberg et al.[80] (1994)	C-C	441	2065	0.8 (0.6-1.0)	Increasing benefit with increasing use
John et al.[121] (1993)	Ovr	110	365		7 case-control studies of black women
Polychronopoulou et al.[122] (1993)	C-C	189			
Whittemore et al.[57] (1992)	Ovr	2197	8,893	0.7 (0.52-0.94) hospital and 0.66 (0.55-0.78) population studies	12 case-control studies of white women
Harris et al.[123] (1992)	Ovr	327	4144	0.80 (0.59-1.1)	9 case-control studies of borderline tumors
Rosenblatt et al.[124] (1992)	C-C	393	2561	0.68 (0.44-1.05) high dose and 0.81 (0.51-1.29) low dose	Protection from high- and low-dose preparations
Gross et al.[125] (1992)	C-C	283	1929	0.6 (0.4-0.9)	Short-term users; no benefit from short-term use if positive family history
Hankinson et al.[89] (1992)	Ovr			0.64 (0.57-0.73)	20 studies
Franceschi et al.[126] (1991)	Ovr	971	2258	0.6 (0.4-0.8)	3 case-control studies
Parazzini et al.[127] (1991)	C-C	91	237	0.3	Borderline tumors
Parazzini et al.[128] (1991)	C-C	505	1375	0.7 (0.5-1.0)	
Booth et al.[78] (1989)	C-C	235	471		
Hartge et al.[129] (1989)	C-C	296	343		
WHO[130] (1989)	C-C	368	2397	0.75 (0.56-1.01)	
Shu et al.[131] (1989)	C-C	172			
Wu et al.[132] (1988)	C-C	299	1011		
Harlow et al.[133] (1988)	C-C	116	158	0.4	Borderline tumors
CASH[67] (1987)	C-C	546	4228	0.6 (0.5-0.7)	Cancer and Steroid Hormone Study
La Vecchia et al.[134] (1986)	C-C	406	1282	0.5 (0.23-1.12)	
Tzonou et al.[135] (1984)	C-C	150	250	0.4 (0.1-1.1)	
Risch et al.[136] (1983)	C-C			0.89	Per year of use
Rosenberg et al.[137] (1982)	C-C	136	587	0.6 (0.4-0.9)	
Cramer et al.[138] (1982)	C-C	144	139		
Franceschi et al.[139] (1982)	C-C	161	544		
Weiss et al.[69] (1981)	C-C			0.57	
Hildreth et al.[140] (1981)	C-C				
Willett et al.[141] (1981)	C-C		470	0.8 (0.4-1.5)	
Ramcharan et al.[142] (1980)	Coh				

C-C, case-control study; Coh, cohort study.

mechanism of the protective effect of the oral contraceptive pill:

- The effect results from a reduction in the number of lifetime ovulations. However, the effect appears to be greater than that expected purely by the reduction in number of ovulations alone. Siskind[92] suggested that there is a 9% reduction in relative risk of ovarian cancer for each year of oral contraceptive use. Even after controlling for the expected decrease in risk due to a reduction in the number of lifetime ovulations, there remained a 7% reduction for each year of use. It is reasonable therefore to presume that there are other mechanisms at work.
- High gonadotrophin levels act directly or indirectly on the steroid-producing stroma of the ovary and induce neoplastic changes in ovarian epithelial cells, especially those entrapped in inclusion cysts.[93] The oral contraceptive pill is known to reduce gonadotrophin levels. However, HRT also results in a reduction in gonadotrophin levels, but there is no evidence of a protective effect against ovarian cancer, and this does not therefore support the role of high gonadotrophin levels in ovarian carcinogenesis.[57,94]
- High androgen or low progesterone levels are responsible for increasing the risk of ovarian cancer.[95] All oral contraceptives contain progestogens, and they suppress androgens.
- Toxins may reach the upper genital tract through the vagina, causing inflammation and predisposing to malignant change. The oral contraceptive pill alters the viscosity of the mucous plug of the cervix and therefore may prevent these toxins from reaching the ovaries.

Studies looking at the association between oral contraceptive use and cancer are summarized in Table 26-5.

Progesterone. Evidence for the protective effect of progesterone is limited. However, analysis of the data of a large, case-control trial looking at oral contraceptive pill use and ovarian cancer had sufficient numbers of women taking the progestogen-only pill to find a statistically significant reduction in ovarian cancer in this group. Relative to never users, the relative risks were 0.39 for less than 3 years of use and 0.21 for 3 years of use or longer.[80] Because up to 40% of women ovulate while taking the progestogen-only pill, this suggests that the mechanism of protection extends beyond that of ovulation suppression. Whether depot medroxyprogesterone acetate (DMPA) offers protection is less clear. The WHO international collaborative case-control study showed a significantly reduced risk for ever users,[96] but this was not the case in a follow-up study of 5000 black American women.[97] It has also been hypothesized that the greatly increased progestogen levels that occur during pregnancy may be the mechanism by which pregnancy protects against ovarian cancer rather than only a reduction in the number of ovulations.

Retinoids. Retinoids are a group of compounds that includes vitamin A, its natural derivatives, and thousands of synthetic analogs. They have been the focus of much interest and investigation into their ability to prevent cancer. Encouraging results with the use of fenretinide (4-HPR), a synthetic retinoid, were obtained by an Italian study looking into its use for the reduction in incidence of second breast cancers.[98,99] During the 5 years of intervention, no patients in the 4-HPR group developed ovarian cancer, compared with six patients in the control group. This was a statistically significant difference ($P = .0162$). Two patients in the 4-HPR group did develop an ovarian cancer in the follow-up period after the intervention, suggesting that any protective effect is restricted to the intervention period. Subsequently, several in vivo and in vitro studies showed that retinoids could effectively inhibit ovarian cancer growth and induce apoptosis at clinically relevant concentrations.

What should we aim for in the future?

The prevention and early diagnosis of ovarian cancer appears to be a promising way to reduce mortality from this disease. It is therefore important to establish the goals for future research:

- Completion of the randomized, controlled trials of ovarian cancer screening using the current screening methods to confirm a reduction in mortality from ovarian cancer screening, as well as documentation of the morbidity and cost involved in an ovarian cancer screening program
- Continued refinement in the way we use the current screening modalities, looking for improved ways of interpreting data from CA 125 determinations and imaging
- Development of new serum markers and imaging modalities and optimization of screening strategies to define risk groups within the population.
- Investigation and verification of new methods of early detection such as proteomics
- Better understanding of ovarian carcinogenesis and identification of premalignant ovarian conditions

REFERENCES

1. Teneriello MG, Park RC: Early detection of ovarian cancer. CA Cancer J Clin 1995;45:71-87.
2. Nguyen HN, Averette HE, Hoskins W, et al: National survey of ovarian carcinoma. VI. Critical assessment of current International Federation of Gynecology and Obstetrics staging system. Cancer 1993;72:3007-3011.
3. Skates SJ, Pauler DK, Symecko HL, et al: Estimated duration of pre-clinical ovarian cancer from longitudinal CA 125 levels. In AACR, 1999. Massachusetts General Hospital, Boston, MA 02114; St. Bartholomew's Hospital, London, UK; and Harvard Medical School, Boston, MA 02115.
4. Urban N, Drescher C, Etzioni R, Colby C: Use of a stochastic simulation model to identify an efficient protocol for ovarian cancer screening. Control Clin Trials 1997;18:251-270.
5. Law MR, Morris JK, Wald NJ: The importance of age in screening for cancer. J Med Screen 1999;6:16-20.
6. Goff BA, Mandel L, Muntz HG, Melancon CH: Ovarian carcinoma diagnosis. Cancer 2000;89:2068-2075.
7. Le T, Krepart GV, Lotocki RJ, Heywood MS: Clinically apparent early stage invasive epithelial ovarian carcinoma: Should all be treated similarly? Gynecol Oncol 1999;74:252-254.

8. Ahmed FY, Wiltshaw E, A'Hern RP, et al: Natural history and prognosis of untreated stage I epithelial ovarian carcinoma. J Clin Oncol 1996;14:2968-2975.

9. McIndoe WA, McLean MR, Jones RW, Mullins PR: The invasive potential of carcinoma in situ of the cervix. Obstet Gynecol 1984;64:451-458.

10. Lu KH, Bell DA, Welch WR, et al: Evidence for the multifocal origin of bilateral and advanced human serous borderline ovarian tumors. Cancer Res 1998;58:2328-2330.

11. Caduff RF, Svoboda-Newman SM, Ferguson AW, et al: Comparison of mutations of Ki-RAS and p53 immunoreactivity in borderline and malignant epithelial ovarian tumors. Am J Surg Pathol 1999;23:323-328.

12. Trope C, Kaern J: Management of borderline tumors of the ovary: State of the art. Semin Oncol 1998;25:372-380.

13. Darai E, Walker-Combrouze F, Mlika-Cabanne N, et al: Expression of p53 protein in borderline epithelial ovarian tumors: A clinicopathologic study of 39 cases. Eur J Gynaecol Oncol 1998;19:144-149.

14. Kupryjanczyk J, Bell DA, Dimeo D, et al: P53 gene analysis of ovarian borderline tumors and stage I carcinomas. Hum Pathol 1995;26:387-392.

15. Lodhi S, Najam S, Pervez S: DNA ploidy analysis of borderline epithelial ovarian tumours. J Pak Med Assoc 2000;50:349-351.

16. Crayford TJ, Campbell S, Bourne TH, et al: Benign ovarian cysts and ovarian cancer: A cohort study with implications for screening. Lancet 2000;355:1060-1063.

17. Hartge P, Hayes R, Sherman M, et al: Complex ovarian cysts in postmenopausal women are not associated with ovarian cancer risk factors: Preliminary data from the prostate, lung, colon, and ovarian cancer screening trial. Am J Obstet Gynecol 2000;183:1232-1237.

18. van Nagell JR Jr, Gallion HH, Pavlik EJ, DePriest PD: Ovarian cancer screening. Cancer 1995;76(Suppl):2086-2091.

19. Bast RC Jr, Feeney M, Lazarus H, et al: Reactivity of a monoclonal antibody with human ovarian carcinoma. J Clin Invest 1981;68:1331-1337.

20. Zurawski VR Jr, Orjaseter H, Andersen A, Jellum E: Elevated serum CA 125 levels prior to diagnosis of ovarian neoplasia: Relevance for early detection of ovarian cancer. Int J Cancer 1988;42:677-680.

21. Einhorn N, Sjovall K, Knapp RC, et al: Prospective evaluation of serum CA 125 levels for early detection of ovarian cancer. Obstet Gynecol 1992;80:14-18.

22. Skates SJ, Xu FJ, Yu YH, et al: Toward an optimal algorithm for ovarian cancer screening with longitudinal tumor markers. Cancer 1995;76(Suppl):2004-2010.

23. Jacobs I, Stabile I, Bridges J, et al: Multimodal approach to screening for ovarian cancer. Lancet 1988;1:268-271.

24. Jacobs I, Davies AP, Bridges J, et al: Prevalence screening for ovarian cancer in postmenopausal women by CA 125 measurement and ultrasonography. BMJ 1993;306:1030-1034.

25. Jacobs IJ, Skates S, Davies AP, et al: Risk of diagnosis of ovarian cancer after raised serum CA 125 concentration: A prospective cohort study. BMJ 1996;313:1355-1358.

26. Jacobs IJ, Skates SJ, MacDonald N, et al: Screening for ovarian cancer: A pilot randomised controlled trial. Lancet 1999;353:1207-1210.

27. Skates SJ, Singer DE: Quantifying the potential benefit of CA 125 screening for ovarian cancer. J Clin Epidemiol 1991;44:365-380.

28. Skates SJ, et al: Screening based on the risk of cancer calculation from Bayesian hierarchical change-point and mixture models of longitudinal markers. J Am Stat Assoc 2001;96:429-439.

29. Xu Y, Shen Z, Wiper DW, et al: Lysophosphatidic acid as a potential biomarker for ovarian and other gynecologic cancers. JAMA 1998;280:719-723.

30. Bast RC Jr, Xu FJ, Yu YH, et al: CA 125: The past and the future. Int J Biol Markers 1998;13:179-187.

31. Petricoin EF, Ardekani AM, Hitt BA, et al: Use of proteomic patterns in serum to identify ovarian cancer. Lancet 2002;359:572-577.

32. Campbell S, Bhan V, Royston P, et al: Transabdominal ultrasound screening for early ovarian cancer. BMJ 1989;299:1363-1367.

33. DePriest PD, Shenson D, Fried A, et al: A morphology index based on sonographic findings in ovarian cancer. Gynecol Oncol 1993;51:7-11.

34. van Nagell JR Jr, DePriest PD, Reedy MB, et al: The efficacy of transvaginal sonographic screening in asymptomatic women at risk for ovarian cancer. Gynecol Oncol 2000;77:350-356.

35. Carter JR, Lau M, Fowler JM, et al: Blood flow characteristics of ovarian tumors: Implications for ovarian cancer screening. Am J Obstet Gynecol 1995;172:901-907.

36. Predanic M, Vlahos N, Pennisi JA, et al: Color and pulsed Doppler sonography, gray-scale imaging, and serum CA 125 in the assessment of adnexal disease. Obstet Gynecol 1996;88:283-288.

37. Bourne TH, Campbell S, Reynolds KM, et al: Screening for early familial ovarian cancer with transvaginal ultrasonography and colour blood flow imaging. BMJ 1993;306:1025-1029.

38. Menon U, Jacobs I: Ovarian cancer screening in the general population. Ultrasound Obstet Gynecol 2000;15:350-353.

39. Prorok PC, Andriole GL, Bresalier RS, et al: Design of the Prostate, Lung, Colorectal and Ovarian (PLCO) Cancer Screening Trial. Control Clin Trials 2000;21(Suppl):273S-309S.

40. Gohagan JK, Prorok PC, Hayes RB, et al: The Prostate, Lung, Colorectal and Ovarian (PLCO) Cancer Screening Trial of the National Cancer Institute: History, organization, and status. Control Clin Trials 2000;21(Suppl):251S-272S.

41. Cottreau CM, Ness RB, Kriska AM: Physical activity and reduced risk of ovarian cancer. Obstet Gynecol 2000;96:609-614.

42. Tavani A, Gallus S, La Vecchia C, et al: Physical activity and risk of ovarian cancer: An Italian case-control study. Int J Cancer 2001;91:407-411.

43. Bertone ER, Willett WC, Rosner BA, et al: Prospective study of recreational physical activity and ovarian cancer. J Natl Cancer Inst 2001;93:942-948.

44. Mink PJ, Folsom AR, Sellers TA, Kushi LH: Physical activity, waist-to-hip ratio, and other risk factors for ovarian cancer: A follow-up study of older women. Epidemiology 1996;7:38-45.

45. Bosetti C, Negri E, Franceshi S, et al: Diet and ovarian cancer risk: A case-control study in Italy. Int J Cancer 2001;93:911-915.

46. Kushi LH, Mink PJ, Folsom AR, et al: Prospective study of diet and ovarian cancer. Am J Epidemiol 1999;149:21-31.

47. La Vecchia C, Decarli A, Negri E, et al: Dietary factors and the risk of epithelial ovarian cancer. J Natl Cancer Inst 1987;79:663-669.

48. Serra-Majem L, La Vecchia C, Ribas-Barba L, et al: Changes in diet and mortality from selected cancers in southern Mediterranean countries, 1960-1989. Eur J Clin Nutr 1993;47(Suppl 1):S25-S34.

49. Tzonou A, Hsieh CC, Polychronopoulou A, et al: Diet and ovarian cancer: A case-control study in Greece. Int J Cancer 1993;55:411-414.

50. Bertone ER, Rosner BA, Hunter DJ, et al: Dietary fat intake and ovarian cancer in a cohort of US women. Am J Epidemiol 2002;156:22-31.

51. Shu XO, Gao YT, Yuan JM, et al: Dietary factors and epithelial ovarian cancer. Br J Cancer 1989;59:92-96.

52. Goodman MT, Wu AH, Tung KH, et al: Association of dairy products, lactose, and calcium with the risk of ovarian cancer. Am J Epidemiol 2002;156:148-157.

53. Yen ML, Yen BL, Bai CH, Lin RS: Risk factors for ovarian cancer in Taiwan: A case-control study in a low-incidence population. Gynecol Oncol 2003;89:318-324.

54. Bertone ER, Hankinson HE, Newcomb PA, et al: A population-based case-control study of carotenoid and vitamin A intake and ovarian cancer (United States). Cancer Causes Control 2001;12:83-90.

55. Engle A, Muscat JE, Harris RE: Nutritional risk factors and ovarian cancer. Nutr Cancer 1991;15:239-247.

56. Fairfield KM, Hankinson SE, Rosner BA, et al: Risk of ovarian carcinoma and consumption of vitamins A, C, and E specific carotenoids: A prospective analysis. Cancer 2001;92:2318-2326.

57. Whittemore AS, Harris R, Itnyre J: Characteristics relating to ovarian cancer risk: Collaborative analysis of 12 US case-control studies. II. Invasive epithelial ovarian cancers in white women. Collaborative Ovarian Cancer Group. Am J Epidemiol 1992;136:1184-1203.

58. Adami HO, Hsieh CC, Lambe M, et al: Parity, age at first childbirth, and risk of ovarian cancer. Lancet 1994;344:1250-1254.

59. Cooper GS, Schildkraut JM, Whittemore AS, Marchbanks PA, et al: Pregnancy recency and risk of ovarian cancer. Cancer Causes Control 1999;10:397-402.

60. Titus-Ernstoff L, Perez K, Cramer DW, et al: Menstrual and reproductive factors in relation to ovarian cancer risk. Br J Cancer 2001;84:714-7121.
61. Parazzini F, Chatenoud L, Chiantera V, et al: Population attributable risk for ovarian cancer. Eur J Cancer 2000;36:520-524.
62. Risch HA, Marrett LD, Howe GR: Parity, contraception, infertility, and the risk of epithelial ovarian cancer. Am J Epidemiol 1994;140:585-597.
63. Chiaffarino F, Pelucchi C, Parazzini F, et al: Reproductive and hormonal factors and ovarian cancer. Ann Oncol 2001;12: 337-341.
64. Chiaffarino F, Parazzini F, Negri E, et al: Time since last birth and the risk of ovarian cancer. Gynecol Oncol 2001;81:233-236.
65. Modan B, Hartge P, Hirsh-Yechezkel G, et al, for the National Israel Ovarian Cancer Study Group: Parity, oral contraceptives, and the risk of ovarian cancer among carriers and noncarriers of a BRCA1 or BRCA2 mutation. N Engl J Med 2001;345: 235-240.
66. Greggi S, Parazzini F, Paratore MP, et al: Risk factors for ovarian cancer in central Italy. Gynecol Oncol 2000;79:50-54.
67. The reduction in risk of ovarian cancer associated with oral-contraceptive use. The Cancer and Steroid Hormone Study of the Centers for Disease Control and the National Institute of Child Health and Human Development. N Engl J Med 1987;316: 650-655.
68. Schneider AP 2nd: Risk factor for ovarian cancer. N Engl J Med 1987;317:508-509.
69. Weiss NS, Lyon JL, Liff JM, et al: Incidence of ovarian cancer in relation to the use of oral contraceptives. Int J Cancer 1981;28: 669-671.
70. Rossing MA, Daling JR, Weiss NS, et al: Ovarian tumors in a cohort of infertile women. N Engl J Med 1994;331:771-776.
71. Shushan A, Paltiel O, Iscovich J, et al: Human menopausal gonadotropin and the risk of epithelial ovarian cancer. Fertil Steril 1996;65:13-18.
72. Potashnik G, Lerner-Geva L, Genkin L, et al: Fertility drugs and the risk of breast and ovarian cancers: Results of a long-term follow-up study. Fertil Steril 1999;71:853-859.
73. Venn A, Watson L, Lumley J, et al: Breast and ovarian cancer incidence after infertility and in vitro fertilisation. Lancet 1995;346:995-1000.
74. Modan B, Ron E, Lerner-Geva L, et al: Cancer incidence in a cohort of infertile women. Am J Epidemiol 1998;147:1038-1042.
75. Mosgaard BJ, Lidegaard O, Kjaer SK, et al: Infertility, fertility drugs, and invasive ovarian cancer: A case-control study. Fertil Steril 1997;67:1005-1012.
76. Lacey JV Jr, Mink PJ, Lubin JH, et al: Menopausal hormone replacement therapy and risk of ovarian cancer. JAMA 2002; 288:334-341.
77. Rodriguez C, Patel AV, Calle EE, et al: Estrogen replacement therapy and ovarian cancer mortality in a large prospective study of US women. JAMA 2001;285:1460-1465.
78. Booth M, Beral V, Smith P: Risk factors for ovarian cancer: A case-control study. Br J Cancer 1989;60:592-598.
79. Hankinson SE, Hunter DJ, Colditz GA, et al: Tubal ligation, hysterectomy, and risk of ovarian cancer: A prospective study. JAMA 1993;270:2813-2818.
80. Rosenberg L, Palmer JR, Zauber AG, et al: A case-control study of oral contraceptive use and invasive epithelial ovarian cancer. Am J Epidemiol 1994;139:654-661.
81. Irwin KL, Weiss NS, Lee NC, Peterson HB: Tubal sterilization, hysterectomy, and the subsequent occurrence of epithelial ovarian cancer. Am J Epidemiol 1991;134:362-369.
82. Rosenblatt KA, Thomas DB: Reduced risk of ovarian cancer in women with a tubal ligation or hysterectomy. The World Health Organization Collaborative Study of Neoplasia and Steroid Contraceptives. Cancer Epidemiol Biomarkers Prev 1996;5: 933-935.
83. Narod SA, Sun P, Ghadirian P, et al: Tubal ligation and risk of ovarian cancer in carriers of BRCA1 or BRCA2 mutations: A case-control study. Lancet 2001;357:1467-1470.
84. Hartge P, Hoover R, McGowan L, et al: Menopause and ovarian cancer. Am J Epidemiol 1988;127:990-998.
85. Kauff ND, Satagopan JM, Robson ME, et al: Risk-reducing salpingo-oophorectomy in women with a BRCA1 or BRCA2 mutation. N Engl J Med 2002;346:1609-1615.
86. Rebbeck TR, Lynch HT, Neuhausen SL, et al: Prophylactic oophorectomy in carriers of BRCA1 or BRCA2 mutations. N Engl J Med 2002;346:1616-1622.
87. Rebbeck TR, Levin AM, Eisen A, et al: Breast cancer risk after bilateral prophylactic oophorectomy in BRCA1 mutation carriers. J Natl Cancer Inst 1999;91:1475-1479.
88. Oral contraceptive use and the risk of ovarian cancer. The Centers for Disease Control Cancer and Steroid Hormone Study. JAMA 1983;249:1596-1599.
89. Hankinson SE, Volditz GA, Hunter DJ, et al: A quantitative assessment of oral contraceptive use and risk of ovarian cancer. Obstet Gynecol 1992;80:708-714.
90. Ness RB, Grisso JA, Klapper J, et al: Risk of ovarian cancer in relation to estrogen and progestin dose and use characteristics of oral contraceptives. SHARE Study Group. Steroid Hormones and Reproductions. Am J Epidemiol 2000;152:233-241.
91. Narod SA, Risch H, Moslehi R, et al: Oral contraceptives and the risk of hereditary ovarian cancer. Hereditary Ovarian Cancer Clinical Study Group. N Engl J Med 1998;339:424-428.
92. Siskind V, Green A, Bain C, Purdie D: Beyond ovulation: Oral contraceptives and epithelial ovarian cancer. Epidemiology 2000;11:106-110.
93. Cramer DW, Welch WR: Determinants of ovarian cancer risk. II. Inferences regarding pathogenesis. J Natl Cancer Inst 1983;71:717-721.
94. Parazzini F, Franceschi S, La Vecchia C, Fasoli M: The epidemiology of ovarian cancer. Gynecol Oncol 1991;43:9-23.
95. Risch HA: Hormonal etiology of epithelial ovarian cancer, with a hypothesis concerning the role of androgens and progesterone. J Natl Cancer Inst 1998;90:1774-1786.
96. Depot-medroxyprogesterone acetate (DMPA) and risk of epithelial ovarian cancer. The WHO Collaborative Study of Neoplasia and Steroid Contraceptives. Int J Cancer 1991;49:191-195.
97. Liang AP, Levenson AG, Layde PM, et al: Risk of breast, uterine corpus, and ovarian cancer in women receiving medroxyprogesterone injections. JAMA 1983;249:2909-2912.
98. De Palo G, Veronesi U, Camerini T, et al: Can fenretinide protect women against ovarian cancer? J Natl Cancer Inst 1995;87:146-147.
99. De Palo G, Mariani L, Camerini T, et al: Effect of fenretinide on ovarian carcinoma occurrence. Gynecol Oncol 2002;86:24-27.
100. van Nagell JR Jr, DePriest PD, Reedy MB, et al: The efficacy of transvaginal sonographic screening in asymptomatic women at risk for ovarian cancer. Gynecol Oncol 2000;77:350-356.
101. DePriest PD, Gallion HH, Pavlik EJ, et al: Transvaginal sonography as a screening method for the detection of early ovarian cancer. Gynecol Oncol 1997;65:408-414.
102. van Nagell JR Jr, Gallion HH, Pavlik EJ, DePriest PD, et al: Ovarian cancer screening. Cancer 1995;76(Suppl):2086-2091.
103. Sato S, Yokoyama Y, Sakamoto T, et al: Usefulness of mass screening for ovarian carcinoma using transvaginal ultrasonography. Cancer 2000;89:582-588.
104. Hayashi H, Yaginuma Y, Kitamura S, et al: Bilateral oophorectomy in asymptomatic women over 50 years old selected by ovarian cancer screening. Gynecol Obstet Invest 1999;47:58-64.
105. Tabor A, Jensen FR, Bock JE, Hogdall CK: Feasibility study of a randomised trial of ovarian cancer screening. J Med Screen 1994;1:215-219.
106. Campbell S, Bhan V, Royston P, et al: Transabdominal ultrasound screening for early ovarian cancer. BMJ 1989;299: 1363-1367.
107. Millo R, Facca MC, Alberico S: Sonographic evaluation of ovarian volume in postmenopausal women: A screening test for ovarian cancer? Clin Exp Obstet Gynecol 1989;16:72-78.
108. Goswamy RK, Campbell S, Whitehead MI: Screening for ovarian cancer. Clin Obstet Gynaecol 1983;10:621-643.
109. Kurjak A, Shalan H, Kupesic S, et al: An attempt to screen asymptomatic women for ovarian and endometrial cancer with transvaginal color and pulsed Doppler sonography. J Ultrasound Med 1994;13:295-301.
110. Vuento MH, Pirhonen JP, Makinen JI, et al: Evaluation of ovarian findings in asymptomatic postmenopausal women with color Doppler ultrasound. Cancer 1995;76:1214-1218.
111. Parkes CA, Smith D, Wald NJ, Bourne TH: Feasibility study of a randomised trial of ovarian cancer screening among the general population. J Med Screen 1994;1:209-214.

112. Holbert TR: Screening transvaginal ultrasonography of post-menopausal women in a private office setting. Am J Obstet Gynecol 1994;170:1699-1703.

113. Schincaglia P, Brondelli L, Cicognani A, et al: A feasibility study of ovarian cancer screening: Does fine-needle aspiration improve ultrasound specificity? Tumori 1994;80:181-187.

114. Grover S, Quinn MA, Weideman P, et al: Screening for ovarian cancer using serum CA125 and vaginal examination: Report on 2550 females. Int J Gynecol Cancer 1995;5:291-295.

115. Adonakis GL, Paraskevaidis E, Tsiga S, et al: A combined approach for the early detection of ovarian cancer in asymptomatic women. Eur J Obstet Gynecol Reprod Biol 1996;65:221-225.

116. Beard CM, Hartmann LC, Atkinson EJ, et al: The epidemiology of ovarian cancer: A population-based study in Olmsted County, Minnesota, 1935-1991. Ann Epidemiol 2000;10:14-23.

117. Beral V, Hermon C, Kay C, et al: Mortality associated with oral contraceptive use: 25 year follow-up of cohort of 46,000 women from Royal College of General Practitioners' Oral Contraception Study. BMJ 1999;318:96-100.

118. Hankinson SE, Colditz GA, Hunter DJ, et al: A prospective study of reproductive factors and risk of epithelial ovarian cancer. Cancer 1995;76:284-290.

119. Vessey MP, Painter P: Endometrial and ovarian cancer and oral contraceptives—findings in a large cohort study. Br J Cancer 1995;71:1340-1342.

120. Purdie D, Green A, Bain C, et al: Reproductive and other factors and risk of epithelial ovarian cancer: An Australian case-control study. Survey of Women's Health Study Group. Int J Cancer 1995;62:678-684.

121. John EM, Whittemore AS, Harris R, Itnyre J: Characteristics relating to ovarian cancer risk: Collaborative analysis of seven U.S. case-control studies. Epithelial ovarian cancer in black women. Collaborative Ovarian Cancer Group. J Natl Cancer Inst 1993;85:142-147.

122. Polychronopoulou A, Tzonou A, Hsieh CC, et al: Reproductive variables, tobacco, ethanol, coffee and somatometry as risk factors for ovarian cancer. Int J Cancer 1993;55:402-407.

123. Harris R, Whittemore AS, Itnyre J: Characteristics relating to ovarian cancer risk: Collaborative analysis of 12 US case-control studies. III. Epithelial tumors of low malignant potential in white women. Collaborative Ovarian Cancer Group. Am J Epidemiol 1992;136:1204-1211.

124. Rosenblatt KA, Thomas DB, Noonan EA: High-dose and low-dose combined oral contraceptives: Protection against epithelial ovarian cancer and the length of the protective effect. The WHO Collaborative Study of Neoplasia and Steroid Contraceptives. Eur J Cancer 1992;28A:1872-1876.

125. Gross TP, Schlesselman JJ, Stadel BV, et al: The risk of epithelial ovarian cancer in short-term users of oral contraceptives. Am J Epidemiol 1992;136:46-53.

126. Franceschi S, Parazzini F, Negri E, et al: Pooled analysis of 3 European case-control studies of epithelial ovarian cancer: III. Oral contraceptive use. Int J Cancer 1991;49:61-65.

127. Parazzini F, Restelli C, La Vecchia C, et al: Risk factors for epithelial ovarian tumours of borderline malignancy. Int J Epidemiol 1991;20:871-877.

128. Parazzini F, La Vecchia C, Negri E, et al: Oral contraceptive use and the risk of ovarian cancer: An Italian case-control study. Eur J Cancer 1991;27:594-588.

129. Hartge P, Schiffman MH, Hoover R, et al: A case-control study of epithelial ovarian cancer. Am J Obstet Gynecol 1989;161:10-16.

130. Epithelial ovarian cancer and combined oral contraceptives. The WHO Collaborative Study of Neoplasia and Steroid Contraceptives. Int J Epidemiol 1989;18:538-545.

131. Shu XO, Brinton LA, Gao YT, Yuan JM: Population-based case-control study of ovarian cancer in Shanghai. Cancer Res 1989;49:3670-3674.

132. Wu ML, Whittemore AS, Paffenbarger RS Jr, et al: Personal and environmental characteristics related to epithelial ovarian cancer. I. Reproductive and menstrual events and oral contraceptive use. Am J Epidemiol 1988;128:1216-1227.

133. Harlow BL, Weiss NS, Roth GJ, et al: Case-control study of borderline ovarian tumors: Reproductive history and exposure to exogenous female hormones. Cancer Res 1988;48:5849-5852.

134. La Vecchia C, Decarli A, Fasoli M, et al: Oral contraceptives and cancers of the breast and of the female genital tract. Interim results from a case-control study. Br J Cancer 1986;54:311-317.

135. Tzonou A, Day NE, Trichopoulos D, et al: The epidemiology of ovarian cancer in Greece: A case-control study. Eur J Cancer Clin Oncol 1984;20:1045-1052.

136. Risch HA, Weiss NS, Lyon JL, et al: Events of reproductive life and the incidence of epithelial ovarian cancer. Am J Epidemiol 1983;117:128-139.

137. Rosenberg L, Shapiro S, Slone D, et al: Epithelial ovarian cancer and combination oral contraceptives. JAMA 1982;247:3210-3212.

138. Cramer DW, Hutchinson GB, Cramer DW, et al: Factors affecting the association of oral contraceptives and ovarian cancer. N Engl J Med 1982;307:1047-1051.

139. Franceschi S, La Vecchia C, Helmrich SP, et al: Risk factors for epithelial ovarian cancer in Italy. Am J Epidemiol 1982;115:714-719.

140. Hildreth NG, Kelsey JL, LiVolsi VA, et al: An epidemiologic study of epithelial carcinoma of the ovary. Am J Epidemiol 1981;114:398-405.

141. Willett WC, Bain C, Hennekens CH, et al: Oral contraceptives and risk of ovarian cancer. Cancer 1981;48:1684-1687.

142. Ramcharan S, Pellegrin FA, Ray RM, Hsu JP: The Walnut Creek Contraceptive Drug Study. A prospective study of the side effects of oral contraceptives. Volume III, an interim report: A comparison of disease occurrence leading to hospitalization or death in users and nonusers of oral contraceptives. J Reprod Med 1980;25(Suppl):345-372.

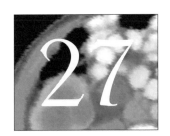

PATHOLOGY OF OVARIAN, FALLOPIAN TUBE, AND PRIMARY PERITONEAL CANCER

Melissa J. Robbie

◆ MAJOR CONTROVERSIES

- How important is specialist gynecologic pathology in managing ovarian cancer, and how should it be defined?
- How valuable is frozen section for ovarian masses?
- Which grading systems should we use?
- Should we measure hormone receptor levels, and if so, how?
- Should we be freezing fresh ovarian tumor tissue for future molecular studies or other research?
- When should the physician suspect familial cancer in an ovarian cancer patient?
- What is the role of *BRCA* and other tumor suppressor genes in sporadic versus hereditary ovarian cancers?
- What is the earliest cancer lesion or precursor in the ovary?
- Do we need to change our pathology methods, and are we examining prophylactic oophorectomy specimens closely enough?
- What features best differentiate metastases from primary ovarian carcinoma?
- What are pseudomyxoma peritonei, disseminated peritoneal adenomucinosis, and peritoneal mucinous carcinomatosis?
- When does endometriosis lead to cancer?
- Do tumor-infiltrating lymphocytes inhibit ovarian cancer?
- How useful are markers and other prognostic factors?
- How can tubal and primary peritoneal cancers be differentiated from ovarian primaries, and how can they be diagnostically categorized?

How important is specialist gynecologic pathology in managing ovarian cancer, and how should it be defined?

It has been established in the United Kingdom that patients referred initially (e.g., for primary diagnosis and treatment) to multidisciplinary centers specializing in ovarian cancer have notably better outcomes. This is at least partly attributable to the quality of debulking and optimal staging by specialist gynecologic oncologists.[1] Accurate frozen section diagnosis facilitates this by avoiding underdiagnosis, understaging, and underuse of chemotherapy. One study found acute frozen section diagnosis to be more common from pathologists in a community hospital than in a teaching hospital.[2]

The clinicopathologic team conference is probably another factor in the better outcome of multi-discipline centers. The clinicopathologic team conference has been regarded as axiomatic in other areas of specialized tumor management, such as bone tumors. Such sessions may facilitate appropriately generous use of chemotherapy. The pathologist's role in this setting is one of communicator regarding all aspects of tumor prognostication.

There have been no studies to quantify other contributions from pathology factors. These are difficult to separate from the effects of using specialist gynecologist-oncologists because quality in pathology tends to coincide with the presence of a specialist gyne-oncology unit. Certainly, in breast cancer, it has been shown that completeness of recording prognostic factors is higher among pathologists who see large numbers of such cancers and who are working in hospital laboratories that see large numbers of such cases.[3]

Training of pathologists. No specific guidelines exist for the extent of training in ovarian cancer and related areas. It seems desirable for pathologists in training to rotate at least for a 3-month period through a laboratory in which there is a significant throughput of gynecologic cancers, with emphasis on learning specimen cut up protocols, because expert review at a later stage cannot compensate for inadequately taken tissue blocks.

Synoptic reporting. There is strong support for the use of standardized reporting protocols.[3,4] They help ensure all relevant prognostic information is assessed and reported, using standardized and therefore more reproducible methods.

Ovarian cancer is an area with a particularly high level of altered diagnosis or grade, or both, on centralized review. Some of this alteration may reflect more experienced or dedicated pathologists' improved assessment, but some alteration results from the poorly defined criteria used, with low reproducibility, especially for grading.[5] Proposals for more reproducible criteria exist and may help to overcome this problem, as detailed in the following sections.

How valuable is frozen section for ovarian masses?

The frozen section analysis aims to separate benign, borderline, and malignant lesions; decide if cancers are primary or metastatic; and pick up special neoplasms such as granulosa cell tumors and lymphomas. Correct diagnosis is most important for the young woman wanting fertility conservation and the older woman for whom unnecessary procedures pose a greater danger. Ovarian lesions produce the highest frozen section error rate in gynecologic surgery (Fig. 27-1).[6]

The overall accuracy of ovarian frozen section has been found to be good for malignant tumors. The sensitivity rate was 92.5%, and a diagnosis of malignancy had a positive predictive power of 99%.[7]

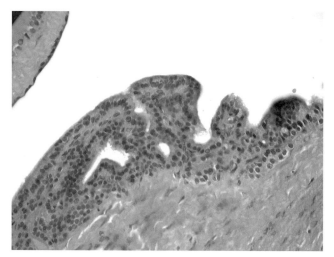

Figure 27–1. Cystic struma ovarii can mimic borderline tumors on frozen section (hematoxylin & eosin stain, magnification ×400).

A study of borderline tumors found a correct frozen section diagnosis in 86% of cases in teaching hospitals but only 58% in the more common community hospital setting.[2] Overdiagnosis of malignancy was twice as common as underdiagnosis.

A study of laparoscopic investigation of isolated ovarian masses included 13 lesions that on final histologic examination were found to be borderline or malignant. Three of these were missed intraoperatively despite frozen section.[8]

Under real-world conditions, frozen section is least accurate at diagnosing malignancy in the lower-grade or borderline and low-stage lesions. One reason for this is inadequate sampling when only one small block is examined, which is the norm. This is particularly risky for very large and for mucinous tumors, in which malignancy tends to be heavily underdiagnosed.[6,9] If this problem is anticipated, several frozen section blocks can be frozen simultaneously and then cut in quick succession to give a more accurate diagnosis with only minor delay.

Differentiating metastases from primaries is expected to be difficult on one small block with no adjuvant stains; there is a limit to what can be expected from frozen sections (Fig. 27-2). Studies showed 13 of 17 and 13 of 16 metastatic tumors were distinguished by frozen section; the experience level of the pathologist was not indicated, but the pathologist was presumed to be from a specialist center.[6,7]

Which grading systems should we use?

Numerous studies show the grade of ovarian carcinomas to be an independent prognostic factor, even when the method is unspecified, despite the fact that many studies have shown poor interobserver correlation.[10]

Some previous methods, such as those of the World Health Organization (WHO), were good at discriminating at the top and bottom ends of the spectrum of

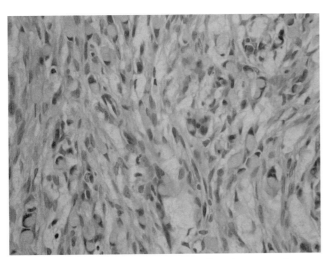

Figure 27–2. Krukenberg tumors can confuse the unwary by mimicking a sarcoma on frozen section (hematoxylin & eosin stain, magnification ×400).

disease, but the findings for grade II tumors tended to be unpredictable.[10] Some methods give great reproducibility but have very little prognostic power.[11]

There is evidence that different features give the best grading prognostication in different histotypes, but some principles apply across most of the common types. From these principles, a universal grading system has been developed that has the advantage of systematic criteria and applicability to mixed histotypes. The authors suggest that reproducibility is good in their hands, although no measures of this are given.[12] There is good predictive power across high and low stages for nearly all types.[13,14] The method combines a mitotic score (0-3), a nuclear atypia score (0-3), and an architectural score based on the dominant pattern (glandular = 1, papillary or sloppy cribriform pattern related to papillae = 2, and solid = 3).

Another group reviewed the universal method and found that, although it did well in their hands, the assessment of nuclear grade alone (by two pathologists jointly assessing the worst area) was even slightly better as a prognostic discriminator than the full three-component grade.[15] One advantage of using nuclear grade alone for clear and transitional cell types is that architecture is known not to discriminate in these two less common types and mitotic cutoffs for clear cell types do not match those for other types[13]; nuclear grade therefore is the most universally relevant. However, because there were few clear cell and no transitional types in the study, the study's results probably reflect the relative precision with which pathologists were able to grade their nuclei as opposed to their architectural or mitotic grading. Close reading of the papers introducing the universal grading system shows that the researchers also found only poor prognostication from mitotic grade, and it is not clear that including it adds any power to the grading system except for the clear cell type, for which a special low cutoff point is needed in any case.

Morphometry has been suggested as a means to improve the accuracy of nuclear grading. Although still requiring decisions about which field and which nuclei to measure, this subjective component is minimized if strict guidelines are followed and multiple areas are visually "sampled."[10]

Mean nuclear area (MNA) has been found to exceed grading as a prognosticator in cases of endometrial cancer,[16] which share many similarities with ovarian epithelial tumors. This suggests that investigation of MNA of ovarian cells is needed. Standard deviation of the MNA (SDMNA), a measure of pleomorphism, was found in one study to be a strong prognosticator in advanced-stage ovarian tumors.[17]

These measures unfortunately require sophisticated, relatively expensive, and time-consuming use of video and software programs that are not likely to become available in most laboratories. However, a study on thyroid neoplasms found that simpler and cheaper methods of assessment using a routine microscope equipped with a micrometer gave results with equally good reproducibility. They assessed percentage of nucleolated nuclei, percentage of nuclei with two or more nucleoli, and mean major nuclear diameter.[18] It may be possible to use these types of measures as a substitute for the subjective nuclear assessment in the universal grading system.

Mitotic activity reproducibility tends to be low in most studies.[16] The rate of reproducibility can be lifted by careful attendance to a strict protocol, good-quality sections, and especially the use of ongoing quality-assurance feedback.[19] Correction for the size of high-power fields (HPFs) is also desirable.[15]

Questions about cellularity and architectural pattern are mixed with the proliferative rate per cell in the assessment of the mitotic index. In breast cancer, the independent prognostic significance of a mitotic count was strengthened by weighting it for an assessment of the cellularity per field (i.e., volume percent epithelium [VPE]). This may also be relevant in studying ovarian cancer. However, evidence suggests that there is only a mild improvement in the predictive power for breast cancer from adding VPE as a compensating variable.[20]

Conclusions on grading methods. The appeal of using nuclear grade alone is that it is simple and predictive across all histotypes. However, it would be undesirable to throw out independent prognostic information from the architectural component of the universal score for most tumors (i.e., serous, mucinous, and endometrioid types) for which it is relevant. A combination of nuclear grade and architectural grade for these and mixed tumors seems desirable, and the use of nuclear grade and mitosis count (cutoff point of 6 mitoses per 10 HPFs imparts significance[21]) is suggested for predominately clear cell tumors. The advantage of morphometry is that a quantitative cutoff can be used rather than a qualitative one, facilitating reproducibility between laboratories. An alternative is for a teaching set of images used as nuclear grading references at the laboratory that determined best prognostic cutoffs to be made available over the

Internet. All other laboratories could then make visual reference to this standard set. Quantitation may be useful for central reference laboratories and external quality-assurance programs. Such an approach is the most practical method of lifting world reporting standards using current technology.

Implications of a universal grading system. Many papers have observed prognostic differences between different histotypes (e.g., serous do worse than endometrioid tumors). A universal grading system subsumes such differences. For example, grade for grade, serous and endometrioid types should have the same prognosis, but there would be more endometrioid tumors in the grade 1 category. So do we need to consider histotype at all? It seems likely that histotypes will be even more important in the future as therapeutic options widen. They already tell us important information about chemotherapy. For instance, the response rate of mucinous and clear cell types to cisplatin is much less than for serous and endometrioid tumors, and endometrioid types respond better to cyclophosphamide, doxorubicin, plus cisplatin than to cyclophosphamide plus cisplatin.[12]

Should we measure hormone receptor levels, and if so, how?

Comparison of the radioligand binding assay on fresh frozen tissue with the semiquantitative method on immunostaining showed poor correlation, especially in the less cellular tissues.[22] The assay is impaired if there is any delay in freezing the specimen. Immunostaining is plagued by batch-to-batch staining variation.

In a study of unselected ovarian carcinomas, progesterone receptor positivity (by assay) was an independent variable favoring good prognosis (RR = 2.3),[23] whereas estrogen receptor (ER) levels showed no correlation. However, a study in patients with optimally cytoreduced stage IIIc serous carcinoma found low ER levels (by assay) gave a better prognosis.[24] This is paradoxical given that previous studies have shown low ER levels (by immunostaining) were associated with a worse prognosis, a finding confirmed for high-stage serous tumors by a refined method using assay scores corrected for percentage of tumor cells from histologic examination of the adjacent block of tissue.[25] The low levels of ERs determined by assay in the study by Zeimet and colleagues[22] might have been a reflection of low tumor cell numbers per gram. It seems that any study using the assay method needs to look at cellularity as a correcting factor before interpretation.

Should we be freezing fresh ovarian tumor tissue for future molecular studies or other research?

DNA fingerprint analysis of ovarian tumors by in situ hybridization (using the satellite probes 33.15, 228S and 216S) has been found in trials to be a sensitive method for detecting changes in tumor DNA and for investigating clonality.[26] cDNA microarray chips have been used to subcategorize tumors, and they show promise as a method for predicting chemosensitivities in the near future.[27]

Although DNA analysis is currently a research method, it may yield valuable results in the future to guide chemotherapy for advanced or recurrent disease. It may be appropriate to "bank" a small (0.5 cm in diameter) segment of the tumor at $-70°C$ in case future analysis is required. This is appropriate only when the tumor tissue is present in marked excess to sampling requirements for the routine histopathologic examination.

Similarly, some fresh frozen tissue may be wanted purely for research purposes. This area needs further clarification, as does using separate paraffin blocks for research purposes. The U.S. Department of Health guidelines permit both of these approaches when the tissue is clearly surplus and specific patient-identifying details are not attached. A diagnosis is obtained, because the sample is otherwise of no research benefit. Such a mechanism would need to be suitable to the laboratory concerned. Primary tumors with an estimated volume of more than 100 cm^3 (i.e., average diameter of 5 cm or larger) could be safely regarded as having "surplus" material to sample.

When should the physician suspect familial cancer in an ovarian cancer patient?

In *BRCA1* cases, the ovarian tumor excess over normal population appears to be almost entirely serous carcinomas (not borderline tumors) from ovarian and peritoneal sites, and the average age at diagnosis is 10 years younger than for sporadic cases.[28] If a woman with a positive family history is of Ashkenazi Jewish descent, the chance of carrying *BRCA1* is much higher. *BRCA2* patients also appear to have an excess of serous papillary tumors and fewer borderline tumors compared with sporadic cases, although this is less well documented.[28]

A breast cancer patient is most likely to carry the *BRCA1* gene if the tumor was found to be medullary or atypical medullary, if it was high grade and ER negative, and if the diagnosis was made before the patient was 36 years old. Adding these features stratifies women much more effectively as likely *BRCA1* carriers or not than does family history alone.[29] Most *BRCA1* carriers have no significant family history. If a patient with ovarian serous carcinoma has a history of breast cancer or any relative with breast cancer, it is important to review the pathology report before assessing her likelihood of genetic disease.

Patients with a genetic defect causing MSI are more likely to have ovarian *mucinous* tumors.[30] For women presenting with mucinous carcinomas, the examiner should look for a kindred with a variety of cancers occurring at high frequency, especially colon cancer at an early age and endometrial cancer.[31]

What is the role of *BRCA* and other tumor suppressor genes in sporadic versus hereditary ovarian cancers?

In patients identified with hereditary ovarian cancer, almost 75% have a mutant *BRCA1* gene. In 15% to 20%, the affected gene is *BRCA2*, and in 10%, it is one of the mismatch repair genes (*MLH1* or *MSH2*).[28]

BRCA1 and *BRCA2* have similar functions, as well as similar gene architecture, and both genes have a large exon 11 region. They are expressed similarly in tissues, and they both seem to combine a role in DNA repair with increasing the transcription rates of other genes (through their zinc finger motif), such as that for p21 (WAF1/CIP1), which also responds to DNA injury. Their DNA repair role includes colocalization with *RAD1*, which has a key role in homologous recombination (i.e., using the matching undamaged DNA strand as template to fix a damaged one).[28]

In cell cultures, complete loss of *BRCA1* or *BRCA2* function causes the cells to die, but only if the pathway of P53 induction of peptide p21 (WAF1/CIP1) is intact. The current view is that if a cell has lost both *BRCA1* copies, it has to also lose at least one link in the P53/21 pathway before it can lead to malignancy.[28] Otherwise, this pathway would cause apoptosis rather than allow mitosis to continue with DNA damage unrepaired. There is evidence that *TP53* loss or inactivation is present in most hereditary ovarian cancers, whereas in sporadic cancers, *TP53* is usually lost only in the high-grade tumors (e.g., those with *BRCA1*).

Entry into the G_1 phase (i.e., DNA replication) of the cell cycle before DNA is repaired is regarded as the dominant cause of accumulating large amounts of random DNA loss (or gain) and therefore causing the onset of malignancy. Loss of the P53 pathway as above is one way this can happen. The retinoblastoma gene (*RB1*) pathway that includes cyclin D1 is also essential to prevent premature DNA replication, and in sporadic tumors, it is often the one inactivated, forming an alternate route to cancer.[32]

In nonhereditary ovarian carcinomas, mutation of *BRCA* genes is uncommon, but newer results show *BRCA* inactivation by hypermethylation of its promoter is reasonably common in sporadic tumors.[33] However, loss of RNA or protein BRCA1 expression in sporadic tumors of the breast and ovary usually occurs only in higher-grade tumors.[29] Although loss of heterozygosity (LOH) in the 17q region occurs in up to 80% of sporadic ovarian tumors, fine deletion studies have shown that this most often affects an area of the chromosome slightly distal to *BRCA1*.[31]

Normal *BRCA1* expression appears to be regulated by steroid hormones.[31] A study on an ovarian tumor cell line with wild-type *BRCA1* showed that the tumor ceased to depend on estrogen for survival after *BRCA1* was inactivated (by transfection with antisense RNA to *BRCA1* to bind up any *BRCA1*-encoded RNA).[34] The cells then showed a growth advantage in vitro and in a mouse model, implying that estrogen had been necessary to suppress a *BRCA1* function that inhibited mitosis. All of this evidence suggests that, in sporadic cases, loss of *BRCA1* is a promoter but not an initiator of malignancy.

What is the earliest cancer lesion or precursor in the ovary?

The first question to be answered is how often borderline tumors, if not excised, evolve into carcinomas. There is wide variation in the percentage of carcinomas diagnosed as having adjacent borderline or benign components, from rare to 56%. Equally, there is controversy about how often small areas of invasion are found in otherwise borderline tumors.[28] Both problems presumably reflect variations in criteria and the number of sections examined. Personal experience suggests that a residual clearly recognizable cystadenofibroma (Fig. 27-3) is more common than residual simple benign or borderline cystadenoma, possibly because the dense stroma makes them harder for the carcinoma to colonize and destroy.

Despite initial enthusiasm for claims of dysplastic lesions being detected in the prophylactic oophorectomy specimens of *BRCA* carriers (and contralateral ovaries of patients with stage I carcinoma), no confirmation of a reproducible difference from age-matched controls has been found on blinded examination, even when they are studied for P53 expression.[28] However, prophylactic oophorectomies have revealed microscopic invasive carcinomas within ovarian cortex, growing as ovarian surface lesions, and more surprisingly, within the fallopian tube.[35]

It seems likely that concentration on studies of *BRCA1/2* carriers will considerably underestimate the degree to which carcinomas arise from borderline tumors, because these patients have a borderline tumor incidence no higher than that of the normal population.[28] Equally, carcinomas with focal, apparently borderline components are more often identified

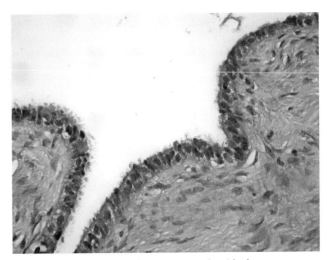

Figure 27–3. Notice the cilia in an area of residual serous cystadenofibroma at one edge of a tumor that elsewhere showed high-grade invasive serous carcinoma (hematoxylin & eosin stain, magnification ×400).

among mucinous and endometrioid than serous tumors.[36]

More sensitive techniques are revealing tiny chromosomal changes that suggest a continuum from benign to fully malignant tumors: a deletion of 300 kb within the D6S149-D6S193 interval at band 6q27 has been found in a borderline tumor, whereas alterations in this interval have previously been found mainly in advanced ovarian carcinoma.[37] The fact that some genetic alterations occur with higher frequency in borderline tumors than invasive tumors[28] suggests only that some (not all) carcinomas arise without a borderline precursor.

Another study[38] showed expression of amphiregulin (a member of the epidermal growth factor [EGF] superfamily) mainly among borderline tumors (i.e., serous and mucinous types) and much less in benign or malignant tumors, interpreted by the investigators as evidence that they have separate origins. However, the finding could equally represent a transient phenotype at that stage in a tumor's development.

It is likely that there are at least two pathways to carcinoma, *carcinoma ab initio* and *carcinoma ex borderline tumor*. This resembles the situation with serous or clear cell tumors in endometrium. Some of these tumors appear to arise from aberrant differentiation within an endometrioid tumor that still has adjacent residual preneoplastic hyperplasia. Some show no evidence of any preceding lower grade conditions (unpublished data).

Do we need to change our pathology methods, and are we examining prophylactic oophorectomy specimens closely enough?

There are several reports of microscopic cancers in the ovaries or fallopian tubes of *BRCA* carriers, and some have been associated with positive washings or subsequent tumor recurrence.[28] In at least one case, the positive washings caused a more vigorous search that uncovered a small tumor in the tube missed on the initial sections.[35] This is not surprising because the tube has tended to be disregarded in the past, with the diagnostic focus solely on the ovary. The recent literature implies that, at a minimum, all of both tubes and ovaries from *BRCA* carriers should be blocked in for histologic examination. Step sectioning at 0.5-mm intervals should also be given consideration.

Where does this leave us regarding taking samples of these tissues for research? After consent is obtained, one possibility is to chill the fresh tissue to improve firmness, divide it at several points, and then take the thinnest block possible with a razor blade at each point and perform frozen sections. If results are negative, tumors larger than 1 mm have been excluded, and the frozen blocks can reasonably be stored for research. This approach imposes a time and cost burden on pathologists, which should be acknowledged in the research planning. If microcancer is found and appropriate consent exists, about 5 to 10 unstained frozen serial sections could be preserved unstained and frozen for research, but the block itself and the rest of the ovary would need to be submitted to paraffin blocks for diagnostic assessment.

Surgical dissection of the omentum. Macroscopically negative omentum often has microscopic deposits (12%), and these are commonly the only evidence for upstaging the patient and giving adjuvant therapy.[39] It is important to look for these microscopic foci carefully.

In a retrospective study,[39] the average number of blocks submitted was only two, and it seems likely that some cases might have been missed because submitting all of the omentum would require hundreds of blocks. This is a considerable undersubmission habit compared with the large number of blocks often taken to assess much less clinically crucial information. It is therefore recommended that an absolute minimum of four blocks be submitted for a macroscopically negative omentum when there is no other macroscopic evidence of high-stage disease.

Special tests on nodes. A study[40] of node-negative breast cancer showed examination of *extra* sections with routine hematoxylin and eosin (H&E) staining revealed a 7% rate of previously undetected tumor, whereas staining with immunoperoxidase to epithelial markers detected even more (20%). The group with occult nodal metastases had a worse prognosis than the truly node-negative group.[40] Similar findings have been made for endometrial cancer.[41] Other groups have used polymerase chain reaction (PCR) as an even more sensitive method for single-cell metastases, but prognostic significance over that of immunohistochemistry is unproved.[42] Although nodal staging is done less often in ovarian cancer, we still need to ask if immunostaining should be done on them (i.e., will it change management?).

In this context, a Medline search revealed no studies on the significance of lymphatic invasion in ovarian carcinoma (Fig. 27-4) despite its considerable importance in prognostication and treatment guidance for other gynecologic cancers. However, one study showed that lymphatic invasion was significant in cases of granulosa cell tumor.[43]

What features best differentiate metastases from primary ovarian carcinoma?

The presence of "dirty" necrosis has been held out as a major criterion for identifying a metastasis,[45] but a study showed endometrioid carcinomas had a similar prevalence of dirty necrosis, although on average it was less extensive (Fig. 27-5).[46] Similarly, other criteria favoring metastasis, such as bilaterality, multiple nodules, and the presence of lymphatic invasion, are relatively soft signs, encouraging the move to immunostaining. Unfortunately, the extensive literature on the subject is complicated by the fact that most study authors do not include their raw data, and the results of different studies cannot be summed to obtain a reliable overview or meta-analysis.

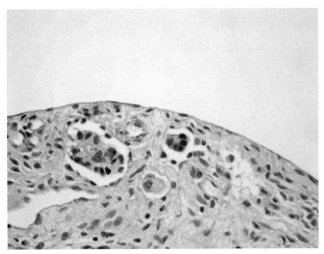

Figure 27–4. Reluctance to quantify lymphatic invasion results partly from the fact that true invasion into an endothelial lined space (upper two spaces in the figure) can be mimicked by pseudo-invasion as the tumor cells secrete fluid, creating a space (lower space in the figure), but with no endothelial lining.

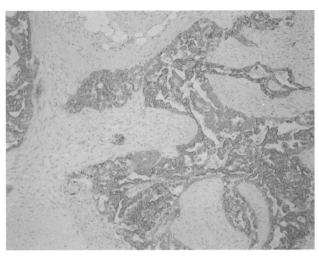

Figure 27–6. This CK7 immunostain is strongly positive, as expected in an ovarian primary tumor (hematoxylin & eosin stain, magnification ×100). See also Color Figure 27-6.

Metastases most often mimic primary carcinoma of the endometrioid type, followed by mucinous-type carcinoma. The many studies comparing immunostaining of ovarian cancers in general (most are serous types) with colonic tumors are less than ideal. One study on this type[47] found 15 of 16 ovarian tumors to be positive for the macrophage marker HAM56, compared with none of the colonic tumors.

Results of vimentin and ER analysis are particularly inconsistent from one study to the next,[48,49] probably because staining tends to occur as a spectrum rather than giving clear cutoffs for positive versus negative.

The most commonly used panel assesses CK7 and CK20 (Fig. 27-6). It discriminates very well for endometrioid (CK7 positive, CK20 negative) compared with colon tumors, but so does any combination of CA 125-positive, MUC2-positive, pCEA-negative, HBME1-positive, and ER- and PR-positive results.[50] Almost any panel will do for this particular distinction. Mucinous ovarian cancers are the problem. Because 5% to 10% are CK7 negative and a full 60% are CK20 positive, this panel is useless or even misleading for this differential diagnosis. MUC5AC positivity and, to a lesser extent, MUC2 negativity are useful markers to show ovarian origin,[51] most reliably when combined with CK7 positivity. Even with this panel, some results are indeterminate. For the determined, CA 125 (positivity favors ovary by 3:1), P53 (positivity favors colon by 3:1), pCEA (negativity favors ovary by 6:1[50]), and HBME1 (positivity strongly favors ovary) can be added and an overall odds ratio calculated (see http://www.immunohistoquery.com by D. Frisman for more details).

Immunostaining to distinguish breast metastases is even more unsatisfactory. CA 125 is the cornerstone, but in some studies, only 60% to 68% of ovarian cancers (more of serous subtype) and only 3% to 20% of breast cancers were positive for CA 125.[50] Fortunately, breast does not mimic well any of the usual histologic patterns of ovarian primaries, tending to a generic ductal pattern or an obvious lobular single file pattern (Fig. 27-7).[44]

The monoclonal antibody GCDFP-15 has been claimed to be relatively specific for a breast cancer metastasis.[30] However, another study concluded that although, compared with breast, most ovarian tumors showed less GCDFP and ER staining, this was a matter of less intense staining rather than absent staining, and grade 1 endometrioid types matched breast for intensity as well.[50] The distinction is therefore fairly subjective because of the batch-to-batch staining variations that can be expected even in the one laboratory.

The latest research concept is to use cDNA microchips to analyze RNA expression patterns into

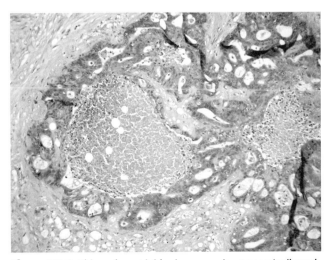

Figure 27–5. This endometrioid primary ovarian tumor (unilateral, CK7 positive, CK20 negative, no bowel primary after 5 years' follow-up) shows focal dirty necrosis with a rim of cribriform pattern (i.e., garlanding). However, this pattern is not as extensive as in many bowel cancer metastases (hematoxylin & eosin stain, magnification ×100).

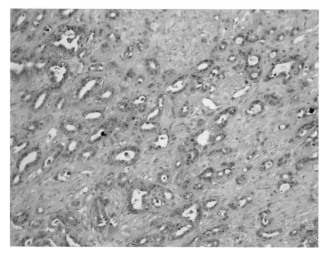

Figure 27–7. This metastasis from breast shows the typical nonspecific ductal pattern (hematoxylin & eosin stain, magnification ×100).

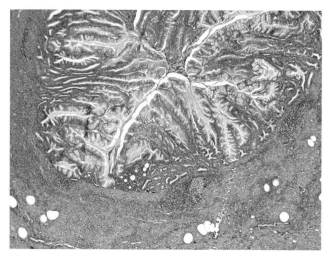

Figure 27–8. The appendix shows the pattern of a hyperplastic polyp.

groups related to tissue of origin. This approach (which requires snap frozen tissue) can effectively separate metastases from ovary, colon, breast, and other sites.[27]

Simultaneous endometrial tumors. It has been suggested that patients with simultaneous ovarian and endometrial cancers have a relatively good prognosis and that the tumors are therefore usually separate primaries rather than one being metastatic.[30] However, a study using several genetic markers found evidence that three of the five cases studied (all endometrioid) were genetically identical, implying that the ovarian tumor was metastatic.[52] It is likely that simultaneous tumors represent a mixture of both conditions, but it is not clear what methods can most reliably separate them.

What are pseudomyxoma peritonei, disseminated peritoneal adenomucinosis, and peritoneal mucinous carcinomatosis?

Pseudomyxoma peritonei has been regarded as a complication of ruptured borderline mucinous tumors of the ovary, but it occurs similarly in men and women. In women, the ovaries are usually involved, particularly the right ovary, which is consistent with direct spread from a lesion of the appendix. Lesions of the appendix can be very subtle and easily missed if it is not step-sectioned; alternatively the right iliac fossa area may be completely replaced by tumor. Allowing for this, one review[53] revealed no convincing cases in which a gastrointestinal tract origin for the pseudomyxoma could not be postulated.

Criteria for assessing the appendix are similar to those for the ovary, but the appendix may also have a lesion resembling hyperplastic polyp of the colon, although in a flat form (Fig. 27-8). This appears to be significantly correlated with pseudomyxoma, even

though it does not fit current criteria for neoplasia. Many other sites in the gastrointestinal tract or pancreaticobiliary system are associated occasionally with pseudomyxoma peritonei.[30]

The ovarian tumor in pseudomyxoma peritonei usually stains with the intestinal pattern of CK7 negative, CK20 positive, and HAM56 negative, but as with colon tumors, CK7-positive cases occasionally are seen.[30,54,55] LOH analysis of 12 appendix and ovarian tumor pairs showed that each exactly matched the LOH pattern of its partner, providing strong evidence of common clonal origin in most pseudomyxoma cases.[56]

The cytologic atypia and architectural features of the mucinous tumor cells in the peritoneal deposits or in the free-floating mucinous ascites correlate very strongly with prognosis.[57] On this basis, a new terminology has been proposed. If the cells show features like those seen in benign or borderline ovarian tumors (not including carcinoma in situ forms), they are labeled disseminated peritoneal adenomucinosis (DPAM) (Fig. 27-9). If they show architectural or cytologic features as expected in a frank malignancy, the lesion is peritoneal mucinous carcinomatosis (PMC). Their 5-year survival rates are 84% and 7%, respectively. DPAM constitutes 80% of cases. PMC is more often associated with nonappendiceal origin. If there is discordance between the features of the appendix or ovary and the peritoneal component, it is suggested that the term *discordant PMC* be used because they have a 5-year survival rate of 38%. Clinically, DPAM spares the bowel loops and is less nodular.

Other researchers have commented that peritoneal mucin can be categorized as free, superficially adherent to peritoneum, organizing (i.e., with granulation tissue growing into it (Fig. 27-10), or as dissecting mucin with surrounding fibrosis. The degree of reaction is thought to correlate with later bowel complication rates.[30] It is not clear whether this is completely superseded by the distinction between DPAM and PMC. It is evident that any literature on the prognosis

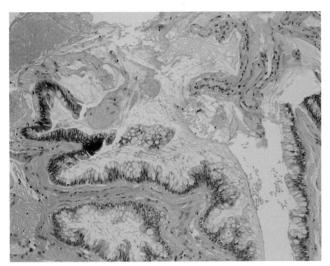

Figure 27–9. Peritoneal tumor with borderline features, i.e., disseminated peritoneal adenomucinosis (DPAM) (hematoxylin & eosin stain, magnification ×400).

of borderline mucinous tumors of the ovary that did not specifically exclude pseudomyxoma peritonei cases must now be disregarded, because true primary borderline mucinous tumors appear to have an excellent prognosis.

When does endometriosis lead to cancer?

If only a direct continuity from endometriotic epithelium to malignancy is counted, this is seen in less than 1% of cancers. However, nearly 9% of cancers (especially clear cell and endometrioid types) show endometriosis in the same ovary.[58] The authors of one study[58] analyzed records of all types of specimens with endometriosis coded in the diagnosis and found 5% of the ovarian specimens also had a cancer, but only 1% of other biopsies had the same result. The investigators concluded that ovarian endometriosis

was more likely to cause cancer. This inference is somewhat speculative because surgeons may do more biopsies of minor endometriotic lesions of the peritoneum than they do of ovary, diluting out the sample with nontumorous biopsies. However, the fact that large chocolate cysts are almost exclusive to the ovary may indicate that local hormone levels cause more stimulation in that site than elsewhere.

A study following 37 women whose endometriotic biopsies had shown cytologic atypia alone and 23 with complex atypical hyperplasia in their endometriosis found that all had no problems at 8 years, whereas 2 of 11 women whose specimens were interpreted as showing early grade 1 carcinoma within endometriosis developed second malignancies within the average 7-year follow-up.[36] Atypia in endometriosis may nevertheless be preneoplastic; it could be that excision removes the only clonal focus. Another group[59] did ploidy studies by image analysis on markedly atypical areas within endometriosis and found aneuploidy in 3 of 6 cases (Fig. 27-11).

Studies have detected LOH (implying small chromosomal deletions) in 28% of endometriotic foci but not in normal endometrium.[60] There were different deletion patterns in different deposits within the one woman, implying that each may represent a different clone, at least in some patients. These investigators also showed the same LOH pattern in tumors arising adjacent to endometriotic tissue as within the endometriosis itself, providing strong evidence of the tumor arising from the endometriotic cells.

New Hypotheses on the Cells of Origin for Common and Rare Carcinomas of the Ovary

Common epithelial tumors. The accepted theory is that mesothelium on the ovarian surface becomes incorporated in the ovarian stroma and that metaplasia then occurs, giving rise to serous inclusion cysts (Fig. 27-12), which have cilia and resemble small benign serous cystadenomas but without the papillary

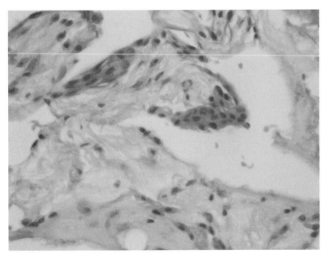

Figure 27–10. Pseudomyxoma peritonei, showing organization of mucin (hematoxylin & eosin stain, magnification ×400). See also Color Figure 27-10.

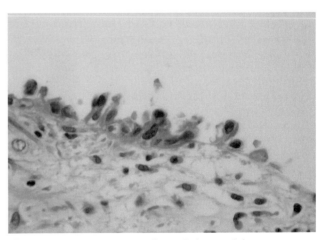

Figure 27–11. Atypia in an endometriotic cyst of the ovary.

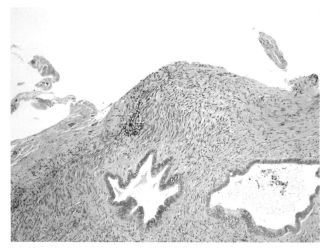

Figure 27–12. Typical serous inclusion cysts. Notice the associated surface adhesions (hematoxylin & eosin stain, magnification ×100).

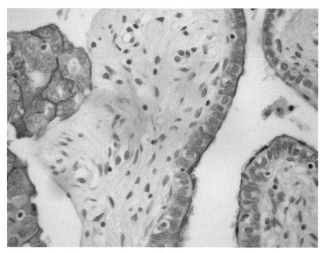

Figure 27–13. The invasive serous tumor on the left shows an immunostaining pattern identical to the normal tubal epithelium on the right (immunoperoxidase to human milk fat globulin, ×400). See also Color Figure 27-13.

infoldings. These are believed to be the cells from which epithelial tumors develop. This metaplasia is thought to occur as a secondary mullerian system. The accumulating weight of evidence favors an origin from endometriosis (and by implication from cells of the endometrium originally) for many endometrioid and clear cell tumors. However, the surface metaplasia theory still prevails for most tumors as the conventional explanation. Recently some criticism of this theory has been made.[61] In addition, the incessant ovulation hypothesis is being questioned by new data.[62]

Another alternative hypothesis is that the serous inclusion cysts are of the same derivation as those seen elsewhere in the pelvic peritoneum, particularly in the pouch of Douglas uterine serosa, which are classified as endosalpingiosis. In this theory both are derived, as the name of the latter implies, from physical adhesion and incorporation of epithelium from the exposed surface of the fallopian tube fimbriae.[63] This would explain why the cells of serous tumors have H&E and immunohistochemical staining features so similar to those of the normal fallopian tube (Fig. 27-13) and very different from those of normal mesothelial cells or the mesotheliomas clearly derived from them.[64] The significance of this alternative hypothesis is that almost all current molecular biology research uses ovarian mesothelium as the control normal tissue, but this gives misleading or nonsense results if the tubal epithelium is the correct normal control tissue.

One study showed a correlation of tubal carcinoma with the presence of salpingitis and atypia in the opposite tube (e.g., dilation, loss of plicae, chronic inflammation) (Fig. 27-14).[65] This is interesting given that tubal ligation or removal appears to halve the risk of ovarian carcinoma. Might ligation be associated with a decreased incidence of inflamed tubes and therefore less subtle premalignant changes already present in the fimbriae?

Transitional cell carcinoma ovary. Because of their morphologic resemblance to urothelial transitional cell carcinomas (TCCs), ovarian TCCs and malignant Brenner tumors have been grouped together (Fig. 27-15). However, there is evidence that only Brenner tumors and not TCCs of the ovary show urothelial differentiation with markers such as uroplakin III.[66] On the contrary, TCCs of ovary show strong CA 125 staining as well as occasional vimentin staining, features typical of serous tumors. This may explain why the histology of high-grade serous and transitional tumors is so hard to differentiate (i.e., TCC is just a variant pattern of serous carcinoma). These findings also provide an intellectual framework for the distinction long drawn between malignant Brenner tumors (with residual benign or borderline Brenner component) and TCCs (with their worse prognosis).

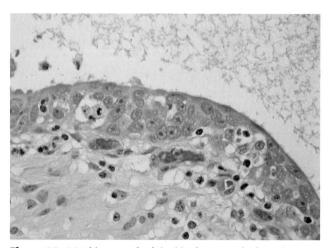

Figure 27–14. This case of salpingitis shows marked atypia, a possible source of cells with preneoplastic changes (hematoxylin & eosin stain, magnification ×400).

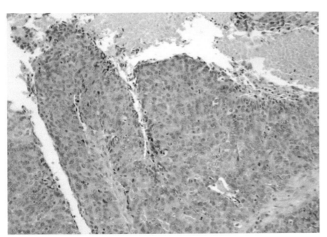

Figure 27–15. Transitional cell carcinoma of ovary (hematoxylin & eosin stain, magnification ×100). There were areas of typical serous carcinoma elsewhere.

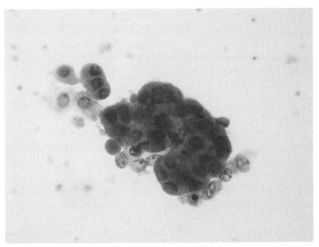

Figure 27–16. This fine-needle aspiration of an ovarian cyst showed a few groupings of papillae with mild atypia. Histologic examination confirmed the diagnosis of a borderline serous tumor. Flow cytometry may help with difficult cytologic results from a screening follow-up test (Papanicolaou stain, magnification ×400).

Small cell carcinoma of ovary. Small cell (hypercalcemic-type) carcinomas of the ovary do not stain for inhibin and therefore have been excluded from the ovarian stromal tumor category and regarded as true epithelial tumors, despite their resemblance on H&E staining to granulosa cell tumors. However, they have been shown to be CD99 (MIC-2) positive, a feature shared with all the other stromal tumors of the ovary tested[55] and various stromal tumors from other organs, suggesting that they may represent a poorly differentiated tumor derived from granulosa or related cells.

Pathology of Screening Tests

Evidence exists that common ovarian cancers sometimes show microscopic spread at a very early stage.[67] It remains to be shown how much earlier diagnosis by screening would change outcomes. Screening probably needs to be very cheap and very specific to be cost-effective, and it would need to be done considerably more frequently than for Papanicolaou (Pap) cervical smears where there is a long latent phase from first acquisition of human papillomavirus (HPV) or dysplasia to surgically incurable cancer.

The best specificity in screening test studies has been obtained by examining only postmenopausal patients (who have fewer false-positive results caused by benign disease), combining serum test results for several markers over a period (to look for a rise) plus results of vaginal ultrasound to assess ovarian masses or "significant" cysts.[68]

We now need to retrieve and store blood taken preoperatively and immediately postoperatively from women who, after histopathologic analysis, turn out to have *very early* ovarian cancer so that these samples can be used as a valid reference set to assess new tests. With screening tests in trials, we need a follow-up procedure that is less invasive than laparotomy or laparoscopy with ovarian biopsy or cystectomy. Fine-needle aspiration may be the answer (Fig. 27-16), but

there is evidence of a high false-negative rate, and there are also case reports suggesting the procedure can spread malignant cells into the peritoneum with adverse effect.[69] The finer the needle, the less likely it is that there will be spillage or seeding problems. The sensitivity and specificity of cytology may be improved by processing some of the specimen by flow cytometry. The presence of any cytokeratin markers (e.g., CK7, CK20) on cells would suggest neoplasia, whereas the cells would nearly all be inhibin positive if from a follicle cyst.

Assessment of Prognostic Features in Nonepithelial Malignancies

Diagnosing malignancy in struma ovarii. The literature on malignant struma reveals much debate about the criteria. It seems that some of the malignancies have a general resemblance to well-differentiated follicular or papillary thyroid carcinoma, but circumscription and mitoses are apparently not useful criteria, whereas large size is a bad sign.[70,71] There is dispute over the significance of atypia and cellularity.[72]

The literature includes references to struma with clear-cut malignant behavior that did not meet standard thyroid-based diagnostic criteria for malignancy.[72,73] These appear to be follicular lesions, which is not surprising because the criteria for these tumors are difficult to apply even in the thyroid, and in the setting of a teratoma, there may not be a capsule between the struma and other tissues with which to demonstrate capsular invasion. Papillary carcinoma, in contrast, has cytologic criteria that can be easily applied in the teratoma setting.

Quantitative morphometry has been found to be reasonably predictive on cytologic examination of thyroid follicular carcinomas.[75] This method could be applied to ovary as long as touch prints or needle aspirates were done after the diagnosis of struma was made (e.g., at frozen section). In thyroid, it has also been found that, unlike the papillary type, follicular carcinomas have extensive LOH.[75] Because this can be studied on paraffin sections and is available in numerous laboratories, it may be helpful to examine future and retrospective cases of possibly malignant struma for this feature.

Immature teratomas, grading, and the relationship to dermoid cysts.

To improve reproducibility of the original grading method, a two-grade system was developed.[76] The section with the greatest cross-sectional area of primitive neural tissue is selected (taken to mean the aggregate area). If this area is greater than a low-power field (4×4 mm^2) in diameter, the tumor is high grade (Fig. 27-17).

Occasionally, dermoid cysts are found histologically to have one to several small foci (1 to 21 mm^2) of primitive neurectoderm. A small series[27] showed an excellent outcome for these lesions at 3 years after oophorectomy. However, the study also found on review that three cases of dermoid cysts treated with cystectomy followed by the later presentation of an ipsilateral immature teratoma had such small foci in their original cyst. Thus cystectomy alone is insufficient for these lesions.

Assessment of Prognostic Features in Granulosa Cell Tumors

Several articles have suggested that some form of grading correlates with prognosis for adult-type granulosa cell tumor. Selecting one as the best is difficult. These tumors tend to late relapse, and survival figures at only 5 years of follow-up are therefore unhelpful.

There has been a consensus that sarcomatoid variants, characterized by sheets of cells lacking Call-Exner body formation and with atypia and numerous mitoses, are associated with a significantly worse prognosis.[30] However, it is probably the mitosis count that matters; this and lymphatic invasion were prognostic independent of stage,[43] and the pattern was not significant (Fig. 27-18).

Another study showed univariate significance of mitotic count[77] and of MNA (i.e., average of 36 mm^2 in tumors that did not recur and 44 mm^2 in tumors that later recurred). A previous study[78] did not show that mitotic count was significant but included seven juvenile granulosa tumors, none of which recurred. The juvenile granulosa tumors have a much higher mitotic rate, which was a confounding factor.

For juvenile granulosa cell tumors, stage is of great importance, and other features have not been shown to contribute significantly after stage is considered.[30] Possibly, this effect is caused by the small number of high-stage cases in any one study, because a trend to significance of the S-phase fraction was observed in a small group.[79]

Leiomyosarcoma versus leiomyoma.

It is believed that high mitotic counts are not clear evidence of malignancy if there are no other major features such as significant atypia.[30] A study of 53 ovarian smooth muscle tumors found that more than five mitoses per 10 HPFs, moderate-to-severe atypia, necrosis, and infiltrative margins favored malignant behavior,[80] which is fairly similar to the uterine criteria that have been used in the past.

Fibrosarcoma versus cellular fibroma.

Features that have been used to diagnose the sarcomas are more than four mitoses per 10 HPFs, at least moderate atypia, and to a lesser extent, hemorrhage and necrosis.[30] One study showed that trisomy 8 (in addition to

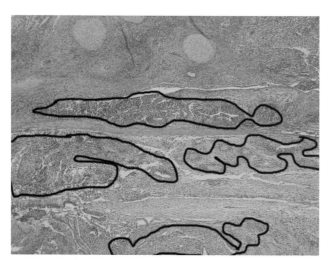

Figure 27–17. The blue areas of primitive neuroepithelium *(outlined)* in this section sum to more than 4 mm^2, indicating a high-grade immature teratoma (hematoxylin & eosin stain, magnification ×40). See also Color Figure 27-17.

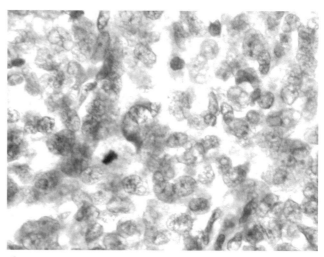

Figure 27–18. Mitosis is evident in this recurrent, diffuse-pattern granulosa cell tumor (hematoxylin & eosin stain, magnification ×400).

the trisomy 12 characteristic of fibroma and other stromal tumors) may be relatively specific for sarcomas.[81]

Any suspected sarcoma at frozen section should have cytogenetic examination because nongynecologic sarcomas often have specific karyotypic anomalies.

Do tumor-infiltrating lymphocytes inhibit ovarian cancer?

In four cases of ovarian carcinoma in which the primary and relapsed tumors were saved for cytokine analysis, the relapses showed more transforming growth factor-β1 (TGF-β1) and a trend to lower levels of interleukin-10 (IL-10) mRNA.[82] The source of these factors on immunostaining was tumor cells. This pattern was associated with a significant reduction in number of tumor-infiltrating lymphocytes (TILs) in general, and CD8-positive lymphocytes and macrophages in particular. Another study showed a cytokine pattern of IL-4 production in TILs versus one of interferon-γ production in peripheral blood lymphocytes (PBLs) of the same patient.[83] This finding is in accordance with the cytotoxic ability of TILs, which is weakened compared with that of PBLs. It seems that ovarian cancers typically produce factors that reduce the numbers and efficacy of responding lymphocytes and that this ability is strengthened in cases of tumor relapse (Fig. 27-19). These findings give a theoretical underpinning to early reports of good results from intraperitoneal interferon treatment.[84]

How useful are markers and other prognostic factors?

In several studies on the immunostain detection of HER2/NEU and P53, detection of either has been a negative predictor in some multivariate analyses.[85]

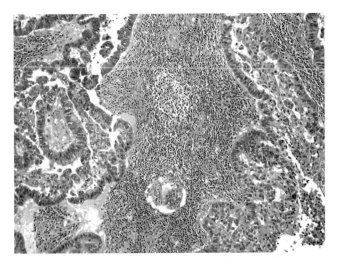

Figure 27–19. This ovarian adenocarcinoma is unusual in the number of infiltrating lymphocytes. Notice the germinal follicle center *(upper center)* (hematoxylin & eosin stain, magnification ×100).

This probably depends on how good the staging and grading quality is in the study and whether other important clinical factors such as degree of debulking achieved, age, symptom score, and CA 125 levels are included in the analysis. When all of these factors are entered in an algorithm, excellent prognostication is possible,[14,86,87] and it is unlikely the molecular factors will add much to survival prediction. If additional markers are to contribute, they may help in tailoring chemotherapy and the newer antibody, gene, or immunologic therapies.

One study[88] showed similar percentages of benign, borderline, and malignant tumors were immunostain positive for BCL2, but positivity did correlate with residual tumor after debulking or with subsequent reduced survival in this group. There was an inverse correlation with P53 immunostaining, suggesting that they represent alternative pathways of oncogenesis.[88] Epidermal growth factor receptor (EGFR) positivity on radioimmunoassay correlated with a much reduced response to chemotherapy.[89]

The serum level of anti-P53 was a negative survival predictor after allowing for stage, grade, and residual tumor, similar to results in breast and lung cancer studies. The presence of the antibody in patients' serum correlated with detectable (presumably mutant-inactivated) P53 in the tumor cells on immunostaining, but correlation with gene status is not yet available.[90]

Overexpression of HER2/NEU (i.e., ERBB2) did not correlate with grade or stage, but it was an independent prognostic factor. It has relevance to possible treatment with Herceptin.[91]

Immune status assessment. Immune status has been studied in patients with advanced disease (a mix including ovarian tumors) who were enrolled in trials of interferon therapy. Assessment of the peripheral blood T4/T8 numbers correlated with outcome and helped with adjustment of dosage regimens. This approach remains investigational.

CA 125 levels. The postoperative CA 125 level is a strong prognostic factor in grade 2, stage I disease.[92] It can be most useful for stratifying grade 2, stage I patients who are otherwise considered borderline for adjuvant therapy.

The best CA 125 cutoff level for prognostication after surgery but before chemotherapy is 65 U/mL for patients with known residual disease and 35 U/mL for those with no known residual disease after resection.[93] Postoperative levels may be followed for some months to see if they fall to within the normal range after adjuvant therapy. The patient's benefit from this testing is controversial, because it is not clear that any management improvement results.

A high CA 125 level (>35 U/mL) before the third course of chemotherapy is a predictor of positive findings at second-look laparotomy, even if the level has subsequently fallen to within the normal range,[93] but the positive and negative predictive power is not sufficient to make the second-look operation redundant.

The single greatest potential benefit from CA 125 is measurement during the preoperative workup of patients with a suspected pelvic mass, ovarian cyst, or ascites. A very high level strongly indicates ovarian malignancy and should lead to preoperative referral to a gynecologist-oncologist at a specialist center, which can improve the patient's overall survival.[1]

How can tubal and primary peritoneal cancers be differentiated from ovarian primaries, and how can they be diagnostically categorized?

There is no doubt that the incidence of ovarian cancer is significantly higher than that of tubal or primary peritoneal tumors, and when there is any ambiguity about which is the primary site, pathologists follow guidelines of exclusion (i.e., it is categorized as an ovarian primary tumor, unless ovarian origin can be excluded). Evidence from review of prophylactic oophorectomy series suggests that this approach may result in significant underdiagnosis of tubal primaries, which were found much more often in the setting of very early preclinical disease.[94] Similarly, in preclinical cancers detected by a CA 125 screening, the ratio of ovarian to tubal was only 6:1, far higher than the incidence after conventional diagnosis.[95]

These studies also suggest that primary peritoneal carcinoma may be overdiagnosed when an ovarian origin is excluded based on previous oophorectomy with negative histologic results. Subsequent review of some "negative" prophylactic oophorectomies has revealed initially overlooked microscopic cancers in the ovary.[28,35] Any subsequent peritoneal recurrence would have been classified in usual practice as a primary peritoneal tumor, and a number of primary peritoneal cancers have been documented after prophylactic oophorectomy. However, contrariwise one study[96] suggested, based on significantly different mutation profiles in 10 of 13 cases, that late recurrence of ovarian carcinoma may in a significant number of cases represent de novo peritoneal carcinoma.[96]

Our current methods are clearly flawed, but no standard better than the exclusion diagnosis yet exists because of the great similarity of the histology of tumor types from all three sites, which is similar to those seen in endometrium and endocervix but different in the frequency of subtypes. At all three sites, serous cancers are most common, particularly for peritoneal primaries, whereas for the fallopian tube, endometrioid cancer is also significantly common.[97] Tubal cancer has been documented arising in association with endometriosis. It is surprising how rare primary peritoneal endometrioid and clear cell cancers are in the literature given that peritoneal endometriosis is so common.

A few studies have looked at the molecular biology markers for fallopian tube and peritoneal tumors, and no striking differences from ovary have emerged. One study[98] comparing peritoneal with ovarian serous carcinomas showed more P53 and HER2/NEU alterations, but this appeared to reflect the higher histologic grade of the peritoneal tumors.

There is contradictory evidence about whether primary peritoneal tumors occur in a significantly older group.[99,100] This probably reflects the comparison group used, with peritoneal tumors manifesting at an age similar to that of the stage III or IV ovarian cancer patients used as controls.[100] These patients do appear to have significantly less history of perineal talc usage than the ovarian cancer patients.[99] The percentage of peritoneal tumor patients carrying *BRCA1/2* gene mutations is very similar to that of ovarian tumor patients.[101]

Finally, it is worth noting that there are site-specific prognostic factors for tubal carcinoma, including disease at the fimbrial end (worse prognosis), hydropic appearance of the tube, and degree of invasion of the tube wall.[102,103]

REFERENCES

1. Junor EJ, Hole DJ, Gillis CR: Management of ovarian cancer: Referral to a multidisciplinary team matters. Br J Cancer 1994;70:363-370.
2. Lin PS, Gershenson DM, Bevers MW, et al: The current status of surgical staging of ovarian serous borderline tumors. Cancer 1999;85:905-911.
3. Bilous M, McCredie M, Porter L: Adequacy of histopathology reports for breast cancer in New South Wales. Pathology 1995;27:306-311.
4. Scully RE, Henson DE, Nielsen ML, Ruby SG: Practice protocol for the examination of specimens removed from patients with ovarian tumors: A basis for checklists. Cancer 1996;78:927-940.
5. Baak JP, Langley FA, Talerman A, Delemarre JF: Interpathologist and intrapathologist disagreement in ovarian tumor grading and typing. Anal Quant Cytol Histol 1986;8:354-357.
6. Wang KG, Chen TC, Wang TY, et al: Accuracy of frozen section diagnosis in gynecology. Gynecol Oncol 1998;70:105-110.
7. Rose PG, Rubin RB, Nelson BE, et al: Accuracy of frozen-section (intraoperative consultation) diagnosis of ovarian tumors. Am J Obstet Gynecol 1994;171:823-826.
8. Ulrich U, Paulus W, Schneider A, Keckstein J: Laparoscopic surgery for complex ovarian masses. J Am Assoc Gynecol Laparosc 2000;7:373-380.
9. Puls L, Heidtman E, Hunter JE, et al: The accuracy of frozen section by tumor weight for ovarian epithelial neoplasms. Gynecol Oncol 1997;67:16-19.
10. Scully RE, Silva E: Pathology of ovarian cancer. In Gershenson DM, McGuire WP, eds., Ovarian Cancer: Controversies in Management. New York, Churchill Livingstone, 1998, pp 425-444.
11. Vacher-Lavenu MC, Le Tourneau A, Duvillard P, et al: Pathological classification and grading of primary ovarian carcinoma: Experience of the ARTAC ovarian study group. Bull Cancer 1993;80:135-141.
12. Silverberg SG: Histopathologic grading of ovarian carcinoma: A review and proposal. Int J Gynecol Pathol 2000;19:7-15.
13. Shimizu Y, Kamoi S, Amada S, et al: Toward the development of a universal grading system for ovarian epithelial carcinoma. I. Prognostic significance of histopathologic features—problems involved in the Architectural grading system. Gynecol Oncol 1998;70:2-12.
14. Shimizu Y, Kamoi S, Amada S, et al: Toward the development of a universal grading system for ovarian epithelial carcinoma: Testing of a proposed system in a series of 461 patients with uniform treatment and follow-up. Cancer 1998;82:893-901.
15. Mayr D, Diebold J: Grading of ovarian carcinomas. Int J Gynecol Pathol 2000;19:348-353.
16. Salvesen HB, Iversen OE, Akslen LA: Prognostic impact of morphometric nuclear grade of endometrial carcinoma. Cancer 1998;83:956-964.
17. Brinkhuis M, Baak JP, Meijer GA, et al: Value of quantitative pathological variables as prognostic factors in advanced ovarian carcinoma. J Clin Pathol 1996;49:142-148.

18. Montironi R, Braccischi A, Scarpelli M, et al: Well differentiated follicular neoplasms of the thyroid: Reproducibility and validity of a "decision tree" classification based on nucleolar and karyometric features. Cytopathology 1992;3:209-222.

19. van Diest PJ, Baak JP, Matze-Cok P, et al: Reproducibility of mitosis counting in 2,469 breast cancer specimens: Results from the Multicenter Morphometric Mammary Carcinoma Project. Hum Pathol 1992;23:603-607; comments 601-602.

20. Jannink I, van Diest PJ, Baak JP: Comparison of the prognostic value of four methods to assess mitotic activity in 186 invasive breast cancer patients: Classical and random mitotic activity assessments with correction for volume percentage of epithelium. Hum Pathol 1995;26:1086-1092.

21. Kennedy AW, Biscotti CV, Hart WR, Tuason LJ: Histologic correlates of progression-free interval and survival in ovarian clear cell adenocarcinoma. Gynecol Oncol 1993;50:334-338.

22. Zeimet AG, Muller-Holzner E, Marth C, Daxenbichler G: Immunocytochemical versus biochemical receptor determination in normal and tumorous tissues of the female reproductive tract and the breast. J Steroid Biochem Mol Biol 1994;49:365-372.

23. Slotman BJ, Nauta JJ, Rao BR: Survival of patients with ovarian cancer. Apart from stage and grade, tumor progesterone receptor content is a prognostic indicator. Cancer 1990;66:740-744.

24. Geisler JP, Wiemann MC, Miller GA, Geisler HE: Estrogen and progesterone receptor status as prognostic indicators in patients with optimally cytoreduced stage IIIc serous cystadenocarcinoma of the ovary. Gynecol Oncol 1996;60:424-427.

25. Kieback DG, McCamant SK, Press MF, et al: Improved prediction of survival in advanced adenocarcinoma of the ovary by immunocytochemical analysis and the composition adjusted receptor level of the estrogen receptor. Cancer Res 1993;53:5188-5192.

26. Boltz EM, Harnett P, Leary J, et al: Demonstration of somatic rearrangements and genomic heterogeneity in human ovarian cancer by DNA fingerprinting. Br J Cancer 1990;62:23-27.

27. Yanai-Inbar I, Scully RE: Relation of ovarian dermoid cysts and immature teratomas: An analysis of 350 cases of immature teratoma and 10 cases of dermoid cyst with microscopic foci of immature tissue. Int J Gynecol Pathol 1987;6:203-212.

28. Werness BA, Eltabbakh GH: Familial ovarian cancer and early ovarian cancer: Biologic, pathologic, and clinical features. Int J Gynecol Pathol 2001;20:48-63.

29. Phillips KA: Immunophenotypic and pathologic differences between BRCA1 and BRCA2 hereditary breast cancers. J Clin Oncol 2000;18(Suppl):107S-112S.

30. Scully RE, Young RH, Clement PB: Tumors of the ovary, maldeveloped gonads, fallopian tube and broad ligament. In Armed forces Institute of Pathology Atlas of Tumor Pathology, no. 23, 3rd series. Washington, DC, AFIP, 1998.

31. Boyd J, Rubin SC: Hereditary ovarian cancer: Molecular genetics and clinical implications. Gynecol Oncol 1997;64:196-206.

32. Hashiguchi Y, Tsuda H, Yamamoto K, et al: Combined analysis of p53 and RB pathways in epithelial ovarian cancer. Hum Pathol 2001;32:988-996.

33. Baldwin RL, Nemeth E, Tran H, et al: BRCA1 promoter region hypermethylation in ovarian carcinoma: A population-based study. Cancer Res 2000;60:5329-5333.

34. Annab LA, Hawkins RE, Solomon G, et al: Increased cell survival by inhibition of BRCA1 using an antisense approach in an estrogen responsive ovarian carcinoma cell line. Breast Cancer Res 2000;2:139-148.

35. Agoff SN, Mendelin JE, Grieco VS, Garcia RL: Unexpected gynecologic neoplasms in patients with proven or suspected BRCA-1 or -2 mutations: Implications for gross examination, cytology, and clinical follow-up. Am J Surg Pathol 2002;26:171-178.

36. Seidman JD: Prognostic importance of hyperplasia and atypia in endometriosis. Int J Gynecol Pathol 1996;15:1-9.

37. Tibiletti MG, Bernasconi B, Furlan D, et al: Chromosome 6 abnormalities in ovarian surface epithelial tumors of borderline malignancy suggest a genetic continuum in the progression model of ovarian neoplasms. Clin Cancer Res 2001;7:3404-3409.

38. Stromberg K, Johnson GR, O'Connor DM, et al: Frequent immunohistochemical detection of EGF supergene family members in ovarian carcinogenesis. Int J Gynecol Pathol 1994;13:342-347.

39. Steinberg JJ, Demopoulos RI, Bigelow B: The evaluation of the omentum in ovarian cancer. Gynecol Oncol 1986;24:327-330.

40. Cote RJ, Peterson HF, Chaiwun B, et al: Role of immunohistochemical detection of lymph-node metastases in management of breast cancer. International Breast Cancer Study Group. Lancet 1999;354:896-900.

41. Yabushita H, Shimazu M, Yamada H, et al: Occult lymph node metastases detected by cytokeratin immunohistochemistry predict recurrence in node-negative endometrial cancer. Gynecol Oncol 2001;80:139-144.

42. Yarbro JW, Page DL, Fielding LP, et al: American Joint Committee on Cancer prognostic factors consensus conference. Cancer 1999;86:2436-2446.

43. Fujimoto T, Sakuragi N, Okuyama K, et al: Histopathological prognostic factors of adult granulosa cell tumors of the ovary. Acta Obstet Gynecol Scand 2001;80:1069-1074.

44. Young RH, Scully RE: Metastatic tumors in the ovary: A problem-oriented approach and review of the recent literature. Semin Diagn Pathol 1991;8:250-276.

45. Young RH, Hart WR: Metastatic intestinal carcinomas simulating primary ovarian clear cell carcinoma and secretory endometrioid carcinoma: A clinicopathologic and immunohistochemical study of five cases. Am J Surg Pathol 1998;22:805-815.

46. DeCostanzo DC, Elias JM, Chumas JC: Necrosis in 84 ovarian carcinomas: A morphologic study of primary versus metastatic colonic carcinoma with a selective immunohistochemical analysis of cytokeratin subtypes and carcinoembryonic antigen. Int J Gynecol Pathol 1997;16:245-249.

47. Younes M, Katikaneni PR, Lechago LV, Lechago J: HAM56 antibody: A tool in the differential diagnosis between colorectal and gynecological malignancy. Mod Pathol 1994;7:396-400.

48. Nolan LP, Heatley MK: The value of immunocytochemistry in distinguishing between clear cell carcinoma of the kidney and ovary. Int J Gynecol Pathol 2001;20:155-159.

49. Vang R, Whitaker BP, Farhood AI, et al: Immunohistochemical analysis of clear cell carcinoma of the gynecologic tract. Int J Gynecol Pathol 2001;20:252-259.

50. Lagendijk JH, Mullink H, Van Diest PJ, et al: Tracing the origin of adenocarcinomas with unknown primary using immunohistochemistry: Differential diagnosis between colonic and ovarian carcinomas as primary sites. Hum Pathol 1998;29:491-497.

51. Albarracin CT, Jafri J, Montag AG, et al: Differential expression of MUC2 and MUC5AC mucin genes in primary ovarian and metastatic colonic carcinoma. Hum Pathol 2000;31:672-677.

52. Fujita M, Enomoto T, Wada H, et al: Application of clonal analysis. Differential diagnosis for synchronous primary ovarian and endometrial cancers and metastatic cancer. Am J Clin Pathol 1996;105:350-359.

53. Ronnett BM, Shmookler BM, Sugarbaker PH, Kurman RJ: Pseudomyxoma peritonei: New concepts in diagnosis, origin, nomenclature, and relationship to mucinous borderline (low malignant potential) tumors of the ovary. Anat Pathol 1997;2:197-226.

54. Guerrieri C, Franlund B, Fristedt S, et al: Mucinous tumors of the vermiform appendix and ovary, and pseudomyxoma peritonei: Histogenetic implications of cytokeratin 7 expression. Hum Pathol 1997;28:1039-1045.

55. McCluggage WG: Recent advances in immunohistochemistry in gynaecological pathology. Histopathology 2002;40:309-326.

56. Chuaqui RF, Zhuang Z, Emmert-Buck MR, et al: Genetic analysis of synchronous mucinous tumors of the ovary and appendix. Hum Pathol 1996;27:165-171.

57. Ronnett BM, Zahn CM, Kurman RJ, et al: Disseminated peritoneal adenomucinosis and peritoneal mucinous carcinomatosis: A clinicopathologic analysis of 109 cases with emphasis on distinguishing pathologic features, site of origin, prognosis, and relationship to "pseudomyxoma peritonei." Am J Surg Pathol 1995;19:1390-1408.

58. Stern RC, Dash R, Bentley RC, et al: Malignancy in endometriosis: Frequency and comparison of ovarian and extraovarian types. Int J Gynecol Pathol 2001;20:133-139.

59. Ballouk F, Ross JS, Wolf BC: Ovarian endometriotic cysts: An analysis of cytologic atypia and DNA ploidy patterns. Am J Clin Pathol 1994;102:415-419.

60. Sato N, Tsunoda H, Nishida M, et al: Loss of heterozygosity on 10q23.3 and mutation of the tumor suppressor gene PTEN in benign endometrial cyst of the ovary: Possible sequence progression from benign endometrial cyst to endometrioid carcinoma and clear cell carcinoma of the ovary. Cancer Res 2000;60:7052-7056.

61. Dubeau L: The cell of origin of ovarian epithelial tumors on the ovarian surface epithelium dogma: does the emperor have no clothes? Gynecol/Oncol 1999;72:437-442.

62. Clow OL, Hurst PR, Fleming JS: Changes in the mouse ovarian surface epithelium with age and ovulation number. Mol Cell Endocrinol 2002;191:105-111.

63. Robbie MJ: Are ovarian surface "epithelial" cells the origin of ovarian cancers or could it be the fimbriae? Int J Gynecol Cancer 2003 (submitted).

64. Ordonez NG: Role of immunohistochemistry in distinguishing epithelial peritoneal mesotheliomas from peritoneal and ovarian serous carcinomas. Am J Surg Pathol 1998;22:1203-1214.

65. Demopoulos RI, Aronov R, Mesia A: Clues to the pathogenesis of fallopian tube carcinoma: A morphological and immuno-histochemical case-control study. Int J Gynecol Pathol 2001;20:128-132.

66. Riedel I, Czernobilsky B, Lifschitz-Mercer B, et al: Brenner tumors but not transitional cell carcinomas of the ovary show urothelial differentiation: Immunohistochemical staining of urothelial markers, including cytokeratins and uroplakins. Virchows Arch 2001;438:181-191.

67. Bell DA, Scully RE: Early de novo ovarian carcinoma: A study of fourteen cases. Cancer 1994;73:1859-1864.

68. Petricoin EF, Ardekani AM, Hitt BA, et al: Use of proteomic patterns in serum to identify ovarian cancer. Lancet 2002;359:572-577.

69. Trimbos JB, Hacker NF: The case against aspirating ovarian cysts. Cancer 1993;72:828-831.

70. Young RH: New and unusual aspects of ovarian germ cell tumors. Am J Surg Pathol 1993;17:1210-1224.

71. Devaney K, Snyder R, Norris HJ, Tavassoli FA: Proliferative and histologically malignant struma ovarii: A clinicopathological study of 54 cases. Int J Gynecol Pathol 1993;12:333-343.

72. Chan SW, Farrell KE: Metastatic thyroid carcinoma in the presence of struma ovarii. Med J Aust 2001;175:373-374.

73. Checrallah A, Medlej R, Saade C, et al: Malignant struma ovarii: An unusual presentation. Thyroid 2001;11:889-892.

74. Frasoldati A, Flora M, Pesenti M, et al: Computer-assisted cell morphometry and ploidy analysis in the assessment of thyroid follicular neoplasms. Thyroid 2001;11:941-946.

75. Gillespie JW, Nasir A, Kaiser HE: Loss of heterozygosity in papillary and follicular thyroid carcinoma: A mini review. In Vivo 2000;14:139-140.

76. O'Connor DM, Norris HJ: The influence of grade on the outcome of stage I ovarian immature (malignant) teratomas and the reproducibility of grading. Int J Gynecol Pathol 1994;13:283-289.

77. Miller BE, Barron BA, Dockter ME, et al: Parameters of differentiation and proliferation in adult granulosa cell tumors of the ovary. Cancer Detect Prev 2001;25:48-54.

78. Costa MJ, Walls J, Ames P, Roth LM: Transformation in recurrent ovarian granulosa cell tumors: Ki67 (MIB-1) and p53 immuno-histochemistry demonstrates a possible molecular basis for the poor histopathologic prediction of clinical behavior. Hum Pathol 1996;27:274-281.

79. Jacoby AF, Young RH, Colvin RB, et al: DNA content in juvenile granulosa cell tumors of the ovary: A study of early- and advanced-stage disease. Gynecol Oncol 1992;46:97-103.

80. Nielsen GP, Young RH: Mesenchymal tumors and tumor-like lesions of the female genital tract: A selective review with emphasis on recently described entities. Int J Gynecol Pathol 2001;20:105-127.

81. Tsuji T, Kawauchi S, Utsunomiya T, et al: Fibrosarcoma versus cellular fibroma of the ovary: A comparative study of their pro-liferative activity and chromosome aberrations using MIB-1 immunostaining, DNA flow cytometry, and fluorescence in situ hybridization. Am J Surg Pathol 1997;21:52-59.

82. Merogi AJ, Marrogi AJ, Ramesh R, et al: Tumor-host interac-tion: Analysis of cytokines, growth factors, and tumor-infiltrat-ing lymphocytes in ovarian carcinomas. Hum Pathol 1997;28:321-331.

83. Schondorf T, Engel H, Lindemann C, et al: Cellular characteris-tics of peripheral blood lymphocytes and tumor-infiltrating lymphocytes in patients with gynaecological tumors. Cancer Immunol Immunother 1997;44:88-96.

84. Windbichler GH, Hausmaninger H, Stummvoll W, et al: Interferon-gamma in the first-line therapy of ovarian cancer: A randomized phase III trial. Br J Cancer 2000;82:1138-1144.

85. Yaziji H, Gown AM: Immunohistochemical analysis of gyneco-logic tumors. Int J Gynecol Pathol 2001;20:64-78.

86. Lund B, Williamson P: Prognostic factors for overall survival in patients with advanced ovarian carcinoma. Ann Oncol 1991;2:281-287; comments 245-247.

87. DiSilvestro P, Peipert JF, Hogan JW, Granai CO: Prognostic value of clinical variables in ovarian cancer. J Clin Epidemiol 1997;50:501-505.

88. Henriksen R, Wilander E, Oberg K: Expression and prognostic significance of Bcl-2 in ovarian tumors. Br J Cancer 1995;72:1324-1329.

89. Fischer-Colbrie J, Witt A, Heinzl H, et al: EGFR and steroid receptors in ovarian carcinoma: Comparison with prognostic parameters and outcome of patients. Anticancer Res 1997;17:613-619.

90. Vogl FD, Frey M, Kreienberg R, Runnebaum IB: Autoimmunity against p53 predicts invasive cancer with poor survival in patients with an ovarian mass. Br J Cancer 2000;83:1338-1343.

91. Meden H, Marx D, Rath W, et al: Overexpression of the onco-gene c-erb B2 in primary ovarian cancer: Evaluation of the prognostic value in a Cox proportional hazards multiple regression. Int J Gynecol Pathol 1994;13:45-53.

92. Nagele F, Petru E, Medl M, et al: Preoperative CA 125: An inde-pendent prognostic factor in patients with stage I epithelial ovarian cancer. Obstet Gynecol 1995;86:259-264.

93. Makar AP, Kristensen GB, Kaern J, et al: Prognostic value of pre- and postoperative serum CA 125 levels in ovarian cancer: New aspects and multivariate analysis. Obstet Gynecol 1992;79:1002-1010.

94. Leeper K, Garcia R, Swisher E, et al: Pathologic findings in prophylactic oophorectomy specimens in high-risk women. Gynecol Oncol 2002;87:52-56.

95. Woolas R, Jacobs I, Davies AP, et al: What is the true incidence of primary fallopian tube carcinoma? Int J Gynecol Cancer 1994;4:384-388.

96. Buller RE, Skilling JS, Sood AK, et al: Field cancerization: Why late "recurrent" ovarian cancer is not recurrent. Am J Obstet Gynecol 1998;178:641-649.

97. Rabczynski J, Ziolkowski P: Primary endometrioid carcinoma of fallopian tube. Clinicomorphologic study. Pathol Oncol Res 1999;5:61-66.

98. Halperin R, Zehavi S, Hadas E, et al: Immunohistochemical comparison of primary peritoneal and primary ovarian serous papillary carcinoma. Int J Gynecol Pathol 2001;20:341-345.

99. Eltabbakh GH, Piver MS, Natarajan N, Mettlin CJ: Epidemiologic differences between women with extraovarian primary peritoneal carcinoma and women with epithelial ovarian cancer. Obstet Gynecol 1998;91:254-259.

100. Ben-Baruch G, Sivan E, Moran O, et al: Primary peritoneal serous papillary carcinoma: A study of 25 cases and com-parison with stage III-IV ovarian papillary serous carcinoma. Gynecol Oncol 1996;60:393-396.

101. Menczer J, Chetrit A, Barda G, et al: Frequency of BRCA muta-tions in primary peritoneal carcinoma in Israeli Jewish women. Gynecol Oncol 2003;88:58-61.

102. Baekelandt M, Jorunn Nesbakken A, Kristensen GB, et al: Carcinoma of the fallopian tube. Cancer 2000;89:2076-2084.

103. Alvarado-Cabrero I, Young RH, Vamvakas EC, Scully RE: Carcinoma of the fallopian tube: A clinicopathological study of 105 cases with observations on staging and prognostic factors. Gynecol Oncol 1999;72:367-379.

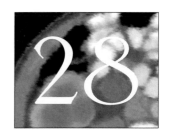

C H A P T E R

MOLECULAR BIOLOGY AND MOLECULAR GENETICS OF OVARIAN, FALLOPIAN TUBE, AND PRIMARY PERITONEAL CANCER

Dusica Cvetkovic, Denise C. Connolly, and Thomas C. Hamilton

 MAJOR CONTROVERSIES

- **Does ovarian cancer fit the histologic/genetic multistep model of carcinogenesis?**
- **Does ovarian cancer arise from the surface epithelium?**
- **Which genes are causal or are likely to provide new targets for diagnosis and therapy of ovarian cancer?**
- **Is there a role for the routine evaluation of tumor suppressor genes in ovarian cancer?**
- **Is there a role for the routine assessment of oncogene status in ovarian cancer?**
- **What are the mechanisms of growth regulation of the normal human ovarian surface epithelium and of ovarian cancer?**

Does ovarian cancer fit the histologic/genetic multistep model of carcinogenesis?

The multistep progression model proposed by Fearon and Vogelstein[1] was one of the early paradigms describing the hypothesis that the accumulation of genetic alterations leads to cancer. This model elegantly illustrated how genetic alterations in normal colonic epithelium lead to the progression of benign lesions to frankly invasive cancer. Although many other solid tumors fit the multistep progression model, epithelial ovarian carcinoma (EOC) has proved to be difficult to categorize in the same way for several reasons. First, invasive EOC comprises several different histologic subtypes, including serous papillary, endometrioid, mucinous, clear cell, and transitional carcinomas. Second, because EOC most frequently is diagnosed at an advanced stage, early ovarian carcinomas are rarely

identified and difficult to obtain for molecular analyses. The fact that disease is usually not identified until advanced stage also has made the identification of precursor lesions of EOC difficult and somewhat controversial. In this chapter, the biology of ovarian cancer is reviewed, along with the genetic and gene expression changes associated with the disease.

Ovarian cancer is the most frequently fatal gynecologic malignancy among women in the Western world.[2] The ovary is a complex endocrine gland consisting of numerous cell types that are responsible for the production of hormones and maintenance and release of ova.[3] In humans, approximately 90% of ovarian cancers are believed to arise from the modified peritoneal mesothelium that covers the ovarian surface (human ovarian surface epithelium, or HOSE).[4-6] The ovarian surface differentiates after invagination of the coelomic mesothelium over the gonadal ridges

385

during early embryonic development. It consists of a single layer of cuboidal, columnar, or simple flat epithelial cells separated from the underlying stroma by basement membrane.[7,8] These cells are important for ovulation in the adult. Morphologically, ovarian carcinomas are similar to those arising from mullerian-derived gynecologic organs, perhaps because of their common embryologic progenitor (i.e., coelomic epithelium). For example, serous ovarian carcinomas are morphologically similar to epithelial tumors that arise in the fallopian tubes; mucinous carcinomas resemble those arising in endocervix; endometrioid ovarian cancers are similar to carcinomas of the endometrium, and clear cell tumors are likewise similar to a variant of endometrial carcinomas.

Because the majority of ovarian tumors are believed to originate from the surface epithelium, they are referred to as common epithelial tumors (see later discussion for controversy in this regard). Clinically, about two thirds of patients present with advanced-stage disease, reflecting the propensity of these tumors for intra-abdominal and peritoneal spread.[9] The mortality rate from ovarian cancer has not changed in the past 3 decades as a result of poor understanding of the underlying biology, lack of reliable biomarkers for disease detection, late stage at presentation, and inaccessible location of the ovary compared with the other portions of the female genital tract. It is difficult to inspect or sample the ovary with the same ease as other cancer-prone epithelia, such as cervix and colon. It is widely hypothesized that the identification of precursor lesions for invasive EOC and the early genetic alterations that contribute to disease development may lead to the identification of targets that can be used in disease detection, prevention, or treatment.

Theories of Ovarian Cancer Development

Does ovarian cancer arise from the surface epithelium? There are few appropriate animal models for ovarian tumors, and the methodology to culture HOSE has become available only recently.[10-12] Another factor that slows progress in unraveling the molecular circuitry of ovarian cancer is the difficulty of working with cells so limited in number (i.e., HOSE). These cells are very fragile and are easily detached by handling of the ovary or allowing it to dry; for this reason, they are commonly absent in human surgical specimens and therefore unavailable for further analysis.[13] As noted earlier, it is also extremely hard to obtain specimens from "early" ovarian carcinomas or premalignant lesions. Therefore, much of the work presented here relates to studies on advanced ovarian cancers.

Although it is widely thought that EOCs arise from the HOSE cells that cover the surface of the ovary, this hypothesis remains somewhat controversial.[14-19] Some investigators believe that evidence for this assumption is lacking and that EOCs more likely arise from secondary mullerian structures.[20] Efforts to understand ovarian cancer are further hampered by controversy concerning ovarian cancer precursors. There are three categories of epithelial neoplasia in the

ovary: benign, borderline (low malignant potential, or LMP) and malignant. It is unclear whether these types represent a biologic continuum of stepwise progression toward malignancy or whether they are distinct entities, each arising de novo.[18] Identification of invasive EOCs that also contain essentially normal epithelium adjacent to benign or borderline neoplastic lesions in archival material has led investigators to hypothesize that epithelial lesions do arise from HOSE cells and that a similar multistep progression paradigm exists for ovarian carcinoma[14-19] as with other cancers. All of the following entities have been proposed as precursors of ovarian cancer: benign tumors,[16] borderline tumors,[15] and HOSE inclusion cysts.[3,21-23] With regard to the latter, Salazar and colleagues,[19] as well as other researchers,[24] evaluated ovaries removed from healthy women who had an inherited risk of ovarian cancer. In addition to increased inclusion cyst formation, they found HOSE pseudostratification, papillomatosis, deep cortical invaginations of the HOSE, stromal abnormalities, and ultrastructural changes in surface epithelial cells (e.g., enlargement of nuclei, presence of nucleoli, dense chromatin). These were suggested to be a fertile substrate from which ovarian cancer could develop. Hyperplastic and metaplastic lesions in the surface epithelium of the contralateral ovaries of women with unilateral ovarian cancer have also been reported.[17]

The incessant ovulation hypothesis of ovarian cancer etiology, proposed in 1971 by Fathalla,[25] is supported by epidemiologic data indicating that the accumulated number of menstrual cycles correlates with the risk of ovarian cancer.[26] Factors that decrease lifetime ovulatory cycles, including use of oral contraceptives and the prostagenic milieu of pregnancy, are protective against ovarian cancer, probably because they decrease lifetime ovulations or increase apoptosis of ovarian epithelial cells, or both, and thereby cleanse the ovary of cells with acquired genetic damage.[27,28] In addition, it has long been known that domestic egg-laying hens have a high incidence of what is believed to be ovarian-derived tumors. These animals are forced to ovulate incessantly by living in 12 hours of light and 12 hours of darkness and tend to develop peritoneal carcinomatosis.[29] The ovarian surface epithelium has not been under strong evolutionary pressure to develop the capacity for repeated wound repair because, in the Darwinian sense, repetitious ovulation is a recent event. Fathalla noted how the human female is extravagant with her ova, compared with most other species that exercise their reproductive potential to the fullest.[25] Females of most species are either pregnant or lactating during the bulk of their adult lives, and this markedly limits the number of ovulatory cycles. Fathalla linked ovulatory damage of the ovarian surface with the initiation of neoplastic growth.[30] To test the idea that the repeated growth of the ovarian epithelium induces its transformation, and in support of Fathalla's hypothesis, surface epithelial cells from rat ovaries (ROSE) were isolated and repeatedly subcultured to produce a series of cell lines. The result was malignant transformation in 10 of 30 attempts.[31,32] Features of this spontaneous in vitro rat transformation model that may mimic ovarian cancer initiation in women are listed in

Table 28–1. Features of a Spontaneous Rat In Vitro Transformation Model of Surface Epithelial Neoplasia

Incidence of transformation is 33% (10/30)

This model provides multiple independent episodes of transformation, all arising from cells with initially identical genetic constitution

Recurrence of genetic changes leading to malignancy can be examined and used to suggest causality and the need for thorough study.

Individual transformed cell lines show innate differences to drug sensitivity, vary in agressiveness, and are nonimmunogenic.

Data from references 31 and 32.

Table 28-1. Use of this model led to the discovery of the so-called lost on transformation-1 gene (*LOT1/PLAGL1*), a candidate tumor-supressor gene. Furthermore, by the technique of genome scanning, it was found that the cathepsin B gene was amplified or overexpressed, or both. There is evidence for the involvement of these genes in human ovarian and other cancers.[33-36]

More recently, consolidative suppression subtractive hybridization (CSSH) technique has been used to identify genes that are differentially expressed in normal ROSE cells compared with their transformed counterparts.[37] This technique allows multiple specimens of distinct phenotypic groups to be compared for consistent differences in gene expression. Northern blot analysis using 14 of 28 nonredundant complementary DNA (cDNA) fragments from this difference library (Table 28-2) showed that the messenger RNA (mRNA) transcripts were present in normal ROSE cells but were

lost or markedly reduced in four related transformed cell lines.[38] Two of the genes downregulated in this ovarian cancer model, retinol-binding protein 4 (*RBP4*) and retinol-binding protein 1, cellular (*CRBP1*), are involved in vitamin A metabolism and transport. As reported by Kuppumbatti and associates,[39] changes in retinol metabolism could be an early event in breast tumorigenesis. Vitamin A derivatives have well-established roles in cancer prevention and treatment. Studies show that the expression of retinol-binding proteins in human ovarian cancer cell lines is lost or markedly reduced relative to their expression in HOSE cells.[38] The clinical relevance of this work was suggested by the examination of a cohort of microdissected frozen serous ovarian cancer samples: expression of CRBP1 was lost in one third of the specimens. The loss of CRBP1 appeared to be an early event in ovarian carcinogenesis, because there was no statistically significant difference in its frequency between tumor stages and grades. This change in the ability of cells to metabolize vitamin A could have implications with regard to ovarian cancer initiation or progression.[38,40]

Genetics of Ovarian Neoplasia

Which genes are causal or are likely to provide new targets for diagnosis and therapy of ovarian cancer?

One of the major controversies in molecular biology and genetics of ovarian, fallopian tube, and primary

Table 28–2. Genes Differentially Expressed in Normal Rat Ovarian Surface Epithelium (ROSE) Cells Versus Transformed ROSE Cells

Clone	GenBank Match	Human Chromosomal Location
A8	Human RGS6	14q24
A9	Human retinol-binding protein	10q23-q24
N10	Human cellular retinol-binding protein	3q21-3q22
C3	Human phospholamban	6q22.1
D4	Rat ASM15/human H19	11p15
A1	Human myosin light chain kinase	3cen-q21
A7	Human serotonin transporter	17q11.1-q12
D1	Human MYBPC1 (protein C—slow)	12(?)
B1	Human myosin heavy chain	—
B6	Human ribosomal protein S4	Xq13.1
D6	Human ephrin-B1	Xp12
E5	Human Pref-1	14q32
A3	Human Wnt-13	1p13
A4	Human angiotensin II receptor	3q21
B2	Human cationic amino acid transporter	13q12-q14
C4	Human LERK-8	17q12
C10	Human rhomboid protein	16p13.3
A6	Unknown	?
C1	Unknown	?
C5	Similar to human transcript 23584	2q34-q35
C6	Unknown	?
D2	Unknown	?
D3	3 human ESTs (similar to AEBP-1)	20p13
D9	Unknown	?
F1	4 overlapping mouse ESTs	?
Q11	Unknown	?
B4	Unknown	?
H5	Unknown	?

Data from references 31 and 32.

EST, Expressed sequence tag.

peritoneal cancers is the question of validity and the real significance of gene expression gains or losses reported in numerous ovarian cancer gene expression studies conducted throughout the world. Ovarian carcinoma does presumably result from the accumulation of genetic alterations, and significant efforts have been made by researchers to identify the genes that are involved in the development and progression of disease.[41-44] Because most ovarian cancers are diagnosed at an advanced stage, numerous genetic alterations are often present, making it difficult to discern the significance of alterations of any single gene. Also, although many studies have been done to identify the molecular changes that may contribute to the development of ovarian carcinoma, not all studies have considered relevant factors such as histologic subtype, grade, and stage of disease in the samples analyzed. In fact, some molecular analyses of ovarian tumors have included not only EOCs but also germ cell and sex cord–stromal tumors as well. These factors have led to some inconsistencies in interpretation of the significance of individual biomarkers and the roles they may play in disease development. As the study of molecular alterations in EOC has matured, it has become apparent that such factors must be considered to identify the genes and molecular pathways that most likely lead to EOC and to determine whether each histologic subtype arises as a result of a distinct set of molecular alterations.

Ovarian cancer, like other types of solid tumors, must result from the accumulation of a number of different genetic and gene expression changes involving two major families of genes, oncogenes and tumor suppressor genes (Table 28-3).[43] Briefly, oncogenes encode proteins of a stimulatory nature, and tumor suppressors encode proteins involved in the negative control of cell growth. For conversion to the neoplastic phenotype, it is generally believed that both activation of oncogenes and deactivation of tumor suppressor

genes are required. DNA mismatch repair (MMR) genes may also be mutated in tumors, and they represent a potential third class of genes involved in cancer development.[45]

Tumor suppressor genes.
Is there a role for the routine evaluation of tumor supressor genes in ovarian cancer? Chromosomal gains and losses throughout the genome of ovarian cancers have been demonstrated, initially by means of classic karyotype analysis and more recently by the technique of comparative genomic hybridization (CGH).[46,47] One of the most useful approaches for locating the tumor suppressor genes is through studying patterns of loss of alleles in tumors with polymorphic markers. This is known as loss of heterozygosity (LOH). A high frequency of allelic loss in a specific region of a chromosome in a tumor type indicates the possible presence of one or more tumor suppressor genes, whose function would then be implicated in the initiation or progression of a particular tumor. LOH has been shown to occur at some level on most chromosome arms in ovarian cancer, but at higher frequency on 6q, 11p, 13q, 14q, 17p, 17q, 18q, 22q, and Xp.[48,49] It is not clear whether these genetic alterations reflect the need to inactivate multiple tumor suppressor genes or are the result of generalized genomic instability in ovarian cancer.

Mutational analyses and LOH studies indicate the significance of chromosome 17 in ovarian tumor development. On the short arm, LOH and mutations at the *TP53* locus as well as LOH at a more distal locus (17p13.3) have been observed in a high percentage of tumors. Similarly, on the long arm, losses in the *BRCA1* region and a more distally located locus (17q22-23) are often found.[50,51] In a study by Pieretti and associates,[52] total chromosome 17 loss was observed in high-grade serous tumors exclusively, suggesting that loss of tumor suppressor genes on chromosome 17 confers a selective

Table 28–3. Tumor Suppressor Genes and Oncogenes Involved in Pathogenesis of Ovarian Cancer

Gene	Class	Activation	Frequency (%)	References
Sporadic				
TP53	Tumor suppressor Transcription factor	Mutation/deletion Overexpression	50-80	Eltabbakh et al.[78]
TP16	Tumor suppressor CDK inhibitor	Homozygous deletion	15	Schultz et al.[88]
LOT1	Tumor suppressor Transcription factor			Abdollahi et al.[33,34,35]
NOEY2	Tumor suppressor, RAS homolog			Yu et al.[91]; Xu et al.[92]
OVCA1, OVCA2	Tumor suppressor			Schultz et al.[97]; Bruening et al.[98]; Prowse et al.[99]
AKT2	Serine-threonine kinase	Amplification	10-20	Thompson et al.[146]; Bellacosa et al.[148]
MYC	Transcription factor	Overexpression	20-30	Boyd et al.[190]
HER2/NEU	Tyrosine kinase	Amplification/ overexpression	15-50	Slamon et al.[113]; Zhang et al.[119]; Berchuck et al.[120]
Hereditary				
BRCA1, BRCA2	Tumor suppressor	Mutation/deletion	3-5	Boyd et al.[190]
MSH2	DNA repair	Mutation	1	Boyd et al.[190]

growth advantage during progression, leading rapidly to the development of a highly malignant tumor. Additionally, chromosome 17 loss was found in only 1 of 22 examined mucinous ovarian tumors, suggesting a different biologic pathway than in the serous tumors.[52] Both LOH and CGH studies have shown that advanced-stage cancers have a greater number of genetic changes than do early-stage lesions.[53] Watson and coworkers[54] reported that borderline tumors have patterns of LOH similar to those of early-stage malignant ovarian tumors, indicating inactivation of the same set of tumor suppressors in the development of malignant and borderline forms.

BRCA1 *and* BRCA2. It is well known that the driving force of tumor development is genetic mutation. Hereditary ovarian cancers are distinguished from sporadic ones by the mechanism through which the requisite mutations occur. In hereditary tumorigenesis, the first rate-limiting genetic alteration is inherited through the germline, and the additional mutations are acquired somatically in the premalignant cell. In sporadic tumorigenesis, all mutations are somatic. Epidemiologic studies have shown that most ovarian cancers occur sporadically, but 10% are hereditary.[55] Among the latter, three distinct autosomal dominant ovarian cancer syndromes are known: breast and ovarian cancer syndrome, associated with mutations in the *BRCA1* and *BRCA2* genes (65% to 75% of all hereditary ovarian cases); site-specific ovarian cancer (10% to 15% of cases); and ovarian cancer associated with Lynch II syndrome or hereditary nonpolyposis colorectal cancer (HNPCC). Lynch syndrome is characterized by predisposition to right-sided colon cancers, cancers of the endometrium, and ovarian cancers; it is caused by mutations in DNA MMR genes.[56,57] Genes that are responsible for familial forms of ovarian cancer may also be involved in sporadic tumors. Sporadic and hereditary ovarian cancers have different characteristics. For example, borderline and mucinous types of tumors are rare in hereditary forms, whereas serous tumors make up a majority of the familial neoplasms.[9,56,58]

BRCA1 and BRCA2 are two tumor suppressor genes that are responsible for the majority of cases of familial breast and ovarian cancer syndrome. They map to chromosomes 17q and 13q, respectively. The discovery of a candidate *BRCA1* gene in 1994[59] was confirmed by several subsequent studies describing the segregation of inactivating mutations in this gene with disease phenotype in many families with the breast and ovarian cancer syndrome.[60,61] The probability of developing cancer after inheriting a mutant *BRCA* allele (penetrance), ranges from 10% to 63% and is lower in *BRCA2* mutant gene carriers than in *BRCA1*-linked families.[62-64] Variable penetrance reflects the effects of various environmental, hormonal, or genetic modifiers, which reduce or increase the risk of ovarian cancer in *BRCA* mutation carriers.[65,66] The fact that somatic allele losses in 17q are also detected in 40% to 75% of sporadic cancers supports the hypothesis that *BRCA1* might also function as a tumor suppressor gene in sporadic ovarian cancers.[50,67] However, the frequency of *BRCA1* somatic mutations in sporadic ovarian tumors is low, suggesting that some other genes on chromosome 17 may contribute to ovarian cancer development.[68]

The *BRCA1* gene consists of 22 coding exons distributed over 100 kb of genomic DNA on chromosome 17q21.[59] The mRNA transcript of 7.8 kb encodes a 220-kd nuclear phosphoprotein and is expressed mostly in testis and thymus, and at lower level in ovary and breast. The majority of mutations are located throughout the gene and represent loss-of-function, nonsense, or frameshift alterations. The *BRCA2* gene consists of 26 coding exons distributed over 70 kb of genomic DNA, encoding a transcript of 11 to 12 kb.[69] BRCA2 is a 460-kd nuclear phosphoprotein. The expression pattern is the same as for BRCA1. An embryonic lethal phenotype is observed in mice with a homozygous null mutation in *Brca1*.[70] The *Brca2* knockout mouse also displays an embryonic lethal phenotype, indicating a critical role for this gene in cellular proliferation during embryogenesis.[71]

These large proteins are primarily involved in transcriptional activation and DNA repair. The presence of the following motifs are consistent with the ability of BRCA1 to activate gene transcription in vitro: an amino-terminal RING-finger domain, a negatively charged region in the carboxyl terminus, and C-terminal sequences known as BRCT domains that are partially homologous to yeast RAD9 and a cloned P53-binding protein.[72-74] BRCA1 is a component of the RNA polymerase II transcription complex.[75] BRCA1 colocalizes in vivo and in vitro with the RAD51 protein, which is known to function in the repair of double-strand DNA breaks.[75]

TP53. The tumor suppressor gene *TP53* is the most frequently mutated gene in human cancer. It is located in the short arm of chromosome 17 and encompasses 16 to 20 kb of DNA, encoding a 393-amino-acid nuclear phosphoprotein that causes arrest of the cell cycle after DNA damage, preventing cell progression into mitosis and triggering apoptosis if the damage is too great to be repaired by normal cellular mechanisms.[43,76] It is well known that *TP53* alterations, including allelic losses, mutation, and overexpression, are the most frequent genetic events in ovarian cancer.[77-79] Frequency of overexpression of mutant *TP53* is significantly higher in advanced ovarian cancer compared with early disease, and *TP53* inactivation is uncommon in benign or borderline tumors.[80,81] Therefore, many investigators consider its mutation to be a late event in ovarian carcinogenesis. Functional wild-type *TP53* has been shown to be required for sensitivity to a variety of chemotherapeutic drugs and radiation, playing a crucial role in the execution of the common end pathway of apoptosis.

Mismatch repair genes. EOC is also recognized as a component of the HNPCC syndrome, which arises from an inherited defect in one of the DNA MMR genes: *MSH2, MLH1, MSH6, PMS2,* or *PMS1,* but most often *MSH2* or *MLH1*.[82] MMR genes function as classic tumor suppressors, because the wild-type allele inherited from the unaffected parent is lost or mutated somatically in HNPCC-linked tumors.[83] The genetic instability phenotype associated with defective MMR genes is observed through somatic length changes in simple repeat sequences located throughout the genome in predominantly noncoding regions of DNA, known as microsatellites. Replication errors in these sequences are common (e.g., insertion-deletion loops, single-base mismatches), and their inefficient repair results in the microsatellite instability phenotype.

PTEN/MMAC1. Several other known tumor suppressor genes, including *PTEN/MMAC1*, have been observed in ovarian cancer. *PTEN/MMAC1*, mapped to chromosome sub-band 10q23.3, is a phosphatase that is mutated in a significant fraction of endometrioid ovarian tumors.[84,85] Frequent loss of *PTEN* expression is linked to increased levels of phosphorylated AKT but is not associated with P27KIP1 and cyclin D1 expression in primary EOCs.[86] Phosphatidylinositol 3-kinase (PI3K) and the *PTEN* tumor suppressor gene product phosphorylate and dephosphorylate the same 3′ site in the inositol ring of membrane phosphatidylinositols.

Other candidate tumor suppressor genes. Cyclin-dependent kinase-4 inhibitor genes (*INK4*) regulate the cell cycle and are candidate tumor suppressor genes. Members of the family are P15 and P16, whose genetic and epigenetic alterations might contribute to the development of ovarian and other human cancers, and P18 and P19, in which somatic mutations are less common.[87] P16 undergoes homozygous deletions in 15% of ovarian cancers[88] and is a potential indicator for poor chemotherapy response and adverse prognosis in ovarian cancer patients.[89] By inactivating MDM2, P19 (ARF) upregulates P53 activities to induce cell cycle arrest and to sensitize cells to apoptosis in the presence of collateral signals.[90] Another gene, *NOEY2/ARHI*, a RAS/RAP homolog mapped to chromosome 1p31, was identified with the use of differential display polymerase chain reaction (PCR). It appears to be a putative imprinted tumor suppressor whose function is abrogated in ovarian and breast carcinomas.[91,92] Unlike RAS or RAP, reintroduction of the *ARHI* gene induces P21[WAF1/CIP1] (CDKN1A), downregulates expression of cyclin D1, truncates signaling through RAS/MAP, and inhibits the growth of cancer cells that lack its expression. The *ARHI* gene is inactivated through maternal imprinting, which silences one allele from conception, and subsequent deletion of the contralateral allele in 30% to 40% of breast and ovarian cancers. In addition, expression of this gene is transcriptionally regulated, accounting for loss of expression in an even higher fraction of cancers at these sites.

As noted earlier, another candidate tumor suppressor gene was identified based on lost expression in transformed rat ovarian surface epithelium. *LOT1*, a growth suppressor gene downregulated by the EGF-R ligands, encodes a nuclear zinc-finger protein.[33,34,36]

DAB2 (disabled homolog 2), another candidate ovarian tumor suppressor gene, is thought to function in the organization of epithelial cell positioning. Its inactivation has been proposed to be an early event in ovarian tumorigenicity that enables the disorganized growth of tumor cells.[93-95] It has been shown by immunohistochemistry that the expression of DAB2 is lost in 80% of ovarian carcinomas.[96]

Finally, *OVCA1* and *OVCA2* are two more candidate tumor suppressor genes that have been mapped to the region most commonly lost in ovarian and breast tumors, chromosome 17p13.3.[97,98] *OVCA2* is evolutionarily conserved and shows regional homology with dihydrofolate reductases, specifically with hydrolase folds found in α/β-hydrolases. Although the functions of *OVCA1* and *OVCA2* are yet to be elucidated, initial evidence suggests their fundamental role in the majority of malignant ovarian tumors. It was most recently reported that *OVCA2* but not *OVCA1* mRNA and protein are downregulated in response to retinoid treatment.[99]

Oncogenes.
Is there a role for the routine assessment of oncogene status in ovarian cancer? The alterations that lead to neoplastic growth occur in oncogenes, tumor suppressors, and DNA repair genes encoding proteins that are involved in normal cell growth and regulation as well as the maintenance of genomic integrity. The normal cellular counterparts of oncogenes, referred to as protooncogenes, are involved in the stimulation of normal cellular growth. There are several classes of molecules involved in growth stimulatory pathways, including peptide growth factors and their receptors, cytoplasmic cell-signaling proteins, cell cycle control proteins, and transcription factors. Activation of protooncogenes by mutation, amplification, or chromosomal rearrangement can lead to disregulated growth and cellular transformation. Unlike the case with tumor suppressor genes, mutation of one copy of a protooncogene can be a dominant genetic alteration that results in loss of controlled cellular growth. There is extensive literature regarding the potential involvement of protooncogenes in the initiation and progression of EOC. The discussion here focuses on the oncogenes that are most frequently associated with EOC, with a particular emphasis on those associated with a certain histologic subtype and those whose alterations can be used to prove or disprove the association of LMP tumors to frankly invasive cancers.

Peptide growth factors and receptors.
What are the mechanisms of growth regulation of the normal human ovarian surface epithelium and of ovarian cancer? Peptide growth factors are secreted from cells and transmit growth stimulatory signals in a local environment.[100,101] Growth factors bind to cognate cell surface receptors, which relay the extracellular mitogenic signal via a series of cytoplasmic signaling proteins to the nucleus, where transcription factors mediate gene transcription.[100,101] Structurally, peptide growth factor receptors consist of an extracellular ligand-binding domain, a hydrophobic transmembrane, and a cytoplasmic domain with intrinsic

Table 28–4. Peptide Growth Factors and Receptors Expressed in Ovarian Carcinomas

Peptide Growth Factor	Cognate Receptor	References
Epidermal growth factor (EGF)	EGF-R	Kimmos et al.[180]; Morishige et al.[181]; Rodriguez et al.[182]
Transforming growth factor-α (TGF-α)	EGF-R	Kimmos et al.[180]; Morishige et al.[181]; Rodriguez et al.[182]
Insulin-like growth factor-1 (IGF-1)	IGF1-R	Yee et al.[183]
Platelet-derived growth factor (PDGF)	PDGF-R	Sariban et al.[184]; Henriksen et al.[185]
Fibroblast growth factor (FGF)	FGF-R	Di Blasio et al.[186]
Colony stimulating factor-1 (CSF-1)	CSF1-R	Ramakrishnan et al.[187]; Kacinski et al.[188,189]

tyrosine kinase activity. Ovarian carcinomas express a variety of growth factors and their cognate receptors,[102,103] as shown in Table 28-4. Because normal HOSE has also been shown to produce and respond to several of the same growth factors, it is unclear whether the expression of growth factors or their receptors is cause or consequence of malignant transformation of the ovarian surface epithelium.

Recent studies have led some investigators to propose a role for soluble forms of the EGF-R (ERBB1) and the ERBB2 receptor in the etiology of ovarian carcinoma (reviewed by Maihle and colleagues[104]). The soluble form of the EGF-R has been shown to inhibit activity of the intact receptor in vitro, and to be significantly reduced in metastatic ovarian carcinomas, compared with the primary cancers.[105] Conversely, the increased levels of the ERBB2 receptor have been found in patients with EOC and correlated to overexpression of the ERBB2 receptor and poor clinical outcome.[106-110] Further investigations are required to determine the biologic significance and potential clinical utility of these observations.

HER2/NEU. HER2/NEU (also referred to as ERBB2) is a 185-kd transmembrane glycoprotein that was initially identified as the transforming gene present in a chemically induced model of neuroglioblastoma in rat.[111] The HER2/NEU protein was found to have a high degree of homology to the EGF-R (encoded by ERBB1) and other members of the ERBB family of growth factor receptors, including HER3 (ERBB3) and HER4 (ERBB4). Activation of HER2/NEU has been reported in a variety of solid tumors including EOC,[112-114] and it is thought to occur by amplification of the gene or overexpression of the protein, perhaps as a result of the production of alternative transcripts that have increased stability.[115] Activating structural mutations of the *HER2/NEU* gene have not been identified in human cancers.[113,116-118]

There have been many reports of HER2/NEU overexpression in EOCs, with the percentage of positive cases varying from 15% to 50%, depending on the study.[113,119,120] The reasons for these inconsistencies remain unclear, but Slamon and associates[113] proposed they may reflect the different experimental means by which alterations are detected. Specifically, because contaminating stromal, vascular, and inflammatory cells are often present in EOC specimens, the contaminating normal component can obscure alterations in HER2/NEU expression. In addition, a common method of detection of HER2/NEU expression is by

immunohistochemical staining of tissues, which is exquisitely sensitive to variations in methods of tissue fixation and preparation. A consistently cited estimate of overexpression of HER2/NEU in EOCs is 20%. In studies of both breast and ovarian tumors, *HER2/NEU* gene amplification has been demonstrated for 20% to 30% of cases, with an additional 10% overexpressing the protein in the absence of gene amplification.[113] HER2/NEU overexpression in EOCs has not been correlated to histologic subtype, grade, or International Federation of Gynecologists and Obstetricians (FIGO) stage, but some reports do indicate that overexpression is more common in invasive cancers than in benign lesions or borderline tumors.[110,121-123] A comparison of specimens from newly diagnosed tumors with malignant ascites and tumors obtained at second surgeries showed that, although the primary cancers exhibited HER2/NEU in fewer than 25% of cases, all of the tumors and ascites obtained at subsequent surgery exhibited overexpression.[124] Based on these observations, the investigators suggested that overexpression of the HER2/NEU protein confers a selective growth advantage for tumor cells. Several studies have suggested that there is a significant correlation of HER2/NEU overexpression and poor prognosis,[113,120,125,126] but this association was not observed in several others.[127-129] This issue remains controversial, although there is some suggestion that statistical methods used in analysis may explain these results.[130] Several,[120,131,132] but not all,[133] studies have also suggested that chemotherapy is more likely to fail in patients with EOCs that overexpress HER2/NEU. Although there seems to be a consensus that HER2/NEU is overexpressed in approximately 20% of EOCs, further investigation is required to resolve issues regarding its prognostic significance and potential role in chemoresistance.

Intracellular signaling proteins.
RAS. The RAS family of cellular oncogenes encodes cell membrane–bound proteins with guanosine triphosphatase activity. Mutations in KRAS, HRAS, ad NRAS (*Harvey, Kirsten,* and *Neuroblastoma,* respectively) are common in a variety of human epithelial cancers.[134] These genes encode proteins that are normally activated by growth factor receptors and stimulate a cascade of serine-threonine kinases involved in cell signaling from the cell membrane to the nucleus. Activation by point mutation (most commonly at codons 12, 13, or 61) results in constitutive activation of the protein and chronic stimulation of downstream signaling events. Mutations of c-Ki-*ras* are observed most commonly in

mucinous tumors.[52,135-137] Several independent investigations have suggested not only a correlation with histologic subtype but also that K-*ras* mutation is an early event in the progression of mucinous tumors.[136,138-140]

There has been some discordance in reports relating to the frequency of mutation of K-*ras* in serous tumors. Mutation of K-*ras* occurs more frequently in serous borderline ovarian tumors and in those with LMP than in invasive serous carcinomas.[136,141] Ortiz and coworkers[142] analyzed K-*ras* mutations in a series of serous borderline ovarian tumors and subsequently occurring invasive serous carcinomas and found that most cases had different mutations in the invasive cancer than in the primary tumor. In light of these findings, it appears that serous borderline tumors arise via a molecular pathway that is distinct from that of invasive serous carcinomas and that these lesions are perhaps unrelated. Singer and colleagues[143] proposed that serous borderline ovarian tumors are related to, and potentially a precursor of, a recently recognized class of serous carcinomas consisting of micropapillary serous carcinomas (MPSCs) and invasive MPSCs, as opposed to common invasive serous carcinomas.

PIK3CA. PIK3CA encodes the p110α catalytic subunit of PI3K. PI3K is recruited by activated growth factor receptors and, in turn, activates the downstream effectors AKT1 and AKT2. The *PIK3CA* gene maps to chromosomal region 3q26, a region that is frequently amplified in EOCs. Investigation of *PIK3CA* as a candidate oncogene involved in ovarian tumorigenesis revealed an increased copy number of the gene; copy increase was associated with increased transcription, p110α protein expression, and PI3K activity.[144]

AKT2. The *AKT1* and *AKT2* genes encode serine-threonine kinases that share homology with the virally transduced oncogene *v-Akt*, which induces lymphomas in mice.[145] *AKT1* and *AKT2* encode proteins with serine-threonine kinase activity that lie downstream of PI3K in growth-stimulatory cell-signaling processes. Amplification of the *AKT2* gene in human ovarian carcinoma has been reported by several investigators,[49,146,147] and overexpression has been associated with higher grade and poor prognosis.[148]

Transcription factors.
MYC. The MYC family of protooncogenes, B-*myc*, c-*myc* (*MYC*), L-*myc*, N-*myc*, and s-*myc*, encode nuclear transcription factors that stimulate gene expression as a final result of the transduction of growth-stimulatory signals emanating from the cell surface. Alterations of MYC protooncogenes can occur via gene rearrangement or translocation or, as in most solid tumors, by gene amplification. The c-*myc* (*MYC*) gene is amplified or overexpressed in 25% to 37% of EOCs.[55,149-153] It has been mapped to chromosome 8q24, a chromosomal region that is frequently amplified in ovarian carcinomas.[154-156] Studies using fluorescen in situ hybridization (FISH) analysis have demonstrated amplification of *MYC* by an oncogene:centromere (chromosome 8)

ratio analysis[157] and have found that *MYC* is the origin of the homogeneous staining region (hsr) in ovarian carcinomas.[155]

β-Catenin. Studies have revealed a potential role for alterations of the *CTNNB1* gene, which encodes β-catenin, in the endometrioid subtype of ovarian cancer.[158-162] The β-catenin protein is involved in both cell adhesion via interactions with E-cadherin at the cell membrane and T-cell factor (TCF)–regulated transcription mediated by WNT signaling.[163] Several groups of investigators reported a high frequency of mutations in the *CTNNB1* gene and nuclear accumulation of the β-catenin protein in endometrioid carcinomas.[158-161] A later study confirmed frequent mutations of *CTNNB1* and further demonstrated alterations in members of the β-catenin/TCF signaling pathway (including AXIN1, AXIN2, APC, cyclin D1, MMP7, PPAR-Δ, connexin 43, and ITF2) in cases where mutations of the *CTNNB1* gene were absent but expression of the β-catenin was aberrant.[162,164] These studies indicate the likely significance of β-catenin, WNT signaling, or both in the development and progression of ovarian endometrioid carcinoma.

Molecular profiling for classification of epithelial ovarian carcinomas. A significant effort is now under way to characterize tumors by molecular profiling. Molecular profiling uses high-throughput technologies to assess genomic, gene expression, and protein expression alterations in an effort to characterize and classify tumors en masse. CGH and spectral karyotyping (SKY) are used to identify gross alterations (chromosomal gains, losses, and translocations) in genomic structure in tumors. Gene expression profiles of tumors are investigated by the comparison of tumor to normal tissue using serial analysis of gene expression (SAGE) and cDNA microarray technologies. Large-scale analysis of cellular protein profiles of normal and tumor tissue are also being used to reveal quantitative changes in expression and post-translational modifications of proteins that can be important hallmarks of disease. Investigation of molecular alterations using multiple modalities to analyze DNA, RNA, and protein is advantageous in that important molecular alterations are not likely to be missed, and in some cases they may be validated by two or more of the methods used for analysis. The use of high-throughput technologies allows for relatively rapid data acquisition for a large number of specimens. The hope is to compare large numbers of tumor specimens and ultimately to classify tumors by tissue type and histologic subtype as well as to identify important biomarkers that can assist in diagnosis, detection, and clinical management of disease.

Molecular profiling is particularly attractive with regard to ovarian cancer. If, as most investigators hypothesize, EOCs of each different histologic subtype arise by genetic alterations affecting distinct molecular pathways, then analysis of large numbers of tumors of each subtype may yield molecular signatures that are unique to each. In the process, genes may be identified that contribute to disease initiation or progression. Another question that may be answered in the process of molecular profiling of ovarian carcinomas is whether benign, borderline (LMP), and invasive cancers of each histologic subtype are related to one another by molecular signature, which would indicate a progression of disease through this pathway. By comparison of early-stage invasive cancers with those that are more advanced, molecular profiling may reveal biomarkers that are hallmarks of early disease, providing targets for early diagnosis and chemotherapeutic treatments.

Early investigations using profiling strategies with EOCs have already begun to meet some of these goals. Moreover, independent studies conducted at individual institutions have identified similar biomarkers, effectively providing independent validation of each study. For example, several independent analyses of gene expression (using SAGE and cDNA microarrays) have identified similar genes that are either upregulated or downregulated in EOC.[47,165-167] Examples of genes that are consistently identified as upregulated in EOCs are mucin-1, claudin-3 and -4, and the *WFDC2* gene, which encodes the epididymal-specific whey acidic protein, a secreted protease inhibitor that holds significant promise as a tumor marker.[47,165-167] As large datasets are obtained and mined, gene expression patterns begin to emerge, such as groups of genes that are coordinately regulated.[168] In addition, analysis of large numbers of EOCs has allowed investigators to reduce the complexity of arrays used for gene expression analyses by eliminating large subsets of genes that are not expressed or whose expression does not change in EOCs compared with normal ovarian tissue.[169] Molecular profiling of EOCs undoubtedly will contribute greatly to understanding of the individual histologic subtypes of EOCs and of the development of ovarian carcinomas in general.

Cancers With Phenotypes Similar to Ovarian Cancer

There are two malignancies in the female that have a clinical behavior similar to that of ovarian cancer and are treated similarly. These are cancer of the oviduct and primary peritoneal cancer. The fallopian tube is the least common site of origin for malignant neoplasms of the female genital tract. In contrast to ovarian cancer, tubal tumors cause early clinical signs and symptoms. They tend to metastasize intra-abdominally in a manner similar to ovarian cancer and therefore are assumed to have the same biologic characteristics.[170] The most common histologic type of tubal malignancy is papillary serous carcinoma.

The literature on molecular biology and molecular genetics of fallopian tube cancers is scarce. The data are insufficient to offer conclusions about the significance or frequency of oncogene and tumor suppressor gene alterations. In one study of *HER2/NEU* using a real-time PCR assay, no tumors displayed amplification of the oncogene.[171] In a second study of 43 women

with fallopian tube carcinomas, the gene products of *HER2/NEU* and *TP53* were identified in 26% and 61% of the tumors, respectively, frequencies similar to those seen in ovarian carcinoma. However, in contrast to ovarian tumors, their expression was not associated with a worse prognosis.[172] A genetic epidemiologic study of carcinoma of the fallopian tube concluded that this type of tumor should be considered a clinical component of the hereditary breast and ovarian cancer syndrome, and it may be associated with *BRCA1* and *BRCA2* mutations. It is important to consider the risk of fallopian tube carcinoma when prophylactic oophorectomy is performed in high-risk women.[173,174]

Primary peritoneal carcinoma is a recently recognized disease entity that is characterized by carcinomatosis in the peritoneal cavity, with minimal to no involvement of the ovary, and by the lack of an identifiable primary tumor.[175] This is a relatively rare disease that occurs uniquely in women and has been reported in women who have undergone prophylactic oophorectomy.[175] Primary peritoneal carcinomas most frequently exhibit serous histology. Papillary serous carcinoma of the peritoneum (PSCP) is a malignant tumor that is widespread in the peritoneum but present in the ovary only on the surface, if at all. These tumors are identical to serous papillary ovarian carcinoma in presentation, appearance, and response to treatment. PSCP may have acquired many of the same molecular alterations that are observed in papillary serous ovarian carcinomas, but, because of its infrequent diagnosis, relatively few cases are available for study. Despite the many similarities in molecular alterations (e.g., loss of WT1[176]) observed in PSCPs and papillary serous ovarian carcinomas and the accumulation of P53,[177] it is proposed that the diseases are distinct entities. Support for this hypothesis lies in studies reporting that, although primary EOCs are usually unifocal in origin, PSCP is likely to have a multifocal origin, as evidenced by distinct patterns of allelic loss and both the presence and absence of *TP53* mutations in samples from multiple tumor sites in the same patient.[178,179]

Conclusions

This chapter summarized studies on the molecular biology and molecular genetics of ovarian cancer. These studies address several controversies with regard to the disease. The question was raised as to whether ovarian cancer follows the multistep model of carcinogenesis that is characteristic of most cancers. It seems rational, on the basis of available data and lack of conclusive proof in the alternative, to suggest that preneoplasia precedes overt disease, as in other solid tumor types. There is no reason why ovarian cancer should be different. There has also been some controversy as to whether ovarian cancer arises from the surface epithelium. In this regard, data on the ability to experimentally transform rat, mouse, and human surface epithelium supports the long-held view that ovarian cancer arises from this cell type. With the advent of modern molecular biology techniques, much information has been generated concerning gene expression and genetic alterations in ovarian cancer. The difficulty remains in proving which ones are causal to some aspect of the disease phenotype. The most conclusive answers to these questions may require the use of transgenic ovarian cancer models. The question has also been posed as to whether any of the molecular changes in ovarian cancer thus far discovered warrant routine analysis. With the exception of those genes documented to be involved in the inheritance of risk of ovarian cancer (i.e., *BRCA1*, *BRCA2*, and MMR genes), routine analysis is not justified. Even for these genes, a family history of ovarian or ovarian/breast cancer is generally considered important before germline analysis of mutation in these genes is undertaken. The last area discussed relates to how growth of HOSE and its transformed counterpart is controlled. Here, cell line models are clearly yielding information. The question remains whether perturbation of these pathways will yield clinical benefit. In summary, much progress is being made with regard to understanding ovarian cancer etiology and progression. It is hoped that this information will lead to more effective prevention, diagnosis, and treatment.

REFERENCES

1. Fearon ER, Vogelstein B: Genetic model for colorectal tumorigenesis. Cell 1990;61:759-767.
2. Cancer Facts and Figures. Atlanta: American Cancer Society, 2002.
3. Hamilton TC: Ovarian cancer. Part I: Biology. Curr Probl Cancer 1992;16:1-57.
4. Bast RC Jr, Boyer CM, Jacobs I, et al: Cell growth regulation in epithelial ovarian cancer. Cancer 1993;71(4 Suppl):1597-1601.
5. Godwin AK, Testa JR, Hamilton TC: The biology of ovarian cancer development. Cancer 1993;71(2 Suppl):530-536.
6. Hamilton TC, Johnson SW, Godwin AK: Molecular biology of gynecologic malignancies. Cancer Treat Res 1998;95:103-114.
7. Auersperg N, Maclaren IA, Kruk PA: Ovarian surface epithelium: Autonomous production of connective tissue-type extracellular matrix. Biol Reprod 1991;44:717-724.
8. Auersperg N, Wong AS, Choi KC, et al: Ovarian surface epithelium: Biology, endocrinology, and pathology. Endocr Rev 2001;22:255-288.
9. Piver MS, Baker TR, Jishi MF, et al: Familial ovarian cancer: A report of 658 families from the Gilda Radner Familial Ovarian Cancer Registry 1981-1991. Cancer 1993;71(2 Suppl):582-588.
10. Kruk PA, Maines-Bandiera SL, Auersperg N: A simplified method to culture human ovarian surface epithelium. Lab Invest 1990;63:132-136.
11. Auersperg N, Maines-Bandiera S, Booth JH, et al: Expression of two mucin antigens in cultured human ovarian surface epithelium: Influence of a family history of ovarian cancer. Am J Obstet Gynecol 1995;173:558-565.
12. Auersperg N, Maines-Bandiera SL, Dyck HG: Ovarian carcinogenesis and the biology of ovarian surface epithelium. J Cell Physiol 1997;173:261-265.
13. Clement PB: Histology of the ovary. Am J Surg Pathol 1987;11:277-303.
14. Scully RE: Definition of precursors in gynecologic cancer. Cancer 1981;48(2 Suppl):531-537.
15. Puls LE, Powell DE, DePriest PD, et al: Transition from benign to malignant epithelium in mucinous and serous ovarian cystadenocarcinoma. Gynecol Oncol 1992;47:53-57.
16. Powell DE, Puls L, van Nagell J Jr: Current concepts in epithelial ovarian tumors: Does benign to malignant transformation occur? Hum Pathol 1992;23:846-847.
17. Resta L, Russo S, Colucci GA, Prat J: Morphologic precursors of ovarian epithelial tumors. Obstet Gynecol 1993;82:181-186.
18. Scully RE: Pathology of ovarian cancer precursors. J Cell Biochem Suppl 1995;23:208-218.
19. Salazar H, Godwin AK, Daly MB, et al: Microscopic benign and invasive malignant neoplasms and a cancer-prone phenotype in prophylactic oophorectomies. J Natl Cancer Inst 1996;88:1810-1820.
20. Dubeau L: The cell of origin of ovarian epithelial tumors and the ovarian surface epithelium dogma: Does the emperor have no clothes? Gynecol Oncol 1999;72:437-442.
21. Radisavljevic SV: The pathogenesis of ovarian inclusion cysts and cystomas. Obstet Gynecol 1977;49:424-429.
22. Bell DA, Scully RE: Early de novo ovarian carcinoma: A study of fourteen cases. Cancer 1994;73:1859-1864.
23. Aoki Y, Kawada N, Tanaka K: Early form of ovarian cancer originating in inclusion cysts: A case report. J Reprod Med 2000;45:159-161.
24. Werness BA, Afify AM, Bielat KL, et al: Altered surface and cyst epithelium of ovaries removed prophylactically from women with a family history of ovarian cancer. Hum Pathol 1999;30:151-157.
25. Fathalla MF: Incessant ovulation: A factor in ovarian neoplasia? Lancet 1971;2:163.
26. Riman T, Persson I, Nilsson S: Hormonal aspects of epithelial ovarian cancer: Review of epidemiological evidence. Clin Endocrinol (Oxf) 1998;49:695-707.
27. Whittemore AS, Harris R, Itnyre J: Characteristics relating to ovarian cancer risk: Collaborative analysis of 12 US case-control studies. IV. The pathogenesis of epithelial ovarian cancer. Collaborative Ovarian Cancer Group. Am J Epidemiol 1992;136:1212-1220.
28. Rodriguez GC, Walmer DK, Cline M, et al: Effect of progestin on the ovarian epithelium of macaques: Cancer prevention through apoptosis? J Soc Gynecol Investig 1998;5:271-276.
29. Fredrickson TN: Ovarian tumors of the hen. Environ Health Perspect 1987;73:35-51.
30. Fathalla MF: Factors in the causation and incidence of ovarian cancer. Obstet Gynecol Surv 1972;27:751-768.
31. Godwin AK, Testa JR, Handel LM, et al: Spontaneous transformation of rat ovarian surface epithelial cells: Association with cytogenetic changes and implications of repeated ovulation in the etiology of ovarian cancer. J Natl Cancer Inst 1992;84:592-601.
32. Testa JR, Getts LA, Salazar H, et al: Spontaneous transformation of rat ovarian surface epithelial cells results in well to poorly differentiated tumors with a parallel range of cytogenetic complexity. Cancer Res 1994;54:2778-2784.
33. Abdollahi A, Roberts D, Godwin AK, et al: Identification of a zinc-finger gene at 6q25: A chromosomal region implicated in development of many solid tumors. Oncogene 1997;14:1973-1979.
34. Abdollahi A, Godwin AK, Miller PD, et al: Identification of a gene containing zinc-finger motifs based on lost expression in malignantly transformed rat ovarian surface epithelial cells. Cancer Res 1997;57:2029-2034.
35. Abdollahi A, Getts LA, Sonoda G, et al: Genome scanning detects amplification of the cathepsin B gene (CtsB) in transformed rat ovarian surface epithelial cells. J Soc Gynecol Investig 1999;6:32-40.
36. Abdollahi A, Bao R, Hamilton TC: LOT1 is a growth suppressor gene down-regulated by the epidermal growth factor receptor ligands and encodes a nuclear zinc-finger protein. Oncogene 1999;18:6477-6487.
37. Diatchenko L, Lau YF, Campbell AP, et al: Suppression subtractive hybridization: A method for generating differentially regulated or tissue-specific cDNA probes and libraries. Proc Natl Acad Sci U S A 1996;93:6025-6030.
38. Roberts D, Williams SJ, Cvetkovic D, et al: Decreased expression of retinol-binding proteins is associated with malignant transformation of the ovarian surface epithelium. DNA Cell Biol 2002;21:11-1 9.
39. Kuppumbatti YS, Bleiweiss IJ, Mandeli JP, et al: Cellular retinol-binding protein expression and breast cancer. J Natl Cancer Inst 2000;92:475-480.

40. Cvetkovic D, Williams SJ, Hamilton TC: Loss of cellular retinol-binding protein 1 gene expression in microdissected human ovarian cancer. Clin Cancer Res 2003;9:1013-1020.

41. Gallion HH, Pieretti M, DePriest PD, van Nagell JR Jr: The molecular basis of ovarian cancer. Cancer 1995;76(10 Suppl):1992-1997.

42. Berchuck A, Kohler MF, Bast RC Jr: Molecular genetic features of ovarian cancer. Prog Clin Biol Res 1996;394:269-284.

43. Matias-Guiu X, Prat J: Molecular pathology of ovarian carcinomas. Virchows Arch 1998;433:103-111.

44. Aunoble B, Sanches R, Didier E, Bignon YJ: Major oncogenes and tumor suppressor genes involved in epithelial ovarian cancer [review]. Int J Oncol 2000;16:567-576.

45. Kinzler KW, Vogelstein B: Cancer-susceptibility genes: Gatekeepers and caretakers. Nature 1997;386:761, 763.

46. Kallioniemi A, Kallioniemi OP, Sudar D, et al: Comparative genomic hybridization for molecular cytogenetic analysis of solid tumors. Science 1992;258:818-821.

47. Shridhar V, Lee J, Pandita A, et al: Genetic analysis of early- versus late-stage ovarian tumors. Cancer Res 2001;61:5895-5904.

48. Cliby W, Ritland S, Hartmann L, et al: Human epithelial ovarian cancer allelotype. Cancer Res 1993;53(10 Suppl):2393-2398.

49. Cheng PC, Gosewehr JA, Kim TM, et al: Potential role of the inactivated X chromosome in ovarian epithelial tumor development. J Natl Cancer Inst 1996;88:510-518.

50. Saito H, Inazawa J, Saito S, et al: Detailed deletion mapping of chromosome 17q in ovarian and breast cancers: 2-cM region on 17q21.3 often and commonly deleted in tumors. Cancer Res 1993;53:3382-3385.

51. Godwin AK, Vanderveer L, Schultz DC, et al: A common region of deletion on chromosome 17q in both sporadic and familial epithelial ovarian tumors distal to BRCA1. Am J Hum Genet 1994;55:666-677.

52. Pieretti M, Cavalieri C, Conway PS, et al: Genetic alterations distinguish different types of ovarian tumors. Int J Cancer 1995;64:434-440.

53. Iwabuchi H, Sakamoto M, Sakunaga H, et al: Genetic analysis of benign, low-grade, and high-grade ovarian tumors. Cancer Res 1995;55:6172-6180.

54. Watson RH, Neville PJ, Roy WJ Jr, et al: Loss of heterozygosity on chromosomes 7p, 7q, 9p and 11q is an early event in ovarian tumorigenesis. Oncogene 1998;17:207-212.

55. Claus EB, Schildkraut JM, Thompson WD, Risch NJ: The genetic attributable risk of breast and ovarian cancer. Cancer 1996;77:2318-2324.

56. Bewtra C, Watson P, Conway T, et al: Hereditary ovarian cancer: A clinicopathological study. Int J Gynecol Pathol 1992;11:180-187.

57. Boyd J, Rubin SC: Hereditary ovarian cancer: Molecular genetics and clinical implications. Gynecol Oncol 1997;64:196-206.

58. Schildkraut JM, Thompson WD: Familial ovarian cancer: A population-based case-control study. Am J Epidemiol 1988;128:456-466.

59. Miki Y, Swensen J, Shattuck-Eidens D, et al: A strong candidate for the breast and ovarian cancer susceptibility gene BRCA1. Science 1994;266:66-71.

60. Castilla LH, Couch FJ, Erdos MR, et al: Mutations in the BRCA1 gene in families with early-onset breast and ovarian cancer. Nat Genet 1994;8:387-391.

61. Simard J, Tonin P, Durocher F, et al: Common origins of BRCA1 mutations in Canadian breast and ovarian cancer families. Nat Genet 1994;8:392-398.

62. Ford D, Easton DF, Bishop DT, et al: Risks of cancer in BRCA1-mutation carriers. Breast Cancer Linkage Consortium. Lancet 1994;343:692-695.

63. Easton DF, Ford D, Bishop DT: Breast and ovarian cancer incidence in BRCA1-mutation carriers. Breast Cancer Linkage Consortium. Am J Hum Genet 1995;56:265-271.

64. Ford D, Easton DF, Stratton M, et al: Genetic heterogeneity and penetrance analysis of the BRCA1 and BRCA2 genes in breast cancer families. The Breast Cancer Linkage Consortium. Am J Hum Genet 1998;62:676-689.

65. Narod SA, Goldgar D, Cannon-Albright L, et al: Risk modifiers in carriers of BRCA1 mutations. Int J Cancer 1995;64:394-398.

66. Narod SA, Risch H, Moslehi R, et al: Oral contraceptives and the risk of hereditary ovarian cancer. Hereditary Ovarian Cancer Clinical Study Group. N Engl J Med 1998;339:424-428.

67. Russell SE, Hickey GI, Lowry WS, et al: Allele loss from chromosome 17 in ovarian cancer. Oncogene 1990;5:1581-1583.

68. Jacobs IJ, Smith SA, Wiseman RW, et al: A deletion unit on chromosome 17q in epithelial ovarian tumors distal to the familial breast/ovarian cancer locus. Cancer Res 1993;53:1218-1221.

69. Tavtigian SV, Simard J, Rommens J, et al: The complete BRCA2 gene and mutations in chromosome 13q-linked kindreds. Nat Genet 1996;12:333-337.

70. Hakem R, de la Pompa JL, Sirard C, et al: The tumor suppressor gene Brca1 is required for embryonic cellular proliferation in the mouse. Cell 1996;85:1009-1023.

71. Suzuki A, de la Pompa JL, Hakem R, et al: Brca2 is required for embryonic cellular proliferation in the mouse. Genes Dev 1997;11:1242-1252.

72. Koonin EV, Altschul SF, Bork P: BRCA1 protein products: Functional motifs. Nat Genet 1996;13:266-268.

73. Chapman MS, Verma IM: Transcriptional activation by BRCA1. Nature 1996;382:678-679.

74. Monteiro AN, August A, Hanafusa H: Evidence for a transcriptional activation function of BRCA1 C-terminal region. Proc Natl Acad Sci U S A 1996;93:13595-13599.

75. Scully R, Chen J, Plug A, et al: Association of BRCA1 with Rad51 in mitotic and meiotic cells. Cell 1997;88:265-275.

76. Lane DP: Cancer: p53, guardian of the genome. Nature 1992;358:15-16.

77. Kohler MF, Kerns BJ, Humphrey PA, et al: Mutation and over-expression of p53 in early-stage epithelial ovarian cancer. Obstet Gynecol 1993;81(5 Pt 1):643-650.

78. Eltabbakh GH, Belinson JL, Kennedy AW, et al: p53 overexpression is not an independent prognostic factor for patients with primary ovarian epithelial cancer. Cancer 1997;80:892-898.

79. Bennett M, Macdonald K, Chan SW, et al: Cell surface trafficking of Fas: A rapid mechanism of p53-mediated apoptosis. Science 1998;282:290-293.

80. Mazars R, Pujol P, Maudelonde T, et al: p53 mutations in ovarian cancer: A late event? Oncogene 1991;6:1685-1690.

81. Berchuck A, Kohler MF, Hopkins MP, et al: Overexpression of p53 is not a feature of benign and early-stage borderline epithelial ovarian tumors. Gynecol Oncol 1994;52:232-236.

82. Peltomaki P, Vasen HF: Mutations predisposing to hereditary nonpolyposis colorectal cancer: Database and results of a collaborative study. The International Collaborative Group on Hereditary Nonpolyposis Colorectal Cancer. Gastroenterology 1997;113:1146-1158.

83. Leach FS, Nicolaides NC, Papadopoulos N, et al: Mutations of a mutS homolog in hereditary nonpolyposis colorectal cancer. Cell 1993;75:1215-1225.

84. Obata K, Morland SJ, Watson RH, et al: Frequent PTEN/MMAC mutations in endometrioid but not serous or mucinous epithelial ovarian tumors. Cancer Res 1998;58:2095-2097.

85. Fujii H, Matsumoto T, Yoshida M, et al: Genetics of synchronous uterine and ovarian endometrioid carcinoma: Combined analyses of loss of heterozygosity, PTEN mutation, and microsatellite instability. Hum Pathol 2002;33:421-428.

86. Kurose K, Zhou XP, Araki T, et al: Frequent loss of PTEN expression is linked to elevated phosphorylated Akt levels, but not associated with p27 and cyclin D1 expression, in primary epithelial ovarian carcinomas. Am J Pathol 2001;158:2097-2106.

87. Gemma A, Takenoshita S, Hagiwara K, et al: Molecular analysis of the cyclin-dependent kinase inhibitor genes p15INK4b/MTS2, p16INK4/MTS1, p18 and p19 in human cancer cell lines. Int J Cancer 1996;68:605-611.

88. Schultz DC, Vanderveer L, Buetow KH, et al: Characterization of chromosome 9 in human ovarian neoplasia identifies frequent genetic imbalance on 9q and rare alterations involving 9p, including CDKN2. Cancer Res 1995;55:2150-2157.

89. Kudoh K, Ichikawa Y, Yoshida S, et al: Inactivation of p16/CDKN2 and p15/MTS2 is associated with prognosis and response to chemotherapy in ovarian cancer. Int J Cancer 2002;99:579-582.

90. Tsuji K, Mizumoto K, Sudo H, et al: p53-independent apoptosis is induced by the p19(ARF) tumor suppressor. Biochem Biophys Res Commun 2002;295:621-629.

91. Yu Y, Xu F, Peng H, et al: NOEY2 (ARHI), an imprinted putative tumor suppressor gene in ovarian and breast carcinomas. Proc Natl Acad Sci U S A 1999;96:214-219.

92. Xu F, Xia W, Luo RZ, et al: The human ARHI tumor suppressor gene inhibits lactation and growth in transgenic mice. Cancer Res 2000;60:4913-4920.

93. Xu XX, Yang W, Jackowski S, Rock CO: Cloning of a novel phosphoprotein regulated by colony-stimulating factor 1 shares a domain with the *Drosophila* disabled gene product. J Biol Chem 1995;270:14184-14191.

94. Fazili Z, Sun W, Mittelstaedt S, et al: Disabled-2 inactivation is an early step in ovarian tumorigenicity. Oncogene 1999;18:3104-3113.

95. Sheng Z, Sun W, Smith E, et al: Restoration of positioning control following Disabled-2 expression in ovarian and breast tumor cells. Oncogene 2000;19:4847-4854.

96. Yang DH, Smith ER, Cohen C, et al: Molecular events associated with dysplastic morphologic transformation and initiation of ovarian tumorigenicity. Cancer 2002;94:2380-2392.

97. Schultz DC, Vanderveer L, Berman DB, et al: Identification of two candidate tumor suppressor genes on chromosome 17p13.3. Cancer Res 1996;56:1997-2002.

98. Bruening W, Prowse AH, Schultz DC, et al: Expression of OVCA1, a candidate tumor suppressor, is reduced in tumors and inhibits growth of ovarian cancer cells. Cancer Res 1999;59:4973-4983.

99. Prowse AH, Vanderveer L, Milling SW, et al: OVCA2 is downregulated and degraded during retinoid-induced apoptosis. Int J Cancer 2002;99:185-192.

100. Schlessinger J, Schreiber AB, Levi A, et al: Regulation of cell proliferation by epidermal growth factor. CRC Crit Rev Biochem 1983;14:93-111.

101. Yarden Y, Ullrich A: Growth factor receptor tyrosine kinases. Annu Rev Biochem 1988;57:443-478.

102. Bauknecht T, Kiechle M, Bauer G, Siebers JW: Characterization of growth factors in human ovarian carcinomas. Cancer Res 1986;46:2614-2618.

103. Berchuck A, Olt GJ, Everitt L, et al: The role of peptide growth factors in epithelial ovarian cancer. Obstet Gynecol 1990;75:255-262.

104. Maihle NJ, Baron AT, Barrette BA, et al: EGF/ErbB receptor family in ovarian cancer. Cancer Treat Res 2002;107:247-258.

105. Ilekis JV, Gariti J, Niederberger C, Scoccia B: Expression of a truncated epidermal growth factor receptor-like protein (TEGFR) in ovarian cancer. Gynecol Oncol 1997;65:36-41.

106. Yazici H, Dolapcioglu K, Buyru F, Dalay N: Utility of c-erbB-2 expression in tissue and sera of ovarian cancer patients. Cancer Invest 2000;18:110-114.

107. Wu JT, Astill ME, Zhang P: Detection of the extracellular domain of c-erbB-2 oncoprotein in sera from patients with various carcinomas: correlation with tumor markers. J Clin Lab Anal 1993;7:31-40.

108. McKenzie SJ, DeSombre KA, Bast BS, et al: Serum levels of HER-2 neu (C-erbB-2) correlate with overexpression of p185neu in human ovarian cancer. Cancer 1993;71:3942-3946.

109. Molina R, Jo J, Filella X, et al: Serum levels of C-erbB-2 (HER-2/neu) in patients with malignant and non-malignant diseases. Tumour Biol 1997;18:188-196.

110. Cheung TH, Wong YF, Chung TK, et al: Clinical use of serum c-erbB-2 in patients with ovarian masses. Gynecol Obstet Invest 1999;48:133-137.

111. Shih C, Padhy LC, Murray M, Weinberg RA: Transforming genes of carcinomas and neuroblastomas introduced into mouse fibroblasts. Nature 1981;290:261-264.

112. Slamon DJ, Clark GM, Wong SG, et al: Human breast cancer: Correlation of relapse and survival with amplification of the HER-2/neu oncogene. Science 1987;235:177-182.

113. Slamon DJ, Godolphin W, Jones LA, et al: Studies of the *HER-2/neu* proto-oncogene in human breast and ovarian cancer. Science 1989;244:707-712.

114. Wright C, Mellon K, Neal DE, et al: Expression of c-erbB-2 protein product in bladder cancer. Br J Cancer 1990;62:764-765.

115. Doherty JK, Bond CT, Hua W, et al: An alternative HER-2/neu transcript of 8 kb has an extended 3′UTR and displays increased stability in SKOV-3 ovarian carcinoma cells. Gynecol Oncol 1999;74:408-415.

116. Greenlee RT, Hill-Harmon MB, Murray T, Thun M: Cancer statistics, 2001. CA Cancer J Clin 2001;51:15-36.

117. Kraus MH, Popescu NC, Amsbaugh SC, King CR: Overexpression of the EGF receptor-related proto-oncogene *erbB-2* in human mammary tumor cell lines by different molecular mechanisms. Embo J 1987;6:605-610.

118. Lemoine NR, Staddon S, Dickson C, et al: Absence of activating transmembrane mutations in the *c-erbB-2* proto-oncogene in human breast cancer. Oncogene 1990;5:237-239.

119. Zhang X, Silva E, Gershenson D, Hung MC: Amplification and rearrangement of *c-erb B* proto-oncogenes in cancer of human female genital tract. Oncogene 1989;4:985-989.

120. Berchuck A, Kamel A, Whitaker R, et al: Overexpression of HER-2/neu is associated with poor survival in advanced epithelial ovarian cancer. Cancer Res 1990;50:4087-4091.

121. Rubin SC, Finstad CL, Federici MG, et al: Prevalence and significance of HER-2/neu expression in early epithelial ovarian cancer. Cancer 1994;73:1456-1459.

122. Afify AM, Werness BA, Mark HF: HER-2/neu oncogene amplification in stage I and stage III ovarian papillary serous carcinoma. Exp Mol Pathol 1999;66:163-169.

123. Kim YT, Kim JW, Lee JW: c-erbB-2 oncoprotein assay in ovarian carcinoma and its clinical correlation with prognostic factors. Cancer Lett 1998;132:91-97.

124. Hellstrom I, Goodman G, Pullman J, et al: Overexpression of HER-2 in ovarian carcinomas. Cancer Res 2001;61:2420-2423.

125. Kacinski BM, Mayer AG, King BL, et al: NEU protein overexpression in benign, borderline, and malignant ovarian neoplasms. Gynecol Oncol 1992;44:245-253.

126. Hengstler JG, Lange J, Kett A, et al: Contribution of c-erbB-2 and topoisomerase IIalpha to chemoresistance in ovarian cancer. Cancer Res 1999;59:3206-3214.

127. Rubin SC, Finstad CL, Wong GY, et al: Prognostic significance of HER-2/neu expression in advanced epithelial ovarian cancer: A multivariate analysis. Am J Obstet Gynecol 1993;168(1 Pt 1):162-169.

128. Singleton TP, Perrone T, Oakley G, et al: Activation of c-erbB-2 and prognosis in ovarian carcinoma: Comparison with histologic type, grade, and stage. Cancer 1994;73:1460-1466.

129. Ross JS, Yang F, Kallakury BV, et al: *HER-2/neu* oncogene amplification by fluorescence in situ hybridization in epithelial tumors of the ovary. Am J Clin Pathol 1999;111:311-316.

130. Fajac A, Benard J, Lhomme C, et al: *c-erbB2* gene amplification and protein expression in ovarian epithelial tumors: Evaluation of their respective prognostic significance by multivariate analysis. Int J Cancer 1995;64:146-151.

131. Meden H, Marx D, Rath W, et al: Overexpression of the oncogene *c-erb B2* in primary ovarian cancer: Evaluation of the prognostic value in a Cox proportional hazards multiple regression. Int J Gynecol Pathol 1994;13:45-53.

132. Felip E, Del Campo JM, Rubio D, et al: Overexpression of c-erbB-2 in epithelial ovarian cancer: Prognostic value and relationship with response to chemotherapy. Cancer 1995;75:2147-2152.

133. Goff BA, Ries JA, Els LP, et al: Immunophenotype of ovarian cancer as predictor of clinical outcome: Evaluation at primary surgery and second-look procedure. Gynecol Oncol 1998;70:378-385.

134. Kiaris H, Spandidos DA: Mutations of *ras* genes in human cancers. Int J Oncol 1995;7:413-421.

135. Enomoto T, Weghorst CM, Inoue M, et al: K-ras activation occurs frequently in mucinous adenocarcinomas and rarely in other common epithelial tumors of the human ovary. Am J Pathol 1991;139:777-785.

136. Mok SC, Bell DA, Knapp RC, et al: Mutation of *K-ras* protooncogene in human ovarian epithelial tumors of borderline malignancy. Cancer Res 1993;53:1489-1492.

137. Scambia G, Masciullo V, Benedetti Panici P, et al: Prognostic significance of ras/p21 alterations in human ovarian cancer. Br J Cancer 1997;75:1547-1553.

138. Cuatrecasas M, Villanueva A, Matias-Guiu X, Prat J: *K-ras* mutations in mucinous ovarian tumors: A clinicopathologic and molecular study of 95 cases. Cancer 1997;79:1581-1586.

139. Morita K, Ono Y, Fukui H, et al: Incidence of P53 and K-ras alterations in ovarian mucinous and serous tumors. Pathol Int 2000;50:219-223.

140. Garrett AP, Lee KR, Colitti CR, et al: *K-ras* mutation may be an early event in mucinous ovarian tumorigenesis. Int J Gynecol Pathol 2001;20:244-251.

141. Haas CJ, Diebold J, Hirschmann A, et al: In serous ovarian neoplasms the frequency of *Ki-ras* mutations correlates with their malignant potential. Virchows Arch 1999;434:117-120.

142. Ortiz BH, Ailawadi M, Colitti C, et al: Second primary or recurrence? Comparative patterns of *p53* and *K-ras* mutations suggest that serous borderline ovarian tumors and subsequent serous carcinomas are unrelated tumors. Cancer Res 2001;61:7264-7267.

143. Singer G, Kurman RJ, Chang HW, et al: Diverse tumorigenic pathways in ovarian serous carcinoma. Am J Pathol 2002;160:1223-1228.

144. Shayesteh L, Lu Y, Kuo WL, et al: *PIK3CA* is implicated as an oncogene in ovarian cancer. Nat Genet 1999;21:99-102.

145. Bellacosa A, Testa JR, Staal SP, Tsichlis PN: A retroviral oncogene, *akt*, encoding a serine-threonine kinase containing an SH2-like region. Science 1991;254:274-277.

146. Thompson FH, Nelson MA, Trent JM, et al: Amplification of 19q13.1-q13.2 sequences in ovarian cancer: G-band, FISH, and molecular studies. Cancer Genet Cytogenet 1996;87:55-62.

147. Yuan ZQ, Sun M, Feldman RI, et al: Frequent activation of AKT2 and induction of apoptosis by inhibition of phosphoinositide-3-OH kinase/Akt pathway in human ovarian cancer. Oncogene 2000;19:2324-2330.

148. Bellacosa A, de Feo D, Godwin AK, et al: Molecular alterations of the *AKT2* oncogene in ovarian and breast carcinomas. Int J Cancer 1995;64:280-285.

149. Zhou DJ, Gonzalez-Cadavid N, Ahuja H, et al: A unique pattern of proto-oncogene abnormalities in ovarian adenocarcinomas. Cancer 1988;62:1573-1576.

150. Baker VV, Borst MP, Dixon D, et al: C-myc amplification in ovarian cancer. Gynecol Oncol 1990;38:340-342.

151. Sasano H, Garrett CT, Wilkinson DS, et al: Protooncogene amplification and tumor ploidy in human ovarian neoplasms. Hum Pathol 1990;21:382-391.

152. Tashiro H, Miyazaki K, Okamura H, et al: C-myc overexpression in human primary ovarian tumors: Its relevance to tumor progression. Int J Cancer 1992;50:828-833.

153. Diebold J, Suchy B, Baretton GB, et al: DNA ploidy and MYC DNA amplification in ovarian carcinomas: Correlation with p53 and bcl-2 expression, proliferative activity and prognosis. Virchows Arch 1996;429:221-227.

154. Sonoda G, Palazzo J, du Manoir S, et al: Comparative genomic hybridization detects frequent overrepresentation of chromosomal material from 3q26, 8q24, and 20q13 in human ovarian carcinomas. Genes Chromosomes Cancer 1997;20:320-328.

155. Abeysinghe HR, Cedrone E, Tyan T, et al: Amplification of C-MYC as the origin of the homogeneous staining region in ovarian carcinoma detected by micro-FISH. Cancer Genet Cytogenet 1999;114:136-143.

156. Sham JS, Tang TC, Fang Y, et al: Recurrent chromosome alterations in primary ovarian carcinoma in Chinese women. Cancer Genet Cytogenet 2002;133:39-44.

157. Wang ZR, Liu W, Smith ST, et al: C-myc and chromosome 8 centromere studies of ovarian cancer by interphase FISH. Exp Mol Pathol 1999;66:140-148.

158. Palacios J, Gamallo C: Mutations in the beta-catenin gene (*CTNNB1*) in endometrioid ovarian carcinomas. Cancer Res 1998;58:1344-1347.

159. Gamallo C, Palacios J, Moreno G, et al: Beta-catenin expression pattern in stage I and II ovarian carcinomas: Relationship with beta-catenin gene mutations, clinicopathological features, and clinical outcome. Am J Pathol 1999;155:527-536.

160. Sagae S, Kobayashi K, Nishioka Y, et al: Mutational analysis of beta-catenin gene in Japanese ovarian carcinomas: Frequent mutations in endometrioid carcinomas. Jpn J Cancer Res 1999;90:510-515.

161. Wright K, Wilson P, Morland S, et al: Beta-catenin mutation and expression analysis in ovarian cancer: Exon 3 mutations and nuclear translocation in 16% of endometrioid tumors. Int J Cancer 1999;82:625-629.

162. Wu R, Zhai Y, Fearon ER, Cho KR: Diverse mechanisms of beta-catenin deregulation in ovarian endometrioid adenocarcinomas. Cancer Res 2001;61:8247-8255.

163. Cadigan KM, Nusse R: Wnt signaling: A common theme in animal development. Genes Dev 1997;11:3286-3305.

164. Zhai Y, Wu R, Schwartz DR, et al: Role of beta-catenin/T-cell factor-regulated genes in ovarian endometrioid adenocarcinomas. Am J Pathol 2002;160:1229-1238.

165. Schummer M, Ng WV, Bumgarner RE, et al: Comparative hybridization of an array of 21,500 ovarian cDNAs for the discovery of genes overexpressed in ovarian carcinomas. Gene 1999;238:375-385.

166. Welsh JB, Zarrinkar PP, Sapinoso LM, et al: Analysis of gene expression profiles in normal and neoplastic ovarian tissue samples identifies candidate molecular markers of epithelial ovarian cancer. Proc Natl Acad Sci U S A 2001;98:1176-1181.

167. Hough CD, Sherman-Baust CA, Pizer ES, et al: Large-scale serial analysis of gene expression reveals genes differentially expressed in ovarian cancer. Cancer Res 2000;60:6 281-6287.

168. Hough CD, Cho KR, Zonderman AB, et al: Coordinately up-regulated genes in ovarian cancer. Cancer Res 2001;61:3869-3876.

169. Sawiris GP, Sherman-Baust CA, Becker KG, et al: Development of a highly specialized cDNA array for the study and diagnosis of epithelial ovarian cancer. Cancer Res 2002;62:2923-2928.

170. Berg JW, Lampe JG: High-risk factors in gynecologic cancer. Cancer 1981;48(2 Suppl):429-441.

171. Stuhlinger M, Rosen AC, Dobianer K, et al: *HER-2* oncogene is not amplified in primary carcinoma of the fallopian tube. Austrian Cooperative Study Group for Fallopian Tube Carcinoma. Oncology 1995;52:397-399.

172. Lacy MQ, Hartmann LC, Keeney GL, et al: C-erbB-2 and p53 expression in fallopian tube carcinoma. Cancer 1995;75:2891-2896.

173. Aziz S, Kuperstein G, Rosen B, et al: A genetic epidemiological study of carcinoma of the fallopian tube. Gynecol Oncol 2001;80:341-345.

174. Hebert-Blouin MN, Koufogianis V, Gillett P, Foulkes WD: Fallopian tube cancer in a *BRCA1* mutation carrier: Rapid development and failure of screening. Am J Obstet Gynecol 2002;186:53-54.

175. Eltabbakh GH, Piver MS: Extraovarian primary peritoneal carcinoma. Oncology (Huntingt) 1998;12:813-819; discussion 820, 825-826.

176. Schorge JO, Miller YB, Qi LJ, et al: Genetic alterations of the *WT1* gene in papillary serous carcinoma of the peritoneum. Gynecol Oncol 2000;76:369-372.

177. Moll UM, Valea F, Chumas J: Role of p53 alteration in primary peritoneal carcinoma. Int J Gynecol Pathol 1997;16:156-162.

178. Muto MG, Welch WR, Mok SC, et al: Evidence for a multifocal origin of papillary serous carcinoma of the peritoneum. Cancer Res 1995;55:490-492.

179. Schorge JO, Muto MG, Welch WR, et al: Molecular evidence for multifocal papillary serous carcinoma of the peritoneum in patients with germline BRCA1 mutations. J Natl Cancer Inst 1998;90:841-845.

180. Kommoss F, Wintzer HO, Von Kleist S, et al: In situ distribution of transforming growth factor alpha in normal human tissues and in malignant tumors of the ovary. J Pathol 1990;162:223-230.

181. Morishige K, Kurachi H, Amemiya K, et al: Evidence for the involvement of transforming growth factor alpha and epidermal growth factor receptor autocrine growth mechanism in primary human ovarian cancers in vitro. Cancer Res 1991;51:5322-5328.

182. Rodriguez GC, Berchuck A, Whitaker RS, et al: Epidermal growth factor receptor expression in normal ovarian epithelium and ovarian cancer. II. Relationship between receptor expression and response to epidermal growth factor. Am J Obstet Gynecol 1991;164:745-750.

183. Yee D, Morales FR, Hamilton TC, Von Hoff DD: Expression of insulin-like growth factor I, its binding proteins, and its receptor in ovarian cancer. Cancer Res 1991;51:5107-5012.

184. Sariban E, Sitaras NM, Antoniades HN, et al: Expression of platelet-derived growth factor (PDGF)-related transcripts and synthesis of biologically active PDGF-like proteins by human malignant epithelial cell lines. J Clin Invest 1988;82:1157-1164.

185. Henriksen R, Funa K, Wilander E, et al: Expression and prognostic significance of platelet-derived growth factor and its receptors in epithelial ovarian neoplasms. Cancer Res 1993; 53:4550-4554.

186. Di Blasio AM, Cremonesi L, Vigano P, et al: Basic fibroblast growth factor and its receptor messenger ribonucleic acids are expressed in human ovarian epithelial neoplasms. Am J Obstet Gynecol 1993;169:1517-1523.

187. Ramakrishnan S, Xu FJ, Brandt SJ, et al: Constitutive production of macrophage colony-stimulating factor by human ovarian and breast cancer cell lines. J Clin Invest 1989;83:921-926.

188. Kacinski BM, Carter D, Kohorn EI, et al: Oncogene expression in vivo by ovarian adenocarcinomas and mixed-mullerian tumors. Yale J Biol Med 1989;62:379-392.

189. Kacinski BM, Carter D, Mittal K, et al: Ovarian adenocarcinomas express fms-complementary transcripts and fms antigen, often with coexpression of CSF-1. Am J Pathol 1990; 137:135-147.

190. Boyd JA, Hamilton TC, Berchuck A: Oncogenes and tumor-suppressor genes. In: Hoskins WJ, Perez CA, Young RC (Eds.): Principles and Practice of Gynecologic Oncology, 3rd ed. Philadelphia: Lippincott Williams & Wilkins, 2000, pp 103-128.

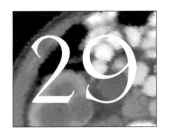

PRIMARY SURGERY FOR OVARIAN CANCER

Jonathan Carter

MAJOR CONTROVERSIES

- **What is optimal surgical management for the high-risk mass?**
- **What constitutes optimal surgical staging in a patient with apparent early-stage ovarian cancer?**
- **What is the role of laparoscopy in the staging of patients with early ovarian cancer?**
- **What are the potential benefits of cytoreductive surgery?**
- **Who is best qualified to perform primary cytoreductive surgery?**
- **What are the potential criticisms of cytoreduction surgery?**
- **What is the optimal approach to cytoreduction?**
- **Is there a role for extended techniques in cytoreductive surgery?**
- **What is the optimal management for patients referred after a "peek and shriek"?**

Ovarian malignancy comprises a variety of tumors arising from the germ cells, stroma, or surface epithelium. Germ cell and stromal tumors can usually be easily separated from the more common epithelial tumors by symptoms, age at presentation, specific tumor marker determinations, and morphology at imaging. Epithelial tumors arising from the epithelium of retention cysts are classified as benign, borderline, and malignant varieties. When ovarian cancer is mentioned, the malignant epithelial variety is implied by default. This chapter specifically deals with the surgical management of epithelial ovarian cancer.

Epithelial ovarian cancer continues to hold the dubious distinction as the most deadly gynecologic cancer, with more women dying each year from it than from cervical and endometrial cancers combined. Advances in surgical techniques, chemotherapy options, and greater community awareness have resulted in an increase in relapse-free survival, although overall survival has not appreciably changed during the past 3 decades. The reasons for this are many and varied, but an important one is that most patients present with nonspecific symptoms and with advanced-stage disease. In such circumstances, the combination of surgery and chemotherapy produces clinical remission in most patients. Although surgery alone in cases of advanced disease is not curative, neither is chemotherapy alone. Unlike other solid tumors, combined surgery and chemotherapy can eradicate disease in most patients, resulting in prolonged periods of remission. The goal for the future is to convert these patients into long-term survivors.

Early Ovarian Cancer

Early ovarian cancer is defined by the International Federation of Gynecologists and Obstetricians (FIGO) as growth limited to the ovaries (stage I) and subclassified as stage Ia (no ascites), stage Ib (both ovaries), and stage Ic (one or both ovaries with tumor rupture, with positive ascites or washings of ovarian surface disease).

A common mode of presentation of patients with early ovarian cancer is with nonspecific symptoms of a short duration, usually 3 to 6 months. Specific evaluation can document a complex pelvic mass. An elevated serum tumor marker, commonly CA 125, is identified in up to one half of such patients. Although preoperative assessment is sensitive for ovarian cancer, it is not specific. Symptoms are nonspecific and may be the result of many other, nonmalignant diagnoses. Findings at physical examination, which may include the presence of an irregular, even fixed mass with cul-de-sac nodularity, may equally be detected in patients with endometriosis and those with ovarian cancer. Endometriosis is called the great mimicker because patients may have suspicious physical examination findings and have an elevated CA 125 level. Likewise, complex masses on ultrasound and radiologic examination, although probably caused by malignancy, may also be caused by endometriomas or cystic teratomas (Fig. 29-1). To enhance the diagnostic accuracy, a variety of "risk of malignancy" indices have been developed. Irrespective of the system used, the rationale is to reduce the number of false-positive evaluations while maximizing the true positives—optimizing the exclusion of all benign cases while identifying all malignant cases.

There are many reasons why it is important to optimize the sensitivity and positive predictive value in the evaluation of a complex pelvic mass thought to be an early ovarian cancer:

1. Should a conservative (wait-and-see) approach be undertaken, or should immediate surgical intervention be advocated?
2. Should laparoscopy or laparotomy be the appropriate method of surgical intervention and management?
3. Should the surgical approach be undertaken by a general gynecologist or referred to a subspecialist board certified gynecologic oncologist?
4. If laparotomy is performed, should a transverse or midline incision be used?

5. Should a conservative surgical procedure, such as an ovarian cystectomy or unilateral oophorectomy, be undertaken?
6. Should frozen section be performed with its inherent inaccuracies, and should this influence the intraoperative decision-making process?

What is optimal surgical management for the high-risk mass? The goal of surgical management of a high-risk, complex mass is to remove the lesion safely and without rupture and, if malignancy is confirmed, to provide timely surgical staging to define the extent of disease. Although issues such as scar size, postoperative recovery, and cost effectiveness influence the decision-making process, the fact remains the tumor needs to be removed safely and intact.

The laparoscopic approach to the surgical excision of a complex and high-risk mass is increasing in popularity.[1-3] When the goals of management can be achieved (i.e., removal without rupture), the laparoscopic approach seems reasonable. However, even the most ardent supporters of this approach have raised concerns regarding the appropriateness of laparoscopic surgery in the management of patients with high-risk adnexal masses.[3] Childers and colleagues[2] reported their experience of laparoscopy in the initial management of patients with high-risk adnexal masses. They reported 138 masses with elevated CA 125 levels or abnormal ultrasound morphology. Malignancy was confirmed in 14% of cases. Eight percent of these procedures were converted to laparotomy, and there were three major complications. Of grave concern were two early recurrences in patients with stage I cancer.[2] Canis and colleagues[3] stated that all masses suspected of being malignant should be managed by laparotomy. When the surgeon cannot ensure that the tumor can be removed without rupture, the decision not to perform a laparotomy is inappropriate and verges on negligence.

Although the impact on rupture can be debated on an academic level, most gynecologic oncologists have patients in their practice who have suffered ill effects from rupture of a complex mass thought to be benign, with a subsequent finding of malignancy.[4] Mature cystic teratomas containing malignancy that rupture intraoperatively result in local spread. The irritating sebaceous material from within dermoids, despite irrigation, results in widespread chemical peritonitis not unlike carcinomatosis or tuberculosis.[4,5] Apparently benign endometriomas containing clear cell or endometrioid carcinoma that rupture during excision may result in local spread, and mucinous ovarian tumors that rupture intraoperatively may result in pseudomyxoma peritonei (Fig. 29-2).

Irrespective of the mode of entry to the abdominal cavity, the operative procedure (laparotomy or laparoscopy) should be the same. Any peritoneal fluid should be aspirated for cytologic assessment; otherwise, warm saline should be instilled into the peritoneal cavity and aspirated as washings. An inspection of the pelvis and abdomen should follow. In resecting an ovarian mass, it is imperative that the ureter is identified and mobilized laterally to allow safe clamping

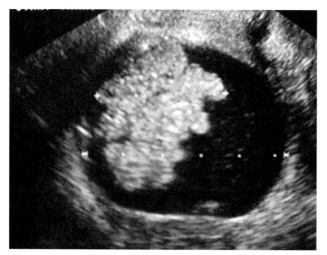

Figure 29–1. Typical transvaginal ultrasound appearance of an early ovarian cancer with prominent internal excrescences or papillations. See also Color Figure 29-1.

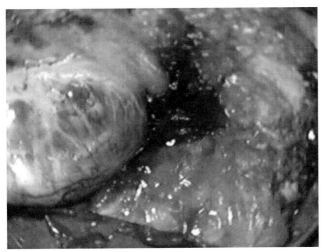

Figure 29–2. Appearance of the gelatinous mucinous ascites typically found with pseudomyxoma peritonei. See also Color Figure 29-2.

and ligation of the infundibulopelvic ligament (Fig. 29-3). With the ureter under direct vision, the posterior leaf of the broad ligament is incised parallel and superior to the ureter, heading toward the ovarian ligament and its attachment to the uterus. The ovarian ligament, the only medial attachment remaining, is clamped, cut, and tied, and the mobile ovarian or adnexal mass is then readily removed. In the case of the laparoscopic approach, removal should be accomplished with an appropriately sized laparoscopic bag to reduce the risk of intraperitoneal spill.

What constitutes optimal surgical staging in a patient with apparent early-stage ovarian cancer? After an ovarian mass has been confirmed as malignant, appropriate and thorough surgical staging is mandatory. Ideally, this should be confirmed at the same surgical procedure with frozen section analysis. Immediate staging can then be performed, saving the patient

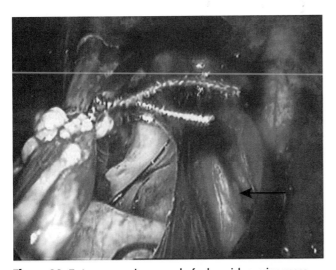

Figure 29–3. Laparoscopic removal of a low-risk ovarian mass. The infundibulopelvic ligament has been tied with extracorporeal knots. The ureter *(arrow)* has been identified and mobilized. See also Color Figure 29-3.

unnecessary delays. Not all complex ovarian masses should be referred to a gynecologic oncologist; however, general gynecologists undertaking the resection of high-risk masses should have a board-certified gynecologic oncologist on call if necessary to complete the surgery or refer the patient within a safe period. Patients often wait for weeks for such referrals and the completion of surgery.[6]

Surgical staging studies of apparent early-stage ovarian cancers have confirmed that up to 22% of patients will have their disease upstaged if a thorough surgical staging procedure is undertaken.[7] Surgery on patients suspected of having ovarian cancer should be performed by a surgeon with the surgical skill to perform the extended staging and a thorough knowledge of the natural history of the disease. The abdomen is entered through a vertical midline incision, extended above the umbilicus. Access to the upper abdomen is mandatory, and this cannot be achieved through a transverse lower abdominal or Pfannenstiel incision. On entering the abdomen, any fluid is collected, or washings are performed for exfoliative cytology. A thorough inspection of all peritoneal surfaces and systematic evaluation of the abdomen and pelvis follows. Attention is then directed toward the pathology within the pelvis. An effort should be made to remove adnexal pathology without rupture, because rupture and release of malignant cells within the peritoneal cavity may increase the patient's stage, may increase the need for adjuvant chemotherapy, and can affect the prognosis. Frozen section analysis of the lesion that confirms malignancy mandates performance of total abdominal hysterectomy and contralateral salpingo-oophorectomy. An omentectomy is performed along with pelvic and para-aortic lymph node assessment and multiple peritoneal biopsies. When such a staging procedure is performed, a significant number of patients thought to have localized disease are found to have disease of a more advanced stage.[7] The importance of performing a thorough and bilateral nodal assessment is highlighted by Cass and colleagues.[8] Of 96 patients with gross disease confined to one ovary, 14 (15%) had microscopically positive lymph nodes on pathologic review. All had grade 3 tumors. Pelvic nodes were positive in seven patients (50%), para-aortic nodes in five patients (36%), and both in two patients (14%). Of the 54 patients who had bilateral node dissections performed, 10 (19%) had positive nodes, and 3 (30%) of these cases had contralateral disease.[8]

In patients with apparent stage I ovarian cancer, the two procedures most likely to yield results are cytology and aortic node dissection. As many as 30% of patients with apparent stage I and II disease whose tumor appears confined to the pelvis have occult metastatic disease in the upper abdomen or the retroperitoneal lymph nodes.[9,10] Young and coworkers[7] showed that 31% of patients are upstaged after a careful staging laparotomy. Their study involved a group of 100 patients operated on elsewhere and initially assessed as having stage I or II disease.

When the intraoperative diagnosis of malignancy is in doubt in young patients, not performing an immediate surgical staging procedure is appropriate. This is particularly important when the pathologist reports a borderline tumor. These tumors are more common in young women and are appropriately managed with conservative surgery until childbearing is completed. It is important to discuss these issues preoperatively with the patient. A conservative staging procedure is appropriate in some patients. It consists of a unilateral oophorectomy only, leaving an apparently normal uterus and contralateral adnexa. This approach is appropriate only if an otherwise thorough staging has confirmed no extraovarian spread in a young patient who desires to retain her fertility potential. She must understand the risks associated with such an approach before providing informed consent. Only if the patient has been fully staged and appears to have stage Ia cancer can the uterus and opposite ovary be retained. There must be no ascites, no dense adhesions, and no surface excrescences. The tumor must be unruptured and unilateral. Only if the final pathology report confirms a borderline or grade 1 tumor with negative washing findings, disease-negative omentum, negative evaluation of the opposite ovary, and negative endometrial biopsy result can the surgeon and patient be reassured that more extensive surgery may not be necessary.[11]

General gynecologists should avoid the temptation of replacing the skills of a gynecologic oncologist with those of a general surgeon. Most general surgeons are unfamiliar with the retroperitoneal anatomy in the pelvis, particularly around the side wall and vessels. The evidence demonstrates that the performance of an adequate surgical staging is most likely to be compromised if performed by a general surgeon (65%) rather than a general gynecologist (48%).[12]

What is the role of laparoscopy in the staging of patients with early ovarian cancer?

In a large, comparative French study conducted across 17 centers and assessing 105 cases of ovarian cancer, 13% of which were staged laparoscopically and 74% by laparotomy, it was concluded that the laparoscopic staging of patients with ovarian cancer is "significantly less accurate" than laparotomy.[13] Canis and colleagues[3] stated that all masses that might be malignant should be managed by laparotomy and that laparoscopic treatment of ovarian cancer should be considered experimental.

Advanced Ovarian Cancer

Locally advanced ovarian cancer with growth involving one or both ovaries and with pelvic extension is by definition stage II disease. Advanced ovarian cancer consists of stage III disease with implants outside the pelvis, and stage IV disease includes distant metastases. Advanced ovarian cancer, more than any of the female genital cancers, requires a multimodal approach to management. The team involved in the treatment includes the gynecologic oncologist, medical oncologist, radiation oncologist, gynecologic pathologist, and palliative care and clinical nurse specialists.

Although surgery may be the cornerstone of initial management, it rarely produces remission, let alone cure in cases of advanced disease. Surgery allows irradiation or, more commonly, chemotherapy to finish the job of killing tumor cells. The extent to which surgery can achieve cytoreduction has been quantified. A reduction of 1 kg of tumor to 1 g of residual disease reduces the total number of cells from 10^{12} to 10^9. This 3-log kill of tumor represents only a one-eighth reduction of tumor. Taking into consideration the repopulation that occurs after surgery and regrowth that occurs between chemotherapy cycles, it has been estimated that approximately seven additional 3-log kills would be needed to eliminate the last surviving cancer cell. Because of the high probability of developing chemoresistance during therapy, it is likely that the role of surgical cytoreduction is removal of resistant clones of cells and regions of poor blood supply rather than a dramatic reduction in tumor volume.[14-16] This concept is supported by Hunter and colleagues,[17] who reviewed 58 studies that encompassed 6962 patients with advanced ovarian cancer. Multiple linear regression showed that maximum cytoreductive surgery was associated with only a small improvement in median survival time.

Spread patterns. Crucial to the surgical management of ovarian cancer is an understanding of the spread patterns of the disease. Ovarian cancer arises from the surface epithelium. This epithelium is often entrapped below the ovarian surface within inclusion cysts.

Ovarian cancer spreads by a variety of mechanisms, including by local extension and by transperitoneal, lymphatic, hematogeneous, and transdiaphragmatic routes. After capsular invasion occurs, disease directly involves adjacent structures such as anterior and posterior cul-de-sacs, sigmoid colon, omentum, small bowel, pelvic wall peritoneum, uterus, fallopian tubes, and the broad ligament. Transperitoneal dissemination ensures spread as exfoliated malignant cells are washed around the peritoneal cavity in the normal flow of fluid within the abdomen. Fluid usually moves with respiration from the pelvis up the paracolic gutters, especially the right gutter, along the intestinal mesenteries to the right hemidiaphragm.

Lymphatic spread occurs by a number of routes. Lymphatic capillaries and vessels of the parenchyma converge on the hilus of the ovary to form the subovarian lymphatic plexus. From this plexus, there are three available routes of lymphatic drainage. The main route continues by a group of six to eight large collecting trunks, which are seen bilaterally along the ovarian blood vessels and terminate in the para-aortic group of lymph nodes between the bifurcation of the aorta and the renal arteries. The second route of spread occurs in less than 50% of women. These lymphatic trunks course within the broad ligaments toward the lateral and posterior pelvic wall and terminate in the uppermost external iliac and hypogastric nodes. From there, the lymph drains along external, internal, and common iliac vessels to the para-aortic region. The third route of efferent lymphatic drainage runs along the round ligament and drains into the external iliac and inguinal lymph nodes. It has been reported that 78% of patients with stage III disease have metastases to the pelvic lymph nodes.[18-21] Chen[9] reported the rate of positive para-aortic lymph nodes was 18% in stage I, 20% in stage II, 42% in stage III, and 67% in stage IV disease.

Another significant drainage pathway is through the diaphragmatic lymphatics to the mediastinal lymph nodes. Supraclavicular, inguinal, and axillary nodes may also be involved. Hematogeneous spread is uncommon and tends to occur only in advanced disease. Common sites of spread include lung and liver, and uncommon sites are the brain and skin. Transdiaphragmatic spread accounts for the presence of ascitic fluid in the right chest and positive cytologic findings. Diaphragmatic lymph channels enter the cisterna chyle and pass to the thoracic duct. Cancer cells can obstruct these afferent lymph-collecting vessels that pass from the diaphragm through the mediastinum to the venous circulation, producing ascites.

Cytoreductive surgery. The current management of patients with presumed advanced ovarian cancer is surgical exploration and cytoreductive surgery. Despite the lack of prospective studies, the substantial weight of retrospective evidence attests to the advantages of such surgery.[22-24] In other advanced epithelial malignancies, an attempt at surgical resection is only undertaken if it is thought that all tumor can be removed with an adequate tumor-free margin and that surgical resection is potentially curative. However, in advanced ovarian cancer, despite the best surgeon and the most exhaustive surgery, rarely is all cancer resected with an appropriate disease-free margin. Surgery is not considered curative, and additional therapy is required to complete the job. Strong evidence exists that this approach is beneficial to the patient, even in the absence of complete tumor removal.[25]

What are the potential benefits of cytoreductive surgery? The benefits of cytoreductive surgery include making the patient feel better after removing ascites and large tumor masses, particularly in the omentum. In the short term, removing large tumor masses alleviates the associated nausea and satiety these patients feel. Moreover, cytoreductive surgery may improve tumor perfusion and increase the growth fraction. Large tumor masses are composed of areas in which the cells are in the resting phase of the cell cycle and therefore relatively resistant to chemotherapy. Areas of necrosis are also present because of the tumor mass outstripping its blood supply. By debulking large masses and leaving only small tumors that tend to have a higher growth fraction and better vascularization and perfusion, the surgeon can enhance the ability of the chemotherapist to maximize cell kill. The *fractional cell kill hypothesis* indicates that a constant proportion of cancer cells are destroyed with each chemotherapy treatment. Treatment that reduces a population of tumor cells from 10^9 to 10^4 also reduces a population of 10^5 cells to a single cell. Pharmacologic sanctuaries are eliminated by removal of poorly perfused, bulky tumor masses.

Another benefit of cytoreduction is related to nonclinical evidence that cytoreductive surgery results in an enhanced immunologic competence. Animal data suggest that large tumor masses are more immunosuppressive than small masses. Bulky tumors are less amenable to host defense mechanisms, and the normal mechanism of recognition of abnormal antigens may be overwhelmed by large numbers of tumor cells. Their removal results in an improved host immune surveillance.[26]

In the 1970s, Griffith and colleagues[27] observed that patients who underwent surgical cytoreduction of bulky disease to small-volume disease had longer survival times than patients with larger-diameter disease. They proposed that their observation supported the *Goldie-Coldman hypothesis*, which states that small-volume tumors are less likely to develop chemotherapy resistance and more likely to be influenced by combination chemotherapy.[14,27] The definition of the amount of residual disease regarded as distinguishing between optimal and suboptimal cytoreduction has varied over time. Traditionally, this meant cytoreduction of all visible tumor down to a 2-cm maximum diameter. Later, a 1-cm tumor diameter was accepted as the norm.[28] In the 1980s, Berek and Hacker[29] noticed patients with small-volume residuum of less than 5 mm had even better survival times. Table 29-1 demonstrates the survival advantage of optimal debulking compared with suboptimal debulking. The median survival can be doubled from 17 months to 39 months by aggressive surgery rendering the tumor down to small-volume residuum. A meta-analysis of 6885 patients found that maximal cytoreduction was one of the most powerful determinants of survival of patients with advanced ovarian cancer. Each 10% increase in maximal cytoreduction was associated with a 5.5% increase in median survival time.[22-24]

Table 29–1. Effect of the Amount of Residual Tumor after Primary Cytoreduction on Survival of Patients with Advanced Ovarian Cancer Treated with Chemotherapy

Study	Year	Optimal (months)	Suboptimal (months)
Hacker et al.[29]	1983	18	6
Vogl et al.[69]	1983	40+	16
Delgado et al.[70]	1984	45	16
Pohl et al.[71]	1984	45	16
Conte et al.[72]	1985	25+	14
Posada et al.[73]	1985	30+	18
Louie et al.[74]	1986	24	15
Redman et al.[75]	1986	37	26
Neijt et al.[76]	1987	40	21
Hainsworth et al.[77]	1988	72	13
Piver et al.[78]	1988	48	21
Sutton et al.[79]	1989	45	23
Bertelson[80]	1990	30	18
Eisenkop et al.[23]	1992	31	18
Michel et al.[81]	1996	24	14
Mean		**39**	**17**

Who is best qualified to perform primary cytoreductive surgery? It is clear from the literature that board-certified gynecologic oncologists are the most qualified and capable surgeons for tackling aggressive pelvic resection and omentectomy, perhaps supplemented with bowel resection, pelvic and para-aortic node dissection, and even diaphragm stripping and splenectomy. Compared with community physicians, general gynecologists, and general surgeons, board-certified gynecologic oncologists are more likely to adequately stage patients, to achieve optimal cytoreduction, and to have a greater proportion of patients surviving and surviving for longer.[12,23,30-32]

What are the potential criticisms of cytoreduction surgery? Despite the enormous body of evidence suggesting a role and survival advantage for maximal surgical effort and optimal cytoreduction, some still question its role in the surgical management of advanced ovarian cancer. Their arguments include the following concepts:

1. No prospective comparative data exist to confirm the benefits of such surgery.
2. The measurement of residual disease, the criteria by which surgical success is marked, is inaccurate with tumor residuum underestimated more likely than overestimated.[33]
3. The ability to optimally cytoreduce disease is more a function of tumor biologic aggressiveness than surgical skill.
4. Tumor volume is more important than maximum largest diameter.[34] For example, although the patient with one isolated lesion 1.5 cm in diameter does not have optimally cytoreduced disease, she does have a better prognosis than the patient with optimally cytoreduced disease with multiple, widespread, 0.5-cm tumors.
5. The morbidity of cytoreductive surgery may be unacceptably high.
6. The initiation of chemotherapy is delayed.
7. Newer chemotherapy agents have a greater effect on log kill than surgery.
8. Smaller metastatic masses are more likely to be resectable but offer a better prognosis, regardless of cytoreduction.
9. Quality of life is worse after radical surgery.

Hacker[29,35] eloquently reported that patients with initially large tumor masses (>10 cm), irrespective of the amount of residual disease left after cytoreduction, did not fare as well as patients with initially small tumor volumes. These findings have been substantiated by Hoskins and colleagues,[36] who undertook a reanalysis of a Gynecologic Oncology Group study (GOG 52) and declared that there was a differential survival for patients with optimal surgical debulking (<1 cm of residual disease), favoring patients with initial small-volume disease and those with less than 20 residual nodules. They further concluded that factors other than cytoreductive surgery were important in predicting survival.[36] Webb and associates[37] and Berek[38] demonstrated that if bowel resection or urinary

tract resection is required to achieve optimal cytoreduction, the patients had a poorer prognosis compared with those not having such surgery. Hunter and colleagues[17] performed a meta-analysis of 58 suitable studies comprising 6962 patients with advanced ovarian cancer. Multiple linear regression was used to analyze the effects of a number of variables on survival. These included the proportion of each cohort undergoing maximum cytoreductive surgery, the use of platinum-containing chemotherapy, the dose intensity of chemotherapy, the proportion of each cohort with stage IV disease, and the year of publication of the study. The study results suggest that only a small improvement in median survival is achieved by maximum cytoreductive surgery. In contrast, the use of platinum-containing chemotherapy appears to be associated with a much greater prolongation of median survival.

What is the optimal approach to cytoreduction?

To increase the rate of optimal cytoreduction, ultra-radical surgery has been performed and proposed. With technologic advances such as the Cavitron ultrasonic surgical aspirator and argon beam coagulator and methods such as peritoneal stripping, splenectomy, and modified posterior exenteration, optimal cytoreduction rates in these series have approached 90%. Despite this level of aggressiveness, comparative data do not exist to show that this sort of extended surgery translates into significant prolongation in survival.[39]

Preoperative considerations. It has been traditional teaching that all patients undergoing exploratory surgery for advanced ovarian cancer should undergo an antibiotic and mechanical bowel preparation. The rationale is that if bowel resection is performed during the process of cytoreduction, infectious morbidity and anastomotic leaks will be reduced. However, this paradigm has been questioned, and in a prospective study of mechanical bowel preparation, van Geldere and colleagues[40] found that it was not a sine qua non for safe colorectal surgery. In their series of 255 colorectal operations involving colectomies, two thirds of which were left sided, relatively few complications were encountered. Three patients had a leak from an extraperitoneal colorectal anastomosis, with an overall anastomotic failure rate of 1.2%.

Operative procedure. An examination under anesthesia should always be performed. This allows assessment of cul-de-sac involvement and the potential for rectosigmoid resection. In such cases, patients are placed in Allen's stirrups to facilitate low rectal anastomotic surgery. Ureteric stents are usually not needed because ovarian cancer rarely invades extraperitoneally and because identification and mobilization of the pelvic ureters is usually easily accomplished.

A generous midline incision is made from the symphysis pubis to above the umbilicus, sufficient to allow adequate inspection of the entire peritoneal

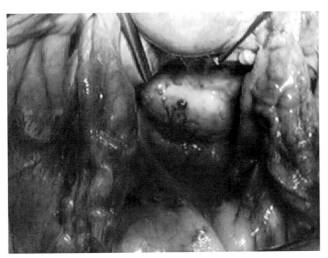

Figure 29–4. Large tumor "drop metastasis" in the cul-de-sac. If such a lesion cannot be shaved off the surface of the rectosigmoid, resection and reanastomosis of the bowel are needed. See also Color Figure 29-4.

cavity. When appropriate, washings or peritoneal fluid is collected and stored for cytologic assessment. In the face of gross intraperitoneal disease, such a maneuver is unnecessary. After inspecting the peritoneal cavity, a systemic evaluation is performed. Although many have their own systems, the important principle is to palpate all peritoneal surfaces, including bowel and mesentery, and the suprahepatic space, including the liver and spleen surface and diaphragm surface.

Depending on the sites and bulk of the pelvic disease, a type I, II, or III hysterectomy may be needed to clear the pelvis of disease. Cul-de-sac disease and disease on the bowel surface, if unable to be resected, require bowel resection (Fig. 29-4).

Omentectomy. Omentectomy is an integral part of the staging process for early ovarian cancer, and in advanced cancer, it is often involved with gross tumor requiring resection to complete cytoreduction. Even when the entire supracolic omentum is replaced by tumor (Fig. 29-5), a tumor-free space can often be developed above the transverse mesentery. In most cases, the omentum can be elevated, displaying the plane between its undersurface and the transverse colon (Fig. 29-6). Incisions through this thin layer gains access to the primarily avascular plane (i.e., lesser sac), which can be developed with sharp and blunt dissection. After the omentum is fully mobilized, it is removed from the greater curvature of the stomach by dividing the small branches arising from the left and right gastroepiploic vessels. Particular attention should be directed toward the splenic tail because it is often involved with bulky tumor.[41]

Node dissection. Despite awareness of the potential for retroperitoneal spread of ovarian cancer, mandatory nodal dissection in cases of advanced ovarian cancer is not routinely performed, and the prognostic benefit remains contested. Surgical studies have confirmed that the retroperitoneal lymph nodes contain disease in up to 50% to 70% of patients with advanced ovarian cancer.[20,21,42,43] Surgical-radiologic studies have also confirmed the difficulties or impossibility of performing a complete pelvic lymphadenectomy.[44,45]

Despite ovarian cancer being primarily an intraperitoneal disease, some believe that ignoring retroperitoneal spread may reduce the likelihood of attaining remission with first-line therapy and increase the rate of early relapse. They argue that the pelvic and para-aortic lymph nodes may harbor occult tumor and act as sanctuary sites, preventing the effect of systemic therapy from reaching them.[43,46] Some retrospective studies have shown benefit for performing lymphadenectomy in patients with advanced ovarian cancer.[47] Others have shown that a proper retroperitoneal evaluation requires complete lymphadenectomy and that the possible therapeutic intent of lymph node

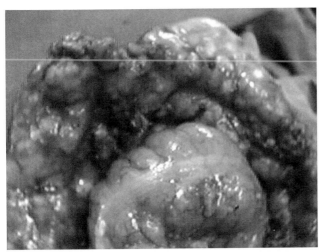

Figure 29–5. The greater omentum is completely replaced by tumor. Usually, an avascular plane can be developed between the tumor-infiltrated omentum and the transverse mesentery. Transverse colectomy is rarely required. See also Color Figure 29-5.

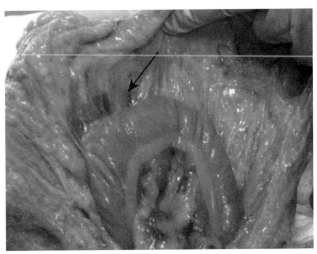

Figure 29–6. The omentum is elevated, showing the underneath side of the transverse colon and the avascular plane to be divided (arrow). See also Color Figure 29-6.

resection cannot be realized if only a sampling is performed.[48]

Although removal of isolated enlarged retroperitoneal nodes is a mandatory process of the debulking procedure, the role of elective, systematic pelvic and para-aortic lymphadenectomy in patients with no palpable enlargement of the retroperitoneal structures is unclear. There is some evidence that a complete nodal dissection in advanced ovarian cancer may offer a survival advantage.[49-51] However, even the most ardent supporters admit there appears to be little survival advantage in performing an aortic and pelvic lymphadenectomy in patients with macroscopically normal-appearing nodes.[43] There does appear to be an advantage in removing bulky, disease-positive retroperitoneal nodes if it can help render patients optimally debulked.[43] However, in a large, randomized clinical trial on advanced ovarian cancer, Parrazzini and colleagues[52] found no survival advantage for patients undergoing selective pelvic and para-aortic lymphadenectomy. This study reanalyzed the data set from a large, multicenter clinical trial. Of the 456 women entered into the trial, a total of 161 (35%) had positive nodes. Grade 3 tumors and stage IV disease were more likely to be associated with positive nodes. They found no difference in the 3-year survival rates between the groups with negative and positive nodes. In particular, nodal status was not a prognostic factor for survival in the subgroup of women with residual disease smaller than 1 cm.[52]

Until definitive data exist, it does not seem logical to inflict the potential morbidity of a pelvic and para-aortic lymph node dissection on a patient with palpably normal retroperitoneal nodes in an attempt to by chance detect microscopic tumor deposits.

Is there a role for extended techniques in cytoreductive surgery?

Bowel surgery. Intestinal surgery is often indicated as part of the initial surgical procedure. In an attempt to render patients optimally debulked of disease, small and large bowel resections may be needed. Surgery also is used to manage an obstructing lesion resulting from direct tumor invasion.

Many series[53-56] have confirmed that optimal cytoreduction to less than 1 cm of residual disease results in improved survival of patients undergoing bowel resection at the time of primary cytoreduction. The technique of modified posterior exenteration as described by Hudson and Chir[58] is extremely useful for removing seemingly unresectable pelvic disease (Fig. 29-7). Knowledge of and experience in operating in the avascular retroperitoneal planes and spaces is the key.[57,58]

Criticisms have been raised regarding the extent of initial surgery, particularly involving bowel resection and the potential for increased morbidity with little or no prolongation of life. Opponents of such surgery argue that the impact of tumor biology and initial

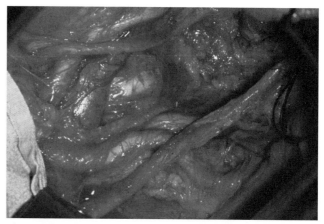

Figure 29–7. Typical appearance of the pelvis after posterior exenteration is performed to clear pelvic disease in a woman with advanced ovarian cancer. See also Color Figure 29-7.

tumor volume is more important than the radicalism of surgery performed.[39] Hammond and Houghton[59] showed no difference in survival between patients undergoing initial bowel resection compared with a group not undergoing bowel resection. Similarly, Jaeger and colleagues,[60] in a retrospective analysis of 194 patients, found no survival advantage when affected segments of bowel were resected. They showed that macroscopic bowel involvement portends a poor prognosis, and even when resected to no or minimal residual disease, the prognosis remained poor.

Splenectomy. Although not commonly performed, removal of the spleen is occasionally required to effect optimal debulking if bulky parenchymal metastases are present or hilar disease is present as a result of extension of bulky omental disease. Occasionally, traumatic rupture of the splenic capsule resulting from excessive tension on the omentum during omentectomy results in uncontrollable bleeding and the need for the removal of a normal spleen.[61]

Surgery can be accomplished with a medial or lateral approach. In either case, the vital steps in the operation involve securing the blood supply without damage to the pancreas and mobilization from the diaphragm and retroperitoneum by dividing the splenophrenic and splenocolic ligaments. The gastrosplenic ligament containing the short gastric arteries also requires division. The splenic bed probably should be drained, and Pneumovax is given postoperatively to reduce the subsequent development of potential serious infections.

Diaphragm stripping. Resectable lesions of the diaphragm may be removed by stripping the peritoneum or superficial or full-thickness diaphragm resection if invasion of the muscularis has occurred. Performance of such surgery requires adequate exposure by extending the incision to the xiphoid process. Further exposure can be obtained by incising laterally the incision under the costal cartilage. The liver is retracted manually and with moist laparotomy packs. The anesthetist should be aware that maneuvers such as occlusion of the vena cava that may result in sudden hypotension and inadvertent entry into the pleural space may occur.[62]

Argon beam coagulator. The argon beam coagulator is an electrosurgical instrument like a diathermy, except that it conducts current to the tissue through a stream of argon gas rather than air. The advantages of the argon beam coagulator are that it allows more predictable tissue desiccation and thermal coagulation. The stream of argon gas provides a dry field by blowing away blood. The blowing effect also cools the tissue, and as the argon spreads out over the tissue, it provides a more homogeneous distribution of energy.[63] The net effect is that there is less thermal injury and necrosis using the argon beam coagulator. It has been used for ovarian cancer debulking, lymph node dissection, and vulvectomy.[64]

Cavitron ultrasonic surgical aspirator. Ultraradical debulking of ovarian cancer has been studied using the Cavitron ultrasonic surgical aspirator (CUSA, Valleylab, Boulder, CO). The handpiece of the CUSA system has a vibrating tip that oscillates at a very high frequency of 23,000 Hz. Tissue is destroyed by cavitation by means of selective tissue fragmentation.[65] The operative field is kept clean by an irrigation and aspiration system built into the handpiece. Tissue with a high water content is more easily damaged than tissue with a high collagen content. In a small, comparative study, van Dam and colleagues[66] were able to show indirectly a more successful cytoreduction using the CUSA, although this did not translate into improved disease-free or overall survival rates.

What is the optimal management for patients referred after a "peek and shriek"?

Despite the availability of board-certified gynecologic oncologists, many patients with complex ovarian masses, ascites, and elevated CA 125 levels are primarily explored by general gynecologists with little or no training in surgical oncology techniques.[67] Exploration and an unexpected finding of advanced ovarian cancer, the so-called peek and shriek, pose a number of questions. For example, should immediate surgery be undertaken or delayed after the delivery of three or more cycles of combination chemotherapy? Because there is little evidence to direct the clinician, the patient's status and other factors often help guide the clinician. In a structured trial setting of patients with suboptimally debulked disease who underwent induction chemotherapy and were then randomized to further debulking surgery compared with patients receiving no further treatment, those having additional surgery had significant prolongation of survival.[68]

REFERENCES

1. Childers J, Lang J, Surwit E, Hatch K: Laparoscopic surgical staging of ovarian cancer. Gynecol Oncol 1995;59:25-33.
2. Childers J, Nasseri A, Surwit E: Laparoscopic management of suspicious adnexal masses. Am J Obstet Gynecol 1996;175: 1451-1459.
3. Canis M, Pouly J, Wattiez A, et al: Laparoscopic management of adnexal masses suspicious at ultrasound. Obstet Gynecol 1997; 89:679-683.
4. Mayer C, Miller D, Ehlen T: Peritoneal implantation of squamous cell carcinoma following rupture of a dermoid cyst during laparoscopic removal. Gynecol Oncol 2001;84:180-183.
5. Ranney B: Iatrogenic spillage from benign cystic teratoma causing severe peritoneal granulomas and adhesions: Report of a case. Obstet Gynecol 1970;35:562-564.
6. Maiman M, Seltzer V, Boyce J: Laparoscopic excision of ovarian neoplasms subsequently found to be malignant. Obstet Gynecol 1991;77:563-565.
7. Young R, Decker D, Wharton JT: Staging laparotomy in early ovarian cancer. JAMA 1983;250:3072-3076.
8. Cass I, Li A, Runowicz C, et al: Pattern of lymph node metastases in clinically unilateral stage I invasive epithelial ovarian carcinomas. Gynecol Oncol 2001;80:56-61.
9. Chen S, Lee L: Incidence of para-aortic and pelvic lymph node metastasis in epithelial carcinoma of the ovary. Gynecol Oncol 1983;16:95-100.
10. Piver M, Barlow J, Lele S: Incidence of subclinical metastasis in stage I and II ovarian carcinoma. Obstet Gynecol 1978;52: 100-108.
11. Morrow C: Malignant and borderline epithelial tumors of ovary: Clinical features, staging, diagnosis, intraoperative assessment and review of management. In Coppleson M, Monaghan J, Morrow C, Mattersall M (eds): Gynecologic Oncology, vol 2, 2nd ed. London, Churchill Livingstone, 1992, pp 889-915.
12. McGowan L, Lesher L, Norris H, Barnett M: Misstaging of ovarian cancer. Obstet Gynecol 1985;65:568-572.
13. Lecuru F, Desfeux P, Camatte S, et al: Role of laparoscopy on staging and survival after early ovarian cancer [abstract]. Gynecol Oncol 2002;84:505.
14. Griffiths C: Surgery at the time of diagnosis in ovarian cancer. In Blackledge G, Chan K (eds): Management of Ovarian Cancer. London, Butterworth, 1986, pp 67-70.
15. Griswold D, Chavel F, Wilcox W: Success and failure in the treatment of solid tumors. 1. Effects of cyclophosphamide (NSCO26271) on primary and metastatic plasmacytoma in the hamster. Cancer Chemother Rep 1968;52:345-387.
16. Hoskins W, Rubin S: Surgery in the treatment of patients with advanced ovarian cancer. Seminars in Oncology 1991;18:213-221.
17. Hunter R, Alexander N, Soutter W: Meta-analysis of surgery in advanced ovarian carcinoma: Is maximum cytoreductive surgery an independent determinant of prognosis? Am J Obstet Gynecol 1992;166:504-511.
18. Wu P, Lang J, Huang R, et al: Lymph node metastasis and retroperitoneal lymphadenectomy in ovarian cancer. In Burghardt E, Monaghan J (eds): Bailliere's Clinical Obstetrics and Gynaecology, vol 3. Operative Treatment of Ovarian Cancer. London, Bailliere Tindall, 1989, pp 143-155.
19. Wu P, Qu J, Lang J, et al: Lymph node metastasis of ovarian cancer: A preliminary survey of 74 cases of lymphadenectomy. Am J Obstet Gynecol 1986;155:1103-1108.
20. Burghardt E, Pickel H, Lahousen M, Stettner H: Pelvic lymphadenectomy in operative treatment of ovarian cancer. Am J Obstet Gynecol 1986;155:315-319.
21. Burghardt E, Girardi F, Lahousen M, et al: Patterns of pelvic and paraaortic lymph node involvement in ovarian cancer. Gynecol Oncol 1991;40:103-106.
22. Bristow R, Tomacruz R, Armstrong D, et al: Survival effect of maximal cytoreductive surgery for advanced ovarian carcinoma during the platinum era: A meta-analysis. J Clin Oncol 2002;20:1248-1259.
23. Eisenkop S, Spirtos N, Montag T, et al: The impact of subspecialty training on the management of advanced ovarian cancer. Gynecol Oncol 1992;47:203-209.

24. Eisenkop S, Friedman R, Wang H: Complete cytoreductive surgery is feasible and maximizes survival in patients with advanced epithelial ovarian cancer: A prospective study. Gynecol Oncol 1998;69:103-108.

25. Le T, Krepart G, Lotocki R, Heywood M: Does debulking surgery improve survival in biologically aggressive ovarian carcinoma? Gynecol Oncol 1997;67:208-214.

26. Bookman M, Berek J: Biologic and immunologic therapy of ovarian cancer. Hematol Oncol Clin North Am 1992;6:941-965.

27. Griffiths C, Parker L, Fuller A: Role of cytoreductive surgical treatment in the management of advanced ovarian cancer. Cancer Treat Rep 1979;63:235-240.

28. Omura G, Brady M, Homesley H, et al: Long term follow-up and prognostic factor analysis in advanced ovarian carcinoma: The Gynecologic Oncology Group experience. J Clin Oncol 1991;9:1138-1150.

29. Hacker N, Berek J, Lagasse L, et al: Primary cytoreductive surgery for epithelial ovarian cancer. Obstet Gynecol 1983;61:413-420.

30. Puls L, Carrasco R, Morrow M, Blackhurst D: Stage I ovarian cancer: Specialty-related differences in survival management. South Med J 1997;90:1097-1100.

31. Junor E, Hole D, McNulty L, et al: Specialist gynaecologists and survival outcome in ovarian cancer: A Scottish national study of 1866 patients. Br J Obstet Gynaecol 1999;106:1130-1136.

32. Mayer A, Chambers S, Graves E, et al: Ovarian cancer staging: Does it require a gynecologic oncologist. Gynecol Oncol 1992;47:223-227.

33. Prefontaine M, Gelfand A, Donovan J, Powell J: Reproducibility of tumor measurements in ovarian cancer: A study of interobserver variability. Gynecol Oncol 1994;55:87-90.

34. Covens A: A critique of surgical cytoreduction in advanced ovarian cancer. Gynecol Oncol 2000;78:269-274.

35. Hacker N (ed): Controversial aspects of cytoreductive surgery in epithelial ovarian cancer. Bailliere's Clinical Obstetrics and Gynaecology, vol 3. Operative Treatment of Ovarian Cancer. London, Bailliere Tindall, 1989.

36. Hoskins W, Bundy B, Thigpen J, Omura G: The influence of cytoreductive surgery on recurrence-free interval and survival in small-volume stage III epithelial ovarian cancer: A Gynecologic Oncology Group study. Gynecol Oncol 1992;47:159-166.

37. Berek J, Hacker N, Lagasse L, Leuchter R: Lower urinary tract resection as part of cytoreductive surgery for ovarian cancer. Gynecol Oncol 1982;13:87-92.

38. Webb M: Cytoreduction in ovarian cancer: Achievability and results. In Burghardt E, Monaghan J (eds): Bailliere's Clinical Obstetrics and Gynaecology, vol 3. Operative Treatment of Ovarian Cancer. London, Bailliere Tindall, 1989, pp 83-94.

39. Potter M, Partridge E, Hatch K, et al: Primary surgical therapy of ovarian cancer: How much and when. Gynecol Oncol 1991;40:195-200.

40. van Geldere D, Fa-Si-Oen P, Noach L, et al: Complications after colorectal surgery without mechanical bowel preparation. J Am Coll Surg 2002;194:40-47.

41. Heintz A, Hacker N, Berek JS, et al: Cytoreductive surgery in ovarian carcinoma: Feasibility and morbidity. Obstet Gynecol 1986;67:783-788.

42. Onda T, Yoshikawa H, Yokota H, et al: Assessment of metastases to aortic and pelvic lymph nodes in epithelial ovarian carcinoma. Cancer 1996;78:903-908.

43. Spirtos N, Gross G, Freddo J, Ballon S: Cytoreductive surgery in advanced epithelial cancer of the ovary: The impact of aortic and pelvic lymphadenectomy. Gynecol Oncol 1995;56:345-352.

44. Kolbenstvedt A, Kolstad P: The difficulties of complete pelvic lymph node dissection in radical hysterectomy for carcinoma of the cervix. Gynecol Oncol 1976;4:244-258.

45. Kolbenstvedt A, Kolstad P: Pelvic lymph node dissection under perioperative lymphographic control. Gynecol Oncol 1974;2:39-59.

46. Hacker N: Systematic pelvic and paraaortic lymphadenectomy for advanced ovarian cancer—therapeutic advance or surgical folly? Gynecol Oncol 1995;56:325-327.

47. Allen D, Planner R, Grant P: Maximum effort in the management of ovarian cancer, including pelvic and paraaortic lymphadenectomy. Aust N Z J Obstet Gynaecol 1992;32:50-53.

48. Carnino F, Fuda G, Ciccone G, et al: Significance of lymph node sampling in epithelial carcinoma of the ovary. Gynecol Oncol 1997;65:467-472.

49. Scarabelli C, Gallo A, Visentin M, et al: Systematic pelvic and para-aortic lymphadenectomy in advanced ovarian cancer patients with no residual intraperitoneal disease. Int J Gynecol Cancer 1997;7:18-26.

50. Benedetti P, Scambia G, Baiocchi G, et al: Technique and feasibility of radical paraaortic and pelvic lymphadenectomy for gynecologic malignancies. A prospective study. Int J Gynecol Cancer 1991;1:133-140.

51. di Re F, Baiocchi G, Fontanelli R, et al: Systemic pelvic and paraaortic lymphadenectomy for advanced ovarian cancer: Prognostic significance of node metastases. Gynecol Oncol 1996;62:360-365.

52. Parazzini F, Valsecchi G, Bolis G, et al: Pelvic and paraaortic lymph nodal status in advanced ovarian cancer and survival. Gynecol Oncol 1999;74:7-11.

53. Spirtos N, Eisenkop S, Schlaerth J, Ballon S: Second look laparotomy after modified posterior exenteration: Patterns of persistence and recurrence in patients with stage III and IV ovarian cancer. Am J Obstet Gynecol 2000;182:1321-1327.

54. Gillette-Cloven N, Burger R, Monk B, et al: Bowel resection at the time of primary cytoreduction for epithelial ovarian cancer. J Am Coll Surg 2001;193:626-632.

55. Weber A, Kennedy A: The role of bowel resection in the primary surgical cytoreduction of carcinoma of the ovary. J Am Coll Surg 1994;179:465-470.

56. Scarabelli C, Gallo A, Franceschi S: Primary cytoreductive surgery with rectosigmoid resection for patients with advanced epithelial ovarian carcinoma. Cancer 2000;88:389-397.

57. Eisenkop S, Nalick R, Teng N: Modified posterior exenteration for ovarian cancer. Obstet Gynecol 1991;78:879-885.

58. Hudson C, Chir M: Surgical treatment of ovarian cancer. Gynecol Oncol 1973;1:370-378.

59. Hammond R, Houghton C: The role of bowel surgery in the primary treatment of epithelial ovarian cancer. Aust N Z J Obstet Gynaecol 1990;30:166-169.

60. Jaeger W, Ackermann S, Kessler H, et al: The effect of bowel resection of survival in advanced epithelial ovarian cancer. Gynecol Oncol 2001;83:286-291.

61. Nicklin J, Copeland L, O'Toole R: Splenectomy as part of cytoreductive surgery for ovarian carcinoma. Gynecol Oncol 1995;58:244.

62. Fiorica J, Hoffman M, LaPolla J, et al: The management of diaphragmatic lesions in ovarian cancer. Obstet Gynecol 1989;74:927-929.

63. Morrow C, Curtin J: Gynecologic Cancer Surgery. New York, Churchill Livingstone, 1996.

64. Brand E, Pearlman N: Electrosurgical debulking of ovarian cancer: A new technique using the argon beam coagulator. Gynecol Oncol 1990;39:115-118.

65. Deppe G, Malviya V, Boike G, Malone JJ: Use of Cavitron surgical aspirator for debulking of diaphragmatic metastases in patients with advanced ovarian carcinoma. Surg Gynecol Obstet 1989;165:455-456.

66. van Dam P, Tjalma W, Weyler J, et al: Ultraradical debulking of epithelial ovarian cancer with the ultrasonic surgical aspirator: A prospective randomized trial. Am J Obstet Gynecol 1996;174:943-950.

67. Carney M, Lancaster J, Ford C, et al: A population-based study of patterns of care for ovarian cancer: Who is seen by a gynecologic oncologist and who is not? Gynecol Oncol 2002;84:36-42.

68. van der Burg M, van Lent M, Buyse M, et al: The effect of debulking surgery after induction chemotherapy on the prognosis in advanced epithelial ovarian cancer. N Engl J Med 1995;332:629-634.

69. Vogl S, Pagano M, Kaplan B, et al: Cisplatin based combination chemotherapy for advanced ovarian cancer: High overall response rate with curative potential only in women with small tumor burdens. Cancer 1983;51:2024-2030.

70. Delgado G, Oran D, Petrilli E: Stage III epithelial ovarian cancer: The role of maximal surgical reduction. Gynecol Oncol 1984;18:293-298.

71. Pohl R, Dallenbach-Hellweg G, Plugge T, Czernobilsky B: Prognostic parameters in patients with advanced ovarian malignant tumors. Eur J Gynecol Oncol 1984;5:160-169.
72. Conte P, Sertoli M, Bruzzone M, et al: Cisplatin, methotrexate and 5-fluorouracil combination chemotherapy for advanced ovarian cancer. Gynecol Oncol 1985;20:290-297.
73. Posada J, Marantz A, Yeung K, et al: The cyclophosphamide, hexamethylmelamine, 5-fluorouracil regimen in the treatment of advanced and recurrent ovarian cancer. Gynecol Oncol 1985; 20:23-31.
74. Louie K, Ozols R, Myers C, et al: Long term results of a cisplatin containing combination chemotherapy regimen for the treatment of advanced ovarian carcinoma. J Clin Oncol 1986; 4:1579-1585.
75. Redman J, Petroni G, Saigo P, et al: Prognostic factors in advanced ovarian carcinoma. J Clin Oncol 1986;4:515-523.
76. Neijt J, ten Bokkel Juinink W, van der Burg M, et al: Randomized trial comparing two combination chemotherapy regimens (CHAP-5 vs CP) in advanced ovarian carcinoma. J Clin Oncol 1987;5:1157-1168.
77. Hainsworth J, Grosh W, Burnett L, et al: Advanced ovarian cancer: Long term results of treatment with intensive cisplatin-based chemotherapy of brief duration. Ann Intern Med 1988; 108:165-170.
78. Piver M, Lele S, Marchetti D, et al: The impact of aggressive debulking surgery and cisplatin-based chemotherapy on progression-free survival in stage III and IV ovarian carcinoma. J Clin Oncol 1988;6:983-989.
79. Sutton G, Stehman F, Einhorn L, et al: Ten year follow-up of patients receiving cisplatin, doxorubicin, and cyclophosphamide chemotherapy for advanced epithelial ovarian carcinoma. J Clin Oncol 1989;7:223-229.
80. Bertelson K: Tumor reduction surgery and long-term survival in advanced ovarian cancer: A DACOVA study. Gynecol Oncol 1990;38:203-209.
81. Michel G, De Iaco P, Castaigne D, et al: Extensive cytoreductive surgery in advanced ovarian carcinoma. Eur J Gynecol Oncol 1997;18:9-15.

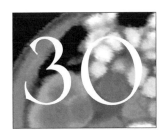

C H A P T E R

Adjuvant Treatment for Early-Stage Epithelial Ovarian Cancer

Claes Tropé   and   Janne Kaern

✦ MAJOR CONTROVERSIES

- **Should comprehensive surgical staging be done for all early-stage epithelial ovarian carcinomas?**
- **Is lymph node assessment a technical gimmick or the standard care at the beginning of the third millennium?**
- **Should all improperly surgically staged patients be restaged?**
- **Is it gambling to perform conservative surgery for stage I epithelial ovarian carcinoma in women of childbearing age?**
- **What have we learned from prospective, randomized clinical trials of early-stage epithelial ovarian cancer during the past 25 years?**
- **Is there a place for pelvic radiotherapy, whole abdominal radiotherapy, or radiolabeled isotopes in the management of early epithelial ovarian carcinoma?**
- **Is watch and wait adequate after comprehensive surgical staging of low-risk early-stage epithelial ovarian cancer?**
- **Is high-risk early-stage epithelial ovarian cancer overtreated surgically and systemically?**
- **Can classic and clinical prognostic factors help separate high-risk disease from low-risk disease?**
- **Can molecular biologic parameters replace the classic prognostic factors?**
- **Is it possible to develop new adjuvant therapeutic strategies that translate into enhanced survival?**

Ovarian cancer is the second most common gynecologic cancer, with an incidence rate of about 15 cases per 100,000 women in Western countries and approximately 141,000 new cases and 106,000 deaths worldwide annually. Because there is no effective screening method for ovarian cancer, more than 70% of cases are diagnosed after the tumor has already spread beyond the ovaries.

Although the incidence varies from one study to another, approximately one third of the patients present with localized (early-stage) disease, classified

as International Federation of Obstetrics and gynecology (FIGO) stage I and II epithelial ovarian cancer (EOC) (Table 30-1).[1] The prognosis for these women is much better than for women with spread of disease outside the ovaries at the time of diagnosis. The 5-year survival rates reported for patients with EOC vary, in part because of differences in surgical staging, from 50% to 90% and from 30% to 80% for patients with stage I and II disease, respectively.[2,3,4] In Norway, the population-based overall relative 5-year survival rate improved between 1975 and 1990 from 60% to

Table 30–1. Carcinoma of the Ovary: FIGO Nomenclature

Stage	Description
I	Growth limited to the ovaries
Ia	Growth limited to one ovary; no ascites containing malignant cells
	No tumor on the external surface; capsule intact
Ib	Growth limited to both ovaries; no ascites containing malignant cells
	No tumor on the external surface; capsule intact
Ic*	Tumor either stage Ia or Ib, but with tumor on surface of one or both ovaries, or with capsule ruptured, or with ascites present containing malignant cells, or with positive peritoneal washings
II	Growth involving one or both ovaries with pelvic extension
IIa	Extension and/or metastases to the uterus and/or tubes
IIb	Extension to other pelvic tissues
IIc*	Tumor either stage IIa or IIb, but with tumor on surface of one or both ovaries, or with capsule(s) ruptured, or with ascites present containing malignant cells, or with positive peritoneal washings
III	Tumor involving one or both ovaries with histologically confirmed peritoneal implants outside the pelvis and/or positive retroperitoneal or inguinal nodes. Superficial liver metastases equals stage III. Tumor is limited to the true pelvis, but with histologically proven malignant extension to small bowel or omentum
IIIa	Tumor grossly limited to the true pelvis, with negative nodes, but with histologically confirmed microscopic seeding of abdominal peritoneal surfaces or histologically proven extension to small bowel or mesentery
IIIb	Tumor of one or both ovaries with histologically confirmed implants, peritoneal metastasis of abdominal peritoneal surfaces, none exceeding 2 cm in diameter; nodes are negative
IIIc	Peritoneal metastasis beyond the pelvis > 2 cm in diameter and/or positive retroperitoneal or inguinal nodes
IV	Growth involving one or both ovaries with distant metastases. If pleural effusion is present, there must be positive cytology to allot a case to stage IV. Parenchymal liver metastasis equals stage IV

*To evaluate the impact on prognosis of the different criteria for allotting cases to stage Ic or IIc, it would be of value to know if rupture of the capsule was spontaneous or caused by the surgeon and if the source of malignant cells detected was peritoneal washing or ascites.

82% for stage I and from 42% to 62% for stage II disease.[5]

Patients with EOC who suffer a relapse after surgery do so because of subclinical metastases at time of surgery, most commonly in the peritoneal cavity but occasionally in extraperitoneal locations such as lymph nodes. Identification of patients with such micrometastases is crucial to be able to offer additional treatment.[6-9] The risk for early peritoneal seeding depends on stage and on biologic factors not included in the current FIGO 1988 staging system.[10]

Adjuvant chemotherapy most often involves the systemic administration of chemotherapeutic agents to patients without evidence of residual tumor after removal of the primary tumor. This approach is based on data from 1950 to 1960, which found an inverse relationship between response to chemotherapy and number of tumor cells. The possibility of improved survival in patients with minimal disease after surgery, coupled with a poorer response in advanced disease, provided a good rationale for the use of adjuvant chemotherapy. EOC signifies localized disease and is equivalent to FIGO stage Ia, Ib, and Ic (sometimes including stage IIa). Truly localized disease is curable by surgery. Two problems are encountered with regard to adjuvant therapy in EOC.[11] The first is to find prognostic factors that can predict the presence of micrometastasis (i.e., disease is no longer localized) and the second is to find adjuvant therapies that are effective in controlling micrometastatic disease and tolerable in terms of short- and long-term side effects.

Patients with a significant statistical risk for having persistent disease are treated with adjuvant therapy.

This means that only a fraction of the patient population treated actually has micrometastatic disease and can potentially benefit from the treatment, which is why the role of adjuvant treatment in patients with EOC remains controversial.

Should comprehensive surgical staging be done for all early-stage epithelial ovarian carcinomas?

It has been postulated that neoplasms originating in the ovary have two major routes of spread. The first is migration of exfoliated cells within the normal circulation of peritoneal fluid, reaching the domes of the diaphragm and omentum through the paracolic gutters, followed by local stromal activation and then invasion. Stage I tumors have evidence of ovarian stromal invasion and "drop metastases" on the local serosal surfaces, such as seen in stage II disease.[12,13]

The second route is by lymphatic permeation.[13,14] Six to eight lymphatic channels originate on the ovarian surface and drain by three main routes: along the infundibulopelvic ligament to the supracaval and intercavoaortic nodes, along the broad ligament to the interiliac and upper gluteal nodes, and by the round ligament to the external iliac and inguinal nodes. Lymphatic involvement, which is common in patients with advanced-stage disease, can be explained in part by local invasive activity and local blood and lymph vessel angiogenesis, but it may be considered a step earlier in metastatic activity, occurring before parenchymal involvement. There are no data indicating that the presence of lymph node disease is a marker for or a precursor of synchronous or late-manifesting parenchymal disease.

There is evidence of a third route. Although rare (1.9%), hematogenous circulation of EOC cells has been shown in blood and bone marrow studies.[15,16] Controversy exists about the prognostic importance of these findings because at least two large studies have not documented a worse outcome in cases of ovarian cancer cells in bone marrow or blood.[15,16]

In the 1980s, surgery remained the cornerstone of treatment of ovarian cancer, and the need for a comprehensive surgical staging of apparent EOC was clear. The staging system of FIGO incorporates surgical evaluation of the previously mentioned anatomic areas in its staging criteria.[17] Nevertheless, most published series regarding the survival of patients with EOC include many women who did not undergo such comprehensive staging,[4,18-29] and the problems of understaging are well documented. A report by Young and colleagues[7] showed that staging was often carelessly performed. They performed prospective, systematic restaging of 100 patients referred as EOC cases within 4 weeks. Only 25% of the patients were found to have an initial surgical incision large enough for complete examination of the abdomen. Of the 68 patients restaged by laparotomy, 61 were referred by their physician as free of residual cancer, but at the time of restaging laparotomy, 22 of these patients were upstaged. Of a total of 100 patients, 31 were upstaged, and 23 of these had stage III disease. The most common missing pieces of information are the status of the omentum, the status of the retroperitoneal nodes, and the peritoneal-diaphragmatic biopsies. The most common sites of occult cancer are within peritoneal fluid or washings, the pelvic peritoneum or omentum, and in the subdiaphragmatic areas or nodes.[7]

In a 1985 publication, McGowan and coworkers[28] compared the stage distribution of 157 patients properly staged with data from the FIGO annual report of the same period. There was a reduction of stage I rates from 28% to 16%, reduction of stage II rates from 17% to 4%, and a reallocation to stage III from 55% to 80% when a thorough staging procedure was adopted.

Le and associates[29] demonstrated in their retrospective series of 138 patients with EOC that lack of proper staging at surgery led to overtreatment and to undertreatment of patients with significant potential to be cured with chemotherapy. When all potential confounding variables known to predict for recurrent disease are controlled, lack of proper staging at surgery by itself almost triples the risk for disease recurrence. In a multivariate analysis, Zanetta and colleagues[30] showed in 351 patients with stage I ovarian cancer that the extent of the surgical staging was a statistically independent prognostic factor for disease-free survival and overall survival. The completeness of staging depends on the type of specialist performing the procedure: gynecologic oncologists (97% complete), obstetrician-gynecologists (53%), and general surgeons (35%).[28] The conclusion from McGowan and coworkers[28] was that general gynecologists should have better oncologic surgery education

or patients should be referred to a center for gynecologic cancer.

Is lymph node assessment a technical gimmick or the standard care at the beginning of the third millennium?

The emphasis on surgical staging has increased our awareness of retroperitoneal nodal involvement associated with EOC. Bergman[12] first provided some data concerning the incidence of node involvement in ovarian cancer from autopsy studies, and in the 1970s and early 1980s, reports appeared on the clinical importance of nodal metastases in patients with ovarian cancer. In 1974, Knapp and Friedman[20] reported their findings of aortic nodal metastases in 19% of 26 patients with apparent stage I ovarian cancer. Data from the literature show that when cancer is apparently confined to the ovaries and sampling of macroscopically enlarged nodes only is performed, positive nodes can be found in 4% to 25% of the cases (mean, 8%).[8,14,20,31-37] When data only from systematic pelvic and para-aortic lymphadenectomy of apparently normal nodes are considered, the node-positivity rate is between 10% and 25% (mean, 16%),[32-35] underscoring the inaccuracy in using palpation to determine nodal status. For this reason, a systematic lymphadenectomy seems to be more accurate in an apparent EOC than selective lymphadenectomy or random samplings.[34,35]

The integration of lymphadenectomy in the management of EOC cancer has been hampered by the belief that the first group of nodes involved by retroperitoneal metastases will be those in the para-aortic region, away from the pelvis and therefore beyond the reach of conventional surgery and irradiation. Many groups, however, have shown the importance of pelvic nodes as a site for metastases and have demonstrated that the external iliac and obturator nodes are more likely to be involved than the common iliac nodes.[14] When systematic lymphadenectomy (median number of nodes removed is more than 20) was performed, the median number of positive nodes was 2 (range, 1 to 46), and in more than two thirds of the cases, metastases occurred in both the pelvic and para-aortic regions.[14] This means that a considerable number of patients with apparent EOC would be upstaged to stage IIIc as a result of lymphadenectomy. However, the 5-year survival (60%) for stage IIIc with only retroperitoneal spread is clearly higher than for stage IIIc with intra-abdominal dissemination, which varies between 20% and 30%.[31,39] Nodal disease correlates with unfavorable histology (more frequent in serous or clear cell tumors than in mucinous or endometrioid types),[35,37] poor differentiation (more frequent in grade 3 than in grade 1 and 2),[35,37] and intraperitoneal spread.[31,35] The possible benefits from lymphadenectomy include a more appropriate treatment for upstaged patients, the excision of retroperitoneal disease, a possibility to assess the appropriateness of intraperitoneal treatment, and possible survival benefits associated with the removal of occult

Table 30–2. Lymphatic Spread in Stage I Ovarian Cancer Apparently Limited to One Ovary

Study	No. of Patients	No. of Lymph Nodes Involved (%)		
		Unilateral	Contralateral	Bilateral
Wu et al.[8]	6	3 (50.0)	3 (50.0)	—
Benedetti-Panici et al.[45]	5	5 (100)	—	—
Petru et al.[34]	6	5 (83.3)	1 (15.7)	—
Onda et al.[35]	6	4 (66.6)	—	2 (33.3)
Baiocchi et al.[37]	22	16 (72.7)	3 (13.6)	3 (13.6)
Total	45	33 (73.3)	7 (15.5)	5 (11.2)

Adapted from DiRe F, Baiocchi G: Value of lymph node assessment in ovarian cancer: Status of the art at the end of the second millennium. Int J Gynecol Cancer 2000;10:435-442.

disease.[7] It has also been suggested that platinum-based treatment may be less effective against nodal disease.[39,40]

Several investigators have studied the distribution of lymphatic metastases when the tumor is macroscopically localized to one ovary (i.e., stage Ia or stage Ib with macroscopic cancer on one side and microscopic on the other).[30,33-35,37,39] As indicated in Table 30-2 from the findings of DiRe and Baiocchi,[14] lymph node metastases were limited to the ipsilateral node groups in a high percentage of patients (73%). However, in 16% of patients, isolated contralateral metastases can be observed.[14,21,33,41] Li and associates[41] conclude that bilateral lymph node sampling significantly increased the identification of nodal metastases in patients with apparent stage Ia invasive EOC.

Despite all these data, there is a lack of convincing evidence that survival benefit is gained from lymphadenectomy. In a retrospective study from 1994, Petru and colleagues[34] reported no significant differences in the 5-year survival rates for patients undergoing radical lymphadenectomy (82%) compared with no lymphadenectomy (87%). Bolis and coworkers[42] and Tropé and associates[43] found in their prospective studies that complete or more aggressive staging as defined by FIGO[17] 1986 lymphadenectomy guidelines did not appear to play an important prognostic or therapeutic role. Overall, the disease-free survival was the same in the suboptimally staged group as in the optimally staged group. The only way to find out the role of radical lymphadenectomy is to perform prospective randomized studies.

Maggioni and colleagues[44] (later updated by Benedetti-Panici and coworkers[45]) performed the only prospective, randomized study comparing radical lymphadenectomy (LY) with sampling (SA) or resection of bulky nodes (RBN) as the primary surgical procedure for EOC. From January 1992 to April 1996, 202 patients (103 LY, 99 SA or RBN) were enrolled by six Italian institutes. Positive nodes were detected in 14% of patients undergoing LY versus 8% of patients undergoing SA or RBN (P = .07). With a median follow-up of 32 months, 18 (17.5%) relapsed in the LY group, and 21 (21%) of the SA or RBN group relapsed. No significant difference in time to relapse was observed. Sixteen deaths (15.5%) occurred in the LY group, and 13 (13%)

occurred in the SA or RBN group. The events observed are still not sufficient to highlight significant differences between patients who undergo radical lymphadenectomy and those who undergo lymph node sampling. No difference in disease-free survival (P = .644) or overall survival (P = .699) was observed, but the follow-up time is too short to make a final conclusion. The complication rates were significantly higher in the LY group (i.e., more injury to the third part of duodenum, vena cava, and mesenteric vessels; more lymph cyst formation, infection, and leg edema).

Should all improperly surgical staged patients be restaged?

We agree with Le and associates,[29] who think that there is a major dilemma facing gynecologists when a patient with apparent EOC is referred to the reference gynecologic oncologic center and has had an incomplete staging procedure. It is not clear from the literature whether these patients should be reoperated to collect data that can accurately stage their cancers, followed by chemotherapy if needed, or they should be treated based on already known risk factors for recurrence. Proper staging may benefit true high-risk patients with EOC by limiting the duration of adjuvant chemotherapy or postponing the adjuvant chemotherapy until a relapse occurs.

At the Norwegian Radium Hospital (NRH), improperly staged EOC patients have their pathologic slides reviewed, DNA ploidy determined with flow cytometry and image cytometry, and postoperative 3-week CA 125 determinations, liver ultrasound, and pelvic and abdominal MRI or CT performed.[46] After the tumor has been reviewed by our pathologist and if it appears to be grade 3 or grade 1 or 2 and aneuploid or clear cell tumor or with an elevated CA 125 value 3 weeks postoperatively, we perform a second laparotomy within 3 weeks with a complete restaging procedure. In our experience, 35% of these patients have positive nodes, and 32% of these high-risk patients relapse despite adjuvant chemotherapy. At the NRH, we have performed complete restaging procedures in low-risk, stage I patients and found only 1% with positive nodes. We believe that performing repeat

■ **Table 30-3.** Restaging of FIGO Stage I Tumors

Table 30-3. Restaging of FIGO Stage I Tumors

FIGO Stage I Tumors for Which Restaging Is Not Indicated
Stage Ia, Ib, grade 1 mucinous, serous or endometrioid tumors
Stage Ia, Ib, grade 2 diploid mucinous, serous or endometrioid tumors

FIGO Stage I Tumors for Which Restaging Is Indicated
Stage Ia, Ib, Ic, grade 1 and grade 2 aneuploid tumors of mucinous, serous, mixed or endometrioid types
Stage Ia, Ib, Ic, grade 3 and undifferentiated tumors
Stage Ia, Ib, Ic clear cell adenocarcinomas

laparotomy in that particular group of patients is overtreatment and can harm the patient. Table 30-3 lists the criteria that we use to decide when restaging is necessary.

The morbidity associated with a repeat laparotomy can be decreased by laparoscopic techniques done by experienced laparoscopic surgeons.[47-50] Pomel and colleagues[49] have outlined in detail a laparoscopic approach to staging of EOC. However, abdominal dissemination or recurrences at trocar sites have been observed in a few studies.[51,52]

Norwegian Radium Hospital Staging Guidelines

The standards for staging were introduced 20 years ago by the Gynecologic Oncology Group (GOG).[25] Based on the results from Zanetta and coworkers,[30] Benedetti-Panici and associates,[45] and our own experience, the guidelines for proper staging should consist of the following:

1. The vertical abdominal incision is enlarged supraumbilically as much as necessary to complete the upper abdominal staging procedure. In selected cases, laparoscopy can be used to access the external appearance of an ovarian mass and help the surgeon decide which approach (laparoscopy or laparotomy) or incision is the most suitable.[53]
2. For evaluation of ascites, sampling peritoneal fluid is first performed before contamination by blood cells. When no ascites is found, multiple peritoneal washings for cytologic analysis must be performed.
3. The entire peritoneal surface of the abdominopelvic wall, from the pelvis to the diaphragm, is thoroughly inspected and palpated, searching for tumor implants. The abdominal organs are inspected, and the sizes of all lesions are reported.
4. Random biopsies of pelvic peritoneum and abdominal peritoneum (including paracolic gutters) are taken. It does not seem to be necessary to sample the subdiaphragmatic area routinely.[54]
5. Bilateral para-aortic and pelvic node sampling is performed.
6. Resection of primary ovarian cancer is achieved by total hysterectomy plus bilateral salpingo-oophorectomy.
7. Omentectomy is indicated as a staging procedure and as a part of surgical therapy.
8. The benefit of systematic appendectomy is controversial. The appendix is seldom involved (<4% of

EOC cases).[55,56] In cases of mucinous tumors, 8% of appendices are involved.[57] It can be the only site of extraovarian spread in patients with EOC.[58] This suggests that routine appendectomy should be performed as part of the standard staging procedure at least in cases of mucinous tumors and grade 3 tumors.
9. Restaging should be done only in patients at high risk for recurrences (see Table 30-3). The laparoscopic procedure can be safely used for the restaging of apparent EOC by teams that are experienced in ovarian and advanced laparoscopic surgery.[53]

Is it gambling to perform conservative surgery for stage I epithelial ovarian carcinoma in women of childbearing age?

Although most EOCs occur in older women in whom bilateral salpingo-oophorectomy and hysterectomy are standard treatment, a small subset of patients is young and can be managed conservatively with preservation of reproductive potential. Most clinicians are seldom faced with the problem of preserving ovarian function in the presence of malignant ovarian tumors. Common errors in surgical management include incomplete staging and unnecessary bilateral salpingo-oophorectomy. Some patients are mismanaged because of an error in the pathologic diagnosis. Stage I ovarian cancer and borderline tumors can frequently be observed in women of childbearing age for whom preservation of reproductive function is important. Because of the increase in number of such women referred to the NRH during the past 2 decades, it has been necessary to revise some of the earlier radical treatment principles for selected cases of ovarian malignancies found in women younger than 40 years of age.[59] The question of conservative surgery should not be considered in cases of clear cell, grade 3, or undifferentiated carcinomas, and we agree with most gynecologic oncologists that conservative surgery should be performed only in young patients with borderline tumors and endometrioid, mucinous, or serous stage Ia, grade 1 ovarian cancer. However, the literature lacks prospective studies with adequate numbers of patients to assess the cost-benefit ratio of conservative surgery in ovarian cancer.

When is it advisable to perform unilateral oophorectomy in fertile women with one of these types of epithelial malignancy? Well-differentiated serous and endometrioid tumors are frequently bilateral. In a large series of 2800 patients with EOC treated at the NRH, 10% of the mucinous and endometrioid cancers were bilateral, and 30% of the serous cancers were bilateral.[59] Even when the contralateral ovary is macroscopically normal, a microscopic lesion may be found in the stroma. In two series, this risk was estimated to be as low as 2.5%.[60,61] Despite these facts, the surgeon should not perform wedge biopsies of the remaining ovary if it looks normal because this may cause mechanical infertility.[62,63] Because of the possibility of endometrial involvement, we include an endometrial biopsy when performing a conservative procedure. We perform careful inspections of ovarian surfaces and biopsy any suspicious lesion or perform a cystectomy if it can be done radically. If the tumor ruptures during surgery or if ascites is present, our policy at the NRH has been to avoid performing conservative surgery. Peritoneal washings may contain cancer cells. Because the diagnosis of ovarian cancer in young women is often unanticipated at the time of laparotomy for an adnexal mass and misdiagnosed as endometriosis or pelvic inflammatory disease, the surgeon in such cases may not have enough experience with oncologic surgery. In such situations, a two-step procedure is always preferable; the first step is extirpation of the adnexal tumor in toto, performed after obtaining cytologic washings. After definitive histopathologic evaluation, a second operation can be performed to obtain optimal staging before a conservative (fertility sparing) attitude is allowed. Using this strategy, we have achieved more than 20 normal pregnancies.

Although no prospective, randomized study on this specific issue has been performed, a very important contribution to the matter has been published by Zanetta and colleagues.[62] In the 10-year period between 1982 and 1992, Zanetta and coworkers[62] treated 99 patients younger than 40 years of age with stage I EOC using a fertility-sparing approach in 56 patients. This approach was carried out in 36 of 56 stage Ia patients (24 grade 1, 8 grade 2, and 4 grade 3), in 1 of 5 stage Ib patients, and 19 of 45 stage Ic patients, and 43 were treated with removal of the internal genital organs. All 99 patients were properly staged and received adjuvant cisplatin treatment. With a median follow-up of 7 years, 5 (9%) of 56 of conservatively managed patients had recurrent disease, including two relapses (3.5%) in the contralateral ovary, whereas 5 (12%) of 46 radically operated patients had recurrent disease. The low rate of contralateral recurrence illustrates, according to Zanetta and associates,[62] the safety of conservative treatment, especially in low-risk patients but also in patients with high-risk tumors (e.g., stage I, grade 3; stage Ic), provided that optimal staging, adjuvant platinum-based treatment, and informed consent are achieved. Seventeen patients desired children, and there were 15 uncomplicated pregnancies with 16 healthy babies. Similar results have been reported by Brown and colleagues.[64]

Controversies still exist concerning the necessity of removal of the internal genital apparatus after completion of childbearing.[65] It is clear that the risk of relapse after conservative treatment is low, particularly for stage Ia grade 1 tumors. More long-term data are needed. We currently discuss the matter with each patient and her husband.

Natural Course of Early Epithelial Ovarian Cancer Without Adjuvant Treatment

Three prospective, observational studies have been published in which patients did not receive adjuvant therapy after surgery.[66-68] Ten Canadian institutions recruited 82 patients (68 eligible) with FIGO stage I EOC. With a median follow-up time of 4 years, only three patients with disease progression were identified (two had clear cell tumors). However, in this study, patients with FIGO stage Ic disease and with grade 3 tumors were underrepresented, presumably because of reluctance to withhold treatment.[66] Trimbos and coworkers[67] demonstrated excellent prognosis with surgery only (100% disease-free survival rate for grade 1, stage I patients), provided adequate surgical staging is performed. The third study by Ahmed and associates[68] from Royal Marsden, London, included 194 consecutive patients with FIGO stage I disease. After a median observation time of 54 months, the 5-year overall survival rates were as follows: stage Ia, 93%; stage Ib, 92%; and stage Ic, 84%. The 5-year disease-free survival rates were 87%, 65%, and 62% according to FIGO substages and 90%, 85%, and 45% for patients with grade 1, grade 2, or grade 3 tumors, respectively. Although these three studies are of moderate size, they are important because no patients received adjuvant treatment and because all patients with stage I were entered prospectively onto these observational studies. This group of patients represents the largest natural history studies of surgically treated stage I ovarian cancer patients.

At the American Society of Clinical Oncologists (ASCO) meeting in San Francisco in 2001, Kolomainen and colleagues[69] discussed the salvageability of the 61 patients who subsequently relapsed following a policy of no adjuvant chemotherapy from an original cohort between 1980 and 1994 of 194 EOC patients. The median follow-up period was 70 months (range, 1 to 190), and the median time from diagnosis to relapse was 17 months (range, 6 to 188). Treatment at relapse was single-agent cisplatin, platinum-based combination therapy, or carboplatin-paclitaxel therapy. The overall response rate to first-line chemotherapy at relapse was 47%. The disease-free survival rates at 3 and 5 years were 26% and 24%, respectively. The overall survival rates at 3 and 5 years were 53% and 46%, respectively. These 61 relapsing patients had about the same outcome as patients with stage IIIa or IIIb ovarian cancer who are given chemotherapy at diagnosis, and the authors of these four studies recommended that prospective, randomized studies of adjuvant versus delayed chemotherapy in properly staged EOC who are most at risk of relapse should be designed.

What have we learned from prospective, randomized clinical trials of early-stage epithelial ovarian cancer during the past 25 years?

In the past, many randomized trials have enrolled patients with EOC to test the value of adjuvant therapies (e.g., external radiotherapy, intraperitoneal installation of radionuclides such as ^{198}Au or ^{32}P, single alkylating agent or combination chemotherapy) in preventing recurrence. Högberg and coworkers[11] reviewed the literature of early trials of such therapies for EOC.

They found 16 randomized studies that included 3130 patients.[42,43,70-82] However, nine of these studies[70-74,77,79-81] were excluded in their review because they had methodologic flaws such as the omission of a control arm, inclusion of borderline tumors, incomplete surgical staging, or the inclusion of patients in stage II and III with minimal residual disease and were too small for conclusive results.

Is there a place for pelvic radiotherapy, whole abdominal radiotherapy, or radiolabeled isotopes in the management of early epithelial ovarian carcinoma?

In 1979, Dembo and associates[71] published a randomized study involving 147 patients with stage Ib, II, or III EOC. The study compared pelvic radiotherapy (PR) plus whole abdominal radiotherapy (WAR) (76 patients) to PR plus chlorambucil (6 mg/day) for 2 years (71 patients) and showed a 27% improvement in survival for patients who had complete surgical resection and were treated with PR + WAR postoperatively ($P = .006$). The study has been criticized because of incomplete surgical staging, unusual patient classification, suboptimal chlorambucil dose, and too few patients. However, this finding spawned two other studies testing the effect of WAR. Klaassen and colleagues[75] randomized 257 patients to PR + WAR (107 patients) versus PR + ^{32}P (44 patients) versus PR + melphalan (106 patients), and the Danish Ovarian Cancer Group (DACOVA)[78] randomized 118 patients with EOC to PR + WAR (60 patients) versus PR + chlorambucil (58 patients). These two trials failed to show an advantage for WAR over the use of alkylating agents and concluded that WAR should not be recommended as adjuvant therapy for EOC.

In the study by Klaassen and coworkers,[75] 29 patients developed secondary cancers, whereas 19 would have been expected ($P = .018$), and PR + melphalan was associated with an increased risk of developing acute myelogenous leukemia and myelodysplastic syndrome compared with the PR + WAR arm ($P = .06$). A long-term follow-up (13.5 years) of the study by Klaassen and associates[83] did not reveal any overall survival difference.

At MD Anderson Cancer Center, Smith and colleagues[80] randomized 156 patients with FIGO stage I, II, or III disease between PR +WAR and melphalan arms. For FIGO stage I disease, the 5-year disease-free survival rates were 85% and 90% and the overall survival rates were 100% and 86 % for WAR (14 patients) and chemotherapy (28 patients), respectively. The differences were not statistically significant. However, this study was criticized for not irradiating the diaphragm adequately, for using liver shielding, for an imbalance in stage distribution between the two treatment arms, and for too few patients. Despite the inadequacies, Smith and coworkers[80] concluded that chemotherapy was the preferred treatment because it was as effective as irradiation but less toxic and less costly. In a later update, two deaths from treatment

complications in the radiotherapy arm were reported, and two patients from the chemotherapy arm had developed acute leukemia. Right or wrong, this study had a great impact in that most institutions in the United States abandoned postoperative external radiotherapy of ovarian cancer in favor of chemotherapy.[80,81] None of the published trials has compared WAR with platinum-based chemotherapy.[11]

Whole abdominal irradiation with chromic phosphate versus chemotherapy. Young and associates[81] reported a trial by the GOG in which 145 patients with high-risk EOCs (grade 1 to 3, stage I or II tumors) were randomized between ^{32}P and melphalan. No difference in survival between the two randomized arms was observed. However, deaths due to alkylating agent–induced leukemia were seen in the melphalan arm, and because of that, ^{32}P was considered the new standard treatment of EOC patients in the United States, Italy, and Scandinavia. At that time, cisplatin combined with cyclophosphamide was considered the standard treatment for advanced ovarian cancer in the United States. In Europe, single-agent cisplatin was the standard therapy.

It was therefore logical in the United States, Italy, and Norway to compare ^{32}P with standard chemotherapy. Three prospective, randomized trials testing ^{32}P versus cisplatin-based regimens as an adjuvant treatment in EOC have been published: one from the NRH in Oslo, Norway[84]; one from the GOG (GOG95)[82]; and one from Italy.[42] The NRH study compared adjuvant intraperitoneal ^{32}P therapy with six cycles of cisplatin (50 mg/m^2 every 3 weeks) in a group of 347 (not comprehensively surgically staged) patients but without residual tumor after primary laparotomy. The NRH study could not discern any differences in treatment results between ^{32}P (169 patients) and cisplatin (171 patients). However, late bowel obstruction occurred more often in the group treated with ^{32}P compared with the cisplatin group. Because of the absence of therapeutic differences in the NRH report between the ^{32}P and cisplatin groups, a low frequency of serious toxicity after cisplatin therapy, the difficulty in administering ^{32}P due to maldistribution of radioisotopes, and a higher occurrence of bowel complications after ^{32}P therapy, the NRH suggested that cisplatin (or other platinum analogs) should be the standard adjuvant treatment in EOC.[84]

The GOG95 study randomized 251 (205 eligible) patients with grade 2 or grade 3 EOC after surgical staging to ^{32}P (98 patients) or to cyclophosphamide (1 g/m^2) plus cisplatin (100 mg/m^2) (106 patients) for three cycles.[82] The cumulative incidence of progression at 10 years was 35% for patients receiving ^{32}P and only 28% for those receiving cyclophosphamide plus cisplatin. The patients treated with cyclophosphamide plus cisplatin had an estimated recurrence rate of 35% lower than those who received ^{32}P ($P = .15$, two-tailed test). If both groups are analyzed together, the cumulative incidence of recurrence at 10 years for all stage I patients was 27%, compared with 44% for stage II patients ($P = .014$).[85] Two of the patients in the GOG95 study had bowel perforation in conjunction with the administration of ^{32}P, and two patients died of treatment complications, one in each arm.[85] After GOG95, the GOG changed their strategy, and because of the longer (although not statistically significant) disease-free survival observed with cyclophosphamide combined with platinum and the late bowel toxicity associated with ^{32}P, cyclophosphamide plus cisplatin was recommended as standard care for adjuvant therapy outside of protocol for this subset of patients.[86]

The Italian study group Gruppo Italiano Collaborative Oncologica Ginecologica (GICOG) performed two multicenter, randomized clinical trials between October 1983 and October 1990.[42] In one of these studies, Bolis and colleagues[42] compared intraperitoneal installation of ^{32}P (75 patients) with cisplatin (50 mg/m^2 every 28 days for six cycles) (77 patients) intravenously after adequate staging surgery of 152 EOCs (FIGO 1973 stage Ia$_{ii}$/Ib$_{ii}$ and Ic). After a median observation time of about 10 years, results still confirm the observation reported in the initial report that cisplatin reduced the rate of progression, with a relative risk of 0.39 (P = .0007). There was no difference in overall survival (79% and 81%).[87] This could be explained by the power of the study being too low. It was the first randomized study to show an impact of chemotherapy on disease-free survival in high-risk EOC patients. The GICOG study showed that cisplatin-treated patients had a poorer outcome at relapse than patients not treated with cisplatin. Alternatively, the adjuvant cisplatin therapy may have selected a resistant population of cells at recurrence. This could indicate that patients failing to respond to cisplatin had more virulent disease or perhaps that they had resistance to cisplatin-containing regimens, whereas in the ^{32}P arm, cisplatin after relapse can still be an active treatment. A more effective second-line treatment might have affected overall survival. The conclusion from these studies in the United States, Italy, and Norway is that cisplatin-conforming regimens are preferable to radiotherapy or intraperitoneal radioisotopes.[9]

Is watch and wait adequate after comprehensive surgical staging of low-risk early-stage epithelial ovarian cancer?

The comparison of survival results in nonrandomized studies using different types of adjuvant treatment and no adjuvant treatment at all is difficult. Most prior randomized trials compared two or three different treatment modalities, and nearly all have had very low power because of the small number of patients and events. However, without an untreated observation group, the efficacy of any adjuvant treatment cannot be firmly established. Only two randomized, prospective studies including a control arm have been published for low-risk EOC.[42,81] In the first study by the GOG, 81 patients with low-risk disease (grade 1 or grade 2 tumors; FIGO 1973 stage Ia or Ib) were randomized between 12 cycles of orally administered adjuvant melphalan therapy and no treatment.[81] Unfortunately,

30% of the patients were, at subsequent central pathology review, found to have tumors of borderline malignancy and were therefore excluded. After a median follow-up period exceeding 6 years, no significant difference in overall survival (94% versus 98%) or disease-free survival (91% versus 94%) could be seen. One patient in the melphalan arm died of aplastic anemia.

The second study by GICOG[42] showed a significant disease-free survival advantage in the cisplatin group (83%, 41 patients) compared with the untreated group (64%, 42 patients) (P = .028). However, when the controls were treated with cisplatin at relapse, they had the same overall 5-year survival as the group receiving immediate cisplatin treatment (82% and 88%, respectively). These results have been confirmed with more than 120 months (median) of observation time.[87] This suggests, however, that 8 of 10 women in the cisplatin group had been overtreated. It was observed that the risk of dying was greater for patients treated with cisplatin up front after progression had occurred.[86]

These two studies did not show any significant overall survival differences between the treatment arm and the control arm. Such a difference would not be expected because approximately 1000 patients are required to detect a difference in survival of 5% at a significance level of 5% and power of 90% when the expected survival is 90%.[88] Because the prognosis is so good in stage Ia, Ib grade 1, and Ib grade 2 ovarian cancer patients (93% to 95% 5-year overall survival),[42,66-68,81] it is generally accepted by all gynecologic oncologists in the world that no adjuvant treatment should be given provided the patient was properly staged.

Is high-risk early-stage epithelial ovarian cancer overtreated surgically and systemically?

Only large, prospective trials of poor-prognosis EOC patients with an untreated control arm (i.e., treat at relapse) will be able to resolve the question of whether adjuvant therapy contributes to survival. Although cyclophosphamide plus cisplatin was the preferred treatment in GOG95, the toxicity and duration of therapy may not be optimal because 26% of the patients had recurrent disease within 5 years.[85] Based on the results of GOG111,[89] cisplatin plus paclitaxel became the new standard of care for advanced ovarian cancer in the United States. The GOG replacement study of EOC (GOG157) was activated in March 1995 and closed in May 1998.[90] In this study, 457 patients with high-risk EOC were randomized after surgical staging to receive carboplatin (AUC = 7.5) and paclitaxel (175 mg/m^2) every 21 days for three cycles or the same chemotherapy regimen every 21 days for six cycles. Carboplatin replaced cisplatin in the combination-chemotherapy regimens because of equal efficacy but less toxicity.[91,92] As in the previous trial, GOG95, the end points for GOG157 were disease-free survival, overall survival, and comparative toxicities.[90] At the UICC (Union Internationale Contre le Cancer) meeting in Oslo in July 2002, Young presented preliminary data that showed no difference in disease-free survival or overall survival between the two arms.[85] The toxicities were, however, significantly worse in the groups receiving six cycles of cyclophosphamide plus cisplatin.

GOG157 reflects a difference in attitude between the United States and Europe. In the United States, it is regarded as ethically and legally necessary to treat patients with poor prognostic factors with adjuvant therapy.[86,93] In Europe, the philosophy has been somewhat different. British gynecologic oncologists[94] have questioned the value of adjuvant chemotherapy. In Scandinavia and the European Organization of Research and Treatment of Cancer (EORTC) countries, ethics committees have approved trials with an observation arm because of lack of documentation for the benefit of adjuvant therapy.[11]

However, it is very difficult to conduct such studies because patients hesitate to be randomized to a control arm when they are informed about the increased disease-free survival with cisplatin. We have found that many patients refuse to participate in a trial that includes a no-treatment control arm.[43] Despite these difficulties, three very important studies have been conducted in Europe to determine whether adjuvant treatment in high-risk patients significantly improves progression-free and long-term survival.

The Nordic Cooperative Ovarian Cancer Group (NOCOVA) study[43] was closed prematurely because of poor accrual. Between 1992 and 1997, 230 adequately operated patients (162 eligible) with FIGO stage I invasive EOC, grade 2 and grade 3, or grade 1 aneuploid or with clear cell histology were randomized to observation (81 patients) or to postoperative carboplatin (AUC = 7) for six courses (81 patients). With a median follow-up of 60 months, progression was registered for 46 patients: 25 in the treatment group and 21 in the control group. The estimated 5-year overall survival and disease-free survival rates were 80% versus 85% and 70% versus 71% for the treatment and control groups, respectively (not significant) (Fig. 30-1A,B).

When the control group patients were treated with carboplatin at relapse, they had a better, although not statistically significant 5-year overall survival rate compared with the group receiving immediate carboplatin: 40% and 18%, respectively (see Fig. 30-1C). This is a repetition of the GICOG study[42] and suggests that 8 of 10 women in the carboplatin group had been overtreated.

The other two prospective, randomized studies addressing this question were presented at the 2001 ASCO meeting in San Francisco.[95] The Adjuvant Clinical Trial in Ovarian Neoplasms (ACTION) is an EORTC-sponsored randomized trial comparing observation with chemotherapy (at least 75 mg/m² of cisplatin or at least 350 mg/m² of carboplatin for a minimum of four cycles). In this trial, 448 patients after adequate surgery with stage Ia, Ib (grade 2 or 3), Ic, and IIa (all grades) were randomized, with 224 in each arm.

The other large trial, the International Collaborative Neoplasm Studies (ICON1), was organized by the British Medical Research Council (MRC). Its inclusion criteria were more liberal, not requiring adequate staging and randomizing any patients. This trial randomized patients to immediate platinum-based chemotherapy (80% with carboplatin, AUC = 5) for six cycles or to observation. More than 447 patients were randomized. Both studies closed in January 2000, and the median follow-up time was 5.5 years. Unfortunately, both studies failed to recruit the target number of patients. Both studies were well balanced concerning prognostic factors. Both studies showed a significant difference in disease-free survival and overall survival in favor of immediate adjuvant treatment.

In the ACTION study, the disease-free survival and overall survival differences were 11% and 8%, respectively ($P < .01$ and $P < .02$). In the ICON1 study, the disease-free survival and overall survival differences were 10% and 7%, respectively ($P = .02$ and $P = .05$). When all 925 patients included in the two studies were analyzed together, a significant improvement was observed in disease-free survival by an absolute difference at 5 years of 11% (range, 65% to 76%; 95% CI: 5%-16%) and overall survival by an absolute difference at 5 years of 7% (range, 75% to 82%; 95% CI: 2%-11%) for high-risk patients receiving chemotherapy compared with follow-up without adjuvant treatment. There was no evidence that the effect of adjuvant chemotherapy is smaller or larger in any of the tested subgroups (e.g., age, differentiation, histologic type, FIGO substages). This is the first evidence that immediate treatment is significantly better than treatment at relapse. However, comprehensiveness of surgical staging was a significant prognostic factor for tumor recurrence in the observational arm. When subset analysis from the ACTION study was performed for 151 adequately staged patients (16%), no difference in disease-free survival or overall survival between immediate treatment and observation was found (Table 30-4). This probably means that there were a number of patients with occult stage III disease in the suboptimally staged patients, which could explain the differences between disease-free survival and overall survival in the two studies.

Looking at the survival benefit of adjuvant chemotherapy for EOC relative to the completeness of surgical staging reveals several interesting results. For the incompletely staged patients in ICON1 (all patients), ACTION (two thirds of patients), and NOCOVA (two thirds of patients), there was a significantly better overall survival for those in the chemotherapy arm in the ICON1 ($P = .05$) and ACTION ($P = .03$) studies, but not in the NOCOVA study.[95] For the completely staged patients in GOG95, ACTION (one third of patients), and GICOG, there was no significant difference between the observation arm and active treatment arm. Does this mean that immediate adjuvant therapy suffices for bad surgical staging? After 30 years and many prospective, randomized studies around the world, we still do not know what therapy, if any, is appropriate for the subset of patients with poor-prognosis EOC. However, there are two

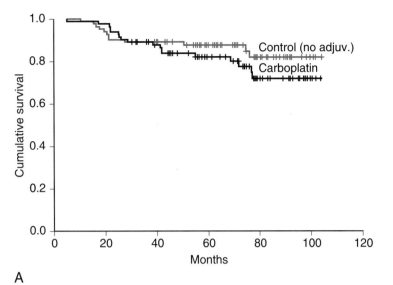

A

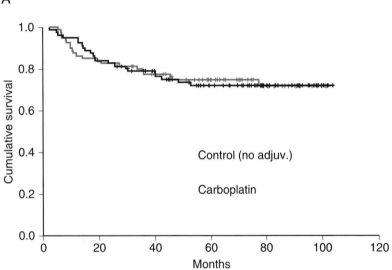

B

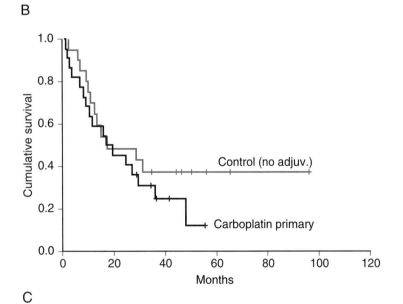

C

Figure 30–1. A, Five-year disease-specific survival in months according to randomization groups: control (n=81) and carboplatin (n=81). **B,** Five-year disease-free survival in months according to randomization group: control (n=81) and carboplatin (n=81). **C,** Five-year cumulative survival for relapsing patients. The control group was treated with carboplatin (AUC=7), and the carboplatin group individually received second-line treatment. (From Tropé C, Kaern J, Högberg T, et al: Randomized study on adjuvant chemotherapy in stage I high-risk ovarian cancer with evaluation of DNA-ploidy as prognostic instrument. Ann Oncol 2000;11:281-288.)

Table 30–4.   Survival Rates for 151 Patients by Staging Performance and Treatment in the ACTION Trial

Treatment and Staging Performance	5-Year Survival Rate	5-Year Disease-Free Survival Rate (Significance)
Observation/optimal staging	87%	75%
		(Not significant)
Chemotherapy/optimal staging	86%	78%
Observation/nonoptimal staging	74%	65%
		(P = .02)
Chemotherapy/nonoptimal staging	86%	75%

From Vergote IB, Trimbos JB, Guthrie D, et al: Results of a randomized trial in 923 patients with high risk early ovarian cancer, comparing adjuvant chemotherapy with no further treatment following surgery [abstract 802]. J Clin Oncol 2001;20:201A.

dominant attitudes, one in the United States and one in Europe (Table 30-5).

Can classic and clinical prognostic factors help separate high-risk disease from low-risk disease?

Earlier reports on EOC have identified FIGO substage, grade of differentiation, histologic type (e.g., clear cell carcinoma), dense adhesions, large-volume ascites, rupture before or during surgery, extracapsular growth, and age as independent prognostic factors.[4,18,22,23,97-99] The independent significance of tumor rupture is still controversial.[18,23,68,97-101] However, the latest FIGO subclassification identified tumor spillage, extracapsular growth, and positive peritoneal cytologic results as one variable for substage Ic (FIGO 1988). The degree of differentiation is the only factor with independent prognostic value in all published multivariate analysis, but it is not used in the new FIGO subclassification.[4]

The reliability of analysis of prognostic factors depends on the number of cases analyzed, the number of prognostic variables analyzed, and the internal consistency of the factors analyzed. Studies of EOC are affected by low statistical power due to small numbers, great heterogeneity of the patients considered in the different trials, and lack of large, prospective, randomized trials. The extent of surgical staging, histopathologic examination, and treatment varies over time and from trial to trial. To get reliable results from multivariate analysis, only patients staged according to the uniform guidelines concerning comprehensive

staging in EOC should be included in multivariate analysis.[9,102,103]

The prognostic significance of tumor rupture and grade were described in a meta-analysis by Vergote and coworkers,[4] who analyzed 1545 patients with stage I disease. The multivariate analysis identified degree of differentiation as the most powerful prognostic factor followed by rupture before surgery or rupture during surgery and FIGO stage (1973). Aside from these three factors, no other variables were of prognostic value. Patients without tumor rupture had a 5-year disease-free survival rate of 83%, compared with 72% and 70% for patients with tumor rupture before or during surgery. However, the studies were done retrospectively and could not distinguish between intraoperative spontaneous rupture and rupture due to surgical needle aspiration. These findings should stimulate surgeons to avoid rupture during surgery. Recommendation from the study was that laparoscopic removal of ovarian cysts should be restricted to patients with preoperative evidence that the cyst is benign.

Can molecular biologic parameters replace the classic prognostic factors?

Grade of differentiation is an independent and important prognostic factor in EOC and should be used in the risk classification of patients for treatment decisions. The histologic grading is, however, hampered by interobserver and intraobserver variations.[103,104] Detailed knowledge of prognostic factors is essential for the clinician to divide patients into risk groups for treatment decisions and to make more individualized

Table 30–5.   Attitudes about Treatment of Poor-Prognosis Epithelial Ovarian Cancer

Attitude in Europe	Attitude in the United States
Selective	Massive
Conservative	Aggressive
There should be clear evidence of benefit of adjuvant chemotherapy necessary.	There is only one chance in ovarian cancer.
Chemotherapy should not be given on a "benefit of the doubt" basis.	We should fire with every gun we have and accept possible "collateral damage."

From Vergote IB, Trimbos JB, Guthrie D, et al: Results of a randomized trial in 923 patients with high risk early ovarian cancer, comparing adjuvant chemotherapy with no further treatment following surgery [abstract 802]. J Clin Oncol 2001;20:201A.

treatment possible. For this purpose, we need more objective and reproducible factors. DNA ploidy has been identified as a strong prognostic factor in EOC.[96,105-108] Cells with abnormal DNA content may represent clones expressing multiple mutations. Genomic instability may affect expression and function of the cell cycle, cell death, or DNA repair pathways that may be responsible for the enhanced aggressiveness of the malignant cells. At the NRH, the prognostic value of DNA ploidy measured by flow cytometry was analyzed in 219 stage I patients.[96] The median follow-up was 60 months, and the 5-year overall survival and disease-free survival rates were 80% and 78%, respectively. Of these, 51% had diploid tumors, and 49% had aneuploid tumors. The 5-year disease-free survival rate for the patients with diploid tumors was 90%, compared with 64% for patients with aneuploid tumors ($P = .0001$). By univariate analysis, the degree of differentiation, DNA ploidy, FIGO substage (1986/1973), histologic type, dense adhesions, age, and extracapsular growth were of prognostic importance. In patients with graded tumors (non–clear cell tumors), multivariate analysis identified the degree of differentiation, DNA ploidy, and FIGO substage (1986) as the only independent prognostic factors. None of the patients with DNA-diploid grade 1 tumors and only 9% of the patients with DNA-diploid grade 2 tumors relapsed. Similar results have been reported by Schueler and associates[108] for 94 stage I patients, identifying by multivariate analysis DNA index and grade as the only independent prognostic factors.

The value of DNA ploidy measurement by image cytometry to predict long-term survival of patients with stage I disease was studied in another large, retrospective analysis from the NRH.[106] The study included 284 patients with a median follow-up of more than 13 years. The 10-year disease-free survival and overall survival rates were 72% and 68%, respectively. Sixty-five percent had diploid or tetraploid tumors, and 35% had aneuploid tumors. The 10-year disease-free survival rates were 92% for the diploid and tetraploid tumors and 33% for the aneuploid tumors. By multivariate analysis, DNA ploidy was the strongest predictor of survival, followed by histologic grade or type and FIGO stage. Clear cell tumors were not graded, but patients with these tumors had the same survival as those with grade 3 tumors, and these groups were therefore categorized together in the analysis. The conclusion from the study was that DNA ploidy measured by image cytometry combined with histologic grade or type allows separation of patients into risk groups. The low-risk group consisted of FIGO stage Ia, Ib, and Ic, grade 1 or 2, non–clear cell tumors with diploid or tetraploid DNA content. This group of patients had an excellent survival (10-year disease-free survival and overall survival rates higher than 95%) and can be cured by surgery alone. An intermediate-risk group consisted of patients with tumors with diploid or tetraploid DNA content, grade 3 or clear cell histologic type, and stage Ib or Ic (10-year disease-free survival rate of 76%). The high-risk group consisted of all aneuploid tumors independent of grade and FIGO substage[106] (Table 30-6).

The only way to confirm the prognostic significance of DNA ploidy is to test this variable in large, prospective, randomized trials of stage I patients with comprehensive surgical staging. The only such study including DNA ploidy was done by the NOCOVA group.[43] No difference in disease-free survival or overall survival were found between the carboplatin-treated patients and the control arm (see Fig. 30-1A, B). All 162 patients could therefore be analyzed together in a multivariate analysis identifying DNA ploidy, grade of differentiation, and FIGO substage as the only independent prognostic factors (Table 30-7). Our results show that DNA ploidy adds objective independent prognostic information regarding disease-free survival and overall survival of patients with EOC and should be included in the FIGO subclassification. At the NRH, we have taken the results from these studies (see Table 30-7) to define low-risk and high-risk EOC. Table 30-8 shows our guidelines for treatment for stage I EOC patients based on these risk groups.

In an attempt to better classify patients into risk groups, a search is needed for additional prognostic factors that can be more objectively and reproducibly

Table 30–6. Stratified Analysis of 10-Year Disease-Free Survival Related to Ploidy Classification, Degree of Differentiation, and FIGO stage

ICM Ploidy	Grade	FIGO Stage	No. of Patients	10-Year Relapse-Free Survival (%)
Diploid Tetraploid	Well/moderately	1A	55	98.2
		1B + C	77	92.8
	Poorly/clear cell	1A	17	91.2
		1B+C	34	76.0
Aneuploid or Polyploid	Well/moderately	1A	9	66.7
		1B+C	25	49.1
	Poorly/clear cell	1A	15	46.7
		1B+C	52	16.4

ICM, image cytometry; FIGO, International Federation of Gynecology and Obstetrics.
Adapted from Kristensen GB, Kildal W, Abeler VM et al: Large-scale genomic instability predicts long-term outcome for women with invasive stage I ovarian cancer. Ann Oncol 2003;14:1494-500.

Table 30–7. Multivariate Analysis of Disease-Free and Disease-Specific Survival from the Prospective, Randomized NOCOVA Study of 162 High-Risk Stage I Patients

Characteristic	DFS		DSS	
	P	RR	P	RR
FIGO substage	ns		0.01	
a + b				1
c				14
Grade	0.05		0.05	
1 (aneuploid)		1		1
2 + 3 + clear cell		2.5		7.3
DNA ploidy	0.03		<0.05	
Diploid		1		1
Nondiploid		6.0		7.7
Extracapsular growth	0.005		ns	
No		1		
Yes		2.8		
Rupture	0.03		ns	
No		1		
Yes		2.0		

DFS, disease-free survival; DSS, disease-specific survival; NOCOVA, Nordic Cooperative Ovarian Cancer Group; ns, not significant; P, significance; RR, relative risk.

From Tropé C, Kaern J, Högberg T, et al: Randomized study on adjuvant chemotherapy in stage I high-risk ovarian cancer with evaluation of DNA-ploidy as prognostic instrument. Ann Oncol 2000;11:281-288.

measured. Several molecular biologic probes, such as P53 protein, platelet-derived growth-factor (PDGF), platelet-derived growth factor α-receptor (PDGFR-α), vascular endothelial growth factor (VEGF), B-cell leukemia/lymphoma-2 protein (BCL-2), and BCL-2–associated X protein (BAX), are under investigation. The data on these factors are still insufficient for decisions about clinical treatment of EOC.

Expression of PDGF and PDGFR-α was studied by Henriksen and colleagues[109] in normal ovaries and in EOC using immunohistochemistry. Ovarian cancer patients with stage I PDGF-α–positive staining have an overall shorter survival time than those with negative staining of the tumor cells.

VEGF antibodies have been shown to inhibit neoplasm vascularization in ovarian cancer cell lines.

Expression of VEGF has been upregulated markedly in ovarian cancer specimens compared with normal and benign ovarian cysts. It has been suggested that VEGF-driven angiogenesis is an early event in ovarian carcinogenesis.[110] Studies of Paley and coworkers[110] and Tempfer and associates[111] showed that patients with EOC with increased VEGF expression had a poorer prognosis and observed that VEGF overexpression might be useful in identifying patients who could benefit from aggressive adjuvant therapy. Paley and colleagues[110] studied 68 patients with EOC. Of these, 29 tissue samples overexpressed VEGF. In the group of patients with VEGF-positive tumors, the median disease-free survival was 18 months, compared with more than 120 months for the VEGF-negative group (P < .001).

The prognostic significance of angiogenesis as demonstrated by the degree of neovascularization has been investigated by Alvarez and coworkers.[112] In 88 patients, tissue microvessel counts were evaluated with antibodies to von Willebrand factor F and CD31. A low microvessel count was associated with better 5-year survival, especially in patients with EOC. The conclusion was that the degree of angiogenesis might allow the selection of women with EOC at high risk for recurrence who might benefit from aggressive adjuvant therapy.[112]

Cell kinetic data are other important indicators of tumor aggressiveness and treatment response. Tumor growth is determined by the balance between tumor cell proliferation and cell loss. Proliferation depends on the fraction of the cells in the cell cycle. Cell proliferative activity measured by Ki-67 expression in EOC specimens was examined by Henriksen and associates[113] and found to be of significant predictive value for overall survival. High proliferation rates were significantly related to high histologic grade and to advanced stage. For reliable information on these variables, Ki-67 expression should be studied further in larger prospective populations.

The P53 protein is a nuclear phosphoprotein discovered in virus-transformed cells[114] and was originally classified as an oncogene product. There is substantial evidence that it has tumor suppressor function. Two studies have shown that *TP53* mutations are quite common in ovarian cancer,[115,116] but the

Table 30–8. Guidelines for Treatment Outside Protocols of Stage I Epithelial Ovarian Cancer Patients Referred to the Norwegian Radium Hospital

DNA Ploidy	Grade of Differentiation	FIGO Substage	Adjuvant Chemotherapy*	
			Comprehensively Staged	Not Comprehensively Staged
Diploid and tetraploid	1-2	a, b	Observation	Observation
	3 + clear cell	a, b	Observation	Restaging,† observation
	3 + clear cell	c	Carboplatin+paclitaxel	Restaging,† carboplatin+paclitaxel
Aneuploid and polyploid	1-2-3 + clear cell	a, b, c	Carboplatin+paclitaxel	Restaging,† carboplatin+paclitaxel

*Follow-up: every 3 months for the first 2 years; palpation under anesthesia, CA 125, and computed tomography every 6 months; and assessment every 6 months for years 2 through 5.
†When positive nodes = stage IIIc: carboplatin + paclitaxel (6 courses).

significance of abnormal P53 protein production for tumor development and survival has not been examined in depth. Overexpression of P53 is more common in advanced ovarian cancer than in EOC (50% versus 15%). Anttila and colleagues[117] found a significant association between tumor grade and P53 overexpression (i.e., P53 positive) in 445 patients with ovarian cancer stage I through IV. In this study, P53 status was significantly associated with overall survival in 132 patients with EOC.

In other studies, P53 status was not significantly associated with survival.[118,119] In a study of 52 cases of EOC in which 29% of the tumors were P53 positive, Kohler and coworkers[120] found that P53 status was not related to an adverse outcome. At the NRH, 374 cases of EOC, including 27 borderline and 347 stage I carcinomas, were investigated immunohistochemically for overexpression of P53. Alterations in P53 were detected in 15% of stage I carcinomas. Mutations in the *TP53* gene (exons 5 through 8) were demonstrated in 29 of the 50 stage I carcinomas studied using denaturing gel electrophoresis followed by direct sequencing. Our results indicated that P53 abnormalities play a crucial role in the development of EOC. There was, however, no significant association between P53 and survival in multivariate analyses.[121]

In contrast, a new study by Skirnisdottir and associates[122] analyzing 109 EOC cases found that P53 and tumor grade were independent and significant prognostic factors for cancer-specific survival. In this study, the combination of P53 and BCL-2 status could be used for classifying patients into risk groups. The worst prognosis was seen for patients with P53-positive and BCL-2–negative tumors, and the best prognosis was for P53-negative and BCL-2–positive tumors. BCL-2 is an oncoprotein that apparently inhibits apoptosis. In one study of EOC, BCL-2 expression was positively correlated with survival.[123] Cell-line experiments have shown that BCLl-2 expression, depending on the cellular content, can result in specific and profound growth suppression. BCL-2 also can delay entry of cells into S phase, and the resulting lower proliferation index may help to explain the favorable prognostic significance of this marker.[123]

The significance of the *ERBB2 (HER2)* oncogene as a prognostic indicator in EOC is controversial.[124,125] Most of the studies done show that HER2 is rarely expressed and does not possess any major prognostic significance in patients with EOC.[126,127] Other oncogenes have been studied, including the *RAS* and *MYC* oncogenes, but protein overexpression or gene amplification of these candidates has not been shown to have any prognostic significance.[127,128]

The role of expression of NME1 (formerly designated nm23-H1) is still controversial. Schneider and colleagues[129] studied 247 EOCs and showed in a multivariate analysis of a subset of 57 grade 1 or 2 tumors that NME1 overexpression was the only significant independent predictor of an ominous prognosis. This result may be of clinical significance if NME1 overexpression can identify patients at high risk for recurrence within this low-risk group of grade 1 or 2 EOC.

Detection of Early-Stage Epithelial Ovarian Cancer Requires New Technologies

EOCs have an excellent prognosis compared with advanced-stage disease. Survival could theoretically be improved by earlier detection of disease (i.e., stage migration) or by prevention. Shridbar and coworkers[130] have attempted to understand early events in ovarian carcinogenesis by exploring the steps in its progression. Twenty-one EOCs were analyzed together with 17 advanced-stage tumors by multiple molecular genetic techniques (e.g., cDNA microarrays, total RNA isolating and labeling, semiquantitative reverse transcriptase–polymerase chain reaction [RT-PCR]). Profound alterations in gene expression were found in EOCs, many of which were similar to those identified in advanced ovarian cancer. However, the differences observed at the genomic level suggest differences between early and advanced ovarian cancer and provide support for a progression model for ovarian cancer development. The screening strategies assume that most advanced ovarian cancers originate from stage I lesions. The results from Shridhar and associates[130] are consistent with this theory. EOCs have most of the genetic changes required for metastatic spread and require aggressive therapy. Future studies of the genes that show consistently high levels of transcription may result in the identification of markers useful for early cancer detection and may further point to potential therapeutic targets.

Another step in the detection of EOC has been performed by Petricoin and colleagues,[131] who hypothesized that complex serum proteomic patterns might reflect the underlying pathologic state of an organ, such as the ovary. A bioinformatics tool was developed and used to identify proteomic patterns in serum that distinguish cancer from benign disease. Proteomic spectra were generated by mass spectroscopy. A preliminary "training" set of spectra derived from analysis of sera from 50 unaffected women and 50 patients with ovarian cancer was analyzed by an iterative searching algorithm, which identified a proteomic pattern that completely discriminated cancer from noncancerous conditions. Thereafter, the same pattern was used to classify an independent set of 116 masked serum samples: 50 from EOC patients and 66 from unaffected women or women with benign disease. Pattern recognition correctly identified each of the 50 cancers, including all 18 stage I tumors. Sixty-three of the 66 nonmalignant cases were recognized as benign. These findings yielded a positive predictive value of 94%, compared with 35% for CA 125 determinations for the same samples. In the future, serum proteomic pattern analysis may be applied in screening clinics as a supplement if the 100% sensitivity and specificity is confirmed by prospective detection of stage I ovarian cancer in trials of high-risk and low-risk women.

Although it is tempting to adopt the newer prognostic factors reviewed in this chapter, they need to be subjected to the same rigorous testing as the traditional clinical and histologic variables. The only way to do this is by performing large, prospective, randomized trials.

Is it possible to develop new adjuvant therapeutic strategies that translate into enhanced survival?

Early local invasion of EOC and its usual late parenchymal dissemination is evident clinically but not well characterized molecularly. The interactive role with the stroma is clear through the demonstration clinically and in the laboratory of the importance of angiogenesis in EOC biology. The production of large numbers of growth factors and cytokines that regulate cellular growth, cellular survival, and invasive potential has led to new directions for basic and translational research in this arena.[132] Invasion and angiogenesis remain important translational targets for research into biomarkers of disease, prognostic factors, molecular targets for therapy, and biomarkers of response to treatment. Progress will be made by investigation of the causes of invasion and angiogenesis in ovarian cancer. A large number of new agents targeted against invasion and angiogenesis reached clinical trials in the final decade of the 20th century. More than 100 agents are under development or in phase I, II, or III clinical trials, including metalloproteinase inhibitors (e.g., marimastat), integrin inhibitors, ion channel inhibitors (e.g., calcium ion inhibitor), growth factor inhibitors (e.g., VEGFR), cytoskeleton inhibitors (e.g., taxane), and some mechanisms (e.g., thalidomide).[133]

The targeting of cell receptor signaling is proving to be a viable method of treating cancer, as shown by use of the anti-HER2 monoclonal antibody trastuzumab (Herceptin) and the tyrosine kinase (TK) inhibitor imatinib mesylate (STI-571 or Gleevec).[134] Because of the clonally heterogenous nature of solid tumors, the targeting of multitasking receptor TKs or the simultaneous targeting of different TKs is likely to be a feature of treatment aimed at ovarian cancer. One such multitasking TK is the epidermal growth factor receptor (EGFR, formerly designated ERBB),[135] which is involved in multiple downstream effects through its dimerization potential with other receptors from the EGFR family (ERBB, ERBB2, ERBB3, ERBB4). Iressa (ZD 1839), a synthetic anilinoquinazoline, is an orally active, selective EGFR-TK inhibitor that blocks EGFR signaling. Iressa has shown in vitro growth inhibition against a range of tumor cell types, including ovarian cancer.[136]

It is not yet clear how to use these agents optimally or how to assess their benefit. Critical questions remain. When is the best time to use these new agents? How do we determine the balance between benefit and risk? With what agents are these families of drugs best suited for combination therapy? Are there cancer types or patient subsets for whom these agents should be used as primary agents or in combinations?

Prior conventional wisdom was that agents to be used in adjuvant treatment would only be active if the agent had produced clinical response when used for advanced disease. This is probably untrue for small-molecule targeted agents because they do not cause marked disease reduction. The hypothesis underlying adjuvant testing is the capacity to maintain stabilization of disease and to reduce angiogenic and invasive potential. If cancer deposits can be maintained in the prevascularized or minimally vascularized and noninvasive state, patients may achieve a prolonged time to detectable relapse. Whether this translates into overall disease survival remains to be seen. In the coming years, the current research initiative on adjuvant treatment of EOC will be undertaken, and several lines of research should be pursued:

- Proteomics and gene expression studies of neovessel development in various in vitro and in vivo models
- Characterization of new ovarian cancer growth factors and cytokines and their regulation of the angiogenic and invasive pathways
- Development of novel reagents to modulate angiogenesis and invasion
- Improved imaging approaches using dynamic MRI and PET approaches
- Drug combination testing using dual anti-invasive and antiangiogenic agents and combinations of anti-invasive plus antiangiogenic agents with conventional chemotherapy
- Assessment of antiangiogenic and anti-invasive activity of conventional chemotherapeutics when administered in different doses and schedules
- Dissection of signaling pathways regulating neovascularization and invasion in ovarian cancer models
- Application of putative surrogate markers of biologically effective dose to current clinical trials
- Evaluation of the implication of circulating or bone marrow–based ovarian cancer cells on time to progression or overall survival

REFERENCES

1. Annual report on the results of treatment in gynaecological cancer, vol 23. Statements of results obtained in patients treated in 1990-1992. J Epidemiol Biostat 1998.3:1-135.
2. Greenlee RT, Murray T, Bolden S, et al: Cancer statistics 2000. CA Cancer J Clin 2000;50:7-33.
3. Ozols RF: Chemotherapy for ovarian cancer. Semin Oncol 1999;26:34-40.
4. Vergote I, De Brabanter J, Fyles A, et al: Prognostic importance of degree of differentiation and cyst rupture in stage I invasive epithelial ovarian carcinoma. Lancet 2001;357:176-182.
5. Bjorge T, Engeland A, Sundfor K, et al: Prognosis of 2,800 patients with epithelial ovarian cancer diagnosed during 1975-94 and treated at the Norwegian Radium Hospital. Acta Obstet Gynecol Scand 1998;77:777-781.
6. Piver MS, Barlow JJ, Lele SB: Incidence of subclinical metastases in stage I and II ovarian carcinoma. Obstet Gynecol 1978;52:100-1004.
7. Young RC, Decker DG, Wharton JT, et al: Staging laparotomy in early ovarian cancer. JAMA 1983;250:3072-3076.
8. Wu P-C, Qu J-Y, Lang J-H, et al: Lymph node metastasis of ovarian cancer: A preliminary survey of 74 cases of lymphadenectomy. Am J Obstet Gynecol 1986;155:1103-1108.
9. Favalli G, Odicino F, Torri V, et al: Early stage ovarian cancer: The Italian contribution to clinical research. An update. Int J Gynecol Cancer 2002;11:9-12.
10. Ozols R, Rubin SC, Thomas G, et al: Epithelial ovarian cancer. In Hoskins W, Perex C, Young RC (eds): Principles and Practice of Gynecologic Oncology, 2nd ed. Philadelphia, Lippincott-Raven, 1996, pp 919-986.

11. Högberg T, Glimelius B, Nygren P: A systematic overview of chemotherapy effects in ovarian cancer. Acta Oncol 2001;40: 340-360.

12. Bergman F: Carcinoma of the ovary: A clinico-pathological study of autopsied cases with special reference to mode of spread. Acta Obstet Gynecol Scand 1966;45:211-232.

13. Tropé C, Makar APH: Unsettled questions regarding ovarian cancer. Acta Obstet Gynecol Scand 1992;71:7-18.

14. DiRe F, Baiocchi G: Value of lymph node assessment in ovarian cancer: Status of the art at the end of the second millennium. Int J Gynecol Cancer 2000;10:435-442.

15. Engel H, Kleespies C, Friedrich J, et al: Detection of circulating tumor cells in patients with breast or ovarian cancer by molecular cytogenetics. Br J Cancer 1999;81:1165-1173.

16. Marth C, Kisic J, Kaern J, et al: Circulating tumor cells in the peripheral blood and bone marrow of patients with ovarian carcinoma do not predict prognosis. Cancer 2002;94:707-712.

17. FIGO Cancer Committee: Staging announcement. Gynecol Oncol 1986;25:383-385.

18. Dembo AJ, Davy M, Stenwig AE, et al: Prognostic factors in patients with stage I epithelial ovarian cancer. Obstet Gynecol 1990;75:263-273.

19. Webb MJ, Drecker DG, Mussey E, et al: Factors influencing survival in stage I ovarian cancer. Am J Obstet Gynecol 1973;116: 222-226.

20. Knapp RC, Friedman EA: Aortic lymph node metastases in early ovarian cancer. Am J Obstet Gynecol 1974;119:1013-1017.

21. Musumeci R, Banfi A, Bolis G: Lymphangiography in patients with ovarian epithelial cancer. Cancer 1997;40:1444-1449.

22. Mayer AR, Chambers SK, Graves E, et al: Ovarian cancer staging: Does it require a gynecologic oncologist? Gynecol Oncol 1992;47:223-227.

23. Sevelda P, Vavra N, Schemper M, et al: Prognostic factors for survival in stage I epithelial ovarian carcinoma. Cancer 1990;65:2349-2352.

24. Helewa ME, Krepart GV, Lotocki R: Staging laparotomy in early epithelial ovarian carcinoma. Am J Obstet Gynecol 1986;154: 282-286.

25. Buchsbaum HJ, Brady MF, Delgado G, et al: Surgical staging of carcinoma of the ovaries. Surg Gynecol Obstet 1989;169: 226-232.

26. Trimbos JB, Schueler JA, van Lent M, et al: Reasons for incomplete surgical staging in early ovarian carcinoma 1990;37: 374-377.

27. Muños KA, Harlan LC, Trimble EL: Patterns of care for women with ovarian cancer in the United States. J Clin Oncol 1997; 15:3408-3415.

28. McGowan L, Lesher LP, Norris HJ, et al: Misstaging of ovarian cancer. Obstet Gynecol 1985;65:568.

29. Le T, Adolph A, Krepart G, et al: The benefit of comprehensive surgical staging in the management of early-stage epithelial ovarian carcinoma. Gynecol Oncol 2002;85:351-355.

30. Zanetta G, Rota S, Chiari S, et al: The accuracy of staging: An important prognostic determinator in stage I ovarian carcinoma: A multivariate analysis. Ann Oncol 1998;9:1097-1101.

31. Burghardt E, Pickel H, Lahousen M, et al: Pelvic lymphadenectomy in operative treatment of ovarian cancer 1986;155:15-19.

32. Burghardt E, Girardi F, Lahousen M, et al: Patterns of pelvic and paraaortic lymph node involvement in ovarian cancer. Gynecol Oncol 1991;40:103-106.

33. Benedetti-Panici P, Greggi S, Maneschi F, et al: Anatomical and pathological study of retroperitoneal nodes in epithelial ovarian cancer. Gynecol Oncol 1993;51:150-154.

34. Petru E, Lahousen M, Tamussino K, et al: Lymphadenectomy in stage I ovarian cancer. Am J Obstet Gynecol 1994;170:656-662.

35. Onda T, Yoshikawa H, Yokota H, et al: Assessment of metastases to aortic and pelvic lymph nodes in epithelial ovarian carcinoma. Cancer 1996;78:803-808.

36. Carnino F, Fuda G, Ciccone G, et al: Significance of lymph node sampling in epithelial carcinoma of the ovary. Gynecol Oncol 1997;65:467-472.

37. Baiocchi G, Raspagliesi F, Grosso G, et al: Early ovarian cancer: Is there a role for systematic pelvic and paraaortic lymphadenectomy? Int J Gynecol Cancer 1998;8:103-108.

38. Dexeus S, Cusido MT, Suris JC, et al: Lymphadenectomy in ovarian cancer. Eur J Gynecol Oncol 2000;21:215-222.

39. Podratz KC, Malkasien GD, Wieland HS, et al: Recurrent disease after negative second-look laparotomy in stages III and IV ovarian carcinoma. Gynecol Oncol 1988;29:274-282.

40. Burghardt E, Winter R: The effect of chemotherapy on lymph node metastases in ovarian cancer. Baillieres Clin Obstet Gynaecol 1989;3:167-171.

41. Li AJ, Cass I, Otero F, et al: Pattern of lymph nodes metastases in apparent stage IA invasive epithelial ovarian carcinomas [abstract]. Gynecol Oncol 2000;76:239.

42. Bolis G, Colombo N, Pecorelli S, et al: Adjuvant treatment for early epithelial ovarian cancer: Results of two randomized clinical trials comparing cisplatin to no further treatment or chromic phosphate (^{32}P). GICOG: Gruppo Interregionale Collaborativo in Ginecologia Oncologica. Ann Oncol 1995;6:887-893.

43. Tropé C, Kaern J, Högberg T, et al: Randomized study on adjuvant chemotherapy in stage I high-risk ovarian cancer with evaluation of DNA-ploidy as prognostic instrument. Ann Oncol 2000;11: 281-288.

44. Maggioni F, Maneschi C, Mangioni F, et al: Randomized trial of lymphadenectomy (LY) vs sampling (SA) or resection of bulky nodes (RBN) as primary surgical procedure in early epithelial ovarian cancer [abstract 130]. J Clin Oncol Cancer 1999;9:43A.

45. Benedetti-Panici P, Angioli R: Role of Lymphadenectomy in ovarian cancer. Best practice research. Obstetrics and Gynaecology 2002;16:529-551.

46. Tropé C, Kaern J, Vergote I: Adjuvant therapy for early-stage epithelial ovarian cancer. In Gershenson DM, McGuire WP (eds): Ovarian Cancer: Controversies in Management. New York, Churchill Livingstone, 1998, pp 41-63.

47. Dottino PR, Tobias DH, Beddoe A, et al: Laparoscopic lymphadenectomy for gynecologic malignancies. Gynecol Oncol 1999;73:383-388.

48. Stitt JC, Elg SA: Laparoscopic lymph node dissection in the evaluation and management of patients with pelvic malignancy. Mil Med 1995;160:462-464.

49. Pomel C, Provencher D, Dauplat J, et al: Laparoscopic staging of early ovarian cancer. Gynecol Oncol 1995;58:301-306.

50. Possover M, Mader M, Zielinski J, et al: Is laparotomy for staging early ovarian cancer an absolute necessity? J Am Assoc Gynecol Laparosc 1995;2:285-288.

51. Leminen A, Lehtovirta P: Spread of ovarian cancer after laparoscopic surgery: Report of eight cases. Gynecol Oncol 1999;75: 387-390.

52. Kohlberger PD, Edwards L, Collins C, et al: Laparoscopic port-site recurrence following surgery for a stage IB squamous cell carcinoma of the cervix with negative lymph nodes. Gynecol Oncol 2000;79:324-326.

53. Leblanc E, Querleu D, Narducci F, et al: Surgical staging of early invasive epithelial ovarian tumors. Semin Surg Oncol 2000;19: 36-41.

54. Bertelsen K. Tumor reduction surgery and long-term survival in advanced ovarian cancer: A DACOVA study. Gynecol Oncol 1990;38:223-227.

55. Bese T, Kosebay D, Kaleli S, et al: Appendectomy in the surgical staging of ovarian carcinoma. Int J Gynaecol Obstet 1996;53: 249-252.

56. Rose PG, Reale FR, Fisher A, et al: Appendectomy in primary and secondary staging operations for ovarian malignancy. Obstet Gynecol 1991;77:116-118.

57. Ayhan A, Tuncer ZS, Tuncer R, et al: Is routine appendectomy beneficial in the management of ovarian cancer? Eur J Obstet Gynecol Reprod Biol 1994;57:29-31.

58. Rose PG, Abdul-Karim FW: Isolated appendiceal metastasis in early ovarian carcinoma. J Surg Oncol 1997;64:246-247.

59. Kolstad P, Tropé C: Preservation of ovarian function in the treatment of epithelial and specialized malignant tumors of the ovary: Convegno internazionale su i tumori delle gonadi. Monduzzi Editore S.p.a.-Bologna, Italy, 987:321-337.

60. Benjamin I, Morgan MA, Rubin SC: Occult bilateral involvement in stage I epithelial ovarian cancer. Gynecol Oncol 1999;72: 288-291.

61. Randall TC, Rubin SC: Surgical management of ovarian cancer. Semin Surg Oncol 1999;17:173-180.

62. Zanetta G, Chiari S, Rota S, et al: Conservative surgery for Stage I ovarian carcinoma in women of childbearing age. Br J Obstet Gynecol 1997;104:1030-1035.

63. Weinstein D, Polishuk WZ: The role of wedge resection of the ovary as a cause for mechanical sterility. Surg Gynecol Obstet 1975;141:417-418.

64. Brown CL, Dharmendra B, Barakat RR: Preserving fertility in patients with epithelial ovarian cancer (EOC): The role of conservative surgery in treatment of early stage disease [abstract]. Gynecol Oncol 2000;76:249.

65. DiSaia PJ, Creasman WT: Epithelial ovarian cancer. In DiSaia PJ, Creasman WT (eds): Clinical Gynecologic Oncology. St. Louis, CV Mosby, 1993, pp 333-525.

66. Monga M, Carmichael JA, Shelley WE, et al: Surgery without adjuvant chemotherapy for epithelial ovarian carcinoma after comprehensive surgical staging. Gynecol Oncol 1991;43:195-197.

67. Trimbos JB, Schueler JA, van den Burg M, et al: Watch and wait after careful surgical treatment and staging in well-differentiated early ovarian cancer. Cancer 1991;67:597-602.

68. Ahmed FY, Wiltshaw E, A'Hearn R, et al: Natural history and prognosis of untreated stage I epithelial ovarian carcinoma. J Clin Oncol 1996;14:2968-2975.

69. Kolomainen DF, A'Hearn R, Gore M: Can patients with relapsed previously untreated stage I epithelial ovarian cancer (EOC) be salvaged? [abstract 803] J Clin Oncol 2001;20:201A.

70. Davy M, Stenwig AE, Kjorstad KE, et al: Early stage ovarian cancer. The effect of adjuvant treatment with a single alkylating agent. Acta Obstet Gynecol Scand 1985;64:531-532.

71. Dembo AJ, Bush RS, Beale FA, et al: Ovarian carcinoma: Improved survival following abdominopelvic irradiation in patients with a completed pelvic operation. Am J Obstet Gynecol 1979;134:793-800.

72. Dembo AJ. The role of radiotherapy in ovarian cancer. Bull Cancer (Paris) 1982;69:275-283.

73. Gronroos M, Nieminen U, Kauppila A, et al: A prospective, randomized, national trial for treatment of ovarian cancer: The role of chemotherapy and external irradiation. Eur J Obstet Gynecol Reprod Biol 1984;17:33-42.

74. Hreshchyshyn MM, Park RC, Blessing JA, et al: The role of adjuvant therapy in stage I ovarian cancer. Am J Obstet Gynecol 1980;138:139-145.

75. Klaassen D, Shelley W, Starreveld A, et al: Early stage ovarian cancer—a randomized clinical trial comparing whole abdominal radiotherapy, melphalan, and intraperitoneal chromic phosphate. A National Cancer Institute of Canada Clinical Trials Group report. J Clin Oncol 1988;6:1254-1263.

76. Kolstad P, Davy M, Hoeg K: Individualized treatment of ovarian cancer. Am J Obstet Gynecol 1977;128:617-625.

77. Redman CW, Mould J, Warwick J, et al: The West Midlands early ovarian cancer adjuvant therapy trial. Clin Oncol (R Coll Radiol) 1993;5:1-5.

78. Sell A, Bertelsen K, Andersen JE, et al: Randomized study of whole-abdomen irradiation vs pelvic irradiation plus cyclophosphamide in treatment of early ovarian cancer. Gynecol Oncol 1990;37:367-373.

79. Sigurdsson K, Johnsson JE, Tropé C: Carcinoma of the ovary, stages I and II. A prospective randomized study of the effects of postoperative chemotherapy and radiotherapy. Ann Chir Gyneacol 1982;71:321-329.

80. Smith JP, Rutledge FN, Delclos L: Postoperative treatment of early cancer of the ovary: A random trial between postoperative irradiation and chemotherapy. Natl Cancer Inst Monogr 1975;42:149-153.

81. Young RC, Walton LA, Ellenberg SS, et al: Adjuvant therapy in stage I and stage II early ovarian cancer. Results of two prospective randomized trials. N Engl J Med 1990;322:1021-1027.

82. Young RC, Brady MF, Nieberg RM, et al: Randomized clinical trial of adjuvant treatment of women with early (FIGO I-IIA high risk) ovarian cancer—GOG #95 [abstract A33]. Int J Gynaecol Cancer 1999;9:11.

83. Dent SF, Klaassen D, Pater JL, et al: Second primary malignancies following the treatment of early stage ovarian cancer: Update of a study by the National Cancer Institute of Canada–Clinical Trials Group (NCIC-CTG). Ann Oncol 2000;11:65-68.

84. Vergote IB, Vergote-De Vos LN, Abeler VM, et al: Randomized trial comparing cisplatin with radioactive phosphorus or whole abdominal irradiation as adjuvant treatment of ovarian cancer. Cancer 1992;69:741-749.

85. Young RC: Controversy in adjuvant chemotherapy of early ovarian cancer [I205]. Reported at the 18th UICC International Cancer Congress, Oslo, July 2002. Int J Cancer 2002;suppl.13:66.

86. Young RC, Pecorelli S: Management of early ovarian cancer. Semin Oncol 1998;25:335-339.

87. Torri V: The state of the art in the treatment of ovarian cancer. Proceedings in Gruppo Espanol de Investicacion en cancer ginecologiclo. El Escola, Madrid 1999:15-17.

88. Freedman LS: Tables of the number of patients required in clinical trials using the long rank test. Stat Med 1982;1:121.

89. McGuire WP, Hoskins WJ, Brady MF, et al: Cyclophosphamide and cisplatin compared with paclitaxel and cisplatin in patients with stage III and stage IV ovarian cancer. N Engl J Med 1996;334:1-6.

90. Park RC: Phase III randomized study of CBDCA/TAX administered for 3 vs 6 courses for selected stages I A-C and stages IIA-C ovarian epithelial cancer. GOG-157 protocol. http://cancernet.nci.nih.gov

91. Bookman MA, McGuire WP III, Kilpatrick D, et al: Carboplatin and paclitaxel in ovarian carcinoma: A phase I study of the Gynecologic Oncology Group. J Clin Oncol 1996;14:1895-1897.

92. Advanced Ovarian Cancer Trialists Group: Chemotherapy in advanced ovarian cancer: An overview of randomised clinical trials. BMJ1991;303:884-893.

93. Young RC: Three cycles versus six cycles of adjuvant paclitaxel (Taxol)/carboplatin in early stage ovarian cancer. Semin Oncol 2000;27:8-10.

94. Finn C, Luesley D, Buxton E, et al: Is stage I epithelial ovarian cancer overtreated both surgically and systemically? Results of a five-year cancer registry review. Br J Obstet Gynaecol 1992;99:54-58.yy

95. Vergote IB, Trimbos JB, Guthrie D, et al: Results of a randomized trial in 923 patients with high risk early ovarian cancer, comparing adjuvant chemotherapy with no further treatment following surgery [abstract 802]. J Clin Oncol 2001;20:201A.

96. Vergote IB, Kaern J, Abeler VM, et al: Analysis of prognostic factors in stage I epithelial ovarian carcinoma: Importance of degree of differentiation and deoxyribonucleic acid ploidy in predicting relapse. Am J Obstet Gynecol 1993;169:40-52.

97. Bertelsen K, Holund B, Andersen JE, et al: Prognostic factors and adjuvant treatment in early ovarian epithelial cancer. Int J Gynecol Cancer 1993;3:211-218.

98. Sjovall K, Nilsson B, Einhorn N: Different types of rupture of the tumor capsule and the impact on survival in early ovarian carcinoma. Int J Gynecol Cancer 1994;4:333-336.

99. Högberg T, Carstensen J, Simonsen E: Treatment results and prognostic factors in a population-based study of epithelial ovarian cancer. Gynecol Oncol 1993;38-49.

100. deSainz IC, Goff BA, Fuller AFJ, et al: Prognostic importance of intraoperative rupture of malignant ovarian epithelial neoplasms. Obstet Gynecol 1994;1-4.

101. Nasu K, Hirota Y, Kawano Y, et al: Characterization of intraoperative rupture of epithelial ovarian cancer at early stage. Nippon Sanka Fujinka Gakkai Zasshi 1995;907-910.

102. Brinkhuis M: Advanced Ovarian Cancer: Quantitative Pathologic Features, Grading, and Prognosis [thesis]. Amsterdam, Amsterdam Free University, 1995.

103. Bertelsen K, Holund B, Andersen JE: Reproducibility and prognostic value of histologic type and grade in early epithelial ovarian cancer. Int J Gynecol Cancer 1993;3:72-79.

104. Baak J, Lindeman J, Overdiep SH, et al: Disagreement of histopathological diagnosis of different pathologists in a ovarian tumor—with some theoretical considerations. Eur J Obstet Gynecol Reprod Biol 1982;13:51-55.

105. Iversen OE, Skaarland E: Ploidy assessment of benign and malignant ovarian tumors by flow cytometry: A clinicopathologic study. Cancer 1987;60:82-87.

106. Kristensen GB, Kildal W, Abeler VM, et al: Large scale genomic instability predicts long-term outcome for women with invasive stage I ovarian cancer. Ann Oncol 2003;14:1490-1500

107. Friedlander ML: Prognostic factors in ovarian cancer. Semin Oncol 1998;25:305-315.

108. Schueler JA, Trimbos JB, Burg M, et al: DNA index reflects the biological behavior of ovarian carcinoma stage I-IIa. Gynecol Oncol 1996;62:59-66.

109. Henriksen R, Funa K, Wilander E, et al: Expression and prognostic significance of platelet-derived growth factor and its receptors in epithelial ovarian neoplasms. Cancer Res 1993;53:4550-4554.
110. Paley PJ, Staskus KA, Gebhard K, et al: Vascular endothelial growth factor expression in early stage ovarian carcinoma. Cancer 1997;80:98-106.
111. Tempfer C, Obermair A, Hefler L, et al: Vascular endothelial growth factor serum concentrations in ovarian cancer. Obstet Gynecol 1998;92:360-363.
112. Alvarez AA, Krigman HR, Whitaker RS, et al: The prognostic significance of angiogenesis in epithelial ovarian carcinoma. Clin Cancer Res 1999;5:587-591.
113. Henriksen R, Strang P, Backstrom T, et al: Ki-67 immunostaining DNA cytometry in epithelial ovarian cancers as determinants of tumor proliferation and prognosis. Anticancer Res 1994;14:603-608.
114. Lane DP, Crawford LV: T antigen is bound to a host protein in SV40-transformed cells. Nature 1979;278:261-263.
115. Jacobs IJ, Kohler MF, Wiseman RW, et al: Clonal origin of epithelial ovarian carcinoma: Analysis by loss of heterozygosity, p53 mutation and X-chromosome inactivation. J Natl Cancer Inst 1992;84:1793-1798.
116. Milner BJ, Allan LA, Eccles DM, et al: P53 mutation is a common genetic event in ovarian carcinoma. Cancer Res 1993;53:2128-2132.
117. Anttila MA, Ji H, Juhola MT, et al: The prognostic significance of p53 expression quantitated by computerized image analysis in epithelial ovarian cancer. Int J Gynecol Pathol 1999;18:42-51.
118. Auer G, Einhorn N, Nilsson B, et al: Biological malignancy in early-stage ovarian carcinoma. Acta Oncol 1996;35:93-98.
119. Fallows S, Price J, Atkinson RJ, et al: P53 mutation does not affect prognosis in ovarian epithelial malignancies. J Pathol 2001;194:68-75.
120. Kohler MF, Kerns BJM, Humphrey PA, et al: Mutation and overexpression of p53 in early-stage epithelial ovarian cancer. Obstet Gynecol 1993;81:643-650.
121. Skomedal H, Kristensen G, Abeler V, et al: TP53 protein accumulation and gene mutation in relation to overexpression of MDM 2 protein in ovarian borderline tumors and stage I carcinoma. J Pathol 1997;181:158-165.
122. Skirnisdottir I, Seidal T, Gerdin E, et al: The prognostic importance of p53, bcl-2, and bax in early stage epithelial ovarian carcinoma treated with adjuvant chemotherapy. Int J Gynecol Cancer 2002;12:265-276.
123. Henriksen R, Wilander E, Oberg K: Expression and prognostic significance of Bcl-2 in ovarian tumors. Br J Cancer 1995;72:1324-1329.
124. Slamon DJ, Godolphin W, Jones LA, et al: Studies of the HER-2/neu proto-oncogene in human breast and ovarian cancer. Science 1989;244:707-712.
125. Makar AP, Holm R, Kristensen GB, et al: The expression of c-erbB-2 oncogene in patients with invasive ovarian malignancies. Int J Gynecol Oncol 1994;4:194-199.
126. Kacinsky B, Mayer AG, King BL, et al: NEU protein expression in benign, borderline and malignant ovarian neoplasms. Gynecol Oncol 1992;44:245-253.
127. Shingleton TP, Niehans GA, Gu F, et al: Activation of c-erbB-2 and prognosis in ovarian carcinoma: Comparison with histologic type, grade, and stage. Cancer 1994;73:1460-1466.
128. Yanginuma Y, Yamasita K, Kusumaki N, et al: RAS oncogene product p21 expression and prognosis of human ovarian tumors. Gynecol Oncol 1992;46:45-50.
129. Schneider J, Pollan M, Jimenez E, et al: Nm23-H1 expression defines a high-risk subpopulation of patients with early-stage epithelial ovarian carcinoma. Br J Cancer 2000;82:1662-1670.
130. Shridhar V, Lee J, Pandita A, et al: Genetic analysis of early-versus late-stage ovarian tumors. Cancer Res 2001;61:5895-5904.
131. Petricoin EF, Ardekani AM, Hitt BA, et al: Use of proteomic patterns in serum to identify ovarian cancer. Lancet 2002;359:572-577.
132. Payley PJ: Angiogenesis in ovarian cancer: Molecular pathology and therapeutic strategies. Curr Oncol Rep 2002;4:165-174.
133. Kohn EC: Angiogenesis in epithelial ovarian cancer: An important biologic event and therapeutic target. In Jacobs IJ, Sheperd JH, Oram DH, et al (eds): Ovarian Cancer. New York, Oxford Press, 2002, pp 363-330.
134. Baselga J, Tripathy D, Medelsohn J, et al: Phase II study of weekly intravenous recombinant humanized anti-p185HER2 monoclonal antibody in patients with HER2/neu-overexpressing metastatic breast cancer. J Clin Oncol 1996;14:737.
135. Ferrandina G, Ranelletti FO, Lauriola L, et al: Cyclooxygenase-2 (COX-2), epidermal growth factor receptor (EGFR), and Her-2/neu expression in ovarian cancer. Gynecol Oncol 2002;85:305-310.

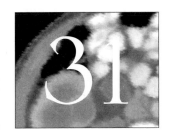

C H A P T E R

PRIMARY CHEMOTHERAPY FOR ADVANCED EPITHELIAL OVARIAN CANCER

Paul A. Vasey

MAJOR CONTROVERSIES

- In scheduling chemotherapy and surgery, is there a role for neoadjuvant therapy?
- Should platinum be used with or without paclitaxel in first-line treatment?
- Which taxane should be used in combination with carboplatin?
- Is there any benefit in adding a third cytotoxic agent in initial chemotherapy, and what is the optimal regimen?
- Does intraperitoneal chemotherapy have a place in the treatment of ovarian cancer?
- How long should initial chemotherapy last?
- What types of trials and integration of novel (biologic) agents will be seen in the future?

The importance of ovarian carcinoma stems not from the fact that it is the fourth most common female cancer in the Western world but from the fact that it is the most lethal gynecologic malignancy, killing more women than uterine and cervical cancer combined.[1] It is predominantly a disease of postmenopausal women, with a median age at diagnosis of 63 years and an increasing incidence thereafter, peaking in the eighth decade. Because of the lack of specific and easily recognizable symptomatology, most women present to their doctors with advanced-stage disease, extended beyond the ovary. Nevertheless, initial treatment is generally surgical, with an attempt at maximal cytoreduction—that is, the surgeon attempts to leave behind no tumor nodules greater than 1 cm in diameter. This unique feature of ovarian cancer treatment—there are no other cancers in which the surgeon attempts to cut through tumor in order to achieve a satisfactory result—is accepted as the best

possible practice. There is overwhelming evidence, albeit indirect, that such attempted cytoreduction is of worthwhile clinical benefit, a fact acknowledged by the U.S. National Institutes of Health (NIH) Consensus Statement in 1994. Although no prospective randomized trials have been performed to evaluate survival in patients after intentional optimal (<1 cm) or suboptimal (≥1 cm) cytoreduction, it is now considered unethical to perform such a study.

After cytoreductive surgery, the mainstay of treatment is chemotherapy, and this (multidisciplinary) approach can produce objective pathologic complete responses in up to 50% of cases. However, most women eventually experience relapse after completion of first-line chemotherapy, and, despite frequently additional, multiple lines of chemotherapy ("salvage therapy"), the acquisition of clinical drug resistance leads to an overall survival rate of only 15% to 20% for patients presenting with advanced disease. This chapter

429

attempts to define the current best practice for first-line therapy for this frustrating but challenging malignancy.

In scheduling chemotherapy and surgery, is there a role for neoadjuvant therapy?

Many patients do not receive maximal cytoreduction with a first (primary) surgical effort. The reasons for this are multifactorial and include the experience of the surgeon, the biologic aggressiveness of the tumor, and the presence of serious coexisting medical problems. The ability of chemotherapy to produce significant cytoreduction was first noted in 1970,[2] and a potential role for a subsequent postchemotherapy attempt at debulking was suggested by Lawton and colleagues in 1989.[3] They described the achievement of maximal cytoreduction in the majority (75%) of patients, who initially had only suboptimal debulking, after first-line chemotherapy. Further evidence of a potential benefit for this interval debulking surgery (IDS) was documented by Neijt and colleagues in 1991.[4] Here, the survival of patients who had received optimal cytoreduction at primary surgery was found to be identical to that of patients treated by chemotherapy followed by IDS that produced optimal cytoreduction.

The European Organization of Research and Treatment of Cancer (EORTC) Gynecological Cancer Cooperative Group performed the only randomized trial on IDS fully reported to date.[5] In their study, 319 women with suboptimal cytoreduction at primary surgery received three initial cycles of cisplatin-cyclophosphamide chemotherapy. Then, those women in whom no progressive disease was documented were randomly assigned to receive either a further three cycles ($n = 138$) or an exploratory laparotomy with a view to cytoreduction ($n = 138$) followed by three more cycles of cisplatin-cyclophosphamide. The group receiving IDS demonstrated 33% reduction (95% confidence interval [CI], 10% to 50%) in risk of death at 2 years, and they also had significant improvements in progression-free and overall survival ($P = .01$).

A further trial of IDS was carried out by the Gynecologic Oncology Group (GOG protocol 152) between June 1994 and January 2001. The study used a paclitaxel-based regimen as initial chemotherapy, followed by IDS for patients who received suboptimal cytoreduction at the first operation. The first results of this trial were presented in 2002[6]; 550 patients with suboptimally cytoreduced advanced-stage ovarian cancer (predominantly stage IIIc by the International Federation of Gynecology and Obstetrics [FIGO] system) were randomly assigned to receive three cycles of chemotherapy with paclitaxel/cisplatin (as per GOG 111) after the initial surgery. Patients whose disease was not progressing at this stage were then randomly assigned either to continue with three further cycles or to have a further attempt at debulking (IDS) followed by three cycles of chemotherapy. The study required 225 events to achieve its survival end

point, and this presentation reported on 252 events. Treatment arms were well balanced with respect to factors such as type of surgeon (e.g., board-certified gynecologic oncologist) and compliance. The results, in contrast to the European study, demonstrated that patients undergoing IDS had a median progression-free survival time (PFS) of 10.5 months, compared with 10.8 months for those receiving chemotherapy without IDS. Likewise, there was no difference in median survival time: 32 months for the chemotherapy plus IDS arm and 33 months for those receiving chemotherapy alone.

It is accepted that a maximal cytoreductive effort at initial laparotomy is of benefit to patients with advanced ovarian cancer, despite the fact that data supporting this practice come from retrospective studies and meta-analyses.[7,8] What remains less clear is whether IDS can improve outcomes for patients who do not receive maximal cytoreduction at their initial operation. There were many intrinsic differences between the EORTC trial and GOG 152, but the most pertinent may have been that the skill level of surgeons varied to differing degrees. It is well known that experienced gynecologic oncologists/specialists can achieve optimal cytoreduction in a high percentage of patients at initial surgery. Trial GOG 152 suggests that patients who are operated on by board-certified gynecologic oncologists without maximal cytoreduction despite a good attempt are unlikely to benefit from a second attempt after a course of chemotherapy. The European study, in which the prevalence of gynecologic oncologist/specialist surgeons was markedly lower, suggests that patients in whom an optimal surgical procedure was not performed may in fact benefit from subsequent IDS. However, the answer is unlikely to be so clear-cut.

Another problem lies in the description "maximal cytoreduction." Frequently, tumor nodules can be left that are less than 1 cm in diameter, but smaller confluent tumor plaques are more difficult to quantify and may represent a poorer prognosis. Documentation of the extent of cytoreduction is often not robust and undoubtedly leads to misclassification. These trial results suggest that further research addressing the timing of surgery is warranted.

Outside of trials, neoadjuvant chemotherapy ("chemical cytoreduction") continues to be offered to many patients whose disease is considered either radiologically or biologically inoperable or who represent a poor surgical risk. However, there are no data from prospective randomized clinical trials that demonstrate equivalent results for neoadjuvant chemotherapy compared with the standard approach of surgery followed by chemotherapy. Nevertheless, many retrospective studies have suggested that this is a feasible option for such patients, with encouraging survivorship statistics.[9,10] There are theoretic advantages to be gained by this approach. Patients who are considered poor operative risks due to the metabolic and mass effects of large intra-abdominal or pelvic tumors can be spared the morbidity and mortality of surgery, saving any operative cytoreductive effort until the tumor has been sufficiently cytoreduced. Subsequent surgery is potentially easier and associated with less risk to the patient and an increased chance of optimal cytoreduction. In addition, in countries where gynecologic oncologic surgeons are still uncommon (e.g., the United Kingdom), neoadjuvant chemotherapy as part of a treatment plan allows for better selection of patients for triage to overextended surgeons. Furthermore, initial planned biopsy followed by chemotherapy and then by "definitive" surgery allows for laboratory evaluation of response markers, giving scientists the opportunity to work with both chemo-naive tumor and postchemotherapy tumor. Given that new molecular targets continue to emerge from laboratories worldwide, biologic studies of this nature will become increasingly important to allow new agents directed against such targets to be efficiently and decisively evaluated in the clinical setting. EORTC trial 55971 (Fig. 31-1) is evaluating the role of neoadjuvant chemotherapy and delayed primary surgery and is collecting tissues taken at surgery for basic research.

To summarize current surgery and chemotherapy timing, the only fully published randomized trial showed that IDS for patients who did not receive optimal cytoreduction at primary surgery and who responded to three initial courses of cisplatin-cyclophosphamide chemotherapy improves PFS and overall survival times. However, a further trial, using paclitaxel/platinum chemotherapy, did not confirm this finding. Analysis of these trials suggests that the most likely reason for this discrepancy is that tumor biology and surgical skill are interlinked; if the initial attempt was made by an experienced surgeon, it may be that no further surgical intervention is likely to improve survival. It may well be that *all* patients could benefit from neoadjuvant chemotherapy and delayed primary surgery, but randomized studies such as EORTC 55971 are required to firmly establish that this scheduling of treatment modalities does not produce inferior outcomes. Entry into such studies should be strongly encouraged.

Should platinum be used with or without paclitaxel in first-line treatment?

An updated meta-analysis of first-line chemotherapy based on individual patient data by the Advanced Ovarian Cancer Trialists Group has been published, succeeding a previous meta-analysis.[11] This analysis, encompassing 5667 patients in 37 randomized trials, suggested that combination chemotherapy was associated with a better outcome compared with single agents, but the results were not significant (hazard ratio [HR], 0.93; 95% CI, 0.83 to 1.05; $P = .23$). A possible improvement in absolute survival, from 25% to 28% at 5 years, was suggested. In addition, the data showed that carboplatin and cisplatin produced equivalent outcomes in combination (HR, 1.02; 95% CI, 0.92 to 1.13; $P = .66$) or as single agents (HR, 1.01; 95% CI, 0.81 to 1.26; $P = .92$).

The taxane era began in the mid-1990s with the publication of GOG trial 111,[12] which demonstrated statistically significant outcome advantages (response, PFS, and overall survival) for the combination of cisplatin 75 mg/m^2 plus Taxol (paclitaxel) 135 mg/m^2 as a 24-hour infusion in patients with bulky FIGO stage III/IV disease, compared with the previous standard regimen of cyclophosphamide 750 mg/m^2 plus cisplatin 75 mg/m^2. Longer-term follow up[13] confirmed these results, with 27% survival at 5 years for those treated with Taxol/cisplatin, compared with 16% for cyclophosphamide/cisplatin (HR, 0.7; 95% CI, 0.57 to 0.87), based on 386 patients with a median duration of follow-up of 6.5 years.

A joint European-Canadian Intergroup trial,[14] designated OV.10, was subsequently performed, and the results essentially replicated those of GOG 111 with regard to all efficacy parameters, despite a different patient population. The main differences were that one third of patients in OV.10 had optimally debulked disease, that OV.10 used a 3-hour infusion of paclitaxel 175 mg/m^2, that patients in OV.10 could receive more than six cycles, and that 20% of the patients in OV.10 had stage Ic or II disease). Again, longer term follow-up has now confirmed the survival advantage for paclitaxel/cisplatin versus cyclophosphamide/cisplatin, with 34% versus 23% survival at 5 years (HR, 0.75; 95% CI, 0.63-0.90; 680 patients, 6.5 years median follow-up).[15] High levels of neurotoxicity were evident

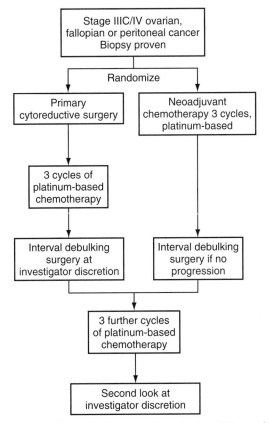

Figure 31–1. Schema for European Organization of Research and Treatment of Cancer (EORTC) randomized trial of interval debulking surgery.

in OV.10, suggesting that the best-tolerated combination of paclitaxel and cisplatin was with the 24-hour infusion schedule of the taxane.

However, two other prospective randomized trials, GOG protocol 132 and the International Collaborative Ovarian Neoplasm (ICON) 3 study, have tested the combination of a platinum agent plus paclitaxel versus platinum without paclitaxel, with results that apparently contradict those of the earlier, pivotal cisplatin/paclitaxel trials. These two studies are worth further discussion and consideration (Table 31-1).

In GOG 132, patients were randomly assigned to receive either the same paclitaxel/cisplatin regimen as in GOG 111 or paclitaxel (200 mg/m^2 over 24 hours) or cisplatin (100 mg/m^2) as single agents.[16] Despite the same patient population as in GOG 111 (i.e., bulky FIGO stage III or any stage IV disease), no statistically significant difference emerged among the three treatment arms with respect to overall survival. In discussing these contradictory results, some GOG investigators suggested that because a significant proportion of patients crossed over to the other treatments before clinical progression—generally as a consolidatory approach to an incomplete response or at second-look laparotomy—these women essentially received a form of sequential chemotherapy. Indeed, 48% of all patients initially assigned to single-agent cisplatin received some form of additional chemotherapy before progression, mostly as "consolidation" after an incomplete response to six cycles of initial chemotherapy; 32% received paclitaxel in this way. In the paclitaxel-only arm, which demonstrated inferiority based on response rate and PFS in comparison with the two cisplatin-containing arms, 50% of patients received additional treatment before progression, with 48% receiving cisplatin. These patients therefore received crossover chemotherapy at a time of microscopic disease bulk, in contradistinction to the timing of treatment in other trials such as OV.10. The notion was therefore put forward by the investigators that, providing paclitaxel is given to the patient after cisplatin but before clinical (bulky) progression, the outcomes are likely to be similar. This study is therefore widely interpreted as a comparison of sequential single agents versus their combination, although it clearly was not designed with this comparison in mind. The paclitaxel-cisplatin combination was preferred by the investigators due to decreased overall treatment duration and less toxicity, particularly when 100 mg/m^2 cisplatin was used.

In the ICON 3 study,[17] a total of 2074 patients were randomly assigned to a research arm, in which they were given six cycles of the combination paclitaxel 175 mg/m^2 over 3 hours plus carboplatin AUC 5/6, or to a control arm using either carboplatin AUC 5/6 as monotherapy or the combination CAP (cisplatin 50 mg/m^2 plus Adriamycin [doxorubicin] 50 mg/m^2 plus Cytoxan [cyclophosphamide] 500 mg/m^2). Carboplatin has since been shown to be at least as efficacious as cisplatin in combination with paclitaxel in three prospective, randomized trials comparing cisplatin/paclitaxel with carboplatin/paclitaxel (Table 31-2).[18-20] Preliminary results from these latter studies indicated no significant difference in PFS (18 versus 17 months in the German trial) or in median time to progression (22 months with either regimen in GOG 158, and 17 months in the Danish-Dutch trial). Overall survival is not yet mature for the larger studies, but early analysis suggested a trend to improved overall survival in GOG 158 for the carboplatin/paclitaxel arm. This interesting feature is further discussed in a later section of this chapter.

In ICON 3, participating institutions were allowed to choose which control arm they would use, a feature

Table 31-1. First-Line Prospective Randomized Trials of Paclitaxel/Platinum versus Platinum-Based (Nonpaclitaxel) Regimens

Comparison	Trial	No. of Patients	Reference	Result
Paclitaxel 135 mg/m^2 over 24 hr + cisplatin 75 mg/m^2 *vs* Cytoxan (cyclophosphamide) 750 mg/m^2 + cisplatin 75 mg/m^2	GOG 111	410	McGuire et al.[12] (1996)	PFS and OS favor paclitaxel arm
Paclitaxel 175 mg/m^2 over 3 hr + cisplatin 75 mg/m^2 *vs* Cytoxan 750 mg/m^2 + cisplatin 75 mg/m^2	OV.10	680	Piccart et al.[14] (2000)	PFS and OS favor paclitaxel arm
Paclitaxel 135 mg/m^2 over 24 hr + cisplatin 75 mg/m^2 *vs* Cisplatin 100 mg/m^2 *vs* Paclitaxel 200 mg/m^2	GOG 132	424	Muggia et al.[16] (2000)	No difference in OS in all three arms
Carboplatin AUC 5/6 + paclitaxel 175 mg/m^2 over 3 hr *vs* Carboplatin AUC 5/6 monotherapy or CAP*	ICON 3	2074	ICON Group[17] (2002)	No difference in PFS or OS

GOG, Gynecologic Oncology Group; ICON, International Collaborative Ovarian Neoplasm [study]; OS, overall survival time; PFS, progression-free survival time.
*Centers could choose whether to use CAP or carboplatin as control arm. (CAP = cisplatin 50 mg/m^2 + Adriamycin [doxorubicin] 50 mg/m^2 + Cytoxan [cyclophosphamide] 500 mg/m^2.)

Table 31–2. Randomized Clinical Trials Comparing Cisplatin/Paclitaxel versus Carboplatin/Paclitaxel

Comparison	Trial	No. of Patients	Inclusion Criteria
Cisplatin 75 mg/m² + paclitaxel 185 mg/m² over 3 hr *vs* Carboplatin AUC 6 + paclitaxel 185 mg/m² over 3 hr	AGO	776	Stage IIb-IV (any)
Cisplatin 75 mg/m² + paclitaxel 135 mg/m² over 24 hr *vs* Carboplatin AUC 7.5 + paclitaxel 175 mg/m² over 3 hr	GOG 158	840	Stage III <1 cm
Cisplatin 75 mg/m² + paclitaxel 175 mg/m² over 3 hr *vs* Carboplatin AUC 5 + paclitaxel 175 mg/m² over 3 hr	Danish-Dutch group	196	Stage IIb-IV (any)

AGO, Arbeitsgemeinschaft Gynakologische Onkologie group; GOG, Gynecologic Oncology Group.

justified by the mature results of a previous ICON study, ICON 2.[21] In ICON 2, approximately 1500 patients were randomly assigned to carboplatin or the CAP regimen and showed no differences in PFS or overall survival at these particular doses. ICON 3 was essentially run as four parallel trials, with four independent randomization centers. Ratios of randomization differed among these four groups, with the United Kingdom and Italian centers randomizing 2:1 in favor of the control arm and the Swiss and Nordic groups randomizing 1:1. This trial has now been fully published, and, as with GOG 132, the results appear to contradict both earlier positive studies. No convincing differences in PFS or overall survival were evident. The absolute difference in 2-year overall survival was 1% in favor of paclitaxel/carboplatin, and no statistically significant benefit for paclitaxel/carboplatin was demonstrated among subgroups defined by age, stage, residual disease status, histologic grade or tumor histology, randomization group, number of patients entered by a center, or choice of control arm.

There continues to be much controversy and heated debate concerning the correct interpretation of these results. ICON 3 has been criticized for the nonrandom allocation of the control arm, the varying ratios of randomization across the randomization groups, and the presence of patients with early-stage disease (approximately 20% of participants). Furthermore, a trend has emerged toward decreased overall survival (not PFS) for centers treating fewer patients (actually the majority, now $P = .05$ [M. K. B. Parmar, personal communication]). However, it must be noted that the number of patients entered by an institution does not always reflect the skills of the investigators or their experience in treating patients who have ovarian cancer. Certainly, the definition of treatment "centers" and correlation with numbers of patients entered by them in the United Kingdom is arbitrary at best.

It has been suggested that a more rigorous examination, or formal audit, of the ICON 3 data is required, to be comparable with GOG studies and EORTC trials, some of which are also audited. For example, ICON 3 data were not audited at the source for histopathology, which raises the question of the inclusion of borderline cases, especially patients with early-stage disease. Of more concern, however, is the possibility of stage misclassification and the question of the true residual volume status of patients reported to have optimal surgical debulking. Because verification of the accuracy of these data from source documents is almost impossible to perform, it has been suggested that the lack of any reported benefit for carboplatin/paclitaxel in important subgroups is in doubt. Nonetheless, given the randomized nature of the trial, it is unlikely that even substantial misclassification of this nature would change the results. ICON 3 had an independently chaired executive committee and an independent data monitoring and ethics committee with expert statisticians that reviewed the trial data carefully and specifically stated that, in their opinion, an audit was unnecessary on scientific grounds. They commented that, to change the results, systematic bias of overwhelming scale would be required (i.e., outcome was systematically overestimated in the control arm or underestimated in the research arm, or both). It is virtually inconceivable that this kind of bias took place collectively by the ICON investigators.

ICON 3 remains an important trial, and the simple fact that more than 2000 patients participated in a randomized, prospective study is a very powerful argument for its validity. It would be disappointing if the scientific community used the lack of a formal audit to ignore the result, which clearly raises many important issues. Certainly, the median survival time in the control arm using single-agent carboplatin (36 months) is comparable to that of almost any other treatment for this heterogeneous patient mix, and indeed this may be the most pertinent feature of the analysis. ICON 3 has been called a "real world" result, with institutions large and small taking part in the study. As suggested by Sandercock and colleagues,[22] the fact that the single-agent platinum arms of ICON 3 and GOG 132 gave overall survival values equal to that of the platinum/paclitaxel combination, and superior to that of the cisplatin/cyclophosphamide combination, in both GOG 111 and OV.10 (Table 31-3) makes a strong case for platinum monotherapy as the most appropriate control arm for future randomized studies. The fact that many patients receiving carboplatin in ICON 3 were able to receive individualized "dose-tailoring" may also have contributed to their excellent outcome. Although such cross-trial comparisons are fraught with difficulties in interpretation, the possibility of an

Table 31–3. Median Survival Time of Control Subjects in Randomized Controlled Trials Described in Table 31-1 (months)

Parameter	Study			
	GOG 111	OV.10	ICON 3	GOG 132
Progression-free survival	12.9	11.5	16.2	16.4
Overall survival	24.4	25.9	36.0	30.2

GOG, Gynecologic Oncology Group; ICON, International Collaborative Ovarian Neoplasm [study]; OV.10, a joint European-Canadian Intergroup trial.

inadequate control arm in GOG 111 and OV.10 is intriguing, and a strong statistical case for this proposal has recently been outlined.[22]

To summarize, the debate continues as to the appropriate first-line "standard-of-care" chemotherapy for patients with advanced ovarian cancer. Many investigators adopt a pragmatic view, giving paclitaxel/carboplatin to younger, fitter patients and carboplatin monotherapy to less fit women and to those reluctant to experience alopecia. However, it is unlikely that single agents will cure solid tumors such as ovarian cancer, given the diverse range of molecular mechanisms of drug resistance that cancers can call upon. Although the ICON 3 collaborators have emphasized that paclitaxel should remain an important option at "some stage of the patient journey," optimization of its integration, sequence, and combination in first-line therapy remains the key consideration for future trial designs. Discussion of the therapeutic options available to patients should be part of the collective decision-making process.

Which taxane should be used in combination with carboplatin?

As a potential alternative to paclitaxel, docetaxel (Taxotere) has demonstrated efficacy in recurrent disease at least equivalent to that of paclitaxel, with an overall response rate of 28% in a meta-analysis of 155 patients with platinum-refractory ovarian cancer.[23] There is documented activity in ovarian cancer patients for whom prior paclitaxel has failed.[24] Moreover, docetaxel is generally delivered as a more convenient 1-hour infusion. Phase II trials of docetaxel/carboplatin combinations, published by the both the Cleveland Clinic and the Scottish Gynaecological Cancer Trials Group (SGCTG), demonstrated adequate safety profiles and good outpatient utility.[25,26] The dose-limiting toxicity with the combination was neutropenia, in addition to diarrhea at higher doses. Low levels (5% to 6%) of significant neuropathy were a noteworthy feature, and antitumor activity was significant, with a median PFS time of more than 17 months for all 139 patients in the SGCTG study.

This potential for a different and potentially advantageous toxicity profile with similar or better levels of efficacy led the SGCTG to perform the only randomized trial to date that has compared docetaxel/carboplatin with paclitaxel/carboplatin in untreated ovarian cancer patients. This trial (Scottish Randomized Trial in Ovarian Cancer, SCOTROC 1) compared paclitaxel (175 mg/m^2 over 3 hours) or docetaxel (75 mg/m^2 over 1 hour) in combination with carboplatin (dosed to AUC 5 with the glomerular filtration rate for dose calculation performed by the chromium 51–labeled ethylene diamine tetraacetic acid [^{51}CrEDTA] isotopic method), given for six cycles every 21 days after initial surgery (Fig. 31-2). The primary end point was PFS, and the study had an 80% power to detect superiority in either arm of 25%, or to detect equivalence within the same limit. In 17 months, 1077 patients from 12 countries and from 83 cancer centers were entered. Different premedications were used before treatment: a standard triple intravenous (IV) cocktail of antihistamines and corticosteroids for paclitaxel, and the now standard 3-day oral dexamethasone regimen for docetaxel. A total of six treatment cycles were planned.

First results focusing primarily on toxicity were presented in 2001,[27] and early survival data in 2002.[28]

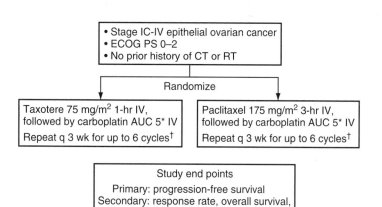

Figure 31–2. Schema of Scottish Gynaecological Cancer Trials Group (SGCTG) 1 randomized trial.

- Stage IC-IV epithelial ovarian cancer
- ECOG PS 0–2
- No prior history of CT or RT

Randomize

Taxotere 75 mg/m^2 1-hr IV, followed by carboplatin AUC 5* IV
Repeat q 3 wk for up to 6 cycles†

Paclitaxel 175 mg/m^2 3-hr IV, followed by carboplatin AUC 5* IV
Repeat q 3 wk for up to 6 cycles†

Study end points
Primary: progression-free survival
Secondary: response rate, overall survival, toxicity, QOL

CT = chemotherapy; RT = radiotherapy
*Calculated according to Calvert formula.
†Interval debulking surgery permitted within 4 weeks of cycle 3 or after cycle 6.

The study arms were well balanced for known prognostic factors. The median age was 59 years, and most patients exhibited Eastern Cooperative Oncology Group (ECOG) performance status 0 or 1 (87%), had advanced-stage disease (80%), and were considered to have received optimal cytoreduction (63%). The main differences in toxicity between the two regimens concerned peripheral neuropathy and myelosuppression, with more neuropathy seen with paclitaxel/carboplatin and more myelosuppression with docetaxel/carboplatin ($P < .001$). There was a marked difference in the incidence of clinically important (National Cancer Institute-Common Toxicity [NCI-CTC] grade II or greater) neurotoxicity, with the results strongly in favor of docetaxel/carboplatin (11% versus 30%, $P < .001$). This was confirmed by two other methods of assessing neurotoxicity: a published neurotoxicity scoring system[29] and individual patient answers to an EORTC quality-of-life questionnaire (QLQ-OV28) developed during the trial.[30] All three methods of neurotoxicity assessment confirmed a statistically significant advantage for the docetaxel/carboplatin combination. In addition, more patients (32 versus 4) came off protocol therapy prematurely because of severe neurotoxicity.

Myelogenous toxicity was greater for docetaxel/carboplatin, with the incidence of grade 3/4 neutropenia being 94%, compared with 82% for paclitaxel/carboplatin ($P < .001$). All patients had weekly hematology checks during treatment, which probably explains the higher than expected level of neutropenia for the paclitaxel/carboplatin combination. There were also more instances of febrile neutropenia and prolonged neutropenia for docetaxel, but, importantly, there were no excess toxic deaths (2 versus 1), and in general neutropenia was managed safely in the community setting. In addition, there was no difference in median dose intensity between paclitaxel/carboplatin and docetaxel/carboplatin (98% versus 98%), and treatment delivery was similar (percentage of patients through six cycles, 79% versus 84%). There were differences in other nonhematologic toxicities, such as more arthralgia, myalgia, and alopecia for paclitaxel/carboplatin and more diarrhea, hypersensitivity, and edema for docetaxel/carboplatin, but the overall incidence of grade 3 or 4 toxicities was less than 8% for both arms.

For the preliminary survival presentation in 2002, 670 events had occurred for PFS, exceeding the required 630 for the primary end point. The data presented were 95% clean, and the median follow-up duration was 23 months, with a maximum of 26 months. No difference in PFS was evident between the paclitaxel-based and docetaxel-based regimens (15.4 versus 15.1 months), and overall survival rates at 2 years were estimated to be 69.8% and 65.4%, respectively. However, there were not enough events in the overall survival analysis to be confident about these curves, and the data require another 12 months or so to mature. In addition, there were no emergent different treatment effects in any of the stratified prognostic groups, such as residual disease, FIGO stage, age, and performance status.

Longer-term data for neurotoxicity using both NCIC-CTC grading and the neurotoxicity scoring system demonstrated that paclitaxel/carboplatin continued to be significantly more neurotoxic after completion of chemotherapy, up to at least to 14 months after randomization. Furthermore, quality-of-life scales using the EORTC QLQ-OV28 questionnaire confirmed these differences in neurotoxicity from the patients' perspective, with statistically significant differences being apparent out to 22 months from randomization. Other positive benefits in quality-of-life scales were demonstrated for aches and pains, weakness, hair loss, body image, insomnia, gastrointestinal symptoms, and general pain. All of these differences were statistically significant, and all favored the docetaxel/carboplatin arm of the study.

The different toxicity profiles demonstrated by the SCOTROC data, in conjunction with a better quality-of-life profile, argue not only that docetaxel is a viable alternative to paclitaxel in combination first-line therapy but also that it could even be considered the taxane of choice. The main toxicity differences—neurotoxicity and myelosuppression—are both important and need careful management. However, in the SCOTROC trial, myelosuppression was transient, was not associated with increased mortality, and was managed successfully by dose reductions and oral antibiotics. In addition, lowering the dose of docetaxel to 60 mg/m^2 is unlikely to adversely affect efficacy and, according to the Cleveland Clinic data,[25] would decrease the incidence of clinically significant bone marrow suppression. Furthermore, there was not an excess of patients stopping chemotherapy early due to myelosuppression in the docetaxel/carboplatin arm, and the levels of overall grade 3 or 4 myelosuppression seen on treatment were high for both arms (74% versus 89%).

For these reasons, neurotoxicity has emerged as the most important determinant of tolerance on this protocol. More patients stopped chemotherapy early and patients had more NCIC-CTC grade II or III toxicity that lasted longer with paclitaxel/carboplatin. If the OV28 quality-of-life findings are factored in (despite more on-treatment gastrointestinal toxicity with docetaxel/carboplatin, OV28 demonstrated a small positive benefit), in addition to a shorter infusion time (meaning less time spent in clinic), it is hard to argue against docetaxel/carboplatin as the superior combination. The caveat regarding immature overall survival data is relevant, but it is considered unlikely, with the existing tight confidence intervals in PFS curves, that a significant divergence in overall survival will appear. Mature overall survival data are likely to be available in 2003, with the definitive publication of this trial.

Is there any benefit in adding a third cytotoxic agent in initial chemotherapy, and what is the optimal regimen?

The incorporation of a new, potentially non–cross-resistant agent into first-line therapy can give rise to greater toxicity, resulting in dose reductions of other active agents. However, the scheduling of all agents in the most effective way is often not straightforward. Currently, there are no conclusive data supporting the routine incorporation of additional agents into the first-line treatment of ovarian cancer. The results of two large meta-analyses (from the Advanced Ovarian Cancer Trialist Group [AOCTG] and the Ovarian Cancer Meta-analysis Project [OCMP]) using data from more than 1700 untreated patients demonstrated that the addition of an anthracycline to platinum chemotherapy (not containing taxanes) significantly improved survival (HR, 0.85; $P = .003$).[31] However, four randomized trials comparing cisplatin/ cyclophosphamide with and without doxorubicin did not demonstrate a convincing survival advantage for the addition of the anthracycline.[32-35] In addition, the ICON 2 trial showed no difference in time to progression or overall survival for single-agent carboplatin or CAP, and, as anticipated, toxicity was greater for the anthracycline-containing regimen.[21]

The Arbeitsgemeinschaft Gynakologische Onkologie (AGO) group have now completed a randomized trial comparing carboplatin/paclitaxel (TC) with carboplatin/ paclitaxel/epirubicin (TEC) as first-line treatment for FIGO stages IIb and IV ovarian cancer.[36] A total of 1281 patients participated, and there were no significant differences in response rate between TEC and TC (75% versus 69%, $P = .122$). Furthermore, no apparent differences between TEC and TC for PFS were noted (18 versus 17 months, $P = .104$), and although overall survival data were relatively immature, no differences were apparent for suboptimally debulked or stage IV disease (28 versus 26 months, $P = .565$). There was a trend toward an improvement in patients with optimal surgical cytoreduction and not stage IV disease (26 versus 21 months, $P = .064$). The three-drug combination produced a markedly higher myelotoxicity (grade 3/4 neutropenia, 74% versus 54%; $P < .001$), which produced an increased demand for supportive care, more dose reductions, and treatment delays. In addition, this arm was associated with more emesis (10% versus 4%, $P < .001$). A further study comparing these regimens at slightly different doses was performed by the Nordic Society Gynecological Oncology (NSGO)/EORTC/NCIC CTG and presented in 2002.[37] In this randomized study of 888 patients, the complete response rate was highest with the triplet arm, although overall response rates were similar. Toxicities were greater in the TEC arm, and early outcome data did not show any advantage.

In today's armamentarium, agents that are active against both platinum- and paclitaxel-resistant disease are likely to be the best candidates for combination therapy. Preclinical models have predicted that platinum combined with agents such as gemcitabine, topotecan hydrochloride, or pegylated liposomal doxorubicin hydrochloride (PLDH) are likely to have at least additive effects on antitumor activity, and all agents have been shown to be active against platinum/ paclitaxel-resistant tumors in the clinic. All have different mechanisms of action and mechanisms of resistance (see the review by Bookman[38]).

Triplets. A triplet composed of gemcitabine, paclitaxel and carboplatin produced a response rate of 100% (complete response, 60%; partial response, 40%) in 25 evaluable previously treated ovarian cancer patients.[39] However, this combination also produced grade IV hematologic toxicity in most patients, and many dose reductions were required. Median time to progression was 16 months, and overall survival time was longer than 30 months.

It was not anticipated that a triplet containing carboplatin/gemcitabine and PLDH would be as toxic, given that the dose-limiting toxicity profile of PLDH is essentially nonhematologic, consisting primarily of plantar-palmar erythrodysesthesia and mucositis. However, a triplet containing standard doses of carboplatin and paclitaxel was not able to be combined with more than 20 mg/m² PLDH every 28 days without excessive bone marrow suppression.[40] The study protocol was revised to administer PLDH every second cycle, and this allowed an active, feasible regimen to be developed, utilizing a dose of 30 mg/m² of PLDH.

Alternating or sequential doublets. Triple-drug combinations have the advantage of exposing all tumors to the three agents simultaneously, thereby theoretically abrogating the emergence of drug-resistant clones. However, doses of the most important agent—in this case, platinum—are often compromised by myelosuppression and other toxicities that result in both dose delays and dose reductions. One alternative is to use sequential or alternating doublets for as many as eight cycles of treatment. This potentially retains the concept of preventing the acquisition of drug resistance, while introducing new agents in a less toxic way.

Topotecan hydrochloride is an agent that is clearly schedule dependent as a single agent, with shorter administration schedules having a substantial negative impact on efficacy.[41] Furthermore, topotecan is very difficult to combine in a triplet with platinum and paclitaxel, as evidenced in trial GOG 9602, where the maximum tolerated dose for topotecan was exceeded at 0.6 mg/m² given on days 1 through 5 because of thrombocytopenia, despite the addition of colony-stimulating factors to abrogate dose-limiting neutropenia.[42] The NCIC-EORTC developed a sequential couplet design whereby patients received four 3-week cycles of cisplatin 50 mg/m² plus topotecan 0.75 mg/m² on days 1 through 5, followed by four 3-weekly cycles of standard cisplatin/paclitaxel chemotherapy.[43] Feasibility was established with 44 chemonaive patients with ovarian cancer, mainly suboptimally cytoreduced, who demonstrated a response rate of 66% after the first four cycles and an overall response rate of 78%. A phase III study with carboplatin/paclitaxel replacing cisplatin/ paclitaxel as the second four couplets, compared with eight cycles of carboplatin/ paclitaxel (trial OV.16), was initiated in August 2001.

The GOG looked at a similar sequential doublet but replaced cisplatin with the potentially less toxic analog, carboplatin. GOG 9906 was an extended-cohort phase I study with expanded accrual at each dose level to assess safety and deliverability over multiple (i.e., the first four) cycles (M. Bookman, personal communication). The first cohorts used a "forward" sequence, in which carboplatin was delivered on day 1 and topotecan was split over days 1 through 3. This sequence was especially hematotoxic, and despite de-escalation of topotecan to 0.75 mg/m² given over days 1 through 3 in combination with carboplatin AUC 5, it was believed to be not feasible. However, a "reverse" sequence was established, with carboplatin administered on day 3, and this time a feasible dosing combination of topotecan 1.25 mg/m² on days 1 through 3 plus carboplatin AUC 5 without colony-stimulating factors was defined.

Gynecologic oncology group study 182 (ICON 5). In 2001, the GOG, in collaboration with the NCIC, key pharmaceutical sponsors, and selected international participants from Australasia (ANZ GOG), the United Kingdom's Medical Research Council, and European EORTC groups, developed a five-arm, prospective randomized trial to evaluate many of these concepts together. With an accrual goal of more than 5000 patients, this study, GOG 182, is comparing an eight-cycle carboplatin/paclitaxel reference arm with four experimental arms, using triplet or alternating doublet three-drug regimens (Fig. 31-3). A specially designed interim analysis based on PFS will be used to select the best regimen to go on to an overall survival analysis compared with the control arm. First results are expected in 2004.

Alternative sequential therapy. Another sequential approach is to deliver the new drug either alone or in combination after initial treatment with carboplatin. This kind of sequential chemotherapy is not a novel concept: four cycles of full-dose, single-agent anthracycline chemotherapy followed by four to eight cycles of cyclophosphamide/methotrexate/5-fluorouracil (CMF) is firmly established as a treatment paradigm for node-positive breast cancer.[44] In ovarian cancer, sequential treatment involving a platinum agent first, followed by a taxoid, might prove superior to combination schedules based on a consideration of molecular targets. In vitro models (fibroblasts) with *p53* mutations have been found to be hypersensitive to paclitaxel but resistant to platinum, whereas cells with normal p53 function are more sensitive to platinum.[45] Hence, it might be expected that initial platinum treatment could eradicate one population of (wild-type p53)

tumor cells, leaving a population of predominately mutant p53 cells amenable to treatment with taxanes. Furthermore, an accumulating body of evidence suggests that not only is there little biologic evidence for synergy between platinum and the taxanes, but there also may actually be antagonistic effects.

The optimal dose of platinum as a single agent remains unclear, although many historical studies have evaluated concepts of dose intensification and cumulative dosing of this agent. Most analyses of the numerous randomized trials that have used approximately twofold systemic differences in platinum dose intensity (all that can be realistically achieved without stem cell support) have failed to show any conclusive benefit for higher doses.[46] For platinum-based cumulative dosing, it is unlikely that there is a significant difference with respect to outcome for patients receiving more than five or six cycles,[47-49] although none of these studies included paclitaxel (see later discussion). Extrapolation of these findings to carboplatin suggests that within the cumulative dose range of AUC 24 to 36, survival would be equivalent, and outside of a clinical trial most investigators using carboplatin as a single agent have dosed to an AUC of 5 to 7 for six cycles administered every 3 to 4 weeks.

The SGCTG SCOTROC 2 program was designed to examine the feasibility of this type of sequential chemotherapy scheduling as first-line chemotherapy (Fig. 31-4). The arms of these three separate studies were randomized in order to assess the feasibility of delivering a planned eight cycles of treatment in comparable groups of patients between studies with similar control arms. Randomization of patients ensured that the feasibility of each regimen was assessed in similar groups of patients. In addition, it provided an unbiased basis for making informal comparisons of the relative merits of the combinations.

In SCOTROC 2A, all patients were scheduled to receive four cycles of carboplatin AUC 7 every 3 weeks (if possible), followed by four cycles of either docetaxel 100 mg/m² every 3 weeks; docetaxel 75 mg/m² on day 8 followed by gemcitabine 1250 mg/m² on days 1 and 8 every 3 weeks; or docetaxel 25 mg/m² followed by gemcitabine 800 mg/m², both drugs given on days 1, 8, and 15 every 3 weeks. In SCOTROC 2B, all patients were to receive four cycles of either (1) docetaxel 100 mg/m² every 3 weeks or (2) docetaxel 60 mg/m² and camptothecin-11 (CPT-11) 200 mg/m² every 3 weeks, following carboplatin. CPT-11 is a DNA topoisomerase I inhibitor with significant antitumor

Figure 31–3. Schema of Gynecologic Oncology Group (GOG) 182 randomized trial.

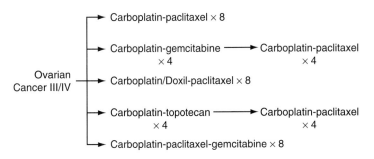

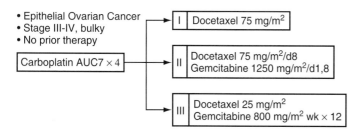

Figure 31–4. Scottish Gynaecological Cancer Trials Group (SGCTG) 2 program.

activity particularly in colorectal cancer, for which it has been found to be more effective than 5-fluorouracil.[50] Moreover, in recurrent ovarian cancer after platinum-based chemotherapy, CPT-11 is active, with a response rate of 23%.[51] Diarrhea, the toxicity most characteristic for CPT-11, is manageable if treatment with loperamide or atropine is promptly initiated. SCOTROC 2C was a single-arm study evaluating carboplatin followed by a paclitaxel/gemcitabine weekly combination.

After completion of this program, the SGCTG intends to consider one or more of these new treatment arms as comparators against the "best" arm of the SCOTROC 1 trial.

Summary for use of a third drug. To date, there is no evidence base for the off-protocol addition of a third drug to a concurrent combination of a platinum analog and a taxane in first-line chemotherapy for ovarian cancer. Many randomized trials are in progress, and results are eagerly awaited.

Does intraperitoneal chemotherapy have a place in the treatment of ovarian cancer?

Direct administration of cytotoxic agents into the peritoneal cavity is a strategy designed to enhance locoregional drug delivery to tumors assumed to be confined there, while concurrently reducing dose-limiting toxicities normally associated with systemic use. This method of administration allows concentrations many times higher than would be tolerated in the systemic circulation to be attained at the site of the tumor, and these can easily exceed concentrations shown in vitro to be required to overcome clinical drug resistance. Clinical studies have not demonstrated any advantage for small (twofold) increases in dose intensity, and two published randomized trials using carboplatin did not show any advantage for AUC 8 over AUC 4 dosing,[52] or for AUC 12 over AUC 6.[53] However, it is feasible to safely deliver fourfold or fivefold increases in platinum dose using peripheral blood stem cell support, and in vitro models predict that overcoming relative drug resistance in vitro requires drug concentrations in excess of fivefold higher than the usual cytotoxic range.[54] Extrapolation to the clinical situation suggests that if the benefit from dose intensification lies in circumventing drug resistance, then dose escalations of this magnitude are likely to be required.

It has also been demonstrated in vitro for many cytotoxic agents that the size of their therapeutic effect is time and concentration dependent. Using two human colorectal carcinoma lines, Link and colleagues[55] demonstrated that the cytotoxicity of drugs such as 5-fluorouracil, cisplatin, and anthracyclines could be significantly increased with higher concentrations and longer exposure times. However, longer exposure times are difficult to achieve with high-dose chemotherapy with stem cell support, and multiple cycles of therapy would be required, with significantly increased risks of associated morbidity and mortality. Currently, clinical trials of high-dose chemotherapy in ovarian cancer are limited mainly to nonrandomized studies delivering at most one or two cycles of a variety of moderately high-dose treatments. Two randomized trials have been performed, one in the United States that failed to recruit successfully and was closed, and an ongoing study in Europe. Most nonrandomized high-dose protocols demonstrated high response rates but short response durations and therefore did not justify the excessive toxicity produced by these treatments. However, intraperitoneal (IP) chemotherapy theoretically delivers high dose intensity of active agents directly to the predominant site of the disease.

The problem with extrapolating preclinical data to this clinical situation lies with the capability to deliver the drug in high therapeutic concentrations into tumor nodules. Using rat peritoneal tumor nodules, Los and colleagues[56] compared the concentration of cisplatin at the periphery of the tumor (≤1.5 mm from tumor surface) with the concentration of cisplatin at the center of the tumor, after both IV and IP administration. Cisplatin was shown to be present at a higher concentration at the tumor periphery when given IP, but there was no difference in concentration at the tumor center with IP versus IV administration. These data suggested that any major therapeutic benefit from IP delivery is likely to be restricted to small tumor nodules.

Three relatively large prospective, randomized trials investigating the benefits of IP chemotherapy in maximally cytoreduced ovarian cancer have now been reported (Table 31-4). The first study, published in 1996, randomly assigned 546 eligible patients, after initial cytoreduction to 2 cm or less residual disease, to six cycles of IV Cytoxan 600 mg/m² in combination with either IV or IP cisplatin at 100 mg/m².[57] Patients obtaining a complete remission underwent a second-look laparotomy. Surgically defined complete responses

Table 31–4. Randomized Trials of Intraperitoneal (IP) versus Intravenous (IV) Chemotherapy

Trial	No. of Patients	Residual Disease after Cytoreduction (cm)	Regimens	Progression-Free Survival (mo)	Overall Survival (mo)	Reference
1	546	≤2	IV Cisplatin 100 mg/m² + IV Cytoxan (cyclophosphamide) 600 mg/m² vs IP Cisplatin 100 mg/m² + IV Cytoxan 600 mg/m²	N/A	41 vs 49 (P < .02)	Alberts et al.[47] (1996)
2	462	≤1	IV Cisplatin 75 mg/m² + IV paclitaxel 135 mg/m² vs IV Carboplatin AUC 9 + IP cisplatin 75 mg/m² + IV paclitaxel 135 mg/m²	22 vs 28 (P = .01)	63 vs 52 (P = .05)	Markman et al.[58] (2001)
3	416	<1	IV Cisplatin 75 mg/m² + IV paclitaxel 135 mg/m² vs IV paclitaxel 135 mg/m² on day 1 + IP cisplatin 100 mg/m² on day 1 + IP paclitaxel 80 mg/m² on day 8	19 vs 24 (P < .29)	N/A	Armstrong et al.[59] (2002)

were seen in 47% of those in the IP arm and 36% of those in the IV arm. Toxicity was reduced for patients receiving IP cisplatin, and survival was significantly better for this group (49 versus 41 months, P < .02). However, accrual was extended to include more patients with residual disease measuring 0.5 cm or less, with the investigators rationalizing that this group would benefit most from IP chemotherapy. Counterintuitively, there turned out to be no statistically significant survival benefit for this group. In addition, because the IV cisplatin/cyclophosphamide combination has been shown to be inferior to cisplatin/paclitaxel in two randomized studies in patients with both suboptimal (GOG 111) and optimal cytoreduction (mix in OV.10), it is not considered an appropriate control arm to gauge any new therapy.

In the second study, 462 evaluable patients with disease surgically cytoreduced to 1 cm or less were randomly assigned to receive either six cycles of the GOG 111 protocol of IV cisplatin 75 mg/m² and paclitaxel 135 mg/m² over 24 hours or a regimen consisting of two cycles of IV carboplatin AUC 9 followed by six cycles of IP cisplatin 75 mg/m² and IV paclitaxel 135 mg/m².[58] The latter research arm was significantly more toxic, with approximately one fifth of the patients actually receiving two cycles or less of IP cisplatin, largely because of persistent toxicity from carboplatin. Nevertheless, median PFS time favored the IP arm (28 versus 22 months, P = .01), as did overall survival time (63 versus 52 months, P = .05).

This second trial had a number of design flaws, not least of which was the fact that delivering two cycles of carboplatin at AUC 9 in addition to six cycles of cisplatin/paclitaxel adds a longer duration of chemotherapy and increased cumulative dose of platinum, thus unbalancing the trial in favor of the research arm,

regardless of the mode of administration. In addition, the timing of salvage therapies (which were not subjected to protocol) is not known and may have influenced the PFS and overall survival end points if administered pre-emptively.

Despite these caveats, the positive results of both trials did hint that IP therapy was a strategy worth pursuing, and therefore the results of the third trial, GOG 172, were awaited with great interest. This study randomly assigned patients who had 1 cm or less residual disease after cytoreduction to receive either six cycles of IV cisplatin plus IV paclitaxel (as in the GOG 111 protocol) or a research arm of six cycles of a 3-week regimen consisting of IV paclitaxel 135 mg/m² on day 1, IP cisplatin 100 mg/m² on day 2, and IP paclitaxel 80 mg/m² on day 8. The study was powered to detect a 50% increase in PFS. At the American Society of Clinical Oncology (ASCO) meeting in 2002, data were presented on 416 randomized and eligible patients, and 213 events were available (208 required).[59] The IP research arm was significantly more toxic, with greater grade 3 or 4 metabolic, infective, neurologic, and gastrointestinal toxicities. In addition, more thrombocytopenia and neutropenia were also present. Nevertheless, the IP regimen was feasible and there was a significant advantage in PFS for IP chemotherapy: 24 versus 19 months (P = .029, one-tailed test; HR, 0.73). This advantage also persisted for patients with gross residual disease: 21 versus 16 months. No data for PFS for the subgroup with truly microscopic residual disease were available, and, in addition, no data were available on overall survival time.

Despite the lack of overall survival data for GOG 172, it is difficult to completely dismiss the fact that there are now three consecutive phase III trials that have all documented outcome advantages for IP therapy. However, it is evident that the increased organ toxicities with the IP research arm reflect a significant contribution from systemic absorption of the chemotherapeutic agents. Approaches aimed at circumventing this problem could involve lower doses of cisplatin or substitution with carboplatin, but it is not certain that modifications of this sort would continue to deliver the same outcome advantages. Nevertheless, when overall survival data from GOG 172 become available (and as of this date there are fewer deaths in the research arm), if they once again show an overall survival benefit for IP chemotherapy in this carefully selected patient population, more widespread adoption of this mode of therapy is extremely likely.

There certainly has been a prevailing belief against IP chemotherapy for a long time, most likely because of the practical and logistic difficulties involved. Catheter-related problems have not made it easy to cross this therapy over into mainstream use, and thus it appears that the required burden of proof for this treatment is greater than for other new systemic therapies. Are any other studies likely to be performed now that would finally convince the oncologic community of the merits of IP treatment? Perhaps not, but an individual patient meta-analysis from all three studies could attempt to evaluate any heterogeneity among these important trials. Even so, the optimal catheter system is still not known, and there remain unanswered questions that many clinicians may want addressed before this therapy moves beyond the setting of clinical trials and into routine clinical practice for fit women with optimally debulked stage III ovarian cancer.

One such interesting and biologically relevant avenue of research would be for IP therapy to be used as consolidation treatment after the induction of a complete clinical response with standard IV treatments. This approach may provide the optimal environment and setting for a maximal antitumor effect of IP delivery by exposing nonbulky residual tumor masses, which are by definition "resistant" to conventional IV doses at this stage, with extremely high local dose intensification. By reviewing the records of 433 patients who received IP chemotherapy as consolidation after a good response to IV chemotherapy, Barakat and colleagues[60] discovered that some patients had exceptionally long survival times after receiving this therapy. It was demonstrated that the size of residual disease correlated with median survival time: patients achieving pathologic complete response to initial IV chemotherapy had a median survival time of 8.7 years, compared with 4.8 years for patients with macroscopic residual disease. Clearly, the heterogeneity of patients considered to be in clinical remission after first-line therapy requires this information to be properly documented and used in the evaluation of new strategies in the setting of "consolidation" treatment. Prolongation of primary chemotherapy, for either "consolidation" or "maintenance," is discussed in the next section.

How long should initial chemotherapy last?

Three randomized trials have been reported that examined the duration of platinum chemotherapy (i.e., number of cycles) in advanced ovarian cancer (Table 31-5).[47-49] None of these studies demonstrated a difference in median survival time, but longer durations were associated with more toxicity, especially neuropathy. These studies were the basis for the current rationale for six cycles of treatment as the convention, although it is noteworthy that none contained a taxane as part of combination treatment.

GOG protocol 178/Southwestern Oncology Group (SWOG) 9701 was set up to test the theory that prolongation of treatment with paclitaxel would have outcome advantages over conventional shorter durations of therapy. In this study, patients with advanced ovarian cancer achieving a complete response to five or six cycles of carboplatin/paclitaxel at standard doses were randomly assigned to further cycles of paclitaxel 175 mg/m^2 given every 4 weeks for either 3 or 12 months. The primary end point, PFS, was achieved early in 2001, after a planned interim efficacy analysis was reported by the data monitoring committee.[61] With 54 events—20 in the 12-month arm and 34 in the 3-month arm—a statistically significant difference in PFS was observed: 28 versus 21 months, respectively (one-sided, $P = .0035$; adjusted Cox model analysis, $P = .0023$; HR, 2.31, 99% CI, 1.08 to 4.94). The study was therefore closed with 262 randomized and eligible patients. At the time of this analysis, a secondary end point, overall survival time, did not demonstrate a similar advantage, although with only 17 deaths on the trial in total (eight on the 3-month arm, nine on 12-month arm, $P = .63/.7$ unadjusted/adjusted), robust conclusions are impossible to draw. With regard to toxicity, overall reported levels by NCIC-CTC grades were considered acceptable.

Despite the significant demonstrated advantage in PFS for 1 year of monthly paclitaxel, this trial has not so far led to its widespread adoption. First, because of the unblinding of results at midstudy, patients were crossed over to the 12-month arm; therefore, the

Table 31-5. Trials Examining Duration of First-Line Chemotherapy (Non–platinum-containing Regimens)

Trial	No. of Patients	Regimens (Cycles)	Reference
MSKCC	84	Cisplatin 100 mg/m^2 + Adriamycin (doxorubicin) 40 mg/m^2 + Cytoxan (cyclophosphamide) 600 mg/m^2 (5 *vs* 10)	Hakes et al.[48] (1992)
DACOVA	202	Cisplatin 60 mg/m^2 + Adriamycin 40 mg/m^2 + Cytoxan 500 mg/m^2 (6 *vs* 12)	Bertelsen et al.[47] (1993)
North Thames	233	Cisplatin 75 mg/m^2 or carboplatin 400 mg/m^2 (5 *vs* 8)	Lambert et al.[49] (1997)

impact of this prolonged course of treatment on overall survival cannot be known. Second, an early protocol amendment required patients to drop to 135 mg/m^2 paclitaxel because of what was considered by the investigators to be an unacceptably high level of toxicity and withdrawal due to neuropathy. Therefore, the advantage in PFS is based on results from a only few patients treated at a mixture of dose levels. If it is acknowledged that the higher dose is not feasible, it is not known whether the lower dose—presumably the "recommended" dose—will have the same effect on outcome. This may be even more important because the majority of reliable evidence for a difference in outcome comes from the first 12 months after registration (i.e., while patients in the 12-month treatment arm were receiving therapy). The PFS curve looks extremely unreliable beyond 18 months, so there is little evidence that any advantage is sustained much beyond completion of treatment.

Furthermore, the low incidence of reported neurotoxicity raises questions as to whether this side effect was underestimated. The NCIC-CTC grading system for neurotoxicity is acknowledged to be prone to errors and interobserver variability, and this effect may be especially evident here. Patients receiving the 12-month treatment would have accumulated a dose of paclitaxel well in excess of that known to produce clinically significant neurotoxicity in most patients, in addition to the neurotoxicity produced by six cycles of the paclitaxel/carboplatin couplet described in the literature, and certainly more than the 33% overall incidence described in this study. Finally, a major flaw and missed opportunity in this protocol was the omission of any comparative quality-of-life data, particularly in light of the fact that continued chemotherapy in the absence of symptoms is recognized to have a detrimental impact on quality of life. This single study has produced much controversy, and it is important that follow-up studies using consolidation or maintenance approaches be performed. Whether cytotoxic chemotherapy is an appropriate choice for maintaining responses is debatable, and this task may fall to novel cytostatic agents or biologic agents in future trial paradigms.

What types of trials and integration of novel (biologic) agents will be seen in the future?

Over the last decade, there has been an explosion of knowledge in understanding of the molecular engineering of the cancer cell. Critical pathways in carcinogenesis have been identified, and key molecular events in important areas such as acquisition of resistance to cytotoxic chemotherapy are being uncovered. The discovery of a diverse array of new molecular targets is now allowing the chemical and pharmacologic construction of novel agents to specifically hit these targets, and this process is accelerating. Genetic and proteomic profiling is anticipated to predict outcome and guide therapies to tumors within the next decade.

The challenge is to put this new knowledge and therapeutic approaches into the clinic in such a way that the potential for efficacy is maximized and the chances of overlooking important treatment advances are minimized.

The problem lies in the sheer diversity and proliferation of these new nonconventional approaches to cancer therapy. Table 31-6 provides an overview of the biologic and genetic therapeutic approaches that are currently undergoing clinical investigation in ovarian cancer. This is by no means an inclusive list. These novel therapies hold great promise for significant treatment advances, and both investigators and patients hold high expectations for meaningful improvements in survival and quality of life. But the key question remains, how do we integrate treatments such as these into clinical practice?

In general, randomized trials are considered to be the definitive source of evidence regarding the utility of any new therapeutic approach. This is particularly relevant when the expected differences in outcome are not thought to be large. Randomized phase III studies have been instrumental in changing oncologic clinical practices, but they are only as good as the questions asked and the quality of data collected. The controversy around the use of paclitaxel in first-line chemotherapy is a prime example of this precept, and it must be remembered that even meta-analyses of trials apparently asking similar questions will potentially have their conclusions blunted by the same issues.

However, it is not going to be feasible to conduct large randomized trials using every interesting agent in every group from Table 31-6. In addition, understanding of the basic science behind these novel therapies is still lacking in many important areas, which will undoubtedly lead to poorly designed clinical

Table 31–6. Novel and Biologic Agents in Ovarian Cancer

Approach	Examples
New Targets	
Growth factor receptors: epidermal growth factor receptor (EGFR), human epidermal growth factor receptor 2 (HER2)	OSI-774, ZD1839, C-225, Herceptin
Cellular kinases	PD173885
Apoptosis mechanisms: Bcl-2, antisense	G3139
Cell cycle inhibitors	RO31-7453
β-Tubulin	Epothilones
Gene Therapies	
Replicating viruses	ONYX-015
Angiogenesis and Metastasis	
Matrix metalloproteinase inhibitors	BY 12-9566
Vascular endothelial growth factor	Bevaczumab
Antibodies	Ovarex
Vaccines	
Immune Modulators	Interferon-γ

trials and potentially disappointing and even misleading results.

It has been suggested that phase II randomized trials could more easily facilitate selection of promising approaches if equivalent pharmacodynamic end points are agreed. It is clear that new strategies are required to efficiently and effectively evaluate the plethora of new targets and agents that are emerging. These smaller studies would still include end points of feasibility and efficacy, although a change away from response rates to time to progression may be warranted given the nature of many of these new agents. However, primary end points would need to be dominated by evaluation of the pharmacodynamic effects on the target.

Ultimately, randomized trials are still likely to be required in ovarian cancer as we continue to be subjected to evidence-based medicine and guideline-related treatment protocols. Given that most of these novel biologic therapies appear to be most effective in microscopic or small-volume disease, there is still going to be a significant role for cytoreductive surgery and cytotoxic chemotherapy. Whether these new therapies should be given in combination with cytotoxic agents (given that synergistic effects are documented for many new agents, such as epidermal growth factor receptor [EGFR] inhibitors) or as consolidation or maintenance therapies remains to be determined.

Multidrug resistance (MDR) is frequently present in ovarian cancer patients as a result of increased expression of the *MDR1* gene and subsequent overactivity of the p-glycoprotein drug efflux pump. PSC 833 (Valspodar) is a nonimmunosuppressive cyclosporin analog that is administered orally as a microemulsion drink solution and was previously shown to alter the pharmacokinetics of paclitaxel, resulting in an increase in the area under the curve and decreased renal clearance.[62] This alteration in drug metabolism required a lower dose of paclitaxel to be administered (70 to 80 mg/m^2), but there were clear responses at this dose in phase II studies of heavily pretreated patients whose cancer was resistant or refractory to paclitaxel.[63,64] The first results of a randomized trial of 762 patients with FIGO stages III and IV ovarian cancer who received six cycles of either (1) paclitaxel 175 mg/m^2 plus carboplatin AUC 6, or (2) paclitaxel 80 mg/m^2 plus carboplatin AUC 6 plus 12 doses (5 mg/kg per dose) of PSC 833 given every 6 hours on days 1 through 3 of each cycle, were presented in 2002.[65] More adverse events were reported in the PSC 833 arm, and response data actually disadvantaged the PSC 833 arm at 33% versus 41% (P = .022), although the number of on-treatment progressions was similar. No differences emerged in median PFS: 13.2 months for PSC 833 plus paclitaxel/carboplatin and 13.5 months with paclitaxel/carboplatin alone.

This negative study leads to more rather than fewer questions, which could perhaps have been better addressed in preclinical models or in smaller, more scientifically driven trials. The mechanisms of resistance in ovarian cancer are multifactorial, and subversion of the resistant phenotype may require a number of different and simultaneous approaches. Inactivation of administered cytotoxic drugs, enhanced DNA repair mechanisms, and increased expression of survival signals are likely to be at least as important as enhanced drug efflux due to overexpression of p-glycoprotein; indeed, MDR may not be clinically relevant in the resistance of ovarian cancer to cytotoxic drugs.

Another illustration of this problem can be shown by the recent study of the EGFR tyrosine kinase inhibitor ZD1839 (Iressa) in combination with chemotherapy in non–small cell lung cancer.[66] Novel agents directed against the EGFR subfamily of tyrosine kinases have tremendous potential, because extensive preclinical data have linked aberrant EGFR signaling with the development of cancers and aggressive malignant behavior (see review by Mendelsohn[67]). Agents such as ZD1839 and OSI-774 (Tarceva) have been shown to selectively target tyrosine kinase domains of EGFR and have demonstrated clinical efficacy in tumors previously treated with chemotherapy. In addition, these agents are generally well tolerated without significant hematologic toxicity.

ZD1839 demonstrated encouraging activity in early phase I clinical studies, particularly in advanced non–small cell lung cancer.[68-70] The level of activity was deemed so encouraging that phase III evaluation proceeded rapidly (INTACT 1 and 2 ["Iressa" NSCLC Trial, assessing combination therapy]), without firm and robust data on crucial matters such as the optimal dose of the inhibitor or how to select patients. First reports from this study indicated that no statistically significant differences in overall survival were achieved with the addition of ZD1839 to standard platinum-based chemotherapy.[71,72]

In ovarian cancer, OSI-774 has shown efficacy in heavily pretreated patients, with 3 (10%) of 30 patients having partial responses and 15 (30%) of 30 having stable disease as their best response.[73] However, as with all agents in this class, more data are required as to which patients are most likely to benefit, which molecular events should be monitored to determine the degree of downregulation achieved, and how this approach can best be integrated with existing cytotoxic therapies.

One such approach with strong preclinical data that could lead to a relevant randomized study is the use of DNA methyltransferase inhibitors to increase the chemosensitivity of tumors resistant to platinum. Decitabine (5-aza-2'-deoxycytidine) has been demonstrated to increase the sensitivity of ovarian (and colon) xenografts known to have promotor methylation of the DNA mismatch repair (MMR) gene *MLH1*.[74] Although this deoxycytidine analog is used as cytotoxic therapy for some hematologic malignancies, it is also known to induce demethylation and re-expression of MLH1 at noncytotoxic dosages.

Earlier retrospective studies demonstrated that many postchemotherapy ovarian cancers had hMLH1 promotor methylation and that the frequency of methylation increased with relapse.[75] Furthermore, increased DNA methylation may have prognostic value, as demonstrated by poorer PFS in patients with higher levels of genome-wide promoter DNA methylation.[76]

Given this strong rationale for decitabine-induced drug sensitization in ovarian cancer and the fact that carboplatin is the cornerstone of treatment for this disease, a clinical study of decitabine in combination with carboplatin was initiated by Cancer Research UK in 2002. The successful completion of this phase I study, with correlative pharmacodynamic data demonstrating the degree of hypomethylation induced by decitabine, will make a subsequent randomized trial in ovarian cancer extremely attractive.

REFERENCES

1. Yancik R: Ovarian cancer: Age contrasts in incidence, histology, disease stage at diagnosis and mortality. Cancer 1993;71 (2 Suppl):S17-S23.

2. Smith JP, Rutledge F: Chemotherapy in the treatment of cancer of the ovary. Am J Obstet Gynaecol 1970;107:691-703.

3. Lawton FG, Redman CW, Leusley DM, et al: Neoadjuvant (cytoreductive) chemotherapy combined with intervention debulking surgery in advanced unresected epithelial ovarian cancer. Obstet Gynaecol 1989;73:61-65.

4. Neijt JP, ten Bokkel Huinink WW, van der Burg MEL, et al: Long term survival in ovarian cancer. Eur J Cancer 1991;27:1367-1372.

5. van der Berg MEL, van Lent M, Buse M, et al: The effect of debulking surgery after induction chemotherapy on the prognosis in advanced epithelial ovarian cancer. N Engl J Med 1995;332:629-634.

6. Rose PG, Nerenstone S, Brady M, et al: A phase III randomized study of interval secondary cytoreduction in patients with advanced stage ovarian carcinoma with suboptimal residual disease: A Gynecologic Oncology Group study [abstract 802]. Proc Am Soc Clin Oncol 2002;21:201a.

7. Hunter RW, Alexander NDE, Soutter WP, et al: Meta-analysis of surgery in advanced ovarian carcinoma: Is maximum cytoreductive surgery an independent determinant of prognosis? Am J Obstet Gynecol 1992;166:504-511.

8. Bristow RE, Tomacruz RS, Armstrong DK, et al: Survival impact of maximum cytoreductive surgery for advanced ovarian carcinoma during the platinum-era: A meta-analysis of 6,848 patients [abstract 807]. Proc Am Soc Clin Oncol 2001;20:202a.

9. Onnis A, Marchetti M, Padovan P, et al: Neoadjuvant chemotherapy in advanced ovarian cancer. Eur J Gynaecol Oncol 1996;17:393-396.

10. Chambers JT, Chambers SK, Voynick IM, et al: Neoadjuvant chemotherapy in stage X ovarian cancer. Gynaecol Oncol 1990; 37:327-331.

11. Advanced Ovarian Cancer Trialists Group: Chemotherapy in advanced ovarian cancer: Four systematic meta-analyses of individual patient data from 37 randomized trials. Br J Cancer 1998; 78:1479-1487.

12. McGuire WP, Hoskins WJ, Brady MF, et al: Cyclophosphamide and cisplatin compared with paclitaxel and cisplatin in patients with stage III and stage IV ovarian cancer. N Engl J Med 1996;334:1-6.

13. McGuire WP, Brady MF, Ozols RF: The Gynecologic Oncology Group experience in ovarian cancer. Ann Oncol 1999;10(Suppl 1): 29-34.

14. Piccart MJ, Bertelsen K, James K, et al: Randomized intergroup trial of cisplatin-paclitaxel versus cisplatin-cyclophosphamide in women with advanced epithelial ovarian cancer: Three year results. J Natl Cancer Inst 2000;92:699-702.

15. Neymark N, Gorlia T, Adriaenssen I, et al: Cost effectiveness of paclitaxel/cisplatin compared with cyclophosphamide/cisplatin in the treatment of advanced ovarian cancer in Belgium. Pharmacoeconomics 2002;20:485-497.

16. Muggia FM, Braly PS, Brady MF, et al: Phase III randomized study of cisplatin versus paclitaxel versus cisplatin and paclitaxel in patients with suboptimal stage III or IV ovarian cancer: A Gynaecologic Oncology Group Study. J Clin Oncol 2000; 18:106-115.

17. The International Collaborative Ovarian Neoplasm (ICON) Group: Paclitaxel plus carboplatin versus standard chemotherapy with either single agent carboplatin or cyclophosphamide, doxorubicin and cisplatin in women with ovarian cancer: The ICON3 randomized trial. Lancet 2002;360:505-515.

18. Neijt JP, Engelholm SA, Tuxen MK, et al: Exploratory phase III study of paclitaxel and cisplatin versus paclitaxel and carboplatin in advanced ovarian carcinoma. J Clin Oncol 2000;18: 3084-3092.

19. du Bois A, Lueck HJ, Meier W, et al: Cisplatin/paclitaxel vs. carboplatin/paclitaxel in ovarian cancer: Update of an Arbeitsgemeinshaft Gynaekologishe Onkologie (AGO) Study Group Trial [abstract 1374]. Proc Am Soc Clin Oncol 1999;18: 356a.

20. Ozols RF, Bundy BN, Fowler J, et al: Randomized phase III study of cisplatin(CIS)/paclitaxel(PAC) versus carboplatin(CARBO)/ PAC in optimal stage III epithelial ovarian cancer (OC): A Gynecologic Oncology Group Trial (GOG 158) [abstract 1373]. Proc Am Soc Clin Oncol 1999;18:356a.

21. ICON Collaborators: ICON2: A randomized trial of single agent carboplatin against the 3-drug combination of CAP (cyclophosphamide, doxorubicin and cisplatin) in women with ovarian cancer. Lancet 1998;352:1571-1576.

22. Sandercock J, Parmar MKB, Torri V, Qian W: First-line treatment for advanced ovarian cancer: Paclitaxel, platinum and the evidence. Br J Cancer 2002;87:815-824.

23. Kaye SB, Piccart M, Aapro M, et al: Phase II trials of docetaxel (Taxotere) in advanced ovarian cancer: An updated overview. Eur J Cancer 1997;33:2167-2170.

24. Vershraegen CF, Sittisomwong T, Kudelka AP, et al: Docetaxel for patients with paclitaxel-resistant mullerian carcinoma. J Clin Oncol 2000;18:2733-2739.

25. Markman M, Kennedy A, Webster K, et al: Combination chemotherapy with carboplatin and docetaxel in the treatment of cancers of the ovary and fallopian tube and primary carcinoma of the peritoneum. J Clin Oncol 2001;19:1901-1905.

26. Vasey PA, Atkinson R, Coleman R, et al: Docetaxel-carboplatin as first-line therapy for epithelial ovarian cancer. Br J Cancer 2001;84:170-178.

27. Vasey PA on behalf of the Scottish Gynaecological Cancer Trials Group: Preliminary results of the SCOTROC Trial: A phase III comparison of paclitaxel-carboplatin (PC) and docetaxel-carboplatin (DC) as first-line chemotherapy for stage IC-IV epithelial ovarian cancer [abstract 804]. Proc Am Soc Clin Oncol 2001;20: 202a.

28. Vasey PA on behalf of the Scottish Gynaecological Cancer Trials Group: Survival and longer-term toxicity results of the SCOTROC study: Docetaxel-carboplatin (DC) vs. paclitaxel-carboplatin (PC) in epithelial ovarian cancer (EOC) [abstract 804]. Proc Am Soc Clin Oncol 2002;21:202a.

29. Cassidy J, Paul J, Soukop M, et al: Clinical trials of nimodopine as a potential neuroprotector in ovarian cancer patients treated with cisplatin. Cancer Chemother Pharmacol 1998;41:161-166.

30. Cull A, Howat S, Greimel E, et al: Development of a European Organization for Research and Treatment of Cancer questionnaire module to assess the quality of life of ovarian cancer patients in clinical trials: A progress report. Eur J Cancer 2001;37:47-53.

31. A'Hern RP, Gore ME: Impact of doxorubicin on survival in advanced ovarian cancer. J Clin Oncol 1995;13:726-732.

32. Gruppo Interregionale Cooperativo Oncologico Ginecologia: Randomized comparison of cisplatin with cyclophosphamide/ cisplatin and cyclophosphamide/cisplatin/doxorubicin in advanced ovarian cancer. Lancet 1987;2:353-359.

33. Conte PF, Bruzzone M, Chiara S, et al: A randomized trial comparing cisplatin plus cyclophosphamide versus cisplatin, doxorubicin and cyclophosphamide in advanced ovarian cancer. J Clin Oncol 1986;4:965-971.

34. Omura GA, Bundy BN, Berek JS, et al: Randomized trial of cyclophosphamide plus cisplatin with or without doxorubicin in ovarian carcinoma: A Gynecologic Oncology Group Study. J Clin Oncol 1989;7:457-465.

35. Bertelsen K, Jakobsen A, Andersen JE, et al: A randomized study of cyclophosphamide and cisplatinum with or without doxorubicin in advanced ovarian carcinoma. Gynecol Oncol 1987;28: 161-169.

36. du Bois A, Weber B, Pfisterer J, et al: Epirubicin/paclitaxel/carboplatin (TEC) vs. paclitaxel/carboplatin (TC) in first-line treatment of ovarian cancer FIGO stages IIb-IV: Interim results of an

AGO-GINECO Intergroup Phase III Trial [abstract 805]. Proc Am Soc Clin Oncol 2001;20:202a.

37. Kristensen G, Vergote I, Stuart G, et al: First line treatment of ovarian cancer FIGO stages IIb-IV with paclitaxel/epirubicin/carboplatin (TEC) vs paclitaxel/carboplatin (TC): Interim results of an NSGO-EORTC-NCIC CTG Gynaecological Cancer Intergroup phase III trial [abstract 805]. Proc Am Soc Clin Oncol 2002;21:202a.

38. Bookman M: Developmental chemotherapy in advanced ovarian cancer: Incorporation of newer cytotoxic agents in a phase III randomized trial of the Gynaecologic Oncology Group (GOG-0182). Semin Oncol 2002;29(S1):20-31.

39. Hansen SW: Gemcitabine in the treatment of ovarian cancer. Int J Gynaecol Cancer 2001;11(S1):39-41.

40. Rose PG, Greer BE, Markman M, et al: A phase I study of pacltiaxel, carboplatin and liposomal doxorubicin in ovarian, peritoneal and tubal carcinoma: A Gynecologic Oncology Group study [abstract 1531]. Proc Am Soc Clin Oncol 19:387a.

41. Hoskins P, Eisenhauer E, Beare S, et al: Randomized phase II study of two schedules of topotecan in previously treated patients with ovarian cancer: A National Cancer Institute of Canada Clinical Trials Group study. J Clin Oncol 1998;16:2233-2237.

42. Armstrong D, O'Reilly S, Bookman M, et al: A phase I study of topotecan, cisplatin, and paclitaxel in newly diagnosed epithelial ovarian cancer: A Gynecologic Oncology Group Study [abstract 1351]. Proc Am Soc Clin Oncol 1998;17:350a.

43. Hoskins P, Eisenhauer E, Vergote I, et al: Phase II feasibility study of sequential couplets of cisplatin/topotecan followed by paclitaxel/cisplatin as primary treatment for advanced epithelial ovarian cancer: A National Cancer Institute of Canada Clinical Trials Group study. J Clin Oncol 2000;18:4038-4044.

44. Bonadonna G, Zambetti M, Valagussa P: Sequential or alternating doxorubicin and CMF regimens in breast cancer with more than three positive nodes: Ten-year results. JAMA 1995;273:542-527.

45. Wahl AF, Donaldson KL, Fairchild C, et al: Loss of normal p53 function confers sensitization to Taxol by increasing G_2/M arrest and apoptosis. Nat Med 1996;2:72-79.

46. Vasey PA, Kaye SB: Dose intensity in ovarian cancer. In Gershenson DM, McGuire WP (eds): Ovarian Cancer: Controversies in Management. New York, Churchill Livingstone, 1997, pp 139-169.

47. Bertelsen K, Jakobsen A, Stroyer J, et al: A prospective randomized comparison of 6 and 12 cycles of cyclophosphamide, adriamycin and cisplatin in advanced epithelial ovarian cancer: A Danish Ovarian Study Group trial (DACOVA). Gynaecol Oncol 1993;49:30-36.

48. Hakes T, Chalas E, Hoskins WJ, et al: Randomized prospective trial of 5 versus 10 cycles of cyclophosphamide, doxorubicin and cisplatin in advanced ovarian cancer. Gynaecol Oncol 1992;45:284-289.

49. Lambert HE, Rustin GJ, Gregory WM, et al: A randomized trial of five versus eight courses of cisplatin or carboplatin in advanced epithelial ovarian carcinoma: A North Thames Ovary Group Study. Ann Oncol 1997;8:327-333.

50. Van Cutsem E, Pozzo C, Starkhammar H, et al: A phase II study of irinotecan alternated with five days bolus of 5-fluorouracil and leucovorin in first-line chemotherapy of metastatic colorectal cancer. Ann Oncol 1991;9:1199-1204.

51. Takeuchi S, Dobashi K, Fujimoto S, et al: A late phase II study of CPT-11 on uterine cervical cancer and ovarian cancer: Research Groups of CPT-11 in Gynecologic Cancers. Gan To Kagaku Ryoho [Japanese Journal of Cancer and Chemotherapy] 1991;18:1681-1689.

52. Jakobsen A on behalf of DACOVA: A dose intensity study of carboplatin in ovarian cancer. Int J Gynaecol Cancer 1995;5:S5.

53. Gore ME, Mainwaring PN, Macfarlane V: A randomized study of high versus standard dose carboplatin in patients (pts) with advanced epithelial ovarian cancer (EOC) [abstract]. Proc Am Soc Clin Oncol 1996;15:284a.

54. Behrens BC, Hamilton TC, Masuda H, et al: Characteristics of cisdiammine-dichloroplatinum(II)-resistant human ovarian cancer cell line and the evaluation of platinum analogues. Cancer Res 1987;47:414-418.

55. Link KH: In vitro pharmacologic rationale for intraperitoneal regional chemotherapy. In Sugarbaker PH (ed): Peritoneal Carcinomatosis: Principles of Management. Boston, Kluwer Academic Publishers, 1996, pp 101-114.

56. Los G, Mutsaers PH, van der Vijgh WJ, et al: Direct diffusion of cis-diamminedichloroplatinum(II) in intraperitoneal rat tumours after intraperitoneal chemotherapy: A comparison with systemic chemotherapy. Cancer Res 1989;49:3380-3384.

57. Alberts DS, Liu PY, Hannigan EV, et al: Intraperitoneal cisplatin plus intravenous cyclophosphamide versus intravenous cisplatin plus intravenous cyclophosphamide for stage III ovarian cancer. N Engl J Med 1996;335:1950-1955.

58. Markman M, Bundy BN, Alberts DS, et al: Phase III trial of standard-dose carboplatin followed by intravenous paclitaxel and intraperitoneal cisplatin in small volume stage III ovarian carcinoma: An intergroup study of the Gynecologic Oncology Group, Southwestern Oncology Group and Eastern Cooperative Oncology Group. J Clin Oncol 2001;19:1001-1007.

59. Armstrong DK, Bundy BN, Baergen R, et al: Randomized phase III study of intravenous paclitaxel and cisplatin versus IV paclitaxel, intraperitoneal cisplatin and IP paclitaxel in optimal stage III epithelial ovarian cancer (OC): A Gynecologic Oncology Group Trial (GOG 172) [abstract 803]. Proc Am Soc Clin Oncol 2002;21:201a.

60. Barakat RR, Sabbatini P, Bhaskaran D, et al: Intraperitoneal chemotherapy for ovarian carcinoma: Results of long term follow-up. J Clin Oncol 2002;20:694-698.

61. Markman M: Paclitaxel consolidation therapy for advanced ovarian cancer: Preliminary findings from GOG 178. SGO 33rd Annual Meeting, March 16-20, 2002.

62. Patnaik A, Warner E, Michael M, et al: Phase I dose-finding and pharmacokinetic study of paclitaxel and carboplatin with oral valspodar in patients with advanced solid tumors. J Clin Oncol 2000;18:3677-3689.

63. Fields A, Hochster C, Runowicz C, et al: SDZ PSC 833/paclitaxel in paclitaxel refractory ovarian carcinoma: A phase II trial with renewed responses [abstract 1254]. Proc Am Soc Clin Oncol 1997;16:351a.

64. Fracasso PM, Brady MF, Moore DH, et al: Phase II study of paclitaxel and valspodar (PSC 833) in refractory ovarian carcinoma: A gynecologic oncology group study. J Clin Oncol 2001;19:2975-2982.

65. Joly F, Mangioni C, Nicoletto M, et al: A phase III study of PSC 833 in combination with paclitaxel and carboplatin (PC-PSC) versus paclitaxel and carboplatin (PC) alone in patients with stage IV or suboptimally debulked stage III epithelial ovarian cancer or primary cancer of the peritoneum [abstract 806]. Proc Am Soc Clin Oncol 2002;202a.

66. Giaccone G, Johnson DH, Manegold C, et al: A phase III clinical trial of ZD1839 ("Iressa") in combination with gemcitabine and cisplatin in chemotherapy-naïve patients with advanced non–small cell lung cancer (INTACT1) [abstract 40]. Ann Oncol 2002;13(S5):2.

67. Mendelsohn J: Epidermal Growth Factor Receptor Blockade as Anticancer Therapy. American Society of Clinical Oncology, New Orleans, Educational Book, 2000, pp 39-46.

68. Nakagawa K, Yamamoto N, Kudoh S, et al: A phase I intermittent dose escalation trial of ZD1839 (Iressa) in Japanese patients with solid malignant tumors [abstract 711]. Proc Am Soc Clin Oncol 2000;19:183a.

69. Baselga J, Herbst R, LoRusso P, et al: Continuous administration of ZD1839 (Iressa), a novel oral epidermal growth factor receptor tyrosine kinase inhibitor (EGFR-TKI) in patients with five selected tumor types: Evidence of activity and good tolerability [abstract 686]. Proc Am Soc Clin Oncol 2000;19:177a.

70. Ferry D, Hammond L, Ransn M, et al: Intermittent oral ZD1839 (Iressa), a novel epidermal growth factor receptor tyrosine kinase inhibitor shows evidence of good tolerability and activity: Final results from a phase I study [abstract 5]. Proc Am Soc Clin Oncol 2000;19:3a.

71. Giaccone G, Johnson DH, Manegold C, et al: ESMO 2002;Ab4.

72. Johnson DH, Herbst R, Giaccone G, et al: ESMO 2002;Ab468.

73. Finkler N, Gordon A, Crozier M, et al: Phase 2 evaluation of OSI-774, a potent oral antagonist of the EGFR-TK in patients with advanced ovarian carcinoma [abstract 831]. Proc Am Soc Clin Oncol 2001;20:208a.

74. Plumb JA, Strathdee G, Sludden J, et al: Reversal of drug resistance in human tumor xenografts by 2′-deoxy-5-azacytidine-induced demethylation of the hMLH1 gene promoter. Cancer Res 2000;60:6039-6044.

75. Strathdee G, MacKean M, Illand M, et al: A role for methylation of the hMLH1 promoter in loss of hMLH1 expression and drug resistance in ovarian cancer. Oncogene 1999;18:2335-2341.

76. Yan PS, Chen CM, Shi H, et al: Applications of CpG island microarrays for high-throughput analysis of DNA methylation. J Nutr 2002;132(8 Suppl):2430S-2434S.

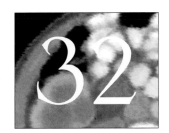

CHAPTER

DECISION-MAKING IN THE MANAGEMENT OF RECURRENT EPITHELIAL OVARIAN CANCER

Maurie Markman

 MAJOR CONTROVERSIES

- **What is the definition of second-line treatment of ovarian cancer?**
- **What are the goals of second-line therapy of ovarian cancer?**
- **What is the difference between potentially platinum-sensitive disease and platinum-resistant disease?**
- **Why reinitiate platinum as the initial second-line treatment option in patients with potentially platinum-sensitive ovarian cancer?**
- **What is the use of nonplatinum therapy in potentially platinum-sensitive recurrent ovarian cancer?**
- **What are additional questions regarding second-line platinum-based therapy in ovarian cancer?**
- **How should platinum-resistant ovarian cancer be treated?**
- **What is the role of radiation therapy in the second-line management of ovarian cancer?**
- **What is the role of surgical cytoreduction in the second-line treatment of ovarian cancer?**
- **What is the treatment for a rising CA 125 antigen level?**

Current state-of-the-art initial chemotherapy for advanced ovarian cancer is based on the results of a series of well-designed and -conducted randomized trials that compared a standard regimen to an experimental chemotherapy program.[1-5] Over the years, cytotoxic agents explored in these phase III ovarian cancer trials in the upfront setting were rationally selected based on prior evidence of objective biologic activity for the drugs in patients with well-characterized resistant disease. For example, cisplatin was examined in randomized trials as a component of initial therapy after it was shown that the agent produced tumor regression in women whose ovarian cancers were found to be refractory to alkylating agents.[6] Similarly, paclitaxel was evaluated in this clinical setting after

documentation of impressive activity in platinum-resistant ovarian cancer.[7,8]

The current large, international, five-arm randomized advanced ovarian trial being led by the Gynecologic Oncology Group (GOG) is exploring several new drugs (i.e., topotecan, liposomal doxorubicin, gemcitabine) added to a carboplatin/paclitaxel program. Justification for the inclusion of each of these drugs in this ambitious study is a previously observed antineoplastic effect in platinum-resistant disease.[9-14]

It is not currently possible to select an optimal treatment program for women with ovarian cancer that has failed to respond to treatment or that has recurred after the attainment of an initial response based on the results of similarly rationally conceived randomized trials. This is due to the fact the vast majority of second-line chemotherapy studies have been phase II, noncomparative trials, which may demonstrate a level of biologic activity for individual agents or combination regimens but do not reveal which program results in a superior clinical outcome (e.g., survival, quality of life).

Further, even the few randomized studies reported in this clinical area have failed to directly address the all-important question of what is optimal therapy for resistant or recurrent ovarian cancer. Rather, they have simply compared drug A with drug B, despite the fact that neither drug may be the appropriate control arm to address superiority or even equivalence of treatment.[9,12]

What is the definition of second-line treatment of ovarian cancer?

Before attempting to address decision-making in the second-line management of ovarian cancer, it is important to define what is meant by second-line treatment.[15] This is truly a misnomer, because currently the typical ovarian cancer patient in the United States receives, and may actually benefit from, multiple lines of chemotherapy during the course of her illness.[16] It is important to recognize that the term *second-line treatment* refers to *all treatment programs employed beyond the initial therapeutic regimen for the malignancy.*

Although this definition encompasses a highly heterogeneous patient population (e.g., a patient who demonstrates a rapidly enlarging pelvic mass after the initial two cycles of carboplatin/paclitaxel; an asymptomatic woman with a rising CA 125 antigen level 3 years after attainment of a surgically documented complete response to six courses of carboplatin/docetaxel), there is one critically important unifying feature associated with the delivery of antineoplastic therapy in this clinical setting: *All such treatment ultimately must be considered palliative in intent, because there is currently no evidence for the legitimate curative potential of any second-line treatment program in ovarian cancer.*

This statement does not preclude the possibility that extended survival may be experienced by individual patients after the initiation of a number of rationally conceived treatment approaches.[15,17,18] Rather, it is a simple (but important) acknowledgment of the fact that currently there are no known strategies that are capable of permanently eliminating ovarian cancer in this clinical setting.

What are the goals of second-line treatment of ovarian cancer?

In my opinion, there are a number of highly clinically meaningful and realistic goals of second-line therapy for ovarian cancer (Table 32-1). This list does *not* include "achieving an objective response" as an independent useful, or clinically meaningful, outcome of treatment

---

Table 32–1. Goals of Second-Line Therapy for Ovarian Cancer

1. Eliminate or reduce symptoms of the disease
2. Prolong symptom-free survival time
3. Optimize overall quality of life (which includes minimizing side effects of therapy)
4. Have a favorable impact on ultimate overall survival time

---

in this setting, despite the documented fact this is the principal feature employed in the large majority of clinical trials that attempt to measure benefit. However, it is appropriate to seriously question whether the mere "shrinkage of a tumor mass" or "a decline in the CA 125 antigen level" has any impact on the clinical course of an individual patient, other than the obvious psychological benefit associated with telling that woman her tumor is responding.

What is the relevance of a change in the diameter of a pelvic mass detected on physical examination or radiographic evaluation from 2.5 cm to 1 cm? What is the importance of a decline in the serum CA 125 concentration from 415 U/mL to 67 U/mL? An extremely strong argument can be advanced that unless such objective changes in tumor volume or burden affect one or more of the outcomes listed in Table 32-1 (e.g., symptoms of disease, survival), then all that has been observed is a biologic effect of the therapy, not a meaningful clinical effect. For example, was that shrinkage of tumor or decline in CA 125 associated with a decrease in pain, an improvement in appetite, or an ability of the patient to increase her level of routine daily activities? Or, did she have the same level of pain, and did she, in fact, become increasingly debilitated secondary to the severe fatigue associated with chemotherapy-induced neutropenia or anemia? The answers to these types of questions should substantially influence the interpretation of whether "achieving an objective response" has been a valid clinical outcome, both for an individual woman with ovarian cancer and for a population of patients treated on an investigative trial.

What is the difference between potentially platinum-sensitive disease and platinum-resistant disease?

Despite the lack of definitive data regarding optimal treatment in the second-line setting for women with ovarian cancer, extensive retrospective data have provided a strong justification for dividing patients being considered for such treatment into two broad categories: those with *potentially platinum-sensitive* disease and those with *platinum-resistant* disease.[15] Although exact definitions may differ, individuals with potentially platinum-sensitive disease include those who have demonstrated a response to prior platinum-based treatment and have not received therapy for a variable period of time. Some investigators have used a platinum-free interval or treatment-free interval of 6 months to separate those patients who are potentially sensitive from those who are considered to be resistant[8,19]; others have used a more stringent definition (e.g., 3-month treatment-free interval) to declare that a patient does or does not have a realistic chance to respond to the reinitiation of a platinum-based program.[20]

Regardless of the precise definition of the treatment-free interval employed in eligibility criteria for clinical trials, it is crucial to remember that the potential for retention of sensitivity to a platinum agent is a continuum, so that patients with an extended period of no treatment (e.g., 24 months) have a far greater probability of achieving a clinical response than do those with a shorter treatment-free interval (e.g., 6 to 9 months).[21-23] However, even patients with a relatively rapid recurrence of disease (e.g., 6 months) after an excellent initial response to combination platinum-based chemotherapy may experience a limited, but clinically meaningful, favorable impact on cancer-related symptoms (e.g., reduction in pain) after the reintroduction of a platinum-agent.[24]

Why reinitiate platinum as the initial second-line treatment option in patients with potentially platinum-sensitive ovarian cancer?

It is appropriate to ask why a platinum drug (carboplatin or cisplatin) should be the first choice for second-line therapy in a patient who might still be sensitive to this class of cytotoxic agents. In fact, all of the statements made in the previous section regarding the potential sensitivity of an individual patient's tumor to platinum (e.g., documented response, extended treatment-free interval) could also be made for taxanes (paclitaxel or docetaxel) as single-agent first-line therapy for ovarian cancer.[1-5] How do we know the patient's tumor does not remain equally (if not more) sensitive to the taxane?

Again, in absence of data from randomized trials in this clinical setting, a definitive answer to this highly clinically relevant question cannot be provided. However, limited existing data provide support for the conclusion that in appropriately selected patients a platinum drug should be considered as initial second-line therapy (Table 32-2).[15,21-28]

What is the use of nonplatinum therapy in potentially platinum-sensitive recurrent ovarian cancer?

To date, randomized phase III trials have not been conducted to demonstrate whether the readministration of a platinum agent as the initial choice for second-line therapy in potentially platinum-sensitive disease is superior, equivalent, or inferior to employment of an alternative cytotoxic drug.

A number of arguments can be presented to support the use of nonplatinum single-agent therapy in this

Table 32–2. Why Should a Platinum Agent Be Considered the Treatment of Choice as Initial Second-Line Therapy for Potentially Platinum-Sensitive Ovarian Cancer?

1. Platinum agents (cisplatin, carboplatin) are the single most active type of cytotoxic drugs in ovarian cancer.
2. Extensive data demonstrate the activity of platinum drugs (cisplatin, carboplatin) when employed in the second-line setting.
3. In the palliative setting, there is a relatively favorable impact of carboplatin on quality of life, such as ease of administration (30-min infusion), convenience of schedule (every 3-4 wk), and acceptable toxicity profile (lack of alopecia or significant emesis) in most patients.
4. A rational choice can be made before treatment is initiated, based on the prior toxicity experienced by the individual patient with this class of agents (e.g., prior emesis, marrow suppression, neurotoxicity from platinum-based therapy).
5. The patient has familiarity with the drug to be given (e.g., known toxicity profile).

clinical setting (Table 32-3).[29,30] However, in the selection of any second-line therapeutic option in ovarian cancer, whether the disease is potentially platinum sensitive or platinum resistant, the ultimate treatment goals (see Table 32-1) and the impact of therapy on quality of life must be seriously considered.

What are additional questions regarding second-line platinum-based therapy in ovarian cancer?

Although retrospective data have provided strong support for the delivery of platinum-based treatment as second-line therapy for ovarian cancer, there remain a number of important issues regarding the use of this class of agents (Table 32-4).

First, although data are now available to demonstrate that the high objective response rate to platinum-containing combination chemotherapy[17,31-33] can favorably affect survival in recurrent ovarian cancer,[34] it remains uncertain if an equivalent outcome might not result from the sequential use of active agents in this clinical setting. This point is particularly important when considering the goals of second-line therapy. If it

Table 32–3. Why Employ a Nonplatinum Strategy as Initial Second-Line Therapy for Potentially Platinum-Sensitive Ovarian Cancer?

1. To avoid the toxicities of platinum agents (e.g., neurotoxicity, emesis, bone marrow suppression)
2. To expose the tumor to a potentially non–cross-resistant cytotoxic drug
3. To extend the platinum-free interval, theoretically improving the chance that the tumor will respond to reintroduction of a platinum agent delivered later in the course of the disease
4. To avoid the potential for platinum hypersensitivity reactions
5. To try another drug, given the patient's knowledge that platinum-based therapy did not eliminate the malignancy

Table 32–4. Issues in the Use of Platinum-Based Second-Line Therapy for Ovarian Cancer

1. Single-agent versus combination platinum-based therapy
2. Duration of treatment in a patient experiencing either an objective response (e.g., decrease in tumor volume) or a subjective response (e.g., improvement in pain)
3. Role of dose intensity (e.g., intraperitoneal cisplatin, high-dose intravenous carboplatin-based regimen with stem cell support)
4. Management of platinum hypersensitivity reactions

is not possible to demonstrate that combination platinum-based chemotherapy results in a superior clinical outcome (e.g., more rapid reduction or complete elimination of symptoms, prolongation of survival), compared with the sequential delivery of single-agent platinum (usually carboplatin) treatment, followed by paclitaxel (or other drugs) how can the additional toxicity (e.g., alopecia, marrow suppression, neurotoxicity) be justified?

Second, in a patient who has exhibited a clinically meaningful response to treatment (e.g., major decrease in tumor volume, significant palliation of pain) and an acceptable tolerance of therapy, how long should the program be continued?[35] Although it may be rational for both the physician and patient to strongly consider treatment until disease progression occurs, the long-term side effect profile of therapy (e.g., persistent marrow suppression, induction of secondary leukemia, cardiac dysfunction) must not be forgotten. Prolonged therapy may also interfere with the administration of future beneficial treatment if it results in chronic marrow dysfunction. Further, there is always the potential that continued treatment can have an overall negative impact on quality of life (e.g., fatigue, alopecia, emesis, time and effort associated with drug delivery).

Third, considerable preclinical data and extensive phase II trial experience have suggested a possible role for dose intensity in the second-line treatment of ovarian cancer.[36,37] Trials have examined both regional (intraperitoneal) and systemic (high-dose chemotherapy with bone marrow or peripheral stem cell support) dose-intensive approaches as second-line treatments of ovarian cancer. At the present time, there are no data from randomized studies to demonstrate that the toxicity, inconvenience, and cost associated with any dose-intensive strategy favorably affect survival when used in this clinical setting. Despite this lack of phase III trial experience, some have argued that, in carefully selected patients (e.g., a physiologically younger woman with extensive intra-abdominal disease who demonstrates major inherent chemosensitivity to platinum-based treatment), the use of a platinum-based dose-intensive approach may be a valid management option. Randomized trials in this area are urgently needed, although a recent failed attempt in the United States to mount a phase III protocol examining high-dose systemic chemotherapy demonstrated the difficulty associated with initiating and completing complex (and controversial) studies in this patient population.

A final concern regarding platinum-based second-line therapy for ovarian cancer is the increasing recognition of the development of platinum-associated hypersensitivity reactions.[38-40] It is now understood that such reactions rarely occur during the initial treatment program (e.g., five or six courses) with either cisplatin or carboplatin. Considerable clinical experience has revealed that multiple treatment exposures, and a possible delay between first- and second-line use, are required for the susceptible patient to become "sensitized." When reactions occur, they can be mild (e.g., skin rash) or severe (e.g., anaphylactic shock). In one series, it was estimated that as many as 25% of patients receiving multiple courses of second-line platinum (mostly carboplatin) could ultimately experience some form of a hypersensitivity reaction, although only half of them would be anticipated to develop severe symptoms (e.g., hypotension, respiratory distress).[38]

There has been debate in the oncology literature as to whether patients who experience a significant platinum hypersensitivity reaction should be re-treated with the agent.[38-41] It is clear that delivery of the drug after documentation of hypersensitivity must be performed with great caution (e.g., use of methods designed to prevent anaphylactic reactions). Further, acknowledging the overall goals of second-line treatment of ovarian cancer, it is important that consideration be given to employing an alternative agent when an individual patient develops a significant platinum-associated hypersensitivity reaction.

How should platinum-resistant ovarian cancer be treated?

As previously noted, essentially all patients who experience recurrence after initial treatment of ovarian cancer eventually become platinum resistant, even if they respond on one (or several) occasions to reintroduction of second-line platinum.[15,16] Most patients with advanced ovarian cancer ultimately fall into this disease management category.

At least in the United States, patients often receive multiple agents during the course of their illness after the demonstration that their cancer is resistant to platinum.[15,16] As a result, the question often is not which agent should be used as second-line therapy for platinum-resistant ovarian cancer, but rather which agent should be attempted now and which agent or agents at a later time in the course of the disease?

The availability of CA 125 as a reliable biologic marker of disease progression has accentuated the problem of decision-making, because the failure of current therapy (or observation) can be known by both patient and physician, often months before the development of cancer-related symptoms.[42,43] Sustained rises in CA 125 frequently lead to a patient's request, and a physician's desire, to change therapy, even in the absence of any other clinical evidence of progressive disease. Although there is an obvious concern that a patient initiating chemotherapy based solely on a rise

Table 32–5. Considerations in the Selection of Second-Line Therapy for Platinum-Resistant Ovarian Cancer

1. Quality of available efficacy data (e.g., a phase III trial versus a single abstract describing a small number of patients treated at a single institution)
2. Individual physician familiarity with the drug (e.g., extensive knowledge of side effect profile)
3. Prior toxicity experienced by the patient (e.g., emesis, neurotoxicity, bone marrow suppression)
4. Established potential toxicity of available agents (e.g., topotecan and marrow suppression, weekly paclitaxel and neurotoxicity)
5. Specific comorbid medical conditions (e.g., known significant cardiac disease)
6. Convenience (e.g., difficulty of making frequent visits for treatment if patient lives far from physician's office)
7. Cost (e.g., refusal of insurance company to pay for oral medications)
8. Patient choice

in this tumor marker may experience the toxicity of treatment without any impact on either symptom-free survival or overall survival, it is understandable that documentation of disease progression may lead to a desire to start therapy in an attempt to delay or prevent the development of symptoms.

A number of clinical features can influence the decision regarding which treatment to use at a particular point in time in a patient's illness (Table 32-5). Individual patients and physicians will almost certainly weigh the importance of these items differently. Further, at a given point in a patient's illness a particular consideration may become more or less relevant for that individual. For example, returning to a physician's office for daily therapy may not be an issue for a nonworking older women who is able to care for herself, but as her health fails and an employed family member is required to leave work to take her to the clinic, this management approach can become quite problematic.

A number of antineoplastic agents have demonstrated biologic activity in women with platinum-resistant ovarian cancer (reported objective response rate greater than 10%) (Table 32-6).[15,9-14,44-55] There is

Table 32–6. Antineoplastic Agents with Documented Activity (>10% Objective Response Rate) in Platinum-Resistant Ovarian Cancer

Altretamine
Docetaxel
Epirubicin
Etoposide (oral, 21 days)
Gemcitabine
Ifosfamide
Irinotecan
Liposomal doxorubicin
Paclitaxel (every 3 weeks, weekly)
Tamoxifen
Topotecan
Vinorelbine

currently no evidence based on the results of randomized trials that one drug is superior to another in achieving an objective response or in prolonging progression-free survival or overall survival. Further, data do not exist to document the superiority of any particular agent in the more subjective parameter of "favorable impact on quality of life." The decision of which drug to use, and at what time in an individual patient's illness, should be made only after consideration of a number of general and specific issues (see Table 32-5).

The eventual use of multiple drugs in the majority of women with platinum-resistant ovarian cancer has led to two general schools of thought regarding the basic approach to selection of antineoplastic therapy. The first argues that patients should initially receive the least toxic and most convenient treatment to optimize their quality of life. As the disease progresses, other agents can then be employed. The counterargument states that the regimens of greater potential toxicity should be attempted as the initial second-line treatment, because at a time the patient has the best possible performance status and is more likely to be capable of withstanding the rigors of therapy. Later, when the disease progresses and the individual has a more limited ability to tolerate treatment (e.g., bone marrow suppression), the less aggressive strategies (e.g., tamoxifen) may be applied.

It also must be remembered that at some point in the course of the disease process, the option of supportive, comfort, or hospice care will need to be discussed. At the right time, the majority of patients will welcome, and many will even initiate, this discussion. However, others will seek to deny the reality of their situation and will continue to prefer the toxicity of therapy rather than accepting the fact that treatment can no longer alleviate symptoms or prolong survival. In such circumstances, judicious use of relatively nontoxic antineoplastic treatments (e.g., tamoxifen, lower-dose cytotoxic chemotherapy) is not an irrational option.

What is the role of radiation therapy in the second-line management of ovarian cancer?

For appropriately selected ovarian cancer patients with significant localized symptoms (e.g., pain due to an enlarging pelvic side wall mass), external beam radiation may be an important management approach.[56,57] This strategy is particularly relevant for individuals with documented platinum-resistant disease for whom the anticipated objective response rate and opportunity to observe clinically meaningful subjective improvement after the administration of additional chemotherapy is very limited. There appears to be little (if any) role for whole abdominal radiation therapy in the second-line treatment of ovarian cancer, because of the limited ability to deliver effective dosing over this large volume and the potential for severe treatment-related morbidity (e.g., bowel obstruction).

It should also be noted that occasionally ovarian cancer behaves in an atypical manner, one that is more characteristic of recurrent endometrial cancer. The tumors of such patients may exhibit chemoresistance, recurring rapidly after completion of chemotherapy, or they may never respond to initial treatment. However, despite this highly unfavorable clinical characteristic, the cancer remains confined to the pelvic region (documented initially on computed tomographic scan of the abdomen/pelvis and confirmed at a subsequent exploratory laparotomy or laparoscopy). In this uncommon clinical setting, it would not be unreasonable to treat the patient with a more intensive approach to the use of external-beam radiation to the pelvis (i.e., curative rather than palliative dosing), designed to reduce the chances of progressive symptomatic disease in this region and possibly to substantially prolong overall survival time. In the rare situation in which a patient experiences several recurrences in the same location (e.g., pelvic lymph nodes), consideration should also be given to local radiation of the area after surgical removal of any mass lesions.

What is the role of surgical cytoreduction in the second-line treatment of ovarian cancer?

One of the most controversial questions in the second-line treatment of ovarian cancer is the possible role of surgery before (or after) initiation of cytotoxic chemotherapy.[58-62] In the setting of a prolonged treatment-free interval (e.g., longer than 24 months), if an isolated mass of several centimeters is present on computed tomographic scanning, surgical removal is not inappropriate before chemotherapy is restarted. The supporting argument is that such a patient has a high probability (greater than 60%) of responding to platinum-based treatment, and removal of gross tumor will enhance the opportunity to deliver active drugs all to sites of residual cancer.[21-23] However, although this is a rational strategy, no controlled trial data currently exist to document the superiority of this approach in comparison with platinum-based chemotherapy alone.

It is more difficult to develop a strong rationale to support the use of aggressive surgical cytoreduction in patients whose cancers are likely to be minimally chemosensitive (e.g., those with a short treatment-free interval before disease progression). Although it may be possible to remove considerable tumor volume, the impact of this surgery on the natural history of such a cancer should be questioned in the absence of evidence that subsequent chemotherapy can successfully interfere with rapid regrowth of the malignancy. Randomized trials are clearly needed to directly address this question.

In the setting of recurrent, persistent, or resistant ovarian cancer, carefully selected patients are appropriate candidates for palliative surgical procedures (e.g., colostomy, ileostomy).[63,64]

What is the treatment for a rising CA 125 antigen level?

As previously noted, the availability of the serum CA 125 antigen level as a highly predictive marker for disease progression in ovarian cancer has led to the relatively common situation in which this laboratory test is the sole evidence of failure of the current management strategy (e.g., ongoing active antineoplastic therapy or observation after the completion of a treatment program).[42,43,65] In the absence of other manifestations of progressive cancer (e.g., measurable symptoms, ascites), what is the optimal approach to patient management?

Should patients be restarted on chemotherapy or switched to alternative drugs with any documented elevation in CA 125 from their prior baseline determination, or after a predefined rate of rise, or after the level has doubled, tripled, or quadrupled? Does institution of such therapy in the absence of symptomatic disease progression favorably affect survival time or time to the development of symptoms? Currently, the answers to these highly clinically relevant questions are unknown. It is hoped that the results of an ongoing randomized trial being conducted in Europe, which examines the issue of treatment of an asymptomatic rise in the CA 125 antigen level, will provide useful guidance to practicing oncologists.

For the present, physicians need to individualize recommendations and actively include patients in the decision-making process. In particular, patients should be informed that there is currently no evidence that altering therapy based solely on small changes in this serum tumor marker favorably affects the course of disease. Further, the negative impact on quality of life associated with treatment of an asymptomatic patient with cytotoxic chemotherapy must be considered.

REFERENCES

1. McGuire WP, Hoskins WJ, Brady MF, et al: Cyclophosphamide and cisplatin compared with paclitaxel and cisplatin in patients with stage III and stage IV ovarian cancer. N Engl J Med 1996; 334:1-6.
2. Piccart MJ, Bertelsen K, James K, et al: Randomized intergroup trial of cisplatin-paclitaxel versus cisplatin-cyclophosphamide in women with advanced epithelial ovarian cancer: Three-year results. J Natl Cancer Inst 2000;92:699-708.
3. Ozols RF, Bundy BN, Fowler J, et al: Randomized phase III study of cisplatin (CIS)/paclitaxel (PAC) versus carboplatin (CARBO)/PAC in optimal stage III epithelial ovarian cancer (OC): A Gynecologic Oncology Group Trial (GOG 158). Proc Am Soc Clin Oncol 1999;18:356a.
4. du Bois A, Lueck HJ, Meier W, et al: Cisplatin/paclitaxel vs carboplatin/paclitaxel in ovarian cancer: Update of an Arbeitsgemeinschaft Gynaekologische Onkologie (AGO) study group trial. Proc Am Soc Clin Oncol 1999;18:356a.
5. Vasey PA on behalf of the Scottish Gynaecological Cancer Trials Group: Survival and longer-term toxicity results of the SCOTROC study: Docetaxel-carboplatin (DC) vs. paclitaxel-carboplatin (PC) in epithelial ovarian cancer (EOC). Proc Am Soc Clin Oncol 2002;21:202a.
6. Katz ME, Schwartz PE, Kapp DS, Luikart S: Epithelial carcinoma of the ovary: Current strategies. Ann Intern Med 1981;95: 98-111.

7. McGuire WP, Rowinsky EK, Rosenshein NB, et al: Taxol: A unique antineoplastic agent with significant activity in advanced ovarian epithelial neoplasms. Ann Intern Med 1989;111:273-279.

8. Thigpen JT, Blessing JA, Ball H, et al: Phase II trial of paclitaxel in patients with progressive ovarian carcinoma after platinum-based chemotherapy: A Gynecologic Oncology Group study. J Clin Oncol 1994;12:1748-1753.

9. ten Bokkel Huinink W, Gore M, Carmichael J, et al: Topotecan versus paclitaxel for the treatment of recurrent epithelial ovarian cancer. J Clin Oncol 1997;15:2183-2193.

10. Bookman MA, Malmstrom H, Bolis G, et al: Topotecan for the treatment of advanced epithelial ovarian cancer: An open-label phase II study in patients treated after prior chemotherapy that contained cisplatin or carboplatin and paclitaxel. J Clin Oncol 1998;16:3345-3352.

11. Muggia FM, Hainsworth JD, Jeffers S, et al: Phase II study of liposomal doxorubicin in refractory ovarian cancer: Antitumor activity and toxicity modification by liposomal encapsulation. J Clin Oncol 1997;15:987-993.

12. Gordon AN, Fleagle JT, Guthrie D, et al: Recurrent epithelial ovarian carcinoma: A randomized phase III study of pegylated liposomal doxorubicin versus topotecan. J Clin Oncol 2001;19:3312-3322.

13. Lund B, Hansen OP, Theilade K, et al: Phase II study of gemcitabine (2',2'-difluorodeoxycytidine) in previously treated ovarian cancer patients. J Natl Cancer Inst 1994;86:1530-1533.

14. Shapiro JD, Millward MJ, Rischin D, et al: Activity of gemcitabine in patients with advanced ovarian cancer: Responses seen following platinum and paclitaxel. Gynecol Oncol 1996;63:89-93.

15. Markman M, Bookman MA: Second-line treatment of ovarian cancer. The Oncologist 2000;5:26-35.

16. Markman M: Why study third-, fourth-, fifth-,. .. line chemotherapy of ovarian cancer? Gynecol Oncol 2001;83:449-450.

17. Rose PG, Fusco N, Fluellen L, Rodriguez M: Second-line therapy with paclitaxel and carboplatin for recurrent disease following first-line therapy with paclitaxel and platinum in ovarian or peritoneal carcinoma. J Clin Oncol 1998;16:1494-1497.

18. Markman M, Kennedy A, Webster K, et al: Continued chemosensitivity to cisplatin/carboplatin in ovarian carcinoma despite treatment with multiple prior platinum-based regimens. Gynecol Oncol 1997;65:434-436.

19. McGuire WP, Blessing JA, Bookman MA, et al: Topotecan has substantial antitumor activity as first-line salvage therapy in platinum-sensitive epithelial ovarian carcinoma: A Gynecologic Oncology Group study. J Clin Oncol 2000;18:1062-1067.

20. Markman M, Hall J, Spitz D, et al: Phase II trial of weekly single-agent paclitaxel in platinum/paclitaxel-refractory ovarian cancer. J Clin Oncol 2002;20:2365-2369.

21. Gore ME, Fryatt I, Wiltshaw E, Dawson T: Treatment of relapsed carcinoma of the ovary with cisplatin or carboplatin following initial treatment with these compounds. Gynecol Oncol 1990;36:207-211.

22. Markman M, Rothman R, Hakes T, et al: Second-line platinum therapy in patients with ovarian cancer previously treated with cisplatin. J Clin Oncol 1991;9:389-393.

23. Hoskins PJ, O'Reilly SE, Swenerton KD: The "failure free interval" defines the likelihood of resistance to carboplatin in patients with advanced epithelial ovarian cancer previously treated with cisplatin: Relevance to therapy and new drug testing. Int J Gynecol Cancer 1991;1:205-208.

24. Markman M, Kennedy A, Webster K, et al: Evidence that a "treatment-free interval of less than 6 months" does not equate with clinically defined platinum resistance in ovarian cancer or primary peritoneal carcinoma. J Cancer Res Clin Oncol 1998;124:326-328.

25. Gershenson DM, Kavanagh JJ, Copeland LJ, et al: Re-treatment of patients with recurrent epithelial ovarian cancer with cisplatin-based chemotherapy. Obstet Gynecol 1989;73:798-802.

26. Seltzer V, Vogl S, Kaplan B: Recurrent ovarian carcinoma: Retreatment utilizing combination chemotherapy including cis-diamminedichloroplatinum in patients previously responding to this agent. Gynecol Oncol 1985;21:167-176.

27. Muggia FM, Braly PS, Brady MF, et al: Phase III randomized study of cisplatin versus paclitaxel versus cisplatin and paclitaxel in patients with suboptimal stage III or IV ovarian cancer: A Gynecologic Oncology Group study. J Clin Oncol 2000;18:106-115.

28. Cantu MG, Buda A, Parma G, et al: Randomized controlled trial of single-agent paclitaxel versus cyclophosphamide, doxorubicin, and cisplatin in patients with recurrent ovarian cancer who responded to first-line platinum-based regimens. J Clin Oncol 2002;20:1232-1237.

29. Bookman MA: Extending the platinum-free interval in recurrent ovarian cancer: The role of topotecan in second-line chemotherapy. Oncologist 1999;4:87-94.

30. Kavanagh J, Tresukosol D, Edwards C, et al: Carboplatin reinduction after taxane in patients with platinum-refractory epithelial ovarian cancer. J Clin Oncol 1995;13:1584-1588.

31. Gronlund B, Hogdall C, Hansen HH, Engelholm SA: Results of reinduction therapy with paclitaxel and carboplatin in recurrent epithelial ovarian cancer. Gynecol Oncol 2001;83:128-134.

32. Dizon DS, Hensley ML, Poynor EA, et al: Retrospective analysis of carboplatin and paclitaxel as initial second-line therapy for recurrent epithelial ovarian carcinoma: Application toward a dynamic disease state model of ovarian cancer. J Clin Oncol 2002;20:1238-1247.

33. Roland PY, Barnes MN, Niwas S, et al: Response to salvage treatment in recurrent ovarian cancer treated initially with paclitaxel and platinum-based combination regimens. Gynecol Oncol 1998;68:178-182.

34. The ICOn and AGO Collaborators. Paclitaxel plus platinum-based chemotherapy versus conventional platinum-based chemotherapy in women with relapsed ovarian cancer: The ICON4/AGO-OVAR-2.2 trial. Lancet 2003;361:2099-2196.

35. Eltabbakh GH, Piver MS, Hempling RE, et al: Prolonged disease-free survival by maintenance chemotherapy among patients with recurrent platinum-sensitive ovarian cancer. Gynecol Oncol 1998;71:190-195.

36. Stiff PJ, Veum-Stone J, Lazarus HM, et al: High-dose chemotherapy and autologous stem-cell transplantation for ovarian cancer: An autologous blood and marrow transplant registry report. Ann Intern Med 2000;133:504-515.

37. Barakat RR, Sabbatini P, Bhaskaran D, et al: Intraperitoneal chemotherapy for ovarian carcinoma: Results of long-term follow-up. J Clin Oncol 2002;20:694-698.

38. Markman M, Kennedy A, Webster K, et al: Clinical features of hypersensitivity reactions to carboplatin. J Clin Oncol 1999;17:1141-1145.

39. Robinson JB, Singh D, Bodurka-Bevers DC, et al: Hypersensitivity reactions and the utility of oral and intravenous desensitization in patients with gynecologic malignancies. Gynecol Oncol 2001;82:550-558.

40. Rose PG, Fusco N, Fluellen L, Rodriguez M: Carboplatin hypersensitivity reactions in patients with ovarian and peritoneal carcinoma. Int J Gynecol Cancer 1998;8:365-368.

41. Zanotti KM, Rybicki LA, Kennedy AW, et al: Carboplatin skin testing: A skin-testing protocol for predicting hypersensitivity to carboplatin chemotherapy. J Clin Oncol 2001;19:3126-3129.

42. Markman M: CA-125: An evolving role in the management of ovarian cancer. J Clin Oncol 1996;14:1411-1412.

43. Rustin GJS, Nelstrop AE, Tuxen MK, Lambert HE: Defining progression of ovarian carcinoma during follow-up according to CA 125: A North Thames Ovary Group study. Ann Oncol 1996;7:361-364.

44. Piccart MJ, Gore M, ten Bokkel Huinink W, et al: Docetaxel: An active new drug for treatment of advanced epithelial ovarian cancer. J Natl Cancer Inst 1995;87:676-681.

45. Verschraegen CF, Sittisomwong T, Kudelka AP, et al: Docetaxel for patients with paclitaxel-resistant müllerian carcinoma. J Clin Oncol 2000;18:2733-2739.

46. Vergote I, Himmelmann A, Frankendal B, et al: Hexamethylmelamine as second-line therapy in platin-resistant ovarian cancer. Gynecol Oncol 1992;47:282-286.

47. Markman M, Blessing JA, Moore D, et al: Altretamine (hexamethylmelamine) in platinum-resistant and platinum-refractory ovarian cancer: A Gynecologic Oncology Group phase II trial. Gynecol Oncol 1998;69:226-229.

48. Hoskins PJ, Swenerton KD: Oral etoposide is active against platinum-resistant epithelial ovarian cancer. J Clin Oncol 1994;12:60-63.

49. Rose PG, Blessing JA, Mayer AR, Homesley HD: Prolonged oral etoposide as second-line therapy for platinum-resistant and platinum-sensitive ovarian carcinoma: A Gynecologic Oncology Group study. J Clin Oncol 1998;16:405-410.

50. Sutton GP, Blessing JA, Homesley HD, et al: Phase II trial of ifosfamide and mesna in advanced ovarian carcinoma: A Gynecologic Oncology Group study. J Clin Oncol 1989;7:1672-1676.

51. Markman M, Kennedy A, Sutton G, et al: Phase 2 trial of single agent ifosfamide/mesna in patients with platinum/paclitaxel refractory ovarian cancer who have not previously been treated with an alkylating agent. Gynecol Oncol 1998;70:272-274.

52. Bajetta E, Di Leo A, Biganzoli L, et al: Phase II study of vinorelbine in patients with pretreated advanced ovarian cancer: Activity in platinum-resistant disease. J Clin Oncol 1996;14:2546-2551.

53. Gershenson DM, Burke TW, Morris M, et al: A phase I study of a daily × 3 schedule of intravenous vinorelbine for refractory epithelial ovarian cancer. Gynecol Oncol 1998;70:404-409.

54. Havsteen H, Bertelsen K, Gadeberg CC, et al: A phase 2 study with epirubicin as second-line treatment of patients with advanced epithelial ovarian cancer. Gynecol Oncol 1996;63:210-215.

55. Perez-Gracia JL, Carrasco EM: Tamoxifen therapy for ovarian cancer in the adjuvant and advanced settings: Systematic review of the literature and implications for future research. Gynecol Oncol 2002;84:201-209.

56. Davidson SA, Rubin SC, Mychalczak B, et al: Limited-field radiotherapy as salvage treatment of localized persistent or recurrent epithelial ovarian cancer. Gynecol Oncol 1993;51:349-354.

57. Corn BW, Lanciano RM, Boente M, et al: Recurrent ovarian cancer: Effective radiotherapeutic palliation after chemotherapy failure. Cancer 1994;74:2979-2983.

58. Segna RA, Dottino PR, Mandeli JP, et al: Secondary cytoreduction for ovarian cancer following cisplatin therapy. J Clin Oncol 1993;11:434-439.

59. Gadducci A, Iacconi P, Cosio S, et al: Complete salvage surgical cytoreduction improves further survival of patients with late recurrent ovarian cancer. Gynecol Oncol 2000;79:344-349.

60. Munkarah A, Levenback C, Wolf JK, et al: Secondary cytoreductive surgery for localized intra-abdominal recurrences in epithelial ovarian cancer. Gynecol Oncol 2001;81:237-241.

61. Bristow RE, Lagasse LD, Karlan BY: Secondary surgical cytoreduction for advanced epithelial ovarian cancer: Patient selection and review of the literature. Cancer 1996;78:2049-2062.

62. Eisenkop SM, Friedman RL, Wang H-J: Secondary cytoreductive surgery for recurrent ovarian cancer: A prospective study. Cancer 1995;76:1606-1614.

63. Rubin SC, Hoskins WJ, Benjamin I, Lewis JL Jr: Palliative surgery for intestinal obstruction in advanced ovarian cancer. Gynecol Oncol 1989;34:16-19.

64. Feuer DJ, Broadley KE, Shepherd JH, Barton DPJ: Systematic review of surgery in malignant bowel obstruction in advanced gynecological and gastrointestinal cancer. Gynecol Oncol 1999;75:313-322.

65. van Dalen A, Favier J, Burges A, et al: Prognostic significance of CA 125 and TPS levels after 3 chemotherapy courses in ovarian cancer patients. Gynecol Oncol 2000;79:444-450.

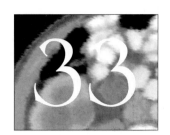

SECONDARY SURGERY FOR EPITHELIAL OVARIAN CANCER

James L Nicklin

- **What is the place of secondary surgery after suboptimal response to primary treatment?**
- **What is the place of second-look surgery?**
- **What is the place of second-look laparoscopy?**
- **What is the place of debulking surgery at the time of second-look surgery?**
- **What is the place for consolidation therapy after negative second-look surgery?**
- **What is the place of secondary cytoreductive surgery?**
- **What is the role of interval cytoreductive surgery?**

Secondary surgery for epithelial ovarian cancer may be defined as surgery undertaken at some time after the completion of primary treatment. This broad definition includes second-look laparotomy and secondary cytoreductive surgery. *Second-look laparotomy* is a comprehensive surgical staging procedure that is performed on patients who are clinically free of disease at the completion of a primary treatment program. *Secondary cytoreductive surgery* is defined as surgical debulking of recurrent malignancy after clinical remission is achieved by primary treatment. *Interval cytoreductive surgery*, typically a part of the primary management of epithelial ovarian cancer, is defined as a surgical attempt at tumor debulking after a limited course of chemotherapy, usually two to four cycles.

What is the place of secondary surgery after suboptimal response to primary treatment?

Few studies have specifically addressed the issue of secondary cytoreductive surgery in the patient population with progressive or chemoresistant, clinically demonstrable disease at the completion of primary therapy.[1-3] These studies report a modest surgical achievement of meaningful tumor debulking. Only

42% to 55% of patients had surgical cytoreduction of tumor down to less than 2 cm of residual disease.[1,2] In the study by Michel and colleagues,[1] the survival characteristics of patients with optimal and suboptimal cytoreduction were almost identical. By contrast, the study by Morris and colleagues[2] did show a survival advantage for patients whose disease could be optimally debulked. The median survival time for patients left with disease smaller than 2 cm was 12 months, compared with 7.8 months for patients with larger residual disease ($P < .03$). However, survival curves converged after 2 years. If the disease could be resected down to a maximum diameter of less than 1 cm, the median survival time was 19.5 months, compared with a median of 8.3 months for patients with residual disease greater than 1 cm ($P < .004$).[2] Given the morbidity of surgery, the low incidence of meaningful cytoreduction, and the limited survival benefit, there is little justification for surgery in this circumstance.

Patients with macroscopic disease at the time of second-look laparotomy are comparable to those patients with clinically evident disease at the completion of chemotherapy. By definition, their disease is chemoresistant, but it typically is of smaller volume and is not detected during the standard workup before second-look surgery (SLS).

What is the place of second-look surgery?

SLS is performed primarily as a means of most accurately establishing disease status at the completion of primary treatment. There is also an opportunity for therapeutic intervention in the form of secondary cytoreduction if macroscopic disease is encountered. The sensitivity of nonoperative imaging modalities in determining disease status has proved inferior to that of surgical evaluation. Computed tomography scanning, ultrasonography, magnetic resonance imaging, positron emission tomography, and even radioimmunoscintigraphy have each been demonstrated to be inferior to surgical evaluation.[4-16]

SLS is a meticulous, systematic surgical evaluation of the entire peritoneal cavity and retroperitoneal areas at risk for metastatic disease. Saline washings are taken from all areas of the peritoneal cavity. After division of any adhesions, multiple biopsies are taken from representative areas of the entire peritoneal cavity, including any scar tissue excised during adhesiolysis. The sites of previous known disease, particularly any residual disease after primary surgery, are at greatest risk for demonstration of persistent disease.[17] These areas warrant careful evaluation and generous tissue sampling.[18] If hysterectomy, salpingo-oophorectomy, omentectomy, appendectomy, and lymph node sampling were not previously performed, they can be completed at the time of SLS. The number of biopsies taken is left to the discretion of the surgeon. Ozols and associates[19] suggested that a SLS with grossly negative findings should produce 20 to 30 biopsy specimens.

The philosophy of SLS is predicated on the belief that early identification of resistant disease can allow instigation of salvage treatment strategies that may alter the long-term course of disease. SLS was enthusiastically embraced particularly during the 1980s; however, in the absence of data from randomized trials, the pendulum has swung away from this as standard therapy.[20,21]

A large number of retrospective studies have attempted to correlate the influence of features of the primary management of disease with findings at SLS.[4-16,22-49] These studies include heterogeneous patient populations, tumor characteristics, chemotherapeutic approaches, and surgical philosophies. Recognizing this, the following clinical features have been found to correlate with second-look findings: tumor stage, residual disease after primary surgery, and tumor grade. The variables of age and chemotherapy type and duration have a weak correlation with SLS findings.

The clinical variable with the strongest influence on second-look findings is stage. For patients with stage I disease, approximately 80% to 95% have negative second-look findings.[22,24,28,29,31,32,34-37,39,40-44,46-48,50-55] Between 70% and 75% of those with stage II disease have negative second-look findings, but only 33% to 50% of those with either stage III or stage IV disease do so.[22,24,28,29,31,32,34-37,39,40,42-44,46-48,50-56] Because earlier studies included patients with stage I and II disease who did

not undergo complete staging (and therefore included some patients with occult advanced disease), it is probable that the true negative second-look rate in this group is closer to the higher rate quoted.

The amount of residual disease after primary surgery has been found to correlate with second-look findings. Patients with no residual disease have a negative second-look rate of approximately 75%. The greater the volume of residual disease at primary surgery, the greater the likelihood of disease at SLS. Patients left with bulky residual disease after primary surgery have an approximately 25% chance of negative findings at SLS.[22-26,29-31,35-37,39,48,49]

Although no study has been able to demonstrate grade of tumor to be independently prognostic of findings at SLS, an inverse trend has been demonstrated consistently between grade of disease and negative findings at second-look laparotomy.[22-24,26,29-31,35-37,39,48,49] Approximately 60% of patients with grade I tumors have a negative second-look laparotomy, compared with 45% for grade II and 42% for grade III.[7,57] Patients with grade I tumors are more likely to have early-stage disease and no residual disease after primary surgery.

Based on the aforementioned correlates, some investigators have developed predictive formulas to identify patients who are most likely to benefit from a second-look procedure.[39,58]

The morbidity and mortality of second-look laparotomy is well established. The surgical mortality has been estimated at 1 per 1000 patients. The rate of infectious, pulmonary, and gastrointestinal complications is predictably less than that observed at primary laparotomy.[59] Minor morbidity rates are 15% to 50% (depending on definition), and major morbidity rates are less than 5%.[18,22-38,40-49,57,60-62] As a generalization, second-look laparotomy is a feasible and safe procedure.[18,22-38,40-49,57,59-62]

In the absence of randomized data demonstrating a survival benefit, there is little place for patients with epithelial ovarian cancer to undergo second-look laparotomy after primary therapy. SLS should therefore be confined largely to patients enrolled in clinical trials.

What is the place of second-look laparoscopy?

There are limited data on the feasibility and efficacy of laparoscopy as an alternative to laparotomy for SLS. By definition, such surgery is conducted on patients who have undergone prior extensive open surgery and may have widespread adhesive disease. There is also a significant learning curve with such surgery. From the published studies, laparoscopic SLS appears feasible, with accuracy rates for recurrent disease approaching those quoted for open surgery and acceptably low morbidity rates. The rate of conversion to laparotomy ranges from 10% to 21%.[63-65] This includes conversion because of extensive adhesions, management of complications, and elective conversion to facilitate secondary cytoreductive surgery. By comparison with open surgery, laparoscopic SLS has been associated with a significantly lower mean blood loss, shorter operating time, shorter hospital stay, lower total hospital charges, and fewer biopsies.[64,65] The rate of positive second-look laparoscopy has been reported to be 54% to 62.5%, which is comparable with most series of patients treated by open surgery.[63-65] In the series by Clough and coworkers,[66] 20 patients were treated with second-look laparoscopy followed immediately by comparative laparotomy. Six of the 20 patients were found to have persistent disease on laparoscopy, but there were 2 false-negative cases among the remaining 14 patients. The rate of "complete intraperitoneal investigation" was 95% for the open group but only 41% for the laparoscopy group.

It is apparent that the role of laparoscopy in SLS is still evolving and that the final place for this technique is yet to be determined. At the very least, the early results suggest that this technique is feasible and safe and may be a part of the armamentarium after complete clinical remission at the completion of primary therapy. Furthermore, laparoscopic SLS may be complementary to laparotomy, particularly for patients found to have bulky disease, who may benefit from elective conversion to laparotomy for cytoreductive surgery. However, in the absence of data to support the routine use of second-look laparotomy for patients with epithelial ovarian cancer, the place of second-look laparoscopy is even less well established. Second-look laparoscopy should be largely limited to patients enrolled in clinical trials.

What is the place of debulking surgery at the time of second-look surgery?

Macroscopic disease encountered at SLS is associated with a poor prognosis.[67] The place of secondary cytoreductive surgery at the time of SLS is controversial. Studies by Hoskins[68] and Potter[69] and their associates, as well as others,[49,70] have demonstrated a statistically significant survival advantage for patients who are left with no macroscopic residual disease, compared with those with any macroscopic disease at the completion of SLS. More recent studies by Obermair and Sevelda[71] and by Gadducci and colleagues[72] could not confirm the results of these earlier studies.

Based on the conflicting evidence from the literature, it seems prudent to make a decision about the appropriateness of debulking surgery at the time of operation. The following factors need to be considered: the extent and distribution of disease, the general health of the patient, the likelihood of achieving a complete macroscopic clearance, and the suitability for further chemotherapy. It seems appropriate to proceed with debulking surgery if there is a high expectation of achieving optimal clearance and a low expectation for significant morbidity. As with patients who have microscopically positive SLS, cytoreductive surgery in this circumstance typically would be followed by further active treatment, such as systemic or intraperitoneal chemotherapy.

What is the place for consolidation therapy after negative second-look surgery?

The prognosis of patients with a negative second-look operation is good, but recurrent disease is not uncommon. The factors that influence findings at the time of SLS also influence the likelihood of recurrent disease after negative SLS.[56] Furthermore, the longer the follow-up period, the greater the incidence of recurrence.[73] The incidence of recurrent disease after negative SLS has been reported to range from 0% to 52%, with a median time to recurrence ranging from 14 to 24 months and median survival time after the diagnosis of recurrence ranging from 11 to 45 months.[56,73-79]

Because of the significant incidence of recurrent disease in this patient population, a number of consolidation therapies have been investigated in an attempt to further improve survival. These include intraperitoneal phosphorus 32, intraperitoneal chemotherapy, whole abdominal radiation therapy, continued systemic chemotherapy, high-dose chemotherapy with stem cell rescue, hormone therapy, and biologic therapies. The Gynecologic Oncology Group (GOG) completed a randomized trial of consolidation intraperitoneal ^{32}P versus no further therapy, but the results are yet to be published. Nonrandomized trials and retrospective series of intraperitoneal ^{32}P have shown conflicting results, with relapse rates ranging from 0% to 47%.[80-82] Intraperitoneal chemotherapy regimens that have been evaluated include three cycles of cisplatin,[83,84] three to six cycles of mitoxantrone,[84,85] and three cycles of cisplatin and etoposide.[86] These studies reported recurrence rates of 21% to 26%. The Southwestern Oncology Group (SWOG) is currently investigating use of intraperitoneal interferon-α. The Royal Hospital for Women in Sydney, Australia, is evaluating the role of high-dose-rate chemotherapy and stem cell rescue, and The Royal Prince Alfred Hospital, Sydney, Australia is investigating the role of tamoxifen as consolidation therapy. Outside a trial setting, the standard of care for patients with negative SLS is expectant observation.

The GOG and SWOG recently presented the findings of a randomized trial of 12 versus 3 months of single-agent paclitaxel in patients with advanced epithelial ovarian cancer who had achieved a complete response to primary surgery and platinum- and paclitaxel-based chemotherapy.[87] Although neither arm of the study represents the currently accepted gold standard of treatment in this circumstance, the 12-month arm showed a median progression-free survival advantage of 28 months, compared with 21 months in the 3-month arm ($P = .0023$). At the time of presentation of the study, with few deaths in the study population, there was no difference in overall survival.

Consolidation treatment with whole abdominal radiation therapy has been reported in a number of small studies.[88-90] Median survival times of 72 to 95 months were reported; however, when comparisons were made with nonirradiated patients, no difference in survival could be demonstrated.[88-90]

With the absence of data to support SLS as part of standard clinical management of patients with ovarian carcinoma, it is likely that future trials of consolidation therapy will follow findings of "clinical complete response" rather than "negative second-look laparotomy."

What is the place of secondary cytoreductive surgery?

Recurrent epithelial ovarian cancer is associated with a poor prognosis. The optimal treatment of recurrent disease is not well established, and the place of secondary cytoreductive surgery is controversial. There is a paucity of studies that address the issue. Most studies have been retrospective and have included heterogeneous patient populations with considerable variation in tumor biology. There has been variability in the extent of previous surgery, the extent and type of previous chemotherapy, the time to diagnosis, and the extent of disease at the time of diagnosis of recurrence. As with primary disease, tumor biology probably significantly influences resectability and certainly influences chemosensitivity.

There are a number of theoretical benefits to secondary cytoreductive surgery. As with primary disease, bulky masses of recurrent tumor may be poorly perfused and hypoxic, with a low growth fraction. This may be associated with relative resistance to chemotherapy. Furthermore, large masses of tumor may be associated with gastrointestinal obstruction, nutritional compromise, metabolic abnormalities, and relative immunosuppression. Secondary debulking also allows the opportunity to collect tumor for in vitro chemosensitivity analysis. Although there is substantial evidence in advanced primary disease that optimal surgical cytoreduction followed by chemotherapy is associated with improved progression-free and overall survival times, the place for this approach in the management of recurrent disease is becoming increasingly established.

A number of retrospective studies[50-52,91-96] and a single large prospective series[97] have addressed the feasibility and outcome of secondary cytoreductive surgery for recurrent epithelial ovarian cancer. Although the volume and distribution of disease partly predetermine some of the outcomes of surgery, the radicality or comprehensiveness of the surgery also has an impact on morbidity and probably on survival. This is largely determined by the training, experience, and philosophy of the surgeon.

The morbidity and mortality rates and length of hospital stay for patients undergoing secondary cytoreductive surgery are comparable to those quoted for patients undergoing primary cytoreductive surgery. Operative times have been reported to range from 45 to 600 minutes, median transfusion rates from 0 to 3 units, and mortality rates from 0% to 3.3%. Depending on definition, morbidity rates approximate 30% and range from 16% to 44%. The surgical morbidity profile is reflective of the nature of the surgery, with prolonged ileus, small-bowel obstruction, pulmonary complications (pneumonia and atelectasis), febrile morbidity, urinary tract infection, and wound infection the most commonly reported complications.[50-54,91-97] These can be managed satisfactorily in subspecialty gynecologic oncology units.

The distribution of disease and the radicality of the surgeon's approach largely determine the extent of surgery. The large prospective series reported by Eisenkop and associates[97] merits special attention. To achieve optimal debulking, this team was prepared to perform such procedures as small- and large-bowel resections, stripping of the diaphragm, splenectomy, distal pancreatectomy, axillary node dissection, inguinal node dissection, pleural implant ablation, partial liver resection, and even partial lung resection. They achieved an impressive optimal cytoreductive rate, with 82% of patients left with no macroscopic evidence of residual disease at the completion of surgery. They had an overall morbidity rate of 32.1%, a mortality rate of 1.9%, and a median survival time of 44.4 months in the group with optimal cytoreduction.

In the two largest reported series, by Scarabelli[93] and Eisenkop[97] and their colleagues, 8.7% and 4.7% of patients, respectively, experienced disease progression or postoperative compromise to the extent that the patient could not proceed with chemotherapy.

Table 33-1 is a summary of the world literature regarding secondary cytoreductive surgery for patients with recurrent ovarian cancer. The definition of optimal cytoreduction ranged from no macroscopic disease to less than 2 cm residual. Optimal cytoreduction rates of 38% to 82% were achieved and resulted in statistically superior median survival times in all except two small retrospective studies. Median survival time in the group with optimal cytoreduction ranged from 18 to 56.9 months, compared with 5 to 23 months in the group with suboptimal cytoreduction. All but the smallest studies were amenable to multivariate analysis, and the extent of residual disease consistently was found to be an independent prognostic variable for survival.[50,51,92,93,95,97] In the larger studies, the disease-free interval was found to be positively associated with overall survival time.[51,93,95,97] A disease-free interval of greater than 12 months was the most common and useful criterion in most studies.[51,92,93,97] In the study by Zang and colleagues,[95] the presence of ascites correlated negatively with survival. Finally, both Eisenkop[97] and Scarabelli[93] showed that chemotherapy before secondary cytoreduction was associated with some survival advantage.

Landoni and coworkers[55] reported a regimen for the treatment of recurrent ovarian cancer that incorporated secondary cytoreductive surgery in a novel manner. In their institution, all patients with recurrent ovarian cancer after primary cytoreduction, platinum-based chemotherapy, and negative SLS were retreated with platinum compounds. A highly selected group of 38 patients who demonstrated a partial response to chemotherapy with an apparently solitary site of disease were offered secondary cytoreduction. The median interval to recurrent disease was 22 months.

Table 33-1. Secondary Cytoreductive Surgery in Patients with Recurrent Epithelial Ovarian Cancer

Reference and Year	No. Patients	Optimal Cytoreduction		Median Survival Time (mo)		Probability Value	Prognostic Factors for Survival on Multivariate Analysis
		Criterion	Rate (%)	Optimal	Suboptimal		
Scarabelli et al.[93] (2001)	149	≤1 cm	70	32	12	<.001	RD, DFI, prior chemotherapy
Munkarah et al.[94] (2001)	25	≤2 cm	72	56.9	15.1	.08	N/A
Eisenkop et al.[97] (2000)	106	0	82	44.4	19.3	.007	RD, DFI, prior chemotherapy
Zang et al.[95] (2000)	106	<1 cm	43	20	8	<.0001	RD, DFI, ascites
Gadducci et al.[96] (2000)	30	0	57	37	19	.04	N/A
Vaccarello et al.[50] (1995)	38	<0.05	37	NR	23	<.0001	RD
Segna et al.[92] (1993)	100	<2 cm	61	27	9	.0001	RD
Janicke et al.[51] (1992)	30	0	47	29	9	.007	RD, DFI, postoperative chemotherapy
Morris et al.[91] (1989)	30	<2 cm	57	18	13.3	>.05	N/A
Berek et al.[52] (1983)	32	1.5 cm	38	20	5	<.01	N/A

DFI, disease-free interval; N/A, not applicable; RD, residual disease; NR, not reported.

All patients had complete surgical cytoreduction with no macroscopic residual disease. No patient received any further alternative adjuvant chemotherapy. There were 2 (5%) perioperative deaths, and the entire group had a median survival time of 29 months. Few conclusions can be drawn from this retrospective series. However, with the number of active salvage chemotherapy agents available, intuitively it seems important to consolidate secondary cytoreductive surgery with some form of chemotherapy.

Palliative surgery and "third-look" laparotomy may be considered under the category of secondary surgery. This aspect of secondary surgery is highly individualized and is beyond the scope of this chapter.

Secondary cytoreductive surgery for recurrent ovarian cancer is feasible with acceptably low morbidity and mortality rates. There is a sound theoretical rationale to support secondary cytoreductive surgery. The appropriate candidates for surgery ideally should have a disease-free interval of at least 12 months from the time of completion of primary treatment. There should be no major medical contraindication to the surgery. The distribution of disease should not preclude a realistic expectation of complete cytoreduction. The surgeon should aim for complete macroscopic clearance if feasible and should be willing to undertake advanced cytoreductive measures such as bowel and urinary tract surgery, splenectomy, limited liver resections, partial gastrectomy, and diaphragmatic and extraperitoneal surgery.

The utility of secondary cytoreductive surgery can be definitively established only by prospective, randomized trials. Given that secondary cytoreductive surgery is rarely curative, quality of life is of paramount importance. There is a dearth of information about quality of life in these circumstances, and any future trials of secondary cytoreductive surgery need

to address this issue. Until such information becomes available, the place of secondary cytoreductive surgery must ultimately be determined on an individual basis, between patient and physician, after the requisite counseling.

What is the role of interval cytoreductive surgery?

The treatment protocol of neoadjuvant chemotherapy and interval cytoreductive surgery (ICS) has been used in a number of clinical contexts.[98] The most common context is that in which primary cytoreduction is attempted but, because of the extent of tumor or limitations in the skill or diligence of the surgeon, significant residual disease remains. This heterogeneous patient group represents a broad spectrum of tumor biologic behavior. At one extreme are patients with imminently resectable disease who are operated on, often in regional centers by general surgeons or gynecologists, with little more than histologic confirmation of the tumor and documentation of the extent of disease. At the other end of the spectrum are patients who have had a concerted and genuine attempt at radical cytoreduction by an experienced gynecologic oncologist in a major surgical unit, whose attempts at optimal cytoreduction were thwarted by the biologically aggressive nature of the tumor.

The second context includes patients who are deemed too medically unfit to tolerate surgery radical enough to accomplish optimal cytoreduction. Neoadjuvant chemotherapy is offered in the hope that tumor regression may either improve the performance status of the patient or reduce the necessary radicality of surgery. This group also potentially represents a range of tumor biologic behavior. Patients who are rendered moribund by their cancer potentially respond differently than patients who have a concurrent unrelated systemic illness. The third context for ICS includes patients who are electively treated with neoadjuvant chemotherapy and interval cytoreduction as primary therapy.[99] These final two contexts include patients who have not had to undergo major surgery, who have had the extent of their disease determined by imaging studies and the disease process confirmed by cytology or Tru-Cut biopsy.

There are several theoretical advantages to ICS. Because survival in part depends on chemosensitivity, a history of neoadjuvant therapy that failed to produce a response may save a small group of patients from surgical intervention that may in fact do little to prolong survival. The corollary is that patients with chemosensitive disease may be targeted for aggressive surgery in the knowledge that they are likely to benefit from further chemotherapy.

A number of retrospective studies have been published regarding neoadjuvant chemotherapy and ICS in patients with epithelial ovarian cancer suboptimally debulked at primary surgery. There was considerable heterogeneity in the type and duration (usually two to four cycles) of neoadjuvant, platinum-based chemotherapy. There was also variation in the training and skill of the primary surgeon and in the criteria for optimal cytoreduction.[100-105] Reports of these retrospective series demonstrated that this approach is technically feasible and may result in optimal cytoreduction in 69% to 77% of patients, with acceptable rates of morbidity and mortality. Where comparisons were made with nonrandomized control subjects treated with no further surgery, a trend toward improved survival in the ICS arm was demonstrated but no statistically significant difference. One study of quality of life in patients treated with neoadjuvant chemotherapy and ICS suggested that patients' overall quality of life and functional status improved after neoadjuvant chemotherapy.[106]

Three randomized prospective trials have evaluated the efficacy of neoadjuvant chemotherapy and ICS.[105,107,108] Redman and colleagues[105] reported on 79 patients with stages II to IV epithelial ovarian cancer with bulky residual disease after primary surgery who were treated with cis-platinum-based chemotherapy. Of the 37 patients randomly assigned to ICS, only 25 (67%) proceeded to secondary surgery, and only 19 of those patients had disease reduced down to less than 2 cm. Using intention-to-treat analysis, the median survival time for the ICS group was 15 months (95% confidence interval [CI], 10 to 20 months), compared with 12 months (95% CI, 8 to 16 months) among those treated with chemotherapy alone. No statistically significant difference in survival was demonstrated. This was a small study with sufficient power to demonstrate only large differences in survival. The criteria for optimal cytoreduction (less than 2 cm) was larger than for the two more recent studies, and fewer patients randomly assigned to ICS actually underwent surgery than in most series.

Van der Burgh and coworkers[107] reported the findings of a European Organization of Research and Treatment of Cancer (EORTC) study in which 319 patients with suboptimal tumor debulking (greater than 1 cm) were randomly assigned, after three cycles of cisplatin and cyclophosphamide chemotherapy, to either ICS or no surgery followed by three further cycles of chemotherapy. Those with progressive disease after neoadjuvant chemotherapy were excluded from the study. ICS was performed on 140 patients and was well tolerated, without severe complications or mortality. Sixty-five percent of patients had residual disease greater than 1 cm after induction chemotherapy, and optimal cytoreduction was achieved for 45% of those patients at the second operation. Median survival time was 26 months for those who underwent ICS and 20 months for those who did not ($P = .04$). Progression-free survival time also showed a statistically significant advantage for the group undergoing ICS (18 versus 13 months).

Finally, the GOG have published the results of a randomized study of ICS in 550 patients with advanced epithelial ovarian cancer suboptimally debulked (residual disease greater than 1 cm) at primary surgery.[108] After three courses of paclitaxel and cisplatin chemotherapy, 425 patients showing either stable disease or a response to treatment were randomly assigned to receive either ICS or no surgery, followed by three further courses of chemotherapy. Patients receiving ICS had a median survival time of 32 months, compared with 33 months for those receiving chemotherapy alone. There was also no difference in progression-free survival time (10.5 versus 10.8 months, respectively).

There were two major differences between the EORTC and GOG studies that may account for their contradictory results. The chemotherapy regimen used in the EORTC study was cisplatin and cyclophosphamide, whereas the regimen used in the GOG study was cisplatin and paclitaxel. Perhaps of greater importance, all patients in the GOG study had their primary surgery performed by a subspecialty-trained gynecologic oncologist, whereas patients in the European study did not necessarily have their primary surgery performed by an expert in gynecologic cancer surgery. In conclusion, it is apparent that there is little place for ICS in patients with advanced ovarian carcinoma that is initially suboptimally debulked by a subspecialty-trained gynecologic oncologist and then treated by standard chemotherapy. However, there may be a place for ICS if there is some question about the adequacy of initial cytoreductive attempts.

In terms of future directions, these randomized studies raise the question of immediate cytoreduction and standard chemotherapy versus neoadjuvant chemotherapy and ICS for all patients with ovarian carcinoma, rather than just for patients suboptimally debulked of disease at primary surgery. The EORTC have now activated a randomized trial of neoadjuvant chemotherapy followed by ICS versus up-front primary debulking surgery followed by chemotherapy with or without ICS in patients with stage IIIc or IV epithelial ovarian, peritoneal, or fallopian tube cancer (EORTC-55971).

REFERENCES

1. Michel G, Zarca D, Castaigne D, Prade M: Secondary cytoreductive surgery in ovarian cancer. Eur J Surg Oncol 1989;15:201-204.
2. Morris M , Gershenson DM, Wharton JT: Secondary cytoreductive surgery in epithelial ovarian cancer: Nonresponders to first-line therapy. Gynecol Oncol 1989;33:1-5.
3. LoCoco S, Covens A, Carney M, et al: Does aggressive therapy improve survival in suboptimal stage IIIc/IV ovarian cancer? A Canadian-American comparative study. Gynecol Oncol 1995;59:194-199.
4. Lund B, Jacobson K, Rasch L, et al: Correlation of abdominal ultrasound and computed tomography scans with second- or third-look laparotomy in patients with ovarian carcinoma. Gynecol Oncol 1990;37:279.
5. De Rosa V, Mangioni di Stefano ML, Brunetti A, et al: Computed tomography and second-look surgery in ovarian cancer patients: Correlation, actual role and limitations of CT scan. Eur J Gynaecol Oncol 1995;16:123.
6. Clarke-Pearson D, Bandy LC, Dudzinski M, et al: Computed tomography in evaluation of patients with ovarian carcinoma in complete clinical remission: Correlation with surgical-pathological findings. JAMA 1986;255:627.
7. Barter JF, Barnes WA: Second-look laparotomy. In Rubin SC, Sutton GP (eds): Ovarian Cancer. New York, McGraw-Hill, 1993, p 269.
8. Brenner DE, Shaff MI, Jones HW, et al: Abdominopelvic computed tomography: Evaluation in patients undergoing second-look laparotomy for ovarian carcinoma. Obstet Gynecol 1985;65:715.
9. Khan O, Cosgrove DO, Fried AM, Savage PE: Ovarian carcinoma follow-up: US versus laparotomy. Radiology 1986;159:111.
10. Murolo C, Constantini S, Foglia G, et al: Ultrasound examination in ovarian cancer patients: A comparison with second look laparotomy. J Ultrasound Med 1989;8:441-443.
11. Nardelli GB, Onnis GL, Lamaina V, Petrillo MR: Ultrasound evaluation in the follow-up of ovarian cancer today. Clin Exp Obstet Gynecol 1987;14:174.
12. Fishman-Javitt M, Stein H, Lovecchio J: Imaging of the Pelvis: MRI with Correlations to CT and Ultrasound. Boston, Little Brown, 1990.
13. Surwit EA, Childers JM, Krag DN, et al: Clinical assessment of 111In-Cyt-103 immunoscintigraphy in ovarian cancer. Gynecol Oncol 1993;48:285-292.
14. Barzen G, Friedmann W, Richter W, et al: The place of radioimmunoscintigraphy in the diagnosis and follow-up of ovarian cancer in comparison with computed tomography and second-look surgery. Nuklearmedizin 1992;31:15.
15. Loboguerrero A, Perault C, Leihn JC: Volume rendering and binocular scale in double isotope studies: Application to immunoscintigraphy and bone landmarking. Eur J Nucl Med 1992;19:201-204.
16. Forstner R, Hricak H, Powell CB, et al: Ovarian cancer recurrence: Value of MR imaging. Radiology 1995;196:715-720.
17. Phibbs GD, Smith JP, Stanhope CR: Analysis of sites of persistent cancer at "second-look" laparotomy in patients with ovarian cancer. Am J Obstet Gynecol 1983;147:611-617.
18. Podratz KC, Kinney WK: Second-look operation in ovarian cancer. Cancer 1993;71(4 Suppl):1551-1558.
19. Ozols RF, Rubin SC, Thomas G, Robboy S: Epithelial ovarian cancer. In Hoskins WJ, Perez CA, Young RC (eds): Principles and Practice of Gynecologic Oncology. Philadelphia, Lippincott-Raven, 1997, pp 919-986.
20. NIH Consensus Conference: Ovarian cancer: Screening, treatment, and follow-up. NIH Consensus Panel on Ovarian Cancer. JAMA 1995;273:491-497.
21. Greer B, Bundy BN, Ozols RF, et al: Implications of second-look laparotomy (SLL) in the context of Gynecologic Oncology Group (GOG) Protocol 158: A non-randomized comparison using an explanatory analysis. Gynecol Oncol 2003;88:156.
22. Barnhill DR, Hoskins WJ, Heller PB, Park RC: The second-look surgical reassessment for epithelial ovarian carcinoma. Gynecol Oncol 1984;19:148-154.
23. Berek JS, Hacker NF, Lagasse LD, et al: Second-look laparotomy in stage III epithelial ovarian cancer: Clinical variables associated with disease status. Obstet Gynecol 1984;64:207-212.
24. Curry S, Zembo M, Nahhas W, Jahshan A: Second-look laparotomy for ovarian cancer. Gynecol Oncol 1981;11:114-118.
25. Gershenson DM, Copeland LJ, Wharton JT, et al: Prognosis of surgically determined complete responders in advanced ovarian cancer. Cancer 1985;55:1129-1135.
26. Dauplat J, Ferriere JP, Gorbinet M, et al: Second-look laparotomy in managing epithelial ovarian carcinoma. Cancer 1986;57:1627-1631.
27. Webster KD, Ballard LJ: Ovarian carcinoma—second-look laparotomy postchemotherapy: Preliminary report. Cleve Clin Q 1981;48:365-371.
28. Roberts WS, Hodel K, Rich WM, DiSaia PJ: Second-look laparotomy in the management of gynecologic malignancy. Gynecol Oncol 1982;13:345-355.
29. Webb MJ, Snyder JJ, Williams TJ, Decker DG: Second-look laparotomy in ovarian cancer. Gynecol Oncol 1982;14:285-293.
30. Cohen CJ, Goldberg JD, Holland JF, et al: Improved therapy with cisplatin regimens for patients with ovarian carcinoma (FIGO stages III and IV) as measured by surgical end-staging (second-look operation). Am J Obstet Gynecol 1983;145:955-967.
31. Phibbs GD, Smith JP, Stanhope CR: Analysis of sites of persistent cancer at "second-look" laparotomy in patients with ovarian cancer. Am J Obstet Gynecol 1983;147:611-617.
32. Ballon SC, Portnuff JC, Sikic BI, et al: Second-look laparotomy in epithelial ovarian carcinoma: Precise definition, sensitivity, and specificity of the operative procedure. Gynecol Oncol 1984;17:154-160.
33. Milsted R, Sangster G, Kaye S, et al: Treatment of advanced ovarian cancer with combination chemotherapy using cyclophosphamide, adriamycin and cis-platinum. Br J Obstet Gynaecol 1984;91:927-931.
34. Rocereto TF, Mangan CE, Giuntoli RL, et al: The second-look celiotomy in ovarian cancer. Gynecol Oncol 1984;19:34-45.
35. Podratz KC, Malkasian G Jr, Hilton JF, et al: Second-look laparotomy in ovarian cancer: Evaluation of pathologic variables. Am J Obstet Gynecol 1985;152:230-238.
36. Smirz LR, Stehman FB, Ulbright TM, et al: Second-look laparotomy after chemotherapy in the management of ovarian malignancy. Am J Obstet Gynecol 1985;152:661-668.
37. Cain J, Saigo P, Pierce V, et al: A review of second-look laparotomy for ovarian cancer. Gynecol Oncol 1986;23:14-25.
38. Miller DS, Ballon SC, Teng NN, et al: A critical reassessment of second-look laparotomy in epithelial ovarian carcinoma. Cancer 1986;57:530-535.
39. Carmichael JA, Shelly WE, Brown LB, et al: A predictive index of cure versus no cure in advanced ovarian carcinoma patients: Replacement of second-look laparotomy as a diagnostic test. Gynecol Oncol 1987;27:269-281.
40. Gallup DG, Talledo OE, Dudzinski MR, Brown KW: Another look at the second-assessment procedure for ovarian epithelial carcinoma. Am J Obstet Gynecol 1987;157:590-596.
41. Ho AG, Beller U, Speyer JL, et al: A reassessment of the role of second-look laparotomy in advanced ovarian cancer. J Clin Oncol 1987;5:1316-1321.
42. McCusker MC, Hoffman JS, Curry SL, et al: The role of second-look laparotomy in treatment of epithelial ovarian cancer. Gynecol Oncol 1987;28:83-88.
43. Podczaski ES, Stevens CJ, Manetta A, et al: Use of second-look laparotomy in the management of patients with ovarian epithelial malignancies. Gynecol Oncol 1987;28:205-214.
44. Sonnendecker EW: Is routine second-look laparotomy for ovarian cancer justified? Gynecol Oncol 1988;31:249-255.
45. de Gramont A, Drolet Y, Varette C, et al: Survival after second-look laparotomy in advanced ovarian epithelial cancer: Study of 86 patients. Eur J Cancer Clin Oncol 1989;25:451-457.
46. Kamura T, Tsukamoto N, Saito T, et al: Efficacy of second-look laparotomy for patients with epithelial ovarian carcinoma. Int J Gynaecol Obstet 1990;33:141-147.
47. Lund B, Williamson P: Prognostic factors for outcome of and survival after second-look laparotomy in patients with advanced ovarian carcinoma. Obstet Gynecol 1990;76:617-622.
48. Ayhan A, Yarali H, Develioglu O, et al: Prognosticators of second-look laparotomy findings in patients with epithelial ovarian cancer. J Surg Oncol 1991;46:222-225.

49. Lippman SM, Alberts DS, Slymen DJ, et al: Second-look laparotomy in epithelial ovarian carcinoma: Prognostic factors associated with survival duration. Cancer 1988;61:2571-2577.

50. Vaccarello L, Rubin SC, Vlamis V, et al: Cytoreductive surgery in ovarian carcinoma patients with a documented previously complete surgical response. Gynecol Oncol 1995;57:61-65.

51. Janicke F, Holscher M, Kuhn W, et al: Radical surgical procedure improves survival time in patients with recurrent ovarian cancer. Cancer 1992;70:2129-2136.

52. Berek JS, Hacker NF, LaGasse LD, et al: Survival of patients following secondary cytoreductive surgery in ovarian cancer. Obstet Gynecol 1983;61:189-193.

53. Rose PG: Surgery for recurrent ovarian cancer. Semin Oncol 2000;27:17-23.

54. Bristow RE, Lagasse LD, Karlan BY: Secondary surgical cytoreduction for advanced epithelial ovarian cancer. Cancer 1996;78:2049-2062.

55. Landoni F, Pellegrino A, Cormio G, et al: Platin-based chemotherapy and salvage surgery in recurrent ovarian cancer following negative second-look laparotomy. Acta Obstet Gynecol Scand 1998;77:233-237.

56. Chu CS, Rubin SC: Second-look laparotomy for epithelial ovarian cancer: A reappraisal. Curr Oncol Rep 2001;3:11-18.

57. Rubin SC: Second-look laparotomy. In Markman M, Hoskins WJ (eds): Cancer of the Ovary. New York, Raven Press, 1993, p 175.

58. Morgan MA, Noumoff JS, King S, Mikuta JJ: A formula for predicting the risk of a positive second-look laparotomy in epithelial ovarian cancer: Implications for a randomized trial. Obstet Gynecol 1992;80:944-948.

59. Venesmaa P, Ylikorkala O: Morbidity and mortality associated with primary and repeat operations for ovarian cancer. Obstet Gynecol 1992;79:168-172.

60. Rome R, Fortune DW: The role of second-look laparotomy in the management of patients with ovarian carcinoma. Aust N Z J Obstet Gynaecol 1988;28:318-323.

61. Pederson IR, Corfitsen MT, Lebech AM, Kaae HH: Komplikationer ved eftersynsoperation [second look operation] for ovariecancer. Ugerskrift for Laeger 1993;155:958.

62. Chambers SK, Chambers JT, Kohorn EI, et al: Evaluation of the role of second-look surgery in ovarian cancer. Obstet Gynecol 1988;72:404-408.

63. Husain A, Chi DS, Prasad M, et al: The role of laparoscopy in second-look evaluations for ovarian cancer. Gynecol Oncol 2001; 80:44-47.

64. Casey AC, Farias-Eisner R, Pisani AL, et al: What is the role of reassessment laparoscopy of gynecologic cancers in 1995? Gynecol Oncol 1996;60:454-461.

65. Abu-Rustum NR, Barakat RR, Seigel PL, et al: Second-look operation for epithelial ovarian cancer: Laparoscopy or laparotomy? Obstets Gynecol 1996;88:549-553.

66. Clough KB, Ladonne JM, Nos C, et al: Durand JC. Second look for ovarian cancer: Laparoscopy for laparotomy? Prospective comparative study. Gynecol Oncol 1999;72:411-417.

67. Creasman WT, Gall S, Bundy BN, et al: Second-look laparotomy in the patient with minimal residual stage III ovarian cancer (a Gynecologic Oncology Group Study). Gynecol Oncol 1989;35:378-382.

68. Hoskins WJ, Rubin SC, Dulaney E, et al: Influence of secondary cytoreduction at the time of second-look laparotomy on the survival of patients with epithelial ovarian carcinoma. Gynecol Oncol 1989;34:365-371.

69. Potter ME, Hatch KD, Soong S-J, et al: Second-look laparotomy and salvage therapy: A research modality only? Gynecol Oncol 1992;44:3-9.

70. Ngan HY, Wong LC, Ma HK: Place of second-look laparotomy after 18 courses of chemotherapy in epithelial ovarian cancer. Aust N Z J Obstet Gynaecol 1989;29:52-54.

71. Obermair A, Sevelda P: Impact of second look laparotomy and secondary cytoreductive surgery at second-look laparotomy in ovarian cancer patients. Acta Obstet Gynecol Scand 2001;80:1-5.

72. Gadducci A, Iacconi P, Fanucchi A, et al: Surgical cytoreduction during second-look laparotomy in patients with advanced ovarian cancer. Anticancer Res 2000;20:1959-1964.

73. Rubin SC, Randall TC, Armstrong KA, et al: Ten-year follow-up of ovarian cancer patients after second-look laparotomy with negative findings. Obstet Gynecol 1999;93:21-24.

74. Friedman RL, Eisenkop SM, Wang HJ: Second-look laparotomy for ovarian cancer provides reliable prognostic information and improves survival. Gynecol Oncol 1997;67:88-94.

75. Gershensen DM, Copeland LJ, Wharton JT, et al: Prognosis of surgically determined complete responders in advanced ovarian cancer. Gynecol Oncol 1985;55:1129-1135.

76. Gadducci A, Sartori E, Maggino T, et al: Analysis of failures after negative second-look in patients with advanced ovarian cancer: An Italian multicenter study. Gynecol Oncol 1998;68:150-155.

77. Podczaski E, Manetta A, Kaminski P, et al: Survival of patients with epithelial ovarian after second-look laparotomy. Gynecol Oncol 1990;36:43-47.

78. Smirz LR, Stehman FB, Ulbright TM, et al: Second-look laparotomy after chemotherapy in the management of ovarian malignancy. Am J Obstet Gynecol 1985;152:661-668.

79. Podratz KC, Malkasian GD, Wieand HS, et al: Recurrent disease after negative second-look laparotomy in stages III and IV ovarian carcinoma. Gynecol Oncol 1988;29:274-282.

80. Varia M, Rosenman J, Venkatraman S, et al: Intraperitoneal chromic phosphate therapy after second-look laparotomy for ovarian cancer. Cancer 1988;61:919-927.

81. Spencer TR Jr, Marks RD, Renn JO, et al: Intraperitoneal P32 after negative second-look laparotomy in ovarian cancer. Cancer 1989;63:2434-2437.

82. Peters W. Smith M, Cain J, et al: Intraperitoneal P-32 is not effective consolidation therapy after negative second-look laparotomy for epithelial carcinoma of the ovary. Gynecol Oncol 1992;47:146-149.

83. Menczer J, Ben-Baruch G, Ritzel S: Intraperitoneal cisplatin chemotherapy in ovarian carcinoma patients who are clinically in complete remission. Gynecol Oncol 1992;46:222-225.

84. Tarraza HM Jr, Boyce CR, Smith G, Jones MA: Consolidation intraperitoneal chemotherapy in epithelial ovarian carcinoma patients following negative second-look laparotomy. Gynecol Oncol 1993;50:287-290.

85. Dufour P, Bergerat JP, Barats JC, et al: Intraperitoneal mitoxantrone as consolidation treatment for patients with ovarian carcinoma in complete remission. Cancer 1994;73:1865-1869.

86. Barakat RR, Almondrones L, Venkatraman ES, et al: A phase II trial of intraperitoneal cisplatin and etoposide as consolidation therapy in patients with stage II-IV epithelial ovarian cancer following negative surgical assessment. Gynecol Oncol 1998;69:17-22.

87. Markman M, Liu PY, Wilczynski S, et al: A randomized trial of 12 versus 3 months of single-agent paclitaxel in patients with advanced ovarian cancer who attained a clinically defined complete response to platinum/paclitaxel-based chemotherapy: A Southwest Oncology Group and Gynecology Group Trial. Gynecol Oncol 2002;84:479.

88. MacGibbon A, Bucci J, MacLeod C, et al: Whole abdominal radiotherapy following second-look laparotomy for ovarian carcinoma. Gynecol Oncol 1999;75:62-67.

89. Fuks Z, Rizel S, Biram S: Chemotherapeutic and surgical induction of pathological complete remission and whole abdominal irradiation for consolidation does not enhance cure of stage III ovarian carcinoma. J Clin Oncol 1988;6:509-516.

90. Goldberg H, Stein ME, Steiner M, et al: Consolidation radiation therapy following cytoreductive surgery, chemotherapy and second-look laparotomy for epithelial ovarian carcinoma: Long-term follow-up. Tumori 2001;87:245-251.

91. Morris M, Gershenson DM, Wharton JT, et al: Secondary cytoreductive surgery for recurrent epithelial ovarian cancer. Gynecol Oncol 1989;34:334-338.

92. Segna RA, Dottino PR, Mandeli JP, et al: Secondary cytoreduction for ovarian cancer following cisplatin therapy. J Clin Oncol 1993;11:434-439.

93. Scarabelli C, Gallo A, Carbone A: Secondary cytoreductive surgery for patients with recurrent epithelial ovarian carcinoma. Gynecol Oncol 2001;83:504-512.

94. Munkarah A, Levenback C, Wolf JK, et al: Secondary cytoreductive surgery for localized intra-abdominal recurrences in epithelial ovarian cancer. Gynecol Oncol 2001;81:237-241.

95. Zang RY, Zhang ZY, Li ZT, et al: Impact of secondary cytoreductive surgery on survival of patients with advanced epithelial ovarian cancer. Eur J Surg Oncol 2000;26:798-804.

96. Gadducci A, Iacconi P, Cosio S, et al: Complete salvage surgical cytoreduction improves further survival of patients with late recurrent ovarian cancer. Gynecol Oncol 2000;79:344-349.

97. Eisenkop SM, Friedman RL, Spirtos NM: The role of secondary cytoreductive surgery in the treatment of patients with recurrent epithelial ovarian carcinoma. Cancer 2000;88:144-153.

98. Nicklin JL, Copeland LJ: Second-look laparotomy and secondary tumor reduction in epithelial ovarian cancer. In Rock JA, Faro S, Grant NF Jr, et al. (eds): Advances in Obstetrics and Gynecology, vol 3. Chicago, Mosby–Year Book, 1996, pp 439-454.

99. Surwit E, Childers J, Atlas M, et al: Neoadjuvant chemotherapy for advanced ovarian cancer. Int J Gynecol Oncol 1996;6:356-361.

100. Wils J, Blijham G, Naus A, et al: Primary or delayed debulking surgery and chemotherapy consisting of cisplatinum, doxorubicin, and cyclophosphamide in stage III-IV epithelial ovarian carcinoma. J Clin Oncol 1986;4:1068-1073.

101. Jacob JH, Gershenson DM, Morris M, et al: Neoadjuvant chemotherapy and interval debulking for advanced epithelial ovarian cancer. Gynecol Oncol 1991;42:146-150.

102. Lawton FG, Redman CWE, Luesley DM, et al: Neoadjuvant (cytoreductive) chemotherapy combined with intervention debulking surgery in advanced, unresected epithelial ovarian cancer. Obstet Gynecol 1989;73:61-65.

103. Neijt JP, Aartsen EJ, Bouma J, et al: Cytoreductive surgery with or without preceeding chemotherapy in ovarian cancer. Prog Clin Biol Res 1985,:201:217-233.

104. Ng LW, Rubin SC, Hoskins WJ, et al: Aggressive chemosurgical debulking in patients with advanced ovarian cancer. Gynecol Oncol 1990;38:358-363.

105. Redman CWE, Warwick J, Leusley DM, et al: Intervention debulking surgery in advanced epithelial ovarian cancer. Br J Obstet Gynaecol 1994;101:142-146.

106. Chan YM, Ng TY, Ngan HY, Wong LC: Quality of life in women treated with neoadjuvant chemotherapy for advanced ovarian cancer: A prospective longitudinal study. Gynecol Oncol 2003;88:9-16.

107. Van der Berg MEL, van Lent M, Buyse M, et al: The effect of debulking surgery after induction chemotherapy on the prognosis in advanced epithelial ovarian cancer. N Engl J Med 1995;332:629-634.

108. Rose P, Nerenstone S, Brady M, et al: A phase III randomized study of interval secondary cytoreduction in patients with advanced stage ovarian carcinoma with suboptimal residual disease: A Gynecologic Oncology Group study [abstract 802]. Program and Abstracts of the American Society of Clinical Oncology 38th Annual Meeting, May 18-21, Orlando, Florida.

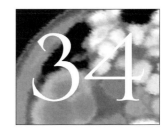

CHEMOTHERAPY FOR REFRACTORY EPITHELIAL OVARIAN CANCER

Franco Muggia

MAJOR CONTROVERSIES

- Is there a role for consolidation after successful initial induction with first-line chemotherapy?
- Should second-line treatment be initiated based solely based on CA 125 levels?
- Should patients be subjected to secondary cytoreduction to improve outcome from chemotherapy?
- Which patients, on recurrence, should receive platinum-based chemotherapy?
- Is there a role for predictive assays in drug selection?
- Is resistance to platinums ever reversible?
- Beyond platinums: single agents or combinations?
- Beyond platinums: a prescribed number of treatment cycles or prolonged maintenance?
- Is there a desirable limit of treatment interventions beyond second-line therapy?
- Is there a salvage role for radiotherapy either alone or in combination with chemotherapy?
- Should emerging noncytotoxic treatments be used outside clinical trials?

Although the initial approach to the treatment of epithelial ovarian cancer after diagnosis has been quite uniform since the introduction of combination therapy with platinum and taxanes,[1-3] the approach to recurrent disease has differed widely. This has given rise to the impression that a vast array of effective treatments is available for these patients. In fact, the dilemmas in selecting the appropriate chemotherapy reflect as much the limited success of these treatments as the lack of reliable comparative trials addressing questions beyond selection of the optimal first-line therapy. Moreover, it is likely that efficacy of and tolerance for any particular agent decline as use occurs later in the sequence of treatments. This chapter focuses on controversies concerning strategy as well as the role of specific therapies. The highlighting of controversies should not obscure the importance of the "platinum-free interval" (the length of time from termination of a platinum-based induction treatment to first evidence of relapse)[4-7] and of clinical studies carefully reporting the efficacy of a drug with attention to known prognostic factors in providing the most relevant information on the management of patients recurrent epithelial ovarian cancer. This chapter reviews these clinical studies within the context of 11 controversies: the first 3 deal with general strategy, the next 3 with platinum versus nonplatinum selection features, the next 3 with what to do "beyond platinum," and the final 2 with emerging general issues.

Refractory ovarian cancer is interpreted here to denote any cancer that has recurred or persists after the initial treatment. The initial treatment is universally "platinum-based," as described in Chapter 30. Within that broad context, this chapter covers first the chemotherapeutic drugs that make up the "second-line lineup" after platinums. After the discovery of paclitaxel's activity in platinum-resistant ovarian cancer, the long drought of searching for agents with reproducible activity in such patients was over.[8] Topotecan, oral etoposide, gemcitabine, pegylated liposomal doxorubicin (PLD, Doxil, Caelyx), and the paclitaxel analog, docetaxel, were subsequently shown to have activity in a resistant setting.[9] Less clear currently is whether "useful" activity (e.g., with a reasonable therapeutic index) exists in platinum-resistant patients for drugs such as altretamine, epirubicin, irinotecan and other camptothecin derivatives, ifosfamide (and other alkylating drugs including cyclophosphamide, melphalan, and treosulfan), and miscellaneous agents such as the vinca alkaloid, vinorelbine, and mitomycin (an alkylating agent under hypoxic conditions). What constitutes a reasonable therapeutic index is subject to debate, but the topic is raised to underscore issues of tolerance that increase after a full exposure to platinum-based induction treatment and with each subsequent therapy. The number of patients entered into published trials of second-line therapy for relapses occurring within 12 months after treatment may be indicative of the investigators' willingness to treat patients with a certain drug. Table 34-1, adapted (by merely including his referencing and adding the one irinotecan study) from Martin Gore's review in an Education Session before the American Society of Clinical Oncology (May 2001),[9] provides such information.

However, for those drugs included in Table 34-1, one must also consider the influence of sponsorship in stimulating trials and their chronology. For example, studies with altretamine were mostly generated when concepts of potential platinum sensitivity and resistance had not been widely applied, and as an oral agent it was not infrequently applied in consolidation (i.e., without intervening relapse). In addition, one must be cognizant that activity may vary with schedule and route of administration (e.g., intravenous, oral). Sponsorship has played a major role in randomized

trials, including single agents for second-line ovarian cancer, because cooperative groups have not adequately addressed these questions. Trials in platinum-sensitive patients have given definitive answers of superiority for platinum-based combinations (Table 34-2). For other drugs, one should consider the results of trials best defined as round-robin trials, because the comparison is meant to position an agent in relation to another that has been granted approval for second-line treatment of ovarian cancer by regulatory agencies (Table 34-2). Efficacy results have been quite similar for the agents being compared, but the studies have also been informative in pointing toward the most responsive subsets of patients (i.e., potentially platinum sensitive, no bulky disease) and in bringing out toxicity differences. A multivariate analysis of predictors of response in 704 patients entered in phase II studies of drugs used in second-line platinum-pretreated patients had already strongly indicated that tumor size, number of sites involved, and serous histology were the only significant independent factors for response.[61] Noteworthy was that the time from last chemotherapy was highly inversely correlated with tumor size: patients being entered on a trial after intervals of 6 months or longer had smaller tumors!

Highlights of each of the major drug families reported to be useful in second-line settings are provided here. Controversies about their use (i.e., single agents versus combinations, maintenance versus no maintenance, and potential utility beyond second-line) are covered later.

Taxanes. Except for a few geographic holdouts, paclitaxel is universally a part of first-line treatments (see Chapter 30). Nevertheless, even in such pretreated patients, paclitaxel's role in second-line therapy remains robust because of (1) demonstrable activity of weekly schedules after failure of every-3-week administration[62] and (2) inability to define resistance to taxanes. Moreover, docetaxel has shown clear activity against disease recurring shortly after paclitaxel treatment.[44] Major *advantages* for these drugs are usually mild,

Table 34–1. Activity of Chemotherapeutic Agents Developed for Epithelial Ovarian Cancer Since the 1990s

Drug	No. of Studies	No. of Patients	Response Rate (%)	References
Paclitaxel	12	1580	22	9
Topotecan	10	882	17	10-19
Doxil/Caelyx	4	428	18	16, 20-22
Altretamine	6	235	18	23-28
Etoposide	7	234	22	29-35
Gemcitabine	6	181	18	36-41
Docetaxel	4	166	31	9, 42-45
Epirubicin	6	132	14	46-51
Oxaliplatin	3	118	23	52-54
Vinorelbine	2	71	23	55, 56
Irinotecan	1	55*	24	57

*Three patients were not pretreated with platinum.
Adapted from Martin Gore, American Society of Clinical Oncology, Educational Session, May 2001.

Table 34–2. Randomized Second-Line Trials Including Single Agents in Epithelial Ovarian Cancer

Drugs	Progression-Free Survival Time	Median Survival Time	Reference
Carboplatin*	14 mo	24 mo	Bolis et al.[58]
Carboplatin + epirubicin	18 mo	28 mo	Bolis et al.[58]
CAP*†	19 mo	24 mo	Columbo et al.[59]
Paclitaxel	7 mo	20 mo	Columbo et al.[59]
Oxaliplatin†	12 wk	42 wk	Piccart et al.[54]
Paclitaxel	14 wk	37 wk	Piccart et al.[54]
Paclitaxel	14 wk	42.6 wk	ten Bokkel Huinink et al.[17]
Topotecan	23.1 wk	61.3 wk	ten Bokkel Huinink et al.[17]
Topotecan	16.1 wk	56.7 wk	Gordon et al.[16]
Doxil/Caelyx	17 wk	60 wk	Gordon et al.[16]
Doxil/Caelyx‡	21.7 wk	45.7 wk	O'Byrne et al.[60]
Paclitaxel	22.4 wk	56.1 wk	O'Byrne et al.[60]

CAP, cyclophosphamide + Adriamycin + Platinol.
*Restricted to platinum-sensitive patients.
†Randomized phase II study.
‡Underpowered phase III study (stopped when paclitaxel became available outside a trial).

subjective intolerance and manageable hematologic toxicities (primarily neutropenia). *Disadvantages* are the potential for aggravation of preexisting neuropathy and the high prevalence of total alopecia. Also, the weekly administration regimen may provide a further deterrent to some patients.

Camptothecins. Topotecan provided the unequivocal demonstration of usefulness against resistant ovarian cancer for the camptothecins (topoisomerase I inhibitors)[9] (see Table 34-1). In trials versus paclitaxel (see Table 34-2), the drug yielded generally similar results but performed better in some aspects. Nevertheless, the impracticality of the once-daily-for-5-days schedule that constituted its basis for approval as a second-line drug, as well as the inability to be combined with cisplatin or carboplatin without major dose and schedule alterations, have hampered its potential to displace paclitaxel in first-line regimens. A number of studies with other schedules have been initiated, but evidence that these should be widely adopted remain unconvincing. In fact, preclinical and some clinical studies clearly suggest the need for continuous exposure to optimize the antitumor effects.[63] Major *advantages* of topotecan are the lack of cumulative toxicity, with the most severe toxicity being experienced during the first cycle, and the unlikelihood of cross-resistance with drugs used in first-line therapy. *Disadvantages* are its schedule of administration and the frequent dose-limiting myelosuppression, particularly in combination use.

Other members of the camptothecin family have shown activity against ovarian cancer, including 9-aminocamptothecin, rubitecan, irinotecan, DX-8915f, and lurtotecan in a liposomal formulation.[64,65] Only irinotecan is currently available outside experimental trials. These agents may have potential advantages over topotecan, but comparative trials are lacking. Use

of irinotecan is associated with a lower incidence of myelosuppression, but gastrointestinal toxicity is frequent. Identification of the breast cancer resistance protein may increase the ability to best select and use these specific drugs. Enhancement of oral bioavailability may render more feasible the protracted exposure scheduling.[66] Another way of enhancing the therapeutic index through prolonged exposures at the tumor site is via liposomes[65] and polymers.[67]

Anthracyclines. Interest in the anthracycline class of drugs was rekindled by (1) reports of activity of Doxil in the second-line setting[68] and (2) a meta-analysis that suggested a positive contribution to outcome in first-line trials when doxorubicin was included in the combination CAP (cyclophosphamide + Adriamycin + Platinol) versus CP (cyclophosphamide + Platinol).[69] In addition, a new generation of studies with epirubicin indicated activity of this drug in second-line therapy (see Table 34-1). However, in the first-line setting, recent phase III studies have suggested no additional benefit from the combination with the addition of doxorubicin or epirubicin versus carboplatin alone or in combination with paclitaxel.[70] An ongoing study by the Gynecologic Oncology Group (GOG 182) includes an arm with Doxil in combination with carboplatin and paclitaxel in first-line, and some results are anticipated in 2004.

Currently, Doxil is viewed increasingly as a preferred drug for salvage treatment because of phase III studies demonstrating similar outcome to paclitaxel or to topotecan with major *advantages* in its toxicity spectrum, avoiding alopecia or severe myelosuppression. In addition, unlike so-called free anthracyclines, Doxil may be suitable for long-term administration generally without concern of cardiomyopathy.[71,72] This renders it suitable for use after failure of high-dose chemotherapy with autologous progenitor cell reconstitution (Fig. 34-1). It has not been established that such maintenance therapy is associated with an improved outcome, but individual patients have been reported to achieve a more prolonged remission after such treatment than from the platinum-based induction regimen that preceded it.[72]

Oral etoposide. Epipodophyllotoxins were reported to have activity in ovarian cancer, but initial trials yielded very erratic results.[73] Accordingly, etoposide enjoyed only a brief period of use, and primarily by the intraperitoneal route.[74] After the introduction of a schedule of continuous exposure at concentrations greater than a threshold that was pharmacodynamically advantageous for antitumor effects, oral etoposide for 14 to 21 days received widespread testing.[75] Phase II trials in patients with ovarian cancer demonstrated reproducible activity in second-line therapy (see Table 34-1). No information exists to compare this with other second-line drugs or in regard to possible cross-resistance to anthracyclines and other topoisomerase II inhibitors. *Disadvantages* include the need for stable gastrointestinal functional status (shared with other oral drugs), universal alopecia, and leukemogenic potential[76];

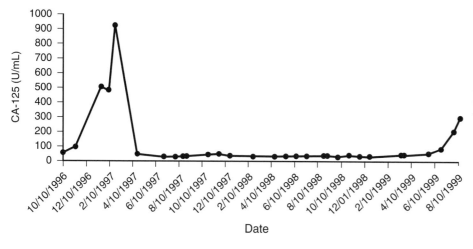

RESPONSE AND PROLONGED REMISSION ON DOXIL
E.Q. 45 YO PAPILLARY SEROUS. DIAGNOSIS 2/1/94.
DOXIL BEGUN 2/97, CUMULATIVE DOSE = 880 mg/m²

Figure 34–1. Patient EQ. The CA 125 pattern reflecting a response lasting slightly more than 2 years after relapse from high-dose chemotherapy that had been given 7 months before the start of Doxil administration. Doxil was tolerated at 40 mg/m² without severe myelosuppression or complications.

the latter finding has dampened enthusiasm for its use in first-line treatment.

Gemcitabine and other antimetabolites. Antifolates and fluoropyrimidines have played only a minor role in the treatment of ovarian cancer, although some antitumor activity has been noted with Tomudex[77] and with 5-fluorouracil[78] or its prodrug, capecitabine.[79] Gemcitabine (difluorodeoxycytidine), on the other hand, is playing an increasing role in salvage settings (see Table 34-1) and is undergoing testing in first-line combinations with carboplatin by the GOG and other groups. The emerging interest in this agent is based on its activity with *advantages* including good subjective tolerance, no neurotoxicity, rapidly reversible myelosuppression, and infrequent alopecia. Synergism with cisplatin or carboplatin has been claimed in preclinical[80] and clinical studies.[81] Activity of such combinations in the face of platinum resistance has been claimed.[82] However, clinical trials to support an advantage over gemcitabine alone under these circumstances are lacking.

Alkylating agents and altretamine. Ifosfamide had demonstrated activity against ovarian cancer up-front and in the refractory setting before the advent of paclitaxel.[83,84] However, enthusiasm for its use, and for the use of cyclophosphamide and melphalan in high doses as consolidation[85-92] or salvage, was tempered by toxicity considerations and by the brevity of remissions, particularly in patients with platinum-resistant disease. High-dose regimens have given inconclusive results in first-line treatment[93-96] and therefore cannot be recommended for salvage. Some interest in use of these drugs in conventional doses has been rekindled in view of the frequent lack of prior exposure to such drugs in current first-line regimens, but as single agents they produced very little activity as second-line agents in older studies.[97] Moreover, the *disadvantages* of myelosuppression, gastrointestinal intolerance, and leukemogenic potential[98] persist with the oxazaphosphorines.

Other alkylating drugs, such as melphalan or treosulfan, are orally active and better tolerated, as is altretamine. Melphalan and treosulfan share the propensity for cumulative marrow damage and induction of leukemias. Myelosuppression is less prominent with altretamine, but this drug is associated with gastrointestinal intolerance and neurotoxicity.[99] Any role of this agent after platinums remains undefined,[100] even if its use as consolidation therapy was promoted by a Southwest Oncology Group pilot study.[101]

Vinca alkaloids and miscellaneous cytotoxic drugs. Vinorelbine (see Table 34-1) and other vinca alkaloids have shown activity against ovarian cancer.[55,56,102] However, a major *disadvantage*, as with other mitotic inhibitors, is the associated neurotoxicity, which may be severe in the presence of preexisting taxane neuropathy.[103] Also, these drugs may lead to ileus in the presence of predisposing factors for bowel dysfunction.

Mitomycin C has been used occasionally to treat ovarian cancer,[104] but its therapeutic index, even if given for no more than four cycles, is inferior to that of any of the drugs discussed earlier.

Oxaliplatin forms platinum-DNA adducts different from those of either cisplatin or carboplatin, and it has shown activity in second-line therapy, although such activity is quite modest in platinum-resistant tumors (see Table 34-1). Its role in the salvage setting is largely undefined, but interest exists in such diaminocyclohexane analogs and also in their combination with cisplatin or carboplatin.[105]

Controversies in Adopting a General Treatment Strategy for Salvage

Is there a role for consolidation after successful initial induction with first-line chemotherapy? This question is addressed elsewhere in regard to first-line therapy and patients who achieve clinical complete responses.

A report by Markman and colleagues to the Society of Gynecologic Oncology in March, 2002, and to the American Society of Clinical Oncology[106] on behalf of the Intergroup Study (SWOG 59701, GOG 178) disclosed reasons for the premature closure of this randomized trial based on a highly significant advantage in progression-free survival (PFS) for 12 months of paclitaxel (175 mg/m^2 every 4 weeks) versus only three such treatments, both after achieving clinical complete response. The reported 7-month advantage in median PFS was accompanied by some increase in neuropathy and patient withdrawal. The early closure renders it unlikely that such an effect will later be reflected in an impact on survival. Nevertheless, the result has highlighted the need to pay attention to issues of consolidation in planning any front-line trial.

The issue of consolidation is also the first issue that arises when a woman is found to have persistent disease at invasive reassessment after induction chemotherapy. Even if only microscopic disease is documented after a remarkable response to platinum-based chemotherapy, such persistence could be an indication of platinum-refractory disease. A number of phase II trials with intraperitoneal platinums proved disappointing, with particularly prompt progression for those patients who had gross residual disease when receiving intraperitoneal treatment.[107] For this reason, and because of theoretical considerations that residual disease represents at least partial platinum resistance, we and others have added other drugs such as etoposide,[74,108,109] fluorodeoxyuridine (FUDR),[110] and topotecan[111] or modalities such as hyperthermia[112] to the platinum compounds for such consolidation. Others have used intraperitoneal cytokines and lymphokine-activated killer cells,[113] radioimmunoconjugates,[114] and gene vectors.[115] As noted earlier, high-dose chemotherapy has also been used under these circumstances.[90] However, there are no phase III data to support the use of any of these modalities.

The GOG 158 protocol revealed that a large number of consolidation regimens were used by the institutions (approximately 50%) that opted to do reassessment after completing the prescribed induction treatment.[116] Not surprisingly, with such variability in applied consolidation treatments, the outcomes of these patients did not differ appreciably from those of patients who did not have reassessments. This result served to reinforce past observations that the strategy of reassessment, not coupled with any consolidation treatment, is not associated with a different outcome, compared with no second-look.[117]

Should second-line treatment be initiated based solely on CA 125 levels? This question must first refer to the specificity of rises in CA 125: if properly defined, are they indicative of ovarian cancer in a patient who was treated for this disease? Rustin and associates[118] provided evidence that doubling of the CA 125 in patients whose baseline level was greater than 23 U/mL had at least a 94% sensitivity for being associated with concomitant or subsequent clinical progression within 12 months. The average lead time of CA

125 progression, so defined, before clinical progression occurred was 72 days in the 80 patients studied. The median survival time for those patients who demonstrated progression was 13 months from the date of CA 125 doubling. This experience was used by the authors to support the stance that "for many patients, there is no urgent need to restart chemotherapy." On the other hand, they went on to state that, "If they delay therapy at least until CA 125 criteria for progression are satisfied, the end point of progression can be used in those patients. Once they have confirmed CA 125 progression, such patients may be good candidates for trials of new cytostatic agents being developed." Figure 34-2 presents what may be the optimum timing for initiation of treatment for recurrence based on CA 125.[9]

Similar views have been expressed by others on treating patients when they are asymptomatic, and generally when disease is suspected from rises in CA 125. According to Armstrong,[119] physicians and patients must balance the potential benefits of deferring therapy in an asymptomatic patient with the increased difficulty of successfully treating larger-volume disease at a later time. Patients with an increased CA 125 concentration as the sole manifestation of disease may be monitored closely with appropriate imaging studies, laboratory evaluation, and physical examination, including pelvic examination. It is entirely appropriate to continue these patients under close observation without therapy.

From Rustin's data,[118] one may deduce that the stances of those who would treat on CA 125-defined progression and those who would wait until clinical progression are not very far apart. In both instances, it is implicit that close follow-up is taking place in order to institute treatment before symptoms occur. Such a therapeutic stance may best be labeled as "preemptive palliation," because beginning salvage chemotherapy

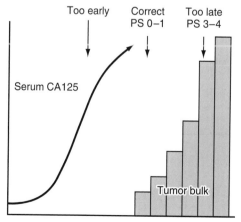

Figure 34–2. Model of the optimum timing for instigation of chemotherapy in patients with relapsed ovarian cancer. (From Gore M: Treatment of relapsed epithelial ovarian cancer. Presented to the American Society of Clinical Oncology Educational Session, May 2001. ASCO, pp 468-476, p 473.)

earlier does not result in cures. Waiting for symptomatic recurrence may lead to complications such as small-bowel obstruction, effusions requiring drainage, life-threatening thromboembolic events, or need to introduce treatment with analgesics. For all of these reasons, and because of the improving therapeutic index of drugs used on recurrence, most specialists would advocate a proactive attitude in the early recognition of refractory disease leading to early, presymptomatic deployment of the appropriate therapeutic intervention. Increasingly, patients manifesting CA 125–only relapses are being considered for clinical trials of interventions with biologic agents. In addition, a large, randomized European trial has been mounted to investigate the therapeutic benefits of monitoring with CA 125 on survival and on quality of life of patients with no evidence of disease.[120]

Should patients be subjected to secondary cytoreduction to improve outcome from chemotherapy?

Strong advocates of secondary cytoreduction in all instances of intra-abdominal recurrence have published highly enthusiastic series.[121] The GOG has planned to activate a study to put such principles of cytoreduction in the salvage setting to a randomized test. At present, cytoreduction may be justified if there is an imminent threat of local complications or if the patient is otherwise subjected to surgery for either diagnostic purposes or relief of symptoms.

Selecting a Platinum Versus a Nonplatinum Treatment

Which patients, on recurrence, should receive platinum-based chemotherapy?

Implicit in this question is the recognition that platinums play a key role not only in first-line therapy but also in circumstances in which retreatment is contemplated. The concept, popularized by Markman and Hoskins,[7] of using a 6-month interval to define patients as having potentially platinum sensitive (recurrence at ≥6 months after cessation of treatment) or platinum resistant (recurrence at <6 months) disease has been widely adopted. Refinements of the definition are often discussed, because there is a continuum of increasing likelihood of response and longer duration of response to retreatment with a platinum compound as the platinum-free interval is extended. But the answer to the question posed must also consider that all active drugs appear to work better against platinum-sensitive compared with platinum-resistant disease. Finally, the appeal of retreatment with platinum drugs in a palliative setting may be considerably less for patients who have sustained some persistent signs of neuropathy or still have vivid recollections of toxicities from these drugs. Therefore, groups such as the GOG have considered a 1-year cutoff satisfactory for trials of nonplatinum interventions in the second-line setting.

Results with cisplatin or carboplatin in patients with "platinum-sensitive" disease have given rise to some impressive results in terms of response rates and PFS (see Table 34-2). The randomized phase II study of the three-drug combination CAP (cyclophosphamide, doxorubicin [Adriamycin], and cisplatin [Platinol]) versus paclitaxel demonstrated median survival times exceeding 2 years, as did the phase III trial of carboplatin versus carboplatin + epirubicin. Single-arm phase II studies using retreatment with carboplatin + paclitaxel also showed impressive results, with more than 60% of patients demonstrating responses and many having complete responses.[122] On the other hand, comparative studies using other drugs, including both platinum-sensitive and platinum-resistant cohorts, have produced usually inferior median survival times (see Table 34-2), and subset analyses show consistent superior outcome and response rates in platinum-sensitive cohorts.[16,60]

The selection of a platinum versus a nonplatinum regimen is most problematic when the interval is between 6 months and 1 year and when there are residual toxicities from the preceding (platinum) regimen. If prolonging the platinum-free interval leads to reversal in platinum resistance, it may be advantageous to interpose another treatment to prolong the interval. This controversy is addressed later.

Is there a role for predictive assays in drug selection?

The previous controversy could move away from a merely theoretical debate if predictive assays for sensitivity to drugs were available. Actually, predictive assays have been in wide use in the treatment of ovarian cancer. Since the initial report using the now obsolete clonogenic assay,[123] ovarian cancer has been the solid tumor for which this approach has most often been used in drug selection.[124] These assays have had a minimal role in selecting the initial treatment, probably because the response to platinum-based chemotherapy often reaches as high as 80%. It would be difficult for an assay to be able to predict response with greater accuracy. In the second-line setting, however, response rates do not exceed 30% for all drugs except retreatment with platinums in the platinum-sensitive subset. Therefore, predictive assays could be useful both in indicating whether there is a role for retreatment with a platinum and in selecting an appropriate regimen for patients whose disease is not sensitive to cisplatin. The available literature contains studies that fall short in validating either of these rationales.

Overviews of various methods of drug resistance testing have been published suggesting a role in cancer treatment.[125] Although much has transpired in terms of methodology and clinical applications since the original reports, rigorous clinical trials have not been conducted to validate the concept. The reported data are analyzed in the following paragraphs from the perspective of state-of-the-art treatment of ovarian cancer.

In regard to correlation of assay findings with response, the pretreatment characteristics that have been related to outcome are response rates, time to failure, and survival. For second-line therapies, as noted earlier, tumor size, number of disease sites, and serous histology have been predictive of response in multivariate analyses.[61] We analyzed factors predictive of response to Doxil on multivariate analyses[126] and found that lack of bulky disease (tumors <5 cm) was the major predictor for a favorable response, time to failure, and survival. Series studying the role of these assays in ovarian cancer do not generally provide this information.

Response as a measure of benefit has been a major objective of such predictive assays. In first-line treatments based on platinums, the superior response rates were indeed associated with substantial gains in progression-free and overall survival in a number of randomized trials. However, the situation in second-line therapy and for previously treated patients is far from clear. Even assuming that the assays are able to accurately predict responsiveness to certain drugs, it is not clear whether such responses will have an impact on survival or will be superior to treatment with other agents that may not produce equivalent objective response rates. With these caveats, some series[127–131] have preferentially studied samples from untreated patients, and the true positive response rate is close to 50%, with a low (12%) false-positive rate. One series confined to platinum-resistant disease,[130] on the other hand, had 6 of 20 samples classified as sensitive to the assay, but only 3 patients responded, suggesting that false-positive results constitute a problem for the assay under these circumstances. All series, nevertheless, suggest a low rate of false-negative results. Overall, the data are consistent with clinical expectations in relation to platinum sensitivity. They also hint at greater problems in obtaining a reliable answer from an assay in the more refractory setting—not an unexpected finding.

A clinical trial showed a strikingly better outcome in 25 patients with assay-directed treatment, compared with 30 concurrent well-matched controls.[131] The encouraging results stimulated the authors to begin a prospective clinical trial. This report is inconclusive because (1) the study is quite small, (2) any such comparison is subject to bias, and (3) the impressive median survival time of almost 2 years (90 weeks, overshadowing the 50-week PFS of the controls) suggests that these patients shared features predicting for good survival, not necessarily reflected by the treatment received.

At present, a clinician considering obtaining such an assay to select a second-line treatment is faced with a number of questions that are difficult to answer: (1) what is the likelihood that the answer will prove helpful, (2) what is the cost of the procedure, and (3) is it worth the added morbidity required in some instances to obtain the sample? The claim that too high a bar is placed against proponents of assay-directed decisions must be contested. The usual requirements of clinical trials—that they address questions of risk versus benefit, avoid reliance on anecdotal reports, and generate the appropriate studies to prove their hypotheses—is applicable to assay-directed determinations in selecting the appropriate therapy for ovarian cancer. In favor of chemosensitivity assays, one might consider that the selection of therapy for retreatment is

guided primarily by the likelihood of responsiveness to platinums. In circumstances in which cures are highly unlikely, platinums could be avoided and toxicity would be spared. A clinical trial is required to prove this premise and has been under discussion in the GOG. On the other hand, if a patient's disease is empirically deemed platinum insensitive, the assay is unlikely to reliably enhance the prospect of a favorable outcome over what might result from empiric selections. Under these circumstances, a low percentage of responses and a substantial percentage of false-positive results may be anticipated from the assay.

Is resistance to platinums ever reversible? Molecular causes of clinical resistance to platinum compounds have defied easy identification and appear to be multifactorial, spanning abnormal uptake, enhanced intracellular detoxification of active platinum species, abnormal tolerance of platinum-DNA adducts, and ability to repair the adducts.[132,133] This complexity has thwarted attempts at restoring sensitivity to platinum compounds, because it is still far from clear what determines sensitivity (or resistance) to cisplatin. Drugs that "modulate" cisplatin antitumor effects, such as pentoxyphylline,[134] cyclosporine,[135] tirapazamine,[136] bryostatin 1, and others, have periodically made their way into phase II trials in ovarian cancer but have not proceeded further to phase III studies. A difficulty in enhancing the viability of such a resistance-reversal or efficacy-enhancing strategy is the formidable toxicity of cisplatin as one continues to treat with this compound in the absence of a proven net therapeutic gain.

Efforts to establish molecular markers of chemosensitivity in ovarian cancer have also been made, but they do not currently guide clinical decisions. The presence of BCL2 and p53 by immunohistochemistry did not correlate with results of the adenosine triphosphate (ATP) tumor chemosensitivity assay.[137] On the other hand, P53 positivity by immunohistochemistry predicted poor survival in patients with minimal residual disease entering a Southwest Oncology Group trial of intraperitoneal consolidation with nonplatinum drugs.[138] Many patients in this study were treated subsequently with carboplatin or cisplatin, so the poor outcome in the P53-positive patients could also have resulted from poorer response to subsequent exposure to these agents, although no difference in response according to P53 status is apparent in first-line therapy.

A hypothesis has been advanced that increasing the platinum-free interval by interposing another treatment, even a less effective treatment, would enhance the chances of responding again to the platinum.[139] If exposure to platinums in fact promotes expression of DNA repair pathways, the platinum-free interval could lead to downregulation of relevant genes and restoration of sensitivity. To test such a treatment strategy would require interposing an active, nonplatinum regimen without overt progression before crossing over to the platinum. A trial could readily be designed, with one arm interposing a treatment for a specified period before the platinum therapy and the other proceeding directly to it. Such a hypothesis has not been formally tested, either through purely clinical end points or through combined clinical and laboratory studies. Nevertheless, it has stimulated the use of agents other than platinums for patients with a potentially platinum-sensitive relapse.

Controversies Regarding Treatment Beyond Platinums

Beyond platinums: single agents or combinations?
This question faces the clinician quite often, but it has not received much attention in clinical trials and therefore remains largely unanswered. In patients with platinum-sensitive disease who are undergoing second-line treatment, a phase III trial showed no advantage of combinations over single-agent platinums (epirubicin + carboplatin versus carboplatin).[58] On the other hand, paclitaxel[122] was tested in combination with carboplatin in second-line therapy, and the response rates to the combinations were generally higher than with either drug alone, as indicated for gemcitabine. If a survival benefit is forthcoming from such combinations, one must be reminded that the proper comparator is sequential treatment, in view of similar findings in the first-line trial of cisplatin versus paclitaxel versus the combination (GOG 132).[140] Doxil in combination with carboplatin has special appeal as a combination for platinum-sensitive recurrences, because toxicity to combined treatment is likely to be quite acceptable, with a high degree of efficacy. An example is shown in Figure 34-3. A phase III trial of this combination versus single-agent carboplatin is planned within the Southwest Oncology Group.

Combinations of two nonplatinum second-line drugs (Doxil + topotecan, Doxil + gemcitabine, topotecan + oxaliplatin, gemcitabine + etoposide, and ifosfamide + paclitaxel)[141-145] have also been investigated in pilot studies, with good results reported in preliminary abstracts. Despite high response rates, such combinations cannot now be advocated outside the context of clinical trials. Other combinations are being proposed based on activity in chemosensitivity assays. Again, as noted earlier, there are considerable shortcomings to the data reported for such predictive assays. Some combinations, such as gemcitabine + cisplatin, are frequently predicted by assay results. Others, such as Doxil + vinorelbine, have been proposed based on patterns of activity from specimens of ovarian cancer subjected to the ATP chemosensitivity assay,[137] compared with little additivity with Doxil + treosulfan or Doxil + 5-FU, or Doxil + cisplatin.

Beyond platinums: a prescribed number of treatment cycles or prolonged maintenance?
There is no clinical trial support for the usual practice of delivering six cycles of treatment in second-line therapy (or thereafter). Current regimens only exceptionally lead to complete responses in second-line treatment, and even patients who achieve complete response exhibit a pattern of continued relapse. Such a pattern is also seen with second-line intraperitoneal therapy (i.e., consolidation), although small series have identified some patients with prolonged disease-free status at last report. Some drugs have little cumulative toxicity, and administration of continued cycles in the face of partial responses or stable disease appears desirable. Specifically, we employed continued treatment with paclitaxel when it was first used in the salvage setting,[146] as long as a response was maintained. Justification for such practice was reinforced by the recent finding that prolonging paclitaxel administration after platinum + paclitaxel induction leads to improved PFS.[106] A similar policy was adopted in our studies with Doxil.[126] Because of concerns about cardiotoxicity under such continued treatment, we reviewed the safety of this maintenance policy across several of our trials.[71] Specifically, with regard to cardiotoxicity, no clinical events were registered, and left ventricular ejection fractions declined from baseline only in patients who had previously received cardiotoxic drugs. The longest period of treatment on Doxil has been 5 years, in a patient whose CA 125 concentration rose steadily within 6 months after the initial carboplatin + paclitaxel treatment (Fig. 34-4).

RESPONSE AND PROLONGED REMISSION ON DOXIL
30 mg/m^2 WITH CARBOPLATIN AUC4 q 3 WEEKS
× 6 CYCLES BEGUN 4/01 FOLLOWED BY DOXIL 30 mg/m^2
q 5 WEEKS BEGUN 9/01. CUMULATIVE DOXIL DOSE 540 mg/m^2

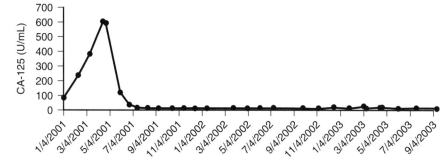

Figure 34–3. Patient CL. Pattern of CA 125 response to Doxil + carboplatin in a patient with platinum-sensitive disease, accompanied by regression of pelvic mass, that persists for longer than 2 years on Doxil maintenance.

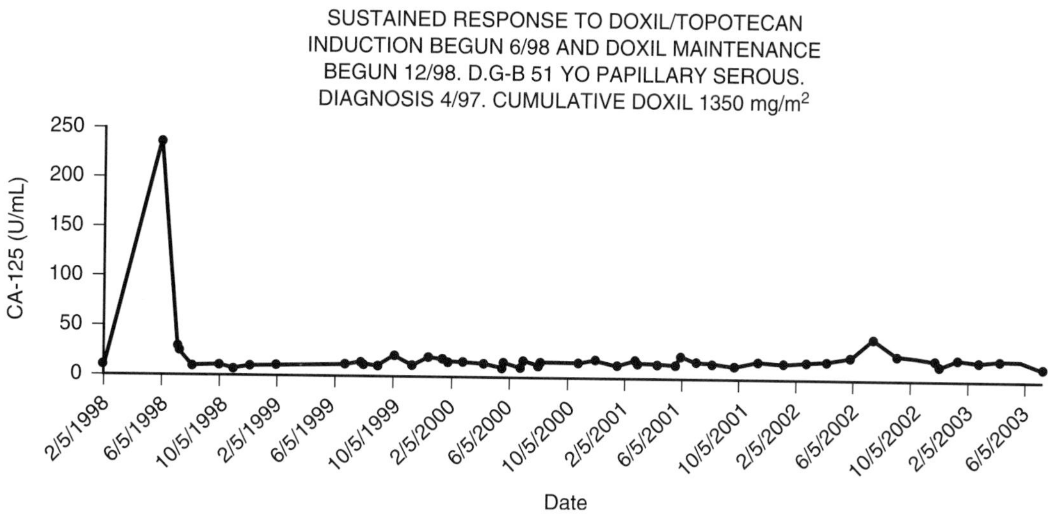

SUSTAINED RESPONSE TO DOXIL/TOPOTECAN
INDUCTION BEGUN 6/98 AND DOXIL MAINTENANCE
BEGUN 12/98. D.G-B 51 YO PAPILLARY SEROUS.
DIAGNOSIS 4/97. CUMULATIVE DOXIL 1350 mg/m^2

Figure 34–4. Patient GB. Pattern of CA 125 response to Doxil + topotecan in a patient with platinum-resistant disease that persists longer than 5 years on every-6-weeks Doxil maintenance. Cardiac function was stable.

Is there a desirable limit in treatment interventions beyond second-line therapy? The large number of drugs available for salvage treatments has encouraged the use or cycling of several regimens, one after another. This practice has justly been criticized as being unsupported by data that benefit is forthcoming for any treatment beyond second-line. In addition, most treatments are tolerated with increasing difficulty, although several of the drugs (i.e., Doxil, gemcitabine, topotecan) appear to have no cumulative toxicities. Currently, it is not uncommon for patients to continue to receive a number of drug trials after one or more platinum-based regimens. New chemotherapeutic agents, such as epothilone B and analogs, have been reported to show useful activity under such circumstances.[147–152]

Emerging General Issues

Is there a salvage role for radiotherapy either alone or in combination with chemotherapy? This is a fertile area for investigation. At present, however, radiation has yielded disappointing results against residual disease after an initial induction. This may in part be related to the emergence of resistance to radiation after platinum failure, as is suggested from preclinical studies.[153] However, one cannot exclude a role for radiation in localized recurrences, whether given by itself or in combination with other drugs. Specifically, topotecan, gemcitabine, or paclitaxel may be attractive radiosensitizers. Conversely, "chemosensitization" by radiation has been described, and a clinical trial with paclitaxel and whole-abdominal radiation in low doses has been initiated in a GOG pilot.

Should emerging noncytotoxic treatments be used outside clinical trials? Trials with pharmacodynamic end points and randomized trials with or without signal transduction or angiogenesis inhibitors have been initiated in patients with ovarian cancer, but results are not yet reported. The use of drugs such as tamoxifen in second-line therapy is supported by a low and variable percentage (0% to 17%) of objective responses after such treatment.[154–158] Notwithstanding the popularity of such approaches in patients with rising CA 125 only, there is no solid support for their use. In addition, the relationship of receptor status to response has been inconsistently studied and has given rise to conflicting results. The GOG is planning a randomized trial in patients with CA 125–only relapse, comparing tamoxifen with the antiangiogenic drug, thalidomide. Signal transduction inhibitors directed to the epidermal growth factor tyrosine kinase[159] and/or HER2[160] are also to be studied in this cohort of patients, with the hope of identifying antitumor effects in the most favorable circumstances. Other available noncytotoxic drug classes include other hormonal agents, agents to circumvent drug resistance, matrix metalloproteinase inhibitors (MMPIs), and immunotherapeutic modalities.[161]

Beyond these clinical circumstances in which the chances of symptomatic problems are few and a noninvasive end point is available, there is little justification for the use of laboratory-supported noncytotoxic agents (e.g., celecoxib, other cyclooxygenase-2 inhibitors), either alone or in combination with chemotherapy, outside clinical trials. A similar statement may be made regarding the addition of antiangiogenic compounds, modulators of drug activity, vaccines, or other stimulators of immunity. It was only through clinical trials that the lack of effect of MMPIs was demonstrated, after they were introduced with very high expectations.[161] Agents to circumvent paclitaxel resistance,[162,163] when given with paclitaxel, have not been shown to be superior to paclitaxel by itself, and pharmacodynamic modulators such as estramustine phosphate[164] have not been subjected to phase III trials together with paclitaxel.

Conclusion

Many of the issues concerning second-line therapies are mirrored in first-line trials, but clinical trials are more difficult to interpret beyond initial induction. Therefore, guidance for treatment strategies must continue to be based in part on findings from clinical trials of first-line treatments. Strategies that are unanswered in second-line treatments concern not only the need for surgical debulking but issues of use of a single agent versus a combination, and a prescribed number of treatment cycles versus maintenance therapy. The principal decision points remain whether to initiate therapy in the presence of a rising CA 125 and whether a platinum-based compound should be used. Such decisions are more critical than the actual selection of a particular non–platinum-containing regimen.

The array of chemotherapeutic agents that are active in the face of platinum resistance has been described, with indications of features that might favor use of one agent over another. The results in second-line therapy, based on randomized clinical trials and many phase II studies, appear equivalent for topotecan, Doxil, gemcitabine, and the taxanes. Areas ripe for clinical trials have been highlighted. Presently, many practices are also ongoing that lack a solid rationale, and this may be the major message of this chapter.

References

1. McGuire WP, Hoskins WJ, Brady MF, et al: Cyclophosphamide and cisplatin compared with paclitaxel and cisplatin in patients with stage III and stage IV ovarian cancer. N Engl J Med 1996;334:1-6.
2. Piccart MJ, Bertelsen K, James K, et al: Randomized intergroup trial of cisplatin-paclitaxel versus cisplatin-cyclo-phosphamide in women with advanced epithelial ovarian cancer: Three-year results. J Natl Cancer Inst 2000;92:699-708.
3. Ozols RF, Bundy BN, Fowler J, et al: Randomized phase III study of cisplatin/paclitaxel versus carboplatin/paclitaxel in optimal stage III ovarian cancer: A Gynecologic Oncology Group study (GOG 158) [abstract 1373]. Proc Am Soc Clin Oncol 1999;18:356a.
4. Blackledge G, Lawton F, Redman C, Kelly K: Response of patients in phase II studies of chemotherapy in ovarian cancer: Implications for patient treatment and the design of phase II trials. Br J Cancer 1989;59:650-653.
5. Markman M, Rothman R, Hakes T, et al: Second-line platinum therapy in patients with ovarian cancer previously treated with cisplatin. J Clin Oncol 1991;9:389-393.
6. Markman M, Reichman B, Hakes T, et al: Responses to second-line cisplatin-based intraperitoneal therapy in ovarian cancer: Influence of a prior response to intravenous cisplatin. J Clin Oncol 1991;9:1801-1805.
7. Markman M, Hoskins W: Responses to salvage chemotherapy in ovarian cancer: A critical need for precise definitions of the treated population. J Clin Oncol 1992;10:513-514.
8. McGuire WP, Rowinsky EK, Rosenshein NB, et al: Taxol: A unique antineoplastic agent with significant activity in advanced epithelial neoplasms. Ann Intern Med 1989;111:273-279.
9. Gore M: Treatment of relapsed epithelial ovarian cancer. American Society of Clinical Oncology Educational Book, McPerry (ed.), Alexandria, VA, May 2001. ASCO, pp 468-476.
10. Armstrong D, Rowinsky E, Donehower R, et al: A phase II trial of topotecan as salvage therapy in epithelial ovarian cancer [abstract 769]. Proc Am Soc Clin Oncol 1995;14:275a.
11. Creemers GJ, Bolis G, Gore M, et al: Topotecan, an active drug in the second-line treatment of epithelial ovarian cancer: Results of a large European phase II study. J Clin Oncol 1996;14:1552-1557.
12. Kudelka AP, Tresukosol D, Edwards CL, et al: Phase II study of intravenous topotecan as a 5-day infusion for refractory epithelial ovarian carcinoma. J Clin Oncol 1996;14:1552-1557.
13. Swisher EM, Mutch DG, Rader JS, et al: Topotecan in platinum and paclitaxel-resistant ovarian cancer. Gynecol Oncol 1997;66:480-486.
14. Malmstrom H, Ridderheim M, Sorbe B, et al: Salvage treatment of advanced ovarian cancer with Hycamtin [abstract]. Proc Am Soc Clin Oncol 1999;18:1462a.
15. Bookman MA, Malmstrom H, Bolis G, et al: Topotecan for the treatment of advanced epithelial ovarian cancer: An open-label phase II study in patients treated after prior chemotherapy that contained cisplatin or carboplatin and paclitaxel. J Clin Oncol 1998;16:3345-3352.
16. Gordon AN, Fleagle JT, Guthrie D, et al: Interim analysis of a phase II randomized trial of doxil/caelyx (D) versus topotecan (T) in the treatment of patients with relapsed ovarian cancer [abstract]. Proc Am Soc Clin Oncol 2000;19:1504a.
17. ten Bokkel Huinink W, Gore M, Carmichael J, et al: Topotecan versus paclitaxel for the treatment of recurrent epithelial ovarian cancer. J Clin Oncol 1997;15:2183-2193.
18. Gore M, Rustin G, Calvert H, et al: A multicenter, randomized, phase III study of topotecan (T) administered intravenously or orally for advanced epithelial ovarian carcinoma [abstract]. Proc Am Soc Clin Oncol 1998;17:1346a.
19. Hoskins P, Eisenhauer E, Beare S, et al: Randomized phase II study of two schedules of topotecan in previously treated patients with ovarian cancer: A National Cancer Institute of Canada Clinical Trials Group study. J Clin Oncol 1998;16:2233-2237.
20. Gordon AN, Granai CO, Rose PG, et al: Phase II study of liposomal doxorubicin in platinum- and paclitaxel-refractor epithelial ovarian cancer. J Clin Oncol 2000;18:3093-3100.
21. Israel VP, Garcia AA, Roman L, et al: Phase II study of liposomal doxorubicin in advanced gynecologic cancers. Gynecol Oncol 2000;78:143-147.
22. Markman M, Kennedy A, Webster K, et al: Phase 2 trial of liposomal doxorubincin (40 mg/m²) in platinum/paclitaxel-refractory ovarian and fallopian tube cancers and primary carcinoma of the peritoneum. Gynecol Oncol 2000;78:369-372.
23. Markman M, Blessing JA, Moore D, et al: Altretamine (hexamethylmelamine) in platinum-resistant and platinum refractory ovarian cancer: A Gynecologic Oncology Group phase II trial. Gynecol Oncol 1998;69:226-229.
24. Manetta A, MacNeill C, Lyter JA, et al: Hexamethylmelamine as a single second-line: Agent in ovarian cancer. Gynecol Oncol 1990;36:93-96.
25. Moore DH, Valea F, Crumpler LS, et al: Hexamethylmelamine/altretamine as second-line therapy for epithelial ovarian carcinoma. Gynecol Oncol 1993;51:109-112.
26. Rustin GJ, Nelstrop AE, Crawford M, et al: Phase II trial of oral altretamine for relapsed ovarian carcinoma: Evaluation of defining response by serum CA125. J Clin Oncol 1997;5:172-176.
27. Schink JC, Harris S, Grosen R, et al: Altretamine (Hexalen) an effective salvage chemotherapy after paclitaxel (Taxol) in women with recurrent platinum resistant ovarian cancer [abstract]. Proc Am Soc Clin Oncol 1995;14:770a.
28. Vergote I, Himmelmann A. Frankendal B, et al: Hexamethylmelamine as second-line therapy in platinum-resistant ovarian cancer. Gynecol Oncol 1992;47:282-286.
29. Hansen F, Malthe I, Krog H: Phase II clinical trial of VP-16-213 (etoposide) administered orally in advanced ovarian cancer. Gyncol Oncol 1990;36:369-370.
30. Hoskins PJ, Swenerton K: Oral etoposide is active against platinum-resistant epithelial ovarian cancer. J Clin Oncol 1994;2:60-63.
31. de Wit R, van der Burg AE, van den Gaast A, et al: Phase II study of prolonged oral etoposide in patients with ovarian cancer refractory to or relapsing within 12 months later platinum-containing chemotherapy. Ann Oncol 1994;5:656-657.
32. Markman M, Hakes T, Reichman B, et al: Phase 2 trial of chronic low-dose oral etoposide as salvage therapy of platinum-refractory ovarian cancer. J Cancer Res Clin Oncol 1992;119:55-57.

33. Marzola M, Zucchetti M, Colombo N, et al: Low-dose oral etoposide in epithelial cancer of the ovary. Ann Oncol 1993;4:517-519.

34. Rose PG, Blessing JA, Mayer AR, et al: Prolonged oral etoposide as second-line therapy for platinum-resistant and platinum-sensitive ovarian carcinoma: A Gynecologic Oncology Group study. J Clin Oncol 1998;16:405-410.

35. Seymour MT, Mansi JL, Gallagher CJ, et al: Protracted oral etoposide in epithelial ovarian cancer: A phase II study in patients with relapsed or platinum-resistant disease. Br J Cancer 1994;69:191-195.

36. Coenen M, Bertellot P, Amant F, et al: Gemcitabine in platinum-paclitaxel resistant ovarian carcinoma [abstract]. Proc Am Soc Clin Oncol 2000;19:603a.

37. Friedlander M, Millward MJ, Bell D, et al: A phase II study of gemcitabine in platinum pre-treated patients with advanced epithelial ovarian cancer. Ann Oncol 1998;9:1343-1345.

38. Kaufmann M, Bauknecht T, Jonat W, et al: Gemcitabine (GEM) in cisplatin-resistant ovarian cancer [abstract]. Proc Am Soc Clin Oncol 1995;14:758.

39. Lund B, Hansen OP, Theilade K, et al: Phase II study of gemcitabine (2',2'-difluorodeoxycitidine) in previously treated ovarian cancer patients. J Natl Cancer Inst 1994;86:530-533.

40. von Minckwitz G, Bauknecht T, Visseren-Grul CM, et al: Phase II study of gemcitabine in ovarian cancer. Ann Oncol 1999;10:853-855.

41. Silver DF, Piver MS: Gemcitabine salvage chemotherapy for patients with gynecologic malignancies of the ovary, fallopian tube and peritoneum. Am J Clin Oncol 1999;22:450-452.

42. Francis P, Schneider J, Hann L, et al: Phase II trial of docetaxel in patients with platinum-refractory advanced ovarian cancer. J Clin Oncol 1994;12:2301-2308.

43. Kavanagh J, Kudelka AP, de Leon CG, et al: Phase II study of docetaxel in patients with epithelial ovarian carcinoma refractory to platinum. Clin Cancer Res 1996;2:837-842.

44. Kavanagh JJ, Winn R, Steger M, et al: Docetaxel for patients with ovarian cancer refractory to paclitaxel: An update [abstract]. Proc Am Soc Clin Oncol 1999;18:1423a.

45. Piccart MJ, Gore M, ten Bokkel Huinink W, et al: Docetaxel: An active new drug for treatment of advanced epithelial ovarian cancer. J Natl Cancer Inst 1995;87:676-681.

46. Coleman R, Towlson K, Wiltshaw E, et al: Epirubicin for pre-treated advanced ovarian cancer. Eur J Cancer 1990;26:850-851.

47. Hurtloup P, Cappelaere P, Armand JP, et al: Phase II clinical evaluation of 4'-epi-doxorubicin. Cancer Treat Rep 1983;67:337-334.

48. Locatelli M, D'Antona A, Vinci M, et al: Second-line chemotherapy with epirubicin (EDR) in ovarian carcinoma [abstract]. Ann Oncol 1990;1(Suppl):15.

49. Simonsen E, Bengtsson C, Hogberg T, et al: A phase II study of the effect of 4' epi-doxorubicin, administered in high dose 150 mg in 24 hours intravenous infusion in advanced ovarian carcinoma. Proc Eur Conf Clin Oncol 1987;4:226.

50. Trope C, Christiansson H, Johnsson JE, et al: A phase II study of 4'-epidoxorobucin in advanced ovarian carcinoma: Anthracyclines and cancer therapy. Proceedings of a Symposium in Ronneby Brunn, Sweden, Oct 6-7, 1982, pp 216-221.

51. Vermorken JB, Kobierska A, Chevallier B, et al: A phase II study of high-dose epirubicin in ovarian cancer patients previously treated with cisplatin: EORTC Gynecological Cancer Cooperative Group. Ann Oncol 2000;11:1035-1040.

52. Bougnoux P, Dieras V, Petit T, et al: A multicenter phase II study of oxaliplatin (OXA) as a single agent in platinum (PT) and or taxanes (TX) pretreated advanced ovarian cancer (AOC): Final results [abstract]. Proc Am Soc Clin Oncol 1999;18:1422a.

53. Chollet P, Bensmaine MA, Brienza S, et al: Single agent activity of oxaliplatin in heavily pretreated advanced epithelial ovarian cancer. Ann Oncol 1996;7:1065-1070.

54. Piccart MJ, Green JA, Lacave AJ, et al: Oxaliplatin or paclitaxel in patients with platinum-pretreated advanced ovarian cancer: A randomized phase II study of the European Organization for Research and Treatment of Cancer Gynecology Group. J Clin Oncol 2000;18:1193-1202.

55. Bajetta E, Di Leo A, Biganzol L, et al: Phase II study of vinorelbine in patients with pretreated advanced cancer: Activity in platinum-resistant disease. J Clin Oncol 1996;14:2546-2551.

56. Burger RA, DiSaia PJ, Roberts JA, et al: Phase II trial of vinorelbine in recurrent and progressive epithelial ovarian cancer. Gynecol Oncol 1999;72:148-153.

57. Takeuchi S, Dobashi K, Fujimoto S, et al: A late phase II study of CPT-11 on uterine cervical cancer and ovarian cancer: Research groups of CPT-11 on gynecologic cancer. Gan Kagehe Ryoho 1991;18:1681-1689.

58. Bolis G, Scarfone G, Giardina G, et al: Carboplatin alone vs carboplatin plus epidoxorubicin as second-line therapy for cisplatin- or carboplatin-sensitive ovarian cancer. Gynecol Oncol 2001;81:3-9.

59. Cantu MG, Buda A, Parma G, et al: Randomized controlled trial of single-agent paclitaxel versus cyclophosphamide, doxorubicin, and cisplatin in patients with recurrent ovarian cancer who responded to first-line platinum-based regimens. J Clin Oncol 2002;20:1232-1237.

60. O'Byrne KJ, Bliss P, Graham JD, et al: A phase III study of Doxyl/Caelyx versus paclitaxel in platinum-treated, taxane-naïve relapsed ovarian cancer [abstract 808]. Proc Am Soc Clin Oncol 2002;21:203a.

61. Eisenhauer EA, Vermorken JB, van Glabbeke M: Predictors of response to subsequent chemotherapy in platinum pretreated ovarian cancer: A multivariate analysis of 704 patients. Ann Oncol 1997;8:963-968.

62. Fenelly D, Aghajanian C, Shapiro F, et al: Phase I and pharmacologic study of paclitaxel administered weekly in patients with relapsed ovarian cancer. JClin Oncol 1997;15:187-192.

63. O'Leary J, Muggia FM: Clinical oncology update. Camptothecins: A review of their development and schedules of administration. Eur J Cancer 1998;34:1500-1508.

64. Muggia F, Liebes L, Potmesil M, et al: Intraperitoneal topoisomerase-I inhibitors: Preliminary findings with 9-aminocamptothecin. Ann N Y Acad Sci. 2000;922:178-187.

65. Calvert H, Grimshaw R, Poole C, et al: Randomized trial of two intravenous schedules of the liposomal topoisomerase I inhibitor, OSI-211 (NX211), in women with relapsed ovarian cancer: An NCIC CTG study [abstract 830]. Proc Am Soc Clin Oncol 2002;21:208a.

66. Kruijtzer CM, Beijnen JH, Rosing H, et al: Increased oral bioavailability of topotecan in combination with the breast cancer resistance protein and P-glycoprotein inhibitor GF 120918. J Clin Oncol 2002;20:2943-2950.

67. Muggia FM: Doxorubicin-polymer conjugates: Further demonstration of the concept of enhanced permeability and retention [editorial]. Clin Cancer Res 1998;5:7-8.

68. Muggia FM, Hainsworth J, Jeffers S, et al: Phase II study of Doxil in refractory ovarian cancer: Antitumor activity and toxicity modification by liposomal encapsulation. J Clin Oncol 1997;15:987-993.

69. Garcia A, Muggia FM: Activity of anthracyclines in refractory ovarian cancer: Recent experience and review. Cancer Invest 1997;15:329-334.

70. Du Bois A, Weber B, Pfisterer J, et al: Epirubicin/paclitaxel/carboplatin vs paclitaxel/carboplatin in first-line treatment of ovarian cancer FIGO stages IIb-IV: Interim results of an AGO-GINECO Intergroup phase III trial [abstract 805]. Proc Am Soc Clin Oncol 2001;20:202a.

71. Safra T, Muggia F, Jeffers S, et al: Pegylated liposomal doxorubicin (doxil): Reduced clinical cardiotoxicity in patients reaching or exceeding cumulative doses of 500 mg/m². Ann Oncol 2000;11:1029-1033.

72. Muggia FM: Management of ovarian cancer after front-line combinations [abstract 35]. Cancer Invest 2001;19(Suppl 1):39-40.

73. Muggia FM, Russell CA: New chemotherapies for ovarian cancer: Systemic and intraperitoneal podophyllotoxins. Cancer 1991;67:225-230.

74. Muggia FM, Groshen S, Russell C, et al: Intraperitoneal carboplatin and etoposide for persistent epithelial ovarian cancer after platinum-based regimens. Gynecol Oncol 1993;50:232-238.

75. Clark PI: Clinical pharmacology and schedule dependency of the podophyllotoxin derivative. Semin Oncol 1992;19(Suppl 6):20-27.

76. Whitbook JA, Greep, Lukens JN: Epipodophyllotoxin-related leukemia. Cancer 1991;68:600-604.

77. Muggia FM, Blessing JA, Homesley HD, Sorosky J: Tomudex (ZD1694, NSC 639186) in platinum-pretreated recurrent epithelial

ovarian cancer: A phase II study by the Gynecologic Oncology Group. Cancer Chemother Pharmacol 1998;42:68-70.

78. Morgan RJ Jr, Speyer J, Doroshow JH, et al: Modulation of 5-fluorouracil with high-dose leucovorin calcium: Activity in ovarian cancer and correlation with CA-125 levels. Gynecol Oncol 1995;58:79-85.

79. Wolf JK, Sun CC, Vershraeggen CF, et al: A phase II study of Xeloda in patients with chemotherapy resistant recurrent ovarian cancer [abstract 893]. Proc Am Soc Clin Oncol 2002; 21:224a.

80. Kroep JR, Peters GJ, van Moorsel CJ, et al: Gemcitabine-cisplatin: A schedule finding study. Ann Oncol 1999;10:1503-1510.

81. Safra T, Jeffers, Sorich J, et al: Gemcitabine plus cisplatin combination given with amifostine (GAP) to heavily pretreated patients with gynecologic and peritoneal cancers: Tolerance and activity in ovarian cancer. Anticancer Drugs 1998;9:511-514.

82. Strauss E: Pretesting tumors. Sci Am 1999;280:19-20.

83. Perren TJ, Wiltshaw E, Harper P, et al: A randomized study of carboplatin vs sequential ifosfamide/carboplatinum for patients with FIGO stage III epithelial ovarian carcinoma. Br J Cancer 1993;68:1190-1194.

84. Sutton GP, Blessing JA, Homesley HD, et al: Phase II trial of ifosfamide and mesna in advanced ovarian carcinoma: A Gynecologic Oncology Group Study. J Clin Oncol 1989;7: 1672-1676.

85. Markman M, Hakes T, Reichman B, et al: Ifosfamide and mesna in previously treated advanced epithelial ovarian cancer: Activity in platinum-resistant disease. J Clin Oncol 1992;10: 243-248.

86. Ledermann JA, Herd R, Maraninchi D, et al: High-dose chemotherapy for ovarian carcinoma: Long-term results from the Solid Tumor Registry of the European Group for Blood and Bone Marrow Transplantation (EBMT). Ann Oncol 2001;12: 693-700.

87. Stiff PJ, Veum-Stone J, Lazarus HM, et al: High-dose chemotherapy and autologous stem-cell transplantation for ovarian cancer: An autologous blood and marrow transplant registry report. Ann Intern Med 2000;133:504-515.

88. Lotz JP, Machover D, Malassagne B, et al: Phase I-II study of two consecutive courses of high-dose epipodophyllotoxin, ifosfamide, and carboplatin with autologous bone marrow transplantation for treatment of adult patients with solid tumors. J Clin Oncol 1991;9:1860-1870.

89. Legros M, Dauplat J, Fleury J, et al: High-dose chemotherapy with hematopoetic rescue in patients with state III to IV ovarian cancer: Long-term results. J Clin Oncol 1997;15:1302-1308.

90. Stiff PJ, Bayer R, Kerger C, et al: High-dose chemotherapy with autologous transplantation for persistent/relapsed ovarian cancer: A multivariate analysis of survival for 100 consecutively treated patients. J Clin Oncol 1997;15:1309-1317.

91. Viens P, Maraninchi D, Legros M, et al: High dose melphalan and autologous marrow rescue in advanced epithelial ovarian carcinomas: A retrospective analysis of 35 patients treated in France. Bone Marrow Transplant 1990;5:227-233.

92. Thigpen JT: Dose-intensity in ovarian carcinoma: Hold, enough? J Clin Oncol 1997;15:1291-1293.

93. McGuire W: How many more nails to seal the coffin of dose intensity. Ann Oncol 1997;8:311-313.

94. Fennelly D, Schneider J, Spriggs D, et al: Dose escalation of paclitaxel with high-dose cyclophosphamide, with analysis of progenitor-cell mobilization and hematologic support of advanced ovarian cancer patients receiving rapidly sequenced high-dose carboplatin/cyclophosphamide courses. J Clin Oncol 1995;13:1160-1166.

95. Schilder R, Shea T, Fennelly D, et al: A pilot evaluation of sequential courses of high dose carboplatin and paclitaxel followed by high dose melphalan rescued with cyclosphosphamide/paclitaxel primed peripheral progenitor cells in patients with advanced ovarian cancer: A Gynecologic Oncology Group pilot #9501. Gynecol Oncol 2003;88:3-8.

96. Cure H, Battista C, Guastalla J, et al: Phase III randomized trial of high-dose chemotherapy (HDC) and peripheral blood stem cell (PBSC) support as consolidation in patients with responsive low-burden advanced ovarian cancer (AOC): Preliminary report of a GINECO/FNCLCC/SFGM-TC study [abstract 815]. Proc Am Soc Clin Oncol 2001;20:204a.

97. Pater JL, Carmichael JA, Krepart GV, et al: Second-line chemotherapy of stage III-IV ovarian carcinoma: A randomized comparison of melphalan to melphalan and hexamethylmelamine in patients with persistent disease after doxorubicin and cisplatin. Cancer Treat Rep 1987;71:277-281.

98. Reimer RR, Hoover R, Fraumeni JF, Young RC: Acute leukemia after alkylating agent therapy in ovarian cancer. N Engl J Med 1977;297:117-122.

99. Weiss RB: The role of hexamethylmelamine in advanced ovarian carcinoma. Gynecol Oncol 1981;12:141-149.

100. Muggia FM: Hexamethylmelamine in platinum-resistant ovarian cancer: How active? [editorial]. Gynecol Oncol 1992;47:279-281.

101. Alberts DS, Rothenberg ML, Liu PY, et al: Altretamine (Hexalen) consolidation for patients with stage III epithelial ovarian cancer in clinical complete remission: A Southwest Oncology Group study [abstract 1520]. Proc Am Soc Clin Oncol 2000;19:384a.

102. Spanu P, Ferrero A, Fuso L, et al: Gemcitabine and vinorelbine in relapsed ovarian cancer: A phase II study [abstract 848]. Proc Am Soc Clin Oncol 2001;20:212a.

103. Parimoo D, Jeffers S, Muggia FM: Severe neurotoxicity from vinorelbine-paclitaxel combinations [letter]. J Natl Cancer Inst 1996;88:1079-1080.

104. Creech RH, Shah MK, Catalano RB, et al: Phase II study of low-dose mitomycin in patients with ovarian cancer previously treated with chemotherapy. Cancer Treat Rep 1985;69:1271-1273.

105. Laadem A, Cvitkovic E: Oxaliplatin: A first DACH-platinum in oncology. Bull Cancer 2001;88:S9-S13.

106. Markman M, Liu PY, Wilczynski S, et al: Phase III randomized trial of 12 versus 3 months of maintenance paclitaxel in patients with advanced ovarian cancer after complete response to platinum and paclitaxel-based chemotherapy: a Southwest Oncology Group and Gynecologic Oncology Group trial. J Clin Oncol. 2003; 21(13):2460-2465.

107. Guastalla JP, Lhomme C, Kerbrat P, et al: Phase II trial of intraperitoneal carboplatin in ovarian carcinoma patients with macroscopic residual disease at second-look laparotomy: A multicenter study of the French Federation Nationale des Centres de Lutte Contre le Cancer. Ann Oncol 1994;5:127-132.

108. Markman M, Reichman B, Hakes T, et al: Phase II trial of intraperitoneal carboplatin and etoposide as salvage treatment of advanced epithelial ovarian cancer. Gynecol Oncol 1992;47:353-357.

109. Reichman B, Markman M, Hakes T, et al: Intraperitoneal cisplatin and etoposide in the treatment of refractory/recurrent ovarian carcinoma. J Clin Oncol 1989;7:1327-1333.

110. Muggia FM, Liu PY, Alberts DS, et al: Intraperitoneal mitoxantrone or floxuridine: Effects on time-to-failure and survival in patients with minimal residual ovarian cancer after second-look laparotomy. Gynecol Oncol 1996;61:395-402.

111. Muggia F, Liebes L, Potmesil M, et al: Intraperitoneal topoisomerase-I inhibitors: Preliminary findings with 9-aminocamptothecin. Ann N Y Acad Sci 2000;922:178-187.

112. Panteix G, Beaujard A, Garbit F, et al: Population pharmacokinetics of cisplatin in patients with advanced ovarian cancer during intraperitoneal hyperthermia chemotherapy. Anticancer Res 2002;22:1329-1336.

113. Edwards RP, Gooding W, Lembersky BC, et al: Comparison of toxicity and survival following intraperitoneal recombinant interleukin-2 for persistent ovarian cancer after platinum: Twenty-four-hour versus 7-day infusion. J Clin Oncol 1997; 15:3399.

114. Epenetos AA, Hooker G, Krausz T: Antibody-guided irradiation of malignant ascites ovarian cancer: A new therapeutic method possessing specificity against cancer cells. Obstet Gynecol 1986;68:71s-74s.

115. Santoso JT, Tang DC, Lane SB, et al: Adenovirus-based p53 gene therapy in ovarian cancer. Gynecol Oncol 1995;50:171-178.

116. Ozols RF, Bundy BN, Fowler J, et al: Randomized phase III study of cisplatin/paclitaxel versus carboplatin/paclitaxel in optimal stage III epithelial ovarian cancer: A Gynecologic Oncology Group Study (GOG 158) [abstract 1373]. Proc Am Soc Clin Oncol 1999;8:356A.

117. Muderspach L, Muggia FM, Conti PS: Second-look laparotomy for stage III epithelial ovarian cancer: Rationale and current issues. Cancer Treat Rev 1996;21:499-511.

118. Rustin GJ, Marples M, Nelstrop AE, et al: Use of CA-125 to define progression of ovarian cancer in patients with persistently elevated levels. J Clin Oncol 2001;19:4054-4057.

119. Armstrong DK: Long-term strategies for the treatment of relapsed ovarian cancer: A chronic disease [abstract 33]. Cancer Invest 2002;20(Suppl 1):42-43.

120. Vanderburg MEL: Symptomless rise in CA 125. In: Ledermann JA, Hoskins WA, Kaye SB, Vergote IB (Eds.): Clinical Management of Ovarian Cancer. London: Martin Dunitz, 2001, pp 189-200.

121. Eisenkop SM, Friedman RL, Spirtos NM: The role of secondary cytoreductive surgery in the treatment of patients with recurrent epithelial ovarian carcinoma. Cancer 2000;88:144-153.

122. Dizon D, Hensley M, Sabbatini P, et al: Carboplatin and paclitaxel as initial second-line therapy in recurrent epithelial ovarian carcinoma [abstract 809]. Proc Am Soc Clin Oncol 2001;20:203a.

123. Alberts DS, Chen HS, Salmon SE, et al: Chemotherapy of ovarian cancer directed by the human tumor stem cell assay. Cancer Chemother Pharmacol 1981;6:279-275.

124. Ness RB, Wisniewski SR, Eng H, et al: Cell viability assay for drug testing in ovarian cancer: In vitro kill versus clinical response. Anticancer Res 2002;22:1145-1149.

125. Weisenthal LM, Kern DH: Prediction of drug resistance in cancer chemotherapy: The Kern and DISC assays. Oncology (USA) 1991;5:93-103.

126. Safra T, Groshen S, Jeffers S, et al: Treatment of patients with ovarian carcinoma with pegylated liposomal doxorubicin: Analysis of toxicities and predictors of outcome. Cancer 2001;91:90-100.

127. Blackman KE, Fingert HJ, Fuller AF, et al: The fluorescent cytoprint essay in gynecological malignancies and breast cancer: Methodologies and results. In Koechli OR, Sevin B-U, Haller U (Eds.): Chemosensitivity Testing in Gynecological Malignancies and Breast Cancer. Basel: Karger, 1994, pp 53-63.

128. Wilson JK, Sargent JM, Elgie AW, et al: A feasibility study of the MTT assay for chemosensitivity testing in ovarian malignancy. Br J Cancer 1990;62:189-194.

129. Ohie S, Udagawa Y, Kazu A, et al: Cisplatin sensitivity of ovarian cancer in the histoculture drug response assay correlates with clinical response to combination chemotherapy with cisplatin, doxorubicin, and cyclophosphamide. Anticancer Res 2000;20:2049-2054.

130. Ng TY, Ngan HYS, Chang DKL, Wonj LC: Clinical applicability of the ATP cell viability assay as a predictor of chemo response in platinum resistant epithelial ovarian cancer using nonsurgical tumor cell sample. Gynecol Oncol 1998;68:45-46.

131. Kurbacher CM, Cree IA, Bruckner HW, et al: Use of an ex vivo ATP luminescence assay to direct chemotherapy for recurrent ovarian cancer. Anticancer Drugs 1998;9:51-57.

132. Los G, Muggia FM: Platinum resistance: Experimental and clinical status. Hematol Oncol Clin North Am 1994;8:411-429.

133. Chaney SG, Vaisman A: DNA adduct tolerance and bypass. In Kelland LR, Farrll N (Eds.): Platinum-based Drugs in Cancer Therapy. Totowa, NJ: Humana Press, 2000, pp 129-148.

134. Mannel RS, Blessing JA, Boike G: Cisplatin and pentoxifylline in advanced or recurrent squamous cell carcinoma of the cervix: A Phase II trial of the Gynecologic Oncology Group. Gynecol Oncol 2000;79:64-66.

135. Manetta A, Blessing JA, Hurteau JA: Evaluation of cisplatin and cyclosporin A in recurrent platinum-resistant ovarian cancer: A phase II study of the Gynecologic Oncology Group. Gynecol Oncol 1998;68:45-46.

136. Brown JM, Wang LH: Tirapazamine: Laboratory data relevant to clinical activity. Anticancer Drug Des 1998;13:529-539.

137. Di Nicolantonio F, Neale MH, Knight LA, et al: Use of an ATP-based chemosensitivity assay to design new combinations of high-concentration doxorubicin with other drugs for recurrent ovarian cancer. Anticancer Drugs 2002;13:625-630.

138. Hawes D, Liu PY, Muggia FM, et al: Correlation of p53 immunostaining in primary and residual ovarian cancer at the time of positive second-look laparotomy, and its prognostic role: A Southwest Oncology Group ancillary study. Gynecol Oncol 2002;87:17-23.

139. McGuire WP: Sequencing therapies in relapsed ovarian cancer [abstract 26]. Chemo Foundation Symposium XX Innovative Cancer Therapy for Tomorrow, Nov. 2002, Cancer Investigation 2003 (Suppl 1); 21:34.

140. Muggia FM, Braly PS, Brady MF, et al: Phase III randomized study of cisplatin versus cisplatin and paclitaxel in patients with suboptimal stage III or IV ovarian cancer: A Gynecologic Oncology Group Study. J Clin Oncol 2000;18:106-115.

141. Hamilton A, Hochster H, Rosenthal M, et al: Continuous infusion topotecan with Doxil: A phase I study of dual topoisomerase inhibition [abstract 777]. Proc Am Soc Clin Oncol 2000;19:200a.

142. Tobias DH, Runowicz C, Mandeli J, et al: A phase I trial of gemcitabine and Doxil in recurrent epithelial ovarian cancer [abstract 1551]. Proc Am Soc Clin Oncol 2000;19:392a.

143. Lu MJ, Hochster H, Escalon J, et al: Oxaliplatin and continuous infusion topotecan regimen for refractory ovarian cancer. [Abstract 1860] Proc Am Soc Clin Oncol 2003;22:463.

144. Lentz S, Garcia A, Bookman M, et al: Phase I trial of gemcitabine and protracted oral etoposide in recurrent gynecological tumors: A Gynecologic Oncology Group study [abstract 1604]. Proc Am Soc Clin Onc 2000;19:405a.

145. Markman M, Spriggs D, Burger RA, et al: Phase I trial of ifosfamide and 24-h infusional paclitaxel in pelvic malignancies: A Gynecologic Oncology Group study. Gynecol Oncol 2001;80:359-363.

146. Uziely B, Groshen S, Jeffers S, et al: Paclitaxel (Taxol) in heavily pretreated ovarian cancer: Antitumor activity and complications. Ann Oncol 1994;5:827-833.

147. Altmann KH, Wartmann M, O'Reilly T: Epothilones and related structures: A new class of microtubule inhibitors with potent in vivo antitumor activity. Biochem Biophys Acta 2000;14770:M79-M91.

148. Lee FY, Borzilleri R, Fairchild CR, et al: BMS-2475509: A novel epothilone analog with a mode of action similar to paclitaxel but possessing superior antitumor efficacy. Clin Cancer Res 2001;7:1429-1437.

149. Bollag DM, McQueney PA, Zhu J, et al: Epothilones, a new class of microtubule-stabilizing agents with a taxol-like mechanism of action. Cancer Res 1995;55:2325-2333.

150. McDaid HM, Mani S, Shen H-J, et al: Validation of the pharmacodynamics of BMS-247550, an analog of epothilone B, during a phase I clinical study. Clin Cancer Res 2002;8:2035-2043.

151. Rubin EH, Siu LL, Beers S, et al: A phase I and pharmacologic trial of weekly epothilone B in patients with advanced malignancies [abstract 270]. Proc Am Soc Clin Oncol 2001;20:68a.

152. Mani S, McDaid H, Shen H-J, et al: Phase I evaluation of an epothilone B analog (BMS-247550): Clinical findings and molecular correlates. Proc Am Soc Clin Oncol 2001;20:269.

153. Vaisman A, Chaney SG: Induction of UV damage recognition protein by cisplatin treatment. Biochemistry 1995;34:105-114.

154. Shirey DR, Kavanagh JJ Jr, Gershenson DM, et al: Tamoxifen therapy of epithelial ovarian cancer. Obstet Gynecol 1985;66:208-213.

155. Weiner SA, Alberts DS, Surwit EA, et al: Tamoxifen therapy in recurrent epithelial ovarian carcinoma. Gynecol Oncol 1987;27:208-213.

156. Hatch KD, Beecham JB, Blessing JA, et al: Responsiveness of patients with advanced ovarian carcinoma to tamoxifen: A Gynecologic Oncology Group study of second line therapy in 105 patients. Cancer 1991;68:269-271.

157. Ahlgren JD, Ellison NM, Gottlieb RJ, et al: Hormonal palliation of chemoresistant ovarian cancer: Three consecutive phase II trials of the Mid-Atlantic Oncology Program. J Clin Oncol 1993; 11:1957-1968.

158. Markman M, Iseminger KA, Hatch KD, et al: Tamoxifen in platinum-refractory ovarian cancer: A Gynecologic Oncology Group Ancillary Report. Gynecol Oncol 1996;62:4-6.

159. Finkler N, Gordon A, Crozier M, et al: Phase II evaluation of OSI-774, a potent oral antagonist of the EGFR-TK in patients with advanced ovarian cancer [abstract 831]. Proc Am Soc Clin Oncol 2001;20:abstr 831.

160. Meden H, Kuhn W: Overexpression of the oncogene c-erB-2 (Her 2/neu) in ovarian cancer: A new prognostic factor. Eur J Obstet Gynecol Reprod Biol 1997;71:173-179.

161. Kaye SB, Eisenhauer EA, Hamilton TC: New non-cytotoxic approaches to ovarian cancer. Ann Oncol 1999;10(Suppl 1): 65-68.
162. Seiden MV: A phase II study with the MDR inhibitor Incel™ (Biricodar, VX-710) with paclitaxel in strictly defined paclitaxel refractory ovarian cancer patients [abstract 36]. Cancer Invest 2001;19(Suppl 1):41-42.
163. Joly F, Mangioni C, et al: A phase 3 study of PSC833 in combination with paclitaxel and carboplatin (PC-PSC) versus paclitaxel and carboplatin (PC) alone in patients with stage IV or suboptimally debulked stage III epithelial ovarian cancer or primary cancer of the peritoneum [abstract 806]. Proc Am Soc Clin Oncol 2002;21:202a.
164. Garcia AA, Keren-Rosenberg S, Parimoo D, et al: Phase I and pharmacologic study of estramustine phosphate and short infusions of paclitaxel in women with solid tumors. J Clin Oncol 1998;16:2959-2963.

C H A P T E R

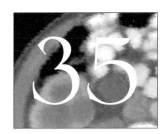

DOSE INTENSITY IN THE TREATMENT OF ADVANCED EPITHELIAL OVARIAN CANCER

Hervé Cure

 MAJOR CONTROVERSIES

- **What is the rationale for dose intensification?**
- **What are the clinical results of dose intensification based on the French experience?**
- **What are the clinical results of dose intensification based on the European experience?**
- **What are the clinical results of dose intensification based on the American experience?**

Ovarian cancer has been known to be a chemosensitive tumor for more than 30 years. However, long-term results in patients with advanced stages of disease remain low, with 5-year overall survival rates of about 20%. There are a number of reasons why high-dose chemotherapy is a reasonable strategy. This chapter reports the French, European, and American experiences with high-dose chemotherapy in three clinical settings: (1) consolidation after complete or very good partial response, (2) after relapse or for refractory disease, (3) as first-line therapy to increase clinical and pathologic complete responses and improve prognosis. The most promising results are in the consolidation setting. Preliminary results from the French multicenter randomized phase III study (high versus conventional dose) show a trend in favor of high-dose chemotherapy as consolidation treatment. This unique trial could establish the place of high-dose chemotherapy as first-line treatment for advanced epithelial ovarian cancer if these results are confirmed on longer follow-up.

Ovarian cancer remains asymptomatic for a long time and therefore is usually diagnosed at an advanced stage. In fact, two thirds of all women with ovarian cancer present with International Federation of Gynecology and Obstetrics (FIGO) stages III and IV. In spite of the efficacy of multimodality treatment including surgery and chemotherapy, the median survival time of patients with advanced disease ranges from 20 to 38 months in most studies, and the overall 5-year survival rate does not exceed 15%.[1-3]

These results have barely improved over the last few decades; however, surgery has become more aggressive because minimal residual disease after laparotomy is acknowledged to be a good prognostic factor. The results of chemotherapy have improved with the introduction of platinum-taxane combinations, and dose intensification has become easier with the use of hematopoietic growth factors.[4] Despite these improvements, median survival time ranges from 12 to 16 months, and most patients still have active tumor at second-look operation (SLO). Furthermore, even if SLO findings are negative, the probability of a recurrence of the disease is estimated to be 10% per year.[5-6]

In the context of such a poor outcome, several strategies have been developed to complete or consolidate the antitumoral effect obtained by first-line treatment. Among these is intensive chemotherapy, a means of increasing the intracellular concentration of anticancer agents, thereby increasing their cytotoxicity on tumor

479

cells and overcoming the potential resistance of the cells to these drugs.

What is the rationale for dose intensification?

Laboratory data. The idea of therapeutic intensification has progressively emerged from experimental data demonstrating the existence of a dose-response relationship for most cytotoxic agents. The dose-response curve is usually sigmoid-shaped, with a threshold, a linear phase, and a plateau. In animal experiments, Skipper[7] demonstrated the importance of dose by showing that a reduction in dose during the linear phase of the dose-response curve provoked a reduction in the rate of cure, even before a significant reduction in the complete remission rate was noted. Norton and Simon[8] enlarged the model by assuming that the rate of tumor regression is directly proportional to the chemotherapy dose administered and the rate of tumor growth. Finally, Goldie and colleagues[9] suggested that the longer it takes for a therapeutic response, the greater the increase in the rate of mutation and resistance to cytotoxic drugs.

Chemosensitivity of ovarian cancer. Standard first-line chemotherapy includes six treatment cycles combining paclitaxel and platinum, providing a clinical response of 75% to 85%, with 40% negative SLO for patients presenting with FIGO stages III-IV.[10]

Dose intensity as applied to ovarian cancer. The effect of dose intensity in ovarian cancer was retrospectively analyzed by Levin and Hryniuk.[11] This retrospective analysis of 75 randomized trials compared the dose intensity of drugs administered with that of a reference protocol, the CHAP by Gréco. A close link between the clinical response or median survival time and the dose intensity of cisplatin was observed. The effect of the dose intensity of platinum given as monotherapy on the response was statistically significant ($P < .02$). The relative dose intensity effect of combination platinum-based therapy decreased below a threshold of 25 to 30 mg/m^2 of cisplatin per week. The difference between a combination platinum regimen and platinum alone was not found to be statistically significant for a given dose intensity of platinum. However, combination therapy with CAP or CHAP resulted in a significantly higher rate of response than platinum alone. The dose intensity effect of cyclophosphamide and the dose intensity effect of Adriamycin were found to be at the limit of statistical significance. A threshold of the dose intensity effect was also found for carboplatin.[12] In 128 patients treated with carboplatin alone, two thirds of whom received 300 to 400 mg/m^2 (range, 40 to 1000 mg/m^2), the rate of response did not increase significantly beyond an AUC (Area Under Curve) of 5 to 7 mg/mL × minute, while the toxicities increased (almost 100% of patients developed leukopenia and thrombocytopenia at an AUC ≥10 mg/mL × minute).

The dose-response of cisplatin is limited.

Meta-analysis. A meta-analysis of 61 prospective, randomized or nonrandomized trials (4118 patients) published between 1976 and 1993 studied the relative roles of the dose intensity of platinum, the dose intensity of associated drugs, and the overall doses administered.[13] There was no link between median survival time and dose intensity of cisplatin at each cycle or the overall dose intensity of cisplatin. However, the overall dose intensity of chemotherapy (considering all of the drugs and treatments administered) was of prognostic significance. An overall dose intensity consisting of fewer than six treatments of 75 mg/m^2 cisplatin associated with 750 mg/m^2 of cyclophosphamide every 3 weeks was associated with a significantly higher risk of recurrence.

Randomized trials. A great many prospective, randomized trials have been carried out to test the dose intensity of platinum, some of which have investigated the total dose of platinum administered. The median survival of patients is always improved by higher doses of platinum if only the trials that use a minimum dose intensity of 50 mg/m^2 every 4 weeks (or carboplatin equivalent) are considered. This holds true even though the increase in the dose intensity of platinum is often low, not more than about a factor of two. However, the differences in survival are not always statistically significant, because the trials are underpowered. Only four trials have had statistically significant results (Table 35-1).[14-17] Among them, the study by Kaye and associates[14] demonstrated that the benefits of the dose intensity of platinum on survival decreased with time, especially in the group of patients with residual disease smaller than 2 cm; the 4-year survival rate in the cisplatin 100 mg/m^2 arm was 44%, compared with 41% for the cisplatin 50 mg/m^2 arm. The benefits were better maintained in the group with residual disease greater than 2 cm (4-year survival rate, 24% versus 14%). Murphy and colleagues[16] in Manchester halved the dose intensity of platinum while maintaining the same total dose. The response rates were 76% in the full-dose-intensity arm and 48% in the half-dose-intensity arm ($P = .009$); the rates of progression during chemotherapy were 8% and 42%, respectively ($P = .0003$). Finally, Bella and coworkers[17] increased the dose intensity without modifying the total dose of cisplatin and showed a survival benefit at 8 years ($P = .03$).

The Gynecologic Oncology Group (GOG) treated 485 patients with either intensive therapy (100 mg/m^2 of cisplatin plus 1000 mg/m^2 of cyclophosphamide × 4 cycles) or conventional therapy (50 mg/m^2 of cisplatin plus 500 mg/m^2 of cyclophosphamide × 8 cycles) but did not find any differences in survival.[18]

Attempts to intensify the dose of platinum are hampered by side effects, in particular neurotoxicity. For instance, most of the 50 patients treated by the National Cancer Institute with twice the normal dose of cisplatin (40 mg/m^2/day × 5 days) plus cyclophosphamide (200 mg/m^2/day × 5 days) every 4 to 6 weeks

Table 35–1. Randomized Studies of Platinum Dose Intensity That Showed a Statistically Significant Survival Advantage

Reference	Dose (mg/m²)	n	No. of Cycles	Cycle Length (wk)	Total Identical Dose	Response Rate (%)	Survival
Ngan et al.[15] (1989)	CDDP: 120 vs 60	50	—	3-4 vs 3-4	No	55 vs 30	3-yr OS: 60% vs 30% (significant)
Kaye et al.[14] (1996)	CDDP: 100 vs 50	159	6 vs 6	3 vs 3	No	61 vs 34	Median survival: 114 vs 69 wk 4.9-yr OS: 32.4% vs 26.6% (NS)
Bella et al.[17] (1994)	CDDP: 100 vs 100	99	(3) × 2 vs 6	1 vs 3	Yes	55 vs 48	8-yr OS ($P = .03$)
Murphy et al.[16] (1993)	CBDCA: 300 vs 150	99	6 vs 12	8 vs 12	Yes	76 vs 48	Follow-up too short

CBDCA, carboplatin; CDDP, cisplatin; NS, not significant; OS, overall survival.

were able to receive only three cycles because of disabling peripheral neuropathy.[19]

Cisplatin-carboplatin combinations. The toxicity of cisplatin (neurologic and renal) differs greatly from that of carboplatin (hematologic). As a result, these two drugs can be combined to intensify the total dose of platinum. Several trials have demonstrated the feasibility of this combination, but the main toxicities are hematologic (leukocytes and platelets) and neurologic (in particular, hearing loss).[20-22] A randomized study comparing cisplatin 100 mg/m² plus cyclophosphamide 600 mg/m² versus cisplatin 100 mg/m² plus carboplatin 300 mg/m² and cyclophosphamide 300 mg/m² was carried out by the gynecology group of the Fédération Nationale des Centres de Lutte Contre le Cancer from February 1992 to December 1996 in 195 patients with residual disease after initial surgery. The intensification of the dose of platinum obtained by the combination of the two platinum compounds significantly increased the median survival time and the 3-year progression-free survival rate (17.4 months and 22% versus 13 months and 11%, $p = .01$).[23] However, there was no impact on overall survival, and because of the hematologic and auditory toxicities, this combination could not be recommended.

Intensive chemotherapy with hematopoietic stem cell support may apply to ovarian cancer.

Intensive chemotherapy has been studied mainly in patients with non-Hodgkin lymphoma, testicular cancer, or breast cancer. A high rate of complete remission has been observed in patients with a partial response after first- or second-line chemotherapy, thereby demonstrating an increase in antitumor activity with this approach.

Ovarian cancer is a good model to study the benefits of dose intensification, and intensive chemotherapy with hematopoietic stem cell support may apply to ovarian cancer.[24] It is chemosensitive, especially to alkylating agents, and a dose-effect relationship has been demonstrated, particularly with platinum compounds. Furthermore, the prognostic factors and long-term results of standard treatment have been well established,

and peripheral contamination of the marrow and blood by malignant cells is not detected by conventional means.[25] However, this last point needs to be qualified, because three studies using newer immunohistochemical detection methods have described micrometastases in bone marrow or blood of patients with ovarian cancer.[25-27] Nevertheless, bone metastases are exceptional in this disease; in a series examined by Dauplat and colleagues,[28] 4 (1.6%) of 255 epithelial ovarian cancer patients had secondary tumors in bone.

What are the clinical results of dose intensification based on the French experience?

Intensification as consolidation. The use of high-dose chemotherapy as consolidation therapy for patients with platinum-sensitive advanced epithelial ovarian cancer was reviewed by Curé and colleagues in 2000.[29]

Retrospective experience of Centre Anticancéreux de Clermont-Ferrand. Between August 1984 and July 1995 (the date of initiation of a prospective randomized phase III consolidation chemotherapy trial of intensive versus standard treatment), 80 grafts of autologous stem cells were carried out at Centre Anticancéreux de Clermont-Ferrand on 77 patients (3 patients had two grafts more than 1 year apart for recurrence). All patients presented with advanced ovarian cancer (60 stage III, 16 stage IV, and 1 stage IIc with multiple recurrences). Their mean age was 49 years, with a range of 23 to 65 years. They all received the same initial treatment, consisting of cytoreductive surgery (15 had no residual disease, 26 had optimal debulking, 22 had suboptimal debulking, and 14 had incomplete surgery) followed by an average of six cycles of chemotherapy with a platinum compound. Approximately one third of the patients also received paclitaxel.

SLO was carried out in 71 cases; 6 patients refused SLO, and their initial surgery was either complete (3) or optimal (3). Forty-three (60.5%) of 71 SLO results were positive, and usually further reduction in tumor burden was performed. Twenty-six SLO (39.5%) were negative, but these patients had well-recognized poor prognostic features: poor histopathologic characteristics, or residual mass after first surgery of 2 cm or larger, or both before intensive chemotherapy, the vast majority of the patients had less than 2 cm residual disease (28 patients had negative SLO; 37 patients had fully excised lesions or ≤2 cm residual disease; 6 patients had ≥2 cm residual disease; 6 patients were non-assessable but were in complete clinical remission).

The intensive chemotherapy consisted of either high-dose melphalan (140 mg/m²) in 26 of 80 grafts or the combination of carboplatin (1000 to 1500 mg/m² per treatment) and cyclophosphamide (6000 mg/m² per treatment) fractionated over 4 days in 54 of 80 grafts. The hematologic support for this high-dose chemotherapy consisted of hematopoietic stem cells only. Hematopoietic growth factors in the postautograft phase were not used. Until 1992, bone marrow taken under general anesthesia from the posterior iliac crest (about 1 L of marrow per patient) was used (37 of 80 grafts). Since 1992, the hematopoietic stem cells have been taken from the peripheral blood by leukapheresis (an average of 2 leukaphereses per patient) after mobilization consisting of 3 g/m² cyclophosphamide on day 1 or combining 200 mg/m²/day etoposide on days 1 and 2 and 2 g/m²/day cyclophosphamide on days 3 and 4, followed by 5 µg/kg/day granulocyte colony-stimulating factor (G-CSF) until the day of the last leukapheresis (39 of 80 grafts). In 4 patients, a bone marrow sample was used to complete an insufficient peripheral blood harvest.

There were no failures of graftment. Full hematologic reconstitution (granulocytes ≥1 × 10⁹/L and platelets ≥50 × 10⁹) after bone marrow transplantation required a median period of 3 weeks, with an average transfusion requirement of 5 units of blood and 5 units of platelets per patient. After the introduction of leukapheresis,

this period was reduced to 11 days and the need for transfusions was reduced by 30% to 50%. However, patients had prolonged thrombocytopenias (with high-dose melphalan). There were only four episodes of severe infection while patients were neutropenic—three patients had meningitis with cytomegalovirus, and one patient had perineal cellulitis due to enterococci—but no long-term sequelae were seen. However, one case of toxic death was reported 5 days after the end of intensive therapy due to multiorgan failure. The toxic death rate was therefore 1.25%. Also, two patients experienced acute cardiomyopathies from high-dose cyclophosphamide, but both had complete resolution.

The median follow-up for this study is now more than 7 years (87 months; range, 2 to 186 months). Sixteen patients (21%) are still alive and in complete remission without any other treatment, 7 patients (9%) have relapsed but are still alive, and 54 patients (70%) have died of progressive disease. In addition, 1 patient died from toxicity and 2 from secondary acute leukemias caused by melphalan. It should be noted that the recurrences (58 of 77 patients) occurred on average 19 months after the high-dose procedure. This did not prevent further chemotherapy, and complete responses were seen with subsequent treatments. The median overall and progression-free survival times were 44 and 19 months, respectively. The overall 5-year survival rate (after the procedure) was 39%, and the 5-year survival rate without recurrence was 18% (Fig. 35-1). The overall survival rate 5 years from diagnosis was 51%, with a median survival time of 60.5 months; the 5-year rate of survival without recurrence after diagnosis was 23%, with a median of 31 months. Among the prognostic factors, the most significant was disease status at SLO: complete pathologic remission was associated with a 5-year survival rate of 54% and a median survival time of 62 months, (Fig. 35-2). These

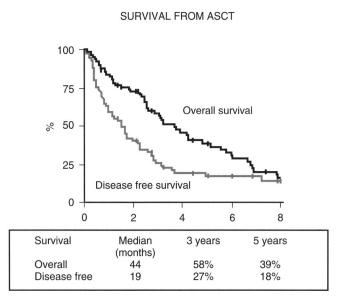

SURVIVAL FROM ASCT

Survival	Median (months)	3 years	5 years
Overall	44	58%	39%
Disease free	19	27%	18%

Consolidation chemotherapy (80 patients from the Clermont-Ferrand data
Survival after the date of the graft: overall survival *vs* disease free survival
ASCT: Autologous stem cell transplant

Figure 35–1. Clermont-Ferrand experience: consolidation chemotherapy. Overall and progression-free survival in 80 patients. Survival figures refer to time after the date of the graft. ASCT, autologous stem cell transplantation.

Figure 35–2. Clermont-Ferrand experience: consolidation chemotherapy. Overall survival based on results of the second-look operation (SLO) in 71 patients, either negative (microscopic disease only) or positive. ASCT, autologous stem cell transplantation.

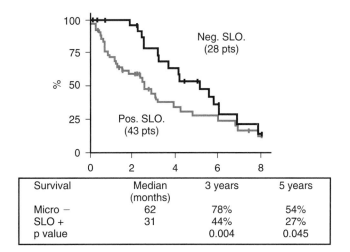

OVERALL SURVIVAL FROM ASCT
(ACCORDING TO SLO RESULTS)

Survival	Median (months)	3 years	5 years
Micro −	62	78%	54%
SLO +	31	44%	27%
p value		0.004	0.045

Consolidation chemotherapy in Clermont-Ferrand
Overall survival as a result of the second look (n = 71 patients) = negative *versus* positive
ASCT: Autologous stem cell transplant

results are updated from the previously published report by Legros and colleagues in 1997.[30]

Retrospective French experience of six French centers. A total of 180 files on patients who received high-dose chemotherapy between 1982 and 1995 were collected from six centers (Hôpital Saint-Louis, Hôpital Tenon, and Institut Curie, Paris; Institut Paoli-Calmettes, Marseille; Centre Léon Bérard, Lyon; Centre Jean Perrin, Clermont-Ferrand). The median age was 47 years; 137 patients (76%) had stage III disease, and 44 (24%) had stage IV. This retrospective study completes and updates the data from the French experience on high-dose chemotherapy and bone marrow/stem cell support in patients with ovarian cancer that was published in 1993.[31] The data set was closed in 1995 when it was decided to initiate a prospective, randomized phase III consolidation chemotherapy trial of intensive versus standard therapy by the Groupe des Investigateurs Nationaux pour l'Etude des Cancers Ovariens (GINECO) in July 1995.

It is difficult to draw specific conclusions from this study, because the indications for grafting varied from one center to the next and a variety of treatments were used. A total of 10 regimens were used, the main one being high-dose melphalan, and the second one, followed by a carboplatin-cyclophosphamide schedule and irradiation, which was given to 23% of the patients (Hôpital Saint-Louis). Nevertheless, this study provides some interesting data:

- The toxic death rate was 2.5%. This is acceptable considering the gravity of the disease and the severity of the intensive treatment.
- There were three deaths, at 70, 82, and 54 months, from a second cancer (one breast cancer and two acute leukemias).

- The median duration of remission was 102 months (range, 61 to 209 months).
- The median overall survival time was 33 months (46 months after diagnosis), and the median survival time without recurrence was 16 months (28 months after diagnosis).
- The 5-year overall survival rate was 37%, and the 5-year survival rate without recurrence was 21%. The corresponding figures for survival 5 years after diagnosis were 41% and 23%, respectively; after 10 years, both rates were 14% (Fig. 35-3).

OVERALL AND PROGRESSION FREE SURVIVAL
FROM HDC IN THE OVERALL FRENCH EXPERIENCE (*n* = 181)

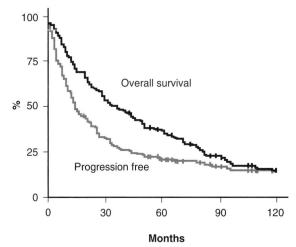

Figure 35–3. Overall and progression-free survival from high-dose chemotherapy in the overall French experience (*n* = 181).

Prognostic factors were analyzed, and the only statistically significant features associated with 5-year overall survival were the quality of the initial surgery, the attainment of a complete clinical response with first-line chemotherapy, and the finding of a complete histopathologic response at SLO. These same prognostic factors were also determinants for the 5-year probability of survival without recurrence.

Three prognostic groups can be distinguished:

- SLO completely negative (46 patients): the 5-year survival rate was 54%, and the 5-year recurrence-free survival rate was 43%. There was no difference in outcome depending on initial surgery (5-year survival rate with optimal debulking, 58%; with suboptimal debulking, 50%). However, among the 18 patients who received intensified therapy with melphalan, 76% were still alive after 5 years, compared with 39% of patients treated with other regimens (with $p = 0.0004$) (Fig. 35-4).
- Optimal initial surgery but SLO positive (48 patients): the 5-year survival rate was 44%, but the 5-year recurrence-free survival rate was 25%.
- Suboptimal initial surgery and positive SLO (71 patients): the overall 5-year survival rate was 18%, and the 4-year recurrence-free survival rate was 6%.

Prospective randomized phase III trial of consolidation chemotherapy (intensive versus standard).
A randomized trial was set up in the summer of 1995 as a collaboration between GINECO, FNCLCC (Fédération Nationale des Centres de Lutte Contre le Cancer), and SFGM-TC (Société Française de Greffe de Moelle et Thérapie Cellulaire). It was a multicenter, phase III consolidation chemotherapy trial, performed in France and in Naples, in which patients were randomly assigned to receive either three cycles of conventional doses of carboplatin-cyclophosphamide (300 and 600 mg/m^2, respectively) or a single high-dose cycle (1600 and 6000 mg/m^2, respectively) with an autograft of peripheral stem cells. The randomization occurred after SLO, and all patients had disease sensitive to first-line chemotherapy. This is the only randomized trial of intensive consolidation chemotherapy in ovarian cancer. Accrual was halted in October 2000 for planned interim analysis, after 70 patients had been accrued. The number of cases required was revised to yield a difference in 3-year recurrence-free survival of 25%; this made the new target 100 patients instead of 140. The characteristics of the patients in the two randomization arms (intensive and standard) are set out in Table 35-2. The preliminary results seem to indicate that the intensive arm is superior in terms of median survival without recurrence, compared with the standard arm (22 versus 11 months; $p = 0.033$) (Fig. 35-5).[32]

A parallel study on the type of mobilization of peripheral stem cells (3 g/m^2 cyclophosphamide + 5 μg/kg/day filgrastim versus filgrastim alone 10 μg/kg/day), which was supported by AMGEN S.A.S (Study 940186), was carried out at the same time. This study assessed whether it was possible to mobilize stem cells by G-CSF alone in patients with ovarian cancer. Mobilization of stem cells by G-CSF alone provides several potential advantages: it is safe (myelosuppressive chemotherapy is accompanied by adverse reactions of variable intensity that may require hospitalization); it takes less time than chemotherapy followed by G-CSF (7 days versus 10 to 18 days); and it is more practical because it can be preplanned, with the leukaphoresis taking place 5 to 7 days after administration of the hematopoietic growth factors. The variability of time required for hematologic recovery after chemotherapy makes it much more difficult to plan the leukaphoresis. Analysis of this study[33] did not reveal any difference in terms of mobilization (CD34+ T-lymphocyte count >2 × 10^6/kg) or hematologic recovery after grafting, whether cyclophosphamide was used or not.

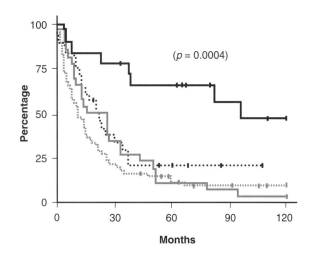

PROGRESSION FREE SURVIVAL FROM HDC
ACCORDING TO PATHOLOGICAL RESPONSE AT SECOND-LOOK
AND HDC REGIMEN IN THE OVERALL FRENCH EXPERIENCE

($p = 0.0004$)

pCR with Melphalan ($n = 18$)

pCR without Melphalan ($n = 28$)

non pCR without Melphalan ($n = 92$)

non pCR without Melphalan ($n = 27$)

Figure 35–4. Progression-free survival from high-dose chemotherapy, according to pathologic response at second-look operation and chemotherapy regimen, in the overall French experience PCR, pathological complete response (no tumoral cells on histologic examination).

Table 35–2. Characteristics of Patients in the GINECO/ FNCLCC/SFGM-TC Randomized Phase III Trial

Characteristic	Intensive Treatment	Standard Treatment %
No. of patients	52	50
Median age (years range)	48 (26-59)	50 (28-60)
Stratification		
Stage III		
No disease	30	32
Microscopic	23	17
<2 cm	21	23
>2 cm	19	19
Stage IV	7	9
FIGO stage		
IIIa	7	3
IIIb	5	9
IIIc	78	77
IV	10	11
Grade		
1	17	20
2	32	34
3	32	31
Not known	19	15
Histologic type		
Serous	83	83
Nonserous	17	17
Performance status		
0	64	67
1	33	30
2	3	3
Prior taxane	34	29

FIGO, International Federation of Gynecology and Obstetrics; FNCLCC, Fédération Nationale des Centres de Lutte Contre le Cancer; GINECO, Groupe des Investigateurs Nationaux pour l'Etude des Cancers Ovariens; SFGM-TC, Société Française de Greffe de Moelle et Thérapie Cellulaire.

An additional study of circulating tumor cells was carried out at the Hôpital Saint-Louis by L. Dal-Cortivo and J. P. Marolleau.[27] In this investigation, 4 of 11 aliquots obtained from the first 11 leukaphereses appeared to be contaminated by clonogenic tumor cells, challenging the dogma that ovarian cancer is a locoregional abdominopelvic disease.

Intensification for chemoresistant or recurrent disease. In patients with chemoresistant or recurrent disease, intensified therapy is sometimes associated with a high response rate. However, these responses are short, and prolonged survival without further recurrence is rare. High-dose chemotherapy is not indicated in these circumstances except when new drugs are being investigated. A phase I trial assessing increasing doses of topotecan (first as monotherapy, then in association with cyclophosphamide 120 mg/kg) was established more than 2 years ago in France (ITOV 01 protocol of FNCLCC). The standard regimen for topotecan is 1.5 mg/m^2/day intravenously over 30 minutes × 5 days every 21 days.[34-35] The toxicity is mainly hematologic, and therefore several high-dose regimens have been investigated.[36] In the ITOV 01 trial, topotecan was administered in daily 30-minute infusions for 5 consecutive days, after which hematopoietic stem cells were reinfused. Increasing doses of topotecan were examined; the first dose level was 4 mg/m^2/day, and the maximum tolerated dose was found to be 9.5 mg/m^2/day × 5.[36] This study is ongoing with the addition of increasing doses of cyclophosphamide.

First-line intensification. First-line intensification regimens consist of sequentially administered drugs that have different mechanisms of action and also are not cross-resistant. This therapeutic approach involves growth factors and sequential reinfusions of stem cells collected toward the end of the first chemotherapy cycle or cycles. The application of this strategy to ovarian tumors is currently being assessed as first-line therapy in patients with poor prognostic features.

Figure 35–5. GINECO/FNCLCC/SFGM-TC trial: three cycles of standard-dose carboplatin-cyclophosphamide (CBCY) versus one cycle of high-dose carboplatin-cyclophosphamide (HD).

3 CYCLES OF CARBOPLATIN-CYCLOPHOSPHAMIDE (STANDARD DOSE) VERSUS 1 CYCLE OF HIGH DOSE CARBOPLATIN CYCLOSPHOSPHAMIDE

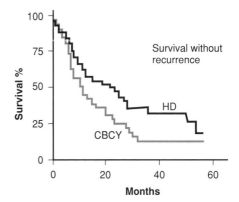

Treatment	Total	Median	p
CBCY	50	10 m	
HD	52	22 m	0.033

In 1998, Schilder and colleagues[37] reported their experience in a small series of patients at the annual meeting of the American Society of Clinical Oncology (ASCO). The regimen consisted of three cycles of carboplatin (AUC = 16), paclitaxel (250 mg/m² over 24 hours), and topotecan (10 to 15 mg/m²). At the same meeting, Möbus and colleagues[38] reported their experience with paclitaxel (250 mg/m² over 24 hours) and cyclophosphamide (3000 mg/m²) plus filgrastim for two cycles with stem cell rescue. These two cycles were followed by two cycles of carboplatin (AUC 18 to 20) and paclitaxel (250 mg/m²), then an intense cycle consisting of melphalan (140 mg/m²), carboplatin (AUC = 18 to 20), and etoposide (1600 mg/m²). These two trials demonstrated the feasibility of an intensive approach as first-line therapy.

In France, the ITOV 02 trial by FNCLCC involves patients with stage IIIc-IV ovarian cancer, whatever their volume of the residual tumor after initial surgery. The treatment consists of eight cycles of intensive chemotherapy with G-CSF. The chemotherapy begins with two cycles of cyclophosphamide (6000 mg/m²) and epirubicin (100 mg/m²), with collection of hematopoietic stem cells. The following sequence is then administered twice: one cycle of carboplatin (AUC = 18), then two cycles of paclitaxel (200 mg/m² over 3 hours). The stem cells collected after the first two cycles of combination therapy are reinfused after the two administrations of carboplatin. Thirty-five patients were accrued to this study, but the main goal of increasing the pathologic complete response rate at SLO to 50% was not achieved because only 35% of patients obtained a complete remission. The trial was therefore prematurely closed (not published).

What are the clinical results of dose intensification based on the European experience?

Ledermann and colleagues[39] published data from the European Bone Marrow Transplant Solid Tumor Registry. This was an analysis of 254 patients with an average age of 46 years (range, 22 to 63 years) who had stage III (70%) or stage IV (21%) disease. The data were obtained from 39 European centers between 1982 and 1996. A total of 105 patients received intensification while in complete remission or very good partial remission; 27 patients were in a second remission. More than 50% of the patients had macroscopic disease before intensive chemotherapy. The median survival time of patients in complete or good partial remission was 33 months, compared with 14 months for the other patients. Median survival from diagnosis for all 105 patients in remission who received intensification was 76 months. For patients with stage III disease, the median survival time without recurrence was 42 months, and the median overall survival time was 59 months; for those with stage IV disease, these times were 26 and 40 months, respectively.

What are the clinical results of dose intensification based on the American experience?

At the 1995 ASCO annual meeting, Shpall and colleagues[40] reported the American experience of intensive chemotherapy for ovarian cancer. Based on the data provided by the Autologous Blood and Marrow Transplant Registry (ABMTR), 249 grafts were reported in January 1995 from 51 American centers. Intensification was carried out as consolidation therapy in 17% of the cases (83% of patients had disease present). The treatment-related death rate was reported to be 9%. The probability of survival at 2 years for patients undergoing intensified chemotherapy who were in complete remission was 68%; for those with disease present, it was 33%. The workers also indicated that the South-Western Oncology Group (SWOG) began a phase II trial of intensive consolidation chemotherapy for residual disease after induction chemotherapy with platinum-based chemotherapy (SWOG 9106). The patients were to be randomly assigned to receive either thiotepa/cyclophosphamide/cisplatin or mitoxantrone/cyclophosphamide/carboplatin.[41] This trial was prematurely closed due to a lack of accrual.

Stiff and colleagues[42] published the only American retrospective study to date. It consisted of 100 patients (median age, 48 years; range, 23 to 65 years) who were treated between 1989 and 1996 for stage III and IV disease (66 and 16 patients, respectively). At the time of intensification, 13 patients were considered to be disease-free, 6 had microscopic disease, 20 had residual disease of less than 1 cm, and 61 had residual disease greater than 1 cm. The median time of survival without recurrence and median overall survival time were 7 and 13 months, respectively, for the entire population. For platinum-sensitive patients with a residuum of 1 cm or less, these medians were 19 and 30 months, respectively.

Conclusion

Therapeutic intensification in ovarian cancer is still limited to a small series of selected patients. About 180 patients have been included in trials in France, 250 in the rest of Europe, and about 250 in the United States. Nevertheless, analysis of the data confirms that intensive chemotherapy for refractory ovarian cancer provides a high rate of responses, about 70%, including 20% complete remissions,[39,42-48] whereas the probability of a response to standard second-line chemotherapy does not usually exceed 30%. However, the early morbidity is high (5% to 20%) in this pretreated population, and the duration of the responses is short, about 3 to 8.5 months (Table 35-3). In a consolidation situation, the overall life expectancy and 5-year recurrence-free survival rate are about 40% and 20%, respectively, after high-dose chemotherapy, and this treatment does not appear to prejudice the delivery of subsequent chemotherapy in the event of a recurrence (Table 35-4).[39,42,48-51]

Table 35-3. Intensive Chemotherapy in Patients with Refractory Ovarian Cancer

Reference	Dosage (mg/m²)	No. of Patients	OR (n)	CR (n)	Response Duration (mo)
Shpall et al.[43] (1990)	CTX (5600) P (90-150) Thio (300)	8	6	—	6
Viens et al.[48] (1990)	Mel (140-240)	12	9	4	3
McKenzie et al.[46] (1991)	CTX (90-120 mg/kg) Cb (1500) Mito (39-75)	6	5	4	—
Collins et al.[47] (1992)	CTX (6840) Thio (900) Cb (400-800)	7	4	1	8
Lotz et al.[44] (1993)	IFOS (7,500-10,000) Cb (875-100) VP 16 (650-1000)	16	9	2	—
Broun et al.[45] (1994)	Cb (1500) IFOS (7,500-10,000)	8	7	5	6
Stiff et al.[42] (1997)	Cb (1500) CTX (1206) NVT (75) or Mel (180) or P (165) CTX (5625)	61	—	—	NVT (90) 7 TTP (600)
Ledermann et al.[39] (2001)	Not specified	122	—	—	9
Total		**240**	**72%**	**31%**	

CR, full clinical response; Cb, carboplatin; CTX, cyclophosphamide; IFOS, ifosfamide; Mel, melphalan; Mito, mitoxantrone; NVT, Novantrone; OR, overall response; P, cisplatin; Thio, thiotepa; VP 16, etoposide.

Table 35-4. Intensive Chemotherapy as Consolidation Treatment after Second-Look Laparotomy in Ovarian Cancer

Reference	Dosage (mg/m²)	No. of Patients	Recurrence-free Survival Time (mo)	Overall Survival Time (mo)
Mulder et al.[49] (1989)	CTX (7000) VP 16 (900-1000)	11	ND	23
Largos et al.[50] (1992)	Mel (140) or Cb (1000-1500) CTX (6000)	18 13	27	47
Viens et al.[48] (1990)	Mel (140) or CTX (120 mg/kg) Mel (140) or Cb (1600) CTX (6400) VP 16 (1750)	12	ND	36
Extra et al.[51] (1993)	CTX (440) TBI + Mel (140) or Cb (600-1500)	37	13	32
Stiff et al.[42] (1997)	Cb (1500) CTX (1206) NVT (75) or NVT (90) Mel (180) or Thio (600) P (165) CTX (5625)	39	19	30
Ledermann et al.[39] (2001)	Not specified	132	18	33

Cb, carboplatin; CTX, cyclophosphamide; Mel, melphalan; NVT, Novantrone; P, cisplatin; TBI, total body irradiation; Thio, thiotepa; VP 16, etoposide; ND, No data.

These results seem to be better than those for conventional treatments, but they need to be confirmed in randomized trials. Such a study was carried out in a French prospective, multicenter, randomized phase III study by GINECO/FNCLCC/SFGM-TC that ended in October 2000. The preliminary results are encouraging and seem to support the role of high-dose chemotherapy for consolidation of the antitumor effect obtained after first-line treatment. As for intensive sequential induction chemotherapy with repeated grafts of peripheral hematopoietic stem cells and hematopoietic growth factors,[52-53] this technique has not fulfilled expectations, at least in the ITOV 02 trial performed by FNCLCC. The goal of a 50% complete histopathologic remission rate at SLO was not achieved, and the trial was prematurely closed.

The still too frequent problem of chemosensitive relapse may perhaps be solved by an approach involving intensive chemotherapy. However, it is highly likely that intensification only delays the development of further recurrences of ovarian cancer by an average of 18 months. It is therefore important to continue to develop treatments that may potentially eliminate the last cancer cell,[54] such as cytokine therapy with intraperitoneal γ-interferon[55] or interleukin 12, intraperitoneal adoptive cellular immune therapy using monocytes, or activated macrophages,[56] vaccinations, and antiangiogenic agents.

References

1. Friedlander ML, Dembo AJ: Prognostic factors in ovarian cancer. Semin Oncol 1989;25:205-212.
2. Marsoni S, Torri V, Valsecchi MG, et al: Prognostic factors in advanced epithelial ovarian cancer. Br J Clin Oncol 1990;62:444-450.
3. Omura GA, Brady MF, Homesley HD, et al: Long-term follow-up and prognostic factor analysis in advanced ovarian carcinoma: The Gynecologic Oncology Group experience. J Clin Oncol 1991;9:1138-1150.
4. Curé H, Dauplat J, Chollet P: First line chemotherapy for advanced ovarian cancer in 2000: Standards and questions. Bull Cancer 2000;87:189-199.
5. Dauplat J, Ferrière JP, Gorbinet M, et al: Second look laparotomy in managing epithelial ovarian carcinoma. Cancer 1986;57:1627-1631.
6. De Gramont A, Droley Y, Varette C, et al. (GERCOD): Survival after second look laparotomy in advanced ovarian epithelial cancer: Study of 86 patients. Eur J Cancer Clin Oncol 1989;25:451-457.
7. Skipper HE: Dose intensity versus total dose of chemotherapy: An experimental basis. In De Vita VT, Hellman S, Rosenberg SA (eds): Cancer: Principles and Practice of Oncology. Philadelphia, JB Lippincott, 1990, pp. 43-64.
8. Norton L, Simon R: Tumor size, sensitivity to therapy, and design of treatment schedule. Cancer Treat Rep 1977;61:1307-1317.
9. Goldie JH, Goldman AJ, Gudauskas GA: Rationale for the use of alternating cross-resistant chemotherapy. Cancer Treat Rep 1982;66:439-449.
10. Rubin SC: Second laparotomy in ovarian cancer. In Markmann M, Hoskins WJ (eds): Cancer of the Ovary. New York, Raven Press, 1993.
11. Levin L, Hryniuk WM: Dose intensity analysis of chemotherapy regimens in ovarian carcinoma. J Clin Oncol 1987;5:756-767.
12. Jodrell DI, Egorin MJ, Canetta RM, et al: Relationships between carboplatin exposure and tumor response and toxicity in patients with ovarian cancer. J Clin Oncol 1992;10:520-528.

13. Ben-David Y, Rosen B, Franssen E, et al: Meta-analysis comparing cisplatin total dose intensity and survival. Gynecol Oncol 1995;59:93-101.
14. Kaye SB, Paul J, Cassidy J, et al: Mature results of randomized trial of two doses of cisplatin for the treatment of ovarian cancer. Scottish Gynecology Cancer Trials Group. J Clin Oncol 1996;14:2113-2119.
15. Ngan HY, Choo YC, Cheung M, et al: A randomized study of high-dose versus low-dose cisplatin combined with cyclophosphamide in the treatment of advanced ovarian cancer. Hong Kong Ovarian Carcinoma Study Group. Chemotherapy 1989;35:221-227.
16. Murphy D, Crowther D, Renninson J, et al: A randomized dose intensity study in ovarian carcinoma comparing chemotherapy given at four week intervals for six cycles with half dose chemotherapy given for twelve cycles. Ann Oncol 1993;4:377-383.
17. Bella M, Cocconi G, Lottici R, et al: Mature results of a prospective randomized trial comparing two different dose-intensity regimens of cisplatin in advanced ovarian carcinoma. Ann Oncol 1994;5(Suppl 8):2.
18. McGuire WP, Hoskins WJ, Brady MF, et al: Assessment of dose-intensive therapy in suboptimally debulked ovarian cancer: A Gynecologic Oncology Group study. J Clin Oncol 1995;13:1589-1599.
19. Rothenberg ML, Ozols RF, Glatstein E, et al: Dose-intensive induction therapy with cyclophosphamide, cisplatin and consolidative abdominal radiation in advanced-stage epithelial ovarian cancer. J Clin Oncol 1992;10:727-734.
20. Grem J, O'Dwyer P, Elson P, et al: Cisplatin, carboplatin, and cyclophosphamide combination chemotherapy in advanced-stage ovarian carcinoma: An Eastern Cooperative Oncology Group pilot study. J Clin Oncol 1991;9:1793-1800.
21. Piccart MJ, Nogaret JM, Marcelis L, et al: Cisplatin combined with carboplatin: A new way of intensification of platinum dose in the treatment of advanced ovarian cancer. Belgian Study Group for Ovarian Carcinoma. J Natl Cancer Inst 1990;82:703-707.
22. Fanning J, Hilgers RD: High dose cisplatin carboplatin chemotherapy in primary advanced epithelial ovarian cancer. Gynecol Oncol 1993;51:182-186.
23. Joly F, Heron JF, Kerbrat P, et al: High-dose platinum versus standard dose in advanced ovarian carcinoma: A randomized trial from the Gynecologic Cooperative Group of the French comprehensive cancer centers (FNCLCC). Gynecol Oncol 2000;78:361-368.
24. Thigpen T: High-dose chemotherapy with autologous bone marrow support in ovarian carcinoma: The bottom line, more or less [editorial]. Gynecol Oncol 1995;57:275-277.
25. Cain JM, Ellis GK, Collins C, et al: Bone marrow involvement in epithelial ovarian cancer by immunocytotechnical assessment. Gynecol Oncol 1990;38:442-445.
26. Ron AA, Miller GW, Moss TJ, et al: Immunocytochemical detection of tumor cells in bone marrow and peripheral blood stem cell collections from patients with ovarian cancer. Bone Marrow Transplant 1995;15:929-933.
27. Dal Cortivo L, Orfeuvre H, Dumont C, et al: Micrometastatic cells (MC) in peripheral blood stem cells (PBSC) of patients with advanced ovarian cancer (AOC) in complete clinical remission (CCR) after initial therapy [abstract 22]. Proc Am Soc Clin Oncol 2001;20:6a.
28. Dauplat J, Hacker NF, Nieberg R, et al: Distant metastases in epithelial ovarian carcinoma. Cancer 1987;60:1561-1566.
29. Curé H, Extra JM, Viens P, et al: High-dose chemotherapy as consolidation therapy for patients with platinum-sensitive advanced epithelial ovarian cancer. Bone Marrow Transplantation 2000;26:S27-S29.
30. Legros M, Dauplat J, Fleury J, et al: High-dose chemotherapy with hematopoietic rescue in patients with stage III to IV ovarian cancer: Long-term results. J Clin Oncol 1997;15:1302-1308.
31. Extra JM, Curé H, Viens P, et al: High dose chemotherapy with autologous bone marrow transplantation in ovarian adenocarcinoma. Bull Cancer 1993;80:156-162.
32. Curé H, Battista C, Guastalla JP, et al: Phase III randomized trial of high-dose chemotherapy (HDC) and peripheral blood stem cell (PBSC) support as consolidation in patients (pts) with responsive low-burden advanced ovarian cancer (AOC): Preliminary

results of a GINECO/FNCLCC/SFGM-TC study [abstract 815]. Proc Am Soc Clin Oncol 2001;20:2041.

33. Curé H, Marolleau JP, Biron P, et al, for the GINECO: Randomized phase II study of peripheral blood progenitor cell (PBPC) mobilization in patients with advanced ovarian cancer (OVCA) treated with high-dose (HD) consolidation chemotherapy: comparison of filgrastim used alone or in combination with cyclophosphamide [abstract 1560]. Proc Am Soc Clin Oncol 2000;394a.

34. Creemers GJ, Bolis G, Gore M, et al: Topotecan, an active drug in the second line treatment of epithelial ovarian cancer: results of a large European phase II study. J Clin Oncol 1996;14:3056-3061.

35. Rowinsky EK, Grochow LB, Sartorius SE, et al: Phase I and pharmacologic study of high doses of the topoisomerase I inhibitor topotecan with granulocyte colony-stimulating factor in patients with solid tumors. J Clin Oncol 1996;14:1224-1235.

36. Lhomme C, Lotz JP, Fabbro M, et al: High dose (HD) topotecan (TPC) with blood stem cells support (BSCS) in ovarian carcinoma (OC): A phase I study (ITOV 01 protocol) [abstract 861]. Proc Am Soc Clin Oncol 2002;216a.

37. Schilder RJ, Gallo JM, Johnson JW, et al: Phase I study of multiple cycles of high dose topotecan, carboplatin and paclitaxel with peripheral blood stem cell support [abstract 290]. Proc Am Soc Clin Oncol 1998;17:75a.

38. Möbus VJ, Koenigsmann M, Opri F, et al: Sequential high dose chemotherapy with hematopoietic progenitor cell support as first line treatment of patients with advanced ovarian cancer [abstract 1423]. Proc Am Soc Clin Oncol 1998;17:369a.

39. Ledermann J, Herd R, Maraninchi D, et al: High dose chemotherapy for ovarian carcinoma: Long-term results from the solid tumor registry of the European Group for Blood and Marrow Transplantation (EBMT). Ann Oncol 2001;12:693-699.

40. Shpall EJ, Cagnoni PJ, Bearman SI, et al: High dose chemotherapy with autologous hematopoietic cell support (AHCS) for the treatment of epithelial ovarian cancer. Presented at the 31st Annual Meeting of the American Society of Clinical Oncology, May 20–23, 1995, Los Angeles, CA (Educational Book), pp. 360-364.

41. Stiff P, Bayer R, Camarda M: A phase II trial of high-dose mitoxantrone, carboplatin and cyclophosphamide with autologous bone marrow rescue for recurrent epithelial ovarian carcinoma: Analysis of risk factors for clinical outcome. Gynecol Oncol 1995;57:278-285.

42. Stiff P, Bayer R, Kerger C, et al: High-dose chemotherapy with autologous transplantation for persistent/relapsed ovarian cancer: A multivariate analysis of survival for 100 consecutively treated patients. J Clin Oncol 1997;4:1309-1317.

43. Shpall EJ, Clarke-Pearson D, Soper TJ, et al: High-dose alkylating agent chemotherapy with autologous bone marrow support in patients with stage III-IV epithelial ovarian cancer. Gynecol Oncol 1990;38:386-391.

44. Lotz JP, Bouleuc C, André T, et al: Tandem high dose chemotherapy with ifosfamide, carboplatin and teniposide with autologous

bone marrow transplantation for the treatment of poor prognosis common epithelial ovarian carcinomas. Cancer 1996;77:2550-2559.

45. Broun ER, Belinson JL, Berek JS, et al: Salvage therapy for recurrent and refractory ovarian cancer high-dose chemotherapy with autologous bone marrow support: A Gynecologic Oncology Group pilot study. Gynecol Oncol 1994;54:142-146.

46. McKenzie RS, Alberts DA, Bishop MR, et al: Phase I trial of high-dose cyclophosphamide (CY), mitoxantrone (MX), and carboplatin (CB) with autologous bone marrow transplantation (ABMT) in female malignancies: Pharmacologic levels of mitoxantrone and high response rate in refractory ovarian cancer [abstract 605]. Proc Am Soc Clin Oncol 1991;10:186.

47. Collins RH, Pineiro L, Fay JW: High-dose chemotherapy and autologous bone marrow transplantation for advanced ovarian cancer [abstract 745]. Proc Am Soc Clin Oncol 1992;11:233.

48. Viens P, Maraninchi D, Legros M, et al: High-dose melphalan and autologous marrow rescue in advanced epithelial ovarian carcinomas: A retrospective analysis of 35 patients treated in France. Bone Marrow Transplant 1990;5:227-233.

49. Mulder POM, Willemse PHB, Aalders JG, et al: High-dose chemotherapy with autologous bone marrow transplantation in patients with refractory ovarian cancer. Eur J Cancer Clin Oncol 1989;25:645-649.

50. Legros M, Fleury J, Curé H, et al: High-dose chemotherapy (HDC) in autologous bone marrow transplantation (ABMT) in 31 advanced ovarian cancers: Long-term results [abstract 700]. Proc Am Soc Clin Oncol 1992;11:222.

51. Extra JM, Curé H, Viens P, et al: High-dose chemotherapy with autologous bone marrow transplantation in ovarian adenocarcinoma. Bull Cancer 1993;80:156-162.

52. Shea TC, Mason JR, Storniolo AM, et al: Sequential cycles of high-dose carboplatin administered with recombinant human granulocyte-macrophage colony-stimulating factor and repeated infusions of autologous peripheral-blood progenitor cells: A novel and effective method for delivering multiple courses of dose-intensive therapy. J Clin Oncol 1992;10:464-473.

53. Tepler I, Cannistra SA, Frei E III, et al: Use of peripheral-blood progenitor cells abrogates in myelotoxicity of repetitive outpatient high-dose carboplatin and cyclophosphamide chemotherapy. J Clin Oncol 1993;11:1583-1591.

54. Curé H, D'Incan C, Bignon YJ, et al: Immunothérapie du cancer de l'ovaire, passé, présent, futur. Références en Gynécologie Obstétrique 1997;5:161-168.

55. Pujade-Lauraine E, Guastalla JP, Colombo N, et al: Intraperitoneal recombinant interferon gamma in ovarian cancer patients with residual disease at second look laparotomy. J Clin Oncol 1996;14:343-350.

56. Faradji A, Bohbot A, Frost H, et al: Phase I of liposomal MTP-PE activated autologous monocytes administered intraperitoneally to patients with peritoneal carcinomatosis. J Clin Oncol 1991;9:1251-1260.

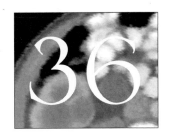

HORMONAL TREATMENT OF OVARIAN CANCER

Peter E. Schwartz

 MAJOR CONTROVERSIES

- Are physiologic levels of sex hormones deleterious to the health of women with ovarian cancer?
- Is there a role for hormonal therapy in the treatment of epithelial ovarian cancer?
- Can estrogen, progestin, and androgen receptor analyses predict the response to hormone therapy for epithelial ovarian cancer?
- What is the future role for hormonal therapy in the treatment of epithelial ovarian cancer?

Ovarian cancer is the major pelvic reproductive organ cancer health hazard for women in the United States.[1] Approximately 70% of ovarian cancers are identified as advanced-stage disease, and available treatment is overwhelmingly palliative rather than curative.[2] Because of the inability to detect this cancer early or to recognize it in a premalignant state, physicians treating ovarian cancer frequently exhaust effective cytotoxic chemotherapy. Hormonal therapy has been used for the management of ovarian cancer for the past 40 years. The concept of hormonal therapy is based on two observations. The first is that most ovarian cancers occur after women enter menopause, suggesting that excessive circulating gonadotropins may be associated with the development of ovarian cancer.[3,4] The second observation is the efficacy of hormonal and antihormonal therapy in the management of uterine and breast cancers, cancers that occur in women with demographic features similar to that seen in women who develop ovarian cancer.[5-7]

The use of hormone therapy occurs almost invariably after conventional cytotoxic chemotherapy has been exhausted.[8] Realistically, patients who receive hormonal therapy or any other form of treatment late in the course of the disease have little likelihood of achieving objective clinical responses.[9] The selection of hormonal therapy and the expectations for the effectiveness of hormonal therapy in women with ovarian cancer have been compared with the experience when hormone therapies are used in the treatment of breast cancer.[9] However, hormonal therapy for patients with breast cancer is now routinely employed as part of the initial therapy. Comparisons of the effectiveness of hormone therapy for previously untreated breast cancer and advanced, recurrent ovarian cancer are not valid.[9]

Several controversies are discussed in this chapter. Are physiologic levels of sex hormones deleterious to the health of women with ovarian cancer; is there a role for hormonal therapy in the management of ovarian cancer; and can estrogen, progestin, and androgen receptor analyses predict response to hormone therapy for women with ovarian cancer? This chapter covers experiences with hormonal therapy for epithelial and nonepithelial ovarian cancers.

Are physiologic levels of sex hormones deleterious to the health of women with ovarian cancer?

There are few data to suggest that physiologic levels of sex hormones are deleterious to the health of women with ovarian cancer. Small series of women are available in which the contralateral ovary has been left in place when an epithelial ovarian cancer has been diagnosed to preserve fertility.[10,11] These series suggest that women who have early-stage epithelial ovarian cancer limited to one ovary do not have their lives compromised by leaving the contralateral ovary in place.[10,11] Malignant germ cell tumors of the ovary most often occur in women of reproductive age.[12] It is now routine to leave the contralateral ovary in place and preserve fertility in the management of women with this disease.[11] Sex cord–stromal tumors occurring in women in the reproductive age frequently are found to be limited to one ovary (i.e., stage I).[13] Removing the involved ovary and retaining the normal contralateral ovary does not appear to jeopardize the patient's life.[13]

From clinical observations, physiologic levels of sex hormones present in reproductive-age women are not deleterious to the health of women with ovarian cancer. Preservation of ovarian function and fertility has become a routine part of the management of early-stage epithelial and nonepithelial ovarian cancers.

Is there a role for hormonal therapy in the treatment of epithelial ovarian cancer?

Many hormonal therapies have been employed in the management of ovarian cancer. These include estrogens, progestins, estrogen agonists, and antagonists, androgens, antiandrogens, leuteinizing hormone–releasing hormone (LHRH) agonists, and corticosteroids.[7] Many of these approaches were employed before steroid receptor analyses were available.

Estrogen therapy. Diethylstilbestrol was one of the first hormone-like agents used in the management of recurrent ovarian cancer.[3] It was used primarily as a means of inhibiting gonadotropin production. In a series of 14 patients treated with 15 to 30 mg daily of diethylstilbestrol for recurrent ovarian cancer, 2 patients reportedly had objective responses (clinical complete or partial responses) lasting more than 1 year, and 2 patients had disappearance of ascites and an increased sense of well-being.[3] Remarkably, this approach has not been reported in any other series of women.

Progestin therapy. Progestins have been used for at least 40 years in the management of recurrent ovarian cancer.[14-26] The progestins employed for recurrent disease included 17α-hydroxyprogesterone caproate (Delalutin), medroxyprogesterone acetate (Provera), megestrol acetate (Megace), and 6α-dimethylprogesterone (NSC12301A). Although no consistent group of patients has been identified to have recurrent ovarian cancer responsive to progestin therapy, Wilailak and colleagues[26] reported that three of nine patients treated with high-dose megestrol acetate for platinum-refractory endometrioid ovarian cancers had complete responses, with one of the responses persisting more than 3 years. Unfortunately, Wiernik and coworkers[27] were unable to substantiate any objective responses

among 33 stage III or IV ovarian cancer patients who had recurrent disease when they were treated with high-dose megestrol acetate. Only four of the patients in the latter study had endometrioid carcinomas. Similarly, Hamerlynck and colleagues[25] documented only one partial response among 41 patients treated with high-dose medroxyprogesterone acetate, and that response lasted only 20 weeks.

Three series investigated the use of progestin therapy in previously untreated ovarian cancer patients.[28-30] The progestins used were medroxyprogesterone acetate and gestonorone caproate (Depostat). The most compelling data for a role for progestins in the management for previously untreated epithelial ovarian cancer come from Rendina and colleagues.[29] In that report, 17 (55%) of 31 patients with endometrioid adenocarcinomas of the ovary had objective responses to their treatment. This study was unique in that so many of the patients had well-differentiated endometrioid carcinoma. Among 30 patients with stage III or IV disease, 26 had well-differentiated endometrioid carcinomas. Bergqvist and associates[28] reported that three of four women with mucinous carcinomas experienced objective responses to medroxyprogesterone acetate. Timothy[30] reported that two of seven patients with stage III or IV ovarian cancer experienced complete responses when treated with gestonorone caproate. These responses lasted 9 and 18 months. The small number of patients in these series precludes any firm conclusions regarding the role of progestins in the primary management of epithelial ovarian cancers.

Schwartz and coworkers[8] reviewed 13 studies of women treated with progestin therapy for refractory ovarian cancer. The median response rate was 9% (range, 0% to 32%). Differences in criteria of response rate, the small number of patients in each study (median, 23; range, 6 to 33) and the different hormones used make these reports difficult to assess.

Estrogen and progestin therapy. Sixty-five women have been treated with a combination of ethinyl estradiol and medroxyprogesterone acetate in the management of ovarian cancer.[31,32] Nine had objective responses. Ethinyl estradiol doses used in the initial study had to be reduced because of the severe nausea associated with this regimen.

Tamoxifen therapy. Schwartz and associates[33] were the first to demonstrate a possible role for tamoxifen, an estrogen agonist-antagonist, in the treatment of women with recurrent ovarian cancer who had failed standard therapy, including chemotherapy and radiation therapy. In that series, 4 of 13 patients had stabilization of rapidly progressive disease for 3 to 9 months, and 1 patient had a partial clinical response. A literature review by Perez-Garcia and colleagues[9] revealed that of 648 women treated with tamoxifen therapy for recurrent ovarian cancer, 13% had objective responses (range, 0% to 38%). As with progestin therapy, tamoxifen has been overwhelmingly employed in the management of patients with advanced recurrent disease who had failed conventional therapy.[33-50]

Tamoxifen and progestin therapy. Combinations of cyclic tamoxifen with progestins were employed in two studies.[51,52] Unfortunately, no objective responses have been observed, although stabilization of disease has been identified for periods of 4 to 16 months.

Tamoxifen combined with cytotoxic chemotherapy. Schwartz and coworkers[53] employed tamoxifen in combination with cytotoxic chemotherapy as part of initial treatment of women with stage III or IV ovarian cancer participating in a prospective, randomized trial. Patients were randomized to receive the combination of Adriamycin and cisplatin or Adriamycin, cisplatin, and tamoxifen therapy. The tamoxifen-containing regimen was not demonstrated in this trial to have any effect on survival. This study result has been questioned because the tamoxifen dose (20 mg/day) was believed by some to be too low despite being the standard dose used in the management of breast cancer.[9] It has also been criticized because tamoxifen was used only while the patients received the primary cytotoxic chemotherapy regimen. The concern was that cytostatic drugs might require much longer use to achieve a survival benefit.[9]

Despite the negative results of the prospective, randomized trial reported by Schwartz and coworkers,[53] Ercoli and colleagues[54] demonstrated in the laboratory that the combination of tamoxifen and cisplatin results in synergistic antiproliferative activity and a complete reversal of the acquired cisplatin-resistant phenotype, suggesting that patients with cisplatin-refractory disease might benefit from this combination therapy. The latter investigators also showed that the steroidal pure antiestrogen ICI 182,780 and tamoxifen significantly inhibited the growth of the estrogen receptor (ER)–negative ovarian cancer cell line A2780 in a dose-dependent fashion.[55] Both agents also induced apoptosis in a dose-dependent fashion.[55] Investigators from the same institution subsequently reported the results of a study combining cisplatin or carboplatin with tamoxifen in patients with recurrent or progressive ovarian cancer.[56] Sixty-four percent of the platinum-sensitive and 39% of the platinum-resistant patients demonstrated objective responses to the combination of this chemotherapy plus hormonal therapy regimen. The overall median survival was 23 months (range, 3 to 48 months), including 20 months for the platinum-resistant group. This clinical observation strongly supported the laboratory findings previously made by these investigators and their colleagues that there is a therapeutic role for platinum agents in combination with tamoxifen in recurrent or progressive epithelial ovarian cancers. Only one patient in this series had an endometrioid carcinoma.[56]

Progestins combined with cytotoxic chemotherapy. Three reports have combined progestins with cytotoxic chemotherapy.[28,57,58] One series combined melphalan and medroxyprogesterone acetate.[28] The treatment details were incomplete. The second report failed to demonstrate an objective response when medroxyprogesterone acetate was combined with cytotoxic chemotherapy in five women.[57] The third trial, a phase I trial, treated 44 patients with epithelial ovarian cancer or primary peritoneal cancers with paclitaxel (135 to 175 mg/m^2 over 3 hours) plus an oral loading dose (800 to 9600 mg over 24 hours) and subsequent maintenance dose (800 to 3200 mg/day for 3 days) of micronized megestrol acetate. Therapy was repeated every 21 days. Four patients developed major venous blood clots, and one suffered a stroke. Three patients experienced significant declines in CA 125 values. In one patient, malignant ascites disappeared. No patient achieved an objective response (partial or complete response) of measurable disease.[57]

Androgen therapy. Conflicting laboratory data exist regarding the effect of androgens on ovarian tumor cell proliferation in vitro. One report demonstrated that testosterone and androstenedione inhibited proliferation of ovarian tumor cells in vitro and led the investigators to suggest that the development of epithelial ovarian cancer might be facilitated when the postmenopausal ovary fails to produce adequate androgen in the postmenopausal era.[59] A later study demonstrated that androgens promote the growth of ovarian cancer cell lines in vitro, in part by inhibiting transforming growth factor-β (TGF-β) receptor levels and allowing ovarian cancer cells to escape TGF-β1 growth inhibition.[60] However, at a clinical level, androgen therapy for the management of refractory ovarian cancer did not demonstrate any objective responses in two studies reported.[17,61]

Antiandrogen therapy. Ovarian cancer cell lines containing androgen receptors show a dose-dependent inhibitory effect to antiandrogens in vitro.[62] Antiandrogen therapy has been evaluated by the European Organization for Research and Treatment of Cancer (EORTC) Gynaecological Cancer Cooperative Group.[63] Two (6.3%) of 32 patients who received a minimum treatment of 2 months of oral flutamide and had previously received at least one regimen of platinum-based chemotherapy and a median of two chemotherapy regimens experienced objective responses (one complete and one partial). Nine (28%) patients in this series had disease stabilization.

Luteinizing hormone–releasing hormone agonists. LHRH agonists have been employed in the management of advanced, recurrent ovarian cancer based on the hypothesis that gonadotropins are elevated in postmenopausal women, the group in whom ovarian cancer is most commonly found, and that in at least one study premenopausal women receiving hormone replacement therapy had an improved survival, suggesting that a reduction in gonadotropins might enhance survival.[44] Gonadotropin receptors (i.e., follicle-stimulating hormone receptor [FSHR] and luteinizing hormone receptor [LHR]) are present in normal ovarian surface epithelium, ovarian epithelium inclusions, and most ovarian epithelial neoplasms, including borderline epithelial tumors and invasive cancers.[64-66] Zheng and coworkers[64] showed that FSH acts directly as a mitogen on ovarian epithelial cells and that its activity can be blocked by luteinizing hormone. FSH stimulates ovarian epithelial cell growth by upregulating cyclin B1 expression.[67] FSH also upregulates vascular epithelial growth factor (VEGF) expression in ovarian cancer and cancer cells.[68,69] VEGF levels have been elevated in tissue extracts and in ascites from women with stage III or IV ovarian cancers compared with those with stage I or II disease. High VEGF levels have been associated with a poorer survival in those cases.[70] Other investigators have shown a reduction in ovarian cancer cell line growth when human epithelial ovarian cancer cells were transplanted into nude mice and the mice were treated with LHRH agonists.[71,72] Suppression of endogenous gonadotropins was believed to be the mechanism for cell growth reduction.

Four series have employed gonadotropin-releasing hormone agonists in the management of women with refractory ovarian cancer.[73-75] For 107 patients, 1 complete and 12 partial responses (12.2%) have been reported. Patients most likely to respond were those with well-differentiated epithelial ovarian cancers that were initially optimally cytoreduced and those who had delayed (>18 months) first recurrences. The duration of responses varied from 6 to 24 months in these series, perhaps reflecting the natural history of well-differentiated cancers.

Luteinizing hormone–releasing hormone agonists combined with cytotoxic chemotherapy. Emons and colleagues[76] reported a multi-institutional, phase III, prospective, placebo-controlled, randomized trial in which women with previously untreated stage III or IV ovarian cancer received first-line chemotherapy containing at least 50 mg/m^2 of cisplatin or an equivalent dose of carboplatin with or without an LHRH agonist (i.e., triptorelin). Treatment of drug was started within 14 days of cytoreductive or diagnostic surgery. Injections of the triptorelin or placebo were continued until the patients' deaths or the end of the trial. Sixty-nine patients received the monthly injections of the LHRH agonist, and 66 patients received placebo. No significant difference could be established in progression-free survival or overall survival between the triptorelin group and the placebo group, despite the fact that the triptorelin-treated patients consistently experienced suppression of endogenous gonadotropins.[76]

Erickson and associates[77] reported a phase II study combining leuprolide acetate with cyclophosphamide and cisplatin after cytoreductive surgery for stage III or IV ovarian cancer. The investigators found that the use of an LHRH agonist with platinum-based combination chemotherapy did not alter the toxicity profile or the efficacy of chemotherapy when comparisons were made with historical controls. Although the regimen was well tolerated, the LHRH agonist had no apparent effect on the overall outcome of the patients.[77]

Corticosteroid therapy. Only one series using corticosteroid therapy in the management of refractory ovarian cancer has been reported.[17] No objective responses were observed in these patients.

Can estrogen, progestin, and androgen receptor analyses predict the response to hormone therapy for epithelial ovarian cancer?

If hormone therapy for epithelial ovarian cancer is effective, it should be used as part of the initial treatment of the ovarian cancer.[9] Efficacy potentially would be enhanced if the clinician knew whether the presence of estrogen, progestin, or androgen receptors were predictive of response to hormonal manipulation. The presence of ER proteins in epithelial ovarian cancers, mixed mesodermal tumors, and sex cord–stromal tumors were initially identified by biochemical techniques and subsequently confirmed by immunohistochemical techniques.[8,78] The presence of progestin receptors (PRs) in epithelial ovarian cancers and in nonepithelial ovarian cancers was also identified after ER proteins were confirmed to be present in epithelial ovarian cancers.[8,78] Although there were differences when tissues were analyzed by the biochemical or immunohistochemical techniques, the immunohistochemical technique has become the standard method of evaluating specimens to determine whether tumor cells contain ERs or PRs.[8]

After the identification of ERs and PRs in specimens of epithelial ovarian cancers, androgen receptor assays were performed. Androgen receptors are the most common receptors in epithelial ovarian cancer. Between 70% and 95% of epithelial ovarian cancers assayed are immunohistochemically positive for androgen receptor proteins.[79,80] It has been accepted that ovarian surface epithelium is an androgen-responsive tissue. Androgens can be shown in vitro to cause an increase in cell proliferation of normal epithelial cells and a decrease in cell death.[60,81] Polymorphic variations in the (CAG)$_n$ repeat of the androgen receptor gene suggests that a short androgen receptor allele resulted in a diagnosis of ovarian cancers in patients 7.2 years earlier than in patients who did not carry a short allele. This suggests that length of the androgen receptor allele affects the age of diagnosis of ovarian cancer.[82] The latter information was consistent irrespective of *BRCA* gene mutation status.

Having identified the presence of steroid receptor proteins does not mean that the receptors are active in the ovarian cancer cells. Hua and colleagues[83] found that ER-positive ovarian cancer is often refractory to antiestrogen therapy. In a series of studies involving SKOV3 cells that express ER mRNA and protein at a level similar to that of estrogen-responsive T47D breast cancer cell lines, the researchers observed no expression of the PR gene and noticed that the protein products of the estrogen-responsive genes *HER2/NEU* and *CTS* (cathepsin) were expressed at constitutive levels that were not regulated by estrogen. These study authors concluded that estrogen resistance in SKOV3 cells might be the result of constitutive expression and loss of estradiol regulation of selected growth regulatory gene products rather than a defect in estrogen activation of ER as a transcriptional regulator.[83]

Isoforms of the ER and the PR have been identified.[84] The original ER protein identified biochemically and immunohistochemically is now referred to as estrogen receptor-α (ERα). A second receptor, ERβ, has been identified in epithelial ovarian cancers.[84] The ratio of ERα to ERβ is quite high in ovarian cancers compared with the ratio in normal ovarian epithelial cells.[85,86] ERβ has been associated with apoptosis (i.e., programmed cell death), whereas ERα has been associated with proliferative effects.[85,87]

One problem in using steroid receptor protein evaluations to determine whether the ovarian cancer might be sensitive to hormonal manipulation is the heterogeneity of the cancers. Studies have demonstrated that a person can have steroid receptor protein–positive primary tumors but have steroid receptor–negative metastases.[88] Occasionally, the opposite can occur.[88] Heterogeneity of steroid receptor proteins in ovarian cancer can make it quite difficult to use this approach based on analysis of an isolated piece of tissue as a way of indicating the likelihood of response to hormone therapy.

A review of more than 2500 ovarian cancer patients reported in the literature revealed that 67% of their tumors expressed ER and 47% expressed PR.[89] The combination of ER and PR was measured in more than 1300 ovarian cancer patients. Thirty-six percent of the tumors were ER and PR positive, 26% were ER positive but PR negative, 12% were ER negative but PR positive, and 25% lacked both receptors. Only a few trials have tried to correlate hormone receptor status with response to hormonal manipulation of epithelial ovarian cancers. Schwartz and coworkers[53] reported a prospective, randomized trial comparing Adriamycin and cisplatin with or without tamoxifen in 100 patients. Hormone receptor proteins were identified in 72 of the patients, only 23 of whom were ER positive (at a level of 20 fmol/mg of cytosol protein [cp]). Eleven patients received chemotherapy and tamoxifen, and 12 received chemotherapy alone. Thirty-eight percent expressed PR based on using an arbitrary value of more than 7 fmol/mg cp. There was no correlation between receptor status and response to the hormonal therapy, even when higher cutoff levels for positivity were analyzed. There was no evidence that combining tamoxifen with combination cytotoxic chemotherapy had any impact in a positive or negative fashion on patient survival.

Rowland and colleagues[34] reported no response to tamoxifen in six patients with ER-positive tumors or in three patients with ER-negative tumors. These patients had been heavily pretreated with cytotoxic chemotherapy. Weiner and coworkers[36] found no correlation in 11 patients between steroid receptor protein content

and response to therapy. Shirey and associatates[41] came to a similar conclusion for six patients treated with tamoxifen. The latter data were quite disappointing because Lazo and coworkers[90] were able to demonstrate in vitro that tumors displaying response to tamoxifen all had ER and PR levels higher than 30 fmol/mg cp. None of 14 specimens with ER values less than 30 fmol/mg cp exhibited a significant decline in colony formation in the latter study.

Chu and colleagues[87] studied the presence of ERα and ERβ in a panel of ovarian cancers, including granulosa cell, serous, and mucinous tumors, and in normal ovarian tissue. They found widespread ERα in all tumor types at a very low level. ERβ was expressed predominately in granulosa cell tumors, with lower levels found in mucinous tumors and very low levels in serous tumors. They also identified a C-terminal truncation variant ERβ (cx) that exhibited widespread expression across all tumor types. This variant of ERβ has been shown to be a ligand-independent antagonist of ERα action. These study authors suggest that relative ratios of ERβ (cx), ERα, and ERβ may influence the response of a tumor to antiestrogen treatment.[87]

What is the future role for hormonal therapy in the treatment of epithelial ovarian cancer?

The available data strongly suggest that there is at least a minor role for hormonal therapy in the management of women with epithelial ovarian cancer. Limited experience suggests a possible role for hormonal therapy in the management of women with sex cord–stromal tumors.[77] The available data on using hormonal therapy as part of first-line therapy demonstrate a need for further assessment of this approach in the initial treatment of women with epithelial ovarian cancers.[53,76] It is possible that hormonal therapy may replace one drug in a combination of cytotoxic chemotherapy drugs used for the initial management of ovarian cancers, but there is little support for the addition of hormonal therapy after combination chemotherapy is employed. Nevertheless, the lack of side effects associated with most hormonal treatments would make hormone therapy more acceptable than cytotoxic chemotherapy. As further understanding of the molecular biology of ovarian cancer occurs, hormonal and antihormonal therapy may play a more important role in the management of women with ovarian cancers.

REFERENCES

1. Jemal A, Thomas A, Murray T, et al: Cancer Statistics, 2002. CA Cancer J Clin 2002;52:23-47.
2. McGuire WP, Hoskins WJ, Brady MF, et al: Cyclophosphamide and cisplatin compared with paclitaxel and cisplatin in patients with stage III and IV ovarian cancer. N Engl J Med 1996;334:1-6.
3. Long RTL, Evans AM: Diethylstilbestrol as a chemotherapeutic agent for ovarian carcinoma. Mo Med 1963;60:1125-1127.
4. Cramer DW, Welch WR: Determinants of ovarian cancer risk. II. Inferences regarding pathogenesis. J Natl Cancer Inst 1983;71:717-721.

5. Elit L, Hirte H: Current status and future innovations of hormonal agents, chemotherapy and investigational agents in endometrial cancer. Curr Opin Obstet Gynecol 2002; 14:67-73.

6. Schwartz PE, Chu MC, Zheng W, Mor G: Endometrial stromal tumors—are they hormonally sensitive? In Genazzani AR (ed): Hormone Replacement Therapy and Cancer. The Current Status of Research and Practice. London, Parthenon Publishing Group, 2002, pp 128-154.

7. Chan S: A review of selective estrogen receptor modulators in the treatment of breast and endometrial cancer. Semin Oncol 2002;28(Suppl 11):129-133.

8. Schwartz PE, Chambers JT: Hormone therapy in ovarian cancer. In Markman M, Hoskins WJ (eds): Cancer of the Ovary. New York, Raven Press, 1993, pp 339-348.

9. Perez-Garcia JL, Carrasco EM: Tamoxifen therapy for ovarian cancer in the adjuvant and advanced settings: Systematic review of the literature and implications for future research. Gynecol Oncol 2002;84:201-209.

10. Colombo N, Chiari S, Maggioni A, et al: Controversial issues in the management of early epithelial ovarian cancer: Conservative surgery and role of adjuvant therapy. Gynecol Oncol 1994;55: 347-351.

11. Zanetta G, Chiari S, Rota S, et al: Conservative surgery for Stage I ovarian carcinoma in women of child-bearing age. Br J Obstet Gynaecol 1997;104:1030-1035.

12. Fishman DA, Schwartz PE: Current approaches to diagnosis and treatment of ovarian germ cell malignancies. Curr Opin Obstet Gynecol 1994;6:98-104.

13. Price FV, Schwartz PE: Management of ovarian stromal tumors. In Rubin SC, Sutton GP (eds): Ovarian Cancer. New York, McGraw-Hill, 1993, pp 405-423.

14. Jolles B: Progesterone in the treatment of advanced malignant tumors of breast, ovary and uterus. Br J Cancer 1962;16:209-221.

15. Varga A, Henriksen E: Effect of 17-alpha-hydroxyprogesterone 17-n-caproate on various pelvic malignancies. Obstet Gynecol 1964;23:51-62.

16. Ward HW: Progestogen therapy for ovarian carcinoma. J Obstet Gynaecol Br Commonw 1972;79:555-559.

17. Kaufman RJ: Management of advanced ovarian carcinoma. Med Clin North Am 1966;50:845-856.

18. Malkasian GD, Decker DG, Jorgensen EO, Edmonson JH: Medroxyprogesterone acetate for the treatment of metastatic and recurrent ovarian carcinoma. Cancer Treat Rep 1977;61: 913-914.

19. Mangioni C, Franceschi S, LaVecchia C, D'Incalci M: High-dose medroxyprogesterone acetate (MPA) in advanced epithelial ovarian cancer resistant to first- or second line chemotherapy. Gynecol Oncol 1981;12:314-318.

20. Aabo K, Pedersen AG, Hald I, Dombernowski P: High-dose medroxyprogesterone acetate (MPA) in advanced chemotherapy-resistant ovarian carcinoma: A phase II study. Cancer Treat Rep 1982;66:407-408.

21. Slayton RE, Pagnano M, Creech RH: Progestin therapy for advanced ovarian cancer: A phase III Eastern Cooperative Group trial. Cancer Treat Rep 1981;65:895-896.

22. Trope C, Johnson JE, Sigurdsson K, Simonson E: High-dose medroxyprogesterone acetate for the treatment of advanced ovarian carcinoma. Cancer Treat Rep 1982;66:1441-1443.

23. Geisler HE: The use of high-dose megestrol acetate in the treatment of ovarian adenocarcinoma. Semin Oncol 1985;12: 20-22.

24. Ahlgren JD, Thomas D, Ellison N, et al: Phase II evaluation of high-dose megestrol acetate in advanced refractory ovarian cancer [abstract]. Proc Am Soc Clin Oncol 1985;4:124.

25. Hamerlynck JV, Maskens AP, Mangioni C, et al: Phase II trial of medroxyprogesterone acetate in advanced ovarian cancer: An EORTC Gynaecological Cancer Cooperative Group Study. Gynecol Oncol 1985;22:313-316.

26. Wilailak S, Linasmita V, Srisupundit S: Phase II study of high-dose megestrol acetate in platinum-refractory epithelial ovarian cancer. Anticancer Drugs 2001;12:719-724.

27. Wiernik PH, Greenwald ES, Ball H, et al: High-dose megestrol acetate in the treatment of patients with ovarian cancer who have undergone previous treatment: Eastern Cooperative Oncology Group Study PD884. Am J Clin Oncol 1998;21:565-567.

28. Bergqvist A, Kullander S, Thorell J: A study of estrogen and progesterone cytosol receptor concentration in benign and malignant ovarian tumors treated with medroxyprogesterone acetate. Acta Obstet Gynecol Scand 1981;101(Suppl):75-81.

29. Rendina GM, Donadio C, Giovannini M: Steroid receptors and progestinic therapy in ovarian endometrioid carcinoma. Eur J Gynaecol Oncol 1982;3:241-246.

30. Timothy I: Progestogen therapy for ovarian carcinoma. Br J Obstet Gynaecol 1982;89:561-563.

31. Jolles CJ, Freedman RS, Jones LA: Estrogen and progestogen therapy in advanced cancer: Preliminary report. Gynecol Oncol 1983;16:352-359.

32. Freedman RS, Saul PB, Edwards CL, et al: Ethinyl estradiol and medroxyprogesterone acetate in patients with epithelial ovarian carcinoma: A phase II study. Cancer Treat Rep 1986;70:369-373.

33. Schwartz PE, Keating G, MacLusky N, et al: Tamoxifen therapy for advanced ovarian cancer. Obstet Gynecol 1982;59:583-588.

34. Rowland K, Bonomi P, Wilbanks G, et al: Hormone receptors in ovarian carcinoma [abstract C-456]. Proc Am Soc Clin Oncol 1985;4:117.

35. Quinn MA: Hormonal therapy of ovarian cancer. In Sharp F, Soutter WP (eds): Ovarian Cancer: The Way Ahead. London, Royal College of Obstetricians and Gynaecologists 1987, pp 383-393.

36. Weiner SA, Alberts DS, Surwitt EA, et al: Tamoxifen therapy in recurrent epithelial ovarian carcinoma. Gynecol Oncol 1987; 27:208-213.

37. Landoni F, Bonazzi C, Regallo M, et al: Antiestrogen as last-line treatment in epithelial ovarian cancer. Chemioterapia 1985; 4(Suppl N.2):1059-1060.

38. Hatch KD, Beecham JB, Blessing JA, Creasman WT: Responsiveness of patients with advanced ovarian cancer to tamoxifen: A Gynecologic Oncology Group study of second-line therapy in 105 patients. Cancer 1991;68:269-271.

39. Osborne RJ, Malik ST, Slevin ML, et al: Tamoxifen in refractory ovarian cancer: The use of a loading dose schedule. Br J Cancer 1988;57:115-116.

40. Ahlgren JD, Ellison NM, Gottlieb RJ, et al: Hormonal palliation of chemoresistant ovarian cancer: Three consecutive phase II trials of the Mid-Atlantic Oncology Program. J Clin Oncol 1993;11:1957-1968.

41. Shirey DR, Kavanagh JJ, Gershenson DM, et al: Tamoxifen therapy of epithelial ovarian cancer. Obstet Gynecol 1985;66: 575-578.

42. Slevin ML, Harvey VJ, Osborne RJ, et al: A phase II study of tamoxifen in ovarian cancer. Eur J Cancer Clin Oncol 1986; 22:309-312.

43. Pagel J, Rose C, Thorpe S, Hald I: Treatment of advanced ovarian carcinoma with tamoxifen: A phase II trial. Proceedings of the Second European Conference of Clinical Oncologists [abstract]. Clin Oncol 1983;42.

44. Hamerlynck JV, Vermorken JB, Van der Burgh ME, et al: Tamoxifen therapy in advanced ovarian cancer: A phase II study [abstract]. Proc Am Soc Clin Oncol 1985;4:115.

45. Jager W, Sauerbrei W, Beck E, et al: A randomized comparison of triptorelin and tamoxifen as treatment of progressive ovarian cancer. Anticancer Res 1995;15:2639-2642.

46. Van der Velden J, Gitsch G, Wain GV, et al: Tamoxifen in patients with advanced epithelial ovarian cancer. Int J Gynecol Cancer 1995;5:301-305.

47. Van der Vange N, Greggi S, Burger C, et al: Experience with hormonal therapy in advanced epithelial ovarian cancer. Acta Oncol 1995;34:813-820.

48. Rolski J, Pawlicki M: Evaluation of efficacy and toxicity of tamoxifen in patients with advanced chemotherapy resistant ovarian cancer. Ginekol Pol 1998;69:586-589.

49. Gennatas C, Dardoufas C, Karvouni H, et al: Phase II trial of tamoxifen in patients with advanced epithelial ovarian cancer [abstract]. Proc Am Soc Clin Oncol 1996;15:782.

50. Marth C, Sorheim N, Kaern J, Trope C: Tamoxifen in the treatment of recurrent ovarian carcinoma. Int J Gynecol Cancer 1997;7:256-261.

51. Jakobsen AJ, Bertelsen K, Sell A: Cyclic hormone treatment in ovarian cancer: A phase II trial. Eur J Cancer Clin Oncol 1987;23:915-916.

52. Belinson JL, McClure M, Badger G: Randomized trial of megestrol acetate vs. megestrol acetate/tamoxifen for the management of progressive or recurrent epithelial ovarian carcinoma. Gynecol Oncol 1987;28:151-155.

53. Schwartz PE, Chambers JT, Kohorn EI, et al: Tamoxifen in combination with cytotoxic chemotherapy in advanced epithelial cancer. Cancer 1989;63:1074-1078.

54. Ercoli A, Scambia G, DeVincenzo R, et al: Tamoxifen synergizes the antiproliferative effect of cisplatin in human ovarian cancer cells: Enhancement of DNA platination as a possible mechanism. Cancer Lett 1996;108:7-14.

55. Ercoli A, Scambia G, Fattorossi A, et al: Comparative study on the induction of cytostasis and apoptosis by ICI 182,780 and tamoxifen in an estrogen receptor-negative ovarian cancer cell line. Int J Cancer 1998;76:47-54.

56. Benedetti-Panici P, Greggi S, Amoroso M, et al: A combination of platinum and tamoxifen in advanced ovarian cancer failing platinum-based chemotherapy: Results of a phase II study. Int J Gynecol Cancer 2001;11:438-444.

57. Kahanpaa V, Karkkainen J, Nieminen U: Multi-agent chemotherapy with and without medroxyprogesterone acetate in the treatment of advanced ovarian cancer. Excerpta Medica International Congress Series 1982;611:477-482.

58. Markman M, Kennedy A, Webster K, et al: Phase I trial of paclitaxel plus megestrol acetate in patients with paclitaxel refractory ovarian cancer. Clin Cancer Res 2000;6:4201-4204.

59. Thompson MA, Adelson MD: Aging and development of ovarian epithelial carcinoma: The relevance of changes in ovarian stromal androgen production. Adv Exp Med Biol 1993;330:155-165.

60. Evangelou A, Jindal SK, Brown TJ, Letarte M: Down-regulation of transforming growth factor beta receptors by androgen in ovarian cancer cells. Cancer Res 2000;60:929-935.

61. Kavanagh JJ, Wharton JT, Roberts WS: Androgen therapy in the treatment of refractory epithelial ovarian cancer. Cancer Treat Rep 1987;71:537-538.

62. Slotman BJ, Rao BR: Response to inhibition of androgen action of human ovarian cancer cells in vitro. Cancer Lett 1989;45:213-220.

63. Tumolo S, Rao BR, van der Burg ME, et al: Phase II trial of flutamide in advanced ovarian cancer: An EORTC Gynaecological Cancer Cooperative Group Study. Eur J Cancer 1994;30A:911-914.

64. Zheng W, Lu J, Luo F, et al: Ovarian epithelial tumor growth promotion by FSH and inhibition of the effect by LH. Gynecol Oncol 2000;76:80-88.

65. Zheng W, Magid MS, Kramer EE, Chen YT: Follicle-stimulating hormone receptor is expressed in human ovarian surface epithelium and fallopian tube. Am J Pathol 1996;148:47-53.

66. Lu JJ, Zheng Y, Yuan J-M, et al: Decreased luteinizing hormone receptor mRNA expression in human ovarian epithelial cancer. Gynecol Oncol 2000;21:417-433.

67. Zhou H, Luo M, Schönthal AH, et al: Regulation of ovarian epithelial tumor growth by menstrual cycle hormones. Cancer Biol Ther 2002;1:208-304.

68. Schiffenbauer YS, Abramovitch R, Meir G, et al: Loss of ovarian function promotes angiogenesis in human ovarian carcinoma. Proc Natl Acad Sci U S A 1997;94:13203-13208.

69. Wang J, Luo F, Chen P, et al: VEGF expression and enhanced production by gonadotropins in ovarian epithelial tumors. Int J Cancer 2002;97:163-167.

70. Yabushita H, Narmiya H, Sawaguchi K, Norguchi M: Role of VEGF in peritoneal dissemination of ovarian cancer. Proc Am Soc Clin Oncol 2002;21(Pt 2):175b.

71. Mortel R, Satyaswaroop PG, Schally AV, et al: Inhibitory effect of GnRH superagonist on the growth of human ovarian carcinoma NIH: OVCAR-3 in the nude mouse. Gynecol Oncol 1986;23:254-255.

72. Peterson CM, Ziminiski SJ: A long acting gonadotropin-releasing hormone agonist inhibits the growth of a human ovarian epithelial carcinoma (BG-1) heterotransplanted in the nude mouse. Obstet Gynecol 1990;76:264-267.

73. Parmar H, Rustin G, Lightman SL, et al: Response to D-Trp-6-luteinizing hormone releasing hormone (Decapeptyl) microcapsules in advanced ovarian cancer. Br Med J 1988;296:1229.

74. Kavanagh JJ, Roberts W, Townsend P, Hewitt S: Leuprolide acetate in the treatment of refractory or persistent epithelial ovarian cancer. J Clin Oncol 1989;7:115-118.

75. Bruckner HW, Motwani BT: Treatment of advanced refractory ovarian carcinoma with a gonadotropin-releasing hormone analogue. Am J Obstet Gynecol 1989;161:1216-1218.

76. Emons G, Ortmann O, Teichert H-M, et al: Leuteinizing hormone-releasing hormone agonist triptorelin in combination with cytotoxic chemotherapy in patients with advanced ovarian carcinoma: A prospective double blind randomized trial. Cancer 1996;78:1452-1460.

77. Erickson LD, Hartmann LC, Su JQ, et al: Cyclophosphamide, cisplatin and leuprolide acetate in patients with debulked stage III or IV ovarian carcinoma. Gynecol Oncol 1994;54:196-200.

78. Schwartz PE, MacLusky N, Sakamoto H, Eisenfeld A: Steroid receptor proteins in non-epithelial malignancies of the ovary. Gynecol Oncol 1983;15:305-315.

79. Kuhnel R, deGraaff J, Rao BR, Stolk JG: Androgen receptor predominance in human ovarian carcinoma. J Steroid Biochem 1987;26:393-397.

80. Shaw PA, Rittenberg PV, Brown TJ: Activation of androgen receptor–associated protein 70 (ARA 70) mRNA expression in ovarian cancer. Gynecol Oncol 2001;80:132-138.

81. Edmonson RJ, Monahan JM, Davies BR: The human ovarian surface epithelium is an androgen responsive tissue. Brit J Cancer 2002;86:879-885.

82. Levine DA, Boyd J: The androgen receptor and genetic susceptibility to ovarian cancer: Results from a case series. Cancer Res 2001;61:908-911.

83. Hua W, Christianson T, Rougeot C, et al: SKOV3 ovarian carcinoma cells have functional estrogen receptor but are growth-resistant to estrogen and antiestrogens. J Steroid Biochem Mol Biol 1995;55:279-289.

84. Lau KM, Mok SC, Ho SM: Expression of human estrogen receptor-alpha and -beta, progesterone receptor and androgen receptor mRNA and malignant ovarian epithelial cells. Proc Natl Acad Sci U S A 1999;96:5722-5727.

85. Rutherford T, Brown WD, Sapi E, et al: Absence of estrogen receptor–beta expression in metastatic ovarian cancer. Obstet Gynecol 2000;96:417-421.

86. Pujol P, Rey JM, Nirde P, et al: Differential expression of estrogen receptor-alpha and -beta messenger RNAs as a potential marker of ovarian carcinogenesis. Cancer Res 1998;58:5367-5373.

87. Chu S, Mamers P, Burger HG, Fuller PJ: Estrogen receptor isoform gene expression in ovarian stromal and epithelial tumors. J Clin Endocrinol Metab 2000;85:1200-1205.

88. Schwartz PE, LiVolsi VA, Hildreth N, et al: Estrogen receptors in human ovarian epithelial carcinoma. Obstet Gynecol 1982;59:229-238.

89. Rao BR, Slotman BJ: Endocrine factors in common epithelial ovarian cancer. Endocr Rev 1991;12:14-26.

90. Lazo JS, Schwartz PE, MacLusky NJ, et al: Anti-proliferative actions of tamoxifen to human ovarian carcinomas in vitro. Cancer Res 1984;44:2265-2271.

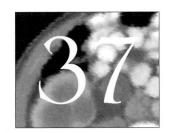

MALIGNANT OVARIAN GERM CELL TUMORS

Stephen D. Williams

 MAJOR CONTROVERSIES

- **What are the roles of surgical staging and cytoreduction?**
- **What is the optimal treatment for patients with early-stage ovarian germ cell tumors: adjuvant chemotherapy or surveillance?**

Ovarian germ cell tumors are rare. Consequently, there have been no randomized trials (nor will there every be). The database from which the modern standard of care has been developed arises from three sources. The first is numerous papers in literature that are retrospective reviews of patients' treatment and outcome. In general, these studies have been conducted at single institutions and span many years. Although these studies provide helpful and sometimes insightful information, they do not provide the level of evidence that is obtained from prospective clinical trials. The second source is prospective trials, some of which have been conducted in cooperative groups. Treatment in these studies is generally uniform, but they are limited by the fact that they are descriptive studies rather than randomized trials. Nonetheless, some have provided very useful information.

The third source is numerous prospective trials, many of them randomized, conducted in male germ cell tumors. These studies, by virtue of their much larger accrual, have added greatly to the body of knowledge that has been extrapolated to female germ cell tumors. They assume that this information is valid in women. This is probably largely true for chemotherapy regimens but less valid for surgical issues.

There are severe limitations to the historic database that clinicians apply to derive a management plan for new patients. Significant controversy exists in several areas, and I address three of these in this chapter.

What are the roles of surgical staging and cytoreduction?

If metastatic disease is encountered at initial surgery, the same principles concerning cytoreductive surgery that have been applied in the surgical management of advanced epithelial ovarian cancer are generally followed, with resection of as much tumor as is technically feasible and safe. There is, however, scant information in the literature about the true value of cytoreductive surgery of malignant germ cell tumors because of their rarity.

In an early study of the Gynecologic Oncology Group (GOG), 15 (28%) of 54 patients with completely resected disease at primary surgery failed chemotherapy with a combination of vincristine, dactinomycin, and cyclophosphamide (VAC regimen), as opposed to 15 (68%) of 22 patients with incompletely resected disease treated with the same regimen.[1] A higher percentage of patients with bulky residual disease (82%) failed chemotherapy compared with those with minimal residual disease (55%). In a subsequent GOG study in which patients received the combination of cisplatin, vinblastine, and bleomycin (PVB regimen), patients with tumors other than dysgerminoma who had clinically nonmeasurable disease had a greater likelihood of remaining free of disease progression than those with measurable disease (65% versus 34%). Patients who had their tumors surgically debulked to optimal disease had an outcome intermediate between patients with suboptimal disease and those with optimal disease without debulking.[2]

Germ cell tumors are much more chemosensitive than epithelial tumors. The advisability of aggressive resections of metastatic disease, especially bulky retroperitoneal nodes, is questionable. On the other hand, significant tumor debulking may result in improved prognosis if it can be accomplished without undue risk of postoperative morbidity and delay of chemotherapy. This situation requires careful surgical judgment, but evidence supports a reasonable attempt at surgical debulking if it can be accomplished with an acceptable amount of surgical morbidity, particularly considering the necessity of prompt initiation of chemotherapy for these patients, some of whom have very rapidly progressive tumors.

Optimal Chemotherapy Regimens

The era of modern chemotherapy began in the mid-1970s with the discovery of the major single-agent activity of cisplatin and its subsequent incorporation into combination chemotherapy regimens. Studies in testis cancer documented the curability of metastatic disease, particularly in patients with small-volume tumors. Several subsequent trials enrolling women with ovarian germ cell tumors confirmed the applicability of this finding to these patients and established a baseline for future studies.[2,3] About 60% to 80% of women with advanced-stage (stage III and IV) tumors are cured with this approach. As in epithelial ovarian cancer, an important prognostic factor appears to be the volume of residual tumor at initiation of chemotherapy. The initial chemotherapy regimen was PVB, but a subsequent randomized trial in testis cancer showed that the substitution of etoposide for vinblastine (BEP) reduced acute toxicity, and it may improve therapeutic outcome in patients with bulky tumor.[4] Subsequent studies seemed to confirm that this observation also is valid for women.[3]

For male germ cell tumors, several institutions and cooperative groups developed various but similar systems to predict the outcome of patients with metastatic disease who were receiving chemotherapy. Ultimately, an international collaboration was developed and validated. This system rather accurately predicts outcome using levels of initial serum markers (i.e., human chorionic gonadotrophin and alphafetoprotein), primary site (i.e., testis and retroperitoneum versus mediastinum), pathology, and the presence or absence of nonpulmonary visceral metastases. Using this information, investigators for clinical trial purposes separate male germ cell tumor patients into two groups. Clinical trials enrolling patients with the most favorable prognosis focus on toxicity reduction. Trials enrolling patients with a less favorable prognosis attempt to increase the likelihood of cure. Unfortunately, there is no such prognostic system for ovarian germ cell tumors. Ovarian germ cell tumor patients are separated into groups with or without residual tumor after initial surgery. Those with residual tumor are further divided into those with small-volume disease (<1 to 2 cm) and those with more extensive residual tumor or stage IV disease.

Recommendations for chemotherapy for ovarian germ cell tumors are derived from experience with testis cancer, which may or may not be totally relevant, but it seems appropriate given the lack of more definitive information. Sequential, large, randomized trials enrolling favorable-prognosis testis cancer patients (i.e., no nonpulmonary visceral metastases and no extreme marker elevations) have shown that three courses of BEP is equivalent to four courses.[5] However, deletion of bleomycin in patients who receive only three courses is associated with a lower complete response rate and a higher risk of recurrence in patients who are complete responders.[6] Until recently, it was thought that four courses of etoposide and cisplatin (EP regimen) was equivalent to three courses of BEP. However, results of a randomized trial in Europe suggest that this may not be the case and that three courses of BEP is marginally superior to four courses of EP.

Prospective, single-arm trials of treatment for ovarian germ cell tumors seem to validate these results and suggest similar and excellent results in patients with no or small-volume residual tumor. Although bleomycin's lung toxicity is a significant consideration and a very serious complication of treatment, it is a rare event in women (and men) who only receive three courses (9 weeks) of treatment.[6,7] Compared with four courses, it is intuitively obvious that three courses of therapy should lessen short-term unpleasantness and minimize late complications. I believe that the appropriate chemotherapy regimen for women with no or small-volume residual tumor after surgery is three courses of BEP. This regimen can preserve the high cure rate and minimize short-term unpleasantness and late toxic effects. Although bleomycin lung disease is a concern, it is uncommon in patients receiving only three courses and can be minimized with careful monitoring. The most important method of monitoring is a careful physical examination of the lungs and discontinuation of bleomycin if the patient develops physical findings of early lung toxicity, which are rales or a lag or diminished expansion of a lung.

Randomized trials enrolling patients with poor-prognosis testis cancer (i.e., liver or brain metastases or very high marker elevations) have not demonstrated a regimen superior to four courses of BEP. Given that, I believe that patients with ovarian germ cell tumors who have bulky residual disease after initial surgery should receive four courses of BEP.

What is the optimal treatment for patients with early-stage ovarian germ cell tumors: adjuvant chemotherapy or surveillance?

For many years, appropriate management of patients with completely resected ovarian germ cell tumors has included adjuvant chemotherapy. Patients with embryonal carcinoma, endodermal sinus tumors, and mixed tumors containing these elements are thought to have a very high risk of recurrence without postoperative therapy. A widely used earlier chemotherapy combination was the VAC regimen. No comparative studies have been done, but many trials suggest that the risk of relapse of patients so treated is less than would be expected if no adjuvant therapy were administered. In a GOG study[1] (Protocol 44), 31 of 50 patients with these tumors remain free of recurrence with adjuvant VAC. In a follow-up study[7] (Protocol 78), 50 of 51 patients remained well with no evidence of disease when BEP was the adjuvant regimen. Although these regimens were not directly compared in a randomized trial, the superiority of BEP is thought to be demonstrated, and there seems little doubt that adjuvant therapy is appropriate. Many other studies using cisplatin-based therapy have given similar results.

The situation for patients with immature teratoma is more complex. Immature teratomas are graded according to the system of Thurlbeck and Scully as modified by Norris and colleagues.[8] These neoplasms are categorized as grade 1, 2, or 3 based on the amount of immature neuroepithelium. Prognosis of patients is related to tumor grade. In this study, only 1 of 14 patients with grade 1, stage I immature teratoma had recurrent disease. However, 9 of 20 patients with grade 2 tumors had recurrences, as did 4 of 6 patients with grade 3 tumors. Because of these data, most clinicians have not recommended adjuvant therapy for patients with stage I, grade 1 tumors but have done so for those with localized tumors of grades 2 and 3. These patients have been eligible for previous GOG trials (Protocols 44 and 78). Forty-two patients with resected high-grade immature teratoma were entered on Protocol 78 and treated with three courses of BEP. Of these, 39 have no evidence of disease.[7]

Unfortunately, the data from which the recommendation for adjuvant therapy is derived was developed in an era before surgical staging was routinely done. It is conceivable that the relatively high risk of recurrence was not because of biologic aggressiveness of high-grade immature teratoma but because of underestimation of extent of disease at the time of initial tumor resection.

In the modern era of surgical staging of ovarian neoplasms, it may be appropriate to re-evaluate the role of routine adjuvant therapy in such patients and perhaps define a patient population that may not have a risk of recurrence sufficiently high to warrant such treatment. Such an approach must be done with great caution, because surgery followed by adjuvant therapy can cure virtually all patients with localized high-grade teratoma. However, it is possible that the risk of relapse will be low in a defined population of well-staged patients and, with careful follow-up, that nearly all relapsing patients can be diagnosed with relatively small-volume tumor and cured with subsequent chemotherapy for metastatic disease. Although some issues are different in testis cancer, a deferral of chemotherapy has been shown to be an appropriate therapeutic alternative for patients with resected stage II tumors and for patients with clinical stage I disease.

At least three groups of investigators have reported results of surveillance of patients with resected immature teratomas. An intergroup study of the Pediatric Oncology Group and the Children's Cancer Group investigated surveillance after surgical resection in 41 girls with ovarian immature teratoma. The median age was 10 years. Central pathology review confirmed that 31 patients had immature teratoma alone (18 grade 1, 9 grade 2, and 4 grade 3 tumors) and that 10 patients had immature teratoma plus identifiable yolk sac tumor. Forty of 41 patients remain continuously disease free, with median follow-up of 33 months for the immature teratoma group and 24 months for the combined group. One patient developed liver metastases, was successfully treated with BEP, and is disease free 30 months after chemotherapy.[9]

Investigators at Mt. Vernon and Charing Cross Hospitals in England have observed 15 patients after initial surgical treatment. All patients had stage Ia tumors, but surgical staging was incomplete in some patients. Nine patients had grade 2 or 3 immature teratomas only, and six also had elements of endodermal sinus tumor. A total of three patients had recurrences, 1 of 9 in the pure immature teratoma group and 2 of 6 in the group that also contained endodermal sinus tumor. One patient died of a pulmonary embolus during chemotherapy; all others are alive and without evident tumor.[10]

Investigators at the University of Milan followed a group of ovarian immature teratoma patients according to a comprehensive prospective protocol. Patients with stage Ia, grade 1 or 2 tumors were assessed with physical examinations and ultrasound studies every 3 months for the first year, every 6 months in the second year, and annually thereafter. Patients with gliomatosis peritonei or with stage Ib, Ic, or II and grade 1 or 2 tumors also underwent laparoscopy every 6 months for the first year. Chemotherapy was to be given to patients with grade 3 or stage III tumors. There were a total of 32 patients, of whom nine had stage Ia, grade 2 or 3 tumors and did not receive adjuvant chemotherapy. Of these, one patient relapsed with a pelvic tumor that was removed surgically and found to be mature teratoma. Another developed gliosis during follow-up. None of these patients ever received chemotherapy, and all are free of evident disease. Four other patients with stage Ic tumors did not receive adjuvant chemotherapy. One had an abdominopelvic relapse that was treated surgically; another developed gliosis during follow-up. None received chemotherapy, and all have no evidence of disease. For these 13 patients, follow-up ranged from 11 to 138 months, and only 2 were followed for less than 2 years.[11]

Considering all of these data, it is hard to know how to manage patients with stage I immature teratoma. We are lacking a prospective trial enrolling well-staged adult patients. It is possible that the routine use of adjuvant chemotherapy is excessive treatment for most patients. It is equally possible that adult patients are different from children and that to not treat such patients increases the amount of treatment that is required for them (i.e., more chemotherapy and further surgery) and possibly the risk of death. I feel that treatment is indicated for most patients. It is very important that a well-designed, prospective trial of surveillance be conducted.

REFERENCES

1. Slayton RE, Park RC, Silverberg SG, et al: Vincristine, dactinomycin, and cyclophosphamide in the treatment of malignant germ cell tumors of the ovary: A Gynecologic Oncology Group study (a final report). Cancer 1985;56:243-248.
2. Williams SD, Blessing JA, Moore DH, et al: Cisplatin, vinblastine, and bleomycin in advanced and recurrent ovarian germ-cell tumors. Ann Intern Med 1989;111:22-27.
3. Gershenson DM, Morris M, Cangir A, et al: Treatment of malignant germ cell tumors of the ovary with bleomycin, etoposide, and cisplatin. J Clin Oncol 1990;8:715-720.
4. Williams SD, Birch R, Einhorn LH, et al. Treatment of disseminated germ-cell tumors with cisplatin, bleomycin, and either vinblastine or etoposide. N Engl J Med 1987;316:1435-1440.
5. Einhorn LH, Williams SD, Loehrer PJ, et al: Evaluation of optimal duration of chemotherapy in favorable-prognosis disseminated germ cell tumors: A Southeastern Cancer Study Group protocol. J Clin Oncol 1989;7:387-391.
6. Loehrer PJ Sr, Johnson D, Elson P, et al: Importance of bleomycin in favorable-prognosis disseminated germ cell tumors: An Eastern Cooperative Oncology Group trial. J Clin Oncol 1995; 13:470-476.
7. Williams S, Blessing JA, Liao SY, et al: Adjuvant therapy of ovarian germ cell tumors with cisplatin, etoposide, and bleomycin: A trial of the Gynecologic Oncology Group. J Clin Oncol 1994;12:701-706.
8. Norris HJ, Zirkin HJ, Benson WL: Immature (malignant) teratoma of the ovary. Cancer 1976;37:2359-2372.
9. Marina NM, Cushing B, Giller R, et al: Complete surgical excision is effective treatment for children with immature teratomas with or without malignant elements: A Pediatric Oncology Group/Children's Cancer Group intergroup study. J Clin Oncol 1999;17:2137-2143.
10. Dark GG, Bower M, Newlands ES, et al. Surveillance policy for stage I ovarian germ cell tumors. J Clin Oncol 1997;15:620-624.
11. Bonazzi C, Peccatori F, Colombo N, et al: Pure ovarian immature teratoma, a unique and curable disease: 10 years' experience of 32 prospectively treated patients. Obstet Gynecol 1994;84:598-604.

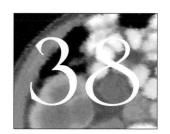

OVARIAN SEX CORD–STROMAL TUMORS

Nicoletta Colombo and Gabriella Parma

 MAJOR CONTROVERSIES

- **Is there a difference between the juvenile and the adult histotype?**
- **What is the most common clinical presentation?**
- **Are there tumor markers that are useful in the diagnosis and follow-up?**
- **How should sex cord–stromal tumors be clinically managed?**
- **Is there a role for chemotherapy?**
- **Are there other therapeutic options besides surgery and chemotherapy?**

Sex cord–stromal tumors account for approximately 7% of all malignant ovarian neoplasms, and their extreme rarity represents a limitation in understanding their natural history, management, and prognosis (Table 38-1). Sex cord–stromal tumors of the ovary are derived from the sex cords and the ovarian stroma or mesenchyme. This category of ovarian neoplasms usually is composed of various combinations of elements, including the "female" cells (granulosa cells, theca cells, and their luteinized derivatives), "male" cells (Sertoli cells and Leydig cells), and fibroblasts of gonadal stromal origin as well as morphologically indifferent cells. A classification of this group of tumors is presented in Table 38-2.

The peak incidence of ovarian sex cord–stromal tumors is in women older than 50 years of age, but a significant proportion occur in premenopausal women. Histologically, these tumors are considered to be malignant neoplasms. However, their natural history is indolent, and the long-term prognosis is very favorable, similar to that of tumors of low malignant potential. The low incidence of these tumors, their multiplicity of histologic patterns, and their variable biologic behavior limit the optimal management of sex cord–ovarian tumors. Contemporary treatment principles have developed based on observations of small groups of patients and on information extrapolated from clinical management of epithelial tumors. Adequate

knowledge of these tumors is imperative to appropriate diagnosis and individual definitive surgical and adjuvant therapy.

Is there a difference between the juvenile and the adult histotype?

Sex cord–stromal tumors include granulosa cell tumors, thecomas, fibroma-fibrosarcomas, and sclerosing stromal cell tumors. Granulosa cell tumors account for approximately 70% of ovarian sex cord–stromal tumors and represent 3% to 5% of all ovarian neoplasms.[1-7] The incidence in developed countries varies from 0.4 to 1.7 cases per 100.000 women.[5,8] The average age at diagnosis is 52 years, but granulosa cell tumors have been diagnosed from infancy through to the tenth decade of life. Because the clinical and pathologic characteristics of the tumors that occur after the menopause are different from those that occur in children and younger patients, the adult and juvenile granulosa cell types are considered separately.

The *adult type* accounts for 95% of all granulosa cell tumors. Hormone production is common, with a predominance of estrogen production, and results in abnormal vaginal bleeding in about two thirds of the patients. The typical endometrial alteration associated with functioning tumors is simple hyperplasia, usually

Table 38–1. Age at Diagnosis of Primary Ovarian Neoplasm (% of Patients)

Tumor Type	<20 yr	20-50 yr	>50 yr
Coelomic epithelium	29	71	81
Germ cell	59	14	6
Sex cord	8	5	4
Nonspecific mesenchyme	4	10	9

Table 38–3. Concomitant Uterine Pathology in Granulosa Cell Tumors (% of Cases)

Reference	Hyperplasia	Adenocarcinoma
Norris[57]	22	9
Fox et al[2]	51	10
Stenwig et al[10]	—	5
Pankratz et al[6]	66	12
Gusberg and Kardon[9]	55	27
Evans et al[1]	55	13

exhibiting some degree of precancerous atypia (Table 38-3). Gusberg and Kardon,[9] in a retrospective study, reported that 13% of 69 patients had cystic glandular hyperplasia, 42% had atypical hyperplasia, 5% had adenocarcinoma in situ, and 22% had invasive adenocarcinoma. Similarly, a study by Evans and colleagues[1] of 76 patients with granulosa cell tumors from whom endometrial tissue was available showed a high incidence of endometrial hyperplasia (55%) and adenocarcinoma (13%).

If strict criteria for the diagnosis of carcinoma are used and all patients are considered, the estimated frequency of associated endometrial adenocarcinoma is about 5%.[10] In addition, granulosa cell tumors are associated with an increased incidence of breast cancer.[11] Granulosa cell tumors are frequently considered to be low-grade malignancies and are prognostically similar to epithelial borderline neoplasm of the ovary. This is reflected in the propensity for the tumor to remain localized and to demonstrate an indolent growth pattern. A large majority of these tumors are diagnosed in stage I, although it must be remembered that accurate and complete surgical staging was not available in most of the published series. In three of the largest series,[1,4,10] the frequency of stage I disease

Table 38–2. Classification of Sex Cord–Stromal Tumors

Granulosa–Stromal Cell Tumors
Granulosa Cell Tumors
Adult type
Juvenile type

Tumors in the Thecoma-Fibroma Group
Thecoma
Fibroma-fibrosarcoma
Sclerosing stromal tumor

Sertoli-Leydig Cell Tumors (Androblastomas)

Sertoli Cell Tumors

Leydig Cell Tumor

Sertoli-Leydig Cell Tumors
Well-differentiated
Of intermediate differentiation
Poorly differentiated
With heterologous elements
Retiform
Mixed

Gynandroblastoma

Sex Cord Tumor with Anular Tubules

Unclassified

ranged from 78% to 91%. Bilateral ovarian involvement is unusual, ranging from 0% to 8%.

The prognosis of this tumor is excellent: the relapse rate ranges from 10% to 33%. The average time to recurrence is between 5 and 10 years,[10] with some recurrences occurring as late as 25 years after the initial diagnosis. The long-term survival rate ranges from 75% to 90% for all stages. A collective assessment of 190 surgically staged patients showed a 5-year survival rate of 92% to 100% for stage I disease.[1,8,12] The earlier presentation, the infrequency of bilaterality, the long median time to recurrence (6.0 years), the long-term survival rate, and the long median survival time after recurrence (5.6 years) demonstrate a behavior very different from that of epithelial ovarian cancer.[4,13] However, stage III disease, although rare, carries a poor prognosis, with a 5-year survival rate of 0% to 22%, similar to that observed for epithelial ovarian cancer.

The *juvenile type* was described by Scully and associates[14] as a variant of granulosa cell tumor that tends to occur in younger women and has a natural history and histologic characteristics that are very different from those of the typical granulosa cell tumor. About 90% of granulosa tumors occurring in prepubertal girls and many of those seen in women before the age of 30 years are of this juvenile type. In Scully's series of 125 cases, 44% of the tumors occurred before 10 years of age and only 3% after the third decade of life. The tumor usually arises in otherwise normal children, although there is a suggestion for a specific association with Ollier's disease (enchondromatosis) and Maffucci's syndrome (enchondromatosis and hemangiomatosis).[15-19] Similar to the adult type, the frequency of bilaterality is 5%[14] and most tumors are diagnosed at an early stage. An extraovarian spread is infrequently observed at exploration, and rupture of the tumor is noted in approximately 10% of cases. Although the juvenile germ cell tumors usually appear to be less well differentiated than those of the adult form, follow-up data indicate a high cure rate. Scully and associates[14] reported that 92% of 95 patients were alive and free of disease after an average follow-up period of 5 years. In contrast to the adult-type disease, in which recurrences occur remotely from the site of initial diagnosis, the juvenile form is characteristically aggressive in advanced stages, and the time to relapse and death is of limited duration. In data extracted from three series,[14,20,21] only 3 (23%) of 13 patients with advanced disease (stage II, III, or IV) were alive and without recurrence after 3 years and the recurrences and deaths occurred within 3 years.

What is the most common clinical presentation?

Granulosa cell tumors are the most common clinically estrogenic ovarian neoplasms. Abnormal uterine bleeding manifests the endometrial changes associated with these tumors, and increased levels of estrogens have been reported in the blood and urine. Rarely, androgenic changes such as oligomenorrhea, hirsutism, and other virilizing signs may be present. The most common clinical symptoms at presentation include abdominal distention and abdominal pain, resulting from the gross size of the tumor and the presence of ascites. The cause of acute severe pain is usually adnexal torsion, hemorrhage into the tumor, or rupture of a cystic component. About 15% of patients who have cystic granulosa cell tumors are first examined for acute abdomen associated with hemoperitoneum. Adult granulosa cell tumors vary in size from microscopic lesions, not detected by pelvic examination (10% to 15% of cases), to very large masses measuring 40 cm in diameter.

In the juvenile granulosa cell tumors, the majority of prepuberal patients present with clinical evidence of isosexual precocious pseudopuberty, which may include breast enlargement, development of pubic and axillary hair, vaginal secretions, irregular uterine bleeding, advanced somatic and skeletal development, and other secondary sex characteristics.[14,20-23] Infrequently, patients present with an androgen-secreting tumor accompanied by a virilization syndrome. If the juvenile germ cell tumor occurs after puberty, patients typically present with abdominal pain, sometimes associated with menstrual irregularities or amenorrhea.

Sertoli-Leydig cell tumors (androblastomas), which represent fewer than 0.2% of ovarian cancers and occur most frequently in the second and third decades, typically produce androgens; clinical virilization is noted in 70% to 85% of patients.[24-25] The androgenic symptoms include oligomenorrhea followed by amenorrhea, breast atrophy, acne, hirsutism, clitoromegaly, a deepening voice, and a receding hairline. The prevalence of androgenic manifestations appears to be independent of the degree of histologic differentiation, but these symptoms are observed less frequently with heterologous and retiform lesions. Measurement of plasma androgens may reveal increased testosterone and androstenedione, with normal or slightly elevated dehydroepiandrosterone sulphate.[24] Surgical excision of the tumor results in a precipitous drop in androgen levels and partial to complete resolution of the clinical signs associated with androgen excess. Approximately 50% of patients with these tumors have no endocrine manifestations; usually, they present with complaints of abdominal swelling or pain. Occasionally, tumors are correlated with various estrogenic syndromes. Sertoli-Leydig tumors are unilateral in 98% of cases and are variable size, averaging about 10 cm in diameter.

In a series of about 200 patients, tumors were stage Ia in 80% of the cases. In 12% of the total, the tumor either had ruptured or involved the external surface of the ovary; in 4%, ascites was present.[26]

Are there tumor markers that are useful in the diagnosis and follow-up?

The identification of a specific tumor marker would facilitate early detection of recurrent disease. Among the proteins derived from granulosa cells, inhibin (a follicle-regulating protein) and mullerian inhibiting substance are assayable in serum. The granulosa cells of the ovary secrete inhibin, a peptide hormone composed of an α subunit and one of two β subunits.[27] Its major physiologic function is to inhibit the secretion of follicle-stimulating hormone (FSH) by the anterior pituitary gland.[28] It functions locally by stimulating progesterone production while inhibiting the production of estradiol and serves as a negative regulator of gonadal cell proliferation.[29]

Inhibin is expressed in excessive quantities by granulosa cell tumors. The first report of elevated serum inhibin levels associated with these tumors was published by Lappohn and colleagues[30] in 1989. In their study, four of six patients with granulosa cell tumors had increased levels of inhibin before surgery, and all six had normal levels after surgery; in the two patients with recurrence, increased serum inhibin levels were observed 5 and 20 months before clinical evidence of disease. Similarly, in a prospective evaluation of 27 patients with granulosa cell tumors, Jobling and coworkers[31] demonstrated a sevenfold elevation of inhibin levels before surgery and rising inhibin levels several months before clinical recurrence.

Inhibin has been demonstrated to be a useful tumor marker in granulosa cell tumors, and further studies are needed to delineate the effects of its use on prognosis, morbidity, and mortality.

How should sex cord–stromal tumors be clinically managed?

Surgery remains the cornerstone of treatment for patients with sex cord–ovarian tumors. The diagnosis of these tumors often is not made until surgery, and a correct frozen-section diagnosis can be a challenge even for experienced gynecologic pathologists. Because frozen-section analysis can frequently be inaccurate, a great deal of experience is needed in the operating room to perform the appropriate surgery. Many reports indicate that more than 90% of these neoplasms are unilateral and more than 90% are confined to the ovary.[1,2,10,14,26,32,33] Therefore, a conservative surgical approach with unilateral salpingo-oophorectomy seems to be reasonable for patients who wish to preserve their fertility, given careful staging and the absence of extraovarian spread. In patients with granulosa cell tumors, endometrial curettage must be performed to rule out concomitant endometrial pathology.

If reproductive potential is not an issue, or if advanced-stage disease or bilateral ovarian involvement is present, abdominal hysterectomy and bilateral salpingo-oophorectomy should be performed. In addition, a careful surgical staging should be undertaken. This includes a thorough exploration of the abdominal cavity, washing for cytologic analysis, multiple biopsies, omentectomy, and pelvic and para-aortic lymph node sampling or dissection. Although no scientific evidence exists regarding the efficacy of cytoreduction, an effort should be made to remove metastatic disease.

An understanding of prognostic factors is essential to select those patients who should receive postoperative therapy. However, available information is controversial and incomplete. For granulosa cell tumors, the only prognostic factor that is consistently significant is the stage of disease; patients with advanced disease have been reported to have a poorer survival rate (Table 38-4).[1,4,6,10] Others factors, such as patient age, tumor size, number of mitoses, and, more recently, DNA ploidy and S-phase fraction determined by cytometry, have been reported to be of prognostic importance. There are no data to support any kind of postoperative adjuvant treatment for patients with stage I granulosa cell tumors, given the indolent nature of this neoplasm and the overall good prognosis for these cases. Evans and colleagues[13] reported a 9% risk of recurrence for stage Ia disease. It would appear that patients with stage I disease who receive optimal surgical therapy have a very low risk of recurrence. In Bjorkholm's retrospective series,[3,4] there was no observed benefit for adjuvant irradiation in early-stage disease.

For Sertoli-Leydig cell tumors, stage, histologic differentiation, and, less frequently, mitotic index, the presence of heterologous elements, and tumor rupture appear to have prognostic significance.[26,32,33] Based on this evidence, postoperative adjuvant therapy should be considered for patients with stage I Sertoli-Leydig cell tumors that are poorly differentiated or contain heterologous elements, and for those with advanced disease of any histologic subtype. For patients with adverse prognostic factors, however, the adjuvant treatment of choice remains unknown. Responses to irradiation, chemotherapy, and hormone therapy have been reported.

Is there a role for chemotherapy?

Information concerning chemotherapy for patients with sex cord–ovarian tumors has been limited by the small number of patients in each report, the varying regimens used, and the tendency for late recurrences, which makes it difficult to draw definitive conclusions. Single alkylating agents were used in the past, with 25% partial response reported.[34-37] In recent years, the few available series suggest a possible advantage for multidrug regimens (combinations of actinomycin-D, 5-fluorouracil, and cyclophosphamide or of vincristine, actinomycin-D, and cyclophosphamide), compared with single alkylating agent monotherapy.[35,38] Since the introduction of cisplatin for the treatment of testicular cancer in the late 1970s, platinum-based chemotherapy became the favored choice. Complete responses have been observed in patients treated with doxorubicin-cisplatin regimens[39] or with doxorubicin-cisplatin-cyclophosphamide combinations.[40-42] Gershenson and associates[40] reported an overall response rate of 63% in eight patients with metastatic sex cord–ovarian tumors treated with Platinol, Adriamycin, and cyclophosphamide (PAC). Overall, durable remissions seem to occur in no more than 50% of patients receiving PAC combination.

The highest activity has been demonstrated with the cisplatin-vinblastine-bleomycin (PVB) regimen: in two separate Italian studies[43,44] and in a European Organization of Research and Treatment of Cancer (EORTC) series,[45] response rates ranged from 57% to 92%. In our series, we observed 6 complete and 3 partial responses in 11 untreated recurrent or metastatic granulosa cell tumors; all 6 clinical complete responses were verified by second-look laparotomy. Zambetti and associates[44] administered the same regimen to seven patients with granulosa cell tumors and observed one complete response and three partial responses. In both series, hematologic and nonhematologic toxicities were considerable, with one and two toxic deaths, respectively.

As for the treatment of germ cell tumors, the substitution of etoposide for the vinblastine could produce lower myelosuppression while retaining similar efficacy. Gershenson and colleagues[46] observed an overall response rate of 83% in a series of nine patients with poor-prognosis sex cord–stromal tumors of the ovary treated with bleomycin-etoposide-cisplatin combination therapy (PEB). Toxicity was acceptable; two patients developed mild bleomycin pulmonary toxicity. Of the seven patients with metastatic disease, only one (14%) had a durable remission. Median progression-free survival time was 14 months, and median survival time was 28 months.

In 1999, Homesley and coworkers[47] reported the results of a Gynecologic Oncology Group (GOG) study on the use of the PEB regimen in the treatment of ovarian granulosa cell tumors and other stromal malignancies. This report represented the largest series of sex cord–ovarian tumors treated with chemotherapy. The patient selection included both primary metastatic (stage II through IV) and recurrent disease. Of the 57 evaluable patients, 48 had granulosa cell tumors, 7 had Sertoli-Leydig cell tumors, 1 had a malignant thecoma, and 1 had an unclassified sex cord tumor. The frequency of negative results on second-look laparotomy was the primary end point for this trial. Thirty-seven

Table 38–4. 10-Year Survival Rate of Patients with Granulosa Cell Tumors by International Federation of Gynecology and Obstetrics (FIGO) Stage

Reference	Stage I	Stage II	Stage III
Evans et al[1]	92	—	33
Bjorkholm[3]	96	—	26
Pankratz et al[6]	75	64	17
Stenwig et al[10]	86	61	—

percent (14/38) of the patients undergoing second-look laparotomy had negative findings. With a median follow-up period of 3 years, 11 (69%) of 16 patients in the primary advanced disease category and 21 (51%) of the 41 patients with recurrent disease were progression free. Although this regimen was active, it was associated with severe toxicity, including two bleomycin-related toxic deaths. Moreover, grade 4 granulocytopenia was observed in 60% of patients, despite reduction of the bleomycin total dose in the latter part of the study.

Therefore, although sex cord–stromal ovarian tumors have been shown to respond to platinum-based therapy, toxicity is considerable. Future strategies should include the search for equally active but less toxic combination regimens, particularly with reduction or deletion of the bleomycin dose. Furthermore, there is a need for alternative treatment after PVB/PEB failure. Some promising antitumor activity has been reported with paclitaxel therapy. The use of single-agent paclitaxel resulted in a dramatic response in a patient with recurrent granulosa cell tumor.[48] Currently, a phase II GOG trial is being conducted by the National Cancer Institute using paclitaxel to treat recurrent ovarian stromal tumors (GOG 0187). The combination of paclitaxel and a platinum drug seems to be a reasonable candidate for future trials. To generate high-quality evidence for the efficacy of chemotherapy in ovarian sex cord–stromal tumors, an international cooperative randomized controlled trial will be necessary.

Are there other therapeutic options besides surgery and chemotherapy?

There is no evidence to support the use of adjuvant radiation therapy for sex cord–stromal ovarian tumors. There are two retrospective studies of patients with metastatic or advanced disease that provide evidence in support of a possible benefit with radiotherapy. In the Royal Marsden Hospital experience,[49] 11 of 62 patients with granulosa cell tumors of the ovary received adjuvant pelvic radiotherapy, with no apparent advantage on recurrence rate or overall survival. For patients with inoperable disease, radiotherapy produced a number of long-term remissions, with an overall response rate of 50%. Wolf and coworkers[50] identified 34 patients with ovarian granulosa cell tumors treated with radiation: 20 patients in the adjuvant setting for minimal residual (<1 cm) or microscopic residual disease and 14 patients with clinically measurable disease after either primary surgery or tumor recurrence. Six of these 14 patients achieved a clinical complete response to radiotherapy, with an overall response rate of 43%. Three responders remained alive and without evidence of disease 10 to 21 years after treatment, whereas three patients who responded had relapses 4 to 5 years later. The eight nonresponders had a median survival time of 12.3 months. Recurrent pelvic disease tended to be more likely to respond to radiotherapy. Finally, there are some case reports concerning the use of radiation treatment for isolated liver, bone, and mediastinal recurrences.[51-53] Despite these data, the lack of uniformity in staging and in treatment programs precludes any definitive conclusion. Radiotherapy may represent an alternative strategy to be considered for patients with localized or metastatic granulosa cell tumors not amenable to surgery, because it can potentially control the disease for several years.

Although considerable rationale exists for the use of hormonal therapy in granulosa cell tumors, the clinical experience with this approach is extremely limited. A proportion of these tumors expresses receptors for FSH, and FSH has been shown to support the growth of granulosa tumors in nude mice.[54] Responses to medroxyprogesterone acetate and to gonadotropin-releasing hormone agonists have been reported. Briasoulis and colleagues[55] observed activity of oral megestrol acetate, 160 mg daily, in the treatment of lung recurrence after platinum chemotherapy. Fishman and associates[56] reported a partial response of 40% (2 out 5 evaulable patients) in a small series of patients with refractory or persistent ovarian granulosa cell tumors without major side effects. The clinical evidence for activity of hormonal treatment in the management of these tumors remains scanty and anecdotal. Hormonal therapy should be used in cases of progressive disease that has failed to respond to chemotherapy or radiation therapy.

REFERENCES

1. Evans AT, Gaffey TA, Malkasian GD, et al: Clinicopathologic review of 118 granulosa and 82 theca cells tumors. Obstet Gynecol 1980;55:231.
2. Fox H, Agrawal K, Langley FA: A clinicopathologic study of 92 cases of granulosa-cell tumor of the ovary with special reference to the factors influencing prognosis. Cancer 1975;35:231.
3. Bjorkholm E: Granulosa cell tumors: A comparison of survival in patients and matched controls. Am J Obstet Gynecol 1980;138:329.
4. Bjorkholm E, Silfversward C: Prognostic factors in granulosa-cell tumors. Gynecol Oncol 1981;11:261.
5. Ohel G, Kaneti H, Schenker JG: Granulosa cell tumors in Israel: A study of 172 cases. Gynecol Oncol 1983;15:278.
6. Pankratz E, Boyes DA, White GW, et al: Granulosa cell tumors: A clinical review of 61 cases. Obstet Gynecol 1978;52:718.
7. Schweppe KW, Beller FK: Clinical data of granulosa cell tumors. J Cancer Res Clin Oncol 1982;104:161.
8. Malmstrom H, Hogberg T, Risberg B, et al: Granulosa cell tumor of the ovary: Prognostic factors and outcome. Gynecol Oncol 1994;52:50.
9. Gusberg SB, Kardon P: Proliferative endometrial response to theca-granulosa cell tumors. Am J Obstet Gynecol 1971;111:633.
10. Stenwig JT, Hazekamp JT, Beecham JB: Granulosa cell tumors of the ovary: A clinico-pathological study of 118 cases with long-term follow up. Gynecol Oncol 1979;7:136.
11. Bridgewater JA, Rustom GJS: Management of non-ephithelial ovarian tumors. Oncology 1999;57:89.
12. Piura B, Nemet D, Yanai-Inbar I, et al: Granulosa-cell tumor of the ovary: A study of 18 cases. J Surg Oncol 1994;55:71.
13. Evans AT, Gaffey TA, Malkasian GD, et al: DNA ploidy of ovarian granulosa cell tumors. Cancer 1995;75:2295.
14. Young RH, Dickersin GR, Scully RE: Juvenile granulosa cell tumor of the ovary: A clinicopathological analysis of 125 cases. Am J Surg Pathol 1984;8:575.
15. Takeuchi H, Hamada H, Sodemoto Y, et al: Juvenile granulosa cell tumor with rapid distant metastases. Acta Pathol Jap 1983;33:537.

16. Tamini HK, Bolen J: Enchondromatosis (Ollier's disease) and ovarian juvenile granulosa cell tumor. Cancer 1984;53:1605.

17. Vaz RM, Turner CH: Ollier's disease (enchondromatosis) associated with ovarian juvenile granulosa cell tumor and precocious pseudopuberty. J Paediat 1986;108:945.

18. Velasco-Oses A, Alonso-Alvaro A, Blanco-Pozo A, et al: Ollier's disease associated with ovarian juvenile granulosa cell tumor. Cancer 1988;62:222.

19. Tanaka Y, Sasaki Y, Nishihira H, et al: Ovarian juvenile granulosa-cell tumor associated with Maffucci's syndrome. Am J Clin Pathol 1992;97:523.

20. Zaloudek C, Norris HJ: Granulosa tumors of the ovary in children: A clinical and pathologic study of 32 cases. Am J Surg Pathol 1982;6:503.

21. Plantaz D, Flamant F, Vassal G, et al: Tumeurs de la granulosa de l'ovaire chez l'enfant et l'adolescente. Arch Fr Pediatr 1992;49:793.

22. Lack EE, Perez-Atayde AR, Murthy ASK, et al: Granulosa theca cell tumors in premenarchal girls: A clinical and pathologic study of 10 cases. Cancer 1981;48:1846.

23. Vassal G, Flamant F, Caillaud JM, et al: Juvenile granulosa-cell tumor of the ovary in children: A clinical study of 15 cases. J Clin Oncol 1988;6:990.

24. Scully RE: Tumors of the ovary and maldeveloped gonads. In Atlas of Tumor Pathology. Washington, DC, 1979.

25. Slayton RE: Management of germ cell and stromal tumors of the ovary. Semin Oncol 1984;11:299.

26. Young RH, Scully RE: Ovarian Sertoli-Leydig cell tumors: A clinicopathological analysis of 207 cases. Am J Surg Pathol 1985;9:543.

27. Burger HG: Inhibin. Reprod Med Rev 1992;1:1.

28. Ying S: Inhibins, activins, and follistatins: Gonadal proteins modulating the secretion of follicle-stimulating hormone. Endoc Rev 1988;9:267.

29. Matzuk MM, Finegold MJ, Su JJ, et al: Alpha inhibin is a tumor suppressor gene with gonadal specificity in mice. Nature 1992;360:313.

30. Lappohn RE, Burger HG, Bouma J, et al: Inhibin as a marker for granulosa-cell tumors. N Engl J Med 1989;321:790.

31. Jobling T, Mamers P, Healy DL, et al: A prospective study of inhibin in granulosa cell tumors of the ovary. Gynecol Oncol 1994;55:285.

32. Roth LM, Anderson MC, Govan ADT, et al: Sertoli-Leydig cell tumors: A clinicopathologic study of 34 cases. Cancer 1981;48:187.

33. Zaloudek C, Norris HJ: Sertoli-Leydig tumors of the ovary: A clinicopathologic study of 64 intermediate and poorly differentiated neoplasms. Am J Surg Pathol 1984;8:405-418.

34. Malkasian JD Jr, Webb MJ, Jorgensen EO: Observations on chemotherapy of granulosa cell carcinomas and malignant ovarian teratomas. Obstet Gynecol 1974;44:885.

35. Schwartz PE, Smith JP: Treatment of ovarian stromal tumors. Am J Obstet Gynecol 1976;125:402.

36. Lusch CJ, Mercurio TM, Runyeon WK: Delayed recurrence and chemotherapy of a granulosa cell tumor. Obstet Gynecol 1978;51:505.

37. Smith JP, Rutledge F: Chemotherapy in the treatment of cancer of the ovary. Am J Obstet Gynecol 1970;107:692.

38. Tavassoli FA, Norris HJ: Sertoli tumors of the ovary: A clinico-pathologic study of 28 cases with ultrastructural observations. Cancer 1980;46:2281.

39. Jacobs HJ, Deppe G, Cohen CJ: Combination chemotherapy of ovarian granulosa cell tumor with cisplatinum and doxorubicin. Gynecol Oncol 1982;14:294.

40. Gershenson DM, Copeland LJ, Kavanagh JJ, et al: Treatment of metastatic stromal tumors of the ovary with cisplatin, doxorubicin and cyclophosphamide. Obstet Gynecol 1987;70:765.

41. Canlibel F, Caputo TA: Chemotherapy of granulosa cell tumors. Am J Obstet Gynecol 1983;154:763.

42. Pectasides D, Alevizakos N, Athanassiou AE: Cisplatin-containing regimen in advanced or recurrent granulosa cell tumors of the ovary. Ann Oncol 1984;3:316.

43. Colombo N, Sessa C, Landoni F, et al: Cisplatin, vinblastine, and bleomycin combination chemotherapy in metastatic granulosa cell tumor of the ovary. Obstet Gynecol 1986;67:265.

44. Zambetti M, Escobedo A, Pilotti S, et al: Cisplatinum/vinblastine/bleomycin combination chemotherapy in advanced or recurrent granulosa cell tumors of the ovary. Gynecol Oncol 1990;36:317.

45. Pecorelli S, Wagenaar HC, Vergote IB, et al: Cisplatin, vinblastine, and bleomycin combination chemotherapy in recurrent or advanced granulosa cell tumor of the ovary: An EORTC Gynecologic Cancer Cooperative Group study. Eur J Cancer 1999;35:1331.

46. Gershenson DM, Morris M, Burke TW, et al: Treatment of poor-prognosis sex cord–stromal tumors of the ovary with the combination of bleomycin, etoposide and cisplatin. Obstet Gynecol 1996;87:527.

47. Homesley HD, Bundy BN, Hurteau JA, et al: Bleomycin, etoposide and cisplatin combination therapy of ovarian granulosa cell tumors and other stromal malignancies: A Gynecologic Oncology Group study. Gynecol Oncol 1999;72:131.

48. Tresukosol D, Kudelka AP, Edwards CL, et al: Recurrent ovarian granulosa cell tumor: A case report of a dramatic response to Taxol. Int J Gynecol Cancer 1995;5:156.

49. Savage P, Constenla D, Fisher C, et al: Granulosa cell tumours of the ovary: Demographics, survival and the management of advanced disease. Clin Oncol 1998;10:242.

50. Wolf JK, Mullen J, Eifel PJ, et al: Radiation treatment of advanced or recurrent granulosa cell tumor of the ovary. Clin Oncol 1999;73:35.

51. Kumar PP, Good RR, Linder J: Complete response of granulosa cell tumor metastatic to liver after hepatic irradiation: A case report. Obstet Gynecol 1986;67(3 Suppl):95S.

52. Dubuc-Lissoir J, Berthiaume MJ, Boubez G, et al: Bone metestasis from granulosa cell tumor of the ovary. Gynecol Oncol 2001;83:400.

53. Wue-Lee I, Levin W, Chapman W, et al: Radiotherapy for the treatment of metastatic granulosa cell tumor in the mediastinum: A case report. Gynecol Oncol 1999;73:455.

54. Davy M, Torjesen PA, Aakaag A: Demonstration of the FSH receptor in a functioning granulosa cell tumor. Acta Endocrinol (copenh) 1977;8:615.

55. Briasoulis E, Karavasilis V, Pavlidis N: Megestrol activity in recurrent adult type granulosa cell tumour of the ovary. Ann Oncol 1997;8:811.

56. Fishman A, Kudelka AP, Tresukosol D, et al: Leuprolide acetate for treating refractory or persistent ovarian granulosa cell tumor. J Reprod Med 1996;41:393.

57. Norris HJ, Taylor HB: Prognosis of giranulosa-theca tumors of the ovary. Cancer 1968;21:255.

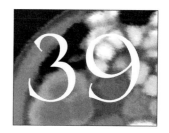

OVARIAN SARCOMAS

Gavin C. E. Stuart   and   Lesa M. Dawson

 MAJOR CONTROVERSIES

- **What are ovarian sarcomas?**
- **How are ovarian sarcomas classified?**
- **Does the available evidence support a histogenesis from a common stem cell population for ovarian sarcomas?**
- **Is the clinical behavior of ovarian sarcomas more aligned with that of other soft tissue sarcomas or that of the more common epithelial ovarian cancers?**
- **Is there a role for fertility-sparing therapy in younger patients with ovarian sarcomas?**
- **What is the optimal postoperative or adjuvant therapy for women with ovarian sarcomas?**

What are ovarian sarcomas?

Primary ovarian sarcomas are rare tumors that in general have a poor prognosis. As a result of their uncommon occurrence, the available evidence to support care of women with these tumors is limited and generally is based on small series and anecdotal case reports. The lack of level I evidence provides the oncologist with challenges for understanding the disease process and recommending appropriate therapy.

Ovarian sarcomas account for approximately 1% to 2% of all ovarian cancers and only 10% of all female genital tract sarcomas.[1] Overall, this diagnosis comprises only 0.1% to 0.3% of all gynecologic malignancies. These tumors may show a single tissue type (pure tumors) or a composite of more than one tissue type (mixed tumors). The pattern may reflect tissue native to the ovary, as in homologous tumors, or tissue not usually found in the ovary, as in heterologous tumors. The most common histologic type is the malignant mixed mesodermal tumor of the ovary, which accounts for the majority of tumors in this category. Less commonly seen are leiomyosarcomas, fibrosarcomas, angiosarcomas, and rhabdomyosarcomas. Ovarian sarcomas have been reported to affect women from the first to the tenth decade of life. Accurate diagnosis and reporting of these rare tumors is essential.

They manifest in a manner similar to epithelial ovarian cancers but tend to have a much poorer prognosis. Surgical management is most common, but there is little evidence or consensus regarding adjuvant therapy or treatment of advanced or metastatic disease. Frequently, management recommendations are extrapolated from experience with other, more common sarcoma types in the adult population.

PATHOLOGY AND PATHOGENESIS

How are ovarian sarcomas classified?

Classification. The subdivision of ovarian sarcomas based on pathologic descriptions can be complex. Historically, authors divided these tumors into subsets of homologous and heterologous types in which the key distinction was the presence of tissues that were not native to the ovary. The heterologous tumors contain unusual components such as chondrosarcoma, rhabdomyosarcoma, liposarcoma, or osteosarcoma. Homologous tumors, in contrast, contained sarcomatous elements of tissue ordinarily found in the ovary, such as angiosarcoma, fibrosarcoma, or leiomyosarcoma.[2]

Another approach to classification of ovarian sarcoma places a division according to the complexity of the lesion. Pure lesions, which contain only one identified tissue type, most commonly include pure leiomyosarcoma, rhabdomyosarcoma, or fibrosarcoma. Pure lesions are quite rare, with fewer than 50 cases reported in the literature for all types combined. Mixed lesions contain more than one type of sarcomatous element or, more frequently, an epithelial malignant component. Classically, the term *carcinosarcoma* was used to describe the subtype with both malignant epithelial (carcinomatous) and mesodermal (sarcomatous) elements when these were all of a homologous type. *Mixed mesodermal tumors* are also mixed tumors, but they were believed to specifically include those tumors with some non-native (heterologous) sarcomatous element. The term *mixed mullerian tumors* has been used in this context but does not distinguish between heterologous and homologous tissues. However, the preferred term for those tumors with both carcinomatous and sarcomatous elements, regardless of their homologous or heterologous nature, is *malignant mixed mesodermal tumors* (MMMT).

Pathology. Grossly, sarcomas of the ovary have a consistent appearance of a pale, tan, solid and cystic tumor with areas of hemorrhage (Fig. 39-1). The size at surgery is variable, but the median diameter has been reported as 6 to 12.5 cm. Leiomyosarcomas may be considerably larger than other sarcomas. Bilaterality is rare. As noted later, most women present with disease beyond the ovary, developing multiple intra-abdominal sites of disease, which may retain gross characteristics similar to those of the primary tumor.

Leiomyosarcoma. Leiomyosarcomas (Fig. 39-2) typically demonstrate spindle cells with cigar- or tobacco-shaped, rounded nuclei. They may be distinguished from their benign counterpart by the presence of nuclear and cytologic pleomorphism and by higher mitotic counts. In general, two or more mitotic figures per 10 high-power fields are required for the diagnosis of leiomyosarcoma.[3] They are not believed to arise from

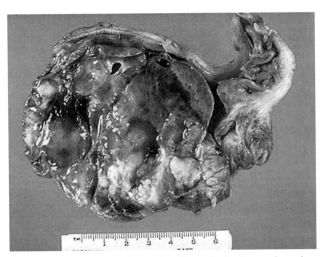

Figure 39-1. Gross specimen of malignant mixed mesodermal tumor of the ovary.

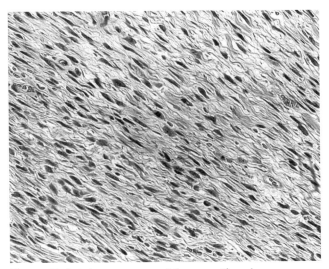

Figure 39-2. Leiomyosarcoma of the ovary. There is a proliferation of mildly atypical spindle cells. A mitosis is present in the center of the proliferation. (Hematoxylin and eosin stain, ×400.)

pre-existing leiomyomas; rather, they seem to develop spontaneously. Inoue and colleagues[3] reported that the tissue of origin may be the vessel wall in the ovarian parenchyma or smooth muscle around follicles or corpus lutea. Other possible origins include smooth muscle in the ovarian ligament as it attaches to the ovary or in the residual Wolffian duct. Immunohistochemistry patterns suggest that leiomyosarcomas will stain positively for actin and desmin, consistent with leiomyosarcomas from other sites.[4]

Angiosarcoma. A highly vascular and often hemorrhagic-appearing tumor, pure angiosarcoma is uncommonly seen. Histologically, angiosarcoma demonstrates anastomosing vascular channels with frequent slitlike vascular spaces that may be filled with red cells.[5] The lining endothelial cells have an atypical appearance, with mitotic activity and abnormal nuclei. Spindle-shaped cells may be seen.[6] The more common benign ovarian hemangiomas are distinguished by the absence of cytologic atypia and mitotic figures.[7] Immunohistochemistry may reveal positivity for CD31 and CD34 or, less commonly, factor VIII–related antibody.[8,9] This profile suggests a vascular endothelial origin. Other tumors that are potentially confused in the pathologic diagnosis include yolk sac tumor, choriocarcinoma, and metastatic melanoma.[10] Angiosarcoma is confirmed with the staining pattern described earlier.

Fibrosarcoma. Fibrosarcomas are solid, pale, yellow-white tumors that are histologically similar to those described in other sites. They are frequently larger than other sarcomas of the ovary, with a median size of 17 cm.[11] The key issue in the pathologic review of fibrosarcoma is the distinction between this lesion and benign cellular fibroma.[12] The marked atypia of fibrosarcoma and the presence of more than four mitotic figures per 10 high-power fields often distinguishes them. Specifically, in a fibrosarcoma, a "herringbone" pattern of cells is often described, and staining is noted by vimentin positivity. Cytogenetic analysis has shown imbalance in chromosome 12, a finding consistent with the known location of several sarcoma-linked oncogenes.[13-15] Cytogenetic analysis using comparative genomic hybridization (CGH) may further characterize these specific tumors. In 2002, Krüger[13] proposed that fibrosarcomas may develop as a result of malignant change within ovarian fibromas, rather than occurring as malignant tumors de novo.

Rhabdomyosarcoma. Grossly, rhabdomyosarcomas are also large tumors, at more than 10 cm. These pure sarcomas may have a solid fleshy or hemorrhagic appearance and may be characterized histologically by either an alveolar or an embryonal pattern.[16,17] The first type is notable for round or spindle-shaped cells with eosinophilic cytoplasm. Cross-striations and "strap" cells may be observed. The embryonal type demonstrates paler cytoplasm and visible nucleoli. Both types stain for actin, desmin, and, most specific to rhabdomyosarcoma, myoglobin.

Rarer types. Pure chondrosarcoma and osteosarcoma of the ovary are extremely rare, with only one or two documented cases known worldwide.[18] These tissue types are more likely to be seen within a mixed tumor. If a primary ovarian tumor is suspected, consideration should first be given to a metastatic lesion from a primary site elsewhere.[19]

Malignant mixed mesodermal tumor. MMMTs comprise two distinct cell types, one epithelial and the other stromal. The epithelial component manifests as a carcinoma and the stromal component as a sarcoma. This mixed tumor is by far the most common manifestation of sarcoma in the ovary. With several hundred cases reported, these tumors are better studied than the pure sarcomas. In 1984, Morrow and coworkers[20] published a series of 30 patients with a diagnosis of MMMT that characterized the tumor well. The carcinomatous component is most often endometrioid, clear cell, or papillary serous, and the sarcoma may demonstrate any of the previously described subtypes (Fig. 39-3). Clinical outcome is linked with the sarcomatous rather than the carcinomatous element. Metastases, however, may demonstrate either pattern.

Metastatic sarcoma. Sarcoma from other primary sites may metastasize to the ovary. Although most of these metastases are from a uterine primary, other sarcomas arising from stomach, small intestine, or bone have been reported to have metastasized to the ovary. Pathologically, the biggest challenge in diagnosis is the distinction between the metastatic endometrial stromal sarcoma and other ovarian primaries, particularly sex cord–stromal tumors. In a review of 21 metastatic lesions, Young and Scully[21] recommended that they may be distinguished from primary lesions by the presence of extraovarian disease, bilaterality, and the characteristic content of small arteries resembling the spiral arteries of late secretory endometrium.

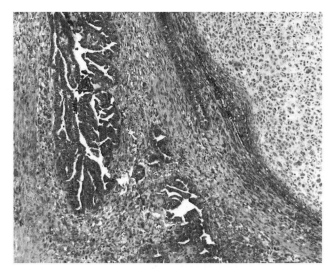

Figure 39–3. Mixed mesodermal tumor of the ovary. On the left side of the picture is an adenocarcinoma formed of irregular glands lined by a malignant tall columnar stratified epithelium. On the right side is a nodule of chondrosarcoma formed of irregular nuclei in lacunae and an acellular matrix. (Hematoxylin and eosin stain, ×200.)

Sarcoma arising from teratoma. Multiple cases of sarcoma, either pure or mixed, arising within a teratoma of the ovary have been described. These represent any of the possible sarcomatous subtypes and are not believed to behave clinically any differently than primary ovarian sarcomas. However, teratomatous transformation may occur at a younger age. Krüger and colleagues[13] reported a pure fibrosarcoma arising in a benign cystic teratoma in a 32-year-old woman. Cases of teratomas with osteosarcoma, leiomyosarcoma, and mixed epithelial/sarcomatous elements have been described.

Pathogenesis. The possibility that radiation plays a role in the pathogenesis of pelvic sarcoma has long been debated. Wei and coworkers[22] reported a case of carcinosarcoma of the ovary that occurred after remote radiotherapy for carcinoma of the cervix. Several case series[23-25] of 20 or more patients with presumed radiation-induced sarcoma have each reported that the median time to development of a sarcoma was 13 years. The lesions described included both soft tissue and extremity sarcomas, particularly osteosarcomas. Wiklund and colleagues[23] reported that the soft tissue types included malignant fibrous histiocytoma and fibrosarcoma. The doses required to consider a causal association ranged from 1600 to 11,000 cGy, with a median of 3500 to 4000 cGy. The secondary tumors were more likely to be of higher grade. Monk and colleagues[24] in 1993, and O'Sullivan and associates[25] in 1998, each reported a case of primary ovarian sarcoma in 12-year-old premenarchal girls. Both patients had previously received pelvic radiotherapy as a component of treatment for a primary medulloblastoma. The similarity of the cases raises the hypothesis of a possible pathogenetic link between the radiotherapy and the sarcoma or perhaps some shared genetic link between medulloblastoma and ovarian sarcoma.

Epithelial ovarian cancer has an increased incidence among women with a genetic predisposition because of *BRCA1/2* mutations. Likewise, those with hereditary nonpolyposis colorectal cancer (HNPCC) mutations also demonstrate higher incidence rates of epithelial cancer. Ovarian sarcoma has not yet been linked to known or suspected mutations. Other hereditary conditions associated with a predisposition to development of sarcomas include neurofibromatosis, retinoblastoma, and Li-Fraumeni syndrome, but these have not demonstrated higher rates of sarcoma arising in the ovary. The rarity of the syndromes themselves, as well as ovarian sarcoma, generally makes these types of connections difficult to study.

Does the available evidence support a histogenesis from a common stem cell population for ovarian sarcomas?

Three hypotheses have been put forward to explain the pathogenesis of ovarian sarcomas. Most of the literature refers to MMMTs or carcinosarcomas because of the relatively greater frequency of these types than the other pure sarcomas. The "collision theory" suggests that these lesions result from the growth of synchronous tumors that derive from separate cell lines and blend together to form their characteristic histologic appearance. The "composition theory" submits that the sarcomatous component represents a nonmalignant reactive process in the stroma in association with a primary carcinoma. The "combination theory" represents the currently held view that these tumors derive from a monoclonal stem cell line with varied phenotypic expression. This last theory has been supported by molecular genetic evidence. Wada and colleagues[26] reported that the patterns of chromosome X activation, K-ras sequence, and P53 expression were similar in both the carcinomatous and the sarcomatous elements of carcinosarcomas. Likewise, Ariyoshi and associates[27] demonstrated similar immunoreactivity for P53 protein in both components of carcinosarcoma tumors.[27] A recent paper by Sonada and coworkers[28] reported a single patient with a *BRCA2* mutation and an ovarian carcinosarcoma in whom they were able to show clonal loss of the wild-type *BRCA2* allele in both histologic elements of the ovarian tumor. This clonal loss is consistent with an etiologic role of *BRCA2* in the carcinogenic process. In this same patient, the same somatic mutation of *TP53* was displayed in both components of the tumor. Although these findings are not definitive, there would appear to be an increasing amount of evidence to support the combination theory, with origin of most MMMTs and carcinosarcomas from a single cell clone.

Clinical-pathologic factors. No specific histologic factors that correlate with prognosis in ovarian sarcoma have been identified. A key issue appears to be whether the presence or absence of heterologous elements in an MMMT has a prognostic relation to clinical outcome. Sood and associates[29] reported

significantly worse survival for those MMMT patients whose tumors contain heterologous elements. This opinion was echoed in a series of 31 cases published by Barakat and colleagues.[30] Muntz and colleagues,[31] however, suggested that this factor had no prognostic significance. Although it appears that homologous tumors may be associated with a more favorable prognosis, this specific question requires further study before being considered as a definitive prognostic factor.

The overexpression of P53 is commonly linked to poorer outcomes in many human cancers. Again, the literature regarding sarcomas is conflicting. In a series of 30 patients with MMMT, Ariyoshi and associates[27] found that only stage carried prognostic significance. Mitotic count, P53 expression, immunoreactivity for Ki67, the presence of heterologous components, and residual tumor were not significant in univariate analysis. Among 37 patients in Britain, Chang and coworkers[32] noted that 70% presented with advanced disease, and again only stage was correlated with outcome. Histology, the distinction between heterologous and homologous types, grade, type, and percentage of the epithelial component had no significant impact on survival. Overall, most authors would concur that stage at the time of diagnosis is the single most significant factor correlating with outcome.

Rasmussen and coworkers[33] reported a case of prolonged survival despite the diagnosis of stage IIIc pure leiomyosarcoma. This tumor demonstrated a relatively low mitotic rate, suggesting that this factor may have contributed to the outcome. The correlation of a high mitotic count with a poorer outcome is often associated most specifically with leiomyosarcoma.[34,35]

CLINICAL FEATURES AND DIAGNOSIS

Is the clinical behavior of ovarian sarcomas more aligned with that of other soft tissue sarcomas or that of the more common epithelial ovarian cancers?

Presentation. The diagnosis of MMMT typically is made only by the pathologist at the time of surgical removal. Preoperative identification is unlikely, because the clinical presentation is indistinguishable from that of epithelial ovarian cancer. The great proportion of patients present with symptoms of abdominal pain or bloating and clinical findings of distention with a pelvic mass. Prendiville and associates[36] reported that symptoms preceded diagnosis by a mean of 3.2 months. This is a relatively short period of symptoms or signs, consistent with an aggressive biologic behavior. Ascites may be noted. Most patients are postmenopausal, with a median age of 59 years. However, this median age at onset in the sixth decade should not deter the clinician from considering this diagnosis in both younger and older cohorts of women, because ovarian sarcomas may be detected in the first or in the tenth decade of life.

No tumor marker is known to be specific for ovarian sarcoma. It is appropriate to obtain a baseline CA 125 serum level before surgery, as in any woman with an adnexal mass suspicious for malignancy. Sood and colleagues[29] suggested that the preoperative CA 125 level may be a prognostic variable, with levels lower than 75 U/mL being associated with a survival advantage. However, an elevated preoperative level may be an excellent marker of treatment response after surgery and adjuvant therapy.

The staging of ovarian sarcomas uses the same criteria as were proposed by the International Federation of Obstetrics and Gynecology (FIGO) for epithelial ovarian cancer.[37] There is no distinction as a result of the sarcoma diagnosis. Notwithstanding the importance of accurate recording of the FIGO stage, the clinically relevant issue is whether the tumor is confined to the ovary or extends beyond it at the time of diagnosis. Given the propensity of these cancers to metastasize, it not surprising that most women are found to have disease outside the ovary. In a series of 47 patients, 41 (87%) had stage III or IV disease at diagnosis.[29] Most authors would concur that fewer than 10% of women with ovarian sarcomas present with disease clinically and surgically confined to the ovary.

Diagnostic imaging has been used in the same manner as for most women with an undiagnosed pelvic mass. Although careful clinical examination and assessment is a prerequisite to accurate diagnosis, ultrasonography and computed tomography may be useful in the identification of extraovarian disease and metastases. Several reports have attempted to define the role of magnetic resonance imaging in the diagnosis of ovarian sarcomas. Wang and colleagues[38] suggested that an MMMT of the ovary may be identified as a heterogeneous mass with solid and cystic components. The solid areas show a relatively high signal intensity and only slight enhancement after contrast injection. However, Saito and colleagues[39] suggested that only when there are specific chondromatous elements will a specific pattern for ovarian sarcomas be suspected. There may be a role for magnetic resonance imaging in defining the response to systemic therapy, as recommended by Kaji and associates.[40]

The pattern of presentation of ovarian sarcomas is quite different from that of other soft tissue sarcomas. There has been frequent debate in the literature as to whether the group of pelvic sarcomas collectively represent a unique subset of those tumors considered as soft tissue sarcomas elsewhere. Most studies have classified uterine and other mullerian tract tumors separately from those arising in extremities, the trunk, or the head and neck area. The proportion of patients presenting with advanced-stage disease is much greater among those women with ovarian sarcoma than among those with other soft tissue sarcomas. This may be affected by a detection bias, because early identification of ovarian pathology is prohibited by both the lack of early symptoms and the lack of effective screening techniques. Biologically, pelvic sarcomas and specifically ovarian sarcomas, should be considered separately.

TREATMENT

Most women who present with ovarian sarcomas have an undiagnosed pelvic or abdominal mass and require a laparotomy for diagnosis and possible treatment. As such, surgical excision of the tumor is the first principle of therapy. Most authors would agree that in the circumstance of histologically proven sarcoma confined to the ovary, the appropriate minimal surgery is a total abdominal hysterectomy and bilateral salpingo-oophorectomy. Some authors have recommended that surgery alone may be appropriate even for recurrent disease without adjuvant therapy. This approach was reported with good outcome in a patient with leiomyosarcoma.[41] There is no evidence to support routine extended surgical staging in patients with disease apparently confined to the ovary, although a careful laparotomy with palpation of the peritoneal surfaces and node-bearing areas should be done. Peritoneal washings for cytology should be obtained, because there have been case reports of documentation of extraovarian disease by this technique.[42] Given that most patients present with clinical evidence of disease beyond the ovary, it is not likely that further evidence will be forthcoming regarding the role of surgical staging in women with stage I tumors.

The role of cytoreductive surgery for women with ovarian sarcomas extending beyond the ovary is not clear. Although most reports in the literature would agree that the FIGO stage at the time of diagnosis can be best correlated with prognosis, it is not clear whether surgical resection of advanced disease improves outcomes. Sood and colleagues[29] reviewed 47 women with a diagnosis of ovarian sarcoma and assessed the role of surgical cytoreduction. In a multivariate analysis, they reported that optimal surgical cytoreduction was the most significant prognostic variable (Fig. 39-4). This applied even to those women

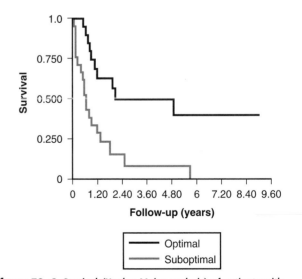

Figure 39-4. Survival (Kaplan-Meier analysis) of patients with advanced-stage (stage III/IV) ovarian sarcoma based on surgical cytoreduction. (Adapted from Sood AK, Sorosky JI, Gelder MS, et al: Primary ovarian sarcoma: Analysis of prognostic variables and the role of surgical cytoreduction. Cancer 1998;82:1736.)

with advanced disease. The 5-year survival rates in their series were 45% for those with optimal cytoreduction and 8% for those with suboptimal cytoreduction. It should be noted, however, that this benefit was achieved with significant surgical morbidity, including long average surgical times (mean, 219 minutes) and with an average blood loss of 1260 mL. This report contrasts with previous reviews by Plaxe[43] and Barakat[30] and their colleagues, who reported no survival advantage for performing optimal cytoreduction. A more recent review by Duska and associates[44] of 28 patients treated with surgery and combination chemotherapy reported that time to recurrence was increased in a statistically significant manner but that overall survival time was not affected by optimal cytoreduction. Furthermore, it is not possible to determine whether the ability to achieve optimal cytoreduction reflects the surgical procedure or the inherent biology (resectability) of the tumor. Regardless of whether optimal cytoreduction is desirable, the question of feasibility is raised. Le and coworkers[45] reported in a series of patients with MMMT of the ovary, stages III/IV, that 22 of 31 patients were left with macroscopic residual despite maximal surgical debulking effort. Other authors have reported similar rates (53%) of optimal surgery in the same population.[29] Despite the conflicting evidence regarding this issue, it seems prudent to attempt optimal cytoreduction whenever possible.

Is there a role for fertility-sparing therapy in younger patients with ovarian sarcomas?

Ovarian sarcomas may manifest in women of childbearing age who remain desirous of fertility. There have been several reports of surgery that preserves the uterus and contralateral ovary, with or without postoperative therapy, with a good long-term outcome. Krüger and associates[13] reported on a 32-year-old woman treated with unilateral salpingo-oophorectomy alone for an ovarian fibrosarcoma who had no evidence of recurrence after 12 months. Fowler and colleagues[46] reported on a 19-year-old woman diagnosed with stage III MMMT of the ovary who underwent a unilateral salpingo-oophorectomy and postoperative chemotherapy with VP-16, cisplatin, and ifosfamide with mesna. She remained free of recurrence at 60 months of follow-up. These case reports suggest that there may be role for fertility-sparing therapy in women with ovarian sarcoma, but such an approach should be considered only after the overall poor prognosis for this group of women is reviewed and well-informed consent is obtained from the patient.

What is the optimal postoperative or adjuvant therapy for women with ovarian sarcomas?

For women with ovarian sarcomas clinically and histologically confined to the ovary (stage I), many authors recommend surgical excision without adjuvant

therapy,[47] based in large part on the lack of evidence of improved outcomes with a more aggressive approach. Other authors reflect on the observed poor outcome in the majority of women with stage II, III, and IV disease and intuitively recommend aggressive treatment of early-stage disease. In any case, effective adjuvant therapy for women with early-stage disease is likely to be guided by identification of the optimal postoperative regimen for women with advanced disease.

The use of systemic therapy after surgical cytoreduction has undergone an evolution over the past 3 decades. Initial postoperative therapy options have included the use of Alkeran (melphalan), hexamethylmelamine, pelvic irradiation with or without abdominal irradiation, and a regimen combining vincristine, dactinomycin, and cyclophosphamide (VAC).[20,48] Although in the report of Morrow's group[20] the recommended Gynecologic Oncology Group (GOG) regimen was a combination of VAC chemotherapy and whole-abdomen radiation therapy, this was not used for all patients in their series. In 1983, Carlson and colleagues[49] reported the MD Anderson Hospital and Tumor Institute experience using this regimen, including a 17% salvage rate. It was apparent however, that this regimen was not associated with long-term benefit for the majority of patients. Subsequently, multiple authors reported use of the combination of cisplatin and Adriamycin (doxorubicin) with improved outcomes. In 1990, Plaxe and colleagues[43] reported on 15 patients treated with this postoperative regimen and demonstrated a median survival time of 16 months. Of the evaluable patients in their series, 85% responded. In a group of 28 women with MMMT of the ovary, Le and associates[45] reported a 3-year survival rate of 35% using a regimen of doxorubicin (50 mg/m^2) and cisplatin (50 mg/m^2) for a maximum of nine cycles. In 1995, Muntz and colleagues[31] reported that the use of cisplatin-based chemotherapy with or without doxorubicin was associated with symptomatic improvement and prolongation of the progression-free interval. Therefore, platinum-based combination therapy appeared to offer an improvement over VAC with or without radiation therapy for the postoperative treatment of women with ovarian sarcomas.

The GOG evaluated the role of ifosfamide and mesna in a phase II trial comprising 32 women with a diagnosis of MMMT of the ovary.[50] A total response rate of 17.6% was reported, suggesting that this regimen had activity. Grade 3 and grade 4 neutropenia was noted in 19.4% and 16.1% of the patients, respectively, showing that the toxicity of the regimen was not insignificant. Ifosfamide has also been combined with cisplatin in a small series of women with MMMT of the ovary.[51] Although this regimen showed activity, 25% of the patients developed significant renal toxicities. The addition of dacarbazine (DTIC) was reported by Baker and coworkers[52] in 1991 in women with both uterine and ovarian MMMTs. This regimen included cisplatin (15 mg/m^2 four times daily for 4 days), DTIC (200 mg four times daily for 4 days), and Adriamycin (20 mg/m^2 on days 1 and 2). This regimen (PAD) was repeated every 28 days and showed a response rate of

40% among the 11 patients with ovarian tumors. Another combination regimen of mesna, doxorubicin, ifosfamide, and DTIC (MAID protocol) was demonstrated to have activity in a patient who had progression after treatment with single-agent cisplatin.[53]

More recent publications have extrapolated the benefit of a cisplatin and paclitaxel regimen among women with advanced epithelial ovarian carcinoma to the population of women with ovarian sarcomas.[54] Sood and associates[29] reported a survival advantage for the inclusion of cisplatin, compared with non–platinum-based regimens (Fig. 39-5). The response rate of 80% among the 27 patients who received platinum combinations was significantly better than that of 12% among the 11 patients who did not. In 2002, Duska and associates[44] reported on a series of 28 women with MMMT of the ovary treated with cytoreductive surgery and combination cisplatin and paclitaxel chemotherapy postoperatively. The regimen included paclitaxel 175 mg/m^2 given over 3 hours and carboplatin administered with an area under the curve of 5. A total response rate of 72% was shown. Grade 3 and 4 toxicities were acceptable, and the treatment was well tolerated as an outpatient regimen. At present, in the balance of efficacy, toxicity, and impact on quality of life, it appears that optimal postoperative or adjuvant treatment for women with ovarian sarcomas is a carboplatin/paclitaxel–based regimen for a minimum of six cycles in dosages as described by Duska and colleagues.[44]

If the available data on the use of chemotherapy for ovarian sarcomas are contrasted with what is known about other soft tissue sarcomas, a difference in the roles of Adriamycin and platinum is noted. As a single agent, Adriamycin has demonstrated the highest activity level, with response rates of 25% to 27%, in the setting of advanced nongynecologic disease. This drug remains very much the central agent in the treatment of these aggressive cancers, although admittedly with unsatisfactory response rates. Cisplatin, in contrast, has demonstrated much less activity at other sites when compared with its utility in the treatment of ovarian sarcoma. This contradiction underscores the importance of clinical trials designed to answer questions for individual disease sites.

Radiation therapy has been reported anecdotally to be of benefit either alone or with combination chemotherapy.[20,49] To date, response rates for women with macroscopic disease treated with radiation therapy have not been comparable to those for similar women receiving combination chemotherapy postoperatively. For those women with no evidence of disease remaining postoperatively, radiation therapy has not been shown to improve survival, even for women with sarcomas of the uterus. There are no prospective data for women with sarcomas of the ovary. The greatest value for external beam radiation therapy may be in palliative relief of symptoms or control of local pelvic recurrences in women with a diagnosis of ovarian sarcoma.

PROGNOSIS

Sarcoma of the ovary has a consistently poor clinical outcome, with long-term survival after advanced disease being virtually unknown. In the larger case series, mean survival times reported are typically less than 2 years despite aggressive chemotherapy. Chang and associates[32] reported a median survival time of 247 days in 37 patients. Among 36 women with MMMT diagnosed in Sweden between 1975 and 1995, the median survival time was 16 months.[55] Topuz and colleagues[56] recorded that 6 of 13 patients had died from their disease after a median follow-up period of 20 months. The GOG experience has also followed this pattern, with a report that 23 of 30 patients died between 1 and 16 months after their initial surgery.[20] Ariyoshi's group[27] published a 5-year survival rate of 27% in 23 patients; the survivors were those women with stage I or II disease. Prendiville and associates[36] also reviewed the experience at the Christie Hospital, where the median survival time was 14 months among 20 patients. In the series reported by Le and colleagues,[45] a better median survival time was noted: 3 years among those women who received chemotherapy. Long-term survival after a diagnosis of ovarian sarcoma is seen almost exclusively among those women with stage I disease.

SUMMARY

Ovarian sarcomas are uncommon tumors and are associated with a poor prognosis. Accurate histopathologic review and interpretation is essential for optimal clinical management. Primary surgery remains the mainstay of diagnosis and initial treatment. Postoperative therapy with combination chemotherapy is recommended. The regimen of paclitaxel and carboplatin

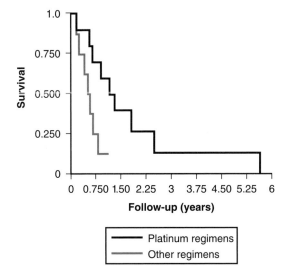

Figure 39–5. Survival (Kaplan-Meier analysis) of patients with ovarian sarcoma treated with platinum-based versus nonplatinum-based regimens. (Adapted from Sood AK, Sorosky JI, Gelder MS, et al: Primary ovarian sarcoma: Analysis of prognostic variables and the role of surgical cytoreduction. Cancer 1998;82:1733.)

has the highest reported response rate and seems to offer promise.

References

1. Piura B, Rabinovich A, Yanai-Inbar I, et al: Primary sarcoma of the ovary: Report of five cases and review of the literature. Eur J Gynaecol Oncol 1998;19:257-261.
2. Russell P: Surface epithelial-stromal tumours of the ovary. In Kurman RJ (ed): Blaustein's Pathology of the Female Genital Tract, 4th ed. New York, Springer-Verlag, 1994, p 705-782.
3. Inoue J, Gomibuchi H, Minoura S: A case of a primary ovarian leiomyosarcoma. J Obstet Gynaecol Res 2000;26:401-407.
4. Rasmussen CC, Skilling JS, Sorosky JI, et al: Stage IIIC ovarian leiomyosarcoma in a premenopausal woman with multiple recurrences: Prolonged survival with surgical therapy. Gynecol Oncol 1997;66:519-525.
5. Lifschitz-Mercer B, Leider-Trejo L, Messer G, et al: Primary angiosarcoma of the ovary: A clinicopathologic, immunohistochemical and electronmicroscopic study. Pathol Res Pract 1998;194:183-187.
6. Nucci MR, Krausz T, Lifschitz-Mercer B, et al: Angiosarcoma of the ovary: Clinicopathologic and immunohistochemical analysis of four cases with a broad morphologic spectrum. Am J Surg Pathol 1998;22:620-630.
7. Nielsen GP, Young RH, Prat J, Scully R: Primary angiosarcoma of the ovary: A report of seven cases and review of the literature. Int J Gynecol Pathol 1997;16:378-382.
8. Furihata M, Takeuchi T, Iwata J, et al: Primary ovarian angiosarcoma: A case report and literature review. Pathol Int 1998;48:967-973.
9. Twu N-F, Juan C-M, Yeng M-S, et al: Treatment of primary pure angiosarcoma of ovary with multiple lung metastases: A case report. Eur J Gynaec Oncol 1999;20:383-385.
10. Platt JS, Rogers SJ, Flynn EA, Taylor RR: Primary angiosarcoma of the ovary: A case report and review of the literature. Gynecol Oncol 1999;73:443-446.
11. Prat J, Scully RE: Cellular fibromas and fibrosarcomas of the ovary: A comparative cliniopathologic analysis of seventeen cases. Cancer 1981;47:2663- 2670.
12. Huang YC, Hsu KF, Chou CY, et al: Ovarian fibrosarcoma with long-term survival: A case report. Int J Gynecol Cancer 2001;11:331-333.
13. Krüger S, Schmidt H, Küpker W, et al: Fibrosarcoma associated with a benign cystic teratoma of the ovary: Case report. Gynecol Oncol 2002;84:150-154.
14. Tsuji T, Kawauchi S, Utsunomiya T, et al: Fibrosarcoma vs cellular fibroma of the ovary: A comparative study of their proliferative activity and chromosome aberrations using MIB-1 immunostaining, DNA flow cytometry and fluorescence in situ hybridization. Am J Surg Pathol 1997;22:52-59.
15. Dal Cin P: Fibrosarcoma vs cellular fibroma of the ovary [letter]. Am J Surg Pathol 1998;22:508-510.
16. Nielsen GP, Oliva E, Young RH, et al: Primary ovarian rhabdomyosarcoma: A report of 13 cases. Int J Gynecol Pathol 1998;17:113-119.
17. Sant'Ambrogio S, Malpica A, Schroeder B, Silva EG: Primary ovarian rhabdomyosarcoma associated with clear cell carcinoma of the ovary: A case report and review of the literature. Int J Gynecol Pathol 2000;19:169-173.
18. Domoto H, Mano Y, Kita T, et al: Chondrosarcomatous differentiation in metastatic deposit of serous papillary cystadenocarcinoma. Pathol Int 2000;50:497-501.
19. Eltabbakh GH, Belinson JL, Biscotti CV: Osteosarcoma metastatic to the ovary: A case report and review of the literature. Int J Gynecol Pathol 1997;16:76-78.
20. Morrow CP, d'Ablaing G, Brady LW, et al: A clinical and pathologic study of 30 cases of malignant mixed mullerian epithelial and mesenchymal ovarian tumours: A gynecologic oncology group study. Gynecol Oncol 1984;18:278-292.
21. Young RH, Scully RE: Sarcomas metastatic to the ovary: A report of 21 cases. Int J Gynecol Pathol 1990;9:231-242.
22. Wei L-H, Huang C-Y, Cheng S-P, et al: Carcinosarcoma of ovary associated with previous radiotherapy. Int J Gynecol Cancer 2001;11:81-84.
23. Wiklund TA, Blomqvist CP, Raty J, et al: Postirradiation sarcoma: Analysis of a nationwide cancer registry material. Cancer 1991;68:524-531.
24. Monk BJ, Nieberg R, Berek JS: Primary leiomyosarcoma of the ovary in a perimenarchal female. Gynecol Oncol 1993;48:89-393.
25. O'Sullivan SG, Narla LD, Ferraro E: Primary ovarian leiomyosarcoma in an adolescent following radiation for medulloblastoma. Pediatr Radiol 1998;28:468-470.
26. Wada H, Enomoto T, Fujita M, et al: Molecular evidence that most but not all carcinosarcomas of the uterus are combination tumours. Cancer Res 1997;57:5379-5385.
27. Ariyoshi K, Kawauchi S, Kaku T, et al: Prognostic factors in ovarian carcinosarcoma: A clinicopathological and immunohistochemical analysis of 23 cases. Histopathology 2000;37:427-436.
28. Sonoda Y, Saigo P, Federici MG, Boyd J: Carcinosarcoma of the ovary in a patient with a germline BRCA2 mutation: Evidence for monoclonal origin. Case report. Gynecol Oncol 2000;76:226-229.
29. Sood AK, Sorosky JI, Gelder MS, et al: Primary ovarian sarcoma: Analysis of prognostic variables and the role of surgical cytoreduction. Cancer 1998;82:1731-1737.
30. Barakat RR, Rubin SC, Wong G, et al: Mixed mesodermal tumour of the ovary: Analysis of prognostic factors in 31 cases. Obstet Gynecol 1992;80:660-664.
31. Muntz HG, Jones MA, Goff BA, et al: Malignant mixed müllerian tumours of the ovary: Experience with surgical cytoreduction and combination chemotherapy. Cancer 1995;76:1209-1213.
32. Chang J, Sharpe JC, A'hern RP, et al: Carcinosarcoma of the ovary: Incidence, prognosis, treatment and survival of patients. Ann Oncol 1995;6:755-758.
33. Rasmussen CC, Skilling JS, Sorosky JI, et al: Stage IIIC ovarian leiomyosarcoma in a premenopausal woman with multiple recurrences: Prolonged survival with surgical therapy. Gynecol Oncol 1997;66:519-525.
34. Friedman HD, Mazur MT: Primary ovarian leiomyosarcoma: An immunohistochemical and ultrastructural study. Arch Pathol Lab Med 1991;115:941-945.
35. Shakfeh SM, Woodruff JD: Primary ovarian sarcomas: Report of 46 cases and review of the literature. Obstet Gynecol Surv 1987;42:331-349.
36. Prendiville J, Murphy D, Renninson J, et al: Carcinosarcoma of the ovary treated over a 10-year period at the Christie Hospital. Int J Gynecol Cancer 1994;4:200-205.
37. Pecorelli S, Benedet JL, Creasman WT, Shepherd JH: FIGO staging of gynecologic cancer. Int J Gynecol Obstet 1999;64:5-10.
38. Wang PH, Lee RC, Lin G, et al: Malignant mixed mesodermal tumours of the ovary: Preoperative diagnosis. Gynecol Obstet Invest 1999;47:69-72.
39. Saito A, Kuwatsuru R, Ogishima D, et al: MR images of ovarian carcinosarcoma. Rad Med 1999;17:447-450.
40. Kaji Y, Sugimura K, Yamamoto N, et al: A case of malignant mixed mesodermal tumour (MMMT) of the ovary: MR features before and after chemotherapy. Rad Med 1999;17:81-83.
41. Dobbs SP, Brown LJR, Hollingworth J, Ireland D: Surgical treatment of recurrent primary ovarian leiomyosarcoma: A case report. Eur J Gynaecol Oncol 1999;20:172-173.
42. Hirakawa E, Kobayashi S, Miki H, et al: Ascitic fluid cytology of adenosarcoma of the ovary: A case report. Diagn Cytopathol 2000;24:343-346.
43. Plaxe SC, Dottino PR, Goodman HM, et al: Clinical features of advanced ovarian mixed mesodermal tumors and treatment with doxorubicin- and cis-platinum-based chemotherapy. Gynecol Oncol 1990;37:244-249.
44. Duska LR, Garrett A, Eltabbakh GH, et al: Paclitaxel and platinum chemotherapy for malignant mixed mullerian tumors of the ovary. Gynecol Oncol 2002;85:459-463.
45. Le T, Krepart GV, Lotocki RJ, Heywood MS: Malignant mixed mesodermal ovarian tumor treatment and prognosis: A 20-year experience. Gynecol Oncol 1997;65:237-240.
46. Fowler JM, Nathan L, Nieberg RK, Berek JS: Mixed mesodermal sarcoma of the ovary in a young patient. Eur J Obstet Gynecol Reprod Biol 1996;65:249-253.

47. Rampaul RS, Barrow S, Naraynsingh V: A primary ovarian leiomyosarcoma with micro-invasive features (stage 1): Is surgical excision enough? [letter]. Gynecol Oncol 1999;73:464.

48. Anderson B, Turner DA, Benda J: Ovarian sarcoma. Gynecol Oncol 1987;26:183-192.

49. Carlson JA, Edwards C, Wharton JT, et al: Mixed mesodermal sarcoma of the ovary. Cancer 1983;52:1473-1477.

50. Sutton GP, Blessing JA, Homesley HD, Malfetano JH: A phase II trial of ifosfamide and mesna in patients with advanced or recurrent mixed mesodermal tumors of the ovary previously treated with platinum-based chemotherapy: A gynecologic oncology group study. Gynecol Oncol 1994;53:24-26.

51. Sit ASY, Price FV, Kelley JL, et al: Chemotherapy for malignant mixed müllerian tumors of the ovary. Gynecol Oncol 2000;79:196-200.

52. Baker TR, Piver MS, Caglar H, Piedmonte M: Prospective trial of cisplatin, Adriamycin and dacarbazine in metastatic mixed mesodermal sarcomas of the uterus and ovary. Am J Clin Oncol 1991;14:246-250.

53. Simon SR, Wang SE, Uhl M, Shackney S: Complete response of carcinosarcoma of the ovary to therapy with doxorubicin, ifosfamide and dacarbazine. Gynecol Oncol 1991;41:161-166.

54. McGuire WP, Hoskins WJ, Brady MF, et al: Cyclophosphamide and cisplatin compared with paclitaxel and cisplatin in patients with stage III and stage IV ovarian cancer. N Engl J Med 1996;334:1-6.

55. Hellström A-C, Tegerstedt G, Silfverswärd C, Pettersson F: Malignant mixed müllerian tumors of the ovary: Histopathologic and clinical review of 36 cases. Int J Gynecol Cancer 1999;9:312-316.

56. Topuz E, Eralp Y, Aydiner A, et al: The role of chemotherapy in malignant mixed müllerian tumors of the female genital tract. Eur J Gynaecol Oncol 2001;22:469-472.

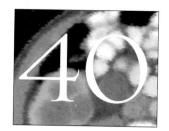

BORDERLINE OVARIAN
TUMORS

Karen H. Lu and Debra A. Bell

✦ MAJOR CONTROVERSIES

- **What is the appropriate surgical management for a woman who is found intraoperatively to have a serous borderline ovarian tumor and who wishes to preserve her fertility?**
- **What is the significance of these three histologic terms on patient prognosis: micropapillary pattern, noninvasive and invasive implants, and microinvasion?**
- **What is the appropriate management for a patient with advanced-stage or recurrent serous borderline ovarian tumor?**

Borderline ovarian tumors, or ovarian tumors of low malignant potential, are distinct from invasive ovarian malignancies clinically and histologically. These tumors account for 15% of all epithelial ovarian cancers. Clinically, women with borderline ovarian tumors are approximately 10 to 15 years younger than women with invasive epithelial ovarian cancer. More than 80% of women with borderline ovarian tumors present with stage I disease. Overall survival for women with borderline ovarian tumors, stage for stage, is also significantly better.[1-3] Histologically, borderline ovarian tumors show complex architecture and nuclear atypia but do not demonstrate invasion of the underlying stroma. Since the 1970s, when the International Federation of Gynecology and Obstetrics (FIGO) and the World Health Organization (WHO) officially recognized borderline tumors as a distinct entity,[4,5] numerous studies have been published describing the clinical and pathologic characteristics of this disease. Borderline ovarian tumors most frequently have serous or mucinous histologic patterns. This chapter primarily focuses on controversies related to serous borderline ovarian tumors.

Challenges to clinicians caring for women with serous borderline ovarian tumors include the following:

- Determining appropriate surgical management with attention to fertility preservation

- Interpreting histologic risk factors that may predict a worse prognosis
- Determining appropriate surgical and medical management for women with advanced-stage or recurrent disease

What is the appropriate surgical management for a woman who is found intraoperatively to have a serous borderline ovarian tumor and who wishes to preserve her fertility?

Most diagnoses of serous borderline ovarian tumor are rendered during intraoperative or postoperative pathologic evaluation. No preoperative tumor markers or radiologic features can accurately identify a pelvic mass as a borderline ovarian tumor. CA 125 levels are elevated in 92% of women with advanced-stage serous borderline tumors, but only 25% of women with stage I serous borderline ovarian tumors have elevated CA 125 levels.[6] In many instances, the diagnosis of a serous borderline tumor is determined by the pathologist during an intraoperative frozen section evaluation. In patients who have completed childbearing, bilateral salpingo-oophorectomy with hysterectomy and staging is recommended. However, many women with serous borderline ovarian tumors are of reproductive age and have not completed child-bearing. In these cases, unilateral oophorectomy with staging is reasonable. This procedure should include visualization of the contralateral ovary, because the risk of bilateral involvement of serous borderline tumors is 25% to 60%.[2] If there is a suspicious mass or lesion, ovarian cystectomy or wedge biopsy may be performed. Random biopsy of the contralateral ovary is not recommended if no gross abnormalities are seen.

Data from a number of series have demonstrated the safety of conservative surgery for patients with borderline ovarian tumors who desire future fertility. Although performing a unilateral oophorectomy or an ovarian cystectomy, or both, does not appear to significantly affect long-term overall survival rates, recurrence rates are higher for women who undergo conservative surgery. Morris and colleagues[7] described 26 women with serous borderline ovarian tumors who underwent conservative surgery with a unilateral oophorectomy or a cystectomy. Eleven (42%) of 26 women developed recurrences. However, only one patient died of disease, and this occurred more than 12 years after her initial diagnosis. Women who undergo conservative surgery should be closely monitored for disease recurrence. Several studies have reported successful pregnancies in women treated conservatively for serous borderline ovarian tumors.[7-9]

For patients who are found to have serous borderline tumors at frozen diagnosis, an adequate staging procedure should be performed, whether the patient undergoes conservative surgery or hysterectomy with bilateral salpingo-oophorectomy. The para-colic gutters and upper abdomen should be thoroughly visualized. Staging should also include washings, omental biopsy, peritoneal biopsies, and lymph node sampling. Lin and associates[10] reviewed a large series of serous borderline tumors and found that only 12% of women had complete surgical staging, defined as having biopsies from pelvic and abdominal peritoneum, omentum, and retroperitoneal lymph nodes. This low rate of surgical staging primarily occurred because the diagnosis of a borderline ovarian tumor was not expected or known intraoperatively. The advantages of performing an adequate staging procedure include the ability to more accurately discuss prognosis, because recurrence rate and survival are associated with stage of disease, and the possibility that the frozen diagnosis of a serous borderline tumor will be upstaged at final review to an invasive carcinoma. Winter and colleagues[11] addressed the question of whether complete surgical staging for serous borderline ovarian tumors affected recurrence rate or survival by examining a group of women who were completely staged and a group of women who did not have full staging. The 5-year overall survival rates for the two groups were similar. The researchers point out in this study that extremely large numbers of patients would be necessary to show a survival difference between staged and unstaged patients because of the overall favorable outcome for these patients. However, 8 of their 93 patients who were diagnosed with a serous borderline tumor at frozen section were upgraded to a carcinoma at final pathology review. We

continue to recommend a thorough evaluation of the peritoneal surfaces in the pelvis and abdomen and retroperitoneal lymph node sampling.

The diagnosis of a serous borderline ovarian tumor often is not made until after the surgery, and a staging procedure has not been performed. For these patients, a CA 125 determination and an abdominopelvic computed tomographic scan can be obtained. In patients with a small Pfannenstiel incision in which there is no documentation of examination of the paracolic gutters and upper abdomen or in patients whose histology shows a micropapillary pattern (discussed later), staging procedures by means of laparotomy or laparoscopy should be considered. If thorough examination of the upper abdomen has been performed with or without staging biopsies, conservative follow-up may be a reasonable option.

For patients with disease apparently confined to the ovaries, adjuvant chemotherapy is not recommended. Barnhill and colleagues[12] reported a Gynecologic Oncology Group prospective study in which 146 women with stage I serous borderline ovarian tumors were observed without adjuvant therapy. With a median follow-up of 42.4 months, no patient developed recurrent disease. Even in patients with stage I disease who have recurrent disease, salvage can often be achieved with surgical debulking alone. For most patients with stage I tumors, long-term disease-free survival can be expected. A large meta-analysis demonstrated a disease-free survival rate of 98.2% and a disease-specific survival rate of 99.5% for women with stage I disease.[13]

What is the significance of these three histologic terms on patient prognosis: micropapillary pattern, noninvasive and invasive implants, and microinvasion?

The category of borderline ovarian tumors or tumors of low malignant potential was formalized as an entity separate from ovarian carcinomas by the FIGO in 1971[5] and accepted by the WHO two years later.[4] The key distinguishing feature between borderline ovarian tumors and invasive ovarian carcinomas is the absence of stromal invasion in borderline tumors. On gross examination, most serous borderline tumors are endophytic cysts; however, surface involvement is present in many cases, especially those with peritoneal involvement.[14-18] Although most serous borderline tumors are definitively treated at the time of initial surgery, a small subset of patients with these tumors develop recurrent disease and may die of their tumor. In an effort to define which patients are at greatest risk for an unfavorable outcome, clinicians and pathologists have attempted to identify risk factors. Stage of disease remains the most important predictor of outcome, but pathologists also have described histologic patterns that may influence risk of recurrence and death from disease. Clinicians caring for women with borderline tumors need to have an understanding of this histologic terminology for appropriate counseling and treatment recommendations to be given. In this

Table 40–1. Histologic Features of Serous Borderline Ovarian Tumors

Classification Characteristics	Micropapillary Pattern	Typical Pattern
Architectural features	Elongate micropapillae arise directly from large papillae or cysts Surface cribriforming Smooth epithelial-stromal interface	"Hierarchical" branching pattern Irregular interface
Cytologic features	Polygonal cells with high nucleus-to-cytoplasm ratio Bland nuclei, often with single nucleolus Mitoses are few and normal	Columnar cells with lower nucleus-to-cytoplasm ratio Bland nuclei Mitoses are few and normal.
Histologic terminology	If ≥5 mm confluent focus: Micropapillary serous borderline tumor or serous tumor of low malignant potential with micropapillary pattern Micropapillary serous carcinoma	If foci <5 mm of micropapillary pattern: Serous borderline tumor Serous tumor of low malignant potential Atypical proliferative serous tumor

section, the terms micropapillary pattern, invasive and noninvasive implants, and stromal microinvasion are discussed, with an emphasis on the clinical implications of each.

Serous borderline ovarian tumors may have two distinct histologic patterns that are often seen in the same neoplasm.[13,19-25] These have been called the *typical pattern* and *micropapillary pattern*. The histologic features and varying nomenclature of each type are compared in Table 40-1 and illustrated in Figure 40-1. It has been suggested that tumors with at least one confluent focus of the micropapillary or cribriform pattern (or both), which measure more than 5 mm pursue a more aggressive clinical course than those that have smaller foci of this pattern or are exclusively of the typical type.[13,19,26,27] Subsequent studies documented that these micropapillary tumors differed from serous borderline tumors of the typical type in that they were more frequently bilateral and more often manifested with peritoneal involvement than typical serous borderline tumors.[21-25,28] Studies have found a higher frequency of invasive implants with micropapillary serous tumors,[20-22,26,28] although a few have not confirmed this

association.[23,25] Controversy exists regarding the prognostic significance of the micropapillary pattern as an isolated feature. Several studies have shown an increased risk of recurrence of tumors of the micropapillary type but have not documented an impact on survival when the implant type is considered (i.e., most deaths in the micropapillary group have been associated with invasive peritoneal implants), and others have not shown an increased risk of relapse (Table 40-2). With longer follow-up intervals, the impact on survival of micropapillary tumors may increase, given that many of the recurrences have been low-grade serous carcinomas. Although some investigators have called such tumors *micropapillary serous carcinoma*,[13,19,26,27] most pathologists classify these tumors as *micropapillary serous borderline tumors* or *tumors of low malignant potential with a micropapillary pattern*.[21-25] Because of the apparent increased association of micropapillary serous tumors with adverse prognostic factors and an increased risk of recurrence as low-grade serous carcinoma, staging should be strongly considered in understaged women with an established diagnosis of a serous borderline tumor of micropapillary type.

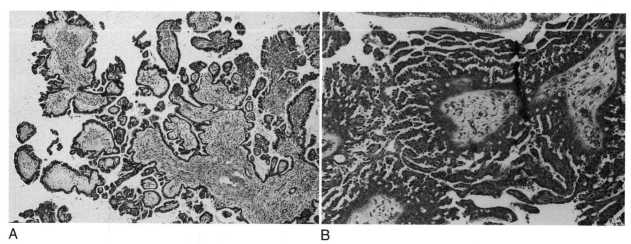

A   B

Figure 40–1. A, Typical serous borderline tumor with irregular, branching papillae. **B,** Serous, borderline tumor with a micropapillary pattern with smooth papillae lined by elongate micropapillae. See also Color Figure 40-1.

Table 40–2. Recurrences in and Survival of Patients with Serous Borderline Tumors

Study	Typical Pattern*		Micropapillary Pattern*	
	No. with Relapse/Total	No. Dead of Tumor/Total	No. with Relapse/Total	No. Dead of Tumor/Total
Slomovitz et al.[25]	1/27[†]	0/27	3/13[†]	0/13
Deavers et al.[22]	25/81[†]	12/81	14/18[†]	6/18
Prat and DeNictolis[23]	4/75	3/75	1/17	1/17
Eichhorn et al.[24]	3/33	0/33	5/33	3/33
Burks et al.[19]	No data	No data	5/13	2/13
Seidman and Kurman[13]	10/54	3/54	7/11	4/11
Gilks et al.[24]	12/36	5/36	2/12	1/12
Total	**55/306 (18%)**	**23/306 (8%)**	**37/117 (32%)**	**17/117 (15%)**

*All stages of tumors with invasive and noninvasive peritoneal implants were combined.
†Statistically significant difference.
‡All cases were stage II or higher.

The peritoneal lesions associated with serous borderline tumors vary in histologic appearance. They are classified as *implants* rather than metastatic carcinoma to emphasize their more favorable prognosis. Implants are subclassifed as noninvasive and invasive subtypes.[13,15,26,29] The histologic features and nomenclature variants of peritoneal implants are outlined in Table 40-3 and illustrated in Figure 40-2. Although the histologic criteria for the diagnosis of invasive implants vary somewhat, patients with noninvasive implants have a lower risk of recurrence and death than patients with invasive implants. Table 40-4 provides a summary of studies in which disease relapse and death were correlated with type of peritoneal implant. These figures represent a minimum estimate of risk because serous borderline ovarian tumors can recur after decades and most studies have only 5 to 10 years of follow-up data. It is unclear whether invasive implants represent a clonal process from the primary ovarian tumor or are separate primary tumors.[30-33]

An unusual finding in serous borderline tumors is the presence of microscopic foci of invasion of the stroma of the tumor by single cells and nests of moderately atypical cells. When such foci measure less than 3 mm in longest linear dimension and 10 mm² or less in area, the tumors are retained in the borderline category and are called *serous borderline tumors* or *serous tumors of low malignant potential with stromal microinvasion.*[34] Several small studies have indicated that the prognosis for these tumors is similar to that for serous

borderline tumors without focal microinvasion.[23,35,36] Clinicians can manage this subset of patients as they do patients with typical serous borderline tumors.

What is the appropriate management for a patient with advanced-stage or recurrent serous borderline ovarian tumor?

Patients with advanced-stage serous borderline tumor are at greatest risk for recurrence and death from disease. Rates of recurrence and death for women with high-stage disease (i.e., stage II and III) vary from 5% to 30%.[13,16,17,19-26,28,29,36-38] Much of the variability in recurrence and death rates results from studies having limited follow-up periods for these patients. Serous borderline ovarian tumors can recur more than 10 years after the initial diagnosis, with a median time to recurrence of 5 to 7 years. However, even with advanced-stage borderline ovarian tumors, the long-term survival rate approaches 70%. This contrasts with the pattern for invasive ovarian cancer, for which 5-year survival rates for advanced disease are less than 30%.

Despite the generally favorable prognosis, women with advanced-stage borderline ovarian tumors present a clinical dilemma for management. Should adjuvant chemotherapy be given postoperatively? Is there a role for conservative surgical management even in the face of peritoneal disease for young women desiring fertility? What is the treatment of women with recurrent

Table 40–3. Classification of Peritoneal Implants Associated with Serous Borderline Tumors

Classification Characteristics	Invasive Implants	Noninvasive Implants
Architectural features	Irregular infiltration of underlying normal tissue	Sharp demarcation from normal tissue
	Fibrotic edematous or myxoid stroma	Fibrotic, inflammatory stroma
	Solid or cribriform nests surrounded by a cleft	Glands, papillary clusters or single cells
	Micropapillary pattern	
Cytologic features	Substantial atypia	Moderate atypia
Alternative histologic terminology	Well-differentiated serous carcinoma	Atypical proliferative serous tumor

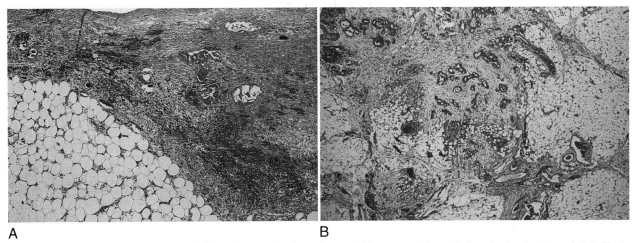

Figure 40–2. **A,** Noninvasive implant, with sharp demarcation from the underlying normal tissue. **B,** Invasive implant irregularly infiltrates and obliterates the underlying omentum. See also Color Figure 40-2.

disease? There are no prospective, randomized clinical trials that address these questions, and therefore much of our practice pattern is based on relatively small, retrospective series.

In general, the diagnosis of advanced-stage serous borderline tumors refers to patients who have peritoneal implants in addition to having serous borderline tumor in one or both ovaries. Peritoneal implants can be histologically categorized as invasive or noninvasive. Regardless of histologic type of implant, multiple investigators have shown that patients with no macroscopic residual disease at initial surgery have better progression-free survival and overall survival rates than patients with any macroscopic disease. As in invasive epithelial ovarian cancer, maximal surgical cytoreduction of visible tumor should be performed. The role of fertility-sparing surgery in women with advanced-stage serous borderline ovarian tumors is less well accepted than for women with early-stage serous borderline ovarian tumors. A study by Zanetta and coworkers[39] reported results for a subset of 25 patients with stage II or III disease who were treated with fertility-sparing

surgery. All 25 were without clinical evidence of disease, but 4 had pathologic persistence of disease. Of the 21 with no evidence of disease, 7 had undergone salvage surgery for recurrent borderline tumor, and 1 had undergone salvage surgery for an invasive carcinoma in the spared ovary. The study authors give a clinical recurrence rate of 40% for women with stage II or III disease after conservative surgery, compared with 12.9% after nonconservative surgery. The investigators conclude that conservative surgery in advanced-stage serous borderline tumors is reasonable, given the high salvage rate in women with recurrences. However, we believe that fertility-sparing surgery in women with advanced-stage serous borderline ovarian tumors should be approached with caution.

The decision to give postoperative chemotherapy to women with advanced-stage serous borderline tumors, whether there is residual disease or none after initial debulking surgery, is unclear. In patients who have had adequate sampling and who have noninvasive implants, surgical debulking may be sufficient.[40] In patients with invasive implants, adjuvant

Table 40–4. Disease Relapse and Death from Tumor in Patients with Stage II through IV Ovarian Serous Borderline Tumors with Invasive and Noninvasive Peritoneal Implants

Study	Invasive Peritoneal Implants		Noninvasive Peritoneal Implants	
	No. with Relapse	*No. Dead of Tumor*	*No. with Relapse*	*No. Dead of Tumor*
Manchul et al.[33]	1/5	0/5	1/7	1/7
Russell[17]	1/2	1/2	1/3	1/6
Michael and Roth[32]	1/8*	1/8*	1/6	0/6
McCaughey et al.[31]	5/11‡	4/11‡	2/19‡	2/19‡
Bell et al.[29]	5/6	2/3	NA	3/50
DeNictolis et al.[38]	4/9	4/9	NA	0/10
Seidman and Kurman et al.[13]	8/13§	6/13§	4/51	1/51
Total	**50/113 (44%)**	**38/119 (32%)**	**64/331 (19%)**	**30/432 (7%)**

*Four patients had been followed for 2 years or less.
†Two patients who did not have a recurrence had been followed for 1 year or less.
‡Six patients who did not have a recurrence had been followed for 1 year or less.
§Eleven patients' primary tumors were classified as "micropapillary serous carcinoma."
NA, not available.

chemotherapy after surgical debulking may be considered. A number of investigators reported pathologic response to platinum-based chemotherapy at the time of second-look surgery. However, no prospective, randomized studies have been performed to determine if postoperative chemotherapy influences survival of women with advanced-stage serous borderline tumors. Gershenson and colleagues[41] reported a complete response to chemotherapy at second-look laparotomy in 8 of 20 patients with macroscopic residual disease after initial debulking surgery and in 5 of 12 patients with microscopic residual disease after initial surgery. Barakat and coworkers[42] reported that 2 of 7 patients with macroscopic borderline tumors and 7 of 8 patients with microscopic disease had pathologic complete remissions at second-look laparotomy after platinum-based chemotherapy. With a mean follow-up of 64 months, only one patient had died of progressive disease. There was no difference in survival between patients who received chemotherapy and those who did not. Sutton and associates[43] reported the Gyneco-logic Oncology Group data using a subset of 32 women with advanced-stage borderline ovarian tumors that were optimally debulked, and the patients were randomized to treatment with cisplatin and cyclophosphamide with or without Adriamycin. Fifteen of 32 patients had second-look surgery, and 9 showed evidence of persistent disease. However, at a median of 31.7 months, 31 of 32 patients were alive, and 1 patient had died of other causes. Because borderline tumors have a low percentage of actively dividing cells, they may be fairly resistant to standard cytotoxic agents. Optimal surgical debulking remains the primary treatment of advanced serous borderline ovarian tumors. Patients must therefore be counseled that the role of adjuvant chemotherapy in advanced-stage serous borderline tumors is unknown. Even with advanced-stage disease, women have excellent overall survival rates.

The median time to recurrence for serous borderline tumors is 5 to 7 years. Recurrence can histologically be similar to the original borderline tumor or can be an invasive carcinoma. Crispens and coworkers[44] reported that of 49 patients who had recurrent disease, 73% of recurrences were low-grade carcinomas. Other groups have also reported that recurrences may be low-grade carcinomas. For patients who develop recurrent borderline tumors, secondary surgical cytoreduction is the treatment of choice. Crispens and associates[44] showed that optimal cytoreduction was significantly associated with improved survival. Of the women who had no gross residual disease after secondary cytoreduction, only one died of progressive disease. In contrast, of 10 women who had more than 2 cm of gross residual disease, 6 (60%) died of disease. Crispens also described the efficacy of chemotherapy in 45 evaluable patients from this same series. Six complete responses and four partial responses were reported with a platinum- or taxane-based regimen. One patient had a partial response to leuprolide, and one patient had a partial response to pelvic irradiation. Overall, 36% of patients with progressive or recurrent serous borderline tumors

died of their disease. Patients who had recurrent, low-grade serous carcinoma were significantly more likely to die of the tumor than those with serous ovarian tumors of low malignant potential. None of the patients presented with a high-grade serous carcinoma at the time of recurrence. It is unclear whether low-grade carcinoma represents a new primary cancer or true recurrence of the serous borderline tumor. Nonetheless, optimal secondary tumor debulking is correlated with long-term survival, and subsequent tumor debulking procedures occasionally must be performed. No randomized, prospective studies have been performed to determine whether chemotherapy confers a survival benefit for women with recurrent serous borderline tumors. There are few data to guide the clinician in deciding whether to give chemotherapy, even in the subgroup of women who have recurrences in the form of low-grade serous carcinoma. Multicenter trials are clearly needed, as well as investigations of biologic or hormonal options.

Mucinous Borderline Ovarian Tumors

Mucinous borderline ovarian tumors often manifest as large, unilateral ovarian masses. The risk of bilateral involvement is low, and peritoneal involvement is rare.[45,46] In women who wish to retain childbearing potential, a unilateral oophorectomy is acceptable. For all mucinous tumors, an appendectomy should be performed with a thorough gastrointestinal evaluation to rule out a primary gastrointestinal tumor.[47] Gross visualization of the appendix is unacceptable to rule out tumor involvement. Pathologists confronted with a probable mucinous borderline ovarian tumor should sample the mass thoroughly. The carcinomatous portion of the tumor often is small and may be missed if thorough sampling is not performed. Risk of recurrent disease for stage I mucinous borderline tumors is exceedingly low, and adjuvant therapy is unnecessary.

Most mucinous borderline ovarian tumors are stage I. Although for many years pseudomyxoma peritonei was thought to result from ovarian mucinous borderline tumors, pathologists now believe that most ovarian tumors associated with pseudomyxoma peritonei are metastatic from appendiceal mucinous neoplasms.[48]

Summary

Our understanding of the natural history of borderline ovarian tumors has greatly increased since FIGO and the WHO officially recognized this category of tumors as distinct from invasive epithelial ovarian cancer. Overall, patients with borderline ovarian tumors (serous and mucinous) have a highly favorable prognosis and can expect to live without recurrence of disease. Because borderline ovarian tumors often occur in reproductive-age women, emphasis at the time of diagnosis should be on performing fertility-sparing procedures.

Even in advanced-stage disease, overall prognosis is favorable. Studies have identified high stage and invasive implants as predictors of recurrence. Further refinement of histologic risk factors for poor outcome is necessary. The development of novel biologic or hormonal therapies with high efficacy and a decreased side-effect profile would be beneficial. Further molecular characterization of these tumors will likely advance our ability to manage women with borderline ovarian tumors.

REFERENCES

1. Trope C, Kaern J: Management of borderline tumors of the ovary: State of the art. Semin Oncol 1998;25:372-380.
2. Trimble CL, Trimble EL: Management of epithelial ovarian tumors of low malignant potential. Gynecol Oncol 1994;55: S52-S61.
3. Leake JF, Currie JL, Rosenshein NB, Woodruff JD: Long-term follow-up of serous ovarian tumors of low malignant potential. Gynecol Oncol 1992;47:150-158.
4. Serov SF, Scully RE, Sobin LH: The World Health Organization International Histological Classification of Ovarian Tumours: Histological Typing of Ovarian Tumors. Geneva, World Health Organization, 1973.
5. International Federation of Gynecology and Obstetrics: Classification and staging of malignant tumors in the female pelvis. Acta Obstet Gynecol Scand 1971;50:1-7.
6. Rice LW, Berkowitz RS, Mark SD, et al: Epithelial ovarian tumors of borderline malignancy. Gynecol Oncol 1990;39:195-198.
7. Morris RT, Gershenson DM, Silva EG, et al: Outcome and reproductive function after conservative surgery for borderline ovarian tumors. Obstet Gynecol 2000;95:541-547.
8. Donnez J, Munschke A, Berliere M, et al: Safety of conservative management and fertility outcome in women with borderline tumors of the ovary. Fertil Steril 2003;79:1216-1221.
9. Morice P, Camatte S, El Hassan J, et al: Clinical outcomes and fertility after conservative treatment of ovarian borderline tumors. Fertil Steril 2001;75:92-96.
10. Lim-Tan SK, Gajiga HE, Scully RE: Ovarian cystectomy for serous borderline tumors: A follow-up study of 35 cases. Obstet Gynecol 1988;72:775-781.
11. Winter WE, Kucera PR, Rodgers W, et al: Surgical staging in patients with ovarian tumors of low malignant potential. Obstet Gynecol 2002;100;671-676.
12. Barnhill DR, Kurman RJ, Brady MF, et al: Preliminary analysis of the behavior of stage I ovarian serous tumors of low malignant potential: A Gynecologic Oncology Group study. J Clin Oncol 1995;13:2752-2756.
13. Seidman JD, Kurman RJ: Ovarian serous borderline tumors: A critical review of the literature with emphasis on prognostic indicators. Hum Pathol 2000;31:539-557.
14. Bell DA: Ovarian surface epithelial-stromal tumors. Hum Pathol 1991;22:750-762.
15. Silva EG, Tornos C, Zhuang Z, et al: Tumor recurrence in stage I ovarian serous neoplasms of low malignant potential. Int J Gynecol Pathol 1998;17:387-389.
16. Katzenstein A-LA, Mazur MT, Morgan TE, Kao M-S: Proliferative serous tumors of the ovary. Histologic features and prognosis. Am J Surg Pathol 1978;2:339-355.
17. Russell P: Borderline epithelial tumors of the ovary: A conceptual dilemma. Clin Obstet Gynaecol 1984;11:259-276.
18. Segal GH, Hart WR: Ovarian serous tumors of low malignant potential (serous borderline tumors): The relationship of exophytic surface tumor to peritoneal "implants." Am J Surg Pathol 1992;16:577-583.
19. Burks RT, Sherman ME, Kurman RJ: Micropapillary serous carcinoma of the ovary. A distinctive low-grade carcinoma related to serous borderline tumors. Am J Surg Pathol 1996;20:1319-1330.
20. Seidman JD, Kurmann RJ: Subclassification of serous borderline tumors of the ovary into benign and malignant types. Am J Surg Pathol 1996;20:1331-1345.
21. Eichhorn JH, Bell DA, Yong RH, Scully RE: Ovarian serous borderline tumors with micropapillary and cribriform patterns: A study of 40 cases and comparison with 44 cases without these patterns. Am J Surg Pathol 1999;23:397-409.
22. Deavers MT, Gershenson DM, Tortolero-Luna G, et al: Micropapillary and cribriform patterns in ovarian serous tumors of low malignant potential. Am J Surg Pathol 2002;26:1129-1141.
23. Prat J, DeNictolis M: Serous borderline tumors of the ovary: A long-term follow-up study of 137 cases, including 18 with a micropapillary pattern and 20 with microinvasion. Am J Surg Pathol 2002;26:1111-1128.
24. Gilks CB, Alkushi A, You JJ, et al: Advanced-stage serous borderline tumors of the ovary: A clinicopathological study of 49 cases. Int J Gynecol Pathol 2003;22:29-36.
25. Slomovitz BM, Caputo TA, Gretz HF, et al: A comparative analysis of 57 serous borderline tumors with and without a noninvasive micropapillary component. Am J Surg Pathol 2002; 26;592-600.
26. Bell KA, Smith Sehdev AE, Kurman RJ: Refined diagnostic criteria for implants associated with ovarian atypical proliferative serous tumors (borderline) and micropapillary serous carcinomas. Am J Surg Pathol 2001;25:419-432.
27. Smith Sehdev AE, Sehdev PS, Kurman RJ: Noninvasive and invasive micropapillary (low-grade) serous carcinoma of the ovary: A clinicopathologic analysis of 135 cases. Am J Surg Pathol 2003;27:725-736.
28. Goldstein NS, Ceniza N: Ovarian micropapillary serous borderline tumors: Clinicopathologic features and outcome of seven surgically staged patients. Am J Clin Pathol 2000;114:380-386.
29. Bell DA, Weinstock MA, Scully RE: Peritoneal implants of ovarian serous borderline tumors: Histologic features and prognosis. Cancer 1988;62:2212-2222.
30. Gershenson DM, Silva EG, Tortolero-Luna G, et al: Serous borderline tumors of the ovary with noninvasive peritoneal implants. Cancer 1998;83:2157-2163.
31. McCaughey WT, Lester KME, Dardick I: Peritoneal epithelial lesions associated with proliferative serous tumors of ovary. Histopathology 1984;8:195-208.
32. Michael H, Roth LM: Invasive and noninvasive implants in ovarian serous tumors of low malignant potential. Cancer 1986;57:1240-1247.
33. Manchul LA, Simm J, Levin W, et al: Borderline epithelial ovarian tumors: A review of 81 cases with an assessment of the impact of treatment. Int J Radiat Oncol Biol Phys 1992;22: 867-874.
34. Scully RE: World Health Organization International Histological Classification of Tumors: Histological Typing of Ovarian Tumours, 2nd ed. New York, Springer Verlag, 1999.
35. Tavassoli FA: Serous tumor of low malignant potential with early stromal invasion (serous LMP with microinvasion). Mod Pathol 1988;1:407-413.
36. Kennedy AW, Hart WR: Ovarian papillary serous tumors of low malignant potential (serous borderline tumors): A long-term follow-up study, including patients with micro-invasion, lymph node metastasis, and transformation to invasive serous carcinoma. Cancer 1996;78:278-286.
37. Bostwick DG, Tazelaar HD, Ballon SC, et al: Ovarian epithelial tumors of borderline malignancy: A clinical and pathologic study of 109 cases. Cancer 1986;58:2052-2064.
38. DeNictolis M, Montironi R, Tommasoni S, et al: Serous borderline tumors of the ovary: A clinicopathologic, immunohistochemical, and quantitative study of 44 cases. Cancer 1992;70:152-160.
39. Zanetta G, Rota S, Chiari S, et al: Behavior of borderline tumors with particular interest to persistence, recurrence, and progression to invasive carcinoma: A prospective study. J Clin Oncol 2001;19:2658-2664.
40. Lackman F, Carey MS, Kirk ME, et al: Surgery as sole treatment for serous borderline tumors of the ovary with noninvasive implants. Gynecol Oncol 2003;90;407-412.
41. Gershenson DM, Silva EG: Serous ovarian tumors of low malignant potential with peritoneal implants. Cancer 1990;65: 578-584.
42. Barakat RR, Benjamin I, Lewis JL, et al: Platinum-based chemotherapy for advanced-stage serous ovarian carcinoma of low malignant potential. Gynecol Oncol 1995;59:390-393.

43. Sutton GP, Bundy BN, Omura GA, et al: Stage III ovarian tumors of low malignant potential treated with cisplatin combination therapy (a Gynecologic Oncology Group study). Gynecol Oncol 1991;41:230-233.

44. Crispens MA, Bodurka D, Deavers M, et al: Response and survival in patients with progressive or recurrent serous ovarian tumors of low malignant potential. Obstet Gynecol 2002;99:3-10.

45. Lee KR, Scully RE: Mucinous tumors of the ovary: A clinico-pathologic study of 196 borderline tumors (of intestinal type) and carcinomas, including an evaluation of 11 cases with "pseudo-myxoma peritonei." Am J Surg Pathol 2000;24:1447-1464.

46. Hart WR, Norris JH: Borderline and malignant mucinous tumors of the ovary. Cancer 1973;31:1031-1045.

47. Young TH, Gilks CB, Scully RE: Mucinous tumors of the appendix associated with mucinous tumors of the ovary: A clinicopathological analysis of 22 cases. Am J Surg Pathol 1991;15:415-429.

48. Misdraji J, Yantiss RK, Graeme-Cook FM, et al: Appendiceal mucinous neoplasms: A clinicopathologic analysis of 107 cases. Am J Surg Pathol 2003;27:1089-1103.

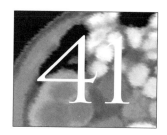

C H A P T E R

PRIMARY PERITONEAL
CANCER

Barbara Goff

 MAJOR CONTROVERSIES

- Is primary peritoneal cancer a variant of mesothelioma?
- Are the risk factors for primary peritoneal cancer the same as for epithelial ovarian cancer?
- Is primary peritoneal cancer unifocal or multifocal in origin?
- Are *BRCA*-related primary peritoneal cancers molecularly different from peritoneal cancers not associated with germline mutations?
- Should patients with primary peritoneal cancer be treated identically to patients with epithelial ovarian cancer?
- Is the clinical outcome for patients with primary peritoneal cancer the same as for patients with epithelial ovarian cancer?
- What is the incidence of primary peritoneal carcinoma in high-risk women, and should screening after prophylactic oophorectomy be offered?

Primary peritoneal carcinoma is a relatively newly defined disease entity that is characterized by abnormal carcinomatosis of the peritoneal cavity with minimal or no involvement of the ovaries. The first case report to document this disease process appeared in 1959. A 27-year-old woman was found to have a tumor of the pelvic peritoneum that resembled a papillary serous carcinoma of the ovary; but the ovaries and fallopian tubes were completely normal.[1] Primary peritoneal carcinoma was initially classified as a variant of mesothelioma, and it was not until the late 1970s that it was recognized as a distinct pathologic entity of mullerian origin.[2] Primary peritoneal carcinoma is similar to papillary serous carcinoma of the ovary in clinical presentation, histologic appearance, and response to treatment.[3,4] In fact, as many as 10% to 15% of advanced "ovarian cancer" cases should be reclassified as primary peritoneal carcinomas.[5] Although there are many similarities between epithelial ovarian carcinoma and peritoneal carcinoma, molecular and epidemiologic studies suggest that these are two distinct entities.[5-8] In addition, it is important for practitioners to know that primary peritoneal carcinoma can occur after bilateral

salpingo-oophorectomy and that it is associated with mutations in *BRCA* genes.

HISTORY

Is primary peritoneal cancer a variant of mesothelioma?

The first case of primary peritoneal carcinoma was reported by Swerdlow in 1959.[1] In this case a 27-year-old woman had a papillary serous carcinoma of the peritoneum with no ovarian involvement. In 1961, Rosenbloom and Foster[9] reported a case of pelvic peritoneal tumor that was called a papillary mesothelioma. Initially, primary peritoneal tumors were classified as mesotheliomas, because the two malignancies were thought to have a common ancestry.[8] However, epidemiologic studies revealed significant differences between the two diseases.[7,8,10-23] Seventy percent of malignant mesotheliomas occur in men, typically in men with asbestos exposure; overall, approximately 85% of patients have known exposure to asbestos.[22,23]

Primary peritoneal carcinoma occurs almost exclusively in women, and no association with asbestos has been reported.

In the 1970s, evidence mounted that the peritoneum of women retains the embryologic potential for mullerian differentiation, with reports of metaplastic and neoplastic transformation (Fig. 41-1).[24-26] Examples included endometriosis, endosalpingosis, borderline tumors of the peritoneum, peritoneal leiomyomatosis, extrauterine sarcomas, and epithelial carcinomas of the peritoneum.[25] Because of this potential, Lauchlan included female pelvic peritoneum as a mullerian structure.[27] Finally, in the 1980s, ultrastructural analysis of primary peritoneal carcinomas and mesotheliomas confirmed that primary peritoneal tumors are ultrastructurally identical to ovarian cancers and quite distinct from mesotheliomas.[26,28]

The first report of primary peritoneal carcinoma arising after bilateral oophorectomy was in 1982 by Tobacman and colleagues.[29] In this study the authors reported intra-abdominal carcinomatosis indistinguishable from papillary serous carcinoma of the ovary in three women, 1, 5, and 11 years after prophylactic oophorectomy for a family history of ovarian cancer. Several additional cases were reported in the 1980s.[30,31] In 1993, Piver and coworkers[32,33] reported on the incidence of primary peritoneal carcinoma in women who had undergone prophylactic oophorectomy from the Gilda Radner Familial Ovarian Cancer Registry. In this study of 324 women, six primary peritoneal cancers developed in women who had at least two family members with ovarian cancer, and three in women who had only one family member with ovarian cancer. In 1997, Bandera and colleagues[34] found BRCA1 germline mutations in 2 (11%) of 17 of women with primary peritoneal carcinoma. These studies have increased the controversy surrounding the benefit of prophylactic oophorectomy.

EPIDEMIOLOGY AND RISK FACTORS

Are the risk factors for primary peritoneal cancer the same as for epithelial ovarian cancer?

The exact incidence of primary peritoneal carcinoma is unknown. If approximately 10% of cases diagnosed as ovarian cancer are truly primary peritoneal, then there are approximately 2000 cases annually in the United States.[3,4] Better recognition of this entity in recent years is probably responsible for a further increase in its relative frequency, so that now up to 18% of laparotomies performed for ovarian carcinoma yield a diagnosis of primary peritoneal malignancy on final pathology review.[5]

Initial studies focused on the epidemiologic differences between malignant mesothelioma and primary peritoneal carcinoma. Significant differences between these two diseases were noted by many authors. Malignant mesothelioma usually occurs in men (60% to 80%), and in more than 80% of these cases there is evidence of asbestos exposure. In addition, malignant mesothelioma responds poorly to chemotherapy, and median survival time is short.[3,4,22,23]

Primary peritoneal carcinoma occurs almost exclusively in women, although two cases in men have been reported.[35,36] Most recent studies have focused on epidemiologic differences between primary peritoneal and ovarian epithelial carcinomas.[5,37,38] A major problem with all of these comparison studies is that they are from single institutions and contain small numbers of

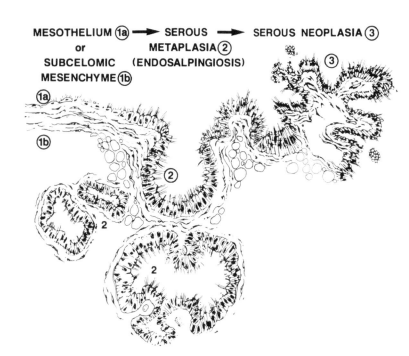

Figure 41-1. A scheme for histogenesis of serous lesions of the peritoneum. A metaplastic or neoplastic change of tubal type (transformation to columnar cells and ciliated cells), similar to that occurring in surface epithelium of the ovary, can occur in the hormonally sensitive female peritoneum, resulting in endosalpingiosis or serous neoplasms. (From Raju U, Fine G, Greenawald KA, Ohorodnik JM. Primary papillary serous neoplasia of the peritoneum: A clinicopathologic and ultrastructural study of eight cases. Hum Pathol 1989;20:434.)

cases; they therefore lack sufficient power to draw meaningful conclusions. The majority of studies have found few epidemiologic differences between peritoneal and epithelial ovarian malignancies. Several studies have shown, although others have not,[3] that women with primary peritoneal carcinoma are significantly older than women with ovarian cancer. Eltabbakh and associates[37] compared epidemiologic factors of 50 women with primary peritoneal carcinoma and 503 women with epithelial ovarian cancer. They found that age at diagnosis was significantly older (64 versus 55 years), menarche was later (13.3 versus 12.8 years), and talc use was less among the women with primary peritoneal carcinoma. A more recent study by Halperin and colleagues[5] found that women with primary peritoneal cancer had a significantly earlier menarche, a higher number of births, and a lower incidence of family history positive for gynecologic malignancies, compared with women with ovarian cancer.[5] Both studies showed no significant differences with regard to race, socioeconomic status, smoking, history of birth control pill use, or hormone replacement. It is not known whether pregnancy and oral contraceptive use decrease the risk of peritoneal cancer, as they do for ovarian cancer. Likewise, it is unclear whether factors that increase the risk of ovarian cancer, such as infertility, also increase the risk of primary peritoneal carcinoma. Women with *BRCA1* mutations are at increased risk for development of primary peritoneal cancer.[34] The risk of primary peritoneal carcinoma for *BRCA1* carriers after prophylactic oophorectomy is unknown but is estimated to be approximately 5% to 10%.[32,33] It is unknown whether *BRCA2* mutations place women at increased risk for primary peritoneal malignancies.

CLINICAL PRESENTATION

The clinical presentation for women with primary peritoneal cancer is identical to that of women with advanced epithelial ovarian cancer. In a study reported by Fowler and colleagues,[39] 75% of women with primary peritoneal cancer had a preoperative diagnosis of ovarian cancer.

The most common presenting symptoms for women with peritoneal cancer are shown in Table 41-1. Bloating, feeling full after small meals, abdominal distention, and change in bowel habits are found in 80% to 90% of patients.[10-21,39,40] Only 6% are asymptomatic. Because ovaries are only minimally involved, pelvic

Table 41–1. Common Symptoms of Peritoneal Cancer

Symptom	Percentage of Cases
Abdominal pain	65
Increase in abdominal size	51
Abdominal bloating	50
Change in bowel habits	30
Dyspepsia	20
Nausea/vomiting	9
Urinary frequency	6

examinations are often normal, which can lead to delays in diagnosis. In patients who have new onset of abdominal and gastrointestinal symptoms that persist beyond 2 to 4 weeks, physicians should have a high index of suspicion of ovarian or peritoneal malignancies; pelvic and abdominal imaging should be performed even if the pelvic examination is normal. Occasionally, peritoneal carcinoma is detected after identification of psammoma bodies on a Papanicolaou smear[25] or during exploratory laparotomy for other indications.[20]

On physical examination, approximately 50% to 80% of patients have evidence of ascites, and 30% have a palpable abdominal or pelvic mass. Normal pelvic examinations are reported in 30% to 50% of cases. CA 125 levels are increased (greater than 35.0 μg/mL) in more than 90% of patients.[10-21,39,40] In a study of 75 women with primary peritoneal carcinoma, the median CA 125 level was 1320 μg/mL.[40]

Primary peritoneal carcinoma spreads mainly transperitoneally; however, lymphatic and blood-borne metastases have been found.[18] Table 41-2 shows the most common sites of disease. The omentum is involved in 90% to 100% of cases. Although ovarian involvement is minimal, when ovaries are present they are involved with disease in more than 90% of cases.[10-21]

PATHOLOGY

Gross Appearance

The typical gross appearance of primary peritoneal carcinoma is similar to that of advanced-stage epithelial carcinoma except that the ovaries are of normal size and have no or minimal surface implants. Typically there is extensive peritoneal studding of the pelvic and abdominal peritoneal implants. Ascites, omental cake, diaphragmatic implants, and pleural effusions are common findings with primary peritoneal cancer.

Diagnostic Criteria

The diagnosis of primary peritoneal cancer can be made only after careful pathologic evaluation of surgical specimens. The central issue in the diagnosis of

Table 41–2. Common Disease Sites of Primary Peritoneal Cancer

Site	Percentage of Cases
Omentum	98
Ovaries	95
Pelvic peritoneum	93
Abdominal peritoneum	88
Diaphragm	84
Malignant ascites	80
Para-aortic lymph nodes	25
Pelvic lymph nodes	20
Pleural cavity	17
Liver parenchyma	10

primary peritoneal carcinoma is distinguishing it from epithelial ovarian cancer. In 1988, Mills and colleagues[41] were the first to establish criteria to separate the two entities. Their definition of primary peritoneal carcinoma specified grossly normal ovaries less than or equal to 3 cm in size, with tumor on the ovaries involving only the surface with minimal invasion. In 1990, Fromm and associates[18] proposed a definition that included ovarian size less than or equal to 4 cm with ovarian implants of 1 to 15 mm. The most widely accepted definition of primary peritoneal carcinoma is the one adopted by the Gynecologic Oncology Group (GOG):

1. Both ovaries must be either physiologically normal in size or enlarged by a benign process.
2. The involvement in the extraovarian sites must be greater than the involvement on the surface of either ovary.
3. Microscopically, the ovarian component must be one of the following:
   - Nonexistent.
   - Confined to ovarian surface epithelium with no evidence of cortical invasion.
   - Involving ovarian surface epithelium and underlying cortical stroma but with any given tumor size less than 5×5 mm.
   - Tumor less than 5×5 mm within ovarian substance associated with or without surface disease.
4. The histologic and cytologic characteristics of the tumor must be predominantly of the serous type that is similar or identical to ovarian serous papillary adenocarcinoma, any grade.

In addition, most authors advocate expanding the criteria to include nonserous histology with histologic appearance identical to other subtypes of epithelial ovarian cancer (e.g., endometrial, mucinous); some also advocate even larger implants than 5×5 mm, as long as the ovaries are otherwise normal and invasion is less than 5 mm.[3,4]

Histology

The histology of primary peritoneal carcinoma is usually indistinguishable from that of papillary serous carcinoma of the ovary. Typically, primary peritoneal carcinomas have a predominantly papillary pattern and often contain psammoma bodies. Necrosis and desmoplastic reactions are common. Tumors are often of high grade, with markedly atypical cells, prominent nucleoli, and high mitotic counts (Fig. 41-2). Although papillary serous histology accounts for more than 90% of peritoneal malignancies, there have been reports of endometrioid histology, extraovarian mucinous tumors, primary peritoneal malignant mixed mullerian tumors, and peritoneal endometrial stromal sarcomas.[42-48] Although the predominant neoplastic differentiation of the female peritoneum is to develop a papillary serous malignancy, it can differentiate into any type of mullerian malignancy.[25]

In contrast, mesotheliomas are generally solid and can have cleft-like spaces. The cells are cubical to polygonal, with abundant dense eosinophilic to pale cytoplasm with centrally placed round nuclei and conspicuous nucleoli (Fig. 41-3).[22] Typically, immunocytochemistry studies are negative for epithelial mucin and carcinoembryonic antigen (CEA), as detailed later.

The ultrastructural appearance of peritoneal papillary serous tumors reveals the presence of focally prominent, slender microvilli on a luminal or papillary surface; cytoplasmic mucin granules can be seen, as well as some degree of nuclear polarization. Mesotheliomas have exuberant, long, slender, undulating microvilli lining several surfaces of the cells. Cytoplasm is abundant, and there is a lack of nuclear polarity.[2]

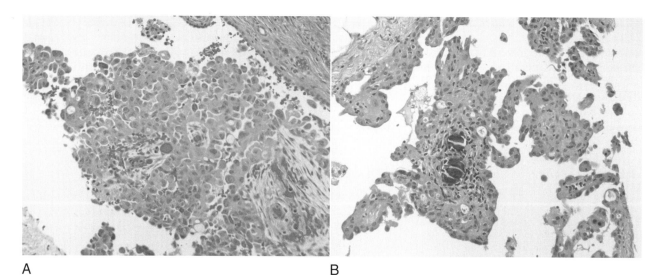

A   B

Figure 41–2. Photomicrograph of primary peritoneal carcinoma: **A,** Showing well-defined papillary structures, psammoma bodies, and nuclear crowding. **B,** Showing psammoma bodies. See also Color Figure 41-2.

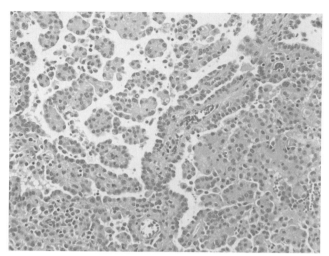

Figure 41–3. Photomicrograph of peritoneal mesothelioma. There are relatively loosely arranged cuboidal cells and poorly defined papillary patterns. The cells have well-spaced nuclei and abundant cytoplasm. There is lack of nuclear crowding. See also Color Figure 41-3.

Immunohistochemistry

Immunohistochemical studies of primary peritoneal cancer show findings similar to those of epithelial ovarian cancer, with positive staining for cytokeratin, epithelial membrane antigen (EMA), and CA 125.[49] Studies that have compared immunohistochemical expression of proteins between epithelial ovarian cancer and peritoneal papillary serous carcinoma have shown that expressions of CEA, estrogen receptor (ER), and progesterone receptor (PR) are significantly lower in primary peritoneal carcinomas; however, HER2/NEU overexpression and Ki-67 (marker of cellular proliferation) were significantly higher in primary peritoneal carcinomas compared with ovarian cancers.[6] P53 overexpression and the incidence of aneuploidy are similar in the two groups. The fact that there are some significant differences in expression of receptors, oncogenes, and proteins between primary peritoneal and epithelial ovarian cancer suggests that the genetic events responsible for malignant transformation may be distinct for each entity.

Comparison of immunohistochemical expression of proteins between mesothelioma and peritoneal carcinoma reveals that the mesothelial markers—calretinin, thrombomodulin, cytokeratin 5/6, and CD44H—are found commonly (50% to 90%) in mesotheliomas but rarely in peritoneal cancers. S100, Ber-EP4, CA 125, and B72.3 are commonly found in ovarian and primary peritoneal cancers and rarely in mesotheliomas (Table 41-3).[25,50,51]

MOLECULAR GENETICS

Epithelial ovarian cancer has been shown in multiple studies to represent a monoclonal expansion of tumor cells.[52-57] Allelic losses at chromosomal loci are commonly found in advanced epithelial ovarian cancer. Analysis of the pattern of allelic loss allows detection of chromosomal deletion in one of two alleles at a specific locus. A pattern of identical loss of heterozygosity (LOH) would be expected in a monoclonal, unifocal tumor. Identical patterns of LOH, *TP53* gene mutation, and X chromosome inactivation have been reported in epithelial ovarian carcinoma. Although primary peritoneal carcinoma resembles advanced epithelial ovarian carcinoma both clinically and histologically, its pathogenesis is not as well understood.

Is primary peritoneal cancer unifocal or multifocal in origin?

There have been two theories as to the origin of this cancer.[58] The first is that the tumor develops in the ovarian surface epithelium and subsequently spreads throughout the peritoneal cavity. The primary tumor is thought to be microscopic and therefore not detectable or to regress completely. The second theory is that the disease starts de novo in the peritoneal mesothelium, which is of mullerian origin. The epithelium of the ovary and peritoneal lining are histologically the same, and factors that induce ovarian epithelium to undergo malignant degeneration may also have the same effect on the peritoneal lining. Evidence in support of this theory is the finding of primary peritoneal carcinoma after prophylactic oophorectomy.

As with ovarian cancer, investigators have evaluated primary peritoneal carcinoma for unifocal versus multifocal origin. Initially, Muto and colleagues[7] evaluated six patients with peritoneal malignancies for clonality. They studied LOH on chromosomes 1, 3, 4, and 17 and the mutational pattern of the *TP53* gene. In three of six cases, different patterns of LOH were found at different tumor sites, suggesting a multifocal origin. In another study, Kupyjanczyk and associates[52] found identical *TP53* mutations in multiple tissues for patients with both advanced ovarian and peritoneal malignancies. They concluded that both ovarian and primary peritoneal malignancy are monoclonal entities. However, their conclusions were based on the evaluation of only two cases of peritoneal cancer. Follow-up studies[59-61]

Table 41–3. Comparison of Immunocytochemistry Staining of Primary Peritoneal (PP) Cancer, Epithelial Ovarian Cancer (EOC), and Malignant Melanoma (MM)

Marker	Percentage Staining Positively		
	PP	EOC	MM
CA 125	75	80	10
S100	100	100	10
CEA	25	60	0
ER	30	72	0
PR	40	80	0
Ber-EP4	50	95	9
Calretin	88	0	0
EMA	100	100	80
B27.3	85	90	0

Data from references 3, 4, 6, 25, 50, 51, and 52.

have looked at unifocal versus multifocal origins in a somewhat larger group of patients. Schorge and coworkers[59] evaluated LOH at the androgen receptor gene and X chromosome inactivation to test the hypothesis that some cases of papillary serous carcinoma of the peritoneum have a multifocal origin. Twenty of 22 cancers were heterozygous at the androgen receptor locus on the X chromosome and thus informative for their analysis. In 5 (25%) of the 20 cases, tumor DNA from different tumor sites showed different patterns of LOH, and 2 of these 5 patients had alternating X chromosome inactivation patterns. This study provides strong evidence that, at least in some cases, peritoneal carcinoma has a multifocal origin.

In the same study, Schroge and colleagues[59] also evaluated the BRCA status of their patients. In three cases a *BRCA1* mutation was identified. All three of these patients had a multifocal origin of disease based on analysis of LOH. The authors concluded that women with *BRCA1* mutations are significantly more likely to have multifocal disease, compared with women without *BRCA1* mutations. However, the generalizability of this finding to all *BRCA1* mutation carriers is limited by the small size of the study.[58]

Are BRCA-related primary peritoneal cancers molecularly different from peritoneal cancers not associated with germline mutations?

In a later study, Schorge and colleagues[60] compared the molecular pathogenesis of *BRCA1*-related primary peritoneal carcinomas with that of wild-type cancers. They evaluated LOH at *BRCA1* and *TP53* loci and immunocytochemical expression of P53, epidermal growth factor, and ERBB2. In their group of 43 patients with primary peritoneal cancer, 11 (26%) were *BRCA1* mutation carriers. *BRCA1* mutation carriers had a higher incidence of *TP53* mutations (89% versus 47%), were more likely to exhibit multifocal or null *TP53* mutations (63% versus 7%), and were less likely to exhibit ERBB2 overexpression. In the authors' opinion, this evidence supports the hypothesis that *BRCA1*-related papillary serous carcinoma of the peritoneum has a unique molecular pathogenesis that is distinct from that of wild-type peritoneal cancers, and the unique molecular pathogenesis of *BRCA1*-related tumors may affect the ability of current methods to reliably prevent or detect this disease before extensive spread occurs.

STAGING

Primary peritoneal carcinoma does not have a distinct staging system. The International Federation of Obstetrics and Gynecology (FIGO) staging system for ovarian cancer is generally applied to women with peritoneal malignancies. However, there can never be a stage I primary peritoneal carcinoma with this staging system. Because patients with peritoneal cancers usually present with extensive peritoneal spread,

the majority of cases (70% to 75%) are stage III. Approximately 25% of patients present with stage IV disease, usually with a malignant pleural effusion or parenchyma liver metastasis.[3,4] There have been only a small number of cases in which disease was limited to the pelvis.

MANAGEMENT

Presurgical Evaluation

Because the clinical presentation of primary peritoneal carcinoma is identical to that of advanced-stage epithelial ovarian cancer, and because the diagnosis of primary peritoneal cancer can be made only after surgical/pathologic evaluation, the preoperative assessment is the same as for women with suspected ovarian cancer. In approximately 75% to 80% of cases, the preoperative diagnosis is ovarian cancer.[39] The presurgical evaluation should include a thorough history, including family history. The physical examination should carefully evaluate the extent of disease in the pelvis, possible rectal involvement, ascites, omental cake, and pleural effusion. Radiographic studies should include a chest radiograph to rule out metastases or pleural effusion and to evaluate potential anesthetic risks. Pelvic ultrasound or abdominal/pelvic computed tomography (CT) scans are helpful in determining extent of disease and in helping the surgeon assess likelihood of optimal cytoreduction. Additional radiographic studies are dictated by the patient's symptoms. Although the diagnosis of primary peritoneal cancer cannot be made preoperatively, it is more likely when radiographic studies reveal evidence of carcinomatosis with normal-size ovaries. In a study of 36 women with primary peritoneal carcinoma, preoperative CT scans revealed ascites in 80%, omental involvement in 78%, peritoneal thickening in 61%, abnormal thickening of the sigmoid in 28%, pleural effusion in 30%, and normal size ovaries in 85%.[62] Laboratory studies should include evaluation of electrolytes, hematology, renal and hepatic function, and serum CA 125. Other tumor markers have not been shown to be clinically useful.

In general, preoperative paracentesis is not indicated unless it is needed for symptomatic relief or for diagnostic purposes in a patient whom it is preferable to treat with neoadjuvant chemotherapy (e.g., poor surgical candidate, extensive disease making optimal cytoreduction very unlikely). In patients with a pleural effusion, thoracentesis is indicated for staging and also for relief of symptoms or to improve pulmonary function preoperatively.

Surgical Management

Because of the clinical and pathologic similarities between epithelial ovarian cancer and primary peritoneal cancer, most authors have advocated a treatment plan identical to that for epithelial ovarian cancer.[3,4,39,40] Surgical exploration is important not only for establishing a diagnosis of primary peritoneal cancer but also for surgical cytoreduction. Because in 98% of cases there is abdominal as well as pelvic disease, extensive cytoreduction or debulking surgery is needed to remove the disease. Surgery should include removal of ovaries and uterus. Even if they are not thought to be primary sites of tumor, they often contain multiple implants, and not infrequently, on histologic review, there is found to be a synchronous primary tumor in either in the ovaries or endometrium. Because the diagnosis can be made only after histologic review, all cases are surgically managed as if they were epithelial ovarian cancers. The omentum is involved with tumor in 80% to 100% of patients and therefore should be resected if possible.[18,39,63] Grossly enlarged pelvic and para-aortic lymph nodes should be removed, but routine diagnostic sampling is not needed. Resection or destruction of peritoneal and diaphragmatic implants is frequently performed for cytoreduction. Bowel resections and splenectomy are often indicated to prevent bowel obstruction and achieve optimal cytoreduction.

Just as the FIGO staging system for epithelial ovarian cancer is applied to primary peritoneal cancers, so are the terms "optimal" and "suboptimal" cytoreduction. Although the definition of optimal residual disease has varied among investigators, the most widely used value is that the largest residual disease nodule should measure less than 1 cm in diameter. The GOG uses this definition of optimal cytoreduction for both ovarian and peritoneal cancers.

There has never been a prospective randomized study to establish the benefit of optimal cytoreduction in advanced epithelial ovarian cancer, but there are considerable retrospective data to indicate a significant survival advantage in those patients for whom optimal cytoreduction can be achieved.[64,65] In a meta-analysis by Bristow and coworkers,[66] a total of 6885 patients were identified from 53 studies; all patients had received platinum-based chemotherapy.[66] These authors found that patients with less than 25% maximal cytoreduction had a median survival time of 22.7 months, and those with more than 75% maximal cytoreduction had a median survival time of 33.9 months (an increase of 50%). Despite the fairly extensive literature evaluating the efficacy of cytoreduction in epithelial ovarian cancer, only a few studies exist for primary peritoneal cancers. These studies are summarized in Table 41-4. In the study by Fromm and associates,[18] there was no significant difference in survival based on residual disease after surgery, but many of these patients were treated in the era before platinum chemotherapy became available. Other authors have reported improved survival in women who obtained optimal cytoreduction, but differences have not been statistically significant because of the small numbers of patients involved.[38,39,67] In a more recent report by Eltabbakh and associates,[40] among 75 women with primary peritoneal cancer, all of whom were treated with platinum, optimal cytoreduction was associated with a median survival time of 40 months, compared with 18.6 months for those with a suboptimal cytoreduction ($P = .0007$). These results were confirmed by Kennedy and coworkers.[68]

The ability to achieve optimal cytoreduction for primary peritoneal cancers varies significantly among studies, ranging from 30% to 70%.[15,18,19,38-40] To some extent, the ability to achieve optimal cytoreduction reflects the extent of disease and the training of the surgeon. With advanced epithelial ovarian cancer, gynecologic oncologists are able to achieve optimal cytoreduction two to three times more frequently than are general surgeons or general gynecologists.[69] Patients with advanced ovarian cancer have a significant survival advantage when their disease is managed surgically by a gynecologic oncologist; therefore, it is recommended that women with suspected ovarian malignancy be referred to a gynecologic oncologist for surgical management.[69,70] Because women with primary peritoneal cancer require the same surgical expertise as women with ovarian cancer, any women with suspected primary peritoneal cancer should also be referred for consultation with a gynecologic oncologist.

Several studies have compared surgical outcomes between primary peritoneal and epithelial ovarian cancers. Many studies have found that patients with primary peritoneal cancer are less likely to achieve an optimal cytoreduction than are those with epithelial ovarian cancer.[5,15,19] Often, optimal cytoreduction for

Table 41-4. Survival Based on Cytoreduction Status

Study	N	Residual Disease (cm)	Median Survival Time (mo)	Probability Value
Strand et al[67]	18	<3	31	NS
		>3	11	
Fromm et al[18]	74	≤2	25	NS
		>2	26	
Fowler et al[39]	36	<1.5	18	NS
		>1.5	17	
Ben-Baruch et al[38]	22	<2	46	NS
		>2	20	
Eltabbakh et al[40]	75	≤1	40	.0007
		>1	18	
Kennedy et al[68]	36	≤1	Not yet reached	.02
		>1	32.8	

NS, not significant.

primary peritoneal cancer was achieved in fewer than 50% of cases.[18,39] The widespread nature of primary peritoneal cancer, especially in the upper abdomen and along the diaphragm, may account for the reduced ability to perform an optimal cytoreduction.

In some situations, surgery is best delayed until after several cycles of chemotherapy. Several studies have investigated the use of neoadjuvant chemotherapy for women with advanced ovarian cancer.[71-73] Neoadjuvant treatment is usually given in the setting of very advanced disease, when the surgeon knows that optimal cytoreduction cannot be achieved. Usually three cycles of chemotherapy are given to reduce the volume of disease, which makes the morbidity of surgery significantly less and the chance of optimal cytoreduction significantly greater. After surgery, additional chemotherapy is given. Retrospective studies have suggested that neoadjuvant treatment may be safer in the setting of very advanced disease because of the decreased morbidity: blood loss, number of days in intensive care, and length of hospital stay can be significantly less compared with upfront cytoreduction.[71,72] Response and cure rates also appear to be similar to what would have been achieved if patients had initially had a suboptimal cytoreduction. However, neoadjuvant therapy has not been studied in prospective randomized trials. Given its success in very advanced ovarian cancer, the use of neoadjuvant chemotherapy in primary peritoneal malignancies is reasonable in the setting of surgically unresectable disease.[68] In patients who respond to chemotherapy, it is still important to perform an exploratory laparotomy and remove the uterus, ovaries, and omental cake, because disease in these sites is rarely sterilized completely by chemotherapy.

Chemotherapy

Should patients with primary peritoneal cancer be treated identically to patients with epithelial ovarian cancer? Most investigators have chosen as chemotherapy for primary peritoneal cancer those drugs that have proved effective in advanced epithelial cancer. In general, response rates for peritoneal cancer are very

similar to those for ovarian cancer. Over the past two to three decades, cisplatin-based regimens have been used most commonly. More recently, recommended chemotherapy has evolved into combination treatment with taxanes and platinum (Table 41-5).

Fromm and colleagues[18] reported the results of 74 patients with primary peritoneal cancer treated at their institution. They found an overall response rate of 64% to various chemotherapy regimens. The pathologic complete response rate was 27%, and the pathologic partial response rate was 45%. These investigators found that patients who received a cisplatin-based regimen had a median survival time of 31.5 months, whereas those who did not receive cisplatin had a median survival time of 19.5 months ($P = .02$). The authors also found that the response rates of peritoneal cancers to chemotherapy were very similar to those of advanced epithelial ovarian cancers that had been treated at their institution during the same time frame. The improved response seen with platinum-based regimens has been confirmed by other investigators.[11,14,15,19-21]

Since Fromm's report,[18] a number of authors have reported response rates of approximately 60% to platinum-based chemotherapy after cytoreduction.[15,18,39] These response rates were comparable to what was achieved by the authors at their own institutions with similar combinations in patients with ovarian carcinomas. Most authors have concluded that primary peritoneal carcinoma should be treated in an identical fashion to ovarian cancer[3,4] (see Table 41-5).

Several case-control studies have compared response rates of ovarian and peritoneal carcinoma to platinum-based chemotherapy. In a case-control study of 33 peritoneal and 33 matched ovarian cancer patients, Bloss and colleagues[15] found no significant differences with respect to response to chemotherapy or overall survival. Complete surgical response rates were 18% for peritoneal and 34% for epithelial ovarian cancer. These findings were not statistically different, but this may be a result of the small study size and the low power to detect differences. Partial surgical response rates were 45% and 48% for peritoneal and epithelial ovarian cancer, respectively. In two other case-control studies, patients with primary peritoneal carcinoma were

---

Table 41–5. Response of Primary Peritoneal Cancer to Chemotherapy

Study	N	Regimen	Response
Fromm et al[18]	44	Melphalan, P, CP	65% OR (23% CR, 41% PR)
Bloss et al[15]	33	CP (n = 29)	63% OR (18% PCR, 45% PPR)
		CAP (n = 4)	
Piver et al[85]	46	CAP (n = 25)	63% OR (CAP)
		TP (n = 21)	70% OR (TP)*
Eltabbakh et al[40]	72	Platinum-based, no paclitaxel (n = 45)	67% OR (20% CR, 47% PR)*
		TP (n = 27)	
Kennedy et al[68]	38	TP(n = 38)	86% OR (68% CR, 18% PR)

CAP, Cisplatin/doxorubicin/cyclophosphamide; CP, cisplatin/cyclophosphamide; CR, complete response; OR, overall response; P, cisplatin; PCR, pathologic complete response; PPR, pathologic partial response; PR, partial response; TP, paclitaxel/platinum.
*No difference in median survival between the two groups.

reported to have reduced response rates to platinum-based chemotherapy, compared with control patients with epithelial ovarian cancer.[6,19] However, all of these studies were retrospective analyses involving small numbers of patients.

The GOG did conduct a prospective phase II trial of cisplatin and cyclophosphamide in 36 patients with primary peritoneal cancer, compared with 130 epithelial ovarian cancer patients treated with the same regimen.[74] The clinical complete response rates were 45% for peritoneal and 35% for ovarian cancers. The pathologic complete response rates were identical at 20% for each group. Based on this study, women with primary peritoneal carcinoma were included in all GOG treatment studies of epithelial ovarian carcinomas.

Because of the improved response rates and improved survival in patients with epithelial ovarian cancer when taxanes are used in combination with platins, these regimens have also become the standard of care for all patients with primary peritoneal cancers.[75] In 1995, paclitaxel was used successfully as salvage therapy in a patient with recurrent peritoneal cancer.[76] Menzin and coworkers[77] reported the first use of paclitaxel and cisplatin as first-line therapy, with a 100% clinical response rate and a 25% pathologic complete response rate in four women with primary peritoneal cancer. Kennedy and colleagues[68] reported a response rate of 87% after treatment with paclitaxel and platinum, with 68% of patients having a complete response. Other authors have found that the addition of paclitaxel to cisplatin does not improve response rates for patients with peritoneal cancer (see Table 41-5).[40,78] As the GOG incorporates patients with primary peritoneal cancer into studies evaluating treatments of epithelial ovarian cancer, subset analysis should allow us to determine whether primary peritoneal cancers respond any differently to first-line treatment.

In 2000, Eltabbakh and colleagues[79] evaluated extreme drug resistance assays in 20 patients with primary peritoneal carcinoma and compared the results to those obtained in women with epithelial ovarian cancer. They found no significant difference in the incidence of extreme drug resistance for nine commonly used drugs (cisplatin, carboplatin, paclitaxel, doxorubicin, cyclophosphamide, ifosfamide, etoposide, hexamethylmelamine, and topotecan). In this study, 19 of 20 patients were treated with paclitaxel and cisplatin. The response rate to chemotherapy for those with peritoneal cancer was 80% and was unrelated to extreme drug resistance to the individual drugs. The response rate for patients with epithelial ovarian cancer was 85.3%. The authors concluded that, because of similarities in drug resistance assays and response to chemotherapy, both peritoneal and epithelial ovarian cancer should be treated similarly.

In the salvage setting, agents that have been used successfully as second- or third-line treatments in ovarian cancer have also been used with varying success in women with primary peritoneal cancer.[3,4] Rose and associates[80] found that patients with primary peritoneal cancer who were sensitive to paclitaxel and platinum with first-line treatment could be successfully retreated with paclitaxel and carboplatinum at the time of recurrence.

Post-Treatment Surveillance

There are no studies that address the best or the most cost-effective method for clinical follow-up of women with primary peritoneal cancer once treatment has been completed. In general, women are monitored in a manner similar to those with advanced epithelial ovarian cancer. Given the very high rates of relapse (70% to 80%), the majority of women have recurrence within the first 2 years after treatment. Post-treatment surveillance in general involves regular examinations, laboratory studies, and radiographic studies, as indicated. Clinical follow-up needs to be individualized for each patient, but usually clinical examinations (including a pelvic examination) are scheduled at 3-month intervals for the first several years, when recurrence rates are highest. The majority of women with peritoneal cancer have an elevated CA 125 level before treatment. Regression of CA 125 levels during treatment usually correlates with response to chemotherapy. Post-treatment levels of CA 125 should be checked at serial intervals as well. Persistent elevations in CA 125 usually indicate recurrence.[41,77] In women without an elevated CA 125 before treatment, measurement of serum levels usually is not indicated. Routine radiographic studies in asymptomatic women with normal CA 125 levels are not indicated. However, if symptoms exist or CA 125 levels are rising, radiographic studies, usually abdominal pelvic CT scans, are indicated. There is some indication that positron emission tomography (PET) scanning may also be valuable when suspicion for disease is high and CT scans are uninformative.

Survival

Is the clinical outcome for patients with primary peritoneal cancer the same as for patients with epithelial ovarian cancer? Many of the early studies in women with primary peritoneal carcinoma revealed a survival rate that was significantly worse than that of women with epithelial ovarian cancer.[12,41,81] Median survival time ranged from 7 to 24 months, and the 5-year survival rate ranged from 0% to 22%. In many of these early studies, optimal cytoreduction was achieved significantly less often in patients with primary peritoneal cancer than in those with epithelial tumors.

In the case-control study by Killackey and Davis,[19] disease-free interval and median survival time were 3.4 and 19 months, respectively, in women with primary peritoneal cancer, compared with 11.7 and 31 months in women with epithelial ovarian cancer. All patients had been treated with platinum-containing regimens. In a study by Halperin and colleagues,[5] median survival time for women with peritoneal cancer was 17 months, compared with 40 months for women with ovarian cancer. In both of these studies, optimal cytoreduction was achieved less frequently in women with peritoneal malignancies. In a case-control study by Bloss and associates[15] in which cases and controls were matched for amount of residual disease after surgery, there were no significant differences in disease-free interval or overall survival time between women with peritoneal versus ovarian malignancies. In the GOG study in which patients with primary peritoneal carcinoma and a suboptimal cytoreduction were compared with patients who had epithelial ovarian cancer with a suboptimal cytoreduction, after both groups were treated with cisplatin and cyclophosphamide, there was no significant difference in survival rate (18% versus 24%, $P = .40$). In a study by Eltabbakh and coworkers[40] of 72 women with peritoneal cancer, the median overall survival time was 23.5 months and the 5-year survival rate was 26.5%. Those who achieved an optimal cytoreduction had a median survival time of 40 months and the 5-year survival was 45%. In a report by Kennedy and colleagues[68] in which all patients were treated postoperatively with paclitaxel and platinums, median survival time was 40 months.

Prognostic Factors

Numerous prognostic factors have been evaluated with regard to impact on survival. Fromm and associates[18] found that use of cisplatin, multiagent chemotherapy, and absence of mitoses was associated with an improved survival. Fowler and colleagues[39] found that survival was independent of age, grade, ascites, and residual disease, although there was a trend toward improved survival in the group that achieved optimal cytoreduction. Eltabbakh and coworkers[40] found that patient age, stage, performance status, and residual tumor after primary cytoreductive surgery were significant factors on univariate analysis. On multivariate analysis, only residual tumor and performance status were independent prognostic factors. Tumor grade, CA 125 level, P53 overexpression, and estrogen and progesterone receptor status did not significantly affect survival. Kowalski and colleagues[16] found that P53, HER-2/NEU overexpression, and flow cytometry had no prognostic significance.

Association with *BRCA* germline mutations

What is the incidence of primary peritoneal carcinoma in high-risk women, and should screening after prophylactic oophorectomy be offered? Reports of women developing primary peritoneal carcinoma after prophylactic oophorectomy performed for a strong family history of ovarian carcinoma led to speculation that peritoneal cancers were part of the familial breast and ovarian cancer syndrome. Piver and associates[32] reported on a series of 324 women who had undergone a prophylactic oophorectomy for a strong family history of ovarian cancer; 6 women

(1.8%) developed peritoneal cancer between 1 and 27 years after ovarian removal. Bandera and coworkers[34] screened 17 patients with peritoneal cancer using single-strand conformation polymorphism analysis and identified 2 patients (11%) with germline mutations in *BRCA1*. Halperin and associates[5] found two *BRCA1* mutations in 28 women with primary peritoneal cancer and no *BRCA2* mutations. They found no significant difference in the incidence of *BRCA1* germline mutations between patients with peritoneal versus ovarian cancer. The fact that women with *BRCA1* and possibly *BRCA2* mutations are at increased risk for primary peritoneal cancer has implications regarding recommendations for screening and prophylactic oophorectomy. In a study of 290 Jewish women who were at risk for ovarian cancer because of their family history, intensive surveillance by CA 125 measurements and ultrasonography did not seem to be an effective means of diagnosing early-stage ovarian cancer.[82] During the study, six women developed stage IIIc peritoneal cancer, and all had had normal ovaries on transvaginal ultrasound imaging. All of the primary peritoneal cancers developed in women with *BRCA1* mutations. The authors concluded that these screening modalities were not effetive in identifying early ovarian cancer and recommended genetic testing with prophylactic bilateral salpingo-oophorectomy to reduce the risk of breast and ovarian cancer. However, they acknowledged that, given the high proportion of cancers with peritoneal origins observed, it is not clear to what extent the risk of cancer is reduced by oophorectomy.

Two recent studies evaluated the benefits of prophylactic oophorectomy and the potential risk of subsequent primary peritoneal cancer. Kauff and coworkers[83] studied 170 women with *BRCA1* and *BRCA2* germline mutations. Of the 72 women who elected surveillance, ovarian/peritoneal cancers developed in 5 (6.9%). Of the 98 who underwent prophylactic oophorectomy, 3 had early tumors diagnosed at surgery, and primary peritoneal cancer developed in 1 patient during follow-up (1%). In the study by Rebbech and associates,[84] there were 551 women with *BRCA* germline mutations. Among 292 women who underwent surveillance, ovarian/peritoneal cancer developed in 58 (19.9%) during a mean follow-up period of 9 years. In contrast, among the 259 women who underwent bilateral prophylactic oophorectomy, stage I ovarian cancer was identified in 6 at the time of surgery, and primary peritoneal cancer subsequently developed in 2 others (0.8%). Each of these studies concluded that bilateral prophylactic oophorectomy significantly reduces the risk of breast and epithelial ovarian cancer. However, the risk of peritoneal cancer remains. Whether the risk of peritoneal cancer increases with time is unknown. It is reassuring to see in the Rebbech study[84] that even after a mean of 9 years, the risk of peritoneal cancer was no greater than 1%. Because the risk of peritoneal cancer remains even after prophylactic oophorectomy, ongoing investigations are studying continued surveillance with CA 125 measurements after prophylactic surgery.

REFERENCES

1. Swerdlow M. Mesothelioma of the pelvic peritoneum resembling papillary cystadenocarcinoma of the ovary. Am J Obstet Gynecol 1959;77:197.

2. Kannerstein M, Churg J, McCaughey WTE, et al. Papillary tumors of the peritoneum in women: Mesothelioma or papillary carcinoma. Am J Obstet Gynecol 1977;127:306-314.

3. Chu CS, Menzin AW, Leonard DG, et al. Primary peritoneal carcinoma: A review of the literature. Obstet Gynecol Surv 1999;54:323-335.

4. Eltabbakh GH, Piver MS. Extraovarian primary peritoneal carcinoma. Oncology (Huntingt) 1998;12:813-819.

5. Halperin R, Zehavi S, Langer R, et al. Primary peritoneal serous papillary carcinoma: A new epidemiologic trend? A matched-case comparison with ovarian serous papillary cancer. Int J Gynecol Cancer 2001;11:403-408.

6. Halperin R, Zehavi S, Hadas E, et al. Immunohistochemical comparison of primary peritoneal and primary ovarian serous papillary carcinoma. Int J Gynecol Pathol 2001;20:341-345.

7. Muto MG, Welch WR, Mok SC, et al. Evidence for a multifocal origin of papillary serous carcinoma of the peritoneum. Cancer Res 1995;55:490-492.

8. Eltabbakh GH, Piver MS, Natarajan N, Mettlin CJ. Epidemiologic differences between women with extraovarian primary peritoneal carcinoma and women with epithelial ovarian cancer. Obstet Gynecol 1998;91:254-259.

9. Rosenbloom MA, Foster RB. Probable pelvic mesothelioma: Report of a case and review of literature. Obstet Gynecol 1961; 18:213-222.

10. Rothacker D, Mobius G. Varieties of serous surface papillary carcinoma of the peritoneum in Northern Germany: A thirty-year autopsy study. Int J Gynecol Pathol 1995;14:310-18.

11. Altaras MM, Aviram R, Cohen I, et al. Primary peritoneal papillary serous adenocarcinoma: Clinical and management aspects. Gynecol Oncol 1991;40:230-236.

12. Gooneratne S, Sassone M, Blaustein A, Taleran A. Serous surface papillary carcinoma of the ovary: A clinicopathologic study of 16 cases. J Gynecol Pathol 1982;1:258-269.

13. Mulhollan TJ, Silva EG, Tornos C, et al. Ovarian involvement by serous surface papillary carcinoma. Int J Gynecol Pathol 1994;13:120-126.

14. Dalrymple JC, Bannatyne P, Russell P, et al. Extraovarian peritoneal serous papillary carcinoma: A clinicopathologic study of 31 cases. Cancer 1989;64:110-115.

15. Bloss JD, Liao SY, Buller RE, et al. Extraovarian peritoneal serous papillary carcinoma: A case-control retrospective comparison to papillary adenocarcinoma of the ovary. Gynecol Oncol 1993; 50:347-351.

16. Kowalski LD, Kanbour AI, Price FV, et al. A case-matched molecular comparison of extraovarian versus primary ovarian adenocarcinoma. Cancer 1997;79:1587-1594.

17. Feuer GA, Shevchuk M, Calanog A: Normal-sized ovary carcinoma syndrome. Obstet Gynecol 1989;73:786-792.

18. Fromm GL, Gershenson DM, Silva EG. Papillary serous carcinoma of the peritoneum. Obstet Gynecol 1990;75:75-89.

19. Killackey MA, Davis AR. Papillary serous carcinoma of the peritoneal surface: Matched-case comparison with papillary serous ovarian carcinoma. Gynecol Oncol 1993;51:171-174.

20. Ransom DT, Patel SR, Keeney GL, et al. Papillary serous carcinoma of the peritoneum: A review of 33 cases treated with platin-based chemotherapy. Cancer 1990;66:1091-1094.

21. Lele SB, Piver MS, Matharu J, Tsukada Y. Peritoneal papillary carcinoma. Gynecol Oncol 1988;31:315-320.

22. Kannerstein M, Churg J. Peritoneal mesothelioma. Hum Pathol 1977;8:83-84.

23. Legha SS, Muggia FM. Pleural mesotheliomas, clinical features and therapeutic implications. Ann Intern Med 1977;87:613-621.

24. Parmley TH, Woodruff JD. The ovarian mesothelioma. Am J Obstet Gynecol 1974;120:234-241.

25. Raju U, Fine G, Greenawald KA, Ohorodnik JM. Primary papillary serous neoplasia of the peritoneum: A clincopathologic and ultrastructural study of eight cases. Hum Pathol 1989;20:426-436.

26. Altaras MM, Aviram R, Cohen I, et al. Primary peritoneal papillary serous adenocarcinoma: Clinical and management aspects. Gynecol Oncol 1991;40:230-236.

27. Lauchlan SC. The secondary müllerian system. Obstet Gynecol Surv 1972;27:133-146.

28. White PF, Merino MJ, Barwick KW. Serous surface papillary carcinoma of the ovary: A clinical, pathologic, ultrastructural, and immunohistochemical study of 11 cases. Pathol Annu 1985; 20:403-418.

29. Tobacman JK, Tucker MA, Kase R. Intraabdominal carcinomatosis after prophylactic oophorectomy in ovarian cancer prone families. Lancet 1982;2:795-797.

30. Chen KTK, Schooley JF, Flam MS. Peritoneal carcinomatosis after prophylactic oophorectomy in familial ovarian cancer syndrome. Obstet Gynecol 1985;66(Suppl):93S-94S.

31. Menczer J, Ben-Baruch G. Familial ovarian cancer in Israeli Jewish women. Obstet Gynecol 1991;77:276-277.

32. Piver MS, Jishi MF, Tsukada Y, Nava G. Primary peritoneal carcinoma after prophylactic oophorectomy in women with a family history of ovarian cancer. Cancer 1993;71:2751-2755.

33. Piver MS. Hereditary ovarian cancer: Lessons from the first twenty years of the Gilda Radner Familial Ovarian Cancer Registry. Gynecol Oncol 2002;85:9-17.

34. Bandera CA, Muto MG, Schorge JO, et al. *BRCA1* gene mutations in women with papillary serous carcinoma of the peritoneum. Obstet Gynecol 1998;92:596-600.

35. Shmeuli E, Leider-Trejo L, Schwartz I, et al. Primary papillary serous carcinoma of the peritoneum in a man. Ann Oncol 2001;12:563-567.

36. Shah IA, Jayram L, Gani OS, et al. Papillary serous carcinoma of the peritoneum in a man: A case report. Cancer 1998;82:860-866.

37. Eltabbakh GH, Piver MS, Natarajan N, Mettlin CJ. Epidemiologic differences between women with extraovarian primary peritoneal carcinoma and women with epithelial ovarian cancer. Obstet Gynecol 1998;91:254-259.

38. Ben-Baruch G, Sivan E, Moran O, et al. Primary peritoneal serous papillary carcinoma: A study of 25 cases and comparison with stage III-IV ovarian papillary serous carcinoma. Gynecol Oncol 1996;60:393-396.

39. Fowler JM, Nieberg RK, Schooler TA, Berek JS. Peritoneal adenocarcinoma (serous) of mullerian type: A subgroup of women presenting with peritoneal carcinomatosis. Int J Gynecol Cancer 1994;4:43-51.

40. Eltabbakh GH, Werness BA, Piver S, Blumenson LE. Prognostic factors in extraovarian primary peritoneal carcinoma. Gynecol Oncol 1998;71:230-239.

41. Mills SE, Andersen WA, Fechner RE, Austin MB. Serous surface papillary carcinoma: A clinicopathologic study of 10 cases and comparison with stage III-IV ovarian serous carcinoma. Am J Surg Pathol 1988;12:827-834.

42. Kuwashima Y, Uehara T, Kurosumi M, et al. Pathological aspects of normal-sized ovarian carcinoma. Eur J Gynaecol Oncol 1996;17:17-23.

43. Shen DH, Khoo US, Xue WC, et al. Primary peritoneal malignant mixed mullerian tumors: A clinicopathologic, immunohistochemical, and genetic study. Cancer 2001;91:1052-1060.

44. Clark JE, Wood H, Jaffurs WJ, Fabro S. Endometroid-type cystadenocarcinoma arising in the mesosalpinx. Obstet Gynecol 1979;54:656-658.

45. Hampton HL, Hufman HT, Meeks GR. Extraovarian Brenner tumors. Obstet Gynecol 1992;79:844-846.

46. Lee KR, Verma U, Belinson JL. Primary clear cell carcinoma of the peritoneum. Gynecol Oncol 1991;41:259-262.

47. Banerjee R, Gough F. Cystic mucinous tumors of the mesentery and retroperitoneum: Report of three cases. Histopathology 1988;12:527-532.

48. Mirc JL, Fenoglio-Preiser CM, Husseinzadeh N. Malignant mixed mullerian tumor of extraovarian secondary mullerian system: Report of two cases and review of the literature. Arch Pathol Lab Med 1995;119:1044-1049.

49. Wick MR, Mills SE, Dehner LP, et al. Serous papillary carcinomas arising from the peritoneum and ovaries:. A clinicopathologic and immunohistochemical comparison. Int J Gynecol Pathol 1989;8:179-188.

50. Khoury N, Raju U, Crissman JD, et al. A comparative immunohistochemical study of peritoneal and ovarian serous tumors, and mesotheliomas. Hum Pathol 1990;21:811-819.

51. Attanoos RL, Webb R, Dojcinov SD, Gibbs AR. Value of mesothelial and epithelial antibodies in distinguishing diffuse

peritoneal mesothelioma in females from serous papillary carcinoma of the ovary and peritoneum. Histopathology 2002; 40:237-244.

52. Kupryjanczyk J, Thor AD, Beauchamp R, et al. Ovarian, peritoneal, and endometrial serous carcinoma: Clonal origin of multifocal disease. Mod Pathol 1996;9;166-173.

53. Pejovic T, Heim S, Mandahl N, et al. et al. Bilateral ovarian carcinoma: Cytogenic evidence of unicentric origin. Int J Cancer 1991;47:358-361.

54. Mok CH, Tsao SW, Knapp RC, et al. Unifocal origin of advanced human epithelial ovarian cancers. Cancer Res 1992;52:5119-5122.

55. Jacobs IJ, Kohler MF, Wiseman RW, et al. Clonal origin of epithelial ovarian carcinoma: Analysis by loss of heterozygosity, *p53* mutation, and X-chromosome inactivation. J Natl Cancer Inst 1992;84:1793-1798.

56. Li S, Han H, Resnik E, et al. Advanced ovarian carcinoma: Molecular evidence of unifocal origin. Gynecol Oncol 1993; 51:21-25.

57. Tsao SW, Mok CH, Knapp RC, et al. Molecular genetic evidence of a unifocal origin for human serous ovarian carcinomas. Gynecol Oncol 1993;48:5-10.

58. Eisen A, Weber BL. Primary peritoneal carcinoma can have multifocal origins: Implications for prophylactic oophorectomy. J Natl Cancer Inst 1998;90:797-799.

59. Schorge JO, Muto MG, Welch WR, et al. Molecular evidence for multifocal papillary serous carcinoma of the peritoneum in patients with germline *BRCA1* mutations. J Natl Cancer Inst 1998;90:841-845.

60. Schorge JO, Muto MG, Lee SJ, et al. *BRCA1*-related papillary serous carcinoma of the peritoneum has a unique molecular pathogenesis. Cancer Res 2000;60:1361-1364.

61. Nishimura M, Wakabayashi M, Hashimoto T, et al. Papillary serous carcinoma of the peritoneum: Analysis of clonality of peritoneal tumors. J Gastroenterol 2000;35:540-547.

62. Zissin R, Hertz M, Shapiro-Feinberg M, et al. Primary serous papillary carcinoma of the peritoneum: CT findings. Clin Radiol 2001;56:740-745.

63. Truong LD, Maccato ML, Awalt H, et al. Serous surface carcinoma of the peritoneum: A clinicopathologic study of 22 cases. Hum Pathol 1990;21:99-110.

65. Griffiths CT. Surgical resection of tumor bulk in the primary treatment of ovarian cancer. Natl Cancer Inst Monogr 1975; 42:101.

65. Hoskins WJ, Bundy BN, Thigpen JT, Omura GA. The influence of cytoreductive surgery on recurrence-free interval and survival in small-volume stage III epithelial ovarian cancer: A Gynecologic Oncology Group study. Gynecol Oncol 1992;47:159-166.

66. Bristow RE, Tomacruz RS, Armstrong DK, et al. Survival effect of maximal cytoreductive surgery for advanced ovarian carcinoma during the platinum era: A meta-analysis. J Clin Oncol 2002;20:1248-1259.

67. Strand CM, Grosh WW, Baxter J, et al. Peritoneal carcinomatosis of unknown primary site in women: A distinctive subset of adenocarcinoma. Ann Intern Med 1989;111:213-217.

68. Kennedy AW, Markman M, Webster KD, et al. Experience with platinum-paclitaxel chemotherapy in the initial management of papillary serous carcinoma of the peritoneum. Gynecol Oncol 1998;71:288-290.

69. Junor EJ, Hole DJ, McNulty L, et al. Specialist gynaecologists and survival outcome in ovarian cancer: A Scottish national study of 1866 patients. Br J Obstet Gynaecol 1999;106:1130-1136.

70. Wolfe CD, Tiling K, Raju KS. Management and survival of ovarian cancer patients in south east England. Eur J Cancer 1997;33: 1835-1840.

71. Schwartz PE, Chambers JT, Makuch R. Neoadjuvant chemotherapy for advanced ovarian cancer. Gynecol Oncol 1994;53:33-37.

72. Surwit E, Childers J, Atlas I, et al. Neoadjuvant chemotherapy for advanced ovarian cancer. Inter J Gynecol Cancer 1996;6: 356-361.

73. Ozols RF, Rubin SC, Thomas GM, Robboy SJ. Epithelial ovarian cancer. In Hoskins WJ, Perez CA, Young RC (eds): Principles and Practice of Gynecologic Oncology, 3rd ed. Philadelphia, Lippincott Williams & Wilkins, 2000, pp 981-1057.

74. Bloss JD, Brady M, Rocereto T, et al. A phase II trial of cisplatin and cyclophosphamide in the treatment of extraovarian peritoneal serous papillary carcinoma with comparison to papillary serous ovarian carcinoma: A Gynecologic Oncology Group study [abstract 150]. Gynecol Oncol 1998;68:109.

75. McGuire WP, Hoskins WJ, Brady MF, et al. Cyclophosphamide and cisplatin compared with paclitaxel and cisplatin in patients with stage III and stage IV ovarian cancer. N Engl J Med 1996; 334:1-6.

76. Wall JE, Mandrell BN, Jenkins JJ 3rd, et al. Effectiveness of paclitaxel in treating serous carcinoma of the peritoneum in an adolescent. Am J Obstet Gynecol 1995;172:1049-1052.

77. Menzin AW, Aikins JK, Wheeler JE, Rubin SC. Surgically documented responses to paclitaxel and cisplatin in patients with primary peritoneal carcinoma. Gynecol Oncol 1996; 62:55-58.

78. Aikins JK, Paulson J, Arnold G, et al. Comparison of paclitaxel/ cisplatin to cyclophosphamide/cisplatinol in incompletely resected papillary serous peritoneal cancer [abstract 143]. Gynecol Oncol 1998;68:107.

79. Eltabbakh GH. Extreme drug resistance assay and response to chemotherapy in patients with primary peritoneal carcinoma. J Surg Oncol 2000;73:148-152.

80. Rose PG, Fusco N, Fluellen L, Rodriguez M. Second-line therapy with paclitaxel and carboplatin for recurrent disease following first-line therapy with palitaxel and platinum in ovarian and peritoneal carcinoma. J Clin Oncol 1998;16:1494-1497.

81. Foyle A, Al Jabi M, McCaughey WTE. Papillary peritoneal tumors in women. Am J Surg Pathol 1981;5:241-249.

82. Liede A, Karlan BY, Baldwin RL, et al. Cancer incidence in a population of Jewish women at risk of ovarian cancer. J Clin Oncol 2002;20:1570-1577.

83. Kauff ND, Satagopan JM, Robson ME, et al. Risk-reducing salpingo-oophorectomy in women with a *BRCA1* or *BRCA2* mutation. N Engl J Med 2002;346:1609-1615.

84. Rebbech TR, Lynch HT, Neuhausen SL, et al. Prophylactic oophorectomy in carriers of *BRCA1* or *BRCA2* mutations. N Engl J Med 2002;346:1616-1622.

85. Piver MS, Eltabbakh GH, Hempling RE, et al. Two sequential studies for primary peritoneal carcinoma: Induction with weekly cisplatin followed by either cisplatin-doxorubicin-cyclophosphamide or paclitaxel-cisplatin. Gynecol Oncol 1997; 67:141-146.

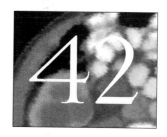

PRIMARY FALLOPIAN TUBE CANCER

Margaret Lorraine Jeune Davy and *Bruce Gordon Ward*

 MAJOR CONTROVERSIES

- **What is the relationship between fallopian tube carcinoma and genetic mutations?**
- **How should fallopian tube cancer be diagnosed and staged?**

Carcinoma of the fallopian tube was previously of interest as a clinical oddity compared with other gynecologic malignancies. It accounts for 0.15% to 1.8% of all primary genital tract malignancies.[1] The cause of the malignancy remains poorly understood. However, with the expansion of clinical genetics and the identification of tumor-associated and predisposing genetic mutations, studies have shed a degree of light on this area. Clinical studies have led to a better understanding of the biologic behavior of the disease, with implications particularly in the area of surgical treatment and staging. Studies comparing chemotherapy responses between ovarian cancer and fallopian tube cancer suggest that response rates and survival are not equivalent, making the distinction between these two conditions important prognostically.

What is the relationship between fallopian tube carcinoma and genetic mutations?

Initially, a series of anecdotal reports linked the diagnosis of fallopian tube cancers with cancer families. The earliest of these was appreciated in 1994, before the cloning of the *BRCA1* gene.[2] In 2000, two such cases were linked to abnormalities in *BRCA1* function,[3] and additional cases have been added in increasingly more impressive detail since then.[4] Histopathologic examination of fallopian tubes removed at prophylactic surgery designed to protect against familial ovarian cancer has demonstrated dysplastic and malignant changes in as many as 50% of the women studied.[5] In one observational study, of 44 women at high risk for ovarian cancer who were undergoing prophylactic surgery, 37% demonstrated dysplastic tubal epithelium, but only 1 of 87 such women examined showed dysplasia in an ovarian inclusion cyst. Based on the ultrastructural findings of the cells from which the dysplastic epithelium arose and particularly the presence of ciliated cells, the researchers postulated an origin of such ovarian dysplasia from tubal epithelium seeding of the ovarian surface.[6] In a similar study, 3 of 30 women undergoing prophylactic pelvic clearance because of a strong probability of developing ovarian cancer had fallopian tube carcinomas; two were in situ carcinomas, and one was invasive.[4]

Although fallopian tube cancer is rare in the general population, in *BRCA1* carriers, a 120-fold increase in risk has been calculated using the Surveillance, Epidemiology and End Results (SEER) database.[7]

Conversely, although the number of women studied has been expectedly small, women diagnosed with fallopian tube cancer have a significantly increased risk of carrying a mutation of *BRCA1* or *BRCA2*. In one study, 16% of 44 women tested carried a mutation, and this risk climbs to 28% if the diagnosis was made before the age of 55 years.[8] Two of three Jewish women in this study carried founder mutations expected in their subpopulation.

There are three consequences of these observations. First, women with a diagnosis of fallopian tube cancer should undergo genetic testing for *BRCA1* and *BRCA2* mutations. Second, prophylactic surgery in *BRCA1* and *BRCA2* mutation carriers should be directed toward preventing fallopian tube cancer and ovarian cancer. Some investigators have suggested that prophylactic surgery should always include hysterectomy on the principle that the intramural portion of the tube remains in situ and potentially at risk if the uterus is left.[3,9,10,11] The benefit of being able to give estrogen replacement alone, without the requirement for progestational protection of the endometrium, is seen as an additional bonus for women requiring hormone replacement therapy. Others, however, argue that this remains to be proved and is unnecessarily invasive,[12,13] particularly because these mutation carriers do not seem to harbor an increased risk of endometrial cancer.[14] Quillin and colleagues[15] attempted to quantify the risk, making the point that although the relative risk is increased, the absolute risk is small—on the order of 3%. The third consequence is that relatives of women diagnosed with fallopian tube cancer are at increased risk for breast and ovarian cancer.

How should fallopian tube cancer be diagnosed and staged?

The impact of the preceding investigations has been an impetus to focus more closely on an accurate diagnosis of fallopian tube cancer so that the lessons learned can be applied in a logical manner. Traditionally, this diagnosis has been restricted to cases that fulfilled the strict criteria established by Hu[16] in 1950. These criteria include the following:

- The bulk of the tumor must be in the tube and have arisen from the endosalpinx.
- The transition from benign to malignant epithelium should be clearly demonstrated.
- There should be no nexus between tubal and ovarian disease.[16]

With the application of these criteria, the diagnosis of fallopian tube cancer has been a rare event, with few institutions able to report series of more than a few cases. Because of this, prognosis for this cancer has been variably reported between dismal[17] and highly optimistic.[18] It is thought that a significant number of cases of disseminated fallopian tube cancer are diagnosed as ovarian or peritoneal carcinomas because of the application of Hu's principles. In 1994, the observation was made that in a large series of women screened for ovarian cancer by a combination of CA 125 estimation and ultrasound of the pelvis, the ratio of ovarian to tubal cancers found was only 6:1, considerably less than that suggested by the literature.[19] A likely cause for the high diagnostic incidence of tubal cancers may have been the presence of a larger than normally seen representation of localized tumors for which the origin of the disease could be more accurately assessed. The default position is that all doubtful cases are diagnosed as *not* being primary fallopian tube cancer.

Does this matter? The link between fallopian tube cancer and genetic mutations would, if proved, be sufficient reason by itself for the implementation of greater accuracy in diagnosis, but there are also emerging biologic reasons to more clearly delineate fallopian tube cancers from ovarian or peritoneal cancers.

Two studies suggest that the survival for women with fallopian tube cancer is superior to that for women with ovarian cancer when standardized for stage.[18,20] Surprisingly, perhaps, other data focus on the importance of lymphatic spread in this disease, with staging lymphadenectomy reporting high rates of pelvic and para-aortic node involvement early in the disease process[21,22] and examination of treatment failures suggesting a higher than previously expected rate of retroperitoneal recurrence. On a more optimistic note, performance of a comprehensive lymphadenectomy in these patients may be associated with a significant lengthening of the median survival time.[22] Earlier reports with inferior survival data may reflect a less vigorous approach to the management of retroperitoneal disease in the women. Although the position of routine lymphadenectomy in ovarian cancer has not been defined clearly, a diagnosis of fallopian tube cancer should lead to such a procedure. It appears that adjuvant chemotherapy should use the combination of carboplatin and paclitaxel. Response rates to this regimen of 80% or higher can be expected.

Future Research

There is an urgent need for a centralized data collection system to analyze and report on these clinical matters. This could be along lines similar to the current hereditary cancer registries that are hospital based or coordinated regionally. Such a registry would collect and collate data on family history, results of genetic screening for *BRCA1/2*, surgical staging (including pelvic and para-aortic node dissection), details of adjuvant therapy, and subsequent clinical outcome. The disease is not sufficiently common to allow large, randomized trials of treatment options, but a large data set of the outcomes of current best practices may convince clinicians who are not gynecologic oncologists to approach these patients in a more curative and positive way.

References

1. Peters WA, Andersen WA, Hopkins MP, et al: Prognostic features of carcinoma of the fallopian tube. Obstet Gynecol 1988; 71:757-762.
2. Sobol H, Jacquemier J, Bonaiti C, et al: Fallopian tube cancer as a feature of BRCA1-associated syndromes. Gynecol Oncol 2000; 78:263-266.
3. Zweemer RP, vanDiest PJ, Verheijen RH, et al: Molecular evidence linking primary cancer of the fallopian tube to BRCA1 germline mutations. Gynecol Oncol 2000;76:45-50.
4. Leeper K, Garcia R, Swisher E, et al: Pathologic findings in prophylactic oophorectomy specimens in high-risk women. Gynecol Oncol 2002;87:52-56.

5. Piek JM, vanDiest PJ, Zweemer RP, et al: Dysplastic changes in prophylactically removed fallopian tubes in women predisposed to developing ovarian cancer. J Pathol 2001;195:451-456.

6. Piek JM, Verheijen RH, Kenemens P, et al: BRCA 1/2–related ovarian cancers are of tubal origin: A hypothesis. Gynecol Oncol 2003;90:49.

7. Brose MS, Rebbeck TR, Calzone KA, et al: Cancer risk estimates for BRCA1 mutation carriers identified in a risk evaluation program. J Natl Cancer Inst 2002;94:1365-1372.

8. Aziz S, Kuperstein G, Rosen B, et al: A genetic and epidemiological study of carcinoma of the fallopian tube. Gynecol Oncol 2001;80:341-345.

9. Paley PJ, Swisher EM, Garcia RL, et al: Occult cancer of the fallopian tube in BRCA-1 germline mutation carriers at prophylactic oophorectomy: A case for recommending hysterectomy at surgical prophylaxis. Gynecol Oncol 2001;80:176-180.

10. Paley PJ: Reply. Gynecol Oncol 2001;83:446-447.

11. Boyd J: BRCA: The breast, ovarian, and other cancer genes. Gynecol Oncol 2001;80:337-340.

12. Morice P, Pautier P, Delaloge S: Prophylactic surgery in patients with inherited risk of ovarian cancer. Gynecol Oncol 2001;83:445-446.

13. Ansink AC, Burger CW, Seynaeve C: Occult cancer in the fallopian tube in patients with a BRCA-1 germline mutation. Gynecol Oncol 2001;83:445.

14. Levine DA, Lin O, Barakat RR, et al: Risk of endometrial carcinoma associated with BRCA mutation. Gynecol Oncol 2001;80:395-398.

15. Quillin JM, Boardman CH, Bodurtha J, Smith T: Preventive gynecologic surgery for BRCA1/2 carriers—Information for decision making. Gynecol Oncol 2001;83:168-170.

16. Hu CY, Taymor ML, Hertig AT: Primary carcinoma of the fallopian tube. Am J Obstet Gynecol 1950;59:58-67.

17. Obermair A, Taylor KH, Janda M, et al: Primary fallopian tube cancer: The Queensland experience. Intl J Gynecol Cancer 2001;11:69-72.

18. Gemignani ML, Hensley ML, Cohen R, et al: Paclitaxel-based chemotherapy in carcinoma of the fallopian tube. Gynecol Oncol 2001;80:16-20.

19. Woolas R, Jacobs I, Davies AP, et al: What is the true incidence of primary fallopian tube carcinoma? Int J Gynecol Cancer 1994;4:384-388.

20. Kosary C, Trimble EL: Treatment and survival for women with fallopian tube carcinoma—A population based study. Gynecol Oncol 2002;86:190-191.

21. Gadducci A, Landoni F, Sartori E, et al: Analysis of treatment failures and survival of patients with fallopian tube carcinoma: A Cooperative Task Force (CTF) study. Gynecol Oncol 2001;81:150-159.

22. Klein M, Graf AH, Rosen A, Lahousen M: Analysis of treatment failures and survival of patients with fallopian tube carcinoma: A cooperative task force study [letter]. Gynecol Oncol 2002;84:351.

GESTATIONAL TROPHOBLASTIC DISEASE

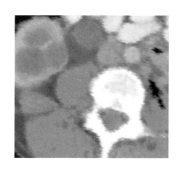

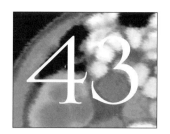

EPIDEMIOLOGY, GENETICS, AND MOLECULAR BIOLOGY OF GESTATIONAL TROPHOBLASTIC DISEASE

Ross S. Berkowitz   and   Donald P. Goldstein

 MAJOR CONTROVERSIES

- Why does the incidence of complete molar pregnancy vary in different global regions?
- Are molar pregnancies generally characterized by an excess dose of paternal genes?
- Do diploid partial moles exist?
- Does relaxation of genomic imprinting occur in gestational trophoblastic disease?
- Do heterozygous complete moles have a higher risk of developing persistent gestational trophoblastic tumor?
- Which protooncogenes, tumor suppressor genes, and growth factors are altered in gestational trophoblastic disease?
- Is there alteration of cell adhesion molecules and proteinases in gestational trophoblastic disease?

The term *gestational trophoblastic disease* (GTD) comprises a group of interrelated diseases, including partial and complete molar pregnancy, invasive mole, placental-site trophoblastic tumor, and choriocarcinoma, that have varying propensities for local invasion and dissemination.[1] During the past decade, important advances have occurred in our understanding of the epidemiology, genetics, and molecular biology of GTD. This chapter reviews areas of controversy in these fields.

Why does the incidence of complete molar pregnancy vary in different global regions?

The reported incidence of complete mole varies dramatically in different regions of the world.[2] The frequency of molar pregnancies in Asian countries is 7 to 10 times greater than the reported incidence in Europe or North America.[3] Whereas the incidence of complete mole in the United States is about 1 in every 1500 live births, complete mole occurs in Taiwan in 1 of every 125 pregnancies. Variations in the incidence of complete molar pregnancy may result in part from differences between hospital-based versus population-based data. The incidence of molar pregnancy may be decreasing in some Asian countries. In South Korea, the hospital-based incidence of GTD decreased from 40.2 per 1000 deliveries during the period 1971-1975 to 2.3 per 1000 deliveries during 1991-1995.[4] In Japan, the incidence of molar pregnancy per 1000 live births declined from 2.70 in 1974 to 1.86 in 1993.[5]

The high incidence of complete molar pregnancy in some populations has been attributed to nutritional and socioeconomic factors. We observed in a case-control study that the risk for complete mole progressively increased with decreasing levels of consumption of animal fat and dietary carotene (vitamin A precursor).[6] Parazzini and colleagues[7] also reported from Italy that an increased risk for GTD was associated with low carotene consumption. Vitamin A deficiency in the rhesus monkey produces degeneration of the seminiferous epithelium with production of primitive spermatogonia and spermatocytes.[8] Global regions with a high incidence of complete molar pregnancy correspond to areas with a high frequency of vitamin A deficiency. Dietary factors such as carotene may partly explain the regional variation in the incidence of complete molar pregnancy.

Are molar pregnancies generally characterized by an excess dose of paternal genes?

Analysis of polymorphic chromosomal markers, such as chromosomal banding heteromorphisms[9] and hypervariable DNA sequences,[10] has shown that complete hydatidiform moles (CHMs) are composed solely of paternal DNA. Complete mole is a unique conception in that all nuclear DNA is paternally derived and all cytoplasmic DNA is maternally derived. Approximately 90% of complete moles have a 46,XX karyotype.[11] It is estimated that 75%[12] to 85%[13] of CHMs are homozygous at all polymorphic markers. This would result from fertilization of an "empty" ovum by a haploid (23,X) sperm that then duplicates its own chromosomes, giving rise to a 46,XX conception. The maternal chromosomes may be either inactivated or absent.[14] The mechanism of loss of the maternal genome is unknown, but possibilities include the exclusion of maternal chromosomes in the cell divisions that follow fertilization. All chromosomes come from the father, whereas the mitochondrial DNA is derived from the mother.[15] Although most complete moles have a 46,XX karyotype, 10% to 15% result from dispermy with fertilization of an "empty" ovum by two sperm. Approximately 6% to 10% of all complete moles have a 46,XY genotype,[16] and another 5%[12] are heterozygous 46,XX cases.

It is important to emphasize that all the chromosomes in CHM are paternal in origin. A CHM is therefore a complete allograft and should stimulate a vigorous immunologic response from the maternal host. However, there is also a maternal contribution to the development of complete mole, because mitochondrial DNA is maternally derived.

At least 90% of partial moles have a triploid karyotype.[17] However, the triploid conceptus has two phenotypes: a partial mole resulting from the fertilization of an apparently normal ovum by two sperm[18] and a more developed fetus without a molar placenta if the extra haploid set is maternally derived.[19] Both complete and partial moles are therefore characterized by an excessive dose of paternal genes.

Completion of normal development requires a genetic contribution from both parents. Perhaps the most compelling evidence of this fact is that asexual reproduction (parthenogenesis and androgenesis) has never produced a viable mammalian offspring. More elaborate evidence of requisite biparental contributions comes from experiments by Surani and associates[20] in which androgenetic or gynogenetic mouse embryos were created by microtransfer of the zygotic pronuclei of fertilized eggs. Gynogenetic embryos transplanted to a foster mother developed only a small placenta with a secondarily stunted embryo, whereas comparable androgenetic embryos had a bulky hypertrophic placenta and a rudimentary embryo,[21] mimicking a human complete molar gestation. The general impression is that both parental genomes are needed for complete development, with the paternal DNA being required for extraembryonic differentiation and maternal DNA for embryonic growth and development.

Do diploid partial moles exist?

Partial moles generally result from fertilization of an apparently normal ovum by two sperm, which results in a triploid conception.[10,17,18] However, some investigators have reported that nontriploid partial moles compose 0.5% to 15% of all partial mole cases.[22-24] Furthermore, diploid partial moles have been reported to carry a particular risk of developing persistent gestational trophoblastic tumor.[25] However, the diagnosis of nontriploid partial mole may potentially be explained by erroneous diagnosis of nontriploidy due to inadvertant sampling of diploid maternal tissues or pathologic misclassification of hydropic nonmolar placenta or early complete mole.

Because of changes in clinical practice, CHM is now diagnosed earlier in pregnancy. Although it was previously diagnosed typically in the second trimester, CHM is now commonly diagnosed in the first trimester.[26,27] The pathologic features of CHM are substantially different in the first trimester.[28,29] First-trimester CHMs have significantly less circumferential trophoblastic hyperplasia, a smaller villous diameter, less necrosis, and more primitive villous stroma. First-trimester complete moles have subtle morphologic alterations that may result in their misclassification as diploid partial moles or nonmolar spontaneous abortions.

Genest and colleagues[30] recently conducted a re-evaluation of pathology and ploidy in 19 putative nontriploid partial moles using standardized histologic diagnostic criteria and repeat flow cytometric testing. On review, 11 were diploid nonpartial moles (initially misclassified as to pathology), 7 were triploid partial moles (initial misclassification as to ploidy), and 1 was a diploid early complete mole (initially misclassified as to pathology). Nontriploid partial moles probably do not exist. Careful re-evaluation of all specimens of presumed nontriploid partial moles is likely to uncover pathologic or ploidy errors in almost all cases.

Does relaxation of genomic imprinting occur in gestational trophoblastic disease?

It appears that some chromosomal regions or specific genes are imprinted such that expression is restricted to one parent's allele.[31-34] *Genomic imprinting* is the process whereby paternal and maternal DNA acquire divergent functions.[34,35] The embryos of normal gestations express H19 (an RNA molecule) only from the maternal allele and insulin-like growth factor 2 (IGF2) only from the paternal allele, whereas both paternal alleles are expressed in androgenetic CHMs. Because the predominant genetic feature of CHMs is the paternal source of the genome, this process of imprinting may play a pivotal role in explaining the molar phenotype.

A change in the biparental balance of the embryonic genome might alter the effective dose of imprinted genes or even the imprinting process itself. Because androgenetic CHMs contain two paternal alleles, these tissues might express a double dose of genes (e.g., *IGF2*). Modification of paternal imprints has been associated with tumor formation. Maternally expressed *H19* gene in the villous cytotrophoblastic cells of the androgenetic CHM represents relaxation of imprinting and may be associated with its malignant potential.[36,37]

It was reported that paternal uniparental disomy in the region of chromosome 11, which contains the imprinted genes *H19* and *IGF2*,[38,39] produces placentomegaly with hydropic villi, including cistern formation, mimicking hydatidiform mole.[40] *H19* is normally expressed in embryos only from the maternal allele.[41] The regulation of *H19* activity is critical for the growth and differentiation of trophoblasts.[42] Indistinct boundaries between abnormal embryogenesis and tumorigenesis serve as a reminder that both may be affected by the imprinting process.

Do heterozygous complete moles have a higher risk of developing persistent gestational trophoblastic tumor?

In some series, complete moles with a heterozygous genotype reportedly have a higher risk of developing persistent gestational trophoblastic tumor (GTT).[13,43] Wake and colleagues[13] reported a persistence rate of 50% after heterozygous complete moles and only 4% for homozygous complete moles.[13] Hypervariable DNA markers permit recognition of heterozygous XX moles, and polymerase chain reaction (PCR) is capable of objectively identifying XY heterozygotes.[10,44] Studies have shown that dispermic (heterozygous) complete moles carry no greater risk than monospermic (homozygous) complete moles do for development of GTT.[10,44] Mutter and coworkers[37] studied the frequency of Y chromosome in complete moles that resulted in metastatic GTT. There was no increased risk for metastatic GTT in Y chromosome–positive compared with Y chromosome–negative complete moles. It therefore appears that heterozygous (dispermic) complete moles are not at greater risk of developing persistent GTT.

Which protooncogenes, tumor suppressor genes, and growth factors are altered in gestational trophoblastic disease?

There is strong evidence that a tumor is a clone of cells derived from a single ancestral cell in which the initiating event (a somatic mutation) has taken place.[45] The clonal nature of tumors has been recognized for many years. The basic mechanism in all cancers is mutation, either in the germline or, much more frequently, in somatic cells. Genes that cause cancer are of two distinct types: oncogenes and tumor suppressor genes. The two types have opposite effects in carcinogenesis. Oncogenes facilitate malignant transformation, whereas tumor suppressor genes, as the name implies, block tumor development by regulating genes involved in cell growth. Both activation of protooncogenes and inactivation of tumor suppressor genes are involved in the genesis and progression of various kinds of human tumors.

Oncogenes have a dominant effect at the cellular level; that is, when activated, a single mutant allele may be sufficient to change the phenotype of a cell from normal to malignant. Structural mutation is only one of the several mechanisms that can induce activation of protooncogenes. Chromosomal translocations are a common mechanism for protooncogene activation in a variety of cancers. If an oncogene is altered or overexpressed, either as a result of a mutation in the gene itself or through altered external control, the cell in which the change occurred can undergo uncontrolled growth, eventually becoming malignant. Most oncogenes are mutated ("activated") forms of normal genes, called protooncogenes, that are involved in the control of cell proliferation and differentiation. Whereas the products of protooncogenes promote growth, the products of tumor suppressor genes contribute to malignancy only if the function of both alleles is lost. One of the surprising findings about tumor progression is that loss or inactivation of the same genes may contribute to development of several different common cancers. Furthermore, several mutations at different loci are required if a tumor is to reach its full malignant potential.

Homozygous deletions usually serve to remove and inactivate tumor suppressor genes, such as *RB1*, *TP53*, *DCC*, *WT1*, and *NF1* genes. Homozygous deletions are rare genetic events but they have played a critical role as molecular markers for the identification of tumor suppressor genes. Studies indicate that the gene encoding P53 is a tumor suppressor in its native form, because the expression of wild-type P53 restrains tumor development.[45]

In several tumor systems, protooncogene or tumor suppressor gene mutations can be implicated in the events leading to neoplastic transformation and tumor progression.[46] There are reports of increased CSF1R (c-fms) RNA in CHM, compared with normal placentas,[47] and increased MYC and RAS RNA in choriocarcinoma.[48] Additionally, BeWo choriocarcinoma cells also express FOS. Oncogenes may play a role in trophoblast proliferation. The β-chain of platelet-derived growth factor (PDGF) is encoded by *SIS* (now called *PDGFB*). PDGF and other mitogens activate MYC and FOS, and detection of PDGFB in the trophoblast in early pregnancy may indicate autocrine growth regulation by placental control of oncogene expression. The significance of such simple quantitative changes in expression by an abnormal trophoblast is in some cases hard to evaluate, because several protooncogenes are already expressed at high levels in normal placentas.[49-51] A study of five choriocarcinoma cell lines showed MYC amplification and CSF1R (formerly c-fms) rearrangement.[52] Choriocarcinoma cell lines contain abnormally high MDM2 protein levels, which could be attributed to enhanced translation of *MDM2* messenger RNA (mRNA). The translational enhancement of MDM2 expression occurs in a variety of human tumor cells. Most of these latter tumor cells—like choriocarcinoma cells—also have high levels of wild-type P53 protein.

There have been several studies of growth factors and their receptors in GTD. Epidermal growth factor receptors (EGFR) are expressed more strongly in molar placentas than in normal placentas of similar gestational age. Tumors with a histologic diagnosis of invasive mole and choriocarcinoma show very strong binding of EGFR. EGFR binds both epidermal growth factor and transforming growth factor (TGF-α), thereby activating several cellular processes. EGFR and its related family of tyrosine kinases consist of EGFR (formerly ERBB), ERBB2, ERBB3, and ERBB4.[53,54] EGFR family products are transmembrane signaling molecules that share close structural homology and have all been implicated in cell transformation and tumor pathogenesis. EGFR expression has been associated with secretion of human chorionic gonadotropin, and after exposure to chemotherapy, EGFR binding sites have been noted to be diminished in choriocarcinoma cells.[55-59]

It was observed that the level of expression of EGFR and ERBB2 in choriocarcinoma was significantly greater in the syncytiotrophoblast and cytotrophoblast of complete mole than in the syncytiotrophoblast and cytotrophoblast of placenta and partial mole.[60,61] This observation was consistent in both immunohistochemical and in situ hybridization studies. In general, expression of ERBB3 and ERBB4 did not differ significantly among placental and GTD tissues.[61] Interestingly, in complete mole the strong expression of EGFR and ERBB3 in the extravillous trophoblasts was significantly associated with the development of persistent postmolar GTT.[61] Yang and coworkers[62] also observed increased expression of ERBB2 in complete moles that developed persistent GTT.[62] Therefore, the EGFR-related family of oncogenes may be important in the pathogenesis of GTD. The increased expression of EGFR, ERBB2, and ERBB3 in complete mole may also influence the development of persistent GTT. Further studies of EGFR and its related family of oncogenes may provide important insights into the biology and clinical behavior of GTD and contribute to the care of patients with these diseases.

BCL2 expression, which is considered an antagonist of apoptosis, was shown to be present in syncytiotrophoblast but not in cytotrophoblast in normal placentas.[63] Apoptosis, a gene-directed program of cell death, is the major mode of cell death. Compared to necrosis, it is an energy-dependent suicidal process that involves a series of well-regulated synthetic events. In addition to prevention of apoptosis, the *BCL2* gene may also play an important role in the path to terminal differentiation. Many drugs currently used in chemotherapy for GTD (e.g., etoposide, methotrexate, vincristine) have also been shown to be effective in the induction of apoptosis in a wide range of cell lines. The trophoblast may be destined to cell death at the end of pregnancy, whereas the trophoblast in GTTs escapes programmed cell death.

Wong and colleagues[63] reported extensive apoptosis in syncytiotrophoblasts, cytotrophoblasts, and villous stromal cells in all hydatidiform mole cases. In normal placentas, positive nuclei for apoptosis were found exclusively in syncytiotrophoblasts. Apoptotic activities were significantly different among various categories of trophoblastic lesions ($P < .001$); in ascending order, normal placentas had less activity than spontaneous abortions, which had less than choriocarcinomas, which had less than hydatidiform moles. In fact, hydatidiform moles had the highest apoptotic activity among various categories of trophoblastic lesions. Furthermore, apoptotic activities of those CHMs that spontaneously regressed was statistically higher than those that developed persistent GTT requiring chemotherapy. This indicates that apoptosis is a crucial event in the regression of hydatidiform moles. In regard to genes regulating apoptosis, apoptotic activities of trophoblastic lesions in general correlated inversely with BCL2 expression, but no significant correlation was found between apoptotic activity and expression of BAX (BCL2-associated X protein). BCL2 protein was significantly more strongly expressed in the syncytiotrophoblast of CHM and choriocarcinoma than in normal placenta or partial mole.[60] The apoptotic index, which reflects apoptotic activity, may be a useful prognostic marker for hydatidiform moles. According to Sakuragi and associates,[64] the relatively low expression of BCL2 in choriocarcinoma cells may render them more susceptible to apoptosis.

Expression of oncogenes, growth factors, and their receptors represents a potentially fruitful area for future investigations. If their role is indeed concerned with control of growth and differentiation, comparison of normal pregnancy with GTD may be worthwhile. Further studies are required to determine whether a specific pattern of oncogene expression is characteristic of invasive trophoblastic neoplasia and could predict malignant potential.

Cellular proliferation is an intricately regulated process that is mediated by the coordinated interactions of critical protooncogenes and tumor suppressor genes. Changes in expression pattern of these genes (e.g., *TP53, MDM2, TP21, RB1*) have been shown to contribute to tumorigenesis in multiple tumor systems. Because the trophoblast develops in an environment that is uniquely rich in hormones and growth factors, interactions among multiple growth factors are also likely.[65]

The *MDM2* oncogene has transforming activity that can be activated by overexpression. The *MDM2* gene has been found to be amplified in several human tumors, indicating that MDM2 overexpression may play a role in tumorigenesis.[66] Investigators found overexpression of MDM2 protein in complete mole and choriocarcinoma specimens.[67] They also found overexpression of P53, P21, and RB1 tumor suppressor gene products in both complete mole and choriocarcinoma. The overexpression of wild-type P53 in cells may lead to the cessation of cell proliferation.[68]

The interaction of P53 and MDM2 proteins may play an important role in regulating cell division.[69] Several tumors, including sarcomas, glioblastomas, anaplastic astrocytomas, and complete moles, have been reported to exhibit increased expression of wild-type P53 protein.[70-72]

In addition to the overexpression of MDM2, 24 of 25 complete moles and all 11 choriocarcinoma cases had overexpression of P53 in the nucleus, and no P53 mutation was detected (one nonsense).[67] The MDM2 gene product is believed to act as a cellular regulator of the P53 protein, because it can bind to wild-type P53 protein. The overexpression of MDM2 can overcome the growth-suppressive properties of wild-type P53 protein and may result in neoplastic transformation.[71] Therefore, it is likely that certain human tumors escape from P53-regulated growth control by amplification and overexpression of MDM2. Overexpression of MDM2 may also promote tumorigenesis by mechanisms other than inactivation of the P53 protein.[72] For example, overexpressed MDM2 proteins may form a complex with RB1 proteins and block RB1 protein suppression of cell activation, which may result in RB1 overexpression in these tumors.[73]

MDM2 may therefore inhibit the action of both P53 and RB1 tumor suppressor gene products.[73] Complete moles and choriocarcinomas, which have high levels of expression of both wild-type P53 protein and MDM2 protein, may represent another type of tumor with abnormal P53 expression.

The *P21* oncogene is regulated by P53, although a P53-independent induction pathway has been identified. Several growth factors such as EGF, fibroblast growth factor (FGF), TGF-α, and granulocyte-macrophage colony-stimulating factor (GM-CSF) can induce P21 expression in cells carrying the wild-type *P53* gene.[74] It was observed that P21 was mainly expressed in syncytiotrophoblast, which has a high concentration of these growth factor receptors.[67,75-78] The expression of P21 was stronger in complete mole and choriocarcinoma than in normal placenta or partial mole.[67] However, whereas P53 was primarily expressed in cytotrophoblast, P21 was mainly expressed in syncytiotrophoblast. Interestingly, the MDM2 protein may also indirectly block the function of P21 through formation of complexes with the RB1 gene product.[73]

In conclusion, altered expression of *TP53*, *TP21*, *RB1*, and *MDM2* may be important in the pathogenesis

of both complete mole and choriocarcinoma. However, unlike complete molar pregnancy, partial mole is not characterized by overexpression of P53. Overexpression of P53 and MDM2 proteins in complete mole and choriocarcinoma may be associated with a more aggressive behavior in GTD.

The development and maintenance of functional tissue structure depends on the balance among cellular proliferation, maturation, and apoptosis. The regulation of trophoblast cell proliferation involves a delicate balance between the expression of proto-oncogenes and tumor suppressor genes. Deregulation of either set of oncogenes may lead to uncontrolled cell proliferation, terminal cell cycle arrest, or enhanced activation of apoptosis.[79]

The *MYC* protooncogene, which is strongly expressed in placental, complete molar, and choriocarcinoma samples,[60] plays an important role in the control of proliferation and differentiation.[47,80] Although it has been shown that MYC mRNA synthesis is increased exclusively in early cytotrophoblast, MYC protein immunoreactivity has been reported in the syncytiotrophoblast.[80] MYC overexpression inhibits differentiation and favors proliferation and tumor formation.[81] The expression of MYC proteins might be induced by growth factors and their receptors.[82] It has been demonstrated that constitutive MYC expression may also help in the induction of apoptotic cell death in cell lines under growth-limiting conditions.[83] Although *KRAS* oncogene mutation appears to represent an early genetic event in several carcinomas, investigators did not detect any *KRAS* mutations in any studied samples of complete mole or choriocarcinoma, suggesting that *KRAS* mutation is not involved in the development of trophoblastic diseases.[60]

The *CSF1R* protooncogene encodes the high-affinity cell surface receptor for macrophage CSF, which plays an important role in the survival, proliferation, and differentiation of cells.[84] Trophoblast cells normally invade adjacent tissue structures, and this process is partially controlled by activation of the CSF1 receptors of implanting trophoblast.[50] Uterine colony stimulating factor-1 (CSF1) may regulate placental and gestational tumor development by interacting with trophoblast CSF1 receptors. Expression of *CSF1R* is detected at similar levels in the syncytiotrophoblastic cells of normal placenta, partial mole, complete mole, and choriocarcinoma, suggesting that overexpression of CSF1R alone may not be important for the development of partial mole, complete mole, and choriocarcinoma.[60] Similar findings were also reported by Pampfer[85] and Jokhi[86] and their colleagues.

In contrast, the ERBB2 protein was overexpressed virtually exclusively in the invading extravillous trophoblast of complete mole and in choriocarcinoma.[60] Overexpression of the *ERBB2* oncogene has been associated with a poor prognosis in several tumors.[87,88] Overexpression of ERBB2 may also be related to an aggressive natural history in both complete mole and choriocarcinoma.

All of these data suggest that synergistic upregulation of MYC, ERBB2, and BCL2 oncoproteins may be important in the pathogenesis of complete mole and choriocarcinoma.[60] However, although both complete mole and choriocarcinoma were characterized by overexpression of MYC, ERBB2, and BCL2, partial mole generally did not strongly express these three oncoproteins. Investigation of oncogene expression in GTD not only may provide important insights into pathogenesis but also may be prognostically useful in guiding therapy.

Genes that show differential expression between normal and tumor tissues are likely to function either directly in growth regulation or cellular differentiation or indirectly as a response to changes in the cellular environment. Several of the tumor suppressor genes characterized to date control growth in epithelial tissues.[89,90] Recent data from a number of groups suggest that additional growth suppressors will be identified in various cell types. One candidate for such a role is the *DOC2/hDAB2* gene, which has been shown to be expressed in all normal ovarian surface epithelial cell lines but was significantly downregulated or absent in all of a series of ovarian carcinoma cell lines tested.[91] Furthermore, the gene has been shown to suppress ovarian tumor growth in vitro and in vivo. The predicted DOC2/hDAB2 protein sequence shows that it is a signal transduction molecule.

High levels of DOC2/hDAB2 expression were demonstrated in normal trophoblastic cells in culture, and downregulation of both DOC2/hDAB2 transcript and the protein was found in choriocarcinoma cells in vitro.[92] Immunohistochemistry showed high levels of DOC2/hDAB2 protein expression in normal placenta. The immunoreactivity in partial mole was significantly less than in placenta, and only low levels of DOC2/hDAB2 expression were observed in complete moles and choriocarcinomas.[92]

Significantly lower levels of DOC2/hDAB2 expression in various trophoblastic diseases suggest that DOC2/hDAB2 may play an important role in growth and differentiation of normal trophoblast cells and that downregulation of DOC2/hDAB2 may be involved in the development of GTD, particularly in complete moles and choriocarcinomas.[92] It was found that the growth rate of the DOC2/hDAB2-transfected choriocarcinoma cells is significantly lower in culture, which suggests that DOC2/hDAB2 can suppress the growth of choriocarcinomas in vitro.

Although differences in expression of oncoproteins may be important in the development of GTD, the precise molecular changes that are critical in the pathogenesis of choriocarcinoma remain unknown.[47,60] Nine genes were found to be differentially expressed between normal trophoblast and choriocarcinoma cells when a complementary DNA (cDNA) expression array technique was used. Six of the genes (for MYC, nuclear factor κB [NF-κB], GATA2, ribosomal protein L6, HIP116, and nerve growth factor [NGF]) were upregulated, and three (for heat shock proteins HSP86 and HSP27 and fibronectin receptor β-subunit [FNRBL]) were downregulated in choriocarcinoma cells.[93] Piao and coworkers[94] showed that GATA2 was expressed strongly in JEG-3 and Jar choriocarcinoma cell lines;

however GATA2 may also have a crucial role in placental trophoblast differentiation. NF-κB transcription factor is a heterodimer molecule composed of two subunits, P50 and P65. The P65 subunit may play an important role in carcinogenesis in several tumor cell lines.[95,96] To confirm this result with the cDNA expression array, overexpression of NF-κB P65, HIP116, and ribosomal protein L6 was also shown in choriocarcinoma cells with Western blot or reverse transcriptase (RT)-PCR analyses.[93] HSP27 was observed to be downregulated in choriocarcinoma cells, and this observation was supported in vitro in cell lines and in vivo with paraffin sections using RT-PCR, Western blot, and immunohistochemical analyses.[93]

HSP27 is expressed in high concentrations in estrogen-sensitive tissues.[97] Padwich[98] and Morrish[99] and their colleagues reported the expression of HSP27 in maternal decidua and the early trophoblast cells, and our data confirm this observation. HSP27 may play a role in placental differentiation during the first trimester of pregnancy. HSP27 may also play a role in the pathogenesis of several human malignancies.[97]

HSP27 expression may also be important in the acquisition of chemotherapeutic drug resistance. Phosphorylation of HSP27 may stabilize the cytoskeleton and thereby increase cellular drug resistance in several malignant cell lines.[100,101] Choriocarcinoma is exceptionally curable with chemotherapy, even in the presence of widespread metastatic disease. The downregulation of HSP27 in choriocarcinoma may contribute to the marked sensitivity of choriocarcinoma to chemotherapy. Further functional studies of HSP27 expression in choriocarcinoma would need to be performed to evaluate its potential relationship with trophoblast differentiation and chemotherapy sensitivity.

The identification of differentially expressed genes may provide important insights into the pathogenesis of GTD and is worthy of further investigation.

Is there alteration of cell adhesion molecules and proteinases in gestational trophoblastic disease?

Placental tissue contains a heterogeneous population of cells, including villous syncytiotrophoblast and cytotrophoblast, as well as extravillous trophoblast. Whereas villous trophoblast does not exhibit invasive behavior, the invasive capacity of the extravillous trophoblast appears to have similarities with the role of malignant cells during tumor invasion.[102,103] However, trophoblast invasion of the endometrium is tightly regulated during the first trimester of normal pregnancy.[103] Extravillous trophoblast cells migrate from the basement membrane of anchoring villi and invade deeply, reaching the myometrium. The process of trophoblast invasion and implantation is dependent on a series of membrane-mediated events that involve complex cell-cell and cell-matrix interactions, as well as the enzymatic degradation of the extracellular matrix. The integrins are a diverse family of glycoproteins that are expressed on cell surfaces as heterodimeric α and β subunits and mediate both cell-matrix and cell-cell interactions. The CD9 molecule has a function connected with the invasive properties of BeWo choriocarcinoma cells, which is partially mediated by integrin $\alpha5\beta1$.[104] The binding of specific extracellular matrix (ECM) components not only anchors the cell to the substratum but activates several signal transduction pathways. The components of ECM such as laminin and fibronectin are glycoproteins that bind to their receptors (integrins) expressed on the cell membrane and thus serve as potent regulators of trophoblast invasion.[105]

The cadherins are a gene superfamily of integral membrane glycoproteins that mediate calcium-dependent cell adhesion. This family of cell adhesion molecules (CAMs) is composed of two evolutionarily distinct subfamilies: type 1 cadherins (also known as classical cadherins) and type 2 cadherins (also known as atypical cadherins). The classical cadherins included the three originally identified entities, E-cadherin (E-cad), N-cadherin, and P-cadherin.[106] The type 2 cadherin subfamily includes the human cadherins known as Cad-5, -6, -8, -11, -12, and -14.[106] Several observations have led to the hypothesis that E-cad is the product of a tumor suppressor gene. Cad-11 expression is restricted to the two types of trophoblast cells (syncytial trophoblasts and extravillous cytotrophoblasts) that form intimate contacts with the underlying maternal tissues. Cad-11 mediates trophoblast-decidual cell interactions and may play a key role in trophoblast differentiation. The expression of Cad-11 and E-cad is regulated during trophoblast differentiation in vitro. Cad-11 is not detectable in JEG-3 or BeWo choriocarcinoma cells. In contrast, E-cad is readily detectable in these cell lines. Cad-11 expression is associated with the fusion of villous mononucleate cytotrophoblasts isolated from the term placenta and with the cyclic adenosine monophosphate (cAMP)-mediated differentiation and fusion of BeWo cells. These differentiation processes have been associated with reduction in trophoblast invasiveness.[106]

Extracellular proteinases are believed to be important in modulating both cell-matrix interactions and the degradation of the basement membrane that is necessary for invasion and metastasis. Different families of matrix-degrading proteases have been found to be involved in trophoblastic invasion into the maternal tissues, including serine proteases and matrix metalloproteinases (MMPs).[107-109] The MMPs are a family of zinc-containing endopeptidases that degrade a wide range of components of the ECM; they are also thought to play an important role in tumor progression and metastasis.[103,107-109] To date, at least 20 members of the MMP family have been reported. They are divided into four main groups according to their substrate specificities: collagenases, gelatinases, stromelysins, and membrane-type MMPs.[110,111] MMPs play important roles in the invasion of the trophoblast cell into the maternal endometrium during placentation. The activity of the MMPs is regulated by several biologic modulators, including tissue inhibitors of metalloproteinases

(TIMPs). These secreted inhibitory proteins bind the active forms of MMPs and inhibit their individual proteolytic activities in the tissue.[110,112,113]

The tissue inhibitor of MMP2 (TIMP2) may be involved in autoregulation of the invasive growth of the trophoblast.[114] The potential interactions among MMPs are currently under active investigation. Both MMP2 and MMP9 degrade type IV collagen, which is a major component of the basement membrane and constitutes an important barrier to tumor cell invasion. In contrast, MMP1 degrades type II and type III collagen. 8-iso-Prostaglandin $F_{2\alpha}$ could reduce invasion of choriocarcinoma cells and MMP2 and MMP9 activity through post-transcriptional regulation.[115] Cytokines also influence the secretion and activity of MMPs. The proinflammatory cytokines (e.g., interleukin-6) exert a stimulating effect, whereas anti-inflammatory cytokines (e.g., interleukin-10) are usually inhibitors of MMPs.[116]

Choriocarcinoma exhibited significantly stronger expression of both MMP1 and MMP2 than did syncytiotrophoblast in normal placenta, partial mole, complete mole, and extravillous trophoblast in placenta. Furthermore, the extravillous trophoblast in partial and complete mole showed significantly stronger staining for MMP2 than did the extravillous trophoblast in normal placenta.[117] Although choriocarcinoma had significantly increased expression of MMP1 and MMP2 compared with placenta, partial mole, and complete mole, choriocarcinoma had significantly less expression of the tissue inhibitor of MMP1 than placenta, partial mole, and complete mole.[117] The increased expression of MMP1 and MMP2 and decreased expression of TIMP1 in choriocarcinoma may contribute to the invasiveness of choriocarcinoma cells.[117]

MMPs and tissue inhibitors may play an important role in the pathogenesis of GTD. Infrequently, patients with drug-resistant GTTs are encountered, and there is a continuing need to develop and evaluate new chemotherapeutic agents. Antineoplastic drugs are currently being developed that modify the activity of MMPs and their inhibitors, and these agents may have activity against GTD.[118,119] Further understanding of the role of MMPs in the biology of GTD may therefore lead to new and novel therapies for patients with these diseases.

REFERENCES

1. Berkowitz RS, Goldstein DP: Chorionic tumors. N Engl J Med 1996;335:1740-1748.
2. Kim SJ: Epidemiology in gestational trophoblastic disease. In Hancock BW, Newlands ES, Berkowitz RS (eds): Gestational Trophoblastic Disease. London, Chapman and Hall, 1997, p 27-42.
3. Palmer JR: Advances in the epidemiology of gestational trophoblastic disease. J Reprod Med 1994;39:155-162.
4. Kim SJ, Bae JN, Kim JH, et al: Epidemiology and time trends of gestational trophoblastic disease in Korea. Int J Gynecol Obstet 1998;60:S33-S38.
5. Hando T, Ohno M, Kurose T: Recent aspects of gestational trophoblastic disease in Japan. Int J Gynecol Obstet 1998;60:S71-S76.
6. Berkowitz RS, Cramer DW, Bernstein MR, et al: Risk factors for complete molar pregnancy from a case-control study. Am J Obstet Gynecol 1985;152:1016-1020.

7. Parazzini F, LaVecchia C, Mangili G, et al: Dietary factors and risk of trophoblast disease. Am J Obstet Gynecol 1988;158:93-99.

8. O'Toole BA, Fradkin R, Warkang J: Vitamin A deficiency and reproduction in rhesus monkeys. J Nutr 1974;104:1513-1516.

9. Kajii T, Ohama K: Androgenetic origin of hydatidiform mole. Nature 1977;268:633-634.

10. Lawler S, Fisher R, Dent J: A prospective genetic study of complete and partial hydatidiform moles. Am J Obstet Gynecol 1991;164:1270-1277.

11. Wake N, Takagi N, Sasaki M: Androgenesis as a cause of hydatidiform mole. J Natl Cancer Inst 1978;60:51-57.

12. Fisher RA, Povey S, Jeffreys AJ, et al: Frequency of heterozygous complete hydatidiform moles, estimated by locus specific minisatellite and Y chromosome-specific probes. Hum Genet 1989;82:259-263.

13. Wake N, Fujino T, Hoshi S, et al: The propensity to malignancy of dispermic heterozygous moles. Placenta 1987;8:319-326.

14. Yamashita K, Wake N, Araki T, et al: Human lymphocyte antigen expression in hydatidiform mole: Androgenesis following fertilization with a haploid sperm. Am J Obstet Gynecol 1979;135:597-600.

15. Azuma C, Saji F, Tokugawa Y, et al: Application of gene amplification by polymerase chain reaction to genetic analysis of molar mitochondrial DNA: The detection of anuclear empty ovum as the cause of complete mole. Gynecol Oncol 1991;40:29-33.

16. Surti U, Szulman AE, O'Brien S: Complete (classic) hydatidiform mole with 46XY karotype of paternal origin. Hum Genet 1979;51:153-155.

17. Lage JM, Mark SD, Roberts DJ, et al: A flow cytometric study of 137 fresh hydropic placentas: Correlations between types of hydatidiform moles and nuclear DNA ploidy. Obstet Gynecol 1992;79:403-410.

18. Lawler SD, Fisher RA, Pickhall VJ, et al: Genetic studies on hydatidiform moles: I. The origin of partial moles. Cancer Gent Cytogenet 1982;5:309-320.

19. Vejerslev LO, Fisher RA, Surti U, et al: Hydatidiform mole: Parental chromosome abberations in partial and complete moles. J Med Genet 1987;24:613-615.

20. Surani MA, Barton SC, Norris ML: Influence of parental chromosomes on spatial specificity in androgenetic-pathenogenetic chimeras in the mouse. Nature 1987;326:395-397.

21. Barton S, Surani MA, Norris M: Role of paternal and maternal genomes in mouse development. Nature 1984;311:374-376.

22. Jeffers MD, Michie BA, Oakes SJ, et al: Comparison of ploidy analysis by flow cytometry and image analysis in hydatidiform mole and non-molar abortion. Histopathology 1995;27:415-421.

23. Fukunaga M: Early partial hydatidiform mole: Prevalence, histopathology, DNA ploidy, and persistence rate. Virchows Arch 2000;437:180-184.

24. Koenig C, Demopoulos RI, Vamuakas EC, et al: Flow cytometric DNA ploidy and quantitative histopathology in partial moles. Int J Gynecol Pathol 1993;12:235-240.

25. Teng NN, Ballon SC: Partial hydatidiform mole with diploid karyotype: Report of three cases. Am J Obstet Gynecol 1984;150:961-964.

26. Soto-Wright V, Bernstein M, Goldstein DP, et al: The changing clinical presentation of complete molar pregnancy. Obstet Gynecol 1995;86:775-779.

27. Paradinas FJ, Browne P, Fisher RA, et al: A clinical, histopathological and flow cytometric study of 149 complete moles, 146 partial moles and 107 non-molar abortions. Histopathology 1996;28:101-109.

28. Mosher R, Goldstein DP, Berkowitz RS, et al: Complete hydatidiform mole: Comparison of clinicopathologic features, current and past. J Reprod Med 1998;43:21-27.

29. Keep D, Zaragoza MU, Harold T, et al: Very early complete hydatidiform mole. Hum Pathol 1996;27:708-713.

30. Genest DR, Ruiz RE, Weremowicz S, et al: Do non-triploid partial hydatidiform moles exist? A histologic and flow cytometric re-evaluation of the non-triploid specimens. J Reprod Med 2002;47:363-368.

31. Cattanach BM: Genome Analysis, vol 2. New York, Cold Spring Harbor Laboratory Press, 1991, pp 41-47.

32. Monk M: Genomic imprinting. Genes Devel 1988;2:921-925.

33. Reik W, Surani MA: Genomic imprinting and embryonal tumors. Nature 1989;338:112-113.

34. Hall JG: Genomic imprinting: Review and relevance to human diseases. Am J Hum Genet 1990;46:857-873.

35. Reik W: Genomic imprinting and genetic disorders in man. Trends Genet 1989;5:331-336.

36. Mutter GL, Stewart CL, Chaponot ML, et al: Oppositely imprinted genes H-19 and insulin-like growth factor 2 are co-expressed in human androgenetic trophoblast. Am J Hum Genet 1993;53:1096-1102.

37. Mutter GL, Pomponio RJ, Berkowitz RS, et al: Sex chromosome composition of complete hydatidiform moles: Relationship to metastasis. Am J Obstet Gynecol 1993;168:1547-1551.

38. Henry I, Bonaiti-Pellie C, Chehensse V, et al: Uniparental paternal disomy in a genetic cancer-predisposing syndrome. Nature 1991;351:665-667.

39. Little M, Van Heyningen V, Hastie N: Dads and disomy and disease. Nature 1991;351:609-610.

40. Lage JM: Placentomegaly with masive hydrops of placental stem villi, diploid DNA content and fetal omphaloceles: Possible association with Beckwith-Wiedemann syndrome. Hum Pathol 1991;22:591-597.

41. Zhang Y, Tycko B: Monoallelic expression of the human H-19 gene. Nat Genet 1992;1:40-44.

42. Mutter GL: Role of imprinting in abnormal human development. Mutat Res 1997;396:141-147.

43. Fisher RA, Lawler SD, Povey S, et al: Genetically homozygous choriocarcinoma following pregnancy with hydatidiform mole. Br J Cancer 1988;58:788-792.

44. Habibian R, Surti S: Cytogenetics of trophoblasts from complete hydatidiform moles. Cancer Genet Cytogenet 1987;29:271-287.

45. Hollstein M, Sidransfy D, Vogelstein B, et al: *p53* mutations in human cancers. Science 1991;253:49-53.

46. Bishop JM: Molecular themes in oncogenesis. Cell 1991;64:235-248.

47. Cheung ANY, Srivastava G, Pittaluga S, et al: Expression of *c-myc* and *c-fms* oncogenes in hydatidiform mole and normal human placenta. J Clin Pathol 1993;46:204-207.

48. Sarkar S, Kacinski BM, Kohorn EI, et al: Demonstration of *myc* and *ras* oncogene expression by hybridization in situ in hydatidiform mole and in the BeWo choriocarcinoma cell line. Am J Obstet Gynecol 1986;154:390-393.

49. Diebold J, Arnholdt H, Lai MD, et al: C-myc expression in early human placenta: A critical evaluation of its localization. Virchows Arch B 1991;61:65-73.

50. Ohlsson R: Growth factors, protoonocogenes and human placental development. Cell Growth Differ 1989;28:1-15.

51. Visvader J, Verma IM: Differential transcription of exon 1 of the human *c-fms* gene in placental trophoblasts and monocytes. Mol Cell Biol 1989;9:1336-1341.

52. Fujino T: Analysis of *c-onc* genes in choriocarcinoma cells. Hokkaido Igaku Zasshi 1987;62:798-807.

53. Prigent SA, Lemoine NR: The type I (EGFR-related) family of growth factor receptors and their ligands. Prog Growth Factors Res 1992;4:1-24.

54. Kraus MH, Issing W, Miki T, et al: Isolation and characterization of erbB-3, a third member of ERB/epidermal growth factor receptor family: Evidence for overexpression in a subset of human mammary tumors. Proc Natl Acad Sci U S A 1989;86:9193-9197.

55. Fisher RA, Newlands ES: Gestational trophoblastic disease: Molecular and genetic studies. J Reprod Med 1998;43:87-97.

56. Cao H, Lei ZM, Rao CV: Transcriptional and posttranscriptional mechanisms in epidermal growth factor regulation of human chorionic gonadotropin (hCG) subunits and hCG receptor gene expression in human choriocarcinoma cells. Endocrinology 1994;135:962-970.

57. Chen F, Goto S, Nawa A, et al: Receptor binding of epidermal growth factor in cultured human choriocarcinoma cell lines: Effects of actinomycin-D and methotrexate. Nagoya J Med Sci 1990;52:5-11.

58. Mulhauser J, Crescimanno C, Kaufman P, et al: Differentiation and proliferation patterns in human trophoblast revealed by c-erbB-2 oncogene product and EGFR. J Histochem Cytochem 1993;41:165-173.

59. Ladines-Llave CA, Maruo T, Manalo AM, et al: Decreased expression of epidermal growth factor and its receptor in the malignant transformation of trophoblasts. Cancer 1993;71:4118-4223.

60. Fulop V, Mok SC, Genest DR, et al: c-myc, c-erbB-2, c-fms and bcl-2 oncoproteins: Expression in normal placenta, partial and complete mole, and choriocarcinoma. J Reprod Med 1998;43:101-110.

61. Tuncer ZS, Vegh GL, Fulop V, et al: Expression of epidermal growth factor receptor related family products in gestational trophoblastic diseases and normal placenta and its relationship with development of postmolar tumor. Gynecol Oncol 2000;77:389-393.

62. Yang X, Zhang Z, Jia C, et al: The relationship between expression of c-ras, c-erbB-2, nm23 and p53 gene products and development of trophoblastic tumor and their predictive significance for the malignant transformation of complete hydatidiform mole. Gynecol Oncol 2002;85:438-444.

63. Wong SYY, Ngan HYS, Chan CCW, et al: Apoptosis in gestational trophoblastic disease is correlated with clinical outcome and bcl-2 expression but not bax expression. Mod Pathol 1999;12:1025-1033.

64. Sakuragi N, Matsuo H, Coukos G: Differentiation-dependent expression of the BCL-2 proto-oncogene in the human trophoblast lineage. J Soc Gynecol Invest 1994;2:164-172.

65. Nelson DM: Apoptotic changes in syncytiotrophoblast of human placental villi where fibrin type fibrinoid is deposited at discontinuities in the villous trophoblast. Placenta 1996;17:387-391.

66. Landers JE, Haines DS, Strauss JF, et al: Enhanced translation: A novel mechanism of mdm2 oncogene overexpression identified in human tumor cells. Oncogene 1994;9:2745-2750.

67. Fulop V, Mok SC, Genest DR, et al: p53, p21, Rb and mdm2 oncoproteins: Expression in normal placenta, partial and complete mole, and choriocarcinoma. J Reprod Med 1998;43:119-127.

68. Momand J, Zambetti GP, Olson DC, et al: The mdm-2 oncogene product forms a complex with the p53 protein and inhibits p53-mediated transactivation. Cell 1992;69:1237-1245.

69. Wu X, Bayle JH, Olson D, et al: The p53-mdm-2 autoregulatory feedback loop. Genes Dev 1993;7:1126-1132.

70. Cheung ANY, Srivastava G, Chung LP, et al: Expression of the p53 gene in trophoblastic cells in hydatidiform moles and normal human placentas. J Reprod Med 1994;39:223-227.

71. Cordon-Cardon C, Latres E, Drobnjak M, et al: Molecular abnormalities of mdm2 and p53 genes in adult soft tissue sarcomas. Cancer Res 1994;54:794-799.

72. Reifenberger G, Liu L, Ichimura K, et al: Amplification and overexpression of the MDM2 gene in a subset of human malignant gliomas without p53 mutations. Cancer Res 1993;53:2736-2739.

73. Xiao Z-X, Chen J, Levine AJ, et al: Interaction between the retinoblastoma protein and the oncoprotein MDM2. Nature 1995;375:694-697.

74. Shimizu T, Miwa W, Nakamori S, et al: Absence of a mutation of the p21/WAF1 gene in human lung and pancreatic cancers. Jpn J Cancer Res 1996;87:275-278.

75. Stellar MA, Mok SC, Yeh J, et al: Effects of cytokines on epidermal growth factor receptor expression by malignant trophoblast cells in vitro. J Reprod Med 1994;39:209-216.

76. Maruo T, Mochizuki M: Immunohistochemical localization of epidermal growth factor receptor and myc oncogene product in human placenta: Implication for trophoblast proliferation and differentiation. Am J Obstet Gynecol 1987;156:721-727.

77. Hampson J, McLaughlin PJ, Johnson PM: Low affinity receptors for tumor necrosis factor–alpha, interferon-gamma and granulocyte-macrophage colony-stimulating factor are expressed on human placental syncytiotrophoblast. Immunology 1993;79:485-490.

78. Ferriani RA, Ahmed A, Sharkey A, et al: Colocalization of acidic and basic fibroblast growth factor (FGF) in human placenta and the cellular effects of bFGF in trophoblast cell line JEG-3. Growth Factors 1994;10:259-268.

79. Williams GT, Smith CA: Molecular regulation of apoptosis: Genetic controls on cell death. Cell 1993;74:777-779.

80. Roncalli M, Bulfamante G, Viale G, et al: C-myc and tumor suppressor gene product expression in developing and term human trophoblast. Placenta 1994;15:399-409.

81. Sach L, Lotem J: Control of programmed cell death in normal and leukemic cells: New implications for therapy. Blood 1993;82:15-21.

82. Lipponen PK: Expression of c-myc protein is related to cell proliferation and expression of growth factor receptors in transitional cell bladder cancer. J Pathol 1995;175:203-210.

83. Alarcon RM, Rupnow BA, Greaber TG, et al: Modulation of c-myc activity and apoptosis in vivo. Cancer Res 1996;56:4315-4319.

84. Springall F, O'Mara S, Shounan Y, et al: C-fms point mutations in acute myeloid leukemia: Fact or fiction? Leukemia 1993;7:978-985.

85. Pampfer S, Daiter E, Barad D, et al: Expression of the colony-stimulating factor-1 receptor (c-fms proto-onocogene product) in human uterus and placenta. Biol Reprod 1992;46:48-57.

86. Jokhi PP, Chumbley G, King A, et al: Expression of the colony stimulating factor–1 receptor (c-fms product) by cells at the human uteroplacental interface. Lab Invest 1993;68:308-320.

87. Wright C, Nicholson S, Angus B, et al: Relationship between c-erbB-2 protein product expression and response to endocrine therapy in advanced breast cancer. Br J Cancer 1992;65:118-121.

88. Pavlidis N, Briassoulis E, Bai M, et al: Overexpression of c-myc, ras and c-erbB-2 oncoproteins in carcinoma of unknown primary origin. Anticancer Res 1995;15:2563-2568.

89. Lee WH, Brookstein R, Hong F, et al: Human retinoblastoma susceptibility gene: Cloning, identification, and sequence. Science 1987;235:1394-1399.

90. Miki Y: A strong candidate gene for the breast and ovarian cancer susceptibility gene BRCA1. Science 1994;266:66-7172.

91. Mok SC, Wong KK, Chan RKW, et al: Molecular cloning of differentially expressed genes in human epithelial ovarian cancer. Gynecol Oncol 1994;52:247-252.

92. Fulop V, Colitti CV, Genest D, et al: DOC-2/hDab2, a candidate tumor suppressor gene involved in the development of gestational trophoblastic diseases. Oncogene 1998;17:419-424.

93. Vegh GL, Fulop V, Liu Y, et al: Differential gene expression pattern between normal human trophoblast and choriocarcinoma cell line: Downregulation of heat shock protein-27 in choriocarcinoma in vitro and in vivo. Gynecol Oncol 1999;75:391-396.

94. Piao YS, Peltoketo H, Vihko P, et al: The proximal promoter of the gene encoding human 17β-hydroxisteroid dehydrogenase type 1 contains GATA, AP-2, and Sp1 response elements: Analysis of promoter function in choriocarcinoma cells. Endocrinology 1997;138:3417-3425.

95. Sharma HW, Narayanan R: The NF-κB transcription factor in oncogenesis. Anticancer Res 1996;16:589-596.

96. Wang W, Abbruzzese JL, Evans DB, et al: The nuclear factor–κB RelA transcription factor is constitutively activated in human pancreatic adenocarcinoma cells. Clin Cancer Res 1999;5:119-127.

97. Ciocca DR, Oesterreich S, Chamness GC, et al: Biological and clinical implications of heat shock protein 27.000(Hsp-27): A review. J Natl Cancer Inst 1993;85:1558-1570.

98. Padwick ML, Whitehead M, King RJB: Hormonal regulation of Hsp-27 expression in human endometrial epithelial and stromal cells. Mol Cell Endocrinol 1994;102:9-14.

99. Morrish DW, Linetsky E, Bhardwaj D, et al: Identification by substractive hybridization of a spectrum of novel and unexpected genes associated with in vitro differentiation of human cytotrophoblast cells. Placenta 1996;17:431-441.

100. Garrido C, Ottavi P, Fromentin A, et al: Hsp-27 as a mediator of confluence-dependent resistance to cell death induced by anticancer drugs. Cancer Res 1997;57:2661-2667.

101. Richards EH, Hickey E, Weber L, et al: Effect of overexpression of small heat shock protein Hsp-27 on the heat and drug sensitivies of human testis tumor cells. Cancer Res 1996;56:2446-2451.

102. Crescimanno C, Foidart JM, Noel A, et al: Cloning of choriocarcinoma cells shows that invasion correlates with expression and activation of gelatinase A. Exp Cell Res 1996;227:240-251.

103. Lala PK, Graham CH: Mechanisms of trophoblast invasiveness and their control: The role of proteases and protease inhibitors. Cancer Metast Rev 1994;9:369-379.

104. Hirano T, Higuchi T, Katsuragawa H, et al: CD9 is involved in invasion of human trophoblast-like choriocarcinoma cell line, BeWo cells. Mol Hum Reprod 1999;5:168-174.

105. Bischof P, Martelli M, Campana A: The regulation of endometrial and trophoblastic metalloproteinases during blastocyst implantation. Contracept Fertil Sex 1994;22:48-52.

106. MacCalman DC, Getsios S, Chen GTC: Type 2 cadherins in the human endometrium and placenta: Their putative roles in human implantation and placentation. Am J Reprod Immunol 1998;39:96-107.

107. Huppertz B, Kerschanska S, Demir AY, et al: Immuno-histochemistry of matrix metalloproteinases (MMP), their substrates, and their inhibitors (TIMP) during trophoblast invasion in the human placenta. Cell Tissue Res 1998;291:133-148.

108. Bischof P, Haenggli L, Campana A: Gelatinase and oncofetal fibronectin expression is dependent on integrin expression on human cytotrophoblasts. Hum Reprod 1995;10:734-742.

109. Castellucci M, Theelen T, Pompili E, et al: Immuno-histochemical localization of serine-protease inhibitors in the human placenta. Cell Tissue Res 1994;278:283-289.

110. Leber T, Boyd R, Balkwill F: Tumour cell-stromal cell interactions: Proteases and protease inhibitors. In Sharp F, Blackett T, Berek J, Bast R (eds): Ovarian Cancer 5. Oxford, Isis Medical Media, 1998, pp 121-129.

111. Sato H, Takino T, Okada Y: A matrix metalloproteinase expressed on the surface of invasive tumor cells. Nature 1994;370:61-65.

112. Murray GI, Duncan ME, Arbucle E: Matrix metalloproteinases and their inhibitors in gastric cancer. Gut 1998;43:791-797.

113. Denhardt DT, Feng B, Edwards DR: Tissue inhibitor of metalloproteinases (TIMP, akaEPA): Structure, control of expression and biological functions. Pharmacol Ther 1993;59:329-341.

114. Ruck P, Marzusch K, Horny HP, et al: The distribution of tissue inhibitor of metalloproteinases-2 (TIMP-2) in the human placenta. Placenta 1996;17:263-266.

115. Staff AC, Ranheim T, Henriksen T, et al: 8-iso-Prostaglandin F(2alpha) reduces trophoblast invasion and matrix metalloproteinase activity. Hypertension 2000;35:1307-1313.

116. Bischof P, Meisser A, Campana A: Paracrine and autocrine regulators of trophoblast invasion: A review. Placenta 2000;21:S55-S60.

117. Vegh GL, Tuncer ZS, Fulop V, et al: Matrix metalloproteinases and their inhibitors in gestational trophoblastic diseases and normal placenta. Gynecol Oncol 1999;75:248-253.

118. Rasmussen HS, McCann PP: Matrix metalloproteinase inhibition as a novel anticancer strategy: A review with specific focus on batimastat and marimastat. Pharmacol Ther 1997;75:69-75.

119. Wojtowitz-Praga S, Torri J, Johnson M, et al: Phase I trial of Marimastat, a novel matrix metalloproteinase inhibitor, administered orally to patients with advanced lung cancer. J Clin Oncol 1998;16:2150-2156.

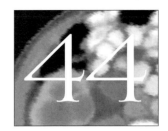

MANAGEMENT OF GESTATIONAL TROPHOBLASTIC DISEASE

Michael J. Seckl   and   *Edward S. Newlands*

✦ MAJOR CONTROVERSIES

- Are false-positive human chorionic gonadotrophin results a problem, and how should physicians deal with this issue?
- How should persistently raised low-level human chorionic gonadotrophin of unknown origin be managed?
- Should twin pregnancies be terminated early?
- Are registration, centralized follow-up, and therapy after uterine evacuation valuable?
- Treating low-risk patients: methotrexate or actinomycin D?
- Treating high-risk patients: EMA/CO regimen or other multiagent treatments?
- When should therapy be discontinued?
- Is there a role for high-dose chemotherapy?
- Does radiotherapy have a role in the management of overt central nervous system disease?
- What is optimal therapy for placental-site trophoblastic tumors?
- Is there a role for a nurse specialist?

The first record of gestational trophoblastic disease (GTD) probably dates to about 400 BC, when Hippocrates and his student, Diocles, described "dropsy of the uterus."[1] In 1276, the attendants of Margaret Countess of Henneberg noticed that her abnormal delivery consisted of multiple hydropic vesicles. They probably believed that each vesicle was a separate conception, which led them to christen one half John and one half Mary. Marie Boivin (1773-1841), who worked as a Parisian midwife, was the first to document the chorionic origin of the hydatids.[1] In 1895, Marchand described a malignant uterine disease of syncytial and cytotrophoblastic origin and made the link between hydatidiform mole and other forms of pregnancy.[1] However, it was not until the mid-20th century that effective therapeutic protocols were developed, which serve as one of the modern success stories in cancer medicine.

The normal gestational trophoblast arises from the peripheral cells of the blastocyst in the first few days after conception. Trophoblastic tissue initially grows rapidly into two layers: an inner cytotrophoblast of mononucleated cells that migrate out and fuse together forming an outer syncytiotrophoblast of large, multi nucleated cells (Fig. 44-1). The latter subsequently aggressively invades the endometrium and uterine vasculature, generating an intimate connection between the fetus and the mother known as the placenta. Invasion is one of the features of malignancy, and normal tro phoblastic cells can be detected by polymerase chain reaction in the maternal circulation.[2] Fortunately, the complex biologic and immunologic mechanisms involved in controlling the relationship between the fetal trophoblast and the maternal host prevent such circulating trophoblasts from producing metastases.

When GTD arises, the normal regulatory mechanisms controlling trophoblastic tissue are lost. The excessively proliferating trophoblast may invade through the myometrium, developing a rich maternal blood supply, with tumor emboli and hematogenous

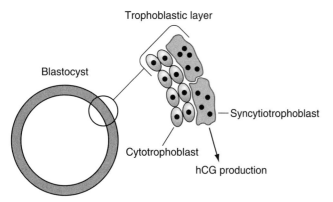

Figure 44–1. The schematic diagram of an embryo at the blastocyst stage demonstrates trophoblast development. hCG, human chorionic gonadotrophin.

spread occurring frequently. The World Health Organization (WHO) has classified GTD as two premalignant diseases called complete and partial hydatidiform mole (CM and PM) and as three malignant disorders (i.e., gestational trophoblastic tumors [GTTs]) called invasive mole, gestational choriocarcinoma, and placental-site trophoblastic tumor.[3] These tumors are important to recognize because they are nearly always curable, and in most cases, fertility can

be preserved. In this chapter, we discuss the current controversies about and management of GTD.

Pathology and Genetics

Complete hydatidiform mole. CMs nearly always only contain paternal DNA and are therefore androgenetic.[4] This occurs in most cases because a single sperm bearing a 23X set of chromosomes fertilizes an ovum lacking maternal genes and then duplicates to form the homozygote, 46XX (Fig 44-2A).[4-9] However, in up to 25% of CMs, fertilization can take place with two spermatozoa, resulting in the heterozygous 46XY or 46XX configuration (see Fig. 44-2B).[10,11] A 46YY conceptus has not yet been described and is presumably nonviable. Rarely, a CM can arise from a fertilized ovum that has retained its maternal nuclear DNA and is therefore biparental in origin.[12]

Macroscopically, the classic CM resembles a bunch of grapes because of generalized (complete) swelling of chorionic villi. However, this appearance is seen only in the second trimester, and the diagnosis is usually made earlier, when the villi are much less hydropic. In the first trimester, the villi microscopically contain little fluid, are branching, and consist of a hyperplastic syncytiotrophoblast and cytotrophoblast with many

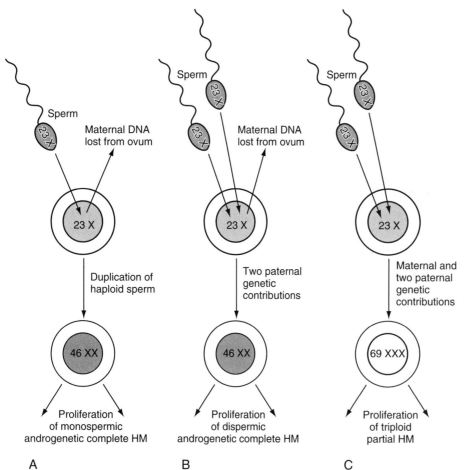

Figure 44–2. The schematic diagram shows that the androgenetic diploid complete hydatidiform mole (HM) is formed by duplication of the chromosomes from a single sperm **(A)** or by two sperm fertilizing the ovum **(B)**, which in both cases has lost its own genetic component. The triploid genetic origin of a partial HM is demonstrated **(C)**.

A

B

C

vessels. Although it was previously thought that CM produced no fetal tissue, histologic examination of 6- to 8-week abortions reveals evidence of embryonic elements, including fetal red blood cells.[13-15] This has resulted in pathologists incorrectly labeling CMs as PMs. Consequently, the reported rates of persistent GTD after PMs has been artificially elevated and is probably less than 0.5%.[16] The presence of embryonic tissue from a twin pregnancy comprising a fetus and a CM is another source of error that can lead to the incorrect diagnosis of PM. Occasionally, it can be very difficult to distinguish an early complete mole from a normal early placenta, and in such cases, the absence of p57[kip2] staining in the CM as opposed to other types of pregnancy can be helpful.[17]

Partial hydatidiform mole. PMs are genetically probably all triploid,[18] with two paternal and one maternal chromosome sets (see Fig 44-2C). Although triploidy occurs in 1% to 3% of all recognized conceptions and in about 20% of spontaneous abortions with abnormal karyotype, triploids due to two sets of maternal chromosome do not become PMs.[19,20] Flow cytometry, which can be done in formalin-fixed, paraffin-embedded tissues,[21] can therefore help in differentiating CM from PM and PM from diploid nonmolar hydropic abortions.

In PMs, villous swelling is less intense and affects only some villi. Swollen and non-swollen villi can have trophoblastic hyperplasia that is mild and focal. The villi have characteristic indented outlines and round inclusions. An embryo is usually present and can be recognized macroscopically or inferred from the presence of nucleated red cells in villous vasculature. It may survive into the second trimester, but in most cases, it dies at about 8 to 9 weeks' gestation, and this is followed by loss of vessels and stromal fibrosis. In PMs evacuated early, villous swelling and trophoblastic excess can be so mild and focal that the diagnosis of PM may be missed.[16] At uterine evacuation for a "miscarriage," it is likely that many PMs are misclassified as products of conception. Fortunately, at the Trophoblastic Screening and Treatment Center at Charing Cross Hospital, London, we only see about one patient per year with persistent GTD related to a previously unrecognized PM. Of the correctly diagnosed PMs, very few patients go on to develop persistent GTD. Of 3000 PMs reviewed and followed at Charing Cross, only 15 (0.5%) patients required chemotherapy.[21]

Other pregnancies mistaken for partial hydatidiform mole. More than one half of first-trimester nonmolar abortions are caused by trisomy, monosomy, maternally derived triploidy, and translocations. They often develop hydrops, but it is small (<3 mm), and PMs can be excluded if the fetuses are diploid on flow cytometry. Turner's, Edward's, and Beckwith-Wiedemann syndromes can cause histologic confusion with PMs.[16,22]

Invasive hydatidiform mole. Invasive mole is common and is clinically identified by the combination of an abnormal uterine ultrasound scan and a persistent or rising human chorionic gonadotrophin (hCG) level after uterine evacuation of a CM or PM. Further pathologic confirmation of invasion is rarely required. Moreover, repeat dilatation and curettage (D&C) is often contraindicated because of the risks of uterine perforation, infection, life-threatening hemorrhage, and subsequent hysterectomy. In some cases for which histologic information is available, invasive mole can be distinguished from choriocarcinoma by the presence of chorionic villi.

Choriocarcinoma. Most choriocarcinomas have grossly abnormal karyotypes, with diverse ploidies and several chromosome rearrangements, none of which is specific for the disease.[23] Studies of the origin of GTTs have confirmed that choriocarcinoma may arise from any type of pregnancy, including a normal term pregnancy[24-27] and from a homozygous or heterozygous CM.[27,28]

Until recently, it was thought that PMs could not give rise to choriocarcinoma. However, there is now incontrovertible genetic evidence proving that PMs can transform into choriocarcinomas.[21] This is important because it is wrongly believed by physicians at some centers that it is safe to discontinue hCG follow-up after a diagnosis of PM.

Choriocarcinoma is highly malignant and appears as a soft purple, largely hemorrhagic mass. Microscopically, it mimics an early implanting blastocyst with central cores of mononuclear cytotrophoblast surrounded by a rim of multinucleated syncytiotrophoblast and a distinct absence of chorionic villi. There are extensive areas of necrosis and hemorrhage and frequent evidence of tumor within venous sinuses. The disease fails to stimulate the connective tissue support normally associated with tumors and induces hypervascularity of the surrounding maternal tissues. This probably accounts for its highly metastatic and hemorrhagic behavior.

Placental-site trophoblastic tumors. Placental-site trophoblastic tumors (PSTTs) have been shown to follow term delivery, nonmolar abortion, and CM. It is conceivable, although unproven, that PSTT may develop after a PM. Like choriocarcinoma, the causative pregnancy may not be the immediate antecedent pregnancy.[29] Genetic analysis of some PSTTs has demonstrated that they are mostly diploid, originating from a normal conceptus and therefore biparental or androgenetic from a CM.[30]

In the normal placenta, placental-site trophoblast is distinct from villous trophoblast and infiltrates the decidua, myometrium, and spiral arteries of the uterine wall. PSTTs are rare, slow-growing, malignant tumors composed mainly of intermediate trophoblast derived from cytotrophoblast, and they therefore produce little hCG. However, they often stain strongly for human placental lactogen (hPL) and β_1-glycoprotein. Elevated Ki-67 levels may help in distinguishing PSTT from a regressing placental nodule.[31] In contrast to other forms of GTT, spread tends to occur late by local infiltration and through the lymphatics, although distant metastases can occur. Although some investigators observed a correlation between mitotic index and the subsequent clinical behavior or outcome,[30,32] a larger single series failed to confirm this association.[33]

The role of imprinting. All autosomal genes consist of two alleles (paternal and maternal). However, some alleles are expressed only from one parent and not the other, a phenomenon called *genomic imprinting.* Three closely related genes that are imprinted may be involved in GTT development and in other overgrowth syndromes. These are *H19,* a putative tumor suppressor gene,[34] *CDKN1C* (also designated P57 and KIP2), a cyclin-dependent kinase inhibitor,[35] which are normally expressed by the maternal allele, and the paternally expressed *IGF2,* a growth factor commonly implicated in tumor proliferation.[36] Although *CDKN1C* showed the expected pattern of expression in CM and choriocarcinoma,[37] CM and postmole tumors were unexpectedly found to express *H19,*[38] and some post-term tumors showed biallelic expression of *H19* and *IGF2.*[39] This suggests that loss of the normal imprinting patterns of these genes may be an important factor in the development of GTT.

The identification of rare families in which several sisters have repeat CMs that are biparental in origin[12] is likely to shed further light on the genes involved in CM formation. Linkage and homozygosity analysis suggested that in two families there is a defective gene located on chromosome 19q13.3-13.4, where at least one imprinted gene is located.[40] However, analysis of another rare family with individuals who have had repetitive biparental CMs has raised the possibility that the genes involved in this disorder may reside on another chromosome.[41] This work has also provided data to support the hypothesis that CMs are a consequence of a global disorder in imprinting in the female germline.

The identification of the genes underlying GTD is a major goal for the coming years. The results will, for example, enable in vitro testing of early embryos before implantation in women with repetitive molar pregnancies.

Human Chorionic Gonadotrophin

Assays for β-human chorionic gonadotrophin. The family of pituitary and placental glycoprotein hormones includes hCG, follicle-stimulating hormone (FSH), luteinizing hormone (LH), and thyroid stimulating hormone (TSH). Each hormone comprises an α-subunit that is common between the family members and a distinct β-subunit. Consequently, assays to measure hCG are directed against the β-subunit. Many β-hCG assays are available. Some detect intact β–hCG, and others are selective for individual fragments or detect various combinations of hCG fragments or hyperglycosylated forms.[42-44] The mechanism of detection is also variable and includes enzyme-linked sandwich assays and radioimmunoassay (RIA). As a result of these differences, great care is required in the interpretation of results obtained. Pregnancy tests employing hemagglutination inhibition or complement fixation methods have a lower limit of sensitivity of only 2000 IU/L and may give false-negative results when values for hCG are very high. In contrast, some assays, including the modern monoclonal or polyclonal sandwich platforms, can give false-positive readings.[45]

Are false-positive human chorionic gonadotrophin results a problem, and how should physicians deal with this issue? Although falsely elevated serum hCG results are rare, they have led clinicians to perform unnecessary medical interventions, including hysterectomy and chemotherapy.[46] The consequences can be disastrous, ranging from infertility to induction of second tumors and even death. Not surprisingly, women who have been subjected to this type of unnecessary treatment have sued their doctors and the companies responsible for the hCG assays used. Features that should make the clinician consider an hCG result as potentially false positive include a well patient, absence of a pregnancy or obvious tumor on imaging, and an hCG concentration that does not significantly rise with time. These false-positive results often arise from human anti-mouse antibodies (hAMAs) cross-reacting with the mouse monoclonal antibodies used to detect hCG. Because hAMAs do not pass into the urine, a simple test for hCG in the urine using the same assay that is used for serum eliminates this cause of false-positive result. An alternative would be to test the serum with a different type of hCG assay, although it is technically possible for hAMAs to interfere in more than one type of serum assay.

The competitive RIA using a polyclonal antibody recognizing all forms of β-hCG remains a gold-standard assay for use in the management of GTD. They are sensitive to 1 IU/L in serum and 20 IU/L in urine and are not generally prone to false-positive readings from heterophilic antibodies such as hAMAs. This is partly because the assays are set up with serial dilutions in which the values for real hCG reduce appropriately but do not in the presence of heterophilic antibodies. However, the competitive RIA is time consuming, requires careful training, and is only as good as the antibodies used. There is general recognition that new assays need to be developed. As we learn more about the various fragments of β-hCG, it may become apparent that certain fragments may be more sensitive for detection of small-volume disease or correlate with poor- or good-prognosis groups.[42] Some work suggests that a hyperglycosylated form of β-hCG may be produced only by GTT, rather than by normal trophoblast.[43] If this work is confirmed in larger studies, it could provide a major new tool to distinguish between malignancy and a normal pregnancy.

Use of human chorionic gonadotrophin as a tumor marker. With a half-life of 24 to 36 hours, hCG is the most sensitive and specific marker for trophoblastic tissue. However, hCG production is not confined to pregnancy and GTD. The hCG is produced by any trophoblastic tissue found, for example, in germ cell tumors and in up to 15% of epithelial malignancies.[47] The hCG levels in such cases can be just as high as those seen in GTD or in pregnancy. Current methods for hCG measurement do not reliably discriminate among pregnancy, GTD, and nongestational trophoblastic tumors. However, serial measurements of hCG have revolutionized the management of GTD for several reasons. The amount of hCG produced correlates with tumor volume so that a serum hCG of 5 IU/L corresponds to approximately 10^4 to 10^5 viable tumor cells. Consequently, these assays are several orders of magnitude more sensitive than the best imaging modalities available today. The hCG levels can be used to determine prognosis.[48,49] Serial measurements allow progress of the disease or response to therapy to be monitored (Fig. 44-3). Development of drug resistance can be detected at an early stage, which facilitates appropriate management changes. Estimates may be made of the time for which chemotherapy should be continued after hCG levels are undetectable in serum to reduce the tumor volume to zero. For these reasons, hCG is the best tumor marker known.

How should persistently raised low-level human chorionic gonadotrophin of unknown origin be managed?

A small subgroup of the population has a persistently raised hCG that is detected by chance on investigation for another disorder or as part of a routine health check. Subsequent intensive workup, including exclusion of pituitary disease, fails to show any abnormality apart from the persistently raised hCG that is proved to be genuine and not a false-positive result. There is debate about how best to manage such individuals. Some have advocated a trial of

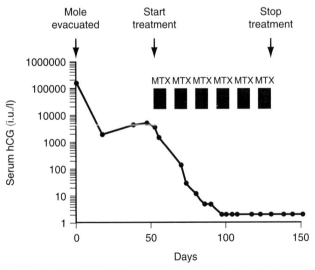

Figure 44–3. The graph demonstrates the use of monitoring serum human chorionic gonadotrophin (hCG) concentrations after evacuation of a hydatidiform mole (HM). In this case, after an initial fall, the hCG level started to rise, indicating the development of an invasive HM or choriocarcinoma, and the patient was called in for disease staging. The prognostic score indicated a low risk (see Tables 44-4 and 44-5), and the patient was successfully treated with methotrexate (MTX) and folinic acid (see Table 44-6).

chemotherapy or a hysterectomy, or both, on the assumption that there must be some hCG-secreting tumor cells present that could include an occult PSTT. However, others have suggested careful surveillance with serial hCG monitoring and repeat investigations that should be intensified if the hCG starts to rise.[50] Although the latter approach is sensible, in women who have completed their families, hysterectomy may be considered to exclude a PSTT, particularly if the hCG level is rising. At Charing Cross, we had one patient with a slowly rising hCG who was found to have a PSTT even though the D&C, hysteroscopy, laparoscopy, transvaginal Doppler ultrasound, gadolinium-enhanced magnetic resonance imaging (MRI) scan of pelvis and brain, computed tomography (CT) of the body, and [^{18}F]fluoro-2-deoxy-D-glucose–enhanced positron emission tomography (FDG-PET) were negative.

Clinical Features

Complete and partial moles. CMs and PMs most commonly manifest in the first trimester as a threatened abortion with vaginal bleeding. If the diagnosis is delayed, patients may notice the passing of grapelike structures (i.e., vesicles), and the entire mole occasionally may be spontaneously evacuated. The uterus may be any size but is commonly large for gestational age. Patients with marked trophoblastic growth and high hCG levels are particularly prone to hyperemesis, toxemia, and the development of theca lutein cysts that may sometimes be palpable above the pelvis. Toxemia was diagnosed in 27% of patients with CMs[51] but is seen less frequently today because of early ultrasound diagnosis.[52,53] Convulsions rarely occur. The high hCG levels may also produce hyperthyroidism because of cross-reactivity between hCG and TSH at the TSH receptor. Although pulmonary, vaginal, and cervical metastases can occur, they may spontaneously disappear after removal of the mole. The presence of metastases does not necessarily imply that invasive mole or choriocarcinoma has developed. Patients rarely present with acute respiratory distress because of pulmonary metastases or anemia and occasionally because of tumor embolization. The risk of embolization is reduced by avoiding agents that induce uterine contraction before the cervix has been dilated to enable evacuation of the CM.

Patients with PMs usually do not exhibit the dramatic clinical features characteristic of CMs.[54] The uterus is often not enlarged for gestational age, and because vaginal bleeding tends to occur later, patients most often present in the late first trimester or early second trimester with a missed or incomplete abortion. The diagnosis is often only suspected when the histology of curettings is available. The pre-evacuation hCG level is less than 100,000 IU/L at diagnosis in more than 90% of cases.

Twin pregnancies. Twin pregnancies comprising a normal fetus and a hydatidiform mole are estimated to occur in 1 of 20,000 to 100,000 pregnancies.[55] Some probably abort in the first trimester and therefore are undiagnosed. However, some are discovered on ultrasound examination routinely or because of complications such as bleeding, excessive uterine size, or problems related to a high hCG level.

Invasive moles. Invasive moles are usually diagnosed because serial urine or serum hCG measurements reveal a plateaued or rising hCG level in the weeks after molar evacuation. Patients may complain of persistent vaginal bleeding or lower abdominal pains and swelling. This may occur as a result of hemorrhage from leaking tumor-induced vasculature as the trophoblast invades through the myometrium or because of vulval, vaginal, or intra-abdominal metastases. The tumor may involve other pelvic structures, including the bladder or rectum, producing hematuria or rectal bleeding, respectively. Enlarging pulmonary metastases or tumor emboli growing in the pulmonary arteries can contribute to life-threatening respiratory complications.[56] The risk of these complications is clearly higher in patients when the initial diagnosis of a molar pregnancy was missed and who therefore are not on hCG follow-up.

Choriocarcinoma. Choriocarcinoma can manifest after any form of pregnancy, but it most commonly occurs after a CM. Histologic proof of choriocarcinoma is usually not obtained after a CM because of the risk of fatal hemorrhage, and it is therefore impossible to distinguish it from invasive mole. Choriocarcinoma after a normal pregnancy or nonmolar abortion usually manifests within a year of delivery but can occur up to 17 years later.[57] The presenting features may be similar to hydatidiform mole with vaginal bleeding, abdominal pain, and a pelvic mass. However, one third of all choriocarcinomas manifest without gynecologic features; patients instead suffer from symptoms associated with their distant metastases. In these cases, lives can be saved by remembering to include choriocarcinoma in the differential diagnosis of metastatic malignancy (particularly in lungs, brain, or liver) manifesting in a woman of childbearing age. Any site may be involved, including skin producing a purple lesion, cauda equina, and the heart. Pulmonary disease may be parenchymal or pleural, or it may result form tumor embolism and subsequent growth in the pulmonary arteries.[58] Respiratory symptoms and signs can include dyspnea, hemoptysis, and pulmonary artery hypertension. Cerebral metastases may produce focal neurologic signs, convulsions, evidence of raised intracranial pressure, and intracerebral or subarachnoid hemorrhage. Hepatic metastases may cause local pain or referred pain in the right shoulder. Although none of these presentations is specific to choriocarcinoma, performing a simple pregnancy test or quantitative hCG assay can provide a vital clue to the diagnosis.

Infantile choriocarcinoma. Choriocarcinoma in the fetus or newborn is rare, with approximately 26 cases reported.[59] Although a primary choriocarcinoma

within the infant is possible, in 11 cases, the mother also had the tumor. The diagnosis was often made in the neonate before the mother. In all cases, the infant was anemic and had a raised hCG level, but the site of metastasis was varied, including brain, liver, lung, and skin. Only six cases have been successfully treated; the rest died within weeks of the initial diagnosis, which might have been delayed. Consequently, serum or urine hCG levels should be measured in all babies of mothers with choriocarcinoma. Because the disease can manifest up to 6 months after delivery, an argument can be made for serial monitoring of hCG levels in these infants.

Placental-site trophoblastic tumor. A PSTT grows slowly and can manifest years after a term delivery, nonmolar abortion, or CM. Unlike choriocarcinoma, it tends to metastasize late in its natural history, and patients frequently present with gynecologic symptoms alone. In addition to vaginal bleeding, the production of hPL by the cytotrophoblastic cells may cause hyperprolactinemia that can result in amenorrhea or galactorrhea, or both. Rarely, patients can develop nephrotic syndrome or hematuria and disseminated intravascular coagulation. Metastases may occur in the vagina, extrauterine pelvic tissues, retroperitoneum, lymph nodes, lungs, and brain. The serum hCG levels can be higher than 50,000 IU/L but are usually low, measuring less than 500 IU/L in 58% of patients in one series.[30,33]

Investigations

Human chorionic gonadotrophin, plain chest radiographs, and pelvic Doppler ultrasonography. All patients who are suspected of having GTTs should have serum and urine hCG level tests, a chest radiograph, and pelvic Doppler ultrasound. The most common metastatic appearance on a chest radiograph is multiple, discrete, rounded lesions, but large and solitary lesions, a miliary pattern, and pleural effusions can occur.[60] Tumor emboli to the pulmonary arteries can produce an identical picture to venous thromboembolism with wedge-shaped infarcts and areas of decreased vascular markings. Pulmonary artery hypertension can cause dilatation of the pulmonary arteries. Routine CT scanning of the chest does not add anything to the management of these cases.[61]

Ultrasound and color Doppler imaging is not diagnostic but is highly suggestive of molar disease[52,53] or persistent GTD[62] when there is a combination of a raised hCG level, no pregnancy, and a vascular mass within the uterus (Fig. 44-4). The latter is seen in more than 75% of patients with persistent trophoblastic disease after initial evacuation of the uterus. The determination of uterine volume correlates with the amount of disease, and uterine volume and the degree of abnormal tumor vasculature independently predict the likelihood of resistance to single-agent methotrexate therapy.[49] The vascular abnormalities within the pelvis and uterus can persist long after the disease has been

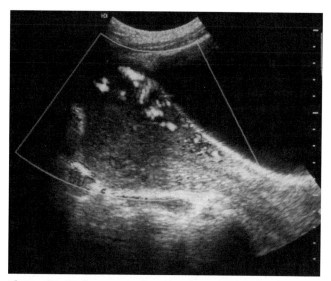

Figure 44–4. Ultrasonography with color Doppler shows persistent gestational trophoblastic disease after removal of a complete hydatidiform mole within the body and wall of the uterus. A typical vesicular or "'snowstorm" appearance of residual molar tissue can be seen within the uterus together with a rich blood supply throughout the endometrium and myometrium. There is no evidence of a fetus. See also Color Figure 44-4.

eradicated with chemotherapy. This is usually of no consequence. However, some patients suffer repeated vaginal hemorrhages from these vascular malformations and require selective arterial embolization. This may need to be repeated on several occasions but is usually successful and does not appear to affect fertility.[63]

A pelvic ultrasound scan can also demonstrate ovarian theca lutein cysts and other ovarian masses. Metastatic spread outside the pelvis, such as to the liver or kidneys, can be identified and shown to have an abnormal Doppler signal.

Investigation of drug-resistant disease. When patients develop drug-resistant disease, further investigation is required to more accurately define where the residual tumor is located because resection can be curative. CT of the chest and abdomen together with MRI of the brain and pelvis is often helpful and can detect deposits not previously seen. If the CT and MRI scans are normal, a lumbar puncture to measure the hCG level in cerebrospinal fluid (CSF) can be useful to detect disease in the central nervous system. An hCG ratio greater than 1:60 (CSF to serum) of that found in the serum is highly indicative of the presence of trophoblastic disease.

Experimental imaging techniques. Radiolabeled anti-hCG antibodies given intravenously can localize tumors producing hCG when the serum hCG level is higher than 100 IU/L.[64] Because false-positive and false-negative results occur, anti-hCG scanning should be regarded as complementary to other imaging investigations. PET has provided a novel way to image many types of tumors using a variety of labels. Whole-body

PET has been reported to distinguish GTT emboli from blood clot in two patients with choriocarcinoma.[65] PET with various compounds, such as FDG, which can identify tumors missed by other techniques,[66] has yet to prove an aid in the location of drug-resistant GTTs.

Genetic analysis. On some occasions, it can be helpful to perform a comparative genetic analysis of the patient's trophoblastic tumor with her normal tissue and, if available, with that of her partner. If the tumor is suspected to be of nongestational origin, this status can be confirmed by the presence of only maternal DNA and the complete absence of paternal DNA. Genetic studies can also determine which of several antecedent pregnancies is the causal pregnancy of the current GTT. This can have an impact on determining appropriate therapy and prognosis.[12]

Management

Molar evacuation. Evacuation of the uterine cavity using suction gives the lowest incidence of sequelae.[67,68] When the molar trophoblast invades the myometrium, it is relatively easy to perforate the uterus if a metal curette is used. Medical induction involving repeated contraction of the uterus induced by oxytocin or prostaglandin or other surgical approaches, including hysterectomy and hysterotomy, increases the risk of requiring chemotherapy by twofold to threefold compared with suction evacuation. This is thought to occur because tumor is more likely to be disseminated by uterine contraction and manipulation. For similar reasons, the use of prostanoids to ripen a nulliparous cervix is not recommended even in nulliparous women.[68] If bleeding is severe immediately after suction evacuation, a single dose of ergometrine to produce one uterine contraction may stem the hemorrhage and does not appear to increase the chance of requiring chemotherapy.

In the past, it has been common practice for gynecologists to perform a second and sometimes a third evacuation of the uterine cavity in patients with a molar pregnancy. However, the chances of requiring chemotherapy after one evacuation is only 2.4% but rises markedly to 18% after two evacuations and to 81% after four evacuations (Table 44-1). Consequently, a second evacuation may be reasonable and should be discussed with the local GTD center if there is vaginal bleeding in the presence of persisting molar trophoblast within the uterine cavity. The use of ultrasound control during this procedure may help to reduce the risk of uterine perforation. Further evacuations are not recommended because of the risk of complications and the high likelihood that the patient will require chemotherapy anyway.

Should twin pregnancies be terminated early? At Charing Cross Hospital in London, we have seen 77 confirmed cases of CM with a separate normal conceptus. The management of twin pregnancies

Table 44–1. Correlation between the Number of Evacuations Performed for a Hydatidiform Mole and the Subsequent Requirement for Chemotherapy at Charing Cross Hospital, 1973-1986

No. of Evacuations	Patients Not Treated	Patients Treated	Patients Treated (%)
1	4481	109	2.4
2	1495	267	18
3	106	106	50
4	5	22	81

Table 44–2. Factors Increasing the Requirement of Chemotherapy after Evacuation of a Hydatidiform Mole

Factor	Study
Uterine size > gestational age	Curry et al.[138] (1975)
Pre-evacuation serum human chorionic gonadotropin (hCG) level > 100,000 IU/L	Berkowitz and Goldstein[51] (1981)
Oral contraceptives given before hCG falls to normal	Stone et al.[74] (1976)
Bilateral cystic ovarian enlargement	Zongfu et al.[139] (1979); Berkowitz and Goldstein[51] (1981)

comprising a normal fetus and a CM is difficult because they can be associated with complications such as fetal death, severe vaginal bleeding, preeclampsia, and a possible increased risk of persistent GTD requiring chemotherapy.[69-71] In our series, although 24 women elected to have an early termination, 53 decided to continue their pregnancies. Nearly 40% of these resulted in live births, most of which occurred beyond 32 weeks' gestation. The remaining women mostly spontaneously terminated their pregnancies before 24 weeks. The risk of severe preeclampsia was 6%. Strikingly, women continuing their pregnancies did not have a significantly increased risk of persistent GTD requiring chemotherapy. Moreover, there were no maternal deaths. It appears reasonably safe to allow patients with twin pregnancies in which one of the conceptions is a CM to continue to term, provided there are no other complications.[55]

Are registration, centralized follow-up, and therapy after uterine evacuation valuable? Most patients require no more treatment after evacuation, but 16% of patients with CM and less than 0.5% with PM develop persistent GTD. It is vital that patients with persistent GTD be rapidly identified because virtually all of them can be cured with appropriate therapy. In 1973, under the auspices of the Royal College of Obstetricians and Gynecologists, a national follow-up service was instituted in the United Kingdom whereby patients with GTD are registered with one of three laboratories located in Dundee, Sheffield, and London. Approximately 1400 women are registered per annum, and 110 to 120 require subsequent chemotherapy, with 85 being treated in the London center and the rest in Sheffield. After registration, the patient's details and pathology together with two weekly blood and urine samples are sent through the mail to one of the reference laboratories for confirmation of diagnosis and serial hCG estimations. This scheme has been very successful and has enabled refinement of treatments that would otherwise not have been possible. Similar centralized registration and treatment has been established in the Netherlands[72] and Korea[73] but has not yet been achieved in the United States or in other European countries. The failure to centralize the registration and subsequent management of GTD patients in these countries has resulted in patchy standards of care. Moreover, despite guidelines, these recommendations can never be detailed enough to substitute for

the experience gained in treating thousands rather than tens of patients.

In most cases, the molar tissue dies spontaneously, the hCG concentration returns to normal (about 4 IU/L), and the patient can start a new pregnancy after another 6 months. If the hCG level has fallen to normal within 8 weeks of evacuation, marker follow-up can be safely reduced to 6 months because none of these patients has required chemotherapy. However, in patients whose hCG levels are still elevated beyond 8 weeks from the date of evacuation, follow-up should continue for 2 years. Because patients who have had a previous mole or GTT are more at risk of having a second, all patients should have a further estimation of hCG at 6 and 10 weeks after the completion of each subsequent pregnancy.

Indications for chemotherapy. Factors associated with an increased risk of requiring chemotherapy are summarized in Table 44-2. The hormones in the oral contraceptive pill (OCP) are probably growth factors for trophoblastic tumors, and for this reason, patients are advised not to use the pill until the hCG levels have returned to normal.[74,75] Prior duration of OCP use may also increase the risk of developing a molar pregnancy.[76]

The indications for intervention with chemotherapy in patients who have had a CM or PM are shown in Table 44-3. The hCG value of 20,000 IU/L 4 weeks after evacuation of a mole or rising values in this range at an earlier stage indicate the patient is at increased

Table 44–3. Indications for Chemotherapy

Any of the following conditions are indications to treat after a diagnosis of gestational trophoblastic disease:
1. Evidence of metastases in the brain, liver, or gastrointestinal tract or radiologic opacities > 2 cm on chest radiograph
2. Histologic evidence of choriocarcinoma
3. Heavy vaginal bleeding or evidence of gastrointestinal or intraperitoneal hemorrhage
4. Pulmonary, vulval, or vaginal metastases unless the human chorionic gonadotropin (hCG) level is falling
5. Rising hCG level after evacuation
6. Serum hCG ≥ 20,000 IU/L more than 4 weeks after evacuation, because of the risk of uterine perforation
7. Raised hCG level 6 months after evacuation, even if the level is still falling

Table 44–4. Scoring System for Gestational Trophoblastic Tumors

Prognostic Factor	Score*			
	0	1	2	6
Age (years)	<39	>39		
Antecedent pregnancy (AP)	Mole	Abortion or unknown	Term	
Interval: end of AP to chemotherapy at CXH† (months)	<4	4-7	7-12	>12
Human chorionic gonadotropin (IU/L)	10^3-10^4	<10^3	10^4-10^5	>10^5
ABO blood group (female × male)		A × O / O × A / O or A × unknown	B × A or O / AB × A or O	
No. of metastases	None	1-4	4-8	>8
Site of metastases	Not detected, lungs, vagina	Spleen, kidney	Gastrointestinal tract	Brain, liver
Largest tumor mass		3-5 cm	>5 cm	
Prior chemotherapy			Single drug	Two or more drugs

*The total score for a patient is obtained by adding the individual scores for each prognostic factor: low risk, 0-5; medium risk, 6-8; high risk, ≥9. Patients scoring 0-8 receive single agent therapy with methotrexate and folinic acid, and patients scoring ≥9 receive combination drug therapy with a regimen consisting of etoposide, methotrexate, and actinomycin D (EMA) alternating weekly with cyclophosphamide and vincristine (Oncovin) (CO).
†Charing Cross Hospital.

risk of severe hemorrhage or uterine perforation with intraperitoneal bleeding. These complications can be life threatening, and their risk can be reduced by starting chemotherapy. Metastases in the lung, vulva, and vagina can be observed only if the hCG levels are falling. However, if the hCG levels are not dropping or the patient has metastases at another site, which can indicate the development of choriocarcinoma, chemotherapy is required.

Prognostic factors and FIGO staging. The principal prognostic variables for GTTs, which were originally identified by Bagshawe[48] and since modified by the WHO and our own experience, are summarized in Table 44-4. They have been combined with the FIGO staging system to give the unified staging and scoring system shown in Table 44-5.[77] Each variable carries a score that, when added together for an individual patient, correlates with the risk of the tumor's becoming resistant to single-agent therapy. The most important prognostic variables carry the highest score and include (1) the duration of the disease, because drug resistance of GTTs varies inversely with time from the original antecedent pregnancy; (2) the serum hCG concentration, which correlates with viable tumor volume in the body; and (3) the presence of liver or brain metastases. ABO blood groups (see Table 44-4) contribute little to the overall scoring and therefore have been removed from the current system (see Table 44-5).

Types of chemotherapy. At Charing Cross, we have used the prognostic scoring system in Table 44-4 to subdivide the patients into three groups, categorized as low, medium, and high risk depending on their overall scores. Formerly, each risk group corresponded with a separate treatment regimen, and there were three types of treatment called low-, medium-, and high-risk therapy. Several years ago, we discontinued

the medium-risk treatment for three reasons. First, the short- and long-term toxicity of this treatment is probably not significantly different from high-risk therapy. Second, some patients treated with medium-risk therapy have developed drug resistance and subsequently required high-risk therapy. Third, about 30% of medium-risk patients can still be cured on low-risk chemotherapy, which is less toxic than medium- or high-risk chemotherapy.[78] Moreover, there is no evidence that prior treatment failure with methotrexate is an adverse prognostic variable.[79,80] Accordingly, patients who score between 0 and 8 (0 to 6 in the unified/FIGO scoring system) receive low-risk chemotherapy. Patients scoring 9 (7 in the unified/FIGO scoring system) are given high-risk treatment. The details of low- and high-risk treatment are discussed later. Patients are admitted for the first 1 to 3 weeks of therapy, principally because the tumors are often highly vascular and may bleed vigorously in this early period of treatment.

Treating low-risk patients: methotrexate or actinomycin D? Most centers in the world treat low-risk patients with single-agent methotrexate plus folinic acid rescue (MTX/FA) or with actinomycin D. A variety of different regimens have been developed for administering these drugs. Many of the reported differences in overall response rates are likely accounted for by differences in total numbers studied, entry criteria, and the decision about when to stop therapy.

Methotrexate has been given as an intravenous bolus with or without folinic acid rescue on a daily, weekly, two-weekly, or even less frequent basis.[81-84] It has also been given intramuscularly with or without folinic acid.[85-87] Oral administration has not been favored because of the variable absorption and bioavailability. In developing countries, omission of folinic acid may be advantageous as a cost-cutting measure.[83]

Table 44-5. WHO Prognostic Scoring System as Modified by FIGO

Scores	0	1	2	4
Age (years)	<40	≥40	—	—
Antecedent pregnancy	Mole	Abortion	Term	
Interval (months) from index pregnancy	<4	4-<7	7-<13	≥13
Pretreatment serum human chorionic gonadotropin (IU/ L) level	$<10^3$	$10^3-<10^4$	$10^4-<10^5$	$≥10^5$
Largest tumor size (including uterus)	—	3-<5 cm	≥5 cm	—
Site of metastases	Lung	Spleen, kidney	Gastrointestinal	Brain, liver
Number of metastases identified	—	1-4	5-8	>8
Previous chemotherapy failed	—	—	Single drug	Two or more drugs

The cure rates with methotrexate are generally more than 60%. Failure to cure is usually caused by the onset of methotrexate resistance or toxicity. Some work has provided further evidence that daily or alternate-daily therapy over 1 week may provide superior antitumor effects and cure rates than weekly or less frequent pulsed administration.[88] Biologically, this observation makes sense because GTT is often rapidly growing and infrequent administration of drugs is likely to allow regrowth of tumor between doses.

The regimen used since 1964 at Charing Cross Hospital and widely followed in other centers is shown in Table 44-6. This schedule is well tolerated and causes no alopecia, and because the folinic acid dose was increased from 7.5 to 15 mg, the incidence of mucosal ulceration has been dramatically reduced from 20%[86] to less than 2%[80] (and our unpublished observations). Methotrexate can induce serositis resulting in pleuritic chest pain or abdominal pain. Myelosuppression is rare, but a full blood cell count should be obtained before each course of treatment. Liver and renal function should also be regularly monitored. Transient elevation of the liver function tests can occur, but in our experience, this has not necessitated a change in therapy. In an evaluation of patients treated between 1992 and 2000, two thirds of 485 treated women were cured with MTX/FA alone. One third required a change of therapy, largely because of drug resistance detected by a plateau or rising serum hCG concentration over three or more values (only 2% changed because of toxicity). The remaining women were subsequently cured with single-agent actinomycin D given intravenously at a dose of 0.5 mg daily for 5 days or by multiagent chemotherapy with EMA/CO (described later).[80]

Table 44-6. Chemotherapy Regimen for Low-Risk and Intermediate-Risk Patients

Drug	Schedule*
Methotrexate (MTX)	50 mg by IM injection, repeated every 48 hr × 4
Calcium folinate	15 mg orally 30 hr after each injection of MTX (folinic acid)

*Courses are repeated every 2 weeks (i.e., days 1, 15, 29, and so on).

Actinomycin D was chosen if the serum hCG level was up to 100 IU/L, and EMA/CO was given when the hCG level was more than 100 IU/L.

Over the past 40 years at our institution, one patient receiving MTX/FA died of concurrent and nontherapy-induced lymphoma, and one died of hepatitis.[80,86] There have been no therapy-induced second tumors.[78]

Like methotrexate, several intravenous actinomycin D regimens have been developed, but the available evidence suggests that daily administration over 5 days every 2 weeks is more efficacious and probably as well tolerated as the pulsed once- or twice-weekly regimens.[80,86,88-91] The overall efficacy is more than 60% and is probably higher than with MTX/FA, although a formal head-to-head study has not been performed. However, the short-term toxicity of actinomycin D is greater. Unlike methotrexate, actinomycin D can induce transient alopecia, although it is usually mild. Actinomycin D also induces nausea, myelosuppression, and oral ulceration that tend to be worse than with methotrexate. The long-term toxicity of actinomycin D probably does not significantly differ from MTX/FA, but this has yet to be fully reported.

In view of the increased short-term toxicity of actinomycin D and the greater ease of community administration of MTX (intramuscularly rather than intravenously), we have continued to favor the MTX/FA regimen as first-line therapy for low-risk GTT patients.

Treating high-risk patients: EMA/CO regimen or other multiagent treatments? Some patients are at high risk for developing drug resistance to single-agent chemotherapy. Since 1979, we have treated them with an intensive regimen consisting of etoposide, methotrexate, and actinomycin D (EMA) alternating weekly with cyclophosphamide and vincristine (Oncovin) (CO) (Table 44-7). The regimen requires one overnight stay every 2 weeks and causes alopecia and myelosuppression, which are reversible. About 70% of patients require granulocyte colony-stimulating factor support during therapy to maintain treatment intensity.[79] Other short-term toxicities include mucositis and vincristine-induced neuropathy.

The cumulative 5-year survival rate for 272 patients treated with this regimen in our center is 86%, with no deaths from GTT beyond 2 years after the initiation of chemotherapy.[79] Although these results are good,

Table 44–7.	Chemotherapy Regimen for High-Risk Patients	
Day	Drug	Schedule*
EMA		
1	Etoposide	100 mg/m² by IV infusion over 30 min
	Actinomycin D	0.5 mg by IV bolus
	Methotrexate	300 mg/m² by IV infusion over 12 hr
2	Etoposide	100 mg/m² by IV infusion over 30 min
	Actinomycin D	0.5 mg by IV bolus
	Folinic acid rescue starting 24 hr after commencing the methotrexate infusion	15 mg IM or orally every 12 hr × 4 doses
CO		
8	Vincristine	1 mg/m² by IV bolus (max. of 2 mg)
	Cyclophosphamide	600 mg/m² by IV infusion over 30 min

*A regimen consisting of etoposide, methotrexate, and actinomycin D (EMA) alternates weekly with cyclophosphamide and vincristine (Oncovin) (CO). To avoid extended intervals between courses caused by myelosuppression, it may occasionally be necessary to reduce the EMA by omitting the day 2 doses of etoposide and actinomycin D.

the presence of liver metastases or brain metastases correlated with 30% or 70% long-term survival, respectively. Patients with both liver and brain involvement appear to fare particularly badly, with only one of five surviving in our series.[92] A later analysis of patients with brain metastases suggested that the survival might not be so poor, with 86% surviving, if those dying within 8 days of admission are excluded.[92] Early deaths accounted for a significant portion of the overall mortality; causes included respiratory failure, cerebral metastases, hepatic failure, and pulmonary embolism. These women did not have preceding moles, were not registered for follow-up, and therefore presented with extensive disease. It will be difficult to improve the survival of this particular subgroup. However, any woman of childbearing age presenting with widespread malignancy should have an hCG measurement, because very high levels of this hormone are highly suggestive of choriocarcinoma.

The long-term risk of chemotherapy-induced second tumors in patients treated for GTTs in our center has been reviewed[78] and is discussed in "Long-Term Complications of Therapy."

EMA/CO is being used in most centers with similar impressive survival results of between 80% and 90%.[93-98] Other regimens that have been used to treat high-risk GTT include combinations of methotrexate, actinomycin D, and etoposide given on a weekly to thrice-weekly basis, combined methotrexate actinomycin D and cyclophosphamide and with hydroxyurea, actinomycin D, methotrexate, folinic acid, cyclophosphamide, vincristine, and doxorubicin (CHAMOCA). Most of these regimens appear in nonrandomized studies to be less effective than EMA/CO,[96] and some increase the exposure to etoposide,[99,100] which although active is clearly proved to induce second tumors.[101] Consequently, we believe that the current optimum therapy for initial treatment of uncomplicated high-risk GTT is EMA/CO therapy. The goal for the future will be to introduce agents that reduce the risk of toxicity such as second tumors without compromising efficacy.

When should therapy be discontinued? After the serum hCG has returned to normal, we estimate that there are still about 10^5 tumor cells left. Consequently, discontinuing therapy when the hCG level is just normal would likely result in higher relapse rates. For this reason, we have elected to continue therapy for 6 weeks after the hCG level is normal, which translates into three courses of MTX/FA or EMA/CO for low-risk or uncomplicated high-risk disease, respectively. Patients with complicated high-risk disease with, for example, overt central nervous system (CNS) or liver metastases or who have a score higher than 12 are usually given 8 rather than 6 weeks of continued therapy with a normal hCG level. Using this protocol, the relapse rate is approximately 3%.[79,80] It is unclear whether this time could be shortened without compromising outcome. At least one group stops therapy after the hCG level is normal in low-risk patients without increasing their relapse rate (D. Goldstein, personal communication, 2002). However, the criteria for treating patients at this center are more inclusive than at our unit; because more patients are treated than necessarily require therapy, comparison of results with the Charing Cross data set is not straightforward. The use of hCG algorithms identifying rates of fall could be helpful. Patients with rapid decreases may need less chemotherapy after the hCG level is normal. Future trials may randomize low-risk patients with a rapid fall in the hCG concentration to fewer courses of MTX/FA by, for example, stopping after one rather than three cycles when the serum hCG level is normal.

Management of drug-resistant disease.
Low-risk disease. Frequent measurement of the serum hCG level is a simple way to detect drug resistance at an early stage because the hormone levels stop falling and may start to rise long before there are other clinical changes. Decisions to alter treatment are not made on the basis of a single hCG result but on a progressive trend over two or three values. In patients receiving MTX/FA for low-risk disease, if the hCG is 100 IU/L when drug resistance occurs, the disease can

often be cured simply by substituting actinomycin D (0.5 mg total dose given intravenously daily for 5 days every 2 weeks). If the hCG is higher than 100 IU/L when developing resistance to MTX/FA, all cases are usually cured with EMA/CO.[80]

If actinomycin D is used as the initial therapy, similar salvage can be achieved by switching to MTX/FA when resistance occurs at a low serum level of hCG. Patients who are treated with once-weekly or alternate-week pulsed actinomycin D can sometimes be salvaged by increasing the frequency of administration to daily actinomycin D for 5 days every 2 weeks.[88]

High-risk disease. Most patients who have failed EMA/CO for high-risk disease can still be salvaged by further chemotherapy or surgery, or both.[79] The combination of surgical removal of the main site of drug resistance (usually uterus, lung, or brain) together with chemotherapy is particularly effective. Preoperative investigations include transvaginal or abdominal ultrasound Doppler of the pelvis, possible repeat D&C or hysteroscopy, CT scan of the whole body, MRI of the brain and pelvis, lumbar puncture to measure hCG levels in the CSF, and experimental imaging techniques such as anti-hCG or FDG-PET scanning. If all these investigations are negative, hysterectomy should be considered. When multiple possible sites of resistant disease are found, anti-hCG or FDG-PET imaging can potentially distinguish the biologically active from dead or necrotic lesions and thereby guide appropriate surgery. After surgery or when surgery is not appropriate, we use the cisplatin-containing regimen of EP (150 mg/m^2 of etoposide and 75 mg/m^2 of cisplatin with hydration) alternating weekly with EMA (omitting day 2, except the folinic acid). Although this regimen is toxic (myelosuppression is common and great care of renal function is required), the outcome has been impressive, with survival rates in excess of 80%.[102]

Other regimens that have been tried but found to be less effective include platinum, vinblastine, and bleomycin (PVB) and bleomycin, etoposide, and cisplatin (BEP).[103-105] Current alternative options include use of some of the new anticancer agents such as the taxanes, topotecan, gemcitabine, irinotecan, and oxaliplatin. Paclitaxel has been shown to have activity in patients with germ cell tumors that have failed on prior treatment.[106] Three cases of drug-resistant GTT responded to paclitaxel, with one remaining in remission,[107,108] and in another report, a fourth patient remains in remission after high-dose paclitaxel (250 mg/m^2 repeated every third week).[109]

Is there a role for high-dose chemotherapy? High-dose chemotherapy with autologous bone marrow or peripheral stem cell transplantation provides another strategy for managing high-risk, EMA/CO-resistant patients. Patient selection is probably important in determining outcome. We know from experience with refractory germ cell tumors that patients with drug-sensitive disease are the ones that stay in remission.[110,111] There have been three encouraging

case reports of remissions after high-dose chemotherapy with cyclophosphamide, etoposide, and melphalan[112] and chemotherapy with carboplatin, etoposide, and ifosfamide[113] or cyclophosphamide.[114] At Charing Cross, we have used high-dose carboplatin etoposide and cyclophosphamide in one and added paclitaxel for three other patients failing EMA/CO or EP/EMA, or both. Despite transient responses, none has achieved a durable remission. Consequently, the jury remains out on the value and timing of high-dose therapy for GTT.

Management of acute, disease-induced complications. ***Hemorrhage.*** Heavy vaginal or intraperitoneal bleeding is the most common immediate threat to life in patients with GTT. The bleeding usually slows down and stops with bed rest and appropriate chemotherapy. However, the bleeding occasionally can be torrential, requiring massive transfusion. In this situation, if the bleeding is coming from the uterus, it may be necessary to consider a vaginal pack or emergency embolization of the tumor vasculature. Fortunately, hysterectomy is rarely required. If the bleeding is intraperitoneal and does not settle with transfusion and chemotherapy, laparotomy may be required. Patients occasionally present this way.

Respiratory failure. Occasionally, patients present with respiratory failure caused by multiple pulmonary metastases or rarely as a result of massive tumor embolism to the pulmonary circulation as shown in Figure 44-5.[56,58] However, in our experience, these patients can be cured with appropriate management. Pulse oximetry and arterial blood gas determinations should be done regularly to allow appropriate adjustment of oxygen therapy and to monitor any deterioration in pulmonary function that may occur after the start of chemotherapy. The latter occurs probably because of edema and inflammation around tumor deposits that are becoming necrotic. To prevent this, we usually commence therapy with only etoposide (100 mg/m^2) and cisplatin (20 mg/m^2) given on days 1 and 2, repeated after 1 week, and we introduce the other drugs after pulmonary function is stable. Oxygen support may be required, including masked continuous positive airway pressure ventilation, but mechanical ventilation is contraindicated because it results in trauma to the tumor vasculature, leading to massive intrapulmonary hemorrhage and death. For this reason extracorporeal oxygenation has been proposed.[115]

Management of cerebral metastases. Involvement of the CNS by GTT may be overt and require intensive therapy or occult and need prophylaxis. Any patient with a GTT who has lung metastases is at risk for CNS disease.[116] The second most common site of metastases in high-risk patients is the CNS, and nearly all of these individuals have had lung deposits.[116] Neurologic symptoms and signs may alert the clinician to the presence of brain metastases. However, some high-risk patients do not have overt pulmonary or CNS disease

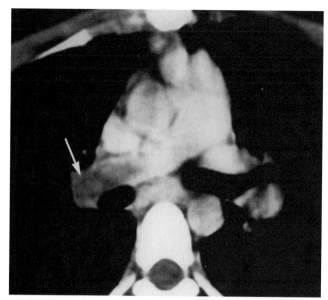

Figure 44–5. Contrast-enhanced computed tomography (CT) of the thorax at the level of the main pulmonary arteries shows a filling defect in the right main pulmonary artery *(arrow)*. The patient presented with a brief history of increasing shortness of breath that had suddenly worsened. During the previous 18 months, she had suffered from irregular, heavy vaginal bleeding; had four separate positive pregnancy tests; and had two pelvic ultrasound investigations with normal results. She was successfully treated with EMA/CO chemotherapy, with some resolution of the changes seen on CT and ventilation-perfusion scanning. Postmortem examinations of similar cases have revealed that the filling defect in the main pulmonary artery is a tumor embolus, not a clot. (From Seckl MJ, Rustin GJS, Newlands ES, et al: Pulmonary embolism, pulmonary hypertension, and choriocarcinoma. Lancet 1991;338:1313-1315.)

at presentation but subsequently develop cerebral metastases that are then drug resistant. Consequently, careful investigation of patients at risk for developing brain metastases is warranted so that appropriate CNS-penetrating chemotherapy is given rather than the standard low- or high-risk treatments. Investigations include contrast-enhanced CT or (preferably) MRI of the brain, and in patients who do not have raised intracranial pressure, the hCG levels in CSF should be measured. A CSF-to-serum ratio of hCG that is greater than 1:60 suggests the presence of CNS disease.

Central nervous system prophylaxis.

At Charing Cross, prophylaxis against possible CNS disease (i.e., MRI of brain is normal) is given to patients from all risk categories with lung metastases and all high-risk patients, regardless of the absence or presence of lung deposits. The prophylaxis consists of 12.5 mg of methotrexate administered intrathecally, followed 24 hours later by 15 mg of folinic acid given orally. This prophylaxis is given with every course of low-risk therapy or with each CO in the high-risk therapy for three doses. Since the introduction of this policy, the development of brain metastases without evidence of drug resistance elsewhere has been rare.[116] Nevertheless, others have not adopted a policy of prophylaxis partly because lumbar punctures are invasive and can induce

headaches in up to 40% of patients. We have been able to eliminate the problem of headaches by using epidural-type spinal needles.[117] In a series of 67 patients who had lung metastases and received no CNS prophylaxis, one patient who was poorly compliant with therapy subsequently developed CNS disease.[118]

Does radiotherapy have a role in the management of overt central nervous system disease?

Overt CNS disease requires careful management because therapy can induce hemorrhage in the tumor, leading to a rise in intracranial pressure and subsequent loss of life.[92,116] We and others have found that early resection of solitary brain deposits in patients with serious neurologic signs can sometimes be lifesaving.[119-121] Alternatively, some have argued that emergency radiotherapy can reduce acute bleeding or the subsequent risk of bleeding.[122] However, there is no biologic mechanism to explain how radiotherapy can acutely stop bleeding, and we do not recommend this approach. To reduce cerebral edema, patients are given 24 mg of dexamethasone in divided doses before starting chemotherapy. By starting chemotherapy gently with low-dose etoposide and cisplatinum over 2 days (as described earlier for severe pulmonary disease), it is possible to reduce the risk of worsening edema and hemorrhage. Subsequently, the EMA/CO regimen is modified by increasing the dose of methotrexate to 1 g/m^2, given as a 24-hour infusion on day 1. The folinic acid rescue is increased to 30 mg, given every 8 hours intravenously for 3 days, commencing 32 hours after the start of the methotrexate infusion. Provided there is no evidence of raised intracranial pressure, 12.5 mg of methotrexate is given intrathecally with each CO dose, with 15 mg of folinic acid rescue 24 hours later, until the serum hCG level is normal. Modified EMA/CO is then continued for another 6 to 8 weeks. Patients who survive the first 8 days of such treatment have a good prognosis, with an 86% chance of cure.[92,121]

Patients who develop cerebral tumor during chemotherapy have a poor prognosis because their disease is almost certainly drug resistant. Nevertheless, a combination of immediate surgery to remove the deposits and modified chemotherapy designed to provide better CNS penetration can be curative in this situation.[92,116,121] Whole-brain radiotherapy alone or in combination with chemotherapy has been advocated as an alternative therapeutic approach in the management of CNS disease.[123,124] However, it has not been shown to eradicate tumor in its own right, and in combination with chemotherapy, it has produced less effective results than chemotherapy alone.[116,121] Moreover, there is potential for more long-term CNS toxicity when combining whole-brain radiotherapy with chemotherapy. Nevertheless, there is probably a role for using stereotactic radiotherapy after chemotherapy for persistent, isolated, deep lesions that cannot be removed surgically.[92]

What is optimal therapy for placental-site trophoblastic tumors?

PSTTs differ from the other forms of GTD and produce little hCG, grow slowly, metastasize late, and are relatively resistant to combination-chemotherapy regimens. Hysterectomy therefore remains the treatment of choice, provided the disease is localized to the uterus. Because the disease usually spreads to local pelvic lymph nodes before distant metastases occur, pelvic lymphadenectomy should be performed. For young women without a family history of ovarian cancer, we recommend conservation of the ovaries. When metastatic disease is present, individual patients can respond and be apparently cured by chemotherapy (EP/EMA) alone or in combination with surgery.[30,32,33,102] Radiotherapy has produced mixed results and has not been proved to cure the disease.

The prognostic scoring system cannot be used to determine the treatment of these patients. However, several prognostic variables have been identified, and probably the most important is the interval from the last pregnancy. When this is less than 4 years, the prognosis is good, and when it is more than 4 years, the outcome is almost universally fatal.[33,125] Because PSTT is rare, it is unlikely that its treatment will ever be optimized.

Patient follow-up after chemotherapy. On completion of their chemotherapy, patients are monitored regularly with hCG estimations (Table 44-8) to confirm that their disease is in remission. At Charing Cross, we review patients 6 weeks after chemotherapy, repeating any initial staging investigations that were positive. Although in most instances pulmonary metastases or uterine vascular malformations disappear, such abnormalities can persist. These are of no consequence unless the serum hCG level rises, and we therefore do not advocate routine repeat chest radiographs or Doppler ultrasound scans to follow these residual abnormalities. Occasionally, persistent uterine vascular malformations can be associated with serious per vaginum (PV) bleeding and require embolization as shown in Figure 44-6. Such procedures may need to be repeated to achieve control of the problem. Fortunately, fertility does not appear to have been compromised in women who have attempted subsequent pregnancies.[63] The risk of GTT relapse is about 3% and is most likely in the first year of follow-up. We continue hCG follow-up for life or until a full set of data are available to more accurately guide us as to when it may be safe to stop.

The optimal follow-up period for PSTT is less clear. The tumor is slow growing and therefore has the potential to relapse late. We have found that all of our patients have shown elevation of serum hCG levels in the presence of disease.[30,33] However, it is possible that these tumors may fail to secrete hCG at relapse despite an extensive tumor burden.[126] Consequently, patients in remission from PSTT should be followed serologically for life, and an argument could be made for regular review in the clinic. After treatment, patients should have baseline MRI of the pelvis and CT or MRI scans of other previously involved areas for future comparison in the event of a relapse.

Timing of pregnancy after treatment and contraceptive advice. Patients are advised not to become pregnant until 12 months after completing chemotherapy. This minimizes the potential teratogenicity of treatment and avoids confusion between a new pregnancy or relapsed disease as the cause of a rising hCG level Despite this advice, 230 women on follow-up at our center between 1973 and 1997 have become pregnant during the first year. Fortunately, this did not appear to be associated with an increased risk of relapse or fetal morbidity, and there were no maternal deaths.[127] Seventy-five percent of women continued their pregnancies to term. Although we continue to advise women to avoid pregnancy for 1 year after completing chemotherapy, those who do become pregnant can be assured of a likely favorable outcome. When a patient becomes pregnant, it is important to confirm by ultrasound and other appropriate means that the pregnancy is normal. Follow-up is then discontinued until 3 weeks after the end of pregnancy, when the hCG level due to the pregnancy should have returned to normal.

OCP use before the hCG level is normal after evacuation of a hydatidiform mole increases the risk of developing persistent GTD.[74] For this reason, patients are advised to avoid OCPs until the hCG level has returned to normal after removal of a hydatidiform mole. Patients who have had chemotherapy for their GTT are advised not to use the OCP until their hCG level is normal and chemotherapy is completed.

Table 44-8. Follow-up of Low- or High-Risk Patients with Gestational Trophoblastic Tumors Treated with Chemotherapy

Follow-up Period	Urine	Blood	Outpatient Follow-up
Year 1			
First 6 wk	Weekly	Weekly	6 wk after chemotherapy
6 wk-6 mo	Every 2 wk	Every 2 wk	—
6 mo-1 yr	Every 2 wk	—	—
Year 2	Monthly	—	—
Year 3	Every 2 mo	—	—
Year 4	Every 3 mo	—	—
Year 5	Every 4 mo	—	—
Rest of Life	Every 6 mo	—	—

Figure 44–6. Arteriographic appearance of a uterine arteriovenous malformation before *(left)* and after *(right)* selective embolization in a patient with repeated vaginal hemorrhages after previous curative treatment for an invasive hydatidiform mole. The patient's bleeding subsequently stopped, and she had a normal pregnancy in 1991.

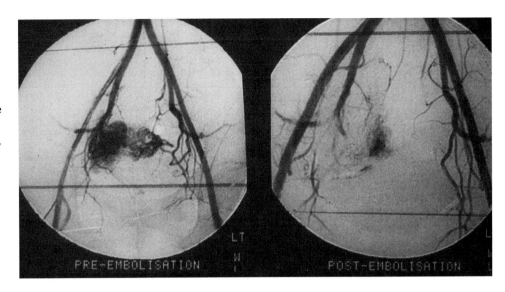

Long-term complications of therapy. Most patients, including those who have received intensive chemotherapy, return to normal activity within a few months, and most side effects, including alopecia, are reversible. Late sequelae from chemotherapy have been remarkably rare. In 15,279 patient-years of follow-up, there was no significant increase in the incidence of second tumors[78] after MTX/FA therapy compared with matched controls (RR = 1.3; 95% CI: 0.6-2.1). Although similar results are not yet published for actinomycin D, this agent when used alone for the treatment of GTT also appears to be unlikely to induce second tumors (D. Goldstein, New England Trophoblastic Disease Center, personal communication, 2002). In contrast, 26 patients receiving combination chemotherapy for GTT developed another cancer when the expected rate was only 16.45, a significant difference.[78] Second tumors included acute myeloid leukemia that was probably related to etoposide[101,128-130] (RR = 16.61; 95% CI: 5.40-38.9; P < .000), colon cancer (RR = 4.59; 95% CI: 1.48-10.7; P < .005), melanoma (RR= 3.41; 95% CI: 0.03-8.75), and at 25 years after treatment, breast cancer (RR= 5.79; 95% CI: 1.19-16.86; P < .016). Consequently, women receiving multiagent chemotherapy must be warned of a small but significant increased risk of treatment-induced second tumors.

Fertility is an important issue in the management of patients with GTTs. Neither MTX/FA nor EMA/CO affected fertility in our predominantly young population of women.[131] Most women can be assured of a likely favorable outcome with regard to future fertility. However, women receiving EMA/CO after the age of 35 years sometimes fail to recover ovarian function. Chemotherapy does move forward the date of the menopause by about 1 year for MTX/FA and 3 years for EMA/CO.[132]

The psychological sequelae of the treatment has until recently been poorly investigated. Ngan and Tang[133] found that women who had a molar pregnancy were less disturbed by the pregnancy loss if they subsequently required chemotherapy. Nevertheless, many women become very depressed after completion of chemotherapy. During treatment, they probably have many different issues to focus on and receive lots of support from various members of staff, and this is lost after treatment is complete. After therapy is over, they often feel physically weakened. A study examining a range of quality of life issues in U.S. and British women treated 5 to 10 years earlier for GTT revealed that 51% would appreciate a counseling program today and that 74% would have appreciated counseling at the time of therapy.[134] Nevertheless, our patients enjoy a good quality of life, with physical, social, and emotional functioning comparable to or better than comparative population norms.[134]

Is there a role for a nurse specialist? In the United Kingdom, both GTT treatment centers have employed a specialist nurse or nurse practitioner. This individual provides continuity of clinical service while junior medical staff rotate and provides counseling and psychological support, gives outpatient and community advice, and is a continuing link for the patient after therapy has been completed. The nurse practitioner also teaches formally and informally at a national and international level. Because the patients, general practitioners, and other medical attendants have all reported an improvement in the level of service, we believe that a nurse practitioner has provided a major advance. A fresh audit of this addition to the GTT service is under way, but it is clear that the employment of nurse practitioners in a variety of health services has led to striking improvements in the level of care delivery.[135,136]

Prognosis

All patients in the low- and middle-risk groups can be expected to be cured of their GTTs.[67,80,137] For high-risk patients, the survival rate has progressively improved and is currently 86%.[79] The diagnosis of choriocarcinoma is often not suspected until the disease is advanced. As a result, some deaths occur before chemotherapy has a chance to be effective. The number of such patients can be diminished by a greater awareness of the possibility that multiple metastases in a woman of childbearing age may be caused by choriocarcinoma. The simple measurement of the hCG level in such individuals is a very strong indicator of choriocarcinoma and could help to hasten referrals for lifesaving chemotherapy.

Summary

In the past, many women died of GTD. However, during the past 50 years, we have learned much about the biology, pathology, and natural history of this group of disorders. Accurate diagnostic and monitoring methods have been developed together with effective treatment regimens. As a result, the management of GTD represents one of the modern success stories in oncology, with few women dying of their trophoblastic tumors.

REFERENCES

1. Ober WB, Fass RO: The early history of choriocarcinoma. Ann N Y Acad Sci 1961;172:299-426.
2. Mueller UW, Hawes CS, Wright AE, et al: Isolation of fetal trophoblast cells from peripheral blood of pregnant women. Lancet 1990;336:197-200.
3. WHO. Gestational trophoblastic diseases. Technical report series 692. Geneva, World Health Organization, 1983, pp 7-81.
4. Kajii T, Ohama K: Androgenetic origin of hydatidiform mole. Nature 1977;268:633-634.
5. Vassilakos P, Riotton G, Kajii T: Hydatidiform mole: Two entities. A morphologic and cytogenic study with some clinical considerations. Am J Obstet Gynecol 1977;127:167-170.
6. Lawler SD, Pickthall VG, Fisher RA, et al: Genetic studies of complete and partial hydatidiform mole [letter]. Lancet 1979;2:580.
7. Lawler SD, Povey S, Fisher RA, Pickthall VG: Genetic studies on hydatidiform moles. II. The origin of complete moles. Ann Hum Genet 1982;46:209-222.
8. Jacobs PA, Wilson CM, Sprenkle JA, et al: Mechanism of origin of complete hydatidiform mole. Nature 1980;286:714-716.
9. Davis JR, Surwit EA, Garay JP, Fortier KJ: Sex assignment in gestational trophoblastic neoplasia. Am J Obstet Gynecol 1984;148:722-725.
10. Ohama K, Kajii T, Okamoto E, et al: Dispermic origin of XY hydatidiform mole. Nature 1981;292:551-552.
11. Fisher RA, Povey S, Jeffreys AJ, et al: Frequency of heterozygous complete hydatidiform moles, estimated by locus-specific minisatellite and Y chromosome-specific probes. Hum Genet 1989;82:259-263.
12. Fisher RA, Newlands ES: Gestational trophoblastic disease: Molecular and genetic studies. J Reprod Med 1998;43:81-97.
13. Paradinas F: The histological diagnosis of hydatidiform moles. Curr Diagn Pathol 1994;1:24-31.
14. Paradinas FJ, Browne P, Fisher RA, et al: A clinical, histopathological and flow cytometric study of 149 complete moles, 146 partial moles and 107 non-molar hydropic abortions. Histopathology 1996;28:101-110.
15. Paradinas FJ, Fisher RA, Browne P, Newlands ES: Diploid hydatidiform moles with fetal red blood cells in molar villi. I. Pathology, incidence and prognosis. J Pathol 1997;181:183-188.
16. Paradinas FJ: The diagnosis and prognosis of molar pregnancy. The experience of the National Referral Centre in London. Int J Gynaecol Obstet 1998;60:S57-S64.
17. Castrillon DH, Sun D, Weremowicz S, et al: Discrimination of complete hydatidiform mole from its mimics by immunohistochemistry of the paternally imprinted gene product p57KIP2. Am J Surg Pathol 2001;25:1225-1230.
18. Genest DR, Ruiz RE, Weremowicz S, et al: Do nontriploid partial hydatidiform moles exist? A histologic and flow cytometric reevaluation of nontriploid specimens. J Reprod Med 2002;47:363-368.
19. Jacobs PA, Hunt PA, Matsuuro JS, Wilson CC: Complete and partial hydatidiform mole in Hawaii: Cytogenetics, morphology and epidemiology. Br J Obstet Gynaecol 1982;89:258-266.
20. Lawler SD, Fisher RA, Pickthall VG, et al: Genetic studies on hydatidiform moles. I. The origin of partial moles. Cancer Genet Cytogenet 1982;4:309-320.
21. Seckl MJ, Fisher RA, Salerno GA, et al: Choriocarcinoma and partial hydatidiform moles. Lancet 2000;356:36-39.
22. Paradinas FJ, Sebire NJ, Fisher RA, et al: Pseudo-partial moles: Placental stem vessel hydrops and the association with Beckwith-Wiedemann syndrome and complete moles. Histopathology 2001;39:447-454.
23. Arima T, Imamura T, Amada S, et al: Genetic origin of malignant trophoblastic neoplasms. Cancer Genet Cytogenet 1994;73:95-102.
24. Wake N, Tanaka K-I, Chapman V, et al: Chromosomes and cellular origin of choriocarcinoma. Cancer Res 1981;41:3137-3143.
25. Chaganti RSK, Kodura PRK, Chakraborty R, et al: Genetic origin of trophoblastic choriocarcinoma. Cancer Res 1990;50:6330-6333.
26. Osada H, Kawata M, Yamada M, et al: Genetic identification of pregnancies responsible for choriocarcinomas after multiple pregnancies by restriction fragment length polymorphism analysis. Am J Obstet Gynecol 1991;165:682-688.
27. Fisher RA, Newlands ES, Jeffreys AJ, et al: Gestational and non-gestational trophoblastic tumours distinguished by DNA analysis. Cancer 1992;69:839-845.
28. Fisher RA, Lawler SD, Povey S, Bagshawe KD: Genetically homozygous choriocarcinoma following pregnancy with hydatidiform mole. Br J Cancer 1988;58:788-892.
29. Fisher RA, Soteriou BA, Meredith L, et al: Previous hydatidiform mole identified as the causative pregnancy of choriocarcinoma following birth of normal twins. Int J Cancer 1995;5:64-70.
30. Newlands ES, Bower M, Fisher RA, Paradinas FJ: Management of placental site trophoblastic tumours. J Reprod Med 1998;43:53-59.
31. Shih IM, Kurman RJ. Ki-67 labelling index in the differential diagnosis of exaggerated placental site, placental site trophoblastic tumour, and choriocarcinoma: A double staining technique using Ki-67 and Mel-CAM antibodies. Hum Pathol 1998;29:27-33.
32. Feltmate CM, Genest DR, Wise L, et al: Placental site trophoblastic tumor: A 17-year experience at the New England Trophoblastic Disease Center. Gynecol Oncol 2001;82:415-419.
33. Papadopoulos AJ, Foskett M, Seckl MJ, et al: Twenty-five years' clinical experience of placental site trophoblastic tumors. J Reprod Med 2002;47:460-464.
34. Hao Y, Crenshaw T, Moulton T, et al: Tumor suppressor activity of H19 RNA. Nature 1993;365:764-767.
35. Matsuoka S, Thompson JS, Edwards MC, et al: Imprinting of the gene encoding a human cyclin-dependent kinase inhibitor, p57kip2, on chromosome 11p15. Proc Natl Acad Sci U S A 1996;93:3026-3030.
36. Ogawa O, Eccles MR, Szeto J, et al: Relaxation in insulin-like growth factor II gene imprinting implicated in Wilms' tumour. Nature 1993;362:749-751.
37. Chilosi M, Piazzola E, Lestani M, et al: Differential expression of p57kip2, a maternally imprinted cdk inhibitor, in normal human placenta and gestational trophoblastic disease. Lab Invest 1998;78:269-276.
38. Walsh C, Miller SJ, Flam F, et al: Paternally derived H19 is differentially expressed in malignant and non-malignant trophoblast. Cancer Res 1995;55:1111-1116.
39. Hashimoto K, Azuma C, Koyama M, et al: Loss of imprinting in choriocarcinoma. Nat Genet 1995;9:109-110.
40. Moglabey YB, Kircheisen R, Seoud M, et al: Genetic mapping of a maternal locus responsible for familial hydatidiform moles. Hum Mol Genet 1999;8:667-671.

41. Judson H, Hayward BE, Sheridan E, Bonthron DT: A global disorder of imprinting in the human female germ line. Nature 2002;416:539-542.

42. Cole LA: hCG, its free subunits and its metabolites. Roles in pregnancy and trophoblastic disease. J Reprod Med 1998;43:3-10.

43. Birken S, Krichevsky A, O'Connor J, et al: Development and characterization of antibodies to a nicked and hyperglycosylated form of a hCG from a choriocarcinoma patient: Generation of antibodies that differentiate between pregnancy hCG and choriocarcinoma hCG. Endocrine 1999;10:137-144.

44. Birken S, Kovalevskaya G, O'Connor J: Immunochemical measurement of early pregnancy isoforms of HCG: Potential applications to fertility research, prenatal diagnosis, and cancer. Arch Med Res 2001;32:635-643.

45. Cole LA, Shahabi S, Butler SA, et al: Utility of commonly used commercial human chorionic gonadotropin immunoassays in the diagnosis and management of trophoblastic diseases. Clin Chem 2001;47:308-315.

46. Rotmensch S, Cole LA: False diagnosis and needless therapy of presumed malignant disease in women with false-positive human chorionic gonadotropin concentrations. Lancet 2000;355:712-715.

47. Vaitukaitis JL: Human chorionic gonadotrophin-a hormone secreted for many reasons. N Engl J Med 1979;301:324-326.

48. Bagshawe KD: Risk and prognostic factors in trophoblastic neoplasia. Cancer 1976;38:1373-1385.

49. Agarwal R, Strickland S, McNeish IA, et al: Doppler ultrasonography of the uterine artery and the response to chemotherapy in patients with gestational trophoblastic tumors. Clin Cancer Res 2002;8:1142-1147.

50. Kohorn EI. Persistent low-level "real" human chorionic gonadotropin: A clinical challenge and a therapeutic dilemma. Gynecol Oncol 2002;85:315-320.

51. Berkowitz RS, Goldstein DP: Pathogenesis of gestational trophoblastic neoplasms. Pathol Annu 1981;11:391-411.

52. Benson CB, Genest DR, Bernstein MR, et al: Sonographic appearance of first trimester complete hydatidiform moles. Ultrasound Obstet Gynecol 2000;16:188-191.

53. Sebire NJ, Rees H, Paradinas F, et al: The diagnostic implications of routine ultrasound examination in histologically confirmed early molar pregnancies. Ultrasound Obstet Gynecol 2001;18:662-665.

54. Goldstein DP, Berkowitz RS: Current management of complete and partial molar pregnancy. J Reprod Med 1994;39:139-146.

55. Sebire NJ, Foskett M, Paradinas FJ, et al: Outcome of twin pregnancies with complete hydatidiform mole and healthy co-twin. Lancet 2002;359:2165-2166.

56. Seckl MJ, Rustin GJS, Newlands ES, et al: Pulmonary embolism, pulmonary hypertension, and choriocarcinoma. Lancet 1991;338:1313-1315.

57. Tidy JH, Rustin GJS, Newlands ES, et al: Presentation and management of choriocarcinoma after nonmolar pregnancy. Br J Obstet Gynaecol 1995;102:715-719.

58. Savage P, Roddie M, Seckl MJ: A 28-year-old woman with a pulmonary embolus. Lancet 1998;352:30.

59. Kishkuno S, Ishida A, Takahashi Y, et al: A case of neonatal choriocarcinoma. Am J Perinenatol 1997;14:79-82.

60. Bagshawe KD, Noble MIM: Cardiorespiratory effects of trophoblastic tumours. Q J Med 1965;137:39-54.

61. Ngan HY, Chan FL, Au VW, et al: Clinical outcome of micrometastasis in the lung in stage IA persistent gestational trophoblastic disease. Gynecol Oncol 1998;70:192-194.

62. Boultebee JE, Newlands ES: New diagnostic and therapeutic approaches to gestational trophoblastic tumours. In Bourne TH, Jauniaux E, Jurkovic D (eds): Transvaginal Colour Doppler. The Scientific Basis and Practical Application of Colour Doppler in Gynaecology. New York, Springer, 1995, pp 57-65.

63. Lim AKP, Agarwal R, Barrett N, et al: Embolization of residual uterine vascular malformations in patients with gestational trophoblastic tumours. Radiology 2002;222:640-644.

64. Begent RHJ, Bagshawe KD, Green AJ, Searle AJ: The clinical value of imaging with antibody to human chorionic gonadotrophin in the detection of residual choriocarcinoma. Br J Cancer 1987;55:657-660.

65. Hebart H, Erley C, Kaskas B, et al: Positron emission tomography helps to diagnose tumor emboli and residual disease in choriocarcinoma. Ann Oncol 1996;7:416-418.

66. Beets G, Penninckx F, Schiepers C, et al: Clinical value of whole body positron emission tomography with [^{18}F]fluorodeoxyglucose in recurrent colorectal cancer. Br J Surg 1994;81:1666-1670.

67. Bagshawe KD, Dent J, Webb J: Hydatidiform mole in the United Kingdom, 1973-1983. Lancet 1986;2:673.

68. Tidy JA, Gillespie AM, Bright N, et al: Gestational trophoblastic disease: A study of mode of evacuation and subsequent need for treatment with chemotherapy. Gynecol Oncol 2000;78(Pt 1):309-312.

69. Matsui H, Iitsuka Y, Ishii J, et al: Androgenetic complete mole coexistent with a twin live fetus. Gynecol Oncol 1999;74:217-221.

70. Matsui H, Sekiya S, Hando T, et al: Hydatidiform mole coexistent with a twin live fetus: A national collaborative study in Japan. Hum Reprod 2000;15:608-611.

71. Steller MA, Genest DR, Bernstein MR, et al: Natural history of twin pregnancy with complete hydatidiform mole and coexisting fetus. Obstet Gynecol 1994;83:35-42.

72. Franke HR, Risse EK, Kenemans P, et al: Plasma human chorionic gonadotropin disappearance in hydatidiform mole: A central registry report from the Netherlands. Obstet Gynecol 1983;62:467-473.

73. Martin BH, Kim JH: Changing face of gestational trophoblastic disease. Int J Gynaecol Oncol 1998;60:S111-S120.

74. Stone M, Dent J, Kardana A, Bagshawe KD: Relationship of oral contraceptive to development of trophoblastic tumour after evacuation of hydatidiform mole. Br J Obstet Gynaecol 1976;86:913-916.

75. Deicas RE, Miller DS, Rademaker AW, Lurain JR: The role of contraception in the development of postmolar gestational trophoblastic tumor. Obstet Gynecol 1991;78:221-226.

76. Palmer JR, Driscoll SG, Rosenberg L, et al: Oral contraceptive use and risk of gestational trophoblastic tumors. J Natl Cancer Inst 1999;91:635-640.

77. Kohorn EI: The new FIGO 2000 staging and risk factor scoring system for gestational trophoblastic disease: Description and critical assessment. Int J Gynaecol Cancer 2001;11:73-77.

78. Rustin GJS, Newlands ES, Lutz J-M, et al: Combination but not single agent methotrexate chemotherapy for gestational trophoblastic tumours (GTT) increases the incidence of second tumours. J Clin Oncol 1996;14:2769-2773.

79. Bower M, Newlands ES, Holden L, et al: EMA/CO for high-risk gestational trophoblastic tumours: Results from a cohort of 272 patients. J Clin Oncol 1997;15:2636-2643.

80. McNeish IA, Strickland S, Holden L, et al: Low risk persistent gestational trophoblastic disease: Outcome following initial treatment with low-dose methotrexate and folinic acid, 1992-2000. J Clin Oncol 2002;20:1838-1844.

81. Berkowitz RS, Goldstein DP, Bernstein MR: Ten years' experience with methotrexate and folinic acid as primary therapy for gestational trophoblastic disease. Gynecol Oncol 1986;23:111-118.

82. Lurain JR, Elfstrand EP: Single-agent methotrexate chemotherapy for the treatment of nonmetastatic gestational trophoblastic tumors. Am J Obstet Gynecol 1995;172(Pt 1):574-579.

83. Wong LC, Ngan HY, Cheng DK, Ng TY: Methotrexate infusion in low-risk gestational trophoblastic disease. Am J Obstet Gynecol 2000;183:1579-1582.

84. Kwon JS, Elit L, Mazurka J, et al: Weekly intravenous methotrexate with folinic acid for nonmetastatic gestational trophoblastic neoplasia. Gynecol Oncol 2001;82:367-370.

85. Dorreen MS, Pennington GW, Millar DR, et al: Results of low-dose methotrexate treatment of persistent gestational trophoblastic disease in Sheffield 1980-1987. Acta Oncol 1988;27:551-556.

86. Bagshawe KD, Dent J, Newlands ES, et al: The role of low dose methotrexate and folinic acid in gestational trophoblastic tumours (GTT). Br J Obstet Gynaecol 1989;96:795-802.

87. Hoffman MS, Fiorica JV, Gleeson NC, et al: A single institution experience with weekly intramuscular methotrexate for nonmetastatic gestational trophoblastic disease. Gynecol Oncol 1996;60:292-294.

88. Kohorn EI: Is lack of response to single-agent chemotherapy in gestational trophoblastic disease associated with dose scheduling or chemotherapy resistance? Gynecol Oncol 2002;85:36-39.

89. Osathanondh R, Goldstein DP, Pastorfide GB: Actinomycin D as the primary agent for gestational trophoblastic disease. Cancer 1975;36:863-866.

90. Twiggs LB: Pulse actinomycin D scheduling in nonmetastatic gestational trophoblastic neoplasia: Cost-effective chemotherapy. Gynecol Oncol 1983;16:190-195.

91. Petrilli ES, Twiggs LB, Blessing JA, et al: Single-dose actinomycin-D treatment for nonmetastatic gestational trophoblastic disease. A prospective phase II trial of the Gynecologic Oncology Group. Cancer 1987;60:2173-2176.

92. Newlands ES, Holden L, Seckl MJ, et al: Management of brain metastases in patients with high-risk gestational trophoblastic tumors. J Reprod Med 2002;47:465-471.

93. Bolis G, Bonazzi C, Landoni F, et al: EMA/CO regimen in high-risk gestational trophoblastic tumor (GTT). Gynecol Oncol 1988;31:439-444.

94. Schink JC, Singh DK, Rademaker AW, et al: Etoposide, methotrexate, actinomycin D, cyclophosphamide, and vincristine for the treatment of metastatic, high-risk gestational trophoblastic disease. Obstet Gynecol 1992;80:817-820.

95. Quinn M, Murray J, Friedlander M, et al: EMACO in high risk gestational trophoblast disease—the Australian experience. Gestational Trophoblast Subcommittee, Clinical Oncological Society of Australia. Aust N Z J Obstet Gynaecol 1994;34:90-92.

96. Kim SJ, Bae SN, Kim JH, et al: Effects of multiagent chemotherapy and independent risk factors in the treatment of high-risk GTT—25 years' experience of KRI-TRD. Int J Gynaecol Obstet 1998;60(Suppl 1):S85-S96.

97. Lurain JR: Management of high-risk gestational trophoblastic disease. J Reprod Med 1998;43:44-52.

98. Xiang Y, Yang X, Han S: [Methotrexate combined chemotherapy for chemorefractory gestational trophoblastic tumor]. Zhonghua Fu Chan Ke Za Zhi 1999;34:97-100.

99. Dobson LS, Lorigan PC, Coleman RE, Hancock BW: Persistent gestational trophoblastic disease: Results of MEA (methotrexate, etoposide and dactinomycin) as first-line chemotherapy in high risk disease and EA (etoposide and dactinomycin) as second-line therapy for low risk disease. Br J Cancer 2000; 82:1547-1552.

100. Matsui H, Suzuka K, Iitsuka Y, et al: Combination chemotherapy with methotrexate, etoposide, and actinomycin D for high-risk gestational trophoblastic tumors. Gynecol Oncol 2000;78:28-31.

101. Boshoff C, Begent RH, Oliver RT, et al: Secondary tumours following etoposide containing therapy for germ cell cancer. Ann Oncol 1995;6:35-40.

102. Newlands ES, Mulholland PJ, Holden L, et al: Etoposide and cisplatin/etoposide, methotrexate, and actinomycin D (EMA) chemotherapy for patients with high-risk gestational trophoblastic tumors refractory to EMA/cyclophosphamide and vincristine chemotherapy and patients presenting with metastatic placental site trophoblastic tumors. J Clin Oncol 2000;18:854-859.

103. Gordon AN, Kavanagh JJ, Gershenson DM, et al: Cisplatin, vinblastine, and bleomycin combination therapy in resistant gestational trophoblastic disease. Cancer 1986;58:1407-1410.

104. DuBeshter B, Berkowitz RS, Goldstein DP, Bernstein M: Vinblastine, cisplatin and bleomycin as salvage therapy for refractory high-risk metastatic gestational trophoblastic disease. J Reprod Med 1989;34:189-192.

105. Azab M, Droz JP, Theodore C, et al: Cisplatin, vinblastine, and bleomycin combination in the treatment of resistant high-risk gestational trophoblastic tumors. Cancer 1989;64:1829-1832.

106. Motzer RJ, Bajorin DF, Schwartz LH, et al: Phase II trial of paclitaxel shows antitumour activity in patients with previously treated germ cell tumours. J Clin Oncol 1994;12:2277-2283.

107. Jones WB, Schneider J, Shapiro F, Lewis JLJ: Treatment of resistant gestational choriocarcinoma with taxol: A report of two cases. Gynaecol Oncol 1996;61:126-130.

108. Gerson R, Serrano A, Del Carmen Bello M, et al: Response of choriocarcinoma to paclitaxel. Case report and review of resistance. Eur J Gynaecol Oncol 1997;18:108-110.

109. Termrungruanglert W, Kudelka AP, Piamsomboon S, et al: Remission of refractory gestational trophoblastic disease with high-dose paclitaxel. Anticancer Drugs 1996;7:503-506.

110. Beyer J, Kramar A, Mandanas R, et al: High-dose chemotherapy as salvage treatment in germ cell tumors: A multivariate analysis of prognostic variables. J Clin Oncol 1996;14: 2638-2645.

111. Lyttelton MP, Newlands ES, Giles C, et al: High-dose therapy including carboplatin adjusted for renal function in patients with relapsed germ cell tumor: Outcome and prognostic factors. Br J Cancer 1998;77:1672-1676.

112. Giacalone PL, Benos P, Donnadio D, Laffargue F: High-dose chemotherapy with autologous bone marrow transplantation for refractory metastatic gestational trophoblastic disease. Gynecol Oncol 1995;58:383-385.

113. van Besien K, Verschraegen C, Mehra R, et al: Complete remission of refractory gestational trophoblastic disease with brain metastases treated with multicycle ifosfamide, carboplatin and etoposide (ICE) and stem cell rescue. Gynaecol Oncol 1997;65:366-369.

114. Knox S, Brooks SE, Wong-You-Cheong J, et al: Choriocarcinoma and epithelial trophoblastic tumor: Successful treatment of relapse with hysterectomy and high-dose chemotherapy with peripheral stem cell support: A case report. Gynecol Oncol 2002;85:204-208.

115. Kelly MP, Rustin GJS, Ivory C, et al: Respiratory failure due to choriocarcinoma: A study of 103 dyspneic patients. Gynaecol Oncol 1990;38:149-154.

116. Athanassiou A, Begent RHJ, Newlands ES, et al: Central nervous system metastases of choriocarcinoma: 23 years' experience at Charing Cross Hospital. Cancer 1983;52:1728-1735.

117. Lo SK, Montgomery JN, Blagden S, et al: Reducing incidence of headache after lumbar puncture and intrathecal cytotoxics. Lancet 1999;353:2038-2039.

118. Gillespie AM, Siddiqui N, Coleman RE, Hancock BW: Gestational trophoblastic disease: Does central nervous system chemoprophylaxis have a role? Br J Cancer 1999;79:1270-1272.

119. Ishizuka T: Intracranial metastases of choriocarcinoma: A clinicopathologic study. Cancer 1983;52:1896-1903.

120. Song HZ, Wu PC: Treatment of brain metastases in choriocarcinoma and invasive mole. In Song HZ, Wu PC (eds): Studies in Trophoblastic Disease in China. Oxford, Pergamon, 1988, pp 231-237.

121. Rustin GJS, Newlands ES, Begent RHJ, et al: Weekly alternating chemotherapy (EMA/CO) for treatement of central nervous systems of choriocarcinoma. J Clin Oncol 1989;7:900-903.

122. Altintas A, Vardar MA: Central nervous system involvement in gestational trophoblastic neoplasia. Eur J Gynaecol Oncol 2001; 22:154-156.

123. Small W Jr, Lurain JR, Shetty RM, et al: Gestational trophoblastic disease metastatic to the brain. Radiology 1996;200:277-280.

124. Schechter NR, Mychalczak B, Jones W, Spriggs D: Prognosis of patients treated with whole-brain radiation therapy for metastatic gestational trophoblastic disease. Gynecol Oncol 1998;68:183-192.

125. Feltmate CM, Genest DR, Goldstein DP, Berkowitz RS: Advances in the understanding of placental site trophoblastic tumor. J Reprod Med 2002;47:337-341.

126. Hopkins MP, Drescher CW, McQuillan A, et al: Malignant placental site trophoblastic tumour associated with placental abruption, fetal distress, and elevated CA-125. Gynecol Oncol 1992;47:267-271.

127. Blagden SP, Foskett MA, Fisher RA, et al: The effect of early pregnancy following chemotherapy on disease relapse and foetal outcome in women treated for gestational trophoblastic tumours. Br J Cancer 2002;86:26-30.

128. Ratain MJ, Kaminer LS, Bitran JD, et al: Acute nonlymphocytic leukemia following etoposide and cisplatin combination chemotherapy for advanced non-small-cell carcinoma of the lung. Blood 1987;70:1192-1196.

129. Whitlock JA, Greer JP, Lukens JN: Epipodophyllotoxin-related leukaemia. Identification of a new subset of secondary leukaemia. Cancer 1991;68:600-604.

130. Pui CH, Ribeiro RC, Hancock ML, et al: Acute myeloid leukemia in children treated with epipodophyllotoxins for acute lymphoblastic lymphoma. N Engl J Med 1991;325:1682-1687.

131. Woolas RP, Bower M, Newlands ES, et al: Influence of chemotherapy for gestational trophoblastic disease on subsequent pregnancy outcome. Br J Obstet Gynaecol 1998;105: 1032-1035.

132. Bower M, Rustin GJS, Newlands ES, et al: Chemotherapy for gestational trophoblastic tumours hastens menopause by 3 years. Eur J Cancer 1998;34:1204-1207.

133. Ngan HYS, Tang GWK: Psychosocial aspects of gestational trophoblastic disease in Chinese residents of Hong Kong. J Reprod Med 1986;31:173-178.

134. Wenzel L, Berkowitz R, Newlands ES, et al: Quality of life after gestational trophoblastic disease. J Reprod Med 2002;47: 387-394.

135. Mundinger MO, Kane RL, Lenz ER, et al: Primary care outcomes in patients treated by nurse practitioners or physicians: A randomized trial. JAMA 2000;283:59-68.

136. Loftus LA, Weston V: The development of nurse-led clinics in cancer care. J Clin Nurs 2001;10:215-220.

137. Newlands ES, Bagshawe KD, Begent RHJ, et al: Development of chemotherapy for medium- and high-risk patients with gestational trophoblastic tumours (1979-1984). Br J Obstet Gynaecol 1986;93:63-69.

138. Curry SL, Hammond CB, Tyrey L, Creasman WT, et al: Hydatidiform moles, diagnosis management and long term follow-up of 347 patients. Obstet Gynaecol 1975;45:1-8.

139. Zongfu X, Hongzhao S, Minyi T: Risk of malignancy and prognosis using a provisional scoring system in hydatidiform mole. China Med J 1979;93:605-612.

COMPLICATIONS OF CANCER TREATMENT

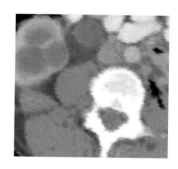

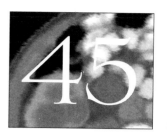

C H A P T E R **45**

MANAGEMENT OF
COMPLICATIONS OF SURGERY

Marcela G. del Carmen,   Robert E. Bristow,   and   F. J. Montz

 MAJOR CONTROVERSIES

- **What is the most appropriate operative management for a colonic injury?**
- **Which radiologic studies are useful in cases of small-bowel obstruction?**
- **Which intestinal tube is preferable in the management of small-bowel obstruction?**
- **How is a small bowel obstruction optimally managed?**
- **When is conservative therapy appropriate in the management of a fistula?**
- **What is the most appropriate surgical repair of bladder serosal and full-thickness injury?**
- **When should suction drains and ureteral stents be used in the repair of a bladder injury?**
- **How should ureteral ligation be managed?**
- **Does repair of a partial ureteral transection require uretero-ureterostomy?**
- **How is an uncomplicated total transection of the upper or middle third of the ureter best managed?**
- **How should the repair be performed if the resected ureteral segments cannot be brought together without tension?**
- **What is the best management option for a ureteral transection involving the lower third of the ureter?**
- **Is the risk of infection higher for an ileal than for a colonic conduit?**
- **How are urinary leaks associated with continent urinary diversions best managed?**
- **Can ureteral strictures or obstruction in reservoirs be managed noninvasively?**
- **How is hemorrhage from the external and internal iliac veins most effectively controlled?**
- **What is the best management strategy for controlling hemorrhage in the parametrial tissue?**
- **How is hemorrhage from the presacral veins controlled?**
- **How is femoral nerve injury best prevented, and how is it managed?**

Gynecologic surgery is reportedly associated with a 0.2% to 26% complication rate.[1-4] Complication rates increase with the degree of surgical difficulty. Part of the treatment of gynecologic malignancies usually involves radical pelvic surgery. This surgical endeavor in turn requires meticulous dissection near the bowel, bladder, ureters, and pelvic vessels and nerves. The more common surgical complications during radical resections are a result of injury to abdominal and pelvic structures when the malignant process distorts normal anatomy. These complications can occur and be recognized at the time of surgery, manifest in the postoperative period, or become a chronic process. The best management strategy continues to be avoidance of complications. It is imperative to commit to memory and practice the basic principles of proper surgical technique. In addition to fundamental knowledge of anatomy, these include ensuring adequate exposure, developing avascular planes and securing the vascular supply of structures before their removal, avoiding blunt dissection, restoring normal anatomy, respectfully handling tissue, and avoiding the use of force whenever possible.[5]

GASTROINTESTINAL INJURY

The most common indications for bowel surgery in gynecologic oncology include the presence of metastatic disease, especially in the case of ovarian cancer, obstruction, fistula, and other radiation-induced injury. The surgical intervention may necessitate resection and reanastomosis, bypass, or an ostomy. Proper planning and preparation maximize the patient's outcome and minimize the incidence of intraoperative injury and postoperative complication. The surgeon should plan the most appropriate procedure for the patient and her disease, aided by the information obtained from preoperative imaging such as upper and lower gastrointestinal (GI) radiologic studies, computed tomography (CT), magnetic resonance imaging (MRI), and fistulograms as indicated.[6] Delineation of the patient's anatomy is also imperative to optimize the surgical outcome. In patients with partial small-bowel obstruction (SBO) and those in whom intestinal surgery is anticipated, a preoperative mechanical and antibiotic preparation and prophylactic antibiotics should be administered.[5] Although a preoperative bowel preparation is contraindicated in patients with complete bowel obstruction, nasogastric (NG) tube decompression and perioperative intravenous antibiotics are still indicated.

Intraoperatively, the same general principles of meticulous surgical technique apply. Once again, the best management of an operative complication is avoidance. It is the surgeon's responsibility to protect the bowel from intraoperative injury. When packing the bowel out of the surgical field, care must be taken to avoid excessive pressure. The bowel should not be traumatized or handled directly with instruments if it obstructs the surgeon's view of the operative field. Bowel adhesiolysis should be performed sharply and not bluntly.

Intraoperative Injury

Gastric and small-bowel injury. The stomach can be injured during laparotomy or laparoscopy. Penetrating injury may be evident either by direct visualization via the laparoscope or from the leakage of digestive tract contents.[7] The small intestine can also be injured at the time of laparotomy or laparoscopy. Jejunal contents are acidic and corrosive, and incidental, undetected, unrepaired injury at this site results in peritonitis, adhesion formation, skin excoriation, and, ultimately, fistula formation. Given the high secretory output in the proximal small bowel, unrecognized intestinal obstruction or fistula at this level leads to severe dehydration and electrolyte abnormalities. Distal small-bowel injury, if

left untreated, can result in fatty acid, bile, and vitamin malabsorption.[7]

Gastric lacerations should be repaired primarily in two layers, with an inner running layer of 3-0 or 4-0 absorbable sutures followed by an outer layer of 3-0 or 4-0 permanent sutures in a Lembert fashion.[8] Given the stomach's generous lumen and blood supply (with the exception of the gastroesophageal junction and the pylorus), the risk of luminal compromise or excessive inversion with the primary repair is usually minimal.[8] Duodenal injury is less common, given the structure's retroperitoneal location. However, duodenal injury has been reported to carry a mortality rate of 15% to 20%.[9] The key to making the diagnosis of duodenal injury intraoperatively relies on exposure. For adequate visualization of its lateral and posterior segments, the duodenum must be mobilized. The lateral peritoneal reflection is incised, and the duodenum can be mobilized from right to left, a procedure known as the Kocher maneuver.[9] The posterior aspect of the proximal segment of the first portion of the duodenum and the medial aspect of the second portion can be exposed by entry into the lesser sac, via the gastrocolic ligament. The third and fourth portions of the duodenum can be exposed by means of the Cattell maneuver. In this procedure, the ligament of Treitz is incised and the right colon is mobilized from right to left to elevate both the small intestine and the colon.[9]

Simple duodenal lacerations or defects can be primarily repaired in two layers, an inner absorbable 3-0 or 4-0 running layer followed by an outer layer with 3-0 or 4-0 permanent suture placed in a Lembert fashion.[8] Luminal compromise is avoided by placing the suture line in a transverse direction to the longitudinal axis. Larger duodenal defects can be repaired with a two-layer primary anastomosis or with a jejunal patch, which is done by bringing a loop of jejunum and placing it onto the injured area, allowing it to reinforce the duodenal repair.[8] Small-bowel serosal tears or small cautery injury can be repaired with a single 3-0 permanent suture layer. If the injured portion of bowel demonstrates mucosal collapse, luminal entry, and leakage of intestinal contents, noncrushing clamps (e.g., linen-shod clamps) should be used to control the leakage while the defect is closed with two layers of continuous 3-0 or 4-0 permanent suture.[7] The first line of suture is placed through all three layers, and the second through the seromuscular segment, placed in a Lembert fashion. Once again, the suture line should be placed transverse to the normal bowel axis to avoid luminal constraint.[7,8] It is critical to inspect the vascular supply of the injured segment of bowel. In the event of ischemic bowel, the recommendation is to perform a resection with a reanastamosis.[7]

Several key principles must be remembered to maximize the outcome from a bowel reanastomosis. The proximal and distal ends of the preserved bowel should be both patent and healthy, and an attempt should be made to preserve the largest possible length of functional bowel. The ends should be free of disease to avoid incorporating tumor in the anastomosis.[5] Distended bowel that may appear avascular should be decompressed and then reassessed for vascularity. The bowel should be resected until a viable segment is ensured. It is important to prevent or minimize the amount of intestinal spillage in the surgical field. Before the transection, the distended bowel can be decompressed with Penrose drain tourniquets or rubber-shod intestinal clamps placed to occlude the proximal and distal bowel.[5] In the event of spillage, the abdomen should be copiously irrigated. The patient should also be given intravenous antibiotics with broad-spectrum coverage. At the conclusion of the surgery, the bowel is returned to its anatomic position, making sure that the mesentery is not twisted. Successful resection and reanastomosis relies on the procurement of healthy and vascular bowel segments, an ample lumen, a tight and tension-free anastomosis, hemostasis, and the exclusion of distal or proximal areas of obstruction.[5]

What is the most appropriate operative management for a colonic injury? The controversy in the intraoperative management of a low-risk colonic injury lies in the decision between primary repair and resection with exteriorization.[8,10] In the presence of hemorrhage exceeding 1 L, significant fecal spillage, hypotension, and elapsed time since injury exceeding 6 hours, the complication rate from primary repair escalates. However, in the absence of these risk factors, primary repair has proved to be safer, in terms of complications, than diversion.[10] Among patients with high-risk injuries, the rate of anastomotic breakdown and leakage is 42%, compared with 3% among those with low-risk injuries. The mortality rate from an anastomotic leak among high-risk patients is reportedly 40%.[11] Prospective series and randomized clinical trials have demonstrated the appropriateness of primary closure for low-risk colonic injury.[12-17] Primary repair can be performed in a two-layer fashion, with an inner layer and an outer layer of permanent suture placed in an interrupted Lembert fashion.[18]

The management of colonic injuries requiring resection remains controversial. High-risk colonic injuries have traditionally been treated with resection and colostomy. Recent data, however, suggest that primary closure may be appropriate even in the presence of certain high-risk factors. In the absence of a large or multiple defects and other medical comorbidities, a primary closure can be performed to repair these intermediate-risk injuries. The closure can be executed using a thoracoabdominal linear stapling instrument and copious irrigation of the surgical field. Careful clinical judgment must be exercised in this setting, because prospective, randomized data supporting primary closure of intermediate-risk colonic injury are currently lacking.[18]

If the colonic injury requires resection, the recommendation is for colostomy.[8,18] The same approach should be taken for patients who are at high risk for development of a suture line leak, such as those with multiple medical comorbidities and significant fecal leakage and blood product transfusion requirements.[8,18]

Rectal injury can be repaired in a two-layer fashion. Care must be taken to ensure that the defect is small,

easily repaired, and without tension.[7] It is critical to assess the entire length of injury to the rectal tube, and mobilization of the rectum is often required to optimize visualization. Large rectal defects and injuries that result in significant fecal contamination require diversion with a defunctioning transverse colostomy, given the inadequacy at obtaining complete fecal stream diversion with a loop colostomy under these circumstances.[7,8]

Ileus and Obstruction

SBO occurs with the interruption of the normal flow of intestinal contents. Bowel obstruction can be categorized as mechanical obstruction or paralytic ileus.[5] An ileus occurs when the propulsive activity of the bowel, including the stomach and the colon, is inhibited. A bowel obstruction results when the propulsive function is lost as a result of a structural abnormality. The incidence of ileus after major gynecologic surgery is 4% to 5% and is not affected by early postoperative feeding.[19,20] An ileus involves the entire length of the GI tract (the stomach, small intestine, and colon), although each segment may be affected differently. Its clinical signs include intolerance of oral intake, abdominal distention, pain, and absence of bowel sounds, flatus, and stool.[5] Ileus can occur as a result of surgery, drugs (anesthetics, opioids), chemotherapy, electrolyte abnormalities, hematomas, abscesses, peritonitis, and carcinomatosis.

An uncomplicated postoperative ileus usually resolves in 2 to 5 days, with the return of normal gastric emptying made evident by the resumption of bowel sounds and the recovery of colonic function manifested by passage of flatus and stool. A paralytic ileus, on the other hand, may last longer than 1 week. Clinically, patients have a history of a prolonged ileus, vomiting, and distention. Radiologically, a flat plate with decubitus and upright views shows air in the GI tract, dilatation of the small bowel, and air-fluid levels.[5] A paralytic ileus should be treated symptomatically with NG tube decompression, intravenous fluid resuscitation and hydration, and bowel rest until return of function occurs.

SBO can result from postoperative adhesions, hernias, and tumors. The morbidity and mortality from SBO are dictated by a number of factors, including the cause of the obstruction, the presence of ischemia, the time interval from surgery to development of the obstruction (time <30 days being worse), partial versus complete obstruction, management strategy, and the patient's health.[5] The primary goal of managing a patient with a SBO is to maximize the outcome of conservative therapy without encountering the increased morbidity that results from an ischemic event. The differential diagnosis of SBO includes ileus, ischemia, fecal impaction, gastroenteritis, and mesenteric thrombosis.[5]

It must be emphasized that the most significant morbidity from SBO occurs secondary to a delay in recognizing the presence of ischemia. Patients develop septic complications from bowel ischemia, with a clinical picture that includes pyrexia, leukocytosis, tachycardia, and peritoneal signs.[5] The obvious goal of treatment is to recognize patients who are at risk for bowel strangulation and ischemia and to intervene appropriately, minimizing the morbidity resulting from a delay in surgical management.

The segment of small intestine that lies proximal to the obstruction dilates as a result of interruption of normal luminal flow and as intestinal secretions are not permitted to pass distally. Patients with a jejunal obstruction present with repeated bouts of nausea and emesis and an intolerance for oral intake. Patients also experience bloating and colicky abdominal pain.[5] Patients with a distal ileal obstruction may be less symptomatic. The bowel dilatation is worsened by the effects of swallowed air and accumulation of bacterial fermentation. The proximal small bowel can become the site of bacterial overgrowth, as may be evident by feculent emesis. The continued process eventually results in edema of the bowel wall, with further sequestration of fluid as the bowel's absorptive function is lost. The proximal dilated bowel continues to secrete fluid into the lumen. As the bowel edema worsens, a transudative loss of fluid into the peritoneal cavity occurs.[21]

In a patient with a suspected SBO, the evaluation should include routine laboratory studies, amylase determination, lipase determination (to exclude acute pancreatitis), and plain abdominal radiographs.[5] Some of the areas of controversy in the management of patients with SBO include the choice of radiologic studies, the choice between NG or nasointestinal (NI) tubes, and the choice between continued conservative management and surgical intervention.

Which radiologic studies are useful in cases of small-bowel obstruction? Plain radiographs of the abdomen, which have a false-negative rate of 5% to 10%, can often be diagnostic of a bowel perforation and can distinguish between a complete and partial SBO. A flat and upright radiograph concurs with the clinical diagnosis of SBO in 75% to 95% of cases.[5] An even pattern of gas distribution along the stomach, small bowel, and colon is usually seen with a paralytic ileus. Dilated loops of bowel, with multiple air-fluid levels, indicate the presence of an SBO.[5,22] Although the presence of air in the colon or rectum makes the diagnosis of complete obstruction less likely, it does not completely exclude it. In an early complete SBO, gas can be seen in the colon if colonic gas has not had enough time to exit. Rectal gas can be introduced at the time of rectal examination.

The plain radiograph is equivocal in 20% to 30% of cases and "normal" or "nonspecific" in 10% to 20%.[22,23] CT can provide information regarding the presence, location, severity, and cause of the obstruction. Other abdominal pathology can also be detected. Dilute barium or a water-soluble contrast agent is given orally or via the NG tube, 30 to 120 minutes before the CT scan. An obstruction is diagnosed if there is a discrepancy in the caliber of proximal and distal small

bowel loops.[22,23] Often a point of transition can be seen. A complete obstruction is seen as absence of air or fluid in the distal small bowel or colon. A closed-loop obstruction is seen on CT scan as a distended, fluid-filled, C- or U-shaped loop of bowel with prominent mesenteric vasculature that converges on the point of incarceration or torsion.[22,23] Hemorrhagic mesenteric changes or intestinal pneumatosis can be seen in cases of advanced strangulation.

Diagnosis and assessment of the degree of SBO can also be made by a small-bowel follow-through series. This upper GI contrast study is the "gold standard" for determining whether the obstruction is partial or complete. However, CT is superior in detecting a closed-loop obstruction or ischemia.[24] Most radiologists recommend a CT scan as the study to be obtained after plain films in difficult-to-diagnose cases. If the CT scan is not diagnostic, a small-bowel series is indicated.[24]

The upper GI series with small-bowel follow-through can be helpful in atypical cases, if the cause for the obstruction is unclear, if plain radiographs and CT scans are inconclusive, in clinically suspected high duodenal or jejunal obstruction, or if a major reason to avoid surgery exists.[5,24] If the upper GI contrast study is diagnostic of SBO and demonstrates a discrete site of obstruction, or if the contrast agent does not reach the colon within 24 hours after its administration, the successful outcome from conservative management alone, without surgical intervention, is very poor.[5,25]

Barium is the contrast medium of choice for many surgeons. Unlike water-soluble contrast agents, it is not diluted by intestinal contents and does not stimulate peristalsis. Water-soluble contrast is favored by those who are concerned with possible impaction in the large bowel. Soluble contrast medium is safer because it is not irritating to the peritoneal cavity. Patients who have an undetected bowel perforation or who develop a perforation during the study are at risk from barium peritonitis if this medium is chosen for the study. Barium-fecal peritonitis is usually a fatal event.[5] Patients receiving barium are also at risk for embolization, aspiration, and appendicitis. Water-soluble contrast, our contrast agent of choice, is a hypertonic solution that requires aggressive patient hydration before its administration to avoid hypovolemia. It is also associated with aspiration and pulmonary edema. In some instances of partial SBO, the hyperosmotic load from the water-soluble contrast can be not only diagnostic but also therapeutic.[5]

It is imperative that patients who are at risk for a distal colonic obstruction in addition to the SBO be evaluated before the upper GI series is obtained (if barium is used) and definitively before surgical intervention. The lower GI tract can be evaluated for the presence of an obstruction via a barium enema or colonoscopy.

Which intestinal tube is preferable in the management of small-bowel obstruction? Both NG and NI tubes carry a 5% complication rate. Commonly reported complications include otitis media, aspiration, sinusitis, nasal/GI hemorrhage, and laryngeal/esophageal trauma.[5] The gastric and intestinal tract is usually decompressed with a 10F sump NG tube. Longer NI tubes, such as the Miller-Abbott and Cantor tubes, require longer time to pass, and are reported to result in more time elapsed between tube insertion and surgery. Adequate tube placement is dependent on peristalsis to carry the tube beyond the pylorus and into the more distal jejunum. NI tubes also have a higher complication rate and are no better at leading to nonsurgical resolution of an SBO, compared with NG tubes.[5,26-29] In the setting of an obstructed intestine, knot formation in the NI tube can occur, as can perforation, mercury aspiration, intussusception, and difficult removal. Neither the Kaslow nor the Cantor tubes can be deflated, and therefore their use can lead to worsening of the obstruction. Intraperitoneal mercury can result in systemic toxicity. Furthermore, if the NI tube is not advanced to the small intestine, it functionally becomes an NG tube, with a marked reduction in its suctioning capacity, given its smaller diameter.[5,27] To ensure that the NI tube is in the small intestine, placement may require fluoroscopic or endoscopic guidance.

Longer intestinal tubes, such as the Baker tube, can be used intraoperatively. Their application includes decompression of the small bowel, stenting of the small bowel in the setting of adhesions, and testing of the diameter of the bowel lumen. The tube is usually passed through a jejunostomy, but it can be advanced from the nose to the stomach and into the intestines. Although the stenting tube may be useful in preventing recurrence of the obstruction postoperatively, it is associated with significant complications, including wound infections, chronic enterocutaneous drainage, and other septic complications.[5]

How is a small-bowel obstruction optimally managed?
In the absence of signs of strangulation, SBO can be managed conservatively—that is, with bowel rest, appropriate intravenous hydration, correction of electrolyte abnormalities, and NG suctioning. Although 50% to 90% of partial obstructions resolve with conservative management, only 15% to 20% of patients with a complete obstruction will show resolution without the need for surgical intervention.[5,30] Much controversy exists regarding the optimal duration of conservative management. Conservative management can be continued as long as the patient demonstrates daily improvement as manifested by symptomatology, physical examination findings, and radiographs. Most patients who respond to nonsurgical interventions show complete resolution of their SBO in 48 to 72 hours.[5,30] It may be reasonable to continue conservative management measures in the patient with a partial SBO during the immediate postoperative period or in the patient with a carcinomatous ileus who may never be a surgical candidate. Patients whose symptoms persist or deteriorate and who show evidence of possible bowel ischemia, such as worsening pain, new-onset pyrexia, and leukocytosis, should undergo surgical intervention.[5]

Patients who have undergone abdominal or extended-field radiation therapy pose a special and difficult management problem. Conservative management is riskier in these patients, because the signs of peritonitis and ischemia may be masked in the irradiated peritoneum. These patients are also at risk for having such extensive radiation enteritis that most of their small intestine needs to be resected at the time of surgery, turning them into so-called "bowel cripples," dependent on parenteral feeding for the remainder of their lives.[5]

Once the decision to proceed with surgical intervention has been made, it is critical to optimize the patient's condition with adequate intravenous resuscitation, electrolyte repletion, and antibiotic prophylaxis. All efforts should be made to avoid spillage of fecal contents into the operative field, to decompress the bowel, and make a thorough assessment of vascular viability of the entire bowel. The surgeon must be prepared to perform any of a wide range of procedures, from a simple lysis of adhesions to resection of an obstructing lesion, resection with a reanastomosis, bypass, diverting colostomy, or ileostomy.[5]

Large-Bowel Obstruction

Colonic obstruction is usually the result of a primary colonic malignancy. However, gynecologic oncology patients can develop a colonic obstruction as a consequence of recurrent ovarian, cervical, or endometrial cancer.[5] Patients with large-bowel obstruction usually have subtle symptoms that range from constipation and thin stools to abdominal distention, vomiting, and pain as the obstruction progresses. On examination, the abdomen is distended and there are high-pitched bowel sounds; tenderness can be appreciated over the right lower quadrant; and the rectal vault is empty or occupied by a mass or stricture.[5] Laboratory findings include hypokalemia and anemia. On plain radiographs, the colon is dilated, with air proximal to the site of obstruction. Gaseous distention of the small bowel can be seen in patients with an incompetent or absent ileocecal valve.[5]

In cases of impending colonic perforation, the bowel must be decompressed by cecostomy or colostomy. These high-risk cases are best managed by aggressive intravenous fluid resuscitation and use of broad-spectrum antibiotics. A mechanical bowel preparation before surgery is contraindicated.[5] Nasogastric tube suction should be offered to patients with emesis. The risk of colonic perforation increases dramatically with increased pain, cecal diameter greater than 10 to 12 cm, and duration of obstruction longer than 4 days.[5] In most instances, the obstruction can be relieved surgically via a diverting transverse colostomy. In patients with only a partial obstruction, use of a mechanical and antibiotic bowel preparation can be entertained. If the decision to proceed with a bowel preparation is made, it should be done over the course of several days and without any stimulant cathartics. In these patients, it is appropriate to proceed with definitive surgical treatment in the form of colonic resection and reanastomosis.[5]

Fistula

A fistula can be defined as an abnormal communication between two epithelial surfaces. In the gynecologic oncology patient, fistulas can result from previous radiation therapy, tumor invasion, or necrosis. Fistulous communications usually involve small bowel and skin (commonly at the cutaneous incision site) or colon or rectum and vagina. However, connections may also be seen to the bladder, ureters, uterus, and peritoneum.[5] Patients with proximal small-bowel fistulas (from the jejunum or proximal ileum) have massive fluid and electrolyte losses as well as excoriation of the skin. Distal ileal fistulas behave like colonic fistulas and do not usually result in massive fluid losses or corrosion of the skin.[5]

The initial management of a fistula is aimed at correction of electrolyte abnormalities, intravascular resuscitation, control of fistula output, treatment of sepsis, and improved nutritional status.[5,7] After these steps have been taken, fistula closure may be attempted. The fistula location can be identified with the aid of any of a number of radiologic studies: plain films, upper/lower GI studies, CT scans, and fistulograms.

When is conservative therapy appropriate in the management of a fistula? The presence of sepsis is the most important factor to consider when deciding between surgical and conservative managements of a fistula.[5,7] Septic patients should be given broad-spectrum antibiotics. Abscesses should be drained under direct CT or ultrasound guidance. Catheters should be left in place until the sepsis has resolved, the cavity has collapsed, the drain output is less than 30 mL/day, and fistula closure is confirmed by a low-pressure fistulogram.[5]

Patients with severe malnutrition have been shown to benefit from total parenteral nutrition (TPN) for 2 to 3 weeks preoperatively as well as postoperatively, until adequate oral nutrition is established.[5,7] The average adult requires approximately 3000 calories of nutritional support daily.[7] However, calculation of the individual patient need is valuable. The somatostatin analog, octreotide, can be administered in an attempt to decrease fistula output during the conservative phase of management.[31] Studies have shown that octreotide is effective in the management of high-output enteric fistulas, accelerating fistula closure, but without increasing the success rate of conservative management.[5,31]

Fistulas can occur spontaneously or as a result of a surgical procedure. Anatomic deterrents, such as foreign bodies (suture, mesh), distal obstruction, tumor, or epithelialization of the tract, can prevent fistula closure. Patients with these high-risk factors for fistula nonclosure inevitably require surgical intervention.[5,7] Sepsis should also be managed surgically. All other patients can be allowed a trial of conservative management.[5,7] High-output fistulas and those resulting from radiation injury are less likely to respond to conservative management.[5,32] Fistulas that do not close after 2 to 3 weeks of conservative management should be treated with surgical correction.

At time of surgery, the fistula can be resected and a primary anastomosis or complete isolation performed. In patients who have a distal obstruction, or are at risk for developing one, and have an isolated fistula should have a mucous fistula created. If a primary anastomosis is performed, an omental flap should be used to protect the suture line and a gastric feeding tube should be placed intraoperatively. Proximal diversion is often the only option for the patient who has an abscess or is in florid sepsis.[5]

In patients with a colocutaneous or colovaginal fistula, in the absence of sepsis, necrosis, and obstruction, local care without bowel rest may be attempted.[5] If a surgical approach is undertaken, the options are a diverting colostomy or primary resection with reanastomosis. Patients who have a diverting colostomy can be returned to the operating room for a takedown at a later date. If the fistula is large or the patient is septic, a diverting colostomy is preferred.[5] Patients who have undergone high-dose external-beam radiation therapy and develop a rectovaginal fistula may need a permanent colostomy, because the compromised blood supply and associated tissue fibrosis often impede the development of a functioning reanastomosis. If conditions are favorable, a diverting colostomy can be performed first, with the patient brought back for repair once the infection, necrosis, and inflammation have resolved.[5] It is critical to use a segment of nonirradiated large bowel and a fresh vascular supply (e.g., muscle, omentum, bulbocavernosus fat pad).

Stoma Complications

The most effective way to avoid a stoma complication is to practice the discipline of attention to creation of the stoma, especially if this part of the operation occurs at the end of a long, arduous surgical procedure. Common stomal complications include prolapse, necrosis, retraction, hernia, leak, and stenosis. Most complications occur within the first 5 years after formation.[8]

Proper site location is critical to development of a successful stoma. Poor location can lead to improper appliance fitting, which in turn can result in leakage of enteric contents and skin breakdown. The site location can be optimized by consulting an enterostomal therapist before the surgery. The intended location can be marked on the abdominal wall, at a site that is functional and comfortable for the patient. The site should be easy for the patient to visualize so as to facilitate patient self-care. The stoma site should also draw the bowel through the rectus muscle to minimize the chance of herniation.[8]

Stomal prolapse can be alarming for the patient, but it usually is functionally insignificant. In certain cases, prolapse can lead to improper appliance fitting, incarceration, and even strangulation. Prolapse occurs in 5% to 25% of patients after transverse loop colostomies.[8] Although mesentery fixation is advocated by some, it does not prevent stomal prolapse. If prolapse occurs, the redundant bowel can be amputated and the mucocutaneous junction reconstructed.[8]

Stomal retraction can be seen in the immediate postoperative period. It can result from obesity (precluding a tension-free anastomosis between the skin and the stoma), from mucocutaneous separation, or as a result of weight gain.[33] Retraction can lead to difficulties with appliance adherence and skin breakdown from enteric content leakage. Initial management interventions include the use of a convex pouching system and the use of a binder/belt.[33] Surgical revision may be necessary if these steps fail. The obese patient should be counseled and encouraged to lose weight before a surgical stomal revision is attempted.

Stomal necrosis and stenosis can result from excessive mesenteric tension or trimming. Stomal ischemia can be seen in 5% of ileostomies and 10% of colostomies. This complication is more common in procedures performed emergently and among obese patients. To avoid ischemia, it is critical to preserve the last vascular arcade of the small bowel mesentery and the marginal artery of the colonic mesentery.[8]

Peristomal hernias occur in 2% to 35% of colostomies and 2% o 25% of ileostomies. Most of these hernias appear within the first 2 postoperative years. Patients who are at increased risk are those who have other abdominal wall hernias; those are obese, older, or malnourished; those who are receiving steroid therapy; and those with active infections.[8] The most critical preventive measure is to bring the stoma through the rectus muscle. If the hernia is asymptomatic and small, it should not be repaired. However, if the patient is symptomatic, the defect is large, bowel is incarcerated or strangulated, or the hernia does not allow proper appliance fitting, the hernia needs to be repaired.

The options for stomal hernia repair are varied and include prosthetic repair, relocation of the stoma to the other side of the abdomen, and primary fascial repair. Approximately 50% of patients with a stomal hernia who undergo relocation have a subsequent incisional hernia.[8] Relocation is the recommended intervention for a first-time stomal hernia. A prosthetic material repair should be considered for the patient with a stomal hernia recurrence.[8]

Stomal stenosis results when narrowing of the stoma is sufficient to interfere with normal function.[33] Stenosis can occur at the level of the skin or of the fascia. Mild stenosis is usually asymptomatic and detected on digitalization of the stoma. Patients with more significant stomal stenosis can experience pain, followed by explosive output. Initial management includes dietary modification (to avoid insoluble fiber) and gentle routine self-dilatation or lavage. Significant stenosis requires surgical correction.

Malabsorption/Maldigestion

Malabsorption denotes the impaired absorption of nutrients. It can be either congenital (primary) or acquired (secondary). Maldigestion can interfere with

nutrient absorption as a result of impaired nutrient digestion within the intestinal lumen or at the brush border membrane of mucosal epithelial cells.[34] Normal nutrient absorption requires three steps: luminal processing, absorption into the intestinal mucosa, and transport into the circulation. Defects in any of these phases can lead to malabsorption. Malabsorption can be either partial or global. Global malabsorption can result from diseases associated with diffuse mucosal damage or reduced absorptive surfaces. Isolated malabsorption is seen with diseases that interfere with absorption of specific nutrients.[34] Ileal resection or damage (as can occur after pelvic-abdominal radiation therapy) usually results in malabsorption due to a luminal phase defect.

The small intestine has an irreplaceable absorptive capacity that can be only partially compensated by the colon.[5,34] The average length of the small bowel in women is 600 to 675 cm, with the jejunum accounting for approximately 40% of this length. As long as the remaining bowel is healthy, a patient can survive removal of 50% of the small bowel without any major nutritional deficits. Serious nutritional deficits result with a small bowel length of 150 to 200 cm, and permanent parenteral feeding is usually required for survival in patients with 100 cm or less of functioning small bowel.[5]

The probability of loss of absorptive function depends on the length and location of resected or damaged bowel. Amino acids are absorbed in the jejunum; sugars are absorbed rapidly, and fatty acids slowly, throughout the small intestine. The terminal 100 cm of the ileum is responsible for the absorption of vitamin B_{12} and bile salts.[5] Fat-soluble vitamins are absorbed slowly in the jejunum and ileum, and water-soluble vitamins are absorbed throughout the length of the small bowel.[34] Because digestion and absorption are a function not only of the bowel's surface area but also of its transit time, loss of the ileum (where the lumen is smaller and intestinal contents are thicker) leads to a marked increase in transit time. Preservation of at least 50% of the colon can result in some compensation for loss of small bowel length and function.[5]

Patients with short bowel syndrome may experience dehydration, diarrhea, electrolyte abnormalities, and nutritional deficiencies.[5,34] Hypertrophy of the bowel wall and mucosa, dilatation, and lengthening of the bowel can be seen as a compensatory response of the small intestine to loss of length.[7] This adaptive measure is seen a few weeks after surgery, is greatest at 12 to 24 months, and can be expedited by the use of enteral feeding, histamine$_2$-blockers, and antimotility agents.[5] Patients without an ileocecal valve may benefit from broad-spectrum antibiotics to treat the diarrhea that results from bacterial overgrowth.[5] In patients with less than 100 cm of ileum remaining after resection, administration of cholestyramine aids the absorption of bile salts.[5,34]

After extensive small-bowel surgery, TPN should be started. Parenteral feeding should be followed by continuous tube feedings (using an isotonic peptide-based formula). Once TPN has been discontinued and an adequate tube feed regimen is established, small oral feeds (low-fat, low-residue diet) can be started. Repletion of specific nutritional deficiencies, either orally or parenterally, may be necessary. Some of these deficiencies include calcium, magnesium, vitamins (B_{12}, folate, K), and iron.[5]

Anastomotic Stricture

Approximately 2% to 3% of proximal rectal anastomoses can be complicated by stricture.[35] Small-bowel anastomotic strictures require surgical management. Colonic strictures, especially high rectal and sigmoid strictures, can be treated by endoscopic dilatation. Hegar or anal dilators can be used to dilate low rectal strictures. Severe rectal strictures may require surgical intervention.[5]

GENITOURINARY INJURY

Operative injury to the urinary tract is not an uncommon complication of gynecologic surgery. Gynecologic oncologists must be cognizant of both the anatomy of all urinary tract structures and the maneuvers to minimize the risk of injury. If injury does occur, it is imperative that the gynecologic oncologist be comfortable with the appropriate reparative procedures. Urinary tract injury complicates 1% to 5% of gynecologic cancer operations. The risk of urinary tract injury is higher in patients with advanced disease and in those who have undergone radiation therapy.[36] Between 26% and 95% of these injuries may be unrecognized intraoperatively.[37] Unrecognized bladder injuries are usually clinically evident in the early postoperative period, whereas unrecognized ureteral injury can lead to permanent loss of renal function.[36]

Intraoperative Bladder Injury

What is the most appropriate surgical repair of bladder serosal and full-thickness injuries? In repairing any bladder injury, it is critical to keep in mind two basic principles: carrying out an exhaustive exploration to identify other genitourinary tract injuries once the first defect has been recognized, and ensuring that neither the defect nor the suture line is ever under tension.

If the bladder injury does not involve the mucosa and there is no extravasation of urine, there is significant liberty as to how the repair can be performed. It can be effected in one or two interrupted or continuous layers, using 2-0 or 3-0 absorbable suture. The denuded detrusor musculature should be imbricated using the extramucosal layer.[36]

Full-thickness injuries can be repaired with the use of two extramucosal layers.[36] It is critical that the defect be closed in the direction that minimizes tension. The first layer should avoid going completely through the mucosa but rather invert the mucosa into the bladder.

This layer can be placed in an interrupted or a running fashion, using 3-0 absorbable suture. The second layer is placed over the first, using 2-0 or 3-0 delayed absorbable suture. This layer can also be placed in a running fashion, provided the defect is less than 4 cm. Larger, multiple, or irregular full-thickness tears should be repaired in an interrupted fashion, using 3-0 delayed absorbable suture.[36] An intentional cystotomy may be useful to identify the location and extent of a bladder tear.[36] A urethral or suprapubic catheter should be left in place for 3 to 10 days, depending on the extent of the tear, to facilitate bladder rest postoperatively.

When should suction drains and ureteral stents be used in the repair of a bladder injury? Suction drains are appropriate in the management of major bladder lacerations and all trigone repairs.[36] Trigone lacerations should be repaired with two layers of 3-0 delayed absorbable suture, using the same technique as described earlier. Either 7F or 8F ureteral catheters should be placed in the bladder transurethrally.[36]

Ureteral Injury

Ureteral injury can occur at one of five locations in pelvic surgery: the tunnel of Wertheim, the intramural portion of the ureter, the cardinal ligament (where the ureter crosses under the uterine artery), dorsal to the infundibulopelvic ligament, and on the lateral pelvic sidewall, above the uterosacral ligament.[38] Intraoperative ureteral injuries are, in general, the result of ureteral ligation, partial or total transection, or thermal or electrical injury. Figure 45-1 illustrates the anatomy and vascular supply of the abdominal and pelvic ureter.

How should ureteral ligation be managed? Although complete ligation of the ureter is uncommon, "kinking" of the ureter with a suture partially placed through the ureter or impinging on the paraureteral tissue is a relatively frequent event.[38] If a suture has been placed in the ureter, the first corrective measure is to remove the suture. Ureteral vascular viability must then be confirmed. Several observational findings are reassuring that viability exists, but none is perfect. Such observations include blanching as the result of gentle manipulation, blood flow through the adventitial sheath blood vessels, peristalsis, and lack of discoloration. The next step involves placing a ureteral stent via ureterotomy (the least preferable approach), cystoscopy, or cystotomy (our preference). After the cystotomy repair, bladder rest for 3 days in the nonirradiated patient and longer in the setting of previous radiation therapy is recommended.[38]

Does repair of a partial ureteral transection require uretero-ureterostomy? Repair of a partial ureteral transection can be carried out by placing a ureteral stent through the inadvertent ureterotomy.[38] The primary

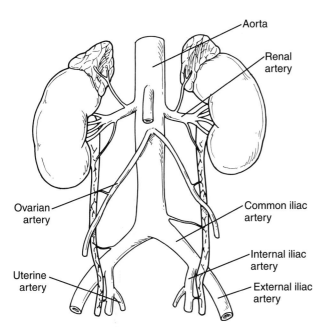

Figure 45-1. Anatomy and vascular supply of the abdominal and pelvic ureter. The ureter derives its blood supply from branches off the hypogastric artery. In most cases, feeders from the uterine artery are present. The ureter crosses over the common iliac artery, diving under the uterine artery as it courses down in the pelvis. (Adapted from Montz FJ: Management of uretal injury. Operative Techniques in Gynecologic Surgery 1998;3:138.)

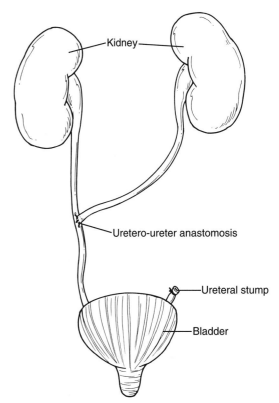

Figure 45-2. Uretero-ureterostomy. Both transected ends of the ureter are spatulated to reduce the risk of ureteral stenosis after anastomosis. The anastomosis is performed with the use of through-and-through interrupted sutures with a ureteral stent in place. (Adapted from Montz FJ: Management of uretal injury. Operative Techniques in Gynecologic Surgery 1998;3:139.)

ureteral defect can be repaired with 5-0 PGA (polyglycolic acid) suture. The temptation to place an excessive number of sutures should be avoided, because this maneuver does not guarantee a watertight seal. In fact, it actually increases the likelihood of devascularization of the ureter and therefore increases the probability of breakdown.[38] An adequate repair usually requires three individual sutures. Placement of a closed-suction drain at the base of the repair is recommended.

How is an uncomplicated total transection of the upper or middle third of the ureter best managed?
The recommended method of repair for this type of injury is a uretero-ureterostomy over a ureteral stent.[38] It is critical to ensure that the uretero-ureterostomy is tension free. Mobilization of the kidney on its vascular pedicle (by dissection of it from Gerota's fascia) allows for additional length of the proximal ureteral segment.[38,39] If this maneuver is performed, the integrity of the renal vascular bundle must be assured. Both ureteral ends are spatulated with the use of Potts or similar scissors. When spatulating the ureter, care must be taken to avoid transecting the vascular supply running in the ureteral sheath. Spatulation is performed on opposing sides of the proximal and distal ureteral ends so as to attain a watertight seal.[38] The uretero-ureterostomy is completed by placing a limited number of 5-0 PGA sutures (three to four sutures) over a ureteral stent (Fig. 45-2). A closed-suction drain should be placed at the site of the repair.[38]

How should the repair be performed if the resected ureteral segments cannot be brought together without tension? This type of complicated upper or middle third ureteral transection injury can be managed in one of two ways. The first method, a transuretero-ureterostomy, necessitates an additional injury to the urinary drainage system and is considered to be of historical interest only (Fig. 45-3). The preferred method is a uretero-enteroneocystostomy[38] (Fig. 45-4). The first step in performing this procedure is the identification and resection of a healthy, viable portion of distal ileum. The resection is performed with the use of a linear stapling device, and the ileo-ileostomy is effected before the ureteral injury repair is continued. Next, the proximal loop of ileum is opened and, over a ureteral stent, the ureteroileal end-to-side anastomosis is executed. Our preference is to bring the ureter through the full thickness of the antimesenteric portion of the ileal segment. Using a 5-0 PGA suture, the full-thickness ureter is splayed open inside the ileal segment. In order to ensure that the anastomosis is tension free, the seromuscular portion of the ureter is attached to the ileal serosa. A PGA linear stapler can be used to close the proximal ileal segment, or a hand-sewn two-layer technique can be used. Metal staples must be avoided, because exposure of a permanent foreign body to urine leads to stone formation.[38]

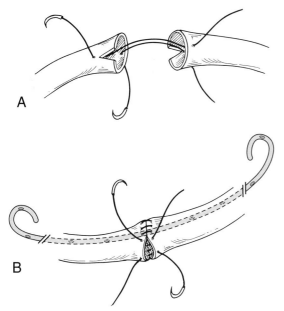

Figure 45-3. Transuretero-ureterostomy. The two ureters are reanastomosed in an end-to-end fashion. (Adapted from Morrow CP, Curtin JP: Gynecologic Cancer Surgery. New York, Churchill Livingstone, 1996, p 318.)

The distal end of the ileal segment is then opened and the ureteroileal anastomosis to the bladder is completed over a stent (which is passed into the bladder in an antegrade fashion). We recommend securing the ileal segment to the psoas muscle tendon so as to maintain a tension-free state and avoid rotation of the mesentery with subsequent vascular compromise. The stent is left in place for at least 6 weeks and is removed

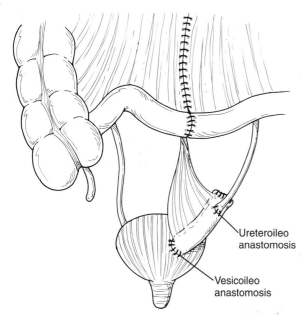

Figure 45-4. Uretero-enteroneocystostomy. The ureter is anastomosed to the small bowel at one end and to the bladder at the other end. An ileo-ileostomy is performed in the area of resection to reanastomose the bowel. (Adapted from Morrow CP, Curtin JP: Gynecologic Cancer Surgery. New York, Churchill Livingstone, 1996, p 106.)

after an intravenous ureterogram rules out the possibility of an occult leak.[38]

What is the best management option for a ureteral transaction involving the lower third of the ureter?
If the ureter is transected within 6 to 8 cm of the ureterovesical junction, the recommended method of repair is a ureteroneocystostomy.[38] The critical first step involves double-ligation of the distal portion of ureter, still attached to the bladder, using silk 2-0 suture. The ventral surface of the bladder is then thoroughly mobilized toward the proximal ureter, with care taken not to compromise the dorsolateral vascular supply. A cystotomy on the ventral bladder dome is then performed, at an angle of 15 to 30 degrees off the sagittal axis toward the side of the ureteroneocystostomy. The ureteroneostomy is then effected using a technique that mimics that described for the ileal interposition. With the use of digital mobilization, the ventrolateral aspect of the bladder is attached to the psoas tendon. Two separate 3-0 nylon/Prolene sutures are used to attach the bladder wall (avoiding the urothelium) to the muscle. A stent is left in the ureter, and the bladder is closed in two layers as described before.[38] We recommend use of a 7F to 8F double-J stent.

Obstruction

Although mild hydronephrosis is frequently evident on postoperative intravenous pyelograms (IVPs), most cases resolve within the first 3 months after surgery. Persistent hydronephrosis beyond this point is usually the result of recurrent cancer, radiation therapy, or surgery.[40] Patients present with abdominal pain or infection. The symptomatology may be so insidious that patients present with unilateral loss of renal function, or in renal failure if the obstruction is bilateral. If there is any concern about the degree of ureteral patency, a renal ultrasound or IVP should be obtained. In the setting of renal failure or compromised renal function, the ultrasound is the preferred imaging study.[41]

Ureteral dilatation can be attempted via retrograde or anterograde stenting through a percutaneous nephrostomy tube. If stenting cannot be achieved, we recommend percutaneous nephrostomy placement.[40,41] Because spontaneous resolution of unstentable ureteral obstructions has been reported, the patient should be observed for 3 to 6 months after nephrostomy placement. If nephrostomy cannot be achieved or the obstruction does not resolve after nephrostomy drainage, surgery with ureteral reimplantation, using a ureteroneocystostomy as previously described, is necessary.[40,41]

Fistula

The presence of a fistula in the urinary tract system is usually recognized early in the postoperative period, although the presenting symptoms can be nondescript. Most patients have a watery, uriniferous vaginal discharge that usually manifests 7 to 10 days after surgery. Most ureteral fistulas are located in the lateral vaginal cuff.[41] In order to differentiate between a vesicovaginal and a ureterovaginal fistula, the bladder can be filled with a methylene blue solution and a sponge stick or tampon placed in the vagina.[40,41] If the sponge stick or tampon is stained blue, the fistula is documented to be from the bladder to the vagina. If the vaginal sponge or tampon is not stained blue, then indigo carmine can be given intravenously. Staining of the vaginal instrument with blue dye in the latter procedure confirms the presence of a ureterovaginal fistula.[41] In the presence of pelvic drains, the fistula may manifest as increased drain output. The diagnosis of a fistula can be made by measuring the urea/creatinine content of the drain output.[41]

Cystoscopy with retrograde pyelography can give information regarding which ureter (or ureters) is involved, whether there is a compound fistula (ureter and bladder), and whether an obstruction is present. Cystoscopy offers the added advantage of the ability to stent the involved ureter. Ureteroscopic guidance of stent placement is recommended if the stent cannot be passed via cystoscopy.[41] If this maneuver also fails, we recommend placement of a percutaneous nephrostomy tube. Most fistulas heal within 14 to 21 days after stent placement. If ureteral stenting fails, the ureter should be reimplanted in the bladder.[41]

The initial management of a vesicovaginal fistula involves bladder rest and adequate drainage with placement of a transurethral catheter. Small bladder fistulas usually heal spontaneously within 30 days after diagnosis.[40,41] Fistulas larger than 1 cm require surgical management. It is critical to allow for all tissue inflammation to subside, and the repair should be delayed for 2 to 3 months after the fistula is diagnosed. Small fistulas at the vaginal apex can be repaired via the Latzko procedure. If the vaginal approach prohibits adequate exposure, the fistula is too close to the ureters, or the fistula is complex, an abdominal approach is preferred.[41]

Continent Diversion Dysfunction and Complications

Is the risk of infection higher for an ileal than for a colonic conduit?

Some authors have documented a higher rate of bacterial growth in ileal than in colonic conduits.[42] It has been reported that approximately 75% of patients with ileal conduits have significant bacterial growth in the loop. In contrast, only 50% of patients with colonic conduits are reported to be infected.[43] The higher infection rate in patients with ileal conduits is thought to be the result of the inherent inability to perform an antireflux anastomosis. Approximately 5% to 20% of patients with urinary conduits develop acute pyelonephritis as a late complication. Patients with transverse colonic conduits and those who have stents placed in the early postoperative period may have a reduction in the risk of developing pyelonephritis.[43]

How are urinary leaks associated with continent urinary diversions best managed?

Urinary leaks can be a severe, early postoperative complication for patients with conduits. Urinary leaks or fistulas are estimated to complicate 2% to 22% of conduits. The patients most commonly affected are those whose conduit is made from irradiated bowel and in whom ureteral stents were not used.[43] Spontaneous leak closure can occur but is not the norm. Although surgical intervention is needed to correct the urinary leak, our recommendation is to resist the temptation to undertake this endeavor in the immediate postoperative period, especially in the setting of a pelvic exenteration.[43] Postoperative urinary leaks are rarely seen with the use of a transverse colon conduit. During the formation of this diversion, the nonirradiated segment of bowel is anastomosed to extrapelvic stented ureters.

Stone Formation

Approximately 2% to 9% of patients with conduits have urinary calculi.[43] The propensity to form stones is thought to be the result of acidosis, chronic urinary stasis, infection, and increased calcium excretion. Some evidence in the literature has attributed stone formation to the use of nonabsorbable (i.e., titanium) staples, and from that has resulted the recommendation to avoid use of staples at the distal end of the conduit to be exposed to urine.

It is important to recognize that conduit diversion is associated with a 17% risk of significant loss of renal function.[43] Chronic renal failure can result from obstruction as strictures at the ureter-bowel anastomosis form. It is imperative to be able to detect biochemical changes in the patient's renal function, or structural changes such as upper tract dilatation, so as to intervene early. Placement of ureteral stents, dilation, or nephrostomy tubes may be necessary to treat the obstruction and prevent permanent renal damage and renal unit loss.

Can ureteral strictures or obstruction in reservoirs be managed noninvasively?

Ureteral strictures can be seen in approximately 13% of patients with a Miami pouch.[44] This problem can be managed via stent placement, balloon dilatation, or nephrostomy placement. Stones can lead to ureteral obstruction, which in turn can be managed with lithotripsy.

HEMORRHAGE

Multiple factors contribute to the increased risk of hemorrhage in gynecologic surgery. Some of these factors are inadequate exposure of the surgical field, obesity, poor operative technique, adhesions, clotting abnormalities, vascularity of tumors, and radical surgery.[45]

Certain basic principles are key in the management of intraoperative hemorrhage. Bleeding vessels should be clearly identified, keeping the ureter and other vital pelvic structures clearly under view during vascular injury repair. Placing clamps in a blind fashion in the setting of pelvic hemorrhage usually results in further blood loss and may lead to nerve, enteric, or ureteral injury. A crushing clamp should be applied only if the bleeding vessel is small and the site clearly visible.[45] Application of a crushing clamp to a major artery or vein can lead to increased bleeding. The initial step in controlling hemorrhage is usually application of pressure with a finger. A sponge stick or other atraumatic instrument may be used if the bleeding space is not easily accessible to the finger or if the surgeon is preparing the injury for repair. Excessive, life-threatening pelvic bleeding can be initially controlled by compression of the aorta below the level of the renal vessels.[45] In the setting of extensive bleeding, packing is appropriate.

After the initial hemorrhage is controlled by either pressure or packing, the surgeon should prepare for the repair. Lighting in the field should be maximized, the anesthesia team allowed to "catch up" with the patient's blood loss, and the proper instruments and suction setup obtained.[45] All other operative action should be halted until adequate vascular access is established, blood loss is replaced, and necessary blood products in an appropriate volume are available for replacement. Optimal exposure may require further dissection to better delineate the patient's anatomy.

Arterial injury can result from an intimal hematoma or from atherosclerotic plaque dissection, which can lead to obstruction and distal ischemia.[45] Initial control of an arterial injury requires digital pressure to control the hemorrhage, followed by application of either vascular clamps or umbilical tapes, proximally and distally, in order to control the bleeding and assess the extent of the injury. A small defect or puncture wound can be repaired with interrupted vascular suture (Prolene 6-0, or similar), making sure that the repair does not compromise the vessel lumen.[45,46] Vascular surgeons should be consulted to manage larger defects, because repair may require arterial grafting or skills that are usually outside the armamentarium of the gynecologic oncologist.

Venous injury is similarly initially managed by digital pressure to control the bleeding.[45,46] If the vessel is adequately mobilized, a Satinsky clamp can be applied to control the hemorrhage proximally and distally and to isolate the injured segment. Another technique is to apply Judd-Allis clamps along the length of the injury and repair the defect with fine Prolene suture.[45] Care must be taken to keep the field under adequate visualization, to use judicious suctioning, and to ensure that the vessel lumen is not compromised.

Serious venous bleeding can be immediately but transiently controlled by packing of the pelvic sidewall, presacral space, or parametria.[45,46] It may be necessary to leave the pack in for 15 minutes or longer, depending on the patient's coagulation status, and then slowly remove it to expose the bleeding areas, identifying the bleeding site or sites carefully.[45] Extensive venous hemorrhage may necessitate leaving the pack in place for 48 hours, transferring the patient to an intensive care unit, and then returning the patient to the operating room for pack removal under general anesthesia.[45,46] Ligation of the hypogastric arteries may help control pelvic hemorrhage but may also have a negative effect on intestinal bowel anastomosis. A bilateral artery ligation distal to the posterior branch is recommended, with the ureter and external iliac artery under direct visualization.[45-47] If ligation of the hypogastric arteries fails to control the bleeding, especially in the setting of an obstetric hemorrhage, ligation of the ovarian vessels may be helpful.[45-47]

Excessive uterine bleeding may be more effectively controlled by ligation of the uterine arteries than by hypogastric artery ligation.[47] Large purchases through the uterine wall are taken at the level of the cervical isthmus, above the bladder flap, with meticulous care taken to avoid injury to the distal ureter as it traverses the space of Morrow.[47]

How is hemorrhage from the external and internal iliac veins most effectively controlled?

Injury to the external iliac vein can result in death or in chronic venous insufficiency of the lower extremity. The external iliac vein is at increased risk of injury at the level of entry of the accessory obturator vein, near the superior pubic ramus.[45] The injured area, on the inferior surface of the vein, needs to be adequately exposed. The vein can be rotated ventrally by passing a sponge around it, or it can be turned with the use of an Allis clamp. The defect can be repaired with a small Prolene suture or a vascular clip, taking care not to obstruct the vessel lumen with the repair.[45-47]

Injury to the internal iliac vein can be catastrophic. This vessel can be injured during a pelvic lymphadenectomy, extensive pelvic sidewall dissection, or ligation of the hypogastric artery.[45,47] The internal iliac vein poses an especially difficult problem in repair given its fragility and immobility. The first step in management of bleeding from this site involves application of pressure for at least 5 to 7 minutes. However, most injuries to the internal iliac vein or its accompanying pelvic venous plexus require further surgical repair.[46,47]

The site of the defect can be identified with careful suctioning and removal of the pressure pack.[47] Small defects may require only the application of vascular clips.[45-47] Larger defects may necessitate repair with 5-0 Prolene or similar suture. It is critical that the surgeon has a clear view of the damaged portion of the vessel before commencing the repair. If the hemorrhage cannot be controlled with these measures, it may be necessary to ligate the internal iliac vein.[45,47] Vascular clamps can be placed proximal and distal to the injured site and the vein ligated with the use of synthetic nonabsorbable suture. Continuous venous bleeding may necessitate intraabdominal packing, with removal in 48 hours, after the patient is adequately resuscitated, and under general anesthesia, as described earlier.[45,47]

Aorta and Inferior Vena Cava Hemorrhage

The massive blood loss that can result from injury to the aorta or the inferior vena cava (IVC) can be fatal. The IVC can be injured during a lymph node dissection or during the Veress needle or trocar insertion at the time of a laparoscopic procedure.[47]

An essential maneuver during the performance of a paraaortic lymph node dissection, in trying to prevent IVC hemorrhage, is identification of a small perforating vessel located anterior to the IVC, just above its bifurcation. By identifying this omnipresent vessel and clamping or clipping it, the surgeon avoids its avulsion and the spectacular blood loss that can ensue if it is injured inadvertently.[47]

If bleeding in these vessels is encountered, the first recommended step is to apply digital pressure. If the injury is large, we recommend placing vasa-loops or vascular clamps.[45] Another option is to place a Judd-Allis clamp over the defect, elevate the vein wall, and then perform the repair with 5-0 Prolene suture.[45,46]

What is the best management strategy for controlling hemorrhage in the parametrial tissue?

Hemorrhage from the cardinal ligaments arises commonly during a radical hysterectomy or pelvic exenteration. The initial step in management of excessive bleeding from this site is once again to apply pressure. After adequate exposure is obtained and suctioning is in place, the area can be reclamped and sutured as the digit or instrument is lifted. If a distinct bleeding site cannot be identified, 2-0 Prolene sutures can be placed to control the bleeding.[45] Care must be taken to avoid sciatic nerve injury, because the roots of this nerve lie under the anterior cardinal ligament at the level of the pelvic side wall.

How is hemorrhage from the presacral veins controlled?

The presacral veins can be injured during mobilization of the rectosigmoid from the retrorectal space or the sacral hollow. The best way to manage bleeding at this site is to avoid it altogether. We recommend leaving Waldeyer's fascia (the fascia between the fascia propria of the rectum and the sacrum) intact during mobilization of the rectosigmoid.[45] Dissection should be done sharply and under direct visualization. Injury to the presacral veins, which are extremely delicate and lie on top of the sacrum, is more likely to result from blunt dissection.[45] Vein branches are at right angles to the middle sacral veins. We discourage the use of clips, cautery, or topical anticoagulants, because they are ineffective and are likely to result in additional injury.[45] If the injured vessel is clearly visualized, suturing can be performed. The bleeding may also be controlled by packing of the presacral space. Another approach is to place a thumbtack into the bone at the site of

hemorrhage.[45] In order to avoid nerve root injury, thumbtack placement in the region of the sacral foramina should be avoided.

▌ NEUROLOGIC INJURY

Neuropathies in gynecologic surgery are usually a result of malpositioning of the patient or a self-retaining retractor injury. Compression is caused by prolonged retraction against the nerve or poor positioning of the patient in stirrups. Hematomas can also induce neuropathies.

How is femoral nerve injury best prevented, and how is it managed?

Femoral nerve neuropathy is the most commonly encountered nerve injury in gynecologic surgery. Certain risk factors are associated with this injury, including wide transverse abdominal incisions, thin body habitus (body mass index <20 kg/m^2), operative time longer than 4 hours, diabetes, general anesthesia, tobacco use, placement of retractor blades that are too deep, and placing pressure on the femoral nerve as it runs under the psoas muscle. In addition, poorly developed rectus muscles and a narrow pelvis have also been implicated with a higher incidence of femoral neuropathy.[48]

Most patients with a femoral neuropathy present with sensory as well as motor deficits. Patients have weakness in the quadriceps femoris muscle of the thigh and are unable to extend their legs at the knee joint or raise their legs straight off the bed.[48] These patients often complain of difficulty in walking or weight bearing when attempting to get out of bed in the early days of recovery. Sensory symptoms include tingling and numbness in the anteromedial aspect of the thigh and the leg. Patients with a nerve transection or ligation may present with neuropathic pain.[48]

The initial workup for a suspected femoral nerve injury includes a thorough physical examination, followed by radiologic studies to investigate for the presence of a hematoma or foreign body.[48] The initial sensory and motor deficits should be clearly documented so as to delineate a proper clinical course of action toward recovery and as preparation for interval assessments. If transection or inadvertent suturing of the nerve is suspected, exploration should be undertaken immediately with neurosurgical expert assistance. A delay in the diagnosis of a nerve injury may result in the need for graft repairs to reconnect the retracted nerve stumps.[49] If the nerve was sharply divided, the best repair is by end-to-end anastomosis.[48] A hematoma compressing the nerve requires appropriate drainage.

The statistically most likely cause of a postoperative femoral neuropathy, once transection and hematoma have been excluded, is a compression injury.[48] It is prudent to consult a neurologist and obtain electromyographic studies. It is critical to initiate immediate physical therapy and rehabilitation, to prevent thrombotic complications from prolonged inactivity and muscle atrophy. Nonnarcotic agents (e.g., carbamazepine, amitriptyline) may alleviate the pain during the recovery period.[48]

Other Nerve Injuries

Obturator nerve injury may result during dissection of the obturator fossa, as part of a pelvic lymph node dissection. A neuropathy in the obturator nerve can also result if tumor-bearing nodal tissue encases the nerve. Symptoms include numbness of the inner thigh and minor ambulatory difficulties, the result of weakened adduction of the thigh.

Both the genitofemoral and the lateral femoral cutaneous nerves can be injured during dissection of the external iliac lymph nodes. Genitofemoral nerve injury leads to numbness over the upper labia and the groin, whereas injury to the lateral femoral cutaneous nerve results in numbness on the front of the thigh. As with other injuries, hematomas should be evacuated if present. It is critical to initiate the proper physical and rehabilitation therapy.

▌ WOUND COMPLICATIONS

Infection

Surgical site infections (SSIs), as labeled by the Centers for Disease Control and Prevention, are the most common nosocomial infections in surgical patients, accounting for approximately 38% of all such infections.[8] Approximately two thirds of SSIs involve the superficial and deep incisional tissues, and one third affect organs or spaces entered during the surgical procedure.[8] Certain factors have been associated with the risk of developing an SSI. Some patient factors include advanced age, poor nutritional status, diabetes, tobacco use, obesity, altered immune status, coexistent infection at a remote body site, colonization with microorganisms, and length of preoperative stay.[50] Operative factors include the duration of surgical scrub, preoperative shaving, duration of the operation, operating room ventilation, use of prophylactic antibiotics, surgical drains, surgical technique, and foreign material in the surgical site.[50]

The classic presenting symptoms of superficial or deep SSIs are *calor* (heat), *rubor* (redness), *dolor* (pain), and *tumor* (swelling).[50] Patients usually present with symptoms in the fifth or sixth postoperative day, with pyrexia and cellulitic changes that worsen if the wound is not opened. After appropriate wound opening, the defect should be packed to allow evacuation of the fluid and prevent premature apposition of the skin edges. Necrotizing fasciitis, a diagnosis made definitively by histologic examination, is suspected when a cloudy gray fluid and frank necrosis of the fascia are noted.[50] We recommend antibiotic therapy in the presence of systemic infection or if the cellulitis is present beyond the wound edges. Initial antibiotic therapy

should cover gram-positive and aerobic gram-negative organisms. This therapy should be broadened if the infection is not remitting in 48 hours or if culture results mandate a change in therapy.[50]

Prevention of SSIs can be attempted through alteration of any of the patient-related preoperative risk factors that are realistically amenable to change.[50] Diabetic patients should try to achieve "tight" glycemic control preoperatively. Tobacco use should be discouraged and, if possible, stopped 2 to 4 weeks before the surgery. Distant sites of infection, such as dental infections, should be treated before surgery. Hair should not be shaved but actually clipped in the operating room immediately before skin preparation.

Operative techniques to reduce the risk of SSIs include compulsive attention to scrubbing and prepping technique and maintenance of a sterile field regardless of the length of the procedure.[50] Adherence to meticulous surgical technique is critical. The surgeon should avoid hypothermia, maintain effective hemostasis, handle tissue gently, remove devitalized tissue, obliterate dead spaces, and use monofilament suture and closed-suction drains when appropriate.[8] Contaminated or dirty wounds should be allowed to close by either delayed primary closure or secondary closure, with the latter being our preference.

Dehiscence

Separation of the fascial layer that occurs early in the postoperative period is called dehiscence. This separation may be partial and undetected or complete. Evisceration occurs when a large fascia defect allows for the protrusion of viscera through the wound. Dehiscence is the result of failure to maintain closure of the fascial layer, secondary to inadequate surgical technique, which in turn is exacerbated by increased tension on the closure (e.g., ascites, bowel distention, coughing, vomiting, straining, obesity).[8]

The incidence of wound dehiscence ranges from 0.5% to 3%, depending on the patient risk pool. The integrity of the fascial tissue is critical for good closure. Malnutrition, obesity, advanced age, immune deficiency, diabetes, renal insufficiency, and malignancy are factors associated with a higher incidence of dehiscence.[8] Other local factors, such as infection, hematoma, and ischemia, also predispose a wound to dehisce.

Partial dehiscence without evisceration manifests with serosanguineous drainage from the wound. If evisceration is seen, the eviscerated tissue should be covered with sterile, saline-soaked gauze or towels and the patient taken emergently to the operating room for closure.[8] A computed tomography scan may be helpful in assessing the integrity of the fascial closure and to ensure that there are no occult additional defects. Bowel loops can be seen protruding through the fascial defect.

Reclosure of a wound dehiscence requires mass closure. All broken sutures should be removed. Antibiotics are indicated in the presence of a wound infection or a break in sterile technique. We recommend the use of extrafascial retention sutures to reapproximate the skin if the wound is clean.[8]

Hernia

Incisional hernias result from late disruption or nonhealing of the fascial layer. Although the incidence of hernia is approximately 1%, it increases to 30% in wounds complicated by a SSI.[8] Multiple previous operations, obesity, and the presence of an underlying collagen formation disorder are all associated with postoperative hernias.

Hernias can manifest as a bulge or painful swelling in the area of a previous incision. Patients may complain of poorly localized pain exacerbated by eating or movement.[8] Computed tomography scans may be helpful in delineating the defect. The defect needs to be repaired surgically. The recommended approach is to achieve a tensionless closure. If the fascial defect is large or not enough viable fascia is present to allow for a tensionless closure, use of a prosthetic material (mesh) may be necessary.[8]

CONCLUSIONS

Intraoperative injures, albeit unpleasant, are an expected reality in the life of an active gynecologic oncologist. Careful attention to certain factors and adherence to the general principles of surgical technique can minimize the risk of intraoperative organ injury. Specifically, it is imperative to be comfortable with the anatomy at hand, to restore normal anatomy, to obtain adequate exposure, to develop avascular planes, and to isolate vascular pedicles controlling the blood supply early in the operation. It is also imperative to be aware of the ureter and knowledgeable of its anatomic course through the pelvis. The temptation to clamp blindly should be resisted, as should the use of force over finesse. Finally, if an intraoperative or perioperative injury or complication occurs, timely recognition of the injury or complication and appropriate repair or intervention will result in the most optimal outcome for the patient.

REFERENCES

1. Dicker RC, Greenspan JR, Strauss LT, et al: Complications of abdominal and vaginal hysterectomy among women of reproductive age in the United States. The Collaborative Review of Sterilization. Am J Obstet Gynecol 1982;144:841-848.
2. Mirhashemi R, Harlow BL, Ginsburg ES, et al: Predicting risk of complications with gynecologic laparoscopic surgery. Obstet Gynecol 1998;92:327-331.
3. Harris WJ: Early complications of abdominal and vaginal hysterectomy. Obstet Gynecol Surv 1995;50:795-805.
4. Lambrou NC, Buller JL, Thompson JR, et al: Prevalence of perioperative complications among women undergoing reconstructive pelvic surgery. Am J Obstet Gynecol 2000;183:1355-1358.
5. Morrow CP, Curtin JP: Surgery on the intestinal tract. In Morrow CP, Curtin JP, De la Osa Lopez E (eds): Gynecologic Cancer Surgery. Philadelphia: Churchill Livingstone, 1996, pp 181-267.
6. Pettit PD, Sevin BU: Intraoperative injury to the gastrointestinal tract and postoperative gastrointestinal malignancies. Clin Obstet Gynecol 2002;45:492-506.
7. Knight M: Intestinal injury and how to cope. In Stanton SL (ed): Principles of Gynaecological Surgery. London, Springer Verlag, 1987, pp 157-170.
8. Angood PB, Gingalewski CA, Anderson DK: Surgical complications. In Townsend CM (ed): Sabiston Textbook of Surgery: The Biological Basis of Modern Surgical Practice. Philadelphia, WB Saunders, 2001, pp 215-219.
9. Levinson MA, Peterson SR, Sheldon GF, et al: Duodenal trauma: Experience of a trauma center. J Trauma 1984;24:475-480.
10. Stone HH, Fabian TC: Management of perforating colon trauma: Randomization between primary closure and exteriorization. Ann Surg 1979;190:430-436.
11. Stewart RM, Fabian TC, Croce MA, et al: Is resection with primary anastomosis following destructive colon wound always safe? Am J Surg 1994;168:316-319.
12. Demetriades D, Charalambides D, Pantowits D: Gunshot wounds of the colon: The role of primary repair. Ann R Coll Surg Engl 1992;74:381-384.
13. Ivatury RR, Gaudino J, Nallathambi NM, et al: Definitive treatment of colon injuries: A prospective study. Am Surg 1993;59:43-49.
14. Cornwell ET, Velhamos GC, Berne JV, et al: The fate of colonic suture lines in high risk trauma patients: A prospective analysis. J Am Coll Surg 1998;187:58-63.
15. Sasaki LS, Allaben RD, Golwala R, et al: Primary repair of colon injuries: A prospective randomized study. J Trauma 1995;39:895-901.
16. Chappuis CW, Frey DJ, Dietzen CD, et al: Management of penetrating colon injuries: A prospective randomized trial. Ann Surg 1991;213:492-497.
17. Gonzales RP, Merlotti GJ, Holevar MR: Colostomy in penetrating colon injury: Is it necessary? J Trauma 1996;41:271-275.
18. Miller PR, Fabian TC, Croce MA, et al: Improving outcomes following penetrating colon wounds: Application of a clinical pathway. Ann Surg 2002;6:775-781.
19. MacMillan SL, Kammerer-Doak D, Rogers RG, Parker KM: Early feeding and the incidence of gastrointestinal symptoms after major gynecologic surgery. Obstet Gynecol 2000;96:604-608.
20. Johnson Casto C, Krammer J, Drake J: Postoperative feeding: A clinical review. Obstet Gynecol Surv 2000;55:571-573.
21. Wright HK, O'Brien JJ, Tilson MD: Water absorption in experimental closed segment obstruction of the ileum in man. Am J Surg 1971;121:96-99.
22. Megibow AJ, Balthazar EJ, Cho KC, et al: Bowel obstruction: Evaluation with CT. Radiology 1991;180:313-318.
23. Balthazar EJ. George W: Holmes lecture: CT of small-bowel obstruction. AJR Am J Roentgenol 1994;162:255-261.
24. Peck JJ, Milleson T, Phelan J: The role of computed tomography with contrast and small bowel follow-through in management of small bowel obstruction. Am J Surg 1999;177:375-378.
25. Brolin RE, Krasna MJ, Mast BA: Use of tubes and radiographs in the management of small bowel obstruction. Ann Surg 1987;206:126-133.
26. Cheadle WG, Garr EE, Richardson JD: The importance of early diagnosis of small bowel obstruction. Am Surg 1988;54:565-569.
27. Bizer LS, Liebling RW, Delany HM, Gliedman ML: Small bowel obstruction: The role of nonoperative treatment in simple intestinal obstruction and predictive criteria for strangulation obstruction. Surgery 1981;89:407-413.
28. Brolin RE: Partial small bowel obstruction. Surgery 1984;95:145-149.
29. Fleshner PR, Siegman MG, Slater GI, et al: A prospective randomized trial of short versus long tubes in adhesive small-bowel obstruction. Am J Surg 1995;170:366-370.
30. Sosa J, Gardner B: Management of patients diagnosed as acute intestinal obstruction secondary to adhesions. Am Surg 1993;59:125-128.
31. Paran H, Neufeld D, Kaplan O, et al: Octreotide for treatment of postoperative alimentary tract fistulas. Worl J Surg 1995;19:430-433.
32. Rose D, Yarborough MF, Canizaro PC, Lowry SF: One hundred and fourteen fistulas of the gastrointestinal tract treated with total parenteral nutrition. Surg Gynecol Obstet 1986;163:345-350.

33. Colwell JC, Goldberg M, Carmel J. The state of the standard diversion. J Wound Ostomy Continence Nurs 2001;28:6-9.

34. Riley SA, Marsh MN: Maldigestion and malabsorption. In Felman M, Scharschmidt BF, Sleisenger MV (eds): Gastrointestinal and Liver Disease. Philadelphia, WB Saunders, 1998, pp 1501-1516.

35. Jex RK, VanHeerden JA, Wolff BG, et al. Gastrointestinal anastomoses: Factors affecting early complications. Ann Surg 1987;206:138-143.

36. Mendez LE: Iatrogenic injuries in gynecologic cancer surgery. Surg Clin North Am 2001;81:897-923.

37. Miyazawa K: Urological injuries in gynecologic surgery. Hawaii Med J 1980;39:11-12.

38. Montz FJ, Bristow RE, del Carmen MG: Operative injuries to the ureter. In Rock JA, Jones HW III (eds): Te Linde's Operative Gynecology, 9th ed. New York, Lippincott Williams & Wilkins, 2003.

39. Morrow CP, Curtin JP: Surgery on the urinary tract. In Morrow CP, Curtin JP, De la Osa Lopez E (eds): Gynecologic Cancer Surgery. Philadelphia, Churchill Livingstone, 1996, pp 269-322.

40. Hatch KD, Parham G, Shingleton HM, et al: Ureteral strictures and fistulae following radical hysterectomy. Gynecol Oncol 1984;19:17-23.

41. Morrow CP, Curtin JP: Surgery for cervical neoplasia. In Morrow CP, Curtin JP, De la Osa Lopez E (eds): Gynecologic Cancer Surgery. Philadelphia, Churchill Livingstone, 1996, pp 511-513.

42. Mundy AR: Urological complications and how to cope. In Stanton SL (ed): Principles of Gynaecological Surgery. London, Springer Verlag, 1987, pp 245-256.

43. Estape R, Mendez LE, Angioli R, Penalver M: Urinary diversion in gynecologic oncology. Surg Clin North Am 2001;81: 781-797.

44. Angioli R, Estape R, Cantuaria G, et al: Urinary complications of Miami pouch: Trend of conservative management. Am J Obstet Gynecol 1998;179:343-348.

45. Morrow CP, Curtin JP: Basic surgical principles. In Morrow CP, Curtin JP, De la Osa Lopez E (eds): Gynecologic Cancer Surgery. Philadelphia, Churchill Livingstone, 1996, pp 1-25.

46. Dormandy J: Haemorrhage and how to cope. In Stanton SL (ed): Principles of Gynaecological Surgery. London, Springer Verlag, 1987, pp 185-193.

47. Tomacruz RS, Bristow RE, Montz FJ: Management of pelvic hemorrhage. Surg Clin North Am 2001;81:925-948.

48. Chan JK, Manetta A: Prevention of femoral nerve injuries in gynecologic surgery. Am J Obstet Gynecol 2002;186:1-7.

49. Kim DH, Kline DG: Surgical outcome for intra-and extrapelvic femoral nerve lesions. J Neurosurg 1995;83:783-790.

50. Mangram AJ, Horan TC, Pearson ML, et al: Guidelines for prevention of surgical site infection 1999. Infect Control Hosp Epidemiol 1999;20:256-278.

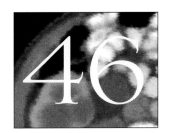

C H A P T E R

Management of Complications of Radiotherapy

Benjamin E. Greer, Ron E. Swensen, Wui-Jin Koh, and Haleigh A. Werner

MAJOR CONTROVERSIES

- **What is the optimal management of radiation-associated small-intestinal injury?**
- **What is the optimal management of radiation-associated rectosigmoid injury?**
- **What is the optimal management of radiation cystitis?**
- **What is the optimal management of radiation-associated ureteral stenosis?**
- **What is the optimal management of radiation-associated enterovesical fistula?**
- **What is the optimal management of radiation-associated vaginal stenosis?**
- **What is the optimal management of radiation-associated lymphedema?**
- **What is the optimal management of radiation necrosis or fibrosis?**
- **What complications are associated with special clinical situations?**

Radiation therapy plays an important role in the treatment of gynecologic malignancies. Radiation complications and toxicities are complex. Many complications redundant from multiple patient variables and radiation therapy algorithms. The toxicities or complications are a result of aggressive treatment with curative intent and need to be balanced against the morbidity of uncontrolled pelvic disease. The management suggestions in this chapter are directed toward pragmatic approaches for symptom control, correction of major tissue damage, and improving quality of life. Consequently, there are not necessarily many controversies.

Primary radiation therapy is used with concurrent chemotherapy in advanced cervical cancers.[1,2] Advanced, unresectable vulvar cancers are also treated with concurrent chemotherapy and irradiation.[3] Vaginal cancers are rare but usually treated with radiation therapy. The use of adjuvant radiation treatment in endometrial cancer is controversial in surgically staged early endometrial cancers, but it is recommended for treating more advanced endometrial cancers.[4] Adjuvant radiation treatment is recommended after radical hysterectomy for cervical cancer with intermediate- or high-risk features.[5] Radiation therapy as a primary treatment modality for ovarian cancer is not commonly recommended in the United States.

Radiation therapy has multiple variables that affect the potential for complications, including the dose of radiation administered and the fraction size, field size (pelvic versus extended field versus whole abdomen), number of fields treated, and treatment position (prone or supine). The energy of the photon beam used determines the depth dose, with higher energy having greater penetration. Most pelvic irradiation is delivered by a high-energy photon beam that is equal to or greater than 15 MV. Brachytherapy, administered with a low dose rate (LDR) or high dose rate (HDR), may contribute to acute and late toxic effects. The addition of concurrent or sequential chemotherapy, as well as surgical procedures before or after radiotherapy, also influences the likelihood of radiation-related toxicity.

Late complications of pelvic field irradiation are most common in patients treated with external beam and brachytherapy. Pretreatment transperitoneal staging as adjuvant therapy before irradiation or irradiation after radical surgery increases bowel complications.[6,7] In a randomized study of radical surgery versus radiotherapy for stage Ib through IIa cervical cancers, the highest complication rate was in the group that received surgery and irradiation.[8] Patient characteristics also play a role in potential complications. These variables include a patient's age, comorbid conditions (e.g., diabetes, hypertension), pelvic inflammatory disease, previous surgery, diverticulitis, inflammatory bowel disease, collagen vascular diseases, and smoking.[9-11] Recurrent disease may contribute to or be the primary cause of local morbidity after radiotherapy.

Radiation-related complications can be classified as acute, late, and consequential late effects. Acute reactions occur in most patients during their initial treatment or in the first several months after treatment. Acute reactions may be severe, although they are usually supportable, and most patients recover. The mild acute reactions that occur during treatment and spontaneously resolve are not included in this chapter. Late complications are less common, but they are important clinically because of the potential of significant long-term morbidity and mortality. The consequential late effects result from acute injury, which links acute and delayed tissue injury. Studies have demonstrated that severe acute injury can contribute to late effects; therefore, decreasing the acute effects may also decrease the severity and incidence of late effects.

The measurement of radiation-induced injuries is usually clinically based on a strong subjective component. There is always a bias toward severe injuries. The question arises of how to quantify subtle injuries, because classifications are mostly based on clinical symptoms rather than on tissue or molecular abnormalities. The rate of complications varies in the literature because of various toxicity criteria, and there probably is underreporting of complications, especially for long-term patients. Despite these shortcomings, this chapter attempts to encapsulate the known complications and strategies for management.

Radiation tolerance is defined as the amount of radiation that a particular organ can receive without developing a serious complication, and it varies from organ to organ and from tissue to tissue. The general concept of dose-response curves for tumor control and tissue or organ damage as a function of total radiation dose is illustrated in Figure 46-1. The probability of tumor control is very small with low doses, rises steeply with moderate doses, and reaches a plateau with high doses. A similar curve is assumed for the percentage of complications as a function of dose. The optimal amount of radiation is the dose that yields the highest probability of tumor control and the lowest probability of complication. Models have been made for the various organs and tissues included in gynecologic cancer radiation treatment fields.[12,13] Clinically, the resulting complications and toxicities observed are more complex because of overlapping tissue and organ radiation

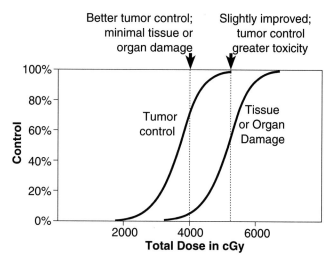

Figure 46-1. Dose-response curves for tumor control and tissue or organ damage as a function of total radiation dose.

doses and because of volume and heterogeneity considerations.

Uniform reporting in the literature of acute and late radiation toxicities or morbidities would allow comparison of treatment algorithm complications. An accurate baseline evaluation before commencement of therapy is necessary. It is important to discriminate between disease- and treatment-related signs and symptoms. Acute toxicity scoring criteria should be used from the commencement of therapy through day 90. Late radiation morbidity scoring is used after day 90.

The Radiation Therapy Oncology Group and European Organization of Research and Treatment of Cancer (RTOG/EORTC) radiation morbidity scoring schema provides relatively uniform scoring of toxicity with well-defined criteria.[14] For the purpose of this chapter, the listings of toxicities are limited to tissues commonly affected by radiation treatment fields for gynecologic cancers. The late effects are outlined in Table 46-1. The scoring schema listed is for grades 1 through 4, but any toxicity that results in death is grade 5. Some of the toxicities listed may only apply to patients with whole abdomen irradiation or to extended-field treatment. There are no criteria listed for vascular radiation damage (Fig. 46-2). The acute and late toxicity profiles for gynecologic cancers change with the addition of concurrent chemotherapy, biologic agents, and newer radiation therapy techniques such as intensity-modulated radiation therapy (IMRT). Table 46-2 outlines the risk of late toxicities or complications after radiation therapy algorithms for gynecologic neoplasms. The estimated risk is based on curative-intent treatments and data reported in the literature.

Reviewing complications or related toxicities in the literature is challenging. Most data are from case reports or small series. There are no level I, evidence-based, randomized data as defined by the U.S. Preventive Task Force regarding reporting and management of irradiation complications.[15] Attention to grading, definitions, technical aspects of radiation

Table 46–1. Modified RTOG/EORTC Late Radiation Morbidity Scoring Schema for Common Organ Tissues Affected by Radiation Treatment for Gynecologic Cancers

Organ Tissue	Grade 0	Grade 1	Grade 2	Grade 3	Grade 4
Skin	None	Slight atrophy, pigmentation change, some hair loss	Patch atrophy, moderate telangiectasia, total hair loss	Marked atrophy, gross telangiectasia	Ulceration
Subcutaneous tissue	None	Slight induration (fibrosis) and loss of subcutaneous fat	Moderate fibrosis but asymptomatic, slight field contracture with < 10% linear reduction	Severe induration and loss of subcutaneous tissue, field contracture with > 10% linear measurement	Necrosis
Mucous membrane (vagina)	None	Slight atrophy and dryness	Moderate atrophy and telangiectasia, little mucus	Marked atrophy with complete dryness, severe telangiectasia	Ulceration
Spinal cord	None	Mild Lhermitte's syndrome	Severe Lhermitte's syndrome	Objective neurologic findings at or below cord level treated	Mono-, para-, quadriplegia
Small or large intestine	None	Mild diarrhea, mild cramping, bowel movement 5 times daily, excessive rectal mucus or intermittent bleeding	Moderate diarrhea and colic bowel movement > 5 times daily, excessive rectal mucus or intermittent bleeding	Obstruction or bleeding requiring surgery	Necrosis, perforation, fistula
Liver	None	Mild lassitude, nausea, dyspepsia, slightly abnormal liver function	Moderate symptoms, some abnormal liver test results, normal serum albumin	Disabling hepatic insufficiency, liver function tests grossly abnormal, low albumin level, edema or ascites	Necrosis, hepatic coma, or encephalopathy
Kidney	None	Transient albuminuria, no hypertension, mild impairment or renal function, urea = 25-35 mg/dL, creatinine = 1.5-2.0 mg/dL, creatinine clearance > 75 mL/min	Persistent moderate albuminuria (2+), mild hypertension, no related anemia, moderate impairment of renal function, urea > 36-60 mg/dL, creatinine clearance = 50-74 mL/min	Severe albuminuria, severe hypertension, persistent anemia (< 10 mg/dL), severe renal failure, urea > 60 mg/dL, creatinine > 4.0 mg/dL, creatinine clearance < 50 mL/min	Malignant hypertension, uremic coma, urea > 100%
Bladder	None	Slight epithelial atrophy, minor telangiectasia (microscopic hematuria)	Moderate frequency, generalized telangiectasia, intermittent macroscopic hematuria	Severe frequency and dysuria, severe generalized telangiectasia (often with petechiae), frequent hematuria, reduction in bladder capacity (< 150 mL)	Necrosis, contracted bladder (capacity < 100 mL), severe hemorrhagic cystitis
Bone	None	Asymptomatic, no growth retardation, reduced bone density	Moderate pain or tenderness, growth retardation, irregular bone	Severe pain or tenderness, complete arrest of bone growth, dense bone sclerosis	Necrosis, spontaneous fracture

delivery, total radiation dose, time-dose relationships, and follow-up time is important. Because of the improvement in irradiation equipment and treatment techniques, the older literature is less relevant or not applicable to current practice. Most of the literature describes toxicity or complications related to radiation treatment for carcinoma of the cervix. However, the principles regarding occurrence, severity, and management of radiation toxicity of carcinoma of the cervix can in great part be applied to other gynecologic malignancies. Other treatment designs and fields may be associated with different toxicities, such as increased small bowel, renal, or hepatic injury with whole abdomen irradiation or increased skin effects in vulvar irradiation.

In general, patients with cervical cancer have an estimated risk of major late radiation-related complications of 5% to 15%. In most of the older literature, calculations of the incidence of complications are accrued with relatively short follow-up. Actuarial methods to calculate and report complication rates are the more current approach. The actuarial methods more accurately reflect a surviving patient's risk of late complications related to treatment. Many reports in

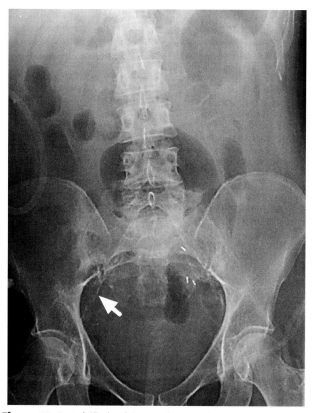

Figure 46–2. Calcified pelvic vessels are indicated by the *arrow* in a 42-year-old woman who had been treated with whole pelvic irradiation for liposarcoma as a teenager. The estimated dose was 6500 cGy to the pelvis.

the literature include patients treated over extended periods. Patterns-of-care studies published over two different periods have suggested a declining complication rate, which is probably related to modern radiation therapy techniques and the increased use of brachytherapy.[16] An actuarial report of major late complications requiring transfusions, hospitalization, or surgical intervention from the University of Texas MD Anderson Cancer Center cited an incidence of 7.7% at 3 years, 9.3% at 5 years, and 14.4% at 20 years.[17] The study consisted of 1784 patients with stage Ib cervical cancer who were treated in a consistent manner between 1960 and 1989. Anterior and posterior opposed fields were used in 98% of patients. In this series, small bowel and rectosigmoid injuries were the most common. Most rectal complications develop in the first 2 years. The incidence of small-bowel obstruction was increased among patients who had pretreatment laparotomy and patients who weighed less than 120 pounds. Fistula rates were increased among patients who underwent extrafascial hysterectomy and pretreatment laparotomy.

Another large series of 1456 patients from Washington University with stage Ib through IVa cervical cancer treated with external beam and two LDR intracavitary insertions to deliver 70 to 90 Gy to point A reported late complications occurring in approximately 8% of stage Ib patients and slightly more than 10% of patients with stage II through IVa disease.[18]

Multivariate analysis demonstrated that rectal and bladder point doses were the factor influencing rectosigmoid sequelae and bladder morbidity.

In an analysis of 517 irradiated cervical cancer patients, a dose-response relationship was demonstrated for increasing bladder and rectum complications with increasing dose.[19] When the combined dose to the bladder or rectum was equal to or greater than 80 Gy, rates of complications involving these organs were 12% and 18%, respectively. Significant late toxicity rates of 10% to 16% in the patterns-of-care study[16,20] and 16% to 21% in the Canadian experience[21] were also shown. One study using expanded pelvic fields had an actuarial 4-year late complication rate of 14.8%.[22] Whole abdomen radiotherapy has been used in the treatment of selected patients with ovarian cancer and endometrial cancer patients with peritoneal dissemination. Late gastrointestinal toxicity rates vary, with a wide range of up to 20%.[23-26]

The symptoms related to radiation complications vary from acute temporary effects to late, long-lasting changes. The spectrum of symptoms varies from one affected tissue or organ to another. Although radiation can affect many different tissue types, severe, late injury is typically manifested (Fig. 46-3). One system often predominates. Except in emergency situations, there should be an evaluation of the patient's general physical condition and comorbid conditions before any definitive treatment. Potential recurrent cancer should always be considered, and it should not be assumed that local tissue injury is caused by radiation without a careful workup. Occasionally, more than one complication may be identified. The best example is an attempt to manage obstruction of the small bowel related to treatment of cervical cancer, only to discover that there was a concurrent rectosigmoid obstruction that was not identified preoperatively. Contrast imaging studies are valuable in preoperative planning for confirmation and localization of fistulas, for the identification of transition points in obstructed areas, for identifying more complex injuries, and for the evaluation of recurrent disease. If the studies suggest a possible recurrence, computed tomography (CT)–directed needle biopsies or positron emission tomography (PET) scanning is indicated for identification.

Gastrointestinal Tract Injuries

The spectrum of symptoms of radiation enteritis includes diarrhea, nausea, rectal bleeding, and rectal and perirectal pain. Imaging studies are rarely indicated to confirm less severe injuries, and management is supportive with antidiarrheals, antiemetics, topical creams, and diet modification. Diagnosis of delayed or late bowel enteropathy is not as straightforward as that of acute enteritis because of the variability of presentation. The mechanisms responsible for symptoms include abnormal absorption, dysmotility, bacterial overgrowth, and stricture.

When a patient presents with a picture of moderate-to-severe abdominal symptoms related to radiation

Table 46-2. Common Radiation Therapy Treatment Algorithms with Potential for Late Toxicities or Complications

Disease Site	Treatment Plan	Risk*
Cervix	Primary treatment	
	Radiation only	M-H
	Radiation + chemotherapy	M-H
	Extended fields radiation therapy	H
	Extended fields radiation therapy + chemotherapy	H
	Radiation with adjuvant hysterectomy	H
	Radiation with interstitial brachytherapy implants	H
	Postsurgical treatment	
	Radical hysterectomy + radiation therapy	M-H
Endometrium	Post primary surgical management with TAH-BSO staging	
	Adjuvant treatment external beam radiation therapy	M
	External beam radiation therapy + LDR brachytherapy	M
	External beam radiation therapy + HDR brachytherapy	M
	Vaginal brachytherapy only, LDR or HDR	L
	Preoperative tandem and ovoids	L
	Whole-abdomen irradiation	M-H
Ovary	Whole-abdomen irradiation	M-H
	Selected cases with limited-field irradiation	L
Vagina	Primary radiation therapy + brachytherapy	M
	Primary radiation therapy with interstitial brachytherapy	M-H
Vulva	Primary radiation	M-H
	Adjunctive radiation after primary surgery for local factors or positive nodes	M-H

*Risk: low (L) = 0% to 5%; medium (M) = 5% to 10%; high (H) ≥10%.
HDR, high dose rate; LDR, low dose rate; TAH-BSO, total abdominal hysterectomy and bilateral salpingo-oophorectomy.

enteropathy, diagnostic tests should be obtained. If the abdominal x-ray films, consisting of upright and supine radiographs, demonstrate areas of significant abnormal gas patterns or a dilated colon without rectal air, the patient should be admitted to the hospital for evaluation (Fig. 46-4). The most common severe regional radiation enteropathy is injury to the terminal ileum. The cause is a relatively fixed anatomic position of the terminal ileum in the pelvis, a lower total-dose tolerance of the small bowel compared with large bowel, and an additional radiation dose from brachytherapy. The second most common gastrointestinal tract complication involves the rectosigmoid. Rectosigmoid injuries are also often caused by the combination of external beam radiotherapy and intracavitary brachytherapy. Occasionally, a perforation of the uterus with the tandem adjacent to the colon occurs, and this extrauterine position increases the rectosigmoid dose. Before any surgical intervention for a radiation-related small-bowel obstruction, a limited barium enema should be performed to rule out a concurrent rectosigmoid obstruction. Additional diagnostic tests such as endoscopy, ultrasound, and transit studies may be useful to determine the cause of the patient's presenting symptoms.

What is the optimal management of radiation-associated small-intestinal injury? The initial management of a hospitalized patient with severe enteropathy should include intravenous hydration and correction of any electrolyte imbalance. The use of nasogastric suction can be beneficial in patients with severe

nausea and vomiting and dilated small-bowel loops. In mild cases of obstruction, conservative management for several days may result in improvement and resolution of a partial obstruction. The patient with diagnostic abdominal radiographs that remain unchanged within 72 hours should be considered for surgical intervention.

The surgical management of small-bowel injuries has evolved over the past several decades. In the mid-1960s, the recommendation for surgical intervention was often to perform a bypass alone.[27] Long-term follow-up of patients managed in this manner revealed a high incidence of infection, abscess, and perforation of the defunctionalized loop of the bowel. The current approach is to do a resection of the injured bowel with anastomosis.[28,29] If possible, one limb of the anastomosis should be nonirradiated bowel to decrease the risk of anastomotic failure. In the case of a perforation and associated walled-off abscess, the bowel potentially can be primarily resected and reanastomosed. When generalized perforation with peritonitis exists, an ileostomy should be performed.[30]

The principles of surgery need to be applied using good surgical judgment. In general, the surgical team should be experienced in dealing with irradiated tissue. Surgical techniques using stapling devices can be employed. In some clinical situations, the use of a hand-sewn anastomosis is indicated and more appropriate. With either technique, the surgeon should be cognizant of the risk of anastomotic leak and consider plication over the staple line or a two-layered closure if the bowel wall is sufficiently mobile.

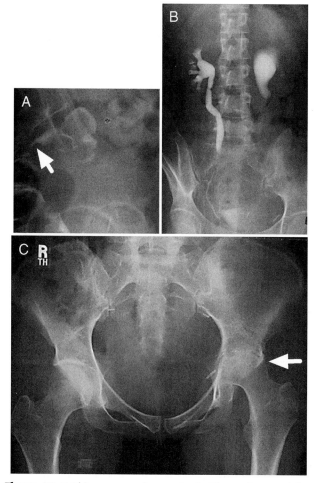

Figure 46-3. This woman, who was treated for carcinoma of the cervix with primary irradiation, developed multiple, late complications. **A,** Sigmoid stricture. **B,** Bilateral hydroureter. **C,** Osteoradionecrosis of the left hip.

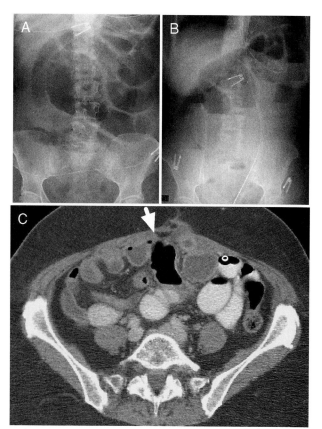

Figure 46-4. A small bowel obstruction occurred after whole abdomen irradiation as an adjunct treatment for endometrial cancer. **A,** Flat plate of the abdomen with dilated loops of small bowel. **B,** Upright radiograph with typical stair-stepping appearance of the loops of the small bowel. **C,** Computed tomography demonstrates the transition point *(arrow)* between dilated small bowl and normal-caliber bowel.

Clinically, irradiated bowel has a pale color, serosal fibrosis, and thickened bowel wall with decreased internal diameter or obstruction (Fig. 46-5). Intraoperatively, the small bowel is often agglutinated and adherent to other loops of the small bowel, large bowel, or pelvic structures such as the uterus, adnexa, or pelvic side wall. This requires tedious dissection. The areas of injured bowel should be resected, with careful evaluation of potential injury to adjacent tissue. Evaluation should start from the ligament of Treitz and progress down to where the bowel is obstructed or nonfunctional. With an injury to the terminal ileum, the surgery often involves removal of the ileocecal segment with an end-to-end, side-to-side, or end-to-side anastomosis of the small bowel to upper ascending colon or transverse colon. If possible, a minimum of 100 cm of small bowel should be left to prevent short-bowel syndrome and resulting nutritional complications. Documentation of the length of residual bowel at the time of surgery is important. Short-bowel syndrome is correlated with extent and location of the resection and with the presence or absence of the ileocecal valve and colon. The clinical result depends on

the function of the remaining gastrointestinal tract. Resection of the ileum can result in problems with bile salt reabsorption, steatorrhea, and absorption of vitamin B_{12}. Loss of colon can result in fluid and electrolyte imbalances. Clinically, patients with more than

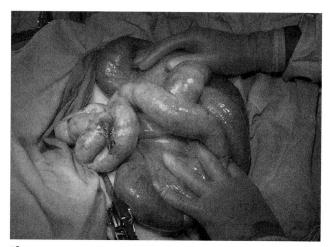

Figure 46-5. Delayed radiation fibrosis of distal small bowel with thickened bowel wall, stenosis of the lumen, and obstruction after pelvic irradiation. See also Color Figure 46-5.

100 cm of remaining small bowel adapt relatively well. Patients occasionally require chronic total parental nutrition.[31]

What is the optimal management of radiation-associated rectosigmoid injury? Rectosigmoid complications from radiation therapy usually manifest with symptoms of proctitis, including rectal bleeding and diarrhea. Patients with mild symptoms can be managed medically with antidiarrheals and steroid suppositories. Patients with significant bleeding from the rectum should undergo endoscopic evaluation of the rectosigmoid and descending colon. Colonoscopy or sigmoidoscopy can confirm the diagnosis of radiation proctitis and rule out other potential causes of bleeding, such as arterial venous malformation, diverticular disease, inflammatory bowel disease, and malignancy. If a specific bleeding point is identified, it can be coagulated at the time of the procedure. Steroid enemas, sucralfate enemas, and short-chain fatty acids have been used as nonsurgical treatment.[32,33] Surgical diversion is indicated as a last resort.

Patients who present with a sigmoid stricture or obstruction usually report progressive bouts of constipation with continued narrowing of the diameter of their stool. Some patients with evidence of total sigmoid obstruction present with obstipation and with abdominal pain, distention, and vomiting. The surgical management of a rectosigmoid stricture requires considerable surgical judgment (see Fig. 46-3A). It is important to review radiation port films and brachytherapy records as part of the clinical evaluation before surgical exploration. In some clinical situations, there is redundant rectosigmoid with a small segment of radiation-induced injury. This may be amenable to resection with anastomosis using a hand-sewn anastomosis or an end-to-end anastomosis stapling device. If possible, the distal resection should be below the level of the radiation field. Some patients have a long segment of sigmoid that is obstructed down into the rectal area, and patients often have significant radiation fibrosis of the pararectal and parametrial tissues that are nonmobile. Depending on the amount of radiation fibrosis to the rectum and adjacent pelvic soft tissues, it may be technically inadvisable and unfeasible to do a resection with anastomosis. If resection and reanastomosis is not possible, a descending loop colostomy should be performed. Gynecologic oncologists are divided over a loop colostomy versus end colostomy.[34] Some surgeons are reluctant to perform a loop colostomy because of concerns about prolapse of the functional end of the loop colostomy or spillage of stool into the descending colon. These concerns are not well founded. Prolapse is predominantly a function of mobility of the mesentery, and the most distal descending colon should be used. This allows minimal mobility of the mesentery. Often, surgeons unfamiliar with managing these patients perform a transverse loop colostomy, which does have problems with prolapse. In managing a rectosigmoid obstruction with a colostomy, if the surgeon elects to do an end colostomy, there must be a

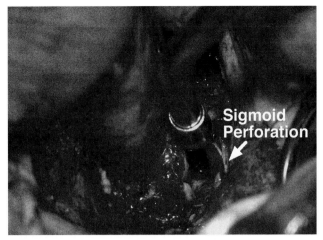

Figure 46–6. Sigmoid perforation with intra-abdominal fecal contamination and abscess after primary irradiation for carcinoma of the cervix in a patient with pelvic inflammatory disease. See also Color Figure 46–6.

defunctionalized stoma formed in addition. Both stomas must be managed. A loop colostomy minimizes stomal management for the patient and the stomal therapist. Usually, a loop colostomy with a bar is performed, and 10 days postoperatively, the stoma bar can be removed. In patients with sigmoid perforations with fecal contamination of the peritoneal cavity, a colostomy is the only surgical option (Fig. 46-6).

Rectovaginal fistulas are rare (Fig. 46-7). Similar surgical principles and judgment for sigmoid or rectal obstruction need to be applied to possible surgical closure. The Bricker-Johnston sigmoid colon graft is a

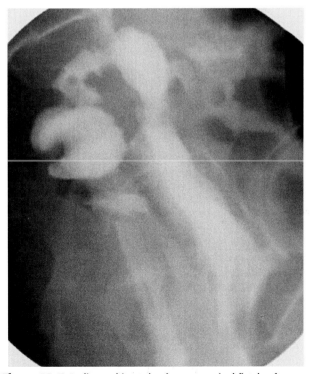

Figure 46–7. Radiographic study of a rectovaginal fistula after surgery and irradiation.

potential technique for the repair of rectovaginal fistulas and stricture.[35]

Urinary Tract Injuries

What is the optimal management of radiation cystitis? Radiation cystitis is the most common urinary tract toxicity, and hematuria is the most frequent symptom. MD Anderson Cancer Center has reported a 6.5% long-term incidence, with most patients having minor symptoms. Actuarial life table analysis demonstrated increasing risk of hematuria of 5.8% at 5 years to 9.6% at 20 years.[36]

Most cases of minor hematuria resolve with antibiotic treatment. Cystoscopy is indicated for persistent bleeding to rule out recurrent cancer or a second primary tumor. Cystoscopic findings after irradiation demonstrate pale mucosa and telangiectasia. Biopsies and cautery should be used sparingly. Severe bleeding requiring admission and transfusion is rare. Based on the MD Anderson Cancer Center data, the risk is 1.0% at 5 years and 2.3% at 20 years.[36] Major bladder complications described in case studies occurred at a rate of 2.5%.[20] Continuous bladder irrigation using a large, three-way Foley catheter is the recommended treatment for a patient with severe bleeding or who is passing clots that could obstruct the urethra. Monitoring the amount of fluid infused and maintaining drainage are important tasks. Bladder distention and rupture can occur. Various agents such as acetic acid, aluminum salts, silver nitrate, and prostaglandins have been added to saline to improve effectiveness.[37] Formalin is considered to be highly effective in stopping hematuria; however, it has many complications and should be used as a last resort. A cystogram should be performed before the use of formalin to rule out perforation or ureteral reflux. Bladder contracture, ureteral fibrosis, papillary necrosis, and delayed fistula formation have been reported with the use of formalin. These complications can be reduced with diluted formalin.[38,39] Invasive procedures such as vascular embolization, bilateral percutaneous nephrostomy tubes, urinary conduit, and cystectomy have been used in cases of severe bleeding or bladder contraction.[40] The Japanese have reported higher severe urologic complications compared with other parts of the world, including an incidence of bladder rupture of 2%. This higher rate of urologic complications may result from HDR brachytherapy.[41]

What is the optimal management of radiation-associated ureteral stenosis? Ureteral stenosis occurs in less than 1% of the patients (see Fig. 46-3B).[17] Ureteral complications are more common in patients who have had combined treatment with surgery and irradiation. After recurrence is ruled out, the function of the affected kidney should be evaluated by renal scan. If the residual function of the affected kidney is reduced to 10% or less, the risks of renal salvage procedures outweigh the benefit. Partial ureteral obstructions can be managed with cystoscopic placement of a

ureteral stent. If cystoscopic insertion is unsuccessful, antegrade placement or percutaneous nephrostomy can be performed. Successful use of these techniques is limited by infection and the need for replacement every 3 months. Surgical options for ureteral obstruction include ureteral neocystostmy with a psoas hitch and bladder-lengthening procedures such as a Biori flap. In patients who have had full-dose, curative-intent irradiation, these procedures may fail. Another option is to use a segment of ileum between the distal ureter and bladder. Transureteroneocystostomy is not advised because it increases the risk to the opposite kidney. If both ureters are obstructed without evidence of recurrence, a urinary conduit is indicated.

What is the optimal management of radiation-associated enterovesical fistula? Enterovesical fistula without recurrent disease is rare (Fig. 46-8). Fourteen cases have been reported in the literature. Six patients had colovesical, five had enterovesical, and three had fistulas involving the small and large bowels.[42] Patients require individualized management. Surgical procedures that resect the necrotic fistulized bowel and result in complete separation of the gastrointestinal and genitourinary tracts provide the best results.

What is the optimal management of radiation-associated vaginal stenosis? Treatments for gynecologic malignancies negatively affect sexual function. For women with endometrial, cervical, and ovarian cancers, sexual desire was diminished in 74% of patients and 42% of their partners.[43-45] Postirradiation treatment for gynecologic cancers often results in vaginal apical atrophy or agglutination resulting in vaginal stenosis. Vaginal stenosis is defined as circumferential fibrosis, which simultaneously diminishes vaginal length and width. Vaginal dilators and intercourse are treatment options, but their efficacy is not documented.

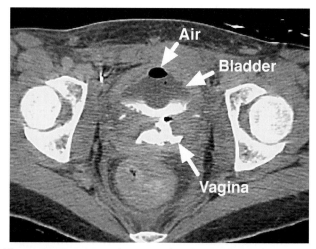

Figure 46–8. Computed tomography of a 33-year-old woman who developed compound rectovaginal, vesicovaginal, and colovesical fistulas after primary irradiation and adjuvant hysterectomy. *Arrows* point to air and contrast in the bladder and to contrast in the vagina.

Prospective studies of a large group of women have not been performed. There may be various degrees of atrophy, telangiectasia, and scarring in the vagina. Vaginal length and vaginal stenosis are related to intracavitary radiation therapy for carcinoma of the cervix.[46,47] Less commonly, vaginal vault necrosis may occur after high-dose radiation therapy.[17]

What is the optimal management of radiation-associated lymphedema? Lymphedema is an additional complication after radiation therapy. It is more common in patients who have had combined surgical management and full-dose radiation therapy, especially with adjuvant therapy for carcinoma of the vulva after radical vulvectomy and groin node dissection. Support hose, physical therapy, and massage treatments are available to ameliorate symptoms, but complete correction of lymphedema is rare. Other management options include intermittent diuretic use and maintenance of overlying skin integrity to prevent infection and tissue breakdown.

What is the optimal management of radiation necrosis or fibrosis? Some patients develop chronic soft tissue radiation necrosis involving the skin and subcutaneous tissue, particularly of the vulva, with or without associated osteoradionecrosis. Surgical management often requires a tri-service approach consisting of gynecologic oncology, orthopedics, and plastic surgery (Fig. 46-9). Some cases require two-stage procedures. The first entails resection of the irradiated and necrotic tissue, resection or reconstruction of fistulized organs, and bony resection, if indicated. One to 2 weeks later, reconstruction is done with flaps. These plastic surgery procedures have used rectus abdominus, gracilis rotational flaps, and latissimus dorsi microsurgical flaps.[48]

Some patients are free of disease but impaired by irradiated wounds that persist despite conservative measures and surgical therapy with well-vascularized flaps. Hyperbaric oxygen has been used for these patients with delayed radiation soft tissue injuries and bony necrosis.[49] Hyperbaric oxygen therapy also has been prescribed for radiation cystitis, enteritis, and proctitis.

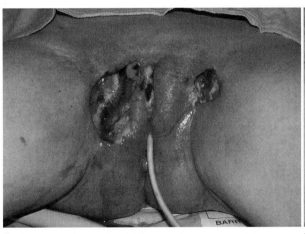

A

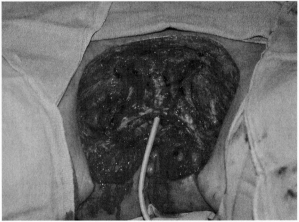

B

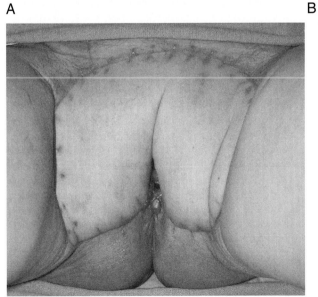

C

Figure 46–9. A, Patient with radiation necrosis of the vulva after primary radiation therapy has secondary infection and osteoradionecrosis, as well as osteomyelitis of the pubis. **B,** Radical vulvectomy and débridement of necrotic tissue with resection of pubis bilaterally back to viable bone of the ischiopubic and ileopubic rami. **C,** After 1 week, pelvic perineal wound reconstruction was performed with a rectus abdominis myocutaneous flap and split-thickness skin graft from the thigh to the abdominal wall. See also Color Figure 46–9.

Medical management of radiation-induced fibrosis or soft tissue necrosis has been reported. A combination of pentoxifylline (800 mg/day) and vitamin E (1000 IU/day) was administered to 43 patients with 50 symptomatic areas of radiation-induced fibrosis for 6 months, and this approach produced clinical regression and functional improvement.[50] These patients had been treated with irradiation for head and neck cancers or breast cancer.

Patients can develop an insufficiency fracture of the femoral head or have microfractures of the pelvis that can look suspicious for recurrent disease (see Fig. 46-3C). CT or magnetic resonance imaging provides the best method of workup for pelvic insufficiency fracture. Bone biopsies should be avoided if possible, because the bone injury may be further enhanced by surgical trauma. Management is typically conservative, with gradual healing occurring over time.[51,52]

Ovarian failure. The ovaries are among the most radiation-sensitive organs in the human body. Radiation-induced castration, with permanent amenorrhea and accompanying pronounced hormonal changes, essentially occurs in all women whose ovaries are exposed to more than 500 to 1500 cGy. This effect is age dependent; women older than 40 years may be rendered postmenopausal by much lower doses, whereas younger women, especially if prepubertal, are somewhat more resistant to the ovarian-ablative effects of radiation.[53] Many patients undergoing cancer therapy before pregnancy receive chemotherapy in addition to radiation therapy, making the specific effects of each treatment modality on fertility and future induction of congenital abnormalities difficult to estimate.

Patients who require high-dose radiation therapy (4000 to 4500 cGy or more) to the whole pelvis in addition to brachytherapy, as is often the case for gynecologic malignancies, should be counseled regarding the loss of reproductive capability. Typically, ovarian function is lost, and irradiation usually results in endometrial ablation, loss of uterine elasticity, and cervical and vaginal stenosis.

Neuropathies. Neuropathies such as lumbosacral plexopathy can develop as a result of treatment.[54] Fortunately, they are rare because treatment is often observational. Neurontin (gabapentin) has been used with some success to address nerve-related pain and dysesthesias.

What complications are associated with special clinical situations?

Special clinical situations that are not common have a different spectrum of complications:

- Interstitial brachytherapy implants such as the Syed-Neblett and the Martinez Universal Perineal Interstitial Template (MUPIT) have been associated with proctitis and with rectovaginal fistulas, with an incidence of 5.1% to 33%.[55-57]

- Intraoperative radiation therapy has been used as an adjunct to pelvic exenteration for recurrent cervical cancer after full-dose radiation therapy, with a 5-year disease-specific survival rate of 43%. Seven out of 22 patients had a peripheral neuropathy related to treatment, and four of these cases resolved.[58] One patient had a vascular complication resulting in a below-knee amputation.
- Single-fraction 10-Gy pelvic radiation therapy for palliation has demonstrated 22% complete tumor response. This treatment was associated with a 33% rate of minor gastrointestinal problems and 6% rate of serious late bowel complications.[59]
- Neutron therapy for cervical cancer is associated with a 19% rate of severe complications.[60] Patients treated with mixed neutron and photons experienced an 11% rate of severe complications.

Future Research

Prospectively, there are treatment strategies that may increase late radiation toxicities. Based on the publication of several landmark randomized clinical trials, there has been widespread acceptance of the concept that, in most cases, when radiotherapy is administered for cervical cancer, it should be given with concurrent platinum-based chemotherapy.[1,2] There has been an increase in use of HDR brachytherapy alone and in combination with external beam radiation therapy.[61] The use of concurrent chemotherapy with radiation, as well as the use of HDR brachytherapy, may result in a different toxicity profile and incidence from that reported in the literature. Chemotherapy should not be administered concomitantly with brachytherapy, unless it is in the context of a controlled clinical trial, because increased rates of complications have been reported.[62]

Newer techniques being employed may decrease the rate of late complications from irradiation. They include patient positioning, better tumor delineation with imaging, and better dose localization. IMRT is a technique that combines high-resolution imaging, advances in computer treatment software and linear accelerator capabilities, inverse planning, and radiation beam flux modulation to produce a highly conformed dose distribution unachievable using conventional approaches. Dosimetric evaluation of its use in gynecologic cancers has demonstrated significantly reduced unwanted radiation exposure to adjacent bowel and bladder while preserving tumor coverage.[63] Early clinical experience has demonstrated a significant reduction in acute gastrointestinal toxicity.[64] In vivo assays are being investigated to determine radiation sensitivity.

Amifostine is being developed as a chemical radioprotector. Limited clinical experience had shown that systemic administration of amifostine, when used in conjunction with pelvic irradiation, reduced gastrointestinal, genitourinary, and perineal toxic effects.[65,66] Amifostine provides cytoprotection against the hematologic, renal, and neurologic effects of cisplatin.[67] In all reported experiences, no sparing of tumor response was observed.

Summary

Radiation complications have proved to be a complex issue. This chapter has provided a broad overview of treatment variables and the principles for managing complications. Many of the severe complications are uncommon and require individualized management.

References

1. Thomas GM: Improved treatment for cervical cancer: Concurrent chemotherapy and radiotherapy. N Engl J Med 1999;340:1198-1200.
2. National Cancer Institute: Concurrent chemoradiation for cervical cancer (clinical announcement). Bethesda, MD, National Institutes of Health, February 1999.
3. Koh W, Wallace H J, Greer B, et al: Combined radiotherapy and chemotherapy in the management of local-regionally advanced vulvar cancer. Int J Radiat Oncol Biol Phys 1993;26:809.
4. Teng N, Greer B, Kapp D, et al: NCCN practice guidelines for endometrial carcinoma. Oncology 1999;13:45.
5. Sedlis A, Bundy B, Rotman M, et al: A randomized trial of pelvic radiation therapy versus no further therapy in selected patients with stage IB carcinoma of the cervix after radical hysterectomy and pelvic lymphadenectomy: A Gynecologic Oncology Group study. Gynecol Oncol 1999;73:177-183.
6. Montz FJ, Holschneider CH, Solh S, et al: Small bowel obstruction following radical hysterectomy: Risk factors incidence and operative findings. Gynecol Oncol 1994;53:114-120.
7. Weiser E, Bundy B, Hoskins W, et al: Extraperitoneal versus transperitoneal selective paraaortic lymphadenectomy in the pretreatment surgical staging of advanced cervical carcinoma (a Gynecologic Oncology Group study). Gynecol Oncol 1989;33:283-289.
8. Landoni F, Maneo A, Colombo A, et al: Randomised study of radical surgery versus radiotherapy for stage Ib-IIa cervical cancer. Lancet 1997;350:535-540.
9. Herold D, Hanlon A, Hanks G: Diabetes mellitus: A predictor for late radiation morbidity. Int J Radiat Oncol Biol Phys 1999;43:475-479.
10. De Naeyer B, De Meerleer G, Braems S, et al: Collagen vascular diseases and radiation therapy: A critical review. Int J Radiat Oncol Biol Phys 1999;44:975-980.
11. Eifel PJ, Jhingran A, Bodurka DC, et al: Correlation of smoking history and other patient characteristics with major complications of pelvic radiation therapy for cervical cancer. J Clin Oncol 2002;20:3651-3657.
12. Potish RA: Prediction of radiation-related small-bowel damage. Radiology 1980;135:219-221.
13. Burman C, Kutcher GJ, Emami B, et al: Fitting of normal tissue tolerance data to an analytic function. Int J Radiat Oncol Biol Phys 1991;21:123-135.
14. Winchester DP, Cox JD: Standards for breast-conservation treatment. CA Cancer J Clin 1992;42:134-162.
15. US Preventive Services Task Force: Guide to Clinical Preventive Services, 2nd ed. Baltimore, Williams & Wilkins, 1995.
16. Komaki R, Brickner TJ, Hanlon AL, et al: Long-term results of treatment of cervical carcinoma in the United States in 1973, 1978, and 1983: Patterns of care study (PCS). Int J Radiat Oncol Biol Phys 1995;31:973-982.
17. Eifel PJ, Levenback C, Wharton JT, et al: Time course and incidence of late complications in patients treated for FIGO stage IB carcinoma of the uterine cervix. Int J Radiat Oncol Biol Phys 1995;32:1289-1300.
18. Perez CA, Grigsby PW, Lockett MA, et al: Radiation therapy morbidity in carcinoma of the uterine cervix: Dosimetric and clinical correlation. Int J Radiat Oncol Biol Phys 1999;44:855-866.
19. Montana GS, Fowler WC: Carcinoma of the cervix: Analysis of bladder and rectal radiation dose and complications. Int J Radiat Oncol Biol Phys 1989;16:95-100.
20. Lanciano RM, Martz K, Montana GS, et al: Influence of age, prior abdominal surgery, fraction size, and dose on complications after radiation therapy for squamous call cancer of the uterine cervix. Cancer 1992;69:2124-2130.
21. Thomas G, Dembo A, Fyles A, et al: Concurrent chemoradiation in advanced cervical cancer. Gynecol Oncol 1990;38:446-451.
22. Greer BE, Koh WJ, Stelzer KJ, et al: Expanded pelvic radiotherapy fields for treatment of local-regionally advanced carcinoma of the cervix: Outcome and complications. Am J Obstet Gynecol 1996;174:1141-1149.
23. Fyles AW, Dembo AJ, Bush RS et al: Analysis of complications in patients treated with abdomino-pelvic radiation therapy for ovarian carcinoma. Int J Radiat Oncol Biol Phys 1992;22:847-851.
24. Firat S, Murry K, Erickson B: High-dose whole abdominal and pelvic irradiation for treatment of ovarian carcinoma: Long-term toxicity and outcomes. Int J Radiat Oncol Biol Phys 2003;57:201-207.
25. Small W, Mahadevan A, Roland P, et al: Whole-abdominal radiation in endometrial carcinoma: An analysis of toxicity, patterns of recurrence, and survival. Cancer J 2000;6:394-400.
26. Lee SW, Russell AH, Kinney WK: Whole abdomen radiotherapy for patients with peritoneal dissemination of endometrial adenocarcinoma. Int J Radiat Oncol Biol Phys 2003;56:788-792.
27. Smith J, Golden P, Rutledge F: The surgical management of intestinal injuries following irradiation for carcinoma of the cervix. Presented at the Eleventh Annual Clinical Conference on Cancer; 1966; Houston, Texas.
28. Hoskins WJ, Burke TW, Weiser EB, et al: Right hemicolectomy and ileal resection with primary reanastomosis for irradiation injury of the terminal ileum. Gynecol Oncol 1987;26:215-224.
29. Smith ST, Seski JC, Copeland LJ, et al: Surgical management of irradiation-induced small bowel damage. Obstet Gynecol 1985;65:563-567.
30. Levenback C, Lucas K, Morris M, et al: Management of small bowel perforation and necrosis following radiotherapy for gynecologic cancer. Gynecol Oncol 1997;64:162.
31. Dudrick SJ, Latifi R, Fosnocht DE: Management of the short-bowel syndrome. Surg Clin North Am 1991;71:625-643.
32. Kochhar R, Sriram PVJ, Sharma SC, et al: Natural history of late radiation proctosigmoiditis treated with topical sucralfate suspension. Dig Dis Sci 1999;44:973-978.
33. Pinto A, Fidalgo P, Cravo M, et al: Short chain fatty acids are effective in short-term treatment of chornic radiation proctitis. Dis Colon Rectum 1999;42:788-796.
34. Segreti EM, Levenback C, Morris M, et al: A comparison of end and loop colostomy for fecal diversion in gynecologic patients with colonic fistulas. Gynecol Oncol 1996;60:49-53.
35. Steichen FM, Barber HKR, Loubeau JM, et al: Bricker-Johnston sigmoid colon graft for repair of postradiation rectovaginal fistula and stricture performed with mechanical sutures. Dis Colon Rectum 1992;35:599-603.
36. Levenback C, Eifel PJ, Burke TW, et al: Hemorrhagic cystitis following radiotherapy for stage IB cancer of the cervix. Gynecol Oncol 1994;55:206-210.
37. DeVries CR, Freiha FS: Hemorrhagic cystitis: A review. J Urol 1990;143:1-9.
38. Fair WR: Formalin in the treatment of massive bladder hemorrhage. Urology 1974;3:573-576.
39. Vicente J, Rios G, Caffaratti J: Intravesical formalin for the treatment of massive hemorrhagic cystitis: Retrospective review of 25 cases. Eur Urol 1990;18:204-206.
40. Cheng C: Management of severe chronic radiation cystitis. Ann Acad Med Singapore 1992;21:368-371.
41. Fujikawa K, Miyamoto T, Ihara Y, et al: High incidence of severe urologic complications following radiotherapy for cervical cancer in Japanese women. Gynecol Oncol 2001;80:21-23.
42. Levenback C, Gershenson DM, McGehee R, et al: Enterovesical fistula following radiotherapy for gynecologic cancer. Gynecol Oncol 1994;52:296-300.

43. Bruner DW, Lanciano R, Keegan M, et al: Vaginal stenosis and sexual function following intracavitary radiation for the treatment of cervical and endometrial carcinoma. Int J Radiat Oncol Biol Phys 1993;27:825-830.

44. Ganz PA, Rowland JH, Desmond K, et al: Life after breast cancer: Understanding women's health-related quality of life and sexual functioning. J Clin Oncol 1998;16:501-514.

45. Bergmark K, Avall-Lundqvist E, Dickman P, et al: Vaginal changes and sexuality in women with a history of cervical cancer. N Engl Med 1999;340:1383-1389.

46. Hartman P, Diddle A: Vaginal stenosis following irradiation therapy for carcinoma of the cervix uteri. Cancer 1972;30:426-429.

47. Seibel MM, Graves WL, Freeman MG: Carcinoma of the cervix and sexual function. Obstet Gynecol 1980;55:484-487.

48. Rand RP, Greer BE, Tamimi HT, et al: Surgical treatment of chronic irradiated pelvic and perineal wounds. Gynecol Oncol 1994;54:111.

49. Feldmeier JJ, Matos LA: Delayed radiation injuries (soft tissue and bony necrosis). The Hyperbaric Oxygen Therapy Committee report. Hyperbaric Oxygen 2003:87-100.

50. Delanian S, Balla-Mekias S, Lefaix JL: Striking regression of chronic radiotherapy damage in a clinical trial of combined pentoxifylline and tocopherol. J Clin Oncol 1999;17:3283-3290.

51. Huh SJ, Kim BK, Kang MK, et al: Pelvic insufficiency fracture after pelvic irradiation in uterine cervix cancer. Gynecol Oncol 2002;86:264-268.

52. Moreno A, Clemente J, Crespo C, et al: Pelvic insufficiency fractures in patients with pelvic irradiation. Int J Radiat Oncol Biol Phys 1999;44:61-66.

53. Gradishar WJ, Schilsky RL: Ovarian function following radiation and chemotherapy for cancer. Semin Oncol 1989;16:425-436.

54. Georgiou A, Grigsby PW, Perez CA: Radiation induced lumbosacral plexopathy in gynecologic tumors: Clinical findings and dosimetric analysis. Int J Radiat Oncol Biol Phys 1993;26:479-482.

55. Martinez A, Edmundson GK, Cox RS, et al: Combination of external beam irradiation and multiple-site perineal applicator (MUPIT) for treatment of locally advanced or recurrent prostatic, anorectal, and gynecologic malignancies. Int J Radiat Oncol Biol Phys 1984;11:391-398.

56. Gaddis O, Morrow CP, Klement V, et al: Treatment of cervical carcinoma employing a template for transperineal interstitial ^{192}Ir brachytherapy. Int J Radiat Oncol Biol Phys 1983;9:819-827.

57. Aristizabal SA, Surwit EA, Hevezi JM, et al: Treatment of advanced cancer of the cervix with transperineal interstitial irradiation. Int J Radiat Oncol Biol Phys 1983;9:1013-1017.

58. Stelzer KJ, Koh WJ, Greer BE, et al: The use of intraoperative radiation therapy in radical salvage for recurrent cervical cancer: Outcome and toxicity. Am J Obstet Gynecol 1995;172:1881-1888.

59. Onsrud M, Hagenn B, Strickert T: 10-Gy single-fraction pelvic irradiation for palliation and life prolongation in patients with cancer of the cervix and corpus uteri. Gynecol Oncol 2001;82:167-171.

60. Maor MH, Gillespie BW, Peters LJ, et al: Neutron therapy in cervical cancer: Results of a phase III RTOG study. Int J Radiat Oncol Biol Phys 1988;14:885-891.

61. Eifel PJ, Moughan J, Owen J, et al: Patterns of radiotherapy practice for patients with squamous call carcinoma of the uterine cervix: Patterns of care study. Int J Radiat Oncol Biol Phys 1999;43:351-358.

62. Nag S, Erickson B, Thomadsen B, et al: The American Brachytherapy Society recommendations for high-dose-rate brachytherapy for carcinoma of the cervix. Int J Radiat Oncol Biol Phys 2000;48:201-211.

63. Portelance L, Chao KSC, Grigsby PW, et al: Intensity-modulated radiation therapy (IMRT) reduces small bowel, rectum, and bladder doses in patients with cervical cancer receiving pelvic and para-aortic irradiation. Int J Radiat Oncol Biol Phys 2001;51:261-266.

64. Mundt AJ, Lujan AE, Rotmensch J, et al: Intensity-modulated whole pelvic radiotherapy in women with gynecologic malignancies. Int J Radiat Oncol Biol Phys 2002;52:1330-1337.

65. Koukourakis MI, Kyrias G, Kakolyris S, et al: Subcutaneous administration of amifostine during fractionated radiotherapy: A randomized phase II study. J Clin Oncol 2000;18:2226-2233.

66. Kemp G, Rose P, Lurain J, et al: Amifostine pretreatment for protection against cyclophosphamide-induced and cisplatin-induced toxicities: Results of a randomized controlled trial in patients with advanced ovarian cancer. J Clin Oncol 1996;14:2101-2112.

67. Pearcey R, Brundage M, Drouin P, et al: Phase III trial comparing radical radiotherapy with and without cisplatin chemotherapy in patients with advanced squamous cell cancer of the cervix. J Clin Oncol 2002;20:966-972.

CHAPTER

MANAGEMENT OF COMPLICATIONS OF CHEMOTHERAPY

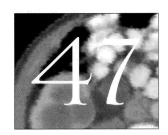

Linda Mileshkin,   Yoland Antill,   and   Danny Rischin

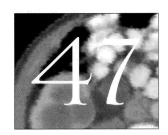 MAJOR CONTROVERSIES

- How should patients with anemia be managed?
- Do the benefits of erythropoietin outweigh the costs and potential side effects?
- How should patients with chemotherapy-induced thrombocytopenia be managed?
- Are alternative approaches to allogeneic platelet transfusions available?
- Should patients with gynecologic malignancies receiving chemotherapy be given prophylactic anticoagulants?
- How should patients with thrombosis occurring during chemotherapy be managed?
- Should vancomycin be used in the initial empirical regimen for treatment of febrile neutropenia?
- Should hematopoietic growth factors be used in the treatment or prevention of febrile neutropenia in patients with gynecologic malignancies?
- Can some patients be safely managed as outpatients with oral antibiotics?
- How should we manage patients developing neuropathy on carboplatin and paclitaxel?
- What supportive care is appropriate for patients with established neuropathy?
- What are the roles of neuroprotectants?
- How should ifosfamide-related neurotoxicity be managed?
- Should patients receiving chemotherapy be warned about possible cognitive effects of treatment?
- Are techniques available to reduce the risk of alopecia?
- Are there useful antidotes that should be delivered if an extravasation occurs?
- What is the appropriate management for a patient who develops a severe hypersensitivity reaction to carboplatin?
- Does monitoring respiratory function help to predict the development of bleomycin-related lung toxicity?
- What is the prognosis for patients with anthracycline-related cardiomyopathy?

The potential toxicities of chemotherapy are many and varied. In this chapter, we focus on the toxic effects that are most relevant to the spectrum of chemotherapeutic agents used to treat gynecologic malignancies, particularly those that are current areas of active controversy and research. We have tried to base any recommendations given on well-conducted clinical trials. In some areas, however, the paucity of data makes this difficult, and our discussion then is based on accepted clinical practice.

Hematologic Complications

Anemia. Anemia is recognized as a complication of cancer and of treatment with chemotherapy that causes considerable morbidity. Anemia is a common problem in patients with gynecologic malignancies receiving chemotherapy. Overall rates of anemia of 67% to 81% have been reported for patients receiving platinum-based chemotherapy, and rates of 47% to 89% have been described for patients receiving non–platinum-based chemotherapy.[1] However, the ways in which rates of anemia were previously reported varies across the literature. Various toxicity grading systems have been used. Some studies have not specified the grade of anemia seen, and others have reported anemia in terms of levels of decrease in hemoglobin seen rather than by the grade.[2] Nevertheless, high rates of anemia are still being reported in trials with more uniform reporting.

In previously untreated patients with ovarian cancer, single-agent carboplatin or cisplatin causes a fairly low incidence of anemia, with grade 3 or 4 anemia occurring in 0% to 7% of patients. However, combination platinum-containing regimens cause higher rates. Phase III trials report rates of grade 3 or 4 anemia of 2% to 42% for platinum/cyclophosphamide and 2% to 8% for platinum/paclitaxel regimens.[2] Hensley and colleagues[3] reported results from a retrospective cohort study of 175 consecutive patients receiving first-line chemotherapy treatment after debulking surgery for epithelial ovarian cancer with carboplatin/paclitaxel or cisplatin/paclitaxel regimens at Memorial Sloan-Kettering Cancer Center. The median nadir hemoglobin level was 9.3 g/dL (range, 6.6 to 11.1 g/dL), with 18% of patients requiring a red blood cell transfusion. Independent risk factors for receipt of transfusion included a hemoglobin level less than 10 g/dL before chemotherapy and the type of chemotherapy received. Among patients with a hemoglobin level of less than 10 g/dL before chemotherapy, 50% of those who received carboplatin plus paclitaxel required a transfusion, compared with 7.7% who received cisplatin plus paclitaxel.

Trials of patients treated with second-line chemotherapy also report significant rates of anemia. For example, in a trial reported by Eisenhauer and coworkers[4] that evaluated patients treated with paclitaxel at doses between 135 and 175 mg/m^2 after failing a first-line platinum-based regimen, grade 1 or 2 anemia was seen in 62% to 73% and grade 3 or 4 anemia in 6% to 12% of patients. Topotecan causes more anemia than paclitaxel when given as second-line treatment. In a phase III trial comparing paclitaxel at a dose of 175 mg/m^2 given over 3 hours with topotecan at a dose of 1.5 mg/m^2 for patients with recurrent, advanced ovarian cancer, 40% of patients developed grade 3 or 4 anemia with topotecan, compared with 6% of those receiving paclitaxel.[5] Similarly, docetaxel used as a single agent to treat patients with relapsed disease after a platinum-containing regimen has been reported to cause grade 1 or 2 anemia in 58% to 60% of patients.[6,7]

Anemia may cause a multitude of symptoms that impair a patient's quality of life. In particular, it may cause fatigue, somnolence, dyspnea, palpitations, and impaired cognitive function.[1] In severe cases or in those with a preexisting cardiac condition, it may cause angina or cardiovascular compromise. Awareness of the potential for transmission of infection through blood transfusion, as well as the shortage of this resource, has led to a common practice of not transfusing patients until significant anemia has developed. As a result, the contribution of anemia to causing fatigue has become increasingly relevant to patients with cancer. In a survey reported by Curt,[8] 76% of 379 patients ranked fatigue as their most significant symptom while receiving chemotherapy. Other factors such as sleep disorders and psychological distress may contribute to fatigue, but anemia may be a major contributor to this problem. There is some evidence that fatigue is a symptom infrequently discussed or addressed by treating clinicians, and it may contribute to some patients withdrawing from potentially curative chemotherapy.[9,10]

The development of anemia during anticancer therapy may compromise the effectiveness of treatment. There is strong retrospective evidence that the development of anemia during radiotherapy treatment for malignancies, including cervical and head and neck tumors, is associated with inferior response rates and overall survival.[11-13] Anemia probably is an indicator of a more aggressive tumor and contributes to resistance to radiotherapy because of an increased hypoxic cell fraction. There has been one published report of similar inferior outcomes for 57 patients receiving chemoradiotherapy treatment for cervical carcinoma.[14] In this study, the nadir hemoglobin level was the most prognostically relevant factor for predicting the response to chemoradiotherapy. Only patients with nadir hemoglobin levels of more than 11 g/dL throughout chemoradiotherapy had a more than 90% chance of achieving a complete clinical response. In this study, similar to those studying radiotherapy alone, the hemoglobin level was not prognostically significant for patients with cervical cancer.

How should patients with anemia be managed?
Given the impact of anemia on patients receiving chemotherapy, it is important that the condition be properly assessed and treated. The clinician should first look for potential contributors to the anemia. Further history regarding known blood loss and concurrent medications should be sought. It is appropriate to

assess the blood film, although blood film changes may sometimes be difficult to interpret for patients receiving chemotherapy. The physician should specifically measure levels of red cell folate, vitamin B_{12}, and iron stores. For example, patients who had chronically increased vaginal blood loss before diagnosis may have become significantly iron deficient. Other factors contributing to anemia that should be considered include ongoing blood loss, hemolysis, bone marrow infiltration, and renal impairment due to prior platinum chemotherapy. Persistent cancer may contribute to anemia of chronic disease with endogenous erythropoietin (EPO) deficiency, impaired iron use, and shortened red blood cell survival.[15] Measurement of serum EPO levels does not seem to be helpful in patients with cancer-related anemia due to solid tumors, because pretreatment levels do not predict response to treatment of anemia.

Until the past decade, blood transfusions had been the only available therapy for treatment of symptomatic anemia. However, there are several potential pitfalls to the use of transfusion, which include the risks of acute reactions, transmission of blood-borne infectious agents, and the limited availability of blood. Moreover, the rise in hemoglobin after transfusion may be only short-lived and will not prevent a subsequent recurrence of anemia that may lead to fatigue or decreased efficacy of chemoradiotherapy.

Recombinant human EPO has been useful treatment for patients with solid tumors who are receiving chemotherapy. Several pivotal randomized, placebo-controlled studies have demonstrated that EPO can increase hemoglobin levels and reduce transfusion requirements in patients receiving platinum-based and non–platinum-based chemotherapy.[16-22] EPO use improved quality of life in two large, community-based, open-label studies of approximately 4700 patients.[23,24] The largest incremental improvement in quality of life was seen in patients whose hemoglobin levels rose from 11 to 12 g/L.[25] Demetri and coworkers[23] reported a retrospective subset analysis of 297 patients with gynecologic malignancies that formed part of one of the open-label studies. In concordance with the results for the total trial group, EPO at a dose of 10,000 IU given subcutaneously three times per week produced a significant, sustained increase in hemoglobin levels.[1] The mean hemoglobin concentration increased by more than 2.0 g/L over the 4-month study period, and overall transfusions were reduced from 36% at baseline to 6% at study completion.

Some concerns have been expressed about the quality of the various trials that have investigated the effectiveness of EPO. For example, some of the trials have been criticized because of a failure to use intent-to-treat analysis. In 2002, the American Society of Clinical Oncology and the American Society of Hematology released evidence-based clinical practice guidelines for the use of EPO in patients with cancer after review of the available literature by an expert panel.[26] Table 47-1 outlines the recommendations given that are relevant to patients with gynecologic malignancies receiving chemotherapy.

Table 47–1. Clinical Practice Guidelines for the Use of Erythropoietin in Patients with Cancer

1. The use of erythropoietin (EPO) is recommended as a treatment option for patients with chemotherapy-associated anemia and a hemoglobin concentration that has declined to a level of ≤ 10 g/dL. Red blood cell transfusion is also an option, depending on the severity of anemia or clinical circumstances

2. For patients with declining hemoglobin levels but less severe anemia (i.e., with a hemoglobin concentration < 12 g/dL but that has never fallen below 10 g/dL), the decision about whether to use EPO immediately or to wait until hemoglobin levels fall closer to 10 g/dL should be determined by clinical circumstances.

3. The recommendations are based on evidence from trials in which EPO was administered subcutaneously thrice weekly. The recommended starting dose is 150 U/kg thrice weekly for a minimum of 4 weeks, with consideration given for dose escalation to 300 U/kg thrice weekly for an additional 4 to 8 weeks in those who do not respond to the initial dose. Although supported by less strong evidence, an alternative weekly dosing regimen (40,000 U/wk), based on common clinical practice, can be considered. Dose escalation of weekly regimens should be under similar circumstances to thrice-weekly regimens.

4. Continued EPO treatment beyond 6 to 8 weeks in the absence of response (e.g., < 1-2 g/dL rise in hemoglobin), assuming appropriate dose increase has been attempted in nonresponders, does not appear to be beneficial. Patients who do not respond should be investigated for underlying tumor progression or iron deficiency. As with other failed therapeutic trials, consideration should be given to discontinuing the medication.

5. Hemoglobin levels can be raised to or near a concentration of 12 g/dL, at which time the dosage of EPO should be titrated to maintain that level or restarted when the levels fall to near 10 g/dL. There is insufficient evidence to support the "normalization" of hemoglobin levels to more than 12 g/dL.

6. Baseline and periodic monitoring of iron, total iron-binding capacity, transferrin saturation, or ferritin levels and instituting iron repletion when indicated may be valuable in limiting the need for EPO, maximizing symptomatic improvement for patients, and determining the reason for failure to respond adequately to EPO. There is inadequate evidence to specify the optimal timing, periodicity, or testing regimen for such monitoring.

Adapted from Rizzo JD, Lichtin AE, Woolf SH, et al: Use of epoetin in patients with cancer: Evidence-based clinical practice guidelines of the American Society of Clinical Oncology and the American Society of Hematology. J Clin Oncol 2002;20:4083-4107.

Folate supplementation is generally recommended for patients receiving EPO during chemotherapy. It is also recognized that inadequate iron stores may impair the response to EPO. Iron use is impaired in patients with cancer-related anemia. Patients with serum ferritin levels less than 40 µg/L or with transferrin saturation levels less than 15% should probably receive concurrent oral iron supplementation.[27,28]

Recommendations about the use of EPO in treating chemotherapy-induced anemia are based on the best available evidence, which includes seven trials (five of which were placebo controlled) that enrolled adult patients with baseline hemoglobin levels of 10 g/dL. In these trials, the difference in the percentage of patients who responded favorably to EPO compared with controls ranged from 28% to 80%, with an absolute difference in the change of mean hemoglobin level between 1.6 and 3.1 g/dL. The difference in the percentage of patients requiring any transfusions between the EPO and control arms in the various trials ranged from 9% to 45% in favor of EPO; this difference was statistically significant in four of the seven trials. Meta-analysis suggested that the use of EPO decreased the relative odds of receiving a blood transfusion by an average of 62%. Further analysis suggested that the number of patients needed to treat to benefit one patient was 4.4 (95% CI: 3.6-6.1). One trial also suggested a survival advantage for patients treated with EPO, but the study was not adequately powered to test this hypothesis.[22]

The guidelines highlight the fact that the evidence for the ability of EPO to improve quality of life is less sound. Most of the data comes from large, phase IV, community-based, single-arm, cohort studies, in which EPO treatment was associated with statistically significant increases in quality of life scores using a variety of measurement instruments. However, many of the trials have large amounts of missing data (10% to 40%), and some have used quality of life instruments for which minimum clinically meaningful differences have not yet been defined. Seven randomized studies (some were not blinded) have made comparisons of quality of life measures before and after treatment with EPO or control. Although the evidence base for an effect on quality of life by EPO has significant limitations, the general thrust of the literature suggests an improvement.

Do the benefits of erythropoietin outweigh the costs and potential side effects?

Although EPO is commonly prescribed to patients in the United States receiving chemotherapy for gynecologic malignancies, the cost of the drug prevents its use in many other areas of the world, with regulatory authorities not accepting the cost-benefit ratio of providing access to the drug. Few data are available about the cost-effectiveness of using the drug in this setting. One study has attempted to examine this issue in 12 consecutive patients receiving chemoradiotherapy with concurrent weekly cisplatin for cervical cancer. The investigators compared the costs of using red blood cell transfusion or EPO to treat anemia in patients with a hemoglobin concentration of less than 10 g/dL. Among the 12 patients, 10 required transfusion of at least 1 unit of red blood cells before or during treatment (average of 3.1 units per patient). Transfusion was most commonly given after the fifth week of treatment. The cost of transfusion was calculated as the cost of the blood itself, laboratory fees, and the expected cost of transfusion-related viral illness (i.e., risk multiplied by cost). The cost of EPO use was calculated as the cost of the drug itself and the cost of supplemental transfusions when the hemoglobin concentration was not maintained. The costs associated with acute reactions to blood transfusion were not included, nor were the costs of person-hours of nursing labor associated with transfusion or EPO injection. The total of the projected average transfusion-related costs was U.S. $990, compared with the total projected EPO-related costs of $3869, suggesting that transfusions were an appealingly less expensive

option. An 80% reduction in the direct cost of EPO would have rendered EPO less costly than transfusions.[29] However, this was a very small study, and more data are required in this area to reach any definitive conclusions.

There have been several reports of patients developing red cell aplasia after treatment with EPO for anemia related to chronic renal failure.[30-32] Development of anti-EPO antibodies has been documented in these patients and is presumed to be the cause of the aplasia. Recovery has been variable, with some patients remaining transfusion dependent for a prolonged time (up to 2 years follow-up) after cessation of EPO, although titers of anti-EPO antibodies have declined. The incidence of this complication is probably extremely low and has not yet been reported in cancer patients treated with EPO. Generally, EPO is very well tolerated, with rarely occurring adverse effects, including hypertension, headache, seizures, and thrombotic events. However, the risk of potentially irreversible complications may deter some patients and clinicians from using EPO during treatment of potentially curable malignancies, such as limited duration chemoradiotherapy for cervical cancer. This risk needs to be balanced against the potential for transfusion-related blood-borne infections, which may also be a long-term complication. The estimated risk of contracting human immunodeficiency virus (HIV) from a single unit of blood transfused is 1 case per 450,000 to 660,000. Risk of contracting hepatitis B from a single unit of blood transfused is estimated to be 1 case per 31,000, and the risk of hepatitis C is 1 case per 28,000.[33,34] Patients also incur the risks of compromised treatment effectiveness if anemia is not treated.

Thrombocytopenia. Thrombocytopenia is a possible complication of chemotherapy for solid tumors. However, major bleeding resulting from this condition is much less of a problem than occurs during treatment of acute leukemia. A retrospective review examined the results for 609 patients with solid tumors or lymphomas who underwent 1262 cycles of chemotherapy that were complicated by chemotherapy-induced thrombocytopenia (platelet count < 50,000/µL). Bleeding occurred during 9% of cycles and caused delays in further chemotherapy in 6% of cycles.[35] Major hemorrhage occurred in 3% of cycles, and there were four hemorrhagic deaths. Several predictors of bleeding were identified, including a baseline platelet count of less than 75,000/µL, a prior bleeding episode, bone marrow metastases, poor performance status, and receipt of carboplatin, cisplatin, carmustine, or lomustine. Major hemorrhage was more common during cycles complicated by febrile neutropenia. The risk of bleeding also increased with the depth of thrombocytopenia; it was more common during cycles in which the platelet count fell below 10,000/µL (7% versus 21%, $P < .0001$).

Twenty-three percent of patients were found to have an inadequate platelet increment after receipt of random-donor platelets, including the four patients with hemorrhagic deaths. Nineteen percent of cycles during which there was a poor response to platelet transfusion ended in the death of the patient, compared with only 3% of cycles in which patients responded to platelet transfusions. Increased costs were associated with patients who had poor responses to platelet transfusions, including increased platelet use and increased hospitalization days.

How should patients with chemotherapy-induced thrombocytopenia be managed? On the basis of studies of patients with leukemia, it is recommended that prophylactic platelet transfusions should be given to asymptomatic patients if the platelet count drops below 10,000/μL, to minimize the risk of major bleeding complications such as intracerebral hemorrhage.[36,37] Some groups have used lower thresholds in patients with solid tumors (e.g., 5000/μL) and described no major bleeding episodes.[38] The threshold for transfusion is often increased to 20,000/μL for patients who are febrile, and transfusions may also be given at higher levels of platelet count to patients who are bleeding. The platelet count should be monitored daily until recovery above the threshold for prophylactic transfusion. For patients who are bleeding, it is important to order a clotting screen to look for other potential causes of coagulopathy and to ensure that an adequate platelet increment has been attained by repeating the platelet count after the transfusion. For patients refractory to random-donor platelets, HLA-matched or single-donor platelets may rarely be required. Infusions of aminocaproic acid can also been used for thrombocytopenic patients with persistent bleeding.

If prolonged or profound thrombocytopenia develops that is not consistent with the expected depth and duration of platelet nadir for the chemotherapy regimen, it is important to look for other contributory factors. For example, it is important to ensure that serum levels of vitamin B$_{12}$ and folate are adequate. It is also appropriate to recheck that the delivered chemotherapy dose is appropriate for the patient's body surface area or renal function (in the case of carboplatin).

Are alternative approaches to allogeneic platelet transfusions available? There are several potential problems with the use of platelet transfusions for thrombocytopenia. Availability is a significant problem, and donor platelets may be stored for only 5 days before they must be discarded. Platelet use has increased over time with the use of more myelosuppressive chemotherapy regimens and has led to associated increased costs. Platelet transfusions also are associated with a risk of transfusion-associated infections similar to that for blood transfusions. The risk with platelet transfusions may be greater if pooled platelets from multiple donors are transfused. Platelet transfusion may also be associated with acute reactions such as fever and rigors in 5% to 30% of cases.[39] These difficulties have led to several developments aimed at limiting the need for allogeneic platelet transfusions.

Several cytokines have been used to stimulate thrombopoiesis in patients who have received chemotherapy.[40] Recombinant human interleukin-11 (rHuIL-11) is approved by the U.S. Food and Drug Administration (FDA) for treatment of severe chemotherapy-induced thrombocytopenia. rHuIL-11 was shown to cause a modest reduction in the need for platelet transfusion in a randomized study of 93 patients receiving chemotherapy who had previously required platelet transfusion (96% versus 70%, $P <$ .05).[41] However, rHuIL-11 is frequently associated with severe side effects such as fluid retention, fatigue, arthralgias, myalgias, and a low incidence of atrial arrhythmias and syncope. A randomized trial of rHuIL-11 in the setting of autologous bone marrow transplantation did not demonstrate convincing efficacy.[42] However, patients in the control group of this study were less likely to be alloimmunized than those who received the rHuIL-11, which may have been a confounding variable.

Thrombopoietin (TPO) is believed to be the primary endogenous platelet-specific growth factor. Initially, a truncated and pegylated derivative of the molecule was produced in *Escherichia coli* (PEG-rHuMGDF, Amgen Inc., Thousand Oaks, CA). However, this molecule proved to be immunogenic in clinical testing, with a subset of cancer patients and normal platelet-donor volunteers developing neutralizing antibodies that led to withdrawal of the molecule from further clinical development.[43] Another bioengineered TPO molecule, rHuTPO (Genentech, Inc., San Francisco, CA, and Pharmacia Corp., Peapack, NJ), has been developed as a full-length, glycosylated molecule. The efficacy and safety of rHuTPO was tested in a phase I/II trial of 29 patients with gynecologic malignancies who were treated with carboplatin.[44] In this study, the need for platelet transfusions, the mean platelet nadir, and the duration of thrombocytopenia were significantly reduced when rHuTPO was given after a second cycle of chemotherapy. The molecule appears to be well tolerated, and neutralizing antibodies have not been detected. Further studies using rHuTPO are in progress.

A different approach has been to collect and store autologous platelets from patients before receipt of chemotherapy. Platelet cryopreservation after apheresis has been found to be safe and feasible, but there are some technical difficulties, including the loss of platelet numbers and function during processing and reactions to the cryoprotectant, which commonly contains dimethyl sulfoxide (DMSO). One report described 20 patients with gynecologic malignancies who were randomly assigned to receive allogeneic fresh donor platelets or autologous cryopreserved platelets during alternate cycles of carboplatin chemotherapy if the platelet count fell below 15,000/μL.[45] The autologous platelets were collected before chemotherapy after two intravenous doses of rHuTPO and cryopreserved in a solution with a low DMSO concentration (2%). The primary end point assessed was the platelet increment after transfusion. The autologous transfusions were well tolerated, and there were no significant differences in the platelet increment obtained after autologous or allogeneic platelet transfusions. There was a decrease in platelet aggregation seen in laboratory studies of the autologous platelets, but there were no major bleeding episodes seen with a median number of days of platelet counts less than 15,000/μL per cycle of 2 days (range, 0 to 11 days). Further studies examining this approach are in progress.

Thrombosis. Thromboembolism is a common problem for cancer patients, and the use of chemotherapy appears to increase the risk of developing thrombosis. However, patients with gynecologic malignancies may be predisposed to developing thromboembolism for a multitude of reasons. Predisposing factors may include recent pelvic surgery, suboptimal postoperative mobilization, increased age, use of central venous catheters, venous stasis due to compression of venous outflow by tumor, and obesity.

The risk seems to be increased while patients are receiving chemotherapy. Most studies that demonstrate this association have assessed women undergoing chemotherapy for breast cancer.[46] The reported rates of thromboembolism depend on whether thrombosis was identified after a clinical diagnosis or after serial monitoring with various imaging techniques, such as venography or duplex ultrasound. In two studies enrolling a total of 130 women receiving platinum-based chemotherapy for ovarian cancer, the rates of venous thromboembolism were 10.6% and 12%.[47,48] It has been suggested that the risk of thromboembolism during chemotherapy may be further increased by additional risk factors, including gross residual tumor bulk,[48] metastatic disease, postmenopausal status,[49] presence of a central venous catheter, increased body mass index, history of venous thromboembolism, and inherited predisposition to thromboembolism such as factor V Leiden mutations.[46]

Various abnormalities in the coagulation pathway have been identified in patients with cancer and those receiving chemotherapy. Figure 47-1 outlines some of the postulated mechanisms by which chemotherapy may increase the risk of thrombosis. However, no test of blood coagulation has been confirmed to predict which patients will develop venous thromboembolism.

Should patients with gynecologic malignancies receiving chemotherapy be given prophylactic anticoagulants? Most patients are not routinely anticoagulated while on chemotherapy. If additional risk factors as outlined previously are present, anticoagulation may be considered. Despite the fact that patients receiving chemotherapy are known to be at increased risk for venous thromboembolism, there is little information about whether prophylactic anticoagulation is helpful. One trial studied 311 women receiving chemotherapy for metastatic breast cancer, who were randomized to receive placebo or warfarin (1 mg daily) for the duration of chemotherapy treatment, aiming to maintain an International Normalized Ratio (INR) of 1.3 to 1.9. The number of thromboembolic events in the warfarin group was one, compared with seven in the placebo group, giving a statistically significant risk reduction of 85% (P = .031).[50]

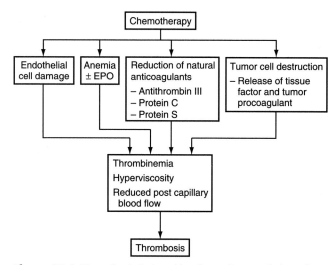

Figure 47-1. Thrombosis induced by chemotherapy. (Adapted from von Tempelhoff GF, Heilmann L: Antithrombotic therapy in gynecologic surgery and gynecologic oncology. Hematol Oncol Clin North Am 2000;14:1151-1169, ix.)

For patients with central venous lines, there is some evidence that anticoagulation may reduce the risk of line-associated thrombosis. Occlusive thrombi associated with central venous lines may lead to the development of pulmonary embolism. Several trials have shown reduced risk of line-associated thrombosis with the use of low-dose warfarin (1 mg daily).[51,52] However, there have also been some trials using low-dose warfarin prophylaxis that showed no protection against the development of line-associated thrombosis.[53] Another trial suggested that low-molecular-weight heparin could reduce the risk of catheter-associated thrombosis compared with placebo.[54] The study was terminated early, when 62% of the placebo group (8 of 13 patients) had developed thrombosis compared with 6% (1 of 16 patients) of those treated with 2500 U per day of dalteparin.[54] Warfarin and low-molecular-weight heparin have not been directly compared to determine the optimal prophylaxis.

How should patients with thrombosis occurring during chemotherapy be managed? The initial treatment of a patient with thrombosis follows the same lines as for patients without cancer. Subcutaneous low-molecular-weight heparin or unfractionated intravenous heparin is initially administered for 5 to 7 days. Options for ongoing anticoagulation for patients with an established thrombosis while receiving chemotherapy include oral anticoagulation with warfarin or subcutaneous low-molecular-weight heparin. There is no definitive evidence available regarding the length of anticoagulation required. However, it is common practice to continue anticoagulation for 3 to 6 months, depending on the severity of the thrombosis. Anticoagulation may be discontinued after chemotherapy has been completed, provided that no active cancer remains.

The use of warfarin in patients receiving chemotherapy may be problematic for several reasons, including variations in diet or gastrointestinal absorption, low platelet nadir counts, and impaired hepatic function.[55] INR levels may also be difficult to stabilize in patients receiving some chemotherapy agents such as capecitabine. Several retrospective studies have suggested a higher risk of bleeding complications on warfarin in cancer patients compared with those without cancer.[56-59] In contrast, two prospective cohort studies suggest that the bleeding risks are comparable.[60,61] However, because of these potential problems with the use of warfarin, some clinicians choose to continue anticoagulation with low-molecular-weight heparin during chemotherapy treatment. A randomized study assessed 146 patients with venous thromboembolism and cancer treated with warfarin for 3 months or enoxaparin sodium (1.5 mg/kg daily). The study suggested that the low-molecular-weight heparin was as effective as the warfarin and appeared to be safer. There were 6 deaths from hemorrhage in the warfarin group and none in the enoxaparin group.[62]

Febrile neutropenia. Febrile neutropenia is a potentially life-threatening complication of chemotherapy that needs to be promptly recognized and treated. It is important that patients receiving chemotherapy are educated to make urgent contact if they develop a fever at anytime during a course of chemotherapy. Patients presenting with a fever should be managed initially as if they may have febrile neutropenia until a blood cell count is available.

Febrile neutropenia is a reasonably common occurrence during chemotherapy treatment for gynecologic malignancies, because many of the chemotherapy agents used produce profound, although short-lived, marrow suppression. It more commonly occurs during treatment of relapsed or refractory disease, because patients who have been previously treated with platinum-based chemotherapy or irradiation, or both, are at greater risk for chemotherapy-induced neutropenia. For example, topotecan during phase II and III trials for relapsed or refractory disease produced grade 4 neutropenia (<500/μL) in 81% of patients, with 26% experiencing associated fever or infection, or both.[63] It is commonly accepted that the risk of infection rises dramatically after a patient's neutrophil count falls below 500/μL and is even greater if the count falls below 100/μL.[64]

In most cases, febrile neutropenia is not associated with any microbiologically proven infection. For cases with positive cultures, the spectrum of causative organisms has changed over time. In the 1960s to mid-1980s, aerobic gram-negative bacilli, particularly *Pseudomonas aeruginosa*, were the most common organisms causing infection in the neutropenic patient.[65] However, gram-positive infections have become more common and account for 60% to 70% of bacteremias, particularly in patients with indwelling central venous lines.[66,67] *Staphylococcus aureus* and coagulase-negative staphylococci predominate. Other organisms that have become a more common cause of infection include viridans streptococci, enterococci, and rarer gram-negative organisms such as *Stenotrophomonas maltophilia*

and *Legionella* species.[68] For patients undergoing chemotherapy for gynecologic malignancies, who are less likely than those receiving treatment for other tumor types to have central venous lines, sustain severe mucositis, or be given prophylactic oral antibiotics, gram-positive infections may be less common.

Various antibiotic regimens may be used in the initial treatment of febrile neutropenia. Appropriate combinations include an antipseudomonal penicillin or cephalosporin combined with an aminoglycoside or ciprofloxacin. Monotherapy with ceftazidime, cefepime, or imipenem may also be safely used, with therapy changed as required by results of any positive cultures.[69-71] Patients with central venous access devices should be carefully assessed for the possibility of a line-associated infection, which may require removal of the venous access device. It is also important that the regimen chosen is appropriate for the local environment in terms of any known local patterns of infection or antibiotic resistance.

Should vancomycin be used in the initial empirical regimen for treatment of febrile neutropenia? Given the increasing frequency of gram-positive infections, some clinicians include vancomycin as part of an initial treatment regimen. Some studies have suggested that initial use of vancomycin is associated with fewer breakthrough bacteremias and local infections due to *S. aureus*.[72] However, later studies have suggested that initial vancomycin can be safely withheld and commenced only in the event of identification of a β-lactamase–resistant, gram-positive infection, without increasing the morbidity or mortality.[72,73] The advantages of this approach include lower expense, decreased risk of nephrotoxicity, and minimizing the potential for development of vancomycin-resistant organisms.

One review[68] suggests that routine initial use of vancomycin is not recommended except in the following instances:

1. Line sepsis is strongly suspected (e.g., a patient shows evidence of infection at the exit site or catheter tunnel of a central venous line).
2. The hospital has a high rate of nosocomial infection with methicillin-resistant *S. aureus* (MRSA) or the patient is known to have been previously colonized or infected with MRSA.
3. There are reasons to suspect overwhelming infection with α-hemolytic streptococcal bacteria, which may be associated with a toxic shock–like syndrome.
4. The patient is at risk for endocarditis because of the presence of a prosthetic heart valve.

Should hematopoietic growth factors be used in the treatment or prevention of febrile neutropenia in patients with gynecologic malignancies? Primary prophylactic administration of the hematopoietic growth factors granulocyte colony-stimulating factor (G-CSF) or granulocyte-macrophage colony-stimulating factor (GM-CSF) is not indicated for patients receiving chemotherapy for gynecologic malignancies. Primary prophylactic use of these growth factors has been shown to reduce the risk of febrile neutropenia only if the involved regimens are likely to be associated with a greater than 40% chance of febrile neutropenia.[74] For patients who have experienced one episode of febrile neutropenia, use of G-CSF or GM-CSF may be considered for subsequent cycles of chemotherapy. A pegylated form of G-CSF (pegfilgrastim) that is available in the United States is a long-acting formulation that may be given once per cycle of chemotherapy.[75] However, there is no evidence in gynecologic malignancies that this is a superior strategy to reducing the dose of chemotherapy for subsequent cycles of treatment.

The commencement of G-CSF or GM-CSF is not generally recommended for patients with established febrile neutropenia. Some trials have suggested that the addition of these growth factors may cause a small reduction in the length of hospital stay or duration of neutropenia. However, a meta-analysis of the available evidence has not shown an overall decline in mortality due to febrile neutropenia with the use of G-CSF or GM-CSF.[76] The mortality due to febrile neutropenia, if appropriately treated with antibiotics, is expected to be low. It is generally considered that the cost of these growth factors does not justify the small additional benefit to be gained by their use for most patients with febrile neutropenia.

Results of a multicenter, randomized trial of these growth factors suggest that there may be a greater benefit if their use is restricted to patients considered to be at high-risk for death or serious medical complications due to febrile neutropenia. The trial randomized 210 solid tumor patients with febrile neutropenia who were considered to be at high-risk to treatment with appropriate antibiotics with or without the addition of G-CSF at a dose of 5 µg/kg per day.[77] Patients were considered to be at high risk if they had at least one of the following: profound neutropenia (<100/µL), short latency from previous chemotherapy cycle (<10 days), sepsis or clinically documented infection at presentation, severe comorbidity, Eastern Cooperative Oncology Group (ECOG) performance status 3 or 4, or prior inpatient status. Patients who received G-CSF were found to have a shorter duration of grade 4 neutropenia and a shorter duration of antibiotic treatment and hospital stay. The G-CSF group also had a reduced risk of the development of serious medical complications, although there was no difference in mortality. Because of these improvements, the median overall cost per patient admission was also reduced. Some clinicians may to choose to commence G-CSF treatment in certain high-risk patients presenting with febrile neutropenia.

Can some patients be safely managed as outpatients with oral antibiotics? Some patients with febrile neutropenia have a lower than average risk of serious complications or death. It has been suggested that such patients may be safely managed at home with oral antibiotic treatment. Several trials have suggested that low-risk patients may be safely managed with oral outpatient regimens such as ciprofloxacin combined with Augmentin-clavulanate. These trials have demonstrated good response to treatment, with overall mortality rates of less than 2%.[68,78,79] Patients considered to be low risk who may be considered for such treatment are those with solid tumors receiving conventional dose chemotherapy, who have no comorbidities, and who are expected to have a short duration of neutropenia (7 days). They should also be carefully assessed to be clinically and hemodynamically stable with only unexplained fever or simple infections such as a urinary tract infection or simple cellulitis.[68] It is also important that patients being assessed for suitability for outpatient treatment be compliant, have good social supports, and have access to basic services such as a telephone to allow 24-hour contact with the treating physician if required. They should not be geographically isolated from a nearby hospital facility.

The potential advantages of outpatient treatment include lower cost of care, enhanced quality of life for patients and their caregivers, reduced rates of nosocomial resistant superinfections, reduced rates of hospital-associated iatrogenic complications, and more efficient use of resources.[68] The potential disadvantages include increased risk for delayed treatment of serious complications of febrile neutropenia such as septic shock or hemorrhage, potential noncompliance with oral antibiotics, and the need to maintain an infrastructure that can safely support such an outpatient program.

Gastrointestinal Complications

Nausea and vomiting. The prospect of nausea and vomiting has been consistently reported as among patients' major concerns about receiving chemotherapy.[80] However, this toxicity is largely preventable with the use of serotonin 5-hydroxytryptamine type 3 receptor (5-HT3) antagonists for moderate or highly emetogenic drugs. Table 47-2 outlines the emetogenicity of commonly used chemotherapy drugs to treat gynecologic malignancies, and Table 47-3 provides the recommendations for appropriate prophylaxis when these drugs are prescribed. The use of such guidelines is extremely effective in preventing emesis for most patients. An optimal antiemetic schedule can prevent acute emesis due to cisplatin in 70% to 90% of cases and acute emesis due to moderately emetogenic drugs in more than 90% of cases. Prophylaxis against delayed emesis due to cisplatin is effective in 60% of cases.[81] Although guidelines are widely available, there is evidence that they are not always followed.[82] Prophylactic measures also tend to be more effective in preventing vomiting rather than nausea. Some patients may still have significant difficulties with nausea and vomiting. Patients who are more likely to have severe emesis include females, younger patients, those with poor control during past chemotherapy, and individuals with a lower alcohol intake.[80] Further research is trying to assess for other risk factors. For example,

Table 47–2. Emetogenic Potential of Chemotherapy Agents Used to Treat Gynecologic Malignancies

Emetic Category	Potential	Chemotherapy Agents
High risk	>90%	Cisplatin $\geq$ 50 mg/m^2
		Cyclophosphamide > 1500 mg/m^2
		Dacarbazine
Moderate risk	>30%	Cisplatin < 50 mg/m^2
		Carboplatin
		Cyclophosphamide (PO or IV)
		$\quad$ $\leq$ 1500 mg/m^2
		Doxorubicin
		Epirubicin
		Ifosfamide
Low risk	>10%	Capecitabine
		Docetaxel
		Etoposide
		Paclitaxel
		Mitomycin
		Topotecan
		Gemcitabine
		Methotrexate 50-250 mg/m^2
		5-Fluorouracil
		Liposomal doxorubicin
Minimal risk	<10%	Bleomycin
		Methotrexate $\leq$ 50 mg/m^2
		Chlorambucil (PO)
		Hydroxyurea
Delayed emetogenic potential		Cisplatin $\geq$ 50 mg/m^2
		Carboplatin $\geq$ 300 mg/m^2
		Cyclophosphamide $\geq$ 600-1000 mg/m^2
		Doxorubicin $\geq$ 50 mg/m^2

Data from Gralla RJ: New agents, new treatments and antiemetic therapy. Semin Oncol 2002;29(Suppl 4):119-124, and from Hesketh PJ: Defining the emetogenicity of cancer chemotherapy regimens: Relevance to clinical practice. Oncologist 1999;4:191-196.

response to 5-HT3 antagonists may vary with cytochrome P-450 genotype.[83]

Delayed emesis is problematic. Although 5-HT3 antagonists have revolutionized the treatment of acute emesis, they tend to be less effective in preventing delayed emesis. Corticosteroids have been found to be helpful in reducing the incidence of delayed emesis

Table 47–3. Recommended Antiemetic Regimen by Emetic Risk Group

Risk Group	Acute Antiemetic Prophylaxis*	Delayed Antiemetic Prophylaxis†
High risk	5HT3 plus Dex $\pm$ lorazepam	Dex plus 5HT3 or Dex plus MCP
Moderate risk	5HT3 plus Dex	Dex alone $\pm$ 5HT3 or MCP
Low risk	Single agent: 5HT3 or Dex or MCP	None
Minimal risk	None	None

*By oral route if tolerated; prophylaxis is started 30 minutes before chemotherapy.
†Days 2 through 4.
5HT3, 5-hydroxytryptamine type 3 receptor antagonists; Dex, dexamethasone (4 to 20 mg/day for acute; 4 to 8 mg/day for delayed cases); MCP, metoclopramide.
Data from references 80, 82, and 85.

and a new class of antiemetics, the neurokinin-1 antagonists, have shown promising activity against delayed emesis in early trials.[84,85] In some patients, 5-HT3 antagonists may cause problematic side effects such as headache and constipation. Patients should be warned about the potential for these side effects and given advice about the appropriate use of laxatives in the event constipation occurs. There is little evidence available about optimal treatment of patients with refractory or breakthrough emesis. General principles include trying antiemetics of a different class from those that have been initially unsuccessful, ensuring that patients are given adequate intravenous hydration to correct dehydration, and considering the possibility of other causes of vomiting such as bowel obstruction or brain metastases.[82]

Neurologic Complications

Peripheral neuropathy. Peripheral neuropathy is an important complication of chemotherapy, particularly for patients with ovarian cancer treated with a combination taxaneplatinum regimen. This troublesome side effect may limit the ability to continue planned chemotherapy and has been documented to affect the quality of life of cancer survivors.[86] Taxanes and platinum compounds can cause peripheral sensory neuropathy, but they are believed to do so by different mechanisms of action.

Cisplatin causes a peripheral sensory neuropathy that is cumulative at doses greater than 300 mg/m^2.[87] The clinical features are most commonly of a "glove and stocking" sensory neuropathy with paresthesia and numbness. Proprioception may also be affected. Patients may demonstrate variable sensory deficits, loss of deep tendon reflexes, and decreased vibratory perception. Other types of neuropathy such as motor and autonomic neuropathy may occur, but they are less common. The neuropathy sometimes may worsen after cessation of cisplatin, and recovery is variable.[88] The mechanism of damage is believed to relate to the alkylating agent accumulating in dorsal root ganglia, where it causes nucleolar damage and alterations in peptide content.[87,89]

Neuropathy may occur with lower doses of cisplatin but is much less common. For example, in the pivotal trials that demonstrated the effectiveness of concurrent chemoradiotherapy for cervical cancer, the reported incidence of neuropathy was low.[90-92] Peripheral neuropathy due to carboplatin may occur but is not common at standard doses. The risk appears to be greater for patients previously treated with cisplatin or those who have preexisting neuropathy due to alcohol or diabetes.

Paclitaxel also causes a cumulative peripheral neuropathy, which proved to be a dose-limiting toxicity in early-phase studies of the drug. The clinical features are similar to those seen with cisplatin. The reported incidence varies across trials. At doses of 135 to 200 mg/m^2, symptoms and signs of neuropathy may be seen in up to 85% of patients, but they are mild in most cases.[93] Severe neuropathy has been reported in 2% to 27%.[94] As with cisplatin, features of neuropathy may worsen for several months after discontinuation of the drug. Paclitaxel-related neuropathy appears to be related to microtubule disruption. In animal studies, the drug has been demonstrated to induce accumulation of intra-axonal neurotubules and inhibit neurite growth, with resultant axonal degeneration in peripheral nerves due to interference with axonal transport.[95,96]

Neuropathy is also a dose-limiting toxicity of docetaxel but is generally less problematic. In phase II studies using doses of 100 mg/m^2, approximately 50% of patients developed mild neuropathy, and 4% had severe neuropathy.[93] Taxane/platinum combinations may cause more peripheral neuropathy than when the drugs are used as single agents. The greatest effect is seen with the combination of cisplatin and paclitaxel. The combination of cisplatin combined with a 3-hour infusion of paclitaxel proved unacceptable because of a very high incidence of neurotoxicity.[97]

Despite the problems with neuropathy, this side effect does tend to abate with time, particularly for patients treated with carboplatin or paclitaxel. In a study that reported long-term effects of first-line chemotherapy for ovarian cancer, 41% of patients had some neuropathy 12 months after completing cisplatin plus paclitaxel, compared with 18% after carboplatin plus paclitaxel. After 24 months, 13% of cisplatin plus paclitaxel patients still had some degree of neuropathy, whereas no carboplatin plus paclitaxel patients had residual features.[98]

How should we manage patients developing neuropathy on carboplatin and paclitaxel? The most commonly used regimen for first-line treatment of ovarian cancer is carboplatin dosed at an area under the curve (AUC) 5/6 plus paclitaxel given as a 3-hour infusion at a dose of 175 mg/m^2. For patients who develop peripheral neuropathy that is causing functional impairment, a change in therapy is appropriate. The dose or schedule of paclitaxel may be altered, or the drug may be ceased altogether and the patient continued on carboplatin alone. Alternatively, docetaxel may be substituted for paclitaxel.

It is generally believed that multiagent chemotherapy is superior to single-agent chemotherapy for ovarian cancer, although no randomized study has conclusively demonstrated a survival difference for this approach. Results of the third International Collaborative Ovarian Neoplasm (ICON3) trial suggest that single-agent carboplatin and paclitaxel plus carboplatin are similarly effective as first-line treatment for women requiring chemotherapy for ovarian cancer.[99] However, one third of women on the carboplatin-alone arm in this trial did cross over to receive paclitaxel. Nevertheless, it seems reasonable to cease the paclitaxel if a patient develops significant peripheral neuropathy and continue on single-agent carboplatin.

The taxane could be modified rather than omitted if a patient has unacceptable neuropathy. Paclitaxel causes less neurotoxicity if given as a 24-hour rather

than 3-hour infusion. However, this benefit is offset by the need to hospitalize the patient for treatment and by an increase in neutropenia.[100] Alternatively, the dose of paclitaxel may be reduced to 135 mg/m^2. A joint European and Canadian randomized trial compared different doses and schedules of paclitaxel in women with recurrent ovarian cancer. Using a 2 × 2 factorial design, the trial evaluated doses of 135 and 175 mg/m^2 given over 3 or 24 hours. No difference in overall survival was observed in any of the four groups. However, there was some increase in time to disease progression for patients treated at the higher dose, with a median of 19 weeks for the higher dose versus 14 weeks for the lower dose ($P = .02$).[101] No difference in quality of life was seen in the different groups, but patients treated with 175 mg/m^2 had significantly more neurosensory symptoms than those treated with 135 mg/m^2. How this finding translates into the initial treatment setting using carboplatin plus paclitaxel is unclear. However, this trial lends some support to the practice of dose reduction of paclitaxel.

Another alternative is to substitute docetaxel for the paclitaxel. The reported Scottish Randomized Trial in Ovarian Cancer (SCOTROC) suggested equivalence in efficacy of treatment using carboplatin plus docetaxel or carboplatin plus paclitaxel for first-line treatment for advanced ovarian cancer. Mature survival data is still awaited. However, when the data were presented at a median follow-up of 21 months for 1077 randomized patients, the response rates and median progression-free survival times were equivalent.[102] The investigators reported a significant reduction in neurotoxicity for patients in the docetaxel arm based on National Cancer Institute common toxicity criteria (NCI-CTC) and on a structured neurotoxicity questionnaire and neurologic examination. The differences seen were statistically significant while patients were receiving treatment ($P < .001$) and at 6 months from randomization ($P < .001$). However, rates of grade 4 neutropenia and febrile neutropenia were increased in the docetaxel arm.

What supportive care is appropriate for patients with established neuropathy? Further management of the patient who develops peripheral neuropathy should include general advice about skin care. This includes the need to monitor affected areas of skin for any injuries that may result in infection if not tended. Supportive shoes without open toes may also reduce the chance of skin injury. The home environment may need to be modified to reduce the chance of falls due to loose objects, such as rugs, by patients with proprioceptive defects or sensory ataxia.[103]

Vitamin B supplementation is sometimes advocated for treatment or prevention of chemotherapy-related peripheral neuropathy. Vitamin supplementation may be helpful in those who have proven B$_{12}$ or folate deficiencies. However, there is little evidence to suggest this approach is helpful in a patient who is not vitamin deficient. In one prospective study that examined the effect of using pyridoxine to try to reduce cisplatin-related neurotoxicity in patients with advanced ovarian carcinoma, the response duration was significantly reduced in the patients who had taken concurrent pyridoxine.[104]

In some patients, peripheral neuropathy may be painful or result in unpleasant abnormal sensation. Patients may describe hypoesthesia (i.e., areas of numbness or decreased feeling), paresthesia (i.e., spontaneous abnormal nonpainful sensations such as tingling), dysesthesia (i.e., spontaneous abnormal painful sensations such as burning, tingling, or electrical sensations), hyperalgesia (i.e., increased perception of painful stimuli), hyperpathia (i.e., exaggerated pain response), and allodynia (i.e., pain induced by nonpainful stimuli). These symptoms may be constant or intermittent.[105]

Various medications have been used as analgesics for painful neuropathy. Tricyclic antidepressants have analgesic efficacy that is independent of their antidepressant effects.[106] They may be helpful in low doses and are usually taken at night. However, side effects such as dry mouth, somnolence, and urinary retention may cause problems, particularly in elderly patients. Anticonvulsants can also be used. Gabapentin, a newer antiepileptic, has been particularly helpful for patients with cancer-related neuropathic pain.[107] It is generally well tolerated but may cause some sedation. It is increasingly used as first-line therapy for cancer-related neuropathic pain because of its favorable toxicity profile and lack of significant drug interactions.

What are the roles of neuroprotectants?

Chemotherapy-induced peripheral neuropathy causes serious morbidity, and many agents have been investigated as potential neuroprotectants. Several have been shown to protect against neurotoxicity in animal models without compromising chemotherapy efficacy. These agents include glutamate,[108] glutathione,[109] amifostine,[110] and leukemia inhibitory factor.[111] One study suggested that glutathione in combination with cisplatin caused less toxicity than cisplatin alone when used to treat ovarian cancer. The addition of glutathione improved patients' quality of life scores, including measures of peripheral neurotoxicity.[109] However, convincing clinical benefit for any of these agents as neuroprotectants has yet to be demonstrated in randomized clinical trials.

The agent most advanced in clinical testing is amifostine. In one randomized trial of 242 patients with advanced ovarian cancer, pretreatment with amifostine was shown to reduce cumulative neurotoxicity due to cisplatin and cyclophosphamide without a reduction in antitumor efficacy.[112] However, in a study evaluating pretreatment with amifostine before high-dose paclitaxel treatment for metastatic breast cancer, no evidence of amifostine protection against paclitaxel neurotoxicity was seen.[113] Problems with the use of amifostine include increased cost, need for intravenous administration, and toxicities related to the drug itself, which include vomiting and hypotension. Many preclinical models have suggested that the agent may reduce antitumor efficacy, although this effect has not been seen in clinical trials of the agent.[114]

The 2002 update of the *Recommendations for the Use of Chemotherapy and Radiotherapy Protectants* by the American Society of Clinical Oncology[115] suggested that "Present data are insufficient to support the routine use of amifostine for the prevention of cisplatin ... or ... paclitaxel-associated neurotoxicity." Clinical trials of various other potential neuroprotectants continue to investigate this issue.

Ifosfamide and encephalopathy. Central neurotoxicity, an important toxic effect of ifosfamide, occurs in up to 10% to 15% of patients treated with the drug.[116] The clinical features include mild effects such as hallucinations in the presence of a clear sensorium.[117] However, a true encephalopathy that includes confusion, drowsiness, amnesia, epileptic seizures, and coma has also been described. Changes in the electroencephalograms of some patients have been reported.[118] In most cases, the encephalopathy is of short duration and reverses within 48 to 72 hours of cessation of the drug. However, some fatalities have been reported. Watkin and colleagues[119] described two patients with longer-term effects that included emotional instability, apathy, and short-term memory problems. However, long-term effects have not been well studied.

Various predisposing factors have been identified. Oral ifosfamide and short-duration intravenous infusions of the drug seem to have a greater risk of causing encephalopathy than lower-dose continuous infusions.[120] Clinical features that have been reported to predispose patients to developing this toxicity include low serum albumin concentrations, prior renal toxicity due to cisplatin, renal dysfunction due to ureteric obstruction by pelvic tumor, decreased hepatic function, brain metastases, and older age.[118,121] Some have suggested that concurrent administration of sedatives, such as antiemetics, benzodiazepines, and alcohol, may increase the risk of encephalopathy.[122] Other retrospective studies have not confirmed this suggestion.[121,123] However, it is common practice to avoid concurrent administration of sedatives with ifosfamide.

How should ifosfamide-related neurotoxicity be managed?

Management of the neurologic toxicity depends on its severity. For patients with hallucinations in the presence of a clear sensorium, reassurance about their cause and self-limited nature may be sufficient. For patients with moderate somnolence, agitation, or worse, further action is required. It is important to search for and exclude other causes of delirium such as sepsis, hypoxia, hypercalcemia, or cerebral metastases.

Several small case series and case reports have described patients treated with methylene blue, producing dramatic resolution of their symptoms. Cessation of the ifosfamide infusion is generally recommended, although this has not always been done in some cases of successful treatment with methylene blue.[116] The use of methylene blue was first based on similarities between ifosfamide-related encephalopathy and a congenital glutaricaciduria with increased urinary levels of glutaric acid and sarcosine.[124] Patients with glutaricaciduria type II have been treated with methylene blue, based on its ability to act as a non-physiologic electron acceptor. Methylene blue may also limit the formation and toxic effects of the metabolite of ifosfamide, chloroacetaldehyde, which is believed to account for some of the neurotoxicity.[118] Methylene blue has been given intravenously or orally at a dose of 50 mg every 4 hours until full recovery occurs. It is recommended that it be given in a 5% glucose solution, because glucose compensates for the derangements in fatty acid metabolism and defects in gluconeogenesis seen in glutaricaciduria type II.[124] The use of hemodialysis has also been described to reverse ifosfamide-related neurologic toxicity in a pediatric patient with chronic renal impairment.[125]

For a patient that has had significant neurologic toxicity with ifosfamide, further discussion about the pros and cons of continued use of the drug is appropriate. If retreatment is to occur, attempts to optimize or reverse potential predisposing factors seems sensible. A few cases have been described with successful prophylactic use of methylene blue to allow retreatment with ifosfamide with reduced or no features of encephalopathy.[116,124] The pharmacokinetics and metabolism of ifosfamide do not appear to be affected by concurrent administration of methylene blue, suggesting that drug efficacy should not be compromised by this approach.[126] However, the scarcity of the literature on this important toxicity makes it difficult to devise definitive recommendations.

Cognitive Effects of Chemotherapy

Should patients receiving chemotherapy be warned about possible cognitive effects of treatment? There has been increasing interest by doctors and patients in possible cognitive impairment resulting from systemic chemotherapy. This topic has not been well studied among sufferers of gynecologic cancer. However, several studies involving patients with other types of solid tumors and a variety of chemotherapy drugs have addressed this issue. Chemotherapy may cause a global decrease in cognitive function, an effect that has been most pronounced in studies of patients who have recently completed chemotherapy.[127-130] Longer-term deficits have also been described in a subset of patients studied up to 10 years after completion of systemic chemotherapy.[131] Most of the studies have come from women receiving adjuvant chemotherapy, including high-dose treatment, for breast cancer.

Schagen and colleagues[130] studied 39 node-positive breast cancer patients treated with adjuvant chemotherapy (i.e., cyclophosphamide, methotrexate, and 5-fluorouracil [CMF]) plus or minus tamoxifen and compared them with 34 age-matched control patients with node-negative breast cancer treated with surgery and local radiotherapy plus or minus tamoxifen but no chemotherapy. Patients underwent a battery of neuropsychological tests 2 years after completion of treatment. Cognitive impairment was seen in 28% of chemotherapy patients compared with 12% of controls. Patients who had received chemotherapy had more problems with concentration and memory than those who had not received chemotherapy. Comparisons between those treated with and without tamoxifen showed no significant difference.[130]

Research in this area has had various methodologic problems. For example, some studies have compared chemotherapy patients only to published norms or to control patients without cancer.[131] No studies have performed assessments of baseline cognitive function. It is known that patients with cancer may have significant cognitive impairment that predates any treatment.[132] The reported cognitive problems are often subtle, with only the patient being aware of them. Self-reported defects have generally been more severe than objective findings on neuropsychological testing.[130] Various deficits may be reported, which most commonly involve problems in the areas of concentration, memory, ability to be focused or organized, and working with numbers.[133]

If a patient complains of cognitive dysfunction while receiving chemotherapy or a caretaker has observed problems, it is important to look for other potential causes of this problem. For example, anxiety or depressive symptoms may contribute to cognitive deficits, which may improve with treatment of these conditions. As with other types of cancer, significant anxiety and depression has been reported in up to one fourth of patients with gynecologic malignancies.[134] However, several studies have identified cognitive impairment due to chemotherapy even after controlling for significant anxiety or depression in patients studied.

Acute emotional distress due to a diagnosis of cancer or its recurrence may also produce significant effects. Various medications, such as antiemetics or analgesics, may result in sedation. Cerebral metastases may cause a variety of cerebral symptoms, often including headache and nausea. Fatigue resulting from anemia may also be an important contributing factor, which can be improved with correction of the anemia. Fatigue has rarely been assessed or controlled for in studies describing cognitive impairment due to chemotherapy.[133] Cognitive dysfunction due to treatment-induced menopause has also been described, and the condition may improve with estrogen replacement. However, defects due to estrogen withdrawal are generally fairly specific for verbal memory rather than the global defects observed with chemotherapy.[135] The potential for cognitive defects due to systemic chemotherapy is an area that requires further study because cognitive problems can have a major impact on survivors' educational and career decisions and general quality of life.[133]

Dermatologic Complications

Management of alopecia. Although not a life-threatening complication of chemotherapy, the prospect of hair loss associated with cancer treatment is one of a patient's most feared side effects.[136,137] It can result in a loss of self-confidence, depression, and humiliation in patients already psychologically distressed as a result of their underlying disease. For many patients, hair loss represents an attack on their body image and self-esteem. In a study of 255 patients undergoing chemotherapy for a variety of malignancies, alopecia was the most feared side effect overall before treatment commenced.[136] In a subanalysis, women ranked hair loss as their number one fear, whereas for men, it was ranked fifth. Subjects with a higher education were more likely to rank breathlessness and fatigue above alopecia, and older subjects (>80 years) were more fearful of weight loss. During the course of their treatment, the percentage of subjects ranking alopecia as their number one fear fell from 51% to 40%. Carelle and coworkers[137] report their findings from a study examining perceived severity of side effects in 100 patients (65 women and 35 men) with advanced cancer receiving chemotherapy in an outpatient setting. Interviews were conducted using randomly ordered prompt cards naming 45 physical and 27 nonphysical side effects. Patients were asked to select all those that reflected the side effects they had experienced and then rank them according to their perceived severity. Women ranked hair loss as the second most severe nonphysical side effect, and men ranked it tenth.

Are techniques available to reduce the risk of alopecia? The degree of hair loss is related to the type of drug and amount used, as outlined in Table 47-4. With the aim of preventing chemotherapy-induced hair loss, many techniques have been tried with few successes. Techniques include the use of scalp tourniquets and scalp hypothermia.[138,139] The rationale for their use is that by causing induced vasoconstriction in the scalp vasculature, there will be a reduction of chemotherapy delivery to the hair follicles. In 1990, the FDA withdrew approval for commercial distribution of these devices on the basis of concern about the potential for scalp metastases, a possible reduction in the delivery of drug to sites beyond the scalp such as the skull and brain, and a consistent paucity of data related to their efficacy in the prevention of alopecia.[139] Cooling devices may still be advocated in some units, but controversies with regard to potential success rates and the possibility of detrimental outcomes should be discussed with the patient before use.

Although hair loss cannot be avoided with certain chemotherapy agents, it is important that women are counseled about ways to cope with this important toxicity. The "Look Good, Feel Better" program is an internationally recognized service dedicated to educating women undergoing treatment for cancer about techniques that help to improve their appearance and restore their self-esteem. Included in the sessions are demonstrations of the use of wigs, hats, turbans, and scarves, along with beauty tips about skin care, makeup, and nails.[140] This type of formal program designed to improve the self-esteem of women undergoing

Table 47–4. Alopecia and Chemotherapeutic Agents Commonly Used in the Treatment of Gynecologic Cancers

Chemotherapeutic Agent	Comment
Bleomycin	Some hair loss common, occasionally diffuse
Carboplatin	Grade 3 or 4 hair loss seen in 2%-3% patients
Chlorambucil	Rare
Cisplatin	Hair thinning common
Cyclophosphamide	Common, complete in up to 33% patients
Docetaxel	Complete in 80% patients at doses > 55 mg/m² ; severe with loss of all body hair in 60%
Doxorubicin	Complete hair loss usual
Etoposide	Complete hair loss in 8%-66% patients (dose dependent)
5-Fluorouracil	Hair thinning common
Gemcitabine	Hair loss in up to 15% patients
Ifosfamide	Total hair loss in 74%-83% treated with ifosfamide alone, 100% in combination with other drugs
Liposomal doxorubicin	Significant hair loss in 9% patients
Methotrexate	Occasional hair loss, usually at high doses
Mitomycin	Up to 4% patients (dose dependent)
Paclitaxel	Complete in 100% patients, may include all body hair
Topotecan	Partial hair loss in 16%, complete in 31%

Data from MIMS Australia: Australia, Medical Publishers Association, August 2002; and from American Hospital Formulary Service Drug Information, 42 ed. 2001.

anticancer therapies has been very helpful and supportive.[141]

Management of the extravasation of chemotherapeutic agents. Extravasation of chemotherapeutic agents, or leakage into the surrounding tissues, during an intravenous infusion can be extremely damaging to the local structures. The extent of injury depends on the type and toxicity of drug, the amount of drug that has leaked into surrounding tissues, the site at which it has occurred, and the general nutritional state of the patient. Although all chemotherapy agents have the capacity to cause damage if extravasation occurs, vesicants are associated with the most destructive local effects (Table 47-5). Significant morbidity, including pain, tissue necrosis, and loss of function, can occur because of an extravasation injury. The long-term effects are often more serious than the acute event and can be underestimated at the time of injury.

Data suggest that up to 5% of patients who receive a course of cytotoxic injections will experience extravasation.[142] The type of delivery system may alter the rates of accidental leakage. In a sample of 500 extravasations, the use of an automated intravenous delivery pump was associated with fewer incidences of leakage compared with not using a pump.[143] Certain patient groups are more likely to experience accidental leakage of infused fluids into surrounding tissues, including infants and children, the elderly, and patients who are confused or who have a decreased level of consciousness.[142,144] Despite ideal placement of

Table 47–5. Chemotherapeutic Agents and Their Association with Extravasation Injury

Vesicants	Exfoliants	Irritants	Inflammants	Neutral
Carmustine	Cisplatin	Carboplatin	Etoposide phosphate	Bleomycin
Dacarbazine	Docetaxel	Etoposide	Fluorouracil	Cyclophosphamide
Dactinomycin	Liposomal daunorubicin		Methotrexate	Gemcitabine
Daunorubicin	Liposomal doxorubicin			Ifosfamide
Doxorubicin	Mitoxantrone			
Idarubicin	Oxaliplatin			
Mitomycin				
Paclitaxel	Topotecan			
Streptozocin				
Vinblastine				
Vinorelbine				

Exfoliant, agent capable of causing skin exfoliation on extravasation; inflammant, agent capable of causing skin inflammation on extravasation; irritant, agent capable of causing skin irritation on extravasation; vesicant, agent capable of causing skin ulceration and tissue necrosis on extravasation.

Data from The Chemotherapy Executive Group: Classification of cytotoxic drugs according to their potential to cause serious necrosis when extravasated. Birmingham, UK, City Hospital, 2002 (http://www.extravasation.org.uk), accessed January 10, 2002, and from MIMS Australia: Australia, Medical Publishers Association, August 2002.

an intravenous infuser device, local factors can also increase the risk of extravasation. Diseases associated with abnormal circulation such as lymphedema, peripheral vascular disease, Raynaud's disease, and diabetes are associated with increased rates of leakage around the intravenous device.[143,144] Conditions associated with vein fragility and alteration to the normal architecture of connective tissue may also increase the risk of extravasation. These conditions include sites of previous trauma or surgery, areas affected by prior irradiation, and patients with known connective tissue disorders such as scleroderma. Inadequate nursing knowledge with regard to venipuncture skills, venous access devices, drugs likely to cause injury if leakage occurs, and signs and symptoms of extravasation can also increase the risk of significant injury associated with extravasation.[144]

Signs and symptoms of extravasation may include pain or a burning sensation at the site of infusion, local swelling, induration, erythema, discoloration or mottling, and early blistering of overlying tissues. In patients with central venous catheter devices, the pain may be experienced in the chest wall, neck, or shoulder region. Long-term effects include desquamation, ulceration, and necrosis.

Are there useful antidotes that should be delivered if an extravasation occurs? Many controversies surround the management of an extravasation. There are, however, several common principles aimed at reducing the amount of tissue damage and preventing necrosis and ulceration. At the first sign of leakage, the infusion must be ceased with disconnection of the giving set and aspiration of any residual fluid attempted. Flushing the local area with saline has been effective in some cases, as has thermoregulation.[144-148] Cold packs have reduced tissue injury and are recommended for all agents except vinca alkaloids, for which warm soaks should be used. DMSO used topically has been useful in reducing extravasation injury from a number of agents, including anthracyclines, cisplatin,

carboplatin, and ifosfamide.[145,147] Early surgical consultation for significant injury should be considered but it should be remembered that management with debridement and skin grafting is often unsuccessful with poor cosmetic results.

Anecdotal reports of the use of specific antidotes to cytotoxics indicate that they may help to reduce the injury when injected into the affected tissue. However, the efficacy for most of these agents remains contentious, and they are not used routinely.[142,145] For example, hyaluronidase has been used as an antidote for extravasation injuries with vinca alkaloids and may have a role in preventing ulceration after etoposide and paclitaxel.[145,146] Intradermal and intravenous isotonic sodium thiosulfate has been used in cases of cisplatin and mechlorethamine seepage but is not the standard of care in most institutions.[142,145,146] Although there is no role for parenteral corticosteroids (originally used on the premise of their anti-inflammatory properties), topical steroids remain of interest.

The administration of chemotherapy should not be taken lightly. Steps aimed at preventing extravasation should be taken with each patient receiving intravenous cytotoxics. These steps should include administration by experienced persons only, use of a fresh cannula into a large vein when possible, avoidance of sites on the hands or near joints, avoidance of limbs with impaired circulation, delivery of drugs by infusion not to be under pressure, and educating the patient to report any pain associated with an infusion immediately.

Management of hand-foot syndrome. Liposomal doxorubicin is a formulation containing the anthracycline doxorubicin that is encapsulated in liposomes having surface-bound methoxypolyethylene glycol groups. The pharmacokinetic properties of the formulation allow longer circulation time with a greater concentration of the drug reaching tumor cells.[149] The safety and toxicity profile of this newer formulation is significantly different from its original counterpart. Improvements in nausea, vomiting, alopecia, cardiotoxicity, and bone marrow suppression have been reported in several studies, but cutaneous side effects, thought to be related to the accumulation of the drug in the skin, are significantly worse and represent one of the dose-limiting toxicities of this drug.[150] The most frequent and severe toxicity experienced by women in these studies was palmar-plantar erythrodysesthesia (PPE).

PPE is characterized by painful, erythematous macular or papular vesicular-like eruptions on the skin. PPE was first described by Lokich and Moore[151] with continuous infusion of 5-fluorouracil (5-FU) in 1984. It is also a recognized dermatologic complication of the oral 5-FU prodrugs, capecitabine and UFT. PPE has been described with the use of cytarabine, doxorubicin, and high-dose vinorelbine.[152] Classically, it is seen on the palms of the hands and soles of the feet, but it can occur in any areas of skin that are subject to constant pressure or friction,[153] including skin folds around the stomach, breasts, armpits, and between the thighs. It appears to be a dose-related toxicity and most commonly occurs after two to three cycles of the drug.

Management of this reaction is not well defined and is somewhat controversial. Most evidence supports treatment delays of 1 week for all grades of reaction apart from grade 1. If the patient has persistent symptoms by week 6 after treatment or has had a grade 3 or 4 reaction, the dose should be reduced by 25% before recommencing. There has been at least one report supporting the use of oral pyridoxine for delaying the onset and amelioration of symptoms.[154,155] Use of systemic steroids and topical DMSO treatment have also assisted in resolution of symptoms of patients with documented PPE.[156,157] Other, more controversial management strategies include placing padding around hard surfaces and in shoes, the use of petroleum jelly as a second skin to reduce friction, and avoiding exposure of skin to very hot temperatures for 4 to 7 days after drug administration and then increasing the exposure after this time with the aim of increasing blood flow to the skin and assisting drug clearance. Generally accepted strategies include avoidance of tight-fitting clothes and shoes or the application of tight dressings or bandages.

Immunologic Complications of Chemotherapy

Hypersensitivity reactions. Chemotherapy drugs, like other medications, can cause hypersensitivity reactions. These may range in severity from mild effects to severe anaphylactic reactions. Virtually all chemotherapy drugs have been reported to cause hypersensitivity reactions, which are estimated to occur in 5% to 15% of patients treated with chemotherapy.[158] Most reactions are thought to be type 1 hypersensitivity reactions. These involve exaggerated or inappropriate immune responses to an allergen to which a patient has been previously exposed. In type 1 reactions, exposure to the allergen results in histamine release

from mast cells stimulated by allergen-specific IgE immunoglobulin. This IgE immunoglobulin is present because of previous exposure to the chemotherapy drug. Some drugs, such as paclitaxel, also seem to cause non–IgE-mediated anaphylactoid reactions by directly inducing histamine release from mast cells.[159] In vitro studies have also suggested that reactions to some drugs may result from uncontrolled activation of the complement cascade.[160]

The two major chemotherapy drug classes used in gynecologic cancer, platinum compounds and taxanes, induce hypersensitivity reactions with somewhat different clinical features. Platinum salts were first reported to produce hypersensitivity reactions after occupational exposure. Bronchial asthma induced by exposure to the compound was reported in platinum-refinery workers in 1945.[161] Subsequently, cisplatin has been reported to cause hypersensitivity reactions in patients previously exposed to the drug. Severe anaphylactic reactions have been reported in approximately 5% of reported case series.[162] However, hypersensitivity reactions are more of a problem with carboplatin because it is used in preference to cisplatin for retreatment of patients with platinum-sensitive disease because of its better tolerance and lack of cumulative neurotoxicity.

Several retrospective series have described the clinical features of these reactions. The reaction always occurred after at least four cycles of the drug. Severe reactions may include acute pruritus, diffuse erythroderma, facial swelling, tachycardia, chest tightness and bronchospasm, dyspnea, and hypertension or hypotension. Mild reactions may manifest only as facial flushing, itch, or erythema, particularly of the palms and soles that occurs up to 3 days after completion of the carboplatin infusion. In a series reported from Markman and colleagues,[163] of 205 patients treated with carboplatin over a 3-year period, 24 patients (12%) developed a carboplatin hypersensitivity reaction, despite routine premedication that included 20 mg of intravenous dexamethasone. In approximately one half of the patients, the hypersensitivity reaction occurred after more than 50% of the carboplatin infusion had been completed. The median number of cycles of platinum chemotherapy received before a reaction occurred was eight. It is uncommon to get a hypersensitivity reaction in a platinum-naive patient, but it has been described. The incidence of hypersensitivity reactions in the Markman series increased from 1% for patients who received fewer than six cycles of carboplatin to 27% for patients who received more than seven cycles of the drug.[164] Fifty percent of the patients had at least moderately severe symptoms. Polyzos and associates[165] reported a series of 240 platinum-naive patients with ovarian cancer treated with carboplatin with or without cyclophosphamide or paclitaxel. Thirty-two (16%) of the 194 patients treated with intravenous carboplatin developed symptoms compatible with a hypersensitivity reaction to carboplatin.[165]

For patients with only mild reactions, treatment usually consists of an intravenous antihistamine, such as diphenhydramine, followed by oral antihistamines until the symptoms have resolved. After a mild reaction, patients have been retreated with carboplatin. For example, in the series reported by Polyzos and associates,[165] 16 of 20 patients who had initially mild reactions were successfully retreated after prophylactic antihistamines. These patients did have similar reactions with repeat exposure that responded to symptomatic management. However, 4 of the 20 patients manifested severe hypersensitivity reactions on repeat challenge with carboplatin. None of the 12 patients with severe initial reactions was able to receive a full subsequent dose of carboplatin without experiencing further severe reaction.

What is the appropriate management for a patient who develops a severe hypersensitivity reaction to carboplatin? For all moderate-to-severe hypersensitivity reactions, initial management involves discontinuation of the infusion and appropriate resuscitation measures as outlined in Table 47-6. Intravenous antihistamines are usually given to counteract the effect of histamine released from mast cells. Corticosteroids are also given to prevent a prolonged or rebound reaction to the drug. For patients with acute respiratory compromise, adrenaline and other resuscitation measures may be required.

After resolution of the acute reaction, various management approaches have been suggested. It is appropriate to discuss the pros and cons of retreatment with a platinum compound in terms of the patient's particular clinical scenario. For patients with relapsed ovarian carcinoma, when the treatment is intended for palliative effect, various second-line agents are available as alternative treatment options. However, for the patient for whom platinum is believed to be an important component of potentially curative treatment, other options may be considered.

Some patients have been safely retreated with cisplatin after a hypersensitivity reaction to

carboplatin.[165-167] However, there have been two reports in the literature of anaphylactic death after treatment with cisplatin in this situation.[168,169] Neither of these patients had undergone skin testing to look for cross-reactivity between carboplatin and cisplatin. crossover to oxaliplatin treatment has also been suggested, given the lower incidence of reports of hypersensitivity reactions with this drug,[170] but there are few data to support this approach, and there was one report of eight patients with hypersensitivity reactions to oxaliplatin who had positive skin reactions to testing with carboplatin, suggesting cross-reactivity between these platinum compounds.[171]

Zanotti and coworkers[164] reported the use of skin testing with an intradermal injection of a small quantity of carboplatin as a means of predicting subsequent hypersensitivity reactions in a group of patients with ovarian or primary peritoneal carcinomas previously treated with at least seven cycles of carboplatin. In this study, a negative skin test result accurately predicted the absence of a hypersensitivity reaction with ongoing carboplatin treatment. However, the positive predictive value of the test could not be determined because only 4 of the 13 patients with a positive skin test went on to receive further carboplatin treatment. Three of these four patients subsequently had mild or moderate hypersensitivity reactions.

Several investigators have reported encouraging results for intravenous and oral desensitization protocols.[172-175] Some patients have had further reactions after completion of these protocols. However, when it is believed that further platinum chemotherapy is important for a patient, the physician can attempt treatment with cisplatin after a negative skin test result and completion of a desensitization protocol.

Hypersensitivity reactions to taxanes are somewhat different. Reactions to paclitaxel are the most common and are believed to be caused by the Cremophor EL (i.e., polyoxyethylated castor oil) in which the drug is dissolved, rather than the drug itself.[176] In initial trials using paclitaxel, hypersensitivity reactions were seen in up to 40% of patients. However, with the use of a premedication regimen using corticosteroids and histamine blockers, the incidence has been reduced to between 1.5% and 3%.[177] It was initially thought that increasing the infusion time from 3 to 24 hours could reduce hypersensitivity reactions, but subsequent trials disproved this idea.[178] The corticosteroids are frequently given as two oral doses of 20 mg, 6 and 12 hours before commencement of the chemotherapy. It has also been demonstrated that a single intravenous dose of 20 mg immediately before the chemotherapy safely and effectively reduces the frequency of reactions.[179]

In contrast to hypersensitivity reactions to platinum drugs, reactions to paclitaxel typically occur within minutes of initiation of the infusion[163] and may occur with the very first exposure to the drug. The classic symptoms and signs include dyspnea with or without bronchospasm, back pain, urticaria, erythematous rashes, and changes in blood pressure. The reaction frequently responds promptly to cessation of the

---

Table 47–6. Management of Hypersensitivity Reactions

1. Stop the chemotherapy infusion.
2. Call a physician to assess the patient with regard to airway, breathing, and circulation.
3. Administer IV normal saline if hypotensive.
4. Administer oxygen if dyspneic or hypoxic.
5. Administer IV antihistamine (e.g., 50 mg IV diphenhydramine, 25-50 mg IV promethazine).
6. Administer 5 mg of nebulized salbutamol if the patient has bronchospasm.
7. Administer IV corticosteroids (e.g., 100 mg of hydrocortisone); this may have no effect on the initial reaction but may prevent rebound or prolonged allergic manifestations.
8. If the patient does not promptly improve or has symptoms of persistent or severe hypotension or persistent bronchospasm or laryngeal edema, administer adrenaline or epinephrine (0.1-0.25 mg IV); further acute resuscitation measures may be required.
9. Reassure the patient that the problem is a recognized and treatable one.
10. Consult physician for a decision on further drug administration.

Data from references 160, 179, and 185.

infusion. Treatment with intravenous fluids, antihistamines, corticosteroids, and adrenaline is sometimes required (see Table 47-6). It has been demonstrated that patients can almost always be safely retreated with paclitaxel after such a reaction.[179-182] This can be done on the same day after at least a 30-minute break. Some physicians administer another dose of intravenous corticosteroids and commence the infusion at a slower rate, which is gradually increased.

There have been reports of patients who fail rechallenge of paclitaxel despite these measures and who are unable to receive further treatment with the drug.[183,184] In patients who fail rechallenge or have an extremely severe initial reaction to paclitaxel, it may be reasonable to consider switching to docetaxel treatment. Docetaxel is dissolved in polysorbate 80 and has a lower incidence of hypersensitivity reactions.[159] Premedication with dexamethasone has substantially reduced the frequency of reactions.[185] One case report described successful treatment using docetaxel in four patients with prior hypersensitivity reactions to paclitaxel.[186]

Pulmonary Complications

Pulmonary fibrosis and bleomycin. Bleomycin has a long and established history in the treatment of germ cell tumors. One of the most serious and long-term toxicities associated with this drug is its potential to cause pulmonary damage. After intravenous administration, bleomycin is found in high quantities in the lungs and the skin, the sites of major toxicity for this drug.[187] Renal excretion is responsible for approximately two thirds of the elimination of the drug. The reported incidence of bleomycin-related pneumonitis has varied from 0% to 46% of patients receiving regimens containing bleomycin.[188] Risk factors that increase the likelihood of pulmonary toxicity include a total dose of the drug exceeding 300 mg,[188] increasing age,[189] decreased renal function,[188] prior and concomitant radiotherapy,[189] smoking,[190] and particularly the use of high-dose oxygen therapy during surgery.[189] More controversial is the hypothesis that G-CSF may contribute to the pathogenesis of pulmonary toxicity in patients receiving bleomycin.[191] Although uncommon, death from pneumonitis can occur and has been reported in up to 3% of cases.[192]

The cytotoxic effect of bleomycin occurs by the induction of DNA damage through chemical interactions between the drug and both oxygen and iron. These reactions allow oxygen free radicals to form, which can result in direct cellular toxicity in tissues where bleomycin accumulates.[193] Pulmonary fibrosis can be the end result of bleomycin pulmonary toxicity. Many postulated mechanisms may lead to upregulation of inflammatory and fibrotic pathways in pulmonary beds, including the involvement of various cytokines (i.e., transforming growth factor-β and tumor necrosis factor-α),[188,194] mast cells, and the occurrence of an imbalance between the protease and antiprotease systems.[195,196] Although the relationship between pulmonary toxicity and bleomycin is well recognized, pathogenesis of the pulmonary changes is not completely understood and remains an area of ongoing research.

Does monitoring respiratory function help to predict the development of bleomycin-related lung toxicity?

The earliest and most common symptoms associated with bleomycin-induced lung damage are shortness of breath, nonproductive cough, and general malaise, although malaise may be difficult to distinguish from the anticipated level of fatigue that usually occurs with chemotherapy. Spiking temperatures may occur, even in the earliest phases of pulmonary reaction. Typically, these symptoms appear and progress over several weeks and months. The evolution of changes that can be used to detect the earliest signs of bleomycin-induced pulmonary toxicity remains controversial. Some studies suggest that the earliest changes, preceding any respiratory symptoms, are a decline in objective pulmonary function test results.[197] However, a retrospective study from a New Zealand group revealed that the diffusing capacity of the lung for carbon monoxide (DLCO) failed to detect serious pulmonary toxicity in some patients and had overdiagnosed pulmonary dysfunction in others (when bleomycin had been continued despite a significant decrease in the DLCO with no long-standing effects).[198] High-resolution computed tomography (CT) is a sensitive investigation for quantitating the degree and extent of pulmonary damage after the use of bleomycin, but studies have not been able to demonstrate a correlation between the changes on CT and physiologic differences in pulmonary function tests.[199,200] However, CT may be used to monitor the effects of treatment. Radiolabeled nuclear studies and [18F]fluoro-2-deoxyglucose–enhanced positron emission tomography (FDG-PET) are being investigated for their potential use in the early clinical diagnosis of bleomycin-induced pulmonary toxicity.[201,202] The gold standard for diagnosis in these patients remains open lung biopsy.

The most important step in the management of bleomycin-related pulmonary toxicity is prevention. Patients at potential risk for bleomycin toxicity should be identified before commencement of the drug, allowing dose reductions or perhaps the elimination of bleomycin in those with very good prognoses. Renal function should be assessed in all patients before each dose, with reductions or elimination of a dose in the event of significantly abnormal results. Most centers recommend the assessment of pulmonary function before each cycle of bleomycin-containing regimens, with dose reductions or cessation of the drug in response to any decrease in function. The development of pulmonary symptoms during the course of bleomycin-containing chemotherapy demands a thorough investigation to ensure that other lung pathologies such as metastases or infection are not the cause. Patients, treating physicians, and anesthetists must be made aware of the potential for pulmonary toxicity precipitated by the use of high-dose oxygen during any required surgical procedures after previous bleomycin chemotherapy.

Despite the fact that there have been no randomized trials to support its efficacy, a trial of corticosteroids is usually warranted for the management of bleomycin-induced pulmonary toxicity, and there have been some case reports supporting its use.[203,204] Although the dose remains controversial, the usual starting dose is 1 mg/kg per day of prednisolone, with slow decrements over an extended period. There have experiments using animal models and different compounds such as L-carnitine, *Ginkgo biloba* extract,[205] melatonin,[206] and nonsteroidal agents,[207] and some have had promising results. One study comparing the use of liposomal bleomycin with standard-formulation bleomycin demonstrated no pulmonary injury when the liposomal preparation was used.[208] There is a need for ongoing research in this area because the use of bleomycin is likely to continue, particularly for germ cell tumors, for which the overall prognosis is excellent.

Cardiovascular Complications

Cardiomyopathy. Cardiomyopathy may occur after anthracycline chemotherapy. Anthracyclines are associated with chronic cardiac toxicity, the risk of which increases with higher total cumulative doses. For doxorubicin, the development of cardiomyopathy is rare below doses of 450 mg/m^2. However, the incidence increases at cumulative doses of 550, 600, and 700 mg/m^2 to 7%, 15%, and 30%, respectively.[209] Certain risk factors are associated with a higher risk of developing cardiomyopathy: extremes of age, prior mediastinal radiotherapy, previous cardiac disease, hypertension, and combinations with paclitaxel.[209,210] A lower incidence of cardiotoxicity has been reported with prolonged intravenous infusions and weekly low doses of doxorubicin compared with standard, rapid infusions given every 3 weeks.[210,211] The anthracycline analog, epirubicin, was introduced because preclinical models showed less myelosuppression and decreased cardiotoxicity compared with doxorubicin. However, the use of epirubicin has not resulted in greatly decreased rates of cardiotoxicity when used at an equimyelotoxic dose to doxorubicin.[209,210]

The mechanism of damage is thought to be action on the myocardium by free radicals associated with the cytotoxic effect of anthracyclines.[209] Various alternatives have been tried to reduce the risk of cardiac toxicity. For example, pegylated liposomal doxorubicin appears to cause significantly less cardiotoxicity than the standard formulation, although a small percentage of cases have still been seen in clinical trials.[212,213] The liposomal preparation ensures that normal tissues such as the myocardium are exposed to reduced concentrations of free drug in the plasma.[209] The chemoprotectant dexrazoxane can chelate intracellular iron and may decrease anthracycline-induced free radical generation.[214] It has been shown to reduce cumulative cardiotoxicity in patients with metastatic breast cancer who are being treated with cumulative

doses of doxorubicin above 300 mg/m^2. At this stage, only limited data are available about the effect of dexrazoxane in patients receiving anthracyclines in other disease settings.

The clinical signs and symptoms of anthracycline-related cardiomyopathy are similar to those of heart failure from other causes. Patients may develop exertional dyspnea, jugular venous distension, an S$_3$ gallop, and tachycardia.[211] Fluid overload is a late finding. It has been suggested that the degree of tachycardia may be disproportionate to other symptoms in anthracycline-related cardiomyopathy. The development of cardiomyopathy may be detected before becoming symptomatic using serial measurements of the left ventricular ejection fraction by gated radionuclide studies. A baseline measurement should be taken before chemotherapy, and repeat measurements are recommended at least every two cycles above a dose of 300 mg/m^2. Characteristic signs include early diastolic dysfunction, followed by global hypokinesis with a normal to slightly enlarged ventricle. Function of the basal posterior wall is best preserved.[211] Other methods of detecting toxicity, including measurement of serum troponins and B-type atrial natriuretic peptide or use of positron emission tomography, remain investigational.[211,215]

What is the prognosis for patients with anthracycline-related cardiomyopathy? Early cases of cardiomyopathy were thought to have a high mortality rate, but by using conventional modern techniques for treating cardiac failure with angiotensin-converting enzyme inhibitors, diuretics, and digoxin, the outcome is much improved.[216] β-Blockers, including carvedilol, have also proved to be beneficial.[217,218] Death from cardiac failure is unusual in adults unless the syndrome is not recognized until it is extremely severe.

Genitourinary Complications

Hemorrhagic cystitis. Hemorrhagic cystitis is a complication specific to use of the alkylating agents cyclophosphamide and ifosfamide. It is believed to occur because of exposure of the urothelium to toxic metabolites of these drugs, which are formed after metabolic activation by liver P-450 microsomes.[219] The resultant damage to the urothelium of the bladder leads to hematuria and clot formation, which may be painful. In more severe cases, the upper urinary system may be affected, causing ureteric obstruction and renal failure.[220] In a study of patients with ovarian cancer without specific prophylaxis, hemorrhagic cystitis occurred in 18% of patients receiving ifosfamide and 6% of patients receiving cyclophosphamide.[219]

Prophylactic use of the uroprotectant sodium 2-mercaptoethanesulfonate (mesna) can significantly reduce the development of hemorrhagic cystitis.[219] After intravenous or oral administration, the thiol compound mesna undergoes rapid oxidation in the plasma to dimesna. Dimesna is very hydrophilic and therefore is rapidly excreted by the kidneys into the urine, where it binds to toxic metabolites of the alkylating agents such as acrolein to form stable nontoxic compounds. Cytotoxic activity is not compromised by the use of mesna because of the rapid excretion of mesna and dimesna into the urine. Intravenous mesna is generally recommended because of its low oral bioavailability, although larger doses of oral mesna have been used. The recommended dose for use with ifosfamide is a daily dose of 60% of the total daily dose of ifosfamide, given as three divided doses 15 minutes before and 4 and 8 hours after administration of each dose of ifosfamide (when the dose used is less than 2.5 mg/m^2 daily).[219] Use of 2 L per day of concurrent intravenous hydration is also recommended, with routine monitoring of the patient for the development of fluid overload or hematuria. A baseline pretreatment urinalysis should also be obtained. More intensive hydration or alkalinization of the urine has not been proved to give further protection. In the event of development of hematuria despite the use of mesna, there are few data on which to base management, but in general, increased mesna doses are sometimes given, and the chemotherapy may be interrupted until the hematuria has resolved.

Treatment of established hemorrhagic cystitis involves general supportive care, including appropriate analgesia and transfusion of blood or platelets, or both, if blood cell counts are low.[220] Further intravenous hydration should be given, and continuous bladder irrigation is recommended to try and remove intravesical clots. If the problem persists despite these measures, various alternative treatments can be tried. These have included local intravesical installations of preparation such as alum, formalin, phenol, silver nitrate, and prostaglandins.[221] However, long-term bladder fibrosis has resulted in some cases after this type of treatment.[222] Surgical options have included cystoscopy with evacuation of clot or various methods of urinary diversion. In refractory cases, hyperbaric oxygen therapy has been useful, and cystectomy rarely is required.[222,223]

REFERENCES

1. Campos S: The impact of anemia and its treatment on patients with gynecologic malignancies. Semin Oncol 2002;29(Suppl 8): 7-12.
2. Groopman JE, Itri LM: Chemotherapy-induced anemia in adults: Incidence and treatment. J Natl Cancer Inst 1999;91: 1616-1634.
3. Hensley ML, Lebeau D, Leon LF, et al: Identification of risk factors for requiring transfusion during front-line chemotherapy for ovarian cancer. Gynecol Oncol 2001;81:485-489.
4. Eisenhauer EA, Bokkel Huinink WW, Swenerton KD, et al: European-Canadian randomized trial of paclitaxel in relapsed ovarian cancer: High-dose versus low-dose and long versus short infusion. J Clin Oncol 1994;12:2654-2666.
5. ten Bokkel HW, Gore M, Carmichael J, et al: Topotecan versus paclitaxel for the treatment of recurrent epithelial ovarian cancer. J Clin Oncol 1997;15:2183-2193.
6. Francis P, Schneider J, Hann L, et al: Phase II trial of docetaxel in patients with platinum-refractory advanced ovarian cancer. J Clin Oncol 1994;12:2301-2308.
7. Kavanagh JJ, Kudelka AP, de Leon CG, et al: Phase II study of docetaxel in patients with epithelial ovarian carcinoma refractory to platinum. Clin Cancer Res 1996;2:837-842.
8. Curt GA: Impact of fatigue on quality of life in oncology patients. Semin Hematol 2000;37(Suppl 6):14-17.
9. Vogelzang NJ, Breitbart W, Cella D, et al: Patient, caregiver, and oncologist perceptions of cancer-related fatigue: Results of a tripart assessment survey. The Fatigue Coalition. Semin Hematol 1997;34(Suppl 2):4-12.
10. Winningham ML, Nail LM, Burke MB, et al: Fatigue and the cancer experience: The state of the knowledge. Oncol Nurs Forum 1994;21:23-36.
11. Thomas G: The effect of hemoglobin level on radiotherapy outcomes: The Canadian experience. Semin Oncol 2001;28(Suppl 8): 60-65.
12. Girinski T, Pejovic-Lenfant MH, Bourhis J, et al: Prognostic value of hemoglobin concentrations and blood transfusions in advanced carcinoma of the cervix treated by radiation therapy: Results of a retrospective study of 386 patients. Int J Radiat Oncol Biol Phys 1989;16:37-42.
13. Grogan M, Thomas GM, Melamed I, et al: The importance of hemoglobin levels during radiotherapy for carcinoma of the cervix. Cancer 1999;86:1528-1536.
14. Obermair A, Cheuk R, Horwood K, et al: Impact of hemoglobin levels before and during concurrent chemoradiotherapy on the response of treatment in patients with cervical carcinoma: Preliminary results. Cancer 2001;92:903-908.
15. Miller CB, Jones RJ, Piantadosi S, et al: Decreased erythropoietin response in patients with the anemia of cancer. N Engl J Med 1990;322:1689-1692.
16. Case DC Jr, Bukowski RM, Carey RW, et al: Recombinant human erythropoietin therapy for anemic cancer patients on combination chemotherapy. J Natl Cancer Inst 1993;85:801-806.
17. Cascinu S, Fedeli A, Del Ferro E, et al: Recombinant human erythropoietin treatment in cisplatin-associated anemia: A randomized, double-blind trial with placebo. J Clin Oncol 1994;12: 1058-1062.
18. Silvestris F, Romito A, Fanelli P, et al: Long-term therapy with recombinant human erythropoietin (rHu-EPO) in progressing multiple myeloma. Ann Hematol 1995;70:313-318.
19. Henry DH, Brooks BJ Jr, Case DC Jr, et al: Recombinant human erythropoietin therapy for anemic cancer patients receiving cisplatin chemotherapy. Cancer J Sci Am 1995;1:252.
20. Kurz C, Marth C, Windbichler G, et al: Erythropoietin treatment under polychemotherapy in patients with gynecologic malignancies: A prospective, randomized, double-blind placebo-controlled multicenter study. Gynecol Oncol 1997;65: 461-466.
21. Oberhoff C, Neri B, Amadori D, et al: Recombinant human erythropoietin in the treatment of chemotherapy-induced anemia and prevention of transfusion requirement associated with solid tumors: A randomized, controlled study. Ann Oncol 1998;9: 255-260.
22. Littlewood TJ, Bajetta E, Nortier JW, et al: Effects of epoetin alfa on hematologic parameters and quality of life in cancer patients receiving nonplatinum chemotherapy: Results of a randomized, double-blind, placebo-controlled trial. J Clin Oncol 2001;19: 2865-2874.
23. Demetri GD, Kris M, Wade J, et al: Quality-of-life benefit in chemotherapy patients treated with epoetin alfa is independent of disease response or tumor type: Results from a prospective community oncology study. Procrit Study Group. J Clin Oncol 1998;16:3412-3425.
24. Glaspy J: The impact of epoetin alfa on quality of life during cancer chemotherapy: A fresh look at an old problem. Semin Hematol 1997;34(Suppl 2):20-26.
25. Cleeland CS, Demetri GD, Glaspy J: Identifying hemoglobin level for optimal quality of life: Results of an incremental analysis [abstract]. Proc Am Soc Clin Oncol 1999;18:574a.
26. Rizzo JD, Lichtin AE, Woolf SH, et al: Use of epoetin in patients with cancer: Evidence-based clinical practice guidelines of the American Society of Clinical Oncology and the American Society of Hematology. J Clin Oncol 2002;20:4083-4107.
27. Henry DH: Supplemental iron: A key to optimizing the response of cancer-related anemia to rHuEPO? Oncologist 1998;3: 275-278.

28. Macdougall IC, Cavill I, Hulme B, et al: Detection of functional iron deficiency during erythropoietin treatment: A new approach. BMJ 1992;304:225-226.

29. Kavanagh BD, Fischer BA, Segreti EM, et al: Cost analysis of erythropoietin versus blood transfusions for cervical cancer patients receiving chemoradiotherapy. Int J Radiat Oncol Biol Phys 2001;51:435-441.

30. Casadevall N, Nataf J, Viron B, et al: Pure red-cell aplasia and antierythropoietin antibodies in patients treated with recombinant erythropoietin. N Engl J Med 2002;346:469-475.

31. Prabhakar SS, Muhlfelder T: Antibodies to recombinant human erythropoietin causing pure red cell aplasia. Clin Nephrol 1997; 47:331-335.

32. Weber G, Gross J, Kromminga A, et al: Allergic skin and systemic reactions in a patient with pure red cell aplasia and anti-erythropoietin antibodies challenged with different epoetins. J Am Soc Nephrol 2002;13:2381-2383.

33. Lackritz EM, Satten GA, Aberle-Grasse J, et al: Estimated risk of transmission of the human immunodeficiency virus by screened blood in the United States. N Engl J Med 1995;333:1721-1725.

34. Schreiber GB, Busch MP, Kleinman SH, Korelitz JJ: The risk of transfusion-transmitted viral infections. The Retrovirus Epidemiology Donor Study. N Engl J Med 1996;334:1685-1690.

35. Elting LS, Rubenstein EB, Martin CG, et al: Incidence, cost, and outcomes of bleeding and chemotherapy dose modification among solid tumor patients with chemotherapy-induced thrombocytopenia. J Clin Oncol 2001;19:1137-1146.

36. Heckman KD, Weiner GJ, Davis CS, et al: Randomized study of prophylactic platelet transfusion threshold during induction therapy for adult acute leukemia: 10,000/microL versus 20,000/microL. J Clin Oncol 1997;15:1143-1149.

37. Rebulla P, Finazzi G, Marangoni F, et al: The threshold for prophylactic platelet transfusions in adults with acute myeloid leukemia. Gruppo Italiano Malattie Ematologiche Maligne dell'Adulto. N Engl J Med 1997;337:1870-1875.

38. Fanning J, Hilgers RD, Murray KP, et al: Conservative management of chemotherapeutic-induced thrombocytopenia in women with gynecologic cancers. Gynecol Oncol 1995;59:191-193.

39. McCullough J: Current issues with platelet transfusion in patients with cancer. Semin Hematol 2000;37(Suppl 4):3-10.

40. Demetri GD: Targeted approaches for the treatment of thrombocytopenia. Oncologist 2001;6(Suppl 5):15-23.

41. Tepler I, Elias L, Smith JW, et al: A randomized placebo-controlled trial of recombinant human interleukin-11 in cancer patients with severe thrombocytopenia due to chemotherapy. Blood 1996;87:3607-3614.

42. Vredenburgh JJ, Hussein A, Fisher D, et al: A randomized trial of recombinant human interleukin-11 following autologous bone marrow transplantation with peripheral blood progenitor cell support in patients with breast cancer. Biol Blood Marrow Transplant 1998;4:134-141.

43. Neumann TA, Foote M: Megakaryocyte growth and development factor (MGDF): An Mpl ligand and cytokine that regulates thrombopoiesis. Cytokines Cell Mol Ther 2000;6:47-56.

44. Vadhan-Raj S, Verschraegen CF, Bueso-Ramos C, et al: Recombinant human thrombopoietin attenuates carboplatin-induced severe thrombocytopenia and the need for platelet transfusions in patients with gynecologic cancer. Ann Intern Med 2000;132:364-368.

45. Vadhan-Raj S, Kavanagh JJ, Freedman RS, et al: Safety and efficacy of transfusions of autologous cryopreserved platelets derived from recombinant human thrombopoietin to support chemotherapy-associated severe thrombocytopenia: A randomized crossover study. Lancet 2002;359:2145-2152.

46. von Tempelhoff GF, Heilmann L: Antithrombotic therapy in gynecologic surgery and gynecologic oncology. Hematol Oncol Clin North Am 2000;14:1151-1169, ix.

47. von Tempelhoff GF, Niemann F, Schneider DM, et al: Blood rheology during chemotherapy in patients with ovarian cancer. Thromb Res 1998;90:73-82.

48. Canney PA, Wilkinson PM: Pulmonary embolism in patients receiving chemotherapy for advanced ovarian cancer. Eur J Cancer Clin Oncol 1985;21:585-586.

49. Levine MN: Prevention of thrombotic disorders in cancer patients undergoing chemotherapy. Thromb Haemost 1997;78:133-136.

50. Levine M, Hirsh J, Gent M, et al: Double-blind randomized trial of a very-low-dose warfarin for prevention of thromboembolism in stage IV breast cancer. Lancet 1994;343:886-889.

51. Boraks P, Seale J, Price J, Bass G, et al: Prevention of central venous catheter–associated thrombosis using minidose warfarin in patients with haematological malignancies. Br J Haematol 1998;101:483-486.

52. Bern MM, Lokich JJ, Wallach SR, et al: Very low doses of warfarin can prevent thrombosis in central venous catheters: A randomized prospective trial. Ann Intern Med 1990;112:423-428.

53. Heaton DC, Han DY, Inder A: Minidose (1 mg) warfarin as prophylaxis for central vein catheter thrombosis. Intern Med J 2002;32:84-88.

54. Monreal M, Alastrue A, Rull M, et al: Upper extremity deep venous thrombosis in cancer patients with venous access devices—prophylaxis with a low molecular weight heparin (Fragmin). Thromb Haemost 1996;75:251-253.

55. Lee AY: Treatment of venous thromboembolism in cancer patients. Thromb Res 2001;102:V195-V208.

56. Hutten BA, Prins MH, Gent M, et al: Incidence of recurrent thromboembolic and bleeding complications among patients with venous thromboembolism in relation to both malignancy and achieved international normalized ratio: A retrospective analysis. J Clin Oncol 2000;18:3078-3083.

57. Wester JP, de Valk HW, Nieuwenhuis HK, et al: Risk factors for bleeding during treatment of acute venous thromboembolism. Thromb Haemost 1996;76:682-688.

58. Gitter MJ, Jaeger TM, Petterson TM, et al: Bleeding and thromboembolism during anticoagulant therapy: A population-based study in Rochester, Minnesota. Mayo Clin Proc 1995;70:725-733.

59. Palareti G, Legnani C, Lee A, et al: A comparison of the safety and efficacy of oral anticoagulation for the treatment of venous thromboembolic disease in patients with or without malignancy. Thromb Haemost 2000;84:805-810.

60. Bona RD, Sivjee KY, Hickey AD, et al: The efficacy and safety of oral anticoagulation in patients with cancer. Thromb Haemost 1995;74:1055-1058.

61. Prandoni P, Lensing AW, Cogo A, et al: The long-term clinical course of acute deep venous thrombosis. Ann Intern Med 1996;125:1-7.

62. Meyer G, Marjanovic Z, Valcke J, et al: Comparison of low-molecular-weight heparin and warfarin for the secondary prevention of venous thromboembolism in patients with cancer: A randomized controlled study. Arch Intern Med 2002;162: 1729-1735.

63. Armstrong D, O'Reilly S: Clinical guidelines for managing topotecan-related hematologic toxicity. Oncologist 1998; 3:4-10.

64. Bodey GP, Buckley M, Sathe YS, Freireich EJ: Quantitative relationships between circulating leukocytes and infection in patients with acute leukemia. Ann Intern Med 1966;64:328-340.

65. Schimpff S, Satterlee W, Young VM, Serpick A: Empiric therapy with carbenicillin and gentamicin for febrile patients with cancer and granulocytopenia. N Engl J Med 1971;284:1061-1065.

66. Zinner SH: Changing epidemiology of infections in patients with neutropenia and cancer: Emphasis on gram-positive and resistant bacteria. Clin Infect Dis 1999;29:490-494.

67. Elting LS, Rubenstein EB, Rolston KV, Bodey GP: Outcomes of bacteremia in patients with cancer and neutropenia: Observations from two decades of epidemiological and clinical trials. Clin Infect Dis 1997;25:247-259.

68. Donowitz GR, Maki DG, Crnich CJ, et al: Infections in the neutropenic patient—new views of an old problem. Hematology (Am Soc Hematol Educ Program) 2001;113-139.

69. Sanders JW, Powe NR, Moore RD: Ceftazidime monotherapy for empiric treatment of febrile neutropenic patients: A meta-analysis. J Infect Dis 1991;164:907-916.

70. Yamamura D, Gucalp R, Carlisle P, et al: Open randomized study of cefepime versus piperacillin-gentamicin for treatment of febrile neutropenic cancer patients. Antimicrob Agents Chemother 1997;41:1704-1708.

71. Winston DJ, Ho WG, Bruckner DA, Champlin RE: Beta-lactam antibiotic therapy in febrile granulocytopenic patients. A randomized trial comparing cefoperazone plus piperacillin, ceftazidime plus piperacillin, and imipenem alone. Ann Intern Med 1991;115:849-859.

72. Karp JE, Dick JD, Angelopulos C, et al: Empiric use of van-comycin during prolonged treatment-induced granulocytope-nia. Randomized, double-blind, placebo-controlled clinical trial in patients with acute leukemia. Am J Med 1986;81:237-242.

73. Vancomycin added to empirical combination antibiotic therapy for fever in granulocytopenic cancer patients. European Organization for Research and Treatment of Cancer (EORTC) International Antimicrobial Therapy Cooperative Group and the National Cancer Institute of Canada Clinical Trials Group. J Infect Dis 1991;163:951-958.

74. Update of recommendations for the use of hematopoietic colony-stimulating factors: Evidence-based clinical practice guidelines. American Society of Clinical Oncology. J Clin Oncol 1996;14:1957-1960.

75. Holmes FA, Jones SE, O'Shaughnessy J, et al: Comparable efficacy and safety profiles of once-per-cycle pegfilgrastim and daily injection filgrastim in chemotherapy-induced neutropenia: A multicenter dose-finding study in women with breast cancer. Ann Oncol 2002;13:903-909.

76. Berghmans T, Paesmans M, Lafitte JJ, et al: Therapeutic use of granulocyte and granulocyte-macrophage colony-stimulating factors in febrile neutropenic cancer patients. A systematic review of the literature with meta-analysis. Support Care Cancer 2002;10:181-188.

77. Garcia-Carbonero R, Mayordomo JI, Tornamira MV, et al: Granulocyte colony-stimulating factor in the treatment of high-risk febrile neutropenia: A multicenter randomized trial. J Natl Cancer Inst 2001;93:31-38.

78. Rubenstein EB, Rolston K, Benjamin RS, et al: Outpatient treat-ment of febrile episodes in low-risk neutropenic patients with cancer. Cancer 1993;71:3640-3646.

79. Malik IA, Khan WA, Karim M, et al: Feasibility of outpatient management of fever in cancer patients with low-risk neutrope-nia: Results of a prospective randomized trial. Am J Med 1995; 98:224-231.

80. Gralla RJ: New agents, new treatments and antiemetic therapy. Semin Oncol 2002;29(Suppl 4):119-124.

81. Licitra L, Spinazza S, Roila F: Antiemetic therapy. Crit Rev Oncol Hematol 2002;43:93-101.

82. Aapro MS: How do we manage patients with refractory or breakthrough emesis. Support Care Cancer 2002;10:106-109.

83. Kaiser R, Sezer O, Papies A, et al: Patient-tailored antiemetic treatment with 5-hydroxytryptamine type 3 receptor antagonists according to cytochrome P-450 2D6 genotypes. J Clin Oncol 2002;20:2805-2811.

84. Van Belle S, Lichinitser MR, Navari RM, et al: Prevention of cisplatin-induced acute and delayed emesis by the selective neurokinin-1 antagonists, L-758,298 and MK-869. Cancer 2002; 94:3032-3041.

85. Hesketh PJ: Defining the emetogenicity of cancer chemotherapy regimens: Relevance to clinical practice. Oncologist 1999;4:191-196.

86. Cavaletti G, Bogliun G, Marzorati L, et al: Long-term peripheral neurotoxicity of cisplatin in patients with successfully treated epithelial ovarian cancer. Anticancer Res 1994;14:1287-1292.

87. Gregg RW, Molepo JM, Monpetit VJ, et al: Cisplatin neurotoxic-ity: The relationship between dosage, time, and platinum concentration in neurologic tissues, and morphologic evidence of toxicity. J Clin Oncol 1992;10:795-803.

88. Grunberg SM, Sonka S, Stevenson LL, Muggia FM: Progressive paresthesias after cessation of therapy with very high-dose cisplatin. Cancer Chemother Pharmacol 1989;25:62-64.

89. Barajon I, Bersani M, Quartu M, et al: Neuropeptides and mor-phological changes in cisplatin-induced dorsal root ganglion neuropathy. Exp Neurol 1996;138:93-104.

90. Keys HM, Bundy BN, Stehman FB, et al: Cisplatin, radiation, and adjuvant hysterectomy compared with radiation and adjuvant hysterectomy for bulky stage IB cervical carcinoma. N Engl J Med 1999;340:1154-1161.

91. Morris M, Eifel PJ, Lu J, et al: Pelvic radiation with concurrent chemotherapy compared with pelvic and para-aortic radiation for high-risk cervical cancer. N Engl J Med 1999;340:1137-1143.

92. Rose PG, Bundy BN, Watkins EB, et al: Concurrent cisplatin-based radiotherapy and chemotherapy for locally advanced cervical cancer. N Engl J Med 1999;340:1144-1153.

93. Amato AA, Collins MP: Neuropathies associated with malig-nancy. Semin Neurol 1998;18:125-144.

94. Spencer CM, Faulds D: Paclitaxel: A review of its pharmaco-dynamic and pharmacokinetic properties and therapeutic potential in the treatment of cancer. Drugs 1994;48:794-847.

95. Rowinsky EK, Chaudhry V, Cornblath DR, Donehower RC: Neurotoxicity of Taxol. J Natl Cancer Inst Monogr 1993;15: 107-115.

96. Cavaletti G, Tredici G, Braga M, Tazzari S: Experimental peripheral neuropathy induced in adult rats by repeated intraperitoneal administration of Taxol. Exp Neurol 1995; 133:64-72.

97. Connelly E, Markman M, Kennedy A, et al: Paclitaxel delivered as a 3-hr infusion with cisplatin in patients with gynecologic cancers: Unexpected incidence of neurotoxicity. Gynecol Oncol 1996;62:166-168.

98. Meier W, duBois S, Olbricht U: Cisplatin/paclitaxel versus car-boplatin/paclitaxel in optimal stage III ovarian cancer: Results of a prospective randomized phase III study [abstract]. Proc Int Gynecol Cancer Soc 1999:48.

99. Paclitaxel plus carboplatin versus standard chemotherapy with either single-agent carboplatin or cyclophosphamide, doxoru-bicin, and cisplatin in women with ovarian cancer: The ICON3 randomized trial. Lancet 2002;360:505-515.

100. Rowinsky EK: The taxanes: Dosing and scheduling considera-tions. Oncology (Huntingt) 1997;11(Suppl 2):7-19.

101. Eisenhauer EA, Bokkel Huinink WW, Swenerton KD, et al: European-Canadian randomized trial of paclitaxel in relapsed ovarian cancer: High-dose versus low-dose and long versus short infusion. J Clin Oncol 1994;12:2654-2666.

102. Vasey P: Survival and longer-term toxicity results of the SCOTROC study: Docetaxel-carboplatin (DC) vs paclitaxel-carboplatin (PC) in epithelial ovarian cancer [abstract]. Proc Am Soc Clin Oncol 2002;21:804a.

103. Almadrones L: Toxicity management for chemotherapeutic agents used in the treatment of ovarian cancer. Memorial Sloan-Kettering Cancer Center, New York 2002 (http: // www.medscape.com/viewarticle/429839_22), accessed April 12, 2002.

104. Wiernik PH, Yeap B, Vogl SE, et al: Hexamethylmelamine and low or moderate dose cisplatin with or without pyridoxine for treatment of advanced ovarian carcinoma: A study of the Eastern Cooperative Oncology Group. Cancer Invest 1992; 10:1-9.

105. Farrar JT, Portenoy RK: Neuropathic cancer pain: The role of adjuvant analgesics. Oncology (Huntingt) 2001;15:1435-1442, 1445.

106. Max MB, Lynch SA, Muir J, et al: Effects of desipramine, amitriptyline, and fluoxetine on pain in diabetic neuropathy. N Engl J Med 1992;326:1250-1256.

107. Caraceni A, Zecca E, Martini C, De Conno F: Gabapentin as an adjuvant to opioid analgesia for neuropathic cancer pain. J Pain Symptom Manage 1999;17:441-445.

108. Boyle FM, Wheeler HR, Shenfield GM: Amelioration of experi-mental cisplatin and paclitaxel neuropathy with glutamate. J Neurooncol 1999;41:107-116.

109. Smyth JF, Bowman A, Perren T, et al: Glutathione reduces the toxicity and improves quality of life of women diagnosed with ovarian cancer treated with cisplatin: Results of a double-blind, randomized trial. Ann Oncol 1997;8:569-573.

110. DiPaola RS, Schuchter L: Neurologic protection by amifostine. Semin Oncol 1999;26(Suppl 7):82-88.

111. Boyle FM, Beatson C, Monk R, et al: The experimental neuro-protectant leukaemia inhibitory factor (LIF) does not compro-mise antitumour activity of paclitaxel, cisplatin and carboplatin. Cancer Chemother Pharmacol 2001;48:429-434.

112. Kemp G, Rose P, Lurain J, et al: Amifostine pretreatment for protection against cyclophosphamide-induced and cisplatin-induced toxicities: Results of a randomized control trial in patients with advanced ovarian cancer. J Clin Oncol 1996;14: 2101-2112.

113. Gelmon K, Eisenhauer E, Bryce C, et al: Randomized phase II study of high-dose paclitaxel with or without amifostine in patients with metastatic breast cancer. J Clin Oncol 1999;17: 3038-3047.

114. Twentyman PR: Modification by WR 2721 of the response to chemotherapy of tumours and normal tissues in the mouse. Br J Cancer 1983;47:57-63.

115. Schuchter LM, Hensley ML, Meropol NJ, Winer EP: 2002 Update of recommendations for the use of chemotherapy and radiotherapy protectants: Clinical practice guidelines of the American Society of Clinical Oncology. J Clin Oncol 2002; 20:2895-2903.

116. Pelgrims J, De Vos F, Van den BJ, et al: Methylene blue in the treatment and prevention of ifosfamide-induced encephalopathy: Report of 12 cases and a review of the literature. Br J Cancer 2000;82:291-294.

117. DiMaggio JR, Brown R, Baile WF, Schapira D: Hallucinations and ifosfamide-induced neurotoxicity. Cancer 1994;73:1509-1514.

118. Kerbusch T, de Kraker J, Keizer HJ, et al: Clinical pharmacokinetics and pharmacodynamics of ifosfamide and its metabolites. Clin Pharmacokinet 2001;40:41-62.

119. Watkin SW, Husband DJ, Green JA, Warenius HM: Ifosfamide encephalopathy: A reappraisal. Eur J Cancer Clin Oncol 1989;25:1303-1310.

120. Cerny T, Castiglione M, Brunner K, et al: Ifosfamide by continuous infusion to prevent encephalopathy. Lancet 1990;335:175.

121. Meanwell CA, Blake AE, Kelly KA, et al: Prediction of ifosfamide/mesna associated encephalopathy. Eur J Cancer Clin Oncol 1986;22:815-819.

122. Goren MP, Wright RK, Pratt CB, Pell FE: Dechloroethylation of ifosfamide and neurotoxicity. Lancet 1986;2:1219-1220.

123. Antman KH, Ryan L, Elias A, et al: Response to ifosfamide and mesna: 124 previously treated patients with metastatic or unresectable sarcoma. J Clin Oncol 1989;7:126-131.

124. Kupfer A, Aeschlimann C, Wermuth B, Cerny T: Prophylaxis and reversal of ifosfamide encephalopathy with methyleneblue. Lancet 1994;343:763-764.

125. Carlson L, Goren MP, Bush DA, et al: Toxicity, pharmacokinetics, and in vitro hemodialysis clearance of ifosfamide and metabolites in an anephric pediatric patient with Wilms' tumor. Cancer Chemother Pharmacol 1998;41:140-146.

126. Aeschlimann C, Kupfer A, Schefer H, Cerny T: Comparative pharmacokinetics of oral and intravenous ifosfamide/mesna/methylene blue therapy. Drug Metab Dispos 1998;26:883-890.

127. Kaasa S, Olsnes BT, Mastekaasa A: Neuropsychological evaluation of patients with inoperable non-small cell lung cancer treated with combination chemotherapy or radiotherapy. Acta Oncol 1988;27:241-246.

128. van Dam FS, Schagen SB, Muller MJ, et al: Impairment of cognitive function in women receiving adjuvant treatment for high-risk breast cancer: High-dose versus standard-dose chemotherapy. J Natl Cancer Inst 1998;90:210-218.

129. Brezden CB, Phillips KA, Abdolell M, et al: Cognitive function in breast cancer patients receiving adjuvant chemotherapy. J Clin Oncol 2000;18:2695-2701.

130. Schagen SB, van Dam FS, Muller MJ, et al: Cognitive deficits after postoperative adjuvant chemotherapy for breast carcinoma. Cancer 1999;85:640-650.

131. Ahles TA, Saykin AJ, Furstenberg CT, et al: Neuropsychologic impact of standard-dose systemic chemotherapy in long-term survivors of breast cancer and lymphoma. J Clin Oncol 2002;20:485-493.

132. Ahles TA, Silberfarb PM, Herndon J, et al: Psychologic and neuropsychologic functioning of patients with limited small-cell lung cancer treated with chemotherapy and radiation therapy with or without warfarin: A study by the Cancer and Leukemia Group B. J Clin Oncol 1998;16:1954-1960.

133. Ahles TA, Saykin A: Cognitive effects of standard-dose chemotherapy in patients with cancer. Cancer Invest 2001;19:812-820.

134. Bodurka-Bevers D, Basen-Engquist K, Carmack CL, et al: Depression, anxiety, and quality of life in patients with epithelial ovarian cancer. Gynecol Oncol 2000;78(Pt 1):302-308.

135. Sherwin BB: Cognitive assessment for postmenopausal women and general assessment of their mental health. Psychopharmacol Bull 1998;34:323-326.

136. Passik SD, Kirsh KL, Rosenfeld B, et al: The changeable nature of patients' fears regarding chemotherapy: Implications for palliative care. J Pain Symptom Manage 2001;21:113-120.

137. Carelle N, Piotto E, Bellanger A, et al: Changing patient perceptions of the side effects of cancer chemotherapy. Cancer 2002;95:155-163.

138. Cline BW: Prevention of chemotherapy-induced alopecia: A review of the literature. Cancer Nurs 1984;7:221-228.

139. Seipp C: Adverse effects of treatment: Hair loss in cancer. In DeVita VT Jr, Hellman S, Rosenberg SA (ed): Principles and Practice of Oncology. Philadelphia, Lippincott-Raven, 1997, pp 2705-2806.

140. Cancer Patients Foundation Ltd: Look Good … Feel Better. Australia, Cosmetic, Toiletry and Fragrance Association of Australia, 2002 (http://www.lgfb.org.au/home_ct.html), accessed October 1, 2002.

141. Williams TR, O'Sullivan M, Snodgrass SE, Love N: Psychosocial issues in breast cancer. Helping patients get the support they need. Postgrad Med 1995;98:97-94, 107.

142. Khan MS, Holmes JD: Reducing the morbidity from extravasation injuries. Ann Plast Surg 2002;48:628-632.

143. The Chemotherapy Executive Group: Classification of cytotoxic drugs according to their potential to cause serious necrosis when extravasated. Birmingham, UK, City Hospital, 2002 (http://www.extravasation.org.uk), accessed October 1, 2002.

144. Camp-Sorrell D: Developing extravasation protocols and monitoring outcomes. J Intraven Nurs 1998;21:232-239.

145. Dorr RT: Antidotes to vesicant chemotherapy extravasations. Blood Rev 1990;4:41-60.

146. Bertelli G, Cafferata MA, Ardizzoni A, et al: Skin ulceration potential of paclitaxel in a mouse skin model in vivo. Cancer 1997;79:2266-2269.

147. Olver IN, Aisner J, Hament A, et al: A prospective study of topical dimethyl sulfoxide for treating anthracycline extravasation. J Clin Oncol 1988;6:1732-1735.

148. Scuderi N, Onesti MG: Antitumor agents: Extravasation, management, and surgical treatment. Ann Plast Surg 1994;32:39-44.

149. Wu NZ, Da D, Rudoll TL, et al: Increased microvascular permeability contributes to preferential accumulation of stealth liposomes in tumor tissue. Cancer Res 1993;53:3765-3770.

150. Waterhouse DN, Tardi PG, Mayer LD, Bally MB: A comparison of liposomal formulations of doxorubicin with drug administered in free form: Changing toxicity profiles. Drug Saf 2001;24:903-920.

151. Lokich JJ, Moore C: Chemotherapy-associated palmar-plantar erythrodysesthesia syndrome. Ann Intern Med 1984;101:798-9.

152. Nagore E, Insa A, Sanmartin O: Antineoplastic therapy–induced palmar plantar erythrodysesthesia ("hand foot") syndrome. Incidence, recognition and management. Am J Clin Dermatol 2000;1:225-234.

153. Lyass O, Uziely B, Ben Yosef R, et al: Correlation of toxicity with pharmacokinetics of pegylated liposomal doxorubicin (Doxil) in metastatic breast carcinoma. Cancer 2000;89:1037-1047.

154. MIMS Australia: St. Leonards, NSW, Australia, Medical Publishers Association, August 2002.

155. Vail DM, Chun R, Thamm DH, et al: Efficacy of pyridoxine to ameliorate the cutaneous toxicity associated with doxorubicin containing pegylated (stealth) liposomes: A randomized, double-blind clinical trial using a canine model. Clin Cancer Res 1998;4:1567-1571.

156. Lopez AM, Wallace L, Dorr RT, et al: Topical DMSO treatment for pegylated liposomal doxorubicin-induced palmar-plantar erythrodysesthesia. Cancer Chemother Pharmacol 1999;44:303-306.

157. American Hospital Formulary Service Drug Information, 42 ed. Am Soc Hlth Sys, Bethesda, MD, 2001.

158. Weiss RB: Hypersensitivity reactions. Semin Oncol 1992;19:458-477.

159. Bernstein BJ: Docetaxel as an alternative to paclitaxel after acute hypersensitivity reactions. Ann Pharmacother 2000;34:1332-1335.

160. Labovich TM: Acute hypersensitivity reactions to chemotherapy. Semin Oncol Nurs 1999;15:222-231.

161. Hunter D, Milton R, Perry KMA: Asthma caused by complex salts of platinum. Br J Ind Med 1945;2:92.

162. Von Hoff DD, Schilsky R, Reichert CM, et al: Toxic effects of cis-dichlorodiammineplatinum(II) in man. Cancer Treat Rep 1979;63:1527-1531.

163. Markman M, Kennedy A, Webster K, et al: Clinical features of hypersensitivity reactions to carboplatin. J Clin Oncol 1999;17:1141.

164. Zanotti KM, Rybicki LA, Kennedy AW, et al: Carboplatin skin testing: A skin-testing protocol for predicting hypersensitivity to carboplatin chemotherapy. J Clin Oncol 2001;19: 3126-3129.

165. Polyzos A, Tsavaris N, Kosmas C, et al: Hypersensitivity reactions to carboplatin administration are common but not always severe: A 10-year experience. Oncology 2001;61:129-133.

166. Weidmann B, Mulleneisen N, Bojko P, Niederle N: Hypersensitivity reactions to carboplatin. Report of two patients, review of the literature, and discussion of diagnostic procedures and management. Cancer 1994;73:2218-2222.

167. Shukunami K, Kurokawa T, Kubo M, et al: Hypersensitivity reaction to carboplatin during treatment for ovarian cancer: Successful resolution by replacement with cisplatin. Tumori 1999;85:297-298.

168. Dizon DS, Sabbatini PJ, Aghajanian C, et al: Analysis of patients with epithelial ovarian cancer or fallopian tube carcinoma retreated with cisplatin after the development of a carboplatin allergy. Gynecol Oncol 2002;84:378-382.

169. Zweizig S, Roman LD, Muderspach LI: Death from anaphylaxis to cisplatin: A case report. Gynecol Oncol 1994;53: 121-122.

170. Gutierrez M, Pautier P, Lhomme C: Replacement of carboplatin by oxaliplatin may be one solution for patients treated for ovarian carcinoma who are hypersensitive to carboplatin. J Clin Oncol 2002;20:353.

171. Meyer L, Zuberbier T, Worm M, et al: Hypersensitivity reactions to oxaliplatin: Cross-reactivity to carboplatin and the introduction of a desensitization schedule. J Clin Oncol 2002;20:1146-1147.

172. Goldberg A, Confino-Cohen R, Fishman A, et al: A modified, prolonged desensitization protocol in carboplatin allergy. J Allergy Clin Immunol 1996;98:841-843.

173. Robinson JB, Singh D, Bodurka-Bevers DC, et al: Hypersensitivity reactions and the utility of oral and intravenous desensitization in patients with gynecologic malignancies. Gynecol Oncol 2001;82:550-558.

174. Broome CB, Schiff RI, Friedman HS: Successful desensitization to carboplatin in patients with systemic hypersensitivity reactions. Med Pediatr Oncol 1996;26:105-110.

175. Kook H, Kim KM, Choi SH, et al: Life-threatening carboplatin hypersensitivity during conditioning for autologous PBSC transplantation: Successful rechallenge after desensitization. Bone Marrow Transplant 1998;21:727-729.

176. Szebeni J, Muggia FM, Alving CR: Complement activation by Cremophor EL as a possible contributor to hypersensitivity to paclitaxel: An in vitro study. J Natl Cancer Inst 1998;90:300-306.

177. Rowinsky EK, Eisenhauer EA, Chaudhry V, et al: Clinical toxicities encountered with paclitaxel (Taxol). Semin Oncol 1993; 20(Suppl 3):1-15.

178. Eisenhauer EA, Bokkel Huinink WW, Swenerton KD, et al: European-Canadian randomized trial of paclitaxel in relapsed ovarian cancer: High-dose versus low-dose and long versus short infusion. J Clin Oncol 1994;12:2654-2666.

179. Micha JP, Rettenmaier MA, Dillman R, et al: Single-dose dexamethasone paclitaxel premedication. Gynecol Oncol 1998;69:122-124.

180. Cormio G, Di Vagno G, Melilli GA, et al: Hypersensitivity reactions in ovarian cancer patients receiving paclitaxel. J Chemother 1999;11:407-409.

181. Markman M, Kennedy A, Webster K, et al: Paclitaxel-associated hypersensitivity reactions: Experience of the gynecologic oncology program of the Cleveland Clinic Cancer Center. J Clin Oncol 2000;18:102-105.

182. Peereboom DM, Donehower RC, Eisenhauer EA, et al: Successful re-treatment with taxol after major hypersensitivity reactions. J Clin Oncol 1993;11:885-890.

183. Del Priore G, Smith P, Warshal DP, et al: Paclitaxel-associated hypersensitivity reaction despite high-dose steroids and prolonged infusions. Gynecol Oncol 1995;56:316-318.

184. Laskin MS, Lucchesi KJ, Morgan M: Paclitaxel rechallenge failure after a major hypersensitivity reaction. J Clin Oncol 1993;11: 2456-2457.

185. Provincial Systemic Program Committee. Acute Hypersensitivity Reactions to Chemotherapy. Vancouver, British Columbia, BC Cancer Agency, 1998 (http://www.bccancer.bc.ca/HPI/DrugDatabase/Appendices/Appendix2/AcuteHypersensitivityReactionstoChemotherapeuticAgentsPolicyIV10.html), accessed August 29, 2002.

186. Lokich J, Anderson N: Paclitaxel hypersensitivity reactions: A role for docetaxel substitution. Ann Oncol 1998;9:573.

187. Chabner BA, Allegera CJ, Curt GA, et al: Antineoplastic agents. In Hardman JG, Limbird LE, Molinoff PB (eds): Goodman and Gilman's the Pharmacological Basis of Therapeutics. New York, McGraw-Hill, 1996.

188. Sleijfer S, Vujaskovic Z, Limburg PC, et al: Induction of tumor necrosis factor-alpha as a cause of bleomycin-related toxicity. Cancer 1998;82:970-974.

189. Comis RL: Bleomycin pulmonary toxicity: Current status and future directions. Semin Oncol 1992;19(Suppl 5):64-70.

190. Strumberg D, Brugge S, Korn MW, et al: Evaluation of long-term toxicity in patients after cisplatin-based chemotherapy for non-seminomatous testicular cancer. Ann Oncol 2002;13:229-236.

191. Adach K, Suzuki M, Sugimoto T, et al: Granulocyte colony-stimulating factor exacerbates the acute lung injury and pulmonary fibrosis induced by intratracheal administration of bleomycin in rats. Exp Toxicol Pathol 2002;53:501-510.

192. Levi JA, Raghavan D, Harvey V, et al: The importance of bleomycin in combination chemotherapy for good-prognosis germ cell carcinoma. Australasian Germ Cell Trial Group. J Clin Oncol 1993;11:1300-1305.

193. Freeman BA, Crapo JD: Biology of disease: Free radicals and tissue injury. Lab Invest 1982;47:412-426.

194. Khalil N, Whitman C, Zuo L, et al: Regulation of alveolar macrophage transforming growth factor-beta secretion by corticosteroids in bleomycin-induced pulmonary inflammation in the rat. J Clin Invest 1993;92:1812-1818.

195. Cooper JA Jr, White DA, Matthay RA: Drug-induced pulmonary disease. Part 1. Cytotoxic drugs. Am Rev Respir Dis 1986;133:321-340.

196. Olman MA, Mackman N, Gladson CL, et al: Changes in procoagulant and fibrinolytic gene expression during bleomycin-induced lung injury in the mouse. J Clin Invest 1995; 96:1621-1630.

197. Villani F, De Maria P, Bonfante V, et al: Late pulmonary toxicity after treatment for Hodgkin's disease. Anticancer Res 1997; 17:4739-4742.

198. McKeage MJ, Evans BD, Atkinson C, et al: Carbon monoxide diffusing capacity is a poor predictor of clinically significant bleomycin lung. New Zealand Clinical Oncology Group. J Clin Oncol 1990;8:779-783.

199. Lynch DA, Hirose N, Cherniack RM, Doherty DE: Bleomycin-induced lung disease in an animal model: Correlation between computed tomography–determined abnormalities and lung function. Acad Radiol 1997;4:102-107.

200. Bellamy EA, Nicholas D, Husband JE: Quantitative assessment of lung damage due to bleomycin using computed tomography. Br J Radiol 1987;60:1205-1209.

201. Ugur O, Caner B, Balbay MD, et al: Bleomycin lung toxicity detected by technetium-99m diethylene triamine penta-acetic acid aerosol scintigraphy. Eur J Nucl Med 1993;20:114-118.

202. Hain SF, Beggs AD: Bleomycin-induced alveolitis detected by FDG positron emission tomography. Clin Nucl Med 2002; 27:522-523.

203. Hartmann LC, Frytak S, Richardson RL, et al: Life-threatening bleomycin pulmonary toxicity with ultimate reversibility. Chest 1990;98:497-499.

204. Kozielski J: Reversal of bleomycin lung toxicity with corticosteroids. Thorax 1994;49:290.

205. Daba M, Abdel-Aziz A, Moustafa A, et al: Effects of L-carnitine and ginkgo biloba extract (EG b 761) in experimental bleomycin-induced lung fibrosis. Pharmacol Res 2002;45:461.

206. Arslan SO, Zerin M, Vural H, Coskun A: The effect of melatonin on bleomycin-induced pulmonary fibrosis in rats. J Pineal Res 2002;32:21-25.

207. Mall G, Zimmermann P, Siemens I, et al: Prevention of bleomycin-induced fibrosing alveolitis with indomethacin: Stereological studies on rat lungs. Virchows Arch A Pathol Anat Histopathol 1991;419:339-347.

208. Arndt D, Zeisig R, Bechtel D, Fichtner I: Liposomal bleomycin: Increased therapeutic activity and decreased pulmonary toxicity in mice. Drug Deliv 2001;8:1-7.

209. Maluf FC, Spriggs D: Anthracyclines in the treatment of gynecological malignancies. Gynecol Oncol 2002;85:18-31.

210. Singal PK, Iliskovic N: Doxorubicin-induced cardiomyopathy. NEJM 1998;339:900-905.

211. Keefe DL: Anthracycline-induced cardiomyopathy. Semin Oncol 2001;28(Suppl 12):2-7.

212. Harris L, Batist G, Belt R, et al: Liposome-encapsulated doxorubicin compared with conventional doxorubicin in a randomized multicenter trial as first-line therapy of metastatic breast carcinoma. Cancer 2002;94:25-36.

213. Safra T, Muddia F, Jeffers S, et al: Pegylated liposomal doxorubicin (Doxil): Reducing clinical cardiotoxicity in patients reaching or exceeding cumulative doses of 500 mg/m². Ann Oncol 2000;11:1029-1033.

214. Henslet ML, Schuchter LM, Lindley C, et al: American Society of Clinical Oncology clinical practice guidelines for the use of chemotherapy and radiotherapy protectants. J Clin Oncol 1999; 17:3333-3355.

215. Sparano JA, Brown DL, Wolff AC: Predicting cancer therapy–induced cardiotoxicity: The role of troponins and other markers. Drug Saf 2002;25:301-301.

216. Moreb JS, Oblon DJ: Outcome of clinical congestive heart failure induced by anthracyclines chemotherapy. Cancer 1992;70: 2637-2641.

217. Matsui H, Morishima I, Numuguchi N, et al: Protective effects of carvedilol against doxorubicin-induced cardiomyopathy in rats. Life Sci 1999;65:1265-1274.

218. Noori A, Lindenfeld J, Wolfel E, et al: Beta-blockade in adriamycin-induced cardiomyopathy. J Card Fail 2000;6:115-119.

219. Hensley ML, Schuchter LM, Lindley C, et al: American Society of Clinical Oncology clinical practice guidelines for the use of chemotherapy and radiotherapy protectants. J Clin Oncol 1999; 17:3333-3355.

220. Wong TM, Yeo W, Chan LW, Mok TS: Hemorrhagic pyelitis, ureteritis, and cystitis secondary to cyclophosphamide: Case report and review of the literature. Gynecol Oncol 2000;76: 223-225.

221. Seber A, Shu XO, Defor T, et al: Risk factors for severe hemorrhagic cystitis following BMT. Bone Marrow Transplant 1998; 23:35-40.

222. Hattori K, Yabe M, Matsumoto M, et al: Successful hyperbaric oxygen treatment of life-threatening hemorrhagic cystitis after allogeneic bone marrow transplantation. Bone Marrow Transplant 2001;27:1315-317.

223. Koc S, Hagglund H, Ireton RC, et al: Successful treatment of severe hemorrhagic cystitis with cystectomy following matched donor allogeneic hematopoietic cell transplantation. Bone Marrow Transplant 2000;26:899-901.

SURGICAL TECHNIQUES

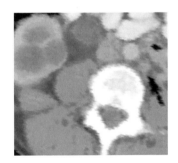

PERIOPERATIVE CARE

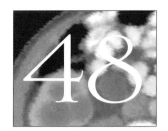

James W. Orr, Jr.,   F. Joseph Kelly,   and   Phillip Y. Roland

---

 MAJOR CONTROVERSIES

- **Are there absolute contraindications to surgery related to cardiac, pulmonary, or renal disease?**
- **What is the optimal method of perioperative deep venous thrombosis prophylaxis?**
- **What constitutes optimal perioperative management of the gastrointestinal tract?**
- **What constitutes the optimal incision or approach for a gynecologic cancer procedure?**

Are there absolute contraindications to surgery related to cardiac, pulmonary, or renal disease?

Gynecologic cancer surgery is frequently required in women with serious comorbidities. High-risk patients and procedures are an inherent, routine part of our practice. These operations may be necessary at diagnosis, during initial treatment, or during post-treatment surveillance. Common procedures, including lymphadenectomy, cytoreductive surgery, and radical resection, result in greater blood loss, often involve multiple organ systems, and typically require longer anesthesia. These treatment factors, individually or combined, contribute to an increased risk of operative morbidity and subsequent poor outcome. Cancer operations undertaken in women with associated medical illness dramatically increase the risk of adverse surgical consequences. Gynecologic oncologists are constantly required to assess risks and weigh benefits during pretreatment planning (even when the recommendation is observation) in an attempt to provide a therapeutic index of the recommended management plan. Perioperative evaluation routinely includes a comprehensive history and physical examination performed to detect the presence of significant medical illness. This information is processed to develop an approach to favorably modify (pharmacologic or otherwise) the potential adverse impact of any existing comorbid variable. In general, diagnostic or therapeutic surgery represents an indicated procedure

most patients managed by gynecologic oncologists. Truly elective surgery (e.g., prophylactic oophorectomy) represents a relatively rare situation. It is within this context of determining the therapeutic index of surgical or other treatment that the pelvic surgeon must attempt to evaluate the existence and effect of an absolute surgical contraindication. During the pretreatment evaluation, the gynecologic surgeon is required to assess overall and individual cardiac, pulmonary, and renal risks of surgery. Only after deciphering this information can we outline the best "routine" or modified plan of care.

Cardiac risk. The classic benchmark for cardiac risk assessment has been the Goldman criteria.[1] This gold standard of perioperative cardiac risk assessment has been modified, tested, and confirmed by Detsky and others.[2,3] The largest and latest validation of a simplified cardiac assessment index for those undergoing noncardiac surgery was repeated by Lee and colleagues,[4] who incorporated high-risk surgical procedure, history of ischemic heart disease (excluding coronary revascularization), history of heart failure, history of stroke or transient ischemic attack, preoperative insulin therapy, and creatinine levels of 152.5 μmol/L (>2 mg/dL) as important indicators suggesting the need for cardiac risk assessment. Their results (Table 48-1) indicate that the risk of a serious perioperative cardiac event can be directly correlated to the presence of an increasing number of these risk factors. Grayburn and Hillis[5] propose that this risk stratification based solely

Table 48–1. Major Cardiac Event Rates by the Revised Cardiac Risk Index

Class*	Events†/Patients	Event Rate (95% CI)
I (0) risk factor	2/488	0.4% (0.05-1.5)
II (1) risk factor	5/567	0.9% (0.3-2.1)
III (2) risk factor	17/258	6.6% (3.9-10.3)
IV (≥ 3) risk factor	12/109	11.0% (5.8-18.4)

*Risk factors include high-risk surgical procedures (intraperitoneal), history of ischemic heart disease (excluding previous revascularization), history of congestive heart failure, history of stroke or transient ischemic attack, preoperative insulin therapy, and preoperative serum creatinine levels greater than 152.5 μmol/L (>2.0 mg/dL).
†Major cardiac events include myocardial infarction, cardiac arrest, pulmonary edema, and complete heart block.
Adapted from Lee TH, Marcantonio ER, Mangione CM, et al: Derivation and prospective validation of a simple index for prediction of cardiac risk of major noncardiac surgery. Circulation 1999;100:1043-1049.

on clinical factors is accurate and beneficial, requiring only a history, physical examination, and measurement of a serum creatinine level. These investigators suggest that noninvasive myocardial perfusion imaging and dobutamine stress echocardiography (DSE) are inaccurate and potentially create an unacceptable harm-benefit ratio. In this schema, invasive coronary angiography is recommended only if it is deemed necessary independent of the proposed need for noncardiac surgery.[5] Conversely, this clinical risk stratification strategy is accurate, beneficial to the patient, and can be easily performed without adding undue delay to patient care.

Further strengthening the role of a modified clinical approach to cardiac risk assessment and avoiding the necessity of preoperative testing are the studies validating the cardioprotective benefit of perioperative β-blocker therapy. Poldermans and coworkers[6] studied perioperative bisoprolol versus placebo in a randomized fashion in high-risk (abdominal aortic aneurysm repair) surgical patients. The study was terminated early after interval analysis demonstrated a significant reduction in cardiac mortality (17% versus 3.4%, $P = .002$) and myocardial infarction (17.4% versus 0%, $P < .001$) in patients receiving perioperative β-blockers. In a randomized, double-blind trial of atenolol versus placebo in patients undergoing noncardiac surgery, Mangano and colleagues[7] detailed a significant ($P < .001$) reduction of acute cardiac events and a decreased incidence of delayed mortality (6 months) associated with the treatment arm. Boersma and associates[8] demonstrated a significant reduction in perioperative morbidity (2.8% to 0.8%) with the addition of β-blockers in patients with low- and intermediate-risk factors (see Table 48-1). These researchers also concluded that DSE contributes to patient evaluation only when three or more high-risk factors are present. For this high-risk subgroup, they reported a reduction in perioperative cardiac events from 11% in patients with DSE-confirmed ischemia to 2% if ischemia was absent on DSE.[8]

Based on this rationale, the American College of Cardiologists/American Heart Association (ACC/AHA) and the American College of Physicians issued guidelines in 2002 for determining the appropriate cardiac evaluation of "at risk" patients before noncardiac surgery. They suggest that no invasive testing is necessary for symptom-free individuals who have undergone cardiac revascularization in the preceding 5 years.[9,10] No clinical benefit is gained by performing preoperative revascularization before noncardiac surgery in patients without prior revascularization, and it may be harmful. Kaluza and colleagues[11] suggested an increase in perioperative cardiac morbidity (i.e., mortality, myocardial infarction, or bleeding) in patients undergoing noncardiac procedures completed soon after percutaneous transluminal coronary angioplasty (PTCA). Further conclusions suggest a benefit of scheduling noncardiac surgery two to four weeks following PTCA may avoid serious postoperative complications (reinfarction).

The lack of obvious benefit of preoperative coronary artery bypass graft (CABG) and PTCA, the preponderance of evidence suggesting a beneficial effect on the therapeutic ratio of using perioperative beta blockade, and the accuracy and ease of clinical stratification of patients based on risk factors prompted Grayburn and Hillis[5] to propose an algorithm (Fig. 48-1) for cardiac risk stratification of patients undergoing noncardiac surgery. They suggest a paradigm shift from extensive preoperative cardiac testing and risk stratification to routine perioperative therapy with β-blockers for those at risk. Other interventions, including the rapid resumption of other cardiac medications, the use of nitrates and other appropriate drugs when indicated, and a thoughtful scheme for postoperative cardiac monitoring (e.g., electrocardiogram, enzymes) are essential in an attempt to minimize perioperative cardiac morbidity. The early, judicious use of subspecialty consultation should always be considered in an effort to maximize surgical outcome.

Pelvic surgeons should find this clinical strategy to be particularly useful in patients with known or suspected gynecologic cancer because it provides an accurate assessment of operative risk in a timely fashion and avoids excessive treatment delay specifically in situations in which obtaining cardiac testing will not affect the decision to proceed with surgery. Some patients have known severe cardiac disease, demonstrating a left ventricular ejection fraction of 20%, evidence of overt right heart failure, severe aortic stenosis, or significant valvular dysfunction or failure. In this situation, it is appropriate to obtain an assessment of the woman's total life expectancy based on the cause and correctibility of the patient's cardiac condition. This information can then be weighed against the benefit of the proposed noncardiac surgical intervention to determine a therapeutic index. We propose careful consideration of the operative approach (i.e., laparoscopic, abdominal, and vaginal), type of anesthesia, and incision placement (i.e., vertical or transverse) as interventions that may favorably affect postoperative cardiac outcome. The extent of the procedure, particularly in those at significant cardiac risk, should be guided or modified as intraoperative

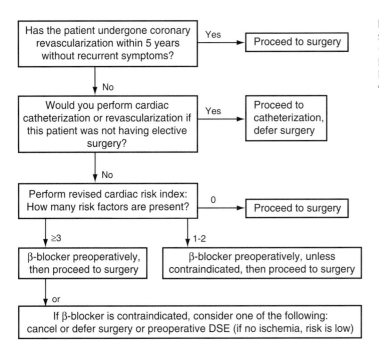

Figure 48–1. Proposed clinical algorithm for risk stratification. DSE, dobutamine stress echocardiography. (Adapted from Grayburn PA, Hillis LD: Cardiac events in patients undergoing noncardiac surgery: shifting the paradigm from noninvasive risk stratification to therapy. Ann Intern Med 2003;138:506-511.)

findings evolve because these perioperative manipulations may result in lessened perioperative cardiac morbidity and mortality. Surgeons need not be reminded that the patient's benefits from an "operative success" are minimized in the presence of perioperative cardiac-related morbidity or mortality. However, a very careful evaluation should be completed before withholding the benefits of surgery from a patient with a gynecologic cancer. It seems appropriate to obtain subspecialty consultation to assist in these sometimes difficult decisions.

Pulmonary risk. Perioperative pulmonary morbidity occurs commonly in women undergoing surgical treatment for a gynecologic cancer, presenting a confusing, frustrating, and occasionally lethal problem. Postoperative pulmonary complications (POPC) after abdominal surgery occur more frequently (10% to 30%) than cardiac complications. Postoperative respiratory failure (frequently requiring prolonged mechanical ventilation), perioperative pneumonia, bronchitis, exacerbation of chronic obstructive pulmonary disease (COPD), asthma, atelectasis, and pleural effusion represent the most frequently encountered problems. When isolated, they contribute significantly to the risk of perioperative morbidity. They frequently contribute to cardiac or other organ decompensation. Alone or in combination, they result in prolonged hospital stays and increased costs.[12-14] These pulmonary risks are exaggerated by the expected postanesthetic changes in vital capacity, functional residual capacity, ventilation-perfusion abnormalities, diaphragmatic dysfunction, decreased number and activity of alveolar macrophages inhibiting mucociliary clearance, increased alveolar-capillary permeability, enhanced pulmonary vascular sensitivity, and

resultant atelectasis.[13] Unfortunately, in contrast to cardiac disease, the clinical epidemiology, value, and role of risk assessment and the benefit of prophylactic perioperative measures to minimize pulmonary morbidity have not been succinctly elucidated in women requiring abdominopelvic surgery. Although formal spirometry may predict risks, this study lacks sensitivity and specificity compared with clinical evaluation. The lack of preoperative predictability and the lack of a widely accepted definition of perioperative pulmonary morbidity contribute to the difficulty in creating an effective plan for the prevention of perioperative morbidity.[15]

Smetana[15,16] delineated pertinent patient risk factors for postoperative pulmonary morbidity (Table 48-2). In his analysis, a smoking history (RR = 3.4) and the presence of COPD (RR = 4.7) were the major risk factors predicting the development of POPC. General health status as assessed by American Society of Anesthesiologists (ASA) classification (RR = 1.7), the

Table 48–2. Potential Patient-Related Factors for Postoperative Pulmonary Complications

Potential Risk Factor	Relative Risk
Smoking	3.4
ASA class > 2	1.7
Age > 70 yr	0.9-2.4
Obesity	0.8-1.3
COPD	2.7-4.7

ASA, American Society of Anesthesiologists; COPD, chronic obstructive pulmonary disease.
Adapted from Smetana GW: Preoperative pulmonary evaluation. N Engl J Med 1999;340:937-944.

Goldman cardiac-risk index score, or poor exercise ability were also predictive of POPC. In his review, age and obesity alone were not determined to be strong indicators for the development of POPC.[15,16]

Although these patient-related risk factors can be easily assessed, this risk index has not been independently reproduced. Even if validated as independent risk factors these clinical morbidities are unlikely to be successfully modified in a time frame that benefits the patient undergoing gynecologic cancer surgery. There is no superior intervention to lessen the potential pulmonary risk associated with age or obesity, and the opportunity to modulate important general health status is small. The presence of COPD with a restrictive or obstructive pattern represents a process whose underlying cause is not reversible. Asthma conveys a similar problem, although airflow may be maximized in the short term with the preoperative combination of physiotherapy, bronchodilators, antibiotics, and corticosteroids. The goal of maximizing airflow should be pursued aggressively in asthmatics, although no validated, uniform strategy has been elucidated. Any nonemergent abdominal surgery in these individuals should be delayed or postponed until a pattern of optimal airflow has been established.

Smoking represents the most modifiable pulmonary risk factor. Unfortunately, the effect of short-term smoking cessation has not been effective in preventing perioperative morbidity. Although some have proposed the postponement of surgery for at least 8 weeks of tobacco abstinence, a report by Warner and collegaues[17] suggests an increase in perioperative morbidity in patients who stop smoking less than 8 weeks before surgery (14.5% vs. 33%) and no benefit after the 8-week period.[15,17] Others disagree about the benefit of long-term cessation. The ability to stop smoking immediately is unusual and associated with increased anxiety. For this reason, we do not "enforce" a smoking cessation policy in the immediate preoperative period.

Smetana[15] also described procedure-related risk factors for developing POPC. Surgical site selection and the duration and type of anesthesia can affect the risk of perioperative pulmonary morbidity. In this study, surgical site was the most predictive factor for the development of POPC. The incidence of POPC increased as the incision approached the diaphragm. The lowest risk of pulmonary morbidity was associated with a laparoscopic approach in a general surgical population.[15] Duration of anesthesia (>3 hours) was also associated with a higher incidence of pulmonary morbidity.[18,19] General anesthesia has been reported to increase morbidity compared with conduction anesthesia, although results have been equivocal.[20,21] For these reasons, it would seem prudent to use the smallest and most inferior placed abdominal (transverse when appropriate) incision possible. The actual duration of anesthesia is related to a number of patient, technical, and disease factors. The pelvic surgeon should incorporate all available aspects of surgical decision-making and technique (i.e., skills and instrumentation) to minimize the need for a prolonged

---

Table 48–3. Perioperative Pulmonary Risk Reduction

Preoperative Measures
Encourage smoking cessation for at least 8 weeks.
Treat airflow obstruction in patients with chronic obstructive pulmonary disease or asthma.
Administer antibiotics if infection is present and delay surgery.
Educate the patient regarding lung-expansion maneuvers.

Intraoperative Measures
Limit surgery duration to 3 hours.
Use conduction anesthesia.*
Avoid pancuronium.
Use laparoscopy when possible.
Limit the procedure to the degree possible.

Postoperative Measures
Use incentive spirometry.
Use continuous positive airway pressure.
Use epidural analgesia.*

*Strategy recommended although variable results have been reported.
Adapted from Smetana GW: Preoperative pulmonary evaluation. N Engl J Med 1999;340:937-944.

---

anesthetic. Although conduction anesthesia alone may not facilitate the completion of an oncologic procedure, its intraoperative and postoperative use may lessen individual risks, particularly for those at high risk for POPC. Other risk reduction strategies (Table 48-3) should always be integrated into the perioperative plan.[15] Although preoperative laboratory or clinical evidence of COPD is a concern, the diagnosis should not be considered an absolute contraindication to the proposed procedure. Preoperative counseling relating the risks of the proposed procedure is vital. Chronic carbon dioxide (CO_2) retainers may benefit from a preoperative arterial blood gas determination and serum bicarbonate (HCO_3^-) or baseline measurement in an attempt to optimize postoperative management.

The question remains: Does a pulmonary condition exist that absolutely precludes surgery in the gynecologic oncology patient? The absence of validated risk assessment strategy and the inability to modify pulmonary risk factors for morbidity suggest not. Preoperative counseling with the patient and her support persons about the therapeutic index is appropriate. Attention to perioperative details is vital. In difficult clinical scenarios, early involvement of a pulmonary consultant may be the best strategy. In most situations, the patient benefits from an intensive postoperative pulmonary program.

Renal disease risk. No validated preoperative risk stratification for the development of renal insufficiency has been devised for patients undergoing noncardiac surgery.[22] A generally accepted definition of renal failure is the rise in serum creatinine over baseline by 0.5 mg/dL or more, a reduction of calculated creatinine clearance of 50%, or the need for dialysis.[23] Although vascular surgery procedures represent the highest risk, the nature of radical gynecologic cancer procedures places our patients at significant risk. Postoperative renal failure is associated with a dramatic increase in morbidity and mortality.[24]

The mortality rate may approach 45%, particularly in the presence of perioperative hypotension, sepsis, and exposure to nephrotoxic drugs.[25,26]

The gynecologic cancer patient undergoing radical surgery is potentially at risk for prerenal, intrinsic renal, or postrenal dysfunction. Dehydration, sepsis, acute blood loss, third-spacing of fluid, and exposure to nephrotoxic agents such as intravenous radiocontrast media, specific antimicrobial agents, cytotoxic agents (e.g., cisplatin), nonsteroidal anti-inflammatory drugs, angiotensin-converting enzyme (ACE) inhibitors, and radical surgery may contribute individually or in combination during a patient's care to significantly increase the incidence of renal failure. Trying to identify a particular high-risk group of patients who may develop renal insufficiency would be fruitless, because many patients would be included and no change in management would occur.

Knowing these facts, what is the optimal strategy to reduce perioperative renal morbidity? Current popular strategies for renal protection include aggressive hydration guided by the use of pulmonary artery catheters, the use of "renal-dose" dopamine, and the induction of mannitol- or furosemide-forced diuresis. Unfortunately, none of these strategies has proved effective.[27-29] Experimental agents, including prostaglandin infusion (PGE$_1$), selective dopaminergic receptor modulators, mixed dopaminergic and β-adrenergic receptor modulators such as dopexamine, growth factors (e.g., insulin-like growth factor 1, fibroblast growth factor 1), and adenosine are being evaluated.[28,30] Review of existing data suggests that no renal protective strategy exists outside of careful preoperative analysis of patients' medications, perioperative supportive care, minimizing exposure to nephrotoxic agents, and maintenance of diligent postoperative surveillance designed to detect and treat postoperative renal insufficiency. Gynecologic oncologists anxiously await the validation of efficacy of new renal protective drugs and strategies for the prevention and treatment of this devastating perioperative condition.

What is the optimal method of perioperative deep venous thrombosis prophylaxis?

Prophylaxis. Preventing the occurrence of venous thromboembolic disease (VTE) is an important aspect of perioperative gynecologic oncology care. The physician who fails to monitor, treat, or provide prophylaxis against this phenomenon will eventually fail the patient. Women undergoing gynecologic procedures for benign or malignant indications are at risk (Table 48-4). Reports suggest that the risk of deep venous thrombosis (DVT) is 1.5% to 38% after routine gynecologic surgery.[31,32] Prophylaxis is estimated to reduce risk in pooled gynecologic patients by 75% (from 0.4% to 0.1%).[31] Cancer patients are the highest-risk patients for VTE because of the fulfillment of each of Virchow's triad. The patient's risk for developing clinical VTE may extend for weeks. Development of delayed VTE is also associated with a poor cancer prognosis and is predictive of postoperative death.[31,33-36]

The Sixth ACCP Consensus Conference on Antithrombotic Therapy has evaluated various risk-reduction strategies (Table 48-5).[31] Pneumatic compression hose have become the classic method of perioperative DVT prophylaxis despite reports suggesting various degrees of success.[32,37-41] Efficacy, ease of use, and a low incidence of side effects (e.g., no postoperative bleeding) confer a high therapeutic index for pulsatile compression stockings, making them an attractive choice of prophylaxis in patients at low or intermediate risk. However, nursing and patient

---

Table 48–4. Levels of Thromboembolism Risk in Surgical Patients without Prophylaxis

Level of Risk and Examples	Calf DVT (%)	Proximal DVT (%)	Clinical PE (%)	Fatal PE (%)	Successful Prevention Strategies
Low Risk Minor surgery in patients < 40 yr with no additional risk factors	2	0.4	0.2	0.002	No specific measure Aggressive mobilization
Moderate Risk Minor surgery in patients with additional risk factors; nonmajor surgery in patients 40-60 yr with no additional risk factors; major surgery in patients < 40 yr with no additional risk factors	10-20	2-4	1-2	0.1-0.4	LDUH q12h, LMWH, ES, or IPC
High Risk Nonmajor surgery in patients > 60 yr or with additional risk factors; major surgery in patients > 40 yr or with additional risk factors	20-40	4-8	2-4	0.4-1.0	LDUH q8h, LMWH, or IPC
Highest Risk Major risk in patients > 40 yr plus prior VTE, cancer, or molecular hypercoagulable state; hip or knee arthroplasty, hip fracture surgery; major trauma; spinal cord injury	40-80	10-20	4-10	0.2-5	LMWH, oral anticoagulators, IPC/ES + LDUH/LMWH, or ADH

ADH, adjusted-dose heparin; DVT, deep venous thrombosis; ES, elastic stockings; IPC, intermittent pneumatic compression; LDUH, low-dose unfractionated heparin; LMWH, low-molecular-weight heparin; PE, pulmonary embolism; VTE, venous thromboembolism.
Adapted from Geerts WH, Heit JA, Clagett GP, et al: Prevention of venous thromboembolism. Chest 2001;119(Suppl):132S-175S.

Table 48-5. Prevention of Deep Venous Thrombosis after Gynecologic Surgery

Regimen	No. of Trials*	No. of Patients	Incidence of DVT (%)	95% CI	Relative Risk Reduction (%)
Untreated control subjects	12	945	16	14-19	—
Oral anticoagulants	5	183	13	8-18	22
IPC	2	132	3	1-8	88
LDUH	47	10339	8	7-8	68
ES	3	196	14	10-20	44

*Data pooled from randomized trials that used routine ^{125}I-fibrinogen uptake test results as the primary outcome.
DVT, deep venous thrombosis; ES, elastic stockings; IPC, intermittent pneumatic compression; LDUH, low-dose unfractionated heparin.
Adapted from Geerts WH, Heit JA, Clagett GP, et al: Prevention of venous thromboembolism. Chest 2001;119(Suppl): 132S-175S.

noncompliance is not uncommon and often frustrating to the physician. Venous compression hose may not represent sufficient prophylaxis for the higher risk patients; women with gynecologic cancer, a history of DVT, or who are older than 60 years of age represent a subgroup of patients most likely to fail intermittent pneumatic compression prophylaxis.[42] This "ultra-high-risk" group may benefit from a more intense combination prophylactic regimen, and a strategy of early postoperative mobilization, initiation of intermittent pneumatic compression hose, and heparin should be considered.[42]

Although in-hospital prophylaxis should be routine, questions remain about the optimal duration of prophylaxis. Patients should be ambulatory before discharge and should be encouraged to increase their ambulatory activities. The postdischarge use of intermittent pneumatic compression may not be feasible and to our knowledge has not been evaluated. Bergqvist and coworkers[43] concluded that continued postdischarge administration of low-molecular-weight heparin (LMWH) might reduce VTE risk in patients with abdominopelvic malignancies. In this trial, 332 patients were given 6 to 10 in-hospital days of LMWH and then randomized to receive subcutaneous placebo or subcutaneous enoxaparin (40 mg) for an additional 21 days. Venography was performed between days 25 and 31. The rate of venous thromboembolism at the end of the double-blind phase was significantly different: 12.0% in the placebo group and 4.8% in the enoxaparin group ($P = .02$). This clinical and statistical significant difference persisted at 3 months (13.8% versus 5.5%, $P = .01$). There were no differences in the incidence of bleeding or other complications during the double-blind or follow-up periods. This report suggests that long-term (4 weeks) postoperative enoxaparin prophylaxis is safe and significantly reduces the incidence of venographically demonstrated thrombosis to a greater degree than does 1 week of enoxaparin prophylaxis.[43] It seems reasonable to offer some form of prophylaxis to all women treated for a gynecologic cancer, using combinations in those at very high risk and consideration of prolonged therapy in those at highest risk.

Treatment of diagnosed venous thromboembolic disease. The management of the patient with the perioperative diagnosis of VTE disease represents a difficult dilemma. A patient whose initial clinical presentation includes active DVT or pulmonary emboli creates the necessity to manage the embolic process as well as the diagnosed malignancy. A prolonged surgical delay may not be feasible or appropriate. The gynecologic oncologist is then forced to artfully combine primary treatment modalities: systemic anticoagulation with unfractionated (UF) or LMWH and the placement of an inferior vena cava (IVC) filter to minimize the risk of embolic phenomena. The use of intravenous or subcutaneous treatment-dose heparin with a temporary discontinuation of therapy 6 hours before surgery and with resumption 6 to 12 hours (or longer) after surgery can be used. Incorporating LMWH with its lower reported incidence of bleeding complications using a strategy of dose reduction in the hours immediately before and after surgery offers the advantage of continuous anticoagulation with minimal risk for the duration of surgery.[44]

Those at highest risk for intraoperative bleeding or propagation of VTE are candidates for IVC filter placement.[45] Disadvantages of IVC filter placement alone include potential intraoperative filter dislodgment and mechanical disruption of hemicorporeal blood flow because of an insufficient azygous system. The latter may result in lower extremity edema, with its severest manifestation a compartment syndrome.[46-48] If possible, it is preferable to delay surgery for up to 1 month after the diagnosis of VTE because of the high rate of thromboembolism. If delay is not feasible, the use of systemic anticoagulation with LMWH or intravenous UF heparin for several days after the diagnosis of VTE to allow clot stabilization is recommended. However, if bleeding (i.e., uterine, intra-abdominal, or systemic) prohibits the use of anticoagulation and surgery is necessary, our second choice involves IVC filter placement with a delay or 24 to 48 hours to allow the filter to settle. Once deemed safe, we begin systemic anticoagulation despite filter placement to prevent clotting of the IVC at the filter site and to promote stabilization of existing thrombi.

Prolonged treatment of patients at risk for recurrence of VTE with warfarin (Coumadin) is appropriate, titrating to an international normalized ratio of 2 to 3 for a planned 6-month treatment. One study suggests a benefit of longer, lower-intensity treatment in noncancer patients.[49] A randomized study comparing LMWH and coumarin suggested a 50% risk reduction for recurrent VTE in cancer patients undergoing treatment.[50] Confirmatory studies are needed, but a benefit of prolonged therapy may exist in cancer patients outside the perioperative period with LMWH during postsurgical irradiation or chemotherapy.

What constitutes optimal perioperative management of the gastrointestinal tract?

Gynecologic surgical procedures are associated with minor, major, and even catastrophic complications involving the gastrointestinal tract. These perioperative events occur more frequently during the extensive procedures often necessary for the initial diagnosis and treatment of women with a pelvic malignancy. Risks of intestinal morbidity are also increased after operations necessary to manage recurrent disease or treatment-related problems. Efforts to minimize the frequency and associated morbidity of gastrointestinal complications require attention to important aspects of preoperative evaluation, preparation, and postoperative care. Although no single management algorithm for gastrointestinal tract care suits all clinical situations, the existing literature can be used to guide the pelvic surgeon in the development of a sound, flexible care plan that results in an increased likelihood of a favorable outcome.

Preoperative screening and evaluation. Colorectal (including anal) cancer will be diagnosed in 77,000 women this year[51] (Table 48-6) representing a significant overall risk in the female population nearly equal to the combined incidence of all reproductive tract cancers. It is of particular importance to the gynecologic oncologist because women diagnosed with reproductive tract cancer, particularly after the diagnosis of endometrial or ovarian disease, carry an increased risk of a concurrent or later diagnosis of gastrointestinal malignancy (Table 48-7).[52,53] The threefold increased risk of colorectal malignancy in this

Table 48–6. Women's Cancers, 2003

Anatomic Site	New Cases	Deaths
Reproductive Tract		
Cervix	12,200	4,100
Corpus	41,100	6,800
Ovary	25,400	14,300
Vulva	4,000	800
Other	2,000	800
Total reproductive tract cancers	84,700	26,800
Breast	211,300	39,800
Gastrointestinal Tract		
Colon	56,500	28,800
Rectum	18,200	3,800
Anus	2,300	300
Total gastrointestinal tract cancers	77,000	32,900
Total for all sites	373,000	99,500

From Jemal A, Murray T, Samuels A, et al: Cancer statistics, 2003. CA Cancer J Clin 2003;52:23-47.

Table 48–7. Risk of Colorectal Cancer in Women with Gynecologic Cancer

Known Gynecologic Cancer	Risks of Colorectal Cancer (RR)*
Cervix	1.0
Endometrial cancer	
< 50 years old	3.39
Ovarian cancer	
< 50 years old	3.67
50-64 years old	1.52

*For 101,754 women in the Surveillance, Epidemiology and End Results (SEER) database, 1974-1995.
From Rex D: Should we colonoscope women with gynecologic cancer? Am J Gastroenterol 2000;95:812-813.

patient subpopulation suggests the need for active surveillance. The incidence of colonic metastases to the reproductive tract is significant and should be in the differential diagnosis when operating on women with an adnexal mass and a previous history of colorectal cancer.[54] Incidentally, significant gynecologic abnormalities are commonly discovered in women during surgical treatment of an intestinal cancer.[55]

Evidence suggests that colorectal cancer screening decreases disease-related mortality,[56-58] which has encouraged efforts of early detection and resulted in the development of numerous screening strategies (Table 48-8).[56-58] Although each organization's recommendation may differ slightly, the consensus opinion is that appropriate screening should be offered to all women. Although individual issues and uncertainly relating to the cost-effectiveness and efficacy of specific screening studies continue to make "absolute" recommendations unavailable, it appears that the use of colonoscopy is becoming the preferred screening strategy.[56-58] The preponderance of scientific information suggests that clinicians have multiple screening options that can be easily and successfully incorporated into routine practice. Although individual recommendations are appropriate, they may differ in relation to patient-risk stratification.[59,60] Women at high risk, defined as those with a previous diagnosis of colorectal cancer or adenomatous polyp, predisposing colorectal disease (e.g., inflammatory bowel disease), or a significant personal or family history (i.e., hereditary nonpolyposis colorectal cancer) may require a different approach or screening strategy.[56-60] New technologies, including virtual colonoscopy, molecular markers, and fecal DNA testing, have great promise but have not yet become a part of accepted testing.[56-60]

Although not necessarily involved with routine colorectal screening, gynecologic oncologists are frequently faced with the option or necessity of preoperative gastrointestinal evaluation. Although the results obtained during screening for primary colon disease or determining the presence of primary or secondary intestinal involvement with a diagnosed pelvic process can be confusing, the decision to offer routine preoperative endoscopic or radiologic evaluation should be simplified. Preoperative gastrointestinal testing should be considered particularly when the

Table 48-8. Colorectal Cancer Screening

Test	Preventative Services Task	Gastrointestinal Consortium*	American College of Gastroenterology†	American Cancer Society‡
Year of screening standards	1996 (revised 2002†)	1997 (revised 2003)	2000	2003
Frequency of 3-sample fecal occult-blood testing alone	Yearly	Yearly	Yearly	Yearly at age 50 yr
Frequency of sigmoidoscopy	Unspecified	5 years	5 years	5 years at age 50 yr
Frequency of 3-sample fecal occult-blood testing plus colonoscopy	Insufficient evidence	Every year and every 5 years, respectively	Every year and every 5 years, respectively	Every year and every 5 years, respectively
Colonoscopy	Insufficient evidence for or against the test	10 years (preferred strategy)	10 years (preferred strategy)	10 years
Barium enema	Insufficient evidence for or against the test	5 years	5-10 years	5 years at age 50 yr

*Data from Winawer S, Fletcher R, Rex D, et al: Colorectal cancer screening and surveillance: Clinical guidelines and rational—update based on new evidence. Gastroenterology 2003;124:544-560.
†Data from Ransohoff D, Sandler R: Screening for colorectal cancer. N Engl J Med 2002;346:40-44.
‡Data from Smith R, Cokkinides V, Eyre H: American Cancer Society guidelines for the early detection of cancer, 2003. CA Cancer J Clin 2003;53:27-43.

findings would significantly alter the treatment approach. It seems logical to obtain the patient's previous history of routine colorectal screening. For those with documented gynecologic cancer and negative stool results for occult blood, additional studies should be based on the patient's risk factors and the presence of significant clinical findings. Available information regarding women with apparent early-stage cervical[61] or uterine[62] malignancy suggests, in the absence of clinical suspicion, that gastrointestinal studies are usually unrevealing (related to involvement with the gynecologic cancer).

Unfortunately, there is little evidence to indicate the benefit of preoperative studies to correctly predict colon involvement or the necessity of colon resection in women with ovarian cancer (Table 48-9).[63-65] Neither endoscopic nor radiologic studies can adequately predict the need for intestinal resection. Normal studies do not preclude the necessity of colonic resection. Although no strict guidelines can be stated, the prudent pelvic surgeon should offer preoperative colon or intestinal evaluation in clinical situations in which abnormalities are likely to be present and when those findings will alter the treatment approach. Colonoscopy can often be obtained without significant delay.[65] This approach may be modified by the presence of other factors, particularly the patient's age.[65] Negative findings may not be reassuring, and the preoperative consenting process should typically include the possibility, rationale, and implications of intestinal surgery regardless of colonoscopic findings. Post-treatment surveillance of the colon can be accomplished according to the patient's risk factors and established guidelines (see Table 48-8).

Preoperative preparation. There are numerous theoretical benefits (Table 48-10) of mechanical bowel preparation. Since its introduction[66] in 1973 and despite the lack of clear scientific proof of benefit, colorectal surgeons typically (99%) use mechanical bowel preparation before elective procedures likely to require intestinal resection (Table 48-11).[67] This dogma has been followed by gynecologic oncologists and other surgeons during the preoperative preparation of individuals deemed at risk for necessary gastrointestinal surgery. A significant volume of scientific literature has been devoted to establishing the optimal method of mechanical preparation.[68] Although numerous options exist, the growing consensus of colorectal surgeons suggests that sodium phosphate (90 mL) combined with clear liquids is a favored, cost-effective, well-tolerated regimen for mechanical bowel cleansing.[68,69] However, a mechanical preparation is not entirely harmless. Patient discomfort, electrolyte imbalance, and dehydration have been frequently described.

The role, benefit, and optimal regimen of perioperative antibiotic administration for colorectal surgery

Table 48-9. Predictive Value of Preoperative Sigmoidoscopy in 30 Patients with Ovarian Cancer

Measurement	Correct Prediction/ No. of Patients	Predictive Value
Satisfactory preparation		70%
Correct prediction to avoid resection	21/25	84%
Correct prediction to resect	5/9	56%

Adapted from Gornall R, Talbot R: Can flexible sigmoidoscopy predict need for colorectal surgery in ovarian carcinoma? Eur J Gynaecol Oncol 1999;20:13-15.

Table 48-10. Potential Benefits of Mechanical Bowel Preparation

Removes fecal material
Lowers the bacterial load
Improves handling
Reduces spillage and contamination
Lessens risk of mechanical disruption
Facilitates intraoperative palpation
Allows intraoperative colonoscopy
Aids laparoscopic handling

Table 48–11. Preferences of 515 Colorectal Surgeons for Bowel Preparation

Preparation	Preference
Routinely use mechanical preparation	99%
Sodium phosphate	47%
Polyethylene glycol	32%
Oral antibiotics: considered essential	50%
Doubtful	41%
Unnecessary	10%
Routinely use oral antibiotics	75% (96% use two antibiotics)
Routinely use intravenous antibiotics	98% (avg. no. of postoperative doses = 2)

Adapted from Zmora O, Wexner S, Hajjar L, et al: Trends in preparation for colorectal surgery: Survey of the members of the American Society of Colon and Rectal Surgeons. Am Surg 2003:69:150-154.

remain controversial. The use of oral, parenteral, or combination prophylaxis has been described and defended.[69] Typically, the oral regimen includes erythromycin and neomycin (sometimes metronidazole), but the lack of prospective randomized data[69] confirming a benefit, combined with the incidence of preoperative nausea and vomiting, raises suspicions about its usefulness. The use of perioperative parenteral antibiotics has been evaluated in a number of randomized studies, and available information strongly suggests their efficacy as a potential substitute (Table 48-12) for oral antibiotics.[69] Although no single drug or regimen has documented superiority, the administration of a short course of a broad-spectrum antibiotic (single dose if the surgery is not twice as long as the drug half-life) is appropriate. Most surgeons continue to combine oral and parenteral antibiotics[70] in an effort to improve outcome.

Despite strict adherence to existing dogma, prospective reports have not confirmed a protective benefit of preoperative mechanical preparation.[69,70] The prospective data (Table 48-13) have specifically failed to demonstrate a lessened risk of wound or abdominal infection. The incidence of anastomotic breakdown was not lowered. Although reports are uncontrolled for surgical indications, perioperative antibiotic regimen, actual procedure (left versus right colon resection), surgical technique, and associated comorbidities (i.e., obstruction, cancer), these results suggest that colonic anastomoses can be safely performed in women even in the absence of a mechanical preparation. As these data mature and additional prospective, randomized studies are reported, it would seem prudent to continue a careful preoperative consenting process and the use of a mechanical preparation if for no other reason than to improve intraoperative handling. These data indicate that, if necessary, the pelvic surgeon can complete a colonic resection and reanastomosis in the presence of an unprepared colon without increasing infectious or breakdown morbidity. It appears that bowel preparation is not a sine qua non for safe colorectal surgery.[71]

The difficulties and concerns of operating on women with a distal colon obstruction have been lessened with the development of expandable colonic stents.[72] Stent placement can be associated with technical failure, perforation, and delayed complications, but stent use in patients with complete or near-complete colonic obstruction may allow stabilization to optimize preoperative preparation. In specific clinical situations, this procedure may offer significant palliation and lessen the need for open operative intervention.

Postoperative care. Optimization of postoperative care of the gastrointestinal tract requires an understanding of normal postoperative recovery of intestinal function. Numerous factors influence intestinal healing (Table 48-14), and the astute pelvic surgeon

Table 48–12. Randomized Clinical Studies Comparing Intravenous Antibiotic Prophylaxis with No Intravenous Prophylaxis for Colorectal Surgery

Study	Year	N	Intravenous Antibiotics/Control	Infections (%)
Barber et al.	1997	59	Gentamicin + clindamycin/placebo	7 vs 1
Eykyn et al.	1997	83	Metronidazole/placebo	6 vs 2*
Wetterfors and Hoejer	1980	118	Doxycycline/placebo	12.4 vs 45*
Hoffmann et al.	1981	65	Cefoxitin/placebo	3 vs 27*
Beggs et al.	1982	97	Metronidazole/oral metronidazole	9.8 vs 13
Portnoy et al.	1983	104	Cefazolin/placebo	35 vs 7*
Condon et al.	1983	1128	Cephalothin/placebo	5.7 vs 7.8
Lewis et al.	1983	44	Cefazolin/oral erythromycin + neomycin	14 vs 2*
Edmondson and Rissing	1983	133	Cephaloridine (IM)/oral erythromycin + neomycin	12.3 vs 1.7*
Gomez-Alonso et al.	1984	188	Gentamicin + metronidazole/placebo	9 vs 39*
Jagelman et al.	1985	68	Metronidazole/placebo	0 vs 22*
Lau et al.	1988	194	Gentamicin + metronidazole/oral erythromycin + neomycin	27 vs 12*
Petrelli et al.	1988	70	Cefamandole/placebo	0 vs 2.8
Schoetz	1990	197	Cefoxitin/placebo	10 vs 22*
Stellato et al.	1990	169	Cefoxitin/oral erythromycin + neomycin	11.4 vs 11.7

*P < .05.
IM, intramuscular, N, number of patients.
Adapted from Zmora O, Pikarsky AJ, Wexner SD: Bowel preparation for colorectal surgery. Dis Colon Rectum 2001;44:1537-1549.

Table 48–13. Randomized, Prospective Studies Considering whether Mechanical Bowel Preparation Is Necessary

Study	No. of Patients	Wound		Abdominal		Anastomotic Breakdown (%)	
		P+	P–	P+	P–	P+	P–
Brownson (1992)	179	5.8	7.5	9.3*	2.2	12.0*	1.5
Burke (1994)	186	4.9	3.4			3.7	4.6
Santos (1994)	149	24.0*	12.0			10.0	0.0
Miettinan (2000)	267	4.0	2.0	2.0	3.0	4.0	2.0
Zmora (2003)	380	6.4	5.7	1.1	1.0	3.7	2.1

*$P < .05$.
P+, mechanical bowel preparation used; P–, no bowel preparation used.
Data from Zmora O, Pikarsky AJ, Wexner SD: Bowel preparation for colorectal surgery. Dis Colon Rectum 2001;44:1537-1549; and from Zmora O, Mahajna A, Bar-Zakai B, et al: Colon and rectal surgery without mechanical bowel preparation: A randomized prospective trial. Am Surg 2003;237: 363-367.

will attempt to manipulate all aspects of the procedure and postoperative care to facilitate recovery and minimize the risk of adverse effects. Although specific patient comorbidities (i.e., previous irradiation, diabetes) may minimize the ability to modulate some factors, preoperative recognition facilitates surgical planning and appropriate discussion during the consenting process.

Although the surgical approach may influence the exact time, normal function returns in the stomach and small intestine, the right colon, and sigmoid colon at 8, 48, and 72 hours, respectively, after an abdominal procedure.[73] Evidence suggests little adverse effect on return of bowel function related to duration of surgery, intestinal manipulation, the use of narcotics, or performing a retroperitoneal dissection. Despite this information, surgical dogma to use nasogastric suction has persisted.[74] A 1999 survey[74] suggested that gynecologic oncologists commonly incorporate nasogastric suction after cytoreductive procedures (57%), lymphadenectomy (34%), radical hysterectomy (29%), and "routine hysterectomy" (15%). They almost always use suction after colon resection (90%) and small bowel resection (97%). The rationale for use was to decrease distention (67%), avoid an anastomotic leak (39%), and lessen nausea (36%).

Table 48–14. Factors Influencing Gastrointestinal Healing

Local Factors	Systemic Factors
Adequate blood supply	Patient nutrition
Absence of anastomotic tension	Sepsis
Healthy tissue edges	Hypovolemia
Bacterial contamination	Medications (e.g., steroids,
Distal obstruction	nonsteroidal anti-inflammatory
Radiation injury	drugs, 5-fluorouracil)
Bowel preparation	Immunocompetence
Hyperthermia	Blood transfusion
	Uremia
	Jaundice

Collective reviews suggest that there is little benefit for the use of nasogastric suction after an abdominal procedure (Table 48-15). A meta-analysis of 3964 patients failed to support a benefit of routine nasogastric decompression. When comparing selective nasogastric suction to routine use after elective laparotomy, there was actually a decreased risk of pneumonia, fever, and overall complication rate when suction was omitted.[75] It appears that approximately 5% of women require some form of postlaparotomy decompression. It makes little clinical sense to routinely use nasogastric suction rather than initiate it only for those in need (1 of 20). This meta-analysis reports no difference in the incidence of death, aspiration, nausea, vomiting, abdominal distention, wound dehiscence, wound infection, anastomotic leak, and length of stay. This information has been reproduced in women undergoing gynecologic cancer procedures,[76] colon resection,[77] and even gastric procedures.[78]

Occasionally, patients may be at extreme risk of a prolonged postoperative ileus (i.e., extensive dissection after irradiation). In those circumstances, intraoperative gastrostomy tube placement should be considered as a comfortable alternative.[79]

During the past decade, in part because of the increased use of laparoscopic surgery, there has been increased attention to the potential benefits of early oral feeding. Although criteria for early feeding differ, the preponderance of evidence (Table 48-16) suggests that in most clinical situations, including those after colorectal surgery, early oral feeding is well tolerated, typically associated with shorter hospital stays, and does not increase the risk of ileus or other complications.[73,80] Although optimal methods of intestinal stimulation remain to be delineated,[73,80,81] it has become evident that the surgical dogma of increasing diet in a graduated manner is no longer a valid dictum of postoperative care. The rapid advancement of oral intake is safe, cost-effective, and well tolerated by most women undergoing abdominal surgery.

Infectious and obstructive complications after gastrointestinal procedures represent serious morbidity.

Table 48–15. Risks and Benefits of Nasogastric Decompression in a Meta-analysis of 3964 Patients*

Factors Considered	Selective Nasogastric Suction	Routine Nasogastric Suction	P Value	RR
No. of patients	1986	1978		
Tubes placed/replaced	103 (5.2%)	36 (1.8%)	<.0001	2.9
Complication	833 (42%)	1084 (55%)	.03	0.76
Pneumonia	53 (2.7%)	119 (6%)	<.0001	0.49
Fever	108 (5.4%)	212 (10.7%)	.02	0.51
Oral feeding (days)	3.53	4.59	.04	

*No difference in deaths, aspiration, nausea, vomiting, abdominal distention, wound dehiscence, wound infection, anastomotic leak, or length of stay.
From Cheatham M, Chapman W, Key S, Sawyers J: A meta-analysis of selective versus routine nasogastric decompression after elective laparotomy. Ann Surg 1995;221:469-478.

It appears that routine drainage does not lessen risks,[82] but clinical suspicion should allow early diagnosis. Infectious complications are frequently controlled with the institution of appropriate broad-spectrum antibiotics. Intra-abdominal abscesses are usually (85%) managed successfully with percutaneous drainage.[83]

After excluding the possibility of strangulation, adhesive postoperative obstruction is typically successfully managed conservatively, with resolution frequently occurring within 48 hours.[84] Early use of contrast-enhanced radiology should be considered for those without resolution in 48 hours because this carries a high predictive value for nonoperative treatment success.[85]

What constitutes the optimal incision or approach for a gynecologic cancer procedure?

Numerous patient-related factors (Table 48-17) can adversely impact surgical outcome. Surgical incision site problems often are significant indicators of morbidity.[86] The classic wound healing paradigm of inflammation, proliferation, and remodeling[87] involves extensive cytokine activity and culminates in a predictable method and time of wound repair. Any number of comorbidities working through different mechanisms can and do dramatically affect the outcome of the wound and recovery as it relates to the abdominal, vaginal, adnexal, retroperitoneal, gastrointestinal, or urogenital incision.

Although preoperative consideration of the patient's preference, habitus, cosmetic outcome, and expected pathology are important, the guiding premise of incision placement or choice of approach should be the goal of providing adequate intraoperative exposure. Regardless of the initial surgical plan, the prudent pelvic surgeon develops alternatives to improve exposure as necessitated by intraoperative findings. These alternatives should be outlined during the preoperative consenting process. Perhaps the only wrong incision or approach is one that prohibits an adequate surgical effort.

The debate on the subject of the benefits of an open operation versus a laparoscopic approach has been ongoing. Advocates of an open (vertical or transverse), laparoscopic, or vaginal approach each have valid arguments.[88-90] The surgeon's experience and bias represent an important factor in decision-making. The

Table 48–16. Prospective, Randomized Trials Considering Early Oral Feeding

Study	Procedure	Comments
Seenu (1995)	Colorectal (open)	No difference in nasogastric tube placement, ileus, or hospital stay; vomiting (21% vs 14%)
Hartsel (1997)	Colorectal	No difference in nausea, vomiting, or hospital stay
Pearl (1998)	Gynecologic oncologic	Decreased time to bowel sounds and decreased hospital stay
Stewart (1998)	Colorectal (open)	80% of patients tolerated a regular diet within 48 hr; no difference in vomiting or nasogastric tube placement; earlier return of bowel function and shorter hospital stay
Cutillo (1999)	Gynecologic oncologic	Less ileus, earlier return of bowel function, decreased time to regular diet
Macmillan (2000)	Gynecologic	No difference in ileus or intestinal function; nausea (23% vs 13%)

Table 48–17. Patient-Related Factors Potentially Influencing Surgical Approach, Incision Placement, and Wound Outcome

Age
Cardiopulmonary disease
Current chemotherapy
Diabetes
Hepatic insufficiency
Hypoxemia
Immunocompetence
Nutritional status
Obesity
Previous incision site, outcome, or current abdominal wall anatomy
Prior radiation therapy
Renal insufficiency
Sepsis
Surgical indication or expectation
Vascular disease

pertinent aspects of laparoscopic surgical adequacy, conversion rates, blood loss, duration of hospitalization, perioperative pain, and time to return to full activity have been reviewed for benign gynecologic procedures and gynecologic cancer operations.[88-94] Although restrictions related to the patient's weight, previous surgery, and the operator's experience are applicable, review of the scientific facts strongly suggests that when appropriate, a minimally invasive or laparoscopic procedure offers specific advantages and can be successfully used in many women during the treatment of cervical, endometrial, and ovarian disease without compromising outcome. Minimally invasive procedures can add diagnostic value in the management of suspicious but undiagnosed disease (i.e., ovarian masses) and may contribute to primary staging or restaging of patients with an incomplete initial procedure or in those with an advanced-stage gynecologic malignancy.[95] Laparoscopy can also add value in the care and management of patients who desire preservation of reproductive potential.[96]

When a laparoscopic approach is not deemed appropriate, it has become apparent that the dogma requiring oncologic procedures to be completed through a vertical incision is no longer valid.[97,98] The transverse incision (muscle or nonsplitting) has been recognized to be safe and adequate to allow a therapeutic procedure in patients with cervical and endometrial disease. Less pain, improved postoperative pulmonary function, shortened hospitalization, and a good cosmetic outcome represent major potential advantages. Minilap procedures have been reported to be as cost-effective as a laparoscopic approach, particularly as it relates to duration of hospitalization and time to full recovery.[99] Although not routine, a primary vaginal approach[100,101] may have value in specific clinical situations (i.e., morbidly obese patients) and should be considered a vital part of the gynecologic oncologists surgical armamentarium.

Myriad intraoperative findings (e.g., during examination under anesthesia, unexpected disease spread) limit the ability to absolutely predict the adequacy of any approach or incision (or extension of a previous incision). However, appropriate preoperative discussion of these plans, their rationales, and additional possibilities forms the groundwork of informed consent and may lessen patient anxiety associated with the proposed procedure.

Regardless of the initial choice of surgical approach, the astute pelvic surgeon evaluates all existing comorbidities (see Table 48-17) and intertwines the surgical indications with the expected findings and the presence and outcome of previous incisions (including indications and actual operative procedures) to approach the abdominal wall in an effort to maximize outcome. Regardless of the designated approach, it is the surgeon's responsibility to ensure the availability of adequate instrumentation and adequate surgical assistance in a manner that will likely optimize outcome.

Age. The elderly, whose demographics mirror the incidence of premalignant or malignant reproductive tract disease, represent the fastest growing segment of the U.S. population.[102] In 10 years, almost 10,000 Americans will celebrate their 65th birthday each day. The older population will double to 70 million, representing almost 20% of the U.S. population in 2030. Age alone should not be the major decision factor determining surgical approach, procedure, or incision placement. However, aging is associated with a gradual attenuation of the inflammatory response and an age-dependent decrease in the proliferative potential of fibroblasts. This population frequently exhibits multiple coexisting medical morbidities, and although the elderly typically tolerate a well-planned procedure, these coexisting processes lower physiologic reserves, rendering them unable to accommodate the demands necessary to recover after the occurrence of significant complications.

Obesity. The epidemic of obesity in this country places a stress on all aspects of the medical system. The risk of wound infection (which can be correlated to the depth of subcutaneous tissue), superficial dehiscence, evisceration, and hernia are all increased.[103] Although weight reduction is desirable, awaiting preoperative weight loss is not typically an option. Successful surgery in obese patients is more likely when special attention is devoted to the technical aspects of incision inscription. Precise efforts to minimize the creation of necrotic tissue (scalpel versus cautery), minimize dead space (single bold stroke), and maximize hemostasis are vital. Although most laparoscopic procedures can be performed in the obese, advanced or complex procedures (e.g., retroperitoneal dissection) are less likely to be successfully completed. Many gynecologic oncologists prefer to avoid transverse incisions during open operations in the morbidly obese, and a vertical incision may be better placed in the supraumbilical part of the abdomen.[104]

Nutritional status. Many women with gynecologic cancer exhibit measurable nutritional deficits.[105] There is ample evidence to suggest a serious adverse effect on the healing process and on recovery.[97,106] Although not clinically apparent, nutritional deficits have an adverse effect on wound outcome, with severe impairment occurring in the seriously malnourished. Although preoperative enteral or parenteral hyperalimentation can be prescribed, most patients require timely surgical intervention, which limits the time frame for "helpful" support.[107] The role of postoperative nutritional support should always be considered as a surgical adjunct for those at risk.

Cardiopulmonary disease. Cardiopulmonary disease (in the absence of a severe hypoxemia) may exert minimal direct effect on surgical-site outcome. However, it may alter surgical approach or incision placement. Anesthesia is not physiologic because it modifies neural tone; it is arrhythmogenic and exerts a depressant effect on myocardial contractility.[108] When significant cardiopulmonary disease is present, it seems appropriate to plan and perform an efficient procedure to minimize the risk of untoward cardiac or pulmonary events. It may be inappropriate to avoid a vertical incision in the woman with severely compromised pulmonary function or to avoid a laparoscopic approach if it will unduly prolong anesthesia.

Diabetes. Postoperative hyperglycemia adversely affects wound outcome.[109] This process may be related to a direct suppression of macrophage activity, but the associated long-term vascular effects of diabetes may alter small-vessel blood supply, rendering the wound at risk.[110] It is prudent to develop a postoperative plan that controls blood sugar levels (<150 mg/dl) and maintains volume replacement to optimize the wound's blood supply. The use of intravenous insulin infusion, when necessary, allows smooth glycemic control.

Renal or hepatic insufficiency. Regardless of cause, renal insufficiency, elevated creatinine levels, and measurable liver function abnormalities correlate with poor wound outcome. Choosing an approach or incision that minimizes trauma to the abdominal wall is imperative. The decision to operate on these individuals with serious dysfunction should be undertaken cautiously.

Chemotherapy and irradiation. Although the use of postoperative chemotherapy (after day 21) does not apparently interfere with short-term and long-term wound outcome, the indirect effects of concurrent chemotherapy, including thrombocytopenia, anemia, and neutropenia, may be disastrous.[97] Growth factor support may assist in minimizing this risk, but these factors predispose to wound infection and poor late wound outcome. Previous ionizing radiation results in microvascular injury, placing the abdominal wound at risk. The choice of incision placement may be affected, and meticulous surgical technique is mandatory to lessen risks of an operation in an irradiated field.[111]

Previous incision site. It is not unusual for women being surgically treated for a gynecologic malignancy to have previously undergone single or multiple operative abdominal procedures. Any reentry abdominal incision carries the risk of encountering increased intra-abdominal adhesive disease with the potential for bowel injury, adding caution to all procedures but particularly to a laparoscopic approach. Although reentry incisions potentially create a less than optimal closure, specific care should be taken to avoid the placement of a new parallel or crossing incision, which may interrupt the abdominal wall blood supply. Intuitively, the operative approach should be carefully considered in situations that signify a poor previous wound outcome and resultant abnormal abdominal wall anatomy. In these situations, the potential need for abdominal wall repair with or without mesh placement becomes an important consideration.

Any operation can be associated with considerable adhesions that result in significant morbidity, hospitalizations, and costs. Although not yet adequately evaluated after radical procedures, the incorporation of techniques (e.g., gentle tissue handling, meticulous

Table 48–18. Surgeon-Related Factors Potentially Influencing Surgical Approach, Incision Placement, and Wound Outcome

Antibiotic prophylaxis
Closure technique
Drains
Dressing
Experience
Incision management
  Placement
  Method
  Hemostasis
Oxygenation
Preoperative stay
Preparation
  Patient
  Staff
Suture material
Temperature homeostasis
Vasoconstrictors

hemostasis, precise treatment) and the addition of specific surgical adjuncts, including oxidized-regenerated cellulose (Intercede), modified hyaluronic acid, carboxymethylcellulose (Seprafilm), and ferric hyaluronate gel (Intergel), should be considered.[112]

Hypoxemia, sepsis, an altered immune status, and coexisting vascular disease have direct adverse effects on wound outcome. The pelvic surgeon must recognize these risks and incorporate strategies that minimize their impact. Although many minimally modifiable, patient-related factors exist, the pelvic surgeon controls a number of very important variables that potentially lessen risks (Table 48-18).

Surgical experience. Surgical technique and outcomes, particularly for extensive surgical procedures, improve in direct relation to previous training and to ongoing experience.[113] Technique-related complications (Table 48-19) represent 24% of all adverse

Table 48–19. Adverse Surgical Events

Type of Event*	Surgical Events (%) (n = 402)	Preventable (%)
Technique-related complication	24.2	68
Wound infection	11.2	23
Postoperative bleeding	10.8	85
Postpartum or neonatal events	8.3	67
Other infections	7.0	38
Drug-related injury	6.5	46
Wound problem	4.0	53
Deep venous thrombosis	3.7	18
Pulmonary embolism	2.3	14
Acute myocardial infarction	2.1	100
Congestive heart failure	1.2	33
Stroke	1.2	0
Total		54

*Of 15,000 nonpsychiatric admissions in Utah and Colorado in 1992, 1 in 7 resulted in permanent disability or death.
From Gawande AA, Thomas EJ, Zinner MJ, Brennan TA: The incidence and nature of surgical adverse events in Colorado and Utah in 1992. Surgery 1999;126:66-75.

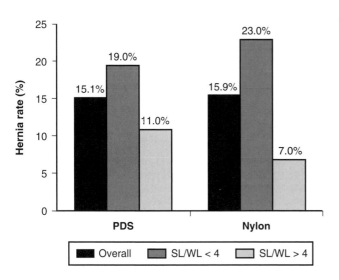

Figure 48–2. Effect of the ratio of suture length (SL) to wound length (WL) on the rate of incisional hernias.

surgical events, and up to 68% are preventable. Wound infection (11%) and wound problems (4%, with 53% of these preventable) contribute significantly to the overall incidence of adverse surgical events.[114] If the premise that gynecologic cancer patients have multiple coexisting morbidities is valid, it may be appropriate to conclude that the patient's best interest is served when cancer procedures are preformed by individuals with appropriate surgical expertise.

Preoperative stay. The risk of surgical-site infection increases in direct proportion to the duration of preoperative stay.[97] Other perioperative complications, including VTE, are also increased. It seems appropriate to minimize preoperative hospital stay to lessen these risks. In specific clinical situations, discharge and later readmission may be justified.

Antibiotic prophylaxis. Preoperative antibiotic prophylaxis reduces the risk of surgical-site infection after extensive surgical procedures. Although most drugs are beneficial, broad-spectrum antimicrobial prophylaxis

may decrease overall costs. In general, single-dose prophylaxis is adequate. Important aspects of administration include appropriate timing (before the incision), adequate (increased) dosing in obese patients, or repeated dosing during prolonged procedures.[115,116]

Incision management. Technical aspects related to incision inscription start with the bold creation of the incision. A single-stoke incision through the skin and subcutaneous tissues lessens the morbidity associated with the creation of excessive dead space. Although achieving appropriate hemostasis is essential, it is important to avoid excessive use of electrocautery and resultant tissue necrosis.[97]

Fascial closure can usually be safely performed with a continuous, nonlocking running stitch. Incorporating a ratio of suture length to wound length of 4:1 (Fig. 48-2) lessens the risk of late wound failure (i.e., hernia).[117] This ratio can be accomplished by placing sutures at least 1.5 cm apart and 1.5 cm from the fascial edge (Fig. 48-3).

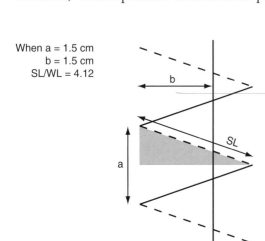

When a = 1.5 cm
b = 1.5 cm
SL/WL = 4.12

An incision (vertical line) sutured in an over-and-over fashion (solid and dashed line). Suture length to wound ratio (SL:WL) may be calculated with the Pythagorean theorem applied to the shaded triangle: $(SL)^2 = (a/2)^2 + (2b)^2$, where a = stitch interval and b = width of tissue bite; WL = a/2.

Figure 48–3. Fascial closure usually can be safely performed by incorporating a suture-to-wound length ratio of at least 4:1.

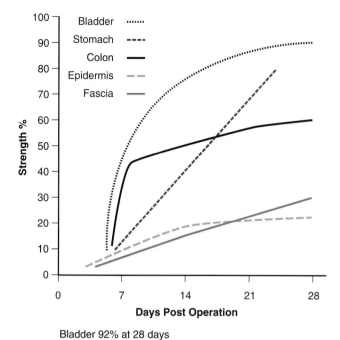

Bladder 92% at 28 days
Stomach 80% at 23 days
Colon 70% at 120 days
Epidermis 100% at 560 days
Fascia 83% at 360 days

Figure 48–4. The return of postoperative wound strength varies for different organs.

Suture material. The return of postoperative tensile strength varies among specific organs (Fig. 48-4). Appropriate selection of suture material for each situation requires an understanding of the healing process and knowledge of suture characteristics. The choice of permanent versus absorbable and monofilament versus multifilament should be individualized. Some specific clinical facts help the decision. The use of the smallest suture size for the desired task reduces foreign body reaction and infection (2-0 sutures are sufficient for most intra-abdominal tasks). Use of chromic suture material compared with synthetic absorbables (i.e., polyglycolic acid suture) is associated with increased inflammatory response and pain. Permanent sutures used for fascial closure lessen the risk of hernia and infection but increase the risk of wound pain and

suture sinus (Fig. 48-5). New suture materials impregnated with antibiotics offer some theoretical benefits.

Vasoconstrictors. There is little use for vasoconstrictors as hemostatic agents in abdominal or vaginal wound incisions.[97,118] Their use has not been documented to reduce clinically relevant blood loss, and the local tissue vasoconstriction potentially increases local hypoxemia and reduces the tissue concentration of antibiotic. The latter situation may predispose the wound to infection.

Drains. There is apparently little role for pelvic drains after major gynecologic procedures.[119] They have not lowered specific risks (i.e., lymphocyst), and they predispose to infection. Although controversial, the use of subcutaneous drains appears to be of little benefit. If a drain is deemed necessary, its duration of use should be minimized. The abdominal wall or groin incision is "sealed" within 24 to 36 hours, and continued drainage allows an avenue for the introduction of bacteria.

Temperature homeostasis. Even small reductions in core body temperature increase the risk of infection and can result in a coagulopathy and poor wound outcome.[120] All attempts to avoid hypothermia should be exercised to lessen wound and other (i.e., cardiac) risks.

Oxygenation. Oxygen is essential to the accelerated metabolic function in the healing wound. Ambient PO_2 levels of 25 mm Hg are necessary for polymorphonuclear neutrophils to produce superoxide radicals for bacterial killing. Other important enzyme systems function optimally at PO_2 levels higher than 50 mm Hg. Local tissue hypoxemia is associated with an increased risk of wound infection and poor outcome in the laboratory and at bedside.[97,121,122] A good perioperative care plan incorporates all methods (e.g., supplemental oxygen, pain control) to maintain or improve tissue oxygenation. Hyperbaric oxygen may be appropriate when existing patient comorbidity further lessens wound vascularity and oxygenation.[123]

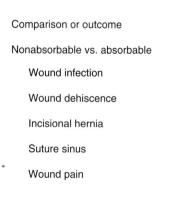

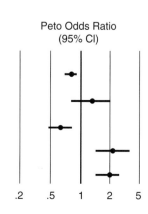

Figure 48–5. Meta-analysis of all outcomes comparing absorbable versus nonabsorbable sutures. *Circles* indicate point estimates of odds ratios, and *horizontal bars* signify 95% confidence intervals. Values less than 1 favor the nonabsorbable group, and values greater than 1 favor the absorbable group. Point estimates are significant at the $P < .05$ level if their confidence intervals exclude the vertical line at 1 (i.e., no effect). (From Hodgson NC, Malthaner RA, Ostbye T: The search for an ideal method of abdominal fascial closure: A meta-analysis. Ann Surg 2000;231:436-442.)

References

1. Goldman L, Caldera DL, Nussbaum SR, et al: Multifactorial index of cardiac risk in noncardiac surgical procedures. N Engl J Med 1977;297:845-850.

2. Detsky AS, Abrams HB, McLaughlin JR, et al: Predicting cardiac complications in patients undergoing non-cardiac surgery. J Gen Intern Med 1986;1:211-219.

3. Detsky AS, Abrams HB, Forbath N, et al: Cardiac assessment for patients undergoing noncardiac surgery: A multifactorial clinical risk index. Arch Intern Med 1986;146:2131-2134.

4. Lee TH, Marcantonio ER, Mangione CM, et al: Derivation and prospective validation of a simple index for prediction of cardiac risk of major noncardiac surgery. Circulation 1999;100:1043-1049.

5. Grayburn PA, Hillis LD: Cardiac events in patients undergoing noncardiac surgery: Shifting the paradigm from noninvasive risk stratification to therapy. Ann Intern Med 2003;138:506-511.

6. Poldermans D, Boersma E, Bax JJ, et al: Bisoprolol reduces cardiac death and myocardial infarction in high-risk patients as long as 2 years after successful major vascular surgery. Eur Heart J 2001;22:1353-1358.

7. Mangano DT, Layug EL, Wallace A, Tateo I: Effect of atenolol on mortality and cardiovascular morbidity after noncardiac surgery. Multicenter Study of Perioperative Ischemia Research Group. N Engl J Med 1996;335:1713-1720.

8. Boersma E, Poldermans D, Bax JJ, et al: Predictors of cardiac events after major vascular surgery: Role of clinical characteristics, dobutamine echocardiography, and beta-blocker therapy. JAMA 2001;285:1865-1873.

9. Eagle KA, Berger PB, Calkins H, et al: ACC/AHA guideline update for perioperative cardiovascular evaluation for noncardiac surgery—executive summary a report of the American College of Cardiology/American Heart Association Task Force on Practice Guidelines (Committee to Update the 1996 Guidelines on Perioperative Cardiovascular Evaluation for Noncardiac Surgery). Circulation 2002;105:1257-1267.

10. Guidelines for assessing and managing the perioperative risk from coronary artery disease associated with major noncardiac surgery. American College of Physicians. Ann Intern Med 1997;127:309-312.

11. Kaluza GL, Joseph J, Lee JR, et al: Catastrophic outcomes of noncardiac surgery soon after coronary stenting. J Am Coll Cardiol 2000;35:1288-1294.

12. Lawrence VA, Hilsenbeck SG, Mulrow CD, et al: Incidence and hospital stay for cardiac and pulmonary complications after abdominal surgery. J Gen Intern Med 1995;10:671-678.

13. Rock P, Preston B: Postoperative pulmonary complications. Curr Opin Anesth 2003;16:1123-1131.

14. Lawrence VA, Dhanda R, Hilsenbeck SG, Page CP: Risk of pulmonary complications after elective abdominal surgery. Chest 1996;110:744-750.

15. Smetana GW: Preoperative pulmonary evaluation. N Engl J Med 1999;340:937-944.

16. Smetana GW: Preoperative pulmonary assessment of the older adult. Clin Geriatr Med 2003;19:35-55.

17. Warner MA, Offord KP, Warner ME, et al: Role of preoperative cessation of smoking and other factors in postoperative pulmonary complications: A blinded prospective study of coronary artery bypass patients. Mayo Clin Proc 1989;64:609-616.

18. Celli BR, Rodriguez KS, Snider GL: A controlled trial of intermittent positive pressure breathing, incentive spirometry, and deep breathing exercises in preventing pulmonary complications after abdominal surgery. Am Rev Respir Dis 1984;130:12-15.

19. Brooks-Brunn JA: Predictors of postoperative pulmonary complications following abdominal surgery. Chest 1997;111:564-571.

20. Williams-Russo P, Charlson ME, MacKenzie CR, et al: Predicting postoperative pulmonary complications. Is it a real problem? Arch Intern Med 1992;152:1209-1213.

21. Yeager MP, Glass DD, Neff RK, Brinck-Johnsen T: Epidural anesthesia and analgesia in high-risk surgical patients. Anesthesiology 1987;66:729-736.

22. Chertow GM, Lazarus JM, Christiansen CL, et al: Preoperative renal risk stratification. Circulation 1997;95:878-884.

23. Thadhani R, Pascual M, Bonventre JV: Acute renal failure. N Engl J Med 1996;334:1448-1460.

24. Levy EM, Viscoli CM, Horwitz RI: The effect of acute renal failure on mortality: A cohort analysis. JAMA 1996;275:1489-1494.

25. Kellerman PS: Perioperative care of the renal patient. Arch Intern Med 1994;154:1674-1688.

26. Sural S, Sharma RK, Singhal M, et al: Etiology, prognosis, and outcome of postoperative acute renal failure. Ren Fail 2000;22:87-97.

27. Friedrich AD: The controversy of "renal-dose dopamine." Int Anesthesiol Clin 2001;39:127-139.

28. Sadovnikoff N: Perioperative acute renal failure. Int Anesthesiol Clin 2001;39:95-109.

29. Hladunewich M, Rosenthal MH: Pathophysiology and management of renal insufficiency in the perioperative and critically ill patient. Anesthesiol Clin North Am 2000;18:773-779.

30. Joseph AJ, Cohn SL: Perioperative care of the patient with renal failure. Med Clin North Am 2003;87:193-210.

31. Geerts WH, Heit JA, Clagett GP, et al: Prevention of venous thromboembolism. Chest 2001;119(Suppl):132S-175S.

32. Schorge JO, Goldhaber SZ, Duska LR, et al: Clinically significant venous thromboembolism after gynecologic surgery. J Reprod Med 1999;44:669-673.

33. von Tempelhoff GF, Heilmann L: Antithrombotic therapy in gynecologic surgery and gynecologic oncology. Hematol Oncol Clin North Am 2000;14:1151-1169, ix.

34. von Tempelhoff GF, Nieman F, Heilmann L, Hommel G: Association between blood rheology, thrombosis and cancer survival in patients with gynecologic malignancy. Clin Hemorheol Microcirc 2000;22:107-130.

35. von Tempelhoff GF, Harenberg J, Niemann F, et al: Effect of low molecular weight heparin (Certoparin) versus unfractionated heparin on cancer survival following breast and pelvic cancer surgery: A prospective randomized double-blind trial. Int J Oncol 2000;16:815-824.

36. von Tempelhoff GF, Pollow K, Schneider D, Heilmann L: Chemotherapy and thrombosis in gynecologic malignancy. Clin Appl Thromb Hemost 1999;5:92-104.

37. Maxwell GL, Synan I, Dodge R, et al: Pneumatic compression versus low molecular weight heparin in gynecologic oncology surgery: A randomized trial. Obstet Gynecol 2001;98:989-995.

38. Madden S, Porter TF: Deep venous thrombosis: Prophylaxis in gynecology. Clin Obstet Gynecol 1999;42:895-901.

39. Clarke-Pearson DL: Prevention of venous thromboembolism in gynecologic surgery patients. Curr Opin Obstet Gynecol 1993;5:73-79.

40. Clarke-Pearson DL, Olt G: Thromboembolism in patients with Gyn tumors: risk factors, natural history, and prophylaxis. Oncology (Huntingt) 1989;3:39-45, discussion 45, 48.

41. Clarke-Pearson DL, Creasman WT, Coleman RE, et al: Perioperative external pneumatic calf compression as thromboembolism prophylaxis in gynecologic oncology: Report of a randomized controlled trial. Gynecol Oncol 1984;18:226-232.

42. Clarke-Pearson DL, Dodge RK, Synan I, et al: Venous thromboembolism prophylaxis: Patients at high risk to fail intermittent pneumatic compression. Obstet Gynecol 2003;101:157-163.

43. Bergqvist D, Agnelli G, Cohen AT, et al: Duration of prophylaxis against venous thromboembolism with enoxaparin after surgery for cancer. N Engl J Med 2002;346:975-980.

44. Merli GJ: Low-molecular-weight heparins versus unfractionated heparin in the treatment of deep vein thrombosis and pulmonary embolism. Am J Phys Med Rehabil 2000;79(Suppl):S9-S16.

45. Hoffman MS, DeCesare S, Fiorica JV, et al: Management of gynecologic oncology patients with a preoperative deep vein thrombosis. Gynecol Oncol 1997;64:76-79.

46. Decousus H, Leizorovicz A, Parent F, et al: A clinical trial of vena caval filters in the prevention of pulmonary embolism in patients with proximal deep-vein thrombosis. Prevention du Risque d'Embolie Pulmonaire par Interruption Cave Study Group. N Engl J Med 1998;338:409-415.

47. Girard P, Tardy B, Decousus H: Inferior vena cava interruption: How and when? Annu Rev Med 2000;51:1-15.

48. Greenfield LJ, Proctor MC: Twenty-year clinical experience with the Greenfield filter. Cardiovasc Surg 1995;3:199-205.

49. Ridker PM, Goldhaber SZ, Danielson E, et al: Long-term, low-intensity warfarin therapy for the prevention of recurrent venous thromboembolism. N Engl J Med 2003;348:1425-1434.

50. Lee AY, Levine MN, Baker RI, et al: Low-molecular-weight heparin versus a coumarin for the prevention of recurrent venous thromboembolism in patients with cancer. N Engl J Med 2003;349:146-153.

51. Jemal A, Murray T, Samuels A, et al: Cancer statistics, 2003. CA Cancer J Clin 2003;52:23-47.

52. Rex D: Should we colonoscope women with gynecologic cancer? Am J Gastroenterol 2000;95:812-813.

53. Weinberg D, Newschaffer C, Topham A: Risk for colorectal cancer after gynecologic cancer. Ann Intern Med 1999;131:189-193.

54. Abu-Rustum N, Barakat R, Curtin J: Ovarian and uterine disease in women with colorectal cancer. Obstet Gynecol 1997;89:85-87.

55. Becker S, Tomacruz R, Kaufman H, et al: Gynecologic abnormalities in surgically treated women with stage II or III rectal cancer. J Am Coll Surg 2002;194:315-323.

56. Ransohoff D, Sandler R: Screening for colorectal cancer. N Engl J Med 2002;346:40-44.

57. Winawer S, Fletcher R, Rex D, et al: Colorectal cancer screening and surveillance: Clinical guidelines and rational—update based on new evidence. Gastroenterology 2003;124:544-560.

58. Smith R, Cokkinides V, Eyre H: American Cancer Society guidelines for the early detection of cancer, 2003. CA Cancer J Clin 2003;53:27-43.

59. Helm J, Choi J, Barthel J, et al: Current evolving strategies for colorectal cancer screening. Cancer Control 2003;10;193-204.

60. Levin B, Brooks D, Smith R, Stone A: Emerging technologies in screening for colorectal cancer: CT colonography, immunochemical fecal occult blood tests, and stool screening using molecular markers. CA Cancer J Clin 2003;53:44-55.

61. Orr J: Cervical cancer. Surg Oncol Clin N Am 1998;7:299-316.

62. Orr J, Orr P, Taylor P: Surgical staging endometrial cancer. Clin Obstet Gynecol 1996;39:656-668.

63. Guidozzi F, Sonnendecker E: Evaluation of preoperative investigations in patients admitted for ovarian primary cytoreductive therapy. Gynecol Oncol 1991;40:244-247.

64. Gornall R, Talbot R: Can flexible sigmoidoscopy predict need for colorectal surgery in ovarian carcinoma? Eur J Gynaecol Oncol 1999;20:13-15.

65. Saltzman A, Carter J, Fowler J, et al: The utility of preoperative screening colonoscopy in gynecologic oncology. Gynecol Oncol 1995;56:181-186.

66. Nichols R, Broido P, Condon R, et al: Effect of preoperative neomycin-erythromycin intestinal preparation on the incidence of infectious complications following colon surgery. Ann Surg 1973;178:453-462.

67. Zmora O, Wexner S, Hajjar L, et al: Trends in preparation for colorectal surgery: Survey of the members of the American Society of Colon and Rectal Surgeons. Am Surg 2003;69:150-154.

68. Nichols R, Smith J, Garcia R, et al: Current practices of preoperative bowel preparation among North American colorectal surgeons. Clin Infect Dis 1997;24:609-619.

69. Zmora O, Pikarsky AJ, Wexner SD: Bowel preparation for colorectal surgery. Dis Colon Rectum 2001;44:1537-1549.

70. Zmora O, Mahajna A, Bar-Zakai B, et al: Colon and rectal surgery without mechanical bowel preparation: A randomized prospective trial. Am Surg 2003;237:363-367.

71. van Geldere D, Fa-Si-Oen P, Noach L, et al: Complications after colorectal surgery without mechanical bowel preparation. J Am Coll Surg 2002;194:40-47.

72. Wong K, Cheong D, Wong D: Treatment of acute malignant colorectal obstruction with self-expandable metallic stents. Aust N Z J Surg 2002;72:385-388.

73. Fanning J, Andrews S. Early postoperative feeding after major gynecologic surgery: Evidence-based scientific medicine. Am J Obstet Gynecol 2001;185:1-4.

74. Brewer M: Routine nasogastric intubation following gynecologic cancer procedures. Gynecol Oncol 1998;68:126.

75. Cheatham M, Chapman W, Key S, Sawyers J: A meta-analysis of selective versus routine nasogastric decompression after elective laparotomy. Ann Surg 1995;221:469-478.

76. Pearl M, Valea F, Fischer M, Chalas E: A randomized controlled trial of postoperative nasogastric tube decompression in gynecologic oncology patients undergoing intra-abdominal surgery. Obstet Gynecol 1996;88:399-402.

77. Wolff B, Pemberton J, van Heerden J, et al: Elective colon and rectal surgery without nasogastric decompression: A prospective, randomized trial. Ann Surg 1989;209:670-673.

78. Wu C, Hwang C, Liu T: There is no need for nasogastric decompression after partial gastrectomy with extensive lymphadenectomy. Eur J Surg 1994;160:369-373.

79. Glesson N, Hoffman M, Fiorica J, et al: Gastrostomy tubes after gynecologic oncologic surgery. Gynecol Oncol 1994;54:19-22.

80. Bisgarrd T, Kehlet H: Early oral feeding after elective abdominal surgery—what are the issues? Nutrition 2002;18:944-948.

81. Asao T, Kuwano H, Morinaga N, et al: Gum chewing enhances early recovery from postoperative ileus after laparoscopic colectomy. J Am Coll Surg 2002;195:30-32.

82. Urbech D, Kennedy E, Cohen M: Colon and rectal anastomoses do not require routine drainage: A systematic review and meta-analysis. Ann Surg 1999;229:174-180.

83. Khurrum B, Hua Z, Batista O, et al: Percutaneous postoperative intra-abdominal abscess drainage after elective colorectal surgery. Tech Coloproctol 2002;6:159-164.

84. Cox M, Gunn I, Eastman M, et al: The safety and duration of non-operative treatment for adhesive small bowel obstruction. Aust N Z J Surg 1993;63:367-371.

85. Onuoe S, Katoh T, Shibata Y, et al: The value of contrast radiology for postoperative adhesive small bowel obstruction. Hepatogastroenterology 2002;49:1576-1578.

86. Orr JW, Taylor PT: Wound healing. In Orr JW, Shingleton HM (eds): Complications of Gynecologic Surgery: Prevention, Recognition, and Management. Philadelphia, JB Lippincott, 1994.

87. Brisset A, Hom D: The effects of tissue sealants, platelet gels, and growth factors on wound healing. Curr Opin Otolaryngol Head Neck Surg 2003;11;245-250.

88. Garry R: The benefits and problems associated with minimal access surgery. Aust N Z J Obstet Gynaecol 2002;42:239-244.

89. Dargent DF: Laparoscopic surgery in gynecologic oncology. Surg Clin North Am 2001,81:949-964.

90. Holub Z: The role of laparoscopic in the surgical treatment of endometrial cancer. Clin Exp Obstet Gynecol 2003;30:7-12.

91. Eltabbakh GH: Analysis of survival after laparoscopy in women with endometrial carcinoma. Cancer 2002;95:1894-1901.

92. Canis M, Rabischong B, Houlle C, et al: Laparoscopic management of adnexal masses: A gold standard? Curr Opin Obstet Gynecol 2002;14:423-428.

93. Mendilcioglu I, Zorlu CG, Trak B, et al: Laparoscopic management of adnexal masses: Safety and effectiveness. J Reprod Med 2002;47:36-40.

94. Hertel H, Kohler C, Elhawary T, et al: Laparoscopic staging compared with imaging techniques in the staging of advanced cervical cancer. Gynecol Oncol 2002;87:46-51.

95. Childers JM, Spirtos NM, Brainard P, Surwit EA: Laparoscopic staging of the patient with incompletely staged early adenocarcinoma of the endometrium. Obstet Gynecol 1994;83:597-600.

96. Schlaerth JB, Spirtos NM, Schlaerth AC: Radical trachelectomy and pelvic lymphadenectomy with uterine preservation in the treatment of cervical cancer. Am J Obstet Gynecol 2003;188:29-34.

97. Orr JW, Orr PJ, Bolen DD, Holimon JL: Radical hysterectomy: Does the type of incision matter? Am J Obstet Gynecol 1995;173:399-406.

98. Horowitz NS, Powell MA, Drescher CW, et al: Adequate Staging for uterine cancer can be preformed through Pfannenstiel incisions. Gynecol Oncol 2003;88:404-410.

99. Hoffman MS, Lynch CM: Minilaparotomy hysterectomy [letter]. Am J Obstet Gynecol 1999;191:1037-1038.

100. Chan JK, Lin TG, Monk BJ, et al: Vaginal hysterectomy as primary treatment of endometrial cancer in medically compromised women. Obstet Gynecol 2001;97(Pt 1):707-711.

101. Lelle RJ, Morley GW, Peters WA: The role of vaginal hysterectomy in the treatment of endometrial carcinoma. Int J Gynecol Cancer 1994:4:342-347.

102. Mion LC: Care Provision for older adults: Who will provide? J Issues Nurs 2003;8:4-9.

103. Wilson JA, Clark JJ: Obesity: Impediment to wound healing. Crit Care Nurs Q 2003;26:119-132.

104. Orr JW, Orr PF: Perioperative care. In Greer BE, Montz FJ (eds): Atlas of Clinical Gynecology. Contemporary Clinical Management of Gynecologic Malignancies. Philadelphia, Appleton & Lange, 1999.

105. Orr JW, Cornwell A, Wilson K, et al: Nutritional status of patients with untreated cervical cancer. I. Biochemical and immunologic assessment. Am J Obstet Gynecol 1985;151:625-631.

106. Orr JR, Shingleton HM: Nutritional complications. In Orr JW, Shingleton HM (eds): Complications in Gynecologic Surgery: Prevention, Recognition, and Management. Philadelphia, JB Lippincott, 1994.

107. Orr JW, Patsner B, Sisson PF: Nutritional support in patients with gynecologic cancer. In Zuspan F (ed): Current Therapy in Obstetrics and Gynecology, 3rd ed. Philadelphia, WB Saunders, 1989.

108. Orr JW, Browne KF Jr: Cardiac complications. In Orr JW, Shingleton HM (eds): Complications of Gynecologic Surgery: Prevention, Recognition, and Management. Philadelphia, JB Lippincott, 1994.

109. Hoogwerf BJ: Postoperative management of the diabetic patient. Med Clin North Am 2001;85:213-228.

110. Marks JB: Perioperative management of diabetes. Am Fam Physician 2003;67:93-100.

111. Roland P, Orr J, Kelly J: Wound healing: The effects of chemotherapy and radiation. Operative Tech Gynecol Surg 2001;6:201-203.

112. Association of Professors of Gynecology and Oncology: The Challenge of Pelvic Adhesions: Strategies for Prevention and Management. APGO Educational Series on Women's Health Issues. Beachwood, OH, Current Therapeutics, 2002.

113. Orr JW, Roland PY, Orr PJ, et al: Subspecialty training: does it affect the outcome of women treated for a gynecologic malignancy? Curr Opin Obstet Gynecol 2001;13:1-8.

114. Gawande AA, Thomas EJ, Zinner MJ, Brennan TA: The incidence and nature of surgical adverse events in Colorado and Utah in 1992. Surgery 1999;126:66-75.

115. Rothenburger S, Spangler D, Bhende S, Burkley D: In vitro antimicrobial evaluation of coated Vicryl plus antibacterial suture (coated polyglactin 910 with triclosan) using zone of inhibition assays. Surg Infect 2002(Suppl 1);3:S79-S87.

116. Orr JW, Montz FJ, Barter J, et al: Continuous abdominal fascial closure: A randomized, controlled trial of poly (L-lactide/glycolide). Gynecol Oncol 2003;90:342-347.

117. Israelsson LA, Jonsson T: Closure of midline laparotomy incisions with polydioxanone and nylon: The importance of suture technique. Br J Surg 1994;81:1606-1608.

118. England GT, Randal HW, Graves WL: Impairment of tissue defences by vasoconstrictors in vaginal hysterectomy. Obstet Gynecol 1983;61:271-274.

119. Jensen J: To drain or not to drain: A retrospective study of closed lymphadenectomy. Gynecol Oncol 1993;51:46-49.

120. Nortcliffe SA, Buggy DJ: Implications of anesthesia for infection and wound healing. Int Anesthesiol Clin 2003;41:31-64.

121. Knighton DR, Halliday B, Hunt TK: Oxygen as an antibiotic: The effect of inspired oxygen on infection. Arch Surg 1984;119:199-204.

122. Greif R, Akca O, Horn EP, et al: Supplemental perioperative oxygen to reduce the incidence of surgical-wound infection. Outcomes Research Group. N Engl J Med 2000;342:161-167.

123. Fine NA, Mustoe TA: Wound healing. In Greenfield LJ, Mulholland M, Oldham K, et al (eds): Surgery: Scientific Principles and Practices. Philadelphia, Lippincott, Williams & Wilkins, 2001.

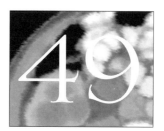

C H A P T E R 49

LYMPHATIC MAPPING OF THE FEMALE GENITAL TRACT

Charles Levenback

 MAJOR CONTROVERSIES

- **How did lymphatic mapping develop?**
- **What are the techniques for sentinel node identification?**
- **What is a sentinel node?**
- **How are sentinel nodes evaluated by pathologists?**
- **Are vulvar and cervix cancers good targets for the lymphatic mapping strategy?**
- **What is the best technique for intraoperative sentinel node identification in patients with vulvar cancer?**
- **Is there a role for preoperative lymphoscintigraphy in treating gynecologic cancers?**
- **How long is the learning curve for lymphatic mapping and sentinel node identification for gynecologic oncologists?**
- **Is ultrastaging of sentinel nodes necessary in patients with squamous carcinomas?**
- **What is the experience with lymphatic mapping in patients with vulvar cancer?**
- **Is lymphatic mapping and sentinel node identification "standard" for patients with vulvar cancer?**
- **Is lymphatic mapping and sentinel node identification a replacement for inguinal lymphadenectomy in patients with vulvar cancer?**

The development of lymphatic mapping and sentinel node identification has the potential to result in the greatest change in the management of solid tumors since the development of radical regional lymphadenectomy by Halsted,[1,2] and others. The development of lymphatic mapping has been accompanied by many controversies regarding how tumors metastasize, the role of lymphadenectomy, the wisdom of tampering with tried and true surgical approaches, the ideal technique for mapping, and clinical applications. This chapter describes the mapping concept, how it developed, and how it is applied to gynecologic cancers.

How did lymphatic mapping develop?

In 1938, the great British anatomist John Gray[3] wrote that study of the mode of spread of solid tumors to lymph nodes was impeded "chiefly by the difficulty demonstrating the lymphatic vessels." Classic anatomists of the 19th century relied on the study of putrefied or fixed tissue. This allowed identification of lymph nodes and their location related to other major structures; however, lymph channels were not visible. Sappey[4] and others injected a variety of compounds, including heavy metals such as mercury, into cadavers to assist in observing lymphatics; however, there were no in vivo techniques, and the process used distorted the anatomy of the fine lymph vessels. In the 20th century, techniques were developed to overcome the problems of studying cadaveric tissue. Hudack and McMaster[5] used small-gauge needles to inject various dyes into the dermis of healthy volunteers to study the microlymphatics of the skin. Gray injected thorostat into fresh tissue taken at surgery for light microscopy studies of the lymphatics of the skin.[3]

For most of the 20th century, the gold standard for surgical management of solid tumors was en bloc removal of the primary tumor in continuity with the regional lymphatic channels and lymph nodes. It was commonly held that spread to lymph nodes was due to mechanical factors and that outcome was determined by resection of all macroscopic and microscopic disease and proper surgical techniques. For example, it was believed that tumor cells could be disseminated during surgery if the tumor was squeezed or otherwise mishandled. At the time, there was no effective nonsurgical adjuvant therapy to accompany surgery, and it was common to see patients with advanced primary tumors. This was an era before there was any emphasis on early detection, screening, or referral to centers or physicians with special interest and skill in caring for patients with cancer. Operative mortality declined with improvements in surgical techniques; however, morbidity rates remained very high. Survival was improved too, and just as today, patients and physicians were willing to accept a high risk of morbidity for even a low chance of long-term cure.

In the last half of the 20th century, many changes in medicine occurred that led to a reduction in mortality and morbidity with an improvement in survival for patients with gynecologic cancers. First was widespread recognition that cancer is curable when detected early. Second was a breakdown of social taboos about gynecologic and breast diseases. Third were many advances in surgical techniques, critical care, transfusion medicine, and antibiotics that improved outcomes in general for surgical patients. With these changes, disfiguring effects of cancer surgery became less acceptable. Lumpectomy and partial vulvectomy[6] were popularized; however, lymphadenectomy remained part of standard treatment and the complications of lymphadenectomy persisted. To this day there is no effective treatment for lymphedema.

Ramon Cabanas' work[7] in patients with penile carcinoma in the 1970s is considered the start of modern lymphatic mapping; however, it was clinicians specializing in the treatment of cutaneous melanoma who embraced and popularized the procedure. There are several reasons why melanoma was the place where mapping took off. First, melanomas of the trunk, which has complex lymphatic drainage, are common. Second, regional node dissection was particularly ineffective in melanoma, making justification of radical regional lymphadenectomy weak. Third, effective adjuvant therapy for node-positive patients was (and is) elusive. These problems led to thinking on how to identify node-positive patients and

avoid regional lymphadenectomy. In 1992, Morton and colleagues[8] described the use of preoperative lymphoscintigraphy and intraoperative lymphatic mapping in 237 patients with cutaneous melanoma. Preoperative lymphoscintigraphy was performed in patients with tumors at sites with ambiguous lymphatic drainage, primarily the trunk, to determine which lymphatic basin to dissect (Fig. 49-1). Peritumoral injection of isosulfan blue was used to identify blue sentinel nodes intraoperatively. At least one sentinel node was successfully identified in 194 of the 237 lymph node basins dissected. All patients underwent regional lymphadenectomy, resulting in resection of over 3000 lymph nodes. Only 2 of 40 lymphadenectomy specimens with positive nodes had falsely negative sentinel nodes.

Interest in applying lymphatic mapping to patients with breast cancer followed quickly after the studies in patients with melanoma and for similar reasons. In the mid-1960s, Dr. Bernard Fisher challenged the Halsted tradition of orderly spread from the primary tumor to regional lymph nodes with a theory that breast cancer was systemic from the outset.[9] This theory coincided with the introduction into clinical practice of systemic therapy (chemotherapy) as an adjuvant to surgery. The most recent theory about the spread of breast

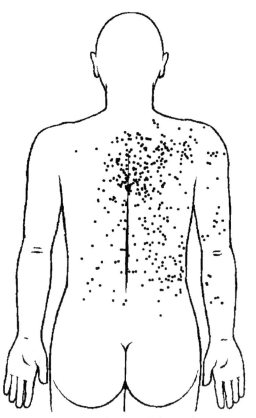

Figure 49–1. Cutaneous melanoma of the trunk presents a serious clinical dilemma regarding identification of the correct draining lymphatic basin. Morton and colleagues[47] demonstrated the wide distribution of tumors with lymphatic drainage to the right axilla. (Adapted from Morton DL: Sentinel lymphadenectomy for patients with clinical stage I melanoma. J Surg Oncol 1997;66:267-269.)

Table 49–1. Models for Spread of Breast Cancer

Halsted[2]
Tumors spread in orderly pattern to lymph nodes.
Lymph node metastases can result in distant spread.
Lymph nodes are barriers to passage of tumor cells.
Hematogenous spread is of minor significance.
Extent of surgery and technique determine outcome.
Operable breast cancer is a locoregional disease.

Systemic[9]
Metastases have no orderly pattern.
Lymph nodes are an ineffective barrier to spread.
Hematogenous spread is very important.
Locoregional therapy does have a small impact on survival.
Operable breast cancer is a systemic disease.

Spectrum[48]
Axillary node spread usually precedes distant spread.
Lymph nodes are ineffective barrier to spread.
Lymph node metastases are not always associated with distant spread.
Hematogenous spread is the route for distant metastases.
Early local treatment is vital to prevent distant spread.
Operable breast cancer is systemic in a small proportion of patients.

Adapted from Gervasoni JE Jr, Taneja C, Chung MA, Cady B: Biologic and clinical significance of lymphadenectomy. Surg Clin North Am 2000;80:1631-1673.

cancer is the "spectrum" theory, which combines elements of the traditional Halsted model and the systemic model of Fisher (Table 49-1). The spectrum theory holds that some patients with metastatic disease have regional (axillary node) involvement only, whereas others have distant spread associated with axillary node metastases.

In the past 10 years, multiple series have been published that essentially validate the observations of Morton and coworkers.[8] In the case of breast cancer, there are almost 4000 published cases (Table 49-2). These data confirm the concept that there is a sentinel node that is the first lymph node draining a primary breast tumor. The sensitivity of the sentinel node—the proportion of patients with any positive axillary node who have a positive sentinel node—is about 93%. The negative predictive value—the proportion of sentinel-node-negative patients in whom the other axillary nodes are also negative—is 96%. In about half of patients, the sentinel node is the only positive lymph node. The specificity—the proportion of patients free of metastases who have a negative sentinel node—is of course always 100%.

What are the techniques for sentinel node identification?

There are several techniques for sentinel node identification that individual clinicians should be familiar with. These can be divided into three categories: blue-dye–based techniques, preoperative lymphoscintigraphy, and intraoperative use of a handheld gamma probe.

In the blue dye technique, the surgeon injects blue dye around the tumor before surgery (Fig. 49-2). During the surgery, the surgeon identifies sentinel nodes by following the path of the blue-stained lymphatics leading away from the tumor. Wong and associates[10] experimented with isosulfan blue, methylene blue, and cyalume in a cat model and found that isosulfan blue performed better than the others. Other mapping materials that have been used include fluorescein and patent blue-V.[11] Isosulfan blue remains the most commonly used dye in North America, and patent blue-V is the most commonly used dye in Europe and Australia. All blue dyes are injected into the dermis or tissue surrounding the primary tumor. Intradermal injection is important in lesions of the vulva to ensure that the dye reaches the superficial dermal lymphatics that communicate with the groin. Deep subcutaneous injection will result in uptake to deep lymphatics that accompany the named vessels of the vulva and perineum to the pelvis. Massage of the injection site might help with uptake to the dermal lymphatics. Transit times to sentinel nodes vary depending on the primary tumor site, the distance to the sentinel node, and the presence or absence of a surrounding inflammatory reaction. In the case of the cervix and vulva, transit time to the sentinel node is under 10 minutes and

Table 49–2. Comparison of Sentinel Node Localization Methods in Multiple Validation Trials of Sentinel Node Biopsy in Breast Cancer

Factor Considered*	Methods of SLN Localization		
	Radioisotope Alone	*Blue Dye Alone*	*Radioisotope plus Blue Dye*
Patients in whom SLNs found at surgery	91% (1768/1934)	80% (790/993)	91% (796/873)
Sensitivity	93% (604/650)	91% (270/296)	95% (256/270)
Negative predictive value	96% (1100/1146)	95% (494/520)	97% (518/532)
Accuracy	97% (1704/1750)	97% (764/790)	98% (774/788)
Patients in whom SLN only site of metastasis	46% (286/624)	61% (120/196)	50% (103/206)

*Sensitivity is the proportion of patients with axillary metastases in whom the sentinel nodes (SLNs) contained tumor (true positive/[true positive + false negative]). The negative predictive value is the proportion of patients without tumor in SLNs in whom the axilla was free of tumor (true negative/[true negative + false negative]). Accuracy is the proportion of patients with successful SLN biopsy in whom the status of the SLN correlated with the status of the axilla ([true positive] + true negative/[true positive + true negative + false positive + false negative]). Adapted from Liberman L, Schneider L: Review of published experience. In Cody HS (ed): Sentinel Lymph Node Biopsy. London, Martin Dunitz, 2002, pp 285-310.

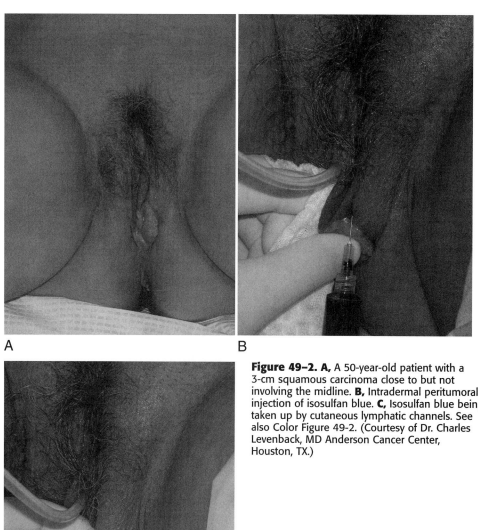

A

B

C

Figure 49–2. A, A 50-year-old patient with a 3-cm squamous carcinoma close to but not involving the midline. **B,** Intradermal peritumoral injection of isosulfan blue. **C,** Isosulfan blue being taken up by cutaneous lymphatic channels. See also Color Figure 49-2. (Courtesy of Dr. Charles Levenback, MD Anderson Cancer Center, Houston, TX.)

usually 5 minutes or less. Isosulfan blue remains visible in the sentinel node for 30-45 minutes.

Toxic reactions to blue dye are uncommon but can be significant. The most common minor reaction is that the urine will turn blue or green for less than 24 hours. Occasionally a patient's skin will appear gray in the recovery room; however, this discoloration fades within the first 24 hours. Allergic reactions are the most serious concern and occur in 1% to 2% of cases.[12] Blue urticaria[13] and full anaphylactic reactions have been described. They appear to be more common in lymphatic mapping for breast cancer, which

requires deep injection of a larger volume of dye, than in lymphatic mapping for melanoma. Unexplained decrease in oxygen saturation measured by pulse oximetry has been reported in a cervix cancer patient.[14]

Sentinel node identification with blue dye injection is quick, inexpensive, and does not require any special technology that might not be available outside major medical facilities. Most experience indicates that the learning curve for sentinel node identification is longer with blue dye alone than with other methods. With blue dye, there is no preoperative phase that allows the surgeon to plan an approach, and the window of opportunity for identifying the sentinel node in the operating room is short.

Lymphoscintigraphy is performed by injecting a weakly radioactive radionuclide around the tumor as described for blue dye and then obtaining an image (a "lymphoscintogram") using a stationary gamma camera. A variety of radiopharmaceuticals is available for use. It appears that particle size is the critical factor that determines the clinical suitability of an agent. If the particles are too small, they will migrate out of the lymphatic vessels before reaching the sentinel node. If the particles are too large, the proportion reaching the sentinel node will be small and the rate of movement will be very slow.[15] In North America, the only radiopharmaceutical clinically available for sentinel node identification is technetium-99m (99mTc) sulfur colloid. In Europe, several other agents are in use, including 99mTc antimony trisulfide colloid and 99mTc nanocolloidial albumin. Although each radiopharmaceutical has slightly different characteristics, all appear to effectively reveal the sentinel nodes.[16,17]

Extensive testing regarding radiation exposure has been performed to determine the safety of lymphoscintigraphy for patients and health care workers. The calculations are complex and depend on multiple factors, including the dose, particle size, washout rate, and any precautions taken. In brief, the amount of radiation exposure from the technique is very small, and the cumulative effects from many cases are still well within acceptable levels.[15,18] It is important, however, to understand that radiation exposure depends on many factors and that all applicable radiation precautions, including proper disposal of contaminated waste, should be observed.

The lymphoscintigram obtained after radionuclide injection (Fig. 49-3) shows the sentinel node near the injection site but does not show the surrounding

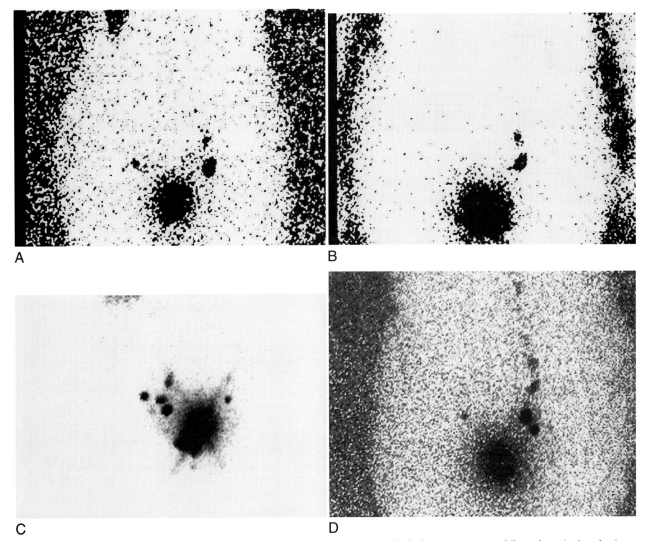

Figure 49-3. Lymphoscintigrams of patients with vulvar cancer demonstrating multiple drainage patterns: bilateral sentinel nodes in a patient with a midline perineal lesion (**A**); unilateral sentinel nodes in a patient with a left labial lesion (**B**); bilateral sentinel nodes in a patient with a right labial lesion close to, but not involving the midline (**C**); multiple second-echelon pelvic, common iliac, and low para-aortic nodes are visible on the right in a patient with cervical cancer (**D**). (Reproduced with permission from Levenback, Coleman, and van der Zee (eds): Clinical Lymphatic Mapping in Gynecologic Cancers, London, Taylor & Francis, 2004.)

structures in any detail. The location of a sentinel node close to the skin may be marked in the nuclear medicine suite to aid the surgeon in identifying the node during surgery. The transit time from the injection site varies depending on the location of the injection and the radiopharmaceutical. The smaller the particle size, the faster the transit time. Radionuclide will begin to reach the sentinel node within 20 minutes, but a wait of up to 2 hours may be required before a satisfactory image can be obtained.

One major use of preoperative lymphoscintigraphy is in the case of tumors that may have drainage to multiple lymphatic basins. For example, a melanoma of the midback could drain to either axilla, either groin, or some combination, and a breast cancer of the medial third of the breast could drain to the axilla or the internal mammary chain. In both cases the preoperative lymphoscintigram could help direct the surgeon to the correct site for the incision and dissection. If the sentinel node is very close to the primary tumor, it may not be possible to distinguish the sentinel node from the tumor. Thyroid and cervix cancers can fall into this category.

The final technique for sentinel node identification is intraoperative use of a gamma probe after injection of a radionuclide around the tumor. There are now several manufacturers of gamma probes for intraoperative use, including laparoscopic probes. These probes are placed in a sterile sheath and can be introduced into the wound to help locate the sentinel node. The gamma probe–based sentinel node identification technique permits identification of a node that is highly radioactive (compared with the background radioactivity) (so-called hot node), and this node is the sentinel node. This technique can be used alone or together with blue-dye–based techniques. The radionuclide can be injected before surgery or in the operating room. Either way, radiation precautions must be strictly observed.

What is a sentinel node?

The definition of a sentinel node proposed by Morton and colleagues[8] in 1992 is "the first draining lymph node on the direct lymphatic pathway from the primary tumor site" (Fig. 49-4). Growing experience with lymphoscintigraphy and intraoperative lymphatic mapping makes it clear that there is a myriad of anatomic variations of sentinel nodes. Thompson and Uren[19] have suggested a slight modification of Morton's definition: "any lymph node that receives lymphatic drainage directly from the primary tumor." This definition helps account for situations in which the primary tumor drains to more than one lymphatic basin or two lymph nodes in the same lymphatic basin have direct lymphatic communication with the primary tumor (regardless of which appeared first on the lymphoscintigram). A practical problem is how to determine whether two blue-stained or radioactive nodes in a single lymphatic basin are both sentinel

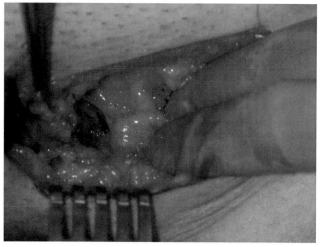

Figure 49–4. Intraoperative appearance of blue-stained sentinel lymph node. See also Color Figure 49–4. (Courtesy of Dr. Charles Levenback, MD Anderson Cancer Center, Houston, TX.)

nodes or one is the true sentinel node and the other is a second-echelon node. A second-echelon node receives its lymphatic drainage from the sentinel node, not the primary tumor. The intensity of blue staining cannot be quantified, so if the blue dye looks more intense in one node than in another, what if anything does that mean? The radioactivity in nodes can be measured; however, Essner and Morton have described 10 different definitions for a sentinel node based on radioactivity.[20] Using any of these definitions, both a sentinel node and a second-echelon node might qualify as sentinel.

From a clinical perspective, what matters? As long as the true sentinel node is removed and analyzed appropriately, it probably does not matter if a second-echelon node is also removed and treated the same way. When the surgeon is confronted with two radioactive or blue nodes in the same lymphatic basin, usually there is little option except to declare both of them sentinel nodes.

How are sentinel nodes evaluated by pathologists?

The traditional approach to histologic analysis of lymphadenectomy specimens is to tease the nodes out of the fat pad, bisect each node and embed the two halves in paraffin, and then prepare one slide from each side of the node. Some nodes too small to be bisected might be submitted in total for fixation. Ten nodes yield perhaps 15 slides. From the pathologist's point of view, each slide has an equal chance of containing metastatic disease.

Lymphatic mapping allows the pathologist to focus the search for metastatic disease on the sentinel nodes, which are the nodes most likely to contain metastases. The primary tools available to the pathologist for evaluation of sentinel lymph nodes are serial sectioning and immunohistochemical staining. Evaluation of lymph nodes using these techniques is commonly referred to as ultrastaging. Gershenwald and coworkers[21] demonstrated the potential benefits of extended histologic sampling of the sentinel nodes in a 1998 series of patients with cutaneous melanoma. In this study, the authors identified a group of 10 patients with melanoma who had a negative sentinel node and had relapse in the lymphatic basin. In 8 of the 10, retrospective analysis with serial sectioning and immunohistochemistry revealed micrometastases within the sentinel node. This study underscored the importance of the pathologist as a member of the lymphatic mapping team.

Melanoma presents a particular challenge to pathologists since melanoma micrometastases can be very difficult to detect on routine hematoxylin-eosin (H&E) staining. Pathologists have experimented with several techniques for rapid intraoperative assessment of sentinel nodes; however, at least in melanoma patients, this has not proved a useful strategy. In a report on 1119 sentinel nodes obtained from 669 patients with melanoma, in 67% of cases a single sentinel node contained tumor, and in 40% of cases immunohistochemical studies were required to confirm the diagnosis of metastatic disease.[22]

Recognition of sentinel node metastases is not as difficult in patients with breast cancer as in patients with melanoma but is nevertheless challenging for the pathologist. Turner and colleagues[23] found that analysis of frozen sections and touch preparations revealed the same findings as analysis with H&E-stained paraffin sections in 93% of patients. In 19 (26%) of 72 patients, the intraoperative assessment was falsely negative. The majority of these cases occurred in patients with small (T1 or T2) lesions. The authors concluded that if sentinel node status was used to determine the need for complete lymphadenectomy, more sensitive intraoperative studies would be needed to avoid a second operation in most patients.

An increasingly important question will be how to treat patients with negative sentinel nodes on traditional H&E staining but positive nodes on immunohistochemical staining or other testing for biochemical markers of metastases. Teng and associates[24] reported that 39 patients with breast cancer out of 519 examined had cytokeratin-positive, H&E-negative sentinel nodes. Twenty-six of these patients underwent complete lymphadenectomy, and three (11.5%) had additional metastases found.

Van Trappen and colleagues[25] used rapid polymerase chain reaction to test for cytokeratin 19 (CK-19) in the lymph nodes of patients who underwent radical hysterectomy. Lymphatic mapping was not performed; however, it appears from the report that the highest concentrations of CK-19–positive nodes corresponded with the most common sites of sentinel nodes. CK-19 was found in only one lymph node from nine patients with benign disease. In contrast, CK-19 was detected in 44% of the H&E-negative lymph nodes from the cervix cancer patients.

Are vulvar and cervix cancers good targets for the lymphatic mapping strategy?

Early vulvar cancer is an excellent target for lymphatic mapping for a number of reasons. The primary tumor is easily accessible for blue dye or radionuclide injection, and the sentinel node can be removed with a minimally invasive surgical technique. Years of observation have shown that systemic metastases in early vulvar cancer are rare and that lymph node metastases in vulvar cancer occur in a predictable sequential pattern. Pelvic node metastases are extremely rare if inguinal metastases are absent. Effective adjuvant therapy is available for node-positive patients, and the morbidity of combined-modality therapy with irradiation is increased in the setting of more extensive surgery. Finally, despite all of the advances in surgical techniques, wound infection, wound breakdown, and lymphedema remain significant problems after complete lymphadenectomy. The extent of long-term lymphedema is very difficult to determine by simple literature review. There is no consistent way to measure lymphedema, and long-term follow-up is required to determine both incidence and severity.

The case for lymphatic mapping in cervix cancer is interesting. The cervix is accessible for injection; however, the sentinel node is more difficult to reach than in the groin. Three techniques are available: laparotomy, retroperitoneal dissection, and laparoscopy. In patients with stage Ib1 and Ib2 disease, knowledge of nodal status is the single most important factor in determining the need for adjuvant therapy. Several recent trials all demonstrate that chemoradiation improves survival in node-positive patients compared with radiation alone. This applies to patients treated with an intact cervix,[26,27] or following radical hysterectomy and node dissection.[28]

On the other hand, lymphedema does not appear to be as common following pelvic lymphadenectomy as it is following groin dissection. The negative impact of radiotherapy on the incidence of lymphedema is not as great with pelvic irradiation as with groin irradiation. Conversely, radiotherapy following pelvic lymphadenectomy and radical hysterectomy results in more bowel complications than pelvic irradiation in an undisturbed pelvis.

Another problem with lymphatic mapping in the cervix relates to the parametrial lymph nodes. One patient in the literature had negative sentinel nodes in the pelvis and multiple small microscopic lymph node metastases in medial parametrial nodes that were resected with the primary tumor.[29] The medial parametrial nodes are too close to the primary tumor to be imaged with lymphoscintigraphy or blue dye. More data will be required to determine if this circumstance occurs regularly or not.

Cervix cancer is an interesting target for lymphatic mapping since lymphatic mapping can be combined with laparoscopy. Dargent and colleagues,[30] Roy and associates,[31] and Malur and coworkers[32] have reported excellent results with laparoscopic identification of sentinel nodes. This technique may allow identification of node-positive patients without laparotomy. Laparoscopy has also been combined with radical vaginal trachelectomy as a fertility-sparing procedure for women with early cervix cancers.[33,34] Patients eligible for this fertility-sparing procedure have a very low rate of node positivity, and lymphatic mapping with sentinel node identification appears to be a natural adjunct to this procedure. Institution of this procedure would permit less dissection in the pelvis and presumably reduce the number of fertility-compromising adhesions.

What is the best technique for intraoperative sentinel node identification in patients with vulvar cancer?

The emerging consensus is that the best technique for intraoperative sentinel node identification in patients with vulvar cancer is the combination of blue dye and radionuclide injections.

Use of blue dye alone, when it works, is quick and easy. It also demonstrates lymphatic channels in a way that lymphoscintigraphy cannot. Unfortunately, with blue dye, the window of opportunity for intraoperative sentinel node identification is brief, making it very difficult to learn lymphatic mapping using blue dye alone. In the largest series of patients with vulvar cancer who underwent lymphatic mapping with blue dye only, the success rate for sentinel node identification reached 100%, but only after a considerable learning period.[35] Advocates of blue dye point out that lymphoscintigraphy adds to the cost and complexity of the procedure but not the accuracy. It is rare for the dye to move to second-echelon lymph nodes, and there is no universal definition of a "hot" sentinel node.

Initial success rates with lymphoscintigraphy, either alone or with blue dye, in patients with vulvar cancer have been outstanding. De Cicco and colleagues[36] identified sentinel nodes in 100% of 37 patients using lymphoscintigraphy alone, and de Hullu and associates[37] identified sentinel nodes in 100% of 59 patients using a combined technique.

In several ongoing clinical trials of lymphatic mapping and sentinel node identification in patients with nongynecologic tumors, several mapping methods are available for use. In the Multicenter Lymphadenectomy Trial in melanoma patients, blue dye alone is acceptable for patients with primary tumors of the extremities, but blue dye plus lymphoscintigraphy is mandatory for truncal tumors. In the American College of Surgeons Oncology Group trials, blue dye alone is acceptable for tumors on the lateral two thirds of the breast but blue dye plus lymphoscintigraphy is mandatory for tumors on the medial third of the breast that may have internal mammary drainage.

In the case of gynecologic cancers, there is a consensus that the combined technique shortens the learning period. A short learning period is especially important since these diseases, especially vulvar cancer, are quite rare. The use of both techniques

provides a little bit of extra insurance for the clinician against unexpected failure of one of the techniques. The final decision depends on the resources at hand, the clinical situation, and the surgeon's skill level.

Is there a role for preoperative lymphoscintigraphy in treating gynecologic cancers?

A major use of preoperative lymphoscintigraphy is in patients with tumors that may have lymphatic drainage to more than one lymphatic basin, such as tumors of the medial third of the breast and the trunk. What about tumors of the vulva? Essentially, all early vulvar tumors drain to the groin, so in such cases is there any use for preoperative lymphoscintigraphy? Some preliminary data suggest that there may be. Our definition of midline versus lateral vulvar cancers is arbitrary and based only on physical examination. De Cicco and colleagues[36] performed preoperative lymphoscintigraphy and gamma probe–guided dissection in 37 patients with vulvar cancer. Eighteen had bilateral lymph node dissections based on location of the tumor within 2 cm of the midline. Five of these 18 patients had unilateral drainage on preoperative lymphoscintigraphy. None of the five had a sentinel node or nodal metastasis on the nondraining side at surgery. De Hullu and associates[37] reported a similar experience. In their well-executed study, 12 patients had midline lesions by clinical criteria and unilateral drainage on preoperative lymphoscintigraphy. All 12 patients had bilateral groin dissections. No sentinel nodes or lymph node metastases were found in the 12 dissected groins that did not have lymphatic drainage from the primary tumor on the preoperative lymphoscintigram. Bowles and coworkers[38] described six patients with tumors located at sites where bilateral drainage would be expected. Five of the six had unilateral drainage on preoperative lymphoscintigraphy. All these studies suggest that preoperative lymphoscintigraphy in patients with vulvar cancer may help determine lymphatic basins at risk for metastases before surgery. Conversely, Stehman and colleagues[39] and Burke and associates[40] each described one patient in whom a vulvar lesion was believed to be unilateral and unilateral dissection was performed and all nodes were negative and relapse occurred in the contralateral groin in the absence of a new vulvar lesion. Presumably these patients had contralateral lymph node metastases that were not recognized.

It is common to see vulvar tumors in which the obviously invasive portion is surrounded by a region of inflammation, preinvasive disease, or vulvar dystrophy. In such cases, it can be difficult to determine if the midline is actually involved or not. Preoperative lymphoscintigraphy may provide a method to determine when bilateral dissection or treatment is needed and when a unilateral approach will suffice (Fig. 49-5).

In the case of cervix cancer, data on the value of preoperative lymphoscintigraphy are even sparser.

Figure 49-5. **A,** Schema for the American College of Surgeons Oncology Group protocol Z-10 for patients with operable breast cancer. **B,** Schema for the American College of Surgeons Oncology Group protocol Z-11 for patients with positive sentinel lymph nodes.

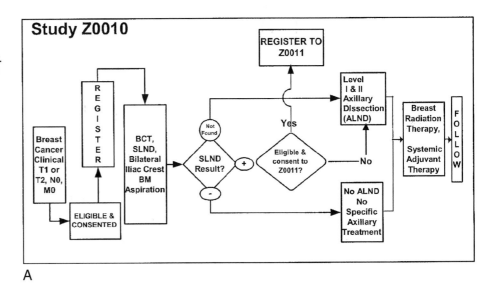

A

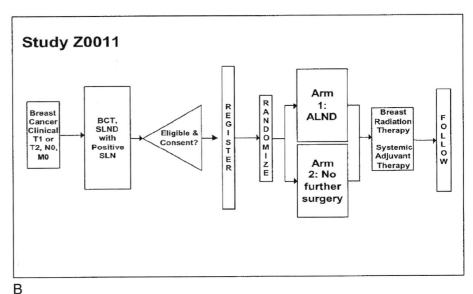

B

The cervix is by definition a midline structure, and therefore bilateral pelvic drainage should be expected in all cases. O'Boyle and colleagues[41] reported successful sentinel node identification in 12 of 20 patients who underwent radical hysterectomy. Five patients had bilateral drainage and seven had unilateral drainage visualized with the use of blue dye only. Levenback and associates[29] reported that 21 (55%) of 39 patients with cervix cancer had bilateral drainage on preoperative lymphoscintigrams. During intraoperative mapping with the gamma probe and blue dye, 28 (72%) of 39 patients had bilateral hot sentinel nodes. Another factor that must be taken into account when considering the role of preoperative lymphoscintigraphy in patients with cervix cancer it that unlike the case with other disease sites, both sides of the pelvis can be reached via a single incision.

It is yet to be seen if the assumption that all cervix cancers have bilateral drainage is accurate. The effects of obstetrical trauma, congenital malformations, pelvic inflammatory disease, prior surgery, and cone biopsy are not known. What role preoperative lymphoscintigraphy will have in cervical cancer remains to be determined.

How long is the learning curve for lymphatic mapping and sentinel node identification for gynecologic oncologists?

Essner and Morton[20] argue that it takes at least 15 and perhaps up to 50 cases for a surgeon to become proficient with lymphatic mapping in patients with melanoma or breast cancer. Cody and associates[42] reported that the false-negative rate in a group of 50 breast cancer patients dropped from 10% to 5% if the first six cases for each surgeon were excluded. Giuliano[43] recommends "see one, do twenty-five, teach one." Krag and coworkers[44] reported a range in accuracy of 82% to 98% among 11 surgeons using radioisotope alone; one surgeon had a false-negative rate of over 20% in a small group of patients. There are no data on accuracy specifically for gynecologic oncologists treating vulvar and cervix cancer;

Table 49–3. Common-Sense Suggestions for Reducing the Learning Curve for Lymphatic Mapping for Gynecologic Oncologists

- Read descriptions of various procedures.
- Perform a lymphatic mapping procedure in an animal laboratory.
- Select the technique you will use.
- Observe melanoma and breast lymphatic mapping cases.
- Invite a surgical oncologist to observe or assist with localization of sentinel nodes.
- Select patients carefully.
- Perform complete lymphadenectomy to determine your own success rate and false-negative rate.

however, there is every reason to believe that accuracy increases and false-negative rates decrease with experience.

There are several common-sense approaches that gynecologic oncologists can use to shorten the learning curve (Table 49-3). First and foremost is to do your homework. Read about the various procedures and find out what is available in your operating room. Perform a lymphatic mapping procedure in an animal laboratory if possible. This can be done in conjunction with laparoscopy courses. Decide which method you will use: blue dye alone, radioisotope alone, or both. Remember, the consensus is that the combined approach is the easiest to learn. In the case of blue dye, find out which one is available. In the case of lymphoscintigraphy, determine who will do the injection and where. It is unreasonable to expect a nuclear medicine specialist who has not done a pelvic examination since medical school to inject radionuclide into your patient while she is in a frog-leg position illuminated with a flashlight on a gamma-camera table. Most nuclear medicine suites are not equipped with a private examination room with a table designed for pelvic examinations. Therefore, alternatives will have to be found. Do the injection yourself as often as possible. Before attempting lymphatic mapping and sentinel node identification, observe at least one and preferably several breast cancer or melanoma cases. In this way you can see how to manage the patient and use the gamma probe for best results. Select your patients carefully. Factors associated with failure to identify sentinel nodes include a prior excisional biopsy, replacement of nodes with tumor, and extensive local inflammation.[35] Consider asking a surgical oncology colleague to look over your shoulder or even assist you during surgery to help you find your first few sentinel nodes. This is especially true for vulvar cases which have a lot in common with melanoma cases. Always do a regional lymphadenectomy following the sentinel node identification, and keep your own scorecard on how you are doing. You should get your sentinel node identification rate up to more than 90% very quickly, and your false-negative rate should be at the most 1 in the first 10.

Is ultrastaging of sentinel nodes necessary in patients with squamous carcinomas?

So-called ultrastaging of sentinel nodes has been useful in patients with breast cancer and melanoma in part because of the difficulty of identifying micrometastases from these tumors using standard H&E staining. In squamous carcinomas, the same difficulty does not exist, so is the extra cost of serial sectioning and immunohistochemical analysis worthwhile? It seems that serial sectioning increases the sampling of the nodal tissue and that this must increase the detection of micrometastases. Should sentinel nodes subjected to serial sectioning and found to be tumor-free be submitted for further study, such as immunohistochemical staining for cytokeratin? The experience in vulvar cancer is very limited. De Hullu and associates[37] performed serial sectioning and immunohistochemical analysis on 102 sentinel nodes that were negative on routine H&E analysis. They found micrometastases in four nodes (4%). Of special interest is the case described by Terada and colleagues.[45] A patient with vulvar cancer with a negative sentinel node had a relapse in the groin. The sentinel node was then reexamined with serial sectioning, and micrometastases were identified. The most recent and informative data from vulvar cancer patients suggest that immunohistochemical staining adds very little to serial sectioning with standard H&E staining. In a series of 89 sentinel nodes (from 30 nodal basins) that were negative on serial sectioning, none of the sentinel nodes were positive on pancytokeratin antibody AE1/AE3 immunostaining.[46]

Data on sentinel node examination in squamous carcinomas are too sparse to permit formulation of specific guidelines. However, it appears prudent to subject sentinel nodes to serial sectioning in patients with vulvar and cervix cancer. The role of immunohistochemical analysis will require more study before firm recommendations can be made.

What is the experience with lymphatic mapping in patients with vulvar cancer?

Table 49-4 summarizes the published literature regarding lymphatic mapping of the vulva. Overall, sentinel nodes were identified in 95.7% of the almost 300 patients included in these series and in 81.8% of the dissected groins. The success rate in groins may be artificially low since not all patients with tumors judged to be midline on clinical grounds have bilateral drainage. In 58% of patients, the sentinel node was the only positive node. False-negative cases were very rare. Routine H&E processing of sentinel nodes revealed metastatic disease in a high proportion of nodes containing metastases on ultrastaging. Serial sectioning or immunohistochemical staining identified metastatic disease in only 6.5% of the sentinel nodes that were negative on routine processing.

Table 49–4. Published Studies of Lymphatic Mapping and Sentinel Node Identification in Patients with Vulvar Cancer

Study	Technique	Technical Success, Patients*	Technical Success, Groins*	Specificity	Sensitivity*	NPV*	Accuracy*	SLN Only Positive LN/Groin	Node (+) Technical Failures (Groin)	Micro Mets on Serial Sections
Barton et al.[50] (1992)	Preop LS	9/10	13/16	6/6	3/3	6/6	9/9	1/3	1	—
DeCesare et al.[51] (1997)	Intraop LS	11/11	17/17	8/8	3/3	8/8	11/11	1/4	0	—
Rodier et al.[52] (1999)	Multiple techniques	7/8	8/10	7/7	1/1	7/7	7/7	1/1	0	—
Echt et al.[53] (1999)	Blue dye	9/12	13/23	6/6	2/2	6/6	8/8	2/3	1	—
Ansink et al.[54] (1999)	Blue dye	NA	52/93	41/41	9/11	41/43	50/52	6/14	1	—
Sideri et al.[55] (2000)	Preop LS Intraop LS	44/44	77/77	31/31	13/13	31/31	44/44	10/13	1	—
Terada et al.[45] (2000)	Preop LS Intraop LS Blue dye	10/10	12/12	8/8	1/2	8/9	9/10	2/2	0	1/15
de Hullu et al.[37] (2000)	Preop LS Intraop LS Blue dye	59/59	95/107	39/39	20/20	39/39	59/59	15/27	0	4/102
Molpus et al.[56] (2001)	Preop LS Intraop LS Blue dye	11/11	13/16	9/9	2/2	9/9	11/11	1/3	1	—
Tavares et al.[59] (2001)	Preop LS Intraop LS Blue dye	15/15	NA	12/12	3/3	12/12	15/15	2/3	0	—
Levenback et al.[35] (2001)	Blue dye	46/52	57/76	35/35	9/9	9/9	44/44	6/11	2	—
Puig-Tintore et al.[57] (2003)	Preop LS Intraop LS Blue dye	25/26	31/39	8/8	8/8	8/8	25/25	6/9	1	3/8
Slutz et al.[58] (2002)	Preop LS Intraop LS	26/26	46/46	17/17	9/9	17/17	26/26	NA	0	—
Total		272/284 (95.7)	434/530 (81.8)	227/227 (100)	83/88 (94.3)	201/204 (98.5)	318/321 (99)	53/93 (57)	8	8/125 (6.5)

*Technical success is the number of patients or groins in which sentinel nodes (SLNs) were found at surgery divided by the total number of patients or groins. Sensitivity is the proportion of patients with lymph node metastases in whom the sentinel nodes (SLNs) contained tumor (true positive/[true positive + false negative]). The negative predictive value is the proportion of patients without tumor in SLNs in whom the groin was free of tumor (true negative/[true negative + false negative]). Accuracy is the proportion of patients with successful SLN biopsy in whom the status of the SLN correlated with the status of the groin ([true positive] + true negative/[true positive + true negative + false positive + false negative]).

Intraop, intraoperative; LS, lymphoscintigraphy; Mets, metastases; NA, not available; NPV, negative predictive value; Preop, preoperative; SLN, sentinel node.

Reproduced with permission from Levenback, Coleman, van der Zee (eds): Clinical Lymphatic Mapping in Gynecologic Cancers. London, Taylor & Francis, 2004.

Is lymphatic mapping and sentinel node identification "standard" for patients with vulvar cancer?

Mounting evidence indicates that the sentinel node concept is valid in patients with vulvar cancer. I believe that lymphatic mapping and sentinel node identification will become a standard part of the surgical management of vulvar cancer in the future, and I recommend the procedure to all of my patients. Lymphatic mapping and sentinel node identification offers several direct benefits to the patient, assurance that the most common site of metastasis is removed, and an opportunity for extended histologic evaluation for metastatic disease with minimal risk.

Is lymphatic mapping and sentinel node identification a replacement for inguinal lymphadenectomy in patients with vulvar cancer?

Although the argument can be made that sentinel node identification is valid in patients with vulvar cancer and should be performed as part of the standard surgical management of vulvar cancer, the relevant data are too sparse to support recommending routine abandonment of inguinal lymphadenectomy. One current trial is designed to answer this question, the Groningen International Sentinel Node in Vulvar Cancer (GROINSV) Study. In this nonrandomized trial, patients with a negative sentinel node are observed. The results of this trial will be known in 2004 or 2005. There are several ongoing large randomized trials in patients with melanoma (Sunbelt Melanoma Trial, Multicentre Lymphadenectomy Trial) and breast cancer (American College of Surgeons Oncology Group trials Z-10 and Z-11 and National Surgical Adjuvant Breast and Bowel Program trial B-32) (see Fig. 49-5) that will help answer questions regarding sentinel node biopsy alone in these groups of patients. There is great interest in the Gynecologic Oncology Group and the European trial groups for a phase III study in vulvar cancer, and there are high hopes that such a trial will be launched in the near future.

In the meantime, inguinal lymphadenectomy must be considered the "standard" procedure for surgical management of the regional lymph nodes in patients with vulvar cancer. There are a few clinical situations in which I consider sentinel node biopsy alone, including early vulvar melanoma, patients at very high risk for lymphedema, patients with comorbid conditions placing them at risk for extended anesthesia time, and the elderly.

REFERENCES

1. Halsted W: The results of operations for the cure of cancer of the breast performed at the Johns Hopkins Hospitals. Ann Surg 1894;20:497.
2. Halsted W: The results of radical operations for the cure of carcinoma of the breast. Ann Surg 1907;46:1.
3. Gray J: The relation of lymphatic vessels to the spread of cancer. Br J Surg 1938;26:462-495.
4. Sappey PC: Anatomie, Physiologie et Pathology, des Vaisseaux Lymphatiques Consideres chez l'Homme et les Vertebres. Paris, A. Délahaye et E. Lecrosnier, 1885.
5. Hudack S, McMaster P: The lymphatic participation in human cutaneous phenomena. J Exp Med 1933;57:751-774.
6. Morris JM: A formula for selective lymphadenectomy: Its application to cancer of the vulva. Obstet Gynecol 1977;50:152-158.
7. Cabanas RM: An approach for the treatment of penile carcinoma. Cancer 1977;39:456-466.
8. Morton DL, Wen DR, Wong JH, et al: Technical details of intraoperative lymphatic mapping for early stage melanoma. Arch Surg 1992;127:392-399.
9. Fisher B, Fisher ER: The interrelationship of hematogenous and lymphatic tumor cell dissemination. Surg Gynecol Obstet 1966;122:791-798.
10. Wong JH: Lymphatic drainage of skin in a sentinel lymph node in a feline model. Ann Surg 1991;214:637-641.
11. Bostick PJ, Giuliano AE: Vital dyes in sentinel node localization. Semin Nucl Med 2000;30:18-24.
12. Leong SP, Donegan E, Heffernon W, et al: Adverse reactions to isosulfan blue during selective sentinel lymph node dissection in melanoma. Ann Surg Oncol 2000;7:361-366.
13. Sadiq TS, Burns WW 3rd, Taber DJ, et al: Blue urticaria: A previously unreported adverse event associated with isosulfan blue. Arch Surg 2001;136:1433-1435.
14. Coleman R, Whitten CW, O'Boyle J, Sidhu B: Unexplained decrease in measured oxygen saturation by pulse oximetry following injection of Lymphazurin 1% (isosulfan blue) during a lymphatic mapping procedure. J Surg Oncol 1999;70:126-129.
15. Eshima D, Fauconnier T, Eshima L, Thornback JR: Radiopharmaceuticals for lymphoscintigraphy, including dosimetry and radiation considerations. Semin Nucl Med 2000; 30:25-32.
16. Wilhelm AJ, Mijnhout GS, Franssen EJ: Radiopharmaceuticals in sentinel lymph-node detection—an overview. Eur J Nucl Med 1999:26(Suppl):S36-S42.
17. Glass EC, Essner R, Morton DL: Kinetics of three lymphoscintigraphic agents in patients with cutaneous melanoma. J Nucl Med 1998;39:1185-1190.
18. Fiorica JV, Grendys E, Hoffman M: Intraoperative radiolocalization of the sentinel node in patients with vulvar cancer. Oper Tech Gynecol Surg 2001;6:27-32.
19. Thompson JF, Uren RF: What is a "sentinel" lymph node? [editorial]. Eur J Surg Oncol 2000:1:103-104.
20. Essner R, Morton DL: The blue-dye technique. In Cody HS (ed): Sentinel Lymph Node Biopsy. London, Martin Dunitz, 2002, pp 91-104.
21. Gershenwald JE, Tseng CH, Thompson W, et al: Improved sentinel lymph node localization in patients with primary melanoma with the use of radiolabeled colloid. Surgery 1998;124:203-210.
22. Cochran AJ: The pathologist's role in sentinel lymph node evaluation. Semin Nucl Med 2000;30:11-17.
23. Turner RR, Hansen NM, Stern DL, Giuliano AE: Intraoperative examination of the sentinel lymph node for breast carcinoma staging. Am J Clin Pathol 1999;112:627-634.
24. Teng S, Dupont E, McCann C, et al: Do cytokeratin-positive-only sentinel lymph nodes warrant complete axillary lymph node dissection in patients with invasive breast cancer? Am Surg 2000;66:574-578.
25. Van Trappen P, Gyselman VG, Lowe DG, et al: Molecular quantification and mapping of lymph-node micrometastases in cervical cancer. Lancet 2001;357:15-20.
26. Morris M, Eifel PJ, Lu J, et al: Pelvic radiation with concurrent chemotherapy compared with pelvic and paraaortic radiation for high-risk cervical cancer. N Engl J Med 1999;340:1137-1143.
27. Rose PG, Adler LP, Rodriguez M, et al: Positron emission tomography for evaluating para-aortic nodal metastasis in locally advanced cervical cancer before surgical staging: A surgicopathologic study. J Clin Oncol 1999;17:41-45.
28. Peters WA 3rd, Liu PYP, Barrett RJ 2nd, et al: Concurrent chemotherapy and pelvic radiation therapy compared with pelvic radiation therapy alone as adjuvant therapy after radical surgery in high-risk early-stage cancer of the cervix. J Clin Oncol 2000;18:1606-1613.

29. Levenback C, Coleman RL, Burke TW, et al: Lymphatic mapping and sentinel node identification in patients with cervix cancer undergoing radical hysterectomy and pelvic lymphadenectomy. J Clin Oncol 2002;20:688-693.
30. Dargent D, Martin X, Mathevet P: Laparoscopic assessment of the sentinel lymph node in early stage cervical cancer. Gynecol Oncol 2000;79:411-415.
31. Roy C, Le Bras Y, Mangold L, et al: Small pelvic lymph node metastases: Evaluation with MR imaging. Clin Radiol 1997; 52:437-440.
32. Malur S, Krause N, Kohler C, Schneider A: Sentinel lymph node detection in patients with cervical cancer. Gynecol Oncol 2001;80:254-257.
33. Roy M, Plante M, Renaud MC, Tetu B: Vaginal radical hysterectomy versus abdominal radical hysterectomy in the treatment of early-stage cervical cancer. Gynecol Oncol 1996;62:336-339.
34. Dargent D, et al: Identification of a sentinel node with laparoscopy in cervical cancer. In Program and Abstracts of the 31st Annual Meeting of the Society of Gynecologic Oncologists, 2000, San Diego, CA.
35. Levenback C, Coleman RL, Burke TW, et al: Intraoperative lymphatic mapping and sentinel node identification with blue dye in patients with vulvar cancer. Gynecol Oncol 2001;83: 276-281.
36. De Cicco C, Sideri M, Bartolomei M, et al: Sentinel node biopsy in early vulvar cancer. Br J Cancer 2000;82:295-299.
37. de Hullu JA, Hollema H, Piers DA, et al: Sentinel lymph node procedure is highly accurate in squamous cell carcinoma of the vulva. J Clin Oncol 2000;18:2811-2816.
38. Bowles J, Terada KY, Coel MN, Wong JH: Preoperative lymphoscintigraphy in the evaluation of squamous cell cancer of the vulva. Clin Nucl Med 1999;24:235-238.
39. Stehman FB, Bundy BN, Ball H, Clarke-Pearson DL: Sites of failure and times to failure in carcinoma of the vulva treated conservatively: A Gynecologic Oncology Group study. Am J Obstet Gynecol 1996;174:1128-1132, discussion 1132-1133.
40. Burke TW, Levenback C, Tornos C, et al: Intraabdominal lymphatic mapping to direct selective pelvic and paraaortic lymphadenectomy in women with high-risk endometrial cancers: Results of a pilot study. Gynecol Oncol 1996;62:169-173.
41. O'Boyle J, Coleman RL, Bernstein SG, et al: Intraoperative lymphatic mapping in cervix cancer patients undergoing radical hysterectomy: A pilot study. Gynecol Oncol 2000;79:238-243.
42. Cody HS 3rd, Hill AD, Tran KN, et al: Credentialing for breast lymphatic mapping: How many cases are enough? Ann Surg 1999;229:723-728.
43. Giuliano AE: See one, do twenty-five, teach one: The implementation of sentinel node dissection in breast cancer. Ann Surg Oncol 1999;6:520-521.
44. Krag D, Harlow S, Weaver D, Ashikaga T: Technique of sentinel node resection in melanoma and breast cancer: Probe-guided surgery and lymphatic mapping. Eur J Surg Oncol 1998;24:89-93.
45. Terada KY, Shimizu DM, Wong JH: Sentinel node dissection and ultrastaging in squamous cell cancer of the vulva. Gynecol Oncol 2000;76:40-44.
46. Moore RG, et al: Pathologic evaluation of inguinal sentinel nodes in vulvar cancer patients: A comparison of immunohistochemical staining versus ultra-staging with hematoxylin and eosin staining. Presented at the Society of Gynecologic Oncologists 34th Annual Meeting, 2003, New Orleans, LA.
47. Morton DL: Sentinel lymphadenectomy for patients with clinical stage I melanoma. J Surg Oncol 1997;66:267-269.
48. Harris J, Hellman S: Natural history of breast cancer. In Harris JR, Morrow M, et al (eds): Diseases of the Breast. Philadelphia, Lippincott-Raven, 1996.
49. Liberman L, Schneider L: Review of published experience. In Cody HS (ed): Sentinel Lymph Node Biopsy. London, Martin Dunitz, 2002, pp 285-310.
50. Barton DP, Berman C, Cavanagh D, et al: Lymphoscintigraphy in vulvar cancer: A pilot study. Gynecol Oncol 1992;46:341-344.
51. DeCesare SL, Fiorica JV, Roberts WS, et al: A pilot study utilizing intraoperative lymphoscintigraphy for identification of the sentinel lymph nodes in vulvar cancer. Gynecol Oncol 1997; 66:425-428.
52. Rodier JF, Janser JC, Routiot T, et al: Sentinel node biopsy in vulvar malignancies: A preliminary feasibility study. Oncol Rep 1999;6:1249-1252.
53. Echt M, Finan MA, Hoffman MS, et al: Detection of sentinel lymph nodes with lymphazurin in cervical, uterine, and vulvar malignancies. South Med J 1999;92:204-208.
54. Ansink AC, Sie-Go DM, van der Velden J, et al: Identification of sentinel lymph nodes in vulvar carcinoma patients with the aid of a patent blue V injection: A multicenter study. Cancer 1999; 86:652-656.
55. Sideri M, De Cicco C, Maggioni A, et al: Detection of sentinel nodes by lymphoscintigraphy and gamma probe guided surgery in vulvar neoplasia. Tumori 2000;86:359-363.
56. Molpus KL, Kelley MC, Johnson JE, et al: Sentinel lymph node detection and microstaging in vulvar carcinoma. J Reprod Med 2001;46:863-869.
57. Puig-Tintore LM, Ordi J, Vidal-Sicart S, et al: Further data on the usefulness of sentinel lymph node identification and ultrastaging in vulvar squamous cell carcinoma. Gynecol Oncol 2003; 88:29-34.
58. Sliutz G, Reinthaller A, Lantzsch T, et al: Lymphatic mapping of sentinel nodes in early vulvar cancer. Gynecol Oncol 2002; 84:449-452.
59. Tavares MG, Sapienza MT, Galeb NA Jr, et al: The use of 99mTc-phytate for sentinel node mapping in melanoma, breast cancer and vulvar cancer: A study of 100 cases. Eur J Nucl Med 2001; 28:1597-1604.

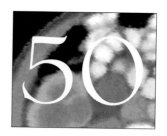

VAGINAL RECONSTRUCTION IN PELVIC EXENTERATION

David E. Cohn and Larry J. Copeland

MAJOR CONTROVERSIES

- **What general category of vaginal reconstruction is appropriate after pelvic exenteration?**
- **Why should vaginal reconstruction be considered? Should reconstruction be performed at the time of pelvic exenteration?**
- **What options exist for women who desire vaginal reconstruction? How does the surgical team select the appropriate technique for reconstruction?**
- **Is there a method to ensure appropriate blood supply to a flap to minimize the risk of necrosis?**
- **What novel surgical techniques have been instituted to modify and improve vaginal reconstruction?**
- **What are the psychological and sexual implications of vaginal reconstruction, and are there methods to minimize their impact?**
- **What oncologic follow-up should be provided for women with vaginal reconstruction after exenteration?**

Since the initial description of pelvic exenteration in the treatment of recurrent gynecologic malignancies by Brunschwig in 1948,[1] improvements in surgical technique, antibiotics, and postoperative care have led to a decrease in both disease- and procedure-related morbidity and mortality. As the technique has continued to be refined, the primary emphasis on disease control has been complemented by consideration of the restoration of patient anatomy and function. Modifications of pelvic exenteration include maintaining continuity in the intestinal and urinary tracts when feasible, performing continent urinary diversions, and reconstructing the vagina. Although vaginal reconstruction is commonly performed in conjunction with pelvic exenteration, some controversy still exists regarding it. This chapter addresses these controversies, reviews the options for vaginal reconstruction, and discusses recent modifications of standard reconstructive techniques.

What general category of vaginal reconstruction is appropriate after pelvic exenteration?

The optimal reconstruction of vaginal defects after pelvic exenteration requires significant preparation before initiation of the procedure. Baseline information regarding a patient's anticipated level of sexual function determines whether vaginal reconstruction will be attempted during the exenterative procedure. Assessment of a patient's preoperative functional status and motivation also guides the operative team in the selection of an appropriate method for vaginal reconstruction, because certain procedures require significant patient-directed care to ensure long-term function. A detailed history of previous surgeries, radiation portals, doses, and complications is imperative in planning appropriate donor sites for vaginal reconstruction. During physical examination, attention to patient size, weight, and fat distribution allows the

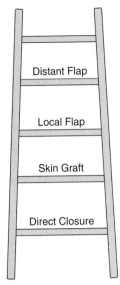

Figure 50–1. The reconstructive ladder. Traditionally, the decision to pursue a more complex reconstructive technique (upper rungs) was made after an inability to perform a simpler technique (lower rungs). However, this concept has now been challenged.

surgical team to predict whether there will be limitations to the ability of the donor site to reach the pelvis for reconstruction. Likewise, previous incisions may direct the surgeon to further investigation of potential vascular disruption to donor sites, such as the inferior epigastric vessels that supply the inferior aspect of the rectus abdominis flap, and obturator artery compromise that may decrease gracilis myocutaneous flap success.

Historically, the appropriate type of reconstruction was assigned according to a "reconstructive ladder" (Fig. 50-1), which described a stepwise ascent

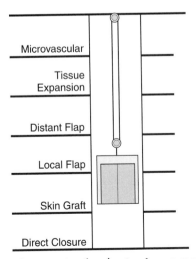

Figure 50–2. The reconstructive elevator. A more modern approach to reconstructive techniques is one described by a "reconstructive elevator," which does not require elimination of simpler techniques before moving to a complex reconstructive technique such as a distant flap or microvascular reconstruction.

from simple procedures (direct closure), through more complex repairs (skin grafting, local flap), to complex reconstruction (distant flaps employing microsurgical anastomosis). More recently, this concept was challenged, and it was recommended that appropriate reconstructive techniques should be assigned according to a "reconstructive elevator" (Fig. 50-2). Because of the significant improvement in safety and reliability of complex vaginal reconstructive techniques, it is appropriate, especially in vaginal reconstruction in the context of pelvic exenteration, to bypass the simple techniques on the lower rungs of the ladder, which may lead to limited function, and move directly to those on the higher rungs that require more technical skill but provide excellent functional results.

Why should vaginal reconstruction be considered? Should reconstruction be performed at the time of pelvic exenteration?

As described earlier, a number of factors influence the decision to perform vaginal reconstruction at the time of pelvic exenteration. Beyond the benefit of providing a functional vagina for sexual activity, there are other, nonsexual benefits to reconstruction that must be considered in planning for the appropriate procedure. Early descriptions of pelvic exenteration without reconstruction of the pelvic floor described a high incidence of postoperative fistula formation. Miller and colleagues[2] reviewed a large series of 533 pelvic exenterations from the MD Anderson Cancer Center over a 33-year period and described a reduction in the rate of intestinal fistula, from 16% to 4.5%, with the introduction of pelvic floor reconstruction with either omental grafts or gracilis flaps to the pelvic exenteration. Similar results were reported by Soper and associates[3] in a series of 69 women who underwent exenteration over a 17-year period and by Cain and coworkers[4] in a series of 24 women undergoing gracilis myocutaneous grafts. Reasons for this decreased complication rate include introducing a new, usually unirradiated, blood supply to the pelvis, and placement of a piece of tissue to physically separate the intestine from the pelvis.

Although vaginal reconstruction may increase operative time, most reconstruction techniques can be done efficiently and without excessive morbidity.[5] The use of a second surgical team for vaginal reconstruction can eliminate this additional time, with the reconstruction performed concurrently with the extirpative portion of the procedure. For patients who have been adequately counseled regarding the implications of pelvic exenteration and vaginal reconstruction, the most appropriate time for repair is at the time of exenteration. However, if reconstruction cannot be performed because of unexpected surgical complications or technical difficulties with reconstructive procedures, delayed vaginal reconstruction is feasible and successful,[6] although it is likely to be more complicated and to carry increased surgical risk. Therefore, if feasible, primary vaginal reconstruction is optimal.

What options exist for women who desire vaginal reconstruction? How does the surgical team select the appropriate technique for reconstruction?

A number of surgical techniques are appropriate for vaginal reconstruction after pelvic exenteration. The selection of one method over another is dictated by a number of factors such as the size and location of the defect, the size and fat distribution of the patient, previous procedures that may have led to disruption of the blood supply to a donor site, and individual skill and bias of the surgical team. It is likely that this last criterion leads most commonly to the selection of one method of reconstruction over others. This section describes options for vaginal reconstruction in detail, and indications for each surgical technique are described.

No vaginal reconstruction. In women undergoing pelvic exenteration who will not become sexually active after surgery, primary closure of the defect is indicated. However, a significant risk of gastrointestinal complications exists in the absence of some form of pelvic floor reconstruction. In this situation, the placement of an omental flap can minimize the risk of fistula formation. This procedure is described later in the chapter. If an omental flap with its independent blood supply cannot be used, other options for reconstruction of the pelvic floor include the placement of material such as a piece of mesh,[7-9] an adhesion prevention barrier, human dura,[10] or other inert materials

to prevent adhesions of the bowel to the denuded pelvic floor and resultant fistula formation.

Omental J-flap and omental neovagina. In women who would benefit from a moderate increase in the length of their native vagina after exenteration, many surgeons recomend the placement of an omental flap at the apex of the residual vagina. Because the arterial blood supply to the omentum is rich (Fig. 50-3), this organ serves as an excellent, well-vascularized flap in pelvic floor and vaginal reconstruction. Other benefits of an omental flap include the short operative time and minimal surgical risk. Because of the small size of an omental flap, this technique is useful only in circumstances in which only a small degree of vaginal augmentation is necessary. The omental flap is created by dividing the right gastroduodenal artery, which supplies this portion of the omentum. Avascular planes are established between the omentum and transverse colon serosa and mesentery. The omentum is mobilized until the appropriate length is established without sacrificing the previously confirmed and present left gastroepiploic artery. The omentum is then repositioned down the paracolic recess into the pelvis. For pelvic reconstruction, the omentum is then sutured to the pelvic wall, separating the intestine from the denuded pelvis. If the omentum is used to lengthen the vagina, the distal end of the omentum is rolled and sutured with fine absorbable suture into a cylinder. The distal end of the omental cylinder is sutured to the apex of the vagina, and the upper end of the cylinder is closed if necessary. This procedure is commonly

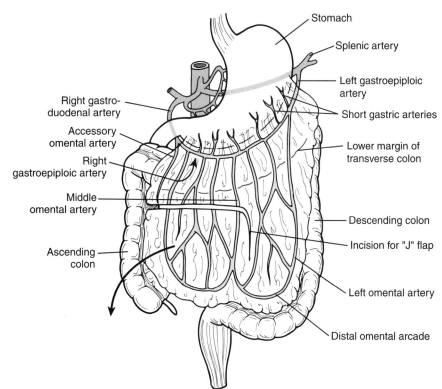

Figure 50–3. Omental J-flap. The vascular supply of the omentum is through the left gastroepiploic artery and right gastroduodenal artery. An omental J-flap is designed by dividing the omentum off of the transverse colon and placing it into the pelvis to cover an exenteration defect or rolling it into a tube for vaginal reconstruction.

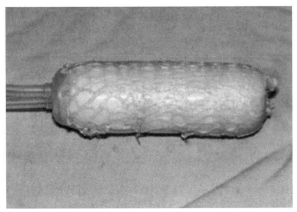

Figure 50–4. Split-thickness skin graft and vaginal stent. After harvest from the donor site, the graft is placed over a stent, which is then placed in the vagina. The stent is left in place for 4 to 7 days and then removed and washed. The patient is instructed in wearing the stent for 3 to 6 months after reconstruction.

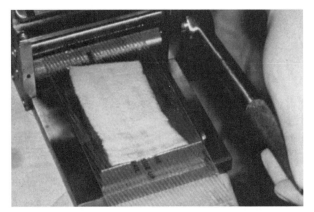

Figure 50–5. Meshing of a split-thickness skin graft. This procedure allows for increased coverage area and minimizes fluid buildup behind the graft.

combined with the application of a split-thickness skin graft (STSG) to the inside of the omental cylinder. In the absence of a skin graft, epithelial cells from the introitus will migrate and lead to epithelialization of the omental flap. After completion of the omental neovagina, the space is filled with a stent. Commonly, this involves packing the vagina with cotton gauze (usually within a condom) or inserting a wood or plastic form to maintain the vaginal lumen (Fig. 50-4). The stent is removed after 4 to 7 days, and the vagina irrigated. Patients are then instructed in the continued use of the stent for 3 to 6 months after surgery to keep the neovagina from contracting.

Split-thickness skin graft. As originally described by McIndoe and Banister[11] for the creation of a neovagina in patients with vaginal agenesis resulting from Mayer-Rokitansky-Kuster-Hauser syndrome, a STSG can be used for vaginal reconstruction after pelvic exenteration. Benefits of STSG include the fact that there is no size limitation for reconstruction, because multiple pieces of skin can be secured together for coverage of a large area. However, like an omental flap, STSG is limited by its thinness, and for this reason it is not appropriate for primary coverage of a sizeable defect. Also, impeccable hemostasis is required before the placement of a STSG, because any bleeding behind the graft will jeopardize graft adherence. If the site to be grafted is not appropriate for immediate reconstruction, a delayed STSG can be performed,[12] assuming that a vaginal stent is placed for the immediate postexenteration period.

A STSG is commonly applied to the inside of an omental neovagina to facilitate epithelialization and is used in patients after pelvic exenteration.[6,13] Donor sites are chosen based on considerations of cosmesis (buttocks and inner thigh sites are well concealed) and an effort to avoid previously irradiated skin. If the STSG technique is to be performed during exenteration, the inner thigh is a more appropriate donor site because of the need for repositioning to access the buttocks for

harvesting. A dermatome is used to harvest a STSG with a thickness of 0.016 to 0.02 inches. Meshing of the graft may allow it to cover a larger area than was harvested and may prevent fluid from building up behind the graft, which would lead to failure (Fig. 50-5). The minimum graft size required for functional vaginal reconstruction is approximately 10 × 20 cm, accounting for the passive contraction of 20% that commonly occurs with STSGs. The grafts are held together with a fine absorbable suture around a vaginal stent, as described for the omental neovagina. Management of the stent is also similar to that described previously for the omental neovagina. Success rates for a STSG with or without an omental flap are variable and are highly dependent on the motivation and compliance of the patient.

The issue of compliance is a particular challenge in women with a recurrent gynecologic malignancy who have just undergone the physical and emotional challenges of pelvic exenteration. This technique should be used in the specific circumstance of a motivated patient with a narrow pelvis who requires lengthening of the vagina. This technique may also be preferred in the obese patient, in whom myocutaneous reconstructive techniques are compromised. Sexual function after placement of a STSG and omental neovagina depends on the preexisting vaginal length and is discussed in a separate section.

Intestinal interposition. The concept of constructing a neovagina from colon or ileum was first proposed in the early 1900s, with minimal modification of the original technique into the 1990s.[14] In general, the substitution of intestine for vagina is not widely used, mainly because of the disadvantages of the production of a malodorous mucoid discharge, contact bleeding, and stricture. Another limitation of this technique is that, because of the thinness of the intestinal wall, this graft is not appropriate for coverage of large defects. Although both ileal and sigmoidal segments have been proposed, the cecum appears to be most reliable and functional when this form of reconstruction is used.[14] Dyspareunia is problematic after intestinal neovaginal reconstruction.

Rectus abdominis myocutaneous flap. The rectus abdominis muscles are paired strap muscles in the abdominal wall with a dual blood supply. Superiorly, the muscle is supplied by the superior epigastric vessels from the internal mammary artery; inferiorly, it is supplied by the deep inferior epigastric artery. This rotational flap can be constructed because the anastomotic vessels cross a watershed in the muscle at its midportion. The sensory and motor innervation is disrupted in raising a rectus flap, so the muscle in the flap is paralyzed and the skin lacks sensation. Tobin and Day[15] described the technique of a distally based rectus abdominis flap for vaginal and pelvic floor reconstruction, and these authors[16] and others[17-20] have continued to describe and refine the technique for use after pelvic exenteration. Compared with other myocutaneous flaps used for vaginal reconstruction, rectus abdominis neovaginas have been demonstrated to have the lowest rate of flap necrosis, as well as a lower rate of prolapse than the gracilis myocutaneous flaps. However, the rectus myocutaneous reconstruction is not an option for patients whose surgery has previously compromised the inferior epigastric vessels. These surgeries include a previous Maylard incision or a retroperitoneal lymphadenectomy in which the epigastric vessels are divided. Previous abdominoplasty can also injure the epigastric vessels. If there is concern as to the nature of any prior surgery, angiographic confirmation of the vascular anatomy should be considered. Because the thickness of the flap is dictated by the thickness of the abdominal wall, the flap may be too bulky for a functional vaginal reconstruction in women with obesity.

Although rectus abdominis flaps can be constructed in either a vertical or a transverse direction, this summary describes the technique of vertical rectus flap, because it is the technique that is most commonly used for vaginal reconstruction. Reasons for the use of a vertical rather than a transverse flap include the fact that only one abdominal incision is required for harvesting the vertical flap; in contrast, a vertical and a transverse incision are required when harvesting a transverse flap during pelvic exenteration through a midline incision. Likewise, Carlson and coworkers[19] described more tension in the closure of the abdominal wall when a transverse flap was used. The paddle of skin overlying the upper portion of the rectus muscle is shaped like an ellipse, with its base beginning just below the umbilicus and its apex ending at the middle of the muscle at the costal margin (Fig. 50-6). The width of the paddle is approximately 15 cm, which allows for a reconstructed vagina that is 4 cm in diameter. Flap length is approximately 10 cm and is limited by the distance between the umbilicus and the costal margin along the course of the rectus abdominis muscle.

Following the skin incision, the anterior rectus sheath is incised, although this incision is narrower than the overlying skin to facilitate closure of the abdominal wall. Here, approximately 1 cm of rectus sheath on the medial aspect and 3 cm of the sheath laterally are preserved. The superior aspect of the muscle is transected at the costal margin, and at this level the

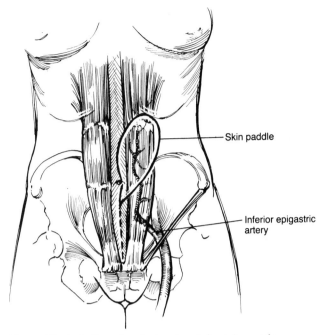

Figure 50–6. Outline of vertical rectus abdominis muscle myocutaneous flap. The base of the flap is oriented at the umbilicus and covers an area 15 cm wide and 10 cm long. A flap this size results in a neovagina approximately 4 cm in width.

superior epigastric vessels are identified and divided. The flap is then mobilized from the posterior rectus fascia until there is adequate mobility to reach the vaginal defect. The flap is then directed to the perineum under the remaining skin bridge on the lower abdomen. The flap is constructed into a vaginal tube by inverting the graft so that the skin surface is on the inside of the cylinder, and the distal end of the tube is sutured closed (Fig. 50-7). The proximal end of the rectus neovagina is then sutured to the perineum (Fig. 50-8). The abdominal wall is closed by suturing

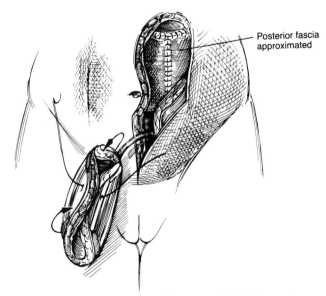

Figure 50–7. After harvesting of the rectus abdominis muscle, overlying skin, and underlying fascia, the flap is rolled into a tube with the skin surface on the inside of the neovagina.

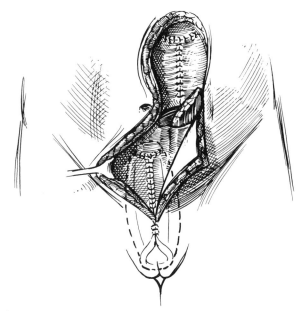

Figure 50–8. Completed vertical rectus abdominis myocutaneous neovagina before delivery through the perineal defect. The top of the flap has been sewn closed with absorbable suture. The completed cylinder is then sewn to the remaining perineal tissues. No vaginal stent is required after myocutaneous vaginal reconstruction.

each side of the residual anterior rectus sheath to the other and reapproximating the skin on completion of the exenteration. A significant advantage of the technique of myocutaneous neovaginal reconstruction is that a vaginal stent is not required to keep the vagina patent, in contrast to the STSG technique. Likewise, patients are not required to perform vaginal dilatation to maintain vaginal patency. Sexual function after rectus abdominis neovaginal reconstruction is variable and is described in a separate section.

Gracilis myocutaneous flap. The technique of gracilis myocutaneous vaginal reconstruction was the first type of myocutaneous graft to be extensively studied in patients who had undergone pelvic exenteration for gynecologic malignancies. McCraw and colleagues[21] pioneered the technique, and many reports including modifications and refinements have been made since the initial description.[22,23] Similar to other myocutaneous grafts, the gracilis flap has the advantage of filling a large defect with a new blood supply, leading to sexual function in many patients, and is easily performed with little added surgical morbidity. However, the gracilis neovagina has been reported to have a relatively high incidence of partial or complete flap necrosis as well as flap prolapse. Initial reports demonstrated a rate of partial flap loss greater than 7%,[4,22-25] with 17% of patients experiencing flap prolapse.[22-24] Likewise, the use of gracilis flaps has been difficult because of their size and bulk. Specifically, the flaps may be too bulky to pass under the pubic arch without tension, causing venous congestion and flap necrosis. Modifications of the technique have included creating smaller gracilis flaps to overcome the limitations of the bulky reconstruction, and ligating the

neurovascular pedicle, thereby increasing the mobility of the flap.[26,27] With these modifications, severe necrosis and prolapse have been decreased.[26] Unchanged, however, remain the bilateral leg scars that are necessary for appropriate reconstruction after pelvic exenteration. Because of the increased rate of necrosis and prolapse compared with rectus abdominis myocutaneous neovaginal reconstruction, gracilis flaps should be used when the skills or anatomy is not feasible for rectus flaps. Advantages of gracilis flaps include the ability for a second operative team to harvest and construct the gracilis neovagina, thereby limiting the extra time necessary for reconstruction.

The gracilis muscle functions as an accessory thigh adductor; it is supplied from a branch of the profunda femoris artery, the medial circumflex femoral artery, that passes between the adductor longus and adductor brevis muscles, approximately 8 cm from the pubis. The flap also gets significant blood supply from the terminal branches of the obturator artery, so the main neurovascular bundle can be divided for increased mobility without an increase in the risk of flap necrosis.[26,28] The gracilis muscle arises from the inferior pubic ramus and inserts onto the medial tibial condyle, along with the sartorius and semitendinosus muscles (Fig. 50-9). The sensory innervation of the gracilis flap comes from branches of the anterior cutaneous nerves of the thigh, which are divided during development of the myocutaneous complex. The gracilis flap can lead to a paddle with dimensions of 12 × 24 cm, although most flaps for vaginal reconstruction require a width of approximately 6 cm.

To develop the gracilis myocutaneous flap, the semitendinosus tendon is palpated as it approaches the posterior aspect of the medial tibial condyle. An incision through the fascia lata is made just above the tendon, and the gracilis tendon is identified and elevated through the incision and pulled to ensure that the correct muscle has been identified. Using the

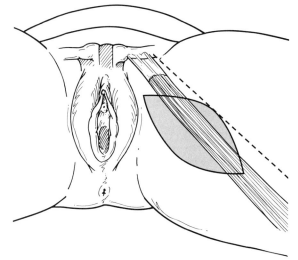

Figure 50–9. Outline of the gracilis muscle before myocutaneous vaginal reconstruction. The muscle is located inferior to a line drawn between the pubic tubercle and the posterior insertion of the semitendinosus muscle at the tibia.

muscle as a landmark, the surgeon designs a skin paddle centered on the muscle belly. The skin supplied by perforators from the gracilis muscle extends to approximately 2 cm above and below the superior and inferior aspects of the palpable muscle. The flap is incised through the skin down to and through the fascia lata. The gracilis muscle and fascia are then separated from the adductor brevis muscle until the neurovascular bundle is identified between the adductor longus and brevis muscles, approximately 8 cm from the head of the gracilis muscle. The flap is then rotated and delivered below the skin flap between the donor site and pelvic defect, and the donor site is closed (Fig. 50-10). If a less bulky flap is desired (the so-called short gracilis flap[26,27]), the main neurovascular bundle is divided and flap viability relies on the distal supply from the obturator artery. With this technique, increased mobility occurs, with resultant decrease in the rate of flap necrosis and prolapse. The bilateral flaps, once delivered through the skin bridges, are brought to the midline and sewn together with fine absorbable suture. The lateral edges are then approximated, creating a tube. The neovagina is rotated posteriorly through the pelvic defect and sutured to the levator muscles and retropubic fascia before the flap is sutured to the perineum (Fig. 50-11).

Tensor fascia lata flap. The use of the tensor fascia lata muscle and fascia for neovaginal reconstruction after pelvic exenteration is not employed widely, despite the ability to create a large, sensate flap.[29,30] Reasons for its rarity in clinical practice include the resultant cosmetic deformity, difficulty in donor site closure, potential for postoperative knee instability, and the options for other myocutaneous flaps without these complications. The tensor fascia lata arises from the anterior 5 cm of the iliac crest, between the gluteus medius and sartorius muscles. The blood supply to the tensor fascia lata muscle is from the terminal ascending branch of the lateral circumflex femoral artery, derived from the profunda femoris artery. Because of the perforators to the skin over the muscle, the skin over the tensor fascia lata muscle as well as the skin over the anterolateral thigh can be used in this myocutaneous flap. The width of the flap therefore can reach at least 15 cm, making primary closure of the donor site challenging (Fig. 50-12). Because of the proximity of this flap to the lateral femoral cutaneous nerve, which supplies the skin overlying the muscle, injury to the nerve can lead to meralgia paresthetica, a syndrome leading to pain and paresthesias similar to that seen in nerve entrapment syndromes. After harvesting, the flap is rotated into the pelvic defect. Because of the location of the flap and its mobility, its utility is limited for neovaginal construction, but it may be appropriate for reconstruction after radical vulvectomy and groin lymphadenectomy.

Bulbocavernosus flap (Martius flap). The repair of urethrovaginal and vesicovaginal fistulas resulting from childbirth was described in 1928 by Martius, who used a bulbocavernosus fat flap as a pedicle graft.[31]

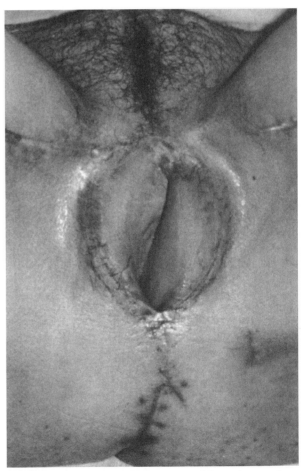

Figure 50–11. Postoperative appearance of the perineum after bilateral gracilis myocutaneous vaginal reconstruction. The donor sites are healed, and the previous drain sites are not visible in this photograph.

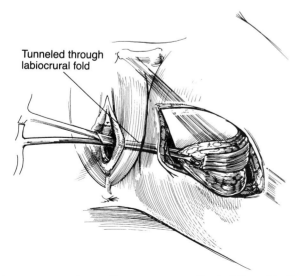

Tunneled through labiocrural fold

Figure 50–10. The gracilis myocutaneous flap is delivered to the perineum through a generous opening between the donor site and the perineum to prevent flap necrosis. The bilateral flaps are then secured together into a tube, and the closed inferior end is drawn up into the pelvic defect and anchored to the levator muscles and retropubic fascia to prevent prolapse.

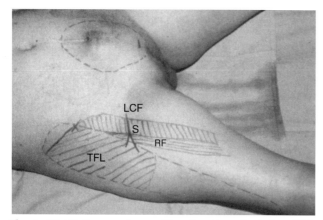

Figure 50–12. Preoperative markings for a tenor fascia lata (TFL) myocutaneous flap. The location of the lateral circumflex femoral (LCF) artery is identified in this photograph, as are the sartorius (S) and rectus femoris (RF) muscles.

In the original description, the preservation of the overlying skin was not a component of this graft. Since then, the Martius technique has been used for vaginal reconstruction after pelvic exenteration because of its reliable blood supply, including that to the overlying epithelium.[32] Advantages of the bulbocavernosus flap include the fact that the external pudendal artery, which supplies this flap, usually is not included in the radiation portals. Limitations include the necessity for redundant donor site vulvar tissue to prevent significant cosmetic deformity and the limited ability to completely reconstruct the vagina. The size of the flap constructed is approximately 4 × 10 cm but varies depending on the amount of vulvar tissue present.

In the procedure to form a bulbocavernosus neovagina, the muscle is first identified on the labia majora, with the lateral margin lying at the lateral aspect of the labia majora, the inner margin between the labia majora and minora, the superior margin above the clitoris, and the lower margin even with the perineal body (Fig. 50-13). The dissection continues and preserves the blood supply from the perineal branch of the external pudendal artery, which enters the flap on the inferior aspect of the pedicle. The flap is then passed through a tunnel into the introitus, and the bilateral flaps are sewn together posteriorly and attached to the levator muscles (Fig. 50-14). Because of the thinness of this flap, it is particularly suited for patients undergoing anterior or posterior exenteration. In cases in which the flap does not create a complete neovagina, the remaining defect is filled with an omental pedicle graft. A vaginal stent is not necessary to ensure preservation of the length and diameter of a bulbocavernosus neovagina.

Pudendal thigh flap (Singapore flap). A fasciocutaneous flap has been described for neovaginal construction using the skin and fascia of the medial thigh supplied by the posterior labial artery.[33] These flaps are constructed from the skin located in the thigh creases, medial to the hair-bearing areas of the perineum. This

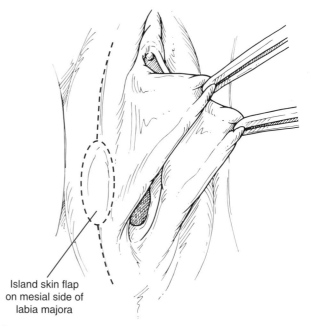

Island skin flap
on mesial side of
labia majora

Figure 50–13. Preoperative markings for a bulbocavernosus (Martius) flap. The major limitation of this flap is the limited volume of tissue available for reconstruction, which limits its utility in the reconstruction of large defects.

flap is sensate, deriving its nervous supply from the posterior labial branches of the pudendal nerve. Although this flap is feasible, its utility is limited by chronic vaginal discharge, neovaginal hair growth, and poor sexual function after reconstruction.[34]

The flap is created by incising a segment of skin on the medial aspect of the thigh, encompassing a region 6 × 15 cm,[34] but preserving the labia majora. The skin, subcutaneous tissues, deep fascia of the thigh, and

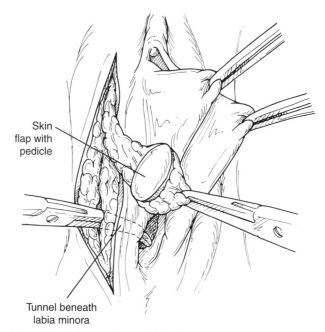

Skin
flap with
pedicle

Tunnel beneath
labia minora

Figure 50–14. Harvesting of the bulbocavernosus muscle and overlying perineal skin.

fascia of the adductor muscles are included in this flap. The flaps are then transposed medially on a subcutaneous pedicle supplied by the posterior labial arteries. The flaps are tunneled under the labia, the posterior aspects of the flaps are sutured in the midline, and the tube is secured to the retropubic fascia.

Posterior thigh (gluteal) fasciocutaneous flap. This neurosensory fasciocutaneous transposition flap is supplied by the terminal descending cutaneous branch of the inferior gluteal artery, a branch of the internal iliac artery. This artery supplies the majority of the posterior thigh, encompassing an area 10×35 cm. Its innervation is derived from the posterior cutaneous nerve of the thigh. Although this flap has been investigated extensively in the repair of defects related to pressure ulceration, its use in neovaginal construction is limited. The flap is designed by connecting a line between the ischial tuberosity and the greater trochanter, which defines the medial and inferior margin of the gluteus maximus muscle. The vascular pedicle supplies this flap from beneath the gluteus muscle, near the midpoint of the line, and should be avoided. The medial and lateral borders of the flap are centered on the midaxial line of the thigh. The dissection of the flap begins at the distal aspect of the posterior skin of the thigh and is brought proximally toward the origin of the neurovascular pedicle. The dissection is taken through the skin, subcutaneous tissues, and fascia lata. If necessary, the gluteus maximus muscle can be divided away from the neurovascular pedicle to improve mobility. The flap is then rotated into the perineal defect through a generous subcutaneous tunnel and secured to the retropubic fascia to prevent prolapse of this heavy flap.

Is there a method to ensure appropriate blood supply to a flap to minimize the risk of necrosis?

The most effective methods to ensure success with vaginal reconstruction after pelvic exenteration include use of the most appropriate flap for the area to be reconstructed, careful tissue handling, strict adherence to the anatomic limitations of the flap, and prevention and treatment of intraoperative and postoperative factors (e.g., infection, hypoperfusion, tension) that increase the risk of flap failure. Despite careful attention to these factors, some flaps are subject to necrosis, occasionally necessitating revision or removal. Although various intraoperative and postoperative techniques to identify flaps at risk for necrosis have been reported, and despite more than 40 years of investigation, none of these methods has consistently been shown to predict a successful reconstruction. In their initial investigation, McCraw and colleagues[35] used intravenous fluorescein (resorcinol phthalein) and detection with a Wood's light and demonstrated that nonfluorescent areas were destined for necrosis; they recommended that these areas not be used in the flap. Although subsequent studies, including those in patients with gynecologic malignancies,[36] have confirmed that

fluorescence demonstrates appropriate arterial blood flow at the time of the test, other investigations have shown some flaps with appropriate fluorescence will still fail. Reasons for these failures include the fact that detection of fluorescein identifies blood flow only at the time of investigation and does not ensure persistent blood flow. Also, flap failures may result from venous congestion and not arterial obstruction, and in these cases fluorescence can be falsely reassuring. The use of Doppler ultrasonography, surface thermometry, photoplethysmography, and other methods to detect fluorescence after fluorescein administration have also been used to demonstrate flow to flaps, but they do not ensure flap viability.[37] The most reliable predictor of a blood supply that will support a flap is the presence of bleeding at the edge of a raised flap. In the absence of this finding, the flap should be investigated for factors that would lead to lack of perfusion or venous congestion, such as flap rotation or tension. Beyond simple inspection of the flap, most investigators do not recommend any adjunct method to evaluate flap blood flow. Debridement of necrotic edges tends to heal very well.

Preoperatively, patients should be strongly encouraged to discontinue smoking. Extensive data exist to support the relationship between delayed healing, flap necrosis, and nicotine use.[38] This association has been demonstrated in vitro, in animal models, and in human studies. Retrospective data indicate that patients who are actively smoking at the time of breast reconstruction after mastectomy have a significantly higher risk for overall complications and specifically for flap necrosis, compared with never-smokers or previous smokers (abstinence for at least 3 weeks before surgery).[39] For this reason, and to minimize other complications, intervention to facilitate smoking cessation should be recommended before exenteration with vaginal reconstruction.

What novel surgical techniques have been instituted to modify and improve vaginal reconstruction?

Although myocutaneous, fasciocutaneous, and STSG techniques are the most commonly employed methods for vaginal reconstruction after pelvic exenteration, others have been investigated that employ novel materials or surgical procedures. As mentioned previously, the insertion of a material between the pelvic floor and the remainder of the pelvic contents is likely to minimize the risk of adhesions, bowel obstruction, and fistula formation even when vaginal reconstruction is performed. Other authors have used fibrin glue to cover the pelvic tissues and suture lines of a pudendal thigh flap to minimize the risk of fistula formation.[40] Likewise, an animal model has been developed that uses buccal mucosa for vaginal reconstruction, with the purpose of identifying a nonkeratinized material that would eliminate the problems of dryness, irritation, and hair growth in flaps and grafts developed from keratinized skin.[41] Commensurate with the increased application of minimally invasive surgical techniques in the armamentarium of gynecologic oncologists, Possover and coworkers[42] developed a technique for the laparoscopic-assisted formation of a sigmoid neovagina.

What are the psychological and sexual implications of vaginal reconstruction, and are there methods to minimize their impact?

The profound psychological implications of pelvic exenteration in gynecologic oncology are without equal when compared with other medical therapies. Patients undergoing exenterative procedures have recently been diagnosed with a recurrence of their malignancy; they have been told that their only chance for cure is radical surgical extirpation and that the surgery will result in the necessity for two stomas and a reconstructed vagina. For these reasons, studies designed to investigate the psychological and sexual impact of pelvic exenteration with vaginal reconstruction are difficult to interpret and compare.[43-46] These studies also vary according to whether patients have undergone vaginal reconstruction and, if so, what type of reconstruction was performed. Nonetheless, consistent findings include the fact that sexual dysfunction is endemic after pelvic exenteration with vaginal reconstruction, suggesting that patients should be counseled preoperatively regarding this possibility. Some of the more common reasons cited for sexual dysfunction include alteration of body image; hesitancy to be seen unclothed; fear of stomas, pain or cancer interfering with intercourse; loss of a sexual partner because of the patient's cancer; and lack of desire after exenteration. The use of intensive preoperative and postoperative sexual counseling has been consistently recommended and has demonstrated improved psychosexual adjustment in women undergoing pelvic exenteration.[45]

Despite the difficulties in returning to baseline psychosexual function after pelvic exenteration, vaginal reconstruction has been shown to significantly improve patient quality of life and body image, compared to no vaginal reconstruction.[46] However, continued improvements in surgical technique and psychosocial intervention are required to improve the sexual function of women undergoing pelvic exenteration with vaginal reconstruction.

What oncologic follow-up should be provided for women with vaginal reconstruction after exenteration?

After pelvic exenteration and vaginal reconstruction, many women are examined on a regular basis with cytology samples obtained from the neovagina. Compared with native cervicovaginal cytology, changes in cytology of a neovagina created from a STSG have been identified that occur in the absence of cancer recurrence. These findings include the presence of anucleated, keratinizing squamous cells and a shift in the maturation index of the sampled cells. As such, it is important that cytopathologists and other physicians involved in postexenteration cancer surveillance recognize these changes to ensure appropriate management of cytology after reconstruction.[47]

Important in the discussion of cancer surveillance in women undergoing vaginal reconstruction is the occurrence of cancer arising in the neovagina. Most cancers arising in patients with a neovagina have been described in the population of women undergoing vaginal reconstruction as a result of vaginal agenesis. Histologically, these malignancies are identical to the cell type of the donor site used for neovaginal construction. A recent review of 16 cancers arising in women with primary vaginal malformations treated with vaginal reconstruction confirmed this finding.[48] Among women undergoing vaginal reconstruction after management of an invasive or in situ gynecologic malignancy, four cases of invasive malignancy of the reconstructed vagina have been described, including one adenocarcinoma arising in a cecal neovagina,[49] two squamous cell carcinomas arising in skin grafts,[50,51] and another squamous cell cancer arising in a rectus abdominis myocutaneous flap.[52] The squamous cell cancer in a rectus flap was thought to arise from extension of disease from the pelvic sidewall, from tumor seeding of the neovagina at the time of exenteration, or, less likely, as a primary neovaginal tumor. Other authors have described carcinoma in situ of a skin graft neovagina in women with primary gynecologic neoplasia. In all of these cases, the histology of the neovaginal malignancy has been that of the origin of the reconstructed vagina. Because of the risk of preinvasive or invasive neoplasia arising in a neovagina, surveillance with examination and cytologic analysis remains important after pelvic exenteration and vaginal reconstruction.

Conclusions

For women undergoing pelvic exenteration, vaginal reconstruction is feasible, beneficial, and often leads to normal sexual rehabilitation. For more detailed descriptions of the techniques used for vaginal reconstruction, the reader is referred to many excellent surgical and anatomy texts written to address this subject. With continued medical and surgical progress, modifications in the techniques and methods used for vaginal reconstruction can be expected to continue to improve on the outcomes experienced by women who undergo the procedure today.

REFERENCES

1. Brunschwig A: Complete excision of pelvic viscera for advanced carcinoma. Cancer 1948;1:177-183.
2. Miller B, Morris M, Gershenson DM, et al: Intestinal fistulae formation following pelvic exenteration: A review of the University of Texas M. D. Anderson Cancer Center experience, 1957-1990. Gynecol Oncol 1995;56:207-210.

3. Soper JT, Berchuck A, Creasman WT, Clarke-Pearson DL: Pelvic exenteration: Factors associated with major surgical morbidity. Gynecol Oncol 1989;35:93-98.

4. Cain JM, Diamond A, Tamimi HK, et al: The morbidity and benefits of concurrent gracilis myocutaneous graft with pelvic exenteration. Obstet Gynecol 1989;74:185-189.

5. Jurado M, Bazan A, Elejabeitia J, et al: Primary vaginal and pelvic floor reconstruction at the time of pelvic exenteration: A study of morbidity. Gynecol Oncol 2000;77:293-297.

6. Berek JS, Hacker NF, Legasse LD: Vaginal reconstruction performed simultaneously with pelvic exenteration. Obstet Gynecol 1984;63:318-323.

7. Buchsbaum HJ, Christopherson W, Lifshitz S, Bernstein S: Vicryl mesh in pelvic floor reconstruction. Arch Surg 1985;120: 1389-1391.

8. Clarke-Pearson DL, Soper JT, Creasman WT: Absorbable synthetic mesh (polyglactin 910) for the formation of a pelvic "lid" after radical pelvic resection. Am J Obstet Gynecol 1988; 158:158-161.

9. Hoffman MS, Roberts WS, LaPolla JP, et al: Use of Vicryl mesh in the reconstruction of the pelvic floor following exenteration. Gynecol Oncol 1989;35:170-171.

10. Delmore JE, Turner DA, Gershenson DM, Horbelt DV: Perineal hernia repair using human dura. Obstet Gynecol 1987;70:507-508.

11. McIndoe AH, Banister JB: An operation for the cure of congenital absence of the vagina. J Obstet Gynaecol Br Empire 1938;5:490-494.

12. Beemer W, Hopkins MP, Morley GW: Vaginal reconstruction in gynecologic oncology. Obstet Gynecol 1988;72:911-914.

13. Kusiak JF, Rosenblum NG: Neovaginal reconstruction after exenteration using an omental flap and split-thickness skin graft. Plast Reconstr Surg 1996;97:775-781.

14. Turner-Warwick R, Kirby RS: The construction and reconstruction of the vagina with the colocecum. Surg Gynecol Obstet 1990;170:132-136.

15. Tobin GR, Day TG Jr: Vaginal and pelvic reconstruction with distally based rectus abdominis myocutaneous flaps. Plast Reconstr Surg 1988;81:62-73.

16. Pursell SH, Day TG Jr, Tobin GR: Distally based rectus abdominis flap for reconstruction in radical gynecologic procedures. Gynecol Oncol 1990;37:234-238.

17. Benson C, Soisson AP, Carlson J, et al: Neovaginal reconstruction with a rectus abdominis myocutaneous flap. Obstet Gynecol 1993;81:871-875.

18. Carlson JW, Soisson AP, Fowler JM, et al: Rectus abdominis myocutaneous flap for primary vaginal reconstruction. Gynecol Oncol 1993;51:323-329.

19. Carlson JW, Carter JR, Saltzman AK, et al: Gynecologic reconstruction with a rectus abdominis myocutaneous flap: An update. Gynecol Oncol 1996;61:364-368.

20. Smith HO, Genesen MC, Runowicz CD, Goldberg GL: The rectus abdominis myocutaneous flap: Modifications, complications, and sexual function. Cancer 1998;83:510-520.

21. McCraw JB, Massey FM, Shanklin KD, Horton CE: Vaginal reconstruction with gracilis myocutaneous flaps. Plast Reconstr Surg 1976;58:176-183.

22. Becker DW Jr, Massey FM, McCraw JB: Musculocutaneous flaps in reconstructive pelvic surgery. Obstet Gynecol 1979;54:178-183.

23. Lacey CG, Stern JL, Feigenbaum S, et al: Vaginal reconstruction after exenteration with the use of gracilis myocutaneous flaps: The University of California, San Francisco experience. Am J Obstet Gynecol 1988;158:1278-1284.

24. Morrow CP, Lacey CG, Lucas WE: Reconstructive surgery in gynecologic cancer employing the gracilis myocutaneous pedicle graft. Gynecol Oncol 1979;7:176-187.

25. Wheeless CR Jr, McGibbon B, Dorsey JH, Maxwell GP: Gracilis myocutaneous flap in reconstruction of the vulva and female perineum. Obstet Gynecol 1979;54:97-102.

26. Copeland LJ, Hancock KC, Gershenson DM, et al: Gracilis myocutaneous vaginal reconstruction concurrent with total pelvic exenteration. Am J Obstet Gynecol 1989;160:1095-1101.

27. Soper JT, Larson D, Hunter VJ, et al: Short gracilis myocutaneous flaps for vulvovaginal reconstruction after radical pelvic surgery. Obstet Gynecol 1989;74:823-827.

28. Soper JT, Rodriguez G, Berchuck A, Clarke-Pearson DL: Long and short gracilis myocutaneous flaps for vulvovaginal reconstruction after radical pelvic surgery: Comparison of flap-specific complications. Gynecol Oncol 1995;56:271-275.

29. Nahai F, Silverton JS, Hill HL, Vasconez LO: The tensor fascia lata musculocutaneous flap. Ann Plast Surg 1978;1:372-379.

30. Temple WJ, Ketcham AS: The closure of large pelvic defects by extended compound tensor fascia lata and inferior gluteal myocutaneous flaps. Am J Clin Oncol 1982;5:573-577.

31. Martius H: Die operative Wiederherstellung der vollkommen fehlenden Harnohre und des Schliessmuskels derselben. Zentralbl Gynakol 1928;52:480-487.

32. Hatch KD: Construction of a neovagina after exenteration using the vulvobulbocavernosus myocutaneous graft. Obstet Gynecol 1984;63:110-114.

33. Wee JT, Joseph VT: A new technique of vaginal reconstruction using neurovascular pudendal-thigh flaps: A preliminary report. Plast Reconstr Surg 1989;83:701-709.

34. Gleeson NC, Baile W, Roberts WS, et al: Pudendal thigh fasciocutaneous flaps for vaginal reconstruction in gynecologic oncology. Gynecol Oncol 1994;54:269-274.

35. McCraw JB, Myers B, Shanklin KD: The value of fluorescein in predicting the viability of arterialized flaps. Plast Reconstr Surg 1977;60:710-719.

36. Magrina JF, Masterson BJ: Evaluation of groin and vulvar flap viability by the use of intravenous fluorescein. Gynecol Oncol 1981;11:96-101.

37. Sloan GM, Sasaki GH: Noninvasive monitoring of tissue viability. Clin Plast Surg 1985;12:185-195.

38. Mosely LH, Finseth F, Goody M: Nicotine and its effect on wound healing. Plast Reconstr Surg 1978;61:570-575.

39. Padubidri AN, Yetman R, Browne E, et al: Complications of postmastectomy breast reconstructions in smokers, ex-smokers, and nonsmokers. Plast Reconstr Surg 2001;107:342-349.

40. Bazan A, Samper A, Lasso JM: The use of fibrin glue in vaginal reconstruction with a pudendal thigh flap. Ann Plast Surg 1999; 43:576.

41. Simman R, Jackson IT, Andrus L: Prefabricated buccal mucosa–lined flap in an animal model that could be used for vaginal reconstruction. Plast Reconstr Surg 2002;109:1044-1049.

42. Possover M, Drahonowski J, Plaul K, Schneider A: Laparoscopic-assisted formation of a colon neovagina. Surg Endosc 2001; 15:623.

43. Andersen BL, Hacker NF: Psychosexual adjustment following pelvic exenteration. Obstet Gynecol 1983;61:331-338.

44. Gleeson N, Baile W, Roberts WS, et al: Surgical and psychosexual outcome following vaginal reconstruction with pelvic exenteration. Eur J Gynaecol Oncol 1994;15:89-95.

45. Ratliff CR, Gershenson DM, Morris M, et al: Sexual adjustment of patients undergoing gracilis myocutaneous flap vaginal reconstruction in conjunction with pelvic exenteration. Cancer 1996;78:2229-2235.

46. Hawighorst-Knapstein S, Schonefussrs G, Hoffmann SO, Knapstein PG: Pelvic exenteration: Effects of surgery on quality of life and body image—a prospective longitudinal study. Gynecol Oncol 1997;66:495-500.

47. Selvaggi SM, Haefner HK, Lelle RJ, et al: Neovaginal cytology after total pelvic exenteration for gynecological malignancies. Diagn Cytopathol 1995;13:22-25.

48. Steiner E, Woernle F, Kuhn W, et al: Carcinoma of the neovagina: Case report and review of the literature. Gynecol Oncol 2002; 84:171-175.

49. Andryjowicz E, Qizilbash AH, DePetrillo AD, et al: Adenocarcinoma in a cecal neovagina—complication of irradiation: Report of a case and review of literature. Gynecol Oncol 1985;21:235-239.

50. Ramming KP, Pilch YH, Powell RD Jr, Ketcham AS: Primary carcinoma in an artificial vagina. Am J Surg 1970;120:108-111.

51. Wheelock JB, Schneider V, Goplerud DR: Malignancy arising in the transplanted vagina. South Med J 1986;79:1585-1587.

52. Carlson JW, Saltzman AK, Carter JR, et al: Recurrent squamous cell carcinoma in a rectus abdominis neovagina. Gynecol Oncol 1995;59:159-161.

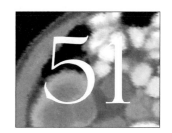

URINARY CONDUITS IN THE PRACTICE OF GYNECOLOGIC ONCOLOGY

Giselle B. Ghurani and Manuel A. Peñalver

◈ MAJOR CONTROVERSIES

- **How did the urinary conduit evolve?**
- **How did the urinary reservoir evolve?**
- **Selecting the appropriate procedure: Who gets what?**
- **When is palliative urinary diversion indicated?**
- **What preoperative preparation is needed to undergo urinary diversion?**
- **What are the most commonly used conduits?**

In the practice of gynecologic oncology, the surgeon must be skilled in performing different techniques of urinary diversion to best manage individual clinical situations. A number of options exist for urinary diversion. Each method comes with its own set of complexities and limitations. Selecting a particular form of diversion for a specific clinical situation can provide a successful outcome for a patient. Despite the many types of urinary diversion available, no one system is perfect or appropriate for every patient. Individualizing treatment options allows the greatest success when performing urinary diversion. Ensuring informed consent, with all risks, benefits, possible complications, and limitations explained to patients, should be a major part of the counseling procedure.

Surgical innovations place great emphasis on developing procedures that minimize the physical and psychological impact on the patient's quality of life without sacrificing cure rates achieved with such extensive surgery. The following sections review the different types of urinary diversion available, their indications, and their complications.

Historical Perspectives of Urinary Diversions

How did the urinary conduit evolve? Surgeons have been challenged for more than a century with the difficult task of substituting the excised urinary bladder. In 1852, Simon[1] reported the first urinary diversion. He treated a patient with exstrophy of the bladder by implanting the ureters into the rectosigmoid. This technique of ureterosigmoidostomy became popular in the first half of the 20th century because of its versatility and ease to perform. However, frequent urinary tract infections, rapid deterioration of renal function, electrolyte abnormalities such as hyperchloremic acidosis, hydronephrosis from stricturing at the ureterocolonic anastomosis, urinary incontinence due to high pressure at the rectal level, and malignancy were frequent complications encountered with the ureterosigmoidostomy. In 1909, Verhoogen and de Graeuve[2] pioneered the use of an isolated segment of ileum and ascending colon as a urinary conduit. However, the high mortality rate from major abdominal surgery performed during this time remained a barrier for widespread application. Despite these innovations in urinary diversion, high complication rates gradually led to their replacement.

In 1950, Bricker first described the ileal conduit diversion.[3] The ileal conduit proved to be a welcome alternative to ureterosigmoidostomy and cutaneous ureterostomy. Because of its acceptable complication rate and its simple and reliable technique, the ileal conduit has become the most common form of urinary diversion. In 1970, Symmonds and Gibbs[4] advocated the use of isolated segments of colon for urinary diversion. They emphasized the advantages of using the terminal end of the sigmoid colon during total pelvic exenterations to obviate small bowel anastomosis. This approach proved favorable, resulting in decreased operating time and decreased morbidity, and it functioned as well as the ileal conduit. The primary disadvantage of these conduits continued to be the lack of continence. The realization that complications such as conduit leaks or fistulas were primarily associated with the use of irradiated segments of bowel led to the introduction of the nonirradiated transverse colon conduits.[5]

Historically, which bowel segment to use for urinary diversion has depended on several factors, including history of previous pelvic radiation therapy, ureteral length, presence of adhesions, and the mobility of bowel segments. Other considerations depend on whether a partial or total exenteration will be done and whether pelvic or vaginal reconstruction is needed.

How did the urinary reservoir evolve? The first attempt at continent urinary diversion with the creation of a catheterizable reservoir using an ileocolonic segment was in 1950 by Gilchrist and colleagues.[6] They used an isolated cecal reservoir with the ileocecal valve to obtain continence. The creation of the reservoir proved to be technically difficult with a higher complication rate. Mansson and coworkers[7] reported that this system had problems with cecal segment hyperactivity causing urinary leakage. In 1978, Kock and associates[8] introduced the continent ileal reservoir. They prepared the reservoir by interrupting the circular muscle fibers of the intestinal wall, thereby accommodating larger volumes of urine at lower pressures than a tubular intestinal segment. This basic principle of bowel detubularization has become the foundation for a low-pressure continent urinary diversion. The Kock pouch used intussuscepted nipple valves to prevent reflux and provide continence. Studies reporting the efficacy of the Kock pouch and the nipple valve system have demonstrated failure rates of 10% to 20% in the efferent nipple mechanism.[9] The search continued for an effective system that would provide lasting urinary continence.

In 1986, Thuroff and colleagues[10] presented the Mainz pouch. This urinary reservoir is created from cecum, ascending colon, and two loops of ileum. Continence is achieved by accomplishing an isoperistaltic intussusception of the distal ileum. The ureters are implanted using a nonrefluxing, submucosal,

tunneled technique into the cecum or ascending colon. In 1987, Rowland and coworkers[11] reported their experience with the Indiana continent reservoir, a right colonic reservoir. This pouch is technically simple to construct with a reliable continence mechanism. Continence is achieved by reinforcing the ileocecal valve by plicating the terminal ileum. Rowland's study reported continence rates of 93% for the daytime and 76% for the nighttime after a mean 14-month follow-up period. In the same year, Lockhart[12] introduced the remodeled right colonic reservoir as an alternative form of urinary diversion. This pouch uses the terminal ileum, cecum, ascending colon, and proximal right transverse colon to construct the reservoir. The continence mechanism consists of plicating the distal ileum with a double row of sutures. Lockhart and Bejany[13] also demonstrated a direct, nontunneled ureteral intestinal implantation technique to prevent ureteral reflux as an alternative to the intussuscepted nipple valve. This design provides a larger reservoir, lower reservoir pressures, and a lower risk of ureteral stenosis than does the Indiana pouch. This Miami pouch was then modified and described by Bejany and Politano in 1988.[14] The goal was to improve the rate of urinary continence, allow for increased flexibility in reimplantation of the ureters, and provide an adequate storage system for urine. By reinforcing the ileocecal valve with three circumferential permanent sutures placed in a purse-string fashion and tapering the distal ileal segment over a 14F catheter, continence was achieved.

Continent urinary diversion has the advantage of not having to wear an external appliance and the effect that has on the patient's self-image. Many types of urinary diversion have been introduced. It is the obligation of the surgeon to become familiar with the different techniques to offer his patient the best opportunity for healthy living.

General Indications for Urinary Diversion

Indications for urinary diversion in the field of gynecologic oncology vary. Most commonly, it is used in the setting of anterior or total pelvic exenterations for the treatment of recurrent cancers of the female genital tract (Fig. 51-1). Most of these patients have received some form of pelvic radiation therapy and have persistent or recurrent cancer, usually of the cervix, vulva, or vagina. The next most common indication is radiation damage causing bilateral ureteral obstruction or vesicovaginal fistulas. Occasionally, a patient with disabling urinary incontinence caused by severe bladder damage from radiation therapy may be managed with urinary diversion. However, bladder augmentation or replacement with a Kock pouch connected to the bladder or urethra may be more appropriate.[15] Rarely, pelvic exenterations necessitating urinary diversion are performed for the treatment of primary gynecologic malignancies or nonirradiated recurrent cancers. Most urinary diversions are performed in women who have had pelvic radiation

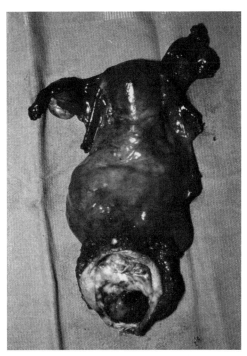

Figure 51–1. Pelvic exenteration specimen from a patient with recurrent cervix cancer. Notice the tumor mass protruding through the vagina.

therapy, which contributes to an increased rate of intraoperative and postoperative morbidity and mortality. In contrast, the surgical and urologic literature primarily focuses on urinary diversion in nonirradiated patients.

Selecting the Appropriate Procedure

Who gets what? When choosing the method of urinary diversion, whether cutaneous or continent, the physician must take into consideration several factors. Ideally, after the operative treatment plan has been chosen, the form of urinary diversion is selected. The surgeon must be cognizant of the surgical goal to provide the most appropriate form of diversion. The patient's life expectancy is also important. A patient who is expected to live several years should be offered a more complex urinary diversion in an attempt to reconstruct the urinary system as best as possible. However, a patient with a poor prognosis or multiple medical problems should be offered the simplest procedure with the quickest recovery and least complications. The patient's age should also influence the type of diversion used. With young patients, the long-term preservation of renal function is especially important. Choosing a diversion with proven lesser complications that lead to the deterioration of renal function is desirable. The patient's current renal function determines her ability to correct the metabolic derangements that occur with the interaction of intestinal mucosa and urine. The surgeon must be aware of the metabolic changes that occur with each type of

diversion. These metabolic abnormalities result from a combination of factors: the segment of intestine used, whether ileum, jejunum, right colon, or rectosigmoid colon; the length of the intestinal segment used; and the kidney's ability to compensate for the metabolic insult. The patient's history of previous treatment is an important consideration. If the patient has previously undergone extensive bowel resection, removing a large segment of intestine to create a urinary reservoir may lead to other complications such as short-bowel syndrome. Perhaps this patient is better served with a urinary conduit that needs only 10 to 15 cm of intestine. Patients with a history of pelvic radiation should receive forms of urinary diversion that avoid using irradiated bowel because of its impaired vascularity and the resulting well-documented complications.

The method of diversion also depends on the patient's physical and psychological state. If the patient is to undergo continent urinary diversion, she must be motivated to self-catheterize and irrigate the stoma. If a urinary conduit is chosen, she must be willing to wear an external appliance for urine collection. Enterostomal nurses and therapists are invaluable in aiding the surgeon in patient education preoperatively and postoperatively. Ostomy associations and other types of support groups should be used to enhance patient education and assistance. However, not all geographic areas are equipped with this type of support system, and the poorly educated patient may not be able to bear the stigma of a stoma. In other parts of the world, the medical supplies necessary to maintain a urinary stoma may be very difficult to obtain or too expensive.

When is palliative urinary diversion indicated? In certain circumstances, palliative urinary diversion may benefit the patient. The decision must be individualized to meet the needs and wishes of the patient after thoroughly and candidly discussing the risks and benefits. The surgeon must consider the morbidity of the procedure, the operative time, and the patient's subsequent quality of life. When pelvic malignancy causes bilateral ureteral obstruction but there is potential for cancer control and a life expectancy of at least 6 months, urinary diversion is indicated. However, a patient with recurrence and intractable pain and with a short life expectancy is not a good candidate for palliative urinary diversion.

Percutaneous nephrostomy tube placement is a reasonable option for palliative urinary diversion in a particular subset of patients. The introduction of percutaneous techniques from the evolving fields of endourology and interventional radiology and the use of ultrasound or computed tomographic (CT) guidance have dramatically reduced the morbidity of ureteral stent placement. Newer stenting biomaterial has contributed to safer urinary diversion. With these developments and the routine use of perioperative antibiotics, the procedure has become simple and has minor associated morbidity.[16] Percutaneous nephrostomies are often useful in patients with malignant ureteral obstruction who are undergoing or plan to undergo pelvic radiation therapy or chemotherapy as treatment of their malignancy. However, what about patients with malignant ureteral obstruction with no further treatment options available for their cancer? Should they be offered percutaneous nephrostomies? Because of the low morbidity, urinary diversion is feasible for most patients. The dilemma facing surgeons is when to intervene and offer it to the patient if no options exist for the treatment of her cancer. The quality of life gained by diversion must be considered along with the wishes of the patient and family. Watkinson and colleagues[17] found that only patients who had treatment options after urinary diversion benefited from percutaneous nephrostomy. The standard is to preserve renal function if chemotherapy or radiation therapy is a feasible option for the patient. Other clinical situations require keen clinical judgment after discussion with the patient and family about the expected outcome.

General Principles of Urinary Diversion

The major goals of urinary diversion are to preserve renal function while providing a convenient route for the disposal of urine with the least impact on the quality and duration of the patient's life. The ideal urinary diversion, while preserving renal function, minimizes infection and complication rates and minimizes the loss of gastrointestinal and sexual function.

What preoperative preparation is needed to undergo urinary diversion? In preparing the patient preoperatively, the physician should focus on psychosocial issues and technical issues. The patient must undergo extensive counseling to address issues of self-image, possible surgical complications, and postoperative self-care. A preoperative consult with an enterostomal therapist is paramount. Nothing is more important to the patient than the stoma that she must live with on a daily basis. Ideally, the skin is marked for the stoma site preoperatively by the stoma nurse. Urinary diversion stomas are most commonly located in the right lower quadrant of the abdomen. The stoma site needs to be visible to the patient so that she can care for the stoma. The site must be clear of bony prominences, the surgical incision, natural skin creases, the belt line, and other skin irregularities. This is especially important in the obese patient, and the site should be checked in the supine, sitting, and standing positions.

Preoperative evaluation of the patient's nutritional status is also important. Many of these patients are debilitated because of their cancers and are unable to meet their daily caloric requirements. Knowing your patient's albumin and total protein levels preoperatively aids in determining nutritional deficiencies and allows time for their correction. Preoperative supplementation with enteral or parenteral nutrition can boost the malnourished patient's immune system and avoid complications in the postoperative course. The 1991 multicenter Veterans Affairs Total Parenteral Nutrition Cooperative Study is recognized as setting the standard for deciding when preoperative nutritional support is indicated.[18] This prospective, randomized study demonstrated that preoperative total parenteral nutrition (TPN) is beneficial only in surgical patients with severe preoperative malnutrition. TPN is not effective in patients who are minimally or moderately malnourished, and using TPN in this group of patients led to increased morbidity with a higher incidence of infectious complications. Using a simplified formula, severe malnutrition is defined by a weight loss of 20% or more or by a serum albumin level of less than 2.8 g/dL.[19] The study also demonstrated that preoperative TPN was beneficial only if given for a minimum of 7 days before surgery and continued for 3 days after surgery.

Bowel preparation and the use of prophylactic antibiotics are essential. Mechanical bowel preparation begins with a clear liquid diet 2 days before surgery. The day before surgery, the patient is instructed to take 1 gallon of polyethylene glycol–electrolyte solution (e.g., GoLYTELY, Colyte, or NuLytely). This is the most commonly prescribed regimen. Another alternative is two 45-mL vials of sodium phosphate (e.g., Fleet Phospho-Soda) taken 3 hours apart. In one study comparing the two alternatives, patients preferred the sodium phosphate to the polyethylene glycol, reporting less abdominal pain, less bloating, less fatigue, and less trouble drinking the preparation.[20] A good mechanical bowel preparation is important because evacuation of the bowel contents and intraluminal bacteria reduces the risk of fecal contamination of the peritoneal cavity and the abdominal incision. A prophylactic antibiotic, usually a second-generation cephalosporin, is given before making the surgical incision. To be effective, the first dose of antibiotic must be given within 2 hours of the start of surgery.[21,22] Prophylactic parenteral antibiotics are also needed if the patient has valvular heart disease or any implant or prosthesis (e.g., knee, pacemaker). In the United States, oral antimicrobial prophylaxis for bowel surgery with neomycin and erythromycin is also commonly used. Outside the United States, oral antimicrobial prophylaxis has been largely replaced by perioperative administration of parenteral antibiotics. Randomized studies have demonstrated a reduction in septic complications in elective colon surgery with the administration of oral or parenteral antibiotics, or both, provided that the antibiotics have aerobic and anaerobic coverage and are administered preoperatively.[23] Many randomized studies have not determined whether oral or parenteral or combination antibiotics are superior.[24-26]

Before surgery, the patient's urinary system must be evaluated using an imaging study with contrast, such as an intravenous pyelogram. These studies are useful to determine the anatomy of each renal collecting system and to identify any anomalies, such as double ureters or hydronephrosis. Baseline information is obtained with these preoperative tests that can later be used in the follow-up management of the patient.

Selecting the Urinary Conduit

Principles of the technique. Certain basic principles should be employed when constructing a urinary conduit. First, a wide ureteroenteric anastomosis should be created to decrease the risk of stenosis. Second, the surgeon must use a segment of intestine that is isoperistaltic. The intestinal segment should be no longer than necessary to ensure quick passage of urine and decrease the reabsorption of solute. This principle is especially important for patients with renal insufficiency. The conduit should be stabilized within the abdominal cavity or to the anterior abdominal wall to prevent tension on the ureteral anastomoses and displacement of the conduit. When creating the tunnel through the anterior abdominal wall, the surgeon must keep in mind the importance of ensuring an adequate diameter for the conduit and a straight tunnel to prevent obstruction. The stoma should also be protuberant to ensure optimal urine collection.

What are the most commonly used conduits?
Ileal conduit. The ileal conduit is traditionally viewed as the most convenient type of urinary diversion (Fig. 51-2). It is probably the most common form of diversion used in gynecologic oncology, although continent diversion is gaining in popularity. The ileal conduit has many advantages over other forms of diversion, including ease of construction and improved stomal preservation when compared with cutaneous urostomies. The ileal segment functions as a ureteral extension to the skin, providing greater flexibility with greater length, an adequate blood supply, and a convenient stomal location in the right lower quadrant. The ileal conduit is associated with a low incidence of infection and metabolic abnormalities, and it provides adequate preservation of renal function.[27] The main disadvantage of the ileal conduit in gynecologic oncology patients is that the bowel segments have been previously irradiated, thereby increasing the complications of ureteral stricture, fistulas, and stomal necrosis. There is a need for anastomosis of small bowel to small bowel because of increased incidences of anastomotic leaks and breakdowns. Consequently, when constructing an ileal conduit in a previously irradiated patient, the ileum and the ureters must be cautiously evaluated intraoperatively for radiation injury. If significant radiation damage exists, the conduit should be constructed from the transverse colon or from proximal ileum or jejunum. If the ureters appear fibrotic or devascularized, they should be trimmed back to healthy ureter above the field of radiation.

Several different types of ileal conduits have been described. The most commonly used is the Bricker ileal conduit and its modifications. A 15- to 20-cm segment of ileum is usually isolated to construct the conduit. Sometimes, the segmental length needs to be longer if the patient is obese, the ureters are short, or the Turnbull stoma (Fig. 51-3) is to be created rather than the end stoma. The segment should end about 20 cm from the ileocecal valve to preserve the ileocecal artery. Stapling devices are used to facilitate the procedure. We prefer to make the stoma before cutting the proximal end of the conduit. This ensures an adequate conduit length, stabilizes the conduit for the ureteral

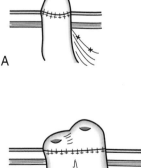

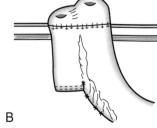

Figure 51–3. Stomal construction. **A,** End stoma. To ensure an adequate bud formation, about 3 to 4 cm of tissue should be pulled through the aperture, above the skin. **B,** Turnbull stoma. The loop of the ileum should protrude above the skin by about 2 cm when completed. The blind end of the loop should be sutured to the underlying peritoneum to prevent prolapse.

Figure 51–2. Ileal conduit.

anastomosis, decreases stomal tension, and ensures an isoperistaltic position. After the stoma is matured, the conduit is measured, usually to the sacral promontory, to ensure sufficient length for a tension-free ureteral anastomosis. Before performing the ureteral anastomoses, bowel continuity should be established. The isolated bowel segment is placed posteriorly, and the ileum reanastomosed anteriorly. The ureters are then anastomosed to the anterior ileal segment in an end-to-side fashion, using single-layer, interrupted, 4-0, absorbable sutures. The left ureter, usually the most difficult to anastomose, should be done first. It is brought under the sigmoid mesentery and the inferior mesenteric artery. Ureteral stents are always used and are inserted before completing the ureteroileal anastomosis. The ureteral stents function to transport the urine past the anastomosis and reduce the flow of urine over the anastomosis. The stents prevent the ureters from becoming kinked.

When creating a urinary conduit stoma, two options usually are available: the end stoma and the Turnbull loop stoma. The original stoma described by Bricker was a simple orifice flush against the skin. Brooke modified the stoma with the construction of the bud, which protrudes above the skin. With the bud formation, stomal complications are significantly reduced by providing a better appliance fit, decreasing skin contact with urine, and decreasing the incidence of stenosis. Surgeons who like to use the end stoma have had good results with few complications. However, the Turnbull loop stoma has advantages and indications that sometimes make it superior to the end stoma.[28] It is advocated for the obese patient with a thick anterior abdominal wall or the patient with a short bowel mesentery. It is also advantageous in the irradiated patient because it permits a longer, better-vascularized loop to reach the skin compared with the end stoma. The main complication with the Turnbull loop stoma has been parastomal hernias. Although studies showing the functional equivalence of the end versus loop ileal conduit stomas have been published,[29] some surgeons recommend the loop stoma for all patients.[30]

Transverse colon conduit. Transverse colon conduits have gained considerable popularity among gynecologic oncologists (Fig. 51-4). The advantages of the transverse colon conduit are many.[31] It is appropriate for the previously irradiated patient because the transverse colon rarely lies within the field of radiation. Although the transverse colon conduit does not avoid a bowel anastomosis, the anastomosis is out of the pelvis and does not involve irradiated tissue. It is indicated for the obese patient or for those with short ureters. Colon conduits are less likely to have stomal complications. The stoma of the transverse colon conduit can be placed almost anywhere on the anterior abdominal wall. The most natural location for an isoperistaltic transverse colon conduit is in the left upper quadrant. Mass peristaltic contractions facilitate the passage of urine in the colon conduit, and it need not be placed in the isoperistaltic direction. The stoma

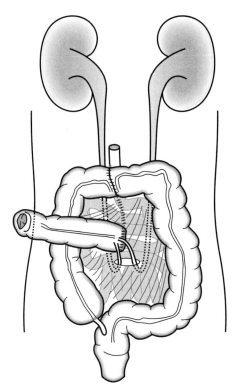

Figure 51–4. Transverse colon conduit.

can be placed in the right upper quadrant in an isoperistaltic or antiperistaltic fashion. As for all types of conduits, the length of the transverse colon conduit, with increased risk of metabolic abnormalities for longer segments, is an issue only in the patient with compromised renal function.

In preparation for the creation of the transverse colon conduit, the omentum is dissected away from its attachment to the colon. Next, the segment of colon is selected by transilluminating the transverse mesocolon and identifying the middle colic artery. Identification of vessel arcades ensures adequate blood supply to the isolated segment. The isolated colon segment is usually about 15 to 20 cm long, depending on the size of the patient and the location of the stoma. Stapling devices are used to transect the bowel and then to later reestablish bowel continuity. The surgeon must remember to reapproximate the mesentery of the anastomosed bowel with interrupted absorbable sutures, thereby preventing small bowel herniation. The ureters are then brought ventrally through the small bowel mesentery for anastomoses to the conduit. End-to-side ureteral anastomoses with interrupted, 4-0, absorbable suture over ureteral stents are then performed. This technique is similar to that used for the ileal conduit. The creation of the stoma is the same as the maturation of a colostomy stoma. The Turnbull loop stoma is not suitable for the transverse colon conduit.

Jejunal conduit. The jejunal conduit is rarely used for urinary diversion in gynecologic oncology. Many studies have been published elaborating the complications associated with this type of conduit.[32] The most characteristic complication is the electrolyte imbalance, known as the jejunal syndrome, resulting from a reabsorption of potassium and urea, a loss of sodium and chloride into the urine, and an increase in aldosterone production.[33] The jejunal syndrome most commonly occurs in patients with preexisting renal insufficiency and long conduits. Contraindications for jejunal conduits include patients with renal compromise, patients on a restricted low-sodium diet, and those needing a long loop for conduit construction. Although the jejunal syndrome is correctable with the administration of salt, this complication renders the jejunal conduit a less favorable choice among the different conduits available. However, some positive reports do support the jejunal conduit. Fontaine and coworkers[34] reported their 20-year experience with jejunal conduits. They found that by using a short length of jejunum (10 to 12 cm), a reliable conduit could be created, giving good long-term renal function with rare electrolyte imbalances. Moreover, the jejunal conduit can be used in almost all situations, especially after pelvic irradiation.

The surgical technique for creating the jejunal conduit is similar to that of an ileal conduit. The major indication today is for the patient whose ileum and large bowel are not suited for urinary diversion. For example, jejunal conduits should be considered in patients with severe radiation damage to the ileum or in those patients with short ureters. It is also an option for patients with inflammatory diseases of the colon such as diverticulitis. To achieve the best outcome for a patient, with the least complications, the shortest possible length of jejunum should be used.

Sigmoid colon conduit.

The sigmoid conduit is used infrequently in gynecologic oncology. Most patients requiring urinary diversion for gynecologic cancer have received pelvic irradiation. It is common to find the sigmoid colon with marked radiation changes such as decreased vascularity and severe fibrosis. This makes it difficult to isolate a segment long enough to reach the right lower quadrant. Ideally, the sigmoid colon conduit is more suited to the left lower quadrant. However, these patients often also need a colostomy, further contributing to the disadvantages of the sigmoid conduit. Sometimes, a low colorectal anastomosis is appropriate for patients undergoing a pelvic exenteration to avoid a colostomy, but by using a segment of sigmoid for urinary diversion, the length of the colon is compromised, making it impossible to reanastomose the rectum. It is rare to find the ideal candidate for the sigmoid conduit among gynecologic cancer patients. This patient should have no prior history of pelvic irradiation and not be suitable for other types of urinary diversion.

The surgical technique of the sigmoid conduit is similar to the previous conduits described. After mobilizing the sigmoid and descending colon to the splenic flexure, the mesentery is transilluminated for identifying the sigmoidal arteries. Usually, a 15- to 20-cm segment of sigmoid is isolated, containing two to three sigmoidal vessels. Stapling devices are used for bowel transection and later on if needed to restore bowel continuity. If bowel continuity is to be reestablished, the anastomosis is performed anterior or posterior to the conduit depending on the location of the stoma. For right lower quadrant stomas, it is best to reanastomose the bowel posterior to the conduit. For left lower quadrant stomas, it is best to reanastomose the bowel anterior to the conduit. The ureters are anastomosed in a similar fashion as described for the ileal conduit. The stoma is brought through the anterior abdominal wall and matured by a series of everting sutures similar to the colostomy.

Cutaneous ureterostomy.

Cutaneous ureterostomy is usually a temporary form of urinary diversion in adult patients. Its associated complications include stomal necrosis, retraction, and stenosis.[35] The propensity for stomal complications in most patients makes this option less desirable. If stomal stricture or stenosis occurs, the ureters need to be chronically stented. The usual indication is for a difficult intraoperative situation for which a quick and temporary solution is needed. Cutaneous ureterostomies should be converted to some form of intestinal segment diversion, especially in patients with normal renal function and a long life expectancy.

When creating cutaneous ureterostomies, it is more favorable for the patient to have a single stoma that can be fitted with a single appliance. The single stoma can be created by using the transureteroureterostomy, in which the narrower ureter is anastomosed in a side-to-end fashion to the other ureter and a single ureter is brought to the skin as an everted stoma (Fig. 51-5). Another option is to create the double stoma by joining the medial borders of the ureteral ends and bringing them through a single opening in the anterior abdominal wall. Despite its lack of popularity among surgeons, it is important to know all options available for urinary diversion to choose the most appropriate technique for a patient in a given clinical scenario.

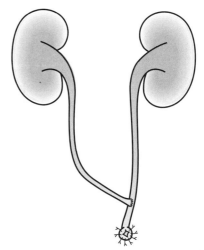

Figure 51–5. Transureteroureterostomy. A single end stoma ureterostomy is created. The narrower ureter is anastomosed in end-to-side fashion to the other ureter, which is brought to the skin as an everted stoma.

Complications of urinary conduits. In general, urinary conduit construction is a safe procedure, although a wide range of complications does occur. They can be divided into early complications, occurring within the first 6 weeks of surgery, and late complications, occurring after 6 weeks of surgery. Several factors influence the incidence of complications, such as the patient's general medical condition, a history of previous radiation therapy, the extent of the surgery performed at the time of urinary diversion, and the type of diversion performed.

Early complications. The most common early complications include postoperative decreased urine output, urinary leakage, infection, small-bowel complications, and stomal complications. Decreased urine output is common in the first 24 to 48 hours of the postoperative period. The most common explanation is that the patient's intravascular volume is depleted from intraoperative blood loss and inadequate fluid and volume replacement. However, other causes of decreased urine output related to the urinary diversion itself must be considered, especially after adequate fluid replacement. The physician must consider obstruction at some level in the conduit. For example, outlet obstruction of the conduit caused by a mucous plug or stomal edema should be considered. This situation can be evaluated by catheterizing and irrigating the conduit with normal saline. Obstruction at the ureteroenteral anastomosis can result from edema at the anastomotic site or from mucous plugging or kinking of the ureteral stents. If oliguria persists, radiographic studies to evaluate the conduit should be performed to rule out ureteral obstruction or urinary leak.

A serious early postoperative complication is leakage of urine from the conduit. Although some urinary leaks spontaneously close, most require some type of intervention to aid in the closing process. The incidence of urinary leaks varies in the literature, ranging from 5% to 20%.[36-39] Factors that predispose patients to leaks include a history of radiation therapy, poor surgical technique, unstented ureters, and poor nutritional status. Conflicting reports exist in the literature about the benefit of placing ureteral stents at the time of urinary diversion. Richie and Skinner[40] reported no significant difference in the incidence of urinary leaks in the stented versus unstented ureters. However, several other reports have demonstrated a significant reduction in urinary leaks with the use of ureteral stents.[41-43] The major disadvantage of ureteral stents is an increased incidence of urinary tract infections. Other disadvantages include occasional stent obstruction from encrustation or mucus, possible stent breakage and retention, and the risk of avulsion. Despite these disadvantages and several conflicting reports in the literature, most surgeons favor ureteral stent placement.

When a urinary leak is suspected, diagnostic workup should include a CT scan to evaluate for a fluid collection and a fluoroscopic loopogram to evaluate the integrity of the conduit. After a urinary leak is confirmed, conservative management is the treatment of choice. In the early postoperative period, repeat surgery after a pelvic exenteration is associated with a mortality rate as high as 50%.[37,38,44] The preferred solution to a urinary leak is the insertion of percutaneous nephrostomies by the interventional radiologist. After complete diversion of the urine, the leaking anastomosis usually closes within a couple of weeks.

Infections are among the most common complications after urinary conduit diversion. Acute pyelonephritis occurs in about 5% to 20% of patients.[38,45,46] It is more common in patients with a history of preexisting obstruction or chronic pyelonephritis. Ureteral stents are associated with increased risk of urinary tract infection. The use of prophylactic parenteral antibiotics, an adequate bowel preparation, and satisfactory hydration may contribute to a reduced risk of postoperative urinary tract infections.

Small-bowel complications after urinary conduit diversion are fairly common. Bowel obstruction, prolonged ileus, and anastomotic breakdown are the most cited complications. The incidence of anastomotic leaks can be reduced significantly by using nonirradiated segments of bowel to construct the conduit. Small-bowel complications may also be associated with other problems, such as a urinary leak. If a bowel anastomosis is leaking, there is increased risk for a leaking urinary conduit. The surgeon must be on high alert and consider these possibilities that can lead to significant patient morbidity and mortality.

Stomal complications occur in approximately 5% of cases and include retraction, necrosis, and stenosis.[38,45,47] Early stomal complications are most commonly the result of ischemia and vascular compromise. After surgery, the stoma often appears dusky or dark, especially if the patient has received prior irradiation or if the mesentery has been dissected to facilitate stoma formation. This usually resolves within a few days. To avoid stomal complications, certain measures should be taken intraoperatively. When making the tunnel in the anterior abdominal wall, care must be taken to follow a straight path, and the fascial aperture should permit the passage of two fingers. This avoids fascial constriction of the segment. Excessive tension on the mesentery or tight closure of the mesenteric window should be avoided. If the stoma turns black or continues to have a dark, dusky appearance, the entire conduit should be evaluated with cystoscopy.

Late complications. Late complications after urinary conduit diversion include stomal complications, ureteroenteric stenosis, infections, stone formation, electrolyte abnormalities, and deterioration of renal function. The incidence of complications usually increases with time, resulting mainly from inherent properties of urinary diversion. The most commonly reported late stomal complications are erosive and erythematous skin changes around the stoma site. This usually is the result of urine leakage causing direct skin irritation, too-frequent appliance changes, or skin reaction to the adhesives used. These peristomal skin problems can be avoided by choosing an appropriate stomal location preoperatively, instructing patients on proper appliance hygiene and technique, and providing the appropriate appliances according to the type of stoma constructed.[48] Another stomal complication is stenosis, which occurs more frequently in small-bowel segments than in colon segments. Using the Turnbull loop stoma rather than the end stoma for small-bowel conduits has decreased the incidence of stenosis.[49] Although the Turnbull loop stoma is associated with a 14% incidence of parastomal hernia, this is easily correctable by meticulously suturing the loop end to the fascia.[49] Stomal stenosis can be managed with periodic dilatation as a temporary solution. However, if the stenosis is resulting in urine outflow obstruction or prevents proper application of the stomal appliance, revision is indicated.

In a literature review by Beckley and associates,[41] the incidence of ureteral stenosis ranged from 1.5% to 18.4%. Most ureteral stenoses occur at the ureteroenteral anastomotic site. Predisposing factors to anastomotic stenosis include poor surgical technique, a history of radiation therapy, and severe inflammation from a urinary leak leading to scarring. Slow deterioration of renal function usually ensues if the ureteral obstruction goes undetected. The patient may be asymptomatic or present with flank pain, pyelonephritis, or evidence of urinary leakage. A radiologic examination should be performed. To preserve renal function and diagnose obstructions early before complications occur, a serum creatinine level and a renal ultrasound or an intravenous pyelogram should be obtained periodically, usually every 6 to 12 months. After the site of obstruction is confirmed by radiographic evaluation, the placement of a ureteral stent antegrade by percutaneous nephrostomy or balloon dilatation performed by the interventional radiologist is a reasonable option. If ureteral stents are placed, they should be exchanged every 4 to 6 months. Surgical revisions are seldom needed and, if considered, should be reserved for the patient with a long life expectancy, preserved renal function, and severe ureteral obstruction.

Urinary tract infections are also a late complication of urinary conduit diversion. Most urinary conduits are permanently colonized by bacteria. This predisposes patients to recurrent infections, especially if ureteral reflux or urinary stasis is present. Hancock and colleagues[37] reported an 18% incidence of urinary tract infections, with no difference in long-term infections found for ileal and colon conduits. Urine cultures are not reliable in these patients because of the bacterial colonization. Although a catheterized urine specimen is somewhat more reliable, patients with clinical signs of acute pyelonephritis should always receive treatment.

Urinary calculi develop in 2% to 9% of patients with urinary conduits.[38,50,51] Approximately one third occur in the conduit, with the remaining developing in the upper urinary tract. Risk factors for stone formation include chronic urinary stasis, recurrent or chronic infections, and increased urinary calcium excretion. Conduit stone formation has also been attributed to the use of nonabsorbable staples during conduit construction.[52] Preventing urinary calculi involves

prompt treatment of urinary tract infections and relief of urinary obstruction. Treatment of patients with recurrent infections caused by stones should entail a plan to remove them.

Electrolyte abnormalities are rare in patients with urinary conduits and normal renal function. The most common electrolyte imbalance is hyperchloremic metabolic acidosis, resulting from increased absorption of solute within the intestinal segment. This usually occurs in patients with compromised renal function or with a longer than usual conduit intestinal segment. Oral sodium bicarbonate is the recommended treatment.

Loss of renal function is a common sequel of urinary diversion. Even patients with no preexisting renal compromise have a 10% to 20% incidence of renal function deterioration. Causes of the loss of renal function include chronic obstruction (from stricture at the ureteroenteral anastomosis, stomal stenosis, or urinary calculi), and chronic or recurrent urinary tract infections.[47,52] Hancock and coworkers,[37] in a study of 212 conduits, reported no significant correlation between the type of conduit used and the subsequent deterioration of renal function. Prevention entails early detection of infections, obstructions, and close surveillance of renal function with serum renal function tests and radiologic studies of the urinary system.

Selecting the Urinary Reservoir

Because of its associated complications and patient dissatisfaction with the external appliance, urinary conduits are often not the procedure of choice for the surgeon or the patient. Consequently, the search continued for the ideal urinary bladder substitute that could provide a low-pressure storage system, prevent ureteral reflux and infection, eliminate the external appliance, and easily empty at the convenience of the patient. Kock[8] was the first to introduce the low-pressure system, created by detubularization of the bowel using a segment of ileum. The ileal reservoir uses an afferent nipple valve to prevent ureteral reflux and an efferent nipple valve to maintain continence. However, the complexity of the Kock pouch with its associated complications led to the development of many different methods of continent urinary diversion with low-pressure reservoirs. Most reservoirs developed in the past 10 to 15 years use the cecum, right colon, and terminal ileum in various ways. The most widely used ileocolonic continent reservoirs include the Miami pouch,[14] Indiana pouch,[11] and the Mainz pouch.[10]

In the practice of gynecologic oncology, the Mainz pouch is not as popular as the Miami pouch or Indiana pouch. The Mainz pouch uses a 12-cm length of cecum and ascending colon, as well as two terminal ileal segments of equal length.[53] The bowel is detubularized, and a side-to-side anastomosis is formed. The ureters are tunneled submucosally in the colonic segment for an anti-refluxing system. The appendix is preferentially used as a continence mechanism. However, if the

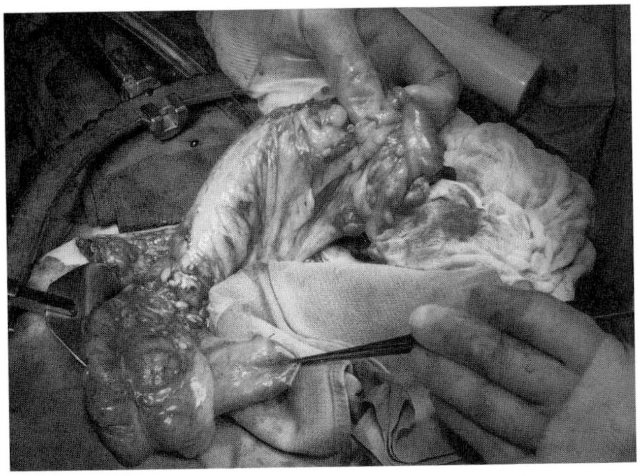

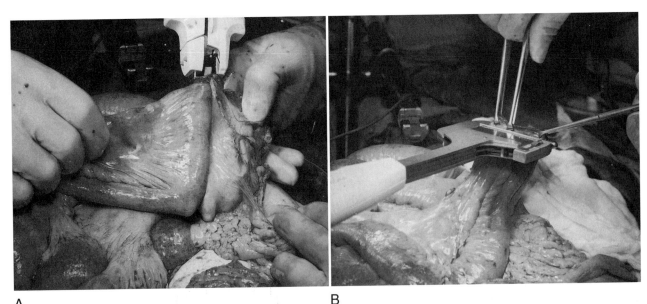

Figure 51–6. The Miami pouch is constructed from the cecum, ascending colon, part of the transverse colon, and 15 cm of distal ileum.

appendix is not suitable, an ileal invaginated nipple fixed to the ileocecal valve is constructed to provide the continent mechanism. Wammack and associates[54] reported their experience with the Mainz pouch in gynecologic cancer patients. Thirty-six patients with a history of gynecologic cancer and prior radiation therapy underwent urinary diversion with the Mainz pouch, usually after pelvic exenteration. This group was compared with 385 nonirradiated patients who underwent urinary diversion with the Mainz pouch for other indications. The Mainz pouch was associated with high complication rates in the irradiated patients, including efferent limb complications in 25% of patients, ureteral complications in 22%, and stomal complications in 39%. They concluded that the Mainz pouch should not be performed in patients with a history of radiation therapy. Because most gynecologic cancer patients have received pelvic radiation, the

following sections focus on the Miami pouch and the Indiana pouch.

The miami pouch. Since 1988, the Gynecologic Oncology Division at the University of Miami has been using a continent ileocolonic reservoir, the Miami Pouch, as the preferred method of urinary diversion.[55] The Miami pouch is one of the most widely used continent urinary reservoirs because it provides a reliable continence mechanism through one of the least technically demanding procedures. To construct the Miami pouch, the distal ileum is transected approximately 10 to 15 cm from the ileocecal valve, depending on the size of the patient and the thickness of her anterior abdominal wall. The cecum, ascending colon, and hepatic flexure are then mobilized, and the transverse colon is transected distal to the middle colic artery (Fig. 51-6). An ileotransverse colon anastomosis is performed to restore bowel continuity (Fig. 51-7). The appendix, if present, should always be removed. The colon is then opened with electrocautery along the taenia and folded onto itself to create a U-shaped intestinal plate (Fig. 51-8). The legs of the U are then reapproximated with absorbable sutures or staples in a side-to-side fashion to form the posterior wall of the reservoir. This step of bowel detubularization creates a low-pressure reservoir. Attention is then turned to the segment of ileum to create the continence mechanism. A 14F rubber catheter is inserted into the distal ileal segment, and Babcock clamps are placed along the antimesenteric border and pulled to provide mild traction (Fig. 51-9). A stapling instrument is then used to reduce the lumen along the antimesenteric border down to the French size of the catheter. At the level of the ileocecal valve, three purse-string sutures of 2-0 silk are then placed in the seromuscular layer to increase the closure pressure. This combination of a tapered distal ileum and purse-string sutures at the

A   B

Figure 51–7. A, The side-to-side anastomosis is created using stapling devices. **B,** Previously irradiated ileum is anastomosed to nonirradiated transverse colon.

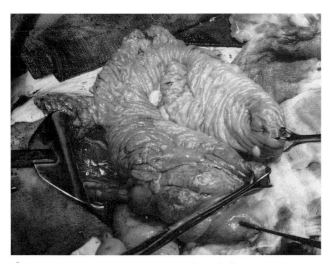

Figure 51–8. Detubularization of the bowel allows creation of a low-pressure reservoir. After opening the bowel along the taenia, it is folded in a U shape to form the reservoir.

ileocecal valve increases the ileal pressure higher than the pressure within the colonic reservoir, thereby achieving continence. The ileal segment is then brought through the right lower quadrant of the anterior abdominal wall, and the stoma is created for future self-catheterization.

The ureters are brought through the posterior wall of the reservoir (Fig. 51-10). The distal 1 cm of ureter is then spatulated and anastomosed to the submucosal layer of the colon with interrupted, 4-0, polyglycolic acid sutures. The anti-reflux mechanism is provided by the low-pressure reservoir and the muscular wall of the colon. This nontunneled ureteral anastomosis has functioned well in the colon. Its main advantage is that it can be performed in any segment of the colon, unlike the tunneled implantation described by Goodwin and colleagues.[56] The incidence of reflux and obstruction

with the nontunneled technique is similar to that reported with other forms of ureteral implantation. The ureters are stented with double-J catheters (Fig. 51-11). Outside the reservoir, the ureteral adventitia is secured to the bowel serosa. The pouch is then completed by closing the anterior wall with interrupted absorbable sutures (Fig. 51-12). The reservoir is secured to the anterior abdominal wall.

In the immediate postoperative period, close attention to urine output is paramount. Pouch irrigations with warm normal saline every 2 to 4 hours to prevent outlet obstruction from a mucus plug should be carefully taught to the nursing staff. Between 2 and 3 weeks after surgery, radiographic studies of the upper urinary tract and the reservoir are performed to search for urinary leaks, ureteral reflux, or obstruction. If the studies are normal, the ureteral stents and the catheter are removed. The patient is taught intermittent catheterization and pouch irrigation. At first, catheterization is necessary every 2 to 4 hours and irrigations every 4 hours. The patient may gradually decrease the frequency of irrigations and catheterizations if mucous obstruction and continence are not a problem. Self-catheterization is usually needed five or six times each day. A full reservoir is usually heralded by a fullness or cramping sensation in the right lower quadrant. An interval longer than 6 hours is not recommended between catheterizations because of the risk of infection and outlet obstruction from overdistention of the reservoir. Close follow-up of renal function and serum electrolytes is essential. Radiographic studies to evaluate for ureteral obstruction are needed every 6 months. Urine cultures are not performed routinely because most pouches are colonized with bacteria and produce positive culture results.

The Indiana pouch. The Indiana pouch is also an ileocolonic reservoir that provides continent urinary diversion. The pouch is created from approximately

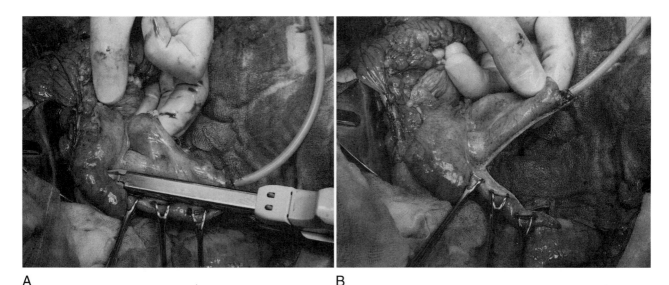

A   B

Figure 51–9. Tapering the distal ileum. **A,** Babcock clamps placed on the antimesenteric border are pulled to provide traction. **B,** A stapling device is then used to taper the lumen to the size of the 14F catheter.

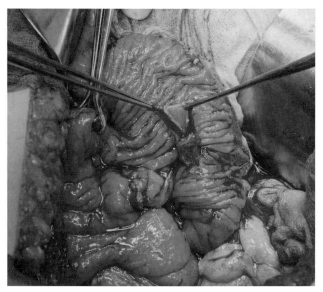

Figure 51–10. The ureters are brought through the posterior wall of the reservoir. The distal 1 cm of ureter is spatulated to facilitate anastomosis and help prevent future stricture.

25 cm of cecum and ascending colon and 15 cm of distal ileum. The large bowel is detubularized and folded on itself. The continence mechanism is achieved by plicating the terminal 4 cm of ileum with two rows of Lembert sutures. The ureters are brought through the posterior wall of the reservoir and anastomosed in a similar fashion as that described previously. The tapered ileum is brought through the anterior abdominal wall, and the stoma is created. The stoma is left intubated for approximately 2 to 3 weeks. The postoperative care and follow-up are similar to what is done for other ileocolonic reservoirs.

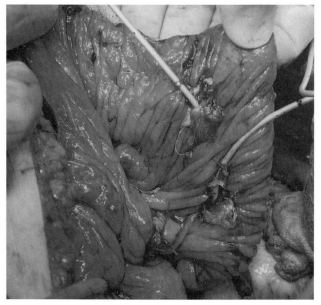

Figure 51–11. Double-J ureteral stents are placed.

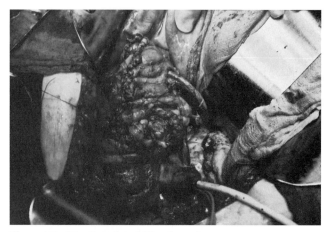

Figure 51–12. Completed Miami pouch.

Complications of urinary reservoirs. The different ileocolonic urinary reservoirs have similar continence rates and similar rates of complications. Because they are technically easier to construct with higher continence rates and fewer complications, the ileocolonic reservoir is preferred over the Kock ileal pouch. In a previously irradiated patient, the ileocolonic reservoir is created from mostly nonirradiated tissue, and bowel continuity is reestablished by connecting nonirradiated large bowel to irradiated small bowel. Consequently, fewer small bowel anastomotic complications should occur with an ileocolonic reservoir than with the ileal pouch. Continent urinary reservoirs have increased risk for complications because of their greater complexity, requiring a longer operative time than urinary conduits. The complications of urinary reservoirs, like those of conduits, can be divided into early and late complications, and many are similar to those seen with urinary conduits.

Early complications. Decreased urine output often occurs in the early postoperative period. The usual causes related specifically to urinary reservoirs include mucous plugs, kinked drainage tubes, and urinary leaks. Physiologic causes of oliguria must also be considered and addressed. The patient's intravascular volume should be replaced adequately during and after surgery. If there is no explanation for the oliguria, the integrity of the reservoir should be evaluated with diagnostic contrast studies. Urinary leaks are reported to occur in approximately 5% of reservoirs.[57,58] Patients can present with low urine output, increased intra-abdominal drain output, ileus, or a pelvic collection. Diagnosis is made by radiologic contrast studies of the pouch. If a leak is diagnosed, conservative management is the preferred approach given the high mortality rate associated with reoperations in the early postoperative period.[37,38,44] A urinoma can be evacuated by an interventional radiologist using CT- or ultrasound-guided drainage.

Urinary tract infections are common after continent urinary diversion, occurring with an incidence of

15% to 30%.[57,58] The use of parenteral antibiotics and mechanical bowel preparation has decreased the infections in these patients. However, given the high bacterial colonization within the reservoirs, pyelonephritis is a constant threat. Patients with clinical signs of pyelonephritis need to be treated immediately with antibiotics and followed closely for signs of ureteral obstruction, outlet obstruction, urinary calculi, or renal compromise. Ureteral stents are removed 2 to 3 weeks after surgery. If the patient requires further stenting, ureteral catheter exchange should occur every 4 to 6 months.

Late complications. As the duration of patient follow-up increases, so does the incidence of late complications for urinary conduits and reservoirs. Common late complications for urinary reservoirs include ureteral stricture, urinary incontinence, infections, urinary calculi, and difficulty with catheterization. Ureteral stenosis is one of the most significant complications of urinary reservoirs. The incidence of ureteral stricture for ileocolonic reservoirs ranges from about 10% to 20%.[57-59] If it persists undetected, it may lead to infections, stone formation, and most importantly, loss of renal function. Periodic evaluation of the urinary system (every 6 months) is important to detect asymptomatic obstruction. Ureteral stricture can temporarily be managed with balloon dilatation and ureteral stent placement retrograde by cystoscopy or antegrade by percutaneous nephrostomy. However, ureteral reimplantation and revision are usually required for the long-term management.

Urinary incontinence can result from incompetence of the ileocecal valve or high-pressure spikes within the reservoir. Urodynamic testing is performed to distinguish between these two causes. When the ileocecal valve is incompetent, the terminal ileum can be replicated, often by revising the stoma without the need for a laparotomy. If reservoir noncompliance is causing incontinence, an ileal patch can be used to augment the pouch and decrease reservoir pressures. More commonly, incontinence is the result of an overdistended pouch. In this case, by increasing the frequency of catheterizations, continence can be achieved.

Most commonly, acute pyelonephritis is associated with outlet obstruction, ureteral obstruction, or an infected pouch with ureteral reflux. If the patient develops recurrent episodes of infection or develops chronic pyelonephritis, a complete evaluation in search of the cause is needed. Urinary calculi are common complications of urinary reservoirs. Pouch calculi usually form within 2 to 3 years after pouch construction. Risk factors for pouch stones are infection, urinary stasis, and the use of stapling devices to construct the pouch. Calculi associated with chronic infections or obstruction should be removed.

Difficulty with self-catheterization can occur with urinary reservoirs. Reports in the literature cite incidences ranging from 5% to 10% of patients with ileocolonic reservoirs.[57,58] The physician must differentiate whether the difficulty in catheterization is related to patient technique or an anatomic problem with the stoma. Enterostomal therapists are critical in patient education and demonstrating proper technique for catheterization. Structural problems with the pouch can be evaluated with radiologic contrast studies. Ultrasound-guided catheter placement can serve as a temporary solution.

Orthotopic Urinary Diversion

Orthotopic urinary diversion is becoming increasingly popular among urologic patients undergoing cystectomy for bladder cancer.[60] The indications for orthotopic reconstruction have expanded over the past decade. It was initially performed on selected men[61] and now is being successfully performed in women.[62] A potential candidate for an orthotopic neobladder must have an intact external urethral sphincter to provide continence and allow conscious voiding through the urethra. The cancer surgery must not be compromised by the orthotopic reconstruction. All surgical margins must be free of tumor. Indications for orthotopic urinary diversion in gynecologic oncology patients are unclear. Because orthotopic reconstruction requires working in a previously irradiated field with poor blood supply, gynecologic cancer patients may not be the best candidates. The most popular orthotopic neobladders use ileum for pouch construction. Using irradiated bowel to form the neobladder would most likely lead to unacceptable complication rates. Exenterative procedures including the vulva eliminate the possibility of orthotopic urinary diversion.

Summary

Many techniques are available for urinary diversion. Despite the absence of a perfect conduit or reservoir, the available techniques allow the surgeon to choose the most appropriate form for a particular patient. With a proper understanding of indications and general principles of urinary diversion, the procedure can be safely performed by the gynecologic oncologist.

REFERENCES

1. Simon J: Ectopia vesica (absence of the anterior walls of the bladder and abdominal parietes): Operation for directing the orifices of the ureters into the rectum; temporary success; subsequent death; autopsy. Lancet 1852;2:568.
2. Verhoogen J, de Graeuve A: La cystectomie totale. Folia Urol 1909;3:629.
3. Bricker EM: Bladder substitution after pelvic evisceration. Surg Clin North Am 1950;30:1511-1521.
4. Symmonds RE, Gibbs CP: Urinary diversion by way of sigmoid conduit. Surg Gynecol Obstet 1970;131:687-693.
5. Schmidt JD, Hawtrey CE, Buchsbaum HJ: Transverse colon conduit: A preferred method of urinary diversion for radiation-treated pelvic malignancies. J Urol 1975;113:308-313.
6. Gilchrist RK, Merricks JW, Hamlin MH, et al: Construction of a substitute bladder and urethra. Surg Gynecol Obstet 1950;90:752-760.
7. Mansson W, Colleen S, Sundin T: Continent caecal reservoir in urinary diversion. Br J Urol 1984;56:359.

8. Kock NG, Nilson AE, Norlen L, et al: Urinary diversion via a continent ileum reservoir. Clinical experience. Scand J Urol Nephrol Suppl 1978;49:23-31.

9. Kock NG, Nilson AE, Nilsson LO, et al: Urinary diversion via a continent ileal reservoir: Clinical results in 12 patients. J Urol 1982;128:469-475.

10. Thuroff JW, Alken P, Riedmiller N, et al: The Mainz pouch (mixed augmentation ileum and cecum) for bladder augmentation and bladder diversion. J Urol 1976116:428-430.

11. Rowland RG, Mitchell ME, Birhrle R, et al: Indiana continent urinary reservoir. J Urol 1987;137:1136-1139.

12. Lockhart JL: Remodeled right colon: An alternative urinary reservoir. J Urol 1987;138:730-734.

13. Lockhart JL, Bejany DE: The antireflux ureteroileal reimplantation in children and adults. J Urol 1986;135:576-579.

14. Bejany DE, Politano VA: Stapled and nonstapled tapered distal ileum for construction of a continent colonic urinary reservoir. J Urol 1988;140:33-38.

15. Kock NG, Ghoneim MA, Lycke KG, Mahran MR: Replacement of the bladder by the urethral Kock pouch: Functional results, urodynamics and radiological features. J Urol 1989; 141:1111.

16. Shekarriz B, Shekarriz H, Upadhyay J, et al: Outcome of palliative urinary diversion in the treatment of advanced malignancies. Cancer 1999;85:998-1003.

17. Watkinson AF, A'Hern RP, Jones A, et al: The role of percutaneous nephrostomy in malignant urinary tract obstruction. Clin Radiol 1992;47:32-35.

18. Buzby GP, for The Veterans Affairs Total Parenteral Nutrition Cooperative Study Group: Perioperative total parenteral nutrition in surgical patients. N Engl J Med 1991;325:525-532.

19. Buzby GP, Williford WO, Peterson OL, et al: A randomized clinical trial of total parenteral nutrition in malnourished surgical patients: The rationale and impact of previous clinical trials and pilot study on protocol design. Am J Clin Nutr 1988;47:357-365.

20. Oliveira L, Wexner SD, Daniel N, et al: Mechanical bowel preparation for elective colorectal surgery: A prospective, randomized, surgeon-blinded trial comparing sodium phosphate and polyethylene glycol-based oral lavage solutions. Dis Col Rectum 1997;40:585-591.

21. Classen DC, Evans RS, Pestotnik SL et al: The timing of prophylactic administration of antibiotics and the risk of surgical-wound infection. N Engl J Med 1992;356:281-286.

22. Orr JW, Sisson PF, Patsner B, et al: Single-dose antibiotic prophylaxis for patients undergoing extended pelvic surgery for gynecologic malignancy. Am J Obstet Gynecol 1990;162: 718-721.

23. Nichols RL: Bowel preparation. In Wilmore DW, Brennan MF, Harken AH, et al (eds): Care of the Surgical Patient, vol 2. New York, Scientific American Medicine, 1990.

24. Condon RE, Bartlett JG, Greenlee H, et al: Efficacy of oral and systemic antibiotic prophylaxis in colorectal operations. Arch Surg 1983;118:496-502.

25. Lau WY, Chu KW, Poon GP, Ho KK: Prophylactic antibiotics in elective colorectal surgery. Br J Surg 1988;75:782-785.

26. Schoetz DJ, Roberts PL, Murray JJ, et al: Addition of parenteral cefoxitin to regimen of oral antibiotics for elective colorectal operations: A randomized prospective study. Ann Surg 1990;212: 209-212.

27. Williams O, Vereb MJ, Libertino JA: Noncontinent urinary diversion. Urol Clin North Am 1997;24:735-744.

28. Emmott D, Noble MJ, Mebust WK: A comparison of end versus loop stomas for ileal conduit urinary diversion. J Urol 1985; 133:588-590.

29. Chechile G, Klein EA, Bauer L, et al: Functional equivalence of end and loop ileal conduit stomas. J Urol 1992;147:582-586.

30. Emmott D, Noble MJ, Mebust WK: A comparison of end versus loop stomas for ileal conduit urinary diversion. J Urol 1985;133:588-590.

31. Schmidt JD, Buchsbaum HJ, Jacob ED: Transverse colon conduit for supravesical urinary tract diversion. Urology 1976;8: 542-546.

32. Klein EA, Montie JE, Montague DK, et al: Jejunal conduit urinary diversion. J Urol 1986;135:244-246.

33. Golimbu M, Morales P: Jejunal conduits: Technique and complications. J Urol 1975;113:787-795.

34. Fontaine E, Barthelemy Y, Houlgatte A, et al: Twenty-year experience with jejunal conduits. Urology 1997;50:207-213.

35. Cukier JM: Ureteral diversion. In Glenn JF (ed): Urologic Surgery, 4th ed. Philadelphia, JB Lippincott, 1991, p 995.

36. Fallon B, Leoning S, Hawtrey CE, et al: Urologic complications of pelvic exenteration for gynecologic malignancy. J Urol 1979;122:158-159.

37. Hancock KC, Copeland LJ, Gershenson DM, et al: Urinary conduits in gynecologic oncology. Obstet Gynecol 1986;67: 680-684.

38. Orr JW Jr, Shingleton HM, Hatch KD, et al: Urinary diversion in patients undergoing pelvic exenteration. Am J Obstet Gynecol 1982;142:883-889.

39. Wrigley JV, Prem KA, Fraley EE: Pelvic exenteration: Complications of urinary diversion. J Urol 116:428-430, 1976.

40. Richie JP, Skinner DG: Complications of urinary conduit diversion. In Smith RB, Skinner DG (eds): Complications of Urologic Surgery: Prevention and Management. London, WB Saunders, 1976, p 209.

41. Beckley S, Wajsman Z, Pontes JE, Murphy G: Transverse colon conduit: A method of urinary diversion after pelvic irradiation. J Urol 1982;128:464-468.

42. Beddoe AM, Boyce JG, Remy JC, et al: Stented versus nonstented transverse colon conduits: A comparative report. Gynecol Oncol 1987;27:305-315.

43. Oakley GJ, Downey GO, Twiggs LB, et al: Urinary diversion in pelvic exenteration: The role of conduit choice in postoperative morbidity. Paper presented at Society of Gynecologic Oncologists 22nd Annual Meeting, February 17-20, 1991, Orlando, FL.

44. Hensle TW, Bredin HC, Dretler SP: Diagnosis and treatment of a urinary leak after ureteroileal conduit diversion. J Urol 1986;116:680-684.

45. Lindenauer SM, Cerny JC, Morley GW: Ureterosigmoid conduit urinary diversion. Surgery 1974;75:705-714.

46. Morales P, Golimby M: Colonic urinary diversion: 10 years of experience. J Urol 1975;113:302-307.

47. Sullivan JW, Gradstald H, Whitmore WF Jr: Complications of ureteroileal conduit with radical cystectomy: Review of 336 cases. J Urol 1980;124:757-763.

48. Nordström GM, Borglund E, Nyman CR: Urostomy appliances and stoma care routines: The relation to peristomal skin complications. Scand J Caring Sci 1990;4:35-42.

49. Bloom DA, Lieskovsky G: The Turnbull loop stoma. In Skinner DG, Lieskovsky G (eds): Diagnosis and Management of Genitourinary Cancer. Philadelphia, WB Saunders, 1988, p 649.

50. Neal DE: Complications of ileal conduit diversion in adults with cancer followed up for at least five years. BMJ 1985;290: 1695-1697.

51. Podratz KC, Angerman NS, Symmonds RE: Complications of ureteral surgery in the non-irradiated patient. In Delgado G, Smith JP (eds): Management of Complications in Gynecologic Oncology. New York, John Wiley, 1982, pp 164-169.

52. Pitts WR, Muecke EC: A 20-year experience with ileal conduits: The fate of the kidneys. J Urol 1979;122:154-157.

53. Lampel A, Fisch M, Stein R, et al: Continent diversion with the Mainz pouch. World J Urol 1996;14:85-91.

54. Wammack R, Wricke C, Hohenfellner R: Long-term results of ileocecal continent urinary diversion in patients treated with and without previous pelvic irradiation. J Urol 2002;167: 2058-2062.

55. Penalver MA, Bejany DE, Averette HE, et al: Continent urinary diversion in gynecologic oncology. Gynecol Oncol 1989;34: 274-288.

56. Goodwin WE, Harris AP, Kaufman JJ, et al: One transcolonic ureterointestinal anastomosis: A new approach. Surg Gynecol Obstet 1953;97:295-300.

57. Penalver MA, Angioli R, Mirhashemi R, Malik R: Management of early and late complications of ileocolonic continent urinary reservoir (Miami pouch). Gynecol Oncol 1998;69: 185-191.

58. Husain A, Curtin C, Brown D, Chi W, et al: Continent urinary diversion and low-rectal anastomosis in patients undergoing

exenterative procedures for recurrent gynecologic malignancies. Gyencol Oncol 2000;78:208-211.

59. Wilson TG, Moreno JG, Weinberg A, Ahlering TE: Late complications of the modified Indiana pouch. J Urol 1994; 151:331-334.

60. Stein JP, Skinner DG: Orthotopic urinary diversion: The new gold standard. Contemp Urol 2001;13:26-45.

61. Elmajian DA, Stein JP, Esrig D, et al: The Kock ileal neobladder: Updated experience in 295 male patients. J Urol 1996;156: 920-925.

62. Stein JP, Grossfeld GD, Freeman JA, et al: Orthotopic lower urinary tract reconstruction in women using the Kock ileal neobladder: Updated experience in 34 patients. J Urol 1997; 158:400-405.

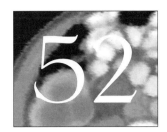

THE ROLE OF LAPAROSCOPY
IN THE MANAGEMENT OF
GYNECOLOGIC CANCERS

Inbar Ben-Shachar   and   Jeffrey M. Fowler

 MAJOR CONTROVERSIES

- **What is the role of laparoscopic surgery in the treatment of cervical cancer?**
- **Can we combine the vaginal and laparoscopic approaches for a conservative treatment of early-stage cervical cancer?**
- **Should laparoscopic surgery be used for staging of advanced disease?**
- **Laparoscopic aortic lymphadenectomy: What is the best approach?**
- **What is the role of laparoscopic surgery in the treatment of endometrial cancer?**
- **Should the laparoscopic approach be used for staging of incompletely staged disease?**
- **What is the role of laparoscopic surgery in the diagnosis and treatment of ovarian cancer?**
- **What is the adequacy and reliability of an intraoperative diagnosis of ovarian cancer?**
- **Is laparoscopy safe and feasible?**
- **What are the risks of rupture and tumor spillage of a malignant ovarian cyst?**
- **How should we manage a malignancy diagnosed during or after a laparoscopic procedure, and what is the influence of delayed staging?**
- **What is the role of laparoscopic staging in clinically apparent early-stage disease?**
- **Is there a role for laparoscopic second-look operations?**
- **Can we evaluate the feasibility of cytoreductive surgery in advanced disease by the laparoscopic approach?**
- **What is the risk for port-site metastasis?**

Operative laparoscopy has been used for several decades by gynecologists for diagnostic procedures and female sterilization. The potential applications for laparoscopy have expanded over the past 15 years with improvements in surgical skills and technologic advancements in instrumentation. Many gynecologic oncologists are using operative laparoscopy in the management of patients with cervical, endometrial, and ovarian cancer for surgical extirpation of the disease and surgical staging. The cornerstone of appropriate surgical staging is accurate pelvic and para-aortic lymph node dissection. Since laparoscopic pelvic and

para-aortic lymph node dissections were first reported (1989 and 1992, respectively) and subsequently perfected, the applications of advanced laparoscopic procedures have widely expanded in the management of patients with gynecologic malignancies.

It is unlikely that the laparoscopic approach will improve the therapeutic effectiveness of surgery applied to women with gynecologic malignancies; therefore, advantages must be seen in other important outcome variables. Potential benefits from the laparoscopic approach include minimization of patient discomfort, shorter length of hospital stay, decreased overall recovery time, improved quality of life, and earlier use of adjuvant therapies. Most data concerning the laparoscopic approach in the surgical treatment of the gynecologic oncology patient are primarily from nonrandomized, retrospective, or feasibility trials in highly selected patients. A few multicenter clinical trials, including Gynecologic Oncology Group (GOG) LAP 2, 9206, and 9402 for endometrial cancer; GOG 9207 for cervical cancer; and GOG 9302 for ovarian cancer, have been initiated to gather information on feasibility, long-term survival, operative times, costs, and complications. Some of these studies compare the laparoscopic approach with conventional surgery performed by laparotomy.

This chapter reviews the data available concerning the role of laparoscopic surgery in the management of the different gynecologic malignancies and discusses common controversies related to the use of this surgical approach.

What is the role of laparoscopic surgery in the treatment of cervical cancer?

The use of laparoscopy in the treatment of cervical cancer has been described in numerous studies in the past decade. The ability to perform the laparoscopic pelvic and para-aortic lymphadenectomy has revived the use of a variety of radical vaginal procedures in women with early-stage disease. Patients with advanced-stage disease may be eligible for pretreatment surgical staging to define disease spread and tailor definitive irradiation and chemotherapy.

Early-stage cervical cancer. The five basic laparoscopic operations that may be performed in the treatment of early-stage (stages Ia through IIa) cervical cancer are laparoscopic simple hysterectomy (total or laparoscopically assisted vaginal hysterectomy), laparoscopically assisted radical vaginal hysterectomy, laparoscopic total abdominal radical hysterectomy, laparoscopic vaginal radical trachelectomy, and laparoscopic pelvic and para-aortic lymph node dissection. (Para-aortic lymph node dissection is discussed with advanced-stage cervical cancer.)

Simple hysterectomies are performed laparoscopically worldwide[1] as laparoscopically assisted vaginal hysterectomy (LAVH) or laparoscopic hysterectomy (LH). Although a criticism by some is that most of these cases could be managed by vaginal hysterectomy, the latter is not considered an adequate approach for most cervical cancer patients and should only be considered for carcinoma in situ or FIGO Ia1 disease.

Because aortic and pelvic lymphadenectomy cannot be performed when using the vaginal approach, an entirely laparoscopic radical hysterectomy (LRH) or the more commonly performed laparovaginal approaches are used to combine laparoscopic lymphadenectomy and radical hysterectomy for stages more advanced than Ia1. There is no standard indication for combining laparoscopic pelvic and para-aortic lymphadenectomy with LAVH or LH in women with cervical cancer.

Laparoscopically assisted radical vaginal hysterectomy.
Numerous reports describe laparoscopically assisted radical vaginal hysterectomy (LARVH),[2-18] but it has not been determined which steps of the operation are best performed vaginally and which should be done laparoscopically. Various modifications of LARVH have been described.[13] The laparoscopic phase of the LARVH ranges from lymph node dissection only to a complete LRH, which is discussed in the following section. Dargent[14] describes the combination of laparoscopic surgery and two variants of vaginal radical hysterectomy (i.e., Schauta operation), the laparoscopically assisted Schauta-Amereich and Schauta-Stoeckel operations. The former is the more radical variant, similar to the Piver[19] type 3 abdominal hysterectomy, and the latter is less radical, the equivalent of Piver type 2 abdominal hysterectomy. Table 52-1 summarizes the recent published experience with the LARVH (i.e., Schauta-Amreich and Schauta-Stoeckel operations).

In the laparoscopically assisted Schauta-Amereich approach, the paracervical ligament is divided during the laparoscopic step. After the completion of lymphadenectomy, the paravesical and pararectal spaces are opened, and the paracervical ligament (parametrium) in between is divided using a laparoscopic endostapler or bipolar cauterization. If an endostapler is used, two or three cartridges are usually enough for dividing the ligament on its whole height to the level of the levator muscles (i.e., pelvic floor). The rest of the procedure is completed vaginally as described for the classic Schauta operation. The main difference between LARVH and the Schauta is that the pararectal and paravesical spaces in the LARVH are defined and opened laparoscopically and the parametria are secured using the endostapler, omitting the need for a Schuchart or lateral vaginal incision.

The data concerning the Schauta-Amreich operation shows clearly that the rate of complications and length of operation are quite high. This negative outcome led Dargent and Mathevet[2] and Schneider and colleagues[16] to develop a laparoscopic modification of the Schauta operation. The rationale for the laparoscopic Schauta-Stockel operation (or modified LAVRH) was to minimize the intraoperative and postoperative complications, mainly bladder and ureteral injuries of the Schauta-Amereich approach, while not reducing the cure rate. The modified LARVH consists of laparoscopic removal of all lymph node–bearing tissue located in the vasculonervous web making up the lateral part of the cervical ligament. First, the obturator nodes are removed, completely opening the paravesical space and exposing the ventral surface of the paracervical ligament. The dorsal aspect of the paracervix is exposed in the second step by opening the pararectal space. After the two aspects of the paracervical ligaments are revealed, the fatty tissue caught up in the paracervical vascular network must be removed, preferably by using the grasping and dissecting forceps. The last step is dissecting the lymphatic tissue between the psoas muscle and the common iliac vessels. After the completion of the

Table 52–1. Laparoscopically Assisted Schauta-Amreich and Schauta-Stockel Operations

Study*	SA/ SS	No. of Pts.	MDS (min)	Complications Patients IOC	Complications Patients POC	EBL (mL)	HS (days)	Comments
Roy et al.[11] (1996)	SA	25	270	BI: 2 VI: 1	Fever: 4 Abscess: 1 Hematoma: 1 Urine retention: 2 Transfusion: 5	400	7	10/25 cases LARVH; 15/25 VRH after laparoscopic pelvic lymphadenectomy (no separate data indicated)
Hatch et al.[15] (1996)	SA	37	225	BI: 2 II: 1	Fistula: 2 Transfusion: 4	525	3	
Schneider et al.[16] (1996)	SS	33	295	BI: 3 UI: 1 VI: 1	Transfusion: 4	NI	11	
Bolger et al.[4] (1998)	NI	17	196	BI: 1	Transfusion: 2 Hematoma: 1	NI	4.3	Incomplete parametrial resection: 2
Sardi et al.[17] (1999)	SS	56	267	UI: 1 BI: 2	Abscess: 1 Hematoma: 1 Lymphedema: 1 Hydronephrosis: 1	NI	4	Procedure not completed: 9
Renaud et al.[18] (2000)	SA	57	270	BI: 3 VI: 1	Transfusion: 2 Hematoma: 1	NI	NI	Pelvic node dissection only
Dargent[14] (2001)	SS	22	194	None	Bleeding: 1 Transfusion: 4	NI	NI	Voiding problems: 4; persistent dysuria: 1
Dargent[14] (2001)	SA	28	204	BI: 1 UI: 2 VI: 1	Transfusion: 8 Bleeding: 1 Incisional evisceration: 1 Intestinal obstruction: 1	NI	NI	Voiding problems: 14; persistent dysuria: 1
Malur et al.[12] (2001)	SS	70	292.9	VI: 2 BI: 5 UI: 1	Transfusion: 6 Minor complication: 15	NI	11.4	
Total		323	345	252.5	8.9%	20.1%	NI	6.78

*All procedures include pelvic and periaortic lymph node dissection.
BI, bladder injury; EBL, estimated blood loss; II, intestinal injury; IOC, intraoperative complications; LARVH, laparoscopically assisted radical vaginal hysterectomy; MDS, mean duration of surgery; NI, not indicated; POC, postoperative complications; SA, Schauta-Amreich; SS, Schauta-Stockel; UI, ureteral injury; VI, vascular injury or bleeding; VRH, Vaginal radical hysterectomy.

paracervical lymphadenectomy, there is no need to divide the cardinal ligament at the level of its origin. This can be done in the midpart and is easier when performed transvaginally. In the vaginal phase of the operation, the vaginal cuff is developed; vesicovaginal, rectovaginal, and paravesical spaces are developed; the ureters are identified and dissected; the uterine arteries are ligated; the bladder pillars, paracervical ligament (parametrium), and uterosacral igaments are isolated, clamped, divided, and ligated; anterior peritoneum and posterior peritoneum are approximated; and the vaginal cuff is sutured.

The laparoscopically assisted Schauta-Stockel operation carries a lesser risk for intraoperative and postoperative complications. In Dargent's series,[14] laparoscopic pelvic lymphadenectomy was followed by Schauta-Amreich or Schauta-Stockel vaginal radical hysterectomy in 95 patients with cervical cancer. The 5-year survival rate was equivalent with the Schauta-Amereich or Schauta-Stockel approach as long as the tumor was less than 2 cm (100%). When the tumor was larger than 2 cm, the Schauta-Amereich operation had a better 5-year disease-free survival rate than the Schauta-Stockel operation (87.7% versus 60.1%,

respectively). The modified laparoscopically assisted approach to vaginal radical hysterectomy may offer a solution for the increased risk of recurrence by a more extensive resection of the cardinal ligament, but there are no data to support this hypothesis, and Bolger's report[4] of 2 of 17 cases with incomplete resection at the parametrial margins in the LARVH group is of concern.

All data comparing laparoscopically assisted vaginal hysterectomy with abdominal radical hysterectomy come from retrospective studies. It seems that the length of surgery and the rate of intraoperative complications, especially in the Schauta-Amreich procedure, are higher in the laparoscopically assisted vaginal approach.[12,20] However, in most of the reports comparing laparoscopically assisted vaginal hysterectomy with abdominal radical hysterectomy, hospital stay was shorter and the blood loss, rates of transfusion, and postoperative complications were all lower in the laparoscopically assisted vaginal approach.[12,15,17]

Laparoscopic radical hysterectomy. LRH was originally described by Canis and colleagues[21] and Nezhat and associates.[22] Spirtos and coworkers[23,27] separate the operation into eight component parts that are all performed laparoscopically: right and left aortic lymphadenectomy; right and left pelvic lymphadenectomy; development of the paravesical and pararectal spaces; ureteral dissection; dissection and ligation of the uterine artery, anterior bladder pillars, and uterosacral ligaments; development of the vesicouterine and rectovaginal spaces; resection of parametria; and resection of the upper vagina. Table 52-2 provides the recent data on experience with LRH in the English literature.

Although the experience with LRH is very limited, possible advantages include better visualization of anatomy and surgical planes; avoiding the need for perineal or vaginal incisions; no limitations of bony configuration, vaginal anatomy, and lack of descent; ability to mimic the standard abdominal radical hysterectomy; decreased blood loss; and shorter hospital stays. Possible disadvantages include expensive laparoscopic equipment and difficult dissection of anterior bladder pillars. The report of Spirtos and coworkers[27] is the first to provide recurrence rates and survival data with a minimum of 3 years of follow-up for stage I cervical cancer patients undergoing LRH and aortic and pelvic lymphadenectomy. The results are promising but they were achieved in a select group of patients: young (average age, 41 years), Quetelet index less than 35, and subclinical or small-volume disease (in 80%, lesion size was less than 4 cm). The average operating time was reduced from 255 minutes in the first 26 patients to 186 minutes for the last 52 patients. Surgical margins were negative, except in three patients, whose disease was microscopically positive or described as "close." The average number of lymph nodes was 34 (10.3 aortic, 23.8 pelvic) and increased to 44 in the last 20 cases. Eight patients (10.3%) had recurrences, and the estimated 5-year disease-free interval after treatment was 89.7%.

There is no doubt that LRH and LARVH are feasible. Operative and postoperative morbidity and mortality may be equivalent or even better compared with that achieved by the open approach as long as the procedure is performed by highly trained and experienced surgeons in a select group of patients.[28,29] Nevertheless, improvements in collective and individual experience in performing the traditional abdominal radical hysterectomy and better perioperative care (especially in the current era), and trends toward decreased hospital stay demonstrate an overall improvement in the outcomes of patients undergoing the open approach.[30,31] Because experience is limited, LRH and LARVH should be performed in a variety of other groups of patients and eventually in randomized controlled trials before a definitive recommendation can be established concerning its role in the treatment of cervical cancer.

Can we combine the vaginal and laparoscopic approaches for a conservative treatment of early-stage cervical cancer? Laparoscopic vaginal radical trachelectomy (LVRT) is one of the most exciting applications of laparoscopy in gynecologic oncology. Radical trachelectomy is a conservative surgical approach for the treatment of young patients with cervical cancer wishing to preserve their childbearing potential. LVRT is the laparoscopic modification of radical vaginal trachelectomy, but most of the procedure is still performed vaginally. The laparoscopic procedure was developed by Dargent[32] in 1987 and performed by others since then.[18,33-36] The technique combines laparoscopic pelvic lymphadenectomy and common iliac node dissection with a radical vaginal trachelectomy. The vaginal approach is a modification of the Schauta-Stoeckel technique for radical vaginal hysterectomy. The main difference is the preservation of the upper portion of the endocervix and the uterine

---

Table 52–2. Laparoscopic Radical Hysterectomy

Study*	No. of Pts.	MDS (min)	Complications Patients		EBL (mL)	HS (days)	Comments
			IOC	POC			
Nezhat et al.[24] (1992)	2	390	None	None	NI	2	First two published cases
Nezhat et al.[22] (1993)	7	315	None	UTI: 1 Bleeding: 1	621	2.1	
Canis et al.[21] (1995)	13	310	UI: 1 BI: 1	None	NI	7.6	
Sedlacek et al.[25] (1995)	14	420	BI: 4	UI/VV fistula: 4	334	5.5	
Spirtos et al.[23] (1996)†	10	253	None	None	300	3.2	
Pomel et al.[26] (1997)	41	270	None	Transfusion: 1	NI	6.5	
Hsieh et al.[28] (1998)	8	298.3	None	None	476	6.5	
Kim and Moon[29] (1998)	18	363	None	None	619	NI	Pelvic lymphadenectomy only
Spirtos et al.[27] (2002)	78	205	BI: 3 UI: 1 VI: 2	UV fistula: 1 DVT: 1 Cuff abscess: 1 Abdominal hematoma: 1	250	2.9	Includes patients reported in ref. 23
Total	181	321	6.6%	5.5%	460	4.7	

*All procedures include pelvic and periaortic lymph node dissection.
†Not included in total statistics because patients' data included in reference 27.
BI, bladder injury; DVT, deep venous thrombosis; EBL, estimated blood loss; II, intestinal injury; IOC, intraoperative complications; MDS, mean duration of surgery. NI, not indicated; POC, postoperative complications; UI, ureteral injury; UV, ureterovaginal; VI, vascular injury or bleeding; VV, vesicovaginal.

corpus. The procedure includes removal of the cervix, vaginal cuff, anterior bladder pillars, paracervical ligament (parametrium), and uterosacral ligaments. The reconstruction phase includes closing the pouch of Douglas, placing a nonabsorbable cerclage suture around the uterine isthmus, and reanastomosing the vaginal cuff to the isthmus. Similar to LARVH, it has not been determined which steps of the operation are best performed vaginally and which should be done laparoscopically. Excellent descriptions of the procedure were published by Dargent and colleagues[32] and Roy and Plante.[34] Lymph node status can be assessed by frozen section or by the results for the embedded nodes. With the first option, the decision whether to perform the vaginal part of the operation is made just after the completion of the laparoscopic part of the procedure. In case of positive nodes, the patient is referred for chemotherapy and irradiation. In cases of upper margin involvement of the vaginal radical trachelectomy specimen in frozen section or in the final pathology result, the whole uterus should be removed. Table 52-3 summarizes the recent published experience with LVRT in the English literature.

In Dargent's[32] series, two patients (4.3%) had tumor recurrence, with a median follow-up of 52 months. Both recurrences were in patients with tumor diameters larger than 2 cm and lymph-vascular space involvement (LVSI). Adenocarcinoma was a third risk factor. Roy and Plante[34] described one recurrence in a patient with stage IIa disease and a tumor size of 3.0 × 2.5 cm. The rates of intraoperative and postoperative complications and 5-year disease-free survival rates in these series are not significantly different from the laparoscopically assisted Schauta-Stoeckel operation[14] and are comparable to those in abdominal or vaginal radical hysterectomy, but the blood loss is significantly lower.[11,16,17,37] There are no prospective randomized trials comparing the oncologic outcome in women undergoing radical vaginal

trachelectomy and radical hysterectomy. However, the results of Covens and associates[35] in a retrospective, case-control study are promising. The outcome of 32 patients who underwent LVRT (all with disease-negative nodes and no prior irradiation) was compared with that of 30 women who underwent radical hysterectomy (matched for age, tumor size, histology, depth of invasion, and presence of LVSI). A second, unmatched control group consisted of all women (556 patients) who underwent radical hysterectomy for tumors smaller than 2 cm, with no node involvement and no perioperative irradiation. The 2-year actuarial recurrence-free survival rates were 95%, 97%, and 100%, respectively, for the patients who underwent LRVT, matched controls, and unmatched controls. These differences were not statistically significant. Shepherd and colleagues[38] reported their experience with 30 patients undergoing radical trachelectomy for early-stage invasive cervical cancer. There were no recurrences, and the mean follow-up period was 23 months (range, 1 to 64 months). Although these preliminary findings are encouraging, there is concern that only parametria to the level of the ureter, with 1- to 2-cm lateral parametria and vaginal margins, can be obtained with this procedure. Two of the three recurrences in the 90 patients discussed by Covens and colleagues[35] occurred in the parametria, which might be a higher rate than expected after radical hysterectomy in similar patient populations.

Rodriguez and coworkers[36] and Ungar and associates[39] reported their experience with abdominal trachelectomy. The main advantages of the abdominal approach are that the operation is technically feasible and uses operative techniques familiar to most gynecologic oncologists and that wider parametrial resection is possible. Rodriguez and colleagues[36] described their experience with three patients with stage Ia1 or Ia2 cervical cancer treated with radical abdominal trachelectomy and lymphadenectomy.

Table 52–3. Laparoscopic Radical Vaginal Trachelectomy

| Study* | No. of Pts. | MDS (min) | Complications Patients | | EBL (mL) | HS (days) | Pregnancies |
			IOC	POC			
Roy and Plante[34] (1998)	30	285	VI: 3 BI: 1	NI	NI	4	6/6 patients conceived, 4/6 delivered
Sheperd et al.[33] (1998)	10	NI	NI	NI	NI	NI	3/7 patients with retained uterus delivered
Covens et al.[35] (1999)	32	180	BI: 6 VI: 1 II: 1	Fistula: 1	400	1-7	4/13 patients conceived, 3 delivered
Renaud et al.[18] (2000)†	34	260	BI: 1 VI: 2	Transfusion: 2 Hematoma: 1	NI	4	NI
Dargent et al.[32] (2000)	47	129	BI: 1	Hematoma or lymphocyst: 6 Bleeding: 1 Transfusion: 3	NI	7	13/25 deliveries among patients seeking pregnancy (6 second-trimester miscarriages)
Total	153	213	11.2%	12.4%	NI	1-7	

*All procedures include pelvic lymph node dissection.
†Pelvic and para-aortic lymph node dissection.
BI, bladder injury; EBL, estimated blood loss; II, intestinal injury; IOC, intraoperative complications; MDS, mean duration of surgery; NI, not indicated; POC, postoperative complications; UI, ureteral injury; VI, vascular injury or bleeding.

The mean duration of surgery was 265 minutes, no intraoperative complication occurred, one patient developed pelvic abscess, and one patient had an isthmovaginal stenosis and needed a dilatation of the outflow tract. Mean estimated blood loss (EBL) was 416 mL, and the mean hospital stay was 4.3 days. One patient conceived spontaneously and delivered an uncomplicated pregnancy at 39 weeks by cesarean section. Unger and associates[39] reported their experience with the first 20 patients undergoing abdominal radical trachelectomy. The operative time was 3.75 hours, average EBL was 1000 mL, and 66% of the patients received a perioperative blood transfusion. One patient had ureteral injury. Considering the higher blood loss, the same rate of intraoperative complications, and equivalent duration of surgery, it seems that the combined laparovaginal approach is superior to the abdominal procedure, although any measured differences between the two surgical approaches could be surgeon dependent. The number of patients enrolling in these studies was too small and the follow-up too short for final conclusions.

Dargent and colleagues[32] and Roy and Plante[34] recommended that LVRT should be offered to young patients who wish to keep their fertility, those with stage Ia2 cervical cancer, and a selected group of patients with stage Ia1 and Ib—those with lesion sizes less than 2 cm, those with limited endocervical involvement at colposcopic evaluation, and those with no evidence of pelvic or para-aortic metastasis. Another relative contraindication is vascular space invasion. It is important that all patients going through LVRT have thorough preoperative workups in to exclude high-risk patients who cannot benefit from the procedure. Dargent and colleagues[32] suggested that the workup should include conization and computed tomography (CT) or magnetic resonance imaging (MRI) of the pelvis and abdomen.

The other primary outcome measure for radical trachelectomy is preserving fertility. Most investigators report excellent results (see Table 52-3). Shepherd and coworkers[38] reported that 8 of 13 patients conceived after LVRT, with a total of 14 pregnancies and nine live births. Dargent and colleagues[32] reported that 13 of 25 patients seeking pregnancy conceived after LVRT. The total number of pregnancies was 25 (including 5 pregnancies at the time of LVRT); 13 delivered, 6 had late second-trimester miscarriages, and 6 had earlier abortions. The elevated rate of second-trimester loss is probably a result of exposure of the membranes to vaginal flora and subclinical chorioamnionitis.

Criticisms of the procedure include inadequate parametrial resection, with increased risk for side wall recurrence and difficulty in performance of the procedure in nulliparous women. It seems, however, that as long as the procedure is performed on patients with clinical stage Ia or Ib1 and the lesion is 2 cm or less, the risk for recurrence is minimal. Women with lesions larger than 2 cm or with LVSI have a higher rate of recurrence, although not necessarily higher than if they had undergone radical hysterectomy. Because experience is limited, it is hard to predict what percentage of the patients would not be able to go through the procedure because of anatomical limitations (e.g., narrow vagina, lack of uterine descensus). With regard to reproductive potential, the results are encouraging, and the vaginal approach is probably superior to the open abdominal one mainly because of fewer abdominal adhesions. There is still concern about the high rate of second-trimester abortions, and different methods are tried to improve the efficacy of the cerclage placed at the time of the initial procedure.

LVRT is one of the best examples of using the combined endoscopic-vaginal approach to treat gynecologic oncology patients who want to minimize the surgical procedure and preserve their fertility. Although the risk of recurrence is not likely to be significantly elevated, this procedure should be offered only to the informed and highly motivated patient willing to accept such undefined risks. To perform LVRT successfully, the surgeon must be trained in radical laparoscopic procedures and radical vaginal surgery, and the pathologist must provide indisputable data.

Laparoscopic pelvic lymph node dissection.
Laparoscopic pelvic lymph node dissection was initially described by Querleu and coworkers[40] at the Second World Congress of Gynecologic Endoscopy in Clermount, France. The ability to perform this procedure is directly responsible for the development of the different types of LRH performed abdominally or in the combined vaginal-abdominal approach for management of women with early-stage cervical cancer. No progress could be made in laparoscopic applications in patients with gynecologic malignancies before laparoscopic dissection of pelvic nodes was feasible. The extraperitoneal approach was the first to be used, and it later was replaced by the transumbilical, transperitoneal approach.[40,41] The transumbilical, transperitoneal laparoscopic approach can be carried out the same way as conventional pelvic lymphadenectomy and therefore is quite widely used by gynecologic oncologists. Querleu and colleagues[40] described the technique in 1991. For the 39 procedures performed on patients with stage Ib through IIb cervical cancer, the mean duration of surgery was 80 minutes. No conversion to laparotomy was needed. Positive nodes were found in 5 patients who were subsequently treated with radiation therapy, and the other 34 patients underwent a radical abdominal or radical vaginal hysterectomy.

There is some debate about the use of laparoscopy for pelvic lymph node dissection, mainly concerning the adequacy and safety of the procedure. Querleu and colleagues[40] reported having recovered an average of only 8.7 nodes. Other studies reported quite variable numbers of retrieved lymph nodes,[8-35] with an average number of 25 nodes, which is comparable to the number of nodes that can be recovered at laparotomy.[5,42-46] Even in elderly[47,48] and obese[49,50] women, adequate numbers of pelvic nodes were obtained. Fowler and associates[42] reported their experience with 12 patients who underwent laparoscopic lymphadenectomy and then immediate laparotomy for radical hysterectomy. Overall, 377 nodes were removed, and 75% of them were obtained on laparoscopy. The retrieval rate improved significantly with experience. No patient with disease-negative nodes on laparoscopy had disease-positive nodes at laparotomy.

In a Gynecologic Oncology Group (GOG) study,[46] 67 patients with cervical cancer (stage Ia through IIa) who were planned for radical abdominal hysterectomy and lymph node dissection underwent laparoscopic removal of pelvic and para-aortic nodes before laparotomy for radical hysterectomy. The two objectives were to gain information on adverse effects and difficulties associated with node removal and to determine the adequacy of the lymph node removal. Seventeen patients did not complete laparoscopic surgery because of metastatic disease or complications, and 10 women could not be evaluated. The median operating time was 170 minutes, and the mean number of resected pelvic nodes was 31.1. There were seven major vascular injuries (10.4%); three required laparotomy for control. There was no way to evaluate the benefits or detriments of laparoscopic lymph node removal in regard to hospital stay, blood loss, or general postoperative complications because laparotomy was subsequently performed in all cases. In 6 (15%) of the 40 evaluable patients, laparoscopic pelvic lymph node dissection was judged incomplete on laparotomy. In all six cases, the residual nodes did not contain metastasis and were all located lateral to the common iliac vessels. The researchers concluded that pelvic lymphadenectomy, although having a reasonable complication rate, demonstrated problems regarding adequacy, which are probably correctable.

In summary, laparoscopic pelvic lymphadenectomy is feasible and is responsible for the major changes in the use of endoscopic techniques in the field of gynecologic oncology. The mean number of nodes retrieved laparoscopically is approximately the same as obtained by laparotomy. Even if the node dissection is not complete, as judged by followed laparotomy, the significant nodes are removed, and there have been no reports of positive pelvic nodes identified at laparotomy in patients with negative nodes at laparoscopy. There has never been a study to measure the adequacy of lymph node dissection by surgeons at laparotomy. There is no question that a complete therapeutic lymph node dissection can be performed laparoscopically and that the extent of that dissection depends on the efforts and skills of the surgeon. Because most cases of lymphadenectomy are combined with additional procedures, it is difficult to assess the specific role of laparoscopic pelvic lymphadenectomy in duration of surgery, intraoperative and postoperative complications, and duration of hospital stay. However, data coming from patients with cervical cancer submitted to laparoscopic lymphadenectomy for staging only[45] show shorter hospital stay, longer mean duration of surgery, and the same rate of intraoperative and postoperative complications compared with the open approach.

Should laparoscopic surgery be used for staging of advanced disease? Patients with advanced-stage disease or even large, bulky early-stage disease (clinical stage Ib2 or higher) are usually treated with a combination of chemotherapy and irradiation without being surgically evaluated. Unfortunately, 30% to 50% of these tumors are inaccurately staged by the clinical methods.[51] Surgical staging has been advocated to define accurately the extent of the disease and guide the extent of subsequent radiation therapy and to allow debulking of grossly involved and otherwise incurable lymph nodes.

Para-aortic lymph node metastases have been diagnosed with open staging in about 6% of stage Ib, 12% of stage II, 30% of stage III, and 25% of patients with positive pelvic nodes.[52-56] The presence of metastases in the common iliac and para-aortic nodes is essential pretherapeutic and prognostic information that can influence clinical decisions.[57-61] Imaging techniques are unfortunately inaccurate in identifying lymphatic spread,[19] and considering the complication rate and costs of laparotomy for aortic lymphadenectomy,[62] a laparoscopic approach has been introduced.

Laparoscopic aortic lymphadenectomy: What is the best approach? The aortic or lumbar lymphatic nodal chain is divided for practical purposes into right and left aortic lymph nodes. The right aortic lymph nodes extend from the front of the inferior vena cava to the right ureter and include the node in the interaortocaval space. The left aortic lymph nodes extend from the front of the aorta and upper part of the left common iliac, lateral to the left ureter. The superior extent of the dissection is the third part of the duodenum or to the renal vein, depending on the primary disease site.[63] The two main approaches to aortic lymphadenectomy are the transumbilical, transperitoneal approach and the extraperitoneal approach.

Laparoscopic transumbilical, transperitoneal aortic lymphadenectomy. The transumbilical, transperitoneal approach was first described by Childers and colleagues,[43] Nezhat and associaates,[24] and Querleu.[64] Table 52-4 summarizes the published experience with transperitoneal para-aortic lymph node dissection for surgical staging in patients with cervical cancer. In some of the studies, pelvic and para-aortic lymph node dissections were performed, and information concerning operating time and complications were not given separately for the two procedures. There are more data in the literature concerning transumbilical, transperitoneal para-aortic lymph node dissection in other malignancies or in combination with other procedures.[5,10,11,15,22,24,42,45,56,64-73]

Extraperitoneal laparoscopic aortic and common iliac dissection. It is accepted that the risk of radiation-induced bowel injury is less after extraperitoneal aortic dissection at laparotomy than with the same procedure performed by transperitoneal laparotomy.[52,54,77] It has also been demonstrated that laparoscopic lymph node dissection is associated with less

Table 52–4. Laparoscopic Transperitoneal Para-aortic Lymphadenectomy for Staging of Cervical Cancer

Study	No. of Pts.	MDS (min)	Complications Patients		EBL (mL)	HS (days)	Nodes Removed (avg. number)
			IOC	POC			
Childers et al.[43] (1992)	16	75-175	None	None	<100	1	NI
Su et al.[74] (1995)	38	77	UI: 1 VI: 1	None	116	NI	15
Kadar[75] (1993)	11	101.5	None	None	NI	1	6
Querleu[64] (1993)	2	95	None	NI	NI	2	6.5
Recio et al.[73] (1996)*	12	176	None	None	60	1	7.0
Chu et al.[5] (1997)	28	95	VI: 1	None	NI	2	8.6
Possover et al.[45] (1998)	26	45	VI: 7	Fever: 1 UTI: 1	<100	3.2	6.8
Dottino et al.[76] (1999)†	64	119.2	VI: 1	None	66	3.6	3.7
Total	197	104.2	5.6%	1.0%	<88	1.97	7.7

*Pelvic and para-aortic node dissection.
†Pelvic and para-aortic node dissection data concern 94 patients: 64 with cervical cancer and 30 with other gynecologic malignancies.
BI, bladder injury; EBL, estimated blood loss; II, intestinal injury; IOC, intraoperative complications; MDS, mean duration of surgery; NI, not indicated; POC, postoperative complications; UI, ureteral injury; UTI, urinary tract infection; VI, vascular injury or bleeding.

adhesions, even compared with extraperitoneal laparotomy in animal models.[78,79] The combination of laparoscopy and extraperitoneal para-aortic lymphadenectomy was shown in a porcine model to generate significantly fewer adhesions than the transperitoneal technique, with equal efficacy.[80] The extraperitoneal approach may offer more advantages compared with the transperitoneal procedure in addition to fewer adhesions formation, including rapid access to the nodes dissection area, because adhesion lysis and bowel mobilization are unnecessary; decreased risk to bowel injury by trocars; decreased risk for electrosurgical or for traction or dissection bowel injury; and decreased risk for hernia formation, especially in lateral ports. Vasilev and McGonigle[81] were the first to publish their experience with laparoscopic extraperitoneal para-aortic lymphadenectomy, followed by Dargant and coworkers[82] and Querleu and associates.[83] The dissection can be performed through a bilateral iliac incision or through a unilateral left side incision. Table 52-5 summarizes the data on laparoscopic extraperitoneal para-aortic lymph node dissection.

No randomized studies have been performed to compare the different approaches of para-aortic lymph node dissection, and it is therefore difficult to compare the results of the different studies. The mean number of nodes retrieved by the three techniques (transperitoneal, bilateral, and left extraperitoneal) is similar[82] and is comparable or even higher than in laparotomy.[85,86] Although in some centers a more radical aortic lymphadenectomy has been advocated and higher node count achieved, there is no evidence that increased radicalism translates into higher cure rates.[87] Dargent and colleauges[82] report a lower mean right aortic node count in the left extraperitoneal approach and recommend a bilateral approach when facing difficulties in the left side approach. The mean duration

Table 52–5. Laparoscopic Extraperitoneal Periaortic Lymphadenectomy in Advanced Cervical Cancer

Study	No. of Pts.	MDS (min)	Complications Patients		EBL (mL)	HS (days)	Nodes Removed (avg. number)
			IOC	POC			
Vasilev and McGonigle[81] (1996)	5	130	None	None	<50	NI	5
Dargent et al.[82] (2000)	35	153 bilat.	None	Phlebitis: 1	NI	2.5	16 7.7 right side
		119 left	None	Lymphocele: 1			15 2.4 right side
Querleu et al.[83] (2000)	42	126	UI-1	Hematoma: 1 Incisional hernia: 1 Lymphocyst: 1	NI	2.5	20
Vergote et al.[84] (2002)	21 extraperitoneal* 21 intraperitoneal	70 55	None	Hematoma: 1	78	2	6†
Total	103‡	115.5	1.0%	5.8%	<64	2.3	11.6

*For 5 of 21 patients in the retroperitoneal approach group, the procedures were converted to transperitoneal procedures after peritoneal tears.
†The procedure was stopped when positive nodes were identified on frozen section; only lower para-aortic nodes were resected.
‡Extraperitoneal lymph node dissection.
BI, bladder injury; EBL, estimated blood loss; II, intestinal injury; IOC, intraoperative complications; MDS, mean duration of surgery; NI, not indicated; POC, postoperative complications; UI, ureteral injury; VI, vascular injury or bleeding.

of surgery, complication rate, and hospital stay were comparable in the three different approaches. The upper level of the dissection was not similar in the different studies and probably varies within many reports secondary to the type of disease and experience of the surgeon.[83] There is no doubt that extending the upper limit of dissection requires increased time to accomplish the necessary exposure and perform the dissection. Vergote and associates[84] reduced the operating time from between 120 and 150 minutes to 70 minutes by omitting the supramesenteric portion of the procedure. The incidence of metastatic para-aortic lymph node involvement was similar in the different studies: 18% to 22%.[83-85]

The only study that has evaluated the adequacy of laparoscopic para-aortic lymph node dissection was performed by the GOG[46]; the mean number of para-aortic nodes removed was six on both the right and left. All cases of bilateral laparoscopic aortic lymph node sampling were judged adequate by all methods of evaluation (i.e., blinded review of video prints or video tape and surgeon opinion at laparotomy), and the investigators concluded that the procedure was reasonably safe and feasible.

The role of surgical staging in the patient with advanced-stage cervical cancer is still being debated. The laparoscopic technique for staging is certainly feasible and somewhat attractive in that most patients would be avoiding a laparotomy before initiating definitive chemotherapy and irradiation. The complication rate and accuracy of the laparoscopic diagnostic procedures should be compared with the additional risk of extended field radiation treatment. The risk of prophylactic para-aortic irradiation (grade 4 or 5 toxicities, mainly gastrointestinal and urinary complications) in randomized controlled trials is 4%.[88,89] Considering the high accuracy and minimal complications rate in the laparoscopic transperitoneal and extraperitoneal para-aortic lymph node dissections (see Tables 52-4 and 52-5), it seems reasonable to use the laparoscopic approach for staging of advanced cervical disease before radiation treatment. The extraperitoneal laparoscopic approach has few advantages, mainly less adhesion formation and a lower risk of bowel injury, but pelvic lymph node dissection is more difficult by this approach. Further studies with larger patient series and longer follow-up are required to assess the safest endoscopic approach and to evaluate the tolerance of the combination of endoscopic staging procedure and extended field radiation. Muti-institutional studies will likely be forthcoming and compare staging of advanced cervical cancer by laparotomy or laparoscopy to imaging methods, including positron emission tomography (PET).

The role of laparoscopy in debulking involved lymph nodes is controversial. Debulking large para-aortic and pelvic nodes not responding to radiotherapy may increase the survival of cervical cancer patients.[90,91] Laparoscopic dissection of nodes obviously involved by metastatic disease is technically feasible, even if vascular adhesions exist, but it is more difficult compared with laparotomy.[45] Dargent and others, [82] however, consider bulky nodes demonstrated by imaging a contraindication to laparoscopic lymphadenectomy because of the hazard of dissemination and the risk of complication. If the prelaparoscopic imaging does not suggest suspicious lymph nodes and an obviously metastatic node is encountered during laparoscopy, three options are suggested: document the metastatic involvement by fine-needle aspiration and refer the patient for radiation treatment; move to laparotomy and debulking of the involved node; or dissect the nodes laparoscopically with an effort not to fragment the nodes and remove them through an endoscopic pouch or colpotomy.

What is the role of laparoscopic surgery in the treatment of endometrial cancer?

Most patients with endometrial cancer present with disease confined to the corpus (stage I). The mainstay of treatment in most patients is based on primary surgery. When surgical staging is performed, at least 20% of clinical stage I tumors are found to have spread beyond the uterus.[92] In 1988, FIGO recommended that staging of endometrial cancer be changed from the clinical to the surgical system. The standard technique is exploratory laparotomy, peritoneal washing for cytology, extrafacial hysterectomy, bilateral salpingo-oophorectomy, and bilateral pelvic and para-aortic lymph node dissection. Although metastatic involvement of pelvic and para-aortic lymph nodes is the most important surgicopathologic staging information, the indications (e.g., invasion, grading, LVSI, histology) and extent (i.e., sampling versus complete) of lymph node dissection have not been established by prospective, randomized clinical trials. Nevertheless, the importance of surgically evaluating the pelvic and para-aortic nodes has been established.

The overall management approach to patients with early-stage endometrial cancer is the least uniform compared with the other types of gynecologic malignancies. Much controversy exists about the treatment of patients with clinically apparent early-stage disease, including who should perform the surgery, the variability of surgical staging performed, use of adjuvant irradiation, and the incorporation of advanced laparoscopic surgery.[93] The two main applications of laparoscopy in the treatment of endometrial cancer patients are laparoscopic staging and laparoscopically assisted vaginal hysterectomy or total laparoscopic hysterectomy for early endometrial cancer and laparoscopic staging of incompletely staged tumors. The primary limitations of the laparoscopic approach applied to patients with endometrial cancer are advanced age; morbid obesity; associated diseases such as diabetes, hypertension, and cardiac disease; tumor extent, such as suspected involvement of the cervix or serosa; risk of tumor seeding due to direct manipulation; and the possibility of associated conditions such as fibroids or adhesions that affect surgical exposure or removal of an intact uterus vaginally.

Laparoscopy in the treatment of early endometrial cancer. Assuming endometrial cancer is confined to the uterus, the curative potential of the vaginal hysterectomy or LAVH and bilateral salpingo-oophorectomy BSO should equal that of the total abdominal hysterectomy. The advent of advanced laparoscopic techniques has made it feasible to perform complete surgical staging of endometrial cancer, including inspection of the peritoneal cavity, obtaining peritoneal washings, ensuring that the adnexa are removed, and pelvic and para-aortic lymph node dissection in selected patients. Childers and Surwit[94] were the first to report laparoscopic treatment of women with early-stage endometrial cancer. Since their report, more studies have been published[67-69,95-99] regarding the feasibility of the combined laparoscopic-vaginal and laparoscopic approaches for management of endometrial cancer (Table 52-6).

Few of the studies compared the laparoscopically assisted vaginal hysterectomy and the abdominal approaches.[48,96,98,100-102] Most of these reports were retrospective reviews of selected groups of patients, usually thin, parous, and with uterine descensus who were treated by several surgeons who were inconsistent in their staging approach (e.g., LAVH only, pelvic and para-aortic sampling versus dissection). The collective retrospective experience demonstrates that laparoscopic management is feasible in selected patients, but no meaningful conclusions can be made regarding outcome measurements when compared with traditional management considering the problems with patient selection and variability in extent of surgical staging.

Only three prospective studies[100-102] have compared the two approaches, and only two of them were randomized trials.[100,102] Table 52-7 shows the patient characteristics and perioperative data.

The data from mainly retrospective studies and three prospective studies show the number of lymph nodes removed by laparoscopy is comparable to that obtained at laparotomy; less blood loss and need for blood transfusion in the laparoscopic approach; similar major and minor complication rates; longer operating time (on average, 1 additional hour with laparoscopy); shorter hospitalization in the laparoscopic group; and possibly superior quality of life in the laparoscopic group.[67,101]

Cost of the procedure is an important variable, but it is quite difficult to track and account for in individual institutions. Eltabbakah and coworkers[101] found that overall cost of laparoscopy was significantly higher than laparotomy, as opposed to decreased cost in other reports.[67,95] Laparoscopic staging combined with vaginal hysterectomy appears to be a feasible alternative surgical approach in women with early-stage endometrial carcinoma. The ability to perform complete surgical staging with this technique is limited by patient factors (i.e., weight, adhesions, and medical comorbidities) and physician factors (i.e., training and experience). The true benefit based on traditional outcome factors has yet to be defined in a well-designed trial. The GOG is conducting a multi-institutional, phase III, prospective, randomized trial (LAP-2) of laparoscopy versus traditional laparotomy for the treatment of endometrial cancer. The number of patients recruited until August 2002 was 1305. Variables that will be assessed include completeness of surgical staging, complications, operative time, hospital stay, costs, quality of life, survival, and recurrence. Results from this important study will definitely shed light on the portion of patients with early-stage endometrial cancer who may benefit from laparoscopic management.

Should the laparoscopic approach be used for staging of incompletely staged disease? Gynecologic oncologists are frequently asked to recommend treatment plans for patients with endometrial cancer referred with an incomplete staging workup. The options are to perform exploratory laparotomy for staging or to consider irradiation based on empiric assessment of known risk factors for recurrence. A therapeutic decision that is not based on surgical staging may lead to undertreatment or overtreatment. An additional option is to perform laparoscopic surgical staging.

Table 52–6. Laparoscopic Staging and Treatment of Endometrial Cancer

Study	No. of Pts.	PLND (%)	Pelvic Nodes Removed (avg. number)	Conversion to Laparotomy (%)	Major Complications, IOC + POC (%)
Fram[100] (2002)	29	55.2	21.3	6.9	10.3
Eltabbakah et al.[101] (2001)	86	83.7	10.8	5.8	10.5
Malur et al.[102] (2001)	37	68	16.1	0	29.7*
Scribner et al.[48] (2001)	67	100	17.8	22	26.9
Margina et al.[99] (1999)	56	98	19.4†	12.5	23.2
Gemignani et al.[95] (1999)	69	16	7	4.3	5.8
Holub et al.[96] (1998)	11	100	NI	0	0
Spirtos et al.[67] (1996)	13	100	20	0	NI
Boike et al.[98] (1994)	23	95	14.5	13	25
Childers et al.[68] (1993)	59	49.2	NI	13.6	5.1
Total	450	76.5	15.9	9.6	15.3

*Two patients died: one of pulmonary embolism and one of vascular injury.
†Pelvic and periaortic nodes were counted together.
IOC, intraoperative complications; NI, not indicated; PLND, pelvic lymph nods dissection; POC, postoperative complications.

Table 52–7. Prospective Trials Comparing Laparoscopy and Laparotomy for the Treatment of Endometrial Cancer: Perioperative Data

Study	Surgery	No. of Pts.	Age (yr, mean)	BMI	PLN (no., mean)	PALN (no., mean)	Blood Loss (mL, mean)	MDS (min.) (mean)	Complications (%) Major	Complications (%) Minor	HS (days)
Fram[100] (2002)	LSS	29	61.2	25.7	21.3	NI	145.5	136.2*	0	10.3	2.3
	LPS	32	60.6	26.2	21.9	NI	501.6*	101.9	3.1	12.5	5.5*
Eltabbakah et al.[101] (2001)	LSS	86	61.2	28.9	10.8	2.7	278.3	190.5	11.6	NI	2.5
	LPS	57	60.5	31.9	4.9*	4.2	307.0	132.8	8.8	NI	5.2*
Malur et al.[102] (2001)	LSS	37	68.3	29.7	16.1	9.6	229.2*	176.4	2.7	27.0	8.6
	LPS	34	67.7	29.7	15.4	8.4	594.2	166.1	2.9	36.4	11.7
Total	LSS	152	63.6	28.1	16.1	6.2	217.7	167.7	7.2	19.7	4.5
	LPS	123	62.9	29.3	14.1	6.3	467.6	133.6	5.7	24.2	7.5

*P < .05.

BMI, body mass index; HS, hospital stay; LPS, laparotomy surgery; LSS, laparoscopic surgery; MDS, mean duration of surgery; NI, not indicated; P, nulliparas; PLN, pelvic lymph nodes; PALN, periaortic lymph nodes.

Childers and associates[103] reported their experience using laparoscopic staging in 13 patients who had been referred with incompletely staged endometrial cancer. Extrauterine disease was found in three (23%) of the patients, and the average number of nodes removed was 17.5. There were no intraoperative complications, the mean blood loss was 50 mL, and the mean hospital stay was 1.5 days. Four of these patients received additional therapy based on the surgicopathologic findings from the restaging procedure. The GOG is also evaluating the feasibility of laparoscopic staging in incompletely staged endometrial cancer.

What is the role of laparoscopic surgery in the diagnosis and treatment of ovarian cancer?

The role of laparoscopic surgery in cases of ovarian cancer is limited to evaluation of the adnexal mass, recognition and staging of early-stage disease, a second-look operation, and evaluation for feasibility of cytoreductive surgery in advanced disease.

Evaluation of adnexal mass. Assessment of the pelvic mass includes pelvic examination, pelvic ultrasound, and in most cases, tumor markers (always assessed in postmenopausal women). Modalities of secondary importance include the CT, MRI, and color flow Doppler ultrasound. Different scoring systems using these tests yield a sensitivity and specificity of 60% to 100% in detecting malignancy.[104-118] Considering that there is no way to identify malignancy preoperatively with 100% sensitivity and specificity, surgical evaluation of the mass is often necessary. The laparoscopic management of adnexal masses is evolving because of increased surgical expertise and technical progress. The advantages of the method include the potential for decreased postoperative pain and recovery time, less adhesion formation, decreased length of stay, and diminished costs. The indications for surgical evaluation of the mass by laparoscopy or laparotomy should be the same. The surgeon should be prepared for the possibility of malignancy and have a surgical plan in case that is the finding.

A few controversies may arise concerning the use of laparoscopy in the management of adnexal mass:

1. Adequacy and reliability of intraoperative diagnosis of ovarian cancer
2. Safety and feasibility of the method
3. Risk of rupture and tumor spillage of a malignant ovarian cyst
4. Proper management of malignancy diagnosed during or after laparoscopic procedure and the effect of delay in the staging procedure

Unfortunately, there are no prospective, randomized trials comparing laparoscopy and laparotomy to answer these questions. Most data are based on a small number of case series, case reports, and retrospective studies.

What is the adequacy and reliability of an intraoperative diagnosis of ovarian cancer? The range of adnexal masses managed by laparoscopy proven to be malignant is between 14% and less than 1% (average of less than 3%).[119-130] Two of the largest series illustrate some of the management problems at the time of the surgical procedure. Canis and colleagues[126] managed 757 patients with 819 masses by laparoscopy. During laparoscopy, peritoneal cytology was performed, and the ovarian masses, pelvis, and abdomen were inspected. In postmenopausal women, both ovaries were removed and extracted with an endobag, and the cyst fluid and the internal cyst wall were inspected. In premenopausal women, puncture placement was decided according to the clinical, ultrasonographic, and laparoscopic data. A puncture with endocystic examination was performed in masses considered to have low malignant potential (LMP), and adnexectomy without a puncture was performed in masses considered to be highly suspicious at ultrasound. Six percent of the masses were identified as likely to be malignant, and 41% of these suspicious masses were found to be malignant or of LMP.

No malignant masses were missed, but 7 of the 15 malignant tumors were punctured during the laparoscopy. In a follow-up study,[129] 230 suspicious masses at ultrasound were evaluated by laparoscopy. At surgery, 62 of the 230 masses, including all of the cancer and LMP cases (25 cases [40.3%]) were diagnosed macroscopically as suspicious or malignant. Three of the 15 invasive cancers and 5 of the 10 LMP cases were punctured before their diagnoses were confirmed. Twelve of 15 invasive cancers were treated by immediate vertical midline laparotomy; the other three invasive cancers were negative for malignancy on frozen section and were staged and treated after permanent section diagnosis.

Dottino and colleagues[127] reported 160 patients referred to their gynecologic oncology clinics who underwent laparoscopy to evaluate an adnexal mass. Patients were excluded if the adnexal mass extended above the umbilicus, if laparotomy was indicated for nonadnexal pathology, or if there was evidence of gross metastatic disease (e.g. omental cake). There were nine ovarian cancers (6%), eight LMPs (5%), and four nongynecologic cancers. Laparoscopic management was successful in 141 patients (88%). Of the nine patients with ovarian cancer, five underwent immediate staging laparotomies, three underwent staging laparoscopy, and one patient originally diagnosed as having a LMP tumor had a second-staging laparoscopy after treatment with chemotherapy. Five (3%) frozen section reports were inconsistent with the corresponding final pathology reports. In all these cases, there was no significant delay in the treatment attributable to the initial frozen section report.

The conclusion of most investigators is that suspicious adnexal masses can be managed laparoscopically. The masses should be carefully assessed externally and internally. The pelvis and abdomen (including paracolic gutters, surface of the bowel, diaphragmatic domes, and omentum) should be inspected. To minimize the risk of intraperitoneal tumor dissemination or upstaging, it is recommended that the mass be removed intact. To prevent a delay in diagnosis, frozen sections of any lesion or suspicious masses are essential so that definitive surgical management can be performed. Considering the limitations of frozen section,[131,132] whenever the tumor is macroscopically suspicious, the entire adnexa should be removed and sent to pathologist. Morcellation of a solid or suspicious tumor should be avoided.

Is laparoscopy safe and feasible? A few studies compared laparoscopy and laparotomy in the management of benign adnexal masses.[130,133] Their conclusions are that the laparoscopic technique is associated with less blood loss, decreased pain and postoperative analgesic demands, shorter hospital stay, and no increase in the complication rate. There are few reports on laparoscopic handling of malignant masses. Childers and associates[128] had 19 patients (14%) with subsequent malignancies in their series of 138 patients with suspicious adnexal masses based on ultrasound or CA 125 levels, or both. Three major complications were reported: rectosigmoid enterotomy, vena cava injury (both repaired laparoscopically without sequelae), and port-site bowel hernia requiring laparotomy and bowel resection. In the series of Dottino and colleagues[127] of 160 patients, only four of the nine cancers were staged laparoscopically. All eight borderline tumors were initially managed laparoscopically, but two patients required conversion to laparotomy because of trocar vascular injuries. There were five operative complications in total: three vascular injuries, one small bowel injury, and one case of persistent bleeding from pelvic adhesions. In neither of these reports were complications divided between benign and malignant cases.

The size of the adnexal mass may be a limiting factor in the use of laparoscopic surgery, especially in solid masses. Dottino and coworkers[127] limited themselves to masses under the umbilicus and drained cysts larger than 10 cm with cyst aspiration apparatus for decompression and prevention of leakage. The resected masses should be placed in bags and removed through laparoscopic port or colpotomy to avoid intraperitoneal spillage of the surgical specimen and contamination of the abdominal wall.

One of the possible risks of the laparoscopic approach is acceleration of malignant spread. There are a few reports in the literature concerning abdominal wall metastasis attributed to laparoscopy.[129,134-136] Most of the cases occurred in patients with advanced disease and ascites, and there are no data to suggest any effect on prognosis in these cases. It is unclear if dissemination reported at restaging laparotomies after laparoscopy was caused by inappropriate staging at the initial laparoscopy or related to the method the mass was removed (i.e., morcellation or not using endobags). There are a few concerning clinical reports of intraperitoneal dissemination after adequate laparoscopic procedures.[129,137,138] It is unclear whether this clinically described phenomenon is related to the surgical technique or more to the biology of the tumor. A few animal models[139-141] suggest that a carbon dioxide pneumoperitoneum may have a growth-stimulating effect on tumor cells and an increased seeding rate. The carbon dioxide may cause diffuse damage to the peritoneum and facilitate the attachment of tumor cells to the basal lamina. Canis and associates,[142] after thoroughly reviewing the animal data, proposed that tumor growth after laparotomy was greater than after endoscopy and that tumor dissemination was worse after carbon dioxide laparoscopy compared with laparotomy.

The conclusion of many investigators[14,119,127,128,143] is that laparoscopic management of early malignancies and LMP cases is possible but should be performed only in controlled clinical trials. The procedure should include washings, random peritoneal biopsies, omentectomy, pelvic and periaortic lymph node dissection, and appendectomy in cases of mucinous histology. Because the risk of dissemination appears high when a large number of malignant cell are present, the following conditions on preoperative evaluation should be considered a contraindication to carbon dioxide laparoscopic procedure: adnexal masses with external vegetation, bulky lymph nodes, and evidence of gross metastatic disease. If an unexpected malignant lesion is found at laparoscopy for a suspicious ovarian mass and documented by frozen section, an immediate staging laparotomy becomes essential unless the patient was recruited initially to a clinical trial and signed an informed consent.[136,144-150]

What are the risks of rupture and tumor spillage of a malignant ovarian cyst?

The main concern about treating suspicious adnexal masses laparoscopically, especially in cancer confined to the ovary, is that rupture may cause dissemination of malignant cells into the peritoneal cavity and adversely affect survival. Laparoscopy is more likely than laparotomy to result in capsular rupture because laparoscopic adnexectomy probably includes more tumor manipulation and masses often must be drained before removal. There are conflicting reports concerning the effect of rupture of a malignant cyst on survival.[151-153] Dembo and colleagues[151] reviewed more than 519 stage I epithelial ovarian cancer cases. Dense adhesions, tumor grade, and large-volume ascites were predictors of relapse; intraoperative cyst rupture did not affect prognosis, but most of these cases did not have comprehensive staging. Multivariate analysis of 394 patients with early-stage ovarian carcinoma by Sjoval and associates[153] showed that there was no difference in survival between patients whose tumors had intact capsules and patients in whom rupture occurred during surgery (i.e., laparotomy). However, a significant reduction in survival was found between patients in whom rupture occurred before surgery compared with a group with intraoperative rupture. Sevelda and coworkers[152] found a 5-year survival rate of 76% for 30 patients with stage I ovarian cancer with capsular rupture and 76% for 30 similar patients who did not have capsular rupture. Webb and colleagues[154] demonstrated a statistically significant difference in survival between patients with stage I carcinoma with capsular rupture and those without capsular rupture (5-year survival of 56% versus 78%). This retrospective univariate analysis did not stratify for tumor adherence or high-grade lesions, both of which were more common in the patients with ruptured cysts. Vergote and coworkers[150] reported from a large retrospective study that rupture before and during surgery had an independent unfavorable impact on disease-free survival (hazard ratios of 2.65 and 1.64, respectively). Because of the retrospective nature of this study, the investigators were not able to distinguish between intraoperative spontaneous rupture and rupture due to surgical needle aspiration. All these studies are related to rupture of cysts before and during laparotomy. There are few data concerning the risk of rupture during laparoscopy. Dottino and associates[127] described one case of intraperitoneal spillage during a laparoscopic removal of "apparent" stage I granulose cell tumor. The patient was observed and had a pelvic recurrence 2 years postoperatively. Childers and colleagues[128] reported one tumor recurrence in nine patients with stage I ovarian carcinoma treated by laparoscopy. The patient had poorly differentiated tumor, and the capsule was ruptured intraoperatively. No frozen section was performed, and therefore staging was delayed.

Canis and associates[129] reported two cases of dissemination possibly related to the laparoscopic approach. One cyst diagnosed on frozen section as benign teratoma was treated by unilateral adnexectomy and morcellation. On permanent section, the diagnosis was changed to immature teratoma. Three weeks later, a stage IV peritoneal gliosis with mature and immature implants was found. One more suspicious ovarian mass with no visible peritoneal implants was diagnosed as uncertain on frozen section with negative peritoneal cytologic results. The adnexa was removed with minimal tumor manipulation and in an endo-bag, and on permanent section, invasive serous cystadenocarcinoma was diagnosed. Three weeks later, diffuse peritoneal metastases less than 1 mm in diameter were found on laparotomy. Mayer and colleagues[155] reported peritoneal implantation of squamous cell carcinoma after rupture of a dermoid cyst during laparoscopic removal.

It is unknown whether the high-pressure pneumoperitoneum, the carbon dioxide gas, or any other factor may influence the outcome if rupture occurs during the laparoscopic procedure. In any case, intraoperative rupture of malignant cyst will upstage tumor from stage Ia to Ic and therefore necessitate the use of adjuvant chemotherapy that otherwise may not have been required. Kadar[143] calculated that for every patient who requires postoperative chemotherapy as a direct consequence of having been treated laparoscopically, 110 to 140 would have been spared a laparotomy.

To minimize the risk of capsular rupture during laparoscopy, Childers and coworkers[128] recommended performing laparotomy in the following cases: masses larger than 10 cm, masses less than 10 cm but adherent to the pelvic sidewall, and masses in which ovarian preservation is desired and cystectomy needs to be performed. It is suggested that all masses should be removed from the abdomen with a commercially available laparoscopic bag or by colpotomy using a transvaginal tube.[156] To reduce the risk of cyst fluid spillage when drainage of a cyst is performed, a Cook needle aspirator (Cook OB/GYN, Spencer, IN) can be used. The aspirator is placed against the cyst wall and connected to wall suction to effect a seal. A needle is inserted through the interior of the aspirator and the capsule pierced. The aspirator can be placed through a pretied surgical Endoloop and after drainage the pretied loop is tightened, sealing the puncture site.[157] If cyst rupture does occur, the abdomen and pelvis should be thoroughly irrigated.

How should we manage malignancy diagnosed during or after a laparoscopic procedure, and what is the influence of delayed staging?

Despite the use of extensive preoperative studies, such as vaginal ultrasonography and tumor markers, it is not always possible to distinguish between benign and malignant ovarian masses before surgical exploration. Even with the most diligent preoperative triage of patients, the gynecologist may encounter unexpected malignancies when undertaking laparoscopic removal of an ovarian mass.

The likelihood of finding signs of malignancy during laparoscopy of benign-appearing ovarian mass is between 4 and 6 per 1000[123,126,147,148] and 1% to 15%[119] for suspicious masses. After malignancy is diagnosed during laparoscopy (usually after frozen section analysis of the specimen), the two main options are to continue with surgical staging or tumor reductive surgery or to stop the procedure and reschedule the patient for definitive surgery. The decision depends on the patient's and the treating physician's circumstances, including the preoperative counseling and the training and experience of the surgeon. A few surgeons evaluated the effect of delaying surgery after laparoscopy on survival in ovarian cancer patients. Lehner and associates[149] reviewed 48 cases of delayed laparotomy after laparoscopy and diagnosis of malignant masses. In one half of the cases, laparotomy was delayed for more than 17 days, and in the other half, laparotomy was performed within 17 days from the time of laparoscopy. The results of this study illustrated that delay in the laparotomy after laparoscopic excision of ovarian masses, later found to be malignant, had a negative prognostic impact on the distribution of disease stage, with the proportion of advanced tumors being significantly higher among patients for whom laparotomy was delayed for more than 17 days after laparoscopy. Although 46 of the 48 patients had tumor restricted to the ovary by laparoscopic evaluation, in 27 of them, advanced disease (stage IIb through IV) was found by staging laparotomy, emphasizing that visual evaluation by laparoscopy should not substitute for a surgical staging procedure. Support for the recommendation not to delay staging laparotomy after the incidental diagnosis of malignancy during laparoscopy comes from a few other studies.[127,147] Kindermann and coworkers[148] showed that even a delay of 8 days from diagnosis to treatment could allow disease progression. Most of the surgical specimens in this study were ruptured or morcellated, possibly causing more rapid tumor dissemination (in only 7.4% of apparent stage Ia cases was an endobag used). It is unclear how early after the diagnosis of ovarian malignancy is made at laparoscopy the tumor Johnson be surgically staged. Most investigators support an "as soon as possible" approach, and Canis and colleagues[142] even consider it an "oncologic emergency." The staging procedure should include all the surgical steps required, regardless of the type of abdominal incision used.

What is the role of laparoscopic staging in clinically apparent early-stage disease? Because of the various potential sites of metastases, surgical staging of clinically apparent early-stage disease requires peritoneal washings, an infracolic omentectomy, pelvic and para-aortic lymph node dissection, and multiple peritoneal biopsies.[158] The laparoscopic approach in staging of

ovarian cancer may limit the surgeon in evaluating the full extent of the bowel and lymph nodes above the inferior mesenteric artery. The first laparoscopic attempt to stage and treat an ovarian cancer patient was reported by Reich and colleagues[70] in 1990. In this case, the procedure did not include para-aortic lymph node dissection. In 1993, Querleu[64] was the first to report an adequate laparoscopic surgical staging procedure. Table 52-8 describes the clinical data available for laparoscopic ovarian staging. Most of these cases were previously diagnosed cancers subsequently referred for definitive management. With no long follow-up and few reported cases, it is unclear whether clinically apparent early-stage ovarian cancer can be adequately and safely staged laparoscopically. Until more information is gathered, laparotomy should be considered the standard approach for ovarian cancer staging and treatment. Laparoscopic staging is likely to be feasible, especially in selected situations, but would be best reserved for clinical trials. The GOG is evaluating the role of laparoscopy for restaging of patients with incompletely staged ovarian cancer.

Is there a role for laparoscopic second-look operations? Second-look operations for patients with advanced ovarian cancers remain controversial.[161,162] The original purpose of a second look was to identify patients who had complete pathologic response to chemotherapy. Traditionally, the procedure was performed through midline vertical incision, with extensive exploration of the abdomen, multiple peritoneal washings, multiple biopsies, and often additional retroperitoneal lymph node sampling.[163] One half of the patients with optimally cytoreduced disease and a complete clinical response to chemotherapy have negative second-look results, and about one half of the patients with negative second-look results develop recurrent disease.[164] The effect of second-look operations on the survival rate is controversial,[165-168] and it is mainly used now for the prospective evaluation of second-line treatment or as part of a clinical trial.

Laparoscopy appears to be an attractive technique as a second-look procedure because of the magnification it provides and the ability to inspect the whole abdominal cavity through a tiny incision. The obvious disadvantage is that the surgeon is not able to palpate and locate disease that may otherwise be difficult to locate. With the development of modern laparoscopic techniques, more groups began to use laparoscopy in second-look operations. The initial studies reported inadequate visualization, high false-negative rates, and a high rate of complications.[169-172] Later studies reported controversial results. Abu-Rustum and colleagues[173] and Casey and associates[174] found that laparoscopy was associated with less blood loss, shorter operative time, and reduced hospital stay. There were more intraoperative and postoperative complications in patients who underwent laparotomy, and the recurrence after negative second-look operation was similar for laparoscopy and laparotomy. Husain and coworkers[175] reported 150 cases of

Table 52–8. Laparoscopic Staging of Ovarian Cancer Patients

Study	No. of Pts.	ORT (min, mean)	PLN (no., mean)	PALN (no., mean)	Blood Loss (mL, mean)	Complications Patients		HS (days)
						IOC	POC	
Reich et al.[70] (1990)	1	300	11, left only	Not done	200	None	NI	2
Querleu[64] (1993)	2	200	12	9	NI	None	Hematoma	2
Querleu and LeBlanc[159] (1994)*	8	227	NI	8.6	<300	None	Hematoma	2.8
Spirtos et al.[56] (1995)†	4	193	20.8	7.9	<100	VI: 2	DVT: 2 SBO: 2	2.7
Childers et al.[71] (1995)	19	120-240	NI	NI	NI	VI: 1	Large ecchymotic area on abdomen	1.6
Pomel et al.[72] (1995)	10	313	6	8	NI	None	Bleeding: 1 PE: 1	4.75
Possover et al.[45] (1997)	13	187	13.4	8.6	<200	VI: 2 II: 1	None	5.6
Dottino et al.[76] (1999)†	3 (94 cases)	130.3	11.9	3.7	83.4	VI: 1	Fever: 1 UTI: 1	3.6
Scribner et al.[169] (2001)†	5 (103 cases)	240.4	18.1	11.9	321.1	BI: 1 UI: 1 VI: 1	DVT: 2 PE: 1	2.8
Total	65	234.5	10.6	8.6	<233	7.5%	12.8%	2.86

*May include patients from a previous report.
†Data derived from studies that have included staging for other malignancies. Operating room time, nodal counts, blood loss, and complications specific to ovarian cancer patients could not be determined from the published reports and were omitted from the total calculation.
BI, bladder injury; EBL, estimated blood loss; II, intestinal injury; IOC, intraoperative complications; MDS, mean duration of surgery; NI, not indicated; PALND, para-aortic lymph node dissection; PE, pulmonary embolism; POC, postoperative complications; SBO, small bowel obstruction; UI, ureteral injury; VI, vascular injury or bleeding.

second-look laparoscopy; the rate for conversion to laparotomy was 12%, and 72% of cases were related to cytoreduction. There were three bowel and one bladder injuries (2.7%), and the researchers concluded that the procedure was safe and accurate. In an Italian retrospective, multicenter study, the disease-free survival rate was lower for patients with negative second-look laparoscopy results compared with negative second-look laparotomy results.[172] Clough and colleagues[176] performed laparoscopic second-look operations immediately followed by laparotomy in 20 patients with advanced ovarian cancer. The positive predictive value of laparoscopy for the diagnosis of residual disease was 100%, and the negative predictive value was 86% (two false negatives of 14). In only 41% of the laparoscopies, complete intraperitoneal investigation could be performed because of postoperative adhesions. The conclusion was that a laparoscopic second-look procedure was less reliable than one performed by laparotomy.

Canis and associates[144] proposed the following management approach for patients with ovarian cancer who need second-look evaluation: The second-look evaluation should begin by laparoscopy. If peritoneal carcinomatosis or metastasis is found, the procedure should be stopped, and second-line treatment should be started as soon as possible. A negative laparoscopic evaluation can be considered reliable only if the entire peritoneal cavity is inspected; complete adhesiolysis is achieved; multiple, random biopsies are taken; and complete staging, including

nodes, is performed before chemotherapy, and no positive nodes are found. If any of these procedures cannot be accomplished, laparotomy should be considered. Patients eligible for a second-look laparotomy usually have had previous extensive surgery for debulking followed by chemotherapy that places them at risk for extensive tenacious adhesions. The laparoscopic second-look operation potentially represents one of the most difficult and tedious endoscopic procedures performed in gynecologic oncology patients, and it should be performed only by surgeons with extensive experience in advanced laparoscopic techniques and expertise in gynecologic oncology.[177]

Can we evaluate the feasibility of cytoreductive surgery in advanced disease by the laparoscopic approach? Treatment of advanced ovarian cancer consists of tumor-reductive surgery followed by platinum- and taxane-based chemotherapy. The amount of residual tumor after the primary surgery is the most important prognostic factor for these patients.[178-181] In the past few years, increasingly radical surgery has been used with the intention to increase the portion of optimally debulked disease. In gynecologic oncology centers, it is possible to achieve complete tumor resection in 40% to 90% of the cases[182-184] Despite advances in surgery, complete debulking is not feasible in many patients. One of the therapy approaches that was tried to improve the prognosis in these patients is neoadjuvant chemotherapy. Neoadjuvant chemotherapy can induce downstaging of the tumor and improve operability.[185-187] Different methods were offered to identify patients with low probability of successful complete tumor resection and hence less likely to benefit from the conventional tumor-reductive surgery and adjuvant chemotherapy approach. Nelson and colleagues[188] proposed CT criteria to predict operability in patients with suspected ovarian mass. Others used the ascitic fluid volume and levels of the tumor marker CA125[189-191] to predict surgical results.

Vegote and Van Dam[192] reported their experience with open laparoscopy to evaluate operability. Seventy-seven patients with clinical and radiologic findings suspected for advanced ovarian carcinoma, which might have been inoperable according to imaging criteria, underwent open laparoscopy. The procedure was proved to be safe, and primary debulking surgery to less than 0.5 cm for the largest residual mass was feasible in 79% of the patients that were subjected to primary surgery.

What is the risk for port-site metastasis? Inoculation of tumor cells into the subcutaneous tissue at the site of previous skin incision is a known phenomenon. The reported rate of recurrences in the abdominal wall after abdominal surgery is 1% to 1.5%.[193,194] There has been increasing concern among surgical oncologists about the apparent increased risk for port-site metastasis after laparoscopic surgeries for a variety of cancers. Although many case reports describing port-site metastases are available (Table 52-9), few studies have been done to define the prevalence of this complication. Recurrence of adenocarcinoma within port sites after laparoscopic resection of gastrointestinal malignancy has been documented at a frequency of 1.0% to 4.5%,[208-212] and ovarian malignancy occurs at a frequency of 1.1% to 16%.[185,188] Manolitsas and Fowler,[119] reviewing the English literature of port-site metastases until 2000, found a reported incidence of 1% to 16% of all laparoscopic procedures for ovarian cancer. A total of 44 cases were reported, 37 in association with ovarian malignancies and 7 associated with LMP tumors. Later studies[135,212] report a lower incidence of abdominal wall metastasis (<1%) if certain precautions are taken, but the true incidence and the actual number of such recurrences are not known, and it is likely that there is underreporting of this complication. Wang and colleagues[213] reviewed the literature of port-site metastases after laparoscopic surgery in gastrointestinal and gynecologic cancers until 1996 and found that most recurrences were in patients with adenocarcinoma cell type, advanced-stage disease, and diffuse peritoneal carcinomatosis. Risk factors contributing to early

Table 52-9. Reported Cases of Port-Site Metastasis in Ovarian Malignancy

Study	No. of Pts.	Stage	Procedure	Ascites	Time to Diagnosis (days)
Dobronte et al.[134] (1978)	1	III	Diagnostic laparoscopy and biopsy	Yes	14
Stockdale et al.[195] (1985)	1	IV	Diagnostic laparoscopy and biopsy	Yes	8
Hsiu et al.[196] (1986)	2	LMP III, LMP III?	Diagnostic laparoscopy and biopsy	NDA	21
Miralles et al.[197] (1989)	1	I?	Laparoscopy after open adnexectomy	NDA	365
Gleeson et al.[198] (1993)	3	LMP Ic III, III	Oophorectomy and morcellation Diagnostic laparoscopy and biopsy	NDA Yes	14 <14
Shepherd et al.[199] (1994)	1	LMP Ia	Laparoscopic cyst aspiration and excision	No	42
Childers et al.[200] (1994)	1	IIa	Second-look procedure (positive for recurrence)	No	56
Kindermann et al.[148] (1995)	14	Ic-III	Diagnostic laparoscopy, laparoscopic biopsies, cystectomies, and morcellation	NDA	8-60
Gungor et al.[201] (1996)	1	IIIb	Third-look procedure	Yes	240
Chu et al.[202] (1996)	1	Ic/IIIc ? Unstaged	Laparoscopic salpingo-oophorectomy	Yes	14
Kruitwagen et al.[203] (1996)	7	IIIc-IV	Diagnostic laparoscopy	Yes	9-35
Van Dam et al.[135] (1999)	9	IIIc-IV	Laparoscopy for tissue diagnosis and assessment of operability	Yes	4-90
Hopkins et al.[204] (2000)	3	LMP I? Unstaged	Laparoscopic drainage and morcellation, partial excision, oophorectomy and ruptured bag	NDA	14-28
Morice et al.[205] (2000)	5	III-IV	Laparoscopic biopsies	Yes	NDA
Haughney et al.[206] (2001)	1	Early stage	Laparoscopic oophorectomy	NDA	3650
Carlson et al.[207] (2001)	1	IIIc	Laparotomy for cancer, recurrence in laparoscopic surgical port for benign disease	Yes	820
Total	52				4-3650

LMP, low malignant potential; NDA, no data available.

occurrence of port-site metastases were ovarian cancer, presence of ascites, and diagnostic or palliative procedures for malignancy.

Although most cases of reported port-site recurrences occur in advanced-staged ovarian cancer patients, a few worrisome reports suggest port-site metastases in early-stage disease,[214,215] LMP tumors,[198,199,204,213] adenocarcinoma of the endometrium,[216-218] and cervical and vaginal cancer patients.[137,204,205,218-224] The most distressing scenario would be a port-site recurrence in a woman with early-stage disease. Most cases of port-site recurrences in early-stage disease were not properly staged[214] or were related to iatrogenic spill of cells into the peritoneal cavity. Spillage can be attributed to the laparoscopic techniques: morcellation, partial excision of ovarian masses,[198] or accidental rupture of the endobag containing the ovarian specimen.[204] Muntz and associates,[217] however, reported a case of port-site recurrence in a patient with early-stage (Ia) endometrial cancer. The woman underwent laparoscopically assisted vaginal hysterectomy, bilateral salpingo-oophorectomy, and lymphadenectomy.

Twenty-one months later, she developed a 5-cm recurrent tumor mass at a lateral laparoscopic port site. The mass was resected and restaging laparotomy was performed without evidence of disease. Two more cases of port-site metastases in patients with early-stage cervical cancer (Ia1 and Ib) and negative lymph nodes were reported.[224,225] In the first case, recurrence was found at the laparoscopic port site 9 months after laparoscopically assisted vaginal hysterectomy, bilateral salpingo-oophorectomy, and bilateral pelvic node dissection for a stage Ia1 adenocarcinoma of the cervix. The latter case was a 31-year-old woman who had a diagnostic laparoscopy for pelvic pain. A grossly abnormal cervix was observed, and a biopsy revealed squamous cell carcinoma. The patient underwent radical hysterectomy and pelvic lymph node dissection through a transverse lower abdominal incision, and 19 months postoperatively, she presented with a port-site metastasis in a suprapubic laparoscopic trocar site.

The period between the laparoscopic surgery and appearance of port-site metastasis varies between 1 week and 3 years in gastrointestinal tract cancers and is usually earlier in gynecologic malignancies.[213,217] It is not clear why some of the recurrences tend to develop so rapidly while others appear after a longer period. It is, however, extremely important to refer patients for complete staging and definitive treatment as soon as the diagnosis of malignancy is made. Delayed referral and treatment increase the risk of port-site metastasis[135] and may worsen the prognosis. There have been only two retrospective studies that have evaluated the effect of port-site metastases on survival in gynecologic cancer patients.[135,203] In these studies, all port-site metastases occurred in stage IIIc or stage IV disease, and there was no statistically significant difference in survival. Kruitwagen and colleagues,[203] in a multivariate analysis, showed that after adjustment for age, stage of disease, histology, grade, ascites, and residual disease after primary debulking, a negative ($P = .14$), although not statistically

significant, correlation existed between port-site metastasis and survival. The investigators assumed that the negative correlation was possibly not statistically significant due to the small sample size (7 of 43 patients who had undergone laparoscopy developed port-site metastasis).

Possible mechanisms for the occurrence of port-site metastasis after surgery in general and specifically after laparoscopic surgery for malignancy. The exact cause of port-site metastasis is unknown and may be multifactorial. Possible mechanisms for the development of port-site metastasis include direct wound implantation by extraction of specimen or instrument contamination; the "chimney effect"; aerosolization of tumor cells; surgical technique; hematogenous spread; and the effect of the pneumoperitoneum (e.g., pressure, carbon dioxide).

Direct contamination of the port site with tumor cells may occur during extraction of the tumor through a small wound or indirectly from instruments contaminated with tumor cells. This is probably an important mechanism in the development of port-site metastasis and is supported by clinical studies and animal models.[213,216,226-230] There is considerable evidence in animals that healing wounds enhance the growth of tumor cells more than unwounded tissues, but only if the tumor cells are inoculated directly into the wound. The greater the size of the tumor inoculum, the greater is the enhancement of tumor growth in the skin incision.[143] Fifty-five percent of port-site metastases found in patients after laparoscopic cholecystectomy for unknown gallbladder carcinoma were found at the port used for extraction of the gallbladder.[229] Bouvy and colleagues,[230] in a tumor model in the rat, showed that the size of the abdominal wall metastases was greater at the port site of extraction of the tumor than at the other port sites and concluded that direct contact between solid tumor and the port site enhances local tumor growth. Laparoscopic instruments and ports contaminated with tumor cells were recognized in clinical studies and animal models,[231-233] and increased manipulation of the ports enhanced tumor cell implantation.[234-236] There is circumstantial evidence in humans that small wounds may promote the growth of tumor cells better than large ones. Carlson and associates[207] reported a case of port-site metastasis of ovarian carcinoma after cytoreductive surgery in a laparoscopic wound site performed a year earlier for benign disease. Other reports[237-239] emphasize the predilection of tumor cells for smaller incision sites. Indirect contamination, such as the chimney effect, has been suggested as a cause for port-site metastasis. In a porcine model, tumor cells were filtered from gas escaping at port sites.[234,240] Tumor cells may exist in aerosol form and be seeded into the wound, especially during desufflation of the pneumoperitoneum,[241] but various studies indicate that aerosolized tumor cells are not viable.[234,241-243] Clinical and experimental data suggest that surgical technique, lack of surgical experience, and not adhering to strict surgical oncologic principles during the development of advanced laparoscopic procedures have contributed to a number of case reports of port-site metastasis. Intraoperative spillage of tumor cells as a cause of port-site metastasis was attributed to morcellation, partial excision, or accidental rupture of the endobag in patients with ovarian cancer[198,204] and manipulation in cases of colorectal cancer.[244,245] Lee and colleagues[246] showed in a murine model that traumatic handling of tumor independent of pneumoperitoneum increased the port-site metastasis rate of colon cancer and that this rate could be decreased with increased laparoscopic experience.[247] The role of the pneumoperitoneum in the development of port-site metastasis was attributed to the pressure and to the use of carbon dioxide. Jacobi and coworkers[248] investigated the effect of different pressures on tumor growth and the port-site metastasis rate using in vitro and in vivo models. In vitro, raised intraperitoneal pressure suppressed tumor growth, and in vivo, intraperitoneal tumor growth was suppressed only by higher pressure (15 mm Hg). Other in vitro studies showed different results,[249-251] and Kruitwagen and colleagues[203] found that abdominal wall recurrences developed with similar frequencies in the paracentesis and trocar tracts, suggesting no pneumoperitoneum effect. The effect of carbon dioxide on tumor growth and proliferation is still unclear. Few studies demonstrated that carbon dioxide directly enhanced cancer cell growth,[139,248] but other work could not confirm such an effect.[252,253] Other reports showed effect of the laparoscopic environment on tumor cell biology.

Upregulation of matrix metalloprotease activity, plasminogen activator activity, urokinase plasminogen activator receptor expression, and other factors may enhance the ability of tumor cells to invade through the reconstituted basement membrane.[213,252,254,255] The laparoscopic environment may also affect the host immune system, as demonstrated by lower cytokines and C-reactive protein levels,[256] impaired tumor necrosis factor secretion, and diminished macrophage function.[257,258]

How to decrease the incidence of port-site metastases. Considering the accumulating data on the possible mechanisms of port-site metastasis, various preventive measures were tested. In an effort to reduce contamination of the incision with viable free exfoliated cancer cells, routine irrigation of the port-site wound is suggested.[200,213,259] The use of bags for the retrieval of specimens during surgery is another procedure used to reduce the risk of wound implantation by tumor cells.[226,260] Different local and intraperitoneal agents have been shown to reduce the incidence of port-site metastasis in animal models, including heparin,[261,262] taurolidine,[261,263] povidone iodine[246,264] and chemotherapeutic agents such as 5-fluorouracil and doxorubicin.[265] Sugarbaker and coworkers[266] demonstrated that the instillation of chemotherapy directly into the peritoneal cavity as part of gastrointestinal surgery decreases cancer spread to the resection site and peritoneal surfaces, significantly improving survival and quality of life. Although data,

mainly from animal models, support the use of local and intraperitoneal agents in the prevention of port-site metastasis, it is not routinely used because the effectiveness is still undetermined.

Few surgical approaches have been proposed to decrease the incidence of port-site metastasis. Gasless laparoscopy and helium pneumoperitoneum may offer some advantage compared with the conventional laparoscopic technique and the use of carbon dioxide as the insufflating gas.[267,268] Slow deflation can decrease the chimney effect, which promotes tumor entrapment on the port site. Van Dam and associates[135] reported that closure of all layers of the laparoscopic wound (i.e., peritoneum, rectus sheath, and skin) followed by chemotherapy or cytoreductive surgery with excision of the trocar wounds within 1 week reduced the incidence of port-site metastasis from 58% to less than 2%. The study group included 104 women with primary advanced or recurrent ovarian cancer undergoing laparoscopy for tissue diagnosis and operability assessment.

The laparoscopic management of malignant disease in humans predisposes patients to port-site metastasis. Port-site recurrences result if the malignancy treated has the propensity to exfoliate cells into the peritoneal cavity and the trocar site remains untreated or if the tumor is resistant to adjuvant treatment. Most gynecologic malignancies are sensitive to adjuvant therapy but differ in their propensity to exfoliate cells; ovarian cancer has the highest such tendency. Endometrial and cervical cancers have a lower propensity to exfoliate tumor cells, are radiosensitive, and usually are diagnosed at an early stage with negative nodes. However, after involved nodes are present and are being extracted through a trocar, there is a considerable risk for port-site metastasis if the port is not within the radiation-treatment fields.

Although experimental data support the theory that laparoscopy and especially carbon dioxide pneumoperitoneum may increase intraperitoneal tumor growth and the risk of port-site recurrences, this phenomenon is not as common as first thought. Meticulous surgical technique to prevent direct contamination of the port site with tumor cells and the use of preventive measures (mainly closing all abdominal layers and early treatment with chemotherapy or cytoreductive surgery) are most probably responsible for this reduction in the incidence of abdominal wall recurrences. The results of ongoing randomized trials will give an indication of the true incidence and the effect on prognosis of port-site metastasis.

Investigational Use of Laparoscopy

Assessment of the sentinel lymph node in cervical cancer.
Lymph node status is the most important prognostic factor for survival in patients with cervical cancer. Removal of the nodes is important for treatment plan and to assess the biology of the disease. The lymph nodes removed from only approximately 10% of patients with early cervical cancer are involved

with disease.[269] This means that about 90% of patients who undergo lymphadenectomy derive no benefit from the procedure but tolerate the associated prolongation in operative time and face the increase risks of blood loss and formation of lymphocyst and lymphedema. All these reasons and the fact that the location of positive nodes cannot be determined based on clinical factors such as location, size of primary tumor, and radiology methods make cervical cancer patients excellent candidates for lymphatic mapping.

The concept of sentinel nodes was first applied in penile cancers,[270] and in melanoma, it was even integrated into the routine surgical staging. The greatest development is in breast cancer, for which large case series showed the validity of the concept.[271,272] The procedure usually involves preoperative lymphoscintigraphy and intraoperative lymphatic mapping with blue dye and technetium 99 radiocolloid. The dye and radiolabeled albumin are injected into the cervix. Some investigators[273,274] found the preoperative lymphoscintigraphy hard to interpret accurately and omitted this stage from the procedure. The intraoperative lymphatic mapping is performed by exposing the retroperitoneum, visually inspecting for blue nodes, and scanning for the radioactive lymph nodes with a hand-held gamma counter. Sentinel nodes are blue or "hot" nodes (e.g., ex vivo count at least 10-fold above background). Detection of the sentinel lymph node in patients with cervical cancer has been described by a few investigators.[273-279] Dargent and colleagues[275] injected patent blue violet into 35 early-stage cervical cancers that were then assessed laparoscopically. Together, 69 pelvic sidewall dissections were performed, and in 59, one or more sentinel nodes were evident and sent for pathologic evaluation. The main reasons for failure to detect a sentinel node were insufficient quantity of injected dye and injection not directly into the cervix. One or more positive pelvic lymph nodes were found in 11 pelvic lymph wall dissections, and the sentinel node was the positive node or one of them in all cases. In the remaining cases, if the sentinel node was not involved, no involved nodes were found in the following systematic dissection. The 100% negative predictive value of the sentinel node is promising, but the investigators estimated that about 400 dissections would be needed before the results are confirmed.

Levenback and coworkers[274] performed sentinel node evaluation with preoperative lymphoscintigraphy and intraoperative lymphatic mapping with blue dye and a hand-held gamma probe in 39 patients with cervical cancer undergoing radical hysterectomy. All 39 patients had at least one sentinel node identified intraoperatively. Eighty percent of sentinel nodes were detected in the iliac, obturator, and parametrial locations. The remaining sentinel nodes were in the common iliac and para-aortic nodal basins. Eight patients had disease metastatic to the lymph nodes. One (12%) of those patients had a false-negative sentinel node. In this patient, four sentinel nodes were identified preoperatively on lymphoscintigraphy. Intraoperatively, all four nodes were hot and blue but with no tumor; however, four nonpalpable metastatic parametrial nodes were identified in the hysterectomy specimen. Twenty-one of the 25 positive nodes were sentinel nodes. The sensitivity of sentinel nodes was 87.5%, and that of the negative predictive value was 97%.

Malur and colleagues[273] reported a 90% detection rate of sentinel nodes after injection of blue dye and radiolabeled albumin, compared with a 55% detection rate in the group injected with only blue dye. Most of the sentinel nodes were located near the origin of the uterine artery or at the division of the common iliac artery. Four of 11 patients with no detected sentinel nodes had pelvic lymph node metastases. The false-negative rate was 16.6% (1 of 6 patients). In this patient, labeling was done with blue dye only. Two blue-stained pelvic nodes were identified that were free of metastases histologically, but 1 of 16 pelvic nodes showed tumor involvement. The overall sensitivity was 83.3%, and the negative predictive value was 97%.

These early reports provided several conclusions:

1. Preoperative lymphoscintigram had little or no impact on clinical decision-making.[273,274]
2. The detection rate of sentinel nodes can be increased by injection of dye and technetium.[273]
3. The dye should be injected into the cervix, and there is a correlation between the volume of the injected dye and the detection rate of sentinel nodes.[275]
4. Positive nodes are located throughout the pelvis and para-aortic regions. The most common locations of the sentinel nodes are near the origin of the uterine artery, the division of the common iliac artery, and in the interiliac area.
5. The sensitivity ranges between 50% and 100%, and the negative predictive value is between 75% and 100%.

The data gathered are not sufficient to abandon the standard practice of pelvic and para-aortic lymphadenectomy and move to sentinel node biopsy. As long as the negative predictive value is not 100% or very close to this number, the method will not be incorporated into clinical practice. New approaches using molecular biologic and immunohistochemical methods for detection of micrometastases in the sentinel lymph nodes are being evaluated. Van Trappen and coworkers,[280] using a fully quantitative, real-time reverse transcriptase–polymerase chain reaction (PCR) assay to document absolute copy numbers of the epithelial marker cytokeratin 19, suggested that 50% of early-stage cervical cancers shed tumor cells to the pelvic lymph nodes. Other studies using immunohistochemical methods detected micrometastases in 9% to 33% of sentinel lymph nodes that were judged as tumor free after hematoxylin and eosin staining.[280-285] Taback and associates[286] developed molecular lymphatic mapping in a rat model to label the sentinel nodes preoperatively with rice gene DNA containing plasmid or linear rice DNA fragment. The molecular marker was detected by PCR in frozen section and paraffin-embedded sentinel nodes.

The potential value of the laparoscopic sentinel node identification is not in the time saved during the dissection but mainly the ability to use this procedure in combination with molecular biologic and immunohistochemical methods as part of the staging of cervical cancer.

Summary

More than 10 years after gynecologic oncologists began to use modern surgical endoscopy for pelvic lymphadenectomy, the role of this approach in the treatment of gynecologic cancer patients is still not clear. The benefits and safety of laparoscopic surgery are questionable. There is no doubt that the possible benefits of the laparoscopic technique are enormous and include less intraoperative blood loss, shorter hospitalization and time to recovery, less adhesion formation and radiation risks, the potential to start chemotherapy earlier after surgery, and the ability to minimize discomfort and analgesic requirements. A few obstacles in the implementation of this technique are related to the longer training period required, the need to establish new protocols for the different operations in use, and lack of data concerning the complications and long-term results.

The evidence from small-scale studies and few randomized, prospective studies (e.g., GOG study of laparoscopic retroperitoneal lymphadenectomy followed by immediate laparotomy in women with cervical cancer) shows promising results for the use of laparoscopy for staging and treatment of cervical and endometrial cancers. In specific groups of patients treated by expert surgeons, the laparoscopic approach is feasible, the intraoperative and postoperative results are comparable or even better, and the risks of recurrence and overall survival are equivalent to those achieved with laparotomy. The role of laparoscopy for surgical staging or restaging of early ovarian malignancies, second-look operations, and assessment of suitability for cytoreductive surgery in advanced-stage disease requires further evaluation in the context of prospective, randomized trials.

The objectives of gynecologic cancer surgery should not be sacrificed for the benefit of a new surgical approach. With this in mind, the adequacy and safety of each laparoscopic procedure should be carefully compared with the conservative alternative in a prospective, randomized trial before applied routinely. The most important factor in surgery is not the extent of the incision or the device, but rather surgical expertise and judgment.

REFERENCES

1. Ottosen C, Lingman G, Ottosen L: Three methods for hysterectomy: A randomised, prospective study of short term outcome. Br J Obstet Gynaecol 2000;107:1380-1385.
2. Dargent D, Mathevet P: Radical laparoscopic vaginal hysterectomy. J Gynecol Obstet Biol Reprod 1992;21:709.
3. Kadar N, Reich H: Laparoscopically assisted radical Schauta hysterectomy and bilateral laparoscopic pelvic lymphadenectomy for the treatment of bulky stage IB carcinoma of the cervix. Gynaecol Endosc 1993;2:135-142.
4. Bolger BS, De Bassor Lopes A, Lavie OD, Monaghan JM: Comparison of laparoscopic-assisted radical vaginal hysterectomy and radical abdominal hysterectomy in the treatment of early stage cervical carcinoma [abstract]. Gynecol Oncol 1998;68:95.
5. Chu KK, Chang SD, Chen FP, Soong YK: Laparoscopic surgical staging in cervical cancer—preliminary experience among Chinese. Gynecol Oncol 1997;64:49-53.
6. Dargent D, Roy M, Keita N, et al: The Schauta operation: Its place in the management of cervical cancer in 1993 [abstract]. Gynecol Oncol 1993;49:109.
7. Hatch K, Hallum A, Nour M, Saucedo M: Comparison of radical abdominal hysterectomy with laparoscopic assisted radical vaginal hysterectomy for treatment of early cervical cancer [abstract]. Gynecol Oncol 1997;64:293.
8. Kadar N: Laparoscopic-vaginal radical hysterectomy. J Am Assoc Gynecol Laparosc 1994;1(Pt 2):S14-S15.
9. Possover M, Krause N, Schneider A: Identification of the ureter and dissection of the bladder pillar in laparoscopic-assisted radical vaginal hysterectomy. Obstet Gynecol 1998;91:139-143.
10. Querleu D: Laparoscopically assisted radical vaginal hysterectomy. Gynecol Oncol 1993;51:248-254.
11. Roy M, Plante M, Renaud MC, Tetu B: Vaginal radical hysterectomy versus abdominal radical hysterectomy in the treatment of early-stage cervical cancer. Gynecol Oncol 1996;62:336-339.
12. Malur S, Possover M, Schneider A: Laparoscopically assisted radical vaginal versus radical abdominal hysterectomy type II in patients with cervical cancer. Surg Endosc 2001;15:289-292.
13. Querleu D, Leblanc E: Gynecologic cancer. In Gomel V, Taylor PJ (eds): Diagnostic and Operative Gynecologic Laparoscopy. Baltimore, Mosby, 1995, pp 277-298.
14. Dargent DF: Laparoscopic surgery in gynecologic oncology [review]. Surg Clin North Am 2001;81:949-964.
15. Hatch KD, Hallum AV 3rd, Nour M: New surgical approaches to treatment of cervical cancer. J Natl Cancer Inst Monogr 1996;21:71-75.
16. Schneider A, Possover M, Kamprath S, et al: Laparoscopy-assisted radical vaginal hysterectomy modified according to Schauta-Stoeckel. Obstet Gynecol 1996;88:1057-1060.
17. Sardi J, Vidaurreta J, Bermudez A, di Paola G: Laparoscopically assisted Schauta operation: Learning experience at the Gynecologic Oncology Unit, Buenos Aires University Hospital. Gynecol Oncol 1999;75:361-365.
18. Renaud MC, Plante M, Roy M: Combined laparoscopic and vaginal radical surgery in cervical cancer. Gynecol Oncol 2000;79:59-63.
19. Piver MS, Rutledge F, Smith JP: Five classes of extended hysterectomy for women with cervical cancer. Obstet Gynecol 1974;44:265-272.
20. Than GN: Wertheim-meigs oder Schauta-Amereich hysterectomy [letter]. Am J Obstet Gynecology 1994;171:287.
21. Canis M, Mage G, Pouly JL, Pomel C, et al: Laparoscopic radical hysterectomy for cervical cancer. Baillieres Clin Obstet Gynaecol 1995;9:675-689.
22. Nezhat CR, Nezhat FR, Burrell MO, et al: Laparoscopic radical hysterectomy and laparoscopically assisted vaginal radical hysterectomy with pelvic and paraaortic node dissection. J Gynecol Surg 1993;9:105-120.
23. Spirtos NM, Schlaerth JB, Kimball RE, et al: Laparoscopic radical hysterectomy (type III) with aortic and pelvic lymphadenectomy. Am J Obstet Gynecol 1996;174:1763-1767, discussion, 1767-1768.
24. Nezhat CR, Burrell MO, Nezhat FR, et al: Laparoscopic radical hysterectomy with paraaortic and pelvic node dissection. Am J Obstet Gynecol 1992;166:864-865.
25. Sedlacek TV, Campion M, Reich H, Sedlacek T: Laparoscopic radical hysterectomy: A feasibility study [abstract 65]. Gynecol. Oncol 1995;56:126.
26. Pomel C, Canis M, Mage G, et al: Laparoscopically extended hysterectomy for cervix cancer: Technique, indications and results. Apropos of a series of 41 cases in Clermont [in French]. Chirurgie 1997;122:133-136, discussion, 136-137.
27. Spirtos NM, Eisenkop SM, Schlaerth JB, Ballon SC: Laparoscopic radical hysterectomy (type III) with aortic and pelvic lymphadenectomy in patients with stage I cervical cancer: Surgical morbidity and intermediate follow-up. Am J Obstet Gynecol 2002;187:340-348.

28. Hsieh YY, Lin WC, Chang CC, et al: Laparoscopic radical hysterectomy with low paraaortic, subaortic and pelvic lymphadenectomy: Results of short-term follow-up. J Reprod Med 1998;43:528-534.

29. Kim DH, Moon JS: Laparoscopic radical hysterectomy with pelvic lymphadenectomy for early, invasive cervical carcinoma. J Am Assoc Gynecol Laparosc 1998;5:411-417.

30. Covens A, Rosen B, Murphy J, et al: Changes in the demographics and perioperative care of stage IA(2)/IB(1) cervical cancer over the past 16 years. Gynecol Oncol 2001;81:133-137.

31. Orr JW Jr: Radical hysterectomy: Lessons in risk reduction. Gynecol Oncol 2001;81:129-132.

32. Dargent D, Martin X, Sacchetoni A, Mathevet P: Laparoscopic vaginal radical trachelectomy: A treatment to preserve the fertility of cervical carcinoma patients. Cancer 2000;88:1877-1882.

33. Shepherd JH, Crawford RA, Oram DH: Radical trachelectomy: A way to preserve fertility in the treatment of early cervical cancer. Br J Obstet Gynaecol 1998;105:912-916.

34. Roy M, Plante M: Pregnancies after radical vaginal trachelectomy for early-stage cervical cancer. Am J Obstet Gynecol 1998;179(Pt 1):1491-1496.

35. Covens A, Shaw P, Murphy J, et al: Is radical trachelectomy a safe alternative to radical hysterectomy for patients with stage IA-B carcinoma of the cervix? Cancer 1999;86:2273-2279.

36. Rodriguez M, Guimares O, Rose PG: Radical abdominal trachelectomy and pelvic lymphadenectomy with uterine conservation and subsequent pregnancy in the treatment of early invasive cervical cancer. Am J Obstet Gynecol 2001;185:370-374.

37. Covens A, Rosen B, Gibbons A, et al: Differences in the morbidity of radical hysterectomy between gynecological oncologists. Gynecol Oncol 1993;51:39-45.

38. Shepherd JH, Mould T, Oram DH: Radical trachelectomy in early stage carcinoma of the cervix: Outcome as judged by recurrence and fertility rates. Br J Obstet Gynaecol 2001;108:882-885.

39. Ungar L, Del priore G, Boyle DC, et al: Abdominal radical trachelectomy (ART) follow-up on the first 20 cases. Paper presented on the 33rd annual meeting of the Society of Gynecologic Oncologists, 2002 [abstract 38].

40. Querleu D, Leblanc E, Castelain B: Laparoscopic pelvic lymphadenectomy in the staging of early carcinoma of the cervix. Am J Obstet Gynecol 1991;164:579-581.

41. Dargent D, Arnould P: Percutaneous pelvic lymphadenectomy under laparoscopic guidance. In Nichols D (ed): Gynecologic and Obstetrics Surgery. St Louis, Mosby, 1993, p 583.

42. Fowler JM, Carter JR, Carlson JW, et al: Lymph node yield from laparoscopic lymphadenectomy in cervical cancer: A comparative study. Gynecol Oncol 1993;51:187-192.

43. Childers JM, Hatch K, Surwit EA: The role of laparoscopic lymphadenectomy in the management of cervical carcinoma. Gynecol Oncol 1992;47:38-43.

44. Kadar N: Laparoscopic pelvic lymphadenectomy for the treatment of gynecological malignancies: Description of a technique. Gynecol Endosc 1992:179-183.

45. Possover M, Krause N, Plaul K, et al: Laparoscopic para-aortic and pelvic lymphadenectomy: Experience with 150 patients and review of the literature. Gynecol Oncol 1998;71:19-28.

46. Schlaerth JB, Spirtos NM, Carson LF, et al: Laparoscopic retroperitoneal lymphadenectomy followed by immediate laparotomy in women with cervical cancer: A gynecologic oncology group study. Gynecol Oncol 2002;85:81-88.

47. Kadar N: Laparoscopic management of gynecological malignancies in women aged 65 years or more. Gynecol Endosc 1995;4:173-176.

48. Scribner DR Jr, Walker JL, Johnson GA, et al: Surgical management of early-stage endometrial cancer in the elderly: Is laparoscopy feasible? Gynecol Oncol 2001;83:563-568.

49. Kadar N: Laparoscopic pelvic lymphadenectomy in obese women with gynecologic malignancies. J Am Assoc Gynecol Laparosc 1995;2:163-167.

50. Scribner DR Jr, Walker JL, Johnson GA, et al: Laparoscopic pelvic and paraaortic lymph node dissection in the obese. Gynecol Oncol 2002;84:426-430.

51. Morrow CP, Curtin JP: Tumors of the cervix. In Synopsis of Gynecologic Oncology. New York, Churchill, Livingston, 1998.

52. Downey GO, Potish RA, Adcock LL, et al: Pretreatment surgical staging in cervical carcinoma: Therapeutic efficacy of pelvic lymph node resection. Am J Obstet Gynecol 1989;160(Pt 1):1055-1061.

53. Michel G, Morice P, Castaigne D, et al: Lymphatic spread in stage Ib and II cervical carcinoma: Anatomy and surgical implications. Obstet Gynecol 1998;91:360-363.

54. Cosin JA, Fowler JM, Chen MD, et al: Pretreatment surgical staging of patients with cervical carcinoma: The case for lymph node debulking. Cancer 1998;82:2241-2248.

55. Goff BA, Muntz HG, Paley PJ, et al: Impact of surgical staging in women with locally advanced cervical cancer. Gynecol Oncol 1999;74:436-442.

56. Spirtos NM, Schlaerth JB, Spirtos TW, et al: Laparoscopic bilateral pelvic and paraaortic lymph node sampling: An evolving technique. Am J Obstet Gynecol 1995;173:105-111.

57. Nelson JH Jr, Boyce J, Macasaet M, et al: Incidence, significance, and follow-up of para-aortic lymph node metastases in late invasive carcinoma of the cervix. Am J Obstet Gynecol 1977;128:336-340.

58. Hughes RR, Brewington KC, Hanjani P, et al: Extended field irradiation for cervical cancer based on surgical staging. Gynecol Oncol 1980;9:153-161.

59. Averette HE, Donato DM, Lovecchio JL, Sevin BU: Surgical staging of gynecologic malignancies [review]. Cancer 1987;60(Suppl):2010-2020.

60. Heller PB, Maletano JH, Bundy BN, et al: Clinical-pathologic study of stage IIB, III, and IVA carcinoma of the cervix: Extended diagnostic evaluation for paraaortic node metastasis—a Gynecologic Oncology Group study. Gynecol Oncol 1990;38:425-430.

61. Podczaski ES, Palombo C, Manetta A, et al: Assessment of pretreatment laparotomy in patients with cervical carcinoma before radiotherapy. Gynecol Oncol 1989;33:71-75.

62. Wharton JT, Jones HW 3rd, Day TG Jr, et al: Preirradiation celiotomy and extended field irradiation for invasive carcinoma of the cervix. Obstet Gynecol 1977;49:333-338.

63. Kadar N: Laparoscopic pelvic and aortic lymphadenectomy [review]. Baillieres Clin Obstet Gynaecol 1995;9:651-673.

64. Querleu D: Laparoscopic paraaortic node sampling in gynecologic oncology: A preliminary experience. Gynecol Oncol 1993;49:24-29.

65. Possover M, Plaul K, Krause N, Schneider A: Left-sided laparoscopic para-aortic lymphadenectomy: Anatomy of the ventral tributaries of the infrarenal vena cava. Am J Obstet Gynecol 1998;179:1295-1297.

66. Childers JM, Hatch KD, Tran AN, Surwit EA: Laparoscopic para-aortic lymphadenectomy in gynecologic malignancies. Obstet Gynecol 1993;82:741-747.

67. Spirtos NM, Schlaerth JB, Gross GM, et al: Cost and quality-of-life analyses of surgery for early endometrial cancer: Laparotomy versus laparoscopy. Am J Obstet Gynecol 1996;174:1795-1799, discussion 1799-800.

68. Childers JM, Brzechffa PR, Hatch KD, Surwit EA: Laparoscopically assisted surgical staging (LASS) of endometrial cancer. Gynecol Oncol 1993;51:33-38.

69. Melendez TD, Childers JM, Nour M, et al: Laparoscopic staging of endometrial cancer: The learning experience. JSLS 1997;1:45-49.

70. Reich H, McGlynn F, Wilkie W: Laparoscopic management of stage I ovarian cancer: A case report. J Reprod Med 1990;35:601-604, discussion 604-605.

71. Childers JM, Lang J, Surwit EA, Hatch KD: Laparoscopic surgical staging of ovarian cancer [review]. Gynecol Oncol 1995;59:25-33.

72. Pomel C, Provencher D, Dauplat J, et al: Laparoscopic staging of early ovarian cancer. Gynecol Oncol 1995;58:301-306.

73. Recio FO, Piver MS, Hempling RE: Pretreatment transperitoneal laparoscopic staging pelvic and paraaortic lymphadenectomy in large (> or = 5 cm) stage IB2 cervical carcinoma: Report of a pilot study. Gynecol Oncol 1996;63:333-336.

74. Su TH, Wang KG, Yang YC, et al: Laparoscopic para-aortic lymph node sampling in the staging of invasive cervical carcinoma, including a comparative study of 21 laparotomy cases. Int J Gynaecol Obstet 1995;49:311-318.

75. Kadar N: Laparoscopic resection of fixed and enlarged lymph nodes in patients with advanced cervical cancer. Gynecol Endosc 1993;2:217-221.

76. Dottino PR, Tobias DH, Beddoe A, et al: Laparoscopic lymphadenectomy for gynecologic malignancies. Gynecol Oncol 1999;73:383-388.

77. Berman ML, Lagasse LD, Watring WG, et al: The operative evaluation of patients with cervical carcinoma by an extraperitoneal approach. Obstet Gynecol 1977;50:658-664.

78. Lanvin D, Elhage A, Henry B, et al: Accuracy and safety of laparoscopic lymphadenectomy: An experimental prospective randomized study. Gynecol Oncol 1997;67:83-87.

79. Chen MD, Teigen GA, Reynolds HT, et al: Laparoscopy versus laparotomy: An evaluation of adhesion formation after pelvic and paraaortic lymphadenectomy in a porcine model. Am J Obstet Gynecol 1998;178:499-503.

80. Occelli B, Narducci F, Lanvin D, et al: De novo adhesions with extraperitoneal endosurgical para-aortic lymphadenectomy versus transperitoneal laparoscopic para-aortic lymphadenectomy: A randomized experimental study. Am J Obstet Gynecol 2000;183:529-533.

81. Vasilev SA, McGonigle KF: Extraperitoneal laparoscopic para-aortic lymph node dissection. Gynecol Oncol 1996;61:315-320.

82. Dargent D, Ansquer Y, Mathevet P: Technical development and results of left extraperitoneal laparoscopic paraaortic lymphadenectomy for cervical cancer. Gynecol Oncol 2000;77:87-92.

83. Querleu D, Dargent D, Ansquer Y, et al: Extraperitoneal endosurgical aortic and common iliac dissection in the staging of bulky or advanced cervical carcinomas. Cancer 2000;88:1883-1891.

84. Vergote I, Amant F, Berteloot P, Van Gramberen M: Laparoscopic lower para-aortic staging lymphadenectomy in stage IB2, II, and III cervical cancer. Int J Gynecol Cancer 2002;12:22-26.

85. Buchsbaum HJ: Extrapelvic lymph node metastases in cervical carcinoma. Am J Obstet Gynecol 1979;133:814-824.

86. Finan MA, DeCesare S, Fiorica JV, et al: Radical hysterectomy for stage IB1 vs IB2 carcinoma of the cervix: Does the new staging system predict morbidity and survival? Gynecol Oncol 1996;62:139-147.

87. Panici PB, Scambia G, Baiocchi G, et al: Technique and feasibility of radical para-aortic and pelvic lymphadenectomy for gynecologic malignancies. J Gynecol Cancer 1991;1:133-140.

88. Rotman M, Pajak TF, Choi K, et al: Prophylactic extended-field irradiation of para-aortic lymph nodes in stages IIB and bulky IB and IIA cervical carcinomas: Ten-year treatment results of RTOG 79-20. JAMA 1995;274:387-393.

89. Haie C, Pejovic MH, Gerbaulet A, et al: Is prophylactic para-aortic irradiation worthwhile in the treatment of advanced cervical carcinoma? Results of a controlled clinical trial of the EORTC radiotherapy group. Radiother Oncol 1988;11:101-112.

90. Hacker NF, Wain GV, Nicklin JL: Resection of bulky positive lymph nodes in patients with cervical carcinoma. Int J Gynecol Cancer 1995;5:250-352.

91. Cosin JA, Fowler JM, Chen MD, et al: Pretreatment surgical staging of patients with cervical carcinoma: The case for lymph node debulking. Cancer 1998;82:2241-2248.

92. Creasman WT, Morrow CP, Bundy BN, et al: Surgical pathologic spread patterns of endometrial cancer. A Gynecologic Oncology Group study. Cancer 1987;60(Suppl):2035-2041.

93. Fowler JM: The role of laparoscopic staging in the management of patients with early endometrial cancer. Gynecol Oncol 1999;73:1-3.

94. Childers JM, Surwit EA: Combined laparoscopic and vaginal surgery for the management of two cases of stage I endometrial cancer. Gynecol Oncol 1992;45:46-51.

95. Gemignani ML, Curtin JP, Zelmanovich J, et al: Laparoscopic-assisted vaginal hysterectomy for endometrial cancer: Clinical outcomes and hospital charges. Gynecol Oncol 1999;73:5-11.

96. Holub Z, Jabor A, Bartos P, et al: Laparoscopic pelvic lymphadenectomy in the surgical treatment of endometrial cancer: Results of a multicenter study. JSLS 2002;6:125-131.

97. Bidzinski M, Mettler L, Zielinski J: Endoscopic lymphadenectomy and LAVH in the treatment of endometrial cancer. Eur J Gynaecol Oncol 1998;19:32-34.

98. Boike G, Laurain J, Burke A: A comparison of laparoscopic management of endometrial cancer and traditional laparotomy [abstract]. Gynecol Oncol 1994;52:105.

99. Magrina JF, Mutone NF, Weaver AL, et al: Laparoscopic lymphadenectomy and vaginal or laparoscopic hysterectomy with bilateral salpingo-oophorectomy for endometrial cancer: Morbidity and survival. Am J Obstet Gynecol 1999;181:376-381.

100. Fram KM: Laparoscopically assisted vaginal hysterectomy versus abdominal hysterectomy in stage I endometrial cancer. Int J Gynecol Cancer 2002;12:57-61.

101. Eltabbakh GH, Shamonki MI, Moody JM, Garafano LL: Laparoscopy as the primary modality for the treatment of women with endometrial carcinoma. Cancer 2001;91:378-387.

102. Malur S, Possover M, Michels W, Schneider A: Laparoscopic-assisted vaginal versus abdominal surgery in patients with endometrial cancer—a prospective randomized trial. Gynecol Oncol 2001;80:239-244.

103. Childers JM, Spirtos NM, Brainard P, Surwit EA: Laparoscopic staging of the patient with incompletely staged early adenocarcinoma of the endometrium. Obstet Gynecol 1994;83:597-600.

104. Finkler NJ, Benacerraf B, Lavin PT, et al: Comparison of serum CA 125, clinical impression, and ultrasound in the preoperative evaluation of ovarian masses. Obstet Gynecol 1988;72:659-664.

105. Roman LD, Muderspach LI, Stein SM, et al: Pelvic examination, tumor marker level, and gray-scale and Doppler sonography in the prediction of pelvic cancer. Obstet Gynecol 1997;89:493-500.

106. Schutter EM, Kenemans P, Sohn C, et al: Diagnostic value of pelvic examination, ultrasound, and serum CA 125 in postmenopausal women with a pelvic mass. An international multicenter study. Cancer 1994;74:1398-1406.

107. Kobayashi M: Use of diagnostic ultrasound in trophoblastic neoplasms and ovarian tumors. Cancer 1976;38(Suppl):441-452.

108. Meire HB, Farrant P, Guha T: Distinction of benign from malignant ovarian cysts by ultrasound. Br J Obstet Gynaecol 1978; 85:893-899.

109. Herrmann UJ Jr, Locher GW, Goldhirsch A: Sonographic patterns of ovarian tumors: Prediction of malignancy. Obstet Gynecol 1987;69:777-781.

110. Benacerraf BR, Finkler NJ, Wojciechowski C, Knapp RC: Sonographic accuracy in the diagnosis of ovarian masses. J Reprod Med 1990;35:491-495.

111. Granberg S, Norstrom A, Wikland M: Tumors in the lower pelvis as imaged by vaginal sonography. Gynecol Oncol 1990;37:224-229.

112. Sassone AM, Timor-Tritsch IE, Artner A, et al: Transvaginal sonographic characterization of ovarian disease: Evaluation of a new scoring system to predict ovarian malignancy [review]. Obstet Gynecol 1991;78:70-76.

113. Jacobs I, Oram D, Fairbanks J, et al: A risk of malignancy index incorporating CA 125, ultrasound and menopausal status for the accurate preoperative diagnosis of ovarian cancer. Br J Obstet Gynaecol 1990;97:922-929.

114. Davies AP, Jacobs I, Woolas R, et al: The adnexal mass: Benign or malignant? Evaluation of a risk of malignancy index. Br J Obstet Gynaecol 1993;100:927-931.

115. Bourne T, Campbell S, Steer C, et al: Transvaginal colour flow imaging: A possible new screening technique for ovarian cancer. BMJ 1989;299:1367-1370.

116. Weiner Z, Thaler I, Beck D, et al: Differentiating malignant from benign ovarian tumors with transvaginal color flow imaging. Obstet Gynecol 1992;79:159-162.

117. Kawai M, Kano T, Kikkawa F, et al: Transvaginal Doppler ultrasound with color flow imaging in the diagnosis of ovarian cancer. Obstet Gynecol 1992;79:163-167.

118. Yamashita Y, Torashima M, Hatanaka Y, et al: Adnexal masses: Accuracy of characterization with transvaginal US and precontrast and postcontrast MR imaging. Radiology 1995;194:557-565.

119. Manolitsas TP, Fowler JM: Role of laparoscopy in the management of the adnexal mass and staging of gynecologic cancers [review]. Clin Obstet Gynecol 2001;44:495-521.

120. Mage G, Canis M, Manhes H, et al: Laparoscopic management of adnexal cystic masses. J Gynecol Surg 1990;6:71-79.

121. Parker WH, Berek JS: Management of selected cystic adnexal masses in postmenopausal women by operative laparoscopy: A pilot study. Am J Obstet Gynecol 1990;163(Pt 1):1574-1577.

122. Mecke H, Lehmann-Willenbrock E, Ibrahim M, Semm K: Pelviscopic treatment of ovarian cysts in premenopausal women. Gynecol Obstet Invest 1992;34:36-42.
123. Nezhat F, Nezhat C, Welander CE, Benigno B: Four ovarian cancers diagnosed during laparoscopic management of 1011 women with adnexal masses. Am J Obstet Gynecol 1992; 167:790-796.
124. Hulka JF, Parker WH, Surrey MW, Phillips JM: Management of ovarian masses. AAGL 1990 survey. J Reprod Med 1992; 37:599-602.
125. Wenzl R, Lehner R, Husslein P, Sevelda P: Laparoscopic surgery in cases of ovarian malignancies: An Austria-wide survey. Gynecol Oncol 1996;63:57-61.
126. Canis M, Mage G, Pouly JL, et al: Laparoscopic diagnosis of adnexal cystic masses: A 12-year experience with long-term follow-up. Obstet Gynecol 1994;83(Pt 1):707-712.
127. Dottino PR, Levine DA, Ripley DL, Cohen CJ: Laparoscopic management of adnexal masses in premenopausal and post-menopausal women. Obstet Gynecol 1999;93:223-228.
128. Childers JM, Nasseri A, Surwit EA: Laparoscopic management of suspicious adnexal masses. Am J Obstet Gynecol 1996;175:1451-1457, discussion 1457-1459.
129. Canis M, Pouly JL, Wattiez A, et al: Laparoscopic management of adnexal masses suspicious at ultrasound. Obstet Gynecol 1997;89(Pt 1):679-683.
130. Hidlebaugh DA, Vulgaropulos S, Orr RK: Treating adnexal masses: Operative laparoscopy vs. laparotomy. J Reprod Med 1997;42:551-558.
131. Twaalfhoven FC, Peters AA, Trimbos JB, et al: The accuracy of frozen section diagnosis of ovarian tumors. Gynecol Oncol 1991;41:189-192.
132. Obiakor I, Maiman M, Mittal K, et al: The accuracy of frozen section in the diagnosis of ovarian neoplasms. Gynecol Oncol 1991;43:61-63.
133. Mais V, Ajossa S, Piras B, et al: Treatment of nonendometriotic benign adnexal cysts: A randomized comparison of laparoscopy and laparotomy. Obstet Gynecol 1995;86:770-774.
134. Dobronte Z, Wittmann T, Karacsony G: Rapid development of malignant metastases in the abdominal wall after laparoscopy. Endoscopy 1978;10:127-130.
135. Van Dam PA, DeCloedt J, Tjalma WA, et al: Trocar implantation metastasis after laparoscopy in patients with advanced ovarian cancer: Can the risk be reduced? Am J Obstet Gynecol 1999;181:536-541.
136. Leminen A, Lehtovirta P: Spread of ovarian cancer after laparoscopic surgery: Report of eight cases. Gynecol Oncol 1999; 75:387-390.
137. Wang PH, Yuan CC, Chao KC, et al: Squamous ceil carcinoma of the cervix after laparoscopic surgery: A case report. J Reprod Med 1997;42:801-804.
138. Cohn DE, Tamimi HK, Goff BA: Intraperitoneal spread of cervical carcinoma after laparoscopic lymphadenectomy. Obstet Gynecol 1997;89(Pt 2):864.
139. Jacobi CA, Sabat R, Bohm B, et al: Pneumoperitoneum with carbon dioxide stimulates growth of malignant colonic cells. Surgery 1997;121:72-78.
140. Volz J, Koster S, Melchert F: The effects of pneumoperitoneum on intraperitoneal tumor implantation in nude mice. Gynaecol Endosc 1996;5:193-196.
141. Volz J, Koster S, Spacek Z, Paweletz N: The influence of pneumoperitoneum used in laparoscopic surgery on an intra-abdominal tumor growth. Cancer 1999;86:770-774.
142. Canis M, Botchorishvili R, Wattiez A, et al: Cancer and laparoscopy, experimental studies: A review. Eur J Obstet Gynecol Reprod Biol 2000;91:1-9.
143. Kadar N: Laparoscopic management of gynecological malignancies [review]. Curr Opin Obstet Gynecol 1997;9:247-255.
144. Canis M, Botchorishvili R, Manhes H, et al: Management of adnexal masses: Role and risk of laparoscopy. Semin Surg Oncol 2000;19:28-35.
145. Berek JS: Ovarian cancer spread: Is laparoscopy to blame? Lancet 1995;346:200.
146. Trimbos JB, Hacker NF: The case against aspirating ovarian cysts. Cancer 1993;72:828-831.
147. Maiman M, Seltzer V, Boyce J: Laparoscopic excision of ovarian neoplasms subsequently found to be malignant. Obstet Gynecol 1991;77:563-565.
148. Kindermann G, Maassen V, Kuhn W: Laparoscopic preliminary surgery of ovarian malignancies. Experiences from 127 German gynecologic clinics [in German]. Geburtshilfe Frauenheilkd 1995;55:687-694.
149. Lehner R, Wenzl R, Heinzl H, et al: Influence of delayed staging laparotomy after laparoscopic removal of ovarian masses later found malignant. Obstet Gynecol 1998;92:967-971.
150. Vergote I, De Brabanter J, Fyles A, et al: Prognostic importance of degree of differentiation and cyst rupture in stage I invasive epithelial ovarian carcinoma. Lancet 2001;357:176-182.
151. Dembo AJ, Davy M, Stenwig AE, et al: Prognostic factors in patients with stage I epithelial ovarian cancer. Obstet Gynecol 1990;75:263-273.
152. Sevelda P, Dittrich C, Salzer H: Prognostic value of the rupture of the capsule in stage I epithelial ovarian carcinoma. Gynecol Oncol 1989;35:321-322.
153. Sjovall K, Nilsson B, Einhorn N: Different types of rupture of the tumor capsule and the impact on survival in early ovarian carcinoma. Int J Gynecol Cancer 1994;4:333-336.
154. Webb MJ, Decker DG, Mussey E, Williams TJ: Factor influencing survival in stage I ovarian cancer. Am J Obstet Gynecol 1973; 116:222-228.
155. Mayer C, Miller DM, Ehlen TG: Peritoneal implantation of squamous cell carcinoma following rupture of a dermoid cyst during laparoscopic removal. Gynecol Oncol 2002;84: 180-183.
156. McCartney AJ, Johnson N: Using a vaginal tube to exteriorize lymph nodes during a laparoscopic pelvic lymphadenectomy. Gynecol Oncol 1995;57:304-306.
157. Boike GM, Graham JE: Ovarian cancer surgery by operative laparoscopy. Oper Tech Gynecol Surg 1997;2:171-179.
158. FIGO Cancer Committee: Staging announcement. Gynecol Oncol 1986;25:383.
159. Querleu D, LeBlanc E: Laparoscopic infrarenal paraaortic lymph node dissection for restaging of carcinoma of the ovary or fallopian tube. Cancer 1994;73:1467-1471.
160. Scribner DR Jr, Walker JL, Johnson GA, et al: Laparoscopic pelvic and paraaortic lymph node dissection: Analysis of the first 100 cases. Gynecol Oncol 2001;82:498-503.
161. Miller DS, Spirtos NM, Ballon SC, et al: Critical reassessment of second-look exploratory laparotomy for epithelial ovarian carcinoma. Minimal diagnostic and therapeutic value in patients with persistent cancer. Cancer 1992;69:502-510.
162. Nicoletto MO, Tumolo S, Talamini R, et al: Surgical second look in ovarian cancer: A randomized study in patients with laparoscopic complete remission—a Northeastern Oncology Cooperative Group–Ovarian Cancer Cooperative Group Study. J Clin Oncol 1997;15:994-999.
163. Ozols RF, Rubin SC, Thomas G, Robboy S: Epithelial ovarian cancer. In Hoskins WZ, Perez CA, et al (eds): Principles and Practice of Gynecologic Oncology, 2nd ed. Philadelphia, Lippincott-Raven, 1997, pp 919-986.
164. Cain JM, Saigo PE, Pierce VK, et al: A review of second-look laparotomy for ovarian cancer. Gynecol Oncol 1986;23:14-25.
165. Creasman WT: Second-look laparotomy in ovarian cancer [review]. Gynecol Oncol 1994;55(Pt 2):S122-S127.
166. Rubin SC, Hoskins WJ, Hakes TB, et al: Recurrence after negative second-look laparotomy for ovarian cancer: Analysis of risk factors. Am J Obstet Gynecol 1988;159: 1094-1098.
167. Rubin SC, Hoskins WJ, Saigo PE, et al: Prognostic factors for recurrence following negative second-look laparotomy in ovarian cancer patients treated with platinum-based chemotherapy. Gynecol Oncol 1991;42:137-141.
168. Rubin SC, Randall TC, Armstrong KA, et al: Ten-year follow-up of ovarian cancer patients after second-look laparotomy with negative findings. Obstet Gynecol 1999;93:21-22.
169. Ozols RF, Fisher RI, Anderson T, et al: Peritoneoscopy in the management of ovarian cancer. Am J Obstet Gynecol 1981; 140:611-619.
170. Quinn MA, Bishop GJ, Campbell JJ, et al: Laparoscopic follow-up of patients with ovarian carcinoma. Br J Obstet Gynaecol 1980;87:1132-1139.
171. Berek JS, Griffiths CT, Leventhal JM: Laparoscopy for second-look evaluation in ovarian cancer. Obstet Gynecol 1981;58: 192-198.

172. Gadducci A, Sartori E, Maggino T, et al: Analysis of failures after negative second-look in patients with advanced ovarian cancer: An Italian multicenter study. Gynecol Oncol 1998; 68:150-155.

173. Abu-Rustum NR, Barakat RR, Siegel PL, et al: Second-look operation for epithelial ovarian cancer: Laparoscopy or laparotomy? Obstet Gynecol 1996;88(Pt 1):549-553.

174. Casey AC, Farias-Eisner R, Pisani AL, et al: What is the role of reassessment laparoscopy in the management of gynecologic cancers in 1995? Gynecol Oncol 1996;60:454-461.

175. Husain A, Chi DS, Prasad M, Abu-Rustum N, et al: The role of laparoscopy in second-look evaluations for ovarian cancer. Gynecol Oncol 2001;80:44-47.

176. Clough KB, Ladonne JM, Nos C, et al: Second look for ovarian cancer: Laparoscopy or laparotomy? A prospective comparative study. Gynecol Oncol 1999;72:411-417.

177. Fowler JM, Twiggs LB: Applications of laparoscopy in gynecologic oncology. Oper Tech Gynecol Surg 1997;2: 132-137.

178. Janicke F, Holscher M, Kuhn W, et al: Radical surgical procedure improves survival time in patients with recurrent ovarian cancer. Cancer 1992;70:2129-2136.

179. Scarabelli C, Gallo A, Franceschi S, et al: Primary cytoreductive surgery with rectosigmoid colon resection for patients with advanced epithelial ovarian carcinoma. Cancer 2000;88: 389-397.

180. McGuire WP, Hoskins WJ, Brady MF, et al: Cyclophosphamide and cisplatin compared with paclitaxel and cisplatin in patients with stage III and stage IV ovarian cancer. N Engl J Med 1996;334:1-6.

181. Hacker NF, Berek JS, Lagasse LD, et al: Primary cytoreductive surgery for epithelial ovarian cancer. Obstet Gynecol 1983;61:413-420.

182. Piver MS, Lele SB, Marchetti DL, et al: The impact of aggressive debulking surgery and cisplatin-based chemotherapy on progression-free survival in stage III and IV ovarian carcinoma. J Clin Oncol 1988;6:983-989.

183. Potter ME, Partridge EE, Hatch KD, et al: Primary surgical therapy of ovarian cancer: How much and when. Gynecol Oncol 1991;40:195-200.

184. Eisenkop SM, Spirtos NM, Montag TW, et al: The impact of subspecialty training on the management of advanced ovarian cancer. Gynecol Oncol 1992;47:203-209.

185. Schwartz PE, Rutherford TJ, Chambers JT, et al: Neoadjuvant chemotherapy for advanced ovarian cancer: Long-term survival. Gynecol Oncol 1999;72:93-99.

186. Vergote IB, De Wever I, Decloedt J, et al: Neoadjuvant chemotherapy versus primary debulking surgery in advanced ovarian cancer. Semin Oncol 2000;27(Suppl 7):31-36.

187. Vergote I, de Wever I, Tjalma W, et al: Interval debulking surgery: An alternative for primary surgical debulking [review]. Semin Surg Oncol 2000;19:49-53.

188. Nelson BE, Rosenfield AT, Schwartz PE: Preoperative abdominopelvic computed tomographic prediction of optimal cytoreduction in epithelial ovarian carcinoma. J Clin Oncol 1993;11:166-172.

189. Kuhn W, Rutke S, Spathe K, et al: Neoadjuvant chemotherapy followed by tumor debulking prolongs survival for patients with poor prognosis in International Federation of Gynecology and Obstetrics stage IIIC ovarian carcinoma. Cancer 2001; 92:2585-2591.

190. Bristow RE, Duska LR, Lambrou NC, et al: A model for predicting surgical outcome in patients with advanced ovarian carcinoma using computed tomography. Cancer 2000;89: 1532-1540.

191. Chi DS, Venkatraman ES, Masson V, Hoskins WJ: The ability of preoperative serum CA-125 to predict optimal primary tumor cytoreduction in stage III epithelial ovarian carcinoma. Gynecol Oncol 2000;77:227-231.

192. Vergote I, De Wever I, Tjalma W, et al: Neoadjuvant chemotherapy or primary debulking surgery in advanced ovarian carcinoma: A retrospective analysis of 285 patients. Gynecol Oncol 1998;71:431-436.

193. Hughes ES, McDermott FT, Polglase AL, Johnson WR: Tumor recurrence in the abdominal wall scar tissue after large-bowel cancer surgery. Dis Colon Rectum 1983;26:571-572.

194. Reilly WT, Nelson H, Schroeder G, et al: Wound recurrence following conventional treatment of colorectal cancer. A rare but perhaps underestimated problem. Dis Colon Rectum 1996;39:200-207.

195. Stockdale AD, Pocock TJ: Abdominal wall metastasis following laparoscopy: A case report. Eur J Surg Oncol 1985;11:373-375.

196. Hsiu JG, Given FT Jr, Kemp GM: Tumor implantation after diagnostic laparoscopic biopsy of serous ovarian tumors of low malignant potential. Obstet Gynecol 1986;68(Suppl):90S-93S.

197. Miralles RM, Petit J, Gine L, Balaguero L: Metastatic cancer spread at the laparoscopic puncture site: Report of a case in a patient with carcinoma of the ovary. Eur J Gynaecol Oncol 1989;10:442-444.

198. Gleeson NC, Nicosia SV, Mark JE, et al: Abdominal wall metastases from ovarian cancer after laparoscopy. Am J Obstet Gynecol 1993;169:522-523.

199. Shepherd JH, Carter PG, Lowe DG: Wound recurrence by implantation of a borderline ovarian tumour following laparoscopic removal. Br J Obstet Gynaecol 1994;101:265-266.

200. Childers JM, Aqua KA, Surwit EA, et al: Abdominal-wall tumor implantation after laparoscopy for malignant conditions. Obstet Gynecol 1994;84:765-769.

201. Gungor M, Cengiz B, Turan YH, Ortac F: Implantation metastasis of ovarian cancer after third-look laparoscopy. J Pak Med Assoc 1996;46:111-112.

202. Chu HS, Jung NW, Kim JH, et al: Tumor implantation along abdominal trocar site after pelviscopic removal of malignant ovarian tumor—a case report. J Korean Med Sci 1996;11:440-443.

203. Kruitwagen RF, Swinkels BM, Keyser KG, et al: Incidence and effect on survival of abdominal wall metastases at trocar or puncture sites following laparoscopy or paracentesis in women with ovarian cancer. Gynecol Oncol 1996;60:233-237.

204. Hopkins MP, von Gruenigen V, Gaich S: Laparoscopic port site implantation with ovarian cancer. Am J Obstet Gynecol 2000;182:735-736.

205. Morice P, Viala J, Pautier P, et al: Port-site metastasis after laparoscopic surgery for gynecologic cancer: A report of six cases. J Reprod Med 2000;45:837-840.

206. Haughney RV, Slade RJ, Brain AN: An isolated abdominal wall metastasis of ovarian carcinoma ten years after primary surgery. Eur J Gynaecol Oncol 2001;22:102-103.

207. Carlson NL, Krivak TC, Winter WE 3rd, Macri CI: Port site metastasis of ovarian carcinoma remote from laparoscopic surgery for benign disease. Gynecol Oncol 2002;85:529-531.

208. O'Rourke N, Price PM, Kelly S, Sikora K: Tumour inoculation during laparoscopy. Lancet 1993;342:368.

209. Fusco MA, Paluzzi MW: Abdominal wall recurrence after laparoscopic-assisted colectomy for adenocarcinoma of the colon: Report of a case. Dis Colon Rectum 1993;36:858-861.

210. Ramos JM, Gupta S, Anthone GJ, et al: Laparoscopy and colon cancer. Is the port site at risk? A preliminary report. Arch Surg 1994;129:897-899.

211. Cirocco WC, Schwartzman A, Golub RW: Abdominal wall recurrence after laparoscopic colectomy for colon cancer. Surgery 1994;116:842-846.

212. Ziprin P, Ridgway PF, Peck DH, Darzi AW: The theories and realities of port-site metastases: A critical appraisal. J Am Coll Surg 2002;195:395-408.

213. Wang PH, Yuan CC, Lin G, et al: Risk factors contributing to early occurrence of port site metastases of laparoscopic surgery for malignancy. Gynecol Oncol 1999;72:38-44.

214. Kindermann G, Masson V, Kuhn W: Laparoscopic management of ovarian tumors subsequently diagnosed as malignant. J Pelvic Surg 1996;2:245-251.

215. Schaeff B, Paolucci V, Thomopoulos J: Port site recurrences after laparoscopic surgery. A review. Dig Surg 1998;15:124-134.

216. Wang PH, Yen MS, Yuan CC, et al: Port site metastasis after laparoscopic-assisted vaginal hysterectomy for endometrial cancer: Possible mechanisms and prevention. Gynecol Oncol 1997;66:151-155.

217. Muntz HG, Goff BA, Madsen BL, Yon JL: Port-site recurrence after laparoscopic surgery for endometrial carcinoma. Obstet Gynecol 1999;93(Pt 2):807-809.

218. Kadar N: Port-site recurrences following laparoscopic operations for gynaecological malignancies. Br J Obstet Gynaecol 1997;104:1308-1313.

219. Gregor H, Sam CE, Reinthaller A, Joura EA: Port site metastases after laparoscopic lymph node staging of cervical carcinoma. J Am Assoc Gynecol Laparosc 2001;8:591-593.

220. Patsner B, Damien M: Umbilical metastases from a stage IB cervical cancer after laparoscopy: A case report. Fertil Steril 1992;58:1248-1249.

221. Naumann RW, Spencer S: An umbilical metastasis after laparoscopy for squamous cell carcinoma of the cervix. Gynecol Oncol 1997;64:507-509.

222. Lane G, Tay J: Port-site metastasis following laparoscopic lymphadenectomy for adenosquamous carcinoma of the cervix. Gynecol Oncol 1999;74:130-133.

223. Carvalho JP, Souen J, Pinotti JA: Trochar site metastasis after laparoscopic pelvic lymphadenectomy for cervical squamous cell carcinoma. Int J Gynaecol Obstet 1999;67:111-112.

224. Kohlberger PD, Edwards L, Collins C, et al: Laparoscopic port-site recurrence following surgery for a stage IB squamous cell carcinoma of the cervix with negative lymph nodes. Gynecol Oncol 2000;79:324-326.

225. Lavie O, Cross PA, Beller U, et al: Laparoscopic port-site metastasis of an early stage adenocarcinoma of the cervix with negative lymph nodes. Gynecol Oncol 1999;75:155-157.

226. Thomas CG: Tumor cell contamination of the surgical wound: Experimental and clinical observations. Ann Surg 1961;153:697-705.

227. Drouard F, Delamarre J, Capron JP: Cutaneous seeding of gallbladder cancer after laparoscopic cholecystectomy. N Engl J Med 1991;325:1316.

228. Russi EG, Pergolizzi S, Mesiti M, et al: Unusual relapse of hepatocellular carcinoma. Cancer 1992;70:1483-1487.

229. Paolucci V, Schaeff B, Schneider M, Gutt C: Tumor seeding following laparoscopy: International survey. World J Surg 1999;23:989-995, discussion 996-997.

230. Bouvy ND, Marquet RL, Jeekel H, Bonjer HJ: Impact of gas(less) laparoscopy and laparotomy on peritoneal tumor growth and abdominal wall metastases. Ann Surg 1996;224:694-700, discussion 700-7001.

231. Doudle M, King G, Thomas WM, Hewett P: The movement of mucosal cells of the gallbladder within the peritoneal cavity during laparoscopic cholecystectomy. Surg Endosc 1996;10:1092-1094.

232. Allardyce R, Morreau P, Bagshaw P: Tumor cell distribution following laparoscopic colectomy in a porcine model. Dis Colon Rectum 1996;39(Suppl):S47-S52.

233. Thomas WM, Eaton MC, Hewett PJ: A proposed model for the movement of cells within the abdominal cavity during CO_2 insufflation and laparoscopy. Aust N Z J Surg 1996;66:105-106.

234. Allardyce RA, Morreau P, Bagshaw PF: Operative factors affecting tumor cell distribution following laparoscopic colectomy in a porcine model. Dis Colon Rectum 1997;40:939-945.

235. Jewell WR, Romsdahl MM: Recurrent malignant disease in operative wounds not due to surgical implantation from the resected tumor. Surgery 1965;58:806-809.

236. Gertsch P, Baer HU, Kraft R, et al: Malignant cells are collected on circular staplers. Dis Colon Rectum 1992;35:238-241.

237. Rieger N, McIntosh N: Port site metastasis from synchronous primaries of the colon and ovary following laparoscopic cholecystectomy. Eur J Surg Oncol 1998;24:144-145.

238. Lane TM, Cook AJ: Port-site metastasis after laparoscopic cholecystectomy for benign disease. J Laparoendosc Adv Surg Tech A 1999;9:283-284.

239. Ugarte F: Laparoscopic cholecystectomy port seeding from a colon carcinoma. Am Surg 1995;61:820-821.

240. Hubens G, Pauwels M, Hubens A, et al: The influence of a pneumoperitoneum on the peritoneal implantation of free intraperitoneal colon cancer cells. Surg Endosc 1996;10:809-812.

241. Whelan RL, Sellers GJ, Allendorf JD, et al: Trocar site recurrence is unlikely to result from aerosolization of tumor cells. Dis Colon Rectum 1996;39(Suppl):S7-S13.

242. Sellers GJ, Whelan RL, Allendorf JD, et al: An in vitro model fails to demonstrate aerosolization of tumor cells. Surg Endosc 1998;12:436-439.

243. Wittich P, Marquet RL, Kazemier G, Bonjer HJ: Port-site metastases after CO(2) laparoscopy. Is aerosolization of tumor cells a pivotal factor? Surg Endosc 2000;14:189-192.

244. Hansen E, Wolff N, Knuechel R, et al: Tumor cells in blood shed from the surgical field. Arch Surg 1995;130:387-393.

245. Hase K, Ueno H, Kuranaga N, et al: Intraperitoneal exfoliated cancer cells in patients with colorectal cancer. Dis Colon Rectum 1998;41:1134-1140.

246. Lee SW, Southall J, Allendorf J, et al: Traumatic handling of the tumor independent of pneumoperitoneum increases port site implantation rate of colon cancer in a murine model. Surg Endosc 1998;12:828-834.

247. Lee SW, Gleason NR, Bessler M, Whelan RL: Port site tumor recurrence rates in a murine model of laparoscopic splenectomy decreased with increased experience. Surg Endosc 2000;14:805-811.

248. Jacobi CA, Wenger FA, Ordemann J, et al: Experimental study of the effect of intra-abdominal pressure during laparoscopy on tumour growth and port site metastasis. Br J Surg 1998;85:1419-1422.

249. Gutt CN, Kim ZG, Hollander D, et al: CO_2 environment influences the growth of cultured human cancer cells dependent on insufflation pressure. Surg Endosc 2001;15:314-318.

250. Wittich P, Steyerberg EW, Simons SH, et al: Retroperitoneal tumor growth is influenced by pressure of carbon dioxide pneumoperitoneum. Surg Endosc 2000;14:817-819.

251. Ishida H, Murata N, Yokoyama M, et al: The influence of different insufflation pressures during carbon dioxide pneumoperitoneum on the development of pulmonary metastasis in a mouse model. Surg Endosc 2000;14:578-581.

252. Ridgway PF, Smith A, Ziprin P, et al: Pneumoperitoneum augmented tumor invasiveness is abolished by matrix metalloproteinase blockade. Surg Endosc 2002;16:533-536.

253. Dorrance HR, Oien K, O'Dwyer PJ: Effects of laparoscopy on intraperitoneal tumor growth and distant metastases in an animal model. Surgery 1999;126:35-40.

254. Yamaguchi K, Hirabayashi Y, Shiromizu A, et al: Enhancement of port site metastasis by hyaluronic acid under CO_2 pneumoperitoneum in a murine model. Surg Endosc 2001;15:504-507.

255. Jones T, Paraskeva P, Peck DH, Darzi A: Exposure to pneumoperitoneum induces tumor invasiveness via an up-regulation of the urokinase plasminogen activator system [abstract]. Br J Surg 2001;88:735.

256. Schwenk W, Jacobi C, Mansmann U, et al: Inflammatory response after laparoscopic and conventional colorectal resections—results of a prospective randomized trial. Langenbecks Arch Surg 2000;385:2-9.

257. West MA, Hackam DJ, Baker J, et al: Mechanism of decreased in vitro murine macrophage cytokine release after exposure to carbon dioxide: Relevance to laparoscopic surgery. Ann Surg 1997;226:179-190.

258. Neuhaus SJ, Watson DI, Ellis T, et al: Influence of gases on intraperitoneal immunity during laparoscopy in tumor-bearing rats. World J Surg 2000;24:1227-1231.

259. Umpleby HC, Fermor B, Symes MO, Williamson RC: Viability of exfoliated colorectal carcinoma cells. Br J Surg 1984;71:659-663.

260. Franklin ME Jr, Rosenthal D, Abrego-Medina D, et al: Prospective comparison of open vs. laparoscopic colon surgery for carcinoma: Five-year results. Dis Colon Rectum 1996;39(Suppl):S35-S46.

261. Jacobi CA, Peter FJ, Wenger FA, et al: New therapeutic strategies to avoid intra- and extraperitoneal metastases during laparoscopy: Results of a tumor model in the rat. Dig Surg 1999;16:393-399.

262. Neuhaus SJ, Ellis T, Jamieson GG, Watson DI: Experimental study of the effect of intraperitoneal heparin on tumour implantation following laparoscopy. Br J Surg 1999;86:400-404.

263. Jacobi CA, Ordemann J, Bohm B, et al: Inhibition of peritoneal tumor cell growth and implantation in laparoscopic surgery in a rat model. Am J Surg 1997;174:359-363.

264. Hoffstetter W, Ortega A, Chiang M, et al: Effects of topical tumoricidal agents on port-site recurrence of colon cancer: An experimental study in rats. J Laparoendosc Adv Surg Tech A 2001;11:9-12.

265. Eshraghi N, Swanstrom LL, Bax T, et al: Topical treatments of laparoscopic port sites can decrease the incidence of incision metastasis. Surg Endosc 1999;13:1121-1124.

266. Sugarbaker PH, Cunliffe WJ, Belliveau J, et al: Rationale for integrating early postoperative intraperitoneal chemotherapy into the surgical treatment of gastrointestinal cancer. Semin Oncol 1989;16(Suppl 6):83-97.

267. Neuhaus SJ, Watson DI, Ellis T, et al: Wound metastasis after laparoscopy with different insufflation gases. Surgery 1998; 123:579-583.

268. Watson DI, Mathew G, Ellis T, et al: Gasless laparoscopy may reduce the risk of port-site metastases following laparoscopic tumor surgery. Arch Surg 1997;132:166-168, discussion 169.

269. Noguchi H, Shiozawa I, Sakai Y, et al: Pelvic lymph node metastasis of uterine cervical cancer. Gynecol Oncol 1987;27: 150-158.

270. Cabanas RM: Anatomy and biopsy of sentinel lymph nodes. Urol Clin North Am 1992;19:267-276.

271. Veronesi U, Paganelli G, Galimberti V, et al: Sentinel-node biopsy to avoid axillary dissection in breast cancer with clinically negative lymph nodes. Lancet 1997;349:1864-1867.

272. Krag D, Weaver D, Ashikaga T, et al: The sentinel node in breast cancer—a multicenter validation study. N Engl J Med 1998;339:941-946.

273. Malur S, Krause N, Kohler C, Schneider A: Sentinel lymph node detection in patients with cervical cancer. Gynecol Oncol 2001;80:254-257.

274. Levenback C, Coleman RL, Burke TW, et al: Lymphatic mapping and sentinel node identification in patients with cervix cancer undergoing radical hysterectomy and pelvic lymphadenectomy. J Clin Oncol 2002;20:688-693.

275. Dargent D, Martin X, Mathevet P: Laparoscopic assessment of the sentinel lymph node in early stage cervical cancer. Gynecol Oncol 2000;79:411-415.

276. Lantzsch T, Wolters M, Grimm J, et al: Sentinel node procedure in Ib cervical cancer: A preliminary series. Br J Cancer 2001;85:791-794.

277. Verheijen RH, Pijpers R, van Diest PJ, et al: Sentinel node detection in cervical cancer. Obstet Gynecol 2000;96:135-138.

278. Kamprath S, Possover M, Schneider A: Laparoscopic sentinel lymph node detection in patients with cervical cancer. Am J Obstet Gynecol 2000;182:1648.

279. O'Boyle JD, Coleman RL, Bernstein SG, et al: Intraoperative lymphatic mapping in cervix cancer patients undergoing radical hysterectomy: A pilot study. Gynecol Oncol 2000;79: 238-243.

280. Van Trappen PO, Gyselman VG, Lowe DG, et al: Molecular quantification and mapping of lymph-node micrometastases in cervical cancer. Lancet 2001;357:15-20.

281. Stitzenberg KB, Calvo BF, Iacocca MV, et al: Cytokeratin immunohistochemical validation of the sentinel node hypothesis in patients with breast cancer. Am J Clin Pathol 2002;117: 729-737.

282. Dowlatshahi K, Fan M, Snider HC, Habib FA: Lymph node micrometastases from breast carcinoma: Reviewing the dilemma. Cancer 1997;80:1188-1197.

283. Pendas S, Dauway E, Cox CE, et al: Sentinel node biopsy and cytokeratin staining for the accurate staging of 478 breast cancer patients. Am Surg 1999;65:500-505, discussion 505-506.

284. Turner RR, Ollila DW, Stern S, Giuliano AE: Optimal histopathologic examination of the sentinel lymph node for breast carcinoma staging. Am J Surg Pathol 1999;23:263-267.

285. McIntosh SA, Going JJ, Soukop M, et al: Therapeutic implications of the sentinel lymph node in breast cancer. Lancet 1999;354:570.

286. Taback B, Hashimoto K, Kuo CT, et al: Molecular lymphatic mapping of the sentinel lymph node. Am J Pathol 2002; 161:1153-1161.

SYMPTOM MANAGEMENT

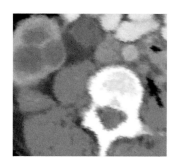

CHAPTER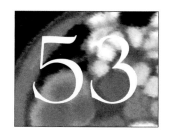

PAIN CONTROL IN PATIENTS WITH GYNECOLOGIC CANCER

J. Norelle Lickiss

 MAJOR CONTROVERSIES

- **What is pain? How does pain relate to pain behavior, to suffering, to human dignity, and to womanhood?**
- **How can pain in a woman with gynecologic cancer be assessed at any phase of her disease and treatment?**
- **How should pain relief be approached, and why are there barriers?**
- **How can reasonable pain relief be ensured for women with gynecologic cancer worldwide? Why do the barriers and inequalities persist?**

In the everyday world, pain is often part of the human condition, especially if cancer complicates the life trajectory. Just as the pain of childbirth can be largely alleviated (despite initial controversy in the 19th century as to whether it was proper to do so), so the pain of women associated with gynecologic cancer can be largely alleviated. Yet pain continues to be experienced—in association with investigations at the time of diagnosis, during and as a result of treatment (surgery, radiotherapy, or chemotherapy), and during periods of relapsing or progressive disease. There is an impressive body of clinical science concerning relief of cancer-related pain,[1-4] as well as material specific for gynecologic cancer.[5,6] Educational interventions can successfully improve cancer pain knowledge and attitudes of health care professionals, but perhaps without much impact on patients' pain levels.[7] Relevant drugs are available, at least in most industrialized nations, yet even in circumstances of affluence patients continue to experience moderate or severe pain.[8,9] Evidence-based guidelines alone have proved inadequate: Carr[10] recently detailed the failure of scientific evidence and guidelines to shift clinicians' attitudes and practices.

The population of patients with cancer pain is heterogeneous. Max and Portenoy[11] listed pain-related, patient-related, and disease-related factors that contribute to the heterogeneity of the population suffering from cancer pain, and warned researchers to take all three types into account. Each patient is unique, and so is the pain experience of each. It is the task of clinicians seeking to relieve the pain experience of a patient to understand as well as possible her unique experience and the place it plays in her life situation.

Controversies with respect to relief of cancer-related pain were outlined by Foley in a classic paper in 1989.[12] Questions still abound in the 21st century, but perhaps with a different focus. This chapter focuses on some of these questions to indicate approaches that may be taken, with the intent to cure or control gynecologic cancer if possible, but at least to relieve the remediable distress associated with this condition.

What is pain? How does pain relate to pain behavior, to suffering, to human dignity, and to womanhood?

More than 2000 years ago, Aristotle described pain as a passion of the soul.[13] Pain was defined by the International Association for the Study of Pain as "an unpleasant sensory and emotional experience associated with actual or potential tissue damage, or described in terms of such damage."[14]

Pain is an experience. It makes little sense to speak of "physical pain" or "psychological pain": pain is an experience of the whole person. Pain is subjective. Only the patient knows the history of her pain, its severity, its location and radiation (if any), the quality of the pain, what increases its severity, and what maneuvers relieve it. For clinicians, the task of understanding all of this is a task of communication.

Pain behavior is not a safe guide to pain severity. More reliable is the patient's own statement of severity (if she can make a statement), codified by the use of validated instruments such as a visual analog scale or numerical rating system. Patients with very severe pain, especially if the pain is chronic (i.e., present for several weeks or longer), may show no external signs of distress but may rate their pain as 8 or 9 on a scale of 10.

Patients with an impaired cognition or communication capacity offer a special challenge. Empathy and keen observation, suspicion, and gentle clinical examination in a "searching" mode, looking for aversive responses, may provide clues to the degree of pain in a patient with severe dementia. This scenario, which is bound to become more common in societies with an aging population, challenges the doctor to make a comprehensive diagnosis of the pain mechanism (and of pain relief), by means of sensitive nonverbal communication techniques and careful, precise drug therapy, often in a context of ethical complexity and emotional distress.

Factors that influence pain behavior (i.e., the patient's expression of pain) may be personal, social, or cultural. If the clinician is to understand a woman's pain experience, the patient herself must be understood. Pain is personal. The following aspects need to be grasped in some way: the patient's current environment (personal, geographical, economic), her history (recent and distant), her cultural and biologic inheritance, and, finally, what she hopes for the present (what she wants to be able to do despite the burden of illness and pain she is bearing). Gradually, as these dimensions are appreciated and taken into a comprehensive assessment, to be combined with adequate clinical examination, investigation, and therapy, pain relief will be facilitated in accord with the patient's priorities.

Pain may be the dominant trigger or an aggravating factor leading to suffering in a woman with gynecologic cancer, or suffering may be centered on other matters, with pain playing a minor part. It is important not to confuse pain with suffering. Cassell[15] formulated an operational definition of suffering as "a sense of impending personal disintegration." Cherny[16] more prosaically define it as "an aversive emotional experience characterized by the perception of personal distress that is generated by adverse factors that undermine quality of life." As Cherny put it, pain is "a phenomenon of conscious human existence." Others have complemented this concept.[17] Schaerer[18] noted also the suffering of a doctor in relation to the deaths of patients, commenting that:

"Suffering is something like crossing a sea, traversing a mountain or a desert; it is an experience, painful indeed, in which the person will become more oneself and will discover oneself; it is an experience in which a person will experience evil, and yet, at the same time, will be led to discover and express the deepest meaning of one's life. This is true also for the suffering of the doctor."

Pain may be well relieved, but the suffering may remain. Medical measures then may (and should) relieve identifiable and treatable components of distress, but suffering, which concerns the human core, may require other measures for its relief—not only psychological interventions[6] but also spiritual dimensions of care.[19]

Suffering is a complex concept; so is human dignity. There is no doubt that unrelieved pain, if it invades consciousness, may compromise at least the expression of dignity, by threatening the cohesiveness of personal activity. Human dignity, in its expression, may be compromised by symptoms and personal circumstances. A woman with gynecologic cancer may be distraught with pain, not only suffering profoundly but also feeling (especially in retrospect) that her dignity has been compromised.

Yet an argument can be sustained that human dignity is intrinsic and that external circumstances cannot wholly delete it. Exploration of dignity appears thus far inadequate in philosophical literature and in the social sciences, yet the notion is fundamental.[20] Levi[21] may have raised this issue most poignantly in the 20th century in his words (about Auschwitz):

Consider if this is a man
Who works in the mud
Who does not know peace
Who fights for a scrap of bread
Who dies because of a yes or no.
Consider if this is a woman,
Without hair and without name,
With no more strength to remember,
Her eyes empty and her womb cold
Like a frog in winter.

Whatever philosophical position may be taken in regard to the concept of human dignity, under all circumstances there is the obligation to ensure relief of severe pain without unnecessarily compromising a patient's other human capacities—her ability to think, to speak, to communicate with those she loves, to stand upright, to explore spiritual issues and the shape of her existential distress, to pray, and to participate in religious ceremony if she wishes—in accord with her uniqueness and irreplaceability. It is startling to realize that a woman undergoing radical treatment for gynecologic cancer in some advanced centers may indeed be "without hair… with no more strength to remember." There is no need for her also to experience unrelieved pain.

Womanhood appears to be especially associated with pain. The pain of childbirth has been a constant presence (however variable its severity, significance, expression, and relief in different times, places, and cultures), and other causes of genital pain abound. Contemporary studies on gender and pain indicate that that females have greater sensitivity to nociceptive stimuli, as well as a higher prevalence of several (nongenital) painful disorders.[22] The field is complex. For example, genetic factors as well as hormonal states may influence responsiveness to opioid drugs. Clinical relevance is as yet unclear, but other factors may be far more relevant to the pain of a woman with gynecologic cancer than genetics or hormones (or even the state of her cancer).

All persons have a threshold for pain, a constellation of factors and circumstances that influence how powerfully a noxious stimulus will give rise to a pain experience, and there is a neurophysiologic basis for this individuality. Pain may be aggravated by factors that affect the pain threshold, and these may relate to a woman's roles as wife or partner, mother, nurturer, caregiver, and lynchpin of a family. Men in most societies have a role as providers, but, despite massive social changes in the last decades, women remain dominant as caregivers even in the Western world. Pain may remind a woman that her role as partner or caregiver is threatened, or it may interfere with her mobility so seriously that she can not fulfill her desired role, precipitating grief. The poignancy of this situation may increase her anxiety or her depression, with consequent worsening of her pain "score." Because of pain, she may feel that her role as a woman in the cohesion of society (in the interlocking of life cycles, the bridging of generations, and the binding together of those in the same generation), is diminished. She may grieve in the face of serious consequences for her family. Actual family disruption may be apparent during extensive treatment directed at cure, as well as during a phase of disease progression; the patient, as mother and central caregiver, may experience anguish because of it, and this may be demonstrated by enhanced pain experience.

How can pain in a woman with gynecologic cancer be assessed at any phase of her disease and treatment?

Assessment remains a crucial step in the path toward pain relief. The assessment of pain is, on one level, simple. There are accepted and validated numerical scales of severity. Publications abound concerning these matters, as usefully reviewed by Caraceni.[23] There are acknowledged pain syndromes that are recognizable by the focused, alert clinician, and a list of syndromes in gynecologic cancer patients is definable.

The views of physicians, nurses, patients, and relatives often differ regarding pain history, characteristics, and severity. It is the patient's view that matters, and the physician needs to understand the pain experience from the patient's point of view. This is really what is entailed by "assessment." Adequate history taking (especially listening to the narrative) and clinical examination, sometimes supplemented by critical investigations, should clarify the mechanisms that most likely are responsible for a patient's pain. Cultural issues, especially in multicultural societies, are being increasingly appreciated. Interpreters, for instance, may be used to diminish language problems.

Why is the assessment process sometimes faulty?

The assessment process involves, first of all, the understanding of a story. The narrative is the diagnostic tool par excellence; the story, if prompted minimally but carefully and listened to attentively, provides information about several of the matters noted previously. The narrative indicates, first, the patient's personal history, against which the pain story is superimposed (with clues to biologic and cultural inheritance), including what stresses she has faced and how she coped with them, as well as her current personal situation and support systems. Second, the narrative should throw light on the history of the pain: how and where it began (and what meaning was laid upon it), how quickly and in what pattern it evolved, how much it began to impinge on other aspects of her life, and what significance she places on the pain. Third, the patient, in her story, can share what clinical interpretations of her pain have been made and by whom, as well as what remedies have been tried and helped, or failed, or gave unacceptable side effects. In the course of listening to the narrative of a patient's cancer saga and concurrent life events, possible pain mechanisms should come to mind and the patient's likely threshold level (high or low) should become apparent. Possible analgesic therapies not yet tried or tried inadequately should also become clear.

The narrative should be followed by relevant clinical examinations, with attention given not only to the whole person but to details concerning possible mechanisms. The site of initial pain and the areas in which it was subsequently felt should be examined carefully. There may be local clues such as palpable tumor, bruising, obvious abscess, or muscle spasm. For example, painful flexion of a hip may indicate psoas spasm as part of the malignant psoas syndrome sometimes caused by retroperitoneal cancer. Attempts to extend the hip in these patients may cause pain (in the absence of hip pathology), and walking is very difficult.

The issue of "back pain" (a relatively meaningless term) is illustrative. Clarity is needed concerning where the pain is felt (spinal or paraspinal), at what level, and with what (if any) radiation. A patient with ovarian cancer and poorly localized back pain who is noted to have a huge supraclavicular mass could well have pain caused solely by enlarged para-aortic nodes—but careful examination of the back to seek for tender areas may reveal sites of pain caused by bony metastases amenable to radiotherapy. Beware of the patient who finds walking difficult because of "back pain": she may well have epidural disease threatening the function of the spinal cord (indicated by equivocal or abnormal plantar reflexes) or cauda equina, and urgent investigation (e.g., magnetic resonance imaging) may be justified. If the patient is well enough for radiotherapy, her mobility may yet be saved. The literature abounds in approaches to spinal cord compression, most stressing the need to suspect the condition long before classic neurologic signs are to be found. The subjective perception of slight power loss or sensory change may be a crucial clue in the absence of any neurologic signs.

How should pain relief be approached, and why are there barriers?

Relief of pain is identified in various studies as a very high priority in patients with cancer, and this is agreed by patients, families, and physicians.[24] However, barriers to pain relief for patients with cancer have been defined,[1] and the literature has been reviewed.[25] Barriers may be related to patients, to physicians, or to institutions, and they need to be understood, as in any task involving navigation toward an identified goal.

Patient-related barriers (apart from any financial considerations) include a patient's reluctance (for many reasons) to report pain, reluctance to follow treatment recommendations, fear of tolerance and addiction, concern about side effects, belief that pain is an inevitable consequence and must be accepted, fear of disease progression, and fear of injections. Family members or friends may share, and therefore reinforce, several of these barriers.

Physician-related barriers relate to inadequate assessment. Demonstrable discrepancy between the patient's and the physician's evaluation of pain severity has been found to be a major predictor of poor pain relief. Knowledge also has been widely found to be deficient. Pain associated with investigative procedures and treatments (surgery, radiotherapy, and chemotherapy) often appears to be poorly relieved and not recognized as worthy of questioning. In addition, physicians may personally share several of the patient-related barriers, although this may be infrequently admitted. Physicians as patients may experience, for many reasons, inadequate pain relief.

Physician-related barriers apply also in instances of poor postoperative pain relief. Despite the advances brought by epidural techniques and patient-controlled analgesia (PCA), the limitations of such procedures must be appreciated. For example, PCA may be inappropriate in the case of a cognitively impaired, anxious or distressed, or very ill patient. Patients going into surgery who are already taking opioid drugs for cancer pain relief require special care to ensure that provision is made for continuing the opioid, unless the surgery in fact removes the major cause for pain entirely (an unusual occurrence).

Institution-related barriers include a tendency to focus almost exclusively on measures designed to cure or control the disease process, with scant attention paid to symptoms such as pain. Flagrant cases of this lack of balance appear to relate not to an uncaring attitude, nor to shortage of time or resources, as much as to difficulty in achieving truly patient-centered rather than tumor-centered care. Clinical leadership is crucial in such matters, but the routine use of pain measurement tools (e.g., vital signs in hospital or clinic charts) may help focus efforts toward recognition of pain relief as an important aspect of care. Institution-related barriers include, in some circumstances, cultural issues and barriers to availability of crucial drugs (see later discussion).

Why these barriers, so clearly defined and documented, still persist is controversial. It may be that they are based on profound issues affecting patients, physicians, and institutions. The so-called myths relating to morphine may illustrate this point and take the discussion further, remembering that myths are human constructions which may embody profound truths.

It is a myth that morphine use may imply imminent death, yet the association is strong in many persons and cultures. Morphine is a reminder of mortality, and denial of the fact of mortality leads to a death-defying approach to antidisease measures, in the name of a life-centered and patient-centered approach. This defiant attitude betrays an inadequate embracing of the human condition as a whole. It is analogous to a music lover's failing to accept that there must be an end to a magnificent symphony, when in fact the end is a crucial part of the pattern, beauty, and core reality of the whole. Failure to grasp the complexity of personhood (and pain is always personal) may be caused by inadequate bridges between medicine and other fields of knowledge and exploration. These issues have been eloquently expressed in the massive and thoughtful report of the U. S. Committee on Care at the End of Life[26] and by individual writers such as Joanne Lynn.[27] Myths concerning the danger of encouraging (or in some countries even permitting) appropriate use of morphine for relief of cancer pain are related to fear of addiction, despite assurances to the contrary by the World Health Organization (WHO).[3] Patients may see symbolic significance in needing a drug to facilitate life and function. There is a streak of independence in many of us, and drugs, however necessary, may be resented. This is particularly true for opioids, because of their emotionally loaded history and their role in drug-related patterns of societal dysfunction. Discussions of such matters may help clarify individual and community attitudes concerning pain relief.

Awareness of all of these barriers is necessary for assessment of patients, but it is even more important in the development of a treatment program. Clearly, the pace of decision-making will be faster in very acute situations, but the principles of cancer pain relief outlined here appear to apply to all situations. A simple approach, which is however in accord with clinical logic, may offer a way through the various controversies about pain and its relief. Over the last decade, a particular approach to the teaching of cancer pain relief has evolved within the Sydney (Australia) Institute of Palliative Medicine, with respect to undergraduates, postgraduates in the West, and doctors in developing countries.[28] Formal evaluation of this educational approach has not been undertaken, but there is indirect evidence that it raises interest in pain relief, enhances competence, and provides a useful conceptual tool (especially for doctors involved in consultation) as a complement to the empiric and well validated WHO ladder. The approach presumes a comprehensive assessment (which may occur in several phases) that takes into account matters stressed earlier in this chapter and includes specific attention to the following: (1) clarifying and reducing noxious stimuli, (2) raising the patient's pain threshold, (3) exploiting the opioid receptor system, and (4) recognizing and treating residual neuropathic pain.

Opioid drugs are only one pharmacologic component of a program for cancer pain relief, but their use continues to remain a matter of controversy. There is extensive recent literature on morphine and alternative opioids.[29-34] Opioid "rotation" or "switching" (a change in the strong opioid being used) may occasionally be of benefit, but change should be undertaken with care and only for good reason. A consensus is emerging as to how and when to undertake such changes.[35] Physicians should not raise the anxiety level of nursing staff, family practitioners, and caregivers, as well as the patient, by unnecessarily introducing an unfamiliar drug. Changing the route of delivery of opioids to a spinal system of delivery is occasionally of benefit to patients with gynecologic cancer, but controversy continues regarding the circumstances in which spinal opioids should be considered.[36]

Controversy also continues concerning the wisdom or necessity of using stimulant drugs such as methylphenidate to ameliorate opioid-induced somnolence.[37] Such somnolence may in fact be evidence of opioid misuse, and particularly of poor dose calibration.

A clinical challenge is presented by the patient who is taking locally acting drugs such as paracetamol or nonsteroidal anti-inflammatory agents, with opioid carefully calibrated up to the level of drowsiness, yet without relief of pain. One of the causes of this combination is so-called morphine-nonresponsive pain, or morphine–partially-responsive pain. Opioid drugs, which alleviate pain by complex methods not wholly understood, do appear to be sometimes only partially effective in relieving pain resulting from certain mechanisms, including pain caused by nerve irritation or nerve injury (neuropathic pain).

There is an extensive evidence base regarding drugs that are effective for neuropathic pain.[38-41] In practice, the choice of drugs may be influenced by the nature of the residual pain. If the residual is clearly flashing and knifelike, a corticosteroid or anticonvulsant agent may be preferred, with the knowledge that improvement is likely within 24 hours or less; but if dysesthesia dominates, antidepressants should be introduced. Selection may also be influenced by the likelihood and gravity of drug side effects in a particular patient. For example, steroids may be withheld in a diabetic patient, or in any patient until the extent and significance of infection is clarified and addressed.

The use of steroids in palliative care, including pain relief, is difficult and controversial.[42] The institution of corticosteroids such as dexamethasone when other measures are readily available is not to be encouraged, because corticosteroid therapy, especially if long continued, has side effects that may mitigate against the quality of life for patients. If corticosteroid therapy is used to the level at which cushingoid features appear, then distressing body image changes may reduce

quality of life. Furthermore, steroid therapy can aggravate infection or diabetes and may induce emotional changes that are either out of character with the previous personality or somehow dissonant in the whole context. Very rarely, patients develop serious emotional consequences such as inappropriate euphoria or depression; the risk of this complication may be suggested by the patient's narrative. Steroid therapy in the context of palliative care should be precise, targeted, evaluated, and discontinued if not proving effective. With these provisos, it is true that corticosteroid therapy can be very valuable in the treatment of neuropathic pain. These drugs should be used at the lowest dose necessary to achieve effect (e.g., dexamethasone 4 mg mane for a few days, then reduced by 2 mg daily or every second day).

Pain therapy, like diabetes therapy, requires continuous vigilance and evaluation. Pain relief is achievable for most of the time, in most patients with cancer, by careful use of the measures described earlier. From time to time, it may be necessary to explore and reconsider further options for therapy by working through the process starting at the beginning again. However, in a small minority of patients some problems do arise. Even more rarely, in possibly 1% of patients at some stage in the course of their cancer, the pain may prove to be refractory to the measures outlined previously. It is mandatory to get assistance from doctors who are experienced in cancer pain management and palliative care under such circumstances.

Evaluation of pain relief is an interesting and clinically significant intellectual task. While trying to assess and measure the level of global relief with the use of validated tools, it is important to delineate the features of what pain is *not* adequately relieved. For example, in a mixed-pain situation, are all the neuropathic features still remaining and clearly unmodified? Or is the burning element in the pain the most obstinate feature? If so, could sympathetically maintained pain be contributing? If such a diagnosis is sustained, relevant therapeutic alternatives exist (e.g., sympathetic blockade). This analytic approach is maintained not only on first assessment but also on all subsequent assessments.

Although extensive reviews of the evidence for efficacy of various drugs for pain have been published, controversy continues in practice concerning which drug or drugs to use in an individual patient. Factors that require consideration include not only evidence of efficacy, availability, cost, and interaction with other drugs in patients with multiple morbidities but also emotional factors. Some patients and families need much counseling and support before morphine is acceptable, especially in ethnic groups in which morphine myths abound. In such circumstances, a strong opioid other than morphine (e.g., oxycodone) may be chosen for the present, with the knowledge that the added flexibility of morphine may be more wisely used in the future, by which time trust may be established in the course of extensive family counseling and support.

Evidence-based medicine is crucial, when adequately understood,[43] but some limitations must be recognized.

One should keep in mind the following provisos relevant to the field of pain relief for women with gynecologic cancer:

- The context of clinical decision-making in which pain relief is being sought is complex and involves cultural, psychological, and social issues, as well as medical facts such as conclusions concerning evidence.
- Each woman's pain is rooted in a unique set of subjective meanings and a unique stance in her life trajectory. The vast array of pain patterns ensures heterogeneity defying reductionism.
- Not all that is known is published, and not all that is published is readily available or in a form amenable to analysis by current methodologies. This is true of all searches for evidence-based clarity in medicine, but it is especially true of pain. In fact, well-focused publications are sparse.

Despite some controversial points, and provided a minimal set of drugs is available, enough is known to ensure good relief from most of the severe pain endured by women with gynecologic cancer, throughout the entire disease trajectory. The question is not what should be done, but why is it not accomplished? The foregoing explorations have indicated the profundity of some of the issues, but at a global level there exists another set of controversies.

How can reasonable pain relief be ensured for women with gynecologic cancer worldwide? Why do the barriers and inequalities persist?

In many countries, a woman with pain related to cancer of the cervix (which is a common affliction and cause of death in the less industrialized nations) can obtain no strong opioid as part of her analgesic regimen: she must die in unrelieved pain—and expects to do so. Data from WHO, the International Narcotics Review Board (INCB), and associated experts continue to demonstrate that, although global morphine use for pain has risen sharply over the last two decades, it has done so almost entirely in Western, affluent countries. With some laudable exceptions, there is a persisting gross global imbalance. Massive efforts have been undertaken to ensure that morphine is available on request, and the drug, at least in immediate-release form, is cheap.[44,45]

Barriers to the use of morphine for pain relief in less industrialized countries include the following:

- The legacy of the opium wars
- Fears that Western values may be imparted with encouragement of the medical use of opioids
- Fears about addiction if medical use is permitted, despite evidence to the contrary
- The conviction that morphine is not needed: "Our women do not feel pain as Western women do"
- Greater importance given to other health priorities on the political agenda

Some of these profound issues are spiritual and philosophical, and they are felt keenly by key persons in developing countries. Questions such as the following may be unspoken, or rarely articulated:

1. Does the adoption of the WHO strategy for cancer pain relief run the risk of damaging the spiritual fabric of our society, destroying our way of thinking about the meaning of life, of suffering, of death?
2. When we are so short of resources, why should we spend time, money, and trouble on pain treatment for those who can no longer work, instead of trying to cure more people?
3. Why is cancer pain relief still so poor in the West, even in prestigious cancer centers?

These matters need discussion—in situations of trust, and in an atmosphere of partnership. It is essential that those seeking to introduce the WHO approach to pain relief be deeply aware of the personal, cultural, and spiritual context into which this new mode of thinking is to be introduced. The beneficial outcome for patients and families is so significant that it may be the key tool for change: like leaven in dough, the change must come from within the community. However, wise leadership from senior administrators and clinicians in partnership with the community can have dramatic consequences, and there have been documented advances.

The eradication of malaria may have failed on a worldwide scale, not because of lack of knowledge, but because of some poorly understood psychological and social factors impeding local implementation of well-researched technology. The challenge now in achieving better levels of global cancer pain relief is a more appropriate understanding of the psychological matrix within which the means to relieve that pain must operate. It is essential to be aware of the total ecological matrix—with its historical, social, economic, psychological, and spiritual components—if cancer pain relief is to be achieved. In some respects, psychological and spiritual development in certain developing countries is far in advance of the rest of the globe, and there is a need for all to recognize exchange-in-partnership as the most promising means of advance for the next century.

In summary, the approach to improving pain relief for women with gynecologic cancer in the developing countries involves the following elements[46]:

- National, state, and local drug policies to ensure adequate supplies of appropriate essential drugs for persons in need
- Education of health professionals and the community with respect to the advantages and possibility of pain relief and the strategies for achieving it
- Careful and sensitive study of the relevant spiritual traditions, values, and practices within each country and subculture
- Recognition of the ethical requirements that cancer pain relief and palliative care be given high priority, be part of mainstream cancer care, and reflect recognition of the value of each woman in the last phase of life (regardless of social circumstances)

- Reasonable goals, including both process measures (e.g., drug availability, education, procedures for drug distribution) and outcome measures (i.e., measured pain relief)
- Dreams: aspiration, not regulation, is the key to rapid human progress. How soon can we achieve relief of severe cancer pain for all?

All of these components are essential so that health professionals, both in the policy arena and at the grass roots of health care, will understand not only the technical aspects but also the cultural and spiritual significance of new approaches to the patient experiencing pain. This includes the need for recognition (not hiding) of the pain and the obligation to relieve relievable distress without denying the precious values forming the fabric of society. Cancer pain relief, and palliative care in general, give expression to compassion, which is one of the basic values within all human societies.

There are controversies indeed regarding adequate relief of the pain so often associated with gynecologic cancer. But controversy may be the stuff of progress. The issues raised concern the human condition, in which physicians as well as patients are participants.

REFERENCES

1. Foley KM: Pain assessment and cancer pain syndromes. In Doyle D, Hanks GW, Macdonald N (eds): Oxford Textbook of Palliative Medicine. Oxford, Oxford University Press, 1998, pp 310-331.
2. Ad Hoc Committee on Cancer Pain of the American Society of Clinical Oncology: Cancer pain assessment and treatment curriculum guidelines. J Clin Oncol 1992;10:1976-1982.
3. World Health Organization: Cancer Pain Relief, 2nd ed. Geneva, World Health Organization, 1995.
4. Ripamonti C, Dickerson ED: Strategies for the treatment of cancer pain in the new millennium [review]. Drugs 2001;61:955-977.
5. Gordin V, Weaver MA, Hahn MB: Acute and chronic pain management in palliative care. Best Pract Res Clin Obstet Gynaecol 2001;15:203-234.
6. Olt GJ: Managing pain and psychological issues in palliative care. Best Pract Res Clin Obstet Gynaecol 2001;15:235-251.
7. Allard P, Maunsell E, Labbe J, Dorval M: Educational interventions to improve cancer pain control: A systematic review. J Palliat Med 2001;4:191-203.
8. Foley KM: Pain relief into practice: Rhetoric without reform. J. Clin Oncol 1995;13:2149-2151.
9. Resnik DB, Rehm M, Minard RB: The undertreatment of pain: Scientific, clinical, cultural, and philosophical factors. Med Health Care Philos 2001;4:277-288.
10. Carr DB: The development of national guidelines for pain control: Synopsis and commentary. Eur J Pain 2001;5(Suppl A):91-98.
11. Max MB, Portenoy RK: Pain research: Designing clinical trials in palliative care. In Doyle D, Hanks GW, Macdonald N (eds): Oxford Textbook of Palliative Medicine. Oxford, Oxford University Press, 1998, pp 173-174.
12. Foley KM: Controversies in cancer pain: Medical perspectives. Cancer 1989;63:2257-2265.
13. Twycross R: Pain Relief in Advanced Cancer. London, WB Saunders, 1994.
14. IASP Subcommittee on Taxonomy: Pain terms: A list with definitions and notes on usage. Pain 1980;8:249-252.
15. Cassell E: The Nature of Suffering and the Goals of Medicine. Oxford, Oxford University Press, 1991.
16. Cherny N. The treatment of suffering in patients with advanced cancer. In Chochinov HM, Breitbart W (eds): Handbook of

17. Chapman RC, Gavrin J: Suffering and its relationship to pain. J Palliat Care 1993;9:5-13.
18. Schaerer R: Suffering of the doctor linked with the death of patients. Palliat Med 1993;7(Suppl 1):27-37.
19. Kearney M, Mount B: Spiritual care of the dying patient. In Chochinov HM, Breitbart W (eds): Handbook of Psychiatry in Palliative Medicine. Oxford, Oxford University Press, 2000, pp 357-373.
20. Street A, Kissane D: Constructions of dignity in end of life care. J Palliat Care 2001;17:93-101.
21. Levi P: If this is a man [trans. Stuart Woolf]. London: The Folio Society, 2000.
22. Stones RW: Female genital pain. In Fillingim RB (ed): Progress in Pain Research and Management. Vol. 17. Sex, Gender and Pain. Seattle, IASP Press, 2001, pp 355-369.
23. Caraceni A: Evaluation and assessment of cancer pain and cancer pain treatment. Acta Anaesthesiol Scand 2001;45:1067-1075.
24. Steinhauser KE, Christakis N, Clipp EC, et al: Factors considered important at the end of life by patients, family, physicians, and other care providers. JAMA 2000;284:2476-2482.
25. Pargeon KL, Hailey BJ: Barriers to effective cancer pain management: A review of the literature. J Pain Symptom Manage 1999;18:358-368.
26. Field MJ, Cassel C (eds): Approaching death: Improving care at the end of life. Report of Committee on Care at the End of Life. Washington, DC, US Institute of Medicine National Academy Press, 1997.
27. Lynn J (ed): Handbook for Mortals: Guidance for People Facing Serious Illness. Oxford, Oxford University Press, 1999.
28. Lickiss JN: Approaching cancer pain relief. Eur J Pain 2001;5(Suppl A):5-14.
29. Lesage P, Portenoy RK: Trends in cancer pain management. Cancer Control 1999;6:136-145.
30. Donnelly S, Davis MP, Walsh D, Naughton M: Morphine in cancer pain management: A practical guide. Support Care Cancer 2000;10:13-35.
31. Sarhill N, Walsh D, Nelson KA: Hydromorphone: Pharmacology and clinical applications in cancer patients. Support Care Cancer 2000;9:84-96.
32. Davis MP, Walsh D: Methadone for relief of cancer pain: A review of pharmacokinetics, pharmacodynamics, drug interactions and protocols of administration. Support Care Cancer 2001;9:73-83.
33. Cairns R: The use of oxycodone in cancer-related pain: A literature review. Int J Palliat Nursing 2001;11:522-527.
34. Loitman JE: Transmucosal fentanyl in ovarian cancer. J Pain Symptom Manage 2002;23:5-7.
35. Indelicato RA, Portenoy RK: Opioid rotation in the management of refractory cancer pain. J Clin Oncol 2002;20:348-352.
36. Mercandante S: Controversies over spinal treatment in advanced cancer patients [review]. Support Care Cancer 1998;6:495-502.
37. Rozans M, Dreisbach A, Lertora JJL, Kahn MJ: Palliative uses of methyphenidate in patients with cancer: A review. J Clinical Oncol 2002;20:335-339.
38. Farrar JT, Portenoy RK: Neuropathic cancer pain: The role of adjuvant analgesics. Oncology (Huntingt) 2001;15:1435-1442.
39. Katz N: Neuropathic pain in cancer and AIDS. Clin J Pain 2000;16(2 Suppl):S41-S48.
40. Rigor BM: Pelvic cancer pain. J Surg Oncol 2000;75:280-300.
41. Wiffen P, McQuay H, Carroll D, et al: Anticonvulsant drugs for acute and chronic pain. Cochrane Database of Systematic Reviews 2000;(2):CD001133.
42. Mercadante S, Fulfaro F, Casuccio A: The use of corticosteroids in home palliative care. Support Care Cancer 2001;9:386-389.
43. Parker M: Whither our art? Clinical wisdom and evidence-based medicine. Med Health Care Philos 2002;5:273-280.
44. Stjernsward J, Colleau SM, Ventafridda V: The World Health Organization Cancer Pain and Palliative Care Program. J Pain Symptom Manage 1996;12:65-72.
45. Stewart BW, Kleihues P (eds): WHO Cancer Report. Lyon, International Agency for Research on Cancer, 2002.
46. Lickiss JN: Cancer pain relief in "developing" countries. Proceedings of the International Working Group on National Cancer Control Programs, 1996 April 28, Sydney, Australia.

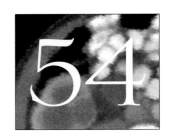

MANAGEMENT OF INTESTINAL OBSTRUCTION IN THE TERMINAL PATIENT AND MANAGEMENT OF ASCITES

Christina S. Chu   and   Stephen C. Rubin

 MAJOR CONTROVERSIES

- **What defines a successful outcome in the treatment of a terminal patient with bowel obstruction?**
- **How does the physician choose between surgical and medical management of bowel obstruction?**
- **What are the surgical options for management, and which patients are good candidates for surgery?**
- **What are the medical options for management?**
- **When is total parenteral nutrition appropriate?**
- **What are the management options for intractable ascites?**

Most patients suffering from ovarian cancer present with advanced disease, and although first-line combination chemotherapy with paclitaxel and platinum-based agents may result in a greater than 70% response rate, most patients ultimately relapse and die of chemotherapy-resistant disease. Because of the tendency of ovarian cancer to spread throughout the abdominal cavity, many patients eventually develop intestinal obstruction.[1] Obstructive symptoms often herald disease progression that results in tumor encasement of the bowel and mesentery, with accompanying alterations of peristalsis, malabsorption, and malnutrition.[2-4]

Because bowel obstruction is a common occurrence in the patient with ovarian cancer, its management has been the focus of much time and attention. Several investigators have reported the incidence of bowel obstruction to range from 5% to 51%.[5-13] One series from the Mayo Clinic included 1295 patients with ovarian cancer undergoing surgery over a 10-year period. Overall, 25% underwent surgery with the indication of intestinal obstruction; 14% were patients experiencing primary surgery, and 34% had surgery for recurrence or palliation.[14] Rubin and colleagues[15] reported that most intestinal surgery for obstruction performed on a gynecologic service is done in patients with ovarian cancer. At the Universities of Milan and Brescia, 79% of intestinal surgery done by gynecologic oncologists was performed on ovarian cancer patients.[16]

A thorough understanding of the causes of intestinal obstruction is necessary to better assess therapeutic options. Bowel obstruction in patients with ovarian cancer may occur through several different mechanisms. Extrinsic occlusion may result from compression by tumor, radiation fibrosis, or postoperative adhesions.[17] Intraluminal occlusion may occur because of annular tumor penetration of the bowel wall.[18] Intestinal motility may also be decreased, causing functional obstruction.[19] Tumor infiltration of the mesentery, retroperitoneal nerve plexuses, bowel muscle or nerves may also promote obstruction.[18,20] The cause is often multifactorial, with bowel inflammation and edema, fecal impaction, and motility-slowing medications all playing contributing roles.[17]

Because most episodes of obstruction are caused by progression of tumor, patients with advanced-stage disease appear more likely to develop bowel obstruction. On average, 12.8% of patients with stage I disease, 15.2% with stage II, 28.0% with stage III, and 30.7% with stage IV disease developed bowel obstruction in two series.[19,21] Along similar lines, Tunca and coworkers[19] reported that patients presenting with advanced stages of disease develop obstruction more rapidly. Among 127 patients with ovarian cancer developing bowel obstruction over an 8-year period at the University of Wisconsin, the median time to obstruction was 332 days from diagnosis for patients with stage I and II disease, 181 days for stage III, and only 72.5 days for stage IV.

Not all intestinal obstruction occurring in ovarian cancer patients is caused by tumor progression. Postoperative adhesions and radiation injury, particularly in older series, are common culprits. A review from Singapore of 92 women with gynecologic malignancies revealed that 31 (34%) suffered from obstruction with a benign cause.[22] Among 26 ovarian cancer patients with radiologically confirmed bowel obstruction undergoing surgery in Birmingham, United Kingdom, 6 (23%) had obstructions unrelated to tumor.[23] Four patients suffered from adhesions, one from radiation stricture, and one from a concurrent ileal carcinoid. Clarke-Pearson and associates[24] examined 49 patients with ovarian cancer undergoing surgery for bowel obstruction. For 33 (67%) patients, ovarian cancer was determined to be the sole cause of the obstruction; for 9 (18%), a combination of cancer and radiation injury was felt to be the cause; and in 7 (14%), obstruction was determined to be a result of benign adhesions or radiation injury alone. Understanding the source of an individual patient's obstruction is key to deciding appropriate therapy. Patients whose symptoms are due to benign disease represent a subset of patients who may potentially benefit from more aggressive surgical intervention.

Location and extent of obstruction may be an important factor when contemplating therapy. In a review of eight series in which site of obstruction could be determined in 420 patients, 54.0% of obstruction was isolated to the small intestine and 31.7% to the large intestine. A significant proportion of patients, 14.3%, suffered from points of obstruction in the large and small intestine.[1,19,21,23-27] Obstruction of the stomach and duodenum appears to be uncommon and is often not discussed in large series of patients with

bowel obstruction in the setting of ovarian cancer. Three case reports[28-30] have documented seven patients with gastric outlet obstruction caused by extrinsic tumor compression or loculated ascites. The patients were treated by various methods, including surgical bypass and drainage of ascites by laparotomy and percutaneously. In one larger series from Leeds, United Kingdom, 11 patients with symptomatic gastroduodenal obstruction were identified from 438 women with ovarian cancer in a 3-year period.[31] They were treated with various regimens, including surgery, percutaneous drainage, and chemotherapy. Only those with obstruction caused by loculated ascites in the lesser sac achieved palliation and longer-term survival. The others died at a median of 5 months after developing symptoms.

Bowel obstruction related to ovarian cancer rarely presents as an acute event or as a surgical emergency.[19] Patients' symptoms depend on the location and extent of gastrointestinal tract involvement. Patients commonly experience nausea and vomiting, distention, borborygmi, anorexia, and overflow diarrhea. Although patients typically present with colicky pain, more than 90% may report constant abdominal pain.[32,33] Despite these symptoms, patients are usually alert and present with relatively normal function of other major organ systems.[34] Initial therapy usually involves admission to the hospital and support with intravenous fluids and gastric drainage. Although some early cases may resolve spontaneously, most persist or recur,[20] and sustained response rates are low (1% to 15%).[35] With rare exceptions, these patients cannot be cured of their tumors.[36] After the diagnosis of bowel obstruction, survival is short.[2] Almost all ovarian cancer patients die within a year of the diagnosis of bowel obstruction, and most live less than 6 months.[37] Gadducci and colleagues[18] reviewed 34 patients with bowel obstruction in the setting of progressive ovarian cancer at the University of Pisa; 22 underwent surgery, and 12 were treated medically. They reported the median time from diagnosis of obstruction to death was only 65.5 days, although the range was 15 to 699 days. For most patients, obstruction presages imminent demise. However, this prognosis is not uniform, and a proportion of patients may experience long-term survival after appropriate intervention. Several factors are important for the physician contemplating treatment options. Treatment decisions must take into consideration the patient's overall medical condition, the extent of tumor present, what antitumor therapy has already been employed, and what options, if any, remain.

For the terminal patient, in light of these issues, what is considered a realistic goal to strive for? Is the problem better managed medically or surgically? What factors can help identify a patient who is likely to experience a successful outcome? When is parenteral nutrition indicated? In this chapter, we hope to examine some of these issues and to highlight particular controversies in the management of bowel obstruction and ascites in the terminal patient.

What defines a successful outcome in the treatment of a terminal patient with bowel obstruction?

To make informed decisions, the patient and physician must have a realistic awareness of the benefits that can result from a given intervention. Successful surgical outcomes have been defined in various ways by different investigators. In the simplest terms, outcome has been examined based on postoperative survival.[23,24,38] In a study conducted in Los Angeles, California, Castaldo and coworkers[39] used postoperative survival of 2 months or longer as their measure of success. This definition was adopted by Krebs and Goplerud[40] at the Medical College of Virginia and used to develop their prognostic scoring index. Although survival is an objective, easy-to-measure variable, the benefit of survival alone as an outcome variable may be questionable if the patient remains obstructed and bedridden in the hospital until death[41] or if intervention causes complications to hasten the patient's demise.

Rubin and associates[1] in New York defined successful palliation of obstruction as discharge from the hospital with the patient able to eat a regular or low-residue diet. Lund and colleagues[27] from Denmark chose instead to examine survival greater than 60 days without symptoms of partial or complete obstruction. Jong and coworkers[41] from the University of Toronto used survival, return home, and relief of obstructive symptoms for longer than 60 days postoperatively. Although these are more restrictive definitions, the investigators made an attempt to account for quality as well as quantity of life.

Because medical interventions for bowel obstruction are diverse, successful palliation has been defined in many ways. Investigators have examined survival[19,23,38,42,43] and obstruction-free survival,[25] but more often, quality of life issues are used as outcome measures. Although formal instruments to measure quality of life have not been employed, investigators have retrospectively examined parameters such as subjective quality of life[44] and more specific factors such as physical and psychological well-being, social interactions, and work or travel ability after institution of home total parenteral nutrition (TPN).[43] Studies of gastric drainage tubes[20,45-48] and pharmacologic strategies[49,50] typically explore relief of symptoms such as nausea, vomiting, and pain, the ability to return home, and the ability to tolerate oral liquids or soft food.

How does the physician choose between surgical and medical management of bowel obstruction?

The decision to approach bowel obstruction surgically or medically in the terminal patient can be problematic. Surgical options have proved to be of value for some patients in nonrandomized, retrospective studies. In series by Rubin and colleagues[1] from New York and Pecorelli and coworkers[16] from Italy, up to 71% to 79% of patients with disease that can be surgically corrected may achieve relief of symptoms and return to adequate oral intake. However, there are no randomized trials comparing surgery with nonsurgical management, nor are there likely any to be conducted in the future. Table 54-1 summarizes the surgical and medical management results from several series.

Several retrospective studies have attempted to compare medical and surgical treatment schemes. Some have shown no difference in survival outcome. Fernandes and associates[51] from Montreal described 62 patients with concomitant ovarian cancer and bowel obstruction. For the 28 patients treated medically (i.e., nasogastric suction, intravenous fluids, antiemetics, and analgesics), the mean 1-year survival rate was 32%, compared with 35% for the 34 surgically treated patients. This difference was not statistically significant. These results are somewhat surprising given that the investigators stated that patients allocated to surgical treatment were more likely to be considered to have a good prognosis and that the study included some patients whose bowel obstruction was the initial presenting sign of their ovarian cancer and were therefore more likely to undergo surgery. Similarly, Larson and colleagues[38] at the Pennsylvania State University examined 14 patients undergoing nonsurgical compared with 19 patients undergoing surgical intervention (i.e., bypass or colostomy, or both, with or without gastrostomy). Median survival was not statistically different at 92 and 102 days, respectively, and surgical intervention incurred an associated operative mortality of 15.8%. The investigators commented that the patients undergoing medical treatment were in worse condition that the patients undergoing surgery, but this bias seemed to be offset by the operative mortality incurred. Lund and coworkers[27] from Copenhagen reported no statistically significant difference in median survival between 16 medically and 25 surgically treated patients (30 versus 68 days). Only 32% of the surgically managed patients achieved successful palliation, defined by the investigators as survival greater than 60 days with total palliation of symptoms. The reported surgical mortality rate was 32%, with an overall complication rate of 64%.

Some studies have reported an improvement in outcome for patients treated surgically. In the study conducted by Tunca and associates,[19] patients deemed inoperable survived an average of 64 days, compared with an average survival of 212 days for those treated surgically, a statistically significant difference. Redman and colleagues[23] compared 12 patients treated medically with 26 patients treated surgically. The median survival of patients who underwent surgery (81 days) was significantly longer than those who did not (30 days). The operative mortality rate was 15%, and major morbidity was observed in 42% of patients. The results of these studies must be interpreted with caution because of the inherent selection bias toward treating more favorable patients surgically. One study by

Table 54–1. Surgical and Medical Management of Intestinal Obstruction in Ovarian Cancer

Study	Number of Patients	Corrected by Surgery	Relief of Obstruction	Survival
Castaldo et al.[39]	23 surgery	100%		80% at 2 mo, 17% at 12 mo
Tunca et al.[19]	90 surgery	100%		Mean, 7.0 mo
	37 no surgery			Mean, 2.1 mo
Piver et al.[2]	60 total surgery:	82%		Median, 2.5 mo
	49 surgical correction			Median, 2.0 mo
	and 11 exploratory only			
Krebs and Goplerud[40]	118 total surgery:	88%		Median, 3.1 mo
	104 surgical correction			All <1 mo
	and 14 exploratory			
Solomon et al.[21]	21 total surgery:	95%		Mean, 8.1 mo
	20 surgical correction			
	and 1 exploratory only			
Clarke-Pearson et al.[24]	49 surgery	100%		Median, 4.7 mo
Fernandes et al.[51]	34 surgery			35%*
	28 no surgery			32%*
Redman et al.[23]	26 total surgery:	92%		Median, 2.7 mo
	24 surgical correction			
	and 2 exploratory only			
Rubin et al.[1]	54 total surgery:	80%	63%	Mean, 5.8 mo
	43 surgical correction		79%	Mean, 6.8 mo
	and 11 exploratory only		0%	Mean, 1.8 mo
Beattie et al.[58]	11 surgery	100%	64%†	Mean, 5.7 mo
	32 no surgery		37%	Mean, 3.1 mo
Lund et al.[27]	25 total surgery:	76%	32%	Median, 2.3 mo
	19 surgical correction		44%	Median, 1.0 mo
	and 6 exploratory only		12%‡	
	16 no surgery			
Larson et al.[38]	19 surgery	100%		Median, 3.4 mo
	14 no surgery			Median, 3.1 mo
Zoetmulder et al.[25]	30 surgery	100%	60%§	Median, 4 mo¶
	28 no surgery		43%	Median, 1 mo¶
Pecorelli et al.[16]	147 total surgery:	80%	56%	Mean, 7.2 mo
	117 surgical correction		71%	Mean, <2 mo
	and 30 exploratory only			
Jong et al.[41]	53 surgery	100%	53%	Median, 2.9 mo

*Estimated 1-year survival probability.
†Includes three patients who presented with bowel obstruction at the time of initial diagnosis.
‡Relief of symptoms for 2 to 3 weeks, then recurrence.
§Includes eight patients who presented with bowel obstruction at the time of initial diagnosis.
¶Median obstruction-free survival.

Zoetmulder and coworkers[25] from the Netherlands attempted to compare surgical and medical treatment after retrospectively dividing patients into poor and favorable prognostic groups. Patients were deemed to have a favorable prognosis if they had no prior treatment for their cancer or if the interval from last treatment to obstruction was longer than 6 months and no ascites was present. Overall results demonstrated a significant difference in median obstruction-free survival of 1 month for those treated medically, compared with 4 months for those treated surgically ($P = .024$). However, when analysis was performed for patients with favorable prognoses, surgery had a only a "marginally significant positive effect" on obstruction-free survival when compared with nonsurgical management, with a P value of .052, which may be interpreted by some as no true difference. Surgical and medical treatments were equivalent in the poor-prognosis group.

Because, with rare exceptions, these patients cannot be cured of their cancer, the potential benefits of any procedure must be balanced against the significant morbidity and mortality associated with major abdominal surgery in this setting, particularly when obstruction may persist[32] or recur[52] in a significant number of patients even after corrective surgery. When postoperative survival is expected to be short, the additional pain and hospitalization, not to mention the real possibility of death in the early postoperative period, may detract from palliative intent. Table 54-2 provides a summary of perioperative morbidity and mortality. In most series, perioperative mortality (usually defined as death within 30 days of surgery) is approximately 15%, with major morbidity occurring in about 50% of patients.

An important consideration in the management of bowel obstruction is the realistic evaluation of an individual patient's remaining treatment options for the disease. For patients who have failed all practical options and then subsequently develop obstruction due to disease progression, medical management with gastric drainage and other measures to alleviate symptoms may be proper. A patient who develops obstruction when potentially effective second-line treatments have yet to be attempted may be a more appropriate

Table 54–2. Perioperative Morbidity and Mortality

Study	Number of Patients	Mortality	Morbidity	Comments on Complications and Outcomes
Castaldo et al.[39]	23	3 (13%)	10 (43%)	Wound infection: 4 Recurrence: 4 Sepsis: 3 Enterocutaneous fistula: 3 Wound dehiscence: 2 Pulmonary embolus: 2 Gastrointestinal bleed: 1
Piver et al.[2]	60	10 (17%)	19 (31%)	Death from sepsis: 5 Enterocutaneous fistula: 4 Anastomotic leak: 2 Short gut syndrome: 2 Myocardial infarction: 1 Pulmonary embolism: 1 Antibiotic nephrotoxicity: 1 Aspiration pneumonitis: 1 Ureteral obstruction: 1
Krebs and Goplerud[40]	118	12 (10%)		Death from anastomotic leak: 4 Gastrointestinal bleed: 2 Persistent obstruction: 2 Sepsis: 1 Pulmonary embolus: 1 Myocardial infarction: 1
Solomon et al.[21]	21	1 (5%)		Persistent obstruction: 3 (2 had additional surgery) Recurrent obstruction: 2 Death from myocardial infarction: 1 Short gut syndrome: 1
Clarke-Pearson et al.[24]	49	7 (14%)	24 (49%)	Wound infection: 12 Enterocutaneous fistula: 9 Sepsis: 6 Abscess: 5 Anastomotic leak: 3 Gastrointestinal bleed: 3 Pneumonia: 4 Pulmonary embolus: 3 Deep venous thrombosis: 3 Wound dehiscence: 2 Adult respiratory distress syndrome: 1 Congestive heart failure: 1 Seizures: 1
Redman et al.[23]	26	4 (15%)	11 (42%)	Sepsis: 4 Persistent obstruction: 2 Pulmonary embolus: 1 Wound dehiscence: 1
Rubin et al.[1]	54	9 (16%)		Enterocutaneous fistula: 6 Pneumonia: 1 Sepsis: 1
Lund et al.[27]	25	8 (32%)	16 (64%)	Wound infection: 3 Wound dehiscence: 3 Deep venous thrombosis: 1 Myocardial infarction: 1
Larson et al.[38]	19	3 (16%)		
Pecorelli et al.[16]	147	23 (16%)		

candidate for aggressive surgical management. Piver and associates[2] examined 44 patients with bowel obstruction who received chemotherapy after surgery to relieve blockage. The investigators found that improved survival was related to response to chemotherapy rather than type of palliative surgery performed. Median survival was 10 months for patients with stable disease or a partial response to therapy and only 3 months for those with progressive disease.

What are the surgical options for management, and which patients are good candidates for surgery?

For the right candidate, surgical management may provide relatively safe and effective palliation, and a reasonable approach to bowel obstruction is initial hospital admission with nasogastric suction and intravenous hydration. For patients who fail a trial of such conservative management, appropriate candidates may be selected and offered surgical intervention. For those declining surgery or for poor candidates, medical palliative measures should be instituted.

A profusion of surgical options have been employed in the alleviation of intestinal obstruction, and the choice of procedure must be tailored individually for each patient. Because only about 0% to 24% of patients were deemed inoperable at the time of laparotomy (see Table 54-1), we conclude that the surgeon's preoperative judgment is relatively good in selecting technically suitable candidates for surgery. For 528 patients reported in various studies, when specified, the most common procedures employed were colostomy (33%), intestinal bypass (27%), bowel resection (16%), jejunostomy or ileostomy (4%), and lysis of adhesions (4%).[1,2,16,19,23,24,27,40]

The difficult question remains: Who is an appropriate candidate for surgical intervention? Unfortunately, there are no uniformly reliable indicators of good prognosis after surgery. Some would propose that patients with limited tumor burden, a single site of obstruction, and additional realistic chemotherapeutic options may benefit from surgery.[36] Conversely, the presence of extensive tumor and multiple sites of obstruction[1,2,22,27] are proposed by many to be poor indicators for surgery. Other investigators have suggested that age, the presence of ascites, distant metastases, parenchymal liver metastases, prior radiation therapy, pleural effusion, palpable masses, and a short time from diagnosis of disease to obstruction may indicate a poor prognosis with surgical intervention.[40,42,51] The site of obstruction in the large or small bowel does not appear to affect prognosis.[23,38]

Fernandes and colleagues[51] retrospectively studied 62 patients with ovarian cancer and the diagnosis of bowel obstruction treated medically and surgically. The investigators examined 20 clinical and biochemical characteristics in an attempt to define useful predictors of survival. On univariate analysis, they found that age at diagnosis of cancer older than 60 years, interval from diagnosis to obstruction of less than 100 weeks, advanced disease stage, the absence of prior radiation therapy, the presence of ascites, evidence of large-bowel obstruction or normal gas patterns on radiologic imaging, serum albumin level less than 3.7 g/dL, blood urea nitrogen concentration greater than 20 mg/dL, and alkaline phosphatase level greater than 110 IU/L were all significant indicators of poor 1-year survival probability. Medical versus surgical intervention, tumor histology, tumor grade, and extent of prior chemotherapy were not statistically related to survival.

In a similar fashion, Zoetmulder and coworkers[25] examined 17 clinical characteristics of 58 patients with bowel obstruction in the setting of advanced ovarian cancer. The patients were treated medically and surgically. On univariate analysis, a statistically significant survival advantage was found for patients who underwent surgical rather than medical intervention, in patients with no prior chemotherapeutic treatment, and for those in whom at least 10 months had elapsed

between their last treatment and the diagnosis of obstruction. Controlling for interval from last treatment to obstruction in the first step of their multivariate analysis, the advantage for patients treated surgically disappeared, but the presence of ascites was revealed as a poor prognostic sign. After controlling for the interval from the last treatment and ascites in the second step of multivariate analysis, no additional prognostic indicators were identified. Stage, interval from diagnosis to obstruction, and type, number of courses, and response to prior chemotherapy did not affect survival outcome.

In 1983, Krebs and Goplerud[40] proposed a prognostic index based on six criteria: age, nutritional status (based on criteria described by Dudrick and coworker[53]), tumor status (presence of palpable intraabdominal masses or the presence of parenchymal liver or distant metastases), ascites, extent of prior chemotherapy, and previous radiotherapy. Each category contributed 0, 1, or 2 points to the cumulative risk score. When applied to their study population of 118 surgical procedures to relieve obstruction in 98 patients, only 20% of patients with a score of 7 or more survived 60 days or longer after surgery. Conversely, 84% of patients with a score of 6 or less survived at least 60 days.

Some investigators confirmed the prognostic value of Krebs and Goplerud's risk score. Larson and associates[38] described 33 patients managed medically and surgically and reported that survival was significantly related to the risk score (P = .002). Gadducci and colleagues[18] assessed 34 patients with intestinal obstruction undergoing surgical and nonsurgical treatment. The only independent prognostic variable for survival identified was Krebs and Goplerud's risk score. Of the patients with a score of 6 or less, 87.5% survived at least 60 days, compared with 16.7% of those with a higher score.

Other investigators have not been able to confirm Krebs and Goplerud's risk score. Lund and colleagues[27] found that 20 of their surgically treated patients had a risk score of 6 or less. Twelve (60%) of these patients did survive more than 60 days, but only 8 patients survived without symptoms. All of the 16 nonsurgically managed patients also had scores of 6 or less, but their median survival was only 30 days. Others have not found the same prognostic value of some or all of the elements in Krebs and Goplerud's score.[13,26,51] Clarke-Pearson and coworkers[26] confirmed that ascites, albumin level, total lymphocyte count, and clinical tumor status were all significantly related to 60-day postoperative survival. However, on multiple regression, only the albumin level and tumor status were found to be significant independent variables.

Unfortunately, based on the retrospective data available, the clinician is left with no clear objective criteria by which to choose patients more likely to achieve palliative gain from surgery. Surgeons must use their best judgment, assisted by experience and the general guidelines provided in the existing literature, when selecting candidates for surgical intervention, and discuss the options in depth with patients to ascertain their wishes.

What are the medical options for management?

Many patients who present with bowel obstruction in this setting are not appropriate candidates for surgical palliation, or they decline surgery. Most patients have failed prior attempts at cytotoxic therapy, and Abu-Rustum and colleagues[54] in New York and Beattie and coworkers[9] in Edinburgh reported no responses to chemotherapy in heavily pretreated patients after bowel obstruction. For these patients, control of symptoms is of paramount importance.

One option for poor surgical candidates suffering from a single accessible site of obstruction is endoluminal stenting. The use of bowel stents for the relief of obstruction caused by gastrointestinal neoplasms has been reported since the early 1990s. In general, these techniques involve endoscopically assisted passage of a guidewire beyond the site of obstruction and placement of an expanding metal stent by the Seldinger technique. Investigators have reported a high success rate for placement to correct malignant colorectal obstruction, with relief of symptoms in 64% to 100% of patients.[55] Similarly, in cases of upper gastrointestinal tract obstruction, greater than 70% success has been reported for stents used in the treatment of gastric outlet, duodenal, and jejunal obstruction.[56] The most common complications associated with this technique are bowel perforation (0% to 15%), stent migration (0% to 40%), and repeat obstruction (0% to 33%).[55] Less common complications include bleeding and infection. Endoluminal stents have primarily been used in the treatment of gastrointestinal malignancies, but Carter and associates[57] from Australia reported the use of stents for the treatment of large-bowel obstruction in two patients with recurrent ovarian cancer. The researchers reported that both patients achieved immediate relief of their symptoms. One patient died 4 weeks after stent placement with symptoms of tenesmus controlled pharmacologically, and the other achieved successful symptom relief until her death 8 months later. Neither suffered any procedure-related complications.

Most strategies for the medical management of bowel obstruction in the terminal patient initially combine plans for long-term decompression proximal to the site of obstruction with interventions to minimize nausea, vomiting, and pain. Gastrointestinal drainage may be accomplished in different ways. "Long tubes," such as Miller-Abbott and Cantor tubes, have been used to successfully drain the proximal small intestine in patients with advanced ovarian cancer,[58] but their use is cumbersome and has not been shown to be superior to simple nasogastric suction.[59-62] In any event, nasogastric tubes should be avoided for the long term. Discomfort is an issue, and nasogastric tubes may predispose to aspiration pneumonia, esophagitis, bleeding, nasal cartilage erosion, and otitis media.[63] nasogastric tubes may severely limit patient mobility by requiring an active suction system.

Gastrostomy eliminates the need for nasogastric tubes and may use gravity for passive drainage, thereby making discharge from the hospital more feasible. Although gastrostomy tubes may be placed by laparotomy,[20,42,47] nonoperative percutaneous approaches for feeding purposes have been described since the early 1980s.[64,65] With these techniques, gastrostomy may be performed with local anesthesia and intravenous sedation, without the need for general anesthesia. Overall, percutaneous placement is usually successful. Inability to place a tube occurs in 7% to 11% of patients with malignant disease,[46,48,66] usually due to tumor infiltration at the proposed site. Complications are generally minor. In a review of six series encompassing 266 patients, leak of ascites or gastric secretions was reported in six patients, mild peritonitis in two, cellulitis in eight, and gastrocolic fistula in two.[45,46,48,66-68] Exploratory laparotomies were performed in two patients for suspected tube complications, which were determined to be unnecessary in retrospect,[68] and one death resulted from severe peritonitis.[48] Of these 266 patients, the investigators reported that tube replacement was necessary in 14 for blockage or dislodgment. The presence of ascites is not a contraindication to gastrostomy tube placement as reported by Lee and colleagues,[67] who successfully placed tubes in 12 patients with extensive ascites. No dislodgments occurred, and pericatheter leakage of ascites only occurred in the three patients who did not undergo paracentesis before the procedure.

Gastrostomy allows patients to be discharged from the hospital in 3 to 4 days[45,66] and to maintain some oral intake of fluids or soft foods despite persistent obstruction, which may be important comfort measures for the terminal patient. Malone and coworkers[45] described 10 patients with ovarian cancer receiving percutaneous gastrostomies who were all discharged to home and taking an oral diet as tolerated. At the time of their report, 7 of the 10 patients had died at a mean of 35 days, but 3 were alive at 77, 150, and 150 days. Similarly, Marks and associates[46] reported that 26 of their 28 patients afflicted with gynecologic cancers were discharged to home and were taking liquids orally. The patients survived 1 to 8 months. Herman and colleagues[48] also studied 26 patients with ovarian cancer who underwent percutaneous gastrostomy placement. Their patients were able to resume oral intake and survived a mean of 47 days.

In conjunction with gastrointestinal decompression, several different pharmacologic approaches for palliation of symptoms are available. Even without the benefit of decompression, aggressive pharmacologic management may control obstructive symptoms. Baines and coworkers[32] reported the aggressive use of narcotics, anticholinergics, antiemetics, phenothiazines, butyrophenones, and tricyclic antidepressants in 38 patients with malignant bowel obstruction deemed to be inappropriate candidates for surgery. In the absence of gastric drainage or intravenous fluids, these patients survived a mean of almost 4 months, and seven patients survived for more than 7 months. Similarly, Isbister and associates[69] from New Zealand reported the successful palliation of 24 patients with bowel obstruction in the setting of advanced cancer managed in a hospice setting with a combination of morphine and metoclopramide administered by a continuous subcutaneous infusion. Patients survived for a mean of 29 days and were encouraged to take free liquids and a low-fiber diet as tolerated without gastric drainage.

Route of administration of medication becomes an important consideration in the patient with bowel obstruction and should be individualized for each patient. Oral medications may not always be an option because of nausea, vomiting, and impaired gastrointestinal absorption. Transdermal, rectal, and sublingual routes are easy to use, but the number of medications able to be delivered in these fashions is limited. Parenteral medications may be necessary, delivered intravenously through a central venous access device or subcutaneously by intermittent injection or pump.

Metoclopramide, a promotility agent, is a common medication used for treatment of nausea and vomiting. Fainsinger and colleagues[70] reported metoclopramide to be the drug of choice in patients with incomplete bowel obstruction when given as a 10-mg dose parenterally every 4 hours. Metoclopramide is not usually recommended in patients with complete obstruction because of its tendency to increase colicky pain,[32,33,71-73] but if complete obstruction occurs below the level of the duodenum, the drug may encourage gastric emptying into a paralyzed reservoir of bowel, thereby relieving some symptoms of nausea.[69]

Haloperidol, prochlorperazine, and promethazine are phenothiazine derivatives commonly used to relieve nausea and vomiting. Haloperidol is one of the drugs of first choice in Europe[17] and is commonly administered by subcutaneous and oral routes, but it may also be dosed as a continuous intravenous drip. Haloperidol may be given with hyoscine in the same syringe subcutaneously. Prochlorperazine and promethazine are more commonly used in the United States, and in addition to being available in oral and parenteral routes, they may be administered in rectal suppositories.

Cyclizine, buclizine, and meclizine are antiemetic medications classified as antihistamines with anticholinergic actions. Although it is rarely used in the United States, cyclizine is the drug of first choice in some palliative care centers in Europe.[17] The drug may be combined with prochlorperazine in suppository form or given with haloperidol subcutaneously.

Scopolamine and hyoscine are anticholinergic and antispasmodic drugs frequently used for vomiting and colicky pain. The anticholinergic activity decreases the tone and peristalsis of the bowel wall[74,75] while also decreasing intestinal secretions. Scopolamine is commonly available as a transdermal patch in the United States, whereas hyoscine butylbromide (which has the advantage of not crossing the blood-brain barrier) is frequently administered by oral, sublingual, and subcutaneous routes in Europe. De Conno and associates[76] reported the use of hyoscine butylbromide administered by subcutaneous pump in three women with malignant bowel obstruction. Nasogastric drainage

was markedly reduced, and after 1 week of treatment, it was possible to discontinue nasogastric tube drainage in all patients. Patients reported good initial relief of colic without the use of narcotics.

Somatostatin and its analogs, octreotide and vapreotide, are also used in the treatment of bowel obstruction. Somatostatin is a polypeptide produced in the gastrointestinal tract that acts by inhibiting the release and action of gastrointestinal hormones.[77] Other actions include reduced gastric acid secretion and bile flow, decreased intestinal motility, increased mucous production, and reduced splanchnic blood flow.[77-79] The half-life of octreotide is only about 1.5 hours, and it is commonly administered as a thrice-daily subcutaneous bolus or continuous infusion.

Octreotide is more powerful than somatostatin[80] and acts to inhibit the secretion of growth hormone, gastrin, vasoactive intestinal peptide, pancreatic polypeptide, insulin, and glucagon, as well as to directly block the secretion of gastric acid, pepsin, pancreatic enzyme, and bicarbonate.[78] Because of its ability to decrease the secretion of intestinal epithelial electrolytes and water, octreotide may provide relief from nausea and pain through reduction in bowel distention.[78] Octreotide has been examined in several palliative studies of malignant disease.[78,79,81-84] Mangili and coworkers[49] from Italy examined its use in 13 patients with bowel obstruction due to advanced ovarian cancer. Octreotide was successful in reducing vomiting in every case to grade 0 on the World Health Organization's emesis scale. Vomiting stopped in most patients within 2 to 3 days of commencing treatment. In eight patients with nasogastric tubes, drainage decreased from 2000 mL to less than 100 mL per day. The investigators reported that all patients were maintained until their death with minimal symptoms.

One major drawback of octreotide is cost, which often results in use of the drug only after conventional antiemetics have failed. Khoo and associates[83] reported its use to treat five patients with intractable vomiting unresponsive to prochlorperazine, metoclopramide, cyclizine, and dexamethasone. Vomiting ceased within 1 hour of the initiation of therapy in all patients. Its use for prolonged treatment must be carefully considered after weighing the cost against the potential improvement in quality of life.

Vapreotide is a microencapsulated preparation with clinical properties similar to somatostatin but with a longer duration of action. Stiefel and Morant[85] administered vapreotide in weekly injections to one patient with advanced pancreatic cancer, with good palliation of nausea and vomiting until the patient's death.

Corticosteroids have been recommended for use in malignant bowel obstruction to reduce inflammation and edema in the area of the tumor, thereby relieving nausea and vomiting.[70,86] However, given the lack of clinical trials using these agents, standard doses and routes of administration are not established. Commonly used steroids include dexamethasone and prednisone. Initial doses are usually tapered after the desired effect is achieved.

Ultimately, many patients require narcotic analgesics to control pain. A wide variety of narcotics are available and may be administered by oral, rectal, parenteral, and transdermal routes. Self-administered methadone has been reported for use in cancer patients with chronic subtotal obstruction in Italy.[50] Patient-controlled analgesia (PCA) pumps have also been used to administer subcutaneous doses of narcotics to control cancer pain.[87] Both of these methods of intermittent administration are useful for treatment of the often fluctuating levels of pain in cases of bowel obstruction and to avoid tolerance through continuous exposure to the drug. Regional anesthesia using narcotics has also been employed to alleviate pain. Chapman and colleagues[88] reported the use of an indwelling epidural catheter to administer continuous infusion morphine from a portable pump. In their report, an ovarian cancer patient whose disease had progressed with recurrent bowel obstruction after five chemotherapeutic and two hormonal regimens still possessed excellent performance status and was maintained for 6 months with good palliation of symptoms until the epidural catheter was removed because of infection. Her therapy was switched to a subcutaneous PCA pump, and she died 3 months later, still with good palliation of symptoms.

Pharmacologic options for palliation in the setting of malignant bowel obstruction are widely varied and highly effective. In combination with gastric drainage, most patients should be able to achieve adequate relief of nausea, vomiting, and pain on an outpatient basis with continued oral intake to maximize quality of life.

When is total parenteral nutrition appropriate?

TPN was developed by Dudrick and colleagues at the University of Pennsylvania in 1968,[89] and its first use in gynecologic cancer patients was reported in 1972.[90] Although malignancy is the most common indication for home TPN in the United States,[91] its use is somewhat controversial. TPN has been shown to be beneficial for the malnourished cancer patient with potentially curable or well-controlled disease in the setting of severe gastrointestinal injury caused by short-gut syndrome, severe chronic radiation-induced enteropathy, or persistent enterocutaneous fistula.[92-96] However, little or no benefit has been demonstrated for well-nourished cancer patients with adequate gastrointestinal function[95,97] and for the patient with widely metastatic disease and poor prognosis.[98] Some have advocated the use of TPN in cancer patients based on improved quality of life, independent of disease status.[44,88,95,99-104] Although TPN support has been shown to increase body weight and to correct metabolic disturbances, it is unclear whether these improvements translate into improved survival and function for the patient.[105-108] Moreover, although body fat may be repleted without difficulty, the protein deficit exhibited by most cachectic cancer patients may be harder to correct.[109]

Frequently, those receiving home TPN are terminally ill patients suffering from malignant bowel obstruction. Case reports have documented long-term survival of patients with high performance status and bowel obstruction when maintained on TPN. Chapman and coworkers[88] described one extensively pretreated patient with excellent performance status who survived 9 months after the diagnosis of obstruction, which was treated with gastrostomy drainage and home TPN. King and associates[43] from the University of Minnesota reported 61 patients with gynecologic malignancies receiving home TPN, 44 of whom suffered from inoperable bowel obstruction. Eleven (25%) of the patients with bowel obstruction survived more than 60 days at home, and four (10%) survived more than 9 months. These data are difficult to interpret because more than 60% of patients in the whole study received additional cancer treatment, and a few patients were able to discontinue TPN and resume oral intake, indicating that these results may not be generalized to a population of terminal, debilitated patients with incurable disease. Complications directly related to TPN treatment were experienced by 18% of patients. No TPN-related mortality occurred, but on average, each patient was rehospitalized twice. The investigators stated that a common denominator in the patients with longer than expected survival was a good performance status before initiation of TPN and that patients with limited survival and poor performance status would probably not benefit.

In the terminally ill patient, the palliative benefits of TPN, expressed as improved survival or quality of life, must justify the expense and potential complications. Aside from the complications related to obtaining and maintaining central venous access, infection, sepsis, metabolic derangements, and volume overload are real concerns. Twelve randomized, controlled trials of TPN use in patients receiving chemotherapy revealed a fourfold increase in significant infections and iatrogenic complications.[94] The North American Home Nutrition Support Registry reported a 1% mortality rate for home TPN.[100]

When weighing the risks, the benefits in regard to prolongation of survival are in question. Abu-Rustum and colleagues[54] described 21 patients treated for bowel obstruction in the setting of advanced ovarian cancer. All were treated with gastrostomy tube and chemotherapy. Eleven patients received TPN. Chemotherapy was ineffective in restoring bowel function in all patients with recurrent or persistent disease. The patients receiving TPN had a median survival of 89 days, compared with 71 days for patients receiving no TPN. This difference of 18 days, although statistically distinct, hardly constitutes a clinically significant difference. The investigators concluded that TPN in the end-stage ovarian cancer patient is of limited value.

Identifying which patients with bowel obstruction in the setting of advanced ovarian cancer will benefit from TPN is difficult. In a study from Yale, 17 patients with inoperable malignant bowel obstruction were discharged from the hospital with home TPN. Of the cancer types studied, median survival was shortest, only 39 days, in the nine patients with ovarian cancer. In comparison, the two patients with appendiceal carcinoma survived 208 and 159 days, and the four patients with colon carcinoma had a median survival of 90 days.[44] Fourteen of the 17 patients and their families perceived TPN therapy as beneficial, but the care providers concurred with this perception for only 11 patients. The investigators concluded that TPN might have palliative benefit in the setting of gastrointestinal tract primary tumors, but that patients with inoperable bowel obstruction due to ovarian cancer derived poorer palliation. Their recommendation was to consider TPN only when patient survival was estimated to be longer than 40 days. Although the recommendation may be sound based on the investigators' data, in practice, determining which patients are likely to survive more than 40 days may be problematic. Cozzaglio and coworkers[110] examined 75 patients with obstruction from various cancers and determined that a high performance status (Karnofsky score greater than 50) predicted an improvement in quality of life for patients receiving TPN, and they concluded that for patients with low performance status, parenteral nutrition should be avoided.

The terminal patient with bowel obstruction may benefit from treatment with TPN in the perioperative setting. Most of the available data regarding this area of inquiry are for the general surgical population and are not specific to patients with ovarian cancer. The largest study was conducted by the Veterans Affairs TPN Cooperative Study Group at several institutions across the United States.[111] The investigators studied 395 malnourished patients who required laparotomy or noncardiac thoracotomy. The patients were randomly assigned to receive TPN for 7 to 15 days preoperatively and 3 days postoperatively or to receive no perioperative TPN. The investigators found that the rates of major complications and mortality were similar between the two groups. However, there were more infectious complications in the TPN group than in the control group, although this increase was limited to patients classified as borderline or mildly malnourished. Patients in these categories received no benefit from TPN. Severely malnourished patients receiving TPN had fewer noninfectious complications than controls (5% versus 43%, $P = .03$), with no concomitant increase in infectious complications. The investigators concluded that the use of preoperative TPN should be limited to patients with severe malnutrition.

In cancer patients, the results are mixed. One prospective study performed at the Memorial Sloan-Kettering Cancer Center[112] examined 117 patients undergoing curative resection for pancreatic cancer who were randomized to receive TPN or intravenous fluids postoperatively. No benefit was demonstrated for routine use of postoperative TPN, but infectious complications were increased among those randomized to TPN. Similarly, Fernandes and associates[51] reported no difference in survival among patients receiving parenteral, enteral, or oral nutrition before surgery for bowel obstruction due to ovarian cancer.

Other investigators have documented a reduction in major surgical complications and operative mortality in cancer patients.[113,114] Krebs and Goperlud[40] described 118 patients undergoing surgery for obstruction due to ovarian cancer and reported that 75% of the 57 patients receiving TPN survived more than 2 months, compared with only 56% of those with no TPN ($P < .025$). The American Society for Parenteral and Enteral Nutrition, the American Society of Clinical Nutrition, and the National Institutes of Health have determined that 7 to 10 days of preoperative TPN in malnourished patients with gastrointestinal cancer results in a 10% reduction in postoperative complications.[92] It seems reasonable to consider these findings when planning palliative surgery for the end-stage ovarian cancer patient.

Aside from considering the scientific evidence, physicians experienced in the care of these patients recognize that patients and families often have strong desires regarding supplemental nutrition. A study performed at the University of Michigan reported that 90% of women undergoing treatment for gynecologic malignancies could envision a time in the future when they would refuse mechanical ventilation, but only 37% could envision refusing nutritional support.[115] Patients and families may be reluctant to refuse parenteral nutrition even when the patient's prognosis is grim because of the perception that withholding nutrition may cause the patient to "starve." Physicians may offer reassurance that terminally ill cancer patients only rarely report hunger or thirst, and those who experience symptoms may achieve relief by small amounts of oral intake.[116] Several investigators have also demonstrated that TPN and intravenous fluids do not improve comfort in terminally ill patients[116-118] and may even add discomfort.[116,119-123] In particular, in the setting of bowel obstruction, intravenous fluids may have a detrimental effect on patient comfort by increasing the volume of ascites and bowel secretions.[124] Patients with extensive cancer are often unable to use hyperalimentation solutions effectively and experience progressive deterioration despite its use.[90]

From the evidence presented, the administration of TPN in the palliative setting for the ovarian patient with bowel obstruction appears to be justified in several instances. Therapy should be initiated in severely malnourished patients for about 7 to 15 days before planned surgery for correction of obstruction. Therapy may be considered for patients with inoperable bowel obstruction who have good performance status or reasonable remaining options for cancer treatment. Before initiation of therapy, discussion with the patient and family is important to ascertain individual preferences for treatment in the palliative setting.

Ascites

Ascites is present in more than two thirds of patients with ovarian cancer. Several factors contribute to its formation. Damaged peritoneal surfaces may produce more fluid, decreased plasma oncotic pressure may favor third spacing of fluid into the peritoneal cavity, and decreased absorption of fluid may occur as a result of obstructed lymphatics.[125,126] Most ascites can be at least initially controlled by treatment with effective chemotherapy, but its persistence or recurrence after cytotoxic treatment heralds a poor outcome and indicates a lack of response to chemotherapy.[127] Although small amounts of ascites rarely cause the patient any significant symptoms, tense and malignant ascites is frequently a source of severe symptoms for the patient with end-stage ovarian cancer. This process can lead to dyspnea, orthopnea, anorexia, nausea, vomiting, severe gastroesophageal reflux, and discomfort from increased abdominal pressure. Quality of life is often severely affected in these patients, and palliative efforts are clearly warranted.

What are the management options for intractable ascites? When systemic chemotherapy has failed to control disease, effective options for the palliation of symptomatic ascites are few. In the past, sodium restriction, bed rest, and diuretics were the standard of care because of the concern about morbidity and mortality associated with large-volume paracentesis.[128] However, diuretic use is ineffective in many patients, and it was eventually shown to have equivalent rates of complications compared with paracentesis.[129]

Large-volume paracentesis is usually the first intervention for the patient with tense, symptomatic ascites. Paracentesis has been demonstrated to be safe. Cardiovascular dynamics, hematocrit, and serum electrolytes in patients with abdominal carcinomatosis were studied after large-volume paracentesis, and no adverse changes were demonstrated during or after the procedure in small series of patients.[130,131] Gotlieb and colleagues[132] prospectively examined clinical parameters and intraperitoneal pressures in 35 sequential total paracenteses performed in Tel-Aviv. The mean volume of ascites drained was 4800 mL. Total paracentesis appeared to improve respiratory and cardiac function. They reported significant decreases in mean pulse (101 to 94 beats/min before and after the procedure) and respiratory rate (29 to 21 respirations/min before and after the procedure). Blood pressure remained stable, and no patients exhibited any signs of hypovolemia during or after the procedure. The investigators concluded that total paracentesis is a safe, inexpensive, and effective method for palliation of symptoms. Unfortunately, although it is very effective in achieving acute relief, ascites inevitably reaccumulates, and palliative benefit is short lived.

More lasting palliative solutions have been sought. Mulvaney[133] initially reported drainage of malignant ascites into the bladder in 1955, and Stehman and Ehrlich[134] reported the use of a peritoneocystic shunt in a patient with ovarian cancer in 1984. Peritoneovenous shunting was first introduced by Smith in 1962,[135,136] but it was not popularized until 1974, with the development of the LeVeen valve for use in patients with cirrhotic ascites.[137,138] In general, the technique involves placement of a plastic catheter leading from the peritoneal cavity, tunneled subcutaneously in a cephalad direction and ending with insertion into a neck vein, allowing ascitic fluid to drain from the peritoneum into the superior vena cava. Valves are pressure sensitive and permit only unidirectional flow of fluid. Two commonly used shunts are the LeVeen[137,138] and the Denver,[139] which differs from the LeVeen in that it incorporates the ability to use a manual pump to clear debris and drain fluid from the peritoneal cavity.

Several reports have been published, almost all originating in Europe, documenting the use of the Denver and LeVeen shunts in patients with malignant ascites.[140-145] Although Battaglia and associates[145] in Italy reported on four patients with ovarian cancer who were all successfully treated with a shunt, in larger series of patients with various peritoneal malignancies, the rate of long-term successful palliation has ranged from 44% to 87%.[140-144] Blockage is a common problem. In a combination of five series from Europe reporting on 104 shunts placed, 35 (34%) became blocked.[140,142-145] In the single series from the United States reported by Straus and colleagues[141] in Chicago, in 2 of their 27 patients with malignant ascites, surgery was abandoned because abdominal ascites was too loculated to allow sufficient drainage and four shunts never functioned. In the remaining 31 patients, four shunts functioned less than 3 months. Of the 129 patients reported in these six combined series, 8 (6%) died as a result of shunt-related complications, including pulmonary embolus, pneumonia, pulmonary edema, disseminated intravascular coagulation, and cerebrovascular accident. Eleven (8%) other patients suffered nonfatal shunt-related complications, including ascites leak, bacteremia, infection, thrombosis, disseminated intravascular coagulation, cerebrovascular accident, and skin necrosis. Draining malignant cells from the ascites into the central venous circulation raises the concern of the development of tumor emboli, particularly in the lungs. However, no patients in these reports died of pulmonary tumor. Straus and coworkers[141] and Souter and associates[142] performed autopsies in 21 patients in their two series and discovered only 5 patients with tumor emboli, all of which were clinically insignificant. In a population of terminal patients who already have very limited survival, the concern for malignant emboli may not be clinically relevant.

Variable success has been reported with the use of intraperitoneal instillation of chemotherapeutics or radioisotopes for the palliation of ascites. Unlike the use of mechanical shunts, almost all reports of intraperitoneal drug therapy originate from the United States. One large series by Ariel and coworkers[146] reported 145 patients with malignant ascites treated with intraperitoneal ^{198}Au or Cr^{32}PO$_4$, or both, and found that 54% of patients experienced complete cessation or appreciable slowing of ascites formation until death (if less than 3 months' survival) or for at least 3 months after treatment. The complications included transient nausea and vomiting, diarrhea, and fever. Noninfectious peritonitis was reported in 1.5% of patients. Another large series by Jackson and Blosser[147] examined 178 patients with various peritoneal malignancies undergoing intracavitary Cr^{32}PO$_4$

therapy. In patients who survived 3 months, 85% experienced symptomatic improvement. Results may be hard to generalize to our population of interest because the patients in this study surviving less than 3 months were not evaluated for symptom relief.

Bleomycin and Adriamycin have been investigated for the palliation of ascites in patients refractory to systemic chemotherapy. Paladine and colleagues[148] reported a response (defined as no or minimal reaccumulation for at least 30 days) to intraperitoneal bleomycin in only 4 of 11 patients (36%) with various peritoneal malignancies, although no significant toxicity was observed. Bitran[149] found a slightly better 60% response rate (defined as greater than 50% shrinkage of measurable tumor or no evidence of ascites for at least 30 days) in his 10 patients treated with intraperitoneal bleomycin with no significant toxicity. In a phase I study of 10 patients with refractory ovarian cancer treated with intraperitoneal Adriamycin,[150] 3 patients demonstrated objective disease response, and 2 achieved resolution of ascites. One trial from Australia compared treatment of intraperitoneal adriamycin, nitrogen mustard, and tetracycline in 11 patients with various peritoneal malignancies.[151] Some patients received several treatments. Nitrogen mustard and tetracycline were deemed ineffective, but all four patients receiving intraperitoneal Adriamycin experienced complete resolution of ascites or an improvement in symptoms for at least 8 weeks.

Other palliative therapies investigated have included various biologic response modifiers. Interferons, which act through tumor antiproliferative effects and host immunomodulatory effects, have been investigated for intraperitoneal use in palliation of malignant ascites. In recurrent ovarian cancer, a 75% rate of palliation has been reported for interferon-β in 8 patients,[152] and a 38% rate of palliation for interferon-α-2b in 13 patients.[153] Side effects for interferon-β included transient fever and hypotension, as well as local pain and moderate nausea and vomiting. Interferon-α-2b also induced transient fever and grade 2 hematologic toxicity, as well as peritonitis in three patients. *Corynebacterium parvum*, a nonspecific immune stimulator, was instilled in the peritoneal cavities of 11 patients with ovarian or endometrial cancer and achieved a 45% response rate.[154] Aside from expected immediate reactions, six patients suffered from ileus (one required laparotomy), four from cellulitis at the injection site, and one from sepsis.

Other immunotherapies that have been employed include intraperitoneal radioiodinated monoclonal antibody 2G3 in patients with breast and ovarian cancer (palliation in 3 of 9 patients who received therapeutic doses)[155] and intraperitoneal allogeneic and autologous lymphokine-activated killer cells that elicited palliation in two patients tested.[156] Both therapies were well tolerated.

A variety of strategies are available for the palliation of malignant ascites. The simplest and most reliable appears to be large-volume paracentesis, although relief is short lived in most patients. Outside of the United States, use of peritoneovenous shunting is a commonly used technique that may provide long-term palliation, although catheter blockage is common and serious side effects may occur. Other intraperitoneal therapies such as chemotherapeutics, immunotherapies, and biologic response modifiers have variable response rates and may induce significant morbidity.

Summary

Most patients with ovarian cancer eventually develop disease resistant to systemic chemotherapy. Tense ascites and bowel obstruction are common occurrences and account for significant morbidity in these terminal patients. The physician must be familiar with the medical and surgical options for palliation and understand how to select appropriate candidates for each to maximize chances for symptom relief. With careful consideration of the available approaches and astute selection of appropriate patients, individual strategies may be developed with thoughtful regard for each patient's wishes.

REFERENCES

1. Rubin SC, Hoskins WJ, Benjamin I, Lewis JL: Palliative surgery for intestinal obstruction in advanced ovarian cancer. Gynecol Oncol 1989;34:16-19.
2. Piver MS, Barlow JJ, Lele SB, Frank A: Survival after ovarian cancer induced intestinal obstruction. Gynecol Oncol 1982;13:44-49.
3. McGowan L: Gynecologic Oncology. New York, Appleton-Century-Crofts, 1978, pp 298-299.
4. DiSaia PJ, Morrow CP, Townsend DE: Synopsis of Gynecologic Oncology. New York, Wiley, 1975, p 161.
5. Ripamonti C, DeConno F, Ventafridda V, et al: Management of bowel obstruction in advanced and terminal cancer patients. Ann Oncol 1993;4:15-21.
6. Dvoretsky PM, Richards, KA, Angel A, et al: Survival time, causes of death, and tumor-treatment-related morbidity in 100 women with ovarian cancer. Hum Pathol 1988;19:1273-1279.
7. Dvoretsky PM, Richards KA, Angel C, et al: Distribution of disease at autopsy in 100 women with ovarian cancer. Hum Pathol 1988;19:57-63.
8. Rose PG, Piver S, Tsukada Y, Lau T: Metastatic patterns in histologic variants of ovarian cancer-an autopsy study. Cancer 1978;64:1508-1513.
9. Beattie GJ, Leonard R, Smyth JF: Bowel obstruction in ovarian carcinoma: A retrospective study and review of the literature. Palliat Med 1989;3:275-280.
10. Paganelli AMM, Leone V, Malagutti V, et al: Intestinal surgery in patients with ovarian carcinoma. Eur J Gynecol Oncol 1990;11:157-160.
11. Ripamonti C: Management of bowel obstruction in patients with advanced terminal cancer. Support Care Oncol 1993;9:10-13.
12. Hogan WM, Boente MP: The role of surgery in the management of recurrent gynecologic cancer. Semin Oncol 1993;20:462-472.
13. Hoskins JW, Rubin SC: Surgery in the treatment of patients with advanced ovarian cancer. Semin Oncol 1991;18:213-221.
14. Tamussino KF, Lim PC, Webb MJ, et al: Gastrointestinal surgery in patients with ovarian cancer. Gynecol Oncol 2001;80:79-84.
15. Rubin SC, Benjamin I, Hoskins WJ, et al: Intestinal surgery in gynecologic oncology. Gynecol Oncol 1989;34:30-33.
16. Pecorelli S, Sartori E, Santin A: Follow-up after primary therapy: Management of the symptomatic patient-surgery. Gynecol Oncol 1994;55:S138-S142.
17. Ripamonti C: Management of bowel obstruction in advanced cancer. Curr Opin Oncol 1994;6:351-357.

18. Gadducci A, Cosio S, Fanucchi AA, Genazzani AR: Malnutrition and cachexia in ovarian cancer patients: Pathophysiology and management. Anticancer Res 2001;21:2941-2948.

19. Tunca JC, Buchler DA, Mack EA, et al: The management of ovarian-cancer-caused bowel obstruction. Gynecol Oncol 1981; 12:186-192.

20. Tsahalina E, Woolas RP, Carter PG, et al: Gastrostomy tubes in patients with recurrent gynaecological cancer and intestinal obstruction. Br J Obstet Gynaecol 1999;106:964-968.

21. Solomon HJ, Atkinson KH, Coppleson JVM, et al: Bowel complications in the management of ovarian cancer. Aust N Z J Obstet Gynaecol 1983;23:65-68.

22. Soo KC, Davidson T, Parker M, et al: Intestinal obstruction in patients with gynaecological malignancies. Ann Acad Med Singapore 1988;17:72-75.

23. Redman CWE, Shafi MI, Ambrose S, et al: Survival following intestinal obstruction in ovarian cancer. Eur J Surg Oncol 1988; 14:383-386.

24. Clarke-Pearson DL, Chin NO, DeLong ER, et al: Surgical management of intestinal obstruction in ovarian cancer. Gynecol Oncol 1987;26:11-18.

25. Zoetmulder FAN, Helmerhorst JM, Coevorden FV, et al: Management of bowel obstruction in patients with advance ovarian cancer. Eur J Cancer 1994;30A:1625-1628.

26. Clarke-Pearson DL, DeLong ER, Chin N, et al: Intestinal obstruction in patients with ovarian cancer-variables associated with surgical complications and survival. Arch Surg 1988;123:42-45.

27. Lund R, Hansen M, Lundvall F, et al: Intestinal obstruction in patients with advanced carcinoma of the ovaries treated with combination chemotherapy. Surg Gynecol Obstet 1989;169: 213-218.

28. Mann WJ, Calayag PT, Muffoletto JP, et al: Management of gastric outlet obstruction caused by ovarian cancer. Gynecol Oncol 1991;40:277-279.

29. Katz LB, Frankel A, Cohen C, Slater G: Ovarian carcinoma complicated by gastric outlet obstruction. J Surg Oncol 1981;18: 261-264.

30. Krebs HB, Walsh J, Goplerud DR: Gastric outlet obstruction caused by ascitic fluid entrapment in the lesser sac-a complication of ovarian cancer: report of two cases. Gynecol Oncol 1982; 14:105-111.

31. Spencer JA, Crosse BA, Mannion RA, et al: Gastroduodenal obstruction from ovarian cancer: imaging features and clinical outcome. Clin Radiol 2000;55:264-272.

32. Baines M, Oliver DJ, Carter RL: Medical management of intestinal obstruction in patients with advanced malignant disease: A clinical and pathological study. Lancet 1985;2:990-993.

33. Ventafridda V, Ripamonti C, Caraceni A, et al: The management of inoperable gastrointestinal obstruction in terminal cancer patients. Tumori 1990;76:389-393.

34. Rubin SC: Surgery for ovarian cancer. Hematol Oncol Clin North Am 1992;6:851-865.

35. Glass RL, LeDuc RJ: Small intestinal obstruction for peritoneal carcinomatosis. Surgery 1980;87:611-615.

36. Rubin SC: Intestinal obstruction in advanced ovarian cancer: What does the patient want? Gynecol Oncol 1999;75:311-312.

37. Piver MS: The Randall/Rubin article reviewed. Oncol 2000; 14:1167-1168.

38. Larson JE, Podczaski ES, Manetta A, et al: Bowel obstruction in patients with ovarian carcinoma: Analysis of prognostic factors. Gynecol Oncol 1989;35:61-65.

39. Castaldo TW, Petrilli ES, Ballon SC, Lagasse LD: Intestinal operations in patients with ovarian carcinoma. Am J Obstet Gynecol 1981;139:80-84.

40. Krebs HB, Goplerud DR: Surgical management of bowel obstruction in advanced ovarian carcinoma. Obstet Gynecol 1983;61:327-330.

41. Jong P, Sturgeon J, Jamieson CG: Benefit of palliative surgery for bowel obstruction in advanced ovarian cancer. Can J Surg 1995; 38: 454-457.

42. van Ooijen B, van der Burg MEL, Planting AST, et al: Surgical treatment or gastric drainage only for intestinal obstruction in patients with carcinoma of the ovary or peritoneal carcinomatosis of other origin. Surg Gynecol Obstet 1993;176:469-474.

43. King LA, Carson LF, Konstantinides N, et al: Outcome assessment of home parenteral nutrition in patients with gynecologic

44. August DA, Thorn D, Fisher RL, Welchek CM: Home parenteral nutrition for patients with inoperable malignant bowel obstruction. JPEN J Parenter Enteral Nutr 1991;15:323-327.

45. Malone JM, Koonce T, Larson DM, et al: Palliation of small bowel obstruction by percutaneous gastrostomy in patients with progressive ovarian carcinoma. Obstet Gynecol 1986;68:431-433.

46. Marks WH, Perkal MF, Schwartz PE: Percutaneous endoscopic gastrostomy for gastric decompression in metastatic gynecologic malignancies. Surg Gynecol Obstet 1993;177:573-576.

47. Hopkins MP, Roberts JA, Morley GW: Outpatient management of small bowel obstruction in terminal ovarian cancer. J Reprod Med 1987;32:827-829.

48. Herman LL, Hoskins WJ, Shike M: Percutaneous endoscopic gastrostomy for decompression of the stomach and small bowel. Gastrointest Endosc 1992;38:314-318.

49. Mangili G, Franchi M, Mariani A, et al: Octreotide in the management of bowel obstruction in terminal ovarian cancer. Gynecol Oncol 1996;61:345-348.

50. Mercadante S, Sapio M, Serretta R: Treatment of pain in chronic bowel subobstruction with self-administration of methadone. Support Care Cancer 1997;5:327-329.

51. Fernandes JR, Seymour RJ, Suissa S: Bowel obstruction in patients with ovarian cancer: A search for prognostic factors. Am J Obstet Gynecol 1988;158:244-249.

52. Ketcham AS, Hoye RC, Pilch YH, Morton DL: Delayed intestinal obstruction following treatment for cancer. Cancer 1970;25: 406-410.

53. Dudrick SJ, Jensen TG, Rowlands BJ: Nutritional support: Assessment and indications. In Dietel M (ed): Nutrition in Clinical Surgery. Baltimore, Williams & Wilkins, 1980, pp 9-27.

54. Abu-Rustum NR, Barakat RR, Venkatraman E, Spriggs D: Chemotherapy and total parenteral nutrition for advanced ovarian cancer with bowel obstruction. Gynecol Oncol 1997;64:493-495.

55. Harris GJC, Senagore AJ, Lavery IC, Fazio VW: The management of neoplastic colorectal obstruction with colonic endoluminal stenting devices. Am J Surg 2001;181:499-506.

56. Soetikno RM, Carr-Locke DL: Expandable metal stents for gastric outlet, duodenal, and small intestinal obstruction. Gastrointest Endosc Clin North Am 1999;9:447-458.

57. Carter J, Valmadre S, Dalrymple C, et al: Management of large bowel obstruction in advanced ovarian cancer with intraluminal stents. Gynecol Oncol 2002;84:176-179.

58. Krebs HB, Goplerud DR: The role of intestinal intubation in obstruction of the small intestine due to carcinoma of the ovary. Surg Gynecol Obstet 1984;158:467-471.

59. Randall TC, Rubin SC: Management of intestinal obstruction in the patient with ovarian cancer. Oncology 2000;14:1159-1163.

60. Brolin RE: Partial small bowel obstruction. Surgery 1984;95: 145-149.

61. Douglas DD, Morissey JF: A new technique for rapid endoscope-assisted intubation of the small intestine. Arch Surg 1978;113: 196-198.

62. Munro A, Jones PF: Operative intubation in the treatment of complicated small-bowel obstruction. Br J Surg 1978;65:123-127.

63. Pictus D, Marx MV, Weyman PJ: Chronic intestinal obstruction: value of percutaneous gastrostomy tube placement. Am J Radiol 1988;150:295-297.

64. Gauderer MWL, Ponsky JL, Izant RJ: Gastrostomy without laparotomy: A percutaneous endoscopic technique. J Pediatr Surg 1980;15:872-875.

65. Wills JS, Oglesby JT: Percutaneous gastrostomy. Radiology 1983;149:449-453.

66. Adelson MD, Kasowitz MH: Percutaneous endoscopic drainage gastrostomy in the treatment of gastrointestinal obstruction from intraperitoneal malignancy. Obstet Gynecol 1993;81:467-471.

67. Lee MJ, Saini S, Brink JA, et al: Malignant small bowel obstruction and ascites: Not a contraindication to percutaneous gastrostomy. Clin Radiol 1991;44:332-334.

68. Ponsky JL, Gauderer MWL, Stellato TA: Percutaneous endoscopic gastrostomy-review of 150 cases. Arch Surg 1983;118: 913-914.

69. Isbister WH, Elder P, Symons L: Non-operative management of malignant intestinal obstruction. J R Coll Surg Edinb 1990;35: 369-372.

70. Fainsinger RL, Spachynski K, Hanson J, Bruera E: Symptom control in terminally ill patients with malignant bowel obstruction. J Pain Symptom Manage 1994;9:12-18.
71. Baines M: The pathophysiology and management of malignant intestinal obstruction. In Doyle D, Hanks GWC, MacDonald N (eds): Oxford Test Book of Palliative Medicine. Oxford, Oxford Medical Publication, 1993, pp 311-316.
72. Reid DB: Palliative management of bowel obstruction. Med J Aust 1988;148:54-57.
73. Twycross RG, Lack SA: Gastrointestinal obstruction. In Twycross RG, Lack SA (eds): Symptom Control in Advanced Cancer: Alimentary Symptoms, vol 11. London, Pitman, 1986, pp 239-257.
74. Bauer VR, Gross E, Scarselli V, et al: Uber wirkungunterchiede van atopin, scopolamin und einigen ihren quartaren eviate nach subcutaner und enteralen gabe unter besonderer berucksichtigung des scopolamine-n-butylbromids. Arzneimittelforschung 1968;18:1132-1137.
75. Weiner N: Atropine, scopolamine and related antimuscarinic drugs. In Goodman-Gilman A, Goodman L, Gilman A (eds): The Pharmacological Basis of Therapeutics. New York, Macmillan, 1980, pp 120-137.
76. DeConno F, Caraceni A, Zecca E, et al: Continuous subcutaneous infusion of hyoscine butylbromide reduces secretions in patients with gastrointestinal obstruction. J Pain Symptom Manage 1991; 6:484-486.
77. Reichlin S: Medical progress: Somatostatin. N Engl J Med 1983; 309:1495-1501.
78. Mercadante S, Maddaloni S: Octreotide in the management of inoperable gastrointestinal obstruction in terminal cancer patients. J Pain Symptom Manage 1992;7:496-498.
79. Mercadante S: The use of octreotide in bowel obstruction. Palliat Med 1993;7:78.
80. Kutz K, Muesh E, Rosenthaler J: Pharmacokinetics of SMS 201-995 in healthy subjects. Scand J Gastroenterol 1986;21(Suppl 119): 65-72.
81. Khoo D, Hall E, Motson R, Riley J, et al: Palliation of malignant intestinal obstruction using octreotide. Eur J Cancer 1994;30A: 28-30.
82. Mercadante S, Spoldi E, Carceni A, et al: Octreotide in relieving gastrointestinal symptoms due to bowel obstruction. Palliat Med 1993;7:295-299.
83. Khoo D, Riley G, Waxman J: Control of emesis in bowel obstruction in terminally ill patients. Lancet 1992;339:375-376.
84. Dean A, Bridge D, Lickiss JM: The palliative effects of octreotide in malignant disease. Ann Acad Med Singapore 1994;23:212-215.
85. Stiefel F, Morant R: Vapreotide, a new somatostatin analogue in the palliative management of obstructive ileus in advanced cancer. Support Care Cancer 1993;1:57-58.
86. Farr WC: The use of corticosteroids for symptom management in terminally ill patients. Am J Hospice Care 1990;1:41-46.
87. Bruera E, Schoeller T: Patient-controlled analgesia in cancer pain. In DeVita VT, Helman S, Rosenberg SA (eds): Principles and Practice of Oncology. Philadelphia: Lippincott, 1992, p 7.
88. Chapman C, Bosscher J, Remmenga S, et al: A technique for managing terminally ill ovarian carcinoma patients. Gynecol Oncol 1991;41:88-91.
89. Dudrick SJ, Wilmore DW, Vars HM, Rhoads JE: Long term parenteral nutrition with growth, development, and positive nitrogen balance. Surgery 1968;64:134-142.
90. Ford JH, Dudan RC, Bennett JS, Averette HE: Parenteral hyperalimentation in gynecologic oncology patients. Gynecol Oncol 1972;1:70-75.
91. Oley/ASPEN Information System (OASIS). Home nutritional support patient registry: Annual report, 1986 data. Albany, NY, Oley Foundation, 1988.
92. Schattner MA, Shike M: Nutritional Support of Patients with Gynecologic Cancers. In Hoskins WJ, Perez CA, Young RC (eds): Principles and Practice of Gynecologic Oncology, 3rd ed. Philadelphia: Lippincott Williams & Wilkins, 2000. pp 611-627.
93. Wesley JR: Home parenteral nutrition: indications, principles, and cost-effectiveness. Compr Ther 1983;9:29-36.
94. American College of Physicians: Position paper: Parenteral nutrition in patients receiving cancer chemotherapy. Ann Intern Med 1989;110:734-736.
95. Howard L: Home parenteral nutrition in patients with a cancer diagnosis. JPEN J Parenter Enteral Nutr 1992;16(Suppl):93-99.
96. Howard L, Ament M, Fleming CR, et al: Current use and clinical outcome of home parenteral and enteral nutrition therapies in the United States. Gastroenterology 1995;109:355-365.
97. Copeland EM: Intravenous hyperalimentation and chemotherapy: An update. JPEN J Parenter Enteral Nutr 1982;6:236-239.
98. Sharp JW, Roncagli T: Home parenteral nutrition in advanced cancer. Cancer Pract 1993;1:119-124.
99. Scribner BH, Cole JJ, Christopher TC: Long term total parenteral nutrition: the concept of an artificial gut. JAMA 1970; 212:457-463.
100. Byrne WJ, Ament ME, Burke M, Fonkalsrud E: Home parenteral nutrition. Surg Gynecol Obstet 1979;149:593-599.
101. Fainsinger RL, Chan K, Bruera E: Total parenteral nutrition for a terminally ill patient? J Palliat Care 1992;8:30-32.
102. Schwartz GF, Green HL, Bendon ML, et al: Combined parenteral hyperalimentation and chemotherapy in the treatment of disseminated solid tumors. Am J Surg 1971;121:169-173.
103. Copeland EM, MacFayden BV Jr, Lanzotti VJ, Dudrick SJ: Intravenous hyperalimentation as an adjunct to cancer chemotherapy. Am J Surg 1975;129:167-173.
104. Hopkins MP, Roberts JA, Morley GW: Outpatient management of small bowel obstruction in terminal ovarian cancer. J Reprod Med 1987;32:827-829.
105. Baker JP, Detsky AS, Wesson DE: Nutritional assessment: A comparison of clinical judgment and objective measurements. N Engl J Med 1982;306:969-972.
106. Lowry SF, Smith JC Jr, Brennan MF: Zinc and copper replacement during total parenteral nutrition. Am J Clin Nutr 1981;34:1853-1860.
107. Kirkemo AK, Burt ME, Brennan NJ: Serum Vitamin level maintenance in cancer patients on TPN. Am J Clin Nutr 1982;35; 1003-1009.
108. Shike M, Russel DM, Detsky AS, et al: Changes in body composition in patients with small cell lung cancer: The effect of TPN as an adjunct for chemotherapy. Ann Intern Med 1984; 101:303-309.
109. Clarke-Pearson DL, Rodriguez GC, Boente M: Palliative surgery for epithelial ovarian cancer. In Rubin SC, Sutton GP (eds): Ovarian Cancer, 2nd ed. Philadelphia, Lippincott Williams & Wilkins, 2001, pp 329-344.
110. Cozzaglio L, Balzola F, Cosentino F, et al: Outcome of cancer patients receiving home parenteral nutrition. J PEN 1997;21: 339-342.
111. The Veterans Affairs Total Parenteral Nutrition Cooperative Study Group: Perioperative total parenteral nutrition in surgical patients. N Engl J Med 1991;325:525-532.
112. Brennan MF, Pisters PWT, Posner M, et al: A prospective randomized trial of total parenteral nutrition after major pancreatic resection for malignancy. Ann Surg 1994;220:436-441.
113. Klein S, Simes J, Blackburn GL: Total parenteral nutrition and cancer clinical trials. Cancer 1986;58:1378-1386.
114. Smale BF, Mullen JL, Buzby GP, Rosato EF: The efficacy of nutritional assessment and support in cancer surgery. cancer 1981;47:2375-2381.
115. Brown D, Roberts JA, Elkins TE, et al: Hard choices: The gynecologic cancer patient's end-of-life preferences. Gynecol Oncol 1994;55:355-362.
116. McCann RM, Hall WJ, Groth-Juncker A: Comfort care for terminally ill patients. JAMA 1994;272:1263-1266.
117. Fletcher JC, Spencer EM: Incompetent on the slippery slope. Lancet 1995;345:271-272.
118. Waller A, Adunski A, Hershkowitz M: Terminal dehydration and intravenous fluids. Lancet 1991;337:745.
119. Cranford RE: Neurologic syndromes and prolonged survival: When can artificial nutrition and hydration be forgone? Law Med Health Care 1991;19:13-22.
120. Dunlop R, Ellershaw JE, Baines MJ, et al: On withholding nutrition and hydration in the terminally ill: Has palliative medicine gone too far? A reply. J Med Ethics 1995;21:141-143.
121. Printz LA: Is withholding hydration a valid comfort measure in the terminally ill? Geriatrics 1988;43:84-88.
122. Schmitz P: The process of dying with and without feeding and fluids by tube. Law Med Health Care 1991;19:23-26.
123. Zerwekh JV: The dehydration question. Nursing 1983;13:47-51.
124. Parker MC, Barnes MJ: Intestinal obstruction in patients with advanced malignant disease. Br J Surg 1996;83:1-2.

125. Feldman GB, Knapp RC, Order SE, Hellman S: The role of lymphatic obstruction in the formation of ascites in a murine ovarian carcinoma. Cancer Res 1972;32:1663-1666.

126. Holm-Nielsen P: Pathogenesis of ascites in peritoneal carcinomatosis. Acta Pathol Microbiol Scand 1953;33:10-21.

127. Appelqvist P, Silvo J, Salema L, Kostianien S: On the treatment and prognosis of malignant ascites: Is the survival time determined when the abdominal paracentesis is needed? J Surg Oncol 1982;20:238-242.

128. Knauer CM, Lowe HM: Hemodynamics in the cirrhotic patient during paracentesis. N Engl J Med 1967;276:491-496.

129. Gines P, Arroyo V, Quintero E, et al: Comparison of paracentesis and diuretics in the treatment of cirrhosis with tense ascites—results of a randomized study. Gastroenterology 1987;93:234-241.

130. Halpin TF, McCann TO: Dynamics of body fluids following the rapid removal of large volume ascites. Am J Obstet Gynecol 1971;110:103-106.

131. Cruikshank DP, Buchsbaum HJ: Effects of rapid paracentesis-cardiovascular dynamics and body fluid composition. JAMA 1973;225:1361-1362.

132. Gotlieb WH, Feldman B, Feldman-Moran O, et al: Intraperitoneal pressures and clinical parameters of total paracentesis for palliation of symptomatic ascites in ovarian cancer. Gynecol Oncol 1998;71:381-385.

133. Mulvaney D: Vesicocoelomic drainage for relief of ascites. Lancet 1955;2:747-749.

134. Stehman FB, Ehrlich CE: Peritoneo-cystic shunt for malignant ascites. Gynecol Oncol 1984;18:402-407.

135. Smith AN: Peritoneocaval shunt with a Holter valve in the treatment of ascites. Lancet 1962;1:671-62.

136. Smith AN, Preshaw RM, Bisset WH: The drainage of resistant ascites by a modification of the Spitz-Holter valve technique. JR Coll Surg Edinb 1962;7:289-294.

137. LeVeen HH, Christoudias G, Moon IP, et al: Perioneo-venous shunting for ascites. Ann Surg 1974;180:580-591.

138. LeVeen HH, Wapnick S, Grosberg S: Further experience with peritoneo-venous shunts for ascites. Ann Surg 1976;184:574-581.

139. Lund RH, Newkirk JB: Peritoneo-venous shunting system for surgical management of ascites. Contemp Surg 1979;14:31-45.

140. Gullstrand P, Alwmark A, Borjesson B, et al: Peritoneovenous shunting for intractable ascites. Scand J Gastroenterol 1982;17:1009-1012.

141. Straus AK, Roseman DL, Shapiro TM: Peritoneovenous shunting in the management of malignant ascites. Arch Surg 1979;114:489-491.

142. Souter RG, Wells C, Tarin D, Kettlewell MGW: Surgical and pathologic complications associated with peritoneovenous shunts in management of malignant ascites. Cancer 1985;55:1973-1978.

143. Sonnenfeld T, Tyden G: Peritoneovenous shunts for malignant ascites. Acta Chir Scand 1986;152:117-121.

144. Oosterlee J: Peritoneovenous shunting for ascites in cancer patients. Br J Surg 1980;67:663-666.

145. Battaglia GB, Levi D'Ancona V, Farsi N, Boffi L: Preliminary experience in the treatment of rebel ascites from ovarian cancer with the peritoneo-venous shunt of LeVeen. Eur J Gyneacol Oncol 1982;3:88-90.

146. Ariel IM, Oropeza R, Pack GT: Intracavitary administration of radioactive isotopes in the control of effusions due to cancer—results in 267 patients. Cancer 1966;19:1096-1102.

147. Jackson GL, Blosser NM: Intracavitary chromic phosphate ^{32}P colloidal suspension therapy. Cancer 1981;48:2596-2598.

148. Paladine W, Cunningham TJ, Sponzo R, et al: Intracavitary bleomycin in the management of malignant effusions. Cancer 1976;38:1903-1908.

149. Bitran JD: Intraperitoneal bleomycin-pharmacokinetics and results of a phase 2 trial. Cancer 1985;56:2420-2423.

150. Ozols RF, Young RC, Speyer JL, et al: Phase 1 and pharmacological studies of Adriamycin administered intraperitoneally to patients with ovarian cancer. Cancer Res 1982;42:4265-4269.

151. Kefford RF, Woods RL, Fox RM, Tattersall MHN: Intracavitary adriamycin, nitrogen mustard, and tetracycline in the control of malignant effusions—a randomized study. Med J Aust 1980;2:447-448.

152. Cherchi PL, Campiglio A, Rubattu A, et al: Endocavitary beta-interferon in neoplastic effusions. Eur J Gynaecol Oncol 1990;11:477-479.

153. Bezwoda WR, Seymour L, Dansy R: Intraperitoneal recombinant interferon-alpha 2b for recurrent malignant ascites due to ovarian cancer. Cancer 1989;64:1029-1033.

154. Currie JL, Gall S, Weed JC Jr, Creasman WT: Intracavitary *Corynebacterium parvum* for treatment of malignant effusions. Gynecol Oncol 1983;16:6-14.

155. Buckman R, DeAngelis C, Shaw P, et al: Intraperitoneal therapy of malignant ascites associated with carcinoma of ovary and breast using radioiodinated monoclonal antibody 2G3. Gynecol Oncol 1992;47:102-109.

156. Kamada M, Sakamoto Y, Furumoto H, et al: Treatment of malignant ascites with allogeneic and autologous lymphokine-activated killer cells. Gynecol Oncol 1989;34:34-37.

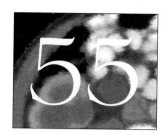

CHAPTER

DEATH AND DYING

Robert Buckman and Walter Baile

 MAJOR CONTROVERSIES

- **Why is end-of-life care still a difficult topic?**
- **Does the process of dying have identifiable stages?**
- **Do most patients react to the prospect of dying in the same way?**
- **Must we tell patients the bad news and take away hope?**
- **Are communication skills innate, or can they be acquired, and can empathy be taught?**
- **Is support an indefinable concept?**
- **Is a patient's death synonymous with medical failure, and is cure the only worthwhile goal of gynecologic oncology?**
- **Is the improvement of communication in palliative care an ineffective use of time and expertise?**
- **How can physicians deal with a patient's unrealistic hopes?**

Why is end-of-life care still a difficult topic?

The process of dying has never been an easy subject for physicians to discuss or to think about, and this awkwardness contributes to the difficulty surrounding end-of-life care problems in gynecologic oncology, perhaps more commonly than in other areas of oncology.[1-3] Oncologists have been trained in the details of therapeutic interventions and options, and until recently, they have customarily equated the end of a patient's life with therapeutic failure. Because of this, the prospect of a patient's death commonly produces feelings—or at least overtones and associations—of failure in the physician. This chapter highlights eight of the key areas in end-of-life care that still create difficulty and contention for most of us and that present obstacles to our improving end-of-life care in gynecologic oncology.

Factors Influencing the Perception of Dying

Many factors contribute to the atmosphere of tension, distress, and discomfort that surrounds conversation about dying.[4,5] As has been suggested,[6] it is helpful to consider the contributory factors under five major

headings: societal, patient-related, physician-related, and family issues and those originating within the medical community. It is worth discussing these points in some detail, because being aware of the sources of the difficulties often makes it easier to cope with them and to consider strategies for reducing them.

Societal factors. The attitudes and expectations of physicians, patients, and family alike are shaped by and reflect prevailing social expectations. Our society is emerging from many decades of death denial, during which private and public discussions of death were almost forbidden or taboo topics.[7,8] Things have changed considerably in recent years, but the prospect of death and dying commonly precipitates deeply rooted distress, including fear, dread, anxiety, disappointment, worry about impending loss, and grief. These are normal and expected reactions and are heightened by preexisting factors from at least four sources. A lengthier discussion of these topics is available elsewhere.[9]

Lack of previous experience of death or dying in the family. Most adults have not witnessed the death of a family member at home when they themselves were

743

young and still forming their view of life. Whereas a century ago approximately 90% of deaths occurred in the home, for the past few decades, more than 65% (varying with regional demographics) occur in hospitals or institutions. This means that, unlike the norm a century ago, contemporary childhood and adolescence do not usually include any personal experience of a death in the family occurring in the home. This change has occurred over the same period as a change in the structure of the average family itself. The norm has changed from the extended family to the nuclear family. Elderly people are now less likely to be living with their grandchildren and may well have no fit, young relatives to support them at the time of their last illness.

This does not mean that the past was a golden era when a death in the family produced a moving and beneficial experience in the survivors. Witnessing a death at home in the past was not always a serene or tranquil experience, particularly before the era of powerful analgesics and other symptom-controlling agents. However, even if a death at home was not a pleasant event, a child growing up in such a home would be imprinted with a sense of the continuity of life, the process of aging, and the natural inevitability of death (i.e., when you are older, you look like dad; when you are much older, you look like granddad; when you are very, very old, you die). As the extended family has disappeared, dying has become the province of the health care professional or institution; most people do not have a sense of continuity and regard the process of dying as intrinsically alien and divorced from the business of living.

Another factor in determining the place of most deaths is the rise and range of modern health services and the increase in facilities and treatments offered. Although these services provide undoubted advantages in medical and nursing care for the person dying in an institution, there is also disruption of family support for the patient. In general, most people have come to regard end-of-life care as being fundamentally within the province of the experts. The feeling that all aspects of the patient's death are in the domain of— and under the professional control of—the hospital or physician adds to the family member's sense that they may not be important or have any significant role at the end of the patient's life.

High expectations of health and life. Advances in medical science are often overreported in the media and hailed as major breakthroughs. The constant bombardment of the public with news of apparently miraculous advances in the fight against disease subconsciously raises expectations of health and offers tantalizing hopes of a cure for all major diseases. This public expectation makes it even harder for an individual to face the fact that he or she will not be cured despite the many miracles reported on television or in print. Sometimes, the information may seem to be irresponsibly optimistic. Data publicly available on the Internet, for example, may detail findings that may be years away from being translated into clinical interventions. From whatever source, hopes that have been falsely raised tend to deepen the sense of disappointment and despair experienced during discussions about transition.

Material evaluation. It is beyond the scope of this chapter to assess the materialistic values of the modern world, except to point out that our society routinely evaluates a person's worth in material and tangible terms. This is our current social system of values and is neither good nor bad. However, it is universally accepted in our society that dying means that the person will be parted from his or her material possessions. A society that places a high and almost exclusive value on material possessions implicitly increases the psychological penalty of dying for its members.

The changing role of religion. The role of religion has changed, and the previously near-universal view of a single exterior, anthropomorphic God is now fragmented and individualized. Religion is much more of an individual philosophical stance than it was in the last century. It is no longer possible to assume that everyone shares the same ideas about God or an afterlife. Whereas a Victorian physician might have said to a patient, "Your soul will be with its Maker by the ebbtide," and might have meant it genuinely as a statement of fact and of consolation, we cannot now assume that such a statement will bring relief to all patients.

For all these reasons, our society is passing through a phase of development during which the process of dying is perceived as alien and fearsome and during which the dying person is marginalized and distanced from the living. This increases the discomfort that surrounds any conversation about dying. This means that even before a discussion about a particular subject between patient and physician begins, the psychological temperature may already be raised to uncomfortable levels. Recognizing the significant impact of these societal factors often makes it easier for health care professionals to avoid feeling that the difficulty in the discussion is somehow their fault.

Patient factors. Individuals facing the prospect of dying experience mixtures of emotions, including fear (about many aspects of the process), guilt, the stigma of bad luck, a sense of failure, diminishing control and independence, increasing dependence on others, and an enhanced awareness of their own unfinished business.

Fear. Fear is perhaps the first and most common emotion. It is almost universal; although very few patients can contemplate their own dying with equanimity, most experience a mixture of fears originating from many sources (Table 55-1). In practice, a patient's fear is as often couched in questions about how she will die as whether she will die. If a patient does not express some measure of fear, physicians should ask whether the patient genuinely understands the situation.

Unfinished business. Underlying the attitude of many individuals about the end of life is the sense of their own unfinished business. It is a common observation

Table 55–1. Three-Stage Concept of Dying

Beginning (Acute Phase)	Middle (Chronic Phase)	End (Final Phase)
Patient's responses are characteristic of the person, not the stage. They may include fear, shock, disbelief, denial, guilt, humor, anger, displacement, and bargaining.	Resolution of the resolvable reactions occurs. Depression is common.	Acceptance is common, although not universal.

that people who are most comfortable with their own state of living tend to be relatively comfortable when it comes to the process of dying. All of us have hopes for the future and our own personal agendas of objectives, and the greater the list of unfulfilled expectations, the harder it is to accept that time is running out. Usually, the issue of unfinished business plays a greater part in the considerations of younger cancer patients.

Guilt. A sense of personal responsibility about the medical situation—whether warranted or not—is very common, although it is often deeply rooted and camouflaged. It is often important to be aware of the possibility of guilt underlying anger or fear. Guilt is often made worse by prevalent views that a positive attitude can enhance survival. Even though several studies have shown that this is not the case, the feeling that advancing disease somehow represents a failure of the patient's willpower or determination adds to the burden.

Denial. Denial is in itself a major topic. In general, denial is not pathologic and can legitimately be regarded as a normal coping strategy in that it allows the person to come to terms with the situation gradually without being overwhelmed by it. However, avoidance of medical facts, false hopes and expectations, and focusing on only the positive things that the patient has heard may lead to misunderstandings about the purpose of treatment or about the chances of cure or remission. A patient with lung cancer metastatic to the brain whose doctor told her he was optimistic about treatment later may report that this meant she had a good chance for cure.

Physician factors.
Therapeutic failure. Physicians' expectations of themselves, engendered by training that disproportionately values cure over care and by attitudes of society at large, make it uncomfortable to confront the fact that treatment for the disease process is not working. When broaching the subject of transition to palliative care for the first time, it is easy for physicians to make a subconscious move from "curative treatment has failed" to "my treatment has failed," which frequently makes oncologists feel they have failed or are themselves failures. In recent years, the much-needed expansion of the palliative care discipline has helped somewhat by demonstrating that good symptom control can be an important goal in itself. However, the sense of therapeutic failure has not yet been totally extinguished.

Attachment. When physicians have been involved in a patient's care over a prolonged period, they may become psychologically invested in the goal of a successful medical outcome. This is intensified when patients are likable or when physicians identify with patients. The patient and physician may experience personal disappointment. Sometimes, this sense of "letting the patient down" can be almost overwhelming and needs to be acknowledged.

Dislike of unpreparedness. When discussing an issue such as end-of-life care or the process of dying, most physicians appropriately feel that they have received inadequate training for the task. Only a small fraction of clinicians have had specific training in the communication skills that are helpful, and this feeling of unpreparedness increases the urge to avoid or parry such conversations. Oncologists are naturally unwilling to enter into a situation or conversation for which they feel unprepared, and they are wary in case they precipitate a reaction from the patient, including something as simple as crying, if they do not know how to deal with it. Clinicians are unaccustomed to answering questions with "I don't know" and find it difficult to discuss situations in which there is a not a clear and immediate medical action that can fix the problem.

Family factors. Family members almost always have their own agendas.[10-12] Sometimes, their expectations and emotions are synchronous with the patient's, but often they are not. This dissonance may occur when the patient has reached acceptance of the prognosis and transition but a relative (frequently an adult son or daughter) has not. (Sometimes, this situation is reversed.) Moreover, family dynamics may create situations such as a strong need on the part of the family member to "rescue" or "protect" the patient, and in these situations, family members or friends may feel hostile toward the professionals. This dissonance may make discussion and planning difficult and needs to be dealt with ("I realize that it is very difficult for you, and it is hard to accept, as your mother has, that the disease is progressing.").

Medical community factors. One source of discomfort is rarely discussed or acknowledged: the feeling that other professionals might have done things differently or better. The feeling that colleagues or some unknown specialist elsewhere might have handled this case differently and that there might have been a better outcome is quite common. This feeling is further exacerbated by the high degree of patient information readily accessible, for example, on the Internet.[13]

Any or all of these factors may contribute to the discomfort that arises during discussions between physicians and patients or their family members. Being aware of some of them at work in the background may allow physicians to be better prepared for these emotional difficult discussions and to acknowledge that the emotional intensity of the conversations is to be expected in today's social values and is not a condemnation of their professional abilities.

Does the process of dying have identifiable stages?

The controversy over the best and most practical way of conceptualizing the process of dying is of great importance. How the health care professional thinks of and views the process affects the way in which she or he prepares strategies to support the patient. It also changes what physicians each regard as normal in a patient's response and what can be regarded as abnormal or pathologic. The conceptual framework also affects the criteria by which physicians judge the status and the progress of the patient in psychological terms and according to many other factors. In many respects, controversies over the most useful conceptual framework for the process of dying affect all other issues.

Decades ago, the process of dying seemed to be impenetrably mysterious and so wrapped up in social taboos and silence that even if physicians wanted to help, there seemed to be no way of doing so. Until the 1960s, there were few published sources that touched on this area, and the books that were available were universally based on anecdotal experience and personal philosophy. None of them proposed a conceptual framework that could be applied by clinicians to the practicalities of end-of-life care.

In 1969, *On Death and Dying* by Kübler-Ross provided a major and much needed change of approach.[14] Based on her experience as a psychiatrist, she divided the process of dying into five stages (Table 55-2), constructing a medical model of the process of dying which made it more accessible and intelligible to clinicians. The Kübler-Ross staging system has been widely viewed as imperfect in several ways; for example, it did not include commonly seen responses such as fear or guilt, and it did not touch on the concept of coping strategies (although bargaining is one, as are

displacement behaviors and humor). Even so, Kübler-Ross' book and its successors achieved the valuable result of presenting the process of dying as a clinical process, comparable to any progressive incurable condition such as amyotrophic lateral sclerosis (i.e., Lou Gehrig's disease). The process of dying became more accessible to the clinician as analogous to other medical processes and one in which therapeutic interventions were legitimate and part of medical management.

It may be more useful and more practical from the point of view of end-of-life care to use a simpler concept of the process of dying, considering it pragmatically as a process that has a beginning, a middle, and an end (see Table 55-1). This three-stage conceptual framework has been set out in detail in several publications and has the merit of being easy to remember and understand and of providing simple markers that act as the basis for the clinician's assessment, intervention, and prediction of what is likely to happen next. The fundamental communication skills involved are described later in this chapter.

The two conceptual frameworks discussed here present fundamentally different views of the process of dying. The five-stage system of Kübler-Ross suggests that the prospect of dying imposes a degree of conformity on the patient. The three-stage system suggests that, faced with a crisis, each individual reacts with a mixture of responses taken from an individual, even idiosyncratic, repertoire characteristic of that person and of his or her coping strategies. It is possible that the latter view has more practical applications to the management of the dying process.

Do most patients react to the prospect of dying in the same way?

As conventional wisdom has it, people are no more uniform in their way of dying than they are in their way of living. An individual's reactions to dying may seem almost imponderable because every patient has a different set of attitudes and responses to disease progression, deterioration, and the prospect of dying. When faced with any serious reverse of fortune or major setback, people tend to react with a mixture of responses and emotions that are to some extent characteristic of their personalities and coping styles. Some people use denial readily and extensively; others exhibit rage; many feel guilt and some degree of self-recrimination; and most (depending on the circumstances, but particularly if faced with a new and serious medical crisis) feel fear. Each patient facing the prospect of dying is likely to react in a way that is characteristic of the individual rather than a fixed pattern of reactions. What health care professionals see as the patient's reactions is more likely to be similar to that patient's responses to previous moments of crisis. Some individuals are easily roused to anger and customarily become angry many times in a day over matters that would not disturb others. Such people are very likely to be angry when confronting a major reverse. Similarly, other people use denial as an initial

---

Table 55–2. Kübler-Ross Five-Stage Concept of Dying

Denial
Anger
Bargaining
Depression
Acceptance*

*Many common reactions, such as fear, shock, and guilt, are not included in these five stages, and coping strategies, including humor, are not incorporated.

reaction and will do so to a greater extent, commensurate with the perceived threat. The same can be said of any reaction to a sudden threat; reactions include fear, disbelief, guilt, humor, and displacement behaviors. The resulting mixture of responses is a personal recipe made up of the commonly used ingredients in that person's repertoire. In other words, the patient's initial response to a crisis can be likened to a portrait in miniature of that person's strategies of response and coping—the "palette of colors" that is characteristic of that person, not of the stage of the response. People are, in this way of thinking, better compared with mosaics, complex patterns composed of elements of many different colors, than with chameleons, changing from one color to the next in a fixed or predetermined sequence.

Viewing the patient's initial reaction to the prospect of dying as a characteristic portrait in miniature of that person's reactions to crisis and her or his coping strategies offers useful insight into the person's psychological makeup. It allows the professional to make a preliminary assessment of the person's coping style and to predict in a general way what reactions will be seen in the immediate future.

Must we tell patients the bad news and take away hope?

Ethical aspects. The issue of hope is often presented as an ethical dilemma. The issue is typically framed by awkward questions: "If by telling the truth you drive a patient to suicide, are you ethically obliged to lie?" The real problem at the center of this particular controversy is not one of ethics, but of communication skills and techniques. Telling the truth is not a simple procedure that is done or not done. It may be done well, supportively, interactively, and therapeutically. Some professionals demonstrate all of these attributes, and a few occasionally demonstrate none of them.[16] There are almost as many ways of approaching this task as there are of taking a clinical history. If one approach does carry a risk of the patient's suicide (and there is some doubt even of that), what is required is a different and better technique, not a retreat to deception.

More than any other rationale, the principle of *do no harm* has been used for centuries by physicians as a reason or perhaps an excuse for not discussing adverse medical news with the patient. It is based on the idea that telling the truth or part of it may inflict harm on an already ill and suffering person. This argument has been used traditionally as a defense for secrecy and deception. As far back as the 16th century, the physician de Sorbiere discussed the prospect of telling the truth to a patient and then concluded that it was not worth the effort![17] In the past few decades, moral, ethical, and medicolegal precedents have settled the issue of the patient's rights beyond dispute. Every mentally competent adult patient is entitled to exercise his or her right to receive all relevant medical information.

There is universal acceptance by the public and by the health care and legal professionals in North America, Europe, Australia, and elsewhere that the patient's rights to information have primacy. The problem is that some measure of psychological damage or harm may be added to the existing burden by ineffective or antagonistic communication. As Billings explains,[18] "insensitive truth-telling may be as harmful—and counterproductive—as insensitive deception."

Communication aspects. The argument that telling a patient bad news will necessarily take away all hope reflects a narrow view of the various dimensions of hope. Although physicians typically define hope in terms of biomedical outcomes such as cure of disease or response to treatment, patients, when given the opportunity, conceptualize hope much more broadly, as has been illustrated in some studies.

In one study,[19] cancer patients were asked to define the most and the least hopeful behaviors of their oncologists. Appropriately, the provision of effective medical care was high on the list, reflecting the patients' desires to have treatment to combat the disease. However, other behaviors not related to anticancer therapy were considered almost equally important in providing hope. These included providing continuity of care and answering the patient's questions. Behaviors and communications that undermined hope included refusing to answer questions about the cancer and giving important medical news over the telephone. A study[20] of patients with acquired immunodeficiency syndrome (AIDS) focused on hope and identified three categories of behaviors that patients found hopeful: giving accurate information, expressing compassion, and understanding and using lay language.

A paper[21] that asked cancer patients about their preferences when receiving bad news revealed that patients want their doctors to provide them with detailed information about their illness, to be honest with them about their condition, and to support them when they got upset.

When narrowly focused on the concept of hope solely as cure of disease, physicians often forget that many patients are able to prepare for the worst and hope for the best.[22] The percentage of cancer patients who overtly state that they wish to know the diagnosis has risen from 50% in a British study in 1981[23] to more than 95% in two later studies.[24,25] Patients may also value knowing how much time they have left to take care of business. A case history provides a useful illustration. A patient with advanced ovarian cancer was seen because of "denial of her illness." Apparently, the patient was thought to have unrealistic expectations of her medical situation. When allowed to express her concerns, it became clear that she was hoping that she had enough time left to divide up her property among her five children so they would not have to litigate over it after she had died.

Often, it is in the way in which physicians communicate bad news that the issue of preserving hope becomes a problem. Giving patients the accurate information that they want while telling them that—even if the prognosis is poor—they will be provided with the best treatment available in the context of continuity of care may provide an important sense of optimism in the face of advanced disease. Moreover, while discussing with patients their perceptions of the illness and their expectations, physicians may be able to identify individual sources of hope, resources that vary among patients. Physicians can explain to patients that cure of their cancer is unlikely but that they will still be provided the best treatment possible, and oncologists can acknowledge secondary goals or objectives that patients may have (e.g., pain control, time to see grandchildren graduate from college, celebration of a wedding anniversary). In this way, it is possible for the physician to support realistic hopes and goals even in the context of bad news.[26]

In some respects, this controversy over the ethics of hope is settled. The rights of mentally competent and adult patients to any information that has a significant bearing on their future are well established. In disclosing information concerning dying and end-of-life care, the question of "whether to tell" has been decided. The important issue is now how to tell the patient.

Are communication skills innate, or can they be acquired, and can empathy be taught?

Until recently, it was a widely held belief that good communication skills were entirely intuitive abilities ("I've always been good at talking to my patients."); they were present or not. Everyone values a good listener, and physicians who smile, are friendly, and take a personal interest in their patients are rated highly by their patients. These physicians have been considered to have a good "bedside manner." However, these basic skills are just one small part of the techniques needed by physicians in their interactions with patients.[27,28] In the task of breaking bad news, for example, at least 20 skills are important in giving information in a sensitive and empathic way. Table 55-3 illustrates the steps involved in a practical protocol for giving bad news and the skills necessary to accomplish them.

Although some practitioners show considerable flair and ability even at an early stage in their careers, it has been shown in many studies over a long period that communication skills can be acquired and may be retained for years.[29-32] The quality that we recognize as empathy is largely determined by a person's ability to acknowledge, address, and handle another person's emotional responses. In many respects, empathy depends heavily on and may be considered as identical with the skill of emotion handling.[33] To deal with a patient's emotion is not the same as experiencing it oneself. As has been said, "You do not need to have pain in your right iliac fossa to diagnose a patient's appendicitis."[34] The ability of a professional to handle emotions in an interview is not the same as that person's ability to experience the same emotion that the patient is manifesting or experiencing.

Dealing with a patient's emotions is identified by most oncologists as the most difficult aspect of patient communication.[35] In practice, the techniques that are most valuable in this situation are relatively straightforward and are learnable.[36-38] The central and most easily learned technique, the empathic response, consists of three steps: the emotion is identified, the cause of the emotion is identified, and the professional responds in a way that demonstrates that he or she has made this connection (i.e., "Clearly, this news about the ultrasound is a big shock to you.").[34] Videotaped illustrations of the use of the empathic response in difficult situations in oncology are available.[39]

In some respects, it may be of greater practical value not to consider empathy as an innate skill but instead to look at the problem of why some physicians "block out" feelings for others and have difficulty in being sensitive to them. In many cases, this occurs because physicians tend to repress their own feelings and awareness of important attitudes. The psychiatric literature describes how certain personalities and professions (e.g., engineers) may find feelings irrelevant or inconvenient. Medical education discourages (inappropriately) the exploration and expression of feelings on the

Table 55-3. Communication Skills Needed for Delivery of Bad News

Step of Giving Bad News	Purpose	Necessary Skills
Setting up (preparing for) the interview	To ensure the physician is ready To ensure the patient is ready To facilitate information exchange	Self-reflection Determining barriers to a discussion (e.g., beeper going off) Assessing whether the patient is able to assimilate information
Finding out the patient's perception (what is already known and understood)	To assess educational gaps and denial	Asking open-ended questions Active listening
Getting an invitation from the patient to give the information	To assess how much the patient wants to know	Asking open-ended questions
Giving information and knowledge	To educate the patient	Knowing how to warn the patient Giving information in small quantities Checking for understanding
Handling emotional reactions	To help the patient deal with the bad news	Validating the patient's feelings Making empathic responses Clarifying thoughts and feelings
Strategy and summary	To map out a treatment plan	Understanding obstacles to treatment Negotiating skills Involving patients in treatment decisions

grounds that it interferes with the ability to be "objective" toward the patient.[40,41] However, the case may be made that feelings such as guilt may create communications that thwart having a good rapport with the patient by leading to false expectations. Identifying such factors will make it easier for the professional to use emotion-handling skills, including the empathic response, in everyday practice.

Is support an indefinable concept?

Through overuse, the word *support* unfortunately has become a cliché and almost devoid of real meaning. To many clinicians, the word has become almost as meaningless as a superficial catch phrase such as "try to be there for your patient." As with "being there," the word *support* in its current usage gives no clue about what type of activities or transactions are implied and no clue about how or whether clinicians are actually providing it.

Despite the fact that many of the skills and activities that comprise support are difficult to delineate precisely and that many of them merge with one another, it is still helpful to consider support as having three many components: *acknowledgment* of emotions (i.e., the supporter has to be able to and willing to acknowledge the person's feelings or responses and not necessarily share them); *validation* of patients' major worries and wants (i.e., the supporter comprehends what the person is concerned about and accepts it as a concern that has genuine meaning for the person, without judging whether it is warranted by the circumstances); and assisting in *making a plan*, often involving *advocacy*. The major components of support are identifiable, and they can be reinforced among supporters by the person who can also distinguish those who are offering genuine and pragmatic support from those who are not. Taking these three elements as the central components of *support* is of practical use.

Although support may be a vague concept, various definitions of support have been identified with important health outcomes. For example, a study by House and colleagues[42] illustrated the value of community and companionship; individuals who are married and who are active members of their community church have better health outcomes. Cancer patients who see their physicians as caring and providing education tend to be better adjusted over the long term.[43]

Counseling techniques for providing support are not vague or foggy and have been employed by physicians long before there were many effective medical cures. Some of these techniques are delineated in Table 55-4.

The attempt to reduce medical care to its technical aspects ignores the fact that patients in health care crisis often regard their physician as an important source of support. Because patients in crisis tend to reach out to caregivers in a disproportionate way, poor communication by emotionally disengaged and aloof physicians can be perceived as uncaring. The medical adage that it is best not to get "emotionally involved" with patients has been widely misinterpreted by

Table 55–4. Counseling Techniques for Providing Support

Technique	Impact on the Patient
Listening (most clinicians interrupt the patient after about 20 seconds[44])	Feels regarded
Clarifying ("Did you mean to say...?")	Feels doctor is listening
Reassurance	Decreases anxiety
Encouragement	Bolsters optimism
Validates the patient's feelings	Thwarts embarrassment
Praise	Feels effort is recognized
Empathetic responses to emotions	Feels doctor is concerned
Exploring ideas and feelings ("Can you tell me why it will be so hard to tell your husband?")	Feels doctor is interested
Forecasting bad news	Allows patient to psychologically prepare
Negotiating	Patient feels views are respected

Adapted from Frankel RM, Beckman HB: The pause that refreshes. Hosp Pract 1988;23:62-67 and Baile WB, Buckman R, Lenzi R, et al.[35]

physicians to mean that they must stay detached and emotionally controlled. On the contrary, when physicians use techniques to provide support and enhance the trust of the patient, they can have positive effects on patient compliance, anxiety about treatment, and satisfaction with care.[44,45] These outcome measures in themselves argue for strategies to support the patient.

Is a patient's death synonymous with medical failure, and is cure the only worthwhile goal of gynecologic oncology?

Undeniably, cure is the ultimate objective in the treatment of any cancer if it is achievable at a cost that is acceptable to the patient in terms of side effects and quality of life. In many clinical situations, that is not the central issue. Commonly, the basic problem in gynecologic oncology, as with most areas of solid-tumor oncology, is that cure for most advanced-stage disease is frequently unachievable. This would not present such a serious problem if physicians' training had alerted them to this reality from the beginning, but unfortunately, for most in clinical practice, training tended to focus on cure, even in circumstances when cures are in the minority. It could be argued that medical training should include a greater number of skills and techniques that are useful in the management of and communication with the incurable patient.

The stance that pursuit of cure is the only worthwhile goal would be a compelling argument if cure were achieved frequently and if the percentage of cures were curtailed by limitations of physicians' time. If patients were not being cured solely because their physicians were spending their time in other activities, there would be no good reason for clinicians doing anything other than curative procedures! In reality, this is not the case; the high proportion of cases that are not curable reflects the natural history of the gynecologic cancer and the limitations of current therapy, not the apportioning of physicians' time and effort.

However, the perception of the quality of care by patients and their relatives is frequently related to the quality of physicians' communication. It is genuinely worthwhile for physicians to demonstrate that they are paying attention to "caring."

Many physicians have commented on public and physicians' attitudes toward death and dying that contribute to the idea that death is therapeutic failure. In the United States, many individuals are unprepared for death. In a study of 16,678 persons, only 9.8% had a living will.[46] Many have unrealistic beliefs about the power of medical technology to prolong life. Medical education is focused on cure and devalues other important outcomes such as improving quality of life and "dying a good death." Unfortunately, the pursuit of cure at all costs has its own price, including the fact that medical care expenditures are highest at the end of life and that patients often linger in intensive care units with little prospect of improvement. Physicians have great difficulty in discussing futility with patients, resulting in the fact that patients do not have do not resuscitate orders written. Families also have difficulty in letting go of relatives and may insist that "everything be done."

It is essential to teach young physicians the communication skills required to discuss a poor prognosis and to acknowledge the patient's hope "for the best" while at the same time preparing the patient for the transition from curative therapy to palliative care. Unless these skills are fostered, health care professionals inadvertently create unrealistic expectations on the part of the patient and family. As a foundation for learning these skills, young physicians need to examine their own attitudes toward death and dying and begin to understand the comprehensive therapeutic role of the physician in providing comfort and support. Physicians entering oncology commonly think that death is synonymous with medical failure. Even though 50% of their patients will not survive for more than 5 years, data indicate that almost 25% of cancer patients receive chemotherapy in the last 3 months of their lives.[47] Fortunately, attitudes seem to be changing. The still emerging specialty of palliative care has focused attention on the important role of good symptom management, and the role of palliative care physicians in teaching has begun to diminish the association of end-of-life care with failure.

Is the improvement of communication in palliative care an ineffective use of time and expertise?

Medicine has moved away from the authoritarian doctor-centered approach to patient care in which treatment is dictated, little information shared, and decisions are not negotiated. In the modern medical climate of better-informed patients, poor physician communication skills constitute an area of medical care that patients complain most bitterly about. This is not surprising when we consider the important outcomes of communication with patients and families. These include understanding the nature of the patient's problem and concerns (data show that physicians interrupt patients within 22 seconds after asking a question); establishing trust and rapport; understanding barriers to care; giving bad news in a compassionate and supportive way; giving patients treatment options when they exist (in some cases, this is required by law); negotiating medical care; using the supportive techniques discussed earlier to enhance patient quality of life; addressing anxiety and depression; and ensuring that consent for treatment is informed. However, when communication is poor, there are several undesirable consequences. These include complaints and litigation by patients (even against technically competent physicians), poor understanding of the purpose of treatment, distrust of the physician, and poor rapport between the patient and physician.

A medical intervention has value if it improves or prevents exacerbation of a clinical situation. The value of enhanced communication may be assessed to some extent against the consequences of poor or ineffective communication. These end points fall under two headings: complaints (including litigation) and personal consequences, including burnout.[48,49]

How can physicians deal with a patient's unrealistic hopes?

Handling a person's hopes about his or her clinical situation is a vitally important component of end-of-life care. For the purposes of this discussion, hope is defined as a positive emotion accompanying the expectation of a beneficial outcome, whether it is justified or not. Hope is an emotional state; it is a feeling that accompanies the assessment of the outcome. For example, a patient may be told that the chance of success of a particular therapy is, say, 10%, but this patient may feel that she definitely will be one of the lucky ones. It is not the statistic itself that engenders the hope; another patient may be crushed or overwhelmed by precisely the same data. Hope is best seen as an attribute of a particular person's emotional reaction to a specific situation. As such, it is neither a good thing nor a bad thing. As with any experience, there is not necessarily an appropriate or correct level or intensity of emotion.

A useful comparison can be made with the sensation of pain. When a patient has, for example, renal colic, there is no correct level for the subjective experience of pain or for its expression. Some patients may feel moderate pain and may be accustomed to voluble expression of it; others may feel more severe pain but have been conditioned by their society not to express it if possible. The same is true of hope. The amount and the intensity of hope experienced by an individual are largely determined by his or her emotional and affective repertoire (i.e., reactions to bad news), and the outward expression of those feelings depends on the person's customary style of sharing and discussing emotions.

Hope can be viewed as a personal experience in response to some uncertainty in the future. It was until recently accepted as a maxim by most of the medical profession that discussion of the future would inevitably take away hope. This was regarded as an argument in defense of concealment or deception. Conventional wisdom was that because "discussion of the facts takes away hope, we should simply not hold those discussions." The important point is that physicians can achieve the latter without resorting to the former. It is feasible to discuss the prognosis and to prepare plans for all eventualities without destroying every hope. The key is to realize that hope is not a single monolithic entity that is present or totally absent. Hope is the sum total of many components, including the hope that the disease will be cured or stabilized for a long time.

Progressing disease and declining function are almost invariably causes of great distress, fear, and disappointment for many patients. How health care professionals handle that distress and disappointment greatly affects the patients' perception of their medical management, of their symptoms, of physicians and all the health care personnel, and probably their friends and family. The main objective should be to identify problems that may be improved and to attempt improvement of them while developing the patient's coping strategies for facing all the other problems. It is essential that physicians acknowledgment of the patient's feelings—including hope—with techniques such as the empathic response and strategizing to provide as many hoped-for outcomes as possible (i.e., providing support).

Strategies for Communication at the End of Life

Communication has been neatly and appropriately compared with a medication.[50] It has a threshold dose below which no therapeutic effects occur, and suboptimal dosing is unfortunately fairly common. It has several interactions with other aspects of therapy, many palliative effects on many symptoms, and is handled differently by different patients (perhaps comparable with pharmacokinetics). At the end of life, all palliative agents have to be used with care regarding the dose and frequency of administration. In the case of communication, overdose is rare (or as pharmacologists might phrase it, "communication has a wide therapeutic index"), and suboptimal dosing with overly long time intervals is common.

Communication skills in end-of-life care are skills, not intuitive or inherited abilities, and they can be taught and retained by anyone. Improvement in the dialogue between the gynecologic oncologist and the patient may well offer the greatest single means of improving the quality of medical care at the end of the patient's life. Practical details and examples of how to do this are available and in current use. Improvement in these aspects of end-of-life care in gynecologic oncology may offer the most immediate and far-reaching changes in the quality of care—and in the quality of life—of patients.

REFERENCES

1. Maguire P: Barriers to psychological care of the dying. BMJ 1985; 291:1711-1713.
2. Houts PS, Yasko JM, Harvey HA, et al: Unmet needs of persons with cancer in Pennsylvania during the period of terminal care. Cancer 1988;62:627-634.
3. Wilkes E: Dying now. Lancet 1984;2:950-952.
4. Seravalli EP: The dying patient, the physician and the fear of death. N Engl J Med 1988;319:1728-1730.
5. Schulz R: The Psychology of Death, Dying and Bereavement. Reading, MA, Addison Wesley, 1978.
6. Buckman R: Breaking bad news: Why is it still so difficult? BMJ 1984;288:1597-1599.
7. Rando TA: Death and the dying patient. In Grief, Dying, and Death. Chicago, Research Press, 1984, pp 199-223.
8. Becker E: The Denial of Death. New York, Free Press, 1973.
9. Buckman R: I Don't Know What to Say—How to Help and Support Someone Who is Dying. London, Macmillan, 1988.
10. Hockley JM, Dunlop R, Davies RJ: Survey of distressing symptoms it dying patients and their families in hospital and the response to symptom control team. BMJ 1988;296: 1715-1717.
11. Kristjanson U: Quality of terminal care: Salient indicators identified by families. J Palliat Care 1989;5:21-28.
12. Stedeford A: Couples facing death. II. Unsatisfactory communication. BMJ 1981;283:1098-1101.
13. Helft PR, Hlubocky F, and Daugherty CK: American oncologists' view of Internet use by cancer patients: A mail survey of American Society of Clinical Oncology members. J Clin Oncol 2003, 21(5): 942-947.
14. Kübler-Ross E: On Death and Dying. London, Tavistock Publications, 1970.
16. Holland J: Now we tell—but how well? J Clin Oncol 1989;7: 557-5559.
17. Katz J: The Silent World of Doctor and Patient. New York, Free Press, 1984, pp 10-12.
18. Billings A: Sharing bad news. In Billings A (ed): Out-Patient Management of Advanced Malignancy. Philadelphia, JB Lippincott, 1985, pp 236-259.
19. Sardell AN, Trielweiler SJ: Disclosing the cancer diagnosis: Procedures that influence patient hopefulness. Cancer 1993;72: 3355-3365.
20. Wong-Wylie G, Jevne RF: Patient hope: Exploring the interactions between physicians and HIV seropositive individuals. Qual Health Q 1997;7:32-56.
21. Parker PA, Baile WF, de Moor C, et al: Breaking bad news about cancer: Patients' preferences for communication. J Clin Oncol 2001; 19:2049-2056.
22. Back AL, Arnold RM, Quill TE: Hope for the best, and prepare for the worst. Ann Intern Med 2003;138;439-443.
23. Jones S: Telling the right patient. BMJ 1981;283:291-292.
24. Benson J, Britten N: How much truth and to whom? Respecting the autonomy of cancer patients when talking with their families—ethical theory and patients' views. BMJ 1996;313; 729-731.
25. Meredith C, Symonds P, Webster L, et al: Information trends in cancer patients in the west of Scotland. BMJ 1996;313: 724-726.
26. Baile WF, Glober GA, Lenzi R, et al: Discussing disease progression and end-of-life decisions. Oncology 1999;13:1021-1031.
27. Maguire P, Pitceathly C: Key communication skills and how to acquire them. BMJ 2002;325:697-700.
28. Luck J, Peabody JW: Using standardised patients to measure physicians' practice: Validation study using audio recordings. BMJ 2002;325:679-682.
29. Suchman AL, Markakis K, Beckman HB, et al: A model of empathic communication in the medical interview. JAMA 1997;277:678-682.

30. Fallowfield L, Jenkins V, Farewell V, et al: Efficacy of a Cancer Research UK communication skills training model for oncologists: A randomized controlled trial. Lancet 2002;359:650-656.

31. Skinner JB, Erskine A, Pearce R, et al: The evaluation of a cognitive behavioural treatment programme in outpatients with chronic pain. J Psychosom Res 1990;34:13-19.

32. Razavi D, Delvaux N: Communication skills and psychological training in oncology. Eur J Cancer 1997;33(Suppl 6):S15-S21.

33. Levinson W, Roter D: The effects of two continuing medical education programs on communication skills of practicing primary care physicians. J Gen Intern Med 1993;8:318-324.

34. Buckman R: Communications and emotions [editorial]. BMJ 2002;325:672.

35. Baile WB, Buckman R, Lenzi R, et al: SPIKES: A six-step protocol for delivering bad news: Application to the patient with cancer. Oncologist 2000;5:302-311.

36. Maguire P, Fairbairns S, Fletcher C: Consultation skills of young doctors: Benefit of feedback training in interviewing as students persists. BMJ 1986;292:1573-1576.

37. Fogerty LA, Curbow BA, Wingard JR, et al: Can 40 seconds of compassion reduce patient anxiety? J Clin Oncol 1999;17: 371-379.

38. Fallowfield L, Lipkin M, Hall A: Teaching senior oncologists communication skills: Results from phase I of a comprehensive longitudinal program in the United Kingdom. J Clin Oncol 1998;16:1961-1968.

39. Buckman R, Baile W: A Practical Guide To Communication Skills in Cancer Care (CD-ROM set). Toronto, Medical Audio-Visual Publishing, 2001.

40. Novack DH, Suchman AL, Clark W, et al: Calibrating the physician: Personal awareness and effective patient care. Working Group on Promoting Physician Personal Awareness, American Academy on Physician and Patient. JAMA 1997;278:502-509.

41. Meier DE, Back AL, Morrison RS: The inner life of physicians and care of the seriously ill. JAMA 2001;286:3007-3014.

42. House JS, Landis KR, Umberson D: Social relationships and health. Science 1988;241:540-545.

43. Roberts CSF, Cox CE, Reintgen DS, et al: Influence of physician communication on newly diagnosed breast cancer patients' psychological adjustment and decision making Cancer 1994; 74:336-341.

44. Cousins N: How patients appraise physicians. N Engl J Med 1985;313:1422-1425.

45. Butow PN, Dunn SM, Tattersall KH: Communication with cancer patients: Does it matter? J Palliat Care 1995;11:34-38.

46. Hanson LC, Rodgman E: The use of living wills at the end of life: A national study. Arch Intern Med 1996;13:1018-1022.

47. Emanuel EJ, Young-Xu Y, Levinsky NG, Gazelle G, Saynina O, and Aoh AS, Chemotherapy use among Medicare beneficiaries at the end of life, Ann Int Med 2003;138(8):639-643.

48. Levinson W, Roter DL, Mullooly JP, et al: Physician-patient communication: The relationship with malpractice claims among primary care physicians and surgeons. JAMA 1997;277: 553-559.

49. Ramirez AJ, Graham J, Richards MA, et al: Burnout and psychiatric disorder among cancer clinicians. Br J Cancer 1995; 71:1263-1269; see comments.

50. Simpson M: Clinical Psycholinguistics: The Language of Illness and Healing. New York, Irvington, 1980.

Life During and After Cancer Treatment: Physical, Psychosocial, and Sexual Health

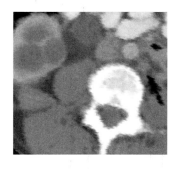

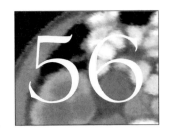

THE GYNECOLOGIC CANCER PATIENT AND HER FAMILY

Hilary Jefferies   and   Jane Groves

 MAJOR CONTROVERSIES

- **What is the impact of cancer services and specialist nurses on the quality of patient care?**
- **What are the communication challenges for clinical practice?**
- **Why is psychosocial support essential for the patient and her family?**
- **What is the impact of gynecologic cancer on a woman's sexuality, and how may this be addressed?**
- **Menopause and hormone replacement therapy: What are the issues?**
- **What effect does gynecologic cancer have on a woman's body image?**
- **Do complementary and alternative therapies have a role in holistic care?**
- **Is there care for the carers?**

Few people go through life without experiencing events that can change their perspective on how they see themselves, their role within their society, and their relationship with those around them. Because people are multidimensional, and more than the sum of their parts,[1] a person who has a physical illness is also affected spiritually, psychologically and sociologically.[2] Cancer is a common illness, affecting 1 in 3 people in the United Kingdom, and it is the second most common cause of death in the United States.[3] It is also considered within Western cultures as the most feared disease and is linked with death. Although 1 in 3 affected individuals can expect to be cured of their illness, it is inevitable that cancer and its treatment can have a life-changing and life-defining effect on them and their families.[4] This chapter explores some of the factors that influence the way in which the gynecologic cancer patient and her family unit face the complexities of the disease and the effects it can have on them and their quality of life.

What is the impact of cancer services and specialist nurses on the quality of patient care?

The organization of cancer services in the United Kingdom has undergone radical changes in the last few years in an attempt to improve clinical outcomes and the patient/family experience. It is now advocated that patients should be looked after in specialist centers by a multidisciplinary team of experts including gynecologic oncology surgeons, clinical oncologists, medical oncologists, specialist nurses, palliative care teams, radiologists, histopathologists, dieticians, and physiotherapists. It is believed that dealing with high numbers of women with gynecologic cancer will allow such teams to develop and maintain the necessary skills and expertise. Indeed, Junor and associates[5] concluded that, when treated by surgeons who specialize in gynecologic cancer, women have a better prognosis and survive longer. Studies have also indicated that a multidisciplinary team working together to provide the highest level of expertise leads to improved communication and coordinated care and ensures that patients are offered the most clinically effective treatment.[6]

The needs of the patient and their family must be the central focus, and although it is essential that patients have access to the best clinically effective treatment available, delivered and coordinated by clinical experts, they must also have a choice about where they have their treatment. Efforts must also be made to ensure that services are accessible and within traveling distance wherever possible. Physical difficulties and expense can cause huge anxieties for patients and their families, beyond the cancer diagnosis and treatment itself.

Nurses are an essential and integral part of the multidisciplinary team.[7] Their role is crucial in facilitating effective communication and offering social, sexual, spiritual, emotional, and psychological support to the patient and the family from the time of diagnosis and throughout the natural history of the disease and the course of its treatment. The role of the Clinical Nurse Specialist (CNS) can vary according to the needs of the user population, but the multifaceted components are education, facilitation, collaboration, research, and coordination of services, as well as ensuring that support and nurture are available for patients and their families. Above all they are there to provide specialist advice, accurate information, support, and continuity of care. Nurses have a critical role to play in improving the quality of survival throughout the patient journey, from diagnosis through treatment to rehabilitation.[8] In collaboration with the multidisciplinary team, nurses can assist the patient and her family in adjusting to significant alterations in bodily function and appearance resulting from the disease and its treatment. However, although nurses are an important resource for the patient and the family, have a vital role as members of the multidisciplinary team, and are essential to ensure quality of patient care delivered, the issues discussed are not solely the responsibility of the nurse. The central philosophy of the multidisciplinary team must be a commitment by all members to the provision of a service that reflects the needs of individual patients and their families, ensuring that issues such as communication, support, and rehabilitation are addressed.

What are the communication challenges for clinical practice?

Communication is the imparting or exchange of information, ideas, or feelings. Communicating openly with cancer patients is particularly important because of the devastation that can be caused by both diagnosis and treatment; it is also central in promoting high-quality patient care. Communication is pivotal in offering support, assessing need, encouraging exploration and expression of distress related to the diagnosis, and facilitating adjustment to what may be an uncertain future. It ensures interaction rather than direct transmission and should reduce unnecessary uncertainty.

Communication is complex and involves more that just the spoken word. It is also about listening to patients and their families and attempting to understand their knowledge, concerns, and expectations in relation to the diagnosis and any further investigations or treatments required.[9] Both verbal and nonverbal activities are integral to this process. Health care professionals should give consideration to body language, body movement, facial expression, and the use of touch as well as verbal content. There is evidence that good communication improves patient satisfaction, recall of information, understanding, and treatment compliance.[10] Insensitive and inadequate communication can be the source of much distress for patients and their families and may hinder their adjustment to the diagnosis of cancer.[11] Despite the need for effective communication, there is evidence that this area of clinical practice is at times extremely poor. This occurs in part because of time pressures, lack of privacy, and interruptions. However, it can also be a result of inadequate training and understanding, and it continues to be a potential cause of anxiety for health care professionals.[12]

Specific challenges to health care professionals have been identified as breaking bad news, handling difficult questions, and collusion. Factors that might create communication difficulties in these areas include the following[13]:

- Previous experiences of patients and family
- Cultural issues
- Blocking behaviors
- Poor symptom control
- Age of patient

Breaking bad news. The goal of health care professionals is to improve or cure patients of their illness, and it is particularly difficult to impart news of a condition that might be life-threatening or cause harm and distress. It is essential, however, that all patients have access to the relevant information, given in a clear and concise manner, so that they can make informed decisions about their care. Health care professionals also have a legal, moral, and ethical duty to inform patients of all developments in their progress, even if it is personally distressing to do so.[12] However, it must be remembered that not all patients want the same amount of information or wish to be involved in the decision-making process. Women with various preferences must be identified and their wishes in relation to information and the devolving of management decisions respected.

Bad news may be defined[14] as any information that drastically alters a patient's view of her future. It is not for us to decide on the patients' behalf what constitutes bad news. For example, a patient may feel relieved when a diagnosis of cancer is finally made, particularly if she has felt unwell for some time, although this degree of acceptance can be difficult to understand. A number of authors have proposed

Table 56–1. Techniques for Breaking Bad News

Buckman[15] (1992)	Kaye[14] (1996)	Faulkner[16] (1998)
Getting starting	Preparation	Identify current knowledge or suspicions
Find out how much the patient knows	What does the patient know?	Warn of impending news (warning shot)
Find out how much the patient wants to know	Is more information wanted?	Give news at patient's pace and in
Share the information (align and educate)	Give a warning shot	manageable chunks
Respond to the patient's feelings	Allow denial	Allow patient to choose when she has
Plan and follow through	Explain if requested	heard enough
	Listen to concerns	Give space
	Encourage ventilation of feelings	Handle reactions
	Summary-and-plan	
	Offer availability	

frameworks for communication that highlight the principles of breaking bad news in a structured way[14-16] (Table 56-1).

Emphasis is placed on careful assessment and preparation, sensitivity, and allowing the patient and the family to determine the pace of the consultation. Individual anxieties and responses are encouraged. Attention should also be given to who breaks the bad news. It is not appropriate to delegate this task to the most junior member of the team, who will undoubtedly lack the skill required to communicate effectively and to handle the strong emotional responses that some patients and families exhibit, including grief, isolation, anger, despair, and shock. Junior team members may also lack the experience and knowledge necessary to answer questions relating to further treatment and disease outcomes, as well as the coping mechanisms required to deal with the consultation from a personal perspective.

Handling difficult questions. Breaking bad news is usually a planned scenario, and communication needs can be anticipated and prepared for.[13] This is not the same as handling difficult questions, which may be spontaneous, potentially leaving the health care professional feeling vulnerable and anxious. Although it is not possible to predict difficult questions, it is possible to identify why a particular question might be perceived as difficult. The answer may not be known, the practitioner may have time or resource restrictions, or the health care professional may not feel that he or she has the skills necessary to handle the question, the subsequent issues that may arise, or the accompanying emotions such as anger, anxiety, or distress.

It has been suggested[13] that the best method of addressing awkward questions lies in the sensitive application of a set of principles that are designed to elicit the most crucial issues beneath the question, thus ensuring that exploration precedes response. These principles include the following[13]:

- Acknowledging the importance of the question by giving your undivided attention
- Using skillful questioning to facilitate ventilation of feelings and elicit what the real issues are
- Listening
- Summarizing to clarify the nature of the problem
- Deciding on the appropriate response

It may become apparent at some point that the patient does not want the question answered. It is important to establish this attitude before answering any questions, because the answers may potentially devastate the patient or family.

Collusion. Collusion, which has been defined as protecting another from bad news,[16] can be an enormous communication challenge. Within the health care setting, the two most common forms of collusion involve the relatives and the health care professionals themselves. Despite the patient's legal right to information regarding her diagnosis and prognosis, the practice of informing the family before the patient still takes place. Once the family has been informed, they inevitably will wish to protect their relative from harm, and to this end, they may request that the information be withheld, presenting a dilemma for the heath care professional. It is also common for the patient to request that the family not be informed. This can evoke a different type of anxiety for the health care professional, particularly if the patient is extremely unwell, because the patient may require increasing amounts of support from a family who are not informed. The family may become increasingly angry at what they perceive to be the unexplained deterioration in their relative, and this anger may be directed at the health care professional. It is important to handle collusion in a sensitive and systematic manner, avoiding situations that might lead to acts or requests for collusion and gently confronting and exploring issues with those involved. Collusion can lead to missed opportunities; it can deprive individuals of the chance to say and do things that are important to them.

Why is psychosocial support essential for the patient and her family?

A diagnosis of cancer has huge ramifications for both the patient and her family. It is a devastating shock that can leave the patient, family, and friends feeling isolated and uncertain about what to expect. Gynecologic cancer can be particularly traumatic,[17] as Corney and associates[18] stated: "A woman who has a diagnosis of gynecologic cancer is worried about more than the general concerns shared by other oncology patients." A diagnosis of gynecologic cancer penetrates to the very core of womanhood. It can affect not only a woman's perception of herself, but also the way in which she perceives and interacts with those around her. This is followed by a potential role transition, if her role as provider, protector, wife, mother, daughter, or lover is threatened. Holistic support at the point of diagnosis and throughout the cancer journey is crucial to the well-being of the patient and her family. Emotional and psychosocial support can have a positive effect on physical health, mental well-being, and social functioning.[19] There is evidence to show that newly diagnosed women benefit from robust psychological support and suffer less anxiety and depression.[20]

The meaning of a cancer diagnosis is unique to the individual and is derived from numerous sources, including past experiences of cancer, cultural biases, and information gained from the media.[8] The patient and/or family may express a range of emotions after a cancer diagnosis; these may include fright, guilt, frustration and helplessness, anger, and denial.[21] A variety of coping styles and strategies may also be exhibited. There can be feelings of stigmatization, associated with society's misconceptions in linking the cancer with promiscuity.[22] The nature of gynecologic cancer and its treatments predisposes women to have a variety of concerns relating to the impact of the disease and its treatment. The loss of fertility also has an impact on body image and sexuality. Many women who have undergone treatment for gynecologic cancer would welcome more emotional support and counselling.[18] Studies have also concluded that psychological interventions and support are likely to reduce the amount of sexual morbidity experienced by these women.[23]

Uncertainty is an emotion experienced by most patients after a diagnosis of cancer, and living with it poses a major challenge to the individual and the family. They may experience uncertainty about the efficacy of treatments, the financial burdens, and, above all, the future. When viewed within the context of a cancer diagnosis, the future, which may once have seemed to hold such potential, immediately becomes limited.[8] A therapeutic relationship between the patient, her family, and the health care professional will help to facilitate a climate that enables the individual to explore her thoughts and feelings about her cancer diagnosis and to develop a sense of control over events. It provides an opportunity to discuss the investigations, subsequent treatments, and potential effects on the body and bodily functions. This may be achieved through accurate verbal and written information and by answering questions on several different occasions, over a period of time and throughout the course of the disease. Anticipatory information also needs to be provided before the next phase of illness. Contact telephone numbers should be made available for the woman and her family and time allocated to respond to further needs and concerns. A comprehensive reassessment of the support needs of the patient and her family is a continuous process from diagnosis onward, because these needs fluctuate throughout the cancer journey.

Role of the family. The impact of cancer on an individual is invariably a life-changing experience, and the impact on those close to them also needs to be addressed. The family will experience distress and anxiety, which will be perceived as a threat to the family network. Family members have a unique role to play in the support of their loved ones. Health care professionals should view the support needs of family members as integral to those of the patient. Families are one of the most important resources to provide informal support to patients, although support cannot be assumed just because of the presence of family members. It is important to ascertain who is available to provide practical help. A family member may accompany the patient to clinic appointments so as to share the experience and understanding of the treatment. Practical ways of allowing families to access support in the community also needs to be explored. These may include referral to district nurses, hospice teams, or social services. It is known that coping by using adaptive strategies, such as seeking emotional and social support, appears to moderate the experience of distress from the cancer diagnosis and treatment.[24,25] Families may also help a woman to adjust to her altered body image and change in family dynamics, ensuring that she feels loved and accepted and still able to contribute to family commitments.

What is the impact of gynecologic cancer on a woman's sexuality, and how may this be addressed?

Sexual function and sexuality are part of being human and can be an important part of quality of life for all people, male and female, young and old, healthy and ill. Although the terms are often used in the same context, sexuality and sexual dysfunction are separate entities, and both can be affected by a diagnosis of cancer and its subsequent treatment. Sexuality is a highly complex phenomenon that engages the biologic basis for experiencing sexual pleasure, involves giving and receiving sensual pleasure, and influences people's relationships with others.[26] It is shaped by society, which teaches us how to interpret the changes that occur over time in our bodies. Religious teachings, laws, popular culture, and social policies also inform us about the nature of sexuality. Just as the term "sexuality" can mean different things to different people, the extent to which patients are affected varies markedly, and health care professionals should assess each patient carefully to ensure that care is adapted and individualized according to her needs.[19]

Corney and colleagues[27] and Burbie and Polinsky[28] described the negative effects that all cancers and cancer treatments have on sexuality and feelings of sexuality and sexual function. A more recent study by Green and associates[29] stated that the extent of the surgery does not always correspond to the degree of postoperative sexual dysfunction. This is important in women who have undergone surgery for vulval cancer and can feel traumatized after a small local excision. Patients who have had a Wertheim's hysterectomy have a shortened vagina that can lead to coital discomfort. The loss of estrogen after an oophorectomy can lead to vaginal dryness and loss of lubrication, causing dyspareunia. Radiotherapy can cause stromal dryness, vascular changes to the vaginal canal, and the laying down of fibrosis in the canal, with a decrease in elasticity.[30] However, it is important that vaginal patency be maintained, not only so that the patient may resume normal sexual activity but also so that a vaginal examination can be undertaken by the doctor at follow-up appointments. The importance and effectiveness of vaginal dilators, together with verbal and written information on their use, has been described in the literature.[31,32] However, it has also been noted that patients are reluctant to use them, particularly patients younger than 50 years of age.[33] Although Robinson and coworkers[34] noted that attendance at a psychoeducational group increased patient compliance, this approach has cost implications for service delivery.[19]

Sexuality and expressing one's sexuality include more than just "having sex,"[35] and just because a patient has a life-threatening disease does not mean that she no longer wishes to express her sexual feelings or to convey expressions of her sexuality.[36] It is important that all health care professionals increase their own knowledge and develop the skills that will enable them to feel comfortable when discussing issues related to sexuality with their patients. This includes taking a full history, using language that is easily understood, listening carefully, and taking care not to assume foreknowledge of the problem. It is also necessary to take account of the patient's body language. There may be a physical cause for sexual dysfunction, or there may be a psychological cause such as loss of libido or loss of femininity. It is important to involve the woman's husband or partner in trying to understand the problem and remedy the underlying cause.[37] There may be a need to acknowledge the woman's cancer treatment and the implications for the patient and her partner as a couple, for example if there is a loss of fertility or a limited prognosis. In some cases, advice may be needed on alternative positions for intercourse. Couples may also need to be reminded of the importance of intimacy. Referral to a specialist psychosexual counselor or sex therapist may be necessary, and all members of the multidisciplinary team should know to whom to refer patients.

Menopause and hormone replacement therapy: what are the issues?

As a result of treatment, whether it involves surgery, radiotherapy or chemotherapy, women with gynecologic cancer may have to contend with a premature or induced menopause. There may be menopausal symptoms such as hot flushes, mood swings, atrophic vaginitis, and night sweats.

The role of hormone replacement therapy (HRT) in the management of gynecologic cancer is often controversial and poorly understood. It is not usually contraindicated in women with gynecologic malignancies, except those with endometrial cancer, which is an estrogen-sensitive tumor. For women who are below the age of the natural menopause, it is important that their estrogen levels be maintained to minimize the risks of ischemic heart disease and osteoporosis in later life.

For some women, there are anxieties that HRT is a risk factor for the development of cancer; this idea is often debated in the media, which adds further uncertainty. This confusion can be extremely worrying for gynecologic cancer patients and their families. Having survived one cancer diagnosis, they are reluctant to expose themselves to the risk of a second cancer. It is important, therefore, that women have access to accurate information, enabling them to make an informed choice.

What effect does gynecologic cancer have on a woman's body image?

Today's society places much emphasis on the physical body, the necessity to have a healthy attractive appearance and to be acceptable to others in everyday life. The ideal body is said to represent youth, vigor, intactness, and health, and there is likely to be a decrease in self-esteem and an increase in insecurity and anxiety among those who deviate significantly from this ideal.[38] The way a woman feels about her body image may be described as having three components: body reality, which represents the body as it is; body ideal, which is how the person wants it to be; and body presentation, which represents the efforts the person has to take to find a compromise between body reality and body ideal.[39] The symptoms of a gynecologic cancer (e.g., ascites, weight loss) can cause physical changes to a person's body before a definitive diagnosis is made. An offensive vaginal discharge or vulval tumor may deter women from seeking help from their family doctor for fear of embarrassment and feelings of loss of femininity. Even the nature of diagnostic procedures and tests makes a woman feel that her body and personal privacy are being invaded. The diagnosis of the cancer itself may cause fear or uncertainty or be seen as a punishment for perceived wrongdoing, and these feelings also can cause an altered body image.

Most treatments for cancer involve surgery. The resulting scar, which may be hidden from other people, can have a profound affect on the woman herself and is a permanent reminder of her sense of loss. Surgical removal of the ovaries equates with premature aging and loss of sexual attractiveness. The surgery may alter a bodily function, with the formation of a stoma or urostomy, or both after a pelvic exenteration, causing revulsion. Stomas can often require considerable attention, and coping with the difficulties of caring for it and returning to a normal lifestyle can have a huge impact. After surgery for a vulval tumor and groin node dissection, and subsequent radiotherapy, lymphedema of the lower limbs may occur, affecting mobility and a normal lifestyle.

Radiotherapy treatment can also have an effect on a woman's body image. The marking of the skin with tattoos can cause distress and can be a permanent reminder of the nature and need of treatment. Some women have a fear of the treatment itself; they may worry that they will be burnt and think that they will become radioactive. Generalized fatigue, nausea, diarrhea, and cystitis may make the patient unable to care for her family and fulfill her normal household duties, compounding her sense of low esteem. Local treatment to the pelvis can cause skin changes, such as erythema, moist and dry desquamation, and permanent loss of pubic hair. Radiotherapy also has an effect on the ovaries, causing the onset of menopausal symptoms such as hot flushes and night sweats. Chemotherapy can cause temporary alopecia, which may include the eyebrows and eyelashes. Loss of hair has a profound effect on most women, and in some cultures a hairstyle indicates an individual's social standing and religious convictions.[38] Alterations in appearance may become more distressing as the cancer progresses. A woman may have to face alopecia during two or more courses of chemotherapy, which often becomes harder to bear on each occasion. She may develop a pelvic mass, ascites, and cachexia. A fistula may develop, causing a continuous offensive discharge, heightening her loss of control over her bodily functions. A fungating vulval lesion can also make women feel dirty, causing them to withdraw from society.

All the members of the multidisciplinary team have a role to play in assisting patients to come to terms with their altered body image. They need to be content with their own image and have a healthy acceptance of themselves, before they can help the patient and her family.[38] After surgery, nursing care involves attention to personal hygiene, including hair and mouth care, and dressings need to be changed as required. The attitude of every member of the multidisciplinary team is crucial in helping the patient adapt to her new circumstance. Specific help may be available to women with alopecia, such as the "Look good, Feel better" cosmetic programs that provide advice on wigs, scarves, and cosmetics, and attention to personal appearance may also help.

Do complementary and alternative therapies have a role in holistic care?

Interest in alternative and complementary therapies has been increasing in recent years. *Alternative therapies* have been defined by Cassileth[40] as "therapies that usually lie outside the health sector," whereas the term *complementary therapies* is "an umbrella term for treatments used to enhance nursing or medical interventions." It is important for the two terms to be defined correctly, because it is the way in which the intervention is used, and not the intervention itself, that makes it alternative or complementary.[41] Patient surveys have shown that it is mainly women of working age with a higher level of education and income who are likely to consult a complementary or alternative therapist. This may be a result of disillusionment with conventional medicine and an increasing desire to take a more holistic approach to their care, involving the body, mind, and spirit. There may also be a need to take control of their disease. They may believe that their health is determined by their own behavior and that they can influence the course of their illness. A more worrying concern, discussed by DeKeyser and associates,[42] is dissatisfaction with the physician-patient relationship, accompanied by the belief that the complementary therapist will devote more time to the patient and that there will be an increased level of communication between them. Many patients do not inform their doctor of their use of complementary therapies. Conversely, how many times are patients asked about this use when a medical history is obtained?

It is known that in palliative care some complementary therapy is helpful, such as acupuncture and aromatherapy to relieve pain. Other therapies, such as relaxation and massage, are known to improve quality of life and to decrease the discomforts associated with treatment (e.g., depression, anxiety, insomnia). These therapies can add an "extra dimension" to a woman's overall experience of treatment. However, there remains a lack of scientific data on the efficacy of these treatments. Surveys of nurses in America, Israel, and the United Kingdom show that increasing numbers of health care professionals are advising patients on complementary therapies.[42,43] However, if advice is to be given, there is a need to conduct both retrospective and prospective quantitative and qualitative studies to explore the effects of these therapies on the patient's response to cancer treatment and on their quality of life. These studies would also ensure that there is no harm to the patients and that the health care professionals are fulfilling their duty of care.

Survivorship Challenges

From the time of diagnosis and for the remainder of her life, an individual with cancer is considered a survivor.[8] As a result of research, screening programs, earlier detection, genetic counseling, and developments in treatments and clinical trials, mortality rates are declining and an increasing number of patients survive.[44] An increasing number of long-term survivors have a normal life expectancy, and others, although not cured, may live for some considerable time with their disease.[45] However, the detrimental effects of cancer and its treatments have been neglected, and little effort has been made to identify acceptable levels of disability, distress, or disfigurement caused by treatments or the emotional demands a cancer diagnosis places on an individual and her family.[46]

A cancer diagnosis is known to drastically erode a person's quality of life.[47] Because the impact of gynecologic cancer on quality of life is multidimensional, women can be left with chronic physical problems[48] and psychological consequences.[49] These may affect their ability to function in their normal social roles, and, although women may be cured of their disease, little is known about their quality of life and survivorship. Health care professionals must be aware that women live with fear and uncertainty and that their survival represents a continual struggle with the long-term effects of the disease and its treatment. They must deal with a range of emotions as they struggle to adjust to life after cancer, including guilt, particularly if there are issues surrounding hereditary risk factors. They may feel that their life has become dominated by the disease, including frequent hospital visits, and they may have a sense of being taken over.[50] A good result from surgery or other treatment does not necessarily translate to a good outcome for the patient. Physical survival should not be assumed to mean social and sexual survival.[50] Sometimes survival may not be enough if perceived quality has gone; for example, a woman who has lost the chance of a family or further children may feel that her future has also been removed.

Rehabilitation is a process that seeks to minimize the physical, psychological, social, sexual, and spiritual dysfunction that may result from cancer or its treatment. As treatments become more toxic and radical and survival improves, issues faced by women will become more complex. Health care professionals must make every effort to understand the survivorship issues those women and their families face, in order to assist with their rehabilitation needs (Table 56-2). This will have a positive impact on the quality of life of patients. Long-term surveillance is required if we are to have a broad understanding of the physical, psychological, sexual, occupational, and social effects of cancer.

Cancer support and self-help groups for patients with the same diagnosis provide support to patients and their families and friends. Support groups are said to reduce the sense of isolation, loneliness, and fear, and to empower patients through sharing their experiences and feelings with others and regaining their "fighting spirit" and sense of control over their illness.[51] However, some patients may not attend because of a reluctance to share feelings with strangers, and in some cases support groups may have a negative effect.[52]

Palliative and Terminal Care

For some women, their diagnosis of gynecologic cancer is made when it is already at an advanced stage. Palliative care provides for all the medical and nursing needs of the patient for whom cure is not possible and for all the psychological, social, and spiritual needs of the patient and the family, for the duration of the patient's illness, including bereavement care.[21] It is concerned with quality of life and making the most of the time left, enabling the woman to come to terms with her limited prognosis and preparing the family for her death. It involves good listening and communication skills to explain the options available, as well as monitoring and advising on symptom control and providing emotional, psychological, and spiritual support. Information should be provided in a sensitive way, and questions should be answered honestly. It is also important for woman to express her choice about her own treatment and care. Although there needs to be a sense of "hope" and achieving goals, these should also be realistic and attainable.

Some families are able to look after their relative at home with help, but for some women it is not possible to be at home, even if would be her place of preference. This can be very disappointing, and care needs to be taken to ensure that time is given for the patient and her family to discuss the reasons, so that she does not feel rejected and isolated. Some patients choose to be cared for in a hospice, where there is a quieter atmosphere and a greater ratio of nurses to patients. However, many patients are inpatients in acute hospitals for the terminal phase of their life. Assessment and control of pain and other symptoms needs to be maintained so that it does not detract from the quality of life. Ethnic, racial, religious, and cultural factors also need to be considered, and a religious advisor or cultural leader should be involved in the care if the patient wishes. Some patients prepare for the end of their life by preparing their will, organizing their funeral, and writing letters to loved ones. This can provide a sense of achievement and "putting one's house in order." Children also need to be fully informed and their questions answered. Some mothers are able to prepare their children by collecting special items for a "memory box." Health care professionals must inform parents where they can obtain advice about how to

---

Table 56–2. Rehabilitation Needs

Physical Function
Strength—Loss of muscle bulk, tiredness, fatigue, immobility, lymphedema
Nutrition—Taste change, loss of appetite, anorexia, malabsorption, changes in metabolism
Control—Altered bladder or bowel function, movement disorders, odor, ascites, bleeding, discharge
Sexuality—Infertility, altered sexual function, menopause, loss of desire

Psychological Function
Changes in body image—Mutilation, loss of function and control, alopecia, conflict with self-image and relationships, role transition
Anxiety—Fear of the unknown, uncertainty, pain and treatment, loss of income
Depression—Due to treatment, fears for the future, genetic risk for family members/guilt

Occupational Function
Work—Loss of job and income, loss of identity, stigma of cancer, attitudes of society
Self-care—Need for job, insecurity, dependence on others
Finance—Supporting self and family, insurance premiums (life/holiday), mortgage cover

Social Function
Self-esteem—Independence and confidence, worth to society
Body Image—Coping with others, stigma of cancer
Communication—Emotion, collusion
Family—Stress, loyalties, collusion, guilt

Adapted from David J. Cancer Care: Prevention, Treatment and Palliation. London: Champion & Hall, 1996.

deal with the needs of their children, particularly if their mother has incurable disease.

Palliative care also continues after a patient's death. It is often provided informally by the community in which the family lives or through their religious organizations. In addition, bereavement support may be available through local palliative services.

A dilemma that often arises is when to introduce the idea of palliative care. In the United Kingdom, the general trend is to inform patients about a fatal prognosis. Although many people associate the words "terminal," "palliative," and "hospice" with the last few days of life, such care should be accessible throughout the cancer experience. It should never be withheld until all modalities of treatment are exhausted.[21] In some parts of the world, however, the patient is part of the family which assumes responsibility for health-seeking and decision-making and shields the sick person from the truth about the diagnosis and prognosis of their terminal illness.[53] This can cause ethical difficulties for the health care professionals involved in maintaining a good therapeutic relationship with the patient and continued support for the family.

Is There Care For the Caregivers?

The challenges of caring for cancer patients and their families place huge demands on health care professionals, and we must ensure that we have effective coping strategies in place and a network of support. During times of stress, they can help us cope with the demands placed on us, relieving us of pressures or providing an avenue for the discussion of feelings. Members of the multidisciplinary team must therefore make it a priority to support each other. It is also essential that health care professionals have interests and hobbies outside the workplace.

Conclusion

Gynecologic cancers are a very diverse group, with different presentations and prognoses affecting a wide age group of women. They can have far-reaching effects on the patient and her family, not only in terms of the treatment modalities and outcome but also in regard to associated factors such as fertility and sexuality. The challenge for all health care professionals is to take a holistic approach toward the patient and her family, while keeping up to date with new medical advances. The multidisciplinary team is the link between the therapeutic model of care and the patient's experience of cancer; by working together with the team, the patient and her family may feel nurtured and supported from the time of her diagnosis onward.

ACKNOWLEDGMENTS: Thanks to Mr. Nigel Acheson and Ms. Jacky Cotton (Birmingham Women's Healthcare NHS Trust) and Miss Cath Finn (Good Hope Hospital NHS Trust) for their support and encouragement.

References

1. Torres G: Theoretical Foundations of Nursing. Norwalk: Appleton-Century-Crofts, 1990.
2. Selanders LC: The life and times of Florence Nightingale. In McQuiston CM, Webb AA (Eds.): Foundation of Nursing Theory. London: Sage Publications, 1995.
3. American Cancer Society: Cancer Facts and Figures. Atlanta: The American Cancer Society, 1996.
4. Corner J, Bailey C: Cancer Nursing: Care in Context. Oxford: Blackwell Science, 2001.
5. Junor E, Hole D, Gillis C: Management for ovarian cancer: Referral to a multi-disciplinary team matters. Br J Cancer 1994; 70:363-370.
6. Redmond K: Meeting the unique needs of cancer patients. The World of Irish Nursing 1997;5:26-27.
7. Carson M, Williams T, Everett A, Barker S: The nurses role in the multi-disciplinary team. Eur J Palliative Care 1997;4:96-98.
8. Otto S: Oncology Nursing, 3rd ed. St. Louis: Mosby, 1997.
9. Jarman E: Communication problems: A patient's view. Nursing Times 1995;91:30-31.
10. Gull S: Communication skills: Recognizing difficulties. The Obstetrician and Gynaecologist 2002;4:107-110.
11. Knuijver I, Kerkstra A, Bensing J, Van der Wiel H: Nurse/patient communication in cancer care: A review of the literature. Cancer Nursing 2000;23:20-31.
12. Franks A: Breaking bad news and the challenge of communication. Eur J Palliative Care 1997;4:61-65.
13. Kinghorn S: Communication in advanced illness: Challenges and opportunities. In Kinghorn S, Gamlin R. (Eds.): Palliative Nursing—Bringing Comfort and Hope. London: Harcourt, 2001.
14. Kaye P: Breaking Bad News: A Ten-step Approach. Northampton: EPL Publications, 1996.
15. Buckman R: How to Break Bad News: A Guide to Health Care Professionals. London: Papermac, 1992.
16. Faulkner A: When the News Is Bad: A Guide for Professionals. Cheltenham: Stanley Thornes, 1998.
17. Wills J: Womanise cancers. Nursing Times 1997;93:26-29.
18. Corney R, Everett H, Howells A, et al: The care of patients undergoing surgery for gynaecological cancer: The need for information, emotional support and counselling. The J Adv Nurs 1992;17:667-671.
19. Jefferies H: The psychosocial care of a patient with cervical cancer. Cancer Nurs Pract 2002;1, 5,19-25.
20. Department of Health: Guidance on Commissioning Cancer Services: Improving Outcomes in Gynaecological Cancers. London: NHS Executive, 1999.
21. Woodruff R: Psychological issues. In Woodruff R (Ed.): Palliative Medicine. Melbourne: Asperula Pty, 1993.
22. Montazeri A, Gillis CR, McEwen J, et al: Tak Tent: Studies conducted in a cancer support group. Support Cancer Care 1997;5:118-125.
23. Kew F, Nevin J, Cruickshank D: Psychosexual impact of gynaecological malignancy. R Coll Obstet Gynaecol 2002;4: 193-196.
24. Lutgendorf S, Anderson B, Larsen K, et al: Cognitive processing, social support coping, and distress in gynaecologic cancer patients. Cancer Res Control 1999;8:123-137.
25. Kubler-Ross E: On Death and Dying. London: Tavistock Publications, 1970.
26. Webb C, O'Neill J: Sexuality and cancer. In Tiffany R, Webb P (Eds.): Oncology for Nurses and Health, Vol. 2. London: Harper Row, 1988, p 26.
27. Corney R, Crowther M, Everett H, et al: Psychosexual dysfunction in women with gynaecological cancer following radical pelvic surgery. Br J Obstet Gynaecol 1993;100:73-78.
28. Burbie G, Polinsky M: Intimacy and sexuality after cancer treatment: restoring a sense of wholeness. J Psychological Oncol 1992;10:19-33.
29. Green M, Wendel-Naumann R, Elliott M, et al: Sexual dysfunction after vulvectomy. Gynecol Oncol 2000;77:73-77.

30. Cartwright-Alcarese F: Addressing sexual dysfunction gynaecologic malignancy following radiation therapy for a gynaecologic malignancy. Oncol Nurs Forum 1995;22:1227-1231.
31. Hassey Dow K: Altered patterns of sexuality. In Hassey-Dow K, Hilderly L (Eds.): Nursing Care in Radiation Oncology. Philadelphia: WB Saunders, 1992.
32. Rice A: Sexuality in cancer and palliative care: Effects of disease and treatment. Int J Palliative Care 2000;6:392-397.
33. Robinson J, Scott CB, Faris PD, et al: Sexual rehabilitation for women with gynaecological cancer: Information is not sufficient. Can J Hum Sexual 1994;3:131-142.
34. Robinson JW, Faris PD, Scott CB: Psycho-educational group increases vaginal dilatation for younger women and reduces sexual fears for women of all ages with gynaecological carcinoma treated with radiotherapy. Int J Radiat Oncol Biol Phys 1999;44:497-506.
35. CancerLink. Close Relationships and Cancer, 2nd ed. London: Macmillan Cancer Relief, 1998.
36. Wells P: No sex please, I'm dying: A common myth explored. Eur J Palliative Care 2002;9:119-122.
37. Wakley G: Sexual dysfunction. Curr Obstet Gynaecol 2002;12:35-40.
38. Salter M: Altered Body Image. London: Bailliere-Tindall, 1997.
39. Price B: Body Image: Nursing Concepts and Care. London: Prentice-Hall, 1990.
40. Cassileth BR: Complementary therapies: Overview and state of the art. Cancer Nurs 1999;22:85-90.
41. Richardson J: Integrating complementary therapies into health care education: A cautious approach. J Clin Nurs 2001;10:793-798.
42. DeKeyser F, Bar Cohen B, Wagner N: Knowledge levels and attitudes of staff nurses in Israel towards complementary and alternative medicine. J Adv Nurs 2001;36:41-48.
43. Sohn P, Loveland-Cook C: Nurse practitioner knowledge of complementary alternative health care: Foundation for practice. J Adv Nurs 2002;39:9-16.
44. McCaffrey D: Surviving cancer. Nurs Times 1991;87:26-30.
45. O'Neill J, Leedham K: Rehabilitation and long term effects of cancer. In Corner J, Bailey C (Eds.): Cancer Nursing: Care in Context. Oxford: Blackwell Science, 2001.
46. Corner J: Cancer nursing as therapy: The contribution of specialist nurses. Oncology Nurses Today 1997;2(3):11-14.
47. Ainslie S: Sexuality and the cancer sufferer. Nursing Mirror 1984;159:38-40.
48. Anderson BL, Anderson B, de Prosse C: Controlled prospective longitudinal study of women with cancer: Sexual functioning outcomes. J Consult Clin Psychol 1989;57:683-691.
49. Maughan K: The effect of a clinical nurse specialist in gynaecological oncology on quality of life and sexuality. J Clin Nurs 2001;10:221-229.
50. David J: Cancer Care: Prevention, Treatment and Palliation. London, Champion & Hall, 1996.
51. Lang S, Path RB: You Don't Have to Suffer. Oxford: Oxford University Press, 1994.
52. Galinsky MJ, Schopler H: Negative experiences in support groups. Social Work Health Care 1994;20:77-95.
53. Pellegrino ED: Emerging ethical issues in palliative care. JAMA 1998;279:1521-1522.

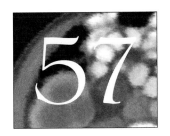

C H A P T E R

SEXUALITY AND
GYNECOLOGIC CANCER

Susan V. Carr

✦ MAJOR CONTROVERSIES

- **Is sexuality important, and should the issue be approached with all gynecologic cancer patients?**
- **Should treatment decisions be made on survival predictions alone without taking account of the woman's views of her sexuality?**
- **Should the issue of sexuality be raised with the woman undergoing colposcopy, a relatively minor and routine procedure?**
- **How can the psychosexually aware approach be managed in a busy health care setting, and who should address the issue of sexual problems with the patients?**

Cancer is a disease that causes mixed and dramatic emotions in the sufferers and their families. There have been extensive advances in the diagnosis and treatment of many of the conditions, and there is increasing interest in quality of life rather than survival alone. Gynecologic cancer directly affects the genital and reproductive areas of the body, the area most directly connected to the sexuality of the woman. Despite its obvious potential importance, the topic of sexuality within gynecologic cancer is underrecognized. This chapter aims to highlight the issues and discuss controversies in this area.

Sexuality

To understand sexuality and recognize and treat sexual disorders, we can consider the separate component parts, which are gender identity, sexual orientation, sexual attitudes, and sexual behavior.

Sexual identity. Sexual identity is the feeling of "who you are" in relation to gender. Approximately one half the world's population is identified as male and one half as female, individuals who have a clear gender identity. There are transsexuals, men or women who

feel they have been born into the wrong body[1] and a small number of people whose gender identity falls somewhere within the wide spectrum of human sexuality.

Sexual orientation. Sexual orientation is the definition of a person's sexual preference in relation to whom the person is sexually attracted in a physical sense. More than 90% of people are heterosexual (i.e., attracted to individuals of the opposite sex), 5% to 10% of men are homosexual (i.e., attracted to men), 2% to 4% of women are lesbian (i.e., attracted to other women), and 7% to 8% of the population are bisexual (i.e., attracted to men and women). In a probability sample of residents between the ages of 16 and 44 years who were living in the United Kingdom, 5.4% of men and 4.9% of women had ever had homosexual sex, but when asked about same-sex partners in the past 5 years, the figures went down to 2.6% for both sexes.[2]

Sexual attitudes. Sexual attitudes are feelings about sex. These attitudes develop throughout the life cycle as the woman develops[3] and can alter quite considerably during a lifetime. Any major life change can cause a woman to feel differently about her body, herself, sex, and relationships, and the impact of gynecologic cancer can have a profound effect on her sexual attitudes, leading to behavior changes.

Sexual behavior. Sexual behavior is determined not only by sexual attitudes, orientation, and gender identity, but by culture, circumstance, and individual choice. Sexuality is inherent in every human being, and everyone should have the right to express or repress it in her or his own way, as long as the activity is consensual.

Gynecologic cancer cannot change a woman's gender identity or sexual orientation, because these components of sexuality have biopsychosocial origins[4] and are set at around 4 or 5 years of age. Sexual attitudes and feelings, and consequently sexual behavior, can change dramatically due to gynecologic cancer, and it is for this reason that it is important to examine these issues.

Prevalence of Sexual Problems

Sexual problems fall into two categories: problems of function and problems of desire. Even if sexual difficulties develop as a result of physical problems, there is almost inevitably an emotional overlay because sex involves the most intimate area of the relationship between the woman and her partner. If the patient is in an ongoing relationship, it is important to involve the partner if the patient wishes. The partner may be male or female, or the woman may be bisexual. In discussing sexual matters, it is important to acknowledge different cultural and religious practices and to be able to accept the sexuality of individuals with disability and the sexuality of people regardless of age. Even gynecologists in their twenties or thirties should be able to accept that there is sexual life right to the end of the natural lifespan!

General population. Most people have untroubled sexual lives most of the time, but there are always individuals who have problems of a sexual nature. The early scientific studies of sex were published by Havelock Ellis 1933,[5] followed by Kinsey and colleagues[6,7] in 1948 and 1953. In 1999, Laumann and coworkers[8] published an epidemiologic survey of sexual problems in the United States. This showed that 43% of women and 31% of men had sexual dysfunction. This is more likely in individuals with poor physical and emotional health and in those with negative experiences in sexual relationships and poor general well-being.[8]

People with cancer. Cancer and its treatment frequently cause sexual problems.[9] Depending on gender, diagnosis, and treatment, studies show between 10% and 90% of people with cancer had a sexual problem. In a survey of 400 survivors and matched noncancer controls,[10] cancer survivors had poorer sexual function than controls, and sexual function was worse after treatment compared with before treatment. The most likely group to have problems of a sexual nature are

menopausal women. More than 50% of women having hematopoietic stem cell transfer reported loss of libido, 30.8% suffered dyspareunia, and 23.1% were unable to achieve orgasm, whereas of the men in the sample, 41.7% had erectile dysfunction, and 16.7% ejaculatory problems.[11] In men with prostatic cancer, erectile dysfunction rates vary from 0% to 84%, depending on the method of radiation treatment; the cause of this is not clearly understood.[12] Women with breast cancer also report psychosexual problems; even though their genitalia are intact, body image and visions for the future are dramatically changed.[13] In one study of 863 women, one third said that breast cancer had a negative impact on their sex life.[14] They experience loss of sensation in the breast, even after reconstruction, which is unexpectedly distressing.[15]

Women with gynecologic cancer. Sexual dysfunction rates after gynecologic cancer surgery range from 20% to 100%.[16] In a study of 105 women with cancer of the cervix or the vulva who were being treated by radical pelvic surgery, 76% of women had sexual problems after surgery, and 66% of these still had problems 6 months later, and 15% remained apareunic.[17] A Canadian study of 73 women at a gynecologic cancer follow-up clinic showed that just over 50% had sexual problems, mainly dyspareunia or loss of libido.[18] Loss of libido has been reported in 52% and 57% of women after irradiation for invasive cervical cancer.[19] A group of German clinic attendees for treatment for invasive carcinoma of the cervix had loss of libido (53% of 168 women), and 61% were anorgasmic.[20]

Is sexuality important, and should the issue be approached with all gynecologic cancer patients?

Sexuality in gynecologic cancer and quality of life. Sexuality is a health issue that has an impact on quality of life.[21] In assessing quality of life in survivors of gynecologic cancers, problems with sexuality had a significant negative impact on quality of life after treatment.[22] Individual differences in sexual self-views are important in predicting sexual difficulty or dysfunction.[23] Sexual problems have been observed in patients with all types of gynecologic cancer and can reduce the positive effects of survivorship. Many women say the experience of cancer has enriched their lives in many ways, but among a group of American and Canadian survivors of ovarian cancer, 57% said their sex lives had been negatively affected by the cancer and remained a concern, particularly for the premenopausal women.[24]

After treatment for cervical cancer, most women return to their precancer life with the exception of sexual functioning, which remains an area of morbidity.[25] A group of women from northeast Thailand identified stigmatization by friends and family and problems with sex as the main problems. This was a group with little knowledge of the disease, and it was felt that education for the women and their families would lead to better understanding and coping with their cancer.[26] Among Chinese survivors of gynecologic cancers, despite positive evaluation of their lives, sexual and marital problems were described, and one third of the husbands were having extramarital relationships. Because all the women in the study reported sexual problems, sexual and psychosexual rehabilitation was proposed.[22]

Ovarian cancer patients may experience serious disruptions in quality of life, including sexual dysfunction.[27] Sexuality is one of the integral factors in the complex interrelationship of many factors affecting quality of life in survivors.[28]

Physical problems. Gynecologic cancer and its treatments can cause physical changes in the woman that can alter her sexual functioning. Added to the emotional and social changes, this can have an enormous impact on her quality of life. An awareness of the patient's sexuality before treatment may spare her some distressing sexual problems later on. Issues such as preservation of the clitoris and the importance of the cervix to the woman's sexual pleasure, as well as the final cosmetic appearance of the vulva, may have an enormous impact on her quality of life after treatment.

Treatment-induced sexual problems. Many women with gynecologic cancer have problems of a sexual nature, but this is rarely part of their treatment plan. The treatment period can be one of the most difficult times for the woman. She is usually in pain or discomfort, suffers overwhelming fatigue, and is still coming to terms with the initial diagnosis. There are also underlying fears about survival and the anxiety that the treatment "will not work." Anxiety, depression, and fear of dying have often been described in cancer patients, all of which can have a major negative effect on sexual function. Women treated for vaginal cancer have persistent vaginal changes that can lead to sexual dysfunction.[29] Vaginal problems, fatigue, pain, and bladder dysfunction were noted as distressing in an Australian survey of gynecologic cancer patients.[30] After radiation therapy for stage I and II cervical cancers, there was decreased frequency of penetrative sex and masturbation and less satisfaction with sex and intercourse compared with before the cancer diagnosis and treatment.[31] In Edinburgh, 61 previously sexually active women who were successfully treated for stage Ib cervical cancer said that sex was poorer after treatment, and radiotherapy-treated women were more likely to report dyspareunia and lack of pleasure in sex.[32] In women treated for invasive cervical carcinoma by irradiation alone, 57% had loss of libido, 50% had dyspareunia, and only 33% had sexual intercourse within the first 3 months after treatment.[19]

Among Swedish women with stage Ib or IIa cervical cancer, reduced orgasmic frequency was found distressing by those treated with surgery plus intracavity radiotherapy or by surgery alone. Surgery plus external radiotherapy caused dyspareunia in about a fourth of the sample, and in those treated with radiotherapy alone, loose stools and dyspareunia were the most distressing symptoms, although less so than in the other groups.[33] After radical pelvic surgery, including Wertheim's hysterectomy, radical vulvectomy, and pelvic exenteration, only one fourth of the women did not have sexual difficulties postoperatively,[17] and 82% of those younger than 50 years who had radiotherapy had sexual dysfunction. Conversely, a small study showed that radical hysterectomy for stage Ib cervical cancer without adjuvant therapy had little impact on sexual functioning.[34] These reports can be compared with outcomes of hysterectomy for nonmalignant conditions, in which there is no change or some improvement in sexual function,[34,35] emphasizing the impact of the diagnosis in each of appropriate counseling or both.

Stomas. Having a stoma can cause sexual problems and enormous problems with body image. The eventual sexual outcome depends on the quality of the woman's relationship before surgery. Although many partners are very supportive, a dramatic change in the body of a sexual partner can cause her partner to be repelled by the thought of sexual contact with someone he used to find desirable. It can be very difficult to recognize and address this problem, because the partner may feel too ashamed and disloyal if he admits his dislike of the stoma. The patient often says that her partner is very supportive, but sexual activity may have lessened. Conversely, the partner may be genuinely accepting of the stoma, but the woman herself has suffered dramatic loss of confidence and self esteem due to the surgery, and she is unable to see herself any longer as an attractive sexual being and cannot believe that her partner can wish to make love to her. This can lead to avoidance of sex altogether. In both scenarios, someone ends up feeling hurt and rejected, which lowers the quality of life for the couple. The imaginative couple can use the stoma for penetrative intercourse, but this is not an option for many couples. For a single woman, a stoma can cause even greater anxiety, and she will despair of ever finding a partner. For all of these women, a chance to discuss sexuality will help to prevent ongoing sexual problems.

Continence. Managing issues of incontinence inevitably raises issues of sexuality.[36] Women who suffer incontinence find it very embarrassing, and it can be particularly distressing during sex. The fear of wetting herself or the bed while with her partner may cause the woman to avoid sexual activity altogether. Fecal incontinence can be even more distressing and is talked about even less than urinary incontinence. She may wish to sleep in a separate bed, which will have a major negative impact on intimacy between the couple. Having to use a catheter can also interfere with sexual activity. Pelvic organ prolapse is more likely than incontinence itself to cause sexual dysfunction, but appropriate behavioral or surgical treatment for the incontinence can improve sexual confidence.[37]

Endocrine changes. Sometimes, the effect of treatments causes a sudden menopause. Along with hot flashes, mood swings, deterioration of memory, and skin changes, vaginal dryness can be a feature of the sudden drop in estrogen levels. Appropriate hormone replacement therapy will help the lubrication problem. Many of these women suffer loss of libido, and the addition of testosterone to hormone replacement therapy can improve their interest in sex. If, however the loss of libido predates the procedures or is caused by social or emotional reasons, testosterone will have no impact. Quality of life in relation to sexuality can also be impaired in relation to prophylactic procedures. Oophorectomy in women with an increased risk of ovarian cancer had no negative effect on the libido of the postmenopausal women. Giving hormone replacement therapy to the premenopausal women helped alleviate the sexual impact of the procedure.[38]

Should treatment decisions be made on survival predictions alone without taking account of the woman's views of her sexuality?

Effect of gynecologic cancer on sexuality in minority groups. When addressing the issues of sexuality in patients, it can be helpful to remember that special characteristics of that woman may change her experience of the illness and her expectations of outcome. Clinicians may also have their own judgmental attitudes about the potential sexuality of their patients, if they think about it at all. "Too old, too young, too fat, or too ugly" for sex are some of the negative stereotypes that may be almost unknowingly imposed on the patient by the treatment team. There are, however, no automatic barriers to sex, and assumptions about patient's intimate lives are dangerous and usually wrong. Allowing the woman to talk about the importance of sex in her life and the effects of treatments can increase her feelings of autonomy and control over her future.

The elderly. The elderly gynecologic cancer patient desires cure as much as the younger patient and is more likely to accept disfiguring treatment than the young. Although sexuality is more important in younger patients, women older than 65 years still consider sexuality an issue when discussing cancer therapy.[39] Difficulty can arise for an older patient in discussing sex, because the doctor may be much younger than she is, and she may find it embarrassing to discuss these issues in front of her family who, if they find it difficult to conceive of their mother being sexual, will find it even harder to accept a grandmother's sexuality. Many more people are in changing relationships in the latter parts of their lives, and sex continues to be vital to quality of life and happiness right into advanced old age.

Young people and adolescents. Young women and adolescents suffering cancer have many issues to deal with such as survival, fertility, and relationships. Sexuality is of vital importance to a young woman in the adolescent and teenage years.

In Finland, in a group of women between the ages of 16 and 26 years who had suffered childhood cancers, one half showed delayed psychosexual maturation.[40] Although not specifically discussing gynecologic tumors, reviews of girls who have suffered childhood cancers state that they have more difficulty with dating and relationships than their peer group,[41] and some found the quality of the relationship disappointing compared with the intense bonds they had with the family and the clinical team when they were being treated for their cancer.[42] Post-treatment psychological interventions in the form of group or individual therapy can improve psychosexual outcomes in this group.

Lesbians. Lesbians may be at higher risk of developing gynecologic cancers than heterosexual women, often due to lifestyle and health-related behaviors. Lesbians may have an increased risk of ovarian cancer because they are less likely to have protective factors such as pregnancies and to use of oral contraceptives.[43] They also have higher rates of obesity, alcohol use, and tobacco use, which puts them at higher risk for other cancers and chronic diseases.[44] Lesbian and bisexual women support ready access to genetic testing for breast and ovarian cancer and believe that testing should be a personal choice. Their attitudes were the same as those of white, African American, and Ashkenazi Jewish women.[45] Although only 3% of lesbians develop cervical dysplasia,[46] most lesbians have had sex with a man at some stage[47] and are therefore at risk of human papillomavirus (HPV) infection. Cervical dysplasia has also been reported in women who have never had heterosexual sex but who have penetrative sexual activity by means of fingers or toys. Lesbians consider themselves to be at lower risk for disease than the heterosexual or bisexual population despite the fact that more than 70% of lesbians have had sex with a man.[48] Negative experiences with health care providers, together with misinformation about the need for Pap smears, in women who have sex with women has led to a reluctance of this group to come forward for screening.[49] Provision of health care services specifically designed to meet the needs of lesbians can encourage attendance for discussion of sexual health needs.[50] If more than 50% of lesbians cannot disclose their sexuality to their general practitioner, discussing issues of sex must be extremely difficult. If the woman's sexuality is disclosed, and her social support systems, which may include a same-sex partner, can be openly used, it makes support in cancer therapy more effective.[50]

Bisexuals. Bisexuals may be reluctant to disclose their embracing sexual orientation for fear of being stigmatized. Although their gynecologic cancer risk is similar to that of heterosexuals, there have been reports that they are more likely to exhibit sexual risk behavior.[2] Their reluctance to discuss sexuality may inhibit them from screening uptake, and they may not understand that HPV can be transmitted to or passed on by female partners, putting themselves and partners at risk of cervical cancer.

Ethnic minorities. Women from different cultures and religions have beliefs and rules about sexuality and illness that influence their sexuality and may influence their wishes for different types of treatment. Vaginal bleeding in some of the major religions is considered "unclean," and sexual relationships are barred during these periods. Any cancer or treatment that causes vaginal bleeding, particularly continuous spotting, will prevent a woman with these beliefs from physical contact of any sort with her husband at a time when she most needs his support and physical closeness. In some cultures, male family members have to be involved in decisions related to medical treatment,[51] and an interpreter often needs to be present. In the "crowded room situation," it is a major problem to ensure that the women is being granted full autonomy and is being permitted some degree of control over her treatment. The discussion of sexual issues should be dealt with at a separate time and with a suitable interpreter,[52] which in this case would be a nonjudgmental female interpreter trained in the language of sexuality and working with a female doctor or nurse.

Women with disabilities. Women with precancer disabilities of any sort, such as physical, learning, sensory, or hidden disabilities, have the same rights to a fulfilling sex life as any other woman. Assumptions about the importance of sex should never be made, and all women should have equal opportunity to discuss their sexuality. Often, these women have developed adaptive strategies to cope with their disability and may well be able to further adapt to the effect that the cancer and treatment will have on their sex lives.

Drug and alcohol users and sex workers. Women with drug and alcohol habits tend to be chaotic in their sexual lives and are at high risk of cervical cancer. They are unlikely to comply with screening programs, although dedicated health care settings can increase the use of cervical screening.[53] Even when they develop cancer, they are unlikely to comply with therapy, unless suitable drug substitution therapy is concurrently prescribed. Many female drug users are prostitutes who earn money for drugs. For these women, discussion of sexuality together with an all encompassing social care package addressing current needs and an addiction program is necessary for treatment compliance. Non–drug-using sex workers who develop gynecologic cancer find it hard to cope with the fact that their means of income has been severely disrupted.

Should the issue of sexuality be raised with the woman undergoing colposcopy, a relatively minor and routine procedure?

Young women and colposcopy. The issue of young people will become more prominent as knowledge and awareness of the link between HPV infection and cervical cancer increases in the general community. With vaccine trials being initiated worldwide, more young women will be faced with the reality that their sexual activity may be linked to potential genital cancer. This infection is so common that the risk of acquiring the virus with only one sexual partner is 46%,[54] but women may feel guilty or dirty when receiving the diagnosis. The link between HPV and cervical cancer means that the patient will experience the fears and anxieties of potentially malignant disease and the conflicting emotions associated with the diagnosis of a sexually transmitted infection. The first question at colposcopy is usually whether the patient has cancer, but when HPV is mentioned, the next questions are usually about the mode of transmission and concerns about her partner's behavior. "'How did I get it, and from whom did I get it?" Initial studies of women with abnormal cytologic results showed that all were frightened of cancer, 22% had sexual difficulties, and another 26% had relationship difficulties.[55]

Loss of libido and sexual interest was found to be higher in women with abnormal smear tests compared with a control group,[56] and it is not unusual to find women unnecessarily abstaining from sex from the time of the initial abnormal smear result until the final "all clear." Often, these girls would like to resume sexual activity but have been too frightened or embarrassed to ask, and the topic of sex has never been mentioned.

Women undergoing investigation for abnormal smears should be allowed to talk about sex. These are generally young, healthy, sexually active women for whom sex is an important part of their lives and relationships. Although the general feeling among clinicians may be that anything to do with sexual discussion is the nurse's domain, women undergoing colposcopy usually do not go on to become cancer patients and may lose contact with clinical settings after they are cured. If the colposcopist discusses the continuation of sexual relationships at the time of the first encounter, the woman can return home with all her queries answered.

Communication about sex. Lack of communication about sex has been cited by patients as a major problem. Because so many women with gynecologic cancer have problems with sex after diagnosis and treatment, it is important for them to have an opportunity to discuss these potential problems. For any rational discussion to take place and for informed consent to treatment that may affect their sexuality, women have to be given information on which to base their consent. This information should be comprehensive, accurate, and comprehensible, but above all, the information should be available!

Several studies have highlighted a lack of information on sex for cancer patients in general[57] and gynecologic cancer patients in particular.[58] Lack of information has been cited as one of the main difficulties women have in dealing with the effect of the cancer on their sexuality, together with changes in feelings about their femininity and problems in communicating these emotions to their partner.[18] Lack of communication about sex in the setting of gynecologic cancer was originally reported less than 20 years ago[59] and has been repeatedly documented since then[32,60] with no obvious improvement in the situation. Cervical cancer patients ask for information regarding side effects of the disease and possible effects on sexual function.[61] Women with ovarian cancer would like to talk about the effects the cancer might have on their sexuality so that "you should know what is going to happen instead of it hitting you like a ton of bricks."[62] However, health care professionals rarely communicate about these issues in a meaningful way.

Of the many psychosocial issues affecting their patients, doctors are most uncomfortable with the topic of sexuality.[63] Even though sexuality is an integral part of every human being, many doctors and health professionals find it difficult to talk to patients about sexual issues, and gynecologic oncologists are no exception. A review of patient self-help web sites confirmed that the word that kept recurring was "communication." Patients were encouraged to communicate with partners and doctors with their patients.[64] There are different opinions about when the information and discussion about sex should take place. Some patients would like the information preoperatively, which is logical in terms of discussing treatment options. It has also been shown that pre-operative discussion of sex leads to a reduction in post-treatment sexual morbidity.[65] Some women, however, prefer a post-treatment discussion.[18]

Communication about sex in the palliative phase. If it is difficult for patients and clinicians to talk about sex after cancer diagnosis, it is infinitely more difficult for them to communicate about sex when the patient may be dying.[66] Sex and death as topics of discussion are two of the greatest taboos in society, and despite calls for more openness, it is still a highly problematic area. There are many issues related to this sensitive area, but the ability to discuss sex and to have meaningful sexual contact with partners in the palliative phase can give much joy to both partners at this key point in their relationship. Sex during the palliative phase can reduce stress and cause physical relaxation and a degree of pain relief in the woman. Although often described by the patient as being tender and poignant or almost violent as a death-defying gesture, sex can also heighten a person's sense of being a complete person and can restore a sense of fun in a relationship that is undergoing enormous stress. The provision of a private room with a double bed for the terminally ill is optimal.

Emotional Themes

A common feature of cancer patients is the increase in levels of psychological distress after treatment and diagnosis. Increased levels of anxiety and depression can cause and be caused by sexual dysfunction. It may seem relatively easy to understand that physical changes in the genital area may cause functional problems, leading to pain or difficulties with sex. These functional sexual problems generally have an emotional overlay and cause distress to the patient. What is harder to understand is that many sexual problems have a purely emotional origin, which may or may not be related to the cancer, and the diagnosis and treatment of the disease may act as a trigger for the emergence of long-standing emotional disruption. Although each patient has her own unique background, social circumstances, and relationships and has her own very personal experience of cancer, there are recurrent emotional themes that appear throughout the individual case histories of gynecologic cancer patients.

Bereavement reactions are common. Fear of dying is one of the first overwhelming emotions felt by the woman and by her family. Feelings of grief and loss can be overwhelming. The natural response to having a life-threatening disease is panic. Women suffer many losses all in one cruel stroke. Loss of health can lead to loss of independence latter and cause dramatic changes in visions for the future.

Women without children who would like to have them are scared that this option will be removed from them. Women suffer mixed and conflicting emotions about desiring a child and leaving a baby or existing children motherless if they are not cured. The desire in humans to leave something of themselves behind is strong, and for many women, this is realized in the form of offspring. The fears about sex are closely linked to anxieties about loss of fertility. When confronted with their own mortality, some women will feel too embarrassed to talk about sex, even though it is a major issue to them, because they think it is regarded as trivial compared with life-and-death issues.

Loss of fertility causes much distress to women. Even if a woman had decided before diagnosis not to have any more children, the fact that the element of choice has been removed can have a profound effect on her perception of herself as a complete woman. Treatment options can often be tailored to fertility preservation, which can greatly improve the emotional impact of the cancer.[67] Loss of self-esteem can follow any major bereavement, leading to lack of sexual confidence and breakdown in emotional and sexual relationships. Discussions about ovum storage, ovarium transposition, or embryo storage are critical in the management of the younger woman when fertility is still an issue.

There is a fundamental link between body image and sexuality, and changes in body image compromise the fundamental sexuality of the woman.[68] Women often have fantasies about the appearance of their genitalia postoperatively, imagining an ugly distorted vulva, a nonexistent introitus, or a gaping vagina, whereas they may have cosmetically intact genitalia. Showing the woman her vulva with a mirror, with the partner present if she chooses, can dispel these myths. Many women have expressed the experience of having the vagina "medicalized" as being invasive, and the loss of the privacy of their genitalia can be profound.

With cervical cancer, there is frequently fear of contamination or being contaminated by the partner. Because cervical cancer is linked in most cases to sexual activity, the woman's feelings often encompass the overlapping impact of cancer and a sexually transmitted infection. Guilt is a common theme. Many blame themselves for "catching" the disease,[32] and they link the diagnosis to previous sexual activity.[69] "Will I infect my partner?" "Can he reinfect me?' These are commonly expressed fears about a cervical cancer diagnosis and treatment. In the patient's mind, one way of ensuring this does not happen is to avoid sex altogether, and apareunia results. Fear of worsening the cancer by any sort of sexual activity is common, particularly so in cervical cancer.

Treatments for Sexual Problems in Gynecologic Cancer

As with all clinical problems, the physician must undertake and complete the relevant investigation of the patient's symptoms. With problems of a sexual nature, the cause may be purely organic, purely psychogenic, or a combination of both. Full physical investigation of the symptoms may reveal an obvious physical cause, such as a shortened or stenosed vagina, both of which can cause dyspareunia or apareunia. Any major distortion of the vulva may render penetrative intercourse impossible.

Menopausal symptoms can be sudden and distressing, causing vaginal dryness and leading to dyspareunia and loss of libido. Appropriate hormone replacement therapy may alleviate these symptoms. After any organic problems have been attended to, including physical, endocrine, biochemical, and hematologic disturbances, if there is still a problem of a sexual nature, the cause may be psychosexual, and an assessment by a trained professional should be carried out. Frequently, even when there is a seemingly obvious organic cause for the sexual disturbance, there is a strong emotional overlay because this strikes at the basis of the lover role that the woman has in relation to her partner.

Chemical treatments. There has been little evidence about the efficacy of drug therapies for female sexual dysfunction. Androgens have an effect on female sexual desire,[70] and testosterone in addition to conventional hormone replacement therapy has been shown to alleviate loss of libido when the diminished sexual interest was caused primarily by menopause.[71] Some positive effect of using sildenafil on women using antidepressants has been found.[72,73] Randomized, controlled trials, however, have shown no overall sexual benefits.[74] In 33 women with various sexual dysfunctions, some degree of increased vaginal lubrication and clitoral sensitivity was observed, but sildenafil use made no significant improvements in the overall sexual satisfaction of the sample.[75]

Behavioral and physical treatments. If most gynecologic oncologists were asked which word sprang to mind when sexuality was discussed, it would be *dilator*. There is an obvious place for the use of this equipment when there is a risk of vaginal stenosis after radiotherapy or surgery. Most women are unlikely to comply with vaginal dilator regimens. Women who did not follow advice on dilatation and did not resume previous sexual practices were more likely to suffer adverse physical and sexual changes.[31] When dilator instruction was combined with behavioral and educational interventions that were tailored to overcome the patients' fears, there was a marked increase in dilator use, especially in younger women.[76] Dilators are used in psychosexual therapy, but because they do not treat organic stenosis, but treat a psychogenic involuntary spasm of the vaginal muscles, they should not be called *dilators*. The current terminology is *vaginal trainer*. The rationale for their use in vaginismus is to allow the woman to learn to allow penetration of her vagina "under her own control." It is easy to make the assumption that painful sex or lack of penetration have physical origins because lack of lubrication or stenosis is assumed. A sensitive genital examination, however, may reveal a well-lubricated and adequate vagina in a patient with persistent complaints of sexual problems. In these cases, the pain may have psychogenic origins, and psychosexual treatment is indicated. The best approach for such a woman is to maximize the therapeutic opportunity and use the dilators or trainers in a combined physical and psychosexual way.

Lubricants have their place in sexual therapy when the patient has drug- or treatment-induced vaginal dryness. The most common cause of vaginal dryness during sex, however, is lack of lubrication due to inadequate sexual arousal. This can be caused by poor or absent foreplay or by a lack of interest or confidence in the partner. If there is no organic disruption to the vaginal skin or secretions, a supply of lubricants will not act as a substitute for passion and good sexual technique.

Psychodynamics. The *sexual self* includes interrelated physical and psychological dimensions that can be conscious or unconscious and that are changing and changeable.[77] Psychological distress is significantly related to physical complaints and functional outcomes.[32] By using the connection between the psyche and physical symptoms, the emotional aspects of sexual problems can be successfully treated.

Psychosexual medicine is body-mind doctoring.[78] The trained clinician uses the "here and now" in the clinical consultation to understand the hidden emotional reasons behind the patient's sexual problem. This is achieved by analyzing the doctor-patient interaction at the time of consultation, recognizing any emotions generated in the room, and by reflecting these feelings to the patient in an attempt to help them understand the root of her own sexual problem. This or any other approach that examines the patient's emotions in a therapeutic way takes time and specialized training, but once learned, these core skills can be used effectively to identify a sexual problem at general consultation. If the problem is recognized, the patient can be brought back at a later date when there is time to spend on the sexual or emotional aspect of her treatment, or she can be referred to a specialist clinic. Some women are too frightened of addressing the emotional issues and are only prepared to talk about the physical aspects of the problem.[79]

Although little research has been done on the impact of treatment of sexual problems in women with gynecologic cancer, one randomized, controlled trial showed that sexual functioning and quality of life improved in women who received specialist psycho-sexual counseling.[80]

Case Scenarios

Scenario 1. Mary, a 34-year-old woman with two children, had been diagnosed with cancer of the cervix and had successfully undergone hysterectomy and irra-diation to the upper vagina. She had been using dilators as requested but was complaining of dyspareunia. On genital examination, her vagina was minimally stenosed and had mild dryness.

Traditional approach. At a busy outpatient clinic, Mary was given a further course of dilators and lubri-cants, and when she returned, there had been no improvement of her symptoms.

Psychosexually aware approach. Mary was encour-aged to talk about her feelings about the sexual problem and her relationship with her partner. She soon revealed that on her diagnosis of cancer, her husband had developed erectile dysfunction, and attempts at penetration were uncomfortable. On further explo-ration, it transpired that he was scared of "stirring up" the cancer again, and this anxiety caused his erectile failure. After some months of couple treatment, the problem was resolved.

Scenario 2. Jean was a 45-year-old woman with treated ovarian cancer. She said she had no interest in sex and would like to improve the situation. Genital examination revealed a healthy, well-lubricated vagina. She requested a change of hormone replacement therapy to "improve things."

Traditional approach. Jean was given hormone replacement therapy with added testosterone. She admitted she felt a little more sexy when watching something erotic on television, but she still had absolutely no interest in sex with her partner.

Psychosexually aware approach. After describing lack of interest in sex with her partner, Jean was prompted to discuss her sexual feelings openly. It transpired that her husband was an alcoholic, who became violent and abusive, and she had lost respect

for him many years before. She said she had no feelings for him but wanted to want sex for the sake of peace in the home. It was only when she developed cancer that she felt there might have been a physical reason for her lack of interest, and it was therefore legitimate to discuss it.

All treatments approaches are valid as long as they are appropriate and the professional has been professionally trained and accredited. The assessment of sexual problems should continue throughout treatment and recovery,[81] and a holistic approach is appropriate.[68]

How can the psychosexually aware approach be managed in a busy health care setting, and who should address the issue of sexual problems with the patients?

The role of the gynecologic oncologist. Doctors frequently claim that they do not have time to deal with sexual problems. This can be because of genuine time constraints, because they themselves are uncom-fortable discussing sexuality, or because they are frightened of the disclosure of a sexual problem they had not been trained to deal with. The treatment of sexual problems cannot take place without initial disclosure and discussion, and all members of the clinical team need to be comfortable with the topic of sexuality, including the doctors. Patients say they would like their doctors to discuss sexual issues with them.[62] If these discussions are carried out before treatment, the implications for the woman's sex life can be addressed. The gynecologist should initiate discussion of the topic at an early stage and should not be expected to perform in-depth psychosexual counseling at this point. With raised awareness of the sexuality of their patients, more sexual problems can be identified at an early stage, and women can then be referred for more specialized treatment. If sex-uality were integrated into core training in gyneco-logic oncology, clinicians would easily be able to incorporate the recognition of sexual problems into their routine consultations.

The role of the nurse. Cancer nurses frequently have extensive contact time with their patients. They see them at different stages of the disease, but more fre-quently in the latter stages. Women often feel more comfortable talking about intimate matters such as sex and relationships with the nurses, who are mainly female and who are seen as more approachable. A frequently heard phrase from the patient is "I didn't like to waste the doctor's time" talking about issues that are vitally important but that she perceives as trivial in the oncologist's eyes. When specialist gynecologic nursing support was provided through individual care and a patient support group, the intervention was positively evaluated.[82] Cancer nurses are uniquely positioned to provide informational support to patients[30]; however, the nurse needs adequate training to incorporate sexuality issues into her routine care of the patient.[83]

The role of the researcher. There are still many unanswered questions about sexuality and gynecologic cancer. Patients who are experiencing sexual problems are the key to the answers. It is feasible to include sexual activity questionnaires in all gynecologic trials requiring ongoing assessment of quality of life.[84] Newer sexual function evaluation tools are available that can help this process.[85]

Barriers to treating sexual problems in gynecologic oncology patients

Because many women with gynecologic cancers have or will develop problems of a sexual nature, it is important to address these issues. This does not always happen because of common barriers.

The patient can be embarrassed to discuss sexual issues with the doctor, and the doctor frequently is too inhibited or too busy to discuss these issues with the patient. Even if the topic of sex is mentioned in the clinical setting, there may be many other people present in a setting totally lacking in privacy. The patient may demonstrate a lack of ability or willingness to communicate with the partner, or the partner may avoid confronting the issue with the woman, particularly if he feels very protective toward her or no longer finds her attractive. There is a lack of trained professionals to treat all those who need therapy.

Summary

Women with gynecologic cancers commonly experience sexual dysfunction. They would like information on possible sexual sequelae of their illness and its treatment; however, this is rarely available. They would also like an opportunity to discuss sexuality with their clinical team, and the doctors in particular are reluctant to do so. If sexuality became an integral part of the core training of gynecologic oncologists and cancer nurses, it would be possible to assess and treat sexual dysfunction throughout the course of a woman's diagnosis, treatment, and recovery. This holistic approach would lead to a high quality of care and improved sexual outcomes for the patient, and it would add a new dimension to survivorship.

REFERENCES

1. Benjamin H: The Transsexual Phenomenon. New York, Jullian Press, 1966.
2. Johnson AM, Mercer CH. Erens B, et al: Sexual behaviour in Britain: Partnerships, practices, and HIV risk behaviours. Lancet 2001;358:1835-1842.
3. Bancroft J: Human sexuality and its problems, 2/e, Edinburgh, Churchill Livingstone, 1989.
4. Stoller RJ, Sex and Gender. London, Hogarth Press, 1968.
5. Ellis H: Psychology of Sex. London, Heinemann, 1933.
6. Kinsey AC, Pomeroy WB Martin CF: Sexual behaviour in the human male. Philadelphia, WB Saunders, 1948.
7. Kinsey AC, Pomeroy WB, Martin CF, et al. Sexual behaviour in the human female. Philadelphia, WB Saunders, 1953.
8. Laumann EO, Paik A, Rosen RC: Sexual dysfunction in the United States. JAMA 1999; 281:537-544.
9. Curdt S, Kamm M: Cancer and Sexuality. Internist Prax 2002;42:531-538.
10. Syrjala KL, Schroeder TC, Abrams JR, et al: Sexual function measurement and outcomes in cancer survivors and matched controls. J Sex Res 2000;37:213-225.
11. Lee HG, Park EY, Kim HM, et al: Sexuality and quality of life after haematopoietic stem cell transplantation. Korean J Intern Med 2002;17:19-23.
12. Incrocci L, Slob AK, Levendag PC: Sexual dysfunction after radiotherapy for prostate cancer. Int J Radiat Oncol Biol Phys 2002;52:681-693.
13. Schover LR: The impact of breast cancer on sexuality, body image, and intimate relationships. Ca: Canc J for Clin 1991; 41: 112-120.
14. Meyerowitz BE, Desmond KA, Rowland JH, et al: Sexuality following breast cancer. J Sex Marital Ther 1999;25:237-250.
15. Wilmot MC, Ross JA: Women's perception. Breast cancer treatment and sexuality. Canc Prac 1997; 5:353-359.
16. Lutgendorf SK, Anderson B, et al: Interleukin-6 and use of social support in gynecologic cancer patients. Inter J Behav Med 2000;7:127-142.
17. Corney RH, Crowther ME, Everett H, et al: Psychosexual dysfunction in women with gynaecological cancer following radical pelvic surgery. Br J Obstet Gynaecol 1993;100:73-78.
18. Bourgeois-Law G, Lotocki R: Sexuality and gynaecological cancer: a needs assessment. Canc J Human Sex 1999;8:231-240.
19. Lasnik E, Tatra G: Sex behaviour following primary radiotherapy of cervix cancer. Geburtshilfe and Frauenheilkunde 1986;46:813-816.
20. Lotze W: Sexual rehabilitation of patients with cervix cancer. Geburtshilfe Frauenheilkd 1990;50:781-784.
21. Butler L, Banfield V, Sveinson T, Allen K: Conceptualising sexual health in cancer care. West J Nurs Res 1998;20:683-699, discussion 700-705.
22. Molassiotis A, Chan CW, Yam BM, Chan SJ: Quality of life in Chinese women with gynaecological cancers. Support Care Cancer 2000;8:414-422.
23. Andersen BL: Surviving cancer: The importance of sexual self-concept. Med Paediatr Oncol 1999;33:15-23.
24. Stewart DE, Wong F, Duff S, et al: What doesn't kill you makes you stronger: An ovarian cancer survivor survey. Gynaecol Oncol 2000;83:537-542.
25. Andersen BL: Stress and quality of life following cervical cancer. J Natl Cancer Inst Monogr 1996;21:65-70.
26. Ratanasiri A, Boonmongkon P, Upayokin P, et al: Illness experience and coping with gynaecological cancer among Northeast Thai female patients. Southeast Asian J Trop Med Public Health 2000;31:547-553.
27. Bodurka-Bevers D, Basen-Engquist K, Carmack CL, et al: Depression, anxiety and quality of life in patients with epithelial ovarian cancer. Gynecol Oncol 2000;78:302-308.
28. Wenzel LB, Donnelly JP, Fowler JM, et al: Resilience, reflection and residual stress in ovarian cancer survivorship: A gynaecologic oncology group study. Psychooncology 2002;11:142-153.
29. Bergmark K, Lundqvist EA, Dickman PW, et al: Vaginal changes and sexuality in women with a history of cervical cancer. N Engl J Med 1999;340:1383-1389.
30. Steginga SK, Dunn J: Women's experiences following treatment for gynaecologic cancer. Oncol Nurs Forum 1997;24:1043-1048.
31. Krumm S, Lamberti J: Changes in sexual behaviour following radiation therapy for cervical cancer. J Psychosom Obstet Gynaecol 1993;14:51-63.
32. Cull A, Cowie VJ, Farquharson DI, et al: Early stage cervical cancer: Psychosocial and sexual outcomes of treatment. Br J Cancer 1993;68:1216-1220.
33. Bergmark K, Lundqvist EA, Dickman PW, et al: Patient-rating of distressful symptoms after treatment for early cervical cancer. Acta Obstet Gynecol Scand 2001;81:443-450.
34. Grumann M, Robertson R, Hacker NF, et al: Sexual functioning in patients following radical hysterectomy for stage IB cancer of the cervix. Int J Gynaecol Cancer 2001;11:372-380.
35. Carlson KJ: Outcomes of hysterectomy. Clin Obst Gynaecol 1997;40:939-946.

36. Sexuality and reproductive issues. Aust Fam Physician 2002;31:102-105.
37. Barber MD, Visco AG, Wyman JF, et al: Sexual function in women with urinary incontinence and pelvic organ prolapse. Obstet Gynecol 2002;99:281-289.
38. Meiser B, Tiller K, Gleeson MA, et al: Psychological impact of prophylactic oophorectomy in women at increased risk for ovarian cancer. Psychooncology 2000;9:496-503.
39. Nordin AJ, Chinn DJ, Moloney I, et al: Do elderly cancer patients care about cure? Attitudes to radical gynaecologic oncology surgery in the elderly. Gynecol Oncol 2001;81:447-455.
40. Kokkonen J, Vainionpaa L, Winqvist S, et al: Physical and psychosocial outcome for young adults with treated malignancy. Paediatr Haematol Oncol 1997;14:223-232.
41. Fritz GK, Williams JR: Issues of adolescent development for survivors of childhood cancer. J Am Acad Child Adolesc Psychiatry 1998;27:712-715.
42. Woolverton K, Ostroff J: Psychosexual adjustment in adolescent cancer survivors. Cancer Invest 2000;18:51-58.
43. Dibble SL, Roberts SA, Robertson PA, Paul SM: Risk factors for ovarian cancer: Lesbian and heterosexual women. Oncol Nurs Forum 2002;29:E1-E7.
44. Cochran SD, Mays VM, Bowen D, et al: Cancer-related risk indicators and preventive screening behaviours among lesbians and bisexual women. Am J Public Health 2001;91:591-597.
45. Durfy SJ, Bowen DJ, McTiernan A, et al: Attitudes and interest in genetic testing for breast and ovarian cancer susceptibility in diverse groups of women in western Washington. Cancer Epidemiol Biomarkers Prev 1999;8(Pt 2):369-375.
46. O'Hanlan KA, Crum CP: Human papillomavirus-associated cervical intraepithelial neoplasia following lesbian sex. Obstet Gynaecol 1996;88:702-703.
47. Bailey JV, Kavanagh J, Owen C, et al: Lesbians and cervical screening. Br J Gen Pract 2000;50:481-482.
48. Price JH, Easton R, Telljohann SK, et al: Perceptions of cervical cancer and Pap smear screening behaviour by women's sexual orientation. J Commun Health 1996;21:89-105.
49. Rankow EJ, Tessaro I: Cervical cancer risk and Papanicolaou screening in a sample of lesbian and bisexual women. J Fam Pract 1998;47:139-143.
50. Carr SV, Scoular A, Elliot L, et al: A community based lesbian sexual health service—clinically justified or politically correct? Br J Fam Plann 1999;25:93-95.
51. Younge D, Mooreau P, Ezzat A, et al: Communicating with cancer patients in Saudi Arabia. Ann N Y Acad Sci 1997;809:309-316.
52. Phelan M, Parkman S: How to do it: Work with an interpreter. BMJ 1995;311:555-557.
53. Carr SV, Goldberg DJ, Elliott L, et al: A primary health care service for Glasgow street sex workers—6 years' experience of the "Drop-in Centre," 1989-1994. AIDS Care 1996;8:489-497.
54. Collins S, Mazloomzadeh S, Winter H, et al: High incidence of cervical human papillomavirus infection in women during their first sexual relationship. BJOG 2002;109:96-98.
55. Beresford JM, Gervaize PA: The emotional mal pap smears on patients referred for colposcopy. Gynaecol Laser Surg 1986;2:83-87.
56. Lerman C, Miller SM, Scarborough R, et al: Adverse psychological consequences of positive cytological cervical screening. Am J Obstet Gynecol 1991;165:658-662.
57. Sanson-Fisher R, Girgis A, Boyes A, et al: The unmet supportive care needs of patients with cancer. Supportive Care Review Group. Cancer 2000;88:226-237.
58. Crowther ME, Corney RH, Shepherd JH: Psychosexual implications of gynaecological cancer. BMJ 1994;308:869-870.
59. Andersen BL, Anderson B, deProsse C: Controlled prospective longitudinal study of women with cancer: 1. Sexual functioning outcomes. J Consulting Clin Psych 1989;57:583-691.
60. Lamb MA, Sheldon TA: The sexual adaptation of women treated for endometrial cancer. Cancer Practice 1994;2:103-113.
61. Bergmark K, Lundqvist EA, Steineck G: A Swedish study of women treated for cervix cancer. Gynaecologic cancer often affects sexuality. Lakartidningen 2000;97:5347-5355.
62. Stead ML, Fallowfield L, Brown JM, et al: Communication about sexual problems and sexual concerns in ovarian cancer: qualitative study. BMJ 2001;323:836-837.
63. Penson RT, Gallagher J, Gioiella ME, et al: Sexuality and cancer: Conversation comfort zone. Oncologist 2000;5:336-344.
64. Yamey G: Online resources on sexuality and cancer. West J Med 2002;176:19-20.
65. Marteau TM, Kidd J, Cuddeford L: Reducing anxiety in women referred by colposcopy using an information booklet. Br J Health Psychol 1996;1:181-189.
66. Gianotten Woet L: Dealing with sexuality in the palliative phase of cancer. Abtract in Proceedings of 6th Congress of the European Federation of Sexology. Limassol, Cyprus, 2002.
67. Trope C, Scheistroen M, Makar AP: Fertility preservation in gynaecologic cancer. Tidsskr Norske Laegeforen 2001;121:1234-1239.
68. Colyer H: Women's experience of living with cancer. J Adv Nurs 1996;23:496-501.
69. Wolff JP, Goldfarb E, Cachelou R: Cervical cancer: Psychology and sexuality. Bull Cancer 1980;67:116-119.
70. Sarrel PM: Psychosexual effects of menopause: Role of androgens. Am J Obstet Gynecol 1999;180:319-324.
71. Sherwin BB: Use of combined estrogen-androgen preparations in the post-menopause: Evidence from clinical studies. Int J Fertil Womens Med 1998;43:98-103.
72. Fava M, Rankin MA, et al: An open trial of oral sildenafilin antidepressant-induced sexual dysfunction. Psychotherapy Psychosom 1998;67:328-331.
73. Nurnberg HG, Lauriello J, Hensley PL, et al: Sildenafil for iatrogenic serotonergic antidepressant medication-induced sexual dysfunction in 4 patients. J Clin Psychiatry 1999;60:33-35.
74. Meston CM, Frohlich PF: Update on female sexual function. Curr Opin Urol 2001;11:603-609.
75. Kaplan SA, Reis RB, et al: Safety and efficacy of sildenafil in postmenopausal women with sexual dysfunction. Urology 1999;53:481-486.
76. Robinson JW, Faris PD, Scott CB: Psychoeducational group increases vaginal dilation for younger women and reduces sexual fears for women of all ages with gynaecological carcinoma treated with radiotherapy. Int J Radiat Oncol Biol Phys 1999;44:497-506.
77. Gill M: Psychosexual Medicine an Introduction, 2/e, (ed) Arnold 2001.
78. Skrine R, Montford H: Psychosexual Medicine an introduction, 2/e, (ed) Arnold 2001.
79. Hutchinson H: Psychosexual medicine for gynaecological oncology patients. Inst Psychosex Med J 2002;30:11-14.
80. Maughan K, Clarke C: The effect of a clinical nurse specialist in gynaecological oncology on quality of life and sexuality. J Clin Nursing 2001;10:221-229.
81. McKee AL Jr, Schover LR: Sexuality rehabilitation [review]. Cancer 2001;92(Suppl):1008-1012.
82. Jeffries H: Ovarian cancer patients: Are their informational and emotional needs being met? J Clin Nurs 2002;11:41-47.
83. Wilmoth MC, Spinelli A: Sexual implications of gynaecologic cancer treatments. J Obstet Gynecol Neonatal Nur 2000;29:413-421.
84. Stead ML, Crocombe WD, et al: Sexual activity questionnaires in clinical trials: acceptability to patients with gynaecological disorders. Brit J Obstet Gynaecol 1999;106;50-54.
85. Quirk FH, Heiman JR, Rosen RC, et al: Development of a sexual function questionnaire for clinical trials of female sexual dysfunction. J Womens Health Gend Based Med 2002;11:277-289.

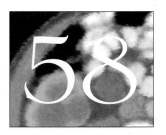

FERTILITY AND GYNECOLOGIC CANCER

Allan Covens

- **What are the options to preserve fertility in patients with cervical cancer?**
- **If the ovaries are to be removed or rendered menopausal by therapy, what are the options to preserve their function?**
- **Can fertility be preserved in patients with endometrial cancer?**
- **Can fertility be preserved in patients with epithelial ovarian cancer?**
- **Can fertility be preserved in patients with ovarian germ cell tumors?**
- **Can ovarian function be protected from chemotherapy?**

The concepts of fertility and gynecologic cancer seem diametrically opposed. Gynecologic cancers usually occur in women who are perimenopausal or post-menopausal. In the uncommon premenopausal scenario, these cancers commonly confer relative infertility. Furthermore, treatment associated with gynecologic cancers, whether surgery or radiation therapy, usually renders the patient sterile or menopausal or both.

For many patients and physicians, the notion of fertility preservation is a small issue; because treatment is thought to be potentially compromised with conservative therapy (as opposed to radical therapy), the prospects for conception are perceived to be remote and the future lifespan of the patient uncertain. Nevertheless, the understanding of gynecologic cancers has dramatically improved over the past several decades. Although much remains to be understood, the identification of prognostic factors, the benefits of adjuvant therapy, and reduction in the morbidity and toxicity of therapy have been incorporated into many approaches to gynecologic cancers.

Fertility preservation can encompass many and varied situations. For example, ovarian conservation at the time of radical hysterectomy may be construed as preservation of fertility, given advances in reproductive technology such as in vitro fertilization (IVF) and surrogacy, or the preservation of the uterus after surgical management of ovarian cancer can allow for subsequent implantation with embryos. Furthermore, the use of gonadotropin-releasing hormone (GnRH) agonists before alkylating agent–based chemotherapy or cryopreservation of oocytes before ovarian ablation (by surgery, chemotherapy, or radiation therapy) may also be construed as fertility preservation.

▍CERVIX CANCER

What are the options to preserve fertility in patients with cervical cancer? Many varied approaches to preserve fertility in cervical cancer have been explored. These include cone biopsy with or without a pelvic lymphadenectomy, cone biopsy followed by intracavitary radiation therapy (in addition to pelvic lymphadenectomy and ovarian transposition), chemotherapy followed by cone biopsy (in addition to a pelvic lymphadenectomy), radical trachelectomy, and pelvic lymphadenectomy. In fact, pregnancies have been reported after radiotherapy for cervical cancer.[1]

Cone biopsy. Cone biopsy alone has proved to be adequate therapy for the SGO (society of gynecologic oncologists) definition of microinvasive cervical cancer (squamous cell, depth <3 mm, linear length <7 mm, no vascular space invasion).[2] More recently, this philosophy has spread to International Federation of Gynaecologists and Obstetricians (FIGO) stages Ia1 and Ia2, both for squamous cell carcinomas and adenocarcinomas.[3] Rationale for this approach stems from the low incidence of pelvic lymph node metastases and the very low incidence of parametrial involvement with such small tumors. At exactly what incidence of node positivity lymphadenectomy should be recommended is an individualized question. For many gynecologic oncologists, this point is reached when the estimated incidence is greater than 1% to 3%. No data are available in the literature regarding fertility and pregnancy outcomes in patients with cervical cancer treated with cone biopsy alone (with or without lymphadenectomy). In any case, the performance of a pelvic lymphadenectomy should not substantially impair fertility, and one would not expect the fertility and obstetric outcomes to be different from those in the general population exposed to cone biopsies and pelvic surgery.

Chemotherapy followed by cone biopsy. At the 2000 International Gynecologic Cancer Society (IGCS) meeting in Buenos Aires, the Italian group of Ospedale San Gerardo from Monza presented data on 12 patients treated between 1996 and 1999 with neoadjuvant chemotherapy, followed in cases of complete clinical response by cone biopsy.[4] The chemotherapy regimen included cisplatin 75 mg/m[2], paclitaxel 175 mg/m[2], epirubicin 90 mg/m[2], and ifosfamide 5 gm/m[2], administered every 3 weeks for three courses. Of 12 patients (9 with lesions of 1 to 2 cm, 3 with lesions of 2.1 to 3 cm), 9 responded, but 1 requested radical therapy. Of the 8 patients submitted to cone biopsy alone, all had confirmed pathologic responses (no residual or minimal residual disease with clear margins). No recurrences were observed after a median of 22 months. Two pregnancies, both resulting in full-term infants, occurred during the follow-up period. Although these data appear very intriguing, the approach must be considered experimental given the low numbers of patients treated and the absence of long-term outcome data.

Cone biopsy followed by intracavitary radiation. In 1996, we reported on a series of three patients with small cervical cancers treated by cone biopsy, laparoscopic pelvic lymphadenectomy, and ovarian transposition.[5] All three patients had negative pelvic lymph nodes and were treated postoperatively with intracavitary radiation therapy. Two patients retained ovarian function, and the third became menopausal after both ovaries slipped back into the pelvis. One patient became pregnant after IVF but aborted during the middle trimester.

In 1998, Morice and colleagues reported on 27 patients with clear cell adenocarcinoma (26 cancers of the cervix, 1 cancer of the vagina) managed between 1974 and 1994 with pelvic lymphadenectomy (all negative), ovarian transposition, and brachytherapy at the Institut Gustave Roussy in Villejuif. The 5-year survival rate was 100% for stage I (10 patients) and 96% for stage II (16 patients). Five pregnancies have occurred, but only one (in the patient with vaginal cancer) resulted in a full-term live birth.

This method is intriguing and has proved to be efficacious in treating cervical cancers and retaining fertility. However, because of the requirements for either IVF or reversal of the transposition for conception to occur and the deleterious effects of radiation therapy on the endometrium and myometrium, we (and others) have abandoned this method of fertility preservation in favor of radical trachelectomy.

Radical trachelectomy. In the mid 1980s, Dargent[7] pioneered the concept and technical aspects of removing just the cervix and its parametrial attachments along with pelvic lymph nodes in patients wishing preservation of fertility. Since that time, a number of other investigators have perfected his work, redefined appropriate patient selection, and reported results.[8-10] The procedure most commonly entails a laparoscopic pelvic lymphadenectomy, followed by a vaginal radical trachelectomy. The theoretical data supporting the procedure include the fact that cervical cancer tends to spread laterally from the cervix (hence the rationale for removal of the contiguous parametrium and vagina, as performed in radical hysterectomy), and it rarely tends to spread superiorly into the uterus in small stage IB cervical cancers. Its spread for the most part tends to be contiguous, rather than discontiguous.

The surgical procedure entails a laparoscopic lymphadenectomy; incision of a vaginal cuff; dissection of the paravesical, rectovaginal, and vesicovaginal spaces; the cardinal and uterosacral ligaments are divided usually in their mid portion; identification of the ureter in the uterovesical ligament, enabling transection of the uterovesical ligament distal to the ureter; ligation of the vaginal branch of the uterine artery; and transection of the cervix at its junction with the uterine isthmus (Figs. 58-1 and 58-2). To prevent cervical

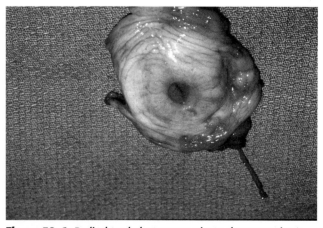

Figure 58–1. Radical trachelectomy specimen demonstrating vaginal cuff resection.

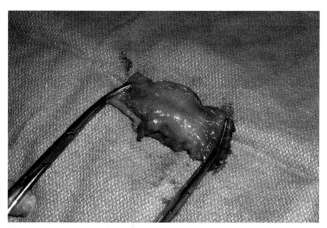

Figure 58–2. Radical trachelectomy specimen demonstrating parametrial resection.

incompetence, a Mersilene (Shirodkar) suture is placed around the lower uterine segment, and the vaginal cuff is sutured to the most lateral portions of the lower uterine segment or "neocervix" while the Mersilene suture is buried (Fig. 58-3). An ideal feature of this procedure is that it can be performed in patients that are pregnant (first trimester).

However, because most gynecologic oncologists are uncomfortable with radical vaginal surgery, some investigators have reported abdominal radical trachelectomies, analogous to abdominal radical hysterectomy.[11]

A comprehensive review of this procedure and literature has recently been published.[12] This summary of the world's four largest series reveals a pooled recurrence rate of 3% among 247 patients reported to have undergone the procedure. Whether some of these patients would have avoided a recurrence had they undergone a radical hysterectomy is unknown. To date, there have been no isolated recurrences reported in the remaining uterus. The recurrence-free survival rate at 36 months in our patients is 96% (Fig. 58-4).

The pooled data from the four series reveal that 92 women have attempted conception after the procedure.[12] A total of 102 pregnancies have resulted (several patients have had more than 1 pregnancy), and

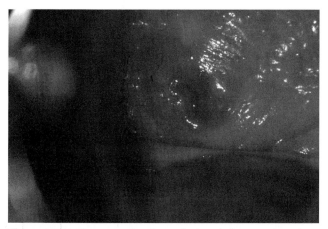

Figure 58–3. Three months after radical trachelectomy. See also Color Figure 58–3.

there have been 65 live births (not including twins). In our center, by 36 months, approximately 55% of patients attempting to conceive have been successful (Fig. 58-5). The majority of pregnancies have gone on to delivery by caesarean section after 34 weeks of gestation; however, we, like the others, found that these pregnancies have a high rate of preterm, premature rupture of the membranes. In our series, 6 of 18 pregnancies that went beyond 15 weeks ended before 36 weeks (2 of these were twin pregnancies). Shepherd[10] found that seven of nine live births in his series were preterm. Dargent[7] believed that these findings may be related to ascending chorioamnionitis resulting from an inadequate mucous plug and began surgically closing the cervix at 14 weeks' gestation. Whether such a maneuver reduces the incidence of preterm rupture of membranes or labor has not yet been elucidated.

It is clear that this surgical procedure is safe and feasible to perform in women with small cervical carcinomas who desire preservation of fertility. Pregnancies resulting in healthy babies are a proven realistic outcome for the majority. It is reassuring that the recurrence rate to date in the four largest series does not appear to be grossly different from that anticipated after radical hysterectomy.

Ovarian Transposition

The most common indication for ovarian transposition is anticipation of definitive radical radiotherapy, or of postoperative adjuvant radiation therapy in a cervical cancer patient undergoing surgery. However, multiple studies have demonstrated that caution must be exercised in cases of advanced cervical cancer, particularly nonsquamous cancer, lest ovarian metastases be transposed.[13-16] The incidence of this phenomenon is difficult to identify but has been estimated to be at least 2%.

Ovarian transposition can commonly be performed via laparoscopy, depending on the patient's surgical requirements and the surgeon's expertise. In 1996, we reported on a series of patients with small cervical cancers treated with cone biopsy, laparoscopic pelvic lymphadenectomy, ovarian transposition, and brachytherapy alone.[5] Recent advances have now made this an outpatient procedure. However, factors to consider before performing an ovarian transposition are as follows: the age of the patient; dose, fractionation, and fields of pelvic irradiation; and the use of systemic chemotherapy.[17] Multiple studies have demonstrated that ovarian tolerance to radiation therapy (and chemotherapy) is highest in young girls and lowest in women close to menopause (Fig. 58-6). Similarly, the location of the transposed ovaries will determine the dose of radiation received by each ovary. In most gynecologic reports, the ovaries have been transposed to the pelvic side walls, a site well within a standard postoperative pelvic irradiation field. It therefore is incumbent on the operator to place the ovaries as far as feasible from the border of an irradiation field, to

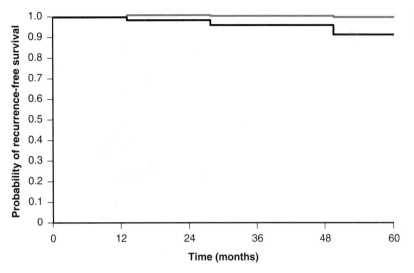

Figure 58-4. Probability of recurrence-free survival after radical trachelectomy.

minimize scatter radiation. In our center, this typically involves placing the ovaries just at the inferior pole of each kidney (Fig. 58-7). Such distances are easily feasible, although care must be taken to avoid torsion of the vascular pedicle and hernia formation under the pedicle, and to achieve an intraperitoneal location for the ovary, to prevent retroperitoneal ovulation and cyst formation.[18]

The largest study with long-term follow-up of hormonal function of transposed ovaries was reported by Buekers and associates.[19] Between 1982 and 1989, 102 patients underwent radical surgery, which included an ovarian transposition in 80 patients. After a mean follow-up period of 87 months for premenopausal women, the following results were observed: the average age at menopause for the 13 patients who received no radiation and no transposition was 50.6 years; 98% of those receiving transposition without radiation retained ovarian function for a mean of 126 months, with menopause occurring at a mean of 45.8 years; and when transposition and radiation therapy were combined, only 41% of patients retained ovarian function for a mean of 43 months, with a mean age at menopause of 36.6 years. The authors' conclusions were that radical hysterectomy with ovarian preservation (without transposition) did not significantly reduce the age at menopause, whereas the addition of ovarian transposition reduced ovarian function appreciably, and the addition of radiation therapy after transposition dramatically shortened the duration of ovarian function.

Morice and coworkers[20] reported on 107 patients treated with ovarian transposition at radical hysterectomy. Without long-term follow-up, ovarian function persisted in 100%, 90%, and 60% of patients treated by surgery only, surgery plus postoperative vaginal brachytherapy, and surgery plus postoperative external radiation therapy, respectively. Similar data were reported from Indiana, where, among patients undergoing ovarian transposition at radical hysterectomy, 97% of those receiving no adjuvant radiation therapy and 50% of those receiving postoperative radiation therapy experienced menopause.[21]

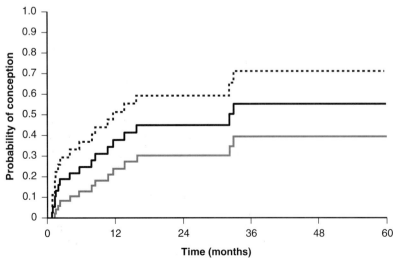

Figure 58-5. Actuarial conception after radical trachelectomy. Upper and lower lines outline the 95% confidence interval.

patient became menopausal within 9 months, and in the latter study no long-term follow-up was given.

Although these data may seem very discouraging, most investigators still consider cryopreservation of ovarian tissue to be a useful endeavor. Because the tissue may not be required for many years, it is quite likely that technologic advances in the future will substantially improve the success rate of regaining ovarian function.

ENDOMETRIAL CANCER

Can fertility be preserved in patients with endometrial cancer? The majority of endometrial cancers occur in perimenopausal and postmenopausal women. However, 5% of endometrial cancers occur in women younger than 40 years of age. Many of these women experience years of anovulation, secondary to either obesity or polycystic ovarian syndrome. Their tumors tend to be well-differentiated endometrioid adenocarcinomas. For the majority of grade 1 tumors, little or no myometrial invasion is present at diagnosis. Cure rates associated with this scenario are greater than 95%.[33] However, given the nonsurgical method of proposed management and concerns listed later in this chapter with respect to the response or regression rate in patients with myometrial invasion, most authors recommend some type of assessment—either transvaginal sonography or magnetic resonance imaging.

Data from several uncontrolled studies have demonstrated regression rates with progesterone therapy approximating 60% (Table 58-1), depending on the grade of tumor.[34-38] The most common formulation of progesterone used has been medroxyprogesterone acetate in the dose range of 300 to 600 mg/day. Furthermore, the literature has many case reports of women that have gone on to achieve pregnancies, usually requiring ovulation induction.[36,39] In fact, there have been case reports of intrauterine pregnancy with concomitant endometrial cancer.[40-42] Importantly, these women need to stay on some form of therapy for life. Cessation of therapy after tumor regression is commonly followed by recurrence of the tumor, given each patient's inherent medical condition associated with the endometrial cancer. Most authors advocate frequent hysteroscopy or endometrial sampling, or both, to confirm response/regression.

Concern must be given to the theoretical possibility that progression of disease may occur while conservative medical management is attempted. Although this is probably an uncommon scenario, it is not inconceivable that a proportion of the 40% of tumors that do not respond will progress. Furthermore, because some of these patients may be harboring subclinical metastases to ovaries or lymph nodes, progression and further metastases may occur. Several authors have documented significant rates (approximating 30%) of ovarian metastases or synchronous primaries in these cohorts.[37] Interestingly, those patients who went on to hysterectomy after progesterone therapy failed demonstrated a high incidence of myometrial invasion.[36] Whether this reflects the biology of the individual tumors or a relative resistance to hormonal management is not clear. However, given this concern and the fact that metastases to lymph nodes and recurrences increase with increasing myometrial invasion, prudence would suggest that patients with grade 2 or 3 tumors, and those with documented myometrial invasion on noninvasive testing, are not appropriate candidates for medical management. As an example, we treated a patient who had a well-differentiated endometrial cancer with progesterone therapy, eradicating the endometrial pathology. Hysterectomy 18 months later after failed attempts to become pregnant revealed viable tumor in the myometrium, with no tumor in the endometrium (unpublished data). Unresolved questions regarding medical management of endometrial cancer are the ideal regimen of therapy, the need for continued therapy after the malignancy is reversed, and whether hysterectomy should be performed on completion of childbearing.

OVARIAN CANCER

Epithelial Ovarian Cancer

Can fertility be preserved in patients with epithelial ovarian cancer? The vast majority (80% to 90%) of epithelial ovarian cancers occur in women who are past childbearing.[43] In many patients, an infertility workup is what leads to the diagnosis.[43,44] Multiple studies have demonstrated stage, grade, and borderline (as opposed to frankly invasive) status as some of the most important prognostic factors in epithelial ovarian cancer. Another important factor is the histology, which has a

| **Table 58-1.** Progesterone as Primary Therapy for Endometrial Cancer

Study	Grade 1		Grade 2	
	No.	% Regression	No.	% Regression
Randall and Kurman[37]	12	75		
Imai et al.[35]	12	58	2	50
Sardi et al.[34]	3	100	1	0
Kim et al.[38]	7	57		
Total	34	76	3	33

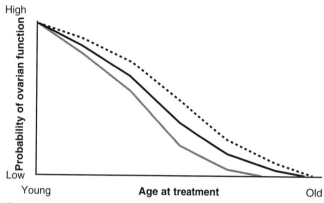

Figure 58–6. Schematic representation of the additive relationship of chemotherapy and radiation and the likelihood of menopause with respect to age at treatment. From Ribosome Communications.

Although the studies cited address hormonal function, pregnancies have been achieved in many patients. Morice and colleagues[6] reported on 18 pregnancies in 12 patients treated for cervical/vaginal cancers, ovarian germ cell tumors, and a pelvic soft tissue sarcoma. All patients received external pelvic radiation or brachytherapy. We reported one pregnancy that required IVF and aborted in the middle trimester due to uterine factors (previous radiation therapy).[5]

Ovarian autotransplantation and cryopreservation.
If the ovaries are to be removed or rendered menopausal by therapy, what are the options to preserve their function? Many options are available for patients who are about to lose ovarian function due to surgery, chemotherapy, or radiation therapy. The most appropriate choice varies with each patient's situation. The patient's age, primary diagnosis, types of planned therapy, urgency of starting therapy,

presence of a partner, and likelihood of malignancy present in the ovary are all influential factors. In some cases, simple methods such as ovarian transposition or GnRH agonists are indicated; in others, ovarian stimulation and retrieval of oocytes before definitive therapy is most appropriate. Advances in reproductive technology have made possible cryopreservation not only of embryos but also of mature oocytes. Although the success rates for both processes are low (implantation rates are approximately 5%), the former is more often successful than the latter.[22] However, because not all patients have identified an appropriate "partner" for IVF, cryopreservation of mature oocytes has been performed for almost as long.[23,24] The difficulty with this plan of management is that a minimum of 1 or 2 months is required before definitive therapy for ovarian stimulation, oocyte maturation, and surgical harvesting before cryopreservation are performed.

Cryopreservation of ovarian tissue is very appealing because of the minimum amount of time and preparation required. Although the first pregnancy associated with cryopreservation of ovarian tissue was in a mouse in 1960, and in 1994 pregnancy in a sheep was achieved, no human pregnancies have yet been reported.[25,26] With modern techniques, at best 70% of the primordial follicles survive the freeze-thaw process.[27] However, these primordial follicles require maturation before fertilization. The three mechanisms to carry out maturation are autografting of cryopreserved ovarian tissue back into the patient (after therapy has been completed), in vitro follicular maturation, and xenografting using animals without functioning immune systems, such as nude mice or severe combined immunodeficiency (SCID) mice.

Autotransplantation of fresh and cryopreserved ovaries has been successfully performed in animals for many years.[28,29] Ovarian tissue has been autotransplanted to its natural location (orthotopic) via microvascular anastomosis and to other areas (heterotopic) at intraperitoneal or subcutaneous sites. However, the latter obviously results in a need for intervention (e.g., IVF) for pregnancy to occur. Ovarian autotransplantation causes some concern with respect to recurrence in cases of malignancy in which the ovary is at risk for metastases or is the primary tumor site. Although in vitro follicular maturation is appealing, particularly if malignancy in the cryopreserved ovary is a concern, it is technically difficult and at present is unsuccessful in humans. Xenografting raises ethical concerns and has not to date been successful.

Callejo and associates[30] performed heterotopic autotransplantation (subcutaneous and intramuscular) in four women before chemotherapy or radiation therapy for malignant disease. Cryopreserved ovarian autografts were used in one patient and fresh tissue in the other three. Despite reestablishment of ovarian function in all cases, premature ovarian failure developed within a short period in all four women. Radford and Oktay[32] and their colleagues described orthotopic and heterotopic autotransplantation of ovarian tissue in oncology patients. In the former study the

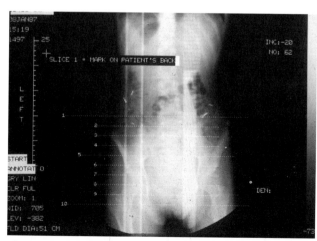

Figure 58–7. Radiograph demonstrating surgical clips (marking ovarian locations) at inferior poles of each kidney (right higher than left).

direct correlation with the incidence of bilateral ovarian involvement. Mucinous tumors are uncommonly bilateral (approximately 5% to 15%), in contrast to serous or endometrioid tumors (approximately 30% to 60%).[45] Another important issue for patients wishing to conceive after a diagnosis of an epithelial ovarian cancer is the use of ovulation-inducing drugs, which have been associated with ovarian cancer.[46]

Approximately 60% of borderline tumors are diagnosed in stage I.[47] In contrast to invasive tumors, the prognosis is excellent in stage I (>95%, 5-year survival rate), and still very good in advanced stages (approximately 90%). However, the optimal management of advanced borderline tumors has not been elucidated.

For early-stage tumors, cystectomy alone may suffice as adequate therapy. Although most case series have indicated higher recurrence rates in patients treated with cystectomy (36%) compared with unilateral adnexectomy (15%) or bilateral adnexectomy (6%), survival rates have not been demonstrated to be different.[44,48-50] It appears that when borderline tumors recur, either in the same ovary (after cystectomy alone) or in the contralateral remaining ovary, they do so as a borderline tumor (not invasive). Therefore, the studies cited have all documented excellent survival rates after re-excision for recurrent borderline tumors in conservatively managed cases.

Although chemotherapy in advanced-stage borderline tumors has not been demonstrated to be efficacious, various researchers have used the presence of invasive implants in advanced borderline tumors as a indicator for postoperative chemotherapy, because those patients with invasive implants have very high rates of recurrence and death (45% and 37%, respectively), compared with patients with noninvasive implants (11% and 6%, respectively).[51]

Fertility after conservative management for borderline tumors has been reported in patients with stage I through III disease. Gotlieb and associates[44] documented 22 pregnancies in 15 patients, Morice and coworkers[48] observed 17 pregnancies in 14 patients (4 infertile), and Duska and colleagues[43] observed 14 pregnancies in 10 patients (4 infertile). Despite the concerns regarding ovulation-inducing drugs and ovarian cancer, they have been used in patients who wished to conceive after such a diagnosis, with no reported recurrences.[43,48,52,53]

In invasive ovarian cancer, excellent survival after surgical management alone has been demonstrated for stage Ia, grade 1 tumors (>95%).[54] As the tumor grade increases, the probability of recurrence increases, even for those patients with surgically documented stage I disease. Although no study has demonstrated a survival advantage with adjuvant chemotherapy after complete surgical staging, most clinicians continue to recommend it for grade 3 tumors, and commonly for grade 2 as well. Equally challenging is the stage II, grade 1 tumor (unilateral adnexal involvement only). Although data on outcomes after preservation of one ovary and postoperative chemotherapy are lacking, these tumors are of concern given the grave prognosis associated with advanced-stage ovarian cancer and

the theoretical issue of the ovary as a sanctuary site from chemotherapy. Although bivalving and biopsy of the contralateral, normal-appearing ovary has been proposed, it is not foolproof in identifying microscopic disease. One study demonstrated a 4% recurrence rate in the remaining ovary.[55] Furthermore, this procedure theoretically may further predispose patients to fertility problems, such as adhesions.[56]

Fertility has been demonstrated in women treated conservatively. Duska and colleagues[43] reported on five patients with stage I disease treated conservatively who attempted to conceive. Three patients were able to get pregnant (one ectopic pregnancy, two full-term deliveries). An important unresolved question is whether the in situ ovary should be removed after childbearing is complete. Removal would seem inherently unwarranted if many years have transpired since the original diagnosis without any evidence of recurrence, but there are no data to support any conclusion at this point.

Germ Cell Ovarian Cancer

Can fertility be preserved in patients with ovarian germ cell tumors?
Germ cell tumors in women, unlike those that occur in men, tend to affect children, adolescents, and young adults. Therefore, preservation of fertility (and hormonal function) is almost always an issue. With modern advances in the management of malignant germ cell tumors (most notably chemotherapy), the overall cure rate is approximately 85%, and even patients with advanced disease can anticipate cure rates greater than 60%.[57] The details concerning which patients should receive chemotherapy versus observation are beyond the scope of this chapter. It is well accepted that the mainstay of therapy for patients with germ cell tumors is chemotherapy. In contrast to epithelial tumors, there is no role for debulking. Furthermore, apart from dysgerminoma (approximately 15%), the incidence of bilateral ovarian involvement is less than 5%.[58] These latter two points are very important for fertility preservation, because there is little role for bilateral adnexectomy in germ cell tumors. Apart from dysgerminomas, a mass on the contralateral ovary is almost universally of another histology rather than being a metastasis or recurrence. Documented cases of bilateral ovarian dysgerminomas treated by biopsy and chemotherapy have been reported in the literature.[59]

An unresolved issue in treated patients is the long-term or late effects on ovarian function. Although studies have been published regarding treatment of Hodgkin's disease and leukemia,[60] no such data exist for modern chemotherapy for germ cell tumors.[60] It would appear from the experience in other tumor sites, mentioned previously, that the chemotherapeutic drugs used do shorten the lifespan of the ovary, and menopause occurs earlier than in the general population. Alkylating agents in particular impair ovarian function. Menstrual function continues during chemotherapy in approximately 33% to 70% of patients, and more than 90% resume menstrual function after completion of chemotherapy.[61,62] Because the prepubertal ovary is more resistant to the adverse effects of chemotherapy, clinicians have attempted to simulate that state of the ovary with oral contraceptives.[63] However, the efficacy of this approach remains questionable. Chapman and associates[63] noted that five of six patients treated with combination chemotherapy and the oral contraceptive pill for Hodgkin's disease had normal menses and serum gonadotrophins at completion of their study. Conversely, in a similar patient population, Whitehead and coworkers[64] found that seven of nine patients were oligomenorrheic. More recently, GnRH agonists have been used for this effect with encouraging results (see next section).

Multiple series have documented full-term pregnancies in a high proportion of women attempting to conceive, with no congenital malformations.[61,62,65,66] The incidence of infertility in the series mentioned does not appear to be significantly different from that in the general population.

USE OF GONADOTROPIN-RELEASING HORMONE AGONISTS BEFORE CHEMOTHERAPY

Can ovarian function be protected from chemotherapy?

The use of agents to prevent premature ovarian failure has been attempted for decades. Early studies, involving the use of oral contraceptive pills, demonstrated mixed results.[63,64] More recently, GnRH agonists have been used with demonstrated efficacy. Blumenfeld and colleagues[67] conducted a nonrandomized, prospective trial in 140 premenopausal women aged 15 to 40 years who were about to undergo chemotherapy. All but 3 of the surviving patients treated with GnRH resumed spontaneous ovulation and menses within 12 months, whereas 45% of the control group did likewise. Of the 45%, one third had temporarily increased levels of follicle-stimulating hormone, suggesting reversible ovarian damage.

A similar study by Pacheco and colleagues[68] demonstrated similar findings. This study was not randomized but involved three groups of patients who were scheduled to receive polychemotherapy. Among five premenarchal girls not given GnRH, all had spontaneous menarche between the ages of 12 and 17.9 years, followed by normal menstrual cycles. Twelve postmenarchal women given GnRH continued normal ovulatory cycles after chemotherapy, whereas four similar women not given GnRH developed hypergonadotropic hypoestrogenic amenorrhea.

Although the numbers of patients in both of these nonrandomized studies were small, the results are intriguing. Further studies, preferably larger and randomized, need to be done to confirm these results.

Another important question, in addition to resumption of ovulatory cycles, is whether these patients will experience a shortened ovulatory lifespan.

CONCLUSIONS

Quality of life has become a significant end point in many therapies for malignancies. No longer are we concerned only with length of life. Particularly in young women with highly curable cancers, quality of life, including reproductive capacity, is very important. There has been massive growth in our knowledge of gynecologic cancers, prognostic factors, and treatment strategies over the past three decades. As advances in these areas have occurred, so have those in reproductive technology. Only three decades ago, the first successful pregnancy from IVF was announced. Such advances, with their resultant consequences and paradigm shifts, require fresh views and reevaluation of our current methods of management of gynecologic malignancies.

References

1. Browde S, Friedman M, Nissenbaum M: Pregnancy after radiation therapy for carcinoma of the cervix. Eur J Gynaecol Oncol 1986;7:63-68.
2. Morris M: Management of stage IA cervical carcinoma. J Natl Cancer Inst Monogr 1996;21:47-52.
3. Schorge JO, Lee KR, Sheets EE: Prospective management of stage IA(1) cervical adenocarcinoma by conization alone to preserve fertility: a preliminary report. Gynecol Oncol 2000;78:217-220.
4. Dargent D: Fertility preserving management of early stage cancer of the cervix. In 8th Biennial Meeting of the International Gynecologic Cancer Society, 2000. Eds. DiPaola G, Sasdi J, Buenos Aires, Monduzzi Editore; 23-30.
5. Covens AL, van der Putten HW, Fyles AW, et al: Laparoscopic ovarian transposition. Eur J Gynaecol Oncol 1996;17:177-182.
6. Morice P, Thiam-Ba R, Castaigne D, et al: Fertility results after ovarian transposition for pelvic malignancies treated by external irradiation or brachytherapy. Hum Reprod 1998;13:660-663.
7. Dargent D, Brun JL, Roy M, et al: La trachélectomie élargie (T.E.): Une alternative à l'hystérectomie radicale dans le traitement des cancers infiltrants développés sur la face externe du col utérin. Journal Obstetrics et Gynecologie 1994;2:285-292.
8. Covens A, Shaw P, Murphy J, et al: Is radical trachelectomy a safe alternative to radical hysterectomy for patients with stage IA-B carcinoma of the cervix? Cancer 1999;86:2273-2279.
9. Roy M, Plante M: Pregnancies after radical vaginal trachelectomy for early-stage cervical cancer. Am J Obstet Gynecol 1998;179:1491-1496.
10. Shepherd JH, Crawford RA, Oram DH: Radical trachelectomy: A way to preserve fertility in the treatment of early cervical cancer. Br J Obstet Gynaecol 1998;105:912-916.
11. Rodriguez M, Guimares O, Rose PG: Radical abdominal trachelectomy and pelvic lymphadenectomy with uterine conservation and subsequent pregnancy in the treatment of early invasive cervical cancer. Am J Obstet Gynecol 2001;185:370-374.
12. Covens A: Preserving fertility in early cervical cancer with radical trachelectomy. Contemporary Obstetrics and Gynecology 2003;48:46-66.
13. Morice P, Haie-Meder C, Pautier P, et al: Ovarian metastasis on transposed ovary in patients treated for squamous cell carcinoma of the uterine cervix: Report of two cases and surgical implications. Gynecol Oncol 2001;83:605-607.

14. Reisinger SA, Palazzo JP, Talerman A, et al: Stage IB glassy cell carcinoma of the cervix diagnosed during pregnancy and recurring in a transposed ovary. Gynecol Oncol 1991;42:86-90.

15. Yamamoto R, Okamoto K, Yukiharu T, et al: A study of risk factors for ovarian metastases in stage Ib-IIIb cervical carcinoma and analysis of ovarian function after a transposition. Gynecol Oncol 2001;82:312-316.

16. Shigematsu T, Ohishi Y, Fujita T, et al: Metastatic carcinoma in a transposed ovary after radical hysterectomy for a stage 1B cervical adenosquamous cell carcinoma: Case report. Eur J Gynaecol Oncol 2000;21:383-386.

17. Covens A: Methods of protecting ovaries from radiation therapy. Journal of the Society of Obstetrians and Gynecologists of Canada 1995;17:975-983.

18. Belinson JL, Doherty M, McDay JB: A new technique for ovarian transposition. Surg Gynecol Obstet 1984;159:157-160.

19. Buekers TE, Anderson B, Sorosky JI, Buller RE: Ovarian function after surgical treatment for cervical cancer. Gynecol Oncol 2001; 80:85-88.

20. Morice P, Juncker L, Rey A, et al. Ovarian transposition for patients with cervical carcinoma treated by radiosurgical combination. Fertil Steril 2000;74:743-748.

21. Feeney DD, Moore DH, Look KY, et al: The fate of the ovaries after radical hysterectomy and ovarian transposition. Gynecol Oncol 1995;56:3-7.

22. Machtinger R, Dor J, Levron J, Mashiach S: The effect of prolonged cryopreservation on embryo survival. Gynecol Endocrinol 2002;16:293-298.

23. Chen C: Pregnancy after human oocyte cryopreservation. Lancet 1986;1:884-886.

24. Trounson A, Mohr L: Human pregnancy following cryopreservation, thawing and transfer of an eight-cell embryo. Nature 1983;305:707-709.

25. Parrott DMV: The fertility of mice with orthotopic ovarian graft derived from frozen tissue. J Reprod Fertil 1960;1:230-241.

26. Gosden RG, Baird DT, Wade JC, Webb R: Restoration of fertility to oophorectomized sheep by ovarian autografts stored at −196 degrees C. Hum Reprod 1994;9:597-603.

27. Newton H, Aubard Y, Rutherford A, et al: Low temperature storage and grafting of human ovarian tissue. Hum Reprod 1996;11:1487-1491.

28. Jeremias E, Bedaiwy MA, Gurunluoglu R, et al: Heterotopic autotransplantation of the ovary with microvascular anastomosis: A novel surgical technique. Fertil Steril 2002;77:1278-1282.

29. Salle B, Demirci B, Franck M, et al: Normal pregnancies and live births after autograft of frozen-thawed hemi-ovaries into ewes. Fertil Steril 2002;77:403-408.

30. Callejo J, Vilaseca S, Ordi J, et al: Heterotopic ovarian transplantation without vascular pedicle in syngeneic Lewis rats: Long-term evaluation of effects on ovarian structure and function. Fertil Steril 2002;77:396-402.

31. Radford JA, Lieberman BA, Brison DR, et al: Orthotopic reimplantation of cryopreserved ovarian cortical strips after high-dose chemotherapy for Hodgkin's lymphoma. Lancet 2001;357: 1172-1175.

32. Oktay K, Economos K, Kan M, et al: Endocrine function and oocyte retrieval after autologous transplantation of ovarian cortical strips to the forearm. JAMA 2001;286:1490-1493.

33. Irvin WP, Rice LW, Berkowitz RS: Advances in the management of endometrial adenocarcinoma: A review. J Reprod Med 2002; 47:173-189.

34. Sardi J, Anchezar Henry JP, Paniceres G, et al: Primary hormonal treatment for early endometrial carcinoma. Eur J Gynaecol Oncol 1998;19:565-568.

35. Imai M, Jobo T, Sato R, et al: Medroxyprogesterone acetate therapy for patients with adenocarcinoma of the endometrium who wish to preserve the uterus-usefulness and limitations. Eur J Gynaecol Oncol 2001;22:217-220.

36. Mitsushita J, Toki T, Kato K, et al: Endometrial carcinoma remaining after term pregnancy following conservative treatment with medroxyprogesterone acetate. Gynecol Oncol 2000; 79:129-132.

37. Randall TC, Kurman RJ: Progestin treatment of atypical hyperplasia and well-differentiated carcinoma of the endometrium in women under age 40. Obstet Gynecol 1997;90:434-440.

38. Kim YB, Holschneider CH, Ghosh K, et al: Progestin alone as primary treatment of endometrial carcinoma in premenopausal women: Report of seven cases and review of the literature. Cancer 1997;79:320-327.

39. Schammel DP, Mittal KR, Kaplan K, et al: Endometrial adenocarcinoma associated with intrauterine pregnancy: A report of five cases and a review of the literature. Int J Gynecol Pathol 1998;17:327-335.

40. Ayhan A, Gunalp S, Karaer C, et al: Endometrial adenocarcinoma in pregnancy. Gynecol Oncol 1999;75:298-299.

41. Schammel DP: Endometrial adenocarcinoma associated with intrauterine pregnancy. Gynecol Oncol 1998;70:153.

42. Schneller JA, Nicastri AD: Intrauterine pregnancy coincident with endometrial carcinoma: A case study and review of the literature. Gynecol Oncol 1994;54:87-90.

43. Duska LR, Chang YC, Flynn CE, et al: Epithelial ovarian carcinoma in the reproductive age group. Cancer 1999;85:2623-2629.

44. Gotlieb WH, Flikker S, Davidson B, et al: Borderline tumors of the ovary: fertility treatment, conservative management, and pregnancy outcome. Cancer 1998;82:141-146.

45. Czernobilsky B: Common epithelial tumors of the ovary. In Kurman RJ (ed): Blaustein's Pathology of the Female Genital Tract. New York, Springer-Verlag, 1987, pp 560-606.

46. Harris R, Whittemore A, Itnyre J: Characteristics relating to ovarian cancer risk: Collaborative analysis of 12 US case-control studies. III. Epithelial tumors of low malignant potential in white women. Am J Epidemiol 1992;136:1204-1211.

47. Heintz AP, Odicino F, Maisonneuve P, et al: Carcinoma of the Ovary. J Epidemiol Biostat 2001;6:107-138.

48. Morice P, Camatte S, El Hassan J, et al: Clinical outcomes and fertility after conservative treatment of ovarian borderline tumors. Fertil Steril 2001;75:92-96.

49. Tazelaar H, Bostwick D, Ballon S: Conservative treatment of borderline ovarian tumors. Obstet Gynecol 1985;66:417-421.

50. Lim-Tan S, Cjigas H, Scully R: Ovarian cystectomy for serous borderline tumors: A follow-up of 35 cases. Obstet Gynecol 1988;72:775-780.

51. Gershenson DM: Contemporary treatment of borderline ovarian tumors. Cancer Invest 1999;17:206-210.

52. Nijman H, Burger CW, Baak JP, et al: Borderline malignancy of the ovary and controlled hyperstimulation: A report of 2 cases. Eur J Cancer 1992;28A:1971-1972.

53. Mantzavinos T, Kanakas N, Genatas C, et al: Five years follow-up in two patients with borderline tumors of the ovary hyperstimulated by gonadotrophin therapy for in-vitro fertilization. Hum Reprod 1994;9:2032-2033.

54. Coukos G, Rubin SC: Early ovarian cancer. Curr Treat Options Oncol 2000;1:129-137.

55. Zanetta G, Chiari S, Rota S, et al: Conservative surgery for stage I ovarian carcinoma in women of childbearing age. Br J Obstet Gynaecol 1997;104:1030-1035.

56. McHale MT, DiSaia PJ: Fertility-sparing treatment of patients with ovarian cancer. Compr Ther 1999;25:144-150.

57. Rustin GJ: Managing malignant ovarian germ cell tumors. Br Med J 1987;295:869-870.

58. DiSaia PJ, Creasman WT: Germ cell, stromal, and other ovarian tumors. In DiSaia PJ, Creasman WT (eds): Clinical Gynecologic Oncology. St. Louis, Mosby, 1997, pp 351-374.

59. Gershenson DM: Management of early ovarian cancer: Germ cell and sex cord-stromal tumors. Gynecol Oncol 1994;55:S62-S72.

60. Horning SJ, Hoppe RT, Kaplan HS, Rosenberg SA: Female reproductive potential after treatment for Hodgkin's disease. N Engl J Med 1981;304:1377-1382.

61. Low JJ, Perrin LC, Crandon AJ, Hacker NF: Conservative surgery to preserve ovarian function in patients with malignant ovarian germ cell tumors: A review of 74 cases. Cancer 2000;89:391-398.

62. Brewer M, Gershenson DM, Herzog CE, et al: Outcome and reproductive function after chemotherapy for ovarian dysgerminoma. J Clin Oncol 1999;17:2670-2675.

63. Chapman RM, Sutcliffe SB, Malpas JS: Cytotoxic-induced ovarian failure in Hodgkin's disease. II. Effects on sexual function. JAMA 1979;242:1882-1884.

64. Whitehead E, Shalet SM, Blackledge G, et al: The effect of combination chemotherapy on ovarian function in women treated for Hodgkin's disease. Cancer 1983;52:988-993.

65. Bakri YN, Ezzat A, Akhtar, Dohami, Zahrani: Malignant germ cell tumors of the ovary: Pregnancy considerations. Eur J Obstet Gynecol Reprod Biol 2000;90:87-91.
66. Perrin LD, Low J, Nicklin JL, et al: Fertility and ovarian function after conservative surgery for germ cell tumors of the ovary. Aust N Z J Obstet Gynaecol 1999;39:243-245.
67. Blumenfeld Z, Dann E, Avivi I, et al: Fertility after treatment for Hodgkin's disease. Ann Oncol 2002;13(Suppl 1):138-147.
68. Pereyra Pacheco B, Mendez Ribas JM, Milone G, et al: Use of GnRH analogs for functional protection of the ovary and preservation of fertility during cancer treatment in adolescents: A preliminary report. Gynecol Oncol 2001;81:391-397.

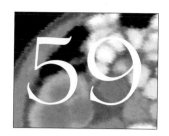

QUALITY OF LIFE IN THE GYNECOLOGIC CANCER PATIENT

Diane C. Bodurka,   Charlotte C. Sun,   and   Karen M. Basen-Engquist

---

 MAJOR CONTROVERSIES

- **Why should quality of life be studied in women with gynecologic cancers?**
- **What do patients expect from palliative chemotherapy?**
- **What is the role of palliative surgery in the treatment of gynecologic cancers?**
- **How do end-of-life issues affect the care of women with gynecologic cancers?**
- **How does the cancer diagnosis affect patients?**
- **Why are patient preferences important to study?**

Why should quality of life be studied in women with gynecologic cancers?

The consideration of quality of life (QOL) information in clinical decision-making is critical to the care of women with gynecologic cancer. QOL is a difficult concept to define. It can mean different things to different people at the same point in time. It can also mean different things to the same person at different points in time. Health care providers to women with gynecologic malignancies must consider the tradeoffs patients make regarding quality versus quantity of life. Issues that might be important to the provider may not be significant to the patient.

QOL is generally recognized as a subjective, multidimensional concept[1] that places emphasis on the subjective experience of various aspects of one's life, including factors such as the safety of the environment, access to health care and health services, and current social status.[2] The phrase QOL is used in a variety of fields; however, the term *health-related quality of life* is often used to describe QOL as it relates to diseases or their treatment. This concept is generally understood to represent an individual's appraisal of his or her QOL as it is affected by a health condition, compared with some internal standard. This concept of health-related QOL differs from the general concept of QOL in that it usually encompasses the psychological, physical, and social functioning of patients but excludes perceptions of environment, housing, or other external dimensions.

A central question in oncology is whether a treatment provides sufficient benefit to compensate for the QOL limitations it brings about. Of course, treatment can improve QOL, as when a treatment successfully eliminates cancer in a patient with a significant symptom or tumor burden. Because of toxicity, however, therapies used to treat cancer may also have a negative effect on QOL, as when sexual functioning is impaired by surgery or radiation therapy,[3-5] or chemotherapy results in extreme fatigue or neuropathy that does not remit after therapy is discontinued.[6] It is in these latter situations that QOL information is critical, especially if the treatment offers limited benefit in terms of increased survival.[7] This chapter discusses in depth three areas of gynecologic oncology in which QOL information should play an important role in clinical decision-making: palliative chemotherapy, palliative surgery, and end-of-life care. Psychosocial effects of the cancer diagnosis and patient preferences for treatment outcomes are also addressed, because these topics are often intertwined with QOL issues.

Two approaches are used to assess QOL outcomes in oncology. The first is a formal measurement of the strength of patients' preferences for a specific treatment or outcome of treatment.[8] Preference (utility) assessment quantitatively measures how patients value QOL in a given state of health. Generally, preferences are measured in three ways.[9] The visual analog scale requires patients to rate a health state on a scale from 0 to 100 (0 = death; 100 = perfect health). The time tradeoff method asks patients to evaluate how much time in a perfect state of health they consider to be equivalent to a longer time in a suboptimal state of health. The standard gamble assesses the preference for a compromised health state by asking patients how much uncertainty they are willing to accept to improve it. All preference scores are converted to a 0-to-1 scale (0 = least preferred; 1 = most preferred). These methods are discussed in greater detail later.

Preference assessments have been demonstrated to be both feasible and well accepted by patients with gynecologic cancers.[10,11] Preference scores are used in clinical decision analysis models to calculate the number of quality-adjusted life years (QALYs) associated with a treatment strategy. The QALY (defined as the preference score multiplied by length of life for a given health state) is a single number that reflects both quantity and QOL. Therefore, quality-adjusted survival outcomes for different treatment strategies can be compared. The strategy that yields the greatest quality-adjusted life expectancy is preferred.

In contrast to the measurement of patient preferences, the psychometric approach to measuring QOL involves the use of multiple-item questionnaires. Rather than evaluating health states and time, respondents rate various aspects of their current QOL using a quantitative scale.

Selecting an appropriate QOL measurement tool is critical to obtaining interpretable QOL data. Attention should be paid to the questionnaire's psychometric characteristics, reliability, and validity. It is also important to ascertain whether the tool measures areas of QOL that are important to patients and whether it measures areas of QOL that are expected to be affected by treatment, if the purpose of measuring QOL is to evaluate a treatment.

Reliability and validity of QOL questionnaires are crucial to interpretation of the data they generate. *Reliability* refers to the lack of measurement error in the questionnaire.[12] Types of reliability often reported for QOL questionnaires include internal consistency (indicates whether the questionnaire items measure the same concept) and test-retest reliability (indicates whether the test scores are stable over time).[13] Theoretically, reliability coefficients can range from 0 (the measure consists of error only) to 1.0 (no error exists in the measure).[14] In general, classification guidelines for reliability are as follows: if the correlation is higher than 0.7, it is considered to have adequate reliability; whereas if the correlation is 0.6 or less, it is considered marginal. Correlations of 0.8 or higher are excellent.[15]

Validity is the degree to which an instrument's scores reflect what is intended to be measured. Procedures for determining test validity usually compare scores on a measure with other related, externally observable facts about the construct being measured.[12] The validity of a measure cannot be considered an absolute; rather, it is relative to a particular situation or use. Questionnaires that have been found to be valid for a particular use in a specific population are not necessarily valid for other uses among other groups. For example, a QOL questionnaire that has been shown to be sensitive to changes in health status over time among stroke patients is not necessarily valid for a clinical trial of salvage chemotherapy in women with cervical cancer. However, as evidence of the validity of an instrument accumulates from multiple studies in a range of populations, one can be more confident that extension of its use to a different population or situation will be valid.

Evidence for validity is classified in three principal categories: content, criterion, and construct validity.[12] Content validity pertains to the issue of whether the scale items are sampled from the domain the instrument intends to measure. Some instruments are expected to cover several domains of content, such as physical, emotional, and social functioning. To have content validity, an instrument must sample items from each of the intended content areas. Content validity is usually addressed in the development of an instrument, such as by having experts in the domain of interest rate the items as to their relevance to the domain.

One difficulty with QOL measures is determining what constitutes a clinically meaningful difference, particularly regarding changes in QOL over time or the effect of a particular treatment on QOL.[16] With a large enough sample size, even very small changes or differences can be statistically significant, but it is unclear whether such differences are clinically meaningful. Two primary approaches have been identified to determine what constitutes a meaningful difference in a particular QOL questionnaire; these are the anchor-based and the distribution-based approaches.[17,18] The anchor-based method involves linking QOL scale score differences or changes to more interpretable variables such as clinical measures (e.g., performance status, response to treatment),[19] functional measures (e.g., ability to walk one block, ability to work),[20,21] or patients' global ratings of health or QOL, or changes in health or QOL.[22,23] Examples include many validation studies of QOL questionnaires, which compare QOL among individuals with differing performance status. For example, a validation study of the Functional Assessment of Cancer Therapy—Ovarian, showed that the scales for patients with a performance status of 0 versus 1 differed by 0.58 to 0.90 standard deviation (SD) units, including 5 points on the physical well-being subscale (0.87 SD units), 3.5 points on the emotional well-being subscale (0.74 SD units), 5.2 points on the functional well-being subscale (.90 SD units), and 3.6 points on the ovarian concerns subscale (0.58 SD units).[24] In a study to identify clinically significant differences or changes in the FACT Anemia and Fatigue Scales, Cella and colleagues[22] used both anchor-based and statistical/distributional methods for identifying clinically significant differences. Effect sizes for differences in scale scores between patients with differing performance status and hemoglobin levels were calculated at baseline and also for changes over time. The effect sizes comparing adjacent categories (e.g., performance status of 0 versus performance status of 1) were larger when the Eastern Cooperative Oncology Group (ECOG) performance status was used as the anchor than when hemoglobin or Karnovsky performance status was used. Effect sizes that indicated clinically significant change over time also tended to be slightly smaller than those calculated cross-sectionally. The effect sizes for cross-sectional comparisons ranged from 0.21 (effect sizes less than 0.20 were not used) to 1.28, whereas for longitudinal comparisons they ranged from 0.25 to 0.81.

A limitation with the use of clinical anchors is that they depart from one of the original intentions in studying QOL, the idea that it is the subjective assessment by the patient that is important. Although anchoring clinically significant changes on externally observed criteria may make the changes seem more valid or "scientific" to an outsider, if the differing levels in the anchor are not important or significant to the patients themselves, this type of anchoring misses the point. An alternative approach that uses the patients' assessment of anchors remedies this situation. A study by Doyle and associates[23] reporting QOL of ovarian cancer patients during palliative chemotherapy provides an example of the second approach. Patients were asked to rate the extent to which their physical condition and QOL had changed since their last visit. Those who responded "a little better" had improvement of 0.30 (on a 0-to-6 scale) on a question from the European Organization for Research and Treatment of Cancer (EORTC) questionnaire about physical functioning, and those who responded "a little worse" showed a 0.36 decrease on the same question. Patients who reported that their QOL was "a little worse" had a 0.42 decrease in a rating of global QOL, whereas those who reported that their QOL was "a little better" had a 0.13 increase in the score.

Statistical criteria may also be used to identify clinically significant change, such as Cohen's definition[25] of small, medium, and large effect sizes (an effect size is a difference divided by the pooled SD). Cohen defined changes of approximately 0.2 SD as small, 0.5 SD as medium, and 0.8 SD as large. Such criteria are somewhat sample-dependent, however, given that the SD can change depending on heterogeneity of the sample.[18] To avoid the problems of sample dependence, some investigators have suggesting using the standard error of measurement (SEM). The SEM indicates the degree to which the score or the change in the score reflects random error in the measurement. Studies that have used both the SEM approach and anchor-based determinations of minimal significant difference have found good agreement between the two.[19,26,27]

What do patients expect from palliative chemotherapy?

The term *palliative chemotherapy* is frequently used to describe chemotherapy prescribed for noncurable disease. Many women with recurrent gynecologic malignancies have limited treatment options and are faced with the choice of palliative chemotherapy or no further treatment. Although this therapy is directed toward both palliation of symptoms and maintenance of QOL, toxicity associated with some palliative regimens may be significant. Justification for such treatments requires some benefit, such as symptom management or improved QOL.

Although more recent studies have begun to incorporate QOL measures as study end points, few investigators have studied the effect of chemotherapy on QOL in gynecologic cancer patients. Additionally, to date, no study has compared palliative chemotherapy versus the best supportive care regimen in this group of patients.

In 1992, Payne reported on QOL in patients with advanced breast or ovarian cancer who received palliative chemotherapy.[28] Fifty-three patients were studied prospectively for 6 months. Of these, 17 patients had recurrent ovarian cancer. The author reported that chemotherapy administered in the hospital was perceived to be more distressing than chemotherapy administered at home. These results indicated that location of chemotherapy administration had a significant impact on patients' QOL. Additionally, regression analyses revealed that anxiety and depression accounted for most of the variance in QOL. From these data, the author recommended that QOL be regarded as an integral part of the clinical evaluation of cancer patients.

To date, no study has been published in the gynecologic oncology literature that examines the complex relationships among palliative chemotherapy, symptoms, and objective response. Such work has been performed in the population of patients with breast cancer. Geels and coworkers,[29] in a study of 300 women with metastatic breast cancer, reported a significant association between symptom improvement and objective tumor response. Symptoms were most improved in patients who demonstrated complete or partial responses to the palliative chemotherapy. Symptoms improved least in those women with progressive disease. In 1993, Guidozzi[30] reported on the QOL of 28 patients with advanced ovarian cancer. Although this study did not focus specifically on the impact of palliative chemotherapy on QOL, the author compared the QOL of patients with persistent disease with that of patients whose disease responded to treatment. All patients complained of decreased QOL during the first year of treatment (surgery followed by chemotherapy). Women with persistent disease rated their QOL much lower than did the responders in all life areas, including activity, daily living, heath support, and outlook.

Relatively little information has been published regarding the impact of palliative chemotherapy on

QOL in patients with gynecologic malignancies, but even less is known about patient expectations in this setting. Doyle and associates[23] recently reported on patient expectations and resource utilization in 27 women with refractory or recurrent ovarian cancer. They developed a questionnaire to assess patient expectations regarding outcomes associated with palliative chemotherapy. The EORTC QLQ 36 and FACT-O were used to evaluate palliative benefit. Despite the fact that all patients met with their own oncologists before the first cycle of chemotherapy and were counseled as to the noncurative intent of this treatment, 65% of them expected that the chemotherapy would extend their lifespan, and 42% expected that this palliative chemotherapy would cure them. QOL was assessed after two cycles of chemotherapy; an improvement in global function was seen in 11 of 21 women. Although the numbers are small, these data are interesting because they demonstrate an improvement in global and emotional-function QOL in half of the study population receiving palliative chemotherapy. A significant discrepancy occurred, however, in terms of information provided and patient expectations regarding the outcome of palliative chemotherapy. Several reasons for this discrepancy exist. First, patients may not wish to acknowledge the possibility of dying from their disease, and they may have high expectations as a mechanism for coping with stress. Second, this disconnect between information and expectations may be the result of poor doctor-patient communication.

Regardless of the reason for this significant difference in expectations, this study raises an unanswered question. When offered palliative chemotherapy, which outcome do patients most value: relief of symptoms, tumor response, or improvement in QOL? Based on the answers, how often are patient expectations met regarding palliative chemotherapy? Once again, discussions about hope and realistic expectations for treatment outcome are key aspects of successful doctor-patient communication.

What is the role of palliative surgery in the treatment of gynecologic cancers?

In the gynecologic oncology literature, the term *palliative surgery* is most often used to describe surgery to relieve bowel obstructions in patients with ovarian cancer. As many as 51% of women with ovarian cancer develop a bowel obstruction during the course of their illness.[31-33] Once this disease progresses, the goal changes from cure to prolongation of life, with an emphasis on QOL during the remaining time. Management of bowel obstruction may include palliative surgery (e.g., colostomy, ileostomy) or medical treatment.

Palliative surgical procedures are performed to restore functioning of the gastrointestinal tract. The overall surgical mortality rate for acute bowel obstruction for all malignant causes is approximately 20%. This rate increases slightly to 23% when surgery is palliative, and it dramatically increases to 72% in patients who are emaciated or malnourished.[34] "Surgical benefit" has traditionally been defined as 8 weeks of survival after surgery.[35] Surgically treated patients have a high likelihood of living with a colostomy or ileostomy for the rest of their lives. Some patients undergo exploration and are found to have unresectable disease. A significant number develop serious complications after surgery, and some die from this intervention. Although several authors have reported significant palliation of symptoms and a surgical benefit in as many as 65% to 80% of patients taken to the operating room,[31,32,36] others point to a lack of survival difference between surgical versus medical management.[37,38] A 1999 review of all studies of intestinal obstruction resulting from advanced gynecologic cancer failed to reach a conclusion regarding the appropriate treatment of bowel obstruction in this patient population.[39]

There is a paucity of data evaluating the medical management of bowel obstruction in patients with ovarian cancer. To our knowledge, Baines and colleagues[40] conducted the only prospective clinical study of the medical management of malignant bowel obstruction; 30% of the study population (14 patients) had ovarian cancer. The authors reported an improvement in the symptoms associated with bowel obstruction (e.g., intestinal colic, vomiting, diarrhea) with intensive medical management and the use of various medications. The mean survival time was 3.7 months.

Attempts have been made to develop a predictive model for appropriate management of bowel obstruction, but these instruments have not been prospectively validated. Krebs and Gopelrud[32] developed a scoring system to determine which patients would possibly benefit from surgical intervention based on six prognostic parameters: advanced age, palpable intra-abdominal tumor, extensive previous chemotherapy, nutritional deprivation, history of pelvic and abdominal radiation therapy, and rapidly reaccumulating ascites. Clarke-Pearson and coworkers[41] attempted to validate this system retrospectively; a stepwise logistical regression analysis to evaluate variables not included in the Krebs and Gopelrud model identified preoperative tumor status and serum albumin level as additional independent significant variables. However, neither of these studies examined the outcomes (e.g., survival, postintervention complications) of patients treated medically; only surgically treated patients were evaluated. Additional research must be conducted that includes outcomes of both surgical and medical treatment strategies. Other limitations with the current body of research include small sample sizes, changes in the standard of care, and inconsistent inclusion of several critical variables, including number of patients who had inoperable disease or required reoperation, performance status, and burden of illness and symptom assessment using validated outcome measures. None of the studies conducted to date has included patient preference or QOL as a defined end point.

Clearly, the medical and surgical treatment strategies for bowel obstruction yield different clinical outcomes, each accompanied by its own QOL implications. As noted by Easson and colleagues in a recent discussion of challenges and opportunities for surgeons in palliative care, "What distinguishes palliative surgery is the palliative surgeon's expansion of clinical outcomes beyond surgical morbidity and mortality outcomes and recurrence of disease to include outcomes that are meaningful to the patient."[42] Because QOL is defined in subjective terms, estimates of caregivers, whether familial or clinical, have been found to correlate poorly with estimates given by the patients themselves.[43] Use of surrogates is not appropriate to measure QOL in ovarian cancer.[44] Members of the health care team must work with patients to set appropriate goals for care. Clinicians and palliative surgeons must understand patients' perspectives on QOL issues regarding treatment for bowel obstruction, as well as symptoms associated with recurrent ovarian cancer and bowel obstruction. Patients must consider the tradeoffs they are willing to make in order to arrive at the clinical outcomes they value most. Clinicians together with patients must establish and study appropriate outcome measures for surgical and medical approaches to the treatment of bowel obstruction. Until this research is performed, the true role of palliative surgery in patients with gynecologic malignancies will not be appropriately defined.

How do end-of-life issues affect the care of women with gynecologic cancers?

Despite advances in early diagnosis and treatment, many women with gynecologic cancer will die from their disease. For this reason, the appropriate care of patients at the end of life is a critical area for training, research, and practice in gynecologic oncology.

Recent trends in the philosophy of end-of-life care have emphasized reducing the aggressiveness of measures taken to extend life and have focused on enhancing the patient's QOL as much as possible through symptom control measures and receiving care at home if possible. Good end-of-life care is broad, encompassing physical concerns as well as emotional and psychological issues, symptom control, family concerns, economic issues, and spiritual needs.[45,46] Providing good end-of-life care is complicated, however, by the fact that cancer patients typically face a more sudden decline in function before death than do people with other life-ending chronic diseases.[47] This makes it difficult to know, for some patients, when the appropriate time has come to reduce the emphasis on curative or life-extending therapy. Curative therapy and supportive care should not be viewed as mutually exclusive, however; there should be a strong emphasis on supportive care throughout the continuum of the illness. Excellent symptom control should be as high a priority for patients receiving potentially curative therapy as for those for patients at the end of their lives.[48]

The literature provides some indications that end-of-life care for gynecologic cancer patients is improving.

Dalrymple and associates[49] reported that at one tertiary cancer care center, a few indicators of quality end-of-life care improved over time. For example, the average length of time between the placement of a "Do Not Resuscitate" (DNR) order and the patient's death increased from 19.2 days during 1992–1994 to 49.4 days during 1995–1997. The presence of a DNR order indicates that the physician and patient have discussed the terminal nature of the disease and the patient does not wish to be resuscitated in the event of cardiopulmonary arrest. It also attempts to eliminate unnecessary procedures and changes the focus of care to "comfort care." Despite the increase in advance discussions about DNR, the proportion of patients who had no DNR order when they were admitted to the hospital did not change. Over the entire study period, 72% of the DNR orders were placed in the chart within 2 weeks of death, and 35% were placed within 72 hours of death.

Results of the Dalrymple study also point to a reluctance on the part of health care providers and patients to discuss end-of-life issues. Although the average time between diagnosis of an incurable condition and death was 11 months, the medical record reflected that patients were informed of the incurable nature of their condition an average of 44 days before death. This result stands in stark contrast to studies indicating that patients with gynecologic cancer prefer honest communication about the severity of their disease from their physician[50-52] and that communication with the health care team at the end of life is associated with better "quality of dying and death" as rated by family members.[53]

Not all patients, however, wish to engage in such frank discussions. Several studies indicate that a substantial proportion of patients who are dying do not want to address specifics of end-of-life care, such as whether they want resuscitation.[54] Many patients with gynecologic cancer remain determined to "fight" their disease, even after it has been deemed incurable.[55] Communication about end-of-life issues with gynecologic cancer patients needs to integrate realism and hope. However, hope does not need to focus solely on curing the disease or extending life; it can also encompass overcoming suffering.[48]

The needs of family members must be considered in the provision of end-of-life care. One of the most important aspects of high-quality end-of-life care from the perspective of family members is knowing that their relative is consistently receiving appropriate care, relieving them of the role of advocate for the relative's needs. The ability to trust the health care team to take appropriate actions in the care of their loved one greatly relieves the family's own suffering. Teno and colleagues[45] describe a "patient-focused, family centered" model of quality medical care of patients at the end of life. The model includes six components: (1) providing physical and emotional support to the patient at the level desired; (2) encouraging shared decision-making; (3) focusing on the individual patient in her social context, with respect for the dignity of the patient and the importance of closure in social relationships; (4) attention to the needs of the family for emotional support before and after the death; (5) coordination of care; and (6) providing information and skills to family members to enable them to care for the patient. This model illustrates the broad nature of care needed by gynecologic oncology patients at the end of life. The emphasis of care must change from specific disease processes to general symptom relief and QOL, and from treating a patient to caring for the patient in the family content.

How does the cancer diagnosis affect patients?

The diagnosis of cancer is a life-changing event for any person. Psychological responses vary substantially depending on the patient population. Past research has indicated that women with breast or ovarian cancer experience higher levels of psychological distress than do men with prostate cancer.[56] For a woman, the diagnosis of cancer, particularly a gynecologic cancer, becomes part of her identity.[57] Consequently, the psychological impact may linger for some time after the diagnosis. Common psychological responses include intrusive thoughts, avoidance, and denial of the cancer diagnosis.[58] Factors shown to influence the psychological impact of a cancer diagnosis include type and severity of the cancer, age at diagnosis, income, education, gender, treatment, and available social support.[59-61] Psychological distress in women occurs during cancer screening procedures as well.[62,63]

A woman diagnosed with gynecologic malignancy may feel a profound sense of loss. The loss may be multifaceted in origin. Many women with newly diagnosed gynecologic cancers face surgeries to remove some or all of their reproductive organs, and the perceived loss of femininity may contribute to the stress of the diagnosis. The physical changes in a woman's body may be a barrier to physical intimacy between the patient and her partner. Age has been shown to be inversely associated with psychological impact, perhaps because a cancer diagnosis in an older woman may be considered to be part of the natural aging process and is not as unexpected. For a woman who is premenopausal at the time of diagnosis, the potential or realized loss of reproductive function can be devastating.[59] For some couples, the loss of reproductive function may affect the purpose of sexual relationships. This feeling of loss may be further compounded by the changes in a woman's role in her family.[64,65] The diagnosis may negatively affect her role as a wife or as a parent. For women with adult children, psychological distress may be present for both parties; a daughter must now meet the needs of her own family while also taking on the role as caregiver to her mother.[66] For families with younger children, a mother with a newly diagnosed gynecologic malignancy not only must come to terms with her new reality but also must face the stresses of how best to convey the information to her children and how her treatment may affect her children's daily routine. Decreased ability or complete inability to continue working may contribute significantly to a woman's distress.[57] A woman's professional role may be diminished because of her treatment schedule or treatment effects. Loss of financial earning power contributes to worries about treatment costs.[57] In summary, a woman may feel a sense of loss on multiple levels that may be characterized as a loss of control over her own life.

Some experts have suggested that a younger age at diagnosis of a gynecologic cancer may be indicative of a greater hereditary predisposition to cancer, causing distress for women who fall into this category.[67] Women with confirmed hereditary cancer syndromes (e.g., ovarian cancer associated with *BRCA1* or *BRCA2* mutations) may experience the emotional burden of guilt because of the increased risks of associated cancers in their daughters and sons.[57] Guilt may also be part of the psychological response for other reasons, including past health behaviors or actions known to be associated with gynecologic cancers, such as noncompliance with routine Papanicolaou smears or sexual behavior leading to cervix cancer associated with human papillomavirus (HPV) infection.

Shock, anger, and frustration are common reactions to a cancer diagnosis.[68,69] Shock may occur because a woman has never considered herself to be at risk for a particular cancer (e.g., no family history of ovarian cancer). Some women may even doubt the accuracy of the diagnosis. Delays in the final diagnosis may contribute to feelings of anger and frustration that are expressed once the diagnosis is confirmed.

Fear and anxiety concerning available treatment options are common responses.[69,70] A woman may also be afraid to disclose her illness to close family members or friends, because she believes that no one can relate to her situation.[57] A cancer diagnosis may alter standing relationships; some may be strengthened and others may be placed at risk.[57] Many women will undergo standard treatment consisting of some combination of surgery, chemotherapy, and radiation, all of which have their own side effects. There may be fear about how the treatment will affect a woman's body (e.g., after loading tandem and ovoid (ALTO), surgery resulting in colostomy). For women who choose clinical trials, the uncertainty concerning the treatment arm or outcome of a phase I study can heighten fear and anxiety.[71] Fear and anxiety associated with clinical outcomes of both standard and experimental treatments should be expected. Furthermore, even after the woman is clinically "cured," the fear and anxiety surrounding a possible recurrence are inevitably present on some level.[57] Finally, a woman with a newly diagnosed cancer may be afraid and anxious about the possibility of dying, perhaps before treatment has even begun.

Feelings of hopelessness and sadness about future health and happiness are also common responses.[56,69,72] For some women, depression persists for some time after a diagnosis and throughout treatment and follow-up. For this reason, the interactions between a woman and her gynecologic oncologist or other members of her treatment team are critical, particularly at the time of diagnosis, because they establish the tone for the rest of treatment and follow-up. Informing a patient of her cancer diagnosis should be done in

Figure 59-1. Example of a visual analog scale.

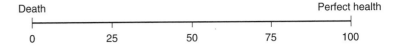

a way that optimizes her well-being.[58,71,73] Every effort should be made to preserve the patient's sense of control over the situation. The gynecologic oncologist should set a reassuring tone, while also acknowledging the patient's feelings about her new diagnosis of cancer. Patients experience lower levels of anxiety when their physicians address such issues as prognosis and treatment plans at or near the time of diagnosis.[59] Establishing a reassuring tone and environment at the time of diagnosis may help to decrease the negative psychological impact on a woman diagnosed with a gynecologic cancer.

Why are patient preferences important to study?

One of the foundations of clinical decision-making in oncology rests on which tradeoffs patients are willing to make to maximize quality and/or quantity of life.

Preference (utility) assessment is the formal measurement of the strength of patients' preferences for a specific treatment or outcome of treatment.[8] Preference assessment quantitatively measures how patients value QOL in a given health state (e.g., clinical condition). Theoretically, preferences are ranked on a scale of 0.0 to 1.0 scale, where 0.0 represents death and 1.0 represents perfect health. The preference metric is used in decision analysis models to determine the quality-adjusted survival of patients undergoing different treatment regimens for a given disease. Decision analysis models are mathematical models that incorporate both QOL and length-of-life outcomes through the outcome measure of a quality-adjusted life year (QALY). Quality-adjusted survival adjusts quantity of life for the quality of time spent in a given health state.[74] The QALY captures both quality and length of life by means of "quality-weighted" health states. A higher weight indicates a more preferred health state, whereas a lower weight reflects a lower preference for the health state. The quality weight, or preference value, for each health state is multiplied by the time spent in each health state. The sum of these numbers indicates the total number of QALYs for a particular intervention. With a common value such as the QALY, comparisons of medical interventions with different outcomes can be made.[9] To determine the quality-adjusted weights for each outcome in a decision analysis model, preference assessments must be conducted. Such models may also be used in cost-effectiveness analyses of disease treatment options and can be used by health policy makers to help determine which treatment costs should be reimbursed.

Three generally accepted preference assessment methods exist. All three methods have been shown to be reliable and valid in both patient and community populations.[75] The simplest instrument to administer is the visual analog scale (VAS). An example is shown in Figure 59-1. The VAS is considered by many researchers to be the most convenient method because it is easily understood by patients and quick to administer. It is particularly useful because it can be used in a clinic setting or at the patient's bedside. For each health state, the patient marks the appropriate position along a scale with clearly defined end points of death (at the zero point) and perfect health (at the maximum point). The placement of the mark indicates the patient's preference relative to these end points. The VAS method aims to have the patient generate an interval scale of preferences, from the worst to the best scenario. Through this ranking, researchers gain an impression of how side effects are ranked in relation to other side effects. The typical VAS asks patients to rank each health state along a 0-to-100 continuum; these scores are then converted to a 0-to-1 scale, where 0 is the worst and 1 is the best.

The second method, the time tradeoff (TTO), assesses the preference for each health state by asking how much time in a perfect state of health the respondent considers to be equivalent to a longer time in a less-than-perfect health state. The TTO framework for permanent health states is shown in Figure 59-2.[9] The

Figure 59-2. Time tradeoffs for two alternative treatment regimens.

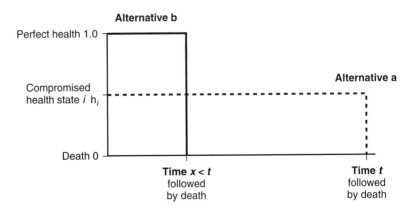

respondent must choose between two alternatives: (1) a compromised health state i (e.g., permanent blindness) for a set length of life (t) followed by death, or (2) a shorter length of life in perfect health (shown as x, where $x < t$) followed by death. Time x is varied until the patient is indifferent between the two scenarios. The preference for the compromised health state i is the ratio of the shorter to the longer life expectancy: $h_i = x/t$. Some researchers have found that the TTO method is more difficult for patients to comprehend than the VAS, but is easier than the third method, the standard gamble. The TTO is suited for clinical situations involving differing times spent in a variety of health states (e.g., duration of side effects). The TTO method can be easily modified to accommodate temporary health states such as toxicities associated with cancer treatment.

The standard gamble (SG) is considered to be the most conclusive way to measure preferences because it is the only method that incorporates decision-making under conditions of uncertainty. The SG is shown in Figure 59-3.[9] The SG assesses the preference for a compromised health state i by asking the respondent how much she would be willing to risk to improve it; specifically, the patient must choose between two alternatives: (1) guaranteed life in health state i with less than perfect QOL, or (2) a gamble between perfect health with probability p and immediate death with the probability of $1 - p$. The probability of death in the gamble is varied until the respondent is indifferent to the outcome. The result is the preference score for health state i ($h_i = p$). Despite its strengths, a major limitation is that some individuals do not grasp the concept of probabilities well enough to adequately understand the preference assessment process.

A significant body of work has been published regarding treatment preferences and desire for aggressive cancer therapy in patients with nongynecologic malignancies. A study of 296 cancer patients, most of whom had breast cancer,[76] found that having children at home and positive social well-being served as predictors of patient willingness to pursue aggressive treatment. Slevin and colleagues[77] evaluated attitudes toward acceptance of chemotherapy among cancer patients, physicians, nurses, and the general public. Patients with cancer were much more likely than other

study participants to chose radical treatment with a minimal chance of benefit.

Formal preference assessments have also been conducted in women with gynecologic cancers. Elit and associates[78] used a decision board at the bedside and reported that patients who were asked to evaluate the poor prognosis situation of advanced epithelial ovarian cancer valued survival more highly than QOL during chemotherapy.

Given these observations, as well as the need for effective physician-patient communication, several groups have begun to further explore preferences for treatment outcomes among caregivers as well as patients. Calhoun and coworkers[79] studied perceptions of cisplatin-related toxicity among women with advanced ovarian cancer (who had received a minimum of six courses of platinum-based chemotherapy) and their gynecologic oncologists. Their data revealed a significant difference in the assessment of the impact of cisplatin-induced toxicities between these two groups. Patients viewed toxic health status more favorably than their physicians did. Additionally, physicians' ratings of the various toxicities were similar to the ratings of patients who had not experienced significant side effects. Physicians' ratings were less favorable than the ratings of patients who had experienced cisplatin-related toxicities. Sun and colleagues[10] studied preferences for health states among women receiving high-dose chemotherapy with stem cell support for advanced ovarian cancer. They reported that chemotherapy-experienced women had consistent preferences for the best and worst health states and that these preferences remained stable over time. They also noted that patients were more averse to nausea and vomiting than to a wide variety of other symptoms.

Sun and associates[80] also evaluated outcome preferences in women at high risk for breast/ovarian cancer and in a control population. A personal history of cancer and the specific method of assessment appeared to influence preference scores. Women in the control group were willing to risk a greater chance of death and to trade more time in order to avoid surgery and cancer.

These studies highlight several important points. First, patients with cancer, women at increased risk for cancer, and physicians appear to have difference preferences for treatment-related side effects. Second, the use of surrogate patient preference scores in decision-analytic models could lead to inaccurate calculations of quality-adjusted survival. Finally, optimal decisions for treatment strategies should incorporate patients' assessments regarding QOL and preferences regarding toxicities and treatment outcomes.

Conclusions

Although the QOL of women with gynecologic malignancies is a complex topic that can be difficult to accurately assess, it is vital that this area of research continue to grow and develop. Because health care providers are aware that patients may have different

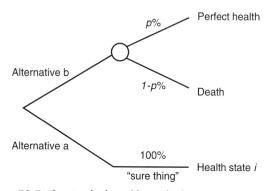

Figure 59-3. The standard gamble method.

preferences for treatment side-effects and outcomes, it is incumbent on them to discuss such issues with their patients. Although the goal is to maximize QOL, it is also critical to remember that some patients may value quantity rather than quality. Only through ongoing dialogue can practitioners work together with patients to optimize decision-making.

REFERENCES

1. Cella DF, et al: The Functional Assessment of Cancer Therapy scale: Development and validation of the general measure. J Clin Oncol 1993;11:570-579.
2. Bonomi AE, et al: Validation of the United States version of the World Health Organization Quality of Life (WHOQOL) instrument. J Clin Epidemiol 2000;53:1-12.
3. Schover LR, Fife M, Gershenson DM: Sexual dysfunction and treatment for early stage cervical cancer. Cancer 1989;63:204-212.
4. Bergmark K, et al: Vaginal changes and sexuality in women with a history of cervical cancer. N Engl J Med 1999;340:1383-1389.
5. Yeo BK, Perera I: Sexuality of women with carcinoma of the cervix. Ann Acad Med Singapore 1995;24:676-678.
6. Portenoy RK, et al: Symptom prevalence, characteristics and distress in cancer population. Qual Life Res 1994;3:189-289.
7. Battista RN, Hodge MJ: Quality of life research and health technology assessment—A time for synergy. Qual Life Res 1996;5:413-418.
8. Stiggelbout AM, DeHaes JCJM: Patient preference for cancer therapy: An overview of measurement approaches. J Clin Oncol 2001;19:220-230.
9. Drummond MF, et al: Methods for the Economic Evaluation of Health Care Pprogrammes, 2nd ed. New York, Oxford University Press, 1997.
10. Sun CC, et al: Patient preferences regarding side-effects of chemotherapy for ovarian cancer: Do they change over time? Gynecol Oncol 2002;87:118-128.
11. Sun CC, et al: A pilot study to assess patient preferences for side effects of chemoradiation. Gynecol Oncol 2001;80:288.
12. Anastasi A: Psychological Testing, 5th ed. New York: MacMillan, 1982.
13. Sax G: Principles of Educational and Psychological Measurement and Evaluation, 4th ed. Belmont, CA: Wadsworth, 1997.
14. Windsor R, et al: Evaluation of Health Promotion, Health Education, and Disease Prevention Programs, 2nd ed. Mountain View, California: Mayfield, 1994.
15. Minium EW: Statistical Reasoning in Psychology and Education, 2nd ed. New York: John Wiley & Sons, 1978.
16. Sloan JA, et al: Assessing clinical significance in measuring oncology patient quality of life: Introduction to the symposium, content overview, and definition of terms. Mayo Clin Proc 2002;77:367-370.
17. Guyatt GH, et al: User's guides to the medical literature XII. How to use articles about health-related quality of life. JAMA members. 1997;277:1232-1237.
18. Guyatt GH, et al: Methods to explaing the clinical significance of health status measures. Mayo Clin Proc 2002;77:371-383.
19. Cella D, et al: Combining anchor and distribution-based methods to derive minimal clinically important differences on the Functional Assessment of Cancer Therapy (FACT) Anemia and Fatigue scales. J Pain Symptom Manage 2002;24:547-561.
20. Ware JE Jr, Kosinski M, Keller SD: SF-36 Physical and Mental Health Summary Scales: A User's Manual. Boston, Massachusetts: The Health Institute, New England Medical Center, 1994, pp 3.2-10.11.
21. Ware JE Jr, et al: SF-36 Health Survey: Manual and Interpretation Guide. Boston: The Health Institute, New England Medical Center, 1997.
22. Cella D, Hahn EA, Dineen K: Meaningful change in cancer-specific quality of life scores: Differences between improvement and worsening. Qual Life Res 2002;11:207-221.
23. Doyle C, et al: Does palliative chemotherapy palliate? Evaluation of expectations, outcomes, and costs in women receiving chemotherapy for advanced ovarian cancer. J Clin Oncol 2001;19:1266-1274.
24. Basen-Engquist K, et al: Reliability and validity of the Functional Assessment of Cancer Therapy—Ovarian (FACT-O). J Clin Oncol 2001;19:1809-1817.
25. Cohen J: Statistical power analysis for the behavioral sciences. Mahway, NJ: Lawrence Erlbaum Associates, 1998.
26. Wyrwich KW, et al: Linking clinical relevance and statistical significance in evaluating intra-individual changes in health-related quality of life. Med Care 1999;37:469-478.
27. Wyrwich KW, Tierney WM, Wolinsky FD: Further evidence supporting an SEM-based criterion for identifying meaningful intra-individual changes in health-related quality of life. J Clin Epidemiol 1999;52:861-873.
28. Payne SA: A study of quality of life in cancer patients receiving palliative chemotherapy. Soc Sci Med 1992;12:1505-1509.
29. Geels P, et al: Palliative effect of chemotherapy: Objective tumor response is associated with symptom improvement in patients with metastatic breast cancer. J Clin Oncol 2000;18:2395-2405.
30. Guidozzi F: Living with ovarian cancer. Gynecol Oncol 1993;50:202-207.
31. Tunca JC, et al: The management of ovarian-cancer-caused bowel obstruction. Gynecol Oncol 1981;12:186-192.
32. Krebs HB, Goplerud DR: Surgical management of bowel obstruction in advanced ovarian carcinoma. Obstet Gynecol 1983;61:327-330.
33. Dvoretsky PM, et al: Survival time, causes of death, and tumor/treatment-related morbidity in 100 women with ovarian cancer. Hum Pathol 1988;19:1273-1279.
34. Meguid MM, et al: Complications of abdominal operations for malignant disease. Am J Surg 1988;156:341-345.
35. Castaldo TW, et al: Intestinal operations in patients with ovarian carcinoma. Am J Obstet Gynecol 1981;139:80-84.
36. Clarke-Pearson DL, et al: Surgical management of intestinal obstruction in ovarian cancer. Gynecol Oncol 1987;26:11-18.
37. Fernandes JR, Seymour RJ, Suissa S: Bowel obstruction in patients with ovarian cancer: A search for prognostic factors. Am J Obstet Gynecol 1988;158:244-249.
38. Lund B, et al: Intestinal obstruction in patients with advanced carcinoma of the ovaries treated with combination chemotherapy. Surg Gynecol Obstet 1989;169:213-218.
39. Feuer DL, et al: Systematic review of surgery in malignant bowel obstruction in advanced gynecological and gastrointestinal cancer. Gynecol Oncol 1999;75:313-322.
40. Baines M, Oliver DJ, Carter RL. Medical management of intestinal obstruction in patients with advanced malignant disease: A clinical and psychological study. Lancet 1985;8:990-993.
41. Clarke-Pearson DL, et al: Intestinal obstruction in patients with ovarian. Arch Surg 1988;123:42-45.
42. Easson AM, et al: Clinical research for surgeons in palliative care: challenges and opportunities. J Am Coll Surg 2003;196:141-151.
43. Present CA: Quality of life in cancer patients: Who measures what? J Clin Oncol 1981;7:571-573.
44. Donovan K, Sanson-Fisher RW, Redman S: Measuring quality of life in cancer patients. J Clin Oncol 1989;7:959-968.
45. Teno JM, et al: Patient-focused, family-centered end of life medical care: Views of the guidelines and bereaved family members. J Pain Symptom Manage 2001;22:738-751.
46. Patrick DL, Engelberg RA, Curtis JR: Evaluating the quality of dying and death. J Pain Symptom Manage 2001;22:717-726.
47. Teno JM, et al: Dying trajectory in the last year of life: Does cancer trajectory fit other diseases? J Palliat Med 2001;4:457-464.
48. Cain JM, et al: Palliative care and quality of life considerations in the management of ovarian cancer. In Livingstone C, Gershenson DM, McGuire WP (eds): Ovarian Cancer: Controversies in Management. Philadelphia: WB Saunders, 1997.
49. Dalrymple JL, et al: Trends among gynecologic oncology inpatient deaths: Is end-of-life care improving? Gynecol Oncol 2002;85:356-361.
50. Roberts JA, et al: Factors influencing views of patients with gynecologic cancer about end-of-life decisions. Am J Obstet Gynecol 1997;176:166-172.
51. Parker PA, et al: Breaking bad news about cancer: Patients' preferences for communication. J Clin Oncol 2001;19:2049-2056.
52. Greisinger AJ, et al: Terminally ill cancer patients: Their most important concerns. Cancer Pract 1997;5:147-154.

53. Curtis JR, et al: A measure of the quality of dying and death: Initial validation using after-death interviews with family members. J Pain Symptom Manage 2002;24:17-31.

54. Hofmann JC, et al: Patient preferences for communication with physicians about end-of-life decisions. Ann Intern Med 1997; 127:1-12.

55. Brown D, et al: Hard choices: The gynecologic cancer patient's end-of-life preferences. Gynecol Oncol 1994;55:355-362.

56. Zabora J, et al: The prevalence of psychological distress by cancer site. Psychooncology 2001;10:19-28.

57. Howell D, Fitch MI, Deane KA: Impact of ovarian cancer perceived by women. Cancer Nurs 2003;26:1-9.

58. Schofield PE, et al: Psychological responses of patients receiving a diagnosis of cancer. Ann Oncol 2003;14:48-56.

59. Auchincloss SS, McCartney CF: Quality of life and psychosocial aspects of gynecologic cancer care. In Hoskins WJ, Perez CA, Young RC (eds.): Principles and Practice of Gynecologic Oncology. Philadelphia: Lippincott-Raven, 1997.

60. Kornblith AB, et al: Hodgkin's disease survivors at increased risk for problems in psychosocial adaptation: The Cancer and Leukemia Group B. Cancer 1992;70:2214-2224.

61. Cella DF Tross S: Psychological adjustment to survival from Hodgkin's disease. J Consult Clin Psychol 1986;54:616-622.

62. Kornblith AB, et al: Quality of life of women with ovarian cancer. Gynecol Oncol 1995;59:231-242.

63. Robinson GE, Rosen BP, Bradley LN: Psychological impact of screening for familial ovarian cancer: Reactions to initial assessment. Gynecol Oncol 1997;65:197-205.

64. Yates P: Family coping: Issues and challenges for cancer nursing. Cancer Nurs 1999;22:63-71.

65. Lowdermilk D, Germino BB: Helping women and their families cope with the impact of gynecologic cancer. J Obstet Gynecol Neonat Nurs 2000;29:653-660.

66. Germino BB, Funk S: Impact of a parent's cancer on adult children: Role and relationship issues. Semin Oncol Nurs 1993;9:101-106.

67. McBride CM, et al: Psychological impact of diagnosis and risk reduction among cancer survivors. Psychooncology 2000;9: 418-427.

68. Ford S, Lewis S, Fallowfield L: Psychological morbidity in newly referred patients with cancer. J Psychosom Res 1995;39: 193-202.

69. American Cancer Society: The emotional impact of a cancer diagnosis. American Cancer Society, 2002.

70. Stark D, et al: Anxiety disorders in cancer patients: Their nature, associations, and relation to quality of life. J Clin Oncol 2002; 20:3137-3148.

71. Zachariae R, et al: Association of perceived physician communication style with patient satisfaction, distress, cancer-related self-efficacy, and perceived control over the disease. Br J Cancer 2003;88:658-665.

72. Ranchor AV, et al: Pre-morbid predictors of psychological adjustment to cancer. Qual Life Res 2002;11:101-113.

73. Ellis PM, Tattersall MHN: How should doctors communicate the diagnosis of cancer to patients? Ann Med 1999;31: 336-341.

74. Torrence GW, Feeney D: Utilities and quality-adjusted-life years. Int J Technol Assess Health Care 1989;5:559-575.

75. Furlong F, et al: Guide to design and development of health-state utility instrumentation. Toronto: Centre for Health Economics and Policy Analysis, 1990.

76. Yellen SB, Cella DF: Someone to live for: Social well-being, parenthood status, and decision-making in oncology. J Clin Oncol 1995;13:1255-1264.

77. Slevin ML, et al: Attitudes to chemotherapy: Comparing views of patients with cancer with those of doctors, nurses, and general public. BMJ 1990;300:1458-1460.

78. Elit LM, et al: Patients' preferences for therapy in advanced epithelial ovarian cancer: Development, testing, and application of a bedside decision instrument. Gynecol Oncol 1996;62: 329-335.

79. Calhoun EA, et al: Perceptions of cisplatin-related toxicity among ovarian cancer patients and gynecologic oncologists. Gynecol Oncol 1998;71:369-375.

80. Sun CC, et al: Patient preferences for outcomes in women at high-risk for breast/ovarian cancer: Who and how you ask matters. In Program/Proceedings of the American Society of Clinical Oncology, 2000.

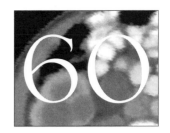

C H A P T E R

60

MENOPAUSE AND HORMONE REPLACEMENT THERAPY

Amanda Vincent   and   Henry Burger

 MAJOR CONTROVERSIES

- What are the indications for the use of hormone therapy?
- What are the adverse effects associated with hormone therapy use?
- Which hormone therapy regimen should be used?
- When should treatment be instituted?
- What is the role of estrogen in the etiology of gynecologic cancer?
- Can hormone therapy be used in women with a history of gynecologic cancer?
- What is the role of androgen therapy in postmenopausal women with a history of gynecologic cancer?
- What is the role of selective estrogen receptor modulators?
- What is the role of phytoestrogens?
- What nonestrogenic therapies are available for the relief of menopausal symptoms?
- What is the role of herbal therapies?
- What alternative therapies are available for management of osteoporosis?

MENOPAUSE

Consideration of the short-term and long-term consequences of the menopause has become an increasingly important issue for women with gynecologic cancer and their treating clinicians due to advances in diagnosis and therapy as well as demographic trends. Increased life expectancy and aging of the "baby boomers" have resulted in a greater proportion of women entering the menopause and therefore an increase in potential cases of gynecologic cancer. In addition, improved disease-free survival rate (the 5-year disease-free survival rate of women with breast cancer or endometrial cancer is now greater than 85% in the United States)[1] and increased use of adjuvant chemotherapy has resulted in more women undergoing premature menopause, creating a larger number of

postmenopausal women with a history of gynecologic cancer than previously.

Definition

Menopause, defined by the World Health Organization (WHO) as the final spontaneous menses, is diagnosed retrospectively after 12 months of amenorrhea. The *perimenopause* delineates the period that begins with the first symptoms of the approaching menopause and ends 12 months after the final menstrual period. Longitudinal studies,[2,3] using a clinical definition of the perimenopause as the period of irregular menses, have documented a median age at onset of 45.5 to 47.5 years (range, 41 to 59 years) and average duration of 4 to 4.8 years (range, 0 to 11 years). Currently, there is no biochemical, hormonal, or symptom cluster marker

795

for the onset of the perimenopause. *Premature menopause*, defined as menopause that occurs before the age of 40 years, may occur spontaneously, as in premature ovarian failure (POF), or as a result of therapeutic intervention.

Spontaneous menopause occurs as a result of the failure of ovarian function. Loss of ovarian follicular activity results in the cessation of ovulation and the characteristic decline in production of ovarian hormones, including estradiol, progesterone, and inhibin, with reciprocal elevation of gonadotrophins (Fig. 60-1). Steroid secretion by the postmenopausal ovary is minimal; estrone (predominantly formed by the aromatization in peripheral tissues of adrenal gland–derived androstenedione) is the main circulating estrogen. Low levels of estradiol may be produced by aromatization of testosterone in adipose tissue. Extragonadal synthesis of estrogens increases with increasing age and body mass index (BMI); however, the mechanisms that regulate estrogen production in postmenopausal women remain unclear.[4] Although the probability of being menopausal increases with the duration of amenorrhea and increasing age,[5] there are no specific predictors of menopause. Population-based studies in Western industrialized societies have determined the average age of spontaneous menopause to be approximately 50 years.[3,6,7] Smoking, single or nulliparous status, low socioeconomic status, and shorter premenopausal cycle

length appear to be associated with an earlier onset of menopause.[6,8]

Causes of Menopause in this Patient Population

Spontaneous physiologic menopause has already occurred in the majority of women at the time of diagnosis of gynecologic malignancy. For example, two thirds of women diagnosed with breast cancer in the United States are postmenopausal.[9] However, in many women diagnosed with gynecologic malignancy, menopause may be a consequence of oophorectomy (surgical menopause), chemotherapy, or may spontaneous occurrence at an earlier age.[10,11] Women younger than 50 years of age who have primary breast cancer derive the greatest benefit from adjuvant chemotherapy[12]; they therefore represent a significant population at risk for chemotherapy-induced premature menopause. The risk of chemotherapy- or radiotherapy-induced POF is increased with age greater than 40 years, use of alkylating agents such as cyclophosphamide, greater cumulative dose of cytotoxic drug, and more extensive irradiation (below the pelvic brim).[11,13,14] The question as to whether conservative hysterectomy (in which one or both ovaries are conserved) is associated with an increased risk of early menopause remains unresolved, but it appears probable[15];

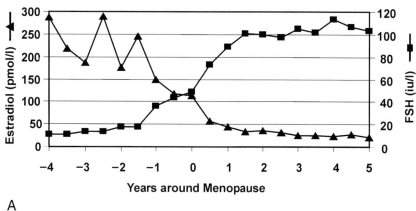

A

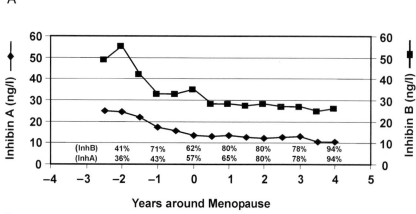

B

Figure 60–1. Hormonal changes that occur during the transition from premenopause to postmenopause. Mean serum levels of (**A**) follicle-stimulating hormone (FSH) and estradiol and (**B**) inhibin A (InhA) and inhibin B (InhB), in relation to the final menstrual period (denoted on the horizontal axis as time 0, with negative and positive numbers indicating years before and after the final menses, respectively). Parentheses above the time scale indicate the percentage of measured InhA or InhB at or below assay sensitivity. (Reproduced with permission of The Endocrine Society from Burger HG, Dudley EC, Hopper JL, et al: Prospectively measured levels of serum follicle-stimulating hormone, estradiol and the dimeric inhibins during the menopausal transition in a population-based cohort of women. J Clin Endocrinol Metab 1999;4025-4030.)

39% of women younger than 39 years develop menopausal symptoms after hysterectomy.[16] Parker and coworkers[17] reported that 20% of women developed ovarian failure after radical hysterectomy for cervical carcinoma.

Clinical Features of Menopause

Consequences of menopausal estrogen deficiency include short-term physical and psychological symptomatology as well as long-term health issues, such as increased risks for osteoporosis, cardiovascular disease, and cognitive decline. The pathophysiologic changes and clinical manifestations associated with androgen and progesterone deficiency are less well defined (Table 60-1). Women with premature menopause may experience more severe symptoms, and their risks for osteoporosis,[18,19] coronary heart disease (CHD),[20-22] and stroke[23] are greater. However, the association between these long-term consequences and menopause induced by chemotherapy or radiotherapy remains unclear. Women with early or premature menopause must also

---

▋ Table 60–1. Clinical Features of Menopause

Symptoms of estrogen deficiency
Vasomotor instability
  Hot flashes/flushes
  Night sweats
Urogenital atrophy
  Vaginal dryness and irritation
  Dyspareunia
  Micturition disorders
Irritability
Mood disturbance/mood swings
Depression
Insomnia
Arthralgia and myalgia
Memory and concentration disturbance
Formication
Dry eyes
Palpitations
Mastalgia
Headache
Paresthesia

Long-term consequences of estrogen deficiency
Osteoporosis
Cardiovascular disease
  Altered lipid metabolism
  Altered vascular reactivity
Cancer
  Colorectal
Cognitive decline

Symptoms of androgen deficiency (?)
Altered sexual function
  Decreased libido
Decreased well-being/energy levels

Long-term consequences of androgen deficiency
Unknown

Symptoms of progesterone deficiency
Unknown

Long-term consequences of progesterone deficiency
Unknown

---

confront issues such as the loss of fertility, altered body image, and "being out of step with their peers."[24,25]

Symptoms associated with menopause. Characteristic symptoms of estrogen deficiency are vasomotor instability and urogenital atrophy. A number of other physical and psychological symptoms are commonly reported in association with menopause (see Table 60-1); however, their relation to hormonal deficiency, psychosocial factors, and environmental influences is less clear. Hot flushes occur in up to 75% of menopausal women, more frequently after surgical menopause; frequent, severe episodes are reported by 10% to 15% of women. The frequency and severity of climacteric symptoms is also greater in hysterectomized women with ovarian conservation.[26] The pathophysiologic cause of hot flushes remains unclear. The onset of symptoms may occur during the perimenopause or within 4 to 6 days after oophorectomy. Variation in the frequency, type, severity, onset, and duration of symptoms occurs between individuals and between ethnic groups.[27]

Osteoporosis. Osteoporosis is a major public health problem associated with significant morbidity, mortality, and financial burden.[28] Although osteoporotic fractures are observed worldwide, geographic variation is demonstrated. The highest incidence occurs in Western countries, where 30% to 40% of women over 50 years of age will suffer an osteoporotic fracture during the remainder of their lifetime.[29] Postmenopausal osteoporosis is characterized by low bone mass, bone fragility resulting from deterioration of bone microarchitecture, and increased risk of fracture.[30] Coexistent independent factors, including inadequate calcium intake, smoking, and concurrent medical problems such as hyperthyroidism or Cushing's syndrome, may further increase the rapidity of bone loss.

Clinical Management of Menopause

A comprehensive evaluation of the patient includes a detailed history, thorough physical examination, and relevant investigations (Table 60-2), including determination of serum lipids for cardiovascular risk assessment, bone densitometry to assess osteoporosis risk, and other measures as indicated by the history (e.g., thyroid function tests, serum iron and coagulation screen). Reproductive hormonal assessment is of little diagnostic value. Discussion with the woman is essential to explore her comprehension, attitude, perceptions, cultural beliefs, and concerns regarding menopause and the potential therapies available, thereby enabling the practitioner to "individualize" management and promote compliance with clinical recommendations.

Management of the menopause includes the following approaches:

1. Dietary advice and lifestyle advice (see later discussion)

Table 60–2. Clinical Evaluation

History	Examination	Laboratory Investigations
Menopausal symptoms Chronologic reproductive history, including age at menarche and menstrual history, gravidity and parity, gynecologic surgical history, date and cause of menopause History of hormonal treatment, both contraceptive and hormone replacement therapy (HRT) Sexual history, including frequency of intercourse, ease of arousal, libido, orgasm, dyspareunia Urogenital symptoms, including bladder dysfunction and prolapse Bone or joint pain, arthritis, fractures, osteoporosis, bone density measurement Loss of height General current and past medical history Gastrointestinal symptoms, including esophageal reflux, and history of achlorhydria, lactose intolerance History of weight fluctuations, physical activity, exercise tolerance Psychiatric history, including premenstrual symptoms and cognitive functioning Family history, especially of early menopause, cardiovascular disease, osteoporosis, cancer, and dementia Social history Dietary history, particularly vitamins, calcium, sodium, alcohol, caffeine, and fiber intake History of smoking Medications, both prescribed and nonprescribed (herbal, "natural therapies") Allergies, including sensitivities to adhesive tapes	General physical examination with particular reference to the following: 　Posture (signs related to the presence of osteoporotic compression fractures), gait, muscle tone, coordination 　Height, body mass index, waist circumference, and body composition 　Heart rate and rhythm, blood pressure Breast examination Cardiovascular examination Pelvic examination, including size and shape of uterus and adnexal structures, estrogenic state of the vagina mucosa and vulva, elasticity of the vaginal wall (discharge, atrophy), integrity of the pelvic floor (cystocele, rectocele) Eyesight and hearing acuity (in terms of fracture risk and quality of life)	Follicle-stimulating hormone (FSH), estradiol (of limited diagnostic use) Serum androgens, including testosterone, free testosterone (or free androgen index), dehydroepiandrosterone sulfate Thyrotropin (TSH) Prolactin if indicated Fasting lipids, glucose Baseline chemistry, including electrolytes and liver function tests Mammogram Papanicolaou (Pap) smear Bone mineral density determination Calcium, phosphate, vitamin D, and parathyroid hormone estimation Vaginal ultrasound and endometrial sampling if indicated Evaluation of clotting profile if indicated

Adapted from American Association of Clinical Endocrinologists: AACE medical guidelines for clinical practice for management of menopause. Endocr Pract 1999; 5:354-366.

2. Use of hormone therapy (HT) and nonhormonal treatments in the management of menopausal symptoms and in prevention and treatment of the long-term complications of menopause (see later discussion)
3. Education of the patient with reference to her previous understanding of menopausal issues, enabling her to make an informed decision regarding the use of various treatments and, particularly, the risk and benefits of HT
4. Exploration and evaluation of relevant psychological issues and the institution of appropriate therapeutic measures (psychosocial distress, mood disorders, anxiety, cognitive impairment, and the complaint of fatigue are commonly experienced by cancer survivors); a multidisciplinary approach involving psychiatrists, psychologists, nurse practitioners, and support groups can be invaluable

Dietary and lifestyle management. Modification of dietary and lifestyle factors assists in control of menopausal symptoms and psychological symptomatology, in addition to reducing the risks of cardiovascular disease and osteoporosis. However, the impact of these modifications on cancer recurrence or mortality is unknown. Evidence from laboratory investigations, epidemiologic studies, and randomized controlled trials (RCTs) supports the following recommendations:

1. Dietary modification incorporating a low trans-saturated fat and low glycemic load, high cereal fiber, and high n-3 fatty acid content with a high ratio of polyunsaturated to saturated fat[31]
2. Calcium, 1000 to 1500 mg/day, with supplemental vitamin D, 400 to 800 U/day[32]
3. Limited caffeine intake
4. Less than 10 g/day of alcohol
5. Cessation of smoking
6. Regular exercise (including aerobic exercise, resistance training, and walking)
7. Maintenance of ideal weight

The use of dietary phytoestrogens is discussed later.

HORMONE THERAPY

The term *hormone therapy* (preferred to the term "hormone replacement therapy"), as discussed here, refers to the use of exogenous estrogen, either alone or in combination with a progestin. Newer agents that exhibit some estrogen-like effects (e.g., tibolone, raloxifene) are discussed separately.

What are the indications for the use of hormone therapy?

Although there is general consensus regarding the short-term use of HT in the management of vasomotor symptoms, controversy exists regarding long-term use, with evidence regarding the benefits of long-term HT counterbalanced by data documenting the risks. Uncertainty also exists regarding the appropriate time at which to initiate long-term therapy and the duration of therapy. Information about the benefits and risks of HT has been derived from studies involving the use of predominately unopposed oral estrogens, mainly conjugated equine estrogens (CEE), in the majority of subjects, with a minority using combined estrogen/progestin therapy (EPT). How the findings of these studies relate to the use of other estrogen preparations is unclear. This issue is further complicated by the exclusion of women with premature menopause or gynecologic cancer from recruitment into the RCTs conducted to evaluate HT use, which reduces the relevance of the study findings to this patient population. The continuing controversy regarding the risks and benefits of HT emphasizes the need to individualize therapy to the particular woman, involving her in the decision-making process. The indications for use of HT and assessment of the adverse effects is discussed in the following sections and summarized in Table 60-3.

Menopausal symptoms. A multitude of studies, both epidemiologic investigations and RCTs, attest to the benefits of estrogen therapy (ET), both alone and in combination with a progestin, in the treatment of vasomotor and urogenital symptoms associated with estrogen deficiency (see Table 60-3).[33] Evidence regarding the benefit of ET in the management of other menopausal-related symptoms, especially psychological symptoms, is less clear.[34] Younger women often require higher doses of estrogen, compared with older postmenopausal women, for relief of their symptoms.[35]

Table 60–3. Benefits and Risks of Hormone Replacement Therapy*

Outcome	Relative Risk (95% CI) from Meta-analysis and Systematic Review	Hazard Ratio (nominal 95% CI) from Women's Health Initiative with 5.2 Yr Follow-up (EPT)
Vasomotor symptom control	77% reduction (58.2-87.5%)	Not measured
Fracture		
Hip	Current use, 0.64 (0.32-1.04)	0.66 (0.45-0.98)
	Ever use, 0.76 (1.56-1.01)	
Vertebral	Ever use, 0.60 (0.36-0.99)	0.66 (0.44-0.98)
Total		0.76 (0.69-0.85)
Colorectal cancer	Current use, 0.66 (0.59-0.74)	0.63 (0.43-0.92)
	Ever use, 0.80 (0.74-0.86)	
Dementia	0.66 (0.53-0.82)	–
Breast cancer		
>5 yr use (all HT)	1.35 (1.21-1.49)	–
>5 yr use (EPT)	1.53	1.26 (1.00-1.59)
Endometrial cancer		
Unopposed estrogen	2.3 (2.1-2.5)	–
EPT	0.8 (0.6-1.2)	0.83 (0.47-1.47)
Coronary heart disease		
Observational studies	0.55-0.97	–
EPT	0.66 (0.53-0.84)	1.29 (1.02-1.63)
HERS	0.99 (0.80-1.22)	–
Stroke (nonhemorrhagic)	1.20 (1.01-1.40)	1.41 (1.07-1.85)
Thromboembolic events		
Current HT use	2.14 (1.64-2.81)	2.11 (1.58-2.82)
<1 Yr use	3.49 (2.33-5.59)	–
Gallbladder disease		
<5 Yr use	1.8 (1.6-2.0)	–
>5 Yr use (all HT)	2.5 (2.0-2.9)	–
HERS	1.44 (1.10-1.90)	–
Total mortality		
Current use >5 Yr	0.54 (0.45-0.63)	0.98 (0.82-1.18)

CI, confidence interval; EPT, combined estrogen and progestin therapy; HT, hormone therapy; HERS, Heart and Estrogen/Progestin Replacement Study.
*Controversy exists as to whether nominal or adjusted CI should be used in relation to each of the study outcomes. If adjusted 95% CI is used, statistical significance is achieved only for decreased risk of total fractures (0.63-0.92) and increased risk of thromboembolic events (1.26-3.55).
Adapted from Nelson HD, Humphrey LL, Nygren P, et al: Postmenopausal hormone replacement therapy: Scientific review. JAMA 2002;288:872-881.

Prevention of osteoporosis. Numerous studies have reported a positive effect of estrogen in regard to maintenance of calcium balance, decreased bone resorption, and increased bone mineral density (reviewed by Compston[32]). The antiresorptive effect appears to be independent of the estrogen formulation used (oral, transdermal, or parenteral) or the addition of a progestin. Although conventional doses of estrogen are considered bone-sparing, the minimal effective dose is undetermined.[36-38] A higher estrogen dose may be required in women with premature menopause.[35] Positive effects are observed regardless of the age at which ET is begun, although the effect may be attenuated if treatment is commenced at a later age.[39]

Data from epidemiologic studies[40] and results of small RCTs[39,41] demonstrate a reduction of approximately 25% in hip fractures and nonvertebral fractures and a 50% decrease in vertebral fractures among ET users (see Table 60-3). Consistent with these earlier studies are data from the Women's Health Initiative (WHI) study,[42] an RCT in which 16,608 women were enrolled in the EPT arm (0.625 mg CEE with continuous 2.5 mg medroxyprogesterone acetate [MPA]) compared with placebo. The WHI results indicated a 34% reduction in hip fracture risk (hazard ratio [HR], 0.66; nominal 95% confidence interval [CI], 0.45 to 0.98) among HT-treated women, with an absolute benefit of 5 fewer fractures per 10,000 women per year (Fig. 60-2; Table 60-4). Reductions in risks of vertebral fractures (HR, 0.66; 95% CI, 0.44 to 0.98) and other osteoporotic fractures (HR, 0.77; 95% CI, 0.69 to 0.86) was also documented (see Table 60-3).

The positive skeletal effects of estrogen decrease rapidly once therapy ceases; therefore, long-term HT use is required for the treatment of osteopenia/osteoporosis. Because most vertebral fractures occur in women who are older than 60 years of age and most hip fractures in those older than 70 years, controversy exists as to when ET should be instituted (i.e., at menopause or at 60 years, when the absolute risk of fracture increases significantly). This question is further complicated by data from the WHI study, which indicate a significantly increased risk of breast cancer, cardiovascular disease, and thromboembolic events in women treated with combined continuous HT, results which precipitated the early cessation of this arm of the trial (see Fig. 60-2 and Table 60-4). These results suggest that the risk/benefit analysis is not supportive of long-term use of this form of HT. Whether such risks and benefits are present with other types of HT (including various EPT preparations), with ET alone (the estrogen-only versus placebo arm of the WHI study continues) or with low-dose HT is unknown.

Prevention of cardiovascular disease. Cardiovascular disease is the leading cause of death among postmenopausal women in industrialized countries.[40] Laboratory studies in animals and humans have documented multiple mechanisms by which estrogens modify cardiovascular risk factors,[43] including improved lipid profile and metabolism, altered vasoreactivity, hemostatic effects, and inflammatory effects. However,

as demonstrated in both animal studies and clinical trials, the addition of a progestin appears to attenuate the beneficial effects of estrogen, an effect that varies with the type of progestin used. The Postmenopausal Estrogen/Progestins Intervention (PEPI) trial documented that treatment with CEE plus MPA (continuous or sequential) raised blood glucose levels and reduced the magnitude of the potentially beneficial rise in high-density lipoprotein, compared with treatment with CEE alone or with CEE plus micronized progesterone.[44]

Previous meta-analyses of observational studies have reported a 35% to 50% decrease in the relative risk (RR) of CHD among women using HT (predominately unopposed estrogen), compared with nonusers.[40,45] However, a recent meta-analysis[46] reported no significant reduction in CHD among current users of estrogen (summary RR, 0.97; 95% CI, 0.82 to 1.16) after excluding poor quality studies and adjusting for socioeconomic status (see Table 60-3). The benefit of ET appeared to be confined to current use of estrogen rather than past use, and the effect of the addition of a progestin on CHD risk was variable.[46] Despite the positive effect noted in many observational studies, the results of RCTs raise questions regarding the use of HT in either secondary or, more recently, primary prevention of cardiovascular events. The Heart and Estrogen/Progestin Replacement Study (HERS), a large, placebo-controlled RCT, assessed the effect of HT (0.625 mg CEE plus 2.5 mg MPA), compared with placebo, in women with known CHD.[47] Although no significant effect of HT on CHD recurrence was observed over the mean 4-year follow-up period (log rank P = .91),[47] or during the subsequently reported 6.8-year follow-up period,[48] an increased RR of CHD was apparent during the first 4 months of the treatment period, with decreased risk present in the final 2 years of the study. The RRs for each individual year were not significantly different, although the trend was (P = .009). The Estrogen Replacement and Atherosclerosis trial also noted no significant difference in progression of angiographically verified coronary atherosclerosis in women with preexisting CHD treated with CEE alone versus combined CEE/MPA versus placebo during a 3-year follow-up period.[49]

The recently published results from the WHI study described earlier also cast doubt regarding the efficacy of HT in primary prevention of CHD. An increase of 29% (nominal 95% CI, 1.02 to 1.63) in CHD events (predominately nonfatal myocardial infarction rather

Figure 60–2. Kaplan-Meier estimates of cumulative hazards for selected clinical outcomes of the Women's Health Initiative (WHI) study. Differences between the treatment and placebo groups became apparent after approximately 4 years and 3 years of follow-up, respectively, for invasive breast cancer and colorectal cancer. Divergence between treatment groups was observed shortly after randomization for coronary heart disease, stroke, and pulmonary embolism. aCI, adjusted confidence interval; HR, hazard ratio; nCI, nominal confidence interval. (Reproduced with permission from Writing Group for the Women's Health Initiative Investigators: Risks and benefits of estrogen plus progestin in healthy postmenopausal women. JAMA 2002;288:321-333.)

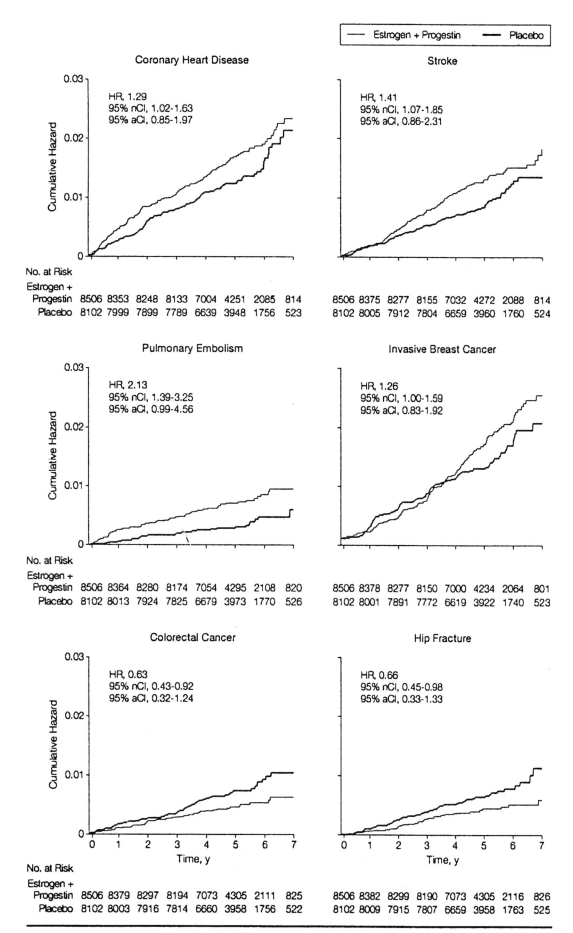

No. at Risk

Coronary Heart Disease

| Estrogen + Progestin | 8506 | 8353 | 8248 | 8133 | 7004 | 4251 | 2085 | 814 |
| Placebo | 8102 | 7999 | 7899 | 7789 | 6639 | 3948 | 1756 | 523 |

Stroke

| | 8506 | 8375 | 8277 | 8155 | 7032 | 4272 | 2088 | 814 |
| | 8102 | 8005 | 7912 | 7804 | 6659 | 3960 | 1760 | 524 |

Pulmonary Embolism

| Estrogen + Progestin | 8506 | 8364 | 8280 | 8174 | 7054 | 4295 | 2108 | 820 |
| Placebo | 8102 | 8013 | 7924 | 7825 | 6679 | 3973 | 1770 | 526 |

Invasive Breast Cancer

| | 8506 | 8378 | 8277 | 8150 | 7000 | 4234 | 2064 | 801 |
| | 8102 | 8001 | 7891 | 7772 | 6619 | 3922 | 1740 | 523 |

Colorectal Cancer

| Estrogen + Progestin | 8506 | 8379 | 8297 | 8194 | 7073 | 4305 | 2111 | 825 |
| Placebo | 8102 | 8003 | 7916 | 7814 | 6660 | 3958 | 1756 | 522 |

Hip Fracture

| | 8506 | 8382 | 8299 | 8190 | 7073 | 4305 | 2116 | 826 |
| | 8102 | 8009 | 7915 | 7807 | 6659 | 3958 | 1763 | 525 |

HR indicates hazard ratio; nCI, nominal confidence interval; and aCI, adjusted confidence interval.

Table 60–4. Outcomes of the Women's Health Initiative Study (Events per 1000 Women during a 5.2-Yr Follow-up Period)*

| | Treatment | | | Significance | |
Outcome	Active	Placebo	Excess/Deficiency	Nominal CI	Adjusted CI
Coronary heart disease	19.3	15.1	+4.2	Yes	No
Stroke	14.9	10.5	+4.4	Yes	No
Venous thromboembolism	17.8	8.3	+9.5	Yes	Yes
Pulmonary embolus	8.2	3.8	+4.4	Yes	No
Invasive breast cancer	19.5	15.3	+4.2	Yes	No
Colorectal cancer	5.3	8.3	−3.0	Yes	No
Total fractures	79	97	−21	Yes	Yes
Hip fracture	5.2	7.7	−2.5	Yes	No
Total deaths	27	27	—	No	No
Global index	88.3	76.9	11.4	Yes	No

CI, 95% confidence interval.

*The active treatment group received conjugated equine estrogen plus medroxyprogesterone acetate (versus a placebo group). The global index summarizes the balance of risks and benefits and includes stroke, pulmonary embolism, endometrial cancer, colorectal cancer, hip fracture, and death due to other causes. Controversy exists as to whether nominal or adjusted CI should be considered in relation to the study outcomes. If the adjusted 95% CI is used, statistical significance is achieved only for decreased risk of total fractures (0.63-0.92) and increased risk of thromboembolic events. Adapted from Writing Group for the Women's Health Initiative Investigators: Risks and benefits of estrogen plus progestin in healthy postmenopausal women. JAMA 2002;288:321-333.

than fatal myocardial infarction or revascularization procedures) was observed in women treated with EPT, compared with placebo (see Fig. 60-2 and Table 60-3).[42] This corresponds to an absolute risk of 7 more CHD events per 10,000 person-years (see Table 60-4). As noted in the HERS study, the difference between the two treatment groups developed within the first year after randomization (see Fig. 60-2). The authors reported that this effect was independent of age, race, BMI, prior hormone use, smoking status, blood pressure, diabetes, statin use, or aspirin use. The discrepancy between the findings of epidemiologic studies and those of RCTs remains speculative but may relate to bias in the observational studies, RCT design regarding the choice of HT regimen, age at initiation of HT, and subject characteristics. Potential biases present in the observational studies include the selection bias "healthy user effect,"[50-52] compliance bias, diagnostic detection bias, and prevalence-incidence bias.[52] In regard to the WHI study, significant cardiovascular disease risk factors were present in the study population at baseline, including a mean age greater than 60 years, past or current smoking status in 50% of subjects, and BMI greater than 25 in most subjects (with one third obese). It is therefore reasonable to conclude that the evidence from RCTs does not support the use of combined oral CEE/MPA for secondary prevention of CHD or primary prevention with initiation of therapy in older women with known risk factors such as obesity and smoking. However, the relevance of these clinical trial findings in relation to younger, nonobese women and the use of other EPT preparations remains unclear. Results from the estrogen-only arm of the WHI study (scheduled to conclude in 2005) are awaited with interest.

Evidence from observational studies suggests that cardiovascular mortality is reduced in ever-users of estrogen (RR, 0.63; 95% CI, 0.55 to 72).[40] Epidemiologic studies have also documented improved survival in women with established CHD.[53-56] Mortality due to CHD was neither increased nor decreased in women treated with HT compared with placebo in the HERS[47] or in the WHI study.[42]

Cancer prevention. Epidemiologic evidence suggests a reduced risk of colorectal cancer among women taking HT (see Table 60-3).[57,58] A meta-analysis[57] of 18 eligible studies published to September 1998 reported a 20% decrease (summary RR, 0.80; 95% CI, 0.74 to 0.86) in the risk of colon cancer and a 19% reduction (summary RR, 0.81; 95% CI, 0.72 to 0.92) in the risk of rectal cancer for women who had ever used HT compared with never-users. Current use of HT was associated with an apparently greater protection from colorectal cancer compared with ever-use (summary RR, 0.66; 95% CI, 0.59 to 0.74). Although a limited number of studies were available for analysis, similar results were observed regardless of the duration of current use, the use of CEE or estradiol compounds, or the use of combined EPT. The association between hormone use and colorectal adenomas (which tend to arise 10 to 15 years before the development of cancer) is ill defined. Consistent with the data from observational studies, WHI study investigators reported a reduction of 37% (95% CI, 0.43 to 0.92) in colorectal cancer risk in the group treated with CEE plus MPA, compared with the placebo group (see Fig. 60-2 and Table 60-3); there was an absolute risk reduction of 6 cancers per 10,000 person-years (see Table 60-4).[42] Biologic mechanisms by which estrogen could exert a protective effect include alteration in bile acid metabolism, direct effects on colonic epithelium, potential tumor suppressor effect of the estrogen receptor, and estrogen-induced suppression of the mitogen designated insulin-like growth factor-1.[57]

Data from epidemiologic studies regarding the association between HT and the prevention of other neoplasms are limited and inconsistent. HT treatment was not associated with reduced cancer risk for any other neoplasm in the WHI study.[42] No reduction in cancer risk or mortality was observed among HT users in HERS.[47]

Prevention of cognitive decline and dementia.

Numerous in vitro and in vivo studies have demonstrated biologic mechanisms by which estrogen may influence brain function. These include neurotrophic and neuroprotective effects, alteration of neurotransmitter systems, antioxidant effects, beneficial alteration of proteins associated with Alzheimer's disease (AD), and indirect favorable changes in cerebral circulation and immune function.[59] Evidence from epidemiologic studies[59,60] indicates a reduction in the risk of AD among postmenopausal estrogen users (summary odds ratio [OR], 0.66; 95% CI, 0.53 to 0.82); this result was reported in a meta-analysis of 12 studies (see Table 60-3).[60] Two meta-analyses, one of combined cohort studies and RCTs[60] and the other a later review of nine RCTs,[46] concluded that HT use was associated with improvement in certain areas of cognitive function (e.g., verbal memory, vigilance, reasoning, motor speed) in symptomatic, but not in asymptomatic, nondemented postmenopausal women. The hypothesis that the estrogen-induced reduction in menopausal symptoms (e.g., alleviation of depression and sleep disturbance) is responsible for cognitive improvement remains controversial.[60] The authors of Cochrane reviews of RCTs investigating the effects of HT on cognitive function in postmenopausal women with[61] and without dementia[62] concluded that there was no overall positive effect of HT. As with the observational studies, methodologic problems limit the interpretation of the RCTs, and the effect of age, type of menopause, type and dose of estrogen, addition of a progestin, and duration of therapy remain unresolved. In regard to the risk of dementia when HT is initiated in women who are many years postmenopausal (in contrast to the data described above obtained in women receiving HT at around the time of menopause), recent results from the Women's Health Initiative Memory Study (WHIMS)[62a] suggest an adverse effect of HT in the risk of dementia. This ancillary study of the WHI involving 4532 postmenopausal women, aged 65 years or older (53% women aged >70 years) and free of probable dementia at the time of recruitment, reported a doubling of the risk probable dementia (HR 2.05; 95% CI 1.21-3.48); with an excess of 23 cases/10000 person-year (45 vs 22 cases/10000 person-year in the EPT and placebo groups respectively; p = 0.01) (see Table 60-3). AD was the most common dementia classification although the authors note that microvascular infarcts may coexist/contribute to AD. No effect of HT on mild cognitive impairment was observed. These data are compatible with the interpretation that delaying of HT until old age is no longer associated with protective effects that may occur when HT is started at the time of declining estrogen levels—the "critical window" of exposure (Victor Henderson 2002, personal communication).

Reduction in mortality. Analysis of data from the Nurse's Health Study,[63] a prospective cohort study, indicated reduced all-cause mortality among current users of HT (mainly CEE), compared with never-users (RR, 0.63; 95% CI, 0.56 to 0.70) (see Table 60-3). This effect appeared to be secondary to a reduction in CHD-associated death (RR, 0.47; 95% CI, 0.25 to 0.49) and, to a lesser extent, in death due to cancer (RR, 0.47; 95% CI, 0.25 to 0.49). Importantly, this study provided information regarding the temporal association of HT use. The protective effect of HT appeared to be lost 5 years after cessation of use, and attenuation of the benefit of HT was observed after 10 years of use. Stratification of risk revealed that women with the lowest risk of CHD derived the least benefit from HT use. The methodologic limitations of this and other observational studies relate to the potential "healthy user" effect[50,51] and the definition of use, raising questions as to whether the observed reduction in mortality actually results from HT use or from characteristics of the user. In contrast to the results of the Nurses Health Study, no differences in mortality or cause of death were observed between women treated with EPT and those treated with placebo in either HERS[47] or the WHI[42] (despite the reported increased risk of cardiovascular and thromboembolic events or breast cancer) (see Table 60-4). The results of the estrogen-only arm of the WHI study may help to further clarify this issue.

What are the adverse effects associated with hormone therapy use?

Endometrial cancer. A causal relationship between unopposed ET and endometrial hyperplasia and carcinoma has been recognized for more than 25 years.[40,64] The risk of endometrial hyperplasia/carcinoma appears to depend on estrogen preparation, dose, and duration. Meta-analyses of 29 observational studies[65] reported a twofold increased risk of endometrial cancer among users of unopposed ET, compared with nonusers (95% CI, 2.1 to 2.5); cancer risk increased to 9.5-fold (95% CI, 7.4 to 12.3) with 10 or more years of use (see Table 60-3). Endometrial cancer risk was greater in users of CEE compared with users of synthetic estrogens (RR, 2.5 versus 1.3, respectively). The elevated risk persisted after cessation of ET for at least 5 years (RR. 2.3; 95% CI, 1.8 to 3.1). A Cochrane review[66] of 18 RCTs reported a significantly increased rate of endometrial hyperplasia among women treated with moderate-dose ET (OR, 8.3; 95% CI, 4.2 to 16.2) or with high-dose ET (OR, 10.7; 95% CI, 4.6 to 25.1), compared with placebo, after 12 months of therapy. However, the risk of endometrial hyperplasia with low-dose ET remains unclear. Longer duration of ET was associated with a further increase in the rate of hyperplasia, with a reported OR of 16.0 (95% CI, 9.3 to 27.5) after 36 months of moderate-dose ET. No increase in endometrial cancer was observed in these RCTs; however, these studies were of limited duration and of insufficient sample size to assess this outcome adequately.[66] Irregular bleeding, nonadherence to therapy, and surgical intervention were more likely with unopposed ET. Despite the increased risk of endometrial cancer associated with unopposed ET, no significant increase in mortality has been observed (RR, 2.7; 95% CI, 0.9 to 8.0).[65]

Use of EPT does not appear to be associated with an elevated risk of endometrial cancer (summary RR, 0.8; 95% CI, 0.6 to 1.2) (see Table 60-3).[65] Although of limited duration (maximum, 5 years), data from RCTs are consistent with the findings of the observational studies, with no demonstrated difference in the rate of endometrial hyperplasia/cancer among women using EPT, compared with placebo.[42,47,66] However, questions remain regarding the long-term protective effect of sequential progestin therapy. Lethaby and coreviewers[65] concluded that, with longer duration, continuous progestin therapy appeared to be more protective than sequential therapy (OR, 0.3; 95% CI, 0.1 to 0.97). At present, the optimal progestin preparation, dose, duration, and regimen for the prevention of endometrial hyperplasia/carcinoma and minimization of side effects are unknown.

Breast cancer. Concern regarding a possible increased risk of breast cancer is a major reason why women choose not to use or continue HT. This issue is complicated by lack of consensus among the many published observational studies. A meta-analysis involving a comprehensive reanalysis of the data from 51 observational studies (incorporating 52,705 women with invasive breast cancer and 108,411 control women) found no significant increased risk of breast cancer with short-term use (less than 5 years) of HT.[67] However, an increased risk of breast cancer was observed with a duration of 5 or more years of ET use (RR, 1.35; 95% CI, 1.21 to 1.49) (see Table 60-3). This increased risk was inversely proportional to weight or BMI and persisted for at least 5 years after cessation of use. Although the data were limited regarding the effects of various hormone preparations, 5 or more years use of EPT was associated with an RR of 1.53 (see Table 60-3). Recently, the Million Women study,[66a] an observational study involving 1,084,110 United Kingdom women aged 50-64 years (average age 55.9 years) who were classified according to their HT use at baseline and with an average follow-up of 2.6 years (breast cancer incidence) and 4.1 years (breast cancer mortality), reported a significant increase in the incidence of breast cancer in current users of ET (RR 1.30, 95% CI, 1.21-1.41; p < 0.0001), EPT (RR 2.00, 95% CI, 1.88-2.12; p < 0.0001) and tibolone (RR 1.45, 95% CI, 1.25-1.68; p < 0.0001). An increased risk of breast cancer was observed regardless of the formulation of ET (oral, transdermal or subcutaneous implant) or EPT (progestin constituent or type of regiman). In contrast to the previous meta-analysis,[67] an increased risk of breast cancer was observed in current HT users who had used HT for less than 5 years (ET RR 1.25, 95% CI, 1.10-1.41 and EPT RR 1.74, 95% CI, 1.60-1.89). However, it is important to note that data regarding duration of hormone use was obtained only at recruitment (several years prior to breast cancer diagnosis). Thus no reliable estimate is really possible of the relationship between duration of HT and cancer risk for this study as actual duration of use could necessarily have been greater than at recruitment for most women.

The results of the WHI are consistent with these data. This RCT was halted prematurely because the test statistic for invasive breast cancer exceeded the predetermined adverse effect boundary. It is noteworthy that 74% of the subjects in the study had not previously used HT while 26% reported varying duration of prior use. After an average of 5.2 years of follow-up, those women without prior HT use had no significant increase in breast cancer risk (HR 1.06; 95% CI, 1.00 to 1.59) compared with placebo (see Fig. 60-2, Table 6-3 and Table 60-4).[42] This difference between the treatment and placebo groups was apparent after approximately 4 years (see Fig. 60-2).[42] Interestingly, no interaction with age, BMI, family history, or age at first birth was observed. The absolute increased risk of breast cancer was therefore calculated as 8 more invasive breast cancers per 10,000 women per year (see Table 60-4).[42] Combined HT appears to be associated with a higher risk of breast cancer compared with estrogen alone, as was demonstrated by evidence derived from observational studies[58,66a,67] and RCTs, including the WHI (the estrogen-only arm of the WHI study currently continues) and the PEPI study (which assessed the effect of combined EPT on mammographic density, a surrogate marker for breast cancer).[68]

Despite a potential increase in the risk of breast cancer with HT use the effect on breast cancer mortality remains unclear; conflicting evidence is provided by the observational studies, some of which show evidence of a reduction in cancer mortality.[69,70] The Million Women study[66a] reported a marginally significant increased risk of fatal breast cancer with current (RR 1.22, 95% CI, 1.00-1.48; p = 0.05) but not past HT use, although the total number of deaths (517) in the follow-up period was small and the authors themselves cautioned regarding the reliability of this section of the data. Mortality due to breast cancer was not assessed in the WHI. Bias present in the observational studies[35] and biologic differences among tumors have been proposed to account for these findings.

Thromboembolic events. Despite methodologic limitations, data from observational studies and RCTs support the association between an increased risk of venous thromboembolism and postmenopausal estrogen use (see Table 60-3). A recent meta-analysis[71] of 12 studies reported an overall RR of 2.14 (95% CI, 1.64 to 2.81) for venous thromboembolic events (VTE) among current estrogen users (see Table 60-3). Significantly, the highest risk was observed during the first year of use (RR, 3.49; 95% CI, 2.23 to 5.59). Limited data also suggest that the risk of VTE is greater with higher estrogen doses and greater with the addition of a progestin (EPT). Consistent with these previous investigations, the WHI[42] demonstrated that women treated with EPT experienced a twofold increase in VTE (HR, 2.11; nominal 95% CI, 1.58 to 2.82), including deep venous thrombosis (HR, 2.07; nominal 95% CI, 1.49 to 2.87) and pulmonary embolism (HR, 2.13; nominal 95% CI, 1.39 to 3.25), compared with the placebo-treated group (see Fig. 60-2, Table 60-3, and Table 60-4). This corresponded to an absolute excess risk of 8 additional pulmonary emboli per 10,000 person-years. As noted in previous studies, the risk of VTE appears to decrease with time.[42] Identified risk factors for VTE in HERS[72] included hip or lower-extremity fracture, cancer, hospitalization, surgery, and later onset of menopause. Interestingly, no interaction was found between the risk of VTE and BMI, smoking status, or blood pressure in either HERS[72] or the WHI.[42] Although aspirin and statin use appeared to be protective in HERS,[47] this effect was not observed in the WHI study.[42] Additional information from the WHI regarding risk factors for VTE is awaited.

The risk of VTE is multiplied in the presence of preexisting thrombophilias or past history of VTE.[73,74] Therefore, the use of HT in women with a known genetic thrombophilia or prior history of VTE is not advocated. Routine coagulation profile screening of women who have no family or personal history of VTE before commencing HT remains controversial. Further investigation is required to delineate risk factors and those who would benefit from screening. The majority of clinical studies have involved the use of oral estrogens. The risk of VTE with transdermal estrogen is unknown, although theoretical and limited clinical data suggest a less procoagulant effect.[75] The efficacy of aspirin or temporary cessation of HT to prevent VTE in the setting of short-term acquired risk factors (e.g., lower-limb fracture, surgery) is unknown. Use of HT with anticoagulation has been reported anecdotally in women at risk for VTE.

The pathophysiology of HT-induced venous thrombosis remains ill defined but appears to involve early activation of coagulation, reduction in circulating anticoagulants, and potential effects on vascular endothelium.[71,76,77]

Stroke. Conflicting results have emerged from epidemiologic research regarding an association between HT and stroke. However, evidence from a recent meta-analysis of epidemiologic studies and from the WHI study suggests that HT is associated with an increased risk of nonhemorrhagic stroke. Nelson and coworkers[46] conducted a meta-analysis of nine observational studies and reported a significantly elevated risk of thromboembolic stroke among ever-users of estrogen (RR, 1.20; 95% CI, 1.01 to 1.40); but this effect was not observed for subarachnoid or intracerebral stroke (see Table 60-3). In addition, overall stroke mortality was slightly reduced (RR, 0.81; 95% CI, 0.71 to 0.92). These findings are consistent with those of the WHI study, which reported an increased rate of nonfatal stroke (but not fatal stroke) among women treated with EPT, compared with placebo (HR, 1.41; nominal 95% CI, 1.07 to 1.85) (see Fig. 60-2, Table 60-3, and Table 60-4). The excess risk of stroke occurred after the first year of HT use and appeared to be independent of age, BMI,

smoking status, prior stroke history, and presence of hypertension.[42] In contrast, two secondary prevention RCTs compared the risk of stroke among women with previous CHD treated with combined CEE plus MPA (HERS)[98] and among women with previous stroke treated with unopposed estradiol (Women's Estrogen and Stroke Trial)[79] with that among placebo-treated women and reported no statistical difference. In those studies, increasing age, atrial fibrillation, hypertension, diabetes mellitus, and smoking status were independent risk factors for stroke events. Therefore, HT does not appear to confer any benefit regarding stroke prevention and may indeed be associated with an increased risk of stroke, particularly in women with vascular risk factors.

Gallbladder disease. With a few exceptions, observational studies have documented an increased risk of gallstones or cholecystectomy in postmenopausal women taking exogenous estrogen. Data from the Nurses' Health Study[80] revealed an increased age-adjusted RR for cholelithiasis of 1.8 (95% CI, 1.6 to 2.0) among current estrogen users, compared with never-users, with a further elevation in risk occurring after 5 years of use (RR, 2.5; 95% CI, 2.0 to 2.0) (see Table 60-3). Past estrogen users continued to demonstrate an increased risk of cholelithiasis. Consistent with the epidemiologic studies, women treated with combined CEE plus MPA in the HERS had a marginally significant increase of 38% (95% CI, 1.00 to 1.92) in the RR of gallbladder disease (89% undergoing biliary tract surgery), compared with the placebo group.[47,81] Information from the WHI regarding gallbladder disease is awaited. The risk of gallbladder disease with nonoral estrogen preparations is unknown.

Experimental studies in animals and humans indicate that estrogen increases bile lithogenicity, leading to cholelithiasis via mechanisms including alteration in hepatic lipoprotein uptake, inhibition of biliary acid synthesis, increased biliary cholesterol, and reduction of cholesterol nucleation time.[82] Limited clinical data suggest that transdermal and oral estrogens exert similar effects.[83]

Ovarian cancer. Data regarding an association between HT and ovarian cancer are inconclusive. Evidence from earlier epidemiologic studies is conflicting[58]; however, results from a cohort study involving 44,241 women suggest an increased risk of ovarian cancer with long-term (>10 years) use of ET (RR, 1.8; 95% CI, 1.1 to 3.0) but not with short-term use of EPT (mean duration, 5.6 years).[84] No increase in ovarian cancer was observed among women using EPT in the WHI study[42] or HERS,[47] compared with placebo.

Other disorders. Observational evidence indicating an association between HT use and systemic lupus erythematosus or Raynaud's disease is inconclusive. Limited, inconclusive data exist regarding an association between HT and other cancers.

Which hormone therapy regimen should be used?

Since the advent of the use of exogenous hormones in the management of menopause, there has been evolution in the preparations available and patterns of use. The most important introduction was the use of EPT after the realization of an increased risk for endometrial malignancy in women with an intact uterus who received ET alone. Administration of estrogen may be via the oral or parenteral route; different preparations demonstrate different degrees of potency, pharmacokinetics, and biologic effects. For example, transdermal estrogen is considered to cause less mastalgia, nausea, and deep vein thrombosis than oral preparations do.[35] Recent research[36-38, 84a, 90] assessing the use of low-dose estrogen regimens (equivalent to 0.3 mg CEE) indicates a positive response in regard to menopausal symptoms, bone mineral density (BMD), lipid profile, and reduction of adverse effects. However, further studies are required to clarify the long-term risks and benefits of these HT regimens. Use of vaginal estrogens has been considered to be associated with minimal systemic absorption. However, variation in serum estrogen levels above pretreatment levels is observed with different vaginal estrogen preparations. Direct comparisons among different preparations are scarce, and long-term safety data are lacking. The dose and type of estrogen used should be individualized depending on the age of the patient, cause of menopause (surgical or nonsurgical), types of menopausal symptoms or conditions requiring therapy, smoking status, presence of concurrent disease (e.g., hepatic disease), and patient acceptance.

The oral progestin preparations that are currently available for use in combined HT include the progesterone-like C21-steroid derivatives, the testosterone-like C19-nortestosterone derivatives, and the antiandrogen, cyproterone acetate. Other modes of delivery include natural progesterone as a vaginal suppository, norethisterone combined with estradiol in a transdermal patch, and the levonorgestrel-releasing intrauterine system. Current evidence indicates that progestin-containing creams (either progesterone or plant-derived "yam" cream) do not provide effective endometrial protection.[85,86] Variation in progestin preparations and sequential regimens is observed among countries. Limited data suggest that the type of progestin may be important in regard to endometrial protection,[87] in addition to duration and dose of progestin therapy. Progestin administration during sequential therapy should continue for at least 10 to 12 days each month[88]; evidence suggests that long-cycle sequential therapy (progestin administered every 3 months) is associated with a higher incidence of endometrial hyperplasia.[66] The long-term protective effect of sequential progestin administration remains in doubt (see earlier discussion). The choice of cyclic or continuous progestin administration depends on the stage of the climacteric; studies suggest that continuous progestin use should be instituted at least 1 year after menopause (reviewed by Marsh and Whitehead[89]). Progestin-related side effects, including both physical and psychological complaints, vary according to the agent used and are a major cause of noncompliance with HT.[89] Irregular bleeding is more likely with continuous combined HT than with sequential combined HT (OR, 2.3; 95% CI, 2.1 to 2.5),[66] although the lower-dose regimens are associated with less bleeding.[90] Evidence from human and animal studies also indicates that progestins may attenuate the beneficial effects of estrogen, particularly in regard to vascular function.

The combined oral contraceptive pill, either conventional dose or low-dose, is a potential therapeutic option particularly for perimenopausal women who require contraception and for women with premature menopause.

When should treatment be instituted?

There is general consensus that treatment should be instituted early for management of menopausal symptoms, particularly in the case of women with surgical menopause or premature menopause. However, for those women without symptoms who are at risk for osteoporosis, the possibility of delayed treatment (low-dose HT beginning at approximately 60 years of age) exists. Potential advantages include reduction in the duration of therapy, facilitation of identification of women at high risk of fracture, and, because most fractures occur in women older than 65 years of age, need to treat fewer women to have a positive outcome.[35] The advantages of delayed or any HT use would need to be evaluated in regard to the adverse effects documented in the WHI.

Tibolone

Tibolone, a synthetic steroid whose metabolites have estrogenic, progestogenic, and androgenic properties, is an alternative to conventional HT. The lack of approval from the Food and Drug Administration (FDA) has restricted its use in the United States, although it is widely used in the rest of the world. After administration, the parent compound is rapidly metabolized to three active compounds: 3α-hydroxytibolone, 3β-hydroxytibolone, and a $\Delta 4$-isomer (Fig. 60-3). These metabolites exhibit differences in steroid receptor affinity, tissue specific metabolism, and concentration. The hydroxytibolone metabolites, binding to the estrogen receptor only, demonstrate estrogenic effects in regard to vasomotor symptoms, bone, and vagina, whereas the $\Delta 4$-isomer, binding to the androgen and progesterone receptors, functions as a progestogen in the endometrium but has androgenic effects in the brain and liver.[91] Interestingly, 3α-hydroxytibolone–induced inhibition of sulphatase activity in breast tissue prevents conversion of estrone to estradiol. Data from in vitro and in vivo studies suggests that tibolone may have antiestrogen and tamoxifen-like effects on the breast.[92] A recent review of RCTs[91] concluded that tibolone significantly reduces

Figure 60–3. Metabolites of tibolone. Tibolone is metabolized into three compounds that exhibit tissue-specific effects. The effects of tibolone can be characterized as stimulatory effects on the receptor (+), suppressive effect on the receptor (–), and unknown effects (?) on postmenopausal women. (Reproduced with permission of The Endocrine Society from Modelska K, Cummings S: Tibolone for postmenopausal women: Systematic review of randomised trials. J Clin Endocrinol Metab 2002;87: 16-23.

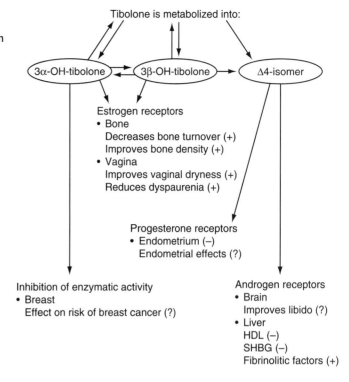

vasomotor symptoms and increases BMD in postmenopausal women. Use of tibolone is also associated with a reduction in abnormal uterine bleeding, compared with conventional continuous EPT, although bleeding rates were higher with a higher dose (5 versus 2.5 mg) and in women with recent onset of menopause. No evidence of endometrial stimulation has been observed in short-term studies. The data also suggest potential beneficial effects on sexual function, hemostasis, and lipid metabolism, but further clarification is required.[91] No increase in the rate of mastalgia or mammographic density with tibolone treatment has been noted in small RCTs.[4,93] However, the long-term effects of tibolone on reduction of fracture, cognitive function, breast cancer risk, and cardiovascular disease remains unclear. The Million Women study[66a] reported that the risk of breast cancer associated with the current use of tiblone lay between ET and EPT (see earlier discussion). However, the total number of incident cases was small (184) including only 88 women who had used tibolone as the sole form of HT. As this was an abservational study, the possibility of bias (or example, tibolone has been advocated as a preferred therapy for women at risk of breast cancer) cannot be excluded. Several RCTs are in progress to address these questions.

What is the role of estrogen in the etiology of gynecologic cancer?

Data regarding a role for estrogen in the etiology of gynecologic cancer are complex and often conflicting. A putative role is suggested by the observed association between increased levels or prolonged exposure to endogenous estrogen and risk of cancer. Earlier onset of menarche, later onset of menopause, nulliparity, delayed childbearing, increased BMI, higher BMD, and chronic anovulation are known risk factors for breast, endometrial, and ovarian cancer. The results of observational studies and RCTs also indicate an association between exogenous estrogen and gynecologic cancer (discussed earlier). Finally, extensive research has been directed at unraveling the biologic basis for this association. Steroid hormone receptors are present in all of these tissues. In vitro studies have reported variable dose-dependent effects of estrogen on cancer cell proliferation, as well as independent local regulation of estradiol levels by breast tumors. Two mechanisms of estrogen-induced carcinogenesis have been proposed (reviewed by Santen[94]): (1) estradiol stimulation of cell proliferation increases the chances of a genetic mutation with subsequent neoplastic transformation, initiation of tumor formation, and promotion of tumor growth; and (2) reactive estradiol metabolites cause depurination, leading to faulty DNA repair, genetic mutations, and tumor initiation. As with estrogen, clinical and laboratory evidence is conflicting regarding an association between progesterone and breast cancer.

Can hormone therapy be used in women with a history of gynecologic cancer?

For many years, the prevailing wisdom has been that HT is contraindicated in women with a history of gynecologic cancer, because of the perceived potential adverse effect of estrogen on disease recurrence or progression and patient survival. However, the large number of postmenopausal gynecologic cancer survivors has

Table 60–5. Use of Hormone Therapy in Women with a History of Gynecologic Cancer

Reference and Year	Study Design	No. of Subjects (Cases/Controls)	Mean Age (Yr)	Tumor Stage	Interval to Treatment after Surgery* (Mo)	Duration of HT (Mo)	Duration of Follow-up (Mo)	No. of Recurrences (Cases/Controls)
A. History of Breast Cancer								
Powles et al.[133] (1993)	Retrospective	35	51	12 Stage T1 14 Stage T2	Mean 31	Mean 14.6	Mean 14.6	2
Wile et al.[100] (1993)	Cohort	25	51	52% Stage I 28% Stage II	Mean 26	Mean 35.2	Mean 25.2	3
Eden et al.[100] (1995)	Case-control	90/180	47	80% Disease limited to breast	Median 60	Median 18	Median 36	7%/17%
Decker[135] (1996)	Cohort	61	52	39 Stage T1 or less	44.4	26.4	26.4†	5
DiSaia et al.[136] (1996)	Case-control	41/82	50	56% Stage I 22% Stage II	NS	NS	48	6/7
Peters & Jones[137] (1996)	Cohort	56	42	40 Stage 0-II	Mean 57	Mean 37	Mean 37	0
Vassilopoulou-Sellin et al.[138] (1997)	Cohort	39	45	—	Median 84	Mean 40	Mean 40	1
Beckman et al.[139] (1998)	Case-control	64	NS	56 Stage T1-T2	0	Mean 15	Mean 32	6
Espie et al.[140] (1999)	Cohort	120	45	>60% Stage T0-T2 15 Stage I 8 Stage II	Mean 96	Mean 28.8	Mean 28.8†	5
Guidozzi[141] (1999)	Cohort	24	48		Mean 34	Mean 32	Mean 68	0
Ursic-Vrscaj & Bebar[142] (1999)	Case-control	21/42	47	66% Disease limited to breast	Mean 62	Mean 28	Mean 108	4/5 19%/11%
DiSaia et al.[143] (2000)	Case-control	125/362	52	42% Stage I 22% Stage II	Mean 46	Median 22	180	Risk of all-cause mortality odds ratio, 0.28 (95% confidence interval, 0.1-0.71)
O'Meara et al.[97] (2001)	Case-control	174/695	Range 35-74	>50% Stage I or II	Range 12- > 96	Median 15	Median 44	16/101 9%/15%
HABITS	RCT in progress							

B. History of Endometrial Cancer

Creasman et al.[144] (1986)	Case-control	47/174	—	30 Stage Ia / 17 Stage Ib / 0 Stage II	Median 26	—	Range 25-150	1/26 2.1%/14.9%
Baker[145] (1990)	Cohort	31	Range 29-69	NS	Range 0-120	NS	Up to 16 years	0
Bryant[146] (1990)	Cohort	20	NS	19 Stage Ia / 1 Stage II	Range 18-24	Range 12-132	Range 42-168	0
Lee et al.[147] (1990)	Case-control	44/99	—	24 Stage Ia / 20 Stage Ib / 0 Stage II	Median (1 > 60)	—	Range 24-84	0/8 0%/8%
Gitsch et al.[148] (1995)	Retrospective	8‡	40	NS	NS	Range 12-78	Range 12-78†	0
Chapman et al.[149] (1996)	Retrospective case-control	62/61	Mean 57.6/69.3	54 Stage Ia + Ib / 6 Stage Ic / 2 Stage II	Median 8	NS	Median 39.5	26 3.2%/9.8%
Gynecologic Oncology Group	RCT	Projected 1054/1054	—	All	<3	—	60	Pending

C. History of Ovarian Cancer

Eeles et al.[103] (1991)	Retrospective case-control	78/295	Cases younger than controls	50% Stage I-II	40	28	42	17/147 deaths
Guidozzi & Daponte[105] (1999)	Nonblinded RCT	59 ERT / 66 No ERT	Range 27-59	65-70% Stage III	6-8 weeks	NS (minimum 48?)	Minimum 48	ERT: 32 (54%) Non-ERT: 41 (62%)
Ursic-Vrscaj et al.[104] (2001)	Case-control	24/4	41/43	Stage IV excluded	1-25	—	1-70	5 (21%)/15 (31%)

HT, hormone therapy; NS, not stated; RCT, randomized controlled trial.
*For breast cancer patients, interval after diagnosis/primary therapy.
†Assumed to be equal to the duration of HT use.
‡Eight of 15 patients accepted HT.

necessitated a reevaluation of this dictum. Responses to questionnaires indicate that menopausal symptoms are common among breast cancer survivors; symptom intensity rather than long-term health risks influence a woman's decision to use HT.[95] The advent of effective nonhormonal therapies for the management of certain menopausal symptoms, osteoporosis, and cardiovascular disease in postmenopausal women, in addition to concerns regarding the risks associated with HT use, has meant that HT may be considered as "second-line" therapy in some instances. Before any treatment is instituted, consideration should be given to cancer prognosis, patient age, premenopausal or postmenopausal status, clinical symptoms, and patient concerns and wishes.

Hormone therapy use in women with a history of breast cancer. A number of observational studies have attempted to address the question of HT use in women with previous breast cancer (Table 60-5A). However, methodologic limitations, including retrospective design, lack of randomization, small sample size, lack of a control group, selection bias, short duration of follow-up, concurrent tamoxifen use, and differing estrogen doses or preparations (vaginal or oral predominantly) mean that cautious interpretation of the results is required. Col and coinvestigators[96] conducted a review and meta-analysis of 11 eligible studies from among 28 published reports to 1999. They reported no significant increase in the risk of recurrence among breast cancer survivors using HT (RR, 0.82; 95% CI, 0.58 to 1.15) (Fig. 60-4). They concluded that their findings "may be limited to women who have been disease free for several years and who take HT for 2 years or less."[96] A subsequent case-control study[97] reported a decreased risk of recurrence (RR, 0.5; 95% CI, 0.3 to 0.85) and mortality (RR, 0.48; 95% CI, 0.29 to 0.78) among women with previous breast cancer using HT. No difference was observed between oral and vaginal estrogen use, or with unopposed versus combined therapy. Data from biologic studies suggests that

continuous progestin may be preferable to sequential progestin use.[98] Vasomotor symptom control, efficacy in the treatment of advanced breast cancer, and in vitro antiproliferative effects[99] provided the basis for the decision to use a moderate-dose (equivalent to 50 mg MPA) continuous progestin regimen as described in the Australian cohort.[100,101] However, the optimal HT regimen for this patient population remains unknown. Further clarification will be obtained from the Hormones After Breast Cancer: Is It Safe (HABITS) RCT.

Hormone therapy use in women with a history of endometrial cancer. The few studies that have investigated the question of HT use in women with a history of endometrial cancer have failed to demonstrate any increase in recurrence or in death rate among HT users (see Table 60-5, part B). However, these studies were limited by a number of methodologic flaws, including small sample size, retrospective design, selection bias, and variations in HT preparation used, time before institution of HT, cancer diagnosis, and disease severity. Therefore the data, although encouraging, do not provide definitive support for the use of HT in women with a history of gynecologic cancer. The patients treated with HT were often younger and included those with significant estrogen deficiency symptoms, earlier-stage disease, and fewer intercurrent illnesses (where assessed). Oral or vaginal estrogens (or both) were the predominant preparations used, and 30% to 50% of patients were treated with additional progestin. The results of the prospective Gynecologic Oncology Group study, a double-blind, placebo-controlled RCT investigating the effects of CEE treatment on recurrence-free and overall survival in women with a history of stage I or II endometrial cancer, will help to clarify this issue. The American College of Obstetrics and Gynecologists[102] concluded that there is insufficient evidence to support specific recommendations regarding the use of HT in women with a history of endometrial cancer. They commented that, although the indications for use of HT in this population are similar

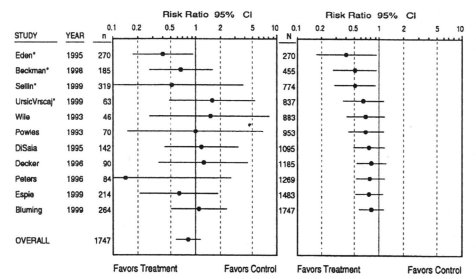

Figure 60-4. Relative risks (RR) of recurrent breast cancer associated with hormone replacement therapy. The left side of the figure represents each study individually, whereas the right side represents a cumulative meta-analysis. (This analysis appeared before the publication of the report by O'Meara and coworkers.[97]) The RR of recurrent breast cancer is denoted by the ● symbol, and the 95% confidence interval by the solid lines. Studies that included a control group are indicated by an asterisk. (Reproduced with permission from Col NF, Hirota LK, Orr RK, et al: Hormone replacement therapy after breast cancer: A systematic review and quantitative assessment of risk. J Clin Oncol 2001;19:2357-2363.)

to those for other women, candidates should be selected on the basis of prognostic indicators such as depth of invasion, degree of differentiation and cell type, and the risk the patient is willing to assume.[102] Despite theoretical advantages, whether the addition of continuous progestin to ET or the use of tibolone provides any advantage over the use of unopposed estrogen in these women who have undergone previous hysterectomy is unknown.

Hormone therapy use in women with a history of ovarian cancer. The two observational studies and one RCT (see Table 60-5, part C) that have investigated the use of HT in women with a history of epithelial ovarian carcinoma reported no adverse effect on recurrence or survival rate. The retrospective study of Eeles and coworkers[103] was limited by small sample size, selection bias to patients with earlier-stage disease, and short follow-up. The small case-control study[104] compared 24 women with significant menopausal symptoms who were treated with oral estrogen (combined with a progestin in 30% of subjects) with 48 control women matched for age, disease stage, cancer treatment, and follow-up. HT was initiated at an average of 21 months after diagnosis and continued for approximately 2 years. The RCT of ovarian cancer survivors,[105] in which women were randomly assigned to CEE treatment or no ET, was also limited by small sample size. Within each group, recurrence was more likely among those with poorly differentiated tumors, more advanced disease, and suboptimal primary surgery. The use of transdermal estrogens or tibolone has not been investigated in this patient population.

Hormone therapy use in women with a history of cervical cancer. Limited evidence from observational studies suggests that noncontraceptive hormone use is associated with a decreased risk of carcinoma of the cervix.[106,107] In addition, HT was not associated with increased risk of virus carriage or replication in a study of human papilloma virus (HPV) infection in postmenopausal women.[108] No published studies specifically addressing the question of HT use in women with previous cervical cancer could be found.

What is the role of androgen therapy in postmenopausal women with a history of gynecologic cancer?

Androgen deficiency, as a clinical entity, has been recognized mainly in women with hypopituitarism, adrenal insufficiency, or ovarian failure (premature menopause or therapeutic intervention including oophorectomy).[109] The occurrence of clinical androgen insufficiency (and the perceived benefits of testosterone therapy) in women who have undergone spontaneous physiologic menopause remains controversial. The presence of characteristic symptoms, including diminished well-being, decreased sexual function, dysphoric mood, and fatigue, in the setting

of a low serum testosterone concentration is required for the diagnosis of female androgen deficiency.[110] Improvement in sexual function, well-being, and energy levels with maintenance of BMD has been reported in small studies of postmenopausal women treated with pharmacologic doses of testosterone plus estrogen, compared with placebo or estrogen-only therapy.[109] The largest study[111] investigated 75 women who had undergone oophorectomy and hysterectomy before menopause and were receiving conventional ET; they were randomly assigned to treatment with either transdermal testosterone patches (150 or 300 μg/day) or placebo for 12 weeks. A significant increase in well-being and parameters of sexual function was observed in women treated with the higher testosterone dose, compared with placebo. The lack of specific androgen formulations for women has necessitated the adaption and use of testosterone preparations designed for men.[109] Recognized side effects of androgen therapy include virilization (which is minimized if testosterone levels approximate the physiologic range) and unfavorable lipid changes (associated with oral androgen use). There are no data regarding the use of androgen therapy in postmenopausal women with a history of gynecologic cancer. Potential disadvantages of androgen therapy in this clinical setting include the requirement for concurrent ET with testosterone therapy to avoid virilization and the potential for aromatization of testosterone to estradiol. However, there is abundant clinical evidence that androgens normally inhibit mammary epithelial proliferation,[80] and clinical trials to assess the effects of combined estrogen/androgen therapy on breast cancer risk and recurrence are needed. Tibolone, with its reported beneficial effects on libido and well-being, is a potential alternative to testosterone therapy, although its efficacy in the treatment of androgen deficiency has not been studied.

USE OF OTHER THERAPIES IN POSTMENOPAUSAL WOMEN WITH A HISTORY OF GYNECOLOGIC CANCER

What is the role of selective estrogen receptor modulators?

Raloxifene, a serum estrogen receptor modulator (SERM) (Fig. 60-5), displays estrogen agonist effects on bone, brain, and lipids and antagonist effects on the uterus and breast. The Multiple Outcomes of Raloxifene (MORE) study, a double-blind, placebo-controlled RCT involving 7705 postmenopausal women with osteoporosis (based on dual-energy x-ray absorptiometry [DEXA] or fracture criteria), reported a 39% decrease (95% CI, 0.43 to 0.88) in new vertebral fracture risk among women treated with 60 mg raloxifene after 4 years of follow-up.[112] Although an increase in BMD was observed, nonvertebral fracture risk was not significantly reduced. Importantly, use of raloxifene was associated with a significant decrease in the risk of estrogen receptor–positive breast cancer

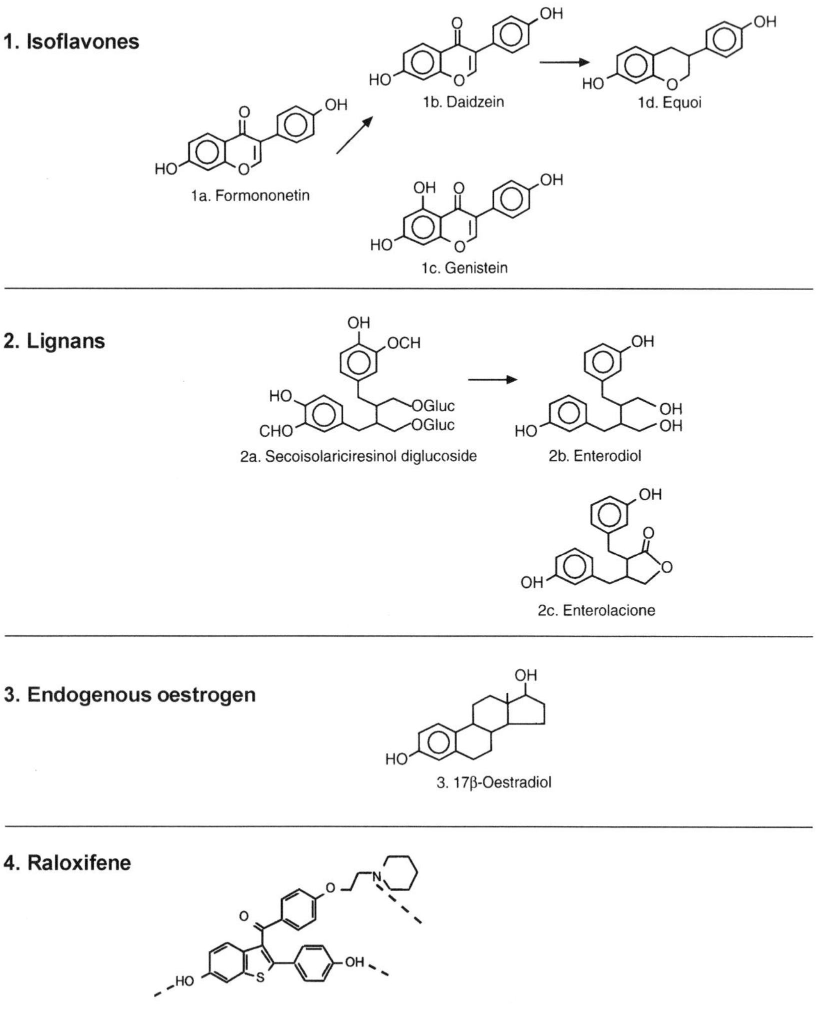

Figure 60–5. A comparison of the chemical structures of estrogen, phytoestrogens and the selective estrogen receptor modulators (SERMs). Structural similarities to 17β-estradiol can be observed in the phytoestrogens (isoflavones and lignans) and in the SERM, raloxifene. (Adapted from Warren M, Shortle B, Dominguez J: Use of alternative therapies in menopause. Best Prac Res Clin Obstet Gynecol 2002;16:411-448.)

(RR, 0.24; 95% CI, 0.13 to 0.44), corresponding to an absolute risk reduction of 7.9 cases per 1000 women over the 40-month follow-up period.[113] No effect of raloxifene on endometrial cancer risk[113] or on overall cognitive scores was demonstrated in the MORE study after 3 years.[114] Beneficial effects of raloxifene treatment on surrogate markers for cardiovascular disease have been reported,[115,116] including altered lipid profile (reduction in low-density lipoprotein, increased high-density lipoprotein, no increase in triglycerides), reduction in lipoprotein(a), decrease in serum homocysteine, and reduction in fibrinogen. In addition, secondary analysis revealed that the risk of cardiovascular events (coronary and cerebrovascular events) was significantly reduced in the subset of women with high cardiovascular risk (RR, 0.60; 95% CI, 0.38 to 0.95), although no significant effect was observed in the overall MORE cohort.[117] The effect of raloxifene on primary and secondary prevention of cardiovascular disease is being investigated in the ongoing Raloxifene Use in the Heart (RUTH) RCT. Raloxifene does not relieve menopausal symptoms and may induce or exacerbate vasomotor symptoms. Other adverse effects of raloxifene include an increase

in the risk of VTE (similar to that with HT) and leg cramps.

Studies investigating tamoxifen, the first-generation SERM used in the management of breast cancer, have demonstrated favorable effects on lipid profile and BMD but increased risks for endometrial cancer, VTE, and vasomotor and urogenital symptoms.[118] Information regarding the combined use of estrogen and tamoxifen is obtained from the tamoxifen prevention studies, in which approximately 25% of subjects were receiving ET and tamoxifen. Beneficial effects on vasomotor symptoms and BMD without detrimental effects on coagulation parameters were observed.[119] In addition, subgroup analysis of the Italian Tamoxifen Prevention Study revealed a significant decrease in breast cancer incidence among women using ET who were treated with tamoxifen, compared with those using ET who were treated with placebo (HR, 0.36; 95% CI, 0.14 to 0.91).[118] The Study of Tamoxifen and Raloxifene (STAR) trial is an ongoing RCT designed to compare the efficacy of tamoxifen or raloxifene in prevention of primary breast cancer in high-risk postmenopausal women. Preliminary evidence suggests that a new SERM, arzoxifene, is active in the treatment of advanced endometrial and breast cancer.[120]

What is the role of phytoestrogens?

Phytoestrogens are plant-derived, estrogen-like compounds that exhibit both agonist and antagonist properties and have been the subject of several recent reviews.[121,122] There are three main classes of phytoestrogens: isoflavones, lignans, and coumestans (see Fig. 60-5). Genistein and diadzein, found in soybeans, possess the greatest estrogenic activity. Laboratory research indicates that phytoestrogens exhibit both estrogen receptor–dependent and independent effects on multiple biologic systems. Despite observational studies indicating potential benefits of phytoestrogens in regard to cardiovascular risk factors, vasomotor symptoms, and urogenital atrophy, data from interventional studies are inconclusive.[122] Evidence regarding phytoestrogen effects on bone and cognition is limited and inconsistent. Epidemiologic evidence suggests an inverse association between phytoestrogen intake and the risk of breast or endometrial cancer, but human and animal interventional studies have demonstrated conflicting results with respect to breast cancer.[121,122] More research is required to establish the efficacy and safety of phytoestrogens before recommendations can be made for their use in the management of menopause in women with previous gynecologic cancer.

What nonestrogenic therapies are available for the relief of menopausal symptoms?

The existence of effective nonestrogenic therapies increases the therapeutic options available to clinicians for the management of mild to moderate vasomotor symptoms in women with a history of gynecologic cancer. Loprinzi and coworkers[123] reported a significant reduction in vasomotor symptoms among postmenopausal breast cancer survivors randomly assigned to treatment with the selective serotonin- and noradrenaline-reuptake inhibitor, venlafaxine, compared with placebo. Low-dose therapy (37.5 and 75 mg) was as effective as the higher 150 mg dose and was associated with a lower rate of side effects. Fluoexetine[124] and paroxetine,[125] selective serotonin reuptake inhibitors, also appear to decrease hot flush frequency and severity. High-dose progestins including megestrol acetate, MPA, and norethisterone are effective in relieving vasomotor symptoms in approximately 60% of patients. Limited clinical evidence suggests that high-dose progestin therapy is associated with a reduction in the risks of secondary breast cancer and spread of endometrial cancer.[99] A significant reduction in hot flush frequency was observed with the administration of clonidine; however, use of this medication is limited by adverse effects, including dry mouth, constipation, and drowsiness.

Nonhormonal therapy for urogenital atrophy consists of vaginal moisturizers, used chronically to improve symptoms, and lubricants, used before sexual intercourse. Use of a vaginal moisturizer decreases vaginal pH, improves vaginal elasticity, and reverses vaginal atrophy, albeit to a lesser extent than vaginal estrogen cream.[126]

What is the role of herbal therapies?

Considerable interest has been expressed by women regarding the use of herbal therapies. This may relate in part to their availability without prescription and also the misconception that these compounds are "natural" and therefore safe. However, these remedies exhibit medicinal properties and there is increasing recognition of adverse effects, including interaction with conventional pharmaceuticals. As denoted by Germany's Commission E, specific herbs that are purported to be efficacious for particular menopausal symptoms (e.g., vasomotor instability, urogenital atrophy, psychological symptoms, sexual functioning) include ginseng, passion flower, St. John's wort, valerian, balm, black cohosh, chaste tree, and ginkgo (reviewed by Warren and colleagues[122]). Although estrogen-like effects have been observed with the use of black cohosh,[122] a short-term RCT conducted to assess the efficacy this herb on vasomotor symptoms in women with breast cancer demonstrated no difference from placebo.[127] The safety of these therapies in women with previous gynecologic cancer is unknown. However, a recent in vitro study demonstrated that ginseng and dong quai (but not black cohosh) increased the growth of a human breast cancer cell line.[128]

What alternative therapies are available for management of osteoporosis?

Drugs that act to inhibit bone resorption include the bisphosphonates, synthetic analogs of pyrophosphate, and calcitonin. In RCTs, oral bisphosphonates, including cyclic etidronate, alendronate, and risedronate, were demonstrated to increase BMD; a significant reduction in hip, spine, and nonvertebral fractures was observed among postmenopausal women with osteoporosis treated with the latter two agents (reviewed by Compston[32]). More recently, an RCT involving the intravenously administered bisphosphonate, zoledronic acid, also demonstrated antifracture efficacy in postmenopausal women with osteopenia/osteoporosis.[129] Inhibition of bony metastases and treatment of malignancy associated hypercalcemia are additional relevant clinical effects of bisphosphonates. Antifracture efficacy has also been demonstrated for intranasal calcitonin. Subcutaneous parathyroid hormone therapy stimulates bone formation; significant increases in BMD and reductions in vertebral and nonvertebral fractures were demonstrated in short-term RCTs involving postmenopausal women (reviewed by Rosen and Bilezikian[130]).

Summary

Demographic trends combined with therapeutic interventions have meant that a greater number of women with a history of gynecologic cancer are experiencing menopause. Although the evidence is encouraging, definitive data regarding HT use and disease recurrence or mortality are lacking. Recent studies also raise questions regarding the long-term use of HT. For most women, climacteric symptom control, rather than long-term disease prevention, is the primary concern and reason for considering HT. A prudent approach would advocate risk factor management through dietary and lifestyle changes and the initial use of nonhormonal therapies for the control of vasomotor symptoms, cardiovascular disease, and osteoporosis. If such agents are ineffective, and after informed patient consent, a trial of HT could be instituted. Introduction of the lowest effective estrogen dose and use of drugs, such as tibolone, that have theoretical advantages over conventional HT are reasonable choices. However, there are no data on the safety of tibolone in women with gynecologic cancer. The SERMS offer future promise in regard to osteoporosis, cardiovascular disease, and breast cancer prevention. The efficacy and safety of phytoestrogens, herbal therapies, and homeopathic preparations have yet to be determined. The 1998 Consensus Statement[9] regarding breast cancer patients is applicable to women with gynecologic cancer: "We should seek other established symptomatic or health promoting interventions before considering the use of estrogens. When estrogen is used as a last resort, it should be used in the lowest dose for the shortest duration of time and only after full discussion of concerns regarding potential risks with respect to breast cancer outcomes. When estrogen is being considered, the role of the informed woman as the final decision maker should be accepted by the health care practitioner."

REFERENCES

1. Landis SH, Murray T, Bolden S, et al: Cancer statistics. CA Cancer J Clin 1998;48:6-29.
2. Treloar AE: Menstrual cyclicity and the premenopause. Maturitas 1981;3:249-264.
3. McKinley S, Brambilla DJ, Posner JG: The normal menopause transition. Maturitas 1992;14:103-115.
4. Gruber C, Tschugguel W, Schneeberger C, et al: Production and action of estrogens. N Engl J Med 2002;346:340-352.
5. Wallace RB, Sherman BM, Bean JA, et al: Probability of menopause with increasing duration of amenorrhea in middle aged women. Am J Obstet Gynecol 1979;135:1021-1024.
6. McKinley SM, Bifano NL, McKinley JB: Smoking and age at menopause. Ann Intern Med 1985;103:350-356.
7. Whelan EA, Sandler DP, McConnaughey DR, et al: Menstrual and reproductive characteristics and age at natural menopause. Am J Epidemiol 1990;131:625-632.
8. Richardson SJ The biological basis of the menopause. Bailliere's Best Pract Res Clin Endocrinol Metab 1993;7:1-16.
9. Santen RJ: Consensus statement: Treatment of oestrogen deficiency symptoms in women surviving breast cancer. J Clin Endocrinol Metab 1998;83:1993-2000.
10. Santen RJ, Pritchard K, Burger HG: The consensus conference on treatment of estrogen deficiency symptoms in women surviving breast cancer. Obstet Gynecol Surv 1998;53:S1-S83.
11. Goodwin PJ, Ennis M, Pritchard KI, et al: Risk of menopause during the first year after breast cancer diagnosis. J Clin Oncol 1999;17:2365-2370.
12. Early Breast Cancer Trialists' Collaborative Group: Polychemotherapy for early breast cancer: An overview of the randomized clinical trials. Lancet 1998;352:930-942.
13. Reichman BS, Green KB:. Breast cancer in young women: Effect of chemotherapy on ovarian function, fertility, and birth defects. Monogr Natl Cancer Inst 1994;125-129.
14. Bines J, Oleske DM, Cobleigh MA: Ovarian function in premenopausal women treated with adjuvant chemotherapy for breast cancer. J Clin Oncol 1996;14:1718-1729.
15. Siddle N, Sarrel P, Whitehead MI: The effect of hysterectomy on the age at ovarian failure: Identification of a subgroup of women with premature loss of ovarian function and literature review. Fertil Steril 1987;47:94-100.
16. Riedel HH, Lehmann-Willenbrock E, Semm K: Ovarian failure after hysterectomy. J Reprod Med 1986;31:597-600.
17. Parker M, Bosscher J, Barnhill D, et al: Ovarian management during radical hysterectomy in the premenopausal patient. Obstet Gynecol 1993;82:187-190.
18. Cann CE, Martin MC, Genant HK, et al: Decreased spinal, mineral content in amenorrhoeic women. JAMA 1984;251:626-629.
19. Jones KP, Ravnikar VA, Tulchinsky D, et al: Comparison of bone density in amenorrhoeic women due to athletics, weight loss and premature menopause. Obstet Gynecol 1985;66:5-8.
20. Rosenburg L, Hennekens CH, Rosner B: Early menopause and the risk of myocardial infarction. Am J Obstet Gynecol 2002;139:47-51.
21. Gordon T, Kannel WB, Bjortland MC, et al: Menopause and coronary heart disease: The Framingham study. Ann Intern Med 1978;89:157.
22. Sznajderman M, Oliver MF: Spontaneous premature menopause, ischaemic heart disease and serum lipids. Lancet 1963;1:1962.
23. Paganini-Hill A, Ross RK, Henderson BE: Post-menopausal oestrogen treatment and stroke—a prospective study. BMJ 1988;297:519-522.
24. Muscari L, Aikin J, Good B: Premature menopause after cancer treatment. Cancer Pract 1999;7:114-121.
25. Boughton M: Premature menopause: Multiple disruptions between the woman's biological body experiences and her lived body. J Adv Nurs 2002;37:423-430.
26. Oldenhave A, Jaszmann LJ, Everaerd WT, et al: Hysterectomized women with ovarian conservation report more severe climacteric complaints than do normal climacteric women of similar age. Am J Obstet Gynecol 1993;168:765-771.
27. Clinical Synthesis Panel on HRT: Hormone replacement therapy. Lancet 1999;354:152-155.
28. De Laet CEDH, Pols HAP: Fractures in the elderly: Epidemiology and demography. Bailliere's Best Pract Res Clin Endocrinol Metab 2000;14:171-179.
29. World Health Organization: Assessment of fracture risk and its application to screening for postmenopausal osteoporosis. Geneva: WHO, 1994.
30. Anonymous. Consensus development conference: diagnosis, prophylaxis and treatment of osteoporosis. Am J Med 1993;94:646-650.
31. Stampfer M, Hu F, Manson J, et al: Primary prevention of coronary heart disease in women through diet and lifestyle. N Engl J Med 2000;343:16-22.
32. Compston J: Prevention of osteoporotic fractures in postmenopausal women. Bailliere's Best Pract Res Clin Endocrinol Metab 2000;14:251-264.
33. MacLennan A, Lester S, Moore V: Oral oestrogen replacement therapy versus placebo for hot flushes. Cochrane Library 2002;1-20.
34. Greendale G, Reboussin B, Hogan P, et al: Symptom relief and side effects of postmenopausal hormones: Results from the

Postmenopausal Estrogen/Progestin Interventions trial. Obstet Gynecol 1998;92:982-988.

35. Barrett-Connor E: Hormone replacement therapy. BMJ 1998;317: 457-461.

36. Ettinger B, Genant HK, Cann CE: Postmenopausal bone loss is prevented by treatment with low-dosage estrogen with calcium. Ann Intern Med 1987;106:40-45.

37. Genant HK, Lucas J, Weiss S, et al: Low-dose esterified estrogen therapy: Effect on bone, plasma oestradiol concentrations, endometrium, and lipid levels. Estratab/Osteoporosis Study Group. Arch Intern Med 1997;157:2609-2615.

38. Lindsay R, Gallagher JC, Kleerekoper M, et al: Effect of lower doses of conjugated equine estrogens with and without medroxy-progesterone acetate on bone in early postmenopausal women. JAMA 2002;287:2668-2676.

39. Torgerson DJ, Bell-Syer SEM: Hormone replacement therapy and prevention of nonvertebral fractures. A meta-analysis of randomized trials. JAMA 2001;285:2891-2897.

40. Grady D, Rubin SM, Petitti DB, et al: Hormone therapy to prevent disease and prolong life in postmenopausal women. Ann Intern Med 1992;117:1016-1037.

41. Nachtigall L, Nachtigall R, Beckman E: Estrogen replacement therapy. I. A 10-year prospective study in the relationship to osteoporosis. Obstet Gynecol 1979;53:277-281.

42. Writing Group for the Women's Health Initiative Investigators: Risks and benefits of estrogen plus progestin in healthy postmenopausal women. JAMA 2002;288:321-333.

43. Teede H: Hormone replacement therapy and the prevention of cardiovascular disease. Hum Reprod Update 2002;8: 201-215.

44. Writing group for the PEPI: Effects of estrogen or estrogen/progestin regimens on heart disease risk factors in postmenopausal women: The Postmenopausal Estrogen/Progestin Interventions Trial. JAMA 1995;273:199-208.

45. Barrett-Connor E, Grady D: Hormone replacement therapy, heart disease and other considerations. Annu Rev Pub Health 1998;19:55-72.

46. Nelson HD, Humphrey LL, Nygren P, et al: Postmenopausal hormone replacement therapy: Scientific review. JAMA 2002; 288:872-881.

47. Hulley S, Grady D, Bush T, et al: Randomized trial of estrogen plus progestin for secondary prevention of coronary heart disease in postmenopausal women. JAMA 1998;280:605-613.

48. Grady D, Herrington D, Bittner V, et al: Cardiovascular disease outcomes during 6.8 years of hormone therapy: Heart and Estrogen/Progestin Replacement study follow-up (HERS II). JAMA 2002;288:49-57.

49. Herrington D, Reboussin B, Brosnihan KB, et al: Effects of estrogen replacement on the progression of coronary-artery atherosclerosis. N Engl J Med 2000;343:522-529.

50. Sturgeon S, Schairer C, Brinton L, et al: Evidence of a healthy estrogen user survivor effect. Epidemiology 1995;6:227-231.

51. Grodstein F: Can selection bias explain the cardiovascular benefits of estrogen replacement therapy. Am J Epidemiol 1996; 143:979-982.

52. Barrett-Connor E, Stuenkel C: Hormones and heart disease in women: Heart and estrogen/progestin replacement study in perspective. J Clin Endocrinol Metab 1999;84:1848-1853.

53. Henderson B, Paganini-Hill A, Ross RK: Estrogen replacement therapy and protection from acute myocardial infarction. Am J Obstet Gynecol 1988;159:312-317.

54. Stampfer M, Willett W, Colditz G, et al: A prospective study of postmenopausal estrogen therapy and coronary heart disease. N Engl J Med 1985;313:1044-1049.

55. Newton KM, LaCroix AZ, McKnight B, et al: Estrogen replacement therapy and prognosis after first myocardial infarction. Am J Epidemiol 1997;145:269-277.

56. Sullivan J, El-Zeky F, Vander Zwagg R, et al: Effect of survival of estrogen replacement therapy after coronary bypass grafting. Am J Cardiol 2002;1997:847-850.

57. Grodstein F, Newcomb PA, Stampfer M: Postmenopausal hormone therapy and the risk of colorectal cancer: A review and meta-analysis. Am J Med 1999;106:574-582.

58. La Vecchia C, Brinton L, McTiernan A: Menopause, hormone replacement therapy and cancer. Maturitas 2001;39:97-115.

59. Henderson VW: Oestrogens and dementia. In Chadwick DJ, Goode JA (eds.): Neuronal and Cognitive Effects of Oestrogens. Chichester, UK: John Wiley & Sons, 2000 (pp. 254-274).

60. LeBlanc E, Janowsky J, Chan BKS, et al: Hormone replacement therapy and cognition: Systematic review and meta-analysis. JAMA 2001;285:1489-1499.

61. Hogervorst E, Yaffe K, Richards M, et al: Hormone replacement therapy to maintain cognitive function in women with dementia (Cochrane review). Cochrane Library (AB003799) 2002.

62. Hogervorst E, Yaffe K, Richards M, et al: Hormone replacement therapy for cognitive function in postmenopausal women (Cochrane review). Cochrane Library (AB003122) 2002.

62a. Schumaker SA, Legault C, Rapp SR et al: Estrogen plus progestin and the incidence of dementia and mild cognitive impairment in postmenopausal women. JAMA 2003;289:2651-2662.

63. Grodstein F, Stampfer M, Colditz G, et al: Postmenopausal hormone replacement therapy and mortality. N Engl J Med 1997; 336:1769-1775.

64. Ziel HK, Finkle WD: Increased risk of endometrial carcinoma among users of conjugated estrogens. N Engl J Med 1975; 293:1167-1170.

65. Grady D, Gebretsadik T, Kerlikowske K, et al: Hormone replacement therapy and endometrial cancer risk: A meta-analysis. Obstet Gynecol 1995;85:304-313.

66. Lethaby A, Farquhar C, Sarkis A, et al: Hormone replacement therapy in postmenopausal women: Endometrial hyperplasia and irregular bleeding. Cochrane Library (AB000402) 2002.

66a. Million Women Study Collaborators. Breast cancer and hormone-replacement therapy in the million women study. Lancet 2003;362:419-427.

67. Collaborative Group on Hormonal Factors in Breast Cancer:. Breast cancer and hormone replacement therapy: Collaborative reanalysis of data from 51 epidemiological studies of 52705 women with breast cancer and 108411 women without breast cancer. Lancet 1997;350:1047-1059.

68. Greendale G, Reboussin B, Sie A, et al:. Effects of estrogen and estrogen-progestin on mammographic parenchymal density. Ann Intern Med 1999;130:262-269.

69. Bergkvist L, Adami H, Persson I, et al: Prognosis after breast cancer diagnosis in women exposed to estrogen and estrogen-progestogen replacement therapy. Am J Epidemiol 1989;130: 221-228.

70. Henderson BE, Paganini-Hill A, Ross RK: Decreased mortality in users of estrogen replacement therapy. Arch Intern Med 1991;151:75-78.

71. Miller J, Chan BKS, Nelson HD: Postmenopausal estrogen replacement and risk for venous thromboembolism: A systematic review and meta-analysis for the U.S. Preventative Services Task Force. Ann Intern Med 2002;136:680-690.

72. Grady D, Wenger N, Herrington D, et al: Postmenopausal hormone therapy increases risk for venous thromboembolic disease. The Heart and Estrogen/progestin Replacement Study. Ann Intern Med 2000;132:689-696.

73. Hoibraaten E, Qvigstad E, Arneson H, et al: Increased risk of recurrent thromboembolism during hormone replacement therapy: Results of a the randomized double-blind, placebo-controlled estrogen in venous thromboembolism trial (EVTET). Thromb Haemost 2000;84:961-967.

74. Lowe G, Woodward M, Vessey M, et al: Thrombotic variables and risk of idiopathic venous thromboembolism in women aged 45-64 years: Relationships to hormone replacement therapy. Thromb Haemost 2000;83:530-535.

75. Hoibraaten E, Os I, Seljeflot I, et al: The effects of hormone replacement therapy on hemostatic variables in women with angiographically verified coronary artery disease: Results from the estrogen in women with atherosclerosis study. Thromb Res 2000;98:19-27.

76. Teede H, McGrath B, Smolich J, et al: Postmenopausal hormone replacement therapy increases coagulation activity and fibrinolysis. Arterioscler Thromb Vasc Biol 2000;20:1404-1409.

77. Hoibraaten E, Qvigstad E, Anderson T, et al: The effects of hormone replacement therapy (HRT) on hemostatic variables in women with previous venous thromboembolism: Results from a randomized double blind, clinical trial. Thromb Haemost 2001; 85:775-781.

78. Simon J, Hsia J, Cauley J, et al: Postmenopausal hormone therapy and the risk of stroke: The Heart and Estrogen-progestin Replacement Study (HERS). Circulation 2001;103:638-642.

79. Viscoli C, Brass L, Kernan W, et al: A clinical trial of estrogen-replacement therapy after ischemic stroke. N Engl J Med 2001; 345:1243-1249.

80. Grodstein F, Colditz G, Stampfer M: Postmenopausal hormone use and cholecystectomy in a large prospective study. Obstet Gynecol 1994;83:5-11.

81. Simon J, Hunninghake D, Agarwal S, et al: Effect of estrogen plus progestin on risk for biliary tract surgery in post-menopausal women with coronary artery disease. The Heart and Estrogen/progestin Replacement Study. Ann Intern Med 2001;135:493-501.

82. Everson G, McKinley C, Kern FJ: Mechanisms of gallstone formation in women. J Clin Invest 1991;87:237-246.

83. Uhler M, Marks J, Voigt B, Judd H: Comparison of the impact of transdermal versus oral oestrogens on biliary markers of gallstone formation in postmenopausal women. J Clin Endocrinol Metab 1998;83:410-414.

84. Lacey JV, Mink PJ, Lubin JH, et al: Menopausal hormone replacement therapy and risk of ovarian cancer. JAMA 2002; 288:334-347.

84a. Utian WH, Shoupe D, Bachmann G, et al: Relief of vasomotor symptoms and vaginal atrophy with lower doses of conjugated equine estrogens and medroxyprogesterone acetate. Fertil Steril 2001;75:1065-1079.

85. Cooper A, Spencer C, Whitehead MI, et al: Systemic absorption of progesterone from progest cream in postmenopausal women. Lancet 1998;351:1255-1256.

86. Wren B, McFarland K, Edwards L, et al: Effect of sequential transdermal progesterone cream on endometrium, bleeding pattern, and plasma progesterone and salivary progesterone levels in postmenopausal women. Climacteric 2000;3:155-160.

87. Weiderpass E, Adami H, Baron J, et al: Risk of endometrial cancer following oestrogen replacement with and without progestins. J Natl Cancer Inst 1999;91:1131-1137.

88. Pike M, Peters R, Cozen W, et al: Estrogen-progestin replacement therapy and endometrial cancer. J Natl Cancer Inst 1997; 89:1110-1116.

89. Marsh MS, Whitehead MI: The practicalities of hormone replacement therapy. Bailliere's Best Pract Res Clin Endocrinol Metab 1993;7:183-202.

90. Archer DF, Dorin M, Lewis V, et al: Effects of lower doses of conjugated equine estrogens and medroxyprogesterone acetate on endometrial bleeding. Fertil Steril 2001;75:1080-1087.

91. Modelska K, Cummings S: Tibolone for postmenopausal women: Systematic review of randomised trials. J Clin Endocrinol Metab 2002;87:16-23.

92. Rymer J: The effects of tibolone. Gynecol Endocrinol 1998;12: 213-220.

93. Colacurci N, Mele P, Costa V, et al: Effects of tibolone on the breast. Eur J Obstet Gynaecol Reprod Biol 1998;80:235-238.

94. Santen RJ: To block estrogen's synthesis or action: That is the question. J Clin Endocrinol Metab 2002;87:3007-3012.

95. Couzi RJ, Helzlsouer KJ, Fetting JH: Prevalence of menopausal symptoms among women with a history of breast cancer and attitudes toward estrogen replacement therapy. J Clin Oncol 1995;13:2737-2744.

96. Col NF, Hirota LK, Orr RK, et al: Hormone replacement therapy after breast cancer: A systematic review and quantitative assessment of risk. J Clin Oncol 2001;19:2357-2363.

97. O'Meara E, Rossing M, Daling J, et al: Hormone replacement therapy after a diagnosis of breast cancer in relation to recurrence and mortality. J Natl Cancer Inst 2001;93:754-762.

98. Eden J, Wren B: Hormone replacement therapy after breast cancer: A review. Cancer Treat Rev 1996;22:335-343.

99. Wren B: Hormone therapy following breast and uterine cancer. Balliere's Clin Endocrinol Metab 1993;7:225-242.

100. Eden J, Bush T, Nand S, et al: A case-control study of combined continuous estrogen-progestin replacement therapy among women with a personal history of breast cancer. Menopause 1995;2:67-72.

101. Dew J, Eden J, Beller E, et al: A cohort study of hormone replacement therapy given to women previously treated for breast cancer. Climacteric 1998;1:137-142.

102. American College of Obstericians and Gynecologists: Hormone replacement therapy in women treated for endometrial cancer. Int J Obstet Gynecol 2001;73:283-284.

103. Eeles RA, Tan S, Wiltshaw E, et al: Hormone replacement therapy and survival after surgery for ovarian cancer. BMJ 1991;302:259-262.

104. Ursic-Vrscaj M, Bebar S, Primic Zakelj M: Hormone replacement therapy after invasive ovarian serous cystadenocarcinoma treatment: The effect on survival. Menopause 2001;8: 70-75.

105. Guidozzi F, Daponte A: Estrogen replacement therapy for ovarian carcinoma survivors: A randomized controlled trial. Cancer 1999;86:1013-1018.

106. Parazzini F, La Vecchia C, Negri E, et al: Case-control study of oestrogen replacement therapy and risk of cervical cancer. BMJ 1997;315:85-88.

107. Lacey JV, Brinton L, Barnes WA, et al: Use of hormone replacement therapy and adenocarcinomas and squamous cell carcinomas of the uterine cervix. Gynecol Oncol 2000;77: 149-154.

108. Ferenczy A, Gelfand MM, Franco E, et. al: Human papillomavirus infection in postmenopausal women with and without hormone therapy. Obstet Gynecol 1997;90:7-11.

109. Burger HG, Davis S: The role of androgen therapy. Best Prac Res Clin Obstet Gynecol 2002;16:383-393.

110. Bachmann G, Bancroft J, Braunstein G, et al: Female androgen insufficiency: The Princeton consensus statement on definition, classification and assessment. Fertil Steril 2002;77:660-665.

111. Shifren J, Braunstein G, Simon J, et al: Transdermal testosterone therapy in women with impaired sexual function after oophorectomy. N Engl J Med 2000;343:682-688.

112. Delmas P, Ensrud K, Adachi J, et al: Efficacy of raloxifene on vertebral fracture risk reduction in postmenopausal women with osteoporosis: Four-year results from a randomised clinical trial. J Clin Endocrinol Metab 2002;87:3609-3617.

113. Cummings SR, Eckert S, Krueger K, et al: The effect of raloxifene on risk of breast cancer in postmenopausal women: Results from the MORE randomized trial. JAMA 1999;281: 2189-2197.

114. Yaffe K, Krueger K, Somnath S, et al: Cognitive function in postmenopausal women treated with raloxifene. N Engl J Med 2001;344:1207-1213.

115. Walsh BW, Kuller LH, Wild RA, et al: Effects of raloxifene on serum lipids and coagulation factors in healthy postmenopausal women. JAMA 1998;279:1445-1451.

116. Walsh BW, Paul S, Wild RA, et al: The effects of hormone replacement therapy and raloxifene on C-reactive protein and homocysteine in healthy postmenopausal women: A randomized controlled trial. J Clin Endocrinol Metab 2000;85:214-218.

117. Barrett-Connor E, Grady D, Sashegyi A, et al: Raloxifene and cardiovascular events in osteoporotic postmenopausal women. JAMA 2002;287:847-857.

118. Kinsinger L, Harris R, Woolf S, et al: Chemoprevention of breast cancer: A summary of the evidence for the US Preventive Task Force. Ann Intern Med 2002;137:59-69.

119. Swain S, Santen RJ, Burger HG, et al: Treatment of estrogen deficiency symptoms in women surviving breast cancer. Part 5: Selective estrogen receptor modulators and hormone replacement therapy. Oncology 1999;13:721-735.

120. Chan S: A review of selective estrogen receptor modulators in the treatment of breast and endometrial cancer. Semin Oncol 2002;29:129-133.

121. Glazier M, Bowman M: A review of the evidence for the use of phyto-oestrogens as a replacement for traditional oestrogen replacement therapy. Arch Intern Med 2001;161:1161-1172.

122. Warren M, Shortle B, Dominguez J: Use of alternative therapies in menopause. Best Prac Res Clin Obstet Gynecol 2002;16:411-448.

123. Loprinzi C, Kugler JW, Sloan J, et al: Venlafaxine in management of hot flashes in survivors of breast cancer: A randomized controlled trial. Lancet 2000;356:2059-2063.

124. Loprinzi C, Quella S, Sloan J, et al. Preliminary data from a randomized evaluation of fluoexetine (Prozac) for treating hot flashes in breast cancer survivors [abstract]. Breast Cancer Res Treat 1999;57:34.

125. Stearns V, Isaacs C, Crawford J, et al: A pilot trial assessing the efficacy of paroxetine hydrochloride (Paxil) in controlling hot flashes [abstract]. Breast Cancer Res Treat 1998;50:308.

126. Nachtigall LE: Comparative study: Replens versus local estrogen in menopausal women. Fertil Steril 1994;61:178-180.

127. Jacobsen J, Troxel A, Evans J, et al: Randomized trial of black cohosh for the treatment of hot flashes among women with a history of breast cancer. J Clin Oncol 2001;19:2739-2745.

128. Amato P, Christophe S, Mellon PL: Estrogenic activity of herbs commonly used as remedies for menopausal symptoms. Menopause 2002;9:145-150.

129. Reid I, Brown JP, Burckhardt P, et al: Intravenous zoledronic acid in postmenopausal women with low bone mineral density. N Engl J Med 2002;346:653-661.

130. Rosen CJ, Bilezikian JP: Anabolic therapy for osteoporosis. J Clin Endocrinol Metab 2001;86:957-964.

131. Burger HG, Dudley EC, Hopper JL, et al: Prospectively measured levels of serum follicle-stimulating hormone, estradiol and the dimeric inhibins during the menopausal transition in a population-based cohort of women. J Clin Endocrinol Metab 1999;4025-4030.

132. American Association of Clinical Endocrinologists: AACE medical guidelines for clinical practice for management of menopause. Endocr Pract 1999;5:354-366.

133. Powles TJ, Hickish T, Casey S, et al: Hormone replacement therapy after breast cancer. Lancet 1993;342:60-61.

134. Wile AG, Opfell RW, Margileth DA: Hormone replacement therapy in previously treated breast cancer patients. Am J Surg 1993;165:372-375.

135. Decker D, Cox T, Burdakin J, et al: Hormone replacement therapy (HRT) in breast cancer survivors. Proc Am Soc Clin Oncol 1996;15:136.

136. DiSaia PJ, Grosen EA, Kurosaki T, et al: Hormone replacement therapy in breast cancer survivors: A cohort study. Am J Obstet Gynecol 1996;174:1494-1498.

137. Peters GN, Jones SE: Estrogen replacement in breast cancer patients: A time for change? Proc Am Soc Clin Oncol 1996; 15:121.

138. Vassilopolou-Sellin R, Theriault R, Klein MJ: Estrogen replacement therapy in women with prior diagnosis and treatment for breast cancer. Gynecol Oncol 1997;65:89-93.

139. Beckman MW, Mohrmann T, Kuschel B, et al: Hormonersatztherapie (HRT) nach mammakarzinomerkrankung-ergebnisse einer beobachtungs-studie. Gerburtsh u Frauenheilik 1998;58: 193-196.

140. Espie M, Gorins A, Perret F, et al: Hormone replacement therapy (HRT) in patients (pts) treated for breast cancer: Analysis of a cohort of 120 patients. Proc Am Soc Clin Oncol 1999;19:586a.

141. Guidozzi F: Estrogen replacement therapy in breast cancer survivors. Int J Gynecol Obstet 1999;64:59-63.

142. Ursic-Vrscaj M, Bebar S: A case-control study of hormone replacement therapy after primary surgical breast cancer treatment. Eur J Surg Oncol 1999;25:146-151.

143. DiSaia PJ, Brewster WR, Ziogas A, Anton-Culver H: Breast cancer survival and hormone replacement therapy: A cohort analysis. Am J Clin Oncol 2000;23:541-545.

144. Creasman WT, Henderson D, Hinshaw W, et al: Estrogen replacement therapy in the patient previously treated for endometrial cancer. Obstet Gynecol 1986;67:326-330.

145. Baker DP: Estrogen-replacement therapy in patients with previous endometrial carcinoma. Compr Ther 1990;16:28-35.

146. Bryant GW: Administration of estrogens to patients with a previous diagnosis of endometrial adenocarcinoma. South Med J 1990;83:726.

147. Lee RB, Burke TW, Park RC. Estrogen replacement therapy following treatment for stage I endometrial carcinoma. Gynecol Oncol 1990;36:189-191.

148. Gitsch G, Hanzal E, Jensen D, et al: Endometrial cancer in premenopausal women 45 years and younger. Obstet Gynecol 1995;85:504-508.

149. Chapman JA, DiSaia PJ, Osann K, et al: Estrogen replacement in surgical stage I and II endometrial cancer survivors. Am J Obstet Gynecol 1996;175:1195-1200.

MISCELLANEOUS

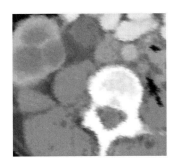

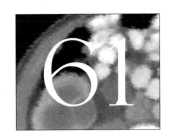

C H A P T E R

INVESTIGATIONAL APPROACHES TO THE TREATMENT OF GYNECOLOGIC CANCERS

Judith K. Wolf

 MAJOR CONTROVERSIES

- What are the most promising targets for treatment of gynecologic malignancies?
- How can gene therapy be used in the treatment of gynecologic cancers?
- What vehicles are available to deliver genes for gene therapy?
- Can genes be expressed in the cancer using specific promoters?
- What is the ideal target for gene therapy in gynecologic cancers?
- What are other mechanisms for targeting abnormalities in gynecologic cancers?

What are the most promising targets for treatment of gynecologic malignancies?

The current treatment of gynecologic malignances has been established over many years of study combining the best results of randomized clinical trials, when available, with single-arm prospective treatment studies or, for rare diseases, retrospective case series. As with the treatment of most other cancers, therapy has focused on what is the best for the most—that is, the treatment that has been identified to work in more patients than any other treatment. Although this is the best approach found to date, it has not been entirely successful for most tumor types, including most gynecologic malignancies. In fact, broadly cytotoxic therapies used to treat most cancers are notoriously associated with systemic toxicities. This approach to cancer treatment has been quite successful in a few types of cancers, such as gestational trophoblastic disease, and treatment of this disease can be viewed as an excellent example of targeted therapy. The front-line chemotherapy (methotrexate or actinomycin-D) used to treat and cure most patients with this disease

targets a specific enzyme, folate dehydrogenase, that is overexpressed in the cancer cells compared with the normal cells, making them more sensitive to chemotherapy than normal cells. Although this treatment is a targeted therapy, it was not developed in what would be considered today as a targeted manner; it was not developed specifically to target the disease but was found by serendipity to target the cancer. Cure rates for low-risk gestational trophoblastic disease today are near 100%.[1]

An example of a true targeted therapy might be the development of imatinib mesylate (Gleevec) for chronic myelogenous leukemia (CML). Gleevec is a protein tyrosine kinase inhibitor that selectively inhibits the kinase action of Abl, platelet-derived growth factor receptor (PDGFR), and c-Kit.[2] The hallmark of CML is the presence of the Philadelphia (Ph) chromosome, which results from a reciprocal translocation between chromosomes 9 and 11.[2] The Ph chromosome encodes for a tyrosine kinase, Bcr-Abl. The activated form of Bcr-Abl then initiates downstream pathways leading to CML. Gleevec inhibits adenosine triphosphate (ATP) binding to Bcr-Abl and thereby interferes with the downstream cascade. Phase II studies have confirmed the safety and efficacy of Gleevec in CML. More than 90% of patients with interferon-resistant chronic-phase CML had a complete hematologic response, and almost all had a major cytogenetic response.

Whereas Gleevec is a success story for the treatment of a specific malignancy related to a specific genetic defect, finding a specific therapy for each type of malignancy presents a much more difficult problem, for several reasons. First, most malignancies are associated with numerous genetic changes, and not one specific change. Second, even malignancies of the same histologic type (e.g., high-grade epithelial papillary serous carcinoma of the ovary) can have different genetic and epigenetic abnormalities. This can be visualized by noting how different these cancers can look under the microscope or even in their gross growth patterns throughout the abdomen and pelvis during surgical exploration. Third, malignancies grow and respond differently in different patients. For example, immunocompromised patients are at higher risk for certain malignancies. Also, in general, malignancies can not be transmitted from patient to patient. Even within a patient, malignancies have preferential growth in certain areas. This is the "seed and soil" hypothesis. Fourth, as a malignancy grows, it adapts to its environment in order to continue surviving. For example, genetic and epigenetic changes can occur that allow a cancer to become resistant to a treatment, to grow in a relatively hypoxic area, or to stimulate blood vessel formation or inhibit immunity. These issues leave a dilemma. If all the genetic changes in a malignancy at the time of diagnosis are identified, unless the context of the patient's internal environment and immunity are known and changes that may occur in the malignancy over time and with exposure to treatments are known, therapy may still not be able to be targeted effectively. This is not to say that targeted therapy will never work, but only that all of these issues need to be considered in the development of targeted therapies. For gynecologic malignancies, most investigations into targeted therapies are preclinical, although there have been a few trials of therapy targeted toward one or more abnormalities. This chapter summarizes what is known and what results of clinical trials are available, if any.

The major lesions detected in cancer cells occur in dominant oncogenes and tumor suppressor genes. Tumor suppressor genes require homozygous loss of function by mutation, deletion, inactivation, or a combination of these events for transformation to occur. The study of genetic abnormalities in cancers must include information about common chromosomal abnormalities, mutations and deletions of specific oncogenes and tumor suppressor genes, the role of angiogenesis and angiogenic factors, and the role of the body's own immune function. The topics covered here include gene therapy and the use of small molecules, kinases, or antibodies to target cancer abnormalities. It is impossible to be comprehensive in a single chapter, so the focus is on topics that are in or nearing clinical trials. Because more clinical research has been completed for gene therapy than for other agents in gynecologic malignancies, a larger proportion of the chapter focuses on gene therapy.

How can gene therapy be used in the treatment of gynecologic cancers?

Gene therapy is therapy performed to correct a known genetic defect. It can target a deleted or mutated gene, and it typically targets only one genetic alteration. In general, gene therapy consists of three components: a delivery system, the promoter for gene expression, and the complementary DNA (cDNA) of the gene being delivered. Gene therapy has been studied in many types of cancer and is currently in clinical trials for lung cancer and for head and neck cancer. In regard to gynecologic malignancies, research has pertained mostly to ovarian cancer, including several clinical trials and preclinical investigations in cervical cancer.

Ovarian cancer tends to remain and recur in the peritoneal cavity in most patients. This regionalization allows for relative ease of gene therapy delivery intraperitoneally, and it theoretically allows vector concentrations sufficiently high for efficient gene transfer. Furthermore, a significant safety advantage is achieved, because most data show the peritoneum to be an effective "container" of transferred genetic material. There are many known genetic defects in ovarian cancer that are targets of gene therapy. Studies done to date have all been early (mostly phase I) trials evaluating the safety and feasibility of delivering genes with the use of various viral and nonviral vectors or other systems to patients with advanced or recurrent ovarian cancer. Presented or published studies have looked at the effectiveness of (1) manipulation of drug-resistance genes, (2) suicide gene therapy, (3) inhibition or downregulation of growth factor receptors, and (4) reintroduction of tumor suppressor genes. Table 61-1 summarizes these trials.

Deisseroth and colleagues[3] published one of the first gene therapy trials for ovarian cancer. Overexpression of the multidrug-resistance gene (MDR) is one of the most common known mechanisms by which cancer becomes resistant to chemotherapy. In addition, one of the most common dose-limiting toxic effects of chemotherapy is bone marrow suppression. The premise of the Deisseroth study was to transfect (ex vivo) the MDR gene into the CD34+ bone marrow cells of patients with ovarian cancer and then to reinfuse these cells to allow delivery of higher doses of systemic paclitaxel. The study was done in the early 1990s, when standard primary chemotherapy for ovarian cancer did not yet include taxanes. All patients had a good performance status, were considered to have platinum-resistant disease, and had received no previous taxane therapy. In this study, CD34+ cells were obtained from the patient, the MDR gene was delivered in a nonreplicative retroviral vector in an ex vivo manner, infected cells were given back to the

Table 61–1. Clinical Trials of Gene Therapy for Ovarian Cancer

Reference	Gene Targeted	Mechanism	Delivery System
Deisseroth et al.[3]	MDR gene	Drug resistance	Retrovirus
Robinson et al.[11]	HSV/TK gene	Suicide gene therapy	Vaccine
Alvarez et al.[12]	HSV/TK gene	Suicide gene therapy	Adenovirus
Hasenburg et al.[13]	HSV/TK and topotecan	Suicide gene therapy with chemotherapy	Adenovirus
Alvarez et al.[19]	HER-2/NEU antibody	Growth factor receptor	Adenovirus
Hortobagyi et al.[20]	E1A against HER-2/NEU	Growth factor receptor	Liposomes
Buller et al.[25]	TP53	Tumor suppressor gene	Adenovirus
Wolf et al.[26]	TP53	Tumor suppressor gene	Adenovirus
Tait et al.[28,29]	BRCA1	Tumor suppressor gene	Retrovirus

patient, and then patients were given high doses of paclitaxel. Importantly, no patients had any toxicity attributable to the retrovirus; however, transduction of the gene was low. After one course of paclitaxel, transduction of CD34+ cells was 2.3% to 20%; after two courses, there was no appreciable MDR expression. Some patients did respond to therapy, however, and the dose-limiting toxicity was thrombocytopenia.[3] This early study was innovative and revealed problems that have continued to be encountered in other studies.

Another approach studied is suicide gene therapy. The goal of suicide gene therapy is to deliver a viral enzyme to cancer cells that makes them susceptible to antibiotic therapy. The herpes simplex virus (HSV)/thymidine kinase (TK)/ganciclovir system has been a focus in ovarian cancer gene therapy research. TK is present in all mammalian and viral cells. The viral equivalent, however, has greater affinity for acyclovir and its analogs, including ganciclovir, preferentially producing the phosphorylated product. Subsequent modification to a triphosphorylated form and incorporation during replication halts growth of the developing DNA strands and inhibits RNA polymerase activity. Mammalian TK exhibits a much lower affinity for the drug, such that tumor cells once transduced are selectively killed in the presence of ganciclovir.[4,5]

The efficacy of this approach is amplified by a "bystander effect," reported initially by Culver et al.[6] Multiple studies have achieved magnified tumor cell death resulting from basal transduction efficiencies.[7-9] In fact, incorporation of the viral enzyme by 10% of tumor cells yielded a 70% tumor cell kill in some studies.[7,10] Therefore, suicide gene therapy theoretically obviates targeting 100% of tumor cells for effective treatment.

Several clinical trials using the HSV/TK system for patients with ovarian cancer have been completed. Robinson and associates[11] published a phase I study of vaccine therapy using the HSV/TK gene. This study relied heavily on the bystander effect. The ovarian cancer cell line PA-1 was transfected with the HSV/TK gene ex vivo, irradiated, and then given intraperitoneally to patients with recurrent ovarian cancer. Patients were then given ganciclovir, and when the HSV/TK-transfected PA-1 cells died, the gene was allowed to infect other cells and cause a toxic immune

response in neighboring cells. This study found a high incidence of fever and abdominal pain but no dose-limiting toxicity, and several patients had resolution of ascites or decreased CA 125 levels.[11] A recently published phase I trial employed an adenoviral vector for intraperitoneal delivery of viral HSV/TK DNA (AdHSV-TK).[12] Fourteen patients with recurrent ovarian cancer were treated with a nonreplicative adenovirus containing the HSV/TK gene at doses ranging from 1×10^9 to 1×10^{11} plaque-forming units. After being given AdHSV-TK, patients were treated with ganciclovir. No dose-limiting toxic effects were noted, and five patients (38%) experienced stable disease. Transient fever was noted in 29% of the patients. Most patients had evidence of transgene DNA and RNA in ascites samples 2 days after AdHSV-TK administration. Most patients also had evidence of adenovirus antibodies.

Building on the results of this trial, Hasenburg and coworkers[13] published a trial combining AdHSV-TK with topotecan for patients with recurrent ovarian cancer after secondary cytoreduction. Ten patients underwent secondary debulking surgery, with less than 0.5 cm residual disease. Two intraperitoneal catheters were placed, and, once bowel function resumed after surgery, patients were given AdHSV-TK. Beginning 24 hours after vector injection, acyclovir therapy was started. At the same time, patients were given intravenous topotecan, 1.0 mg/m² daily for 5 days. No dose-limiting side effects were seen, and the most common side effect was myelosuppression secondary to the chemotherapy. The results of this study led the researchers to an ongoing phase II study of the combination.

Another approach has been inhibition or downregulation of growth factor receptors. HER-2/NEU (also known as c-ErbB/2) encodes a 185-kd protein with tyrosine kinase activity. Overexpression of the HER-2/NEU receptor is known to enhance tumorigenicity, metastasis, and resistance to chemotherapy.[14-17] This growth factor receptor is overexpressed in 10% to 15% of ovarian cancers and confers a poor prognosis.[18] Alvarez and associates[19] published the results of a phase I trial using an adenovirus containing an anti-ErbB-2 single-chain antibody (Ad21). They treated 15 patients with intraperitoneal Ad21 in doses ranging from 1×10^9 to 1×10^{10} plaque-forming units. No dose-limiting toxic effects were seen, and the most common side effects were constitutional. Five patients had stable disease. Analysis of ascites samples after treatment revealed expression of the antibody in 10 (71%) of 14 patients 2 days after treatment. Most patients had evidence of an antiadenovirus immune response.

Hortobagyi and colleagues,[20] in a phase I trial, tried to target HER-2 using a liposome containing the adenovirus E1A gene. E1A was found in preclinical testing to downregulate HER-2 expression and inhibit the growth of cells overexpressing it.[21] In this trial, patients with recurrent ovarian or breast cancer had placement of an intraperitoneal catheter and then were given liposomal E1A weekly for 3 weeks. Again, the most common side effects were constitutional, and abdominal pain was the dose-limiting toxicity. Peritoneal fluid obtained after treatment from several patients showed expression of E1A with a concurrent downregulation of HER-2 expression. Stable disease was noted in 3 (17%) of 18 patients.[20] This study led to further evaluation of this agent in patients with smaller volume disease.

Reintroduction of tumor suppressor genes has also been studied. The most extensively studied tumor suppressor gene is *TP53*. TP53 is a 53-kd nuclear phosphoprotein that binds DNA and functions to regulate transcription, control the cell cycle, and initiate apoptosis. TP53 is abnormal in 30% to 79% of malignant ovarian tumors and is the most common genetic abnormality detected to date. Mutation of one allele commonly results in deletion of the remaining allele. Similarly, binding of the altered gene product inactivates the wild-type allele. Regardless of mechanism, overexpression of this dominant negative allele mediates breakdown of normal genome surveillance, such that apoptosis is not triggered and cells with significant DNA damage are allowed to accumulate.[22-24]

Two clinical trials of a replication-deficient adenovirus delivering wild-type TP53 (Adp53) to patients with recurrent ovarian cancer have been presented. First, Buller and coworkers[25] presented a phase I/II trial of 43 patients who received either intraperitoneal Adp53 alone or in combination with intravenous chemotherapy. Successful gene transfer was detected via reverse-transcriptase polymerase chain reaction in some patients. Toxicity effects included known chemotherapy side effects and constitutional toxic effects thought to be caused by the virus. It is difficult to determine responses, because patients received several different regimens, with or without chemotherapy.[25]

Wolf and associates[26] presented a similar study of Adp53 alone for patients with chemotherapy-refractory ovarian cancer. The study was designed to determine the maximum tolerated dose of intraperitoneally delivered Adp53. Patients with platinum- and paclitaxel-resistant metastatic epithelial ovarian cancer with a Zubrod status of 0, 1, or 2 and adequate bone marrow, liver, and renal function were eligible. All but one patient had been previously treated with two or more chemotherapy regimens. Patients underwent laparoscopy, peritoneal washings, biopsies, and placement of an intraperitoneal catheter. Administration of

Adp53 was begun within 7 days, and the agent was delivered daily for 5 days every 3 weeks at one of four dosing levels: 3×10^{10}, 3×10^{11}, 1×10^{12}, or 3×10^{12} viral particles. Seventeen patients were enrolled in the trial. Fifteen (88%) of 17 patients were evaluable for toxicity. No dose-limiting toxicity was observed, and the most common grade 3 toxic effects were fatigue (6 patients) and abdominal pain (3 patients). Eleven (73%) of 15 patients were evaluable for response. Two (18%) of 11 patients had a partial response, and 4 patients (36%) had stable disease for up to four courses. All patients showed evidence of an antiadenovirus immune response. The conclusion from this study was that multiple dosing of intraperitoneal Adp53 is feasible and well tolerated in this group of patients. TP53 expression could not be confirmed, because most patients did not have ascites and peritoneal washings did not provide enough cells for evaluation.[26]

Another tumor suppressor gene that has been studied in clinical trials for ovarian cancer patients is *BRCA1*. *BRCA1* mutations are implicated in a large number of hereditary cases of ovarian cancer (estimated at 10% of total ovarian cancer cases) with a resultant loss of tumor suppressor activity. Loss of heterozygosity of *BRCA1* is also noted in up to 70% of sporadic ovarian cancers, with an associated decrease in the secreted protein product.[27]

Tait and colleagues[28,29] showed 90% growth inhibition and increased survival with BRCA1 gene therapy in a nude mouse xenograft model. They employed a retroviral vector expressing a *BRCA1* splice variant that produces tumor reduction and cure at markedly higher rates, compared with the wild-type gene. A stable adenoviral vector for use with *BRCA1* has not yet been identified. A phase I study using intraperitoneal delivery of this retroviral construct showed partial responses in 3 (25%) of 12 patients with ovarian cancer, and the majority of patients had stable disease. Three patients developed sterile peritonitis, which resolved in 48 hours. A phase II study in patients with less extensive disease showed no disease stabilization or response and poor vector stability. The authors hypothesized that the difference in response may have resulted from the development of neutralizing antibodies in patients with more intact immune systems.

The relatively recent understanding of the connection between human papillomavirus (HPV) and cervical neoplasia has brought about a new paradigm of research in the prevention, detection, and treatment of cervical intraepithelial neoplasia, as well as invasive cervical cancer. Research spans the spectrum from understanding the epidemiology of HPV infection, including the natural history of these infections, to understanding the molecular biology of cervical cancer. The role of HPV in cervical cancer is illuminated elsewhere in this book. For the discussion of gene therapy research in cervical cancer, it is important to understand the role of the HPV early genes E6 and E7 (Table 61-2). Although HPV has many actions in the infected cell, two of the more pertinent and more studied in cancer are its effects on the cellular genes *TP53* and retinoblastoma, *RB*. The TP53 gene is present in all

Table 61–2. Functions of the Products of Human Papillomavirus Early Region Open Reading Frames (ORFs)

Early Region ORF	Protein Function
E1	1. Two proteins required for extrachromosomal DNA replication and completion of the viral life cycle 2. These work with E2 products
E2	1. Two proteins required for extrachromosomal DNA replication 2. These work with E1 products 3. Full-length protein acts as a transcriptional activator and binds to DNA to increase transcription of the early region 4. Smaller protein inhibits transcription of the early region
E4	1. Protein important for the maturation and replication of the virus 2. Expressed in later stages of infection, when complete virions are being assembled
E5	1. Protein interacts with cell membrane receptors, such as EGF-R and platelet-derived growth factor (PDGF) 2. May stimulate cell proliferation in infected cells
E6	1. Protein critical for viral replication, host cell immortalization, and transformation 2. Binds to TP53 and stimulates TP53 degradation through ubiquitin-dependent proteolytic pathway
E7	1. Protein critical for viral replication, host cell immortalization, and transformation 2. Binds to RB protein and dissociates E2F-RB complex, stimulating transcription of cellular genes

cells and is known as the "housekeeping gene" or cell cycle regulator. One of the important functions of TP53 is to recognize when DNA damage has occurred in a cell and arrest the growth of that cell in the G_1 period of the cell cycle to allow for DNA repair or, if repair is not possible, to lead that cell into cell-mediated death or suicide, called apoptosis. TP53 performs these functions by activating a number of downstream genes.[30,31] Mutation or deletion of TP53 is one of the most common abnormalities in cancers of all types. In cervical cancer, TP53 mutations are less common. Instead, the HPV early gene, E6, inactivates TP53 in these cells by causing its degradation through the ubiquitin system. The RB gene was first recognized as mutated or deleted in retinoblastomas, and it is also a tumor suppressor. It functions to allow or disallow progression through the cell cycle, depending on its state of phosphorylation and interaction with downstream genes. HPV inactivates RB by binding of its early gene, E7, to RB, which blocks these interactions. Both of these events, E6 promoting TP53 degradation and E7 blocking RB function, allow for unregulated growth of cells, in particular cells with DNA abnormalities.[32,33]

One potential gene therapy for cervical cancer is to add additional TP53 to cervical cancer cells infected with HPV. To evaluate the effect of replacing TP53 into cervical cancer cells with HPV infection, researchers used an E1-deleted, replication-deficient adenovirus to deliver human TP53 cDNA under a cytomegalovirus (CMV) promoter (Adp53) to cervical cancer cell lines

in vitro and in a nude mouse model. This is the same delivery system used in the ovarian cancer clinical trial. Cell lines studied included those with HPV-16 infection, HPV-18 infection, or an intrinsic TP53 mutation with no HPV infection. Both in vitro and in the mouse model, treatment with Adp53 inhibited cell growth and tumor growth. TP53 was overexpressed, and infected cells underwent G_1 arrest.[34] Using the Rhesus monkey cervix as a model similar to human cervical epithelium, it was found that the adenovirus could best be delivered via direct injection into the cervical epithelium.[35] These results are similar to those found in squamous epithelial carcinomas of the head and neck. Clinical trials of Adp53 in patients with head and neck disease using direct tumor injection have shown safety, and currently an international phase III study of chemotherapy with Adp53 is ongoing in head and neck cancer patients. As to the future of gene therapy in cervical cancer, the preclinical evidence supports clinical trials of Adp53 in cervical cancer. Development of better delivery systems for gene therapy, as well as the placement of genes under specific promoters so that expression of the transgene occurs only in the targeted cell, are also areas of active investigation. In addition, with the identification of new biomarkers specific for cervical cancer, gene therapy could potentially specifically target one of these markers.

The adenovirus containing TP53 has also been investigated in a preclinical model of uterine papillary serous carcinoma (UPSC). UPSC is the most aggressive type of endometrial cancer, and TP53 mutations are often detected in this tumor type. Ramondetta and associates[36] infected the human UPSC cell line, SPEC-2, which has a known TP53 mutation, with Adp53 in vitro. After infection, they found a greater than 95% inhibition of growth of these cells, increased apoptosis, increased TP53 expression, and loss of anchorage-independent growth, suggesting that TP53 may be a target for this uncommon but aggressive endometrial cancer.

The completion of the Human Genome Project and the development of powerful new molecular genetic technologies have advanced our capabilities to the point that meaningful human application of gene techniques is now possible. However, there are several areas in gene therapy technology that need to be addressed before further clinical trials are instituted in patients with gynecologic cancer. These include the lack of an efficient delivery system, lack of tissue-specific promoters, and lack of tissue-specific targets.

What vehicles are available to deliver genes for gene therapy?

Current delivery systems for gene therapy include viral and nonviral vectors. Advantages and disadvantages of these systems are summarized in Table 61-3. Early gene therapy studies and clinical trials employed retroviruses as a vector. Although they have the advantage of permanent integration into cellular DNA, retroviruses have a limited carrying capacity of

Table 61–3. Delivery Systems for Gene Therapy

Vector	Advantages	Disadvantages
Retroviruses	1-30% transduction frequency; permanent; infects hematopoietic and epithelial cells	Unstable; low titer; must integrate into dividing cells for expansion; 9-12 kb limit
Adenoviruses	Infects epithelial cells at high frequency; cellular proliferation not required	Does not infect marrow; immunogenic and temporary
Adeno-associated virus	Stable; integrates into nondividing cells at low frequency	Small capacity for DNA; low titer; requires a helper virus
Herpes simplex virus type I	Infects a wide range of cell types; can achieve high titer; has relatively prolonged expression	No integration into genome of infected cells; cytotoxic; difficult to develop because it is complex
DNA cassettes	No viruses are involved; easy to use and develop	Low integration frequency; temporary expression
Liposomes	No viruses involved	Low frequency of modification; cytotoxic to some cells

roughly 8 to 12 kb, are reproduced at low titers, and are vulnerable to serum complement inactivation. Also, retroviruses permanently infect epithelial and hematopoietic cells, which can be a safety concern. Finally, with stable integration into the host genome, retrovirus vectors can transduce only the solid tumor cells that are actively dividing.[37]

Adenoviruses have a 36-kb chromosome complement with six gene products early in the course of infection and three late gene products at the onset of DNA replication. Intact viral genes limit the level of therapeutic gene expression. E1A, the first early gene, encodes two proteins via alternative splicing that suppress or activate transcription of viral and cellular genes and regulate the cell cycle.[37,38] Therefore, in gene therapy studies, the majority of adenoviral vectors developed have a deletion of the E1-early gene. This allows the virus to be infective but nonreplicative. Adenoviruses infect epithelial cells with a high frequency but do not infect bone marrow cells. Although cellular proliferation is not required for propagation, infection is highly immunogenic, and the virus does not integrate into cellular DNA, making the infection temporary.

Adenoviral entry into cells is dependent on interaction with the coxsackie-adenovirus receptor (CAR) and α-integrins.[39] The near-ubiquitous expression of these receptors confers tissue-nonspecific infection. This may result in extensive ectopic gene transfer into normal cells and decreased transfection of target tumor cells, because there is evidence showing decreased CAR expression in some tumors that are refractory to adenovirus infection.[40] Development of specialized recombinant adenoviruses that achieve more specific cell targeting and greater gene transduction efficiencies is underway to circumvent some of these issues.

To attempt to target the adenovirus, Rancourt and coworkers have tried redirecting to the highly expressed basic fibroblast growth factor (bFGF) receptor. Using an adenovirus to deliver the HSV/TK gene to ovarian cancer cells in a murine model, Rancourt's group showed that targeting the adenovirus to the bFGF receptor enhanced transfection. Specifically, a 10-fold lower dose of bFGF-modified virus achieved survival rates to those achieved with the unmodified vector.[41]

Another example of adenovirus modification is the targeting of a protein that is present only in cancer cells. TAG-72 is a glycoprotein that is absent in normal peritoneal cells but expressed by most ovarian carcinoma cells. By incorporation of an antibody conjugate with specificity for TAG-72, Kelly and associates[40] found that adenovirus-mediated luciferase (Luc) gene transfer increased up to 60-fold in human ovarian cancer cell lines, with a 10-fold reduction in transfer to mesothelial cells.

This same group also produced a modified adenovirus with an amino acid sequence motif in the H1 loop of the fiber knob domain, which directs viral binding to cell-surface integrins. CAR-independent cell entry was demonstrated, with at least a doubling in transduction efficiency.[40] Subsequent work showed the fiber protein to be a region of attack for neutralizing adenovirus antibodies found in patient ascites.[42]

The adeno-associated virus (AAV) has also been investigated as a potential vector for gene delivery. The AAV can integrate stably into the host cell genome, and it has been successfully transfected with the use of plasmids.[43] The AAV integrates at a site-specific area on chromosome 19,[44] after which it remains dormant until infection with a helper virus (usually an adenovirus) allows its replication.[45] Advantages of the AAV are that it is not implicated in any human disease and that integration into the host genome does not affect cell replication. However, the AAV has not been used clinically to date, because it has a small capacity to hold DNA and it has not been produced in high titers.

Another viral vector that has been used is HSV itself. HSV infects a wide range of cell types, with prolonged expression and high titers.[46] The vector is large and can carry multiple genes; it has exhibited gene transfer quantitatively superior to that of adenoviral vectors at a 100-fold lower dose in vitro.[47] However, because of its large genome, HSV is quite complex and can be difficult to manipulate. In addition, the virus itself can be cytotoxic. Because of these difficulties, clinical trials using HSV have not been done in patients with ovarian cancer, but strategies to overcome these shortcomings are under study.[47]

Nonviral vector strategies have employed primarily liposomes, naked DNA, or particle bombardment. The use of liposomes relies on the electrical charge properties of DNA, cationic lipids, and cell surfaces. Several studies have shown the effectiveness of polycationic liposome delivery of DNA in vivo. The advantages of liposomes include no DNA size constraints, easy bulk preparation, and low immunogenicity.[48]

Direct DNA injection can be done with the use of a pure closed circular DNA; it is simple, inexpensive, and nontoxic compared with viral delivery, and it can carry large DNA constructs. However, it has the disadvantage that gene expression is short-lived. A potential use for this method is as a vaccination procedure, because low-level gene expression may be enough to achieve an immune response. It would not be useful in widespread diseases requiring multiple injections, such as ovarian cancer.[49]

Direct particle bombardment involves coating DNA onto the surface of 1- to 3-μm gold or tungsten beads. These particles are accelerated by an electrical discharge device or gas pulse and are "fired" at the tissue. The physical force overcomes the cell membrane barrier. There is a wide variation in gene expression with this method because of variation in tissue rigidity, foreign DNA processing, and transcriptional capacity. The DNA does not integrate and is an unstable episome. This method also is not useful for gene therapy, but it may be used in the laboratory for rapid screening of tissue-specific DNA constructs or as a vaccination.[50,51]

The use of noninfectious agents has obvious advantages of avoiding immunogenicity and nonspecific toxicity from the virus itself, but the problems of low integration frequencies, difficulty of construction, and variable cytotoxicity remain.

Can genes be expressed in the cancer using only specific promoters?

Cancer gene therapy trials done to date have used constitutively active prokaryotic promoters with abundant expression in normal cells but an absence of specificity or selectivity. The most commonly employed promoters are from the CMV or the SV40 virus. Because of their lack of tumor specificity, these promoters have the potential for significant toxicity in normal cells, and because they are of viral origin, they can be downregulated in vivo. The CMV promoter can also be inactivated via methylation.[52] Choosing a promoter that is specifically upregulated in tumor cells compared with normal cells because of upregulation of its gene product may overcome some of these problems. Examples include the prostate-specific promoter in prostate cancer cells and the α-fetoprotein promoter for hepatocellular carcinoma cells, which are active in the prostate and liver, respectively.[53,54]

Several tumor-specific or ovarian cell carcinoma–specific promoters have been investigated in the preclinical setting; Table 61-4 summarizes the findings. The secretory leukoproteinase inhibitor (SLP1) gene is highly expressed in a variety of epithelial tumors, including ovarian cancers.[55] Robertson and colleagues[56] found that a plasmid containing the HSV/TK gene, under the SLP1 promoter, could kill ovarian cancer cells. My own laboratory evaluated the ability of a plasmid containing the Luc gene under the SLP1 promoter to express the gene in a variety of cell lines. We found that SLP1 was successful in increasing Luc production in several types of epithelial cancer cell lines, including ovarian cancer cell lines, and was less active in nonepithelial and immortalized normal cell lines.[57] In the same study, our laboratory evaluates the effect of the promoter activity of the ovarian-specific promoter (OSP1), a retroviral promoter reported to be transcriptionally active in rat ovaries but not in other cell types.[58] We found this promoter to be active, but not specific, because it showed Luc activity in many cell types.

The human epithelium-specific ETS transcription factor (hESE1) is a promoter that is active in many epithelial cancers and at low levels in normal breast epithelium.[59] My colleagues found hESE1 to be epithelial cell-specific and more active than either the SLP1 or the OSP1 promoter, but it did not have organ or tumor specificity. We found the human telomerase promoter (hTERT)[57] to be most active in cancer cell lines compared with immortalized normal cells, whether epithelial or not, but again it was not specific for ovarian cancer cells. Telomerase is a cellular reverse transcriptase that catalyzes the synthesis and

Table 61–4. Tumor-Specific Promoter Candidates for Ovarian Cancer Gene Therapy

Promoter*	Tissue Specificity	Vector	Transgene Expressed	Tested
SLP1	Epithelial carcinomas	Plasmid	HSV-TK and Luc	Ovarian cancer cell lines
OSP1	Many cell types	Plasmid	Luc	Ovarian cancer cell lines
hESE1	Epithelial cells (cancer and normal)	Plasmid	Luc	Ovarian cancer cell lines
hTERT	Epithelial and nonepithelial cancers	Plasmid	Luc	Ovarian cancer cell lines
HAFR	Ovarian cancer	Adenovirus	Luc	Ovarian cancer cell lines
MUC1	Various carcinomas	Adenovirus	LacZ and HSV-TK	Ovarian cancer cell lines and mouse intraperitoneal model
L-plastin	Various carcinomas	Adenovirus	LacZ	Ovarian cancer cell lines, primary tumors, and mouse intraperitoneal model

*See text for discussion of specific promoters.

extension of telomeric DNA, maintaining telomere length during cell division.[60,61] The transcription of hTERT correlates with telomerase activity, suggesting that it is rate-limiting.[62] Telomerase activity is increased in many malignant tumors and cell lines, and it may therefore be a good tumor-specific promoter.[63]

Promoters evaluated by others include the high-affinity folate receptors (HAFR), which are expressed in normal ovaries and in a majority of ovarian cancers. The folate receptor gene contains two tissue-specific promoters, P1 and P4. Goldsmith and associates[64] reported Luc transcription in ovarian cancer cells after infection with a recombinant adenovirus using the P1 promoter. Further, Luc production correlated with HAFR levels.

Another possible specific promoter is the MUC1/Df3 promoter. The MUC1 gene encodes the polymorphic epithelial mucin, which is expressed in glandular epithelium and is overexpressed in many cancer types, including ovarian cancer. Preliminary studies show some promise for this promoter.[65,66]

Finally, the L-plastin promoter has been found to be more active in ovarian cancer cells than in normal mesothelial cells. L-Plastin is a member of the actin-binding proteins and is highly expressed in most epithelial cancer cells.[67,68]

To summarize, clinical trials to date have used nonspecific, ubiquitous promoters, but many tumor- or ovarian-specific promoters are being investigated to try to target transgene expression to tumor cells and therefore decrease toxicity to normal cells.

What is the ideal target for gene therapy in gynecologic cancers?

As discussed later, clinical trials of gene therapy for ovarian cancer so far have generally targeted alterations in the tumor that are not specific to ovarian cancer. An ovarian cancer–specific genetic defect would be an ideal target. Many researchers are currently investigating such targets, although at this time no ovarian cancer–specific target exists.

What are other mechanisms for targeting abnormalities in gynecologic cancers?

Underlying all of the previous discussion is the idea that abnormalities in cellular genes, caused either by amplification or overexpression (oncogenes) or by loss of function (tumor suppressor genes), are required for carcinogenesis. Cancer can also have epigenetic changes that lead to alteration in cell growth or function. Epigenetic changes are clonally inherited changes in gene expression without accompanying genetic changes. DNA methylation may be a mechanism for perpetuating these epigenetic changes. CpG island methylation is an important mechanism of gene silencing in many cancers. Targeting the ability of these genetic or epigenetic changes by the use of small molecules (antibodies of kinases) is a current area of

research in many types of cancer. However, there are few completed clinical trials of such agents in gynecologic cancers, because the existence of known targets in gynecologic cancer makes it reasonable to investigate several of these agents.

Amplification or overexpression of several different growth factor receptors has been implicated in carcinogenesis. Two, in particular, have been studied in gynecologic malignancies: the epidermal growth factor receptor (EGF-R) and the related HER-2/NEU. The EGF-R is a 170-kd transmembrane glycoprotein with an intracellular component. Its ligands are the epidermal growth factor (EGF) and transforming growth factor-α (TGF-α). Overexpression of the EGF-R is usually related to amplification of the gene, and overexpression seems to confer a growth advantage to cells.[69] EGF-R is expressed in a large proportion of cervical carcinomas, but also in normal and premalignant epithelia. Lakshmi and coworkers[70] showed that EGF-R expression in normal squamous epithelium is restricted to the basal and parabasal cell layers, whereas in premalignant and invasive lesions the expression is more diffuse. Between 50% and 70% of advanced ovarian cancers overexpress EGF-R. Several new agents target the activity of the EGF-R.[71] The antibody C-225 is directed at the extracellular portion of the receptor and blocks activation from its ligands.[72] Several tyrosine kinase inhibitors, which target the activation of the receptor intracellularly and downstream, have also been developed. These are the so-called "small molecules." The furthest along in development, and the only FDA-approved agent thus far, is Iressa.[73] Iressa and small-molecule tyrosine kinase inhibitors, as well as C-225, have been evaluated in clinical trials for several different types of cancers (mostly colon, pancreas, lung, and head and neck) and have some activity when the EGF-R is expressed. Iressa has recently been approved as a third-line agent for lung cancer. None of these agents has yet been evaluated in a completed clinical trial for gynecologic cancers, although several studies are in development.

EGF-R inhibitors are not without toxicity. The major toxicity common to all agents tested is skin changes with an acne-like skin rash. Diarrhea has also been a reported effect, especially with Iressa, which is an oral agent. Toxicities do not seem to be cross-reactive with chemotherapy toxicities, because these agents have been safely used in several combination trials.[74]

The HER-2/NEU gene also encodes for a transmembrane glycoprotein with 78% homology to the intracytoplasmic domain of the EGF-R. It is a 185-kd glycoprotein with tyrosine kinase activity and several described possible ligands.[75] HER-2/NEU is overexpressed in approximately 10% of ovarian cancers and a similar number of endometrial cancers, more commonly in UPSC tumors.[76] In both of these tumor types, it is suggested that HER-2/NEU overexpression confers a poor prognosis. Both Lakshmi[70] and Berchuck[76] reported a high percentage of cervical cancers (and squamous epithelium) to stain positive by immunohistochemistry for HER-2/NEU expression; however, the staining is light and correlates with EGF-R expression.[75,76]

Targeting the HER-2/NEU has already been discussed in regard to gene therapy using the E1A gene from the adenovirus to downregulate its expression. Another agent to target this gene is herceptin, which is an antibody to the extracellular domain of HER-2/NEU. Between 20% and 25% of breast cancers overexpress HER-2/NEU, and this feature is associated with a worse prognosis.[77] Herceptin has been found to be active both alone (in some patients) and in combination with chemotherapy in breast cancers that overexpress HER-2/NEU.[78] Herceptin is currently approved for use in breast cancer. The Gynecologic Oncology Group has completed clinical trials of herceptin in both ovarian and endometrial cancer, but the final results are not yet available. Both studies, however, reiterated the low percentage of these cancers that overexpress this growth factor receptor, suggesting that agents targeting HER-2/NEU may be of benefit only for a small proportion of gynecologic cancer patients. Some of the small-molecule tyrosine kinases that target EGF-R may also be effective when HER-2/NEU overexpression occurs and may have wider application for gynecologic cancer patients.[79]

Gleevec was discussed earlier as an excellent example of targeted therapy. Since its discovery, its potential usefulness in gynecologic and other cancers has been under investigation. In addition to CML, Gleevic has now been approved by the FDA for the treatment of a group of gastrointestinal sarcomas called GISTs. Between 70% and 90% of GISTs had a gain of function of the c-Kit tyrosine kinase receptor that is a target of Gleevec. Early clinical trials of Gleevec in the treatment of GIST demonstrated a remission rate of 60%.[80]

Preclinical studies of ovarian cancer indicated that c-Kit and PDGFR may play a role in ovarian tumorigenesis.[81-86] C-Kit, PDGFR and Abl expression have all been demonstrated to varying degrees in ovarian cancers. Tonary and colleagues[86] found that 71% of ovarian cancers expressed c-Kit and 92% expressed its ligand stem cell factor. Dabrow and associates[85] found that PDGF enhances the growth of human ovarian surface epithelial cells in vitro and may play a role in ovarian cancer development. These findings have led to at least three ongoing trials of Gleevec in ovarian cancer patients.

In UPSC, a similar finding has been reported. In a study by Slomovitz and coinvestigators,[87] 81% of UPSC tumors demonstrated c-Abl expression, and 72% were positive for PDGFR expression. At least one clinical trial of Gleevec for patients with UPSC is under development.

Many other new agents aimed at a multitude of genetic and epigenetic targets are in various stages of development. As we gain knowledge about the underlying defects that lead to gynecologic cancers, new targets for therapy will continue to be identified. The future of targeted therapies will necessitate determining the best way to integrate these new therapies with existing treatments. A new paradigm of individualized therapy based on specific tumor and patient factors may be part of the future of cancer therapy.

REFERENCES

1. Feldman S, Goldstein DP, Berkowitz RS: Low-risk metastatic gestational trophoblastic tumors. Semin Oncol 1995;22:1660-171.
2. Druker BJ, Tamura S, Buchdunger E, et al: Effects of a selective inhibitor of Abl tyrosine kinase on the growth of Bcr-Abl positive cells. Nat Med 1996;2:561-566.
3. Deisseroth AB, Kavanagh J, Champlin R: Use of safety-modified retroviruses to introduce chemotherapy resistance sequences into normal hematopoietic cells for chemoprotection during the therapy of ovarian cancer: A pilot trial. Hum Gene Ther 1994;5:1507-1522.
4. Barnes MN, Deshane JS, Rosenfeld M, et al: Gene therapy and ovarian cancer: A review. Obstet Gynecol 1997;89:145-155.
5. Gomez-Navarro J, Siegal GP, Alvarez RD, Curiel DT: Gene therapy: Ovarian cancer as the paradigm. Anat Pathol 1998;109:444-467.
6. Culver K, Ram Z, Walbridge S, et al: In vivo gene transfer with retroviral vector-producing cells for the treatment of experimental brain tumors. Science 1992;256:1550-1552.
7. Alvarez RD, Curiel DT: A phase I study of recombinant adenovirus vector-mediated intraperitoneal delivery of herpes simplex virus thymidine kinase (HSV-TK) gene and intravenous ganciclovir for previously treated ovarian and extraovarian cancer patients. Hum Gene Ther 1997;8:597-613.
8. Rancourt C, Robertson MW, Wang M, et al: Endothelial cell vehicles for delivery of cytotoxic genes as a gene therapy approach for carcinoma of the ovary. Clin Cancer Res 1998;4:265-270.
9. Tong X, Block A, Chen SH, et al: In vivo gene therapy of ovarian cancer by adenovirus-mediated thymidine kinase gene transduction and ganciclovir administration. Gynecol Oncol 1996;61:175-179.
10. Freeman SM, Abboud CN, Whartenby KA, et al: The "bystander effect": Tumor regression when a fraction of the tumor mass is genetically modified. Cancer Res 1993;53:5274-5283.
11. Robinson W, Adams J, Marrogi A, Freeman S: Vaccine therapy for ovarian cancer using herpes simplex virus-thymidine kinase (HSV-TK) suicide gene transfer technique: A phase I study. Gene Ther Mol Biol 1998;2:31-40.
12. Alvarez RD, Gomez-Navarro J, Wang M, et al: Adenoviral-mediated suicide gene therapy for ovarian cancer. Mol Ther 2000;2:524-530.
13. Hasenburg A, Tong XW, Rojas-Martinez A, et al: Thymidine kinase gene therapy with concomitant topotecan chemotherapy for recurrent ovarian cancer. Cancer Gene Ther 2000;7:839-844.
14. Bargmann CI, Hung MC, Weinberg RA: Multiple independent activations of the neu oncogene by a point mutation altering the transmembrane domain of p185. Cell 1986;45:649-657.
15. Hung MC, Schechter AL, Chevray PY, et al: Molecular cloning of the neu gene: Absence of gross structural alteration in oncogenic alleles. Proc Natl Acad Sci U S A 1986;83:261-264.
16. Yu DH, Hung MC: Expression of activated rat neu oncogene is sufficient to induce experimental metastasis in 3T3cells. Oncogene 1991;6:1991-1996.
17. Yu D, Jing T, Lui B, et al: Overexpression of ErbB2 blocks Taxol-induced apoptosis upregulation of p21Cip1, which inhibits p34Cdc2 kinase. Mol Cell 1998;2:581-591.
18. Slamon DJ, Godolphin W, Jones LA, et al: Studies of the HER-2/neu oncogene in human breast and ovarian cancer. Science 1989;244:707-713.
19. Alvarez RD, Barnes MN, Gomez-Navarro J, et al: A cancer gene therapy approach utilizing an anti-erbB-2 single chain antibody-encoding adenovirus (AD21): A phase I trial. Clin Cancer Res 2000;6:3081-3087.
20. Hortobagyi GN, Ueno NT, Xia W, et al: Cationic liposome-mediated E1A gene transfer to human breast and ovarian cancer cells and its biologic effects: A phase I clinical trial. J Clin Oncol 2001;19:3422-3433.
21. Yu D, Matin A, Xia W, et al: Liposome-mediated in vivo E1A gene transfer suppressed dissemination of ovarian cancer cells that overexpress HER-2/neu. Oncogene 1995;11:1383-1388.
22. Berchuck A, Bast RC: P53-based gene therapy of ovarian cancer: Magic bullet? Gynecol Oncol 1995;59:169-170.
23. Santoso JT, Tang DC, Lane SB, et al: Adenovirus-based p53 gene therapy in ovarian cancer. Gynecol Oncol 1995;59:171-178.

24. Wolf JK, Mills GB, Bazzet L, et al: Adenovirus-mediated p53 growth inhibition of ovarian cancer cells is independent of endogenous p53 status. Gynecol Oncol 1999;75:261-266.

25. Buller RE, Pegram M, Runnebaum I, et al: A phase I/II trial of recombinant adenoviral human p53 (SCH58500) intraperitoneal (IP) gene therapy in recurrent ovarian cancer. Proceedings of the 30th Annual Meeting of the Society of Gynecologic Oncologists, San Francisco, CA, March 20-24, 1999.

26. Wolf JK, Bodurka-Bevers D, Gano JB, et al: A phase I study of Adp53 for patients with platinum- and paclitaxel-resistant epithelial ovarian cancer. Proceedings of the 43rd Annual Meeting of the American Society of Clinical Oncology, New Orleans, LA, May 20-23, 2000.

27. Tait DL, Obermiller PS, Jensen RA, Holt JT: Ovarian cancer gene therapy. Hematol Oncology Clin North Am 1998;12:539-552.

28. Tait DL, Obermiller PS, Fraziier SR, et al: A phase I trial of retroviral BRCA1 vs gene therapy in ovarian cancer. Clin Cancer Res 1997;3:1959-1968.

29. Tait DL, Obermiller PS, Hatmaker RA, et al: Ovarian cancer BRCA1 gene: Phase I and II trial differences in immune response and vector stability. Clin Cancer Res 1999;5:1708-1714.

30. Levine AJ, Momand J, Finlay CA: The p53 tumor suppressor gene. Nature 1991;351:453-465.

31. El-Deiry WS, Harper JW, O'Connor PM, et al: WAF1/CIP1 is induced in p53-mediated G_1 arrest and apoptosis. Cancer Res 1994;54:1169-1174.

32. Werness BA, Levine AJ, Howley PM: Association of human papillomavirus types 16 and 18 E6 proteins with p53. Science 1990;248:76-79.

33. Crook T, Tidy JA, Vousden KH: Degradation of p53 can be targeted by HPV E6 sequences distinct from those required for p53 binding and transactivation. Cell 1991;67:547-556.

34. Hamada K, Zhang WW, Alemany R, et al: Growth inhibition of human cervical cancer cells with the recombinant adenovirus p53 in vitro. Gynecol Oncol 1996;60:373-379.

35. Mitchell MF, Hamada K, Jagannadha S, et al: Transgene expression in the rhesus cervix mediated by an adenovirus expressing beta-galactosidase. Am J Obstet Gynecol 1996;174:1094-1101.

36. Ramondetta L, Mills GB, Burke TW, Wolf JK: Adenovirus mediated expression of p53 or p21 in a papillary serous endometrial carcinoma cell line (SPEC-2) results in both growth inhibition and apoptotic cell death: Potential application of gene therapy to endometrial cancer. Clin Cancer Res 2000;6:278-284.

37. Behbakht K, Benjamin I, Chiu HC, et al: Gynecology: Adenovirus-mediated gene therapy of ovarian cancer in a mouse model. Am J Obstet Gynecol 1996;175:1260-1265.

38. Zhang Y, Yu D, Xia W, Hung MC: HER-2/neu-targeting cancer therapy via adenovirus-mediated E1A delivery in an animal model. Oncogene 1995;10:1947-1954.

39. Dmitriev I, Krasnykh V, Miller CR, et al: An adenovirus vector with genetically modified fibers demonstrates expanded tropism via utilization of a coxsackievirus and adenovirus receptor-independent cell entry mechanism. J Virol 1998;72:9706-9713.

40. Kelly JF, Miller CR, Buchsbaum DJ, et al: Selectivity of TAG-72-targeted adenovirus gene transfer to primary ovarian carcinoma cells versus autologous mesothelial cell in vitro. Clin Cancer Res 2000;6:4323-4333.

41. Rancourt C, Rogers BE, Sosnowski BA, et al: Basic fibroblast growth factor enhancement of adenovirus-mediated delivery of the herpes simplex virus thymidine kinase gene results in augmented therapeutic benefit in a murine model of ovarian cancer. Clin Cancer Res 1998;4:2455-2462.

42. Blackwell JL, Hui L, Gomez-Navarro J, et al: Using a tropism-modified adenoviral vector to circumvent inhibitory factors in ascites fluid. Hum Gene Ther 2000;11:1657-1669.

43. Samulski RJ, Berns KI, Tam M, Muzyczka N: Cloning of adeno-associated virus into pBR322: Rescue of intact virus from the recombinant virus in human cells. Proc Natl Acad Sci U S A 1982;79:2077-2081.

44. Kotin RM, Berns KI: Organization of adeno-associated virus vector for high frequency integration, expression and rescue of genes in mammalian cell. Mol Cell Biol 1989;5:3251-3260.

45. Laughlin CA, Jones N, Carter BJ: Effects of deletions in adenovirus early region 1 genes upon replication of adeno-associated virus. J Virol 1982;41:868-876.

46. Ali M, Lemoine NR, Ring CJA: The use of DNA viruses as vectors for gene therapy. Gene Ther 1994;1:367-384.

47. Wang M, Rancourt C, Navarro JG, et al: High-efficacy thymidine kinase gene transfer to ovarian cancer cell lines mediated by herpes simplex virus type I vector. Gynecol Oncol 1998;71:278-287.

48. Alton EWFW, Middleton PG, Caplan NJ, et al: Non-invasive liposome-mediated gene delivery can correct the ion transport defect in cystic fibrosis mutant mice. Nat Genet 1993;5:135-142.

49. Wolff JA, Malone RW, Williams P, et al: Direct gene transfer into mouse muscle in vivo. Science 1990;247:1465-1468.

50. Williams RS, Johnston SA, Reidy M, et al: Introduction of foreign genes into tissues of living mice by DNA-coated microprojectiles. Proc Natl Acad Sci U S A 1991;88:2726-2730.

51. Cheng L, Ziegelhoffer PR, Yang N-S: In vivo promoter activity and transgene expression in mammalian somatic tissues evaluated by using particle bombardment. Proc Natl Acad Sci U S A 1993;90:4455-4459.

52. Verma IM, Somia N: Gene therapy: Promises, problems and prospects. Nature 1997;389:239-242.

53. Lee SE, Jin RJ, Lee SG, et al: Development of a new plasmid vector with PSA-promoter and enhancer expressing tissue-specificity in prostate carcinoma cell lines. Anticancer Res 2000;20:417-422.

54. Huber BE, Richards CA, Krenitsky TA: Retro-viral mediated gene therapy for the treatment of hepatocellular carcinoma: An innovative approach for cancer therapy. Proc Natl Acad Sci U S A 1990;88:8039-8043.

55. Thomson RC, Ohlsson K: Isolation, properties and complete amino acid sequence of human leukocyte proteinase inhibitor, potent inhibitor of leukocyte elastase. Proc Natl Acad Sci U S A 1986;83:6692-6696.

56. Robertson MW III, Wang M, Siegal GP, et al: Use of a tissue specific promoter for targeted expression of the herpes simplex virus thymidine kinase gene in cervical carcinoma cells. Cancer Gene Ther 1998;5:331-336.

57. Tanyi JL, Lapushin R, Eder A, et al: Identification of tissue and cancer specific promoters for the introduction of genes into human ovarian cancer cells. Gynecol Oncol 2002;85:451-458

58. Godwin AK, Miller PD, Getts LA, et al: Retroviral-like sequences specifically expressed in the rat ovary detect genetic differences between normal and transformed rat ovarian epithelial cells. Endocrinology 1995;136:464-469.

59. Neve R, Chang CH, Scott GK, et al: The epithelium-specific Ets transcription factor ESX is associated with mammary gland development and involution. FASEB J 1998;12:1541-1550.

60. Greider CW, Blackburn EH: Identification of a specific telomere terminal transferase activity in *Tetrahymena* extracts. Cell 1985;43:405-413.

61. Greider CW, Blackburn EH: A telomeric sequence in the RNA of *Tetrahymena* telomerase required for telomere repeat synthesis. Nature 1989;337:331-337.

62. Zhang A, Zheng C, Lindvall C, et al: Frequent amplification of the telomerase reverse transcriptase gene in human tumors. Cancer Res 2000;60:6230-6235.

63. Tzukerman M, Shachaf C, Ravel Y, et al: Identification of a novel transcription factor binding element involved in the regulation by differentiation of the human telomerase (hTERT) promoter. Mol Biol Cell 2000;11:4381-4391.

64. Goldsmith ME, Short KJ, Elwood PC, Kowan KH: A recombinant adenoviral vector with selective transgene expression in ovarian cancer cells [abstract]. Proc Am Assoc Cancer Res 1999;40:479.

65. Ring CJ, Blouin P, Martin LA, et al: Use of transcriptional regulatory elements of the MUC1 and ERBB2 genes to drive tumor-selective expression of a prodrug activating enzyme. Gene Ther 1997;4:1045-1052.

66. Tai YT, Strobel T, Kufe D, Cannistra SA: In vivo cytotoxicity of ovarian cancer cells through tumor-selective expression of the BAX gene. Cancer Res 1999;59:2121-2126.

67. Park T, Chen ZP, Leavitt J: Activation of the leukocyte plastin gene occurs in most human cancer cells. Cancer Res 1994;54:1775-1781.

68. Chung I, Schwartz PE, Crystal RG, et al: Use of the L-plastin promoter to develop an adenoviral system that confers transgene

expression in ovarian cancer cells but not normal mesothelial cells. Cancer Gene Ther 1999;6:99-106.

69. Aaronson SA: Growth factors and cancer. Science 1991;254: 1146-1153.

70. Lakshmi S, Balaraman Nair M, Jayaprakash PG, et al: c-ErbB-2 oncoprotein and epidermal growth factor receptor in cervical lesions. Pathobiology 1997;65:163-168.

71. Salomon DS, Brandt R, Ciardiello F, Normanno N: Epidermal growth factor-related peptides and their receptors in human malignancies. Crit Rev Oncol Hematol 1995;19:183-232.

72. Fan Z, Mendelsohn J: Therapeutic application of anti-growth factor receptor antibodies. Curr Opin Oncol 1998;10:67-73.

73. Anderson NG, Ahmad T, Chan K, et al: ZD1839 (Iressa), a novel epidermal growth factor receptor (EGFR) tyrosine kinase inhibitor, potentially inhibits the growth of EGFR positive cell lines with or without erbB2 overexpression. Int J Cancer 2001;94:774-782.

74. Sridhar SS, Seymour L, Shepherd FA: Inhibitors of epidermal-growth factor receptors: A review of clinical research with a focus on non–small-cell lung cancer. Lancet 2003;4:397-406.

75. Kay EW, Walsh CJB, Cassidy M, et al: c-ErbB-2 immunostaining: Problems with interpretation. J Clin Pathol 1994;47:816-822.

76. Berchuck A, Rodriguez G, Kamel A, et al: Expression of the epidermal growth factor receptor and HER-2/neu in normal and neoplastic cervix, vulva and vagina. Obstet Gynecol 1990; 76:381-387.

77. Bilous M, Dowsett M, Hanna W, et al: Current perspectives on HER2 testing: A review of national testing guidelines. Mod Pathol 2003;16:173-182.

78. Arteaga CL: Trastuzumab, an appropriate first-line single-agent therapy for HER2-overexpressing metastatic breast cancer. Breast Cancer Res 2003;5:96-100.

79. Moulder SL, Yakes FM, Muthuswamy SK, et al: Epidermal growth factor receptor (HER1) tyrosine kinase inhibitor ZD1839 (Iressa) inhibits Her2/neu (erbB2)-overexpressing breast cancer cells in vitro and in vivo. Cancer Res 2001;61:8887-8895.

80. Croom KF, Perry CM: Imatinib mesylate in the treatment of gastrointestinal stromal tumors. 2003;63:513-522.

81. Inoue M, Kyo S, Fujita M, et al: Coexpression of the c-kit receptor and the stem cell factor in gynecologic tumors. Cancer Res 1994;54:3049-3053.

82. Versnel MA, Haarbrink M, Langerak AW, et al: Human ovarian tumors of epithelial origin express PDGF in vitro and in vivo. Cancer Genet Cytogenet 1994;73:60-64.

83. O'Neill AJ, Cotter TG, Russell JM, Gaffney EF: Abl expression in human fetal and adult tissues, tumors, and tumor microvessels. J Pathol 1997;183:325-329.

84. Parrott JA, Kim G, Skinner MK: Expression and action of kit ligand/stem cell factor in normal human and bovine ovarian surface epithelium and ovarian cancer. Biol Repro 2000;62: 1600-1609.

85. Dabrow MB, Francesco MR, McBrearty FX, Cardonna S: The effects of platelet-derived growth factor and receptor on normal and neoplastic human ovarian surface epithelium. Gynecol Oncol 1998;71:29-37.

86. Tonary AM, MacDonald EA, Faught W, et al: Lack of expression of c-KIT in ovarian cancers is associated with poor prognosis. Int J Cancer (Pred Oncol) 2000;89:242-250.

87. Slomovitz BM, Broaddus RR, Thornton AD, et al. Expression of Gleevec (imatinib mesylate)-targeted kinases in endometrial carcinoma [abstract]. Gynecol Oncol 2003;88:207.

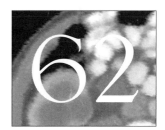

HEREDITARY GYNECOLOGIC CANCER SYNDROMES

Jeffney Boyd

✦ MAJOR CONTROVERSIES

- Is this genetic model relevant to all aspects of human tumorigenesis?
- What is the lifetime risk of ovarian cancer in a *BRCA* mutation carrier?
- Are *BRCA* mutation carriers at increased risk for other cancers?
- Are there genotype-phenotype correlations?
- Are the pathologic and surgical presentations of *BRCA*-linked ovarian cancers distinct from those of sporadic cases?
- Is the early natural history of *BRCA*-linked ovarian cancer unique?
- Are the clinical outcome and treatment effects different for *BRCA*-linked cancers compared with sporadic ovarian cancers?
- What is the cancer risk–reducing surgical procedure of choice?
- To what extent does prophylactic surgery reduce cancer risk?
- Can other medical interventions reduce the risk of ovarian cancer in the population of *BRCA* mutation carriers?
- Is screening for ovarian cancer effective in the high-risk population?
- What is hereditary nonpolyposis colorectal cancer?
- What is the genetic basis of hereditary nonpolyposis colorectal cancer?
- Who should be tested for genetic predisposition to hereditary nonpolyposis colorectal cancer?
- What are the lifetime risks of endometrial and ovarian cancers in mismatch repair gene mutation carriers?
- Are the clinicopathologic features of hereditary nonpolyposis colorectal cancer–associated gynecologic cancers distinct from their sporadic counterparts?
- What is the appropriate clinical management of an individual at risk for hereditary nonpolyposis colorectal cancer?

The molecular genetic bases for all of the clinically significant hereditary gynecologic cancer syndromes have been almost fully elucidated. This knowledge provides new and profound opportunities for the development of novel prevention and early detection strategies that should, in principle, lead to reductions in morbidity and mortality from gynecologic cancers. However, our ability to identify individuals at increased genetic risk for cancer has substantially outpaced the development of

infrastructure and procedures for handling the ethical, legal, and social implications of genetic testing. Clinical interventions (the discussion of which is beyond the scope of this chapter) and data concerning the efficacy of these interventions for cancer prevention are in the early stages, as is any knowledge of the benefit of enhanced surveillance for improved early detection.

This chapter provides brief overviews of cancer genetics in general and the molecular genetic bases of inherited susceptibility to gynecologic cancers in particular. The chapter also discusses the clinical management of individuals at risk for these cancers and highlights some controversies that exist with respect to these topics.

Cancer Genetics

The term *hereditary cancer* is somewhat of a misnomer, because individuals inherit a susceptibility to cancer, not the cancer itself. Although this may seem a trivial or semantic distinction, the reasons underlying this difference have important implications for the clinical management of patients at increased genetic risk for cancer. An introduction to the fundamental principles of cancer molecular genetics provides a necessary conceptual foundation on which to consider the complexities and controversies related to patient management in this context.

All cancers are genetic diseases in the sense that gene mutations are the driving force of cancer development. A tumor may arise through the accumulation of mutations that are exclusively somatic (i.e., acquired) in origin or through the inheritance of a mutation from a parent through the germline, followed by the acquisition of additional somatic mutations. These two genetic scenarios distinguish what are colloquially referred to as *sporadic* and *hereditary* cancers, respectively. In either case, it is the sequential mutation of cancer-related genes and their subsequent selection and accumulation in a clonal population of cells that determine whether a tumor develops and the time required for its development and progression. This multistep, multigenic model of cancer development is among the most robust of all biologic theories and is supported by extensive data from the study of human cancers and model systems.[1-4] Perhaps the most compelling evidence is that the age-specific incidence rates for most solid tumors increase at roughly the fourth to eighth power of elapsed time, consistent with a dependence on four to eight genetic alterations that are rate limiting for cancer development.[5]

Genetic alterations in cancer cells occur in two major families of genes: oncogenes and tumor suppressor genes. Generally, proteins encoded by oncogenes are stimulatory and those encoded by tumor suppressor genes are inhibitory to the neoplastic phenotype. Mutational activation of protooncogenes to oncogenes and mutational inactivation of tumor suppressor genes must occur for cancer development to take place. Protooncogene mutations are usually somatic; two known exceptions affect the *RET* and *MET* protooncogenes, activating mutations of which may be inherited through the germline, predisposing to multiple endocrine neoplasia type II[6] and papillary renal carcinoma,[7] respectively. Tumor suppressor gene mutations may be inherited or acquired somatically. Other than these exceptions, all hereditary cancer syndromes for which predisposing genes have been identified are linked to tumor suppressor genes. Genes encoding proteins involved in various DNA repair pathways have been proposed to represent a third class of genes involved in tumorigenesis, but subclassification of tumor suppressors as "gatekeepers" or "caretakers"[8] would seem more appropriate.

Genetics of cancer predisposition. An understanding of tumor suppressor genetics is essential to a consideration of most hereditary cancer syndromes, including gynecologic cancers. The protein products of tumor suppressor gene function to inhibit malignant transformation and are inactivated through loss-of-function mutations. Knudson's two-hit model established the paradigm for tumor suppressor gene recessivity at the cellular level, wherein both alleles must be inactivated to exert a phenotypic effect on tumorigenesis.[9] This two-hit model is frequently misapplied, especially in the context of hereditary cancers, having become synonymous with the notion that inactivation of both alleles of a single gene is necessary and sufficient for tumorigenesis. It is important to recognize that this theory estimates only the number of events that are rate limiting for cancer development.[10] Most adult solid tumors probably require mutations in multiple genes, many of which may occur at a relatively high frequency compared with the rate-limiting genetic alterations and therefore do not appear in a kinetic analysis such as that performed by Knudson.

The location and type of inactivating mutations in tumor suppressor genes typically vary from one cancer to another. In some cases, most notably for the gene encoding p53 *(TP53)*, missense mutations occur that change a single amino acid in the encoded protein. More often, mutations in tumor suppressor genes alter the base sequence such that the encoded protein product is truncated because of generation of a premature stop codon. Truncated protein products may result from several types of mutational events. Included in this category are nonsense mutations, in which a single base substitution changes a specific amino acid codon to a stop codon. Microdeletions or microinsertions of one or several nucleotides that disrupt the reading frame of the mRNA transcript (i.e., frameshift mutations) also lead to downstream stop codons. This category of mutation is common in *BRCA* and other tumor suppressor genes.

A mutation in one allele, whether germline or somatic, is then revealed after somatic inactivation of the homologous wild-type allele. In theory, the same spectrum of mutational events could contribute to inactivation of the second allele, but what is typically observed in tumors is homozygosity or hemizygosity for the first mutation, indicating "loss" of the wild-type allele. As originally demonstrated for the retinoblastoma susceptibility gene,[11] loss of the second allele may occur through mitotic nondisjunction or recombination mechanisms or through large deletions. This so-called loss of heterozygosity (LOH) has become recognized as the hallmark of tumor suppressor gene inactivation at particular genomic loci.

Several tumor suppressors involved in hereditary predisposition to cancer have been shown to function in the recognition and repair of various forms of DNA damage. The mutational inactivation of DNA repair genes contributes to tumorigenesis indirectly by promoting one or another type of genetic instability that leads to the mutation of additional cancer-related genes. This relatively unique mechanism of tumor suppression has led some to suggest that the DNA repair genes should represent a third cancer gene family. In all cases described, however, the genetic mechanism appears to involve a cellular recessive mechanism involving loss of function, consistent with the tumor suppressor categorization. Perhaps more appropriate is the classification scheme proposed by Kinzler and Vogelstein,[8] in which tumor suppressor genes are subdivided into the categories of *gatekeepers* and *caretakers*. The former category includes genes that function directly to inhibit cell proliferation or promote cell death (e.g., *RB1*, *TP53*, *APC*), whereas the latter category consists of genes that function to maintain genomic integrity (e.g., mismatch repair genes involved in hereditary nonpolyposis colorectal cancer, the nucleotide excision repair genes in involved in xeroderma pigmentosum, *ATM*, *BRCA1*, *BRACA*). Some of these genes do not readily adhere to this distinction; *BRCA1*, for example, may function as gatekeeper and caretaker.

Is this genetic model relevant to all aspects of human tumorigenesis?

This brief exposition of cancer genetics serves as an introduction to the controversies that surround the general applicability of this genetic model to all aspects of human tumorigenesis. There are three noteworthy caveats to this oversimplified genetic model of human cancer development. First, the multistep, multigenic aspect of this model may not apply to some cancer types, including rare embryonal solid tumors such as retinoblastoma. The so-called two-hit model for tumor suppressor gene inactivation in hereditary tumorigenesis was first postulated by Knudson from a theoretical consideration of the kinetics of pediatric retinoblastoma development[12,13] and may apply to this and related tumor types. The model is frequently misinterpreted as applying to all hereditary cancer syndromes, but it clearly does not. Similarly, hematologic malignancies such as chronic myelogenous leukemia (CML) may arise from a single pathogenic chromosomal abnormality, in this case the reciprocal translocation t(9;22) that manifests as the Philadelphia chromosome and produces the *BCR-ABL* oncogene product. It is this very specific genetic scenario that may explain the remarkable efficacy of imatinib mesylate (Gleevec) in treating CML, because the drug specifically targets the central causative molecular defect.[14] The inappropriate extrapolation of this result to the experimental treatment of other cancers is widely underway, but this and similar targeted therapies are unlikely to prove as effective in the treatment of tumors defined by multiple genetic alterations.

Second, this genetic model should not be taken to imply that epigenetic phenomena do not play a role an important role in tumorigenesis. The neoplastic phenotype is partially derived from alterations in gene expression and related molecular phenomena such as alternative splicing of mRNA transcripts or post-translational processing or secretion of proteins. For example, the generation of gene expression profiles or signatures that distinguish clinically relevant subclasses of various tumor types is rapidly becoming recognized as a useful tool for prognostic classification.[15] Similarly, the detection of anonymous proteomic patterns in serum has great potential for the early detection of cancer, as demonstrated for ovarian carcinoma.[16] These phenomena probably represent the downstream effects of a small number of critical genetic mutations, and distinctions must be made between the multiple layers of molecular "causation" in tumorigenesis. It is primarily through stable alterations in DNA structure that a cell maintains and passes to its progeny the molecular blueprint of malignancy.

This leads to the third qualification of the cancer genetic paradigm that pertains to the role of epigenetic alterations in tumorigenesis: gene silencing through promoter hypermethylation and histone modification. Gene silencing is believed to play a critical role in development and tissue-specific gene expression,[17] and aberrations in this process are well described in several genetic disorders,[18] including cancer.[19] These phenomena are said to be epigenetic because they are heritable at the cellular level but do not involve DNA mutations. Despite the very large literature on tumor suppressor gene methylation in human cancers, there remains considerable debate and uncertainty about the mechanisms through which this modification occurs and the characterization of this phenomenon as a cause or consequence of gene silencing.[20] However, it is likely that epigenetic gene silencing, whatever the mechanism, plays a critical role in tumor suppressor gene inactivation in human carcinogenesis.

Genetic Predisposition to Gynecologic Cancers

Epithelial ovarian carcinoma and endometrial carcinoma occur as components of relatively common autosomal dominant cancer predisposition syndromes such as the breast and ovarian cancer (BOC) syndrome and the hereditary nonpolyposis colorectal cancer (HNPCC) syndrome (Table 62-1). There is little evidence to support the occurrence of squamous carcinomas or sarcomas of the female reproductive tract in any common cancer predisposition syndrome. Several

Table 62–1. Hereditary Gynecologic Cancer Syndromes

Syndrome	Cancer	Genes
BOC	Epithelial ovarian carcinoma	*BRCA1*, *BRCA2*
HNPCC	Endometrial carcinoma Epithelial ovarian carcinoma	*MSH2*, *MLH1*, *MSH6*

BOC, breast and ovarian cancer; HNPCC, hereditary nonpolyposis colorectal cancer.

gynecologic neoplasms occur at higher than expected frequencies in rare cancer-predisposition syndromes such as sex cord tumors of the ovary and adenoma malignum of the cervix, which appear to represent integral tumors of the Peutz-Jeghers syndrome. However, these syndromes are not discussed in detail here because there exist few data to guide the clinical management of these individuals.

The proportion of epithelial ovarian carcinomas attributable to autosomal dominant genetic predisposition is approximately 10%,[21] highest of all common forms of adult cancers. Most of these hereditary cases (>90%) occur as part of the BOC syndrome, and the remainder arise in the context of the HNPCC syndrome. A site-specific manifestation of familial ovarian cancer in which an excess of ovarian cancer but not breast or other cancers is observed is also recognized, but genetic analyses have failed to demonstrate linkage of these kindreds to any locus other than the breast and ovarian cancer susceptibility gene *BRCA1*.[22] These families are most appropriately considered as affected by a variant manifestation of the BOC syndrome in which breast cancer is rare or undocumented.

Genetic predisposition to endometrial carcinoma occurs primarily within the context of HNPCC, which probably accounts for less than 5% of all endometrial cancer cases. Descriptions of a site-specific manifestation of familial endometrial carcinoma exist in the literature, but there is no evidence for linkage of these families to any genetic locus other than one of those responsible for HNPCC.[23] Emerging evidence suggests that endometrial carcinoma may also occur as an integral tumor in the Cowden syndrome, a rare autosomal dominant syndrome predisposing to breast and thyroid carcinomas and linked to the *PTEN* tumor suppressor gene.[24] As for Peutz-Jeghers syndrome, there are insufficient data to warrant a discussion of the clinical implications of endometrial cancer occurrence in the Cowden syndrome.

The clinical management of individuals at genetically high risk for gynecologic cancers occurs in a syndrome-specific rather than organ-specific manner. A synopsis of the current knowledge and the major issues and controversies arising in this area is presented according to syndrome.

Breast and Ovarian Cancer Syndrome

What is the lifetime risk of ovarian cancer in a *BRCA* mutation carrier? Estimates for the lifetime risk of ovarian cancer in women with *BRCA* mutations depend on the gene and the population studied. Several initial estimates suggested a lifetime risk of ovarian cancer of 63% for a *BRCA1* mutation carrier,[25] based on data from large breast and ovarian cancer families in which penetrance was likely to be higher than average for reasons that are poorly understood. Later estimates from population-based approaches suggest that the lifetime risk of ovarian cancer is 30% to 40% for *BRCA1* mutation carriers and 15% to 25% for *BRCA2* mutation carriers (Table 62-2).[26-30] There is general consensus

Table 62–2. Lifetime Risks of Cancers Associated with Specific Genes

Cancer	BRCA1*	BRCA2*	MMR†
Breast	35-60%	30-55%	No increase
Ovarian	30-40%	15-25%	6-20%
Endometrial	No increase	No increase	40-60%

*BRCA mutations in the context of the breast and ovarian cancer syndrome.
†Mismatch repair (MMR) gene (MSH2, MLH1, MSH6) mutations in the context of the hereditary nonpolyposis colorectal cancer syndrome.

that the risk associated with *BRCA2* is lower than that with *BRCA1*. These figures contrast markedly with the lifetime risk of ovarian cancer in the general population of 1.4%.

Are *BRCA* mutation carriers at increased risk for other cancers? The lifetime risk of breast cancer in this population is substantial and probably somewhat higher than for ovarian cancer, with estimates ranging from 35% to 60% for *BRCA1* and 30% to 55% for *BRCA2*. This and other issues related to hereditary breast cancer and its clinical management are beyond the scope of this chapter but have been reviewed elsewhere in detail.[31] With respect to other gynecologic malignancies, the molecular evidence indicates that primary peritoneal and fallopian tube carcinomas can be causally linked to *BRCA* mutation,[32-35] and population-based evidence indicates that both tumors should be considered as components of the BOC syndrome.[36,37] It is not uncommon to detect these tumors incidentally in *BRCA* mutation carriers during risk-reducing surgery.[38-43] The relative rarity of these tumors coupled with the difficulty in discerning accurate diagnoses have precluded the calculation of reliable relative risk estimates, but it is reasonable to assume that the risks of these cancers in the *BRCA* population are probably significantly elevated over those in the general population and that the lifetime risks of primary peritoneal and fallopian tube cancers in *BRCA* mutation carriers are considerably less than the risk of ovarian cancer in this group.

Less clear is whether *BRCA* mutation increases the risk of uterine cancer. Several case reports and small case series suggest that endometrial carcinoma, especially the papillary serous histologic subtype,[28,44,45] may be causally linked to *BRCA* mutation, whereas two population-based studies, one focusing on papillary serous tumors specifically[46] and the other on endometrial carcinoma generally,[47] found no evidence for an increased risk in the *BRCA* population. In two large studies of high-risk breast and ovarian cancer families, one concluded that *BRCA1* mutation confers a modest relative risk of uterine cancer,[48] and the other found no evidence of increased risk.[49] In a similar study of *BRCA2*-linked families, no evidence of an increased risk of uterine cancer was observed.[50] When considered together, these studies suggest that some cases of endometrial carcinoma may be causally associated with an inherited *BRCA* mutation but that the

Table 62–3. Other Cancers Attributed to the BOC and HNPCC Syndromes

BOC*	HNPCC†
Fallopian tube	Stomach
Primary peritoneal	Ureter, renal pelvis
Male breast	Small bowel
Pancreas	Brain
Prostate	Hepatobiliary tract
Stomach	Skin (sebaceous)
Gallbladder, bile duct	Breast (?)
Melanoma	
Endometrial (?)	
Colon (?)	

*Cancers most likely to occur at increased frequency in association with a *BRCA* mutation in addition to breast and ovarian.

†Cancers most likely to occur at increased frequency in association with an MMR gene mutation in addition to colorectal, endometrial, and ovarian.

BOC, breast and ovarian cancer; HNPCC, hereditary nonpolyposis colorectal cancer.

penetrance of *BRCA* mutation for endometrial carcinoma is sufficiently low that the relative risk of this malignancy in *BRCA* mutation carriers is not significantly elevated over that of the general population. The clinical implications of all these data are discussed in a later section of this chapter.

The risk of other malignancies in the *BRCA* mutation population are much lower than for breast and ovarian cancer, but data are conflicting with respect to inclusion of various other tumor types in the BOC syndrome and the relative risk of each (Table 62-3). One early and widely quoted study[51] found evidence of increased risks of colorectal and prostate cancers in association with *BRCA1* mutation, but these findings did not prove reproducible. Evidence from two studies of a total of 846 BOC families suggests that *BRCA1* confers a modest risk for cancers of the pancreas (both studies), colon, stomach, and uterus.[48,49] Similarly, a study of 173 BOC families with a *BRCA2* mutation revealed a small but significant increased risks of cancers of the prostate, pancreas, gallbladder, bile duct, and stomach and of malignant melanoma.[50] It is unlikely that these findings will be translated into clinical practice in the immediate future.

Are there genotype-phenotype correlations? Extensive heterogeneity in the *BRCA* mutational spectrum, together with likely functional diversity of the *BRCA* proteins, leads to speculation that phenotypic variation is likely to correlate with the location and type of *BRCA* mutation. Only limited evidence supports this concept. The first study to examine this issue suggested that mutations proximal to exon 13 in the *BRCA1* gene are more strongly associated with ovarian cancer in a series of 30 BOC families linked to *BRCA1*.[52] However, few additional data exist to confirm this observation. In a subsequent study by the same group, an ovarian cancer cluster region (OCCR) was identified in exon 11 of the *BRCA2* gene; mutations in this region are associated with a higher frequency of ovarian cancer than

breast cancer in 25 families with a *BRCA2* mutation.[53] These data are supported by several additional studies. In the largest, confirmation of the existence of the *BRCA2* OCCR was provided by the Breast Cancer Linkage Consortium.[29] Cancer occurrence in 164 breast and ovarian cancer families with *BRCA2* mutations was studied to evaluate genotype-phenotype correlations. Mutations in the OCCR were associated with a significantly higher ratio of cases of ovarian to breast cancers in female carriers than were mutations proximal or distal to this region. The biologic mechanism for this effect remains unknown.

Are the pathologic and surgical presentations of *BRCA*-linked ovarian cancers distinct from those of sporadic cases? Unlike the marked distinction between hereditary and sporadic breast cancers, ovarian cancers associated with *BRCA* mutations appear remarkably similar to their sporadic counterparts, with several subtle exceptions.[28,54-56] With respect to histologic type, serous tumors predominate, and tumors of endometrioid or clear cell histologies are occasionally seen. However, serous tumors are probably somewhat overrepresented, and invasive mucinous tumors and tumors of low malignant potential (or "borderline" tumors) of all types are rarely observed in association with a *BRCA* mutation. With respect to histologic grade, most *BRCA*-linked ovarian cancers are moderately to poorly differentiated; well-differentiated cancers are rare and probably underrepresented compared with the grade distribution for sporadic ovarian cancers.

Similarly, the surgical presentation of *BRCA*-linked ovarian cancer does not appear remarkably different than for sporadic ovarian cancer.[28,54] Most hereditary tumors present at an advanced surgical stage, with approximately three fourths of patients diagnosed with stage II through IV disease. Stage I tumors are sometimes observed, especially in the context of high-risk screening programs and as an incidental finding associated with prophylactic oophorectomy,[40,57] suggesting that these cancers do progress through an identifiable early stage and are amenable to early detection. In terms of surgical cytoreduction of advanced stage ovarian cancers, the ratio of optimal to suboptimal cases does not appear significantly different for *BRCA*-linked compared with sporadic cases.[54] Preoperative serum CA 125 levels are elevated in patients with *BRCA*-linked ovarian cancers, and the mean levels are not significantly different from those in sporadic cases.[58]

Is the early natural history of *BRCA*-linked ovarian cancer unique? Among the requirements for the development of novel screening strategies for ovarian cancer is an understanding of the tumor's early natural history, including characterization of the histologic region of origin and a recognizable premalignant lesion, neither of which has been firmly elucidated with respect to ovarian carcinoma. Increasingly, investigators have attempted to gain insight into these phenomena through the study of ovarian tissues removed prophylactically from women at high risk for ovarian cancer (i.e., *BRCA* mutation carriers). There exist several theories on the histologic origin of ovarian carcinoma. Although it is widely believed that the epithelial component of the ovary gives rise to the common epithelial ovarian carcinomas, it is not clear whether these cancers originate in the single-cell layer of surface epithelium or in architectural aberrations of the surface epithelium. Examples of the latter include surface epithelium-lined clefts, cortical inclusion cysts (postulated to result from postovulatory wound repair), tissue remodeling associated with pregnancy or aging, paraovarian adhesions, and dynamic interactions between surface epithelium and underlying stroma.

Several studies have addressed the hypothesis that these morphologic alterations of surface epithelium are more prevalent in the ovaries of women who have developed ovarian cancer[59,60] or are at high genetic risk for ovarian cancer.[61-65] The consensus from the literature is that these morphologic alterations are common in ovaries from all women and are probably not present at a higher frequency in cancer-prone ovaries. Another histopathology-based theory suggests that ovarian carcinoma may arise in components of the secondary mullerian system, such as rete ovarii, paraovarian or paratubal cysts, endosalpingiosis, endometriosis, and endomucinosis, located within or adjacent to the ovary.[66] This theory gains support through recognition that the ovarian surface epithelium is a modified mesothelium, continuous with and morphologically resembling the peritoneal mesothelial lining. However, typical epithelial ovarian neoplasms are readily distinguishable from primary ovarian mesotheliomas and resemble those arising in other mullerian-derived tissues such as the fallopian tube, endometrium, and endocervix. This suggests a requirement for a metaplastic process during ovarian tumorigenesis if these cancers do arise from the ovarian mesothelium. It is well established that some ovarian cancers, primarily of endometrioid and clear cell histologies, arise within endometriotic implants,[67] and the ovarian cancer risk reduction imparted by tubal ligation (discussed later) is consistent with the possibility that some ovarian cancers may actually represent metastatic fallopian tube cancers.

Similar controversy surrounds the existence of an identifiable premalignant lesion for ovarian carcinoma, a problem compounded by the uncertainty regarding its histologic origin and the fact that most ovarian carcinomas are of advanced stage and associated with little or no evidence of preinvasive or normal epithelium at the time of pathologic diagnosis. It is well accepted that common benign and borderline (or low malignant potential) ovarian tumors are not precursors for invasive ovarian carcinoma.[68] Candidate precursor lesions have included dysplasia, hyperplasia, and more subtle alterations involving cellular or nuclear atypia. Evidence for the development of ovarian carcinoma de novo in the absence of any intermediate precursor lesion has also been presented. The advent of molecular biologic and genetic information and

technologies has begun to allow the study of this problem at a level beyond that of purely morphologic. Examples include the observations of loss of heterozygosity at the *BRCA1* and *TP53* loci in an ovarian carcinoma in situ lesion from a *BRCA1* heterozygote[69] and synuclein expression in ovarian cancers and in some putative precursor lesions, although not in normal ovarian epithelium.[70] In a genetic analysis of ovarian carcinoma histogenesis using ovarian tissues and stage I cancers from *BRCA* mutation carriers, ovarian cancer was found to originate almost exclusively in epithelial inclusion cysts, and invasive cancers invariably arose from a limited field of dysplasia within these cysts.[71] These observations require confirmation with respect to their applicability to sporadic ovarian tumorigenesis, but should provide a conceptual foundation on which to base strategies for the early detection of ovarian cancer.

Are the clinical outcome and treatment effects different for BRCA-linked cancers compared with sporadic ovarian cancers? The original observation that overall survival is improved for *BRCA*-associated compared with sporadic ovarian cancer cases[72] was subsequently confirmed[73] and refuted[74,75] in studies of disparate design. Multivariate analysis of consecutive cases of *BRCA*-linked cancer compared with sporadic ovarian cancer from the same institution revealed that *BRCA* mutation status is an independent predictor of improved survival in advanced-stage ovarian cancer; likewise, a longer recurrence-free interval is observed in hereditary compared with sporadic cases.[54] Similarly, in a large study of Israeli ovarian cancer patients, *BRCA* mutation status was an independent predictor of improved survival.[76] Two population-based studies provide indirect support for improved survival for patients with *BRCA1*-associated ovarian cancer.[28,77] In these studies, the prevalence of *BRCA* mutations increased with time from diagnosis, suggesting that long-term survival was enhanced for *BRCA* mutation carriers.

Emerging data from two lines of laboratory investigation provide a likely mechanistic explanation for the improved response to chemotherapy and overall survival observed for ovarian cancer patients with *BRCA* mutations. First, a higher proliferative index or growth fraction is characteristic of *BRCA*-associated ovarian cancers compared with sporadic cancers of similar histology and grade,[78] a factor possibly associated with an improved response to cytotoxic chemotherapy. Second, consideration of the function of BRCA proteins provides an explanation for an improved response specifically to platinum-based therapy. BRCA1 and BRCA2 proteins are known to function in homology-directed repair of DNA double-strand breaks, a lesion that is produced by the cellular DNA repair machinery in response to mutagenic agents that cause interstrand DNA crosslinks.[79] Among the prototypic agents that cause this type of DNA crosslink are cisplatin, mitomycin C, and γ radiation. As predicted by this model, *BRCA1*-deficient human breast cancer cells, as opposed to those with wild-type

BRAC1, are hypersensitive to all three of these agents but not to others that cause different types of DNA damage.[80] The improved survival and recurrence-free interval observed in cases of *BRCA*-linked ovarian cancer probably reflect the relative hypersensitivity of these tumors to platinum-based therapy, which is standard front-line treatment for epithelial ovarian carcinoma.

What is the cancer risk–reducing surgical procedure of choice? If risk-reducing gynecologic surgery is elected by an asymptomatic *BRCA* mutation carrier, the evidence cited previously indicates bilateral salpingo-oophorectomy (BSO) as the minimal procedure of choice. One study described the detection of positive cytology in the peritoneal lavage specimens obtained from high-risk patients undergoing risk-reducing BSO, and some of these patients were found to have occult ovarian or tubal cancers.[81] These findings suggest that peritoneal lavage and cytologic examination may also be indicated at the time of risk-reducing BSO. Less clear is the indication for hysterectomy. Although *BRCA* mutation carriers are probably not at increased risk for endometrial carcinoma (or other uterine cancers), the intramural portion of the fallopian tube remains within the uterine fundus after salpingo-oophorectomy, presumably with a residual risk of cancer in this tissue remnant. This has led some to suggest that hysterectomy be considered as a component of the risk-reducing procedure in these women.[82] Many *BRCA* mutation carriers may take tamoxifen for the prevention or treatment of breast cancer, with the resultant increase in endometrial cancer risk. Further research on the effect of hysterectomy on cancer risk reduction is important for the development of a consensus standard of care.

To what extent does prophylactic surgery reduce cancer risk? Historically, discussion of the use of risk-reducing BSO in the high-risk population has been profoundly tempered by the knowledge of case reports of primary peritoneal carcinoma after oophorectomy.[83-85] Although *BRCA* mutation carriers are unquestionably at increased risk for primary peritoneal cancer, there have been few published data on the efficacy of BSO in reducing the risk of pelvic (ovarian, fallopian tube, and peritoneal) or breast cancers in women at risk for the BOC syndrome.[86] Retrospective analyses suggest that oophorectomy in *BRCA* mutation carriers reduces the risk of coelomic epithelial cancers by 96% and breast cancer by more than 50%.[87,88] The only prospective study to address this issue similarly found that BSO in *BRCA* mutation carriers reduced the risk of breast or gynecologic cancer by 75%.[41] There are no data to suggest that this procedure is ineffective in significantly reducing the risk of gynecologic and breast cancers in women at risk for the BOC syndrome. The risk of epithelial peritoneal cancer after prophylactic BSO in women with *BRCA* mutations appears to be on the order of 1%.[41,88] Although the efficacy of BSO in reducing cancer risk for *BRCA* mutation carriers is indisputable, many other factors bear on the use and

timing of this procedure in the clinical management of high-risk patients.[89]

Can other medical interventions reduce the risk of ovarian cancer in the population of *BRCA* mutation carriers? The use of oral contraceptives is well established from an epidemiologic perspective to reduce the risk of ovarian cancer in the general population.[90,91] The biologic basis for this association is undoubtedly complex, but it probably involves a reduction in the number of ovulatory cycles, alterations in gonadotropin secretion, and pharmacologic effects on proliferative and apoptotic pathways in the ovarian epithelium.[92-94] Three case-control studies indicate that oral contraceptive use is also protective against ovarian cancer in *BRCA* mutation carriers.[95-97] The magnitude of this protection is similar to that observed in the general population, with more than 5 years of use associated with a greater than 50% reduction in risk. It is understandable that a case-control study from Israel,[98] in which oral contraceptives were found not to protect against ovarian cancer in women with *BRCA* mutations, was met with considerable publicity and discussion in the lay and medical communities. For several reasons discussed elsewhere,[89] in addition to the weight of the available evidence on this topic, this study should not change our view of the utility of oral contraceptives in ovarian cancer prevention. Until further evidence to the contrary emerges, this study is an outlier, and a large body of data supports the protective effect of oral contraceptive use against ovarian cancer in the general and high-risk populations.

Tubal ligation has proved protective against ovarian cancer in the general population.[99,100] The mechanism for this protective effect is obscure; tubal ligation may interrupt blow flow to the ovary or block the passage of carcinogens from the external environment to the ovary, but little evidence exists to support these hypotheses. It was suggested that the cells of origin of ovarian cancer may arise in the fallopian epithelium and undergo transfer to the ovary and that tubal ligation interrupts this passage.[101] With respect to the high-risk population, one study on the role of tubal ligation in *BRCA1* mutation carriers reported a risk reduction of 61%, with the combination of tubal ligation and oral contraceptive use providing a risk reduction of 72%.[96] It is likely that a combination of medical and surgical interventions over a lifetime, such as oral contraceptive use until childbearing is complete, followed by tubal ligation, followed by BSO after menopause, may prove most effective at lowering cancer risk while preserving quality of life.

Is screening for ovarian cancer effective in the high-risk population? Screening for ovarian cancer using serum CA125 measurements or ultrasonography, or both, has been proposed as a method for reducing mortality through early detection.[102] The utility of these procedures has not been proved in prospective trials, but several are underway and should provide definitive evidence soon. It is reasonable to presume that screening may prove more effective in the high-risk population, for whom the prevalence of disease is higher. Data from prospective trials aimed at this population are not yet available, and the findings from several small observational cohort studies are mixed. In one study, several early-stage pelvic cancers were detected in *BRCA* mutation carriers undergoing surveillance.[40] However, the results from another study of a similar cohort were disappointing because the screen-detected cancers were predominantly of advanced stage.[42] Regardless of the results of ongoing screening trials, it is probable that innovative technologies such as the use of serum proteomic patterns to identify early-stage ovarian cancers will supplant existing tools for ovarian cancer detection in the near future. Initial data suggest that the proteomic-based technique is superior in terms of sensitivity and specificity compared with cure and serum known markers in the general and high-risk populations.[16]

Hereditary Nonpolyposis Colorectal Cancer Syndrome

In 1913, Alfred Warthin, a pathologist at the University of Michigan who was reportedly motivated by his seamstress who feared familial cancer, was the first to describe families affected by what was later to become known as *hereditary nonpolyposis colorectal cancer syndrome* (HNPCC).[103] The family of this seamstress, later called *cancer family G*, was observed by Warthin to have an excess of gastric and uterine cancers, but after several generations of study, members have also been documented to suffer from excessive colorectal and extraintestinal tumors.[104] Subsequent studies of similar families by Henry Lynch and colleagues[105] led to a description of the *cancer family syndrome.* In 1984, the terms *Lynch syndrome I* and *Lynch syndrome II* were proposed by Boland and Troncale as corresponding to site-specific familial colorectal cancer and the cancer family syndrome, respectively, without antecedent polyposis.[106] An International Collaborative Group on HNPCC, meeting in Amsterdam in 1991, proposed criteria designed to provide a uniform basis for clinical diagnosis of HNPCC.[107] Recognizing that these so-called Amsterdam criteria (Table 62-4) are likely to lead to the underdiagnosis of HNPCC, other groups have proposed less restrictive criteria that reflect the presence of extracolonic malignancies and genetic information.[108-112] The International Collaborative Group on HNPCC released the revised Amsterdam II criteria in 1999 to reflect these concerns. The definition of HNPCC has evolved considerably and is less than straightforward.

What is hereditary nonpolyposis colorectal cancer?

A survey of the literature on HNPCC reveals considerable discussion of the use of genetic versus clinical criteria for the diagnosis of HNPCC. There is no evidence that an inherited mutation in *MSH2, MLH1,* or *MSH6* confers a genetic predisposition to a cancer syndrome distinct from HNPCC or one of its phenotypic variants. Among the latter is the Muir-Torre syndrome,

Table 62–4. Amsterdam Criteria for Hereditary Nonpolyposis Colorectal Cancer

Amsterdam I Criteria
At least three relatives with colorectal cancer:
  One of whom is a first-degree relative of the other two
  Occurring in at least two successive generations
  At least one of whom was diagnosed with cancer before age 50
  Exclusion of familial adenomatous polyposis
Tumors should be histologically verified whenever possible.

Amsterdam II Criteria
At least three relatives with an HNPCC-associated cancer
  (e.g., colorectal, endometrial, ovarian, stomach, ureter or renal pelvis, brain, small bowel, hepatobiliary tract, sebaceous skin tumor):
  One of whom is a first-degree relative of the other two
  Occurring in at least two successive generations
  At least one of whom was diagnosed with cancer before age 50
  Exclusion of familial adenomatous polyposis for any colorectal cancer case
Tumors should be histologically verified whenever possible.

which is characterized by susceptibility to sebaceous gland tumors and keratoacanthomas in addition to the malignancies seen in HNPCC; this syndrome is associated with mutations primarily in *MSH2* and to a lesser extent in *MLH1*.[113] There is no evidence that HNPCC can result from a mutation in a gene other than one of those in this mismatch repair (MMR) pathway. The distinction between "genetically defined" and "clinically defined" appears largely academic. For the purposes of this discussion, individuals carrying a germline MMR gene mutation are considered at high risk for HNPCC, and those individuals with clinically defined HNPCC are likely to carry an MMR gene mutation. The distinction between Lynch syndromes I and II is probably artificial at the genetic level, and the use of these terms is discouraged. Analogous to the site-specific gynecologic cancer syndromes discussed earlier, there is no recognized genetic basis for Lynch syndrome I apart from that responsible for HNPCC, and Lynch syndrome I probably represents a variant of the HNPCC syndrome in which extracolonic cancers occur with reduced penetrance or simply remain undocumented in the pedigree.

What is the genetic basis of hereditary nonpolyposis colorectal cancer?

Clues to the genetic basis of HNPCC first emerged in 1993, with several independent observations of somatic hypermutability of a class of DNA repetitive elements, known as *microsatellites,* in sporadic and familial colorectal tumors.[114-116] This observation was accompanied by reports of the genetic linkage of HNPCC kindreds to two loci, one on chromosome 2p[117] and another on chromosome 3p.[118] Identification and cloning of the responsible genes at these loci, *MSH2* on chromosome 2[119,120] and *MLH1* on chromosome 3,[121,122] quickly followed, together with the realization that these genes encoded human orthologs of yeast DNA MMR proteins. The microsatellite instability phenotype previously observed in colorectal and other cancer types associated with the HNPCC syndrome could be explained by loss of function of these DNA MMR genes. In HNPCC, one of these genes is inherited in a mutant form through the germline, whereas in sporadic colorectal, endometrial, and gastric carcinomas affected by microsatellite instability, somatic silencing of *MLH1* through promoter hypermethylation appears to be the primary pathogenic mechanism.[123]

Although most HNPCC kindreds appear linked to *MSH2* or *MLH1*, a small fraction are linked to a third MMR gene, *MSH6*. There is some evidence that this gene may account for a substantial number of atypical or low-penetrance HNPCC kindreds and those affected by a disproportionately high number of gynecologic cancers.[23,124-126] Early evidence suggested that the MMR genes *PMS1* and *PMS2* may also play a role in HNPCC,[127] but these observations were not widely confirmed, and a recent report involving the investigators originally linking these genes to HNPCC indicates that these genes are unlikely to be involved in the syndrome after all.[128] Nevertheless, references to *PMS1* and *PMS2* being important in HNPCC are still found in the literature.

Who should be tested for genetic predisposition to hereditary nonpolyposis colorectal cancer? The Amsterdam criteria are very specific for identifying likely MMR gene mutation carriers but are relatively insensitive. They are therefore criticized for being overly exclusive when used as a guide for referring individuals for genetic consultation. Recognizing that there was little consensus with respect to the criteria or threshold for recommending genetic testing for HNPCC, the National Cancer Institute Workshop on HNPCC Syndrome created a set of criteria that, when met, warrant the performance of microsatellite instability testing on the patient's tumor.[110] These criteria have become known as the Bethesda guidelines (Table 62-5), which appear to be substantially more sensitive but less specific than the Amsterdam criteria in identifying HNPCC kindreds with pathogenic mutations.[129] This test is relatively simple and inexpensive, and a negative result translates into a very low probability of the existence of an MMR gene mutation.

Table 62–5. Bethesda Guidelines for Predicting Hereditary Nonpolyposis Colorectal Cancer Genotype

1. Individuals from families that meet the Amsterdam criteria
2. Individuals with two hereditary nonpolyposis colorectal cancer (HNPCC)–related cancers (synchronous or metachronous)
3. Individuals with colorectal cancer and a first-degree relative with colorectal cancer and/or HNPCC-associated extracolonic cancer and/or a colorectal adenoma; one of the cancers diagnosed at less than 45 years and the adenoma diagnosed at less than 40 years
4. Individuals with colorectal or endometrial cancer diagnosed at less than 45 years
5. Individuals with right-sided colorectal cancer with an undifferentiated histologic pattern (solid or cribriform) diagnosed when younger than 45 years
6. Individuals with signet ring cell–type colorectal cancer diagnosed when younger than 45 years
7. Individuals with adenoma diagnosed when younger than 40 years

---

What are the lifetime risks of endometrial and ovarian cancers in mismatch repair gene mutation carriers? The limited available data suggest that the relative risks for extracolonic cancers in the HNPCC syndrome are highest for endometrial and ovarian carcinomas, and there is some evidence to suggest that the risk of endometrial cancer may exceed that of colorectal cancer in females. The lifetime risk estimates for endometrial carcinoma range from 40% to 60%, corresponding to a relative risk of 13 to 20, whereas those for ovarian carcinoma range from 6% to 20%, corresponding to a relative risk of 4 to 8.[130-135] These estimates are not population based but derived from analyses of HNPCC families, and they therefore may be higher than expected for the general population.

Are the clinicopathologic features of hereditary nonpolyposis colorectal cancer–associated gynecologic cancers distinct from their sporadic counterparts? It is reasonably well established that colorectal cancers associated with the HNPCC syndrome are associated with an improved prognosis compared with their sporadic counterparts,[136-138] leading to speculation about the clinical course of HNPCC-associated gynecologic cancers. For endometrial carcinoma, emerging evidence suggests that there is no statistically significant difference in the distribution of histologic subtypes, surgical stage at presentation, or long-term survival compared with endometrial carcinoma in the general population.[139] In contrast, HNPCC-associated ovarian cancer appears to differ markedly from that which occurs in the general population in several respects.[140] In the context of HNPCC, age at diagnosis is significantly younger, tumors are more likely to be of epithelial origin, well or moderately differentiated, and of low surgical stage. Synchronous endometrial carcinoma is also common. There is no evidence for a difference in survival associated with these ovarian cancers that is independent of other established prognostic factors.

What is the appropriate clinical management of an individual at risk for hereditary nonpolyposis colorectal cancer? Consensus recommendations for the clinical care of individuals at risk for HNPCC were offered in 1996 by the International Collaborative Group on HNPCC[141] and in 1997 by the NIH-sponsored Cancer Genetics Studies Consortium.[142] Increased colorectal cancer surveillance in this population decreases mortality from colorectal cancer;[143] the clinical management of gastrointestinal cancer risk in this population is discussed elsewhere.[144,145] Although there are no data on the efficacy of screening for gynecologic cancers, endometrial cancer screening is recommended in light of its presumptive benefit. Screening for ovarian cancer is subject to the same limitations and dubious efficacy discussed earlier.

With respect to risk-reducing surgery, there are no data on the efficacy of hysterectomy and BSO for cancer prevention in women at risk for HNPCC, and no recommendation was made for or against risk-reducing surgery by the Cancer Genetics Studies Consortium[142] that addressed this issue. Nevertheless, it is reasonable to assume that hysterectomy would be completely preventive for endometrial carcinoma, and there are no published case reports to the contrary. Ovarian cancer prevention is subject to the same theoretical caveat related to primary peritoneal carcinoma that is encountered in the context of the BOC syndrome, but evidence of primary peritoneal cancer in the HNPCC syndrome is lacking. Until proven otherwise, hysterectomy and BSO are likely to significantly reduce the incidence of gynecologic cancers in women at risk for HNPCC.

Summary

The cancers of the female reproductive tract that commonly occur in association with autosomal dominant genetic predisposition are ovarian epithelial carcinoma and endometrial carcinoma. Most of these so-called hereditary gynecologic cancers occur in the context of the BOC and HNPCC syndromes, and the molecular genetic bases for these syndromes have been completely elucidated over the past 10 years. Individuals at risk for both syndromes may be identified through genetic testing. For women at risk for the BOC syndrome, evidence is emerging that vigorous surveillance and surgical and medical interventions are likely to prove beneficial for cancer risk reduction. With respect to HNPCC, there are few data to support the efficacy of such risk-reducing strategies, although risk-reducing hysterectomy and BSO are of presumptive benefit until proved otherwise. Future research on the clinical management of these high-risk individuals will allow continued reduction in cancer risk while optimizing quality of life.

REFERENCES

1. Weinberg RA: Oncogenes, antioncogenes, and the molecular basis of multistep carcinogenesis. Cancer Res 1989;49:3713-3721.
2. Boyd J, Barrett JC: Genetic and cellular basis of multistep carcinogenesis. Pharmacol Ther 1990;46:469-486.
3. Vogelstein B, Kinzler KW: The multistep nature of cancer. Trends Genet 1993;9:138-141.
4. Bishop JM: Cancer: The rise of the genetic paradigm. Genes Dev 1995;9:1309-1315.
5. Renan MJ: How many mutations are required for tumorigenesis? Implications from human cancer data. Mol Carcinog 1993;7:139-146.
6. Hofstra RMW, Landsvater RM, Ceccherini I, et al: A mutation in the RET proto-oncogene associated with multiple endocrine neoplasia type 2B and sporadic medullary thyroid carcinoma. Nature 1994;367:375-378.
7. Schmidt L, Duh F-M, Chen F, et al: Germline and somatic mutations in the tyrosine kinase domain of the MET proto-oncogene in papillary renal carcinomas. Nat Genet 1997;16:68-73.
8. Kinzler KW, Vogelstein B: Gatekeepers and caretakers. Nature 1997;386:761-763.
9. Knudson AG: Hereditary cancer, oncogenes, and antioncogenes. Cancer Res 1985;45:1437-1443.
10. Haber DA, Housman DE: Rate limiting steps: The genetics of pediatric cancers. Cell 1991;64:5-8.
11. Cavenee WK, Dryja TP, Phillips RA, et al: Expression of recessive alleles by chromosomal mechanisms in retinoblastoma. Nature 1983;305:779-784.
12. Knudson AG: Mutation and cancer: Statistical study of retinoblastoma. Proc Natl Acad Sci USA 1971;68:820-823.
13. Hethcote HW, Knudson AG: Model for the incidence of embryonal cancers: Application to retinoblastoma. Proc Natl Acad Sci USA 1978;75:2453-2457.
14. Mauro MJ, O'Dwyer M, Heinrich MC, Druker BJ: STI571: A paradigm of new agents for cancer therapeutics. J Clin Oncol 2002;20:325-334.
15. Ramaswamy S, Golub TR: DNA microarrays in clinical oncology. J Clin Oncol 2002;20:1932-1941.
16. Petricoin EF, Ardekani AM, Hitt BA, et al: Use of proteomic patterns in serum to identify ovarian cancer. Lancet 2002;359:572-577.
17. Li E: Chromatin modification and epigenetic reprogramming in mammalian development. Nat Rev Genet 2002;3:662-673.
18. Robertson KD, Wolffe AP: DNA methylation in health and disease. Nat Rev Genet 2000;1:11-19.
19. Jones PA, Baylin SB: The fundamental role of epigenetic events in cancer. Nat Rev Genet 2002;3:415-428.
20. Baylin S, Bestor TH: Altered methylation patterns in cancer cell genomes: Cause or consequence? Cancer Cell 2002;1:299-305.
21. Claus EB, Schildkraut JM, Thompson WD, Risch NJ: The genetic attributable risk of breast and ovarian cancer. Cancer 1996;77:2318-2324.
22. Steichen-Gersdorf E, Gallion HH, Ford D, et al: Familial site-specific ovarian cancer is linked to BRCA1 on 17q12-21. Am J Hum Genet 1994;55:870-875.
23. Wijnen J, de Leeuw W, Vasen H, et al: Familial endometrial cancer in female carriers of MSH6 germline mutations. Nat Genet 1999;23:142-144.
24. Eng C, Parsons R. Cowden syndrome. In Vogelstein B, Kinzler KW (eds): The Genetic Basis of Human Cancer. New York, McGraw-Hill, 1998, pp 519-525.
25. Easton DF, Ford D, Bishop DT: Breast and ovarian cancer incidence in BRCA1-mutation carriers. Breast Cancer Linkage Consortium. Am J Hum Genet 1995;56:265-271.
26. Struewing JP, Hartge P, Wacholder S, et al: The risk of cancer associated with specific mutations of BRCA1 and BRCA2 among Ashkenazi Jews. N Engl J Med 1997;336:1401-1408.
27. Ford D, Easton DF, Stratton M, et al: Genetic heterogeneity and penetrance analysis of the BRCA1 and BRCA2 genes in breast cancer families. Am J Hum Genet 1998;62:676-689.
28. Moslehi R, Chu W, Karlan B, et al: BRCA1 and BRCA2 mutation analysis of 208 Ashkenazi Jewish women with ovarian cancer. Am J Hum Genet 2000;66:1259-1272.
29. Thompson D, Easton D, Consortium BCL: Variation in cancer risks, by mutation position, in BRCA2 mutation carriers. Am J Hum Genet 2001;68:410-419.
30. Satagopan JM, Boyd J, Kauff ND, et al: Ovarian cancer risk in Ashkenazi Jewish carriers of BRCA1 and BRCA2 mutations. Clin Cancer Res 2002;8:3776-3781.
31. Robson ME, Boyd J, Borgen PI, Cody HS: Hereditary breast cancer. Curr Probl Surg 2001;38:377-480.
32. Bandera CA, Muto MG, Schorge JO, et al: BRCA1 gene mutations in women with papillary serous carcinoma of the peritoneum. Obstet Gynecol 1998;92:596-600.
33. Schorge JO, Muto MG, Lee SJ, et al: BRCA1-related papillary serous carcinoma of the peritoneum has a unique molecular pathogenesis. Cancer Res 2000;60:1361-1364.
34. Zweemer RP, van Diest PJ, Verheijen RH, et al: Molecular evidence linking primary cancer of the fallopian tube to BRCA1 germline mutations. Gynecol Oncol 2000;76:45-50.
35. Rose PG, Shrigley R, Wiesner GL: Germline BRCA2 mutation in a patient with fallopian tube carcinoma: A case report. Gynecol Oncol 2000;77:319-320.
36. Aziz S, Kuperstein G, Rosen B, et al: A genetic epidemiological study of carcinoma of the fallopian tube. Gynecol Oncol 2001;80:341-345.
37. Menczer J, Chetrit A, Barda G, et al: Frequency of BRCA mutations in primary peritoneal carcinoma in Israeli Jewish women. Gynecol Oncol 2003;88:58-61.
38. Colgan TJ, Murphy J, Cole DE, et al: Occult carcinoma in prophylactic oophorectomy specimens: Prevalence and association with BRCA germline mutation status. Am J Surg Pathol 2001;25:1283-1289.

39. Leeper K, Garcia R, Swisher E, et al: Pathologic findings in prophylactic oophorectomy specimens in high-risk women. Gynecol Oncol 2002;87:52-56.
40. Scheuer L, Kauff N, Robson M, et al: Outcome of preventive surgery and screening for breast and ovarian cancer in BRCA mutation carriers. J Clin Oncol 2002;20:1260-1268.
41. Kauff ND, Satagopan JM, Robson ME, et al: Risk-reducing salpingo-oophorectomy in women with a BRCA1 or BRCA2 mutation. N Engl J Med 2002;346:1609-1615.
42. Liede A, Karlan BY, Baldwin RL, et al: Cancer incidence in a population of Jewish women at risk of ovarian cancer. J Clin Oncol 2002;20:1570-1577.
43. Agoff SN, Mendelin JE, Grieco VS, Garcia RL: Unexpected gynecologic neoplasms in patients with proven or suspected BRCA-1 or -2 mutations: Implications for gross examination, cytology, and clinical follow-up. Am J Surg Pathol 2002;26:171-178.
44. Hornreich G, Beller U, Lavie O, et al: Is uterine papillary carcinoma a BRCA1-related disease? Case report and review of the literature. Gynecol Oncol 1999;75:300-304.
45. Lavie O, Hornreich G, Ben Arie A, et al: *BRCA1* germline mutations in women with uterine papillary serous carcinoma. Obstet Gynecol 2000;96:28-32.
46. Goshen R, Chu W, Elit L, et al: Is uterine papillary serous adenocarcinoma a manifestation of the hereditary breast-ovarian cancer syndrome? Gynecol Oncol 2000;79:477-481.
47. Levine DA, Lin O, Barakat RR, et al: Risk of endometrial carcinoma associated with *BRCA* mutation. Gynecol Oncol 2001;80:395-398.
48. Thompson D, Easton DF, Consortium BCL: Cancer incidence in BRCA1 mutation carriers. J Natl Cancer Inst 2002;94:1358-1365.
49. Brose MS, Rebbeck TR, Calzone KA, et al: Cancer risk estimates for BRCA1 mutation carriers identified in a risk evaluation program. J Natl Cancer Inst 2002;94:1365-1372.
50. Breast Cancer Linkage Consortium: Cancer risks in BRCA2 mutation carriers. J Natl Cancer Inst 1999;91:1310-1316.
51. Ford D, Easton DF, Bishop DT, et al: Risks of cancer in BRCA1 mutation carriers. Lancet 1994;343:692-695.
52. Gayther SA, Warren W, Mazoyer S, et al: Germline mutations of the *BRCA1* gene in breast and ovarian cancer families provide evidence for a genotype-phenotype correlation. Nat Genet 1995;11:428-433.
53. Gayther SA, Mangion J, Russell P, et al: Variation of risks of breast and ovarian cancer associated with different germline mutations of the *BRCA2* gene. Nat Genet 1997;15:103-105.
54. Boyd J, Sonoda Y, Federici MG, et al: Clinicopathologic features of *BRCA*-linked and sporadic ovarian cancer. JAMA 2000;283:2260-2265.
55. Werness BA, Ramus SJ, Whittemore AS, et al: Histopathology of familial ovarian tumors in women from families with and without germline BRCA1 mutations. Hum Pathol 2000;31:1420-1424.
56. Risch HA, McLaughlin JR, Cole DEC, et al: Prevalence and penetrance of germline BRCA1 and BRCA2 mutations in a population series of 649 women with ovarian cancer. Am J Hum Genet 2001;68:700-710.
57. Lu KH, Garber JE, Cramer DW, et al: Occult ovarian tumors in women with BRCA1 or BRCA2 mutations undergoing prophylactic oophorectomy. J Clin Oncol 2000;18:2728-2732.
58. Leitao M, Boyd J: Preoperative CA-125 levels in patients with hereditary compared with sporadic epithelial ovarian carcinoma. Gynecol Oncol 2002;84:413-415.
59. Westhoff C, Murphy P, Heller D, Halim A: Is ovarian cancer associated with an increased frequency of germinal inclusion cysts? Am J Epidemiol 1993;138:90-93.
60. Tresserra F, Grases PJ, Labastida R, Ubeda A: Histological features of the contralateral ovary in patients with unilateral cancer: A case control study. Gynecol Oncol 1998;71:437-441.
61. Salazar H, Godwin AK, Daly MB, et al: Microscopic benign and invasive malignant neoplasms and a cancer-prone phenotype in prophylactic oophorectomies. J Natl Cancer Inst 1996;88:1810-1820.
62. Stratton JF, Buckley CH, Lowe D, et al: Comparison of prophylactic oophorectomy specimens from carriers and noncarriers of a BRCA1 or BRCA2 gene mutation. J Natl Cancer Inst 1999;91:626-628.
63. Deligdisch L, Gil J, Kerner H, et al: Ovarian dysplasia in prophylactic oophorectomy specimens. Cancer 1999;86:1544-1550.
64. Barakat RR, Federici MG, Saigo PE, et al: Absence of premalignant histologic, molecular, or cell biological alterations in prophylactic oophorectomy specimens from BRCA1 heterozygotes. Cancer 2000;89:383-390.
65. Casey MJ, Bewtra C, Hoehne LL, et al: Histology of prophylactically removed ovaries from BRCA1 and BRCA2 mutation carriers compared with noncarriers in hereditary breast ovarian cancer syndrome kindreds. Gynecol Oncol 2000;78:278-287.
66. Dubeau L: The cell of origin of ovarian epithelial tumors and the ovarian surface epithelium dogma: Does the emperor have no clothes? Gynecol Oncol 1999;72:437-442.
67. Chapman WB: Developments in the pathology of ovarian tumours. Curr Opin Obstet Gynecol 2001;13:53-59.
68. Russell P. Surface epithelial-stromal tumors of the ovary. In Kurman RJ (ed): Blaustein's Pathology of the Female Genital Tract, 4th ed. New York, Springer-Verlag, 1994, pp 705-782.
69. Werness BA, Parvatiyar P, Ramus SJ, et al: Ovarian carcinoma *in situ* with germline BRCA1 mutation and loss of heterozygosity at BRCA1 and TP53. J Natl Cancer Inst 2000;92:1088-1091.
70. Bruening W, Giasson BI, Klein-Szanto AJ, et al: Synucleins are expressed in the majority of breast and ovarian carcinomas and in preneoplastic lesions of the ovary. Cancer 2000;88:2154-2163.
71. Pothuri B, Leitao M, Barakat R, et al: Genetic analysis of ovarian carcinoma histogenesis [abstract]. Gynecol Oncol 2001;80:277.
72. Rubin SC, Benjamin I, Behbakht K, et al: Clinical and pathologic features of ovarian cancer in women with germ-line mutations of *BRCA1*. N Engl J Med 1996;335:1413-1416.
73. Aida H, Takakuwa K, Nagata H, et al: Clinical features of ovarian cancer in Japanese women with germ-line mutations of *BRCA1*. Clin Cancer Res 1998;4:235-240.
74. Johannsson OT, Ranstam J, Borg A, Olsson H: Survival of BRCA1 breast and ovarian cancer patients: A population-based study from southern Sweden. J Clin Oncol 1998;16:397-404.
75. Pharoah PDP, Easton DF, Stockton DL, et al: Survival in familial, *BRCA1*-associated, and *BRCA2*-associated epithelial ovarian cancer. Cancer Res 1999;59:868-871.
76. Ben-David Y, Chetrit A, Hirsh-Yechezkel G, et al: Effect of BRCA mutations on the length of survival in epithelial ovarian tumors. J Clin Oncol 2002;20:463-466.
77. McGuire V, Whittemore AS, Norris R, Oakley-Girvan I: Survival in epithelial ovarian cancer patients with prior breast cancer. Am J Epidemiol 2000;152:528-532.
78. Levine DA, Federici MG, Reuter VE, Boyd J: Cell proliferation and apoptosis in *BRCA*-associated hereditary ovarian cancer. Gynecol Oncol 2002;85:431-434.
79. Hoeijmakers JHJ: Genome maintenance mechanisms for preventing cancer. Nature 2001;411:366-374.
80. Maresco DL, Arnold PA, Bogomolniy F, et al: Role of BRCA1 in response to therapeutic DNA-damaging agents in human breast cancer cells [abstract]. Proc Am Soc Clin Oncol 2001;20:45a.
81. Colgan TJ, Boerner SL, Murphy J, et al: Peritoneal lavage cytology: An assessment of its value during prophylactic oophorectomy. Gynecol Oncol 2002;85:397-403.
82. Paley PJ, Swisher EM, Garcia RL, et al: Occult cancer of the fallopian tube in BRCA-1 germline mutation carriers at prophylactic oophorectomy: A case for recommending hysterectomy at surgical prophylaxis. Gynecol Oncol 2001;80:176-180.
83. Tobacman JK, Tucker MA, Kase R, et al: Intraabdominal carcinomatosis after prophylactic oophorectomy in ovarian cancer prone families. Lancet 1982;2:795-797.
84. Chen KTK, Schooley JF, Flam MS: Peritoneal carcinomatosis after prophylactic oophorectomy in familial ovarian cancer syndrome. Obstet Gynecol 1985;66:93S-94S.
85. Piver MS, Jishi MF, Tsukada Y, Nava G: Primary peritoneal carcinoma after prophylactic oophorectomy in women with a family history of ovarian cancer. A report of the Gilda Radner Familial Ovarian Cancer Registry. Cancer 1993;71:2751-2755.
86. Struewing JP, Watson P, Easton DF, et al: Prophylactic oophorectomy in inherited breast/ovarian cancer families. J Natl Cancer Inst Monogr 1995;17:33-35.
87. Rebbeck TR, Levin AM, Eisen A, et al: Breast cancer risk after bilateral prophylactic oophorectomy in BRCA1 mutation carriers. J Natl Cancer Inst 1999;91:1475-1479.

88. Rebbeck TR, Lynch HT, Neuhausen SL, et al: Prophylactic oophorectomy in carriers of BRCA1 or BRCA2 mutations. N Engl J Med 2002;346:1616-1622.

89. Narod SA, Boyd J: Current understanding of the epidemiology and clinical implications of BRCA1 and BRCA2 mutations for ovarian cancer. Curr Opin Obstet Gynecol 2002;14:19-26.

90. Parazzini F, Franceschi S, La Vecchia C, Fasoli M: The epidemiology of ovarian cancer. Gynecol Oncol 1991;43:9-23.

91. Bosetti C, Negri E, Trichopoulos D, et al: Long-term effects of oral contraceptives on ovarian cancer risk. Int J Cancer 2002; 102:262-265.

92. Whittemore AS, Harris R, Itnyre J: Characteristics relating to ovarian cancer risk: Collaborative analysis of 12 US case-control studies. IV. The pathogenesis of epithelial ovarian cancer. Collaborative Ovarian Cancer Group. Am J Epidemiol 1992;136:1212-1220.

93. Risch H: Hormonal etiology of epithelial ovarian cancer, with a hypothesis concerning the role of androgens and progesterone. J Natl Cancer Inst 1998;90:1774-1786.

94. Rodriguez GC, Nagarsheth NP, Lee KL, et al: Progestin-induced apoptosis in the Macaque ovarian epithelium: Differential regulation of transforming growth factor-beta. J Natl Cancer Inst 2002;94:50-60.

95. Narod SA, Risch H, Moslehi R, et al: Oral contraceptives and the risk of hereditary ovarian cancer. N Engl J Med 1998;339: 424-428.

96. Narod SA, Sun P, Ghadirian P, et al: Tubal ligation and risk of ovarian cancer in carriers of BRCA1 or BRCA2 mutations: A case-control study. Lancet 2001;357:1467-1470.

97. Narod SA, Sun P, Risch HA: Ovarian cancer, oral contraceptives, and BRCA mutations. N Engl J Med 2001;345: 1706-1707.

98. Modan B, Hartge P, Hirsh-Yechezkel G, et al: Parity, oral contraceptives, and the risk of ovarian cancer among carriers and noncarriers of a BRCA1 or BRCA2 mutation. N Engl J Med 2001;345:235-240.

99. Daly M, Obrams GI: Epidemiology and risk assessment for ovarian cancer. Semin Oncol 1998;25:255-264.

100. Ness RB, Grisso JA, Vergona R, et al: Oral contraceptives, other methods of contraception, and risk reduction for ovarian cancer. Epidemiology 2001;12:307-312.

101. Piek JM, van Diest PJ, Zweemer RP, et al: Tubal ligation and risk of ovarian cancer. Lancet 2001;358:844.

102. Menon U, Jacobs IJ: Ovarian cancer screening in the general population. Curr Opin Obstet Gynecol 2001;13:61-64.

103. Warthin AS: Heredity with reference to carcinoma. Arch Intern Med 1913;12:546-555.

104. Lynch HT, Krush AJ: Cancer family G revisited: 1895-1970. Cancer 1971;27:1505-1511.

105. Lynch HT, Shaw MW, Magnuson CW, et al: Hereditary factors in cancer. Study of two large midwestern kindreds. Arch Intern Med 1966;117:206-212.

106. Boland CR, Troncale FJ: Familial colonic cancer without antecedent polyposis. Ann Intern Med 1984;100:700-701.

107. Vasen HFA, Mecklin J-P, Meera Khan P, Lynch HT: The international collaborative group on hereditary non-polyposis colorectal cancer (ICG-HNPCC). Dis Colon Rectum 1991;34: 424-425.

108. Beck NE, Tomlinson IP, Homfray T, et al: Genetic testing is important in families with a history suggestive of hereditary nonpolyposis colorectal cancer even if the Amsterdam criteria are not fulfilled. Br J Surg 1997;84:233-237.

109. Nakahara M, Yokozaki H, Yasui W, et al: Identification of concurrent germline mutations in hMSH2 and/or hMLH1 in Japanese hereditary nonpolyposis colorectal cancer kindreds. Cancer Epidemiol Biomarkers Prev 1997;6:1057-1064.

110. Rodriguez-Bigas MA, Boland CR, Hamilton SR, et al: A National Cancer Institute Workshop on Hereditary Nonpolyposis Colorectal Cancer Syndrome: Meeting highlights and Bethesda guidelines. J Natl Cancer Inst 1997;89:1758-1762.

111. Jass JR, Cottier DS, Jeevaratnam P, et al: Diagnostic use of microsatellite instability in hereditary non-polyposis colorectal cancer. Lancet 1995;346:1200-1201.

112. Muta H, Noguchi M, Perucho M, et al: Clinical implications of microsatellite instability in colorectal cancers. Cancer 1996; 77:265-270.

113. Mathiak M, Rutten A, Mangold E, et al: Loss of DNA mismatch repair proteins in skin tumors from patients with Muir-Torre syndrome and MSH2 or MLH1 germline mutations: Establishment of immunohistochemical analysis as a screening test. Am J Surg Pathol 2002;26:338-343.

114. Ionov Y, Peinado MA, Malkhosyan S, et al: Ubiquitous somatic mutations in simple repeated sequences reveal a new mechanism for colonic carcinogenesis. Nature 1993;363:558-561.

115. Aaltonen LA, Peltomäki P, Leach FS, et al: Clues to the pathogenesis of familial colorectal cancer. Science 1993;260:812-816.

116. Thibodeau SN, Bren G, Schaid D: Microsatellite instability in cancer of the proximal colon. Science 1993;260:816-819.

117. Peltomäki P, Aaltonen LA, Sistonen P, et al: Genetic mapping of a locus predisposing to human colorectal cancer. Science 1993;260:810-812.

118. Lindblom A, Tannergård P, Werelius B, Nordenskjöld M: Genetic mapping of a second locus predisposing to hereditary non-polyposis colon cancer. Nat Genet 1993;5:279-282.

119. Fishel R, Lescoe MK, Rao MRS, et al: The human mutator gene homolog MSH2 and its association with hereditary nonpolyposis colon cancer. Cell 1993;75:1027-1038.

120. Leach FS, Nicolaides NC, Papadopoulos N, et al: Mutations of a mutS homolog in hereditary nonpolyposis colorectal cancer. Cell 1993;75:1215-1225.

121. Bronner CE, Baker SM, Morrison PT, et al: Mutation in the DNA mismatch repair gene homologue hMLH1 is associated with hereditary non-polyposis colon cancer. Nature 1994;368: 258-261.

122. Papadopoulos N, Nicolaides NC, Wei Y-F, et al: Mutation of a mutL homolog in hereditary colon cancer. Science 1994;263: 1625-1629.

123. Peltomaki P: Deficient DNA mismatch repair: A common etiologic factor for colon cancer. Hum Mol Genet 2001;10: 735-740.

124. Miyaki M, Konishi M, Tanaka K, et al: Germline mutation of MSH6 as the cause of hereditary nonpolyposis colorectal cancer. Nat Genet 1997;17:271-272.

125. Akiyama Y, Sato H, Yamada T, et al: Germ-line mutation of the hMSH6/GTBP gene in an atypical hereditary nonpolyposis colorectal cancer kindred. Cancer Res 1997;57:3920-3928.

126. Kolodner RD, Tytell JD, Schmeits JL, et al: Germ-line msh6 mutations in colorectal cancer families. Cancer Res 1999;59: 5068-5074.

127. Nicolaides NC, Papadopoulos N, Liu B, et al: Mutations of two PMS homologues in hereditary nonpolyposis colon cancer. Nature 1994;371:75-80.

128. Liu T, Yan H, Kuismanen S, et al: The role of hPMS1 and hPMS2 in predisposing to colorectal cancer. Cancer Res 2001;61: 7798-7802.

129. Syngal S, Fox EA, Eng C, et al: Sensitivity and specificity of clinical criteria for hereditary non-polyposis colorectal cancer associated mutations in MSH2 and MLH1. J Med Genet 2000; 37:641-645.

130. Watson P, Lynch HT: Extracolonic cancer in hereditary nonpolyposis colorectal cancer. Cancer 1993;71:677-85.

131. Watson P, Vasen HF, Mecklin JP, et al: The risk of endometrial cancer in hereditary nonpolyposis colorectal cancer. Am J Med 1994;96:516-520.

132. Aarnio M, Mecklin JP, Aaltonen LA, et al: Life-time risk of different cancers in the hereditary non-polyposis colorectal cancer (HNPCC) syndrome. Int J Cancer 1995;64:430-433.

133. Vasen HF, Wijnen JT, Menko FH, et al: Cancer risk in families with hereditary nonpolyposis colorectal cancer diagnosed by mutation analysis. Gastroenterology 1996;110:1020-1027.

134. Dunlop MG, Farrington SM, Carothers AD, et al: Cancer risk associated with germline DNA mismatch repair gene mutations. Hum Mol Genet 1997;6:105-110.

135. Aarnio M, Sankila R, Pukkala E, et al: Cancer risk in mutation carriers of DNA-mismatch-repair genes. Int J Cancer 1999;81:214-218.

136. Aarnio M, Mustonen H, Mecklin JP, Jarvinen HJ: Prognosis of colorectal cancer varies in different high-risk conditions. Ann Med 1998;30:75-80.

137. Sankila R, Aaltonen L, Jarvinen HJ, Mecklin JP: Better survival rates in patients with MLH1-associated hereditary colorectal cancer. Gastroenterology 1996;10:682-687.

138. Lynch HT, Smyrk T: Colorectal cancer, survival advantage and hereditary nonpolyposis colorectal cancer. Gastroenterology 1996;110:943-947.

139. Boks DE, Trujillo AP, Voogd AC, et al: Survival analysis of endometrial carcinoma associated with hereditary polyposis colorectal cancer. Int J Cancer 2002;102:198-200.

140. Watson P, Butzow R, Lynch HT, et al: The clinical features of ovarian cancer in hereditary nonpolyposis colorectal cancer. Gynecol Oncol 2001;82:223-228.

141. Weber T: Clinical surveillance recommendations adopted for HNPCC. Lancet 1996;348:465.

142. Burke W, Petersen G, Lynch P, et al: Recommendations for follow-up care of individuals with an inherited predisposition to cancer. I. Hereditary nonpolyposis colon cancer. Cancer Genetics Studies Consortium. JAMA 1997;277:915-919.

143. Jarvinen HJ, Aarnio M, Mustonen H, et al: Controlled 15-year trial on screening for colorectal cancer in families with hereditary nonpolyposis colorectal cancer. Gastroenterology 2000;118:829-834.

144. Lynch HT, de la Chapelle A: Hereditary colorectal cancer. N Engl J Med 2003;348:919-932.

145. Hampel H, Peltomaki P: Hereditary colorectal cancer: Risk assessment and management. Clin Genet 2000;58:89-97.

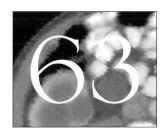

Tumor Markers in the Diagnosis and Management of Gynecologic Cancers

Steven J. Skates

 MAJOR CONTROVERSIES

- Which blood test is the best choice as a first-line test for ovarian cancer screening?
- Is CA 125 recommended as a first-line ovarian cancer screening test?
- Can sensitivity be increased only by decreasing specificity?
- What is the best choice of samples for evaluating multiple putative biomarkers?

Early detection of ovarian cancer is an appealing approach to reducing mortality from this disease. Under usual care, most ovarian cancer is detected in late stage, with consequently poor prognosis, whereas if it is detected in early stage, the prognosis is often excellent. The two target populations under consideration for screening are those in whom most ovarian cancers occur: normal-risk postmenopausal women and women older than a given age from high-risk families. Such families include those in which a close relative has a deleterious *BRCA1* or *BRCA2* mutation and those with a strong history of breast and/or ovarian cancers in relatives close to the subject. Both situations point to the possible presence of a deleterious *BRCA1* or *BRCA2* mutation. In the first target population, the annual incidence of ovarian cancer is less than 1 in 2000, indicating the need to screen many women to detect one ovarian cancer. In the second population, if the subject herself has a *BRCA* mutation, then risk-reducing salpingo-oophorectomy (RRSO) is often advocated after completion of childbearing; it is only when the subject does not know her genetic status (because she does not want to or because she cannot afford the genetic test) that screening is considered.

Despite the increased risk due to familial factors, younger age or distance from the affected relatives may also result in a low incidence, in which case many screening tests will again need to be performed to detect one ovarian cancer.

Given the large number of tests required to detect one cancer, the first-line screening test needs to be inexpensive, well tolerated by both subject and caregiver, sensitive to the presence of most undetected ovarian cancers, and highly specific to the cancer. Candidates for first-line tests include serum/plasma biomarkers,[1-12] transvaginal ultrasound (TVU),[3,13-17] a laparoscopic "Pap" test for high-risk women, and, more recently, urine tests.[18-20] Because of the 5- to 10-fold greater cost of TVU compared with a blood test, the cost and invasiveness of a laparoscopic "Pap" test, and the lack of research on urine tests, this chapter focuses on first-line screening tests that are based on a blood sample, such as plasma and serum biomarkers. If the first-line test is positive, then referral to TVU as a second-line test is likely to be made, followed by referral to a gynecologic oncologist for consideration of surgery if the second-line test is positive. Much debate surrounds the appropriate implementation of second- and third-line components of the screening program, but this subject is beyond the scope of this article.

Which blood test is the best choice as a first-line test for ovarian cancer screening?

One argument against ovarian cancer screening (with any test) is that the incidence of disease is too low to warrant consideration. However, I would submit that incidence is the wrong focus with which to address this issue, and that a far more appropriate statistic is the mortality rate caused by the disease. Although the incidence of breast cancer is nine times higher than that of ovarian cancer, the mortality rate from breast cancer is greater by a factor of 3. In the United States, approximately 14,000 women die annually from ovarian cancer, whereas the annual number of deaths from breast cancer is approximately 44,000. Breast cancer has an accepted first-line screening test, namely mammography, which results in a 20% reduction in disease-specific mortality and furthermore is usually covered by medical insurance. A first-line screening test for ovarian cancer with an equivalent percentage reduction in related mortality would be equally as cost-effective if its cost were one-third that of mammography. In the context of screening programs in a large population with efficiencies of volume driving the economics, the cost of a blood test may well be in that range. If the percentage mortality reduction of an ovarian cancer screening program were in fact 30% (the figure used to determine the size and power of two definitive screening trials), then the cost of the blood test need be only one-half that of mammography to achieve the same cost-effectiveness, and this goal would be even more readily achievable. Therefore, ovarian cancer mortality rates and their refinements (e.g., average years of life saved), rather than the low incidence rates, should drive cost-effectiveness considerations for debating the feasibility of a screening program. In addition, even greater cost-effectiveness could be expected if other cancers were screened for at the same patient visit (e.g., using the same blood sample), perhaps in conjunction with each mammography examination. Although this first-order cost-effectiveness comparison omits many detailed considerations, it does address the critique of ovarian cancer screening based on the assertion that its incidence is too low.

Is CA 125 recommended as a first-line ovarian cancer screening test?

Much criticism has been leveled at CA 125 as a screening test, mostly on the grounds that it is only 50% sensitive for early-stage ovarian cancer.[21] There are three issues with such an assertion. First, the figure of 50% sensitivity for early-stage disease refers to the estimated 50% of patients with clinically diagnosed early-stage disease in which CA125 is elevated higher than 35 U/mL. Because these patients are clinically diagnosed in early stage, they are not the target for a screening program. Instead, the target is the group of patients who are clinically diagnosed in late-stage disease; the screening sensitivity of CA 125 when the disease is in early stage in these patients is unknown and could be much greater than 50%. The CA 125 sensitivity on preoperative samples from late-stage disease is usually in excess of 90%, suggesting that most ovarian cancers clinically detected in late stage produce CA 125, and most probably produce CA 125 during early stages as well.

Second, the sensitivity of 50% is for a reference level of 35 U/mL, a level that was chosen to detect recurrence of previously identified and treated ovarian cancer but was never advocated by the discoverers for first-line testing in a screening program. In fact, longitudinal levels of CA 125 provide information about the presence of undetected ovarian cancer in addition to the absolute level. Because a screening program is designed to test subjects periodically, longitudinal values will be available after the second test. Statistical modeling and analysis has produced a method for calculating the risk of having (undetected) ovarian cancer based on the longitudinal CA 125 profile and the subject's age; this is known as the Risk of Ovarian Cancer Algorithm (ROCA).[22] In retrospective analyses, a screening program in which decisions were made using the ROCA (e.g., referral for a blood test in 3 months rather than 12 months, referral to ultrasound) substantially improved the sensitivity while maintaining the same level of specificity as a first-line test using a reference level of 35 U/mL. Using the risk calculation, referral for an earlier blood test would occur with a single test level of 20 U/mL (depending on the age of the subject). Similarly, subjects with constant low levels of CA 125 (e.g., an average of 6 U/mL) that begin to rise significantly above that baseline (e.g., to 20 U/mL) would be referred to ultrasound under ROCA even if the latest CA 125 measurement was still below the "standard" reference level of 35 U/mL. In this manner, ROCA increases the sensitivity of CA 125 screening, compared with using a global reference level of 35 U/mL. The reference level of 35 U/mL and the sensitivities associated with it therefore are not relevant when using CA 125 as a first-line screening test, whether ROCA or another approach to CA 125 screening for ovarian cancer is used.

Third, even if the screening sensitivity of CA 125 for early-stage disease turned out to be 50%, such a result would be a substantial increase over the 20% of ovarian cancers currently clinically detected in early-stage disease. In fact, given that most ovarian cancers detected in early stage can be cured, whereas most late-stage ovarian cancers cannot be cured, an early-stage screening sensitivity of 50% may result in a 30% reduction in ovarian cancer mortality. If the cost of the blood test in the screening setting can be reduced to less than half that of a mammogram, CA 125 screening for ovarian cancer would approach the cost-effectiveness of mammography.

Two large, definitive screening trials are being performed that will estimate the early-stage screening sensitivity, currently unknown, as well as subsequent disease-specific mortality reduction. The United Kingdom Collaborative Trial of Ovarian Cancer Screening (UKCTOCS)[23] compares ROCA versus annual ultrasound screening versus a control group, with 50,000 subjects randomly assigned to each screened arm and 100,000 to the control arm. This trial is accruing subjects for 3 years, screening subjects for 6 years on average, and providing 1 year of follow-up. The Prostate, Lung, Colorectal, and Ovarian (PLCO) trial[24] is a randomized screening trial of 150,000 men and women. In the ovarian portion of the trial, 37,500 women are being screened with CA 125 ($\geq$35 U/mL) and ultrasound; if either test is positive, the subject is referred to a gynecologist.

Nonetheless, it is known from histology studies of ovarian cancers, that 10% of ovarian cancers do not produce CA 125.[25] For this reason, additional markers will be required to complement CA 125 and maximize the potential for a blood test as a first-line screening instrument for ovarian cancer. Substantial effort is underway to determine complementary markers to CA 125.

To summarize, there are three reasons why it is inaccurate to say that CA 125 is only 50% sensitive for early-stage disease and therefore should not be used for screening. First, the relevant quantity, early-stage screening sensitivity, is unknown and could be completely different from the preoperative early-stage sensitivity of 50% referred to in the assertion. Second, a reference level of 35 U/mL, which was designed for monitoring of recurrence, may not be the best approach to the use of CA 125 as a first-line blood test; instead, a longitudinal approach could provide substantially improved operating characteristics, or a different reference level could be used. Third, even if the early-stage screening sensitivity is estimated to be 50%, it is very possible that this level of sensitivity will provide to a clinically significant reduction in disease-specific mortality.

Nonetheless, it should be emphasized that the spirit of this controversy does contain an important element, and that is that CA 125 screening in the general population outside of clinical research should not be performed. Until at least one of the trials described is completed and the impact on disease-specific mortality is assessed along with other outcome measures, CA 125 screening for ovarian cancer should be performed only in the context of clinical research studies, and not as part of general health care.

Can sensitivity be increased only by decreasing specificity?

It is a common impression, often stated in introductory textbooks on sensitivity and specificity of diagnostic tests, that one of these two operating characteristics can be increased only by decreasing the other. However, this statement is true only if no new information is added. For example, if the CA 125 reference level were decreased from 35 to 20 U/mL for a single test, then the sensitivity would increase and the specificity would decrease. This is the classic example by which changing a reference level improves one of the operating characteristics while necessarily decreasing the other. In contrast, if additional information is gained—such as the value of a new marker or the measurement of CA 125 at a different time point in the same subject—sensitivity can be improved with the same specificity as in the single-marker measurement (or specificity can be improved with the same sensitivity); or, in most cases, both can be increased. Two related issues are addressed in this section, both under the idea that additional information, when utilized appropriately, can increase one or both operating characteristics of screening tests, without detriment to the other.

The naïve approach to combining information in multiple markers is to generalize the approach usually taken with a single marker (at a single time point). A reference level is chosen for a single marker. The sensitivity (for this reference level) is the proportion of subjects with the disease whose marker measurement exceeds the reference level and who are therefore correctly determined to have a positive test result. The specificity is the proportion of subjects without the disease whose marker measurement does not achieve the reference level and who therefore are determined to have a negative test result, also correctly.

There are two naïve generalizations of this approach to the case involving two markers. The first is to define a positive test result as both markers exceeding their respective single-marker reference levels. With this approach, the sensitivity for the combined test is less than that achieved with either marker alone, because more conditions need to be satisfied for the result to be positive. Similarly, the specificity is increased, because a false-positive result (the complement of specificity) needs to satisfy the same additional conditions. The second naïve approach is to define a positive test result as one in which either marker exceeds its respective reference level. Following parallel logic, this approach increases the sensitivity beyond that for either marker alone, whereas the specificity is necessarily decreased, because a false-positive result would occur if either marker were falsely positive. With both of these generalizations, it does appears that an increase in one operating characteristic still requires a decrease in the other. However, the problem here is in the approach taken to combining the information in the two (or more) markers. If one displays the two markers on a two-dimensional plot (i.e., one dimension for each marker) for the cases (subjects with the target disease) and the controls (subjects without disease), it is clear that the only regions in which two measurements can be declared a positive result by these two naïve approaches are those regions defined by lines parallel to the vertical and horizontal axes, corresponding to the individual marker reference levels (Fig. 63-1). This is the case because both approaches first dichotomize the information in each marker and then attempt to combine

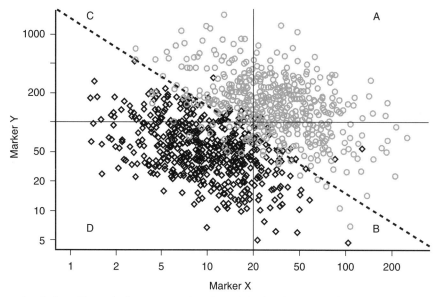

Figure 63–1. Two-dimensional plot with results from two markers (X and Y), showing cases *(diamonds)* and control subjects *(blue circles)*. The vertical line represents the reference level of 20 for marker X, and horizontal line represents the reference level of 100 for marker Y; together they divide the plot into four rectangles (A through D). The requirement that *both* markers must be positive corresponds to points in rectangle A. This requirement increases the specificity (fewer circles in rectangle A), compared with either marker X alone (region formed by rectangles A and B) or marker Y alone (region formed by rectangles A and C). It also decreases the sensitivity (fewer circles in rectangle A) compared with either X alone (rectangles A and B) or Y alone (rectangles A and C). On the other hand, the requirement that *either* marker must be positive corresponds to points in the region formed by rectangles A, B, and C; this requirement increases the sensitivity (more circles in this region), compared with either marker X alone (rectangles A and B) or marker Y alone (rectangles A and C), but it also decreases the specificity (more diamonds in this region) compared with either X (rectangles A and B) or Y (rectangles A and C). A better approach is to combine the information (about being a case based on the two markers), represented here by the diagonal *(dashed line)*. In this way, both the sensitivity (number of circles above the dashed line) and the specificity (number of diamonds below the dashed line) are simultaneously increased over their values for either marker alone.

the information; consequently, both approaches severely restrict the geometry of the region that defines a positive result.

The better approach is to combine the information first, then dichotomize. In the hypothetical example shown in Figure 63-1, the dashed diagonal line (and other lines parallel to it) combine the information first, then dichotomize the test into positive results (above the dashed line) and negative results (below the dashed line). This process simultaneously increases sensitivity and specificity. Sensitivity is increased because more red circles (cases) are above the dashed line than are above either the horizontal or the vertical line. Specificity is increased because more blue circles (controls) are below the dashed line than are below either the horizontal or the vertical line. The approach yields regions of positive results that are entirely unlike the rectangular regions obtained by first dichotomizing each marker. Furthermore, the line of separation does not have to be straight; it can be suitably curved to further improve the operating characteristics.

There are many systematic approaches to combining the information in multiple markers, and active research in statistics and computer science is seeking to improve these methods. Logistic regression[26] is a popular and well-tested statistical method. Restricted logistic regression[27] focuses only on the areas where the circles from the two groups intersect, so that outlying points do not influence the shape of the

separation line. Support vector machines[28] and neural networks, as well as related approaches such as unified maximum separability analysis (UMSA), are derived from the computer science tradition.[2] Mixture discriminant analysis (MDA)[29] describes the distribution for each group using a mixture of bivariate normal distributions; the line of separation is then formed by the ratio of the two densities, one describing the bivariate distribution of the two markers for the cases and the other describing the distribution of the two markers for the controls.

Theoretically, if marker measurements from an extremely large number of subjects in both groups were available, the bivariate distribution of the two markers for each group could be estimated almost without error. The density of the distribution describes a smooth version of a two-dimensional histogram; in the case of Figure 63-1, this would result in ellipses for the contours of the density (or hill) separately for cases and controls, with the summits being at the bivariate mean of the two markers. The ratio of the two densities throughout the entire region gives a series of optimal lines, which in general would be curved, each line describing where the ratios are equal. Tests based on one of these optimal lines would yield the maximum sensitivity theoretically achievable for the corresponding specificity (or vice-versa). As the value of the ratio of the two densities is increased, sensitivity is decreased and specificity is increased, much as with a single marker. In fact, the ratio of the two densities is the best single-number summary of the information provided by the two markers about whether the subject is a case or not.[30] However, given that in any particular study, the number of subjects is never very large, either or both distributions (one for the cases and one for the controls) are estimated with substantial imprecision, and it can be difficult to distinguish which quantitative methods give a more accurate approximation to each distribution or, just as importantly, which methods give the most accurate estimate of the optimal family of separation lines. All statistical and computer science methods for combining the information in multiple markers aim to approximate accurately the two densities and the resulting optimal family of lines of separation formed by the ratio of the two densities.

One approach to combining information in multiple markers is to approximate the case and control distributions through mixtures of multivariate normal distributions; this is called mixture discriminant analysis (MDA). In reality, we do not have the true densities for the biomarkers in cases nor in controls; instead, we have a sample of data from each group. The true densities must be estimated from the data. Linear discriminant analysis estimates the biomarker distributions by fitting bivariate normal distributions; these approximate the distributions well in Figure 63-1, but not in the hypothetical example displayed in the first panel of Figure 63-2. As can be readily imagined, in higher dimensions (i.e., with more markers), the possible distributional shapes and the relationship between cases and controls can become even more complicated. Although the two-dimensional display can guide the choice of analytic methods, similar data can prove difficult to display with three markers (dimensions) and impossible with four or more. Therefore, we need a flexible family of multivariate distributions that can approximate well a variety of multivariate distributions, work in higher dimensions without guidance from data displays, and yet be mathematically tractable for fitting the family to the data. After fitting the data with two members of the flexible family (one

for the case, and one for the controls), we combine the information in the two markers by calculating the ratio of the densities at the point specified by the two (or more) markers. The ratio then forms a test, for which a reference value can be developed in the same way as for a regular biomarker, namely setting the sensitivity or specificity.

Mixtures of multivariate normal distributions, as given by the equation

$$f(x) = \sum_{i=1}^{k} p_i N(x|\mu_i, \Sigma)$$

have been shown to be sufficiently flexible to approximate a wide variety of multivariate distributions.[31,32] Yet they are mathematically tractable for statistical fitting of parameters from data and predictions to be computed, such as heights of the densities $f(x)$ at new combinations of biomarker levels (x) for a new subject. In these equations x represents the panel of biomarkers, so that x is a vector with each element an individual biomarker value. Each mixture component is a multivariate normal distribution with a different mean μ_i and the same covariance matrix Σ. The k mixing proportions p_i sum to 1. The expectation-maximization (EM) algorithm is used to estimate the means of each mixing component, the common covariance matrix, and the mixing proportions. The estimation process is run twice, once to fit the mixture distribution for the controls, and once for the cases.

In a simulation experiment with two biomarkers, it was shown that the mixture of multivariate normal distributions, followed by the ratio of density heights of the cases to the controls, has superior performance characteristics, compared with linear logistic regression, as a method for classifying subjects as positive or negative. In the simulation experiment, 500 data points were simulated as a training sample from each of the bivariate distributions shown by the contour plots on the center panel in Figure 63-2. Each point in the left panel of Figure 63-2 represents the value of two

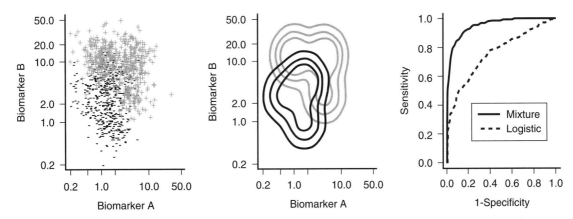

Figure 63–2. *Left panel,* Simulation of two hypothetical biomarkers, A and B, with 500 cases (+) and 500 controls (–). *Center panel,* contours of densities estimated from a mixture of bivariate normal distributions. The family of optimal curves is given by the ratio of densities for cases (+) to controls (–). *Right panel,* the (receiver) operator curves based on a mixture of bivariate normal distributions *(solid line)* and on linear logistic regression *(dashed line),* demonstrating the superiority and flexibility of the nonlinear mixture approach over standard linear methods such as logistic regression.

biomarkers for a subject, the dashed points (–) being controls and the plus points (+) cases. Two rules were then developed for detecting cases, the first using linear logistic regression and the second using a three-component mixture of bivariate normal distributions followed by the ratio of fitted densities to classify a new subject. A further simulation of another set of 500 data points in each group, independent of the previous data set, provided the validation data. The (receiver) operator curve for the mixture of normal distributions was clearly superior to the operator curve for logistic regression, as shown in the right-hand panel of Figure 63-2. This demonstrates the advantage of this flexible, nonlinear approach over linear logistic regression: at any fixed specificity, the sensitivity is higher.

As an example of the application of MDA, we evaluated the combined information in four potential markers for ovarian cancer: CA 125, CA 15.3, and CA 72.4, using Fujirebio assays (Malvern, PA), and macrophage colony-stimulating factor (M-CSF), using a technique previously described.[33] By estimating the sensitivity at a fixed specificity for all combinations of biomarkers, we identified the best panel of markers for any given size. We chose to evaluate the sensitivity at 98% specificity, because the UKCTOCS trial was designed to have 2% of subjects per year referred to ultrasound because of a positive biomarker result. Two data sets were available for this analysis. Samples were obtained from the Duke University Medical Center (Durham, NC), St. Bartholomew's Hospital (London, UK), and the Groningen University Hospital (UK), all with institutional review board approval. The first data set included early-stage cases ($n = 27$), late-stage cases ($n = 36$), and controls ($n = 126$); the second data set had only early-stage cases ($n = 60$) and controls ($n = 98$). Estimation of the parameters in the mixture of multivariate normal distributions was performed on the first set, referred to as the training set, and the resulting MDA method was applied to the independent second data set, or validation set, to give an unbiased estimate of sensitivity at 98% specificity.

The best subpanel of markers of each size is listed in Table 63-1. The best two-marker panel used CA 125II and CA 72-4 to distinguish early cases of ovarian cancer from controls; this panel demonstrated 60% sensitivity at 98% specificity in the mixture model, compared with 45% sensitivity for CA 125II alone at the same specificity. The best three-marker panel included M-CSF, CA 72-4, and CA 125II and achieved 70% sensitivity at 98% specificity. The final line in Table 63-1 indicates that CA 15.3 provides no additional information about the presence of ovarian

cancer after accounting for the information provided by CA 125II, CA 72.4, and M-CSF.

What is the best choice of samples for evaluating multiple putative biomarkers?

Finally, there is debate about which blood samples should be evaluated in assessing biomarker operating characteristics such as sensitivity and specificity. The first choice is preoperative serum samples from late-stage disease cases, compared with blood samples from age-matched control subjects. The rationale is that the cases a screening program aims to detect are women with ovarian cancer who would present clinically with late-stage disease; therefore, the markers shed into the circulation by these cancers are the target markers. The second choice is preoperative serum samples from clinically detected early-stage cases, compared with age-matched controls. The argument for these samples is that the markers should be sensitive for early-stage disease and therefore should be tested on samples from such cases. Nevertheless, such cases are clinically detected under usual care and thus are not the target of screening programs. It is probably safest to state that both sets of samples should be used in reporting the preclinical operating characteristics of each marker and panel of markers and that these samples, more readily available than the "screening samples" referred to later, provide a first hurdle for the biomarkers to be evaluated on the next stage. Another set of comparisons involves the preoperative sample compared with the postoperative sample in the same subject. In these comparisons, true tumor markers would change substantially (usually decreasing) as a result of removal of the tumor.

Finally, a panel of markers, having passed either the early-stage or the late-stage preoperative criteria (i.e., achieving a given sensitivity for a fixed specificity) and having been combined with the use of a systematic statistical or bioinformatic approach, may then be tested on samples from biorepositories formed from prior screening studies. Such studies require 2000 or more subjects to be screened to obtain samples from 1 subject with ovarian cancer. These samples are rare, precious, and expensive, and they should be reserved for testing panels of markers that have clearly met well-established criteria on preoperative samples. These samples also have the added benefit that the status of the subject at the time of sample collection is unknown, which removes any possible bias due to differences in collection and processing that may be in effect for samples collected from ovarian cancer patients compared with healthy subjects (e.g., due to collection at different clinical sites).

Table 63-1. Unbiased Sensitivity at 98% Specificity for Optimal Marker Panels of Size 1 to 4

Marker Panel	Sensitivity (%)
CA125 II	45
CA125 II, CA 72-4	67
CA125 II, CA 72-4, M-CSF	70
CA125 II, CA 72-4, M-CSF, CA 15-3	68

Conclusion

This chapter has discussed the controversies relating to ovarian cancer screening with serum biomarkers. These controversies include methods to combine biomarkers systematically without being penalized for adding additional markers to an existing marker, discussions about the cost-effectiveness of an ovarian cancer screening program with serum markers as a first-line test and comparison with an existing accepted screening program, and sample choice in the evaluation of putative ovarian cancer biomarkers.

REFERENCES

1. Woolas RP, et al: Combinations of multiple serum markers are superior to individual assays for discriminating malignant from benign pelvic masses. Gynecol Oncol 1995;59:111-116.
2. Zhang Z, et al: Combination of multiple serum markers using an artificial neural network to improve specificity in discriminating malignant from benign pelvic masses. Gynecol Oncol 1999;73:56-61.
3. Laframboise S, et al: Use of CA-125 and ultrasound in high-risk women. Int J Gynecol Cancer 2002;12:86-91.
4. Diamandis EP, et al: Human kallikrein 11: A new biomarker of prostate and ovarian carcinoma. Cancer Res 2002;62:295-300.
5. Petricoin EF, et al: Use of proteomic patterns in serum to identify ovarian cancer. Lancet 2002;359:572-577.
6. Robertson DM, et al: Inhibins/activins as diagnostic markers for ovarian cancer. Mol Cell Endocrinol 2002;191:97-103.
7. Ye B, et al: Serum and urine proteomics: Protein profiling and identification of ovarian cancer biomarkers using mass spectrometry and liquid chromatography. Mol Cell Proteomics 2002;1:736.
8. Chen YL, Xu Y: Determination of lysophosphatidic acids by capillary electrophoresis with indirect ultraviolet detection. J Chromatogr B Biomed Sci Appl 2001;753:355-363.
9. Mok SC, et al: Prostasin, a potential serum marker for ovarian cancer: Identification through microarray technology. J Natl Cancer Inst 2001;93:1458-1464.
10. van Haaften-Day C, et al: OVX1, macrophage-colony stimulating factor, and CA-125-II as tumor markers for epithelial ovarian carcinoma: A critical appraisal. Cancer 2001;92:2837-2844.
11. Crump C, et al: Ovarian cancer tumor marker behavior in asymptomatic healthy women: Implications for screening. Cancer Epidemiol Biomarkers Prev 2000;9:1107-1111.
12. Baron AT, et al: Serum sErbB1 and epidermal growth factor levels as tumor biomarkers in women with stage III or IV epithelial ovarian cancer. Cancer Epidemiol Biomarkers Prev 1999;8:129-137.
13. Zanetta G, et al: Ultrasound, physical examination, and CA 125 measurement for the detection of recurrence after conservative surgery for early borderline ovarian tumors. Gynecol Oncol 2001;81:63-66.
14. Modugno F, Weissfeld JL, Hill LM: Reproducibility in the assessment of postmenopausal ovaries with transvaginal ultrasound. Gynecol Oncol 2000;77:289-292.
15. DePriest PD, et al: Transvaginal sonography as a screening method for the detection of early ovarian cancer. Gynecol Oncol 1997;65:408-414.
16. van Nagell JR Jr, et al: Ovarian cancer screening. Cancer 1995;76(10 Suppl): 2086-2091.
17. Bourne TH, et al: The potential role of serum CA 125 in an ultrasound-based screening program for familial ovarian cancer. Gynecol Oncol 1994;52:379-385.
18. Ye B, et al: Preliminary screening and identification of a urinary protein biomarker for ovarian cancer with SELDI-MS technology. Cancer Epidemiol Biomarkers Prev 2002;11:1189S-1189S.
19. Karlan BY, Platt LD: Ovarian cancer screening: The role of ultrasound in early detection. Cancer 1995;76(10 Suppl): 2011-2015.
20. Schwartz M, et al: Utilization of ovarian cancer screening by women at increased risk. Cancer Epidemiol Biomarkers Prev 1995;4:269-273.
21. Bast RC Jr, et al: A radioimmunoassay using a monoclonal antibody to monitor the course of epithelial ovarian cancer. N Engl J Med 1983;309:883-887.
22. Skates S, Pauler D, Jacobs I: Screening based on the risk of cancer calculation from Bayesian hierarchical change-point and mixture models of longitudinal markers. J Am Stat Assoc 2001;96:429-439.
23. Beveridge H, Fallowfield L: UK Collaborative Trial of Ovarian Cancer Screening (UKCTOCS) psychosocial study. Psychooncology 2002;11:547.
24. Gohagan JK, et al: The Prostate, Lung, Colorectal, and Ovarian-Cancer Screening Trial of the National Cancer Institute. Cancer 1995;75:1869-1873.
25. Kabawat SE, et al: Tissue distribution of a coelomic-epithelium-related antigen recognized by the monoclonal antibody OC125. Int J Gynecol Pathol 1983;2:275-285.
26. Cox DR, Snell EJ: Analysis of Binary Data, 2nd ed. Monographs on statistics and applied probability. New York: Chapman and Hall, 1989.
27. McIntosh MW, Pepe MS: Combining several screening tests: Optimality of the risk score. Biometrics 2002;58:657-664.
28. Vapnik V: The Nature of Statistical Learning. New York: Springer, 1995, p 193.
29. Hastie T, Tibshirani R: Discriminant analysis by Gaussian mixtures. J R Statis Soc B- Methodol 1996;58:155-176.
30. Baker SG: The central role of receiver operating characteristic (ROC) curves in evaluating tests for the early detection of cancer. J Natl Cancer Inst 2003;95:511-515.
31. MacLachlan G, Peel D: Finite mixture models. Wiley Series in Probability and Statistics. New York: Wiley, 2000.
32. Titterington DM, Makov UE, Smith AFM: *Statistical analysis of finite mixture distributions.* Wiley series in probability and mathematical statistics. Applied probability and statistics. New York: Wiley, 1985.
33. Xu FJ, et al: Increased serum levels of macrophage colony-stimulating factor in ovarian cancer. Am J Obstet Gynecol 1991; 165:1356-1362.

64

BIOETHICS

Richard E. Ashcroft

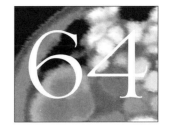

 MAJOR CONTROVERSIES

- **What is bioethics?**
- **What are the bioethical issues related to screening?**
- **What are the bioethical issues related to cancer genetics?**
- **What are the bioethical issues related to primary and secondary prevention of cancer?**
- **What are the bioethical issues related to problems of surgical management?**
- **What are the bioethical issues related to reproductive and sexual health?**
- **What are the bioethical issues related to research and innovative treatment?**
- **What are the bioethical issues related to access to treatment?**
- **What are the ethical issues at the end of life?**

What is bioethics?

Bioethics is a multidisciplinary field primarily concerned with the study and analysis of ethical problems in research and practice in modern medicine, allied health professions (including nursing and public health), and biomedical sciences. It is sometimes considered to include ethical problems in other related areas, such as agriculture, environmental sciences and management, veterinary medicine, and the use of animals in farming, research, and ownership of companion animals.[1,2] However, for the purposes of this chapter, we will restrict our consideration to bioethics narrowly understood as the study of ethical problems in modern biomedical science and clinical practice. As a multidisciplinary field, its research methods include methods in medicine, public health, sociology, anthropology, economics, history of medicine, literature, and theology.[3-8] The central role is held by methods of applied philosophy.[9-11]

Historically, themes in bioethics have been discussed for as long as medicine has been practiced. However, most commentators would point to the 1960s as the period when bioethics became a focus of systematic research.[12,13] Bioethics is a research discipline and increasingly a quasi-clinical discipline, with bioethicists

involved in a number of ways in research, policy-making, support for clinical ethics committees and institutional review boards, and bedside consultation and ward rounds. The roles of clinical ethics consulting and clinical ethics committees are most well established in the United States, but similar activities are found elsewhere and appear to be on the increase throughout Western Europe and North America.[14-17]

The relationships between cancer and bioethics and between health care for women and bioethics are long-standing and complex. Some of the classic controversies in bioethics arise in particularly poignant ways in cancer medicine, and some of the most heated methodologic disputes in bioethics have arisen in the context of discussions of health care for women. This controversial situation continues today.

What are the bioethical issues related to screening?

The aim of a screening program for early diagnosis of disease is to permit early detection of serious disease and appropriate treatment.[18] This form of screening has been defined as "... the systematic application of a test or inquiry to identify individuals at sufficient risk

Box 64–1. Wilson and Jungner Criteria for the Acceptability of a Screening Program

Is the disease an important health problem?
Is there a recognizable latent or early symptomatic stage?
Are facilities for diagnosis and treatment available?
Has the cost of the program been considered in the context of other demands for resources?
Is there an agreed policy on whom to treat as patients?
Does treatment confer benefit?

From Wilson JMG, Jungner G: The Principles and Practice of Screening for Disease. Geneva, World Health Organization, 1968.

of a specific disorder to warrant further investigation or direct preventive action, among persons who have not sought medical attention on account of the symptoms of that disorder."[19] The classic criteria for determining whether a screening program is appropriate for early detection of disease were devised by Wilson and Jungner for the World Health Organization in 1968[20] (Box 64-1).

Over the history of screening for breast and cervical cancer, different aspects of these screening programs have been ethically and socially controversial. One important feature is the image of screening for common gynecologic cancers as "doing something for women's health." Proposals to restrict the availability of such screening are frequently subject to intense public criticism on the grounds that (arguably) women's health care has been relatively poorly funded and that a reduction in the level of screening services compounds, rather than relieves, important gender-based inequalities in health care provision. Access to screening programs was an important part of feminist health campaigns in the 1960s and 1970s, and it continues to be so.[21-23] This argument is based on the principles of distributive justice (i.e., a fair distribution of resources on the basis of equal respect and compelling need) and restorative justice (i.e., positive discrimination in the distribution of resources toward those who have historically been unfairly disadvantaged).[24] At a more specific level, mainstream discussion of screening for cancer tends to focus on the notion of preventable deaths. According to the widely accepted principle of beneficence, we have an obligation to do good where this can be achieved without unreasonable effort, and this obligation to do good would, in most interpretations, involve preventing easily preventable deaths.[9,11,25] Screening apparently offers two advantages to the screened individual: an increased probability of early detection of disease (and the possibility of treatment and the extension of life) and the benefit of knowing that a person's health is being cared for and that if there is a negative test result, the person is probably well.

However, this set of arguments and attitudes has been controversial within and outside medicine. Because any screening test has associated with it probabilities of false-positive results and false-negative results, some women will inevitably be falsely reassured that they are well when in fact they have early signs of disease, and some women will inevitably be told that they are ill when there are no such signs. Periodically, hospitals come into the media spotlight because the pathology or radiology service has failed to identify a number of positive tests or has mistakenly warned some women that they are at risk for disease. In at least some cases, this is no more than statistically expected error, although in many cases poor-quality or negligent care might have been offered. Where a service is offered, it should be performed competently and to a high standard of quality.

Assuming that the quality of the screening service is close to what is theoretically possible, patients are still faced with a double risk: the "natural" risk of having a cancer and the "technical" risk of falsely believing that a person does or does not have the cancer. Screening programs play a part in creating the "worried well" and in generating false reassurance.[26-28] Although arguably false reassurance and the worried well result from any diagnostic test in the ordinary doctor-patient relationship, the particular feature of screening programs that has created ethical and social controversy is the organized and proactive nature of most public health screening programs. To make a significant difference in terms of mortality and morbidity reduction, most screening programs need to identify an at-risk group and to encourage members of that group to present for screening. A number of measures have been used for encouraging the uptake of screening programs, including health information campaigns and capitation payment to primary care physicians.[29] Patients may not always realize that their doctor is reimbursed to encourage the patients' participation.

Sociologic work has tended to be quite critical of the idea that people should be encouraged to think of themselves as "at risk" and as "patients" when they are not ill.[26] However, most bioethicists have tended to concur with the mainstream public health view that people should be encouraged in the direction of personally managed primary prevention and screening. Simplifying this debate somewhat, what seems to be at stake is what is involved in being "autonomous."[30]

In terms of the debate over screening, the controversy about personal autonomy can be understood as an argument about what groups screening is meant to serve. On the face of it, screening is in the interests of those who are tested. Many women agree with this view, particularly those who feel discriminated against or unfairly denied service because they are too young (or too old) for a particular screening program or because the screening program calls them for screening too infrequently. However, those who resent being "forced" into the role of patient-in-waiting regard such screening programs as improper restrictions on their autonomy. Some women in particular resent this policing of their health, and some dislike the invasive nature of particular investigations (notably for carcinoma in situ or cervical cancer). There is some discussion about the degree to which regular radiologic investigation is safe (although mammography now uses much lower doses of ionizing radiation than in the past).[31]

Screening tests can be occasions for a number of inappropriate attitudes on the part of health care staff to be expressed (e.g., attitudes about patients' sexuality). Given that an autonomy-centered ethics seems to be at the heart of modern Western medical ethics, these considerations have led a few commentators, even in state-financed health care systems, to argue that screening proper ought not to be continued for many conditions, but instead offered only on a private, patient-centered basis.[32,33] However, the public health argument that screening can only be effective and cost-effective if a certain take-up rate is met or passed, and the clear public demand for screening services for common gynecologic cancers suggest that a middle way is possible on the basis of "informed choice" about screening.[34] This approach permits women to choose whether to take up an offer of a screening test while ensuring that they have reasonably complete information about the advantages and disadvantages of doing so. Methods for encouraging uptake of the screening program concentrate on making the test as convenient as possible for women but stop short of putting pressure on them to comply.

As can be seen from Table 64-1 of aspects for evaluating a screening program devised by the British public health specialists Donaldson and Donaldson, evaluation of a screening program is highly complex and involves balancing a number of different factors. Sometimes, as with the Norwegian Cochrane collaboration center's systematic review of breast screening by mammography, this balancing can become very controversial.[35] There is no obvious ethical solution to this, other than to note that in the last analysis the decision to run a particular screening program, to decide what rates of false negatives and false positives are acceptable, and to decide at what level issues of cost-effectiveness can determine whether to offer a program is essentially a political one (in state-funded systems) and one of business culture in privately financed systems, such as the managed care systems.[36-38] Some health policy thinkers have placed considerable weight on the idea that evidence-based approaches can resolve whether to provide screening and under what conditions for a particular disease. Table 64-1 indicates that evidence is important, but it is equally important to determine the values and goals underlying the proposed screening program and review the evidence in the light of these goals.[19,35] Classic liberal arguments for interference in patients' choices in the interest of the common good may not apply in screening for noninherited forms of gynecologic cancer.[39] However, they do perhaps apply in the case of inheritable forms.

What are the bioethical issues related to cancer genetics?

Considerable scientific attention has been paid to identifying genetic risk factors for breast and ovarian cancer. Several genes have been identified with mutations known to indicate a significantly raised lifetime risk of the development of breast or ovarian cancer. The most well known are the *BRCA1* and *BRCA2* genes. However, because these are relatively large genes, existing genetic tests can only identify about one half the mutations that are suspected to influence risk of developing cancer. The existing tests are not particularly sensitive, and if a woman is found to test negative for the gene, this information is not very informative. However, if a woman is test positive, this is informative (although there are some false positives). The most reliable way of obtaining an informative genetic test is to identify a woman in a family with a history of breast or ovarian cancer and to identify a mutation in the *BRCA1* or *BRCA2* gene that may be implicated in the family history. After it is established that this mutation is involved in the cancer history of the family, other members of the family may then be tested prospectively for the presence or absence of this mutation. This test is much more sensitive. As such, in many families with a history of disease, it is necessary to investigate not only the putatively at risk patient but other members of the family. In families for which prior genetic or oncologic data are missing, the raw *BRCA1* or *BRCA2* test may be uninformative.[40] Most breast and ovarian cancers are thought not to involve inherited risk factors, although some media representations lead patients to think otherwise.[41]

Table 64–1. Aspects to Consider in Evaluating a Screening Program

Features Evaluated	Benefits and Risks
Priorities and other strategies	Importance of the health problem, whether other control strategies (e.g., primary prevention, treatment) are more appropriate
Properties of the test	Validity (e.g., false positives, false negatives), positive predictive value, convenience, safety, acceptability
Clinical consequences	Effectiveness, acceptability, cost, side effects of diagnosis and treatment after screening positive
Resources	Costs of testing, organization of the program, diagnosis and treatment of the cases of disease detected
Quality assurance	System needed to monitor, ensure, and improve quality of an established program
Ethical and moral aspects	Confidentiality of the data

Adapted from (UK) National Screening Committee: First Report of the National Screening Committee. London, Health Departments of the United Kingdom, 1998.

This situation creates several ethical challenges. For someone who is test positive, there is the problem of knowing how to respond to this information. Part of this problem rests on how to understand the distinction between absolute and relative risk of developing the disease. Before the test, knowing the relative risk of developing a cancer if a person is test positive may be worrying but uninformative. After the test, knowing the absolute risk conditional on a positive test result can be understood as being given information about a person's inevitable fate, even if it is not known when cancer is likely to develop or whether it will develop. Second, if a person tests positive, the range of options facing her can appear very restricted. For many women, the choice between prophylactic mastectomy, long-term prophylactic medication, or watchful waiting may appear to be no choice at all, and acting aggressively against the risk of illness may be a way of taking control in an apparently uncontrollable situation.[42] Third, the classic problem in the ethics of clinical genetics—whether nondirective genetic counseling is possible—arises in this context, although given the clinical uncertainty about the interpretation of genetic tests without other family members' test results and medical history, this is one situation in which nondirectiveness is easier than in the case of the single-gene disorders.[43]

The most poignant and difficult ethical dilemmas in genetic testing for the risk of cancer and genetic testing to make a cellular diagnosis of cancer more precise involve the situation of the woman in her family. One challenging dilemma involves whether the woman (or her physician) incurs a duty to warn others about their possible status as carriers of a cancer risk gene. Research suggests that many women who are positive for a risk gene feel guilt and responsibility for "inflicting" this risk on their children.[43] This can apply when the gene has not been inherited (but the risk of early death of the mother may involve "abandoning" her children) and when it has. Conversely, a woman in a family with a history of disease who is gene negative may be uncertain that her negative result was a "true" negative or feel so-called survivor guilt that she has escaped what other female relatives have not—or she may be simply relieved. These situations can place enormous stress on the woman and her relationships. However, in many families, preexisting stresses may have caused breaches between family members, and in such situations, a woman who is gene positive may not wish to disclose this to other relatives who may be affected and who might wish to be tested if they knew. This becomes even more difficult when the individual who wishes nondisclosure to be adhered to is the only woman who has an identified mutation without which it would be much less likely that a test of her relations would be informative. This situation may license a breach of confidence by a doctor who wishes to inform a possibly affected relative. However, opinion is divided quite sharply on this question. Classic situations in which breach of confidence is permitted normally involve a clear public good (e.g., administration of justice) or the prevention of a serious risk of

significant harm to a third party. It is not clear that disclosure in this situation would prevent harm to another, although it would certainly give them more choices and permit better-informed decisions to be made about whether to be tested and in planning what to do about a positive test.

This situation might be consistent with the liberal theory of personal privacy, although this idea is debatable.[39] However, it is almost certainly consistent with a communitarian theory of moral duty, according to which our obligations to each other can take priority over our personal interests in privacy and self-determination, because it is only through our mutual relationships that our individuality takes shape and has meaning.[44]

Wider public controversies about cancer genetics have some bearing here. According to the well-known theory of geneticization, there is a tendency to reshape all of our disease concepts in genetic terms and to see them in terms of reproduction and destiny. Although this is unfair to the complexity of modern genetic science, it is perhaps not unfair to the ways in which we tend casually to talk about genetics.[45] As with debates about screening but perhaps more intensely because the time interval between a positive genetic test and a detected early cancer may be considerable, the conversion of a woman into a patient-in-waiting may be problematic. When the woman presents herself for testing, it may be considered an understandable exercise of patient autonomy, but this is far from clear when testing one person will directly inform a third party that she is at greatly increased risk of disease, even if she has not been consulted about whether she wants this information. Consider the examples of a homozygous twin of a proband (who will have the same gene) or the children of a proband (who will be at high risk of having the same gene). These difficult situations indicate that very careful genetic counseling is necessary. Further issues concern possible nonmedical uses of the same information (e.g., by insurers or employers). Although most jurisdictions are taking steps to protect their citizens against predatory or unfair uses of their genetic information against them, it is far from clear what public policy ought to be in this area in the long term.[46,47]

What are the bioethical issues related to primary and secondary prevention of cancer?

Most primary prevention measures for cancers are relatively uncontroversial in terms of their impact on patients or on society more generally, although some skeptical challenges have been raised on the grounds that we are creating a "health risk society." The idea is that health promotion and risk reduction strategies combine moralizing concerning particular behaviors (especially tobacco, drugs, and alcohol use or abuse), provoking exaggerated fear and obsession in the population about environmental factors (e.g., diet) and promoting the idea that any death is avoidable.[48] Certainly, there is an ethical dimension to health promotion and to public health, and sometimes, this is not fully thought through by practitioners and policy makers.[49,50] However, although there is room for development in this area, the skeptical challenge to health promotion is rather weak and overgeneralized in content, except when specific measures are subjected to close scrutiny.

An example of close scrutiny devoted to a primary preventive measure is the case of prophylactic hysterectomy or mastectomy to reduce the risk of cervical, uterine, ovarian, or breast cancer. These interventions have been criticized by feminist critics of medicine on a number of grounds, such as their effectiveness, the risks and sequelae of the procedures, the impact on women's self-image, and the lack of investment in research aimed at finding alternative preventive measures. Prophylactic mastectomy and hysterectomy have been challenged because of the complex associations between bodily health, sexuality, and perceptions of health and sexuality by women patients themselves, by others, and by society as a whole.[51,52] Thinking about this from an ethical point of view, some imperatives emerge. Priority needs to be given to the autonomy of the particular woman patient facing the decision about surgical intervention to reduce her risk of cancer. Because almost all women in this situation have good reason to think that their chance of developing cancer is high, the decision to proceed will need to be made with access to high-quality counseling about risk, options, and the evidence regarding the particular interventions being considered (i.e., safety, consequences, and effectiveness).

Similar issues arise when considering secondary prevention, although the debates have been shaped slightly differently because they tend to concern the role of chemoprevention rather than prophylactic surgery. Although the evidence base regarding chemoprevention in breast cancer, for instance, is changing daily, it is difficult to be definitive about the ethical status of chemoprevention. However, some criticism of the way in which chemoprevention may involve women taking long courses of medication on two grounds: safety (pending long-term survival data) and the casting of women who are subjectively well in the role of the permanent patient. Nevertheless, this is a choice many women are willing to make, and a background suspicion of pharmaceutically driven therapeutics presents no specific clinical ethical issue beyond the need to support women's decisions to make informed, autonomous choices.

What are the bioethical issues related to problems of surgical management?

Therapeutic mastectomy and hysterectomy present ethical issues similar to those for prophylactic mastectomy and hysterectomy, although some differences of emphasis apply. The different emphasis when these procedures are conducted therapeutically (for cancerous or precancerous bodies) naturally relates to the need to act to prevent progression of identified disease or neoplasm that possesses a significant risk of becoming disease. Because such procedures may no longer be considered to be elective, the meaning they have for patients may be quite different, and their willingness to undergo these procedures may be greater. However, as with any other serious medical or surgical intervention, this decision needs to be made in an informed way, with complete information about the relative likelihood of success, expected outcomes, and the psychosocial outcome of the procedure. The complexity of this area relates to the intertwining of the medical outcome of the procedure (in treating cancer, extending life, and improving the quality of life for the patient) and the psychosocial outcome (the impact on the woman of having cancer, the alteration in her body image and her experience of her own body, and the impact on her family and other relationships of the disease and the therapeutic procedures).[53] Two principal issues arise. The first is how to help the woman choose among the therapeutic options available to her (e.g., lumpectomy or radical mastectomy in breast cancer) through discussion of expectations, risks, and outcomes. The second issue, which is arguably much more profound, is how to find a way of discussing and listening to her experience and her "voice" in a way which is truly facilitative. Much of contemporary bioethics has observed this problem, but it remains open to criticism in the way that it can present ethical challenges as merely problems of informed choice while paying little attention to how the doctor can best understand and help patients make those choices.[54-56] This is an area where medicine and bioethics can learn much from working with patients and from research in medical sociology and anthropology.

What are the bioethical issues related to reproductive and sexual health?

Much of the complexity in this area is concerned with the intertwining of medical and sexual meanings of the body and bodily experience. This complexity is manifest in some lay and professional theories of disease causation, such as the concept of cervical cancer as a sexually transmitted disease, which can involve cervical screening being seen as a kind of surveillance of sexual activity.[57] This intertwining is even more obviously involved in dealing with the consequences of treatment for cancer. Lumpectomy or mastectomy for cancer has implications for a woman's sense of sexual self and for her relationship with her current or future partner. Hysterectomy in premenopausal women has the effect of ending the woman's capacity to conceive and of causing early menopause. Although the latter can be managed with hormone replacement therapy (HRT), the health consequences of this are somewhat controversial, and feminist critics of HRT have challenged the way HRT may pose health risks to women while constructing a very specific model of what normal female biology is, how it is normative in defining what women's health is, and how the medical management of the female endocrine system may be relatively unresponsive to women's own subjective experience of the physical consequences of HRT. Similar arguments have been raised for many years about the contraceptive pill, and as with the pill, they deserve serious thought, although HRT and the contraceptive pill have large worldwide sales and are widely used by women.[58,59]

Although hysterectomy may end a woman's capacity to conceive a child through natural sexual intercourse, the possibility of removing ovarian tissue before radiotherapy or as part of hysterectomy, freezing this material, and then recovering ova for use with in vitro fertilization techniques at a later date has been available for several years. This procedure has provoked some ethical discussion. When the patient is younger than reproductive age, the issues include whether the child can be competent to consent to this procedure. More generally, there has been discussion of whether infertility should be treated as a medical condition at all, whether infertility caused by hysterectomy or radiotherapy involves creating a right to assistance in conception (in the way that mastectomy may create a right to reconstructive surgery), and whether the attempt to restore or emulate natural fertility is (as with HRT) an imposition of the view that a normal woman should want and be able to have children. In vitro fertilization is itself a controversial technology, involving as it does the creation of some embryos that will not be implanted and subsequently destroyed.[60-63]

Controversial as these issues are socially, from an ethical point of view, it is arguable that these issues really are matters for individual choice and conscience. Although there has been considerable debate about postmenopausal motherhood, in most cases of interest to oncologists, the patient in question who is concerned about the loss of her present fertility is presumably premenopausal, and most of the moral objections to postmenopausal motherhood (however well-founded) are more concerned with age rather than fertility.[62] There are large issues for public policy concerning the ethical and policy acceptability of assisted conception, but in most societies, in vitro fertilization has been accepted, is regulated, and although a choice that can be difficult for would-be parents to make privately, is not controversial for most people.[64,65]

What are the bioethical issues related to research and innovative treatment?

Cancer treatment has made great progress over the past 50 years, and most patients will at some stage in their career as cancer patients be involved in medical or social research into new ways of treating or managing cancer. Considerable debate surrounds research interventions in cancer. The recent revision of the World Medical Association's Declaration of Helsinki has redefined the distinction between therapeutic and nontherapeutic research as a distinction between therapeutic and nontherapeutic procedures, noting that even in what was called therapeutic research, many investigations or procedures were carried out that were not of themselves therapeutic but were done for the purposes of collecting research data.[66] Much debate on the ethics of oncologic research has concentrated on "last chance" therapies, which are not yet licensed (or not for this indication) or which are available only in early (phase I or II) trials. Some commentators have argued that the main problem is one of equity to the dying patient in ensuring access to treatments inside or outside trials that, in the patient's opinion, may be beneficial to her. This argument has drawn on analogies with the acquired immunodeficiency syndrome (AIDS) treatment activist movement of the late 1980s and early 1990s.[67,68] However, much of the argument has been in the opposite direction, arguing that such last chance therapies represent a denial of death, poor-quality treatment at a time when palliative care would be more appropriate, a misleading false hope to patients, and burdensome or toxic treatment of the already gravely ill.[69,70] Some commentators frankly speak of futile, heroic, or extraordinary care.[71] Particularly challenging may be the request from a patient's relative to "do everything" or to "try anything" that will keep the loved one alive, because in most countries relatives have no legal power to consent to treatment for another adult.

Although the principles of research ethics are reasonably well known and long established, the fine detail of when a trial can be said to be ethical can still be difficult to pin down. Debates over placebo or active controls, the meaning of equipoise between two (or more) treatments, the definition of appropriate (and patient-relevant) end points, early stopping of trials (because one or other treatment is thought unsafe or obviously superior on the basis of interim data), and the size of effect that would make clinical use of the treatment under trial worthwhile are all long-standing controversies.[72,73] At their core is a debate about the relationship between justice (i.e., what is fair treatment of a patient in terms of access and of not imposing undue burden), beneficence (i.e., the obligation to do what is best for the patient), and nonmaleficence (i.e., the obligation not to do avoidable harm to a patient).[9] Our ethical review system rests on the twin pillars of informed consent and risk-benefit assessment by investigators and research ethics committees (i.e., institutional review boards), but there remain difficult areas such as research using dying and incompetent patients, and it may be that substantive progress can only effectively be made using more imaginative techniques of patient involvement in research design and priority setting.[74] Most commentators agree that the current review and appraisal system is reasonably reliable in evaluating direct risks and benefits to patients, but more profound problems such as the moral evaluation of the direction of research, the moral purposes pursued in developing new medical treatments, and priority setting between research goals have generally been left out of account as too difficult or as inappropriate for local decision-making.[75,76]

What are the bioethical issues related to access to treatment?

A developing concern worldwide is the ability of private and public sector health services to deliver ever more expensive treatment in a timely and equitable way.[36,77-80] A number of interpretations of the principle of justice have been proposed as solutions to this distribution problem, including frank free-market approaches based on ability to pay, quasi-Marxist approaches based on need, socially conservative approaches based on merit, and liberal approaches based on fair participative decision-making.[81,82] All of these approaches have some validity in particular contexts, without commanding universal assent in any situations. In recent years, much attention has been paid to the quasi-utilitarian approach developed under the themes of quality-adjusted life years (QALYs) and cost-effectiveness. However, in the field of cancer, this approach risks confusion for a number of reasons. First, cancer care is relatively high cost, and the QALY or cost-effectiveness approach may not be all that discriminating within oncology while perhaps placing too little value on the importance of saving life (and striving to save life) when making comparison between oncology and other areas of acute medicine.[11,36] Second, a terminologic confusion exists in the association between quality of life in QALYs and quality of life in treatment outcome assessment, because in the latter context, the point is patients' reported subjective quality of life, which may not be the same thing as objective quality of life, which QALYs purport to measure.[83,84] Third, QALYs are not a particularly useful tool for comparing the value of interventions designed to treat illness with the value of interventions designed to palliate suffering at the end of life, because the latter typically acts over (relatively) short periods, whereas treatment interventions normally are (hoped to be) operative over medium- to long-term periods.[85] Despite these drawbacks, QALYs do have some clear advantages over other proposed allocation tools, because they are clear, measurable, and comparable and have a theoretical basis that is sufficiently well described to make them useful and open to rational criticism as appropriate. For these reasons, they are likely to be with us for some time to come. Terminal care, in particular, consumes a large proportion of any individual's lifetime "spent" (in private health care or by proxy in public health care) on health care. This has been observed and debated for some time, and few serious proposals have come forward to deal with this phenomenon, perhaps because the good of caring for the dying person well is thought to outweigh other competing goods, such as economic efficiency.[38,70,76]

What are the ethical issues at the end of life?

Traditionally, much of the discussion of ethics in oncology turned on appropriate care for patients at the end of life. Detailed analyses are available for much of this field, including the obligation to tell the truth to patients about their diagnosis, the merits and disadvantages of prognosis, the rights and wrongs of euthanasia and assisted suicide, and the roles of palliative care and spiritual support in terminal care.[69,71,85-88] The euthanasia debate is endlessly fascinating, endlessly important, and probably just endless. However, some areas of current controversy include the salience of the distinction between active killing and discontinuation of active life-sustaining treatment and the doctrine of double effect, according to which pain control that results in death may be permissible, provided that death was not the intended but only a foreseen outcome of pain-control medication.[89-92] Standard objections to assisted suicide and active euthanasia remain fairly compelling (e.g., corruption of the role of the doctor, slippery slopes to medical murder of unwilling vulnerable patients), as do standard arguments for patient-requested euthanasia (e.g., patient autonomy, the subjective nature of intolerable pain and suffering). For this reason, states are likely to differ on their public policy in this area, and it is difficult to see any very stable consensus being achieved in the near future.

Related to this debate are the linked debates about "No-Code" or not-for-resuscitation decisions in dying or frail patients and about Advance Directives made out by patients wishing to refuse active treatment in certain circumstances when they will no longer be able to voice their own view. The standing of Advance Directives seems more and more solid, although the number of patients using them to decide about their future care is not growing rapidly. Not-for-resuscitation decisions have been controversial for some time, in that some patients and their relatives regard them as signs of giving up or of discrimination against the patient on grounds of illness or age.[93,94] Conversely, some writers have argued that cardiopulmonary resuscitation itself is so violent and its success rate so relatively low, that not-for-resuscitation directions are not written into notes enough.[95]

A long-standing issue challenges us all. At some point, care of the dying may become care of someone whose pain control medication leaves her in a state of minimal awareness of herself or the environment. When such a patient is about to die, the "death rattle" may be distressing to relatives and other patients on the hospital ward. A number of treatments are being tried to control death rattle. Questions arise about who is being treated and why. As with screening, there is an ambiguity between our obligations to care well for patients and our interests in the welfare of others. Perhaps the most profound problem of all is how to make our obligations to individuals, to families, and to society cohere.

REFERENCES

1. Harris J: Introduction: The scope and importance of bioethics. In Harris J (ed): Bioethics. Oxford, Oxford University Press, 2001, pp 1-22.
2. Singer P, Kuhse H: A Companion to Bioethics. Oxford, Blackwell, 1998.

3. Hope T: Empirical medical ethics. J Med Ethics 1999;24:291-292.
4. Kleinman A, Fox RC, Brandt AM (eds): Bioethics and Beyond. Daedalus 1999;128:v-x, 1-326.
5. Culyer AJ: Economics and ethics in health care. J Med Ethics 2001;27:217-222.
6. Lammers S, Verhey A (eds): On Moral Medicine: Theological Perspectives in Medical Ethics, 2nd ed. Grand Rapids, MI, Wm B Eeerdmans, 1998.
7. Fulford KWM, Dickenson DL, Murray TH (eds): Healthcare Ethics and Human Values: An Introductory Text with Readings and Case Studies. Oxford, Blackwell, 2002.
8. Reverby S (ed): Tuskegee's Truths: Rethinking the Tuskegee Syphilis Study. Chapel Hill, University of North Carolina Press, 2000.
9. Beauchamp TL, Childress JF: Principles of Biomedical Ethics, 4th ed. Oxford, Oxford University Press, 1993.
10. Engelhardt HT: The Foundations of Bioethics, 2nd ed. Oxford, Oxford University Press, 1996.
11. Harris J: The Value of Life: An Introduction to Medical Ethics. London, Routledge, 1985.
12. Rothman DJ: Strangers at the Bedside: How Law and Bioethics Transformed Medical Decision Making. New York, Basic Books, 1991.
13. Jonsen AR: The Birth of Bioethics. Oxford, Oxford University Press, 1998.
14. Jonsen AR, Siegler M, Winslade WJ: Clinical Ethics: A Practical Approach to Ethical Decisions in Clinical Medicine, 5th ed. New York, McGraw-Hill, 2002.
15. LaPuma J, Schiedermayer D: Ethics Consultation: A Practical Guide. Boston, Jones & Bartlett, 1994.
16. Slowther AM, Hope T, Ashcroft RE (eds): Clinical Ethics Committees. J Med Ethics 2001;27(Suppl):i1-i56.
17. Turner L: A career in clinical ethics. Br Med J 2002;325:S105.
18. Donaldson LJ, Donaldson RJ: Essential Public Health, 2nd ed. Newbury, UK, Petroc Press, 2000, pp 118-126.
19. (UK) National Screening Committee: First Report of the National Screening Committee. London, Health Departments of the United Kingdom, 1998.
20. Wilson JMG, Jungner G: The Principles and Practice of Screening for Disease. Geneva, World Health Organization, 1968.
21. Kasper AS: Barriers and burdens: Poor women face breast cancer. In Kasper AS, Ferguson SJ (eds): Breast Cancer: Society Shapes an Epidemic. New York, Palgrave Macmillan, 2000, pp 183-212.
22. Doyal L: What Makes Women Sick. Basingstoke, UK, Palgrave Macmillan, 1995.
23. Philips A, Rakusen J, for the Boston Women's Health Collective: The New Our Bodies, Ourselves: A Health Book By and For Women. London, Penguin, 2000.
24. Tong R, Williams N: Gender justice in the health-care system: Past experiences, present realities and future hopes. In Rhodes R, Battin MP, Silvers A (eds): Medicine and Social Justice: Essays on the Distribution of Health Care. New York, Oxford University Press, 2002, pp 224-234.
25. Kamm FM: Morality, Mortality, vol 1. Death and Whom to Save from It. New York, Oxford University Press, 1993.
26. Petersen A, Lupton D: The New Public Health: Health and Self in the Age of Risk. London, SAGE Publications, 1996.
27. Potts LK (ed): Ideologies of Breast Cancer: Feminist Perspectives. Basingstoke, UK, Macmillan, 2000.
28. Petticrew MP, Sowden AJ, Lister-Sharp D, Wright D: False-negative results in screening programmes: Systematic review of impact and implications. Health Technol Assess 2000;4: 1-51.
29. Jepson R, Clegg A, Forbes C, et al: The determinants of screening uptake and interventions for increasing uptake: A systematic review. Health Technol Assess 2000;4:1-123.
30. O'Neill O: Autonomy and Trust in Bioethics. Cambridge, Cambridge University Press, 2002.
31. Lerner BH: The Breast Cancer Wars: Hope, Fear, and the Pursuit of a Cure in Twentieth-Century America. New York, Oxford University Press, 2001.
32. Thornton JG: Should Health Screening be Private? London, Institute of Economic Affairs, 1999.
33. Shickle D, Chadwick R: The ethics of screening. Is "screeningitis" an incurable disease? J Med Ethics 1994;20:12-18.
34. Dormany E, Hooper R, Michie S, Marteau T: Informed choice to undergo prenatal screening: A comparison of two hospitals conducting testing either as part of a routine visit or requiring a separate visit. J Med Screen 2002;9:109-114.
35. Olsen O, Gøtzsche PC: Cochrane review on screening for breast cancer with mammography. Lancet 2001;358:1340-1342.
36. Ubel PA: Pricing Life: Why It's Time for Health Care Rationing. Cambridge, MA, MIT Press, 2000.
37. Emanuel EJ: Patient v. population: Resolving the ethical dilemmas posed by treating patients as members of populations. In Danis M, Clancy C, Churchill LR (eds): Ethical Dimensions of Health Policy. New York, Oxford University Press, 2002, pp 227-245.
38. Emanuel EJ: The Ends of Human Life: Medical Ethics in a Liberal Polity. Cambridge, MA, Harvard University Press, 1996.
39. Mill JS: On liberty. In Mill JS Three Essays. Oxford, Oxford University Press, 1972.
40. Rose P, Lucassen A: Practical Genetics for Primary Care. Oxford, Oxford University Press, 1999.
41. Henderson L, Kitzinger J: The human drama of genetics: "hard" and "soft" media representations of inherited breast cancer. In Conrad P, Gabe J (eds): Sociological Perspectives on the New Genetics. Oxford, Blackwell, 1999, pp 59-76.
42. Hallowell N: Doing the right thing: Genetic risk and responsibility. In Conrad P, Gabe J (eds): Sociological Perspectives on the New Genetics. Oxford, Blackwell, 1999, pp 97-120.
43. Clarke A: Is non-directive genetic counselling possible? Lancet 1991;338:998-1001.
44. Parker M: Public deliberation and private choice in genetics and reproduction. J Med Ethics 2000;26:160-165.
45. Hedgecoe A: Schizophrenia and the narrative of enlightened geneticization. Soc Studies Sci 2001;31:875-911.
46. Human Genetics Commission: Inside Information: Balancing Interest in the Use of Personal Genetic Data. London, Human Genetics Commission, 2002.
47. Buchanan A, Brock DW, Daniels N, Wikler D: From Chance to Choice: Genetics and Justice. Cambridge, Cambridge University Press, 2000.
48. Skrabanek P: The Death of Humane Medicine and the Rise of Coercive Healthism. London, Social Affairs Unit, 1994.
49. Buchanan DR: An Ethic for Health Promotion: Rethinking the Sources of Human Well-Being. New York, Oxford University Press, 2000.
50. Cribb A, Duncan P: Health Promotion and Professional Ethics. Oxford, Blackwell Scientific, 2002.
51. Kasper AS, Ferguson SJ (eds): Breast Cancer: Society Shapes an Epidemic. Basingstoke, UK, Palgrave Macmillan, 2000.
52. Potts LK (ed): Ideologies of Breast Cancer: Feminist Perspectives. Basingstoke, Macmillan, 2000.
53. Fulford KWM, Dickenson DL, Murray TH (eds): Healthcare Ethics and Human Values: An Introductory Text with Readings and Case Studies. Oxford, Blackwell, 2002.
54. Zaner RM: Ethics and the Clinical Encounter. Englewood Cliffs, NJ, Prentice Hall, 1988.
55. Nelson HL (ed): Stories and Their Limits: Narrative Approaches to Bioethics. London, Routledge, 1997.
56. Tronto JC: Moral Boundaries: A Political Argument for an Ethic of Care. London, Routledge, 1993.
57. Kaufert PA: Screening the body: The pap smear and the mammogram. In Lock M, Young A, Cambrosio A (eds): Living and Working with the New Medical Technologies. Cambridge, Cambridge University Press, 2000, pp 165-183.
58. Oudshoorn N: Beyond the Natural Body: An Archaeology of Sex Hormones. London, Routledge, 1994.
59. Marks L: Sexual Chemistry: A History of the Contraceptive Pill. New Haven, CT, Yale University Press, 2001
60. Pfeffer N, Woollett A: The Experience of Infertility. London, Virago, 1983.
61. Pfeffer N: The Stork and the Syringe: A Political History of Reproductive Medicine. Cambridge, Polity, 1993.
62. Harris J, Holm S (eds): The Future of Human Reproduction: Ethics, Choice, and Regulation. Oxford, Oxford University Press, 1998.
63. Dickenson DL (ed): Ethical Issues in Maternal-Fetal Medicine. Cambridge, Cambridge University Press, 2002.
64. Blank RH: Regulating Reproduction. New York, Columbia University Press, 1992.

65. Lee RG, Morgan D: Human Fertilisation and Embryology: Regulating the Reproductive Revolution. London, Blackstone Press, 2001.

66. World Medical Association: Declaration of Helsinki. Geneva, World Medical Association, 2000.

67. Schüklenk U: Access to Experimental Drugs in Terminal Illness: Ethical Issues. New York, Pharmaceutical Products Press, 1998.

68. Epstein S: Impure Science: AIDS, Activism and the Politics of Knowledge. Berkeley, University of California Press, 1996.

69. Kübler-Ross E: On Death and Dying. London, Routledge, 1970.

70. Callahan D: False Hopes: Overcoming Obstacles to a Sustainable, Affordable Medicine. New Brunswick, NJ, Rutgers University Press, 1998.

71. Zucker MB, Zucker HD (eds): Medical Futility and the Evaluation of Life-Sustaining Interventions. Cambridge, Cambridge University Press, 1997.

72. Edwards SJL, Lilford RJ, Braunholtz DA, et al: Ethical issues in the design and conduct of randomised controlled trials. Health Technol Assess 1998;2:1-128.

73. Ashcroft RE, Chadwick DW, Clark SRL, et al: Implications of socio-cultural contexts for ethics of clinical trials. Health Technol Assess 1997;1:1-65.

74. Dresser R: When Science Offers Salvation: Patient Advocacy and Research Ethics. New York, Oxford University Press, 2001.

75. Evans JH: Playing God? Human Genetic Engineering and the Rationalization of Public Bioethical Debate. Chicago, University of Chicago Press, 2002.

76. Hanson MJ, Callahan D: The Goals of Medicine: The Forgotten Issues in Health Care Reform. Washington, DC, Georgetown University Press, 1999.

77. Danis M, Clancy C, Churchill LR (eds): Ethical Dimensions of Health Policy. New York, Oxford University Press, 2002.

78. Rhodes R, Battin MP, Silvers A (eds): Medicine and Social Justice: Essays on the Distribution of Health Care. New York, Oxford University Press, 2002.

79. Daniels N, Sabin JE: Setting Limits Fairly: Can We Learn to Share Medical Resources? New York, Oxford University Press, 2002.

80. Coulter A, Ham C (eds): The Global Challenge of Healthcare Rationing. Berkshire, UK, Open University Press, 2000.

81. Nozick R: Anarchy, State and Utopia. New York, Basic Books, 1974.

82. Doyal L, Gough I: A Theory of Human Need. Basingstoke, UK, Macmillan, 1991.

83. Fallowfield L: The Quality of Life. London, Souvenir Press, 1994.

84. Ashcroft RE: What is clinical effectiveness? Studies in History and Philosophy of Biological and Biomedical Sciences. 2002;33C:219-233.

85. Randall F, Downie RS: Palliative Care Ethics: A Companion for All Specialties, 2nd ed. Oxford, Oxford University Press, 1999.

86. Katz J: The Silent World of Doctor and Patient, 2nd ed. Baltimore, Johns Hopkins University Press, 2002.

87. Christakis NA: Death Foretold: Prophecy and Prognosis in Medical Care. Chicago, University of Chicago Press, 2000.

88. Keown J (ed): Euthanasia Examined: Ethical, Clinical and Legal Perspectives. Cambridge, Cambridge University Press, 1995.

89. Singer P: Rethinking Life and Death: The Collapse of Our Traditional Ethics. Oxford, Oxford University Press, 1995.

90. British Medical Association: Withdrawing and Withholding Life-Prolonging Medical Treatment, 2nd ed. London, British Medical Association, 2000.

91. Keown J: Euthanasia, Ethics and Public Policy: An Argument against Legislation. Cambridge, Cambridge University Press, 2002.

92. Somerville M: Death Talk: The Case Against Euthanasia and Physician-Assisted Suicide. Montreal, McGill-Queen's University Press, 2002.

93. Ebrahim S: Do not resuscitate decisions: Flogging dead horses or a dignified death? BMJ 2000;320:1155-1156.

94. Cherniack EP: Increasing use of DNR orders in the elderly worldwide: Whose choice is it? J Med Ethics 2002;28:303-307.

95. Timmermans S: Sudden Death and the Myth of CPR. Philadelphia, Temple University Press, 1999.

CHAPTER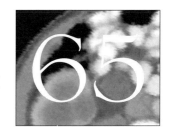

BIOSTATISTICS AND CLINICAL TRIALS

Mark F. Brady   and   Michael W. Sill

 MAJOR CONTROVERSIES

- **Can the conventional approach to phase I drug development be improved?**
- **Why are phase II studies in oncology being misused and abused?**
- **What are the challenges facing chemoprevention studies?**

Can the conventional approach to phase I drug development be improved?

There has been considerable attention given to the statistical design, ethical considerations, and the implementation of phase I studies over the past 10 years. Controversies have arisen from recent research into the methods commonly used to investigate new agents in human populations for the first time. For example, there is evidence that patients often do not entirely understand the purpose of the phase I study in which they are enrolled. Newer study designs that tend to expose fewer patients to subtherapeutic doses than the traditional designs are available, but they have not been widely adopted in oncology practice.

The activity of most cytotoxic agents is assumed to be a nondecreasing function of the dose; that is, the chance of obtaining a clinical benefit or having an adverse side effect does not decrease as the dose increases. If the dose is low, the treatment may not be toxic, but it may also be ineffective. The lowest dose at which an agent is expected to provide a clinically important benefit to the patients is called the minimum effective dose (MED). Drugs are often administered doses higher than the MED to ensure that most patients benefit from the treatment. Unfortunately, when the administered dose is too high, toxicities can occur that are severe and sometimes irreversible. The maximum tolerated dose (MTD) is the highest dose that can be

given without an unacceptable risk of toxicity. A clinically useful treatment is one in which the MTD is greater than the MED (MTD > MED), and the range of doses within these two limits defines the therapeutic window for a particular agent.[1] Regrettably, the definition of the MTD is not consistent throughout the phase I trial literature. This definition is used here, and a more precise definition follows.

The role of a phase I study is to identify a dose within the therapeutic window that can be used in future phase II and phase III clinical trials. The strategy frequently used in oncology has been to evaluate several discrete dose levels considered to be near the MTD in a phase I trial. The highest tolerable dose among those studied is then recommended for further evaluation in a phase II study to determine if the agent is clinically beneficial at this dose. The recommended dose is not necessarily equal to the MTD. If there is insufficient clinical benefit observed at the phase I recommended dose, the MED is assumed to exceed the recommended dose for too many patients. New investigational agents such as chemopreventive agents, vaccines, and cytostatic agents are challenging this tradition approach.

Ethical concerns. The justification for research involving human subjects has been ethically contentious and controversial. Arguably, the most ethically problematic phase of drug development is the phase I study.

The contention arises primarily from three concerns. First, there is concern about an imbalance between the risk and benefit for the patient. Second, there is some concern about the quality of the subject's informed consent.[2] Third, some studies tend to allocate too many patients to inferior dose levels.

The Belmont Report[3] describes the ethical principles underlying clinical research. The cornerstones of these principles are respect for persons, beneficence, and justice. The report explains that beneficence requires maximizing the possible benefits to the patient and minimizing the potential for harm. Clinical research involving human beings should involve only personal risks that are justifiable by the potential personal benefits. However, it is in the phase I trial where risks and benefits are often most imbalanced. A study that has as its goal to identify a drug's MTD must induce toxicities that are otherwise undesirable in any other clinical setting. However, phase I trials seldom involve agents with significant evidence of clinical activity. Although there are societal benefits from phase I research, these benefits cannot provide the rationale for exposing an individual to excessive risk of personal harm.

After evaluating the risk and benefits of treatment, an individual may consent to treatment. Consent is valid when it is informed, competent, and understood. Daugherty and colleagues[4] summarized the results from interviewing 30 subjects who had consented to participate in phase I oncology studies at University of Chicago. Most of these patients indicated that they sought information from their oncologist before making the decision to participate. Moreover, most felt that they understood the information provided to them and found the decision to participate in the trial easy. However, when asked to explain the purpose of the trial, most could not. When asked to state the reasons that contributed to their decision to participate in the trial, all indicated it was for the possibility of medical benefit, 89% felt that they had no better options, and 70% were motivated by trust in their oncologist. Few individuals (22%) were motivated by an altruistic aspiration to increase scientific understanding. When the oncologists who treated these patients were surveyed, they indicated that the most probable benefit to the patient was psychological. In some cases, physicians may overestimate the therapeutic benefit of the new therapies and pass on overly optimistic information to the subjects overtly or inadvertently.[5] This is particularly troubling because Henry Beecher[6] suggested that it was overly enthusiastic investigators who contributed to lapses in ethics in clinical investigations at many U.S. universities reported more than 30 years ago.

Fortunately, over the past 10 years, there has been considerable research into the design of phase I studies intended to increase the potential for benefit while minimizing the risk of harm. To appreciate these newer approaches, it is necessary to review the traditional approach.

Traditional 3 + 3 design. Although there is no universally standard phase I study design, a commonly used design is the one-stage 3 + 3 design. In this case, increasing but discrete dose levels are defined before activating the study. The first dose level is often selected as 10% of the dose that is lethal to 10% of mice (LD_{10}). This dose is not expected to induce significant toxicity in humans. The dose increments are often based on a modified Fibonacci sequence such as 100%, 67%, 50%, 40%, 33%, and so on. There is little justification for this escalation sequence other than it has been used extensively and generally considered practical. Frequently, three patients are treated at the first dose level. If there are no dose-limiting toxicities (DLTs) observed in these three subjects, the dose is escalated to the next higher level, and an additional three patients are treated at this dose. This process continues until all dose levels have been evaluated or a DLT is observed. If one DLT is observed in the three individuals treated at a particular dose level, three additional patients are treated at the same dose level. If there are no more DLTs observed, the current dose is considered safe, and the dose level is escalated again, and the next three patients are evaluated at this dose level. Otherwise, if more than 1 DLT are observed, the current dose level is deemed too toxic, the study is stopped, and the previous dose level is considered the recommended dose.

Traditional 3 + 3 design with de-escalation. There have been several suggested modifications to the traditional 3 + 3 design. First, if an excessive number of DLTs have been observed at a particular dose level, the dose may be stepped down to the previous dose level to ensure that at least 6 patients are treated at the recommended dose and that not more than 1 DLT is observed at this dose. This approach is called a one-stage traditional 3 + 3 design with de-escalation.

Starting dose. If the starting dose is less than the MED, the first patients entered into the study will receive subtherapeutic dose levels. To avoid enrolling an excessive number of patients in these studies, it is important that the starting dose be as close to the MTD dose as possible. When there are no preclinical data and the agent has never been evaluated in humans, the phase I starting dose, expressed as milligrams per meter squared of body surface area, is often based on the dose that is lethal in 10% of the treated mice (murine LD_{10}). Eisenhauer and coworkers[7] reviewed 14 phase I single-agent oncology trials in which the starting dose was based on the murine LD_{10}. A modified Fibonacci scheme was used in each of these studies to define the dose escalation steps. From these studies, they found that when the starting dose was based on 10% of the LD_{10}, the recommended dose was determined after a median of 7 (range, 4 to 14) dose escalations. They speculated that if these studies had used starting doses that were 20% of the murine LD_{10}, the median number of dose escalations required to determine the recommended dose would have been only 5 (range, 3 to 11). Their conclusion is that it is reasonable to consider starting at the 20% of the murine LD_{10} to reduce the number of patients treated at subtherapeutic levels, particularly when preclinical data are available and indicate no interspecies variation in toxicology.[7]

Dose escalation. Two other design modifications that tend to reduce the number of patients treated at subtherapeutic doses are to implement larger escalation steps between consecutive dose levels and to reduce the number of patients treated at each dose level. However, by themselves, these modifications are not recommended for therapies that exhibit life-threatening toxicities. Additional safeguards must be incorporated into the study to prevent escalating too far above the MTD. Designs have been proposed that reduce the number of patients initially treated at each dose level and implement larger increments between doses. Two approaches that implement these modifications with appropriate safeguards are two-stage designs and accelerated titration designs. Both of these designs have been proposed to reduce the number of patients treated at subtherapeutic doses and to accelerate new drug development.

Multistage designs. One modification to the traditional design is to divide the accrual into two stages. During the first stage, typically one or two patients are treated at a particular dose level before escalating to the next dose level. However, after significant but not necessarily dose-limiting toxicities are encountered, the design begins a second stage in which more patients are treated at each dose level. Investigators at the National Cancer Institute (NCI) Cancer Therapeutic Evaluation Program (CTEP) have suggested treating one patient at each dose level during the first stage of accrual.[8] If one first-course DLT or two grade 2 (or worse) toxicities in separate patients are observed, the second stage of the study begins, in which three patients are treated and evaluated at each dose level. That is, two more patients are treated at the current dose level, and the study proceeds like the traditional 3+3 design (Table 65-1, designs 2 though 4). Six individuals are treated at the dose ultimately recommended for future studies.

There are some disadvantages due to designs that treat a single patient at each dose level and base the decision to escalate the dose only on the absence of DLTs. First, these designs are more likely to escalate beyond the MTD, especially when there is significant interpatient variability with regard to tolerance. Second, very limited dose-related pharmacokinetic data are available from designs that involve only one patient observed at each dose level. These concerns must be weighed against designs that require larger cohorts before advancing to the next dose level. Designs that begin with larger cohorts of patients tend to be more cautious but frequently undertreat too many individuals, prolong drug development, and may squander clinic resources. Two-stage study designs attempt to take advantage of the best features from each of these designs. If the initial dose is far from the MTD, the number of patients treated at potentially inferior doses is reduced. Information from non–dose-limiting toxicities are used to switch from the initial, quick dose-escalation phase to the second more cautious dose-escalation phase of the study. The larger cohort sizes used in the second stage reduce the risk of overshooting the MTD. Because more patients are treated at each dose level during the second stage, important pharmacokinetic studies at doses near the MTD may be more feasible.

Titration designs. One additional modification to the traditional design permits dose escalations within each patient. Individuals enter the study, and their first cycle of therapy is administered at the current dose level of the study. If this dose is tolerated, the patient may advance to the next higher dose level. The dose is permitted to escalate at subsequent cycles of therapy, provided the individual experiences no more than grade 1 toxicities[8] (see Table 65-1, design 4). The advantage of these designs is that, if analyzed properly, the estimated incidence of toxicity can account for intrapatient and interpatient variability. The analyses of most phase I studies are based on an assumption that it is primarily the dose that determines the probability of a DLT. There may be important differences between individuals beyond body surface area that are related to metabolism, absorption, distribution, and elimination that may determine an individual's MTD. For example, decreased renal function increases the predictability of a DLT on carboplatin or topotecan, and

Table 65-1. Characteristics of National Cancer Institute/Cancer Therapy Evaluation Program Recommended Accelerated Titration Phase I Study Designs

Design	First-Stage Cohort Size	First-Stage Dose Increment	Intrapatient Dose Escalation	Trigger for Second-Stage to Begin	Second-Stage Cohort Size	Second-Stage Dose Increment
1	3	40%	No	1 DLT*	3-6	40%
2	1	40%	Yes	2 Gr2/1 DLT†	3-6	40%
3	1	100%	Yes	2 Gr2/1 DLT†	3-6	40%
4	1	100%	Yes	2 Gr2/1 DLT‡	3-6	40%

*First dose-limiting toxicity (DLT) during the first course of treatment.
†Second grade 2 (Gr2) or worse toxicity or first DLT during the first course of treatment.
‡Second grade 2 or worse toxicity or first DLT during any course of treatment.
From Simon R, Freidlin B, Rubinstein L, et al: Accelerated titration designs for phase I clinical trials in oncology. J Natl Cancer Inst 1997;89:1138-1147.

older age increases the risk of a DLT on 5-fluorouracil. If the interpatient variability of MTD is small, a single dose can be recommended for future investigations using the study agent. If the interpatient variability is large, using pharmacokinetic measures to predict toxicity and using personalized doses to achieve a targeted concentration are preferred methods. Tracking intrapatient dose escalations and toxicities over consecutive courses of therapy complicates the execution of the study and requires very diligent and careful patient management.[8]

Continual reassessment method. One of the major drawbacks of the traditional phase I study design is that only patients treated at a particular dose level are used to determine whether that dose is safe. If the dose-toxicity relationship is expected to be a nondecreasing function, a model that incorporates this structure with all the available data is preferable. An analysis that uses information from the entire study with an appropriate model can provide a more precise estimate of the MTD. A second drawback of the traditional phase I study is that the study design does not reflect any particular definition of MTD because there is no underlying statistical model, and it is not clear how the study design should be altered when an investigator specifies that the maximum acceptable probability of toxicity is 10% rather than 30%.

One approach that uses data from the entire study to estimate the MTD is the continual reassessment method (CRM). This method begins by selecting a suitable family of models to express the potential relationship between dose and the probability of toxicity.

Although there are several alternatives, a single-parameter logistic family of models is presented here.[9] For this family of models, the probability of a DLT at the ith dose (d_i) can be expressed as follows:

$$\Psi\left(d_i \mid \beta\right) = \frac{\exp\left(3 + |\beta \bullet d_i\right)}{1 + \exp\left(3 + |\beta \bullet d_i\right)} \qquad (1)$$

The dose-toxicity relationships for several values of β are plotted in Figure 65-1. The vertical lines in Figure 65-1 indicate the first 15 consecutive doses from a dose escalation scheme based on a modified Fibonacci series. The doses on the x axis are expressed as the log of the ith dose relative to the 15th dose level. If β is known, a curve such as those in Figure 65-1 can be used to identify the highest dose that is associated with an acceptable probability of toxicity. The assumption underlying the CRM design is that each drug administered by a particular route has a dose-toxicity relationship that is characterized by a particular value of β. The goal of the phase I study is to estimate β, and from this estimate, determine the dose that is associated with the targeted acceptable level of toxicity. Although a Bayesian framework has often been used to estimate the model parameters,[10] a likelihood framework has also been proposed.[11] The Bayesian approach begins with a prior distribution, $f(\beta)$, for the model parameter, which expresses the investigators initial opinion about β, including the degree uncertainty about its true value. This prior distribution is then used to provide an initial prediction of the MTD, and the first patient is treated at this dose level. As data are collected, the posterior density of

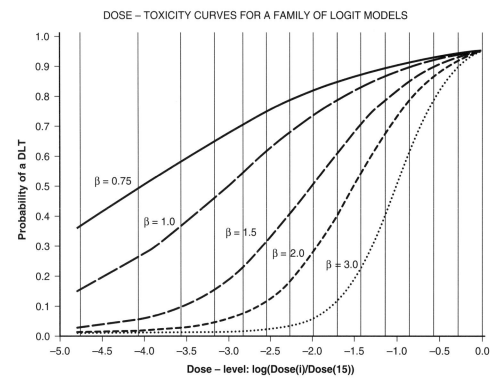

Figure 65–1. Dose-toxicity curves for a family of logit models.

DOSE – TOXICITY CURVES FOR A FAMILY OF LOGIT MODELS

Probability of a DLT (y-axis, 0.0 to 1.0)

Dose – level: log(Dose(i)/Dose(15)) (x-axis, −5.0 to 0.0)

β = 0.75
β = 1.0
β = 1.5
β = 2.0
β = 3.0

β, g(β|D_k) and therefore of the MTD is updated by the Bayes theorem:

$$g(\beta | D_k) = \frac{L(D_k | \beta) f(\beta)}{\int\limits_0^\infty L(D_k | \beta) f(\beta) d\beta} \qquad (2)$$

In Equation 2, the prior distribution for β is $f(\beta)$, and $L(D_k|\beta)$ is the likelihood of the observed data (D_k) from the first k treated patients given β. The vector D_k is composed of data pairs (d_i, t_i) for each of the k patients indicating the dose (d_i) and an indicator for whether the patient experienced a DLT ($t_i = 1$, yes; $t_i = 0$, no). The likelihood is expressed as follows:

$$L(D_k | \beta) = \prod_{i=1}^{k} \left[\Psi(d_i | \beta) \right]^{t_i} \left[1 - \Psi(d_i | \beta) \right]^{1 - t_i} \qquad (3)$$

The prior distribution, $f(\beta)$, expresses the investigator's opinion about the dose-toxicity relationship before the study. Bayes theorem is used to incorporate how this prior opinion should be updated due to the accumulating data from the trial. In practice, each patient is treated and evaluated at the currently predicted MTD, which could be derived from the mode or expectation of the posterior distribution of β, depending on investigator preference. If the current individual experiences a DLT, the updated prediction of β tends toward smaller values, the predicted value of the MTD is smaller, and the next patient receives a lower dose. If the current patient does not experience a DLT, the updated prediction of β tends toward larger values, the expected value of the MTD is assumed to be a higher dose, and the dose for the next patient is escalated. This process is continued until a prespecified number of patients has been treated. With sample sizes of 20 to 25 patients, this procedure has been shown to provide reasonably precise estimates of the MTD.[9,10]

The CRM has several advantages. It provides a statistical basis for identifying a targeted dose based on a specified acceptable probability of toxicity, and as the trial continues, it converges to the targeted dose. It provides a more precise estimate of the targeted dose level than the traditional approach. It allocates fewer patients to very low doses. There is no need to prespecify a dose escalation scheme, because the method automatically escalates and de-escalates the dose. However, the original CRM proposal has been criticized for increasing the overall study duration, escalating the dose too rapidly, tending to treat too many patients at high dose levels, being logistically complicated, and lacking clinical intuitiveness for most clinical investigators.[12,13]

To circumvent these problems, several researchers have recommended modifications,[12] improvements,[13] extensions, and restrictions.[14] The salient recommendations for improving the original CRM design are to use preclinical data as in the traditional design to determine the initial dose level (i.e., 10% to 20% of LD_{10}); prespecify the dose levels as in the traditional design

and limit dose escalation to one dose level at a time; permit investigator discretion in determining the size of any dose reduction; and limit the initial cohort size to one patient per dose level until more than mild toxicities begin to occur, after which cohort sizes should be increased to two or three individuals depending on the degree of toxicity. At least six patients should be evaluated at the final MTD.

As an example of the modified CRM design, consider a phase I study in which the initial dose level is based on 20% of the murine LD_{10}. The subsequent doses are determined from a modified Fibonacci sequence. The probability of a DLT is assumed to follow the logistic family of dose-toxicity indicated by the expression for ψ(d_i|β) provided earlier. A uniform distribution over the values 0 to 5 is used for the prior distribution of β to indicate that there is very little known about the true relationship between dose and toxicity. Suppose the first four patients are treated at each of the first four doses, and no toxicities are observed. However, the fifth patient treated at the fifth dose level experiences a DLT. The solid line in Figure 65-2 displays the posterior density for β (Equation 2) at this time. The most credible value for β given the data is approximately 1.5, which corresponds to the peak of the solid curve in Figure 65-2. Because the last patient treated experienced a DLT, the modified CRM design would indicate that the next two patients should be treated at the same dose level. If the next patient does not experience a DLT, the posterior distribution for β is updated and is displayed as a short dashed line in Figure 65-2. The most credible value (peak of the short dashed line) for β given the data would be 1.6. This drops the expected dose-toxicity curve in Figure 65-1

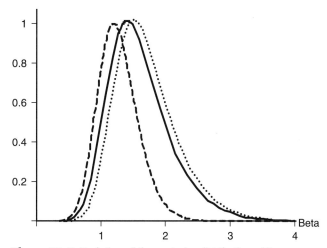

Figure 65–2. Evolution of the posterior distribution of β. Four patients were treated at the first four dose levels and the fifth experienced a dose-limiting toxicity (DLT) *(solid line)*. The update posterior distribution of β if the sixth patient is treated at the same dose level as the fifth patient but does not experience a DLT *(short dashed line)*. The posterior distribution of β if the sixth patient is treated at the same dose level as the fifth patient and does experience a DLT *(long dashed line)*.

slightly toward the lower right corner, indicating that there is less risk of a DLT at the lower doses. On the other hand, if the sixth patient experiences a DLT, the updated prior distribution would resemble the long dashed line in Figure 65-2. The most credible value for β in this case would be 1.2, indicating that there are greater risks of a DLT at the lower doses.

Summary of phase I designs. There are two opposing objectives involved in the design of efficient phase I studies: limiting the number of patients exposed to subtherapeutic doses and ensuring the safety of the study participants. Overly cautious study designs tend to treat too many patients with inferior doses of the study agent, whereas overly aggressive designs treat too many patients at dangerous dose levels. Prudent designs use an initial dose that is generally regarded safe based on one or more preclinical studies. Multistage designs are used to escalate rapidly in the absence of toxicities. During the initial stage, only one patient may be treated at each dose level. During this stage, accelerated dose escalation schemes can be considered that increase the dose 100% at each step. After moderate but not necessarily dose-limiting toxicities are observed, a second stage begins in which two or three patients are evaluated at each dose level. Dose escalation can be scaled back to 40% to 50% increases between consecutive dose levels, and there is no need to limit the size of de-escalation. At least six individuals should be evaluated at the dose finally recommended for further evaluation in subsequent studies. The use of statistical models that use all of the data from the trial to improve the reliability of the estimated MTD is preferable.

It is surprising that although experienced phase I trial investigators seldom recommend traditional phase I study designs, variations of the traditional design are still widely used.[7] The exposure to some agents is often very poorly characterized by data obtained only at the administered dose. This is often caused by variability in absorption, distribution, or elimination rates between individuals. In these cases, alternative measures such as the area under the curve (AUC) for plasma concentration versus time are generally more appropriate measures drug exposure. When a study seeks to assess interpatient variability and evaluate pharmacokinetic data from individuals treated over a broad range of dose levels, it is often desirable to involve several subjects treated at each dose level. In these cases, treating only one individual at each dose level can hinder the goal of obtaining reliable pharmacokinetic estimates for each level of exposure.

Some of the novel agents, such as cytostatic or chemopreventive agents, being considered for phase I study in cancer induce very few serious adverse effects. In these cases, it may not be appropriate to target the MTD. Instead, targeting a dose that inhibits or promotes a specific biologic response may be a more appropriate end point. Designs that use accelerated titration, intrapatient dose escalations, multiple stages, or CRM can still be applied. Rather than selecting doses based on the degree of toxicity, doses are selected based on the degree of biologic response.

Why are phase II studies in oncology being misused and abused?

Phase II studies are important components in the program of drug development. The therapeutic objective of these studies is to benefit the patients enrolled in the study. Toward this end, it is important to limit the number of individuals treated with inactive or excessively toxic agents. The first experimental objective of a phase II trial is to identify treatments worthy of more rigorous assessment in subsequent studies. At the end of a phase I trial, there are typically only a limited number of patients treated at the recommended dose. The second experimental objective of a phase II study is designed to further characterize of the types and the degrees of adverse effects. These studies also provide for a more precise assessment of the treatment activity.

As is the case with phase I studies, there have been several proposals for alternative phase II study designs over the past several years. Unlike phase I trials, however, these newer phase II designs are often used. Although the designs are not controversial, the conclusions from studies in which analysis is not consistent with the original study design are controversial. Controversies in phase II studies arise when there is a mismatch between the study's objectives, design, or final analysis. When this occurs, the conclusions are not commensurate with the original study design. Examples include the use of naïve confidence intervals after multistage designs, hypothesis testing after ranking and selection designs, and interpreting randomized phase II studies as if they were randomized phase III studies.

An overview of phase II clinical trials published in major oncology journals indicates that the quality of the statistical component in these trials is surprisingly poor.[15] Among the 308 publications included in the review that reported results from phase II or pilot trials, only 58 (20%) provided an identifiable statistical design. Among trials with an identifiable statistical design, the quality of reporting was judged good for only 29%. Compliance with the original study design could not be evaluated for 13 of the studies with an identifiable design because of incomplete reporting. When compliance with the original design could be evaluated, it was considered good for 51% (23 of 45) of trials with an identifiable design. Worse, the authors of this survey were unable to identify a trend toward improvement in the quality of reporting among the most recently activated studies. Instead, positive trial results occurred most frequently for studies that lacked an identifiable study design. The researchers concluded that larger biases in study findings might be associated with the lower quality of design or reporting in these phase II or pilot screening studies.

End points. Traditional oncology trials evaluating cytotoxic agents have used reduction in tumor size or, in the case of leukemia, eliminating signs of the disease as the primary indicator of treatment activity. There is no need, however, to be so restrictive in this phase of drug development. For example, response may be some molecular measure of potentiating or inhibiting a particular biologic target. Such surrogate end points are frequently used to identify new agents worthy of further evaluation. The justification for using a surrogate end point in phase II drug development is that these end points typically provide quicker determination of response, are less expensive, and are unaffected by salvage therapies. The usual caveats apply to incorporating surrogate end points into drug screening trials. First, it is necessary to assume that the surrogate end point is in the causal pathway to a truly meaningful clinical end point. If the surrogate end point is not in the causal pathway to a truly meaningful end point, it tends to increase the probability of a false-positive trial result. Second, the etiologic pathways to the clinically relevant end point should frequently involve the surrogate end point; otherwise, the use of that surrogate end point increases the probability of a false-negative trial result.

Phase 1.5 trials. Occasionally, studies that evaluate the activity of single agents are performed in a patient population that is not the target population. This is commonly done in drug development programs evaluating cytotoxic treatments, especially when the standard front-line treatment includes treatments that are generally considered active. Even though the intention in this case is to incorporate newly discovered active agents into the front-line treatment, screening trials may include patients who have already failed standard treatments. The use of this population can be justified for several reasons. First, including potentially inactive experimental agents into the front-line treatment may compromise the activity of the current standard front-line therapy. Second, many patients who have failed standard therapy prefer to try an experimental treatment when one is available. Third, including patients who have failed standard therapy is a reasonable strategy when searching for new agents that are not cross-resistant with the current standard therapy. Although these studies are often designed as if they are phase II studies, some investigators prefer to label them phase 1.5 studies because they can be viewed as bridging the gap between phase I and II study goals.[16] However, the external validity of a study is undermined when it does not involve patients from the target population. For example, if the patients involved in a phase 1.5 trial are debilitated by their disease or prior therapy, it may not be possible to administer adequate doses to detect activity. In this case, an active agent may be dismissed as inactive, which could prevent or delay its development.

Phase IIA designs. The simplest phase II study design is a single-arm design with a fixed sample size. A prespecified number of patients are treated at the same dose and route of administration of the experimental agent. The goal of this design is to reliably identify treatments with activity greater than some minimal threshold and to estimate the probability of response. Even with goals as simple as this, it is useful to distinguish

between phase IIA and IIB studies. When even the best available treatments demonstrate minimal activity, the goal of a phase II study may be to identify agents that have any antitumor activity. For example, a clinical investigator may indicate no interest in agents that would provide responses in no more than 15 of 100 (call this probability P_1) patients treated. Treatments that provide responses in at least 30 of 100 patients (call this probability P_2) may be considered worthy of additional evaluation. If true probability of response to a new agent is P, the design is statistically formulated as two competing hypotheses, H1: $P < P_1$ and H2: $P > P_2$.[17] The number of patients enrolled into the study must provide sufficient precision so that the chance of incorrectly classifying an inactive treatment as active (rejecting H1 when H1 is true) is not greater than α * 100%. The probability of correctly classifying an active treatment (rejecting H1 when H2 is true) must not be less than $(1 - \beta)$* 100%. The α and β values are prespecified study design parameters, type I and type II errors, respectively. Typical (α, β) values used in phase II studies are (0.10, 0.10), (0.05, 0.10), and (0.05, 0.20). In this case, rejecting H1 does not indicate that H2 is true or vice versa. Rejecting H1 implies that the study data support the conclusion that $P > P_1$. More specifically, the probability that the data indicate that H2 is true when in fact H1 is true is not more than α. Likewise, rejecting H2 implies that the study data support the conclusion that $P < P_2$.

The distinguishing feature of a phase IIA design is that the upper limit for the range of inactive response rates (P_1) and the lower limit of the active response rates (P_2) are treated as if they are fixed study parameters. This is in contradistinction to a phase IIB study, in which the intention is to compare the results from the experimental agent with a historical control group, a concurrently randomized control group, or an investigator's vague prior expectation of the probability of responding to standard treatment (e.g., to be used as a prior distribution in a Bayesian analysis). In any case, the phase IIB trial recognizes that P_1 is not known with certainty. Phase IIB studies are described further in the next section.

Single-stage designs. Studies with a fixed sample size are easy to understand and implement. For illustrative purposes, assume that an investigator wishes to screen new agents for a particular disease. Before the study, the investigator may decide that agents with true response probabilities no more than 15% (P_1) should be considered inactive. On the other hand, those with true response probabilities of at least 30% (P_2) are active and warrant further evaluation. Although the true probability of response for a particular treatment is unknown, the goal of a phase II study is to limit the errors caused by misclassifying active and inactive treatments. Table 65-2 summarizes alternative phase IIA study designs for the case when inactive treatments are characterized by true probabilities less than 15%, and active treatments have true response probabilities of at least 30%. To limit the type I and type II errors to no more than 10%, the minimum required sample size

Table 65–2. Comparison of Single-Stage and Some Alternative Two-Stage Phase IIA Designs for Testing H1: $P \leq .15$ versus H2: $P \geq .30$ That Limit α and β to Less Than 0.10

| | Decision Rules for Each Stage Reject Drug if r_i/n_i* | | Study Characteristic When $P = .15$ | |
| | Stage I | Stage II | Expected Sample Size | Probability of Stopping Early |
Design				
Single stage	—	<12/53	53.0	0
Ad hoc	<4/27	<12/53	42.4	0.41
Optimal	<4/23	<12/55	37.7	0.54
Minimax	<6/34	<12/53	41.6	0.60
Flexible	<4/(22-24), 5/(25-29)	<11/53, 12/(54-57), 13/(58-60)	38.3	0.59

*The r_i/n_i term is the cumulative proportion responding out of the number accrued at the end of ith stage of accrual.

is 53 patients for a single-stage design. If fewer than 12 of the 53 patients respond, the agent is classified as being inactive and rejected. Using this decision rule, the investigator accepts that, on average, 10% of the agents that truly provide a 30% chance of responding will be incorrectly classified as inactive and that 10% of those that truly provide a 15% chance of responding will be classified incorrectly as active. If these error rates were unacceptably high, the planned sample size would have to be increased to further limit the chance of misclassification. The acceptability of these errors should be commensurate with the consequences of misclassifying agents. The consequence of misclassifying an active agent is to potentially eliminate it from further evaluation. The consequence of misclassifying an inactive agent is to waste additional time and resources evaluating a clinically useless drug.

Multistage designs. Although single-stage designs are easily understood and implemented, there are practical considerations that limit their usefulness in oncology. Consider the previously described single-stage phase II study. Suppose after completing half of the study ($n_1 = 27$ patients enrolled) that there are only 3 patients who have responded. The estimated probability of response (11.1%) is less than the upper limit of the range considered clinically inactive (15%). Moreover, the upper bound of the 95% confidence interval (29.2%) excludes the lower bound of what is considered the active agents (30%). There are two obvious questions. First, is it reasonable to continue treating patients with what appears to be an inactive and possibly toxic drug? Second, is there sufficient evidence already on hand to reliably classify the drug as inactive? Remarkably, it is justifiable to terminate this study without compromising the original design. Modifying the original single-stage design to permit early termination while still maintaining control of the type I and II errors is desirable.

The general framework for multistage, single-arm phase II studies has been developed.[19] These multistage designs group the accrual into stages. On completing the accrual of n_1 patients during the first stage of accrual, the study results are reviewed. The decision to continue to the next stage is based on the accumulated data from previous stages. Additional patients are entered into the study during subsequent stages provided the drug demonstrates sufficient activity in all of the previous stages. The limits of what is considered sufficient evidence of activity to continue onto the second stage of the study are determined before initiating the study and justified during the study design.

Returning to the example in Table 65-2, the previously proposed modification to the single-stage design requires that there be more than 3 responders among the first 27 patients enrolled into the study before advancing to the second stage of accrual. For the purposes of comparing alternative phase IIA designs, this approach is called the *ad hoc design*. The decision rules and some of the statistical characteristics of this design are summarized in Table 65-2. In this case, if the second stage of accrual is completed, the decision rule for classifying the agent as active is not changed from the single-stage design. If the true probability of response is 0.15, there is a substantial chance (41%) that the study will be closed early. In other words, there is a 41% chance that the sample size will only be 27 patients and a 59% (100% – 41%) chance that it will be 53 patients. If this design were used over and over to screen several agents with a true response probability of 0.15, the *expected sample size* would be 42.4 (0.41 × 27 + 0.59 × 53) patients per trial. Compared with the single-stage design, this design reduces the expected number of patients enrolled by 20%. In general, including an interim analysis in the design of the study decreases the expected number of patients treated with inferior treatments.

Two-stage optimal designs. There is no particular reason to require an interim review after one half of the patients have been entered. This review of the data could occur earlier or later in the overall accrual period. Decreasing the number of patients entered during the first stage of accrual provides an opportunity to reduce the number of patients exposed to inactive agents. However, smaller sample sizes during the first stage mean that the decision to continue is based on less reliable estimates of the probability of response.

Computer programs are available that perform comprehensive searches of all possible two-stage designs to identify the design that minimizes the expected number of patients enrolled when the true probability of response is equal to the upper limit of the range of inactive treatments.[20] Table 65-2 summarizes the characteristics of this so-called optimal design for the experimental conditions used in the current example. The optimal design recommends that 23 patients be accrued in the first stage, and if there are fewer than four responses in this cohort, the agent should be classified inactive. Otherwise, accrual continues until there are 55 patients enrolled. If there are fewer than 12 responses observed at the completion of the second stage of accrual, the agent is classified as inactive. In this case, the expected samples size is 37.7 when the true probability of response is 15%. The optimal design nearly always requires more patients to be entered than the fixed sample size when both stages of accrual are completed. Despite this fact, it is important to realize that when the true probability of response is the value of the upper limit of the inactive range, the expected number of patients entered is the smallest over all possible two-stage designs that limit the type I and type II errors to the specified values.

Two-stage minimax designs. Occasionally, there are designs that provide expected sample sizes nearly as small as the optimal design but do not require a substantial increase in the maximum ($n_1 + n_2$) sample size. The study design that permits an interim assessment of activity but minimizes the maximum sample size while the type I and II errors are limited to specified values is called the *minimax design*.[20] Because there can be several designs that meet this restriction, the one with the smallest expected sample size is usually selected. Even though the expected (average) sample size from the minimax design is never smaller than the comparable optimal design, it may be preferable when the difference in expected sample sizes is small and the overall sample size is smaller. The statistical characteristics of the minimax design for the example study are summarized in Table 65-2. Using this design, a cohort of 34 patients would be accrued during the first stage of the study. If there are fewer than six responses among these patients, the agent is deemed insufficiently active, and the accrual is stopped. Otherwise, the study continues onto the second stage, and accrual is extended to a total of 53 patients. In this case, the decision rule at the end of the second stage is the same as the single-stage design. The expected sample size for this design is 41.6. Whereas the uncurtailed sample size of the minimax design is the same as the fixed and the ad hoc design, the minimax design has a smaller expected sample size. The minimax design delays the interim analysis until there are 34 patients entered; this is much larger than the 27 patients required by the ad hoc design. The benefit of this delay is that when the true probability of response is 0.15, the minimax terminates at the end of the first stage more often (60%) than the ad hoc procedure (41%). The consequence is a slightly smaller *average* sample size when the true

probability of response is 0.15. The minimax design reduces the expected number of patients treated with inferior treatments but never more efficiently than the optimal design. The primary advantage of the minimax design is that for particular studies for which the second stage of accrual is indicated, the overall size of the study is minimized.

Flexible two-stage designs. Because of administrative challenges, multi-institutional phase II studies often require more flexibility in the design than single-institution studies. Several study candidates may be approached to participate in the study simultaneously at different clinics. Occasionally, a few extra patients consent to participate in the study after the accrual goals have been completed but before the clinics are notified that the accrual goals have been met. To accommodate these administrative challenges, optimal but flexible phase II designs have been proposed.[18] Rather than specifying the exact sample size for each stage of accrual, an acceptable accrual range is specified. Chen and Ng[18] provide tables for several two-stage designs in which the accrual for each stage of the study is permitted to range over eight consecutive integers. It is important that the reason for the actual accrual within the permitted range not depend on the underlying response rate. Conceptually, the type I error is calculated as the average of individual type I errors over all permitted combinations of accruals at each stage, assuming that each combination of accrual is equally likely. The type II error is calculated in a similar manner. Limited computer simulations suggest that the statistical errors are not overly sensitive to reasonable alternative distributions of the accrual sizes. Characteristics of an optimal flexible design for the example study are summarized in Table 65-2. The accrual goal for the first stage is between 22 and 29 patients. If fewer than 4 (of 22 to 24) or 5 (of 25 to 29) respond, the accrual stops, and the treatment is considered to have insufficient activity to warrant further evaluation. Otherwise, accrual continues until there are at least 53 but no more than 60 patients entered into the study. If there are fewer than 11 (of 53), 12 (of 54 to 57), or 13 (of 58 to 60) patients responding, the treatment is considered inactive. This flexible design provides expected sample sizes near the more restrictive optimal two-stage design. In their paper, Chen and Ng[18] provide flexible designs based on the optimal or the minimax approach to optimization.

The use of this design is somewhat controversial. Contrarians prefer to emphasize that a study implementing this design and advertising control of type I and II errors to a specific level does not control these errors to these levels for each of the permitted accrual combinations. The type I and type II errors for a particular combination of stage 1 and 2 accrual sizes may be greater than the average error rates advertised by the design. This design only limits the average error rate over all permitted accrual combinations. The proponents of this design emphasize that statistical power is a prestudy concept and does not depend on the data observed at the end of the study. Moreover, the deviations of the actual type I and II errors for a particular accrual combination from their advertised levels tend to be small.

Three-stage designs. One drawback of the optimal two-stage design is that it does not permit study termination when there is a long run of nonresponders among the first patients entering the study. This problem was addressed by one of the earliest proposals of two-stage phase II study designs.[21] Gehan[21] proposed classifying a treatment as inactive when there were no responders among a prespecified number of patients entered during the first stage of accrual. Gehan[21] recommended that the smallest number of patients be entered during the first stage of the study that provides adequate control of type I error. This design has been combined with the optimal design[20] described earlier to form a three-stage design.[22] These designs permit early accrual termination when there are no responses among patients treated during the first stage of accrual together with the optimal two-stage criteria to create efficient three-stage designs that limit the type I and type II errors. Although most of the benefits from multistage phase II studies can be provided with two-stage designs, three-stage designs are worthy of consideration when their additional administrative complexities can be accommodated.

Confidence intervals and hypothesis testing. There is a connection between hypothesis testing and providing confidence intervals for the estimated probability of response. Rejecting H1 at the level α is equivalent to the $100\% \cdot (1 - \alpha)$ one-sided confidence bound for P being greater than P_1 (i.e., upper bound of the inactive drug region). Likewise, rejecting H2 at the level β is equivalent to the upper $100\% \cdot (1 - \beta)$ one-sided confidence bound of P being less than P_2 (i.e., lower bound of the active drug region). This procedure is appropriate for studies with a fixed sample size. However, the inclusion of interim analyses into the study design has implications for estimation. Specifically, using standard procedures for constructing confidence limits after multistage studies can be inaccurate. A "bias" arises from the fact that the decision to stop the study is no longer independent of the study results. The confidence intervals must be adjusted to account for the interim analyses.[23] Applying standard procedures to create confidence limits that ignore the possibility of terminating the study at earlier stages of accrual leads to confidence bounds that do not have the advertised probabilities of coverage. These confidence bounds tend to overstate the precision of the study.

Phase IIB designs. Phase IIB trials usually involve a comparison between a cohort treated with an experimental treatment and some reference group. The reference group may consist of a historical or a concurrently randomized group treated in a standard fashion. If no randomized control group and no historical data are available, the data may be compared with experts' prior expectations of the underlying probability of response. Whereas phase IIA designs compare the probability of response to a prespecified constant, the phase IIB design acknowledges that the true probability of response in the reference group is not known with certainty. If there is uncertainty in the true probability of responding to standard treatment and the study design does not account for this uncertainty, the study will misclassify active treatments and inactive treatments more often than advertised. Moreover, the confidence interval for the estimated difference in the probability of response between the reference group and the experimental treatment group will exaggerate the precision of the study.

Randomized phase IIB clinical studies are not frequently used to screen cytotoxic agents. Their use for this purpose has been discouraged.[24] Randomized phase IIB studies are commonly used for preliminary investigation of chemopreventive agents in which the primary indicator of activity is potentiating or inhibiting a particular molecular marker. In these cases, the underlying probability of response or the other factors that influence these markers typically are unknown. A randomized phase IIB design is often used to control for biases that could arise from these other sources of variability.

Thall and colleagues[25] describe the use of historical controls in the design of phase IIB studies when the response is a binary event. Emrich[26] describes historically controlled study designs when the response is measured as the time to an event.

Randomized phase II designs. Response rates observed in phase II trials may exhibit considerable variability from study to study, even when the same agent is being evaluated. The factors that may contribute to the variability between trials include eligibility criteria, dose, schedule, route of administration, dose modification scheme for toxicities, procedures for evaluating response, schedule for evaluating response, and intraobserver and interobserver variability.[27] To control for some of these sources of variability, Simon and coworkers[27] recommended evaluating several treatments simultaneously within a single, randomized phase II study. Controlling for these sources of variability provides some rationale for interpreting differences in results as representing real differences in toxicity or antitumor activity rather than artifacts of patient selection, study methods, or investigator characteristics.

Ranking and selection designs. Perhaps the simplest randomized phase II design is one based on a single-stage ranking and selection procedure. The goal of this type of study is to select one treatment among several alternatives for further evaluation. The study may involve comparing the same agent being administered with different doses, routes of administration, or schedules. At the completion of the study, the treatment regimens are ranked on the basis of their response rates, and the treatment with the highest response rate is selected for further evaluation. The number of patients treated on each treatment regimen is determined such that if one of the experimental treatments is better than the other treatments by a pre-specified amount, δ, there is at least a (1 − β) • 100% chance that the best treatment will be selected. This design is appropriate when it is planned that only one treatment will be selected at the end of the trial. In the event that two or more treatments tie for the highest rank, one of these treatments may be selected in a random fashion. Although selecting one of the tried agents on the basis of other study end points such as toxicity, cost, or patient convenience may be more pragmatic, estimating the probability of selecting the most active agent becomes more difficult without making additional assumptions regarding the relationships between activity and these other end points.

This approach is frequently used in vaccine development. In this case, there may be several experimental vaccines being considered for evaluation. The vaccines may differ in dose, route of administration, or vector. This type of study provides a rational approach to selecting one vaccine when evaluating multiple vaccines simultaneously is not feasible.

Using this design in inappropriate situations can give rise to considerable confusion. First, suppose more than one treatment is better than the others by the indicated amount, δ. This design can provide a high probability of selecting one of these active regimens, but it does not provide sufficient specificity to permit classifying the unselected treatments as inactive. Second, suppose none of the treatments is active, but there is a nonzero spontaneous response rate. Because it is planned that one treatment will be selected at the end of the trial, it will select out of necessity an inactive agent. In other words, the probability of a type I error for this design is 100%. This design is appropriate in situations when the intention is to select one of several treatments for further evaluation and a rational study design for selecting a regimen among several experimental regimens is needed. Without a significant increase in the samples size, it is inappropriate to classify the unselected treatments as inactive. Moreover, there is often very little justification in this case for declaring the selected treatment as active.

Returning to the hypothetical study described previously, suppose there are several experimental treatments being considered for phase III evaluation, but there are insufficient resources to evaluate all of the agents simultaneously. Suppose the true probability of response is 15% for several experimental treatments under study, except one "best" treatment. Further suppose that the true probability of response to the best study treatment is 30%. A ranking and selection phase II design that provides a 90% chance of correctly selecting the best treatment requires at least 26 patients treated on each treatment regimen of a two–treatment arm trial. It requires 38 patients treated on each treatment regimen for a three–treatment arm trial and 46 patients on each treatment regimen for a four–treatment arm trial. The number of patients required to treat on each treatment arm of the study increases as the number of treatment arms increases. However, the required sample size for each of these studies is considerably smaller than for a phase IIA or IIB trial that

limits the probability of advancing to the next phase of drug development when none of the experimental agents is truly active.

There is an extension to this trial design worth considering. Suppose the difference in response rates between the highest-ranking treatment and the second- or third-ranking treatment is less than an amount considered clinically significant. In this case, an investigator may wish to select one of these agents based on other considerations such as toxicity, cost, or patient convenience. This type of study is described by Sargent and associates,[28] and methods for determining sample size requirements are described by Lui.[29] This additional flexibility at the end of the trial requires a moderate increase in the number of patients treated on each study regimen. Consider again the example in the previous paragraph. If an investigator wished to permit treatment selection based on other factors, such as toxicity, among the treatments that have response rates no more than 5% less than the highest observed response rate, the required samples sizes are 31, 51, and 72 patients in the two-, three- and four-arm trial, respectively.

Summary of phase II designs. Phase II trials provide an opportunity to screen agents for therapeutic activity. There are several approaches worth considering. Selecting the appropriate design requires clearly identifying the goals of the study. The analysis and the conclusions should be commensurate with the study design. A publication that describes the results of a clinical trial should include a description of the study's objectives and design considerations. The conclusions from a study should reflect the study's objective and design.

What are the challenges facing chemoprevention studies?

Justification for chemoprevention when surgery is sufficient. Many chemoprevention trials in the literature discuss the effects of compounds on lesions in or on the body that are considered to be at high risk for developing into an invasive cancer. Examples include trials evaluating Celecoxib to prevent colon cancer in individuals with familial adenomatous polyposis,[30] oral betacarotene for primary prevention of cervical cancer in individuals with high-grade cervical intraepithelial neoplasia (CIN),[31] and 4-hydroxyphenyl retinamide (4-HPR) for secondary prevention in patients with early-stage prostate cancer.[32] For many of these conditions, the disease can be successfully managed with surgical intervention. Conservative procedures such as the large loop excision of the transformation zone (LLETZ) and carbon dioxide laser excision of CIN lesions are about 95% effective,[33] and carbon dioxide laser excision (not vaporization) of vulvar intraepithelial neoplasias (VIN) appears to be about 85% effective.[34] With vigilant surveillance programs such as yearly mammography screening for women and prostate-specific antigen (PSA) screening in conjunction with rectal examinations for men, it is reasonable to believe we could reduce the incidence of death from breast or prostate cancer just as effectively as was done with cervical cancer. The keys, some say, is early detection and surgical elimination of precursor lesions destined to become invasive cancer, and that money spent on developing chemopreventive agents and proving their effectiveness in clinical trials would be better spent on educating the public about the necessity of surveillance because there are no compounds as effective as surgery. Given even a small risk of recurrence and subsequent progression into invasive cancer, a strong argument could be made against substituting chemopreventive agents for surgery on ethical grounds; a patient should be given the best available treatment in the hope of avoiding a devastating disease.

These arguments have merit, but there are more issues to be considered. First, the purpose of many chemoprevention trials is not to demonstrate that a particular agent can substitute for surgery. The men with prostate cancer enrolled to the clinical trial discussed by Urban and colleagues[32] understood that they were going to have a prostatectomy regardless of the drug's effectiveness. The objective of this trial was to determine whether a particular agent could effectively delay progression to a more advanced stage of the disease. However, even if a chemoprevention trial demonstrates that a particular agent provides benefit to only a subset of the population at high risk for a lethal disease, these trials are worthwhile if they can provide future patients more options for the treatment of their disease. Consider the fact that one of the primary motivations for why women participated in a chemoprevention trial against CIN by Follen and colleagues[35] was fear of surgery and the hope to avoid surgery. However, one of the primary motivations for not participating in the trial was a desire to have definitive treatment as soon as possible.[35] If chemopreventive agents that are less effective than surgery are to be integrated into the care of high-risk individuals, large and long-term clinical trials will need to be carried out to provide treatment guidelines. The cost to individuals who choose chemoprevention will likely be greater surveillance.

Perhaps a good analogy is the use of balloon angioplasty in the treatment of coronary heart disease. In the 1980s, bypass surgery was a standard treatment for this disease. Although bypass surgery was considered effective, it was also a very expensive, major surgical procedure with considerable risk of complications. For this reason, many patients were willing to try the less invasive procedure even though the risk of a recurrent restriction of blood flow was greater.

Determining the risk of disease. Many oncologists view invasive, metastatic cancer as the final outcome of a long, chronic disease that progresses over decades in a way similar to the way cardiologists view a myocardial infarction as the final outcome of chronic coronary arterial disease.[36] Like cardiovascular disease, many factors can decrease or increase the risks of developing cancer. Some of these factors are beyond

the control of the individual, such as genetics, but other factors are within the individual's control, such as smoking; eating high-fat, low-fiber diets; and not consuming fruits and vegetables.[36] In an effort to reduce the incidence of cancer, healthy lifestyles have been promoted by the American Cancer Society. These efforts have been prompted by results from numerous epidemiologic studies. Clinical trials have provided evidence that some drugs that control blood pressure or lower cholesterol can reduce the risk of heart disease. There is hope that similar progress can be achieved in oncology with the use of chemopreventive agents. Many chemoprevention trials evaluate the antineoplastic activity of particular agents that may be useful in treating the disease at an earlier stage of development.

There is a practical reason for recruiting patients at high risk for developing a disease: the ability to detect a beneficial impact of a potential agent with statistical significance with relatively few people. For example, an investigator may be interested in testing whether a particular agent reduces the risk of a disease site from spreading, forming new lesions, or otherwise getting worse. (For ethical reasons in oncology, most investigators do not use such an end point; they instead often look for improvements through histologic grade or lesion size.) In such a setting, it may be known that 50% of untreated patients will develop the disease of interest within a particular time interval, and interest may be focused on reducing this risk by 50%. The required sample size that ensures detection of this effect with 80% statistical power (type II error, $\beta = 0.20$) while controlling the probability of a type I error to 5% ($\alpha = 0.05$) is only 31 patients. This is a relatively small sample size. However, as the underlying risk of disease decreases (i.e., π under the null hypothesis, H_0), it becomes increasingly difficult to detect an effect by an agent capable of reducing the risk of progressive disease by one half (Table 65-3). If the same trial is run in a population in which the risk of a particular disease is 1 case per 1000 people, a clinical trial designed to detect whether an agent reduces the risk of disease by 50% requires more than 24,000 individuals. Screening agents in this setting quickly becomes impractical when the costs, resource allocation, and time requirements are considered.

Typically, an agent must demonstrate promising biologic activity in a high-risk population before it is considered for further testing within a population that

Table 65–3. The Required Sample Size for Studies When the Risk of Disease is π_0 and the Intervention Reduces the Risk by 50%

π under H0	π under H1	Required Sample Size
0.50	0.25	31
0.20	0.10	103
0.10	0.05	224
0.02	0.01	1187
0.01	0.005	2390
0.001	0.0005	24053

H0, null hypothesis; H1, alternative hypothesis; π, disease risk.

has less underlying risk of the disease. If an agent continues to show promise, larger trials are conducted in healthier populations using more clinically relevant outcomes such as the development of an invasive cancer. The few studies that have reached this level of development have been enormous. For example, the Prostate Cancer Prevention Trial (PCPT) recruited almost 19,000 men.[37] The subsequent trial, called the Selenium and Vitamin E Cancer Prevention Trial (SELECT), is even larger. It will accrue 32,400 men.[37] Even these large studies restrict the eligibility criteria to a subpopulation of men considered to have an increased risk of developing prostate cancer. The duration each individual is followed on study is also long to study the long-term effects of treatment and to increase the cumulative risk of disease. Although monumental in size, these trials provide the most definitive evidence regarding the activity of a chemopreventive agent.

Weighing the risk of adverse treatment effects. Whether by epidemiologic studies or through screening in clinical trials, the agent needs to show some promise of efficacy. Perhaps even more importantly, the agent needs to be considered reasonably safe. If large segments of the population are going to supplement their diets or apply creams, side effects must be almost nonexistent; otherwise, healthy people will not tolerate the intervention. Not only must the agent exhibit no acute side effects, but it must also cause no long-term adverse effects. Because the risk of developing cancer for an individual from the general population is small, any cost-benefit analysis dictates that the trial must take into account as many potential adverse events as possible, including the possibility of exacerbating existing conditions. In the end, a particular chemopreventive agent may be deemed not useful in preventing cancer (even if it is effective at reducing the incidence of cancer) because the risk of adverse effects outweighs the potential benefits. One such example is the use of estrogen replacement therapy in the treatment of coronary heart disease in asymptomatic postmenopausal women.[38]

It is also possible that the chemopreventive agent is not effective at preventing cancer. Epidemiologic evidence could be misleading if it fails to take into account other confounding variables that are more closely related to the cause of the disease. Agents that prove effective against eliminating precursor lesions may not be effective at preventing invasive disease. Even worse, an agent shown to be effective against the formation of precursor lesions may actually increase the risk of developing invasive disease when used as a chemopreventive agent. Consider the fact that some of the most effective anticancer agents and radiotherapy tend also to be mutagenic, ironically making them likely carcinogens themselves. We may be willing to accept this risk when the consequences of the disease justify it, but it may not be reasonable to advocate daily exposure to radioactive substances for years in the hope of preventing one particular form of cancer. The treatment must be commensurate with the severity of the disease.

Determining the study population. Preliminary chemoprevention trials typically involve individuals from intermediate-risk populations. They have a greater risk of developing cancer than the general population, which makes detecting an effective agent through clinical trials more feasible (i.e., smaller sample sizes). A cost-benefit analysis would not have to be as demanding on the agent's adverse effect profile. Because the risk of developing symptomatic disease is greater, a person is generally willing to accept some risk of treatment side effects, but the risk of disease is not so great that she is fully prepared to have surgery. This essentially would be a compromise between no treatment and an aggressive treatment. An added benefit would likely be greater patient compliance because they are at an increased risk.

How are intermediate-risk populations identified? Several ways are being considered or are being used. Age tends to be a major risk factor for many diseases. A family history of the disease is another. Although a definitive genetic marker of risk is not available for many cancers, genetic testing of *BRCA1* and *BRCA2* has been employed to identify individuals at increased risk for breast and ovarian cancers. Some chemoprevention studies focus recruitment on individuals who had the disease and were treated but are considered to be considerable risk for recurrence. Another approach to identifying high-risk individuals is through the use of biomarkers. If a particular protein in the blood, such as PSA levels for prostate cancer, or immunohistochemical analysis yields results that are associated with the risk of developing a disease, people may be identified as candidates for treatment based on these biomarker results. After these intermediate-risk populations are identified and recruited into clinical trials, the study would usually focus on the development of invasive disease as the primary end point unless the biomarker was also validated as a surrogate end-point biomarker (SEB).

Using surrogate end-point biomarkers. True SEBs can provide many advantages for identifying effective chemopreventive agents because they are more than just risk factors. SEBs such as hypertension and cholesterol levels (with regard to heart disease and stroke) function differently from family history or racial background. Surrogates can be changed, and their modulation reflects true changes in risk. The justification for using SEBs in clinical trials to evaluate therapeutic efficacy are that they can provide the same answers as the large-scale trials in evaluating the true disease state, but they do so with potentially fewer people and in a much shorter period. Although there is no universally accepted definition, most agree that SEBs have the following properties:

1. Useful SEBs tend to be relatively easy to obtain and inexpensive to assess. Examples for cardiovascular disease include blood pressure, triglyceride levels, and low-density lipoprotein counts.
2. SEBs are linked to the risk of developing the true clinical end point of interest such as cancer or a fatal cardiac event.

3. Most importantly, modulation of the SEB is associated with a corresponding change in risk.[39]
4. Ideally, the quantitative relationship between the SEB and the risk of disease is known, so the treatment effects on an SEB predict the treatment effects on the incidence of cancer.

Unfortunately, for all their potential benefits, SEBs have just as many challenges when used in practice. For example, if a biomarker is associated with only one pathway in a disease process, estimates in risk reduction may be larger or smaller than anticipated.[39] If the agent is effective at modulating the biomarker, but the biomarker is not part of a common disease process, the evidence from assessing SEBs will exaggerate the treatment effects on the true clinical end point. If the agent does not significantly affect the biomarker but it is effective at blocking other disease processes, the estimates on risk reduction will be smaller than its true value. Worse is the possibility of unanticipated effects by a drug that exacerbates the disease process despite a favorable SEB outcome.

These kinds of errors are not merely theoretical. They have already occurred. Fleming and DeMets[40] show many examples in which "suspected" or less than ideal surrogate end points have failed to accurately reflect the outcome of interest. One excellent example is the Cardiac Arrhythmia Suppression Trial (CAST). It was discovered that ventricular arrhythmia was associated with an approximately fourfold increase in the cardiac death rate, and it was hypothesized that suppression of these arrhythmias would produce a similar reduction in death. Three drugs were approved by the U.S. Food and Drug Administration (FDA) for use in arrhythmia suppression, but an analysis of CAST showed that two of these drugs actually increased the risk of sudden death from cardiac complications.[40] In another example, a trial was initially designed to detect the effects of interferon-γ on superoxide production by macrophages, which helps the immune system to fight infections. The trial was redesigned before activation to assess the effects of interferon-γ on the clinically relevant outcome, serious infections.[40] The drug was shown to be effective, but its effects on superoxide production were insignificant.[40] These and other examples show that care needs to be taken if clinical evidence of efficacy is based on a surrogate end point. Any positive results demonstrated with surrogate end points should be followed up with a thorough assessment of clinically meaningful end points.

One way to help determine whether a biomarker is likely to yield good surrogate information is with an estimate of its attributable proportion to the disease process, which is often obtained through epidemiologic studies. In the context of classic epidemiology, the attributable proportion of some (putative) causal agent is the proportion of disease occurrence that would be eliminated if the case group were exposed to the same levels as the control group.[41] In the context of SEBs, the attributable proportion of the biomarker is the proportion of cancers that are linked to it.[39] If the biomarker is closely tied to the causal mechanism of all cancers, its attributable proportion should be nearly 100%. A biomarker with an attributable proportion less than 50% would indicate the existence of other causal pathways, perhaps in addition to those involving the biomarker.[39]

Even if a biomarker can serve as a useful surrogate, there are still common problems with its use. Often, biomarkers are estimates of some underlining true process, and it is subject to error. These errors may cause low-risk people to be misclassified as high-risk patients and vice versa. This problem of misclassification tends to produce underestimates of drug efficacy.[39] For example, denote patients with disease (or destined to get disease) by D^+ and those without disease by D^-. Assume a biomarker is positively associated with or predictive of the disease so that E^+ is associated with D^+, and E^- is associated with D^-. The sensitivity of the biomarker, $P(E^+|D^+)$, is indicated by S, and the specificity of the biomarker, $P(E^-|D^-)$, is indicated by SP. The prevalence of the disease, $P(D^+)$, is indicated by P, and the proportion of positive biomarkers, $P(E^+)$, is given by P_+. (Estimates of these parameters would usually be available from epidemiologic studies.) A study that uses the biomarker observes E^+ and E^- only. The relationship of $P(E^+)$ with the other quantities is given by the following equation:

$$P\left(E^+\right) = P\left(E^+|D^+\right) P\left(D^+\right) + \left[1 - P\left(E^-|D^-\right)\right] \bullet \left[1 - P\left(D^+\right)\right]$$

(4)

This is more simply stated as follows:

$$P_+ = S \bullet P + (1 - SP) \bullet (1 - P)$$

(5)

Assuming the prevalence of the disease is 2% and that the biomarker is 95% sensitive and 95% specific, we can expect to observe E^+ about 6.8% of the time. As can be seen, using the biomarker dramatically increases the proportion of "positive" cases (mostly due to errors; 72% of the positive cases are caused by false-positive misclassification). Given all of these facts but assuming the prevalence is only 1%, we can expect to observe E^+ about 5.9% of the time. Next consider a drug that is effective at reducing the incidence of the disease from 2% to 1%. This drug has the ability to reduce the incidence of the disease by 50%, but because the study uses a surrogate, the apparent reduction in the incidence of the disease appears to be only by a factor of 0.87. (An earlier section discussed the need to have observable events to establish an effect by a drug with relatively few patients. Although true, artificially adding observable events through misclassification does not help in the ability to detect an effective agent.) Table 65-4 gives more examples of the disparity between the true risk ratio (TRR) and the observed risk ratio (ORR) associated with taking the drug:

A risk ratio near 1 indicates little difference in the two populations (i.e., indicates that the treatment is not effective at reducing the incidence of the disease). The last row in Table 65-4 shows that a drug truly capable of reducing the incidence of disease by 50%

Table 65–4. True Risk Ratio and Observed Risk Ratios for Different Quality Surrogates

S	SP	$P_{Baseline}$*	P_{Drug}†	TRR	ORR
0.95	0.95	0.50	0.25	0.50	0.55
0.95	0.95	0.10	0.05	0.50	0.68
0.95	0.95	0.02	0.01	0.50	0.87
0.95	0.95	0.01	0.005	0.50	0.92
0.95	0.95	0.001	0.0001	0.10	0.98
0.75	0.95	0.02	0.01	0.50	0.89
0.95	0.75	0.02	0.01	0.50	0.97
0.75	0.75	0.02	0.01	0.50	0.98

*$P_{Baseline}$ is the underlying probability of developing the disease in the untreated population.
†P_{Drug} is the probability of developing the disease among those who take the active treatment.
S, sensitivity; SP, specificity; ORR, observed risk ratio; TRR, true risk ratio.

appears to have virtually no effect (ORR = 0.98) when studied with a surrogate that is 75% sensitive and 75% specific. As seen in the first row, the demands on the biomarker do not have to be very stringent if the prevalence of the disease is fairly high. Unfortunately for scientists studying cancer, the incidence of the disease is usually rare in a chemopreventive setting, and detecting effective compounds with biomarkers is particularly challenging. Rather than helping scientists discover effective agents, biomarkers may obscure the issue. Of the two factors that are commonly described in linking biomarkers to disease, specificity seems to be more important.[39] Figure 65-3 shows the importance of high specificity and near irrelevance of sensitivity when the incidence of the disease is rare. The domain of the graph is the biomarker's sensitivity and specificity. The range is the ORR for a drug that is capable of reducing the incidence of the disease by one half. As can be seen with the surface of this function, most points in the domain yield an ORR near 0.90, which is very close to 1. The ORR is close to 0.50 only when the surrogate's specificity is nearly perfect (>99%). However, even if the sensitivity is perfect (100%) but

the specificity is less than ideal (e.g., 85%), the ORR is quite high (>0.90).

Some investigators have recommended using estimates of the ORR in planning chemoprevention trials that use surrogate end points.[39] This is sound advice, but doing so usually requires larger study sizes than if the true end point were observed.

Despite these challenges, surrogate variables can be useful for several reasons. First, they can provide information about the disease in a much shorter period. Second, the cost of recruiting more patients into a clinical trial that uses surrogate end points is offset by the shorter trial duration. When the prevalence of the disease is high, surrogate variables could be reasonably accurate in discriminating between diseased and disease-free individuals. For example, if a disease had a prevalence rate of 40%, a surrogate with sensitivity of 95% and specificity of 90% would correctly classify 92% of all individuals. This is one reason why surrogate variables are used in precancerous disease settings. It may not be ethical in such settings to ascertain the drug's effectiveness at preventing the development of cancer (i.e., the true end point) when an effective surgical procedure already exists. In this setting, surrogate end points must be used. On the other hand, the usefulness of surrogate end point appears to be limited in areas where the incidence of the disease is smaller than 5% to 30% (depending on the quality of the surrogate). In such situations, evaluating actual clinical end points of interest may be more appropriate.

SEBs are evolving in chemoprevention trials, and as knowledge is gained about the appropriateness of surrogates in use, some will be dropped, and new ones will be added. Many precancerous cervical studies look for an improvement on a histopathologic grading scale (e.g., CIN III to CIN I), called CIN regression. However, this criterion may not be a good predictor of chemopreventive activity for some drugs because the biomarker is a measure of selective destruction of human papillomavirus—infected cells; some useful chemopreventive agents may be effective at stopping the growth of these cells but are ineffective at destroying them. In this case, the biomarker would indicate a higher rate of D^+ when in fact (if they had taken the drug at an earlier time) it would result in a D^- state (i.e., a biomarker event equivalent to $E^+ | D^-$). Investigators aware of these shortcomings may proceed with larger trials despite initially negative results, using more relevant end points and eventually demonstrating the agent's effectiveness. Accurate estimates of the biomarkers' sensitivity are important if we wish to avoid proceeding erroneously into larger chemoprevention trials.

Study compliance. Declining compliance of individuals enrolled into the study poses a serious problem in chemoprevention trials. Unlike cancer patients, who face a life-threatening illness that requires frequent medical care, ostensibly healthy individuals do not necessarily need to follow a rigorous schedule of clinic visits according to protocol guidelines. The fact that

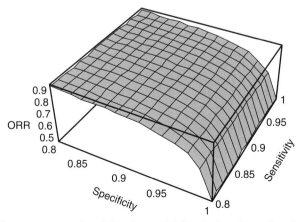

Figure 65–3. A plot of the observed risk ratio (ORR) as a function of the biomarker's specificity and sensitivity when baseline prevalence is 2% and the drug's true risk ratio (TRR) is 0.5.

large chemoprevention trials often require participants to be followed for several years compounds the problem. Attrition can also be a problem in short-term studies. Keefe and colleagues[31] reported a roughly 25% attrition rate after 6 months in a chemoprevention trial involving patients with precancerous cervical lesions. These missing patients were classified as nonresponders for an intent-to-treat analysis,[31] which is a common form of imputation used in clinical trials. In a typical intent-to-treat analysis, patients are listed according to their response, and this includes a category for unknown responses. In calculating the proportion of patients who respond favorably to treatment, those with an unknown response to treatment are included in the denominator. The Response Evaluation Criteria in Solid Tumors (RECIST)[42] also recommends using this approach to estimating the probability of response—that is, to classify patients with an unknown response with the nonresponders. Does this make sense? Most statisticians recognize this method as being conservative, yielding negatively biased estimates against the activity of the drug. How inaccurate is this classification scheme? In some instances, this method probably yields fairly accurate estimates for trials of advanced rapidly progressing diseases because several such studies have shown that patients who fail to return for follow-up assessments do so because of increasing debilitation and have worse survival characteristics than those who remain complaint with the study. If the probability of an unknown response is low (e.g., 5%), the effects of these missing patients on the quality of inference are usually minimal. To illustrate the point, consider a phase II trial that is interested in detecting a 40% response rate in patients treated with a new drug when the baseline response rate is 20% with $\alpha = \beta = 0.10$. A single sample binomial design would require 43 patients under the assumption that all eligible patients entered on the trial are observed. However, when a proportion of the patients cannot be observed because of attrition, the apparent response rate, P_A, is less than the true response rate, P, according to the following equation when the classification scheme described previously is applied:

$$P_A = P \bullet (1 - AR) \qquad (6)$$

In Equation 6, AR is the attrition rate. If the attrition rate is 5%, the apparent response rate is 38% when the drug's true response rate is 40%. Accruing 43 patients gives the design 85% power instead of 90%. This is still a reasonably good design. However, if the attrition rate is 25%, the apparent response rate drops to 30%, giving the design only 47% power. This is unacceptable. Although attrition in randomized, controlled designs does not typically yield as dramatic of an effect, there is loss in power.

One approach to addressing this problem is to increase the sample size until enough evaluable patients are accrued onto the trial. However, the solution may not be so simple. This approach also runs the risk of yielding biased estimates and misleading inferences. Consider, for example, a chemoprevention trial designed to eliminate precancerous lesions. What

factors may influence a patient's compliance? Response to treatment is one possibility. If a patient is not responding to treatment, she may seek treatment at another clinic and avoid the physician associated with the clinical investigation altogether. If that is a major cause for being classified as an unknown response, imputing such patients as nonresponders could be justified. However, if the treatment is very effective, the patient may no longer feel the need to seek further treatment. In such a case, classifying these patients as treatment failures would underestimate the drug's effectiveness, and analysis of the clinical trial could erroneously conclude that the drug is not effective.

In practice, the probability of being missing may depend on treatment assignment (e.g., inconvenience) and treatment efficacy (i.e., response to treatment). It seems that people may be more likely to drop from the study if the treatment was ineffective in addition to being inconvenient. Exactly how these factors affect patient compliance is often unknown. This missing data problem is the most difficult type to handle analytically.[43] To properly handle such problems would require a good understanding of the censoring mechanisms that need to be included into a probabilistic model, and that could be one of the greatest challenges of the study. To avoid these problems, preemptive efforts directed at reducing attrition as much as possible is of paramount importance.

REFERENCES

1. Senn S: Statistical Issues in Drug Development. New York, John Wiley & Sons, 1997.
2. Emanuel E: A phase I trial on the ethics of phase I trials. J Clin Oncol 1995;13:1049-1051.
3. National Commission for the Protection of Human Subjects of Biomedical and Behavioral Research, Belmont Report: Ethical Principles and Guidelines for the Protection of Human Subjects of Research. Washington, DC, Department of Health, Education and Welfare, 1979.
4. Dougherty C, Ratain M, Grochowski E, et al: Perceptions of cancer patients and their physicians involved in phase I trials. J Clin Oncol 1995;13:1062-1072.
5. Rajagopal S, Goodman P, Tannock I: Adjuvant chemotherapy for breast cancer: Discordance between physicians' perceptions of benefit and the results of clinical trials. J Clin Oncol 1994;12:1296-1304.
6. Beecher H: Ethics and clinical research. N Engl J Med 1966;274:1354-1360.
7. Eisenhauer E, O'Dwyer P, Christian M, Humphrey J: Phase I clinical trial design in cancer drug development. J Clin Oncol 2000;18:684-692.
8. Simon R, Freidlin B, Rubinstein L, et al: Accelerated titration designs for phase I clinical trials in oncology. J Natl Cancer Inst 1997;89:1138-1147.
9. Chevret S: The continual reassessment method in cancer phase I clinical trials: A simulation study. Stat Med 1993;12:1093-1108.
10. O'Quigley J, Pepe M, Fisher L: Continual reassessment method: A practical design for phase I clinical trials in cancer. Biometrics 1990;46:33-48.
11. O'Quigley J, Shen L: Continual reassessment method: A likelihood approach. Biometrics 1996;52:673-684.
12. Korn E, Midthune D, Chen T, et al: A comparison of two phase I trials designs. Stat Med 1994;13:1799-1806.
13. Goodman S, Zahurak M, Piantadosi S: Some practical improvements in the continual reassessment method for phase I studies. Stat Med 1995;14:1149-1161.

14. Moller S: An extension of the continual reassessment methods using a preliminary up-and-down design in a dose finding study in cancer patients, in order to investigate a greater range of doses. Stat Med 1995;14:911-922.
15. Mariani L, Marubini E: Content and quality of currently published phase II cancer trials. J Clin Oncol 2000;18:429-436.
16. Thall P, Estey E: A Bayesian strategy for screening cancer treatments before phase II clinical evaluations. Stat Med 1993;12:1197-1211.
17. Storer B: A class of phase II designs with three possible outcomes. Biometrics 1992;48:55-60.
18. Chen T, Ng T: Optimal flexible designs in phase II clinical trials. Stat Med 1998;12:2301-2312.
19. Schultz J, Nichol F, Elfring G, Weed S: Multiple stage procedures for drug screening. Biometrics 1973;29:293-300.
20. Simon R: Optimal two-stage designs for phase II clinical trials. Control Clin Trials 1989;10:1-10.
21. Gehan E: The determination of the number of patients required in a preliminary and follow-up trial of a new chemotherapeutic agent. J Chron Dis 1961;13:346-353.
22. Garnesy-Ensign L, Gehan E, Kamen D, Thall P: An optimal three-stage design for phase II clinical trials. Stat Med 1994;13:1727-1736.
23. Atkinson E, Brown B: Confidence limits for probability of response in multistage phase II clinical trials. Biometrics 1985;41:741-744.
24. Liu PY, LeBlanc M, Desai M: False positive rates of randomized phase II designs. Control Clin Trials 1999;20:343-52.
25. Thall P, Simon R: Incorporating historical controls in planning phase II clinical trials. Stat Med 1990;9:215-228.
26. Emrich L: Required duration and power determinations for historically controlled studies of survival times. Stat Med 1989;8:153-160.
27. Simon R, Wittes R, Ellenberg S: Randomized phase II clinical trials. Cancer Treat Rep 1983;69:1375-1381.
28. Sargent D, Goldberg R: A flexible design for multiple armed screening trials. Stat Med 2001;20:1051-1060.
29. Lui K: A flexible design for multiple armed screening trials. Stat Med 2002;21:627-627.
30. Steinbach G, Lynch PM, Phillips RKS, et al: The effect of Celecoxib, a cyclooxygenase-2 inhibitor in familial adenomatous polyposis. N Engl J Med 2000;342:1946-1952.
31. Keefe KA, Schell M, Brewer C, et al: A randomized, double blind, phase III trial using oral β-carotene supplementation for women with high-grade cervical intraepithelial neoplasia. Cancer Epidemiol Biomarkers Prev 2001;10:1029-1035.
32. Urban D, Myers R, Manne U, et al: Evaluation of biomarker modulation by fenretinide in prostate cancer patients. Eur Urol 1999;35:429-438.
33. Lisowski P, Knapp P, Zbroch T, Kobylec M: The effectiveness of conservative treatment of cervical lesions using the LLETZ and CO_2 laser [in Polish]. Przegl Lek 1999;56:72-75.
34. Sideri M, Spinaci L, Spolti N, Schettino F: Evaluation of CO_2 laser excision or vaporization for the treatment of vulvar intraepithelial neoplasia. Gynecol Oncol 1999;75:277-281.
35. Follen M, Meyskens FL Jr, Atkinson EN, Schottenfeld D: Why most randomized phase II cervical cancer chemoprevention trials are uninformative: Lessons for the future. J Natl Cancer Inst 2001;93:1293-1296.
36. Lieberman R, Nelson WG, Sakr WA, et al: Executive summary of the National Cancer Institute Workshop: Highlights and recommendations. Urology 2001;57(Suppl 1):4-27.
37. Thompson IM Jr, Kouril M, Klein EA, et al: The Prostate Cancer Prevention Trial: Current status and lessons learned. Urology 2001;57(Suppl 1):230-234.
38. Rossouw JE, Anderson GL, Prentice RL, et al: Risks and benefits of estrogen plus progestin in healthy postmenopausal women: Principal results From the Women's Health Initiative randomized controlled trial. JAMA 2002;288:321-333.
39. Trock BJ: Validation of surrogate endpoint biomarkers in prostate cancer chemoprevention trials. Urology 2001;57(Suppl 1):241-247.
40. Fleming TR, DeMets DL: Surrogate end points in clinical trials: Are we being misled? Ann Intern Med 1996;125:605-613.
41. Ahlbom A, Norell S: Introduction to Modern Epidemiology, 2nd ed., Epidemiology Resources, 1990.
42. Therasse P, Arbuck SG, Eisenhauer EA, et al: New guidelines to evaluate the response to treatment in solid tumors. European Organization for Research and Treatment of Cancer, National Cancer Institute of the United States, National Cancer Institute of Canada. J Natl Cancer Inst 2000;92:205-216.
43. Little R, Rubin D. Statistical Analysis with Missing Data. New York, John Wiley & Sons, 1987.

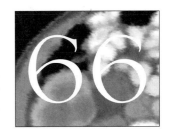

PREVENTION OF GYNECOLOGIC MALIGNANCIES

David S. Alberts, Richard R. Barakat, Mary Daly, Michael W. Method,
Doris M. Benbrook, John F. Boggess, Molly A. Brewer, Louise A. Brinton,
Philip E. Castle, Zoreh Davanipour, Francisco A. R. Garcia, Mark G. Hanly,
Lisa M. Hess, Jeffrey F. Hines, Joseph Kelaghan, Joseph Lucci, Lori Minasian,
Carolyn Muller, George L. Mutter, Janet S. Rader, Gustavo Rodriguez,
Eugene Sobel, and Joan L. Walker

 MAJOR CONTROVERSIES

- What is the importance of intraepithelial neoplasia?
- How do we develop interventions to prevent cancer?
- What is the difference between prevention and treatment research?
- What is the etiology of cervical cancer?
- Is there a genetic predisposition to the development of cervical cancer?
- What is the role of persistent versus transient human papillomavirus infection?
- What is the best method for the detection of pre-invasive cervical cancer?
- What is the best method for the collection of cervical cytology specimens?
- How are the results of cervical cytology interpreted?
- What is the role of human papillomavirus testing?
- Are cervicography and colposcopy useful screening tests?
- What role do disparities play in the effectiveness of screening for cervical cancer?
- What is the best strategy to prevent cervical cancer?
- What is the role of human papillomavirus vaccines in the prevention of cervical cancer?
- Are there promising agents for the chemoprevention of cervical cancer?
- Is hormone replacement therapy associated with an increased risk of endometrial cancer?
- How do exogenous factors affect a woman's risk of developing endometrial cancer?
- Is there a genetic predisposition to the development of endometrial cancer?
- Are all endometrial cancers alike?
- What are the molecular genetic features of type I endometrial cancers?
- What are the molecular genetic features of type II endometrial cancers?
- Is it possible to discriminate between atypical endometrial hyperplasia and in situ carcinoma?
- What is the best management for atypical endometrial hyperplasia?
- What are the relevant genes involved in ovarian carcinogenesis?
- What are the prevalence and penetrance of the ovarian cancer susceptibility genes?
- What are the environmental and physiologic factors associated with ovarian cancer risk?

Continued

- What are the exogenous risk factors for ovarian cancer?
- What is the role of exogenous hormones and ovarian cancer risk?
- Which women should be screened for ovarian cancer?
- What methods are under study for ovarian cancer screening?
- What surgical procedures are indicated in women with a family history of ovarian cancer?
- What is the role of chemopreventive agents in the prevention of ovarian cancer?
- What is the pathogenesis of vulvar cancer?
- What is the natural history of vulvar intraepithelial neoplasia?
- What are the barriers to progress in the prevention of vulvar cancer?

OVERVIEW

Although cancers of the cervix, endometrium, ovary, and vulva are distinctly different disease entities, there is a common pathogenetic pattern, extending from the first carcinogen-initiated cell though mild, moderate, and severe dysplasia to carcinoma in situ (CIS) and invasive cancer. However, this process may not occur in a forward, stepwise sequence, as exemplified by the bidirectional arrows in Figure 66-1. The importance of this multiyear, multistage, multipathway pattern of lesion progression is that each step of carcinogenesis provides an opportunity to intervene with early detection, screening, lifestyle changes, chemoprevention strategies, and supportive care technologies, as well as surgical, radiation, and chemotherapy interventions.

What is the importance of intraepithelial neoplasia?

Preventing gynecologic malignancies requires, at a minimum, a thorough understanding of disease etiology, epidemiology, and risk factors. Defining the etiology of each gynecologic cancer is essential to the ability to sensitively and accurately identify and classify precursor lesions, now referred to as intraepithelial neoplasias (INs or IENs). Knowledge of these IENs is growing rapidly with the identification of specific molecular abnormalities and more general genotypic damage associated with increasingly severe dysplastic histology. Critical steps include inactivation of tumor suppressor genes, such as *BRCA* in ovarian cancers and *PTEN* in

endometrial cancers, and activation of various oncogenes. As discussed in a seminal American Association for Cancer Research Task Force special article in February 2002, "IEN provides a suitable target for treatment intervention because of its phenotypic and genotypic similarities and evolutionary proximity to invasive cancer."[2]

The progression of mild neoplasia to high-grade neoplasia/CIS and, ultimately, invasive cancer is a multiyear process, as exemplified by the carcinogenesis pathway of cervix cancer (Fig. 66-2). Although the sequence of events may not directly follow this exact step-by-step pathway, the progression from grade I cervical intraepithelial neoplasia (CIN I) to CIN III/CIS is estimated to take 10 years, and further progression to invasive cancer may require another 10 to 20 years.[3] This approximately 20- to 30-year duration of IEN transformation to cancer provides multiple opportunities for intervention with standard CIN-ablative treatments and experimental modalities, such as human papillomavirus (HPV) vaccines or chemopreventive agents, or both.

Gynecologic and medical oncologists of the 21st century must focus on all segments of the carcinogenesis pathway for gynecologic malignancies, not just invasive disease; furthermore, these oncologists must be trained in all aspects of cancer prevention disciplines, including basic and translational molecular biology and pharmacology, epidemiology, biostatistics, chemoprevention agent development, and clinical trials. Armed with this strong basic and clinical training background, there are unlimited opportunities to make the gynecologic malignancies preventable diseases in our lifetime.

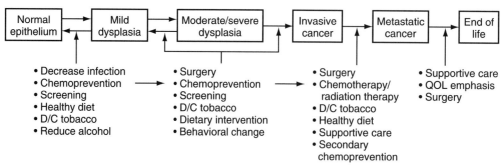

Figure 66–1. A unifying vision of cancer therapy, adapted[1].

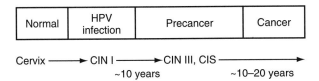

Figure 66–2. Multiyear progress from normal appearing tissue to precancer to cancer: cervix, adapted.[2,3]

This chapter has been conceived and written by members of the Cancer Prevention and Control Committee of the Gynecologic Oncology Group as a comprehensive primer concerning clinical trials and the etiology, epidemiology, early detection, and screening of cervical, endometrial, ovarian, and vulvar intraepithelial neoplasias. Although much research remains to be accomplished over the next few decades, we are confident that gynecologic malignancies will become preventable diseases.

How do we develop interventions to prevent cancer?

Clinical research at universities, cancer centers, and community medical practices is necessary to develop effective interventions to prevent or delay cancer. Relevant interventions include chemoprevention, screening followed by effective treatment, and lifestyle changes related to diet, exercise, and other behaviors. The goal of clinical research is to maximize knowledge concerning the effectiveness, side effects, and secondary benefits of these interventions. An equally important goal is to characterize populations for which the intervention is appropriate and determine their level of risk for developing cancer.

Cancer chemoprevention is the prevention of an initial malignancy or of a second primary or recurrent malignancy. To prevent or reduce the likelihood of developing a malignancy, a chemopreventive agent must either prevent the malignant transformation of a cell or lead to the death or prevention of replication of such a cell (and its progeny) before it becomes established and eventually reaches a diagnosable size.

Epidemiology and basic science (e.g., in vitro studies, animal studies), as well as unanticipated findings from randomized clinical trials, provide the starting points for development of interventions. The final step before approval by the U. S. Food and Drug Administration (FDA) and introduction into general use is demonstration of efficacy and a tolerable side effect profile in a phase III randomized clinical trial with cancer incidence as an endpoint. These studies require large sample sizes (often 10,000 to 30,000 subjects), lengthy exposure to an intervention (several years), and lengthy follow-up (up to 15 years). Because of these requirements, their conduct requires extensive supporting evidence from phase I and pharmacokinetic/metabolic studies to identify a safe dose and schedule and from phase II dose-finding and efficacy studies to demonstrate activity that could potentially interfere with the development of a cancer (i.e., surrogate biomarkers).

The benefits of conducting phase II trials include the precise determination of the optimal chemopreventive agent dose and the ability to gain supportive data in a smaller study population before conducting a more costly, but definitive, phase III randomized trial.

Phase II studies can use either surrogate markers of cancer prevention (which may be different from surrogate markers of activity) or cancer incidence if high-risk subjects are enrolled. Phase II study designs may involve two or more dose levels. Because many biomarkers vary substantially both within and among individuals, many phase II studies also require a randomized, placebo-controlled design (phase IIb), which increases the complexity of the trial and the required sample size. It is important to avoid thinking of phase II studies as "definitive," because by definition they do not have sufficient sample size to demonstrate a protective effect using cancer incidence as an endpoint. However, phase II studies do have adequate sample size to address the hypotheses under investigation in these studies.

Although not yet an option for gynecologic malignancies, a future possible approach to decreasing the size and cost of phase III prevention clinical trials is the use of a validated surrogate as the endpoint, instead of observing subjects until cancer occurs. A measurable biologic phenomenon that occurs earlier than cancer and is documented in a pathway leading to malignant transformation, could be an endpoint in a clinical trial, because reducing the occurrence of such a marker would necessarily decrease the occurrence of the cancer. Potential surrogates for gynecologic malignancies are CIN III and AEH. In the absence of validation for use as endpoints, however, surrogates serve as useful markers in phase II studies to demonstrate that the intervention affects a process associated with the development of cancer. Another approach to decreasing the size of a phase III prevention trial is to conduct the study in subjects who are at very high risk, such as those with a diagnosed precursor lesion or genetic mutation. However, this study design may limit generalizability of the results to lower-risk populations.

A variety of cancer prevention strategies must be developed for populations that differ substantially in their underlying risk of developing cancer. Ideally, some strategies will be suitable for use in a general population at average risk. These strategies must be inexpensive and easy to use, and they can have only rare and minor side effects. It is also important to develop interventions for use by patients who are at high risk for developing cancer. Patients with a well-characterized and substantial risk can tolerate considerably greater costs and side effects. Therefore, phase I through phase III trials for prevention agents must accurately characterize the side effects as well as the degree of protection (to determine the appropriate target population).

Two phase III primary prevention trials sponsored by the National Cancer Institute (NCI) illustrate the application of the results of prevention research. The Breast Cancer Prevention Trial monitored more than 13,000 at-risk women for an average of 3.5 years to detect a 49% decrease in breast cancer incidence for women randomly assigned to treatment with tamoxifen. The results from this trial are applicable to women who meet the risk profile for this study. The Prostate Cancer Prevention Trial recruited more than 18,000 men, each of whom will be monitored for 7 years, to be able to detect a 25% reduction in prostate cancer among men taking finasteride. The results from this trial, available in 2004, will apply to the general population of men older than 55 years of age. The application of results from these two trials will differ because of the slightly higher-risk profile for tamoxifen compared with finasteride. Cancer prevention trials have been successfully conducted through oncology clinical trials networks, and several are scheduled to report results within the next 5 years. A thorough understanding of their unique needs is essential to the development of well-designed cancer prevention trials for gynecologic cancers.

Despite the large amount of information derived from a definitive phase III prevention trial, further information can be derived from phase IV postmarketing evaluation of approved interventions. The difficulty of conducting phase III studies makes further formal clinical trials of efficacy and side effects unlikely. Phase IV studies will be necessary to determine the longer-term safety and efficacy of these interventions for the general population of users. They will also be necessary to derive data on safety and efficacy in patients with coexisting medical conditions and in those who are taking other medications, perhaps even other chemopreventive agents. Phase IV postmarketing studies can take many forms, among them surveillance of reported adverse drug events, case-control studies, and prospective observational studies (including continued follow-up of subjects in a previous phase III study). Exactly how such studies should be designed and conducted is still an open question. Considerations as to continued participation, completeness of information, verification of side effects, and incidence of serious adverse events are vital to chemoprevention study design.

What is the difference between prevention and treatment research?

Prevention research differs substantially from treatment research (Table 66-1). The large sample sizes, length of intervention, and lengthy follow-up for phase III prevention trials contrast with the moderate size and duration of phase III treatment trials. Subjects in prevention trials are usually healthy, and many will never develop the cancer to be prevented, so the significance of side effects differs from that in a treatment trial, in which cancer patients will tolerate greater drug-related toxicities because of the severity of their illness. Many treatment trials are not blinded, whereas all current prevention trials require blinding to preclude a detection bias. Research in community medical practices is particularly important for prevention research. Clinicians in these practices see the majority of patients at risk for cancer, and interventions must be easily implemented in this setting if the goal of reducing the overall burden of cancer is to be achieved.

CERVICAL CANCER

Worldwide, cervical cancer is the second or third most common cancer and cause of cancer-related mortality in women, with approximately 500,000 new cases and 200,000 deaths occurring annually. Eighty percent of cervical cancer cases are diagnosed in developing countries.[4] In the United States, it was estimated that 13,000 new cases of cervical cancer would be diagnosed and 4,000 women would die of this condition in 2002.[5] Much of the reduced incidence of cervical cancer in the last half of the 20th century in the United States is attributed to cancer screening with the use of the Papanicolaou (Pap) smear and cytologic identification of patients with cervical neoplasia or CIS. However, over the past 10 years the incidence rates of cervical cancer have remained relatively stable. A significant discrepancy exists among ethnic groups, with regard to both incidence rates and overall mortality, suggesting a need to readdress current screening and prevention strategies.

What is the etiology of cervical cancer?

A major factor driving cervical carcinogenesis is the deregulation of cell cycle control and response to DNA damage caused by high-risk HPV early proteins, E6 and E7. The normal function of early proteins is to usurp host cellular machinery for replication of viral

Table 66–1. Characteristics of Prevention and Treatment Clinical Trials

Characteristic	Prevention Trials	Treatment Trials
Population	Healthy or at risk	Diagnosed with cancer
Source of subjects	Primary care practices or outside medical practice system	Oncology practices
End point	Incident cancer; surrogates	Response; recurrence; progression-free and overall survival
Placebo	Typically used	Not typically needed
Duration of intervention	Usually years	Months
Duration of follow-up	Defined period, usually years*	Cancer-related mortality
Size of study	Very large (can be 30,000+)	Moderate (100-1000)
		Adjuvant trials (2000-4000)
Side effects	Minimal to low	Moderate or greater

*Extended follow-up beyond original plan requires scientific justification and new hypothesis.

genomic episomes.[6] Initial HPV infection is limited to the basal layer of cervical epithelium, and expression of the E6 and E7 proteins occurs as the cells are pushed into the spinous layer and begin to differentiate. As the cells enter the granular layer and undergo further differentiation, viral DNA replication is turned off and viral capsid proteins encoded by the late genes are synthesized for viral assembly. This manipulation of cellular machinery for viral reproduction normally does not cause cancer and is tightly controlled through regulation of E6 and E7 expression by another HPV early protein, E2.[7] Cervical carcinogenesis occurs when viral genomic episomes integrate into host chromosomes in a manner that disrupts the E2 gene but retains E6 and E7 genes, which results in disregulation of these genes.[8] Although numerous studies have found that the site of chromosomal integration is random, cytogenic and molecular analyses have shown that HPV-16 frequently integrates within common fragile sites (CFSs), including FRA6C and FRA17B.[9] HPV-16 DNA is not always integrated, and it is sometimes present in both episomal and integrated forms in cervical tumors; however, disruption of the HPV-16 E2 gene by integration is associated with significantly shortened disease-free survival time.[10] In contrast, HPV-18 may be integrated more frequently than HPV-16, perhaps in 100% of cervical carcinomas[11]; however, the biologic implications are uncertain, because HPV-16, not HPV-18, is the leading cause of cervical cancer (approximately 50% of cervical cancer cases worldwide are attributable to HPV-16).[10]

Transfection and expression of high-risk HPV E7 alone or in combination with high-risk HPV E6 induces immortalization (unlimited growth potential) and abnormal differentiation in normal human keratinocytes.[12] Immortalization is preceded by periods of increased proliferation and mitotic abnormalities, resulting in aneuploidy and increased telomerase activity.[13,14] However, expression of an additional oncogene, such as ras, is required for complete transformation of the immortalized keratinocytes into cell lines capable of forming tumors in nude mice.[15,16] This reflects the long latency period and requirement for additional genetic mutations needed to develop cervical cancer after initial HPV infection.[17] Combinations of HPV-induced genomic instability with exposure to carcinogens greatly increases the risk of acquiring permanent DNA damage in the appropriate combinations of oncogenes and tumor suppressor genes that can lead to cellular transformation. Evidence that cigarette smoking results in exposure of the cervix to carcinogens is provided by demonstrations that nicotine, its metabolite cotinine, and tobacco-specific carcinogens have been detected in cervical mucus of both active and passive smokers at higher concentrations than in the serum of these individuals.[18,19]

The E6 and E7 proteins control viral replication by intermolecular interactions with host cellular proteins involved in regulation of the cell cycle and DNA damage response (Fig. 66-3). The E6 protein induces ubiquitination (attachment of ubiquitin molecules) and subsequent degradation of p53, a tumor suppressor protein that protects cellular DNA from acquiring permanent mutations.[20] Although the p53 gene is the most frequently mutated gene found in cancers, E6 degradation of p53 apparently bypasses the need for mutation of p53 in primary cervical carcinomas.[21] Mutations in p53 have been found, however, in cervical carcinomas that are HPV negative,[22] are infected with intermediate-risk HPV,[23] or have metastasized.[24] The E7 protein interferes with the ability of cellular Rb and p107 proteins to inhibit the E2F transcription factor from transcribing genes required for DNA synthesis during the G_1 phase or, in the presence of DNA damage, during S phase, respectively.[25] E7 also directly binds and inactivates kinase inhibitors involved in cell cycle progression.[26,27] The high-risk HPV E5 protein induces immortalization, although its role in cervical carcinogenesis is not clear. E5 is a transmembrane protein that inhibits endocytic trafficking from early to late endocytic structures, superinduces signal transduction pathways, changes cellular morphology, and impairs cell motility.[28]

Molecular targets used in developing new strategies to prevent and treat cervical cancer may include epidermal growth factor receptor (EGF-R) and the HPV early proteins. HPV-16 E6 and E7 cooperate to increase EGF-R expression, which overcomes the shortened life span induced by excessive EGF-R signaling in normal human keratinocytes.[29] EGF-R expression levels in cervical carcinoma have a positive correlation with radiation response and an inverse relationship with prognosis.[30,31] Strategies for targeting EGF-R include anti-EGF-R monoclonal antibodies and pharmaceuticals that antagonize EGF-R tyrosine kinase activity.[32,33] The zinc finger of the E6 protein has been targeted by screening for compounds that eject the zinc atoms required for proper formation of the finger domain, a structure that is essential for E6 binding to host cellular proteins.[34] The antigenic properties of several HPV proteins have been identified and targeted in efforts to develop HPV vaccines.[35] Expression of HPV proteins can be repressed by retinoid drugs, which show promise as chemoprevention agents for cervical cancer.[36]

Is there a genetic predisposition to the development of cervical cancer?

Although cervical cancer is not typically associated with an autosomal dominant familial cancer syndrome (with the exception of adenoma malignum in Peutz-Jegers syndrome), well-characterized population studies of first-degree relatives support a modest heritable risk.[37,38] Data obtained from the Swedish Cancer Registry and the National Family Registry demonstrate a 27% genetic heritability effect for cervical tumor development, as compared with a 2% shared environmental effect.[38] In addition, other primary tumors, such as oropharynx, lung, and squamous cell skin cancers that share environmental risk factors (HPV and tobacco exposure), are increased in first-degree relatives of women with cervical tumors.[39,40] These data support the role of modifier genes in the

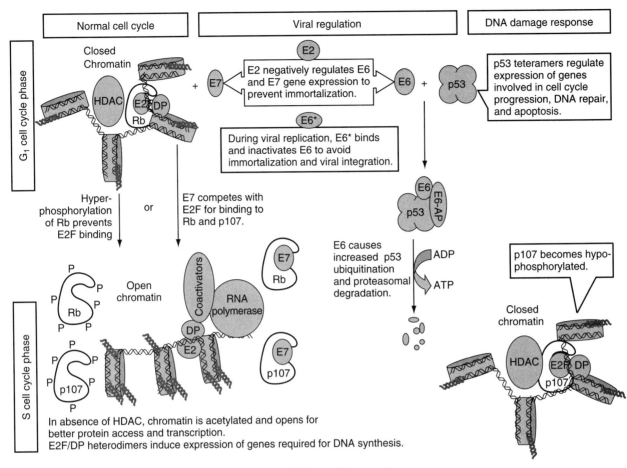

Figure 66–3. Viral replication by intermolecular interactions with host cellular proteins.

natural history of HPV infection leading to cervical carcinogenesis. One pathway by which modifier genes are implicated in the risk for cervical cancer includes human leukocyte antigen (HLA) class I and II genotypes, which are involved in presenting foreign antigens to immune cells and therefore are important in host immune responses to viruses and other pathogens.

There is evidence to suggest HLA haplotypes may affect the risk of high-grade cervical neoplasia, presumably by altering local cervical cellular immune responses to HPV. For instance, in a meta-analysis, HLA class II DQw3 and DR15 were associated with an increased risk of cervical cancer, particularly for HPV-16 infected cases, whereas DR13 demonstrated a decreased risk.[41] Another study found that HLA-DRB1*1301 was associated with decreased risk for high-grade cervical neoplasia.[42] Risk and protective haplotypes may vary among ethnic groups or populations.[42-44] Genetic polymorphisms that alter enzyme function in the metabolic pathways for tobacco carcinogens could also affect the risk of cervical cancer, because smoking is an established HPV cofactor for high-grade cervical neoplasia.[45,46] Many molecular epidemiologic studies support an association of functional polymorphic variants in the cytochrome P-450 (CYP) and glutathione-S-transferase (GST) genes as a susceptibility factor in tobacco-related lung and oropharyngeal cancers.[47,48] Recent studies in cervical cancer and dysplasia suggest that similar susceptibility exists with the risk polymorphism in CYP1A1,[49] particularly in those women with null mutations in both *GSTT1* and *GSTM1*.[50] Although these molecular epidemiologic studies are in their infancy, modifier genetics will likely explain variations in HPV persistence and susceptibility to environmental factors that promote cervical cancer progression. Future studies will be necessary to sort out the complexity of the combined effects of these genetic polymorphisms and will also be important to evaluate response to interventions in vaccine and chemoprevention trials.

Epidemiology of Cervical Cancer

What is the role of persistent versus transient human papillomavirus infection? Cervical infection by one of the 13 cancer-associated (oncogenic) HPV types (16, 18, 31, 33, 35, 39, 45, 51, 52, 56, 58, 59, 68) is generally accepted as the universal cause of cervical cancer.[5,51] (There are inadequate data about the oncogenicity of some HPV types, including HPV-66.) More than 99% of all cervical cancers are positive for HPV DNA.[52] The development of cervical cancer can be summarized as a multistage carcinogenic process (Fig. 66-4). Uninfected women are exposed to infectious HPV virions most often by sexual contact, and some of these

Figure 66–4. Natural history of cervical cancer.

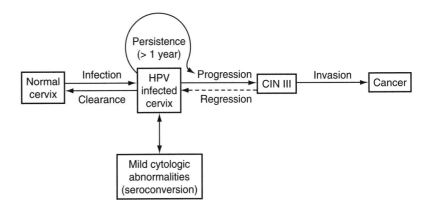

women become detectably infected within the annulus of tissue known as the squamocolumnar junction of the transformation zone. Although HPV infections by oncogenic HPV types can result in precancerous and cancerous lesions of the cervix, more often these infections are self-limiting and resolve within 1 to 2 years. HPV infections often go unnoticed. Productive HPV infections can cause the pleomorphic cellular changes interpreted as abnormal on Pap smear analysis, including some diagnoses of atypical squamous cells of unknown significance (ASCUS) and primarily diagnoses of low-grade squamous intraepithelial lesions (LSIL). Some infected women also develop HPV type-specific antibodies (seroconversion). A few infections persist for 1 year or longer, and it is this subset of women with detectably persistent infections who are at risk for precancer and cancer of the cervix.

The primary risk factor for acquiring HPV infection is the number of male sexual partners, especially the number of recent sexual partners. Some studies have suggested that age at first sexual intercourse is a primary risk factor, but more recent large epidemiologic studies failed to confirm this finding after adjustment for number of sexual partners. The absence of confirmatory data suggests that age at first sexual intercourse is a surrogate for high-risk sexual behavior. However, the more exposed (proximal) positioning of the transformation zone in young women and in women who use oral contraceptives (OCs) should hypothetically lead to greater risk of infection and emphasizes the lack of understanding of the biologic mechanism of viral transmission.

Establishment of HPV as the necessary but not sufficient cause of cervical cancer has led to an epidemiologic search for factors that influence the progression or regression of an HPV infection. HPV cofactors that might alter the natural history of an HPV infection by increasing the likelihood of *progression* of high-grade cervical neoplasia (histologic diagnosis of CIN III) or, conversely, by increasing the *clearance* of an HPV infection are sought. A number of HPV cofactors have been suggested, the most well known being smoking,[45,46] OC use,[53] and parity.[54,55] A prospective study[44] and a nested case-control study[45] demonstrated a twofold to fourfold increased risk of CIN III or cervical cancer among women with HPV infection. A large multicentric study[53] demonstrated a threefold to fourfold

increased association of long-term (5 years or longer) OC use with invasive cervical cancer compared with HPV infection. Other studies have failed to demonstrate this association when adjusted for number of sexual partners. In the same multicentric study,[53] the number of live births was associated with invasive cervical cancer in a dose-dependent manner, with a fourfold increased association among women with 7 or more live births. Multiple case-control comparisons of gravidity and parity showed statistically significantly higher values among those who developed cervical cancer for both measures (gravidity and parity) in women younger than 29 years of age, but not in those 30 years or older, implicating youthful pregnancy (most likely as a surrogate of multiparity) as an etiologic factor in cervical carcinogenesis.[55-59,83-86] Other possible HPV cofactors include genital tract infections (e.g., *Chlamydia trachomatis*, herpes simplex virus-2), cervical inflammation,[60] cell-mediated immunity,[41] micronutrients,[61] and viral load.[62]

What is the best method for the detection of pre-invasive cervical cancer? The Pap smear, the staining of a cellular specimen from the cervix developed by Dr. George N. Papanicolaou more than 50 years ago, has been the principal screening test for cervical cancer in developed countries. Morphologic changes of precancerous cells (CIN) are identified and often treated. Even though there is a lack of randomized studies showing success of this method, it is well accepted that the successful implementation of screening programs using the Pap test has decreased the incidence of cervical cancer. This is based on evidence that the decline in cervical cancer mortality closely parallels the implementation of the Pap smear. However, controversy exists as to the frequency with which the test should be preformed, the accuracy of the traditional Pap test, and the lack of applicability for developing countries.

Observational data suggest that the effectiveness of screening increases when Pap tests are performed more frequently. Although a single Pap test may have a relatively low sensitivity, the cumulative sensitivity of several yearly tests should be high. The American College of Obstetrics and Gynecologist (ACOG) recommends annual Pap test to begin three years after the age of first vaginal intercourse or not later than twenty-one. After the age of thirty, the Pap test maybe performed less frequently in low risk women. Use of the combination of cervical cytology and high-risk HPV testing may be used every three years after the age of thirty. The Canadian Task Force on Preventive Health Care recommends an annual Pap test for women who are sexually active or 18 years of age or older; after two normal smears, screening is recommended every 3 years to age 69 years. The screening frequency may be increased in women with high-risk factors.[64] The National Health Service Cervical Screening Programme in the United Kingdom covers cervical screening for women between 20 and 64 years of age every 3 to 5 years.[65]

Conventional Pap testing detects CIN less effectively than is generally believed: cytologic methods have a mean sensitivity of 58% and a mean specificity of 69% in screening samples.[66,67] The sensitivity of cytology is limited by sampling error, in which the abnormal cells do not get placed on the slide, and reading error, in which a few abnormal cells fail to be identified among the normal cells. The specificity of cytology is also problematic. Screening programs are overburdened by borderline smears of uncertain malignant potential, which are costly to follow-up and cause anxiety to the women involved. Moreover, the multicenter randomized NCI ASCUS and LSIL Triage Study (ALTS), which evaluated triaging methods for mildly abnormal Pap smears, confirmed the poor reproducibility of cytology readings by pathologists: 45% of referral Pap readings were disputed by the pathology quality control group.[68] These studies point to the need to incorporate additional molecular diagnostic markers in screening, either as an ancillary test (e.g., HPV DNA testing) or incorporated into cytology (e.g., molecular Pap test).

What is the best method for the collection of cervical cytology specimens? Cervical cytologic specimens can be collected with a variety of devices. The combined use of an ectocervical spatula and an endocervical brush or swab appears to be the best method for obtaining cervical cells for conventional specimens.[69] Liquid-based cytologic sample collection and analysis is the most common new technology used. The liquid-base, thin-layer preparation system (ThinPrep and AutoCyte Prep) is designed to remove obscuring nonepithelial cells and to distribute cells evenly on a slide. The cervical sample is placed in a small bottle containing fixative solution. The sample is sent to the cytology laboratory, where it is filtered or centrifuged to remove excess blood and debris. The cells are then transferred to the slide in a single layer. The slide is stained and examined manually in the conventional way. Two systems of computer-assisted screening are currently available: AutoPap and AutoCyte Screen. With AutoPap, the device reviews the material on the slide and, based on an algorithm, scores the slide as to the likelihood that an abnormality is present.[70] This algorithm includes a variety of visual characteristics, such as shape and optical density of the cells. The AutoCyte Screen System was developed for primary screening and presents computer images of the 120 most abnormal cells to a human reviewer, who then determines whether manual review is required.[71] After the cytotechnologist has

entered an opinion, the device reveals its determination based on a ranking as to whether manual review is warranted. If the human reviewer and the computer agree that no review is needed, a diagnosis of "within normal limits" is given. Manual review is required for any case that is designated as needing review by either the cytologist or the computer ranking.

How are the results of cervical cytology interpreted?
The Bethesda 2001 workshop updated the terminology used for reporting results of cervical cytology (Table 66-2).[72] These guidelines were developed under the sponsorship of the American Society for Colposcopy and Cervical Pathology (ASCCP). More than 90% of laboratories in the United States use the Bethesda System, as do laboratories in many other countries. The Bethesda System includes a descriptive diagnosis and an evaluation of specimen adequacy (see Table 66-2). The 2001 Bethesda System maintained the "satisfactory for evaluation" and "unsatisfactory for evaluation" categories but eliminated "satisfactory but limited by...," because the term was considered confusing to many clinicians and prompted unnecessary repeat testing. Bethesda 2001 added a new category for atypical cells at higher risk of association with precancer: "atypical squamous cells, cannot exclude a high-grade lesion (ASC-H)." This category highlighted the 5% to 10% of ASCUS cases that are more likely to contain high-grade squamous intraepithelial lesions (HSIL). In addition, the term "atypical squamous cells favor reactive" and "benign cellular changes" were eliminated.

Developing countries lack the infrastructure required for cytology-based screening programs, which require a complex communication system for the identification and recall of patients, a highly skilled and controlled laboratory processing system, and professionally trained cytopathologists. In an attempt to develop alternative methods for identifying women at risk for cervical cancer, the University of Zimbabwe and JHPIEGO evaluated visual inspection of the cervix with acetic acid (VIA) in a large-scale screening program involving 10,934 women.[73] Colposcopy with biopsy, as indicated, was used as the reference test. VIA and Pap smears were done concurrently, and their sensitivity and specificity were compared in 2148 participants. VIA was more sensitive but less specific than cytology. Sensitivity was 76.7% (95% confidence interval [CI], 70.3 to 82.3) for VIA and 44.3% (95% CI, 37.3 to 51.4) for cytology. Specificity was 64.1% (95% CI, 61.9 to 66.2) for VIA and 90.6% (95% CI, 89.2 to 91.9) for cytology. Belinson and colleagues[74] noted similar sensitivity (71%) and specificity (74%) in their study of about 2000 women in rural China using trained gynecologists for the VIA. VIA has a role in areas of the world with limited resources. The procedure does not use technical supplies and allows for screening, diagnosis, and treatment in a single visit. One important caveat is that the low specificity of this test results in overtreatment of screened women.

What is the role of human papillomavirus testing?
Another alternative to cytologic screening is the use of tests for the detection of high-risk HPV in the cervix.

Table 66–2. Bethesda System 2001

Specimen Type

Indicate conventional smear (Pap smear) vs liquid-based vs other

Specimen Adequacy

Satisfactory for evaluation (*describe presence or absence of endocervical/transformation zone component and any other quality indicators, such as partially obscuring blood, inflammation, etc.*)

Unsatisfactory for evaluation (*specify reason*)

    Specimen rejected/not processed (*specify reason*)

    Specimen processed and examined, but unsatisfactory for evaluation of epithelial abnormality because of (*specify reason*)

General Categorization *(optional)*

Negative for intraepithelial lesion or malignancy

Epithelial cell abnormality: see Interpretation/Result (*specify "squamous" or "glandular" as appropriate*)

Other: see Interpretation/Result (*e.g., endometrial cells in a woman >40 years of age*)

Automated Review

If case examined by automated device, specify device and result.

Ancillary Testing

Provide a brief description of the test methods and report the result so that it is easily understood by the clinician.

Interpretation/Result

Negative for intraepithelial lesion or malignancy (*if there is no cellular evidence of neoplasia, state this in the General Categorization and/or in the Interpretation/Result section of the report, whether or not there are organisms or other non-neoplastic findings*)

Organisms

    Trichomonas vaginalis

    Fungal organisms morphologically consistent with *Candida* spp

    Shift in flora suggestive of bacterial vaginosis

    Bacteria morphologically consistent with *Actinomyces* spp.

    Cellular changes consistent with herpes simplex virus

Other Non-neoplastic Findings (optional to report; list not inclusive)

    Reactive cellular changes associated with

        Inflammation (*includes typical repair*)

        Radiation

        Intrauterine contraceptive device

    Glandular cells status post hysterectomy

    Atrophy

Other

Endometrial cells (*in a woman ≥40 years of age*)

(*Specify if "negative for squamous intraepithelial lesion"*)

Epithelial Cell Abnormalities

Squamous Cell

Atypical squamous cells

    Of undetermined significance (ASC-US)

    Cannot exclude HSIL (ASC-H)

Low-grade squamous intraepithelial lesion (LSIL) encompassing HPV/mild dysplasia/CIN I

High-grade squamous intraepithelial lesion (HSIL) encompassing moderate and severe dysplasia, CIS, CIN II and CIN II

    With features suspicious for invasion (if invasion is suspected)

Squamous cell carcinoma

Glandular Cell

Atypical

    Endocervical cells (NOS or specify in comments)

    Endometrial cells (NOS or specify in comments)

    Glandular cells (NOS or specify in comments)

Atypical

    Endocervical cells, favor neoplastic

    Glandular cells, favor neoplastic

Endocervical adenocarcinoma *in situ*

Adenocarcinoma

    Endocervical

    Endometrial

    Extrauterine

    NOS

Other Malignant Neoplasms *(specify)*

Educational Notes and Suggestions *(optional)*

Suggestions should be concise and consistent with clinical follow-up guidelines published by professional organizations (*references to relevant publications may be included*)

CIN, cervical intraepithelial neoplasia; CIS, carcinoma in situ; HPV, human papillomavirus; NOS, not otherwise specified.

From Solomon D, Davey D, Kurman R, et al: The 2001 Bethesda system: Terminology for reporting results of cervical cytology. JAMA 2002;287:2114-2119.

HPV testing could be implemented in a number of ways, such as by primary screening or as a triage test for atypical cytology. Some of these issues were summarized in a consensus conference in September 2001 by the ASCCP that took into account the new Bethesda terminology and the ALTS data.[75] The sensitivity of HPV DNA testing for the detection of biopsy-confirmed CIN II or greater in women with ASC is 83% to 96% and is higher than the sensitivity of a single repeat cervical cytologic test. The negative predictive value of DNA testing for high-risk types of HPV is 98%. Therefore, HPV testing can be used as an alternative approach for the follow-up of ASC to determine who should be referred for further colposcopy. The test is performed on the original liquid-based cytology specimen or a sample co-collected at the original visit to eliminate the need for the patient to return to the clinic. This "reflex HR HPV DNA testing" offers significant advantages because women do not need an additional clinical examination for specimen collection, and 40% to 60% of women are spared a colposcopic examination as a result of the reassurance of a negative HPV test. Presently the only FDA-approved HPV

DNA test in the United States is the Hybrid Capture 2 test (Digene Corporation), which detects the 13 major oncogenic HPV types. Patients with ASC cytology and a positive HPV test result have a 15% prevalence of HSIL, compared with less than 1% for patients with ASC and a negative HPV test, demonstrating the excellent negative reassurance of a sensitive HPV DNA test. Further information on the management of cervical cytology and histology can be found on the American Society for Colposcopy and Cervical Pathology web site.[76] The issue of using HPV testing as a primary screen for cervical cancer was addressed by the Health Technology Assessment Committee of the U. K. Department of Health.[77] They also concluded that HPV testing was more sensitive than cytology but were concerned about the specificity of primary testing, especially in young women, who have a high prevalence, which would lead to excessive follow-up studies. Using the more sensitive, less specific HPV DNA test followed by the less sensitive, more specific cytologic test may be a more efficient screening approach,[78] but it has not yet been tested in clinical trials. The FDA in April 2003 approved the use of the

High-Risk HPV DNA test in conjuntion with the Pap test on women over the age of thirty. The Hybrid Capture test is currently recommended that, a positive HPV DNA test in the presence of a normal Pap test should only prompt a return to annual Pap test in women over 30 years of age should undergo a second HPV test and cytologic evaluation in 6 to 12 months and[80] not prompt immediate intervention.

Are cervicography and colposcopy useful screening tests? Cervicography and colposcopy have been evaluated as primary screening tests, but the accuracy and technical requirements were suboptimal. Cervicography, in which a photograph of the cervix is examined at a central location for atypical lesions, has a sensitivity that is comparable to that of the Pap smear (60%), but with much lower specificity (50%).[79,80] In addition, 10% to 15% of Cervigrams are unsatisfactory. Colposcopy, in which the cervix is examined directly after the application of 4% acetic acid and magnification, is widely performed on women with abnormal Pap smears but has poor sensitivity (34% to 43%) and specificity (68%) when used as a screening test for cervical neoplasia in asymptomatic women.[81] Other disadvantages of colposcopy screening include its cost, the limited availability of the equipment, and the time and skill required to perform the procedure. The ALTS trial also highlighted the lack of precision of colposcopy: 47% of the colposcopically-directed cervical biopsies did not demonstrate pathologic lesions.[68]

What role do disparities play in the effectiveness of screening for cervical cancer? Regular cervical cancer screening needs to be encouraged for all women, especially those who are likely to be exposed to HPV or to human immunodeficiency virus (HIV); infection with HIV increases the risk of HPV infection. Special efforts are needed to reach those women who are less likely to be screened, such as elderly, poor, and less educated women and recent emigrants. The Centers for Disease Control and National Institutes of Health Healthy People 2010 target for cervical cancer screening is to increase from 80% to 90% the proportion of women age 18 years and older who have received a Pap smear within the last 3 years.[82]

Almost 60% of the cervical cancer cases in the United States occur among women who have never had a Pap smear or who have not been screened during the 5 years before diagnosis.[4] The majority of these women come from minority and economically disadvantaged backgrounds.[4] Although disparities in incidence and mortality have decreased in recent years, cervical cancer incidence remains about 50% higher among African-American women (11.2/100,000) compared with Caucasian women (7.3/100,000),[87,88] and mortality among African-American women with cervical cancer (6.7/100,000) is the highest of any racial or ethnic group.[87] Women of Vietnamese origin have the highest age-adjusted incidence rate (43/100,000), whereas women of Japanese origin have the lowest (5.8/100,000).[87] Surveillance Epidemiology and End Results (SEER) data for 1992-1998 showed that

Hispanics continued to have disproportionately higher rates of incidence (14.4/100,000) and mortality (3.3/100,000), compared with non-Hispanic white women (6.9/100,000 and 2.3/100,000, respectively).[89] The gap in incidence and mortality between Caucasian women and women of other racial or ethnic groups increases with age (Figs. 66-5 and 66-6).

Important differences are noted in terms of stage at presentation and prognosis among minority women. African-American women are less likely to present with localized disease (44%, compared with 56% for white women) and are twice as likely to die of their disease.[89] Hispanics are also more likely to present with advanced-stage and invasive disease, compared with their Caucasian peers.[90-92] After controlling for age, adjuvant therapy and race or ethnicity, at least one study has concluded that survival for early-stage carcinoma is most influenced by the type of therapy (surgical versus radiation).[93] Other investigators have found significant differences in treatment modality, with African-American women being less likely to receive surgery (33.5%, versus 48.2% for Caucasian women), more likely to receive radiation (35.3% versus 25.2%), and more likely to die of their disease.[94] Not surprisingly, higher rates of precursor lesions have also been documented for African-American and Hispanic women.[92,95]

Since 1980 in the United States there has been a trend toward significant participation among African-American women (90.9%) in cervical cancer screening programs (compared with 89.3% for Caucasian women).[96] Hispanic women have lagged behind, with the proportion reporting ever having been screened at 82.9%.[96] Women of Mexican ethnicity are less likely to receive regular cervical cancer screening than are women of Puerto Rican origin.[97] Among Mexican-American women, older women and non-English speakers are less likely to be aware of cancer screening recommendations or to be screened.[98] Not surprisingly, lack of acculturation and foreign birth are associated with the lowest utilization levels for cervical cancer screening in the United States.[99,100] Likewise, marital status, insurance coverage, and even domicile in predominantly nonminority census tracts are predictors of better screening.[101] Regardless of age and race or ethnicity, low socioeconomic status and its surrogates are consistently associated with poor outcomes and reduced utilization of screening services.[96,102]

Ultimately, a deeper understanding of the determinants, distribution, and burden of disease in minority populations will not only improve service delivery, but will lead to a better understanding of the biology of the disease through the natural experiments that occur because of the national diversity in the United States.

Prevention of Cervical Cancer

What is the best strategy to prevent cervical cancer? The most successful strategy for cervical cancer prevention has been the implementation of population-based screening programs utilizing the Pap smear.[103] The introduction of screening programs in

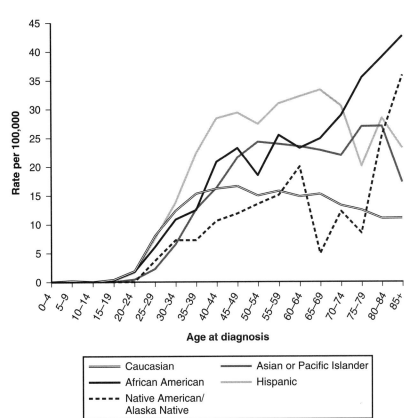

Figure 66–5. SEER Incidence Crude Rates, Cervical Cancer, 11 Registries, 1992-1999.

populations naïve to screening has been shown to reduce cervical cancer rates by 60% to 90% within 3 years after implementation.[104] The Pap test suffers from suboptimal single-test sensitivity, limited reproducibility, and many equivocal results. Its success as a public health intervention reflects three factors: (1) the progression from early cellular abnormalities (low-grade dysplasia), through more severe dysplasia, to CIS and invasive cancer is generally slow, allowing time for detection; (2) associated benign cytomorphic abnormalities can be identified before high-grade disease appears; and (3) effective treatment is available for premalignant lesions. Consequently, invasive squamous cell carcinoma of the uterine cervix is a highly preventable disease. Pap screening has proved ineffective in resource-poor regions throughout the world, including underserved populations in the United States. It is unclear whether new, more sensitive diagnostic techniques (e.g., thin-layer cytology, high-risk HPV DNA testing) will affect cervical cancer incidence and mortality rates in these underscreened populations, because of their associated costs.[51,105,106] Inexpensive interventions that target HPV could significantly reduce the worldwide incidence of cervical cancer.

Infection with HPV plays a central role in the development of cervical cancer. Therefore, prevention of HPV acquisition and transmission could significantly decrease the incidence of cervical cancer. Risk factors relating to sexual behavior that are associated with increased risk, such as onset of intercourse at an early age and a greater number of lifetime sexual partners, may be modifiable through targeted education efforts. Given that the acquisition of HPV by sexually active women occurs early in life, with the peak incidence and prevalence of HPV infection occurring among women younger than 25 years of age, such educational efforts should begin in preadolescent girls.[107] In addition, more than 30% of postmenopausal women have HPV DNA detectable by polymerase chain reaction (PCR) methods. Currently, there are no effective methods to prevent HPV infection outside of avoidance of sexual activity. There is no consistent evidence from population-based studies that any of the current contraceptive methods is associated with lower HPV prevalence, although a careful evaluation of HPV transmission in clinical assessments of condom use is much needed. For these reasons, cervical cancer prevention strategies have primarily targeted the treatment of preinvasive disease.

Smoking is the strongest cofactor for cervical cancer progression in HPV-infected women. Strategies aimed at decreasing smoking are likely to decrease cervical cancer incidence, although this remains unproven. Cigarette smoking is the only nonsexual behavior that is consistently and strongly correlated with cervical dysplasia and cancer; it independently increases the risk twofold to fourfold.[108-110]

What is the role of human papillomavirus vaccines in the prevention of cervical cancer? The viral etiology of cervical carcinoma suggests that a prophylactic vaccine specific for the infecting virus may effectively prevent infection and development of disease. An effective

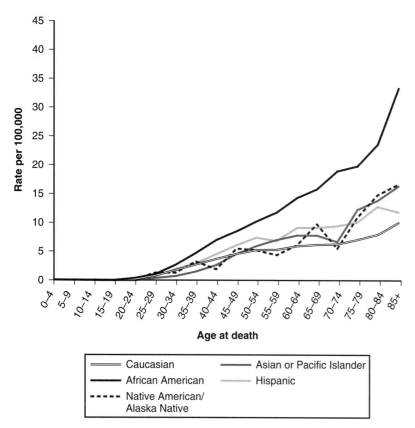

Figure 66–6. SEER Mortality Crude Rates, Cervical Cancer, Total U.S., 1990-1999.

HPV vaccine could ultimately be a more effective and cost-efficient prophylactic measure against cervical cancer than Pap smear screening worldwide, particularly in those places where screening programs are difficult to implement. Use of virus-like particles (VLP) of HPV as the antigenic material in a vaccine holds the greatest promise of success in preventing HPV infection. VLPs are self-assembled viral particles of the main structural HPV protein, L1 protein, in the absence of any viral genetic material. Although these capsid particles structurally resemble HPV virions, they are noninfectious. VLP vaccines have been highly successful in preventing and treating HPV infection in several animal model systems. In humans, the serum antibody response to VLPs is stable over time, even after the HPV infection has cleared.[41] Several trials using VLPs derived from the L1 protein of HPV-16 are ongoing.[111] Although VLPs are able to induce significant systemic immune responses, HPV infection occurs in the genital tract and systemic immunity is only an indirect measure of the utility of the vaccine. Critical to the success of HPV vaccination efforts is the development of type-specific neutralizing antibodies at the cervix to prevent HPV infection of the cervical squamocolumnar junction, where more than 99% of HPV-induced cancers occur in the female lower genital tract. For prophylactic vaccines, antibodies in cervical secretions are likely to be the best indicator of protective immunity. Methods to measure cervical immunity are being perfected and need to be incorporated in future clinical studies examining the efficacy of preventive HPV vaccines.

Therapeutic vaccines for the treatment of HPV infections target the E2, E6, and E7 proteins. Fusions of these proteins VLP have been shown to enhance the immune response produced by these fusion proteins.[112] Because the expression of E6 and E7 is selectively maintained in premalignant and malignant cervical lesions, these proteins are attractive candidates for immunotherapeutic strategies.[113] Cell-mediated immune responses at the cervix will probably be the strongest correlate with the therapeutic efficacy of these vaccines.

Are there promising agents for the chemoprevention of cervical cancer? Chemoprevention is the use of natural and synthetic compounds to intervene in the early precancerous stages of carcinogenesis, before invasive disease begins. Several agents are being investigated in animal and phase I/II human trials as potential chemopreventive agents in cervical cancer and preinvasive disease. Population-based observational studies of diet and cancer can provide clues for new agents to be investigated for safety and efficacy. Other agents have been identified through work done on other tumor sites. What follows is a brief survey of a few of the more promising chemopreventive agents currently being investigated.

The Chemoprevention Working Group to the American Association for Cancer Research considers oral and topical retinoids to be one of the most promising classes of cancer chemoprevention agents.[114] At the molecular level, retinoids decrease expression of HPV E6 and E7 and EGF-R, decrease telomerase activity, and increase transforming growth factor-β (TGF-β).[115-117]

In phase I and II trials, retinoids demonstrated tolerable toxicity and a 50% response rate for topical application of a retinoic acid cream in CIN II.[118-120] A randomized phase III trial demonstrated that this retinoid significantly increased the complete histologic regression rate of CIN II from 27% in the placebo group to 43% in the treatment group.[36] Treatment of CIN II/III with oral administration of a synthetic retinoid, fenretinide (4-HPR), was not effective, which may be related to the low dose used or to the different molecular mechanism of action than conventional retinoids.[121]

Many families of fruits and vegetables contain relatively high concentrations of unique phytochemicals with potential cancer-preventing properties. Diets high in cruciferous vegetables (e.g., broccoli, cabbage, cauliflower, bok-choi, Brussels sprouts) can retard cancer growth in animals, and increased consumption of these vegetables by humans is associated with decreased cancers of the colon, lung, and breast.[122] A specific compound that has been identified in crucifers, indole-3-carbinol (I-3-C), may be able to prevent or halt carcinogenesis.[123] Clinical success has been achieved in the treatment of HPV-induced lesions of the larynx with I-3-C. Further, I-3-C has been shown to strongly induce the activity of an enzyme, found in the liver in humans and other mammals, called CYP1A1/1A2, as well as other P-450 enzymes to a lesser extent. This group of enzymes is known to detoxify or metabolize a variety of chemical carcinogenic substances, and this mechanism may explain its cancer-preventive activity in animals as well as humans.[124] A placebo-controlled pilot study of 27 patients using I-3-C demonstrated a significant regression of CIN at a dose of 400 mg/day, without toxicity (equivalent to the I-3-C present in one-third head of cabbage).[125] A prospective phase III trial is planned to evaluate the efficacy of formulated diindolylmethane (DIM), a biologically active form of I-3-C, in patients with preinvasive cervical cancer.

Serum carotenoid levels have been consistently demonstrated to be negatively associated with cervical dysplasia in epidemiologic studies.[126-128] However, in clinical trials of carotenoids for treatment of high-grade cervical lesions, they have failed to confer protection.[123,129,130] These results may indicate that deficiencies in carotenoids increase the risk of cervical neoplasia but supplementation above threshold levels does not offer significant additional protection. It is possible that supplementation of dietary carotenoids in resource-poor regions may help to reduce the high rates of cervical cancer in endemic areas where diet deficiencies may exist.

Another promising target for chemoprevention is modulation of prostaglandin (PG) production. PGs are arachidonate metabolites that are produced in virtually all mammalian tissues and exhibit diverse biologic activities. Studies suggest that PG synthesis may play a pivotal part in the initiation and promotion of cancer. Prostaglandin E_2 (PGE$_2$) is produced in large amounts by many animal and human tumors, and it appears to support tumor growth by inducing angiogenesis; therefore, targeted inhibition of PGE$_2$ could prevent metastasis.[131] Cervical inflammation may increase the likelihood that HPV infection progresses to high-grade cervical lesions.[60] Cyclooxygenase-2 (COX-2), a PG G/H synthetase that is specifically upregulated in inflammatory processes, has been shown to modulate tumor growth, possibly via inhibition of apoptosis and induction of angiogenesis and proliferation. Moreover, COX-2 is present in the majority of cervical cancers and absent in normal cervical epithelium.[132] The use of selective COX-2 inhibitors (coxibs) for the treatment of low-grade cervical neoplasia may warrant clinical investigation, but they seem unlikely to be therapeutic in high-grade cervical neoplasias, in which genetic damage has already occurred.

Immune modulators could be used to enhance local immunity to HPV and thereby increase the rate of viral clearance. In a placebo-controlled trial of self-administered treatment, 5% imiquimod was able to clear HPV-induced external genital warts in 50% of treated patients, versus 11% in the control arm, with only minimal toxicity.[133] A single preliminary study using topical application of imiquimod to treat cervical dysplasia demonstrated that 50% of patients had elevations in interferon-α (IFN-α) and IFN-γ; 2',5'-oligoadenylate synthetase; and CD4 and CD8 lymphocyte markers.[134] Although such an approach shows promise, it also warrants caution. The nonspecific recruitment of HIV target cells (e.g., dendritic cells) might increase the risk of HIV transmission in high-risk populations, and the extent of vaginal erosion and toxicity has yet to be determined.

Conclusion

In the United States, more than 50% of incident cervical cancer cases occur in women who have never been screened with the Pap smear, suggesting that efforts to improve surveillance in underscreened populations in the United States could be used as a model for targeting underserved populations worldwide. Worldwide, cervical cancer screening and prevention remain a top public health priority, because cervical cancer remains a leading cause of cancer-related deaths in women. Novel screening strategies using DNA probes for detection of high-risk HPV and further development of both prevention and treatment vaccines may have the anticipated impact worldwide, with comparable reductions in incidence and mortality. Clearly, acceptance of this cancer as an infectious disease with the potential for eradication has changed the outlook of public officials, medical personnel, and the scientific community. The identification of HPV as the central cause of cervical cancer has led to the development of new clinical management modalities, treatment strategies, and prophylactic strategies, including large vaccine trials using VLPs as the vaccinogen. Despite these advances, a great deal more research and development are required before the goal of cost-effective cancer prevention is realized.

It is uncertain whether these new advances in screening and triage tests will target or affect those populations that are currently underserved. Specifically, in developing countries where the burden of cervical cancer remains the greatest, and where Pap smear programs cannot be implemented effectively, new and more sensitive assays for HPV (e.g., thin-layer cytology, HPV DNA testing) are unlikely to gain usage because of prohibitive costs. New, low-cost diagnostic techniques are critically needed, but the willingness of pharmaceutical and biotechnology companies to develop such a product is uncertain. Tiered pricing and subsidies from health organizations and governments may be necessary to encourage the development and implementation of new screening diagnostic tools.

Vaccines that prevent HPV infection or promote clearance of an early infection appear promising, but there are a number of concerns. First, the best candidate vaccine, VLPs, is expensive to produce, requires a cold chain for delivery of the vaccine, and requires multiple immunizations. Such a vaccine cannot have worldwide acceptance and implementation until these hurdles are overcome. Second, there is no information about the long-term protection rendered by these vaccines. If the protective immunity lasts months rather than years, there may be little benefit to vaccination. Third, current strategies are primarily targeting HPV-16, but other types are also important causes of cancer, and therefore multivalent vaccines will be needed. In the absence of multitype protection, there will be a continued need for Pap screening.

More specific assays for cervical neoplasia are needed. HPV is a necessary cause of cervical cancer. Most women with an HPV infection do not progress beyond the infection stage. Testing for HPV DNA is highly sensitive but only modestly specific for detection of precancer and cancer, resulting in large numbers of patient referrals. More to the point, most women with LSIL are HPV DNA positive, so there is little advantage to HPV DNA testing these women, and most cases regress in time. If new molecular markers that are linked to progression of HPV to high-grade cervical neoplasia could be identified, they could be used to develop a diagnostic tool that is more specific than an HPV test, thereby reducing referral rates. Potentially, one or more biomarkers could be measured in cervical cells or even in cervical secretions.

Little is understood about the biology of HPV transmission beyond the epidemiologic observation that number of sexual partners is linked to risk of infection. Without a mechanistic understanding of the infectious process, it is likely to be difficult to develop additional strategies for prevention of infection. Most lesions occur on the anterior and posterior portions of the cervix (at 6 and 12 o'clock, respectively), suggesting that the mechanics of intercourse are important for viral transmission, perhaps by means of microtears in epithelia occurring in those locations. If so, it is unknown whether anti-HPV antibodies in cervical secretions developed in response to a vaccine could block the transmission of HPV, because it is uncertain whether virions are exposed to the antibodies in the secretions. New vaginal products (vaginal microbicides) may be similarly ineffective if virions are not exposed to the antimicrobial agent. Finally, it is difficult to interpret a report that

male circumcision is a protective factor for cervical cancer, given the lack of epidemiologic data demonstrating a prophylactic effect of condom use against HPV transmission. Adjudication of these contradictory data will provide a basis for the development of new prophylactic strategies.

ENDOMETRIAL CANCER

Endometrial carcinoma is the most common of all gynecologic cancers. The lifetime risk of being diagnosed with endometrial cancer is approximately 2.7%, and the median age at diagnosis is 65 years. Endometrial cancer is commonly thought of as a "curable cancer," primarily because almost three quarters of cases are diagnosed before disease has spread outside the uterus. The overall 5-year survival rate for all stages is 86%, with disease confined to the uterus having a 97% 5-year survival rate. According to American Cancer Society statistics, 39,300 women developed endometrial cancer, and 6600 died of the disease in 2002.[5] Although the incidence of endometrial cancer is higher in white women than in black women in the United States, the mortality rate is higher in blacks. Endometrial cancer is one of the cancers in which the discrepancy in survival between blacks and whites is the largest.[135,136] This discrepancy is attributable in part to the higher proportion of black women who present with advanced-stage disease and in part to a higher frequency of aggressive, more lethal histologic subtypes (e.g., serous cancers) in black women. Because endometrial cancer is more common among whites, most epidemiologic studies have included few black women. Few studies have conducted centralized pathologic review to determine histologic type or have analyzed results separately by histologic type. Very little is known about risk factors for serous tumors; they do not seem to be related to the hormonal factors that are important for endometrioid tumors. In addition, very few studies have addressed questions of symptoms, recognition of symptoms, and access to care that may result in diagnosis at later stages among black women. In this chapter, the etiology and epidemiology of endometrial cancer are reviewed, along with methods of screening and early detection, and strategies for prevention.

Epidemiology of Endometrial Cancer

Cancer of the endometrium is the most common invasive gynecologic cancer and the fourth most frequently diagnosed cancer among American women. Endometrial cancer is rare before the age of 45 years, but the risk rises sharply among women in their late 40s to middle 60s. The age-adjusted incidence for whites is approximately twice as high as for nonwhites, but mortality rates for nonwhites substantially exceed those of whites. Reasons for these discrepancies are largely unknown.

Rates among American women are among the highest in the world. There is tremendous geographic variation, with an almost fivefold differential in rates from high- to low-risk countries, supporting the notion of a strong influence of environmental factors. Many of these factors have received extensive epidemiologic attention. A number of factors that increase risk have been well defined, including nulliparity, early age at menarche, late age at menopause, obesity, and long-term use of estrogen replacement therapy (ERT). In contrast, multiple births, use of OCs, and cigarette smoking decrease the risk. Many of these factors can be explained by an unopposed estrogen hypothesis, whereby exposure to estrogens unopposed by progesterone or synthetic progestins leads to increased mitotic activity of endometrial cells, increased DNA replication errors, and somatic mutations resulting in malignant phenotype.[137]

Is hormone replacement therapy associated with an increased risk of endometrial cancer? The widespread enthusiasm for use of ERT in the late 1970s led to a major epidemic of endometrial cancers in the United States, which in turn stimulated a series of investigations to assess the specific relationships of risk with usage patterns. Multiple studies showed strong relationships (10- to 20-fold relative risks) with long-term use of ERT.[138] In most studies, cessation of use was associated with a relatively rapid decrease in risk. Results from clinical investigations showing that estrogen-induced endometrial proliferation was reduced by progesterone administration led to a variety of changes in usage patterns, notably to estrogens being prescribed in combination with progestins (particularly for women with intact uteri). Epidemiologic studies have generally shown that the excess risk of endometrial cancer associated with estrogens alone can be counteracted by the addition of a progestin; however, this effect appears to be dependent on the progestin's being given for at least 10 days each month.[139,140] An adverse effect of estrogens on the endometrium is also reflected by studies that show an increased risk of endometrial cancer among breast cancer patients treated with tamoxifen.[141] In contrast to menopausal hormones, users of combination OCs (which contain both an estrogen and a progestin) have been found to have approximately half the risk of nonusers, with long-term users in most studies experiencing even further reductions in risk.[142] This risk reduction appears to persist for at least 3 years after discontinuation, and possibly longer. Several studies suggest that the protective effect of OCs is greatest among nulliparous women and may also be enhanced among nonobese women and among women not exposed to noncontraceptive hormones.[141]

However, the risk/benefit ratio of estrogen plus progestin use must be evaluated. After more than 5 years of follow-up in the Women's Health Initiative (WHI), therapy with estrogen plus progestin was discontinued because of the increased risk of breast cancer and cardiovascular events in the treatment group. This study concluded that the estrogen plus progestin regimen should not be recommended as a viable option for primary prevention of chronic disease.[142]

Users of sequential OCs (which are no longer marketed) have also been found to have substantially higher risks than nonusers of OCs, presumably reflecting that these preparations involve some exposure to a high dose of estrogen unopposed by a progestin.

How do exogenous factors affect a woman's risk of developing endometrial cancer? One of the strongest identified risk factors for endometrial cancer is that of obesity, with studies suggesting a threefold to fourfold differential between women in the highest and lowest quartiles of weight or body mass index (BMI).[144-147] Among postmenopausal women, this association is believed to be largely a result of the conversion of androstenedione to estrone by aromatase in adipose tissue.[137] In premenopausal women, obesity-associated anovulation may be more central. Some studies suggest that body fat distribution may have an independent effect, with high risks seen for women whose weight distributes abdominally rather than peripherally.[145] It has yet to be resolved whether associations with body fat distribution are reflective of unique hormonal profiles. Relationships with timing of obesity and weight cycling are also under scrutiny.

The strong associations with obesity have led to interest in the role of dietary factors.[144,146] Some studies suggest an etiologic role for dietary fat, although inconsistent results prevail. Possibly more consistent are findings relating to effects of micronutrients, with some evidence emerging regarding a possible protective effect of fruits and vegetables. Recent studies have also suggested the possibility that diets high in phytoestrogens or omega-3 fatty acids may reduce endometrial cancer risk,[144,148] although confirmatory results are needed. Given the correlation between BMI, diet, and physical activity, recent studies have assessed risk in relation to levels of activity. Some studies suggest an increased risk associated with inactivity.[144,146,149] Although the hypothesis is biologically appealing given recognized hormonal changes associated with strenuous levels of physical activity, the extent to which physical activity can influence endometrial cancer risk is unclear. Additional studies are needed to address types and timing of physical activity as they relate to risk.

It is likely that there are many pathways to endometrial cancer, and factors that increase risk do not work in isolation from other factors. One central risk factor for endometrial cancer appears to be related to obesity, which affects both the steroid hormone (e.g., estrogen) and the growth hormone (e.g., insulin) pathways. Pathways that involve steroid and growth hormones may unify previously identified isolated risk factors. Existing data suggest a close interrelationship between the estrogen and insulin pathways, in that insulin, insulin-like growth factor (IGF), and estrogen are involved in the regulation of each other. Insulin and IGF-1 appear to be critically involved in the regulation of sex hormone–binding globulin production (SHBP),[150] which in turn modifies the bioavailability of androgens and estrogens.[151] Variations in SHBP are associated with body weight,[152] and obesity increases peripheral estrogen synthesis,[153] which in turn increases the expression of the IGF-1 receptor.[154] Obesity, through effects on different pathways, increases IGF-1 bioavailability and IGF-1 receptor expression, which has the net effect of increasing cell proliferation and decreasing rates of apoptosis, two central events in the development of endometrial cancer.

In several studies, regular consumption of alcoholic beverages has been linked with reductions in endometrial cancer risk. Several of these studies have suggested more pronounced effects among premenopausal or overweight women, suggesting an attenuation in endogenous estrogen levels. An interesting observation is that smokers are at a reduced risk for development of endometrial cancer.[155] In most studies, this effect appears to be restricted to current smokers. This has led to the suggestion that this association may be mediated through changes in hormonal metabolites rather than changes in estrogen levels.

Further support for a role of hormones in the etiology of uterine cancers derives from findings that women with certain endocrine imbalances are at an increased risk.[147] A high risk of endometrial cancer is well established among women with polycystic ovary syndrome, or Stein-Leventhal disease. Women with one of several other diseases (e.g., diabetes, hypertension, thyroid disease) have been suggested as being at elevated risk, although it is unclear whether these effects are independent of those associated with concomitant obesity. There is some evidence that the relationship with diabetes may persist after adjustment for effects of body size.[156] Women with a history of fractures, which are often a reflection of low levels of estrogens, are at a decreased risk for endometrial cancer.[157]

As with breast cancer, there has been recent interest in a possible etiologic role of chemicals known as endocrine disruptors, which include such substances as dichlorodiphenyltrichloroethane (DDT) and polychlorinated biphenyls (PCBs). Given the strong hormonal etiology of uterine cancers, it has been hypothesized there would be an even stronger relationship between these substances and uterine cancers, compared with breast cancer; available studies, however, do not support a relationship.[158] Only limited information is available on other environmental agents, including those received in the occupational setting.

Given the obvious hormonal etiology of endometrial cancer, it is surprising that so few studies have examined the effects of endogenous hormones. The available studies on this topic support the notion that women with higher levels of estrogens and lower levels of sex hormone–binding globulin are at an increased risk for development of postmenopausal endometrial cancers.[137,159] However, the magnitude of association has been moderate and less than would be expected if serum estrogens were the crucial exposure. In addition, estrogen exposure appears to be less important for premenopausal women, for whom anovulation or progesterone deficiency might be paramount. The role of other hormones, including androgens and such

proteins as prolactin and growth factors, is less clear. Also unclear is the extent to which established risk factors might be mediated through hormonal mechanisms. Although it has been widely speculated that the effects of obesity are mediated through high levels of endogenous estrogens, evidence for such pathways remains inconclusive. Tamoxifen and other selective estrogen receptor modulators (SERMs) are used for the prevention of secondary breast cancer among women with estrogen receptor–positive tumors.[160] Although tamoxifen is associated with a 30% to 50% reduction in the development of contralateral breast cancer, it has been associated with up to a threefold increased risk of endometrial cancer.[161] Women undergoing tamoxifen treatment should be screened regularly. Vosse and colleagues[162] suggested an endometrial screening schema that included a baseline assessment before the start of tamoxifen therapy. If the baseline assessment is normal, screening should be performed yearly after 3 years of tamoxifen therapy; if abnormal, yearly surveillance should be done. Symptomatic women should have an immediate investigation.[162]

Is there a genetic predisposition to the development of endometrial cancer? A number of studies suggest an increased risk of endometrial cancer among individuals with a family history of the disease, particularly if affected family members were diagnosed at young ages. Subjects with a family history of colon cancer also have been documented as having an increased risk of endometrial cancer, supporting a role for the dominantly inherited hereditary nonpolyposis colorectal cancer (HNPCC) gene. HNPCC is caused by a germline mutation in one of several identified mismatch repair (MMR) genes and typically presents with microsatellite instability and frequent loss of MMR protein expression in the tumor tissue.[163] Mutation carriers have a lifetime risk of about 50% for endometrial cancer.[164]

Studies are also beginning to emerge regarding effects of several more common genetic polymorphisms, including *p53*, methylenetetrahydrofolate reductase (*MTHFR*) and the cytochrome P-450s (*CYP1A1, CYP17*), with inconclusive results.[165,166] However, there is much enthusiasm that studies that subdivide women according to these genetic markers may be useful in advancing knowledge of poorly understood environmental risk factors. Investigations that pursue obesity-related genes and genes associated with smoking might be particularly informative. Also of interest are effects of tumor-suppressor genes (e.g., *PTEN*) and DNA repair genes (e.g., those silenced by promoter methylation).

Future epidemiologic studies will undoubtedly involve attempts to understand mechanisms underlying many of the established risk factors, to identify biologic markers that allow division of tumors into etiologic distinct subgroups, and to clarify the natural history of the disease, including expansion of knowledge regarding the epidemiology of endometrial hyperplasias.

Etiology of Endometrial Cancer

Are all endometrial cancers alike? Detection of premalignant disease and identification of molecular targets for intervention with chemopreventive agents are major objectives of endometrial cancer prevention. Endometrioid (type I) and nonendometrioid (type II) subtypes of endometrial cancer have fundamentally different mechanisms of carcinogenesis, with profound implications for prevention.[167]

Endometrioid endometrial adenocarcinoma (type I). Endometrioid endometrial adenocarcinoma (type I) may have a premalignant phase that may last months or years.[168] Histologically distinctive aggregates of abnormal endometrial glands are premalignant lesions that increase cancer risk.[169,170] X chromosome inactivation and genetic marker studies have confirmed that these aggregates, often designated as atypical endometrial hyperplasia (AEH),[171] are monoclonal proliferations of genetically altered cells.[172-174] Objective morphometry has more precisely defined their histologic appearance[175] and has led to revised precancer diagnostic criteria designated as endometrial intraepithelial neoplasia (EIN).[176,177] Tracking of those genetic changes that accumulate in stepwise fashion between premalignant and malignant phases of tumorigenesis has confirmed that these putative monoclonal precancers are indeed the physical progenitors of future carcinomas. The premalignant phase is not always linear; it may have branching pathways of genetic diversification yielding a geographic mosaic of related but distinctive epithelial subclones.[178] These subclones have been experimentally resolved using a marker system of altered microsatellites, which are highly informative in those 15% to 20%[179-182] of cases with a microsatellite instability phenotype. A similar process occurs after malignant transformation[183] and is responsible for genesis of tumor heterogeneity, which may confer a nonuniform tumor cell response to systemic therapies. A similar effect is predicted for precancers, in which subclone resistance to systemic therapy may result in chemopreventive failures.

What are the molecular genetic features of type I endometrial cancers? Loss of function of the *PTEN* tumor-suppressor gene occurs very early in endometrioid endometrial neoplasia, allowing use as a marker to track preclinical phases of disease that are attractive targets for chemoprevention. Loss of *PTEN* function is seen in up to 80% of endometrioid endometrial adenocarcinomas,[180,184-187] and a role in carcinogenesis is further supported by *PTEN* inactivation causing endometrial carcinoma in 20% of genetically modified mice.[188] As would be expected for an early genetic event, pathologic loss of PTEN protein occurs in those abnormal gland clusters that comprise histologic precancers (EIN lesions).[187] Somatic inactivation of *PTEN*, however, occurs even before these recognizable histopathologic changes. Forty-three percent of the normal proliferative endogenously cycling endometrium of premenopausal women contains rare PTEN-null glands, in which the basis of inactivation has been shown to be structural alteration of the *PTEN* gene itself (Fig. 66-7).[189] These PTEN-null glands are maintained between menstrual cycles, indicating that at least some affected cells reside in the functional regenerative pool. Clearly, *PTEN* mutation is insufficient for malignant behavior, because only a very small fraction of these initiating events, probably less than 1% to 2%, progress to carcinoma. Chemopreventive reduction of the efficiency by which early "lesions" progress to carcinoma is a possible means of endometrial cancer prevention. Normal endometrial gland PTEN expression increases in an estrogen-rich environment and declines drastically on exposure to progestins.[191] The ambient hormonal environment defines a changing physiologic endometrial gland requirement for PTEN protein, which regulates cell division and enables apoptosis. This is one possible mechanism whereby progestin administration, long known to be antitumorigenic in the endometrium, can obviate the functional consequences of *PTEN* mutation.

Nonendometrioid or papillary serous endometrial cancers (type II)

What are the molecular genetic features of type II endometrial cancers? Nonendometrioid or papillary serous endometrial cancers (type II) are aggressive tumors characterized by defects of the *p53* gene and a paucity of known risk factors. Serous endometrial intraepithelial carcinoma (serous EIC) is a noninvasive form of spread that usually occurs peripheral to a

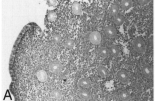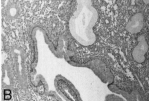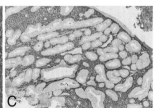

Figure 66–7. PTEN biomarker demarcation of preclinical "latent precancers" and histologically evident premalignant endometrial disease. PTEN-null glands are indistinguishable from PTEN-expressing glands in normal proliferative (Panel A) and anovulatory endometria (Panel B). These constitute subdiagnostic foci that have an extremely high prevalence of 43% and 56%, respectively, in normal cycling and anovulatory women. Progression in inefficient, eventually yielding discrete foci of PTEN-null glands, which are offset from neighbouring PTEN-expressing glands by their crowded architecture and altered cytology (EIN, Panel C). *PTEN* immunohistochemistry with anti-PTEN antibody 6H2.1.[189] (Reprinted with permission of Dr. George L. Mutter[190]).

coexisting invasive focus of tumor.[192,193] Although serous endometrioid carcinomas must begin as a focus of serous EIC, the extreme rarity with which serous EIC is encountered as an isolated finding suggests that this is a very brief phase of tumorigenesis. This is problematic for development of a preinvasive disease screening program, because even if a test were available it would have to be repeated frequently to detect this transient interval. Continuous immune surveillance, such as that which might be invoked by a successful preventative vaccination program, has particular appeal in this disease but has not yet been realized.

Emergent technologies will facilitate discovery of new biomarkers for early detection. High-density microarray comparison of RNA expression between normal and malignant endometrial tissues indicates that about 80% of significant expression differences represent loss in tumors of those genes that are normally transcriptionally active.[194] In contrast, tissue- or fluid-based screening programs best use markers that are uniquely present in pathologic tissues, permitting detection in a sample contaminated by normal tissue. Correspondingly, a unique lesion-associated gene product can confer a high level of therapeutic specificity.

Early Detection of Endometrial Cancer by Image Analysis

Is it possible to discriminate between atypical endometrial hyperplasia and in situ carcinoma?

Histopathologic image analysis refers to a spectrum of techniques that seek to provide objective, quantitative criteria for histopathologic entities. This may occur by the characterization of architectural morphometric features that reflect cellular organization, analysis of the spatial distribution of nuclear chromatin (karyometry), or some combination of the two approaches. Such efforts have a potential for improving knowledge of the neoplastic process, which may lead to improved classification of difficult histopathologic entities (e.g., atypical hyperplasias).

Discriminant analysis using quantitatively derived image analysis features for endometrial disease was first described by Baak and associates in 1981.[195] He and his colleagues measured 12 features related to gland architecture and seven features reflecting nuclear size and shape. In this way, they developed a rule that correctly classified 75% of the test set, which included eight cases each of moderately differentiated and well-differentiated endometrial carcinoma.

Colgan and coworkers,[196] in 1983, applied a similar analytic approach to 24 endometrial curettage specimens from patients with a diagnosis of AEH. They examined three nuclear shape features and developed a discriminant function that identified 83% of cases with a subsequent diagnosis of cancer.

Subsequent work by Baak and coworkers[197] focused on the role of glandular architecture features, specifically volume percent stroma in combination with nuclear axis measurements to identify nonprogressing cases of atypical hyperplasia with an accuracy of 62.5%. Scores derived from a discriminant function that included these terms, as well as a term for outer

surface gland density, could be thresholded to yield a sensitivity of 100% and specificity of 59% for predicting carcinoma.[198] Dunton and associates[199] have applied these analytic techniques to endometrial curettage specimens. They were able to obtain a positive predictive value of 83% and a negative predictive value of 100% for the identification of cases subsequently diagnosed with endometrial carcinoma confirmed at hysterectomy.

More recent work by Mutter and colleagues[187] took these techniques one step further by assessing the expression of *PTEN* tumor-suppressor gene mutations within morphometrically defined endometrial cancer precursors. Such work is crucial because it links quantitatively derived histopathologic features to potential molecular events (i.e., the loss of *PTEN* expression).

Garcia and Bartels focused specifically on nuclear chromatin texture features analysis of endometrial hyperplasias and adenocarcinomas.[200,201] Changes in nuclear chromatin patterns are hypothesized to occur long before any changes in the cellular phenotype, reflecting events earlier in the transformation of the nucleus. Such analysis has yielded curves that quantitatively describe a progression of nuclear abnormality from normal endometrium to simple hyperplasia, atypical hyperplasia, and adenocarcinoma.[200] These investigators further identified statistically distinct populations of nuclei with potentially different risks for malignant progression.[201] Such findings suggest a degree of heterogeneity in the populations of cells involved in these disease entities, as was previously found by Mutter.[187]

Quantitative image analysis is an emerging tool that may assist in the characterization of difficult diagnostic entities (e.g., atypical hyperplasia, grade of adenocarcinoma), as well as advancing the understanding of processes underlying premalignant and malignant endometrial disease.

Prevention of endometrial cancer. The classification of endometrial hyperplasias recognized by the International Society of Gynecological Pathologists is based on the fact that certain endometrial hyperplasias more readily progress to carcinoma.[202] The four classifications—simple hyperplasia, complex hyperplasia, simple hyperplasia with atypia, and complex hyperplasia with atypia—are differentiated based on architectural complexity and the presence of cytologic atypia.[171] Although it is often difficult to distinguish complex atypical hyperplasia from well-differentiated carcinoma,[203] the distinction is important because they exhibit different outcomes. The presence of stromal invasion is the most important histologic criterion for carcinoma.

Kurman and colleagues[171] retrospectively reviewed 170 patients with any degree of endometrial hyperplasia who did not receive any treatment, either medical or surgical, for at least 1 year. The risk of progression to carcinoma was 1% for simple hyperplasia, 3% for complex hyperplasia, 8% for simple atypical hyperplasia, and 29% for complex atypical hyperplasia. The risk for simple atypical versus complex atypical hyperplasia was not statistically different. The most important determinant of risk for progression to carcinoma was the presence of cytologic atypia, with only 2% of hyperplasias without atypia but 23% of atypical hyperplasias progressing to carcinoma. Degrees of atypia, epithelial stratification, and mitotic activity did not predict progression. The time to progression from hyperplasia to carcinoma is long for both nonatypical and atypical hyperplasias, with median times of 9.5 and 4.1 years, respectively. Also, all but 1 of the 13 patients who eventually developed carcinoma were diagnosed with stage I disease. All 13 patients, including one with stage IV disease, were alive without evidence of disease 4 to 25 years after definitive therapy.

What is the best management for atypical endometrial hyperplasia?

In postmenopausal women and in women for whom childbearing is no longer an issue, hysterectomy is the preferred choice of treatment for all atypical hyperplasias because of the relatively high likelihood of an underlying malignancy or of progression to carcinoma. It also effectively eliminates the vaginal bleeding that is almost always associated with endometrial hyperplasia. However, in young, premenopausal women who desire future fertility, a conservative approach may be considered. These women should be initially evaluated with a dilation and curettage (D&C) and contrast-enhanced magnetic resonance imaging. Conservative therapy should also be reserved for those with atypical hyperplasia or with grade 1 endometrioid adenocarcinoma limited to the endometrium who are without evidence of lymphvascular invasion or extrauterine disease. Despite the risk of underlying cancer, most occult malignancies are usually early stage and highly curable and may also respond to conservative therapies.[204-206] Also, atypical hyperplasias tend to either regress or persist, and when they progress they are also usually highly curable.[171] Therefore, in women who desire fertility and who understand all the risks, a conservative approach is acceptable, with many of these women going on to deliver healthy full-term infants.

Chemoprevention of endometrial cancer.

Conservative management of atypical hyperplasia and early-stage endometrial carcinoma has mainly involved the use of progestins, with other agents occasionally used.[204,207-223] Various regimens have been used (Table 66-3) to conservatively treat atypical hyperplasia and well-differentiated early-stage carcinoma, with megestrol acetate (Megace) and medroxyprogesterone acetate (Provera) being the most extensively studied agents. There are only three small retrospective studies on the use of progestins in endometrial carcinoma and equally small retrospective and prospective trials in the treatment of atypical hyperplasia.

Progestin therapy for atypical hyperplasia results in a 50% to 94% rate of complete regression, with the remaining cases exhibiting persistence of hyperplasia and rarely progression to carcinoma.[204,209,211-214] Ferenczy and Gelfand[214] reported a 25% risk (5/20 patients) of developing carcinoma within 2 to 7 years (mean, 5.5 years) after the initial diagnosis while receiving progestin therapy. Perez-Medina and associates[209] reported a 5% risk (1/19 patients) after a 5-year follow-up. All of these cancers were well differentiated with excellent outcomes. The majority of studies with long follow-up have reported no instances of progression to carcinoma.[204,211-213] Recurrences of hyperplasia have been successfully retreated with the same progestins. Median time to treatment response is long (median of 9 months in one study[204]).

The optimal progestin regimen has not been established, but it appears reasonable to start with the most extensively used agent, megestrol acetate, 40 mg/day for at least 14 days every month, and titrate the dosage according to response, keeping in mind that responses may not be seen for many months. Endometrial office sampling should be performed every 3 to 6 months, or sooner if necessary, with a D&C reserved for unclear office results. Continuous progestin therapy may be necessary with close monitoring. Because these conditions are often associated with obesity, exercise and weight loss should also be encouraged.

Table 66–3. Regimens Used for Conservative Treatment of Atypical Endometrial Hyperplasia and Well-Differentiated Early-Stage Endometrioid Carcinoma[203,207-214,217-219]

Agent	Dosage/Schedule (range)	Duration (mo)
Megestrol acetate (Megace)	40-400 mg/day PO continuous followed by nothing, ovulation induction, OCPs, or medroxyprogesterone	2-18
Medroxyprogesterone acetate (MPA, Provera)	10-80 mg/day PO continuous or 10-14 day/mo followed by nothing, ovulation induction, tamoxifen	1.5-24
	500 mg IM q week and triptorelin	3 (MPA)
Hydroxyprogesterone caproate	50-200 mg IM qd then nothing or 500 mg IM 2×/wk	6-12
Cyproterone acetate	50 mg PO 6×/day	1
Norethindrone acetate	1 mg PO qd	2-3
Oral contraceptive pills (OCs)	—	12
Triptorelin	IM q mo in conjunction with MPA	6 (triptorelin)
Danazol	400 mg/day continuous	3-6
Ovulation induction (Clomid)	11-18 cycles followed by IVF in some	—
Bromocriptine	10 mg PO qd	6

The GOG conducted a large, prospective, multi-institutional study to help better define endometrial atypical hyperplasia. It addressed the question of the true incidence of underlying carcinoma in patients diagnosed with atypical hyperplasia on sampling or curettage. Patients underwent immediate hysterectomy within 12 weeks. Among the 302 evaluable cases, there was a greater than 40% incidence of underlying carcinoma.[224] It is clear from this study that the present histopathologic criteria do not provide a distinct separation of AEH from the diagnosis of endometrial carcinoma in situ. The GOG is developing a subsequent study to begin to better classify the precursor lesion of endometrial cancer and to accurately identify women at high risk for coexistent endometrial cancer, based on routine endometrial biopsies. Having a clear diagnostic category that accurately classifies the precursor lesion will provide the target for future chemoprevention trials.

OVARIAN CANCER

Ovarian cancer is the leading cause of death from a gynecologic malignancy among women in the United States, and it is the fourth leading cause of cancer deaths among women overall. In 2002, an estimated 14,000 women died of this disease in the United States alone.[5] The annual incidence of ovarian cancer varies with age, with most diagnoses occurring after menopause. The postmenopausal incidence rate is approximately 5 per 10,000 women; the premenopausal rate is significantly lower.[89] There may also be racial/ethnic differences in age-specific incidence rates. For example, Barnholtz-Sloan and colleagues[225] found that African-American women are younger at the time of diagnosis (61 years, versus 63 years for Caucasian women; $P = .0008$) and tend to have a lower median survival than their Caucasian counterparts (22 versus 32 months, $P < .0001$).

Understanding of the biology of ovarian cancer is slowly advancing, and the molecular events that initiate and promote the carcinogenic process in the ovarian epithelium are the subject of intense scrutiny. This, combined with a growing body of epidemiologic literature that has identified a number of risk factors for the disease, may uncover novel opportunities for primary prevention, screening, and early detection.

Etiology of Ovarian Cancer

Basic understanding of the etiology of epithelial ovarian cancer has to date relied heavily on the epidemiologic literature. In addition to advancing age, reproductive factors and heredity have consistently emerged as important factors in the origin of the disease. The epidemiologic observation that parity and the use of hormonal contraceptives both decreased the risk of ovarian cancer led to the hypothesis that incessant ovulation with subsequent regrowth of the surface epithelium to repair the postovulatory lesion creates an environment for malignant transformation.[226]

More recently, advances in technology and the growing recognition of the importance of genetic change in the process of carcinogenesis has shifted attention from purely epidemiologic studies to analysis of the molecular genetic features of ovarian cancer. If successful, this approach has the potential to produce information that can move forward the efforts to develop more effective prevention and early detection strategies.

It is generally agreed that more than 90% of ovarian cancers arise from the epithelial surface of the ovary, a tissue that is of mesodermal origin. Based on the original "incessant ovulation" theory of Fathalla, studies are now exploring the idea that repeated growth of the surface epithelium results in genetic alterations that can lead to malignant transformation.[227] There is increasing evidence that tumors arise from the sequential accumulation of mutations—either inherited, acquired, or both—which ultimately creates a clonal population of cells that have acquired malignant characteristics.[228] Findings from analysis of human ovarian tumors are also being supported by work in both human and animal cell culture systems. Scientists are now focusing on the genes associated with ovarian cancer and their potential functional significance. The number of genes associated with ovarian cancer continues to grow and represents three major categories: oncogenes, tumor suppressor genes, and MMR genes.

What are the relevant genes involved in ovarian carcinogenesis? Abnormalities in dominant functioning oncogenes, which are often associated with disturbed regulation of cell proliferation, are commonly found in ovarian tumors.[229] The protooncogenes c-*myc*, K-*ras*, and *Akt*, which are involved in cell growth stimulation and cell death pathways, are often overexpressed or mutated in ovarian cancer.[230] *HER2*, a protooncogene that is structurally related to EGF-R, is also overexpressed in ovarian cancer[231]; as with similar findings in breast cancer, it has been suggested to be associated with a poor prognosis.[232] Germline mutations in the tumor suppressor genes *BRCA1* and *BRCA2* are thought to account for up to 10% of all ovarian cancers and up to 85% of hereditary ovarian cancer. Although several hundred mutations in these two genes have been identified, those that appear to be clinically significant lead to premature truncation of protein transcription and defective gene products. These genes appear to function in a complex pathway of cell cycle regulation and gene transcription that also involves the maintenance of genomic stability.[228] The role of *BRCA1* and *BRCA2* in sporadic ovarian cancer is unclear at this time. Another tumor suppressor gene, *p53*, which acts to inhibit inappropriate cellular proliferation by binding to specific areas of DNA, is more commonly mutated in human cancer than any other gene. Although mutations in *p53* are frequent in ovarian cancer, they are acquired as a somatic event rather than being inherited in the germline.[233] Ovarian cancer is also a feature of the HNPCC syndrome, which is attributed to the inheritance of mutations in a family of DNA MMR genes. These genes repair mismatches that occur as a result of nucleotide incorporation errors made during DNA replication. Mutations in these genes result in genomic/microsatellite instability. Approximately 3% of ovarian cancers are thought to be associated with germline mutations of an HNPCC gene.[228]

Despite the progress made in identifying genes associated with ovarian cancer, the underlying molecular mechanisms by which they contribute to the carcinogenic process or to the heterogeneity of histologic subtypes are still largely unknown and are the subject of current research. One family of proteins potentially important to the understanding of ovarian cancer is the family of EGF-Rs. The EGF proteins stimulate a series of mitogenic signaling pathways that alter the activities of kinases, phosphatases, G proteins, and transcription factors. The EGF-R gene is often overexpressed in ovarian cancer; it is postulated to enhance cell growth and adhesiveness and to affect cell-matrix adhesion, integrin expression, protease expression, and migration,[234,235] thereby influencing the proliferative and metastatic potential of the tumor. This is just one example of the kind of genotype/phenotype correlation needed to further understanding of ovarian cancer etiology and to provide new tools for targeted prevention and early detection.

Epidemiology of Ovarian Cancer

Understanding of the factors that increase the risk of developing epithelial ovarian cancer greatly relies on the epidemiologic literature. However, epidemiologic studies vary considerably in size, representative study populations, completeness and accuracy of the data collected, analytic sophistication, sampling error, and a number of other factors (e.g., funding levels, staffing, quality of the instruments, management of data collection and entry) that can affect study findings. Understanding the risk factors for sporadic ovarian cancer may allow physicians to identify women who might benefit from prophylactic oophorectomy, increased surveillance, strategies to reduce risk, or more aggressive screening techniques.

A primary pathway for epithelial ovarian cancer is thought to be oxidative stress and inflammatory processes leading to DNA damage that is not properly repaired.[236-240] Estrogens are known to increase oxidative stress, inflammation, and, of course, epithelial cell turnover. Identified risk factors, particularly estrogen exposure and gene mutations, generally support this theory. Persson[241] concluded from epidemiologic observations and experimental data from animal models that estrogens may have adverse effects, whereas progesterone/progestins may have beneficial effects directly on the ovarian epithelium. DNA damaged induced by reactive oxygen species (ROS) or reactive nitrogen species (RNS) occurs at a position that is not repaired, which leads to malignancy, prevention of apoptosis, cell propagation, and eventual formation of a tumor. ROS and RNS are produced in great numbers in each

cell as a result of aerobic biologic processes required to sustain life. Evolutionarily, several methods and agents have been developed that inhibit the destructive consequences of ROS and RNS. Exogenous and endogenous agents that lower the production of oxidative molecules or neutralize them are clearly candidates for chemopreventive agents.

What are the prevalence and penetrance of the ovarian cancer susceptibility genes? Familial ovarian cancers constitute 5% to 10% of all ovarian cancers.[242] Family history of ovarian cancer is associated with an increased risk, with estimated odds ratios (OR) of 3.1 (95% CI, 2.1 to 4.5) for a woman with a single first-degree relative with ovarian cancer, 4.6 (95% CI, 1.1 to 18.4) for a woman with two or three relatives with ovarian cancer, and 2.9 (95% CI, 1.6 to 5.3) for a woman with second-degree relatives with ovarian cancer.[243,244] Mutations in the BRCA1 and BRCA2 genes have been identified as being associated with the familial risk of breast and ovarian cancer incidence.[232,242] The penetrance of these mutations for ovarian cancer—that is, the likelihood that a carrier of a mutated allele will develop ovarian cancer by a given age—varies considerably. For example, the Anglian Breast Cancer Study Group found ovarian cancer penetrance for BRCA1 and BRCA2 combined to be 22% (6% to 65%) by age 80 years,[245] whereas a Canadian study found that for carriers of BRCA1 mutations, the estimated penetrance by age 80 years was 36%.[246] A British study of 191 women with ovarian cancer diagnosed before 30 years of age found no BRCA1/2 mutations, suggesting that early-onset ovarian cancer may represent an etiologically distinct entity.[247] The reasons for differences in penetrance observed between studies could be methodologic, biologic, environmental, or the result of random chance within populations.[248] Additionally, the lack of knowledge about factors related to penetrance of different mutations (e.g., risk-modifying genes) and the lack of large, well-designed, population-based studies contribute to the current inability to fully understand the role of BRCA1/2 mutations in ovarian cancer.

Published studies indicate that a BRCA1 or BRCA2 mutation has been identified in fewer than 50% of families with aggregation of ovarian or ovarian-breast cancer.[249,250] The current, common assay for mutations misses long deletions, which may account for up to 15% of BRCA1 and BRCA2 mutations.[251] The causes of familial aggregation need to be elucidated. However, it appears that the greater the aggregation, the higher the likelihood that a BRCA1/2 mutation is involved. These genes appear to be tumor suppressors and participate in DNA repair.[250]

What are the environmental and physiologic factors associated with ovarian cancer risk? Reproductive factors that may be associated with an increased risk of ovarian cancer include later age at first full-term pregnancy[252]; factors associated with a decreased risk include increasing lactation,[253] tubal ligation,[254] hysterectomy, late age at menarche, and early menopause.[255] The most established reproductive factor associated with a decreased risk of ovarian cancer is multiparity.[252,255,256] Parity may be an even stronger factor among women with a family history of ovarian cancer.[257] Parity may interact with other protective factors; Ness and colleagues[258] found that tubal ligation and hysterectomy were not protective among nulligravid women.

Polycystic ovary syndrome is the most common endocrine problem among women, affecting approximately 5% of women of reproductive age. Limited data suggest an association between polycystic ovary syndrome and ovarian cancer risk, but further study is required.[259-261]

A significant increased risk of ovarian cancer has been associated with high BMI.[253,262] Purdie and colleagues[262] found that women in the top 15% of the BMI range had an OR of 1.9 (95% CI, 1.3 to 2.6), compared with those in the middle 30%. Stratification by physical activity showed a stronger effect among inactive women (OR, 3.0; 95% CI, 1.3 to 6.9). The relationship between increased BMI and ovarian cancer risk may be related to the fact that increased production of estrogen is associated with increased body fat among both premenopausal and postmenopausal women.

What are the exogenous risk factors for ovarian cancer? The great majority of ovarian cancers are sporadic—that is, there is no history among first- or second-degree relatives, suggesting that environmental factors may play a significant role in ovarian cancer risk. A Finnish nationwide twin study of cancer found that environmental factors (i.e., reproductive and other nongenetic factors) appeared to account for 75% (95% CI, 65% to 85%) of interindividual variation in the risk of cancer in general.[263] Although epidemiologic evidence is generally limited and inconsistent, it is likely the environment (e.g., diet, physical activity) plays a substantial role in the risk of ovarian cancer.

Numerous studies have been conducted that examine dietary risk factors. Generally, high consumption of vegetables and fruits has been associated with a decreased risk, whereas high consumption of animal fat and salted vegetables has been associated with an increased risk.[264,265] However, findings are not consistent. For example, a meta-analysis examining the association between high versus low dietary intake of β-carotene intake and the risk of epithelial ovarian cancer resulted in a summary relative risk (RR) of 0.84 (95% CI, 0.75 to 0.94),[266] but other studies have found no reduction in risk related to β-carotene.[267]

Intense physical activity can affect the menstrual cycle and estrogen levels. For this reason, significant physical activity has been hypothesized to be a potential protective factor. As with dietary factors, study results have been inconclusive. A case-control study in Italy found an adjusted OR of 0.44 for women with the highest level of combined occupational plus leisure-time physical activity,[268] and an American case-control study found leisure-time physical activity to be associated with a reduced risk of ovarian cancer, with the OR ranging from 0.64 to 0.78 at different life periods.[269] After 16 years of follow-up in the Nurses' Health Study, an RR of 0.80 was reported for women with high levels

(>7 hours per week) of physical activity (95% CI, 0.49 to 1.32), but when both frequency and intensity were considered, the activity level was unrelated to the risk of ovarian cancer.[270] The Iowa Women's Health Study, however, found a significant inverse relationship between physical activity and ovarian cancer risk, which is inconsistent with other study findings.[271]

An Australian study found significant increased risk for cigarette smoking (OR, 1.5; 95% CI, 1.2 to 1.9).[272] The risk was greater for ovarian cancers of borderline malignancy (OR, 2.4; 95% CI, 1.4 to 4.1) than for invasive tumors (OR, 1.7; 95% CI, 1.2 to 2.4), and the histologic subtype most strongly associated was the mucinous subtype among both current smokers (OR, 3.2; 95% CI, 1.8 and 5.7) and past smokers (OR, 2.3; 95% CI, 1.3 to 3.9). Similar results were found in the Cancer and Steroid Hormone Study, which showed no overall cancer risk in relation to tobacco smoking, but the OR of mucinous epithelial ovarian cancer for women who had ever smoked was 2.3 (95% CI, 1.4 to 3.9), and for current smokers it was 2.9 (95% CI, 1.7 to 4.9).[273] An American population-based case-control study investigated tobacco exposure in 549 women with newly diagnosed epithelial ovarian cancer and in 516 control women and found that there was no increase in risk for ovarian cancer overall associated with tobacco use.[274]

The use of aspirin and other nonsteroidal anti-inflammatory drugs (NSAIDs) has been associated with a lower risk of ovarian cancer, possibly in relation to inflammatory processes induced during ovulation, but the data again are inconsistent.[264,275-277]

What is the role of exogenous hormones and ovarian cancer risk? The Nurses' Health Study, which monitored subjects between 1976 and 1988, did not find any association between OC use and risk of ovarian cancer.[278] Schildkraut and coworkers[279] found that OC formulations with high progestin potency appeared to be associated with a greater reduction in ovarian cancer risk than those with low progestin potency. This suggests that the underlying mechanisms of OCs may include inhibition of ovulation or some direct biologic effects of progestins. Ness and associates[280] found that the use of low-estrogen/low-progestin pills had a risk reduction that was identical to that for high-estrogen/high-progestin pills (OR, 0.5; 95% CI, 0.3 to 0.6; and OR, 0.5; 95% CI, 0.3 to 0.7, respectively).

ERT and hormone replacement therapy (HRT) with sequential progestins were associated with an increased risk of ovarian cancer in a large, population-based case-control study in Sweden.[281] ERT with continuous progestins was not associated with an increased risk. The ORs were modest (1.43 and 1.54) for ever-use of unopposed estrogen and sequential progestin, respectively. A prospective study of ERT use among postmenopausal women found that estrogen use for 10 or more years was associated with increased risk of ovarian cancer mortality.[282] Results across case-control studies, however, have not been consistent.[256,283] An evaluation of a 1979-1998 cohort study found that women who used estrogen-only replacement therapy, particularly for 10 years or longer, were at significantly increased risk of ovarian cancer, whereas women who used short-term estrogen-progestin replacement therapy were not at increased risk.[284] This result should be further investigated.

Infertility appears to be a significant risk factor for ovarian cancer; furthermore, the risk of ovarian cancer appears to be limited to those women who remain childless despite treatment.[285-290] There may be genetic mechanisms responsible for the increased risk of ovarian cancer among infertile women.[285,289] Others have proposed a potential link between ovarian cancer and fertility drugs.[290]

Early Detection of Ovarian Cancer

Which women should be screened for ovarian cancer?
Ovarian cancer is usually diagnosed in late stages, which are associated with a poorer 5-year survival rate.[291] Many women lack consistent symptoms of ovarian cancer until they have stage III or IV disease. In a review of women younger than 40 years of age with epithelial ovarian cancer, Plaxe and associates[292] found that 44% of the stage I tumors were asymptomatic. The three modalities currently used for early detection of ovarian cancer are ultrasound, CA-125 measurement, and pelvic examination, but the National Institutes of Health consensus report in 1994 stated that there is no single acceptable screening test for ovarian cancer, and there is no evidence that combining these modalities has an acceptable sensitivity and specificity.[293]

In their study on transvaginal ultrasound in asymptomatic women, Van Nagell and colleagues[294] found that only 30% of women with known ovarian masses on ultrasound had an abnormal pelvic examination. Pelvic examination lacks sensitivity, and CA-125 is elevated in only 50% of women with stage I cancers. However, CA-125 frequently is elevated in benign conditions such as endometriosis, benign ovarian cysts, and bowel disease. Ultrasound showed a positive predictive value of only 3.1% in an analysis of five studies, although specificity was on average 95%, which indicates many women will undergo an operative procedure without a diagnosis of malignancy.[295] The ovaries can be visualized 87% of the time in premenopausal patients and 57% of the time in postmenopausal patients.[296]

Noninvasive imaging techniques such as transvaginal ultrasound and color Doppler imaging have been evaluated for their ability to detect organ-confined curable ovarian cancer. Although sensitivities approaching 100% can be achieved by these techniques, their specificities and the frequent invasive procedures required to confirm the abnormal sonographic findings have led to caution regarding the widespread use of transvaginal ultrasound for the early detection of ovarian cancer.[297] Ultrasound findings may predict a higher risk of malignancy. In a series of 240 women, 25% of the ovaries found to have vegetations on ultrasound had a malignancy, whereas 17% of mixed solid and cystic structures had a malignancy.[298] Therefore, high-risk features on ultrasound are not highly predictive of an early malignancy.

Hereditary ovarian cancer syndromes account for approximately 5% to 10% of the cases. Because of the increased risk of ovarian cancer in these families, many studies have focused on this patient population for both screening and early detection. In one study, 180 patients underwent exploratory laparoscopy or laparotomy for ultrasound abnormalities. Seventeen ovarian cancers were detected: 11 at stage I; 3 at stage II; and 3 at stage III. Only three patients with stage I cancers had a palpable ovarian mass on clinical examination.[299] If the ovaries can be visualized with ultrasound, most ovarian enlargements can be found, but the ovary must be enlarged or have abnormal projections to differentiate benign from malignant conditions, and even then they are not reliable findings.[298]

Increased levels of CA-125 are detected in a number of benign conditions, including endometriosis. CA-125 is most consistently elevated in epithelial ovarian cancer, but it can be expressed in a number of other cancers in gynecologic (endometrial, fallopian tube) and nongynecologic (pancreatic, breast, colon, and lung) sites.[300] Muto and colleagues[296] found variations in CA-125 values in premenopausal patients, associated with variations of the menstrual cycle. Ten percent of all premenopausal patients initially had an abnormal CA-125 level, but 84% of these values normalized by the next menstrual cycle.[296] The use of serum tumor markers for the early detection of ovarian cancer has been limited because of their low sensitivity and low positive predictive value. CA-125 levels are elevated in only about one half of women with stage I ovarian cancer, so researchers have focused on using the serial measurement of complementary markers to improve the sensitivity, specificity, and positive predictive value of this approach for screening.[298-301] The Prostate, Lung, Colon and Ovarian (PLCO) screening trial is currently evaluating CA-125 as a potential screening tool to prevent deaths from ovarian cancer. Results from this trial should be available by 2010-2013.

What methods are under study for ovarian cancer screening? Two new technologies that hold promise for improving the accuracy of screening in ovarian cancer are optical spectroscopy and mass spectroscopy. Optical spectroscopy, in particular fluorescence spectroscopy, has been used in the cervix, in head and neck disease, and most recently in the ovary to evaluate the surface and subsurface of the ovary for defects that are not visible normally. Using changes in the redox of cells and the increase in angioneogenesis that develops as cells progress to cancer, small variations can be identified by fluorescence spectroscopy when a probe is placed on the ovary.[302]

An exploratory study using mass spectroscopy to separate serum proteins based on mass and charge revealed five peaks in intensities of molecular weights (mass/charge) that were consistently different in the women with known ovarian cancer and women who were being screened because of their high-risk status. Proteins were selectively bound to protein chips (Ciphergen), and mass spectrometry was conducted with surface-enhanced laser desorption and ionization (SELDI), using pattern detection software (Correlogic Systems) for the analysis. Intriguingly, there was a decrease in the intensity of these peaks in women with cancer. The identified serum protein patterns are not yet associated with individual proteins or protein families, and there may be multiple proteins with molecular weights in five mass/charge positions (534, 989, 2111, 2251, and 2465).[303] Protein identification and sequencing is currently pending. These peaks correctly identified all ovarian cancer cases, including early-stage disease, in a validation set. Complex serum proteomic patterns may indicate a state of cancer, and preliminary results are encouraging, with a sensitivity of 100% and a specificity of 95% in differentiating women with cancer from those who do not appear to have cancer.[303]

To date, screening programs are not feasible because of the very low positive predictive value in the general population of any currently available screening protocol. However, screening for known genetic mutations among members of families with aggregation of ovarian or ovarian-breast cancer is appropriate to determine level of risk.

Prevention of Ovarian Cancer

Epidemiologic studies have identified categories of possible chemopreventive agents for ovarian cancer. These include OCs, dietary antioxidants, and analgesics. All of these are thought to inhibit production of ROS/RNS or to neutralize them in various manners. Epidemiologic studies are seldom definitive. In vitro and animal studies are useful in gaining an understanding of an agent's biologic interactions with ROS/RNS and its possible usefulness in preventing ovarian cancer. However, these studies too are seldom definitive. Different cell lines or even the "same" cell lines in different laboratories give different results, and laboratory animals and humans do not necessarily process proteins, hormones, and chemicals in the same or even similar manners. Therefore, the efficacy of a candidate chemopreventive agent and its side effect profile may not be similar between laboratory animals and humans.

The general population can be divided into three categories with respect to ovarian cancer risk: very high risk (BRCA1/2 mutation); high risk (familial aggregation despite a lack of a segregating BRCA1/2 mutation); medium risk (e.g., nulliparous women who have not taken OCs); "normal" or low risk (the general population). Phase III and phase IV studies that have ovarian cancer incidence as the end point can be smaller and shorter because of the increased expected incidence of ovarian cancer if the subjects come from the very high- or high-risk populations. However, the pathways to ovarian cancer may be different among these various groups, so an agent that is preventive in populations with very high or high risk may not be preventive in the medium- or normal-risk populations. It is also possible that the pathways to ovarian cancer are the same but that members of the very high- or high-risk populations have such a high load of the causative agents, compared with the lower-risk populations, that an agent that may be preventive in the latter populations is overwhelmed in the higher-risk groups. For example, women in the high-risk population may constantly experience significantly more oxidative DNA damage than women in the low-risk population.

Pregnancy confers marked protection against subsequent epithelial ovarian cancer. A first pregnancy lowers the risk of ovarian cancer by 35%, and each subsequent pregnancy lowers the risk by an additional 15%. The protective effect of pregnancy occurs regardless of fertility history, is not age dependent, and is not abrogated in the setting of multiple births.[286,304-307]

The evidence supporting a protective effect of breastfeeding against epithelial ovarian cancer risk is weak. Breastfeeding has not been consistently shown to be associated with lower ovarian cancer risk. Some studies suggest a 10% to 20% decrease in ovarian cancer risk associated with breastfeeding. The impact of breastfeeding on ovarian cancer risk appears to be greatest for the first 6 months of lactation, with no apparent increase in ovarian cancer protection with longer-term lactation.[286,308]

What surgical procedures are indicated in women with a family history of ovarian cancer? Hysterectomy has been shown to be associated with a lower subsequent risk of developing epithelial ovarian cancer. The protective effect of hysterectomy is quite significant. Hysterectomy lowers ovarian cancer risk by 50%, and this protective effect does not wane over time.[286,304] Tubal ligation has not been universally shown to lower ovarian cancer risk. Published studies have demonstrated either no impact of tubal ligation, or a decrease in risk as great as 40%.[242,304,306]

Oophorectomy lowers the risk of subsequent epithelial ovarian cancer by more than 90%. As a method of ovarian cancer prevention, this should be considered only for women who are at extremely high risk for ovarian cancer, such as those who have BRCA1 or BRCA2 mutations, or women with a familial pattern of ovarian cancer incidence that would suggest a very significant risk of developing epithelial ovarian cancer. Even in these high-risk women, oophorectomy is not completely protective, in that a small proportion can subsequently develop intraperitoneal carcinomatosis, indistinguishable from ovarian cancer, arising from the peritoneal surfaces.[309]

The potential benefits of prophylactic oophorectomy must be weighed against its adverse consequences, including surgical risk, the psychological impact of castration, and the potential subsequent risks of cardiovascular and osteoporosis-related complications. One of the most important issues to consider regarding prophylactic oophorectomy in young women is the issue of compliance with subsequent HRT. Oophorectomy not followed by HRT may be associated with a significant risk of cardiovascular and fracture-related morbidity and mortality associated with estrogen deprivation, especially in young women. Using published figures of ERT compliance, Spearoff and colleagues[310] estimated that prophylactic oophorectomy may lead to a shorter life expectancy for low-risk women age 45 years or younger at the time of the operation. A similar analysis in high-risk women is lacking.

What is the role of chemopreventive agents in the prevention of ovarian cancer?

The ovarian epithelium is a hormonally responsive target organ that expresses receptors for most members of the steroid hormone superfamily, including receptors for progestins, retinoids, androgens, and vitamin D. Although little is known regarding the physiologic roles of these steroid hormones within the ovarian epithelium, there is mounting epidemiologic and laboratory evidence to suggest that they have direct and potent biologic effects on the ovarian epithelium relevant to the prevention of ovarian cancer. Progestins, retinoids, and vitamin D have been shown to exert a broad range of common biologic effects in epithelial cells, including induction of apoptosis, upregulation of TGF-β, cellular differentiation, and inhibition of proliferation. It is interesting to speculate that these agents may ultimately work via common molecular pathways in the epithelial cells. In addition to hormonal agents, there is growing evidence that the NSAIDs may have ovarian cancer preventive effects.

Epidemiologic and laboratory evidence suggests a potential role for retinoids as preventive agents for ovarian cancer.[311] Retinoids are natural and synthetic derivatives of vitamin A. They have great potential for cancer prevention because of their broad range of important biologic effects on epithelial cells, including inhibition of cellular proliferation, induction of cellular differentiation, induction of apoptosis, cytostatic activity, and induction of TGF-β. A high dietary intake of β-carotene has been associated with a decreased ovarian cancer risk, whereas low serum retinol levels have been associated with an increased risk of ovarian cancer. In vitro, it has been reported that the growth of human ovarian carcinoma cell lines and normal human ovarian epithelium is inhibited by retinoids.[312] The mechanism underlying this effect may involve induction of TGF-β or apoptosis, or both, in ovarian epithelial cells. The most significant evidence supporting a rationale for retinoids as chemopreventive agents for ovarian cancer is that of an Italian study, which suggests an ovarian cancer preventive effect from the retinoid 4-HPR. Among women randomly assigned to receive either 4-HPR or placebo in a trial designed to evaluate 4-HPR as a chemopreventive agent for breast carcinoma, significantly fewer ovarian cancer cases were noted in the 4-HPR group, compared with controls.[313] Although 4-HPR was protective during the period of administration, the ovarian cancer incidence rose after treatment was discontinued.[314]

Vitamin D is a fat-soluble vitamin that is essential as a positive regulator of calcium homeostasis. In the skin, 7-dehydrocholesterol (provitamin D_3) is photolyzed by ultraviolet light to previtamin D_3, which spontaneously isomerizes to vitamin D_3. Vitamin D_3 (cholecalciferol) is converted into an active hormone by hydroxylation reactions that occur in the liver to produce 25-hydroxyvitamin D_3, which is then converted in the kidneys to produce 1,25-dihydroxyvitamin D_3 (1,25-dihydroxycholecalciferol, or 1,25(OH)$_2$D$_3$, known as calcitriol), which is transported through the blood to target organs containing the vitamin D receptor. 1,25-dihydroxyvitamin D_3 partitions into cells by virtue of its lipophilicity, binds to intracellular receptors, and translocates to the nucleus, where the vitamin D/receptor complex controls the transcription of numerous genes. The vitamin D receptor and the retinoic acid receptors share strong homology and readily dimerize, making it likely that vitamin D and retinoids have common signaling pathways in the cell.[315]

Vitamin D has been shown to have diverse biologic effects in epithelial cells relevant to cancer prevention, including retardation of growth, induction of cellular differentiation, induction of apoptosis, and upregulation of TGF-β.[316] With regard to ovarian cancer, a 1994 study correlated population-based data regarding ovarian cancer mortality in large cities across the United States with geographically based long-term sunlight data reported by the National Oceanic and Atmospheric Administration. The study demonstrated a statistically significant inverse correlation between regional sunlight exposure and ovarian mortality risk.[317] Given that sunlight induces production of native vitamin D in the skin, it is interesting to speculate that vitamin D might confer protection against ovarian cancer via direct biologic effects on nonmalignant ovarian epithelium; for example, through induction of apoptosis or TGF-β in the ovarian epithelium, leading to selective removal of nonmalignant but genetically damaged epithelial cells.

OC use has been shown consistently to be protective against ovarian cancer in observational studies. Routine use of OCs for as little as 3 years is associated with a 30% to 50% reduction in ovarian cancer risk. A protective affect has been described with as little as 6 months of use and increases with the duration of use.[318] The protective effect is independent of fertility status as well as other factors (e.g., prior history of hysterectomy) and persists for as long as 15 to 20 years after discontinuation of use.[286,304,305,318,319] Data are inconclusive with regard to the protective effect of OCs in women who are at genetic risk for ovarian cancer. Results from two case-control studies suggest a protective effect of OC use in women with either a strong family history of ovarian cancer or known *BRCA1* and *BRCA2* mutations[320,321]; however, another study from Israel suggested no protective effect.[322]

Essentially all estrogen/progesterone combination OCs have been shown to be protective. The data regarding progestin-only contraceptives are limited at this time. A World Health Organization (WHO) study evaluating the protective effect of depot medroxyprogesterone acetate (DMPA) did not find an overall reduced risk of ovarian cancer in young women.[323] However, a subsequent reevaluation of the WHO data that excluded mucinous tumors suggested a significant protective effect of DMPA use on ovarian cancer risk.[319] Data with regard to the impact of the hormonal potency and dosage of OCs and subsequent ovarian cancer risk are limited. One study suggested a similar protective effect associated with all combination OCs, regardless of the potency of the estrogen or the progestin component, but another study suggested that progestin-potent combination OCs may be twice as protective against ovarian cancer risk, compared with formulations that contain weak progestins.[279,280]

Although extensive epidemiologic evidence has linked OC use with a reduced risk of ovarian cancer, the biologic mechanisms underlying the protecting effects of OCs have been largely unknown. Previously, it was presumed that the primary mechanism underlying these protective effects related to the inhibitory effects of these agents on ovulation, with the supposition that OCs reduce ovulation-induced damage in the ovarian epithelium, thereby lowering subsequent ovarian cancer risk. More recently, however, an alternative biologic mechanism was suggested. A 3-year study in primates demonstrated that the progestin component of an OC has a potent effect on apoptotic and TGF-β signaling pathways in the ovarian epithelium.[324,325] These two molecular events have been strongly implicated in cancer prevention in vivo and are believed to underlie the protective effects of other well-known chemopreventive agents, such as the retinoids and tamoxifen. The finding that progestins activate these critical pathways in the ovarian epithelium raises the possibility that progestin-mediated biologic effects may underlie the ovarian cancer protective effects of OCs, providing a rationale for examining progestins as potential ovarian cancer preventive agents.

Several epidemiologic studies have suggested that use of NSAIDs may lower ovarian cancer risk.[276,277,326-328] To date, published results have been inconsistent, with some studies suggesting a protective effect associated with use of acetaminophen, but not aspirin or ibuprofen, and others suggesting a protective effect from aspirin use. Several biologic mechanisms have been proposed to account for the chemopreventive effects of NSAIDs, including inhibition of COX, enhancement of the immune response, and induction of apoptosis.[277,329,330] COX-2 is more often expressed in ovarian carcinoma than in tumors of low malignant potential or in normal ovarian tissue. In fact, COX-2 positivity was found in a higher percentage of unresponsive cases (80.0%) than in those responding to chemotherapy (35.7%); this may indicate increased chemopreventive potential of agents that inhibit COX-2.[331,332] The chemopreventive effects of COX inhibitors are related to their ability to inhibit PG synthesis. PGs are suspected to be involved in carcinogenesis through increased mutagenesis, immune suppression, and facilitation of tumor promotion. The anticarcinogenic effects of COX inhibitors may be independent of their effects on PG synthesis and may be related to their ability to induce the apoptotic response.[333]

Summary

The effects of estrogen are implicated in ovarian cancer causation. Nulliparity, *BRCA1* or *BRCA2* deleterious mutations, and family history are established risk factors. Early age at menarche, irregular menstruation, late age at menopause, unopposed or sequential HRT, high BMI, use of talc powder, smoking, and dietary fat intake may be risk factors. Tubal ligation may be a protective factor; hysterectomy and OC use are established protective factors. Dietary vegetables, β-carotene, use of anti-inflammatory medications, and physical exercise may be protective. Environmental exposures need to be studied more thoroughly, with improved study designs.

VULVAR CARCINOMA

Vulvar carcinoma is the fourth most common genital tract malignancy in women, representing 3% to 5% of gynecologic malignancies and affecting an estimated 3600 women in the United States in 2001. The majority of cancers are squamous in origin, with occasional cases of basal cell carcinoma, melanoma, adenocarcinoma, and Paget's disease. Vulvar cancer appears to the clinician to involve two completely different patient populations, with a bimodal age distribution. Younger women typically have a previous history of cervical dysplasia and coexistent HPV-related grade 3 vulvar intraepithelial neoplasia (VIN III). Older women usually have a solitary, often neglected, HPV-negative lesion associated with an underlying benign vulvar chronic irritation. Early detection and prevention strategies must be targeted to the appropriate patient population.

Etiology of Vulvar Cancer

Vulvar cancer tends to be a disease of older women, with a mean age at diagnosis of approximately 65 years. As the population ages, there will be a greater number of elderly women at risk for vulvar carcinoma. Evidence exists for two distinct types of vulvar carcinoma with different etiologies. Tumors in older women are often unifocal and may be associated with chronic vulvar inflammation of long-standing duration, such as lichen sclerosus or hyperplastic dystrophy. These keratinizing squamous cell carcinomas have associated HPV changes in only 6% of cases. Although retrospective studies indicate that up to 50% of vulvar carcinomas are related to hyperplastic dystrophies and lichen sclerosus, it is estimated that only 5% of women with vulvar dystrophies would develop invasive carcinoma. Cancers found in younger women tend to be multifocal with adjacent VIN and to have a basaloid or warty histology. Almost 90% are associated with HPV infection, particularly HPV-16. Thirty-eight percent of women with basaloid-warty carcinoma in Trimble's series were younger than 55 years of age, compared with only 17% of those with classic keratinizing squamous cancers typically found in the elderly.[334] Other associated risk factors are immunosuppression from chronic steroid use, diabetes, HIV infection, smoking, and a history of other lower genital tract dysplasia or neoplasia.

What is the pathogenesis of vulvar cancer? The pathogenesis of vulvar cancer is not well understood. High-grade VIN is the direct precursor lesion, with an estimate cumulative risk of invasive cancer development of 6% per year from the time of diagnosis.[335] HPV is the dominant causative factor in a subset of cases that are more likely to occur in younger individuals who demonstrate multiple vulvar (and other lower genital tract) intraepithelial lesions, supporting the "field effect" of HPV exposure.[336] Infection with HPV-16 is most common, implying that HPV-16 cervical vaccine development may also have a therapeutic or prophylactic role in this disease.[337] HPV-negative tumors usually occur in older women with a history of chronic inflammation or other chronic vulvar dystrophies such as epithelial hyperplasia or lichen sclerosis. In classic epidemiologic studies, conditions that alter the local skin environment, such as heavy smoking, diabetes, and chronic immunosuppression, also increase the risk of vulvar neoplasia. It is clear that all women exposed to HPV or other chronic inflammatory risk factors do not progress to vulvar CIS or to invasive cancer. The additional required steps in the pathogenesis of this disease have yet to be elucidated.

Molecular pathways involved in vulvar carcinogenesis have been explored, although this field is still in its infancy. The discovery of key pathways common to HPV-positive and -negative tumors will permit universal targets for molecular therapeutics or rational chemoprevention strategies. If the molecular mechanisms promoting disease are vastly different between HPV-positive and -negative tumors, then rational therapeutic decisions may be made after clinical HPV testing. Although the molecular studies to date are based on cell line studies in vitro or on predominant archival tissue studies of small sample size, and in some cases on limited techniques, key targets in cell cycle regulation, angiogenesis, tyrosine kinase pathways, and overall genomic instability have been investigated as major molecular targets in vulvar carcinogenesis.

Aberration in genomic DNA, such as chromosomal regional loss or gene amplification, have been described in both HPV-positive and -negative invasive cancers and associated preinvasive lesions. Studies of loss of heterozygosity (LOH) and of comparative genome hybridization (CGH) have been the primary techniques used to identify gene regions involved in loss of suspected tumor suppressor genes or gain of oncogenes as molecular targets in vulvar carcinogenesis. Genomic instability, as measured by chromosome fractional regional loss index (FRL), is more pronounced in HPV-negative tumors,[338,339] suggesting that additional DNA damage is necessary to promote HPV-negative tumors. Genomic lesions that are more common in HPV-negative epithelia include loss of 3p, 4p, and 5q[339]; gain of 3 and 8p[340]; mutations in p53,[338] and microsatellite instability phenotype.[341] The degree of these genomic aberrations increase across the spectrum of lesions, and they are seen both in HPV-positive precursor lesions and in the epithelial hyperplasia and lichen sclerosis lesions adjacent to the vulvar cancers, suggesting these are early events in carcinogenesis.

Loss of cell cycle regulation is a hallmark of neoplasia. Indirect measures of cellular proliferation or direct measures of cyclin proteins or checkpoint proteins have been studied as prognostic indicators for preinvasive and invasive disease. Although limitations of immunohistochemical analyses exist for these studies, cyclin D_1 overexpression was seen in more than one half of invasive vulvar squamous cell carcinomas (VSCCs) and adjacent lichen sclerosis lesions but was less common in the hyperplastic and VIN lesions.[342] Aberrant cyclin D_1 expression may be a viable target for therapeutic antisense development.[343] The prognostic role of aberrant pRb and TP53 expression is less clear. Aberrant expression by immunohistochemistry of pRb and pRb2/p130 is seen in invasive VSCC.[342,344] Aberrant p53 expression is seen in vulvar cancer and in some adjacent lesions.[345-349] Mutations in the p53 gene appear to be more common in the HPV-negative tumors[338,350-355]; however, the role of p53 abnormalities as a prognostic factor for disease progression or death is controversial.[348,355-357] Proliferation as an indirect index of cell cycle dysregulation measured by Ki-67 expression is seen in preinvasive and invasive vulvar lesions.[357-360] The pattern and degree of expression may demonstrate prognostic utility, but this must be confirmed in much larger studies.[357-359,361]

Signal transduction pathways regulate many of the cellular mechanisms for growth and differentiation. Aberrations in these pathways lead to cellular dedifferentiation, aberrant angiogenesis, and metastases. Many kinases involved in these pathways, such as EGF-R and vascular epidermal growth factor receptor (VEGF-R), are targets for small-molecule therapeutics. Aberrations in these receptors and ligands may be therapeutic targets in vulvar cancer and dysplasia. EGF-R expression and overexpression of its ligands, EGF and TGF-α are seen in the majority of invasive vulvar cancers.[362] EGF-R expression increases as disease progresses.[363] Preclinical in vivo studies demonstrate synergistic cytotoxicity when vulvar cancer xenografts are treated with ZD1839, an EGF-R inhibitor, and a platinum derivative.[364] Angiogenesis has been assessed in vulvar lesions using immunohistochemical measures of VEGF, platelet-derived growth factor (PDGF), and microvessel density counts. VEGF is present in the majority of invasive lesions and in the minority of VIN lesions[365]; it has also been measured in the serum of patients with vulvar carcinoma.[366] It appears have increased expression with increasing grade of the lesion, in the presence of HPV-16,[367] and is also associated with increased microvessel density.[368,369] Further understanding of these and similar pathways may lead to therapeutic targets for both invasive cancer and dysplasia.

Similarities exist between cervical cancers and, in particular, the HPV-positive vulvar cancers. The role of local immunity is not well understood in cervical cancer, and even less so for vulvar cancer. Clinical experience suggests some reversal of disease with immune modulators such as imiquimod 5%,[134,370] but the molecular basis is not well understood. Further understanding of the complex pathways involved in local immunity, cell-cell interactions, and complex epithelial cell regulation will help in the development of rational treatment and chemopreventive strategies.

Epidemiology of Vulvar Intraepithelial Neoplasia

What is the natural history of vulvar intraepithelial neoplasia? Vulvar carcinoma theoretically results from malignant transformation of a vulvar CIS, as is seen with cervical squamous lesions. The natural history of VIN is less well understood than that of squamous lesions of the cervix. The incidence of vulvar dysplasia has increased over the last 20 years, particularly among younger women. A recent report from Austria demonstrated a 307% increase in the overall incidence of high-grade VIN, and a 394% increase among women younger than 50 years of age, between 1985 and 1998.[371] In a review of Surveillance, Epidemiology and End Results (SEER) data, Sturgeon and colleagues[372] found that the incidence of VIN III almost doubled between 1973-1976 and 1985-1987, from 1.1 to 2.1 per 100,000 woman-years. Factors implicated in this increase include increased HPV infection, increased surveillance, tobacco use, and immunosuppression (HIV infection, organ transplantation, or diabetes).

Clinical presentation of vulvar intraepithelial neoplasia. Most women present with pruritus and an identifiable lesion. These lesions may appear scaly, white, red, or hyperpigmented. Less common symptoms include pain and bleeding. There is often a delay of many years between onset of symptoms and diagnosis, in part because patients self-medicate with a variety of over-the-counter preparations rather than seeking care, and also because physicians may not biopsy liberally. Any patient with symptoms lasting longer than 2 weeks deserves a thorough examination and biopsy.

To adequately evaluate a patient with a vulvar lesion, 5% acetic acid is applied to the vulva for 5 minutes, and then the area is examined with the naked eye or with a handheld magnifying glass. The entire vulva, including the hair-bearing, perianal, and periclitoral regions, should be examined for suspicious ulcerations and hyperpigmented, acetowhite, or gross warty lesions. An underlying malignancy may be present in 7% to 22% of patients who undergo surgical excision for vulvar CIS. Up to 5% of patients have multifocal disease and may require multiple punch biopsies.

Early Detection of Vulvar Carcinoma

Over the past 40 years, tremendous advances have been made in the prevention of cervical carcinoma.[373,374] However, despite the fact that many vulvar carcinomas are recognized to share a common etiology with cervical carcinomas,[375] the same progress has not been made in vulvar cancer. The incidence of vulvar carcinoma has changed little, and it may be increasing in some populations.

What are the barriers to progress in the prevention of vulvar cancer? Detailed examination of the vulva is often underemphasized during the routine gynecologic examination unless the patient presents with localized symptomatology. This fact is compounded by the both lack of awareness and the reluctance of many women to undertake vulvar self-examination on a regular basis. Although the significance of breast self-examination has been accepted, similar awareness has not been brought to the issue self-examination of the vulva. Vulvar self-examination may provide a key to reducing the incidence of squamous carcinoma and decreasing the mortality associated with other vulvar tumors, if they can be detected at an early stage. Patients should be counseled about the importance of regular vulvar self-examination. Instructions for vulvar self-examination are outlined in Table 66-4.

The sensitivity of self-examination techniques may be enhanced by patient self-collection of vaginal, vulvar, and urine samples with subsequent HPV testing using HPV DNA hybrid capture technology.[376] Vulvoscopy techniques, conceptually similar to colposcopy used in the detection of cervical carcinoma, have also shown some promise.[377,378]

Prevention of Vulvar Carcinoma

The association of vulvar carcinomas with HPV infection, especially in young women,[379,380] suggests that HPV vaccines hold great promise in the prevention and treatment of HPV-associated vulvar carcinoma, but as yet they have not been fully evaluated.[381]

VIN is a precancerous condition that may be surgically treated to prevent the occurrence of invasive squamous cell cancer. The management of VIN III has been modeled on that of CIN, because of their histologic similarities and comparable risk factor profiles. Lesions are usually either surgically excised or vaporized with CO_2 laser. However, because of an overall

Table 66–4. Vulvar Self-Examination

Step	Activity
1	Wash your hands.
2	Lie or sit in a comfortable position in good lighting with a hand mirror (preferentially a magnifying type).
3	Your position may be made more comfortable by propping up on pillows or squatting over the mirror.
4	First look and establish, in your mind, the normal anatomic features of the vulva and perineum.
5	Gently separate the outer lips of the vulva and, starting at the clitoris, inspect and palpate the vulva from front to back on each side.
6	Look for redness, swelling, ulcers, blisters, bumps, lumps, or areas of discoloration.
7	Separate the inner lips of the vulva and look for similar changes.
8	Gently pull the hood of the clitoris back and examine the skin around it.
9	Inspect the area around the urethra, the perineum, and the pubic mound.

field effect for HPV-related change in the vulva, recurrence is common, often multifocal, and repetitive surgeries can often lead to significant scarring and discomfort. Even the use of skin grafting does not preclude recurrence, because there have been reports of recurrences in the grafts.

VIN is an ideal model of HPV-associated neoplasia in which to test chemoprevention drugs for a number of reasons: (1) the disease is very stable, with a long precancerous phase before invasion, and is very resistant to treatment[382]; (2) recurrences are the rule rather than the exception; and (3) the incidence of VIN is increasing and appears to be affecting younger women.[375] Whereas classic squamous cell carcinomas of the vulva are positive for high-risk DNA 60% to 80% of the time, up to 100% of VIN III lesions have been shown to be positive for high-risk HPV DNA.[376,377] The coexistence of HPV-related lesions of the cervix and vulva is common. HPV-related lesions tend to be asymptomatic and often go undetected until surveillance for abnormal cervical cytology is undertaken.

REFERENCES

1. Albert DS: A unifying vision of cancer therapy for the 21st century. J Clin Oncol 1999; 17(11 Suppl): 13-21.
2. O'Shaughnessy JA, Kelloff GJ, Gordon GB, et al: Treatment and prevention of intraepithelial neoplasia: An important target for accelerated new agent development. Clin Cancer Res 2002;8: 314-346.
3. Chanen W: The CIN saga: The biological and clinical significance of cervical intraepithelial neoplasia. Aust N Z J Obstet Gynaecol 1990;30:18-23.
4. Cervical Cancer: NIH Consensus Statement 1996. Apr 1-3; 14(1): 1-38.
5. Jemal A, Thomas A, Murray T, Thun M: Cancer statistics, 2002. CA Cancer J Clin 2002;52:23-47.
6. Alani RM, Munger K: Human papillomaviruses and associated malignancies. J Clin Oncol 1998;16:330-337.
7. Cripe TP, Haugen TH, Turk JP, et al: Transcriptional regulation of the human papillomavirus-16 E6-E7 promoter by a keratinocyte-dependent enhancer, and by viral E2 transactivator and repressor gene products: Implications for cervical carcinogenesis. Embo J 1987;6:3745-3753.
8. Choo KB, Pan CC, Han SH: Integration of human papillomavirus type 16 into cellular DNA of cervical carcinoma: Preferential deletion of the E2 gene and invariable retention of the long control region and the E6/E7 open reading frames. Virology 1987;161:259-261.
9. Thorland EC, Myers SL, Persing DH, et al: Human papillomavirus type 16 integrations in cervical tumors frequently occur in common fragile sites. Cancer Res 2000;60:5916-5921.
10. Vernon SD, Unger ER, Miller DL, et al: Association of human papillomavirus type 16 integration in the E2 gene with poor disease-free survival from cervical cancer. Int J Cancer 1997;74: 50-56.
11. Corden SA, Sant-Cassia LJ, Easton AJ, Morris AG: The integration of HPV-18 DNA in cervical carcinoma. Mol Pathol 1999;52: 275-282.
12. Halbert CL, Demers GW, Galloway DA: The E7 gene of human papillomavirus type 16 is sufficient for immortalization of human epithelial cells. J Virol 1991;65:473-478.
13. Coursen JD, Bennett WP, Gollahon L, et al: Genomic instability and telomerase activity in human bronchial epithelial cells during immortalization by human papillomavirus-16 E6 and E7 genes. Exp Cell Res 1997;235:245-253.
14. Duensing S, Lee LY, Duensing A, et al: The human papillomavirus type 16 E6 and E7 oncoproteins cooperate to induce mitotic defects and genomic instability by uncoupling centrosome duplication from the cell division cycle. Proc Natl Acad Sci U S A 2000;97:10002-10007.
15. Storey A, Banks L: Human papillomavirus type 16 E6 gene cooperates with EJ-ras to immortalize primary mouse cells. Oncogene 1993;8:919-924.
16. Matlashewski G, Schneider J, Banks L, et al: Human papillomavirus type 16 DNA cooperates with activated ras in transforming primary cells. Embo J 1987;6:1741-1746.
17. zur Hausen H: Papillomaviruses in anogenital cancer as a model to understand the role of viruses in human cancers. Cancer Res 1989;49: 4677-4681.
18. McCann MF, Irwin DE, Walton LA, et al: Nicotine and cotinine in the cervical mucus of smokers, passive smokers, and nonsmokers. Cancer Epidemiol Biomarkers Prev 1992;1:125-129.
19. Prokopczyk B, Cox JE, Hoffmann D, Waggoner SE: Identification of tobacco-specific carcinogen in the cervical mucus of smokers and nonsmokers. J Natl Cancer Inst 1997;89:868-873.
20. Scheffner M, Huibregtse JM, Vierstra RD, Howley PM: The HPV-16 E6 and E6-AP complex functions as a ubiquitin-protein ligase in the ubiquitination of p53. Cell 1993;75:495-505.
21. Denk C, Butz K, Schneider A, et al: P53 mutations are rare events in recurrent cervical cancer. J Mol Med 2001;79:283-288.
22. Park DJ, Wilczynski SP, Paquette RL, et al: P53 mutations in HPV-negative cervical carcinoma. Oncogene 1994;9:205-210.
23. Kim HJ, Song ES, Hwang TS: Higher incidence of p53 mutation in cervical carcinomas with intermediate-risk HPV infection. Eur J Obstet Gynecol Reprod Biol 2001;98:213-218.
24. Crook T, Vousden KH: Properties of p53 mutations detected in primary and secondary cervical cancers suggest mechanisms of metastasis and involvement of environmental carcinogens. Embo J 1992;11:3935-3940.
25. Shirodkar S, Ewen M, DeCaprio JA, et al: The transcription factor E2F interacts with the retinoblastoma product and a p107-cyclin A complex in a cell cycle-regulated manner. Cell 1992;68: 157-166.
26. Zerfass-Thome K, Zwerschke W, Mannhardt B, et al: Inactivation of the cdk inhibitor p27KIP1 by the human papillomavirus type 16 E7 oncoprotein. Oncogene 1996;13:2323-2330.
27. Jones DL, Alani RM, Munger K: The human papillomavirus E7 oncoprotein can uncouple cellular differentiation and proliferation in human keratinocytes by abrogating p21Cip1-mediated inhibition of cdk2. Genes Dev 1997;11:2101-2111.
28. Syrjanen SM, Syrjanen KJ: New concepts on the role of human papillomavirus in cell cycle regulation. Ann Med 1999;31: 175-187.
29. Akerman GS, Tolleson WH, Brown KL, et al: Human papillomavirus type 16 E6 and E7 cooperate to increase epidermal growth factor receptor (EGFR) mRNA levels, overcoming mechanisms by which excessive EGFR signaling shortens the life span of normal human keratinocytes. Cancer Res 2001;61: 3837-3843.
30. Nicholson RI, Gee JM, Harper ME: EGFR and cancer prognosis. Eur J Cancer 2001;37(Suppl 4):S9-S15.
31. Kwok TT, Sutherland RM: Differences in EGF related radiosensitisation of human squamous carcinoma cells with high and low numbers of EGF receptors. Br J Cancer 1991;64:251-254.
32. Hambek M, Solbach C, Schnuerch HG, et al: Tumor necrosis factor alpha sensitizes low epidermal growth factor receptor (EGFR)-expressing carcinomas for anti-EGFR therapy. Cancer Res 2001;61:1045-1049.
33. Kelloff GJ, Fay JR, Steele VE, et al: Epidermal growth factor receptor tyrosine kinase inhibitors as potential cancer chemopreventives. Cancer Epidemiol Biomarkers Prev 1996;5:657-566.
34. Beerheide W, Bernard HU, Tan YJ, et al: Potential drugs against cervical cancer: zinc-ejecting inhibitors of the human papillomavirus type 16 E6 oncoprotein. J Natl Cancer Inst 1999;91: 1211-1220.
35. Da Silva DM, Eiben GL, Fausch SC, et al: Cervical cancer vaccines: Emerging concepts and developments. J Cell Physiol 2001; 186:169-182.
36. Meyskens FL Jr, Surwit E, Moon TE, et al: Enhancement of regression of cervical intraepithelial neoplasia II (moderate dysplasia) with topically applied all-trans-retinoic acid: A randomized trial. J Natl Cancer Inst 1994;86:539-543.

37. Magnusson PK, Sparen P, Gyllensten UB: Genetic link to cervical tumors. Nature 1999;400:29-30.
38. Magnusson PK, Lichtenstein P, Gyllensten UB: Heritability of cervical tumors. Int J Cancer 2000;88:698-701.
39. Hemminki K, Li X, Mutanen P: Familial risks in invasive and in situ cervical cancer by histological type. Eur J Cancer Prev 2001; 10:83-89.
40. Horn LC, Raptis G, Fischer U: Familial cancer history in patients with carcinoma of the cervix uteri. Eur J Obstet Gynecol Reprod Biol 2002;101:54-57.
41. Konya J, Dillner J: Immunity to oncogenic human papillomaviruses. Adv Cancer Res 2001;82:205-238.
42. Wang SS, Wheeler CM, Hildesheim A: Human leukocyte antigen class I and II alleles and risk of cervical neoplasia: Results from a population-based study in Costa Rica. J Infect Dis 2001; 184:1310-1314.
43. Zehbe I, Tachezy R, Mytilineos J, et al: Human papillomavirus 16 E6 polymorphisms in cervical lesions from different European populations and their correlation with human leukocyte antigen class II haplotypes. Int J Cancer 2001;94:711-716.
44. Maciag PC, Schlecht NF, Souza PS, et al: Major histocompatibility complex class II polymorphisms and risk of cervical cancer and human papillomavirus infection in Brazilian women. Cancer Epidemiol Biomarkers Prev 2000;9:1183-1191.
45. Castle PE, Wacholder S, Sherman ME, et al: A prospective study of high-grade cervical neoplasia risk among human papillomavirus-infected women. J Natl Cancer Inst 2002;94:1406-1414.
46. Deacon JM, Evans CD, Yule R, et al: Sexual behavior and smoking as determinants of cervical HPV infection and of CIN3 among those infected: A case-control study nested within the Manchester cohort. Br J Cancer 2000;83:1565-1572.
47. Bouchardy C, Benhamou S, Jourenkova N, et al: Metabolic genetic polymorphisms and susceptibility to lung cancer. Lung Cancer 2001;32:109-112.
48. Nair U, Bartsch H: Metabolic polymorphisms as susceptibility markers for lung and oral cavity cancer. IARC Sci Publ 2001;154: 271-290.
49. Goodman MT, McDuffie K, Hernandez B, et al: CYP1A1, GSTM1, and GSTT1 polymorphisms and the risk of cervical squamous intraepithelial lesions in a multiethnic population. Gynecol Oncol 2001;81:263-269.
50. Kim JW, Lee CG, Park YG, et al: Combined analysis of germline polymorphisms of p53, GSTM1, GSTT1, CYP1A1, and CYP2E1: Relation to the incidence rate of cervical carcinoma. Cancer 2000; 88:2082-2091.
51. Bosch FX, Manos MM, Munoz N, et al: Prevalence of human papillomavirus in cervical cancer: A worldwide perspective. International Biological Study on Cervical Cancer (IBSCC) study group. J Natl Cancer Inst 1995;87:796-802.
52. Walboomers JM, Jacobs MV, Manos MM, et al: Human papillomavirus is a necessary cause of invasive cervical cancer worldwide. J Pathol 1999;189:12-19.
53. Moreno V, Bosch FX, Munoz N, et al., and the International Agency for Research on Cancer: Multicentric Cervical Cancer Study. Effect of oral contraceptives on risk of cervical cancer in women with human papillomavirus infection: the IARC multicentric case-control study [see comments]. Lancet 2002;359: 1085-1092.
54. Munoz N, Franceschi S, Bosetti C, et al., and the International Agency for Research on Cancer: Multicentric Cervical Cancer Study. Role of parity and human papillomavirus in cervical cancer: the IARC multicentric case-control study [see comments]. Lancet 2002;359:1093-1101.
55. Yoo KY, Kang D, Koo HW, et al: Risk factors associated with uterine cervical cancer in Korea: A case-control study with special reference to sexual behavior. J Epidemiol 1997;7:117-123.
56. Jordan SW, Key CR, Wright DE: Selected characteristics of cervical cancer incidence cases. Acta Cytol 1982;26:823-832.
57. de Graaff J, Stolte LA, Janssens J: Marriage and childbearing in relation to cervical cancer. Eur J Obstet Gynecol Reprod Biol 1977;7:307-312.
58. Brinton LA, Reeves WC, Brenes MM, et al: Parity as a risk factor for cervical cancer. Am J Epidemiol 1989;130:486-496.
59. Parkin DM, Vizcaino AP, Skinner ME, Ndhlovu A: Cancer patterns and risk factors in the African population of southwestern

Zimbabwe, 1963-1977. Cancer Epidemiol Biomarkers Prev 1994;3:537-547.
60. Castle PE, Hillier SL, Rabe LK, et al: An association of cervical inflammation with high-grade cervical neoplasia in women infected with oncogenic human papillomavirus (HPV). Cancer Epidemiol Biomarkers Prev 2001;10:1021-1027.
61. Giuliano AR: The role of nutrients in the prevention of cervical dysplasia and cancer. Nutrition 2000;16:570-573.
62. van Duin M, Snijders PJ, Schrijnemakers HF, et al: Human papillomavirus 16 load in normal and abnormal cervical scrapes: An indicator of CIN II/III and viral clearance. Int J Cancer 2002;98:590-595.
63. Recommendations on frequency of Pap test screening. Washington, DC: American College of Obstetricians and Gynecologists, 1995.
64. Morrison BJ: Screening for cervical cancer. Canadian Task Force on the Periodic Health Examination, Canadian Guide to Clinical Preventive Health Care. 1994, Ottawa: Health Canada, pp 870-881.
65. NHS Cancer Screening Programmes web site. Available at:http://www.cancer screening.nhs.uk/cervical/index.html. Accessed March 2, 2004.
66. Nanda K, McCrory DC, Myers ER, et al: Accuracy of the Papanicolaou test in screening for and follow-up of cervical cytologic abnormalities: A systematic review. Ann Intern Med 2000;132:810-819.
67. Fahey MT, Irwig L, Macaskill P: Meta-analysis of Pap test accuracy. Am J Epidemiol 1995;141:680-689.
68. Stoler MH, Schiffman M: Interobserver reproducibility of cervical cytology and histologic interpretations: Realistic estimates from the ASCUS-LSIL triage study. JAMA 2001; 285:1500-1505.
69. Sawaya GF, Washington AE: Cervical cancer screening: Which techniques should be used and why? Clin Obstet Gynecol 1999; 42:922-938.
70. Patten SF, Lee JSJ, Wilbur DC, et al: The AutoPap 300 QC system multicenter clinical trials for use in quality control rescreening of cervical smears. I. A prospective intended use study. Cancer Cytopathol 1997;81:337-342.
71. Howell LP, Belk T, Agdigos R, et al: AutoCyte interactive screening system: Experience at a university hospital cytology laboratory. Acta Cytol 1999;43:58-64.
72. Solomon D, Davey D, Kurman R, et al: The 2001 Bethesda system: Terminology for reporting results of cervical cytology. JAMA 2002;287:2114-2119.
73. Visual inspection with acetic acid for cervical-cancer screening: Test qualities in a primary-care setting. University of Zimbabwe/ JHPIEGO Cervical Cancer Project. Lancet 1999;353:869-873.
74. Belinson JL, Pretorius RG, Zhang WH, et al: Cervical cancer screening by simple visual inspection after acetic acid. Obstet Gynecol 2001;98:441-444.
75. Wright TC, Cox JT, Massad LS, et al: 2001 Consensus guidelines for the management of women with cervical cytological abnormalities. JAMA 2002;287:2120-2129.
76. American Society for Colposcopy and Cervical Pathology Home Page. Available at www.asccp.org.
77. Cuzick J, Sasieni P, Davies P, et al: A systematic review of the role of human papillomavirus (HPV) testing within a cervical screening programme: Summary and conclusions. Br J Cancer 2000;83: 561-565.
78. Franco EL: Statistical issues in human papillomavirus testing and screening. Clin Lab Med 2000;20:345-367.
79. Tawa K, Forsythe A, Cove JK, et al: A comparision of the Papanicolaou smear and the cervigram: Sensitivity, specificity, and cost analysis. Obstet Gynecol 1988;71:229-235.
80. Szarewski A, Cuzick J, Edwards R, et al: The use of cervicography in a primary screening service. Br J Obstet Gynaecol 1991; 98:313-317.
81. Olatunbosun OA, Okonofua FE, Ayangade SO: Screening for cervical neoplasia in an African population: Simultaneous use of cytology and colposcopy. Int J Gynecol Obstet 1991;36: 39-42.
82. Cancer Progress Report 2001. http://progressreport.cancer. gov. 2001.
83. Lutz MH, Underwood PB Jr, Rozier JC, Putney FW: Genital malignancy in pregnancy. Am J Obstet Gynecol 1977;129:536-542.

84. Creasman WT, Rutledge FN, Fletcher GH: Carcinoma of the cervix associated with pregnancy. Obstet Gynecol 1970;36:495-501.

85. Hacker NF, Berek JS, Lagasse LD, et al: Carcinoma of the cervix associated with pregnancy. Obstet Gynecol 1982;59:735-746.

86. Norstrom A, Jansson I, Andersson H: Carcinoma of the uterine cervix in pregnancy: A study of the incidence and treatment in the western region of Sweden 1973 to 1992. Acta Obstet Gynecol Scand 1997;76:583-589.

87. Miller BA, Kolonel LN, Bernstein L, et al. (Eds.): Racial/Ethnic Patterns of Cancer in the United States, 1988-1992. Bethesda: National Cancer Institute, 1996.

88. Ries LAG, Kosary LN, Hankey BE, et al. (Eds.): SEER Cancer Statistics Review, 1973-1996. Bethesda: National Cancer Institute, 1999.

89. Ries LAG, Eisner MP, Kosary CL, et al. (Eds.): SEER Cancer Statistics Review, 1973-1998. Bethesda: National Cancer Institute, 2001.

90. Napoles-Springer A, Perez-Stable EJ, Washington E: Risk factors for invasive cervical cancer in Latino women. J Med Syst 1996;20:277-293.

91. Mitchell JB, McCormack LA: Time trends in late-stage diagnosis of cervical cancer: Differences by race/ethnicity and income. Med Care 1997;35:1220-1224.

92. Howe SL, Delfino RJ, Taylor TH, Anton-Culver H: The risk of invasive cervical cancer among Hispanics: Evidence for targeted preventive interventions. Prev Med 1998;27:674-680.

93. Brewster WR, Monk BJ, Ziogas A, et al: Intent-to-treat analysis of stage Ib and IIa cervical cancer in the United States: Radiotherapy or surgery 1988-1995. Obstet Gynecol 2001;97:248-254.

94. Howell EA, Chen YT, Concato J: Differences in cervical cancer mortality among black and white women. Obstet Gynecol 1999;94:509-515.

95. Liu T, Wang X, Waterbor JW, et al: Relationships between socioeconomic status and race-specific cervical cancer incidence in the United States, 1973-1992. J Health Care Poor Underserved 1998;9:420-432.

96. National Center for Health Statistics. Use of selected preventive care procedures—United States, 1982. Vital and Health Statistics. Series 10, No. 157. DHHS Pub No. (PHS)86-1585. Public Health Service, Hyattsville, September 1986.

97. Peragallo NP, Alba ML, Tow B: Cervical cancer screening practices among Latino women in Chicago. Public Health Nurs 1997;14:251-255.

98. Suarez L, Roche RA, Nichols D, Simpson DM: Knowledge, behavior, and fears concerning breast and cervical cancer among older low-income Mexican-American women. Am J Prev Med 1997;13:137-142.

99. Harmon MP, Castro FG, Coe K: Acculturation and cervical cancer: Knowledge, beliefs, and behaviors of Hispanic women. Women Health 1996;24:37-57.

100. Chavez LR, Hubbell FA, Mishra SI, Valdez RB: The influence of fatalism on self-reported use of Papanicolaou smears. Am J Prev Med 1997;13:418-424.

101. Skaer TL, Robison LM, Sclar DA, Harding GH: Cancer-screening determinants among Hispanic women using migrant health clinics. J Health Care Poor Underserved 1996;7: 338-354.

102. Krieger N, Quesenberry C Jr, Peng T, et al: Social class, race/ethnicity, and incidence of breast, cervix, colon, lung, and prostate cancer among Asian, Black, Hispanic, and White residents of the San Francisco Bay Area, 1988-92 (United States). Cancer Causes Control 1999;10:525-537.

103. Papanicolaou GN, Traut HF: The diagnostic value of vaginal smears in carcinoma of the uterus. 1941. Arch Pathol Lab Med 1997;121:211-224.

104. Sasieni PD, Cuzick J, Lynch-Farmery E: Estimating the efficacy of screening by auditing smear histories of women with and without cervical cancer. The National Co-ordinating Network for Cervical Screening Working Group. Br J Cancer 1996;73:1001-1005.

105. Schiffman MH, Bauer HM, Hoover RN, et al: Epidemiologic evidence showing that human papillomavirus infection causes most cervical intraepithelial neoplasia. J Natl Cancer Inst 1993;85:958-964.

106. Munoz N: Human papillomavirus and cancer: The epidemiological evidence. J Clin Virol 2000;19:1-5.

107. Koutsky L: Epidemiology of genital human papillomavirus infection. Am J Med 1997;102:3-8.

108. de Vet HC, Sturmans F, Knipschild PG: The role of cigarette smoking in the etiology of cervical dysplasia. Epidemiology 1994;5:631-633.

109. Winkelstein W Jr: Smoking and cervical cancer—current status: A review. Am J Epidemiol 1990;131:945-957; discussion, 958-960.

110. Lyon JL, Gardner JW, West DW, et al: Smoking and carcinoma in situ of the uterine cervix. Am J Public Health 1983;73:558-562.

111. Harro CD, Pang YY, Roden RB, et al: Safety and immunogenicity trial in adult volunteers of a human papillomavirus 16 L1 virus-like particle vaccine. J Natl Cancer Inst 2001;93:284-292.

112. Greenstone HL, Nieland JD, de Visser KE, et al: Chimeric papillomavirus virus-like particles elicit antitumor immunity against the E7 oncoprotein in an HPV16 tumor model. Proc Natl Acad Sci U S A 1998;95:1800-1805.

113. Daemen T, Pries F, Bungener L, et al: Genetic immunization against cervical carcinoma: Induction of cytotoxic T lymphocyte activity with a recombinant alphavirus vector expressing human papillomavirus type 16 E6 and E7. Gene Ther 2000;7:1859-1866.

114. Prevention of cancer in the next millennium: Report of the Chemoprevention Working Group to the American Association for Cancer Research. Cancer Res 1999;59:4743-4758.

115. Sizemore N, Choo CK, Eckert RL, Rorke EA: Transcriptional regulation of the EGF receptor promoter by HPV16 and retinoic acid in human ectocervical epithelial cells. Exp Cell Res 1998;244:349-356.

116. Ding Z, Green AG, Yang X, et al: Retinoic acid inhibits telomerase activity and downregulates expression but does not affect splicing of hTERT: Correlation with cell growth rate inhibition in an in vitro cervical carcinogenesis/multidrug- resistance model. Exp Cell Res 2002;272:185-191.

117. Borger DR, Mi Y, Geslani G, et al: Retinoic acid resistance at late stages of human papillomavirus type 16-mediated transformation of human keratinocytes arises despite intact retinoid signaling and is due to a loss of sensitivity to transforming growth factor-beta. Virology 2000;270:397-407.

118. Meyskens FL Jr, Graham V, Chvapil M, et al: A phase I trial of beta-all-trans-retinoic acid delivered via a collagen sponge and a cervical cap for mild or moderate intraepithelial cervical neoplasia. J Natl Cancer Inst 1983;71:921-925.

119. Surwit EA, Graham V, Droegemueller W, et al: Evaluation of topically applied trans-retinoic acid in the treatment of cervical intraepithelial lesions. Am J Obstet Gynecol 1982;143:821-823.

120. Weiner SA, Surwit EA, Graham VE, Meyskens FL Jr: A phase I trial of topically applied trans-retinoic acid in cervical dysplasia-clinical efficacy. Invest New Drugs 1986;4:241-244.

121. Follen M, Atkinson EN, Schottenfeld D, et al: A randomized clinical trial of 4-hydroxyphenylretinamide for high-grade squamous intraepithelial lesions of the cervix. Clin Cancer Res 2001;7:3356-3365.

122. Wattenberg LW, Loub WD: Inhibition of polycyclic aromatic hydrocarbon-induced neoplasia by naturally occurring indoles. Cancer Res 1978;38:1410-1413.

123. Grubbs CJ, Steele VE, Casebolt T, et al: Chemoprevention of chemically-induced mammary carcinogenesis by indole-3-carbinol. Anticancer Res 1995;15:709-716.

124. Telang NT, Suto A, Wong GY, et al: Induction by estrogen metabolite 16 alpha-hydroxyestrone of genotoxic damage and aberrant proliferation in mouse mammary epithelial cells. J Natl Cancer Inst 1992;84:634-638.

125. Bell MC, Crowley-Nowick P, Bradlow HL, et al: Placebo-controlled trial of indole-3-carbinol in the treatment of CIN. Gynecol Oncol 2000;78:123-129.

126. Kanetsky PA, Gammon MD, Mandelblatt J, et al: Dietary intake and blood levels of lycopene: Association with cervical dysplasia among non-Hispanic, black women. Nutr Cancer 1998;31:31-40.

127. Nagata C, Shimizu H, Yoshikawa H, et al: Serum carotenoids and vitamins and risk of cervical dysplasia from a case-control study in Japan. Br J Cancer 1999;81:1234-1237.

128. Schiff MA, Patterson RE, Baumgartner RN, et al: Serum carotenoids and risk of cervical intraepithelial neoplasia in Southwestern American Indian women. Cancer Epidemiol Biomarkers Prev 2001;10:1219-1222.

129. Keefe KA, Schell MJ, Brewer C, et al: A randomized, double blind, phase III trial using oral beta-carotene supplementation for women with high-grade cervical intraepithelial neoplasia. Cancer Epidemiol Biomarkers Prev 2001;10:1029-1035.

130. Weiss GR, Liu PY, Alberts DS, et al: 13-cis-Retinoic acid or all-trans-retinoic acid plus interferon-alpha in recurrent cervical cancer: A Southwest Oncology Group phase II randomized trial. Gynecol Oncol 1998;71:386-390.

131. Koki AT, Leahy KM, Masferrer JL: Potential utility of COX-2 inhibitors in chemoprevention and chemotherapy. Expert Opin Investig Drugs 1999;8:1623-1638.

132. Kulkarni S, Rader JS, Zhang F, et al: Cyclooxygenase-2 is overexpressed in human cervical cancer. Clin Cancer Res 2001;7:429-434.

133. Edwards L, Ferenczy A, Eron L, et al: Self-administered topical 5% imiquimod cream for external anogenital warts. Human Papilloma Virus Study Group. Arch Dermatol 1998;134:25-30.

134. Diaz-Arrastia C, Arany I, Robazetti SC, et al: Clinical and molecular responses in high-grade intraepithelial neoplasia treated with topical imiquimod 5%. Clin Cancer Res 2001;7:3031-3033.

135. Hill HA, Eley JW, Harlan LC, et al: Racial differences in endometrial cancer survival: The black/white cancer survival study. Obstet Gynecol 1996;88:919-926.

136. Ries LAG, Eisner MP, Kosary CL, et al. (Eds.): SEER Cancer Statistics Review, 1973-1994. Bethesda: National Cancer Institute, 1997.

137. Akhmedkhanov A, Zeleniuch-Jacquotte A, Toniolo P: Role of exogenous and endogenous hormones in endometrial cancer: Review of the evidence and research perspectives. Ann N Y Acad Sci 2001;943:296-315.

138. Herrinton LJ, Weiss NS: Postmenopausal unopposed estrogens: Characteristics of use in relation to the risk of endometrial carcinoma. Ann Epidemiol 1993;3:308-318.

139. Archer DF: The effect of the duration of progestin use on the occurrence of endometrial cancer in postmenopausal women. Menopause 2001;8:245-251.

140. Pike MC, Peters RK, Cozen W, et al: Estrogen-progestin replacement therapy and endometrial cancer. J Natl Cancer Inst 1997;89:1110-1116.

141. Fisher B, Costantino JP, Wickerham DL, et al: Tamoxifen for prevention of breast cancer: Report of the National Surgical Adjuvant Breast and Bowel Project P-1 Study. J Natl Cancer Inst 1998;90:1371-1388.

142. Voigt LF, Deng Q, Weiss NS: Recency, duration, and progestin content of oral contraceptives in relation to the incidence of endometrial cancer (Washington, USA). Cancer Causes Control 1994;5:227-233.

143. Risks and benefits of estrogen plus progestin in healthy postmenopausal women: Principal results From the Women's Health Initiative randomized controlled trial. JAMA 2002;288:321-333.

144. Goodman MT, Hankin JH, Wilkens LR, et al: Diet, body size, physical activity, and the risk of endometrial cancer. Cancer Res 1997;57:5077-5085.

145. Swanson CA, Potischman N, Wilbanks GD, et al: Relation of endometrial cancer risk to past and contemporary body size and body fat distribution. Cancer Epidemiol Biomarkers Prev 1993;2:321-327.

146. Terry P, Baron JA, Weiderpass E, et al: Lifestyle and endometrial cancer risk: A cohort study from the Swedish Twin Registry. Int J Cancer 1999;82:38-42.

147. Weiderpass E, Persson I, Adami HO, et al: Body size in different periods of life, diabetes mellitus, hypertension, and risk of postmenopausal endometrial cancer (Sweden). Cancer Causes Control 2000;11:185-192.

148. Terry P, Wolk A, Vainio H, Weiderpass E: Fatty fish consumption lowers the risk of endometrial cancer: A nationwide case-control study in Sweden. Cancer Epidemiol Biomarkers Prev 2002;11:143-145.

149. Littman AJ, Voigt LF, Beresford SA, Weiss NS: Recreational physical activity and endometrial cancer risk. Am J Epidemiol 2001;154:924-933.

150. Plymate SR, Hoop RC, Jones RE, Matej LA: Regulation of sex hormone-binding globulin production by growth factors. Metabolism 1990;39:967-970.

151. Lipworth L, Adami HO, Trichopoulos D, et al: Serum steroid hormone levels, sex hormone-binding globulin, and body mass index in the etiology of postmenopausal breast cancer. Epidemiology 1996;7:96-100.

152. Troisi R, Potischman N, Hoover RN, et al: Insulin and endometrial cancer. Am J Epidemiol 1997;146:476-482.

153. Heber D: Interrelationships of high fat diets, obesity, hormones, and cancer. Adv Exp Med Biol 1996;399:13-25.

154. Westley BR, May FE: Role of insulin-like growth factors in steroid modulated proliferation. J Steroid Biochem Mol Biol 1994;51:1-9.

155. Brinton LA, Barrett RJ, Berman ML, et al: Cigarette smoking and the risk of endometrial cancer. Am J Epidemiol 1993;137:281-291.

156. Anderson KE, Anderson E, Mink PJ, et al: Diabetes and endometrial cancer in the Iowa women's health study. Cancer Epidemiol Biomarkers Prev 2001;10:611-616.

157. Newcomb PA, Trentham-Dietz A, Egan KM, et al: Fracture history and risk of breast and endometrial cancer. Am J Epidemiol 2001;153:1071-1078.

158. Weiderpass E, Adami HO, Baron JA, et al: Organochlorines and endometrial cancer risk. Cancer Epidemiol Biomarkers Prev, 2000;9:487-493.

159. Potischman N, Hoover RN, Brinton LA, et al: Case-control study of endogenous steroid hormones and endometrial cancer. J Natl Cancer Inst 1996;88:1127-1135.

160. Zujewski J: Selective estrogen receptor modulators (SERMs) and retinoids in breast cancer chemoprevention. Environ Mol Mutagen 2002;39:264-270.

161. Pukkala E, Kyyronen P, Sankila R, Holli K: Tamoxifen and toremifene treatment of breast cancer and risk of subsequent endometrial cancer: A population-based case-control study. Int J Cancer 2002;100:337-341.

162. Vosse M, Renard F, Coibion M, et al: Endometrial disorders in 406 breast cancer patients on tamoxifen: the case for less intensive monitoring. Eur J Obstet Gynecol Reprod Biol 2002;101:58-63.

163. Planck M, Rambech E, Moslein G, et al: High frequency of microsatellite instability and loss of mismatch- repair protein expression in patients with double primary tumors of the endometrium and colorectum. Cancer 2002;94:2502-2510.

164. Berends MJ, Kleibeuker JH, de Vries EG, et al: The importance of family history in young patients with endometrial cancer. Eur J Obstet Gynecol Reprod Biol 1999;82:139-141.

165. Esteller M, Garcia A, Martinez-Palones JM, et al: Germ line polymorphisms in cytochrome-P450 1A1 (C4887 CYP1A1) and methylenetetrahydrofolate reductase (MTHFR) genes and endometrial cancer susceptibility. Carcinogenesis 1997;18:2307-2311.

166. Haiman CA, Hankinson SE, Colditz GA, et al: A polymorphism in CYP17 and endometrial cancer risk. Cancer Res 2001;61:3955-3960.

167. Sherman ME, Sturgeon S, Brinton L, Kurman RJ: Endometrial cancer chemoprevention: Implications of diverse pathways of carcinogenesis. J Cell Biochem Suppl 1995;23:160-164.

168. Bokhman JV: Two pathogenetic types of endometrial carcinoma. Gynecol Oncol 1983;15:10-17.

169. Hertig A, Sommers S: Genesis of endometrial carcinoma. I. Study of prior biopsies. Cancer 1949;2:946-956.

170. Baak JP, Orbo A, van Diest PJ, et al: Prospective multicenter evaluation of the morphometric D-score for prediction of the outcome of endometrial hyperplasias. Am J Surg Pathol 2001;25:930-935.

171. Kurman RJ, Kaminski PF, Norris HJ: The behavior of endometrial hyperplasia: A long-term study of "untreated" hyperplasia in 170 patients. Cancer 1985;56:403-412.

172. Esteller M, Garcia A, Martinez-Palones JM, et al: Detection of clonality and genetic alterations in endometrial pipelle biopsy and its surgical specimen counterpart. Lab Invest 1997;76:109-116.

173. Mutter GL, Chaponot ML, Fletcher JA: A polymerase chain reaction assay for non-random X chromosome inactivation

identifies monoclonal endometrial cancers and precancers. Am J Pathol 1995;146:501-508.

174. Jovanovic AS, Boynton KA, Mutter GL: Uteri of women with endometrial carcinoma contain a histopathological spectrum of monoclonal putative precancers, some with microsatellite instability. Cancer Res 1996;56:1917-1921.

175. Mutter GL, Baak JP, Crum CP, et al: Endometrial precancer diagnosis by histopathology, clonal analysis, and computerized morphometry. J Pathol 2000;190:462-469.

176. Mutter GL: Histopathology of genetically defined endometrial precancers. Int J Gynecol Pathol 2000;19:301-309.

177. Mutter GL: Endometrial intraepithelial neoplasia (EIN): Will it bring order to chaos? The Endometrial Collaborative Group. Gynecol Oncol 2000;76:287-290.

178. Mutter GL, Boynton KA, Faquin WC, et al: Allelotype mapping of unstable microsatellites establishes direct lineage continuity between endometrial precancers and cancer. Cancer Res 1996;56:4483-4486.

179. Faquin WC, Fitzgerald JT, Lin MC, et al: Sporadic microsatellite instability is specific to neoplastic and preneoplastic endometrial tissues. Am J Clin Pathol 2000;113:576-582.

180. Levine RL, Cargile CB, Blazes MS, et al: PTEN mutations and microsatellite instability in complex atypical hyperplasia, a precursor lesion to uterine endometrioid carcinoma. Cancer Res 1998;58:3254-3258.

181. Duggan BD, Felix JC, Muderspach LI, et al: Microsatellite instability in sporadic endometrial carcinoma. J Natl Cancer Inst 1994;86:1216-1221.

182. Risinger JI, Berchuck A, Kohler MF, et al: Genetic instability of microsatellites in endometrial carcinoma. Cancer Res 1993;53: 5100-5103.

183. Faquin WC, Fitzgerald JT, Boynton KA, Mutter GL: Intratumoral genetic heterogeneity and progression of endometrioid type endometrial adenocarcinomas. Gynecol Oncol 2000;78:152-157.

184. Risinger JI, Hayes AK, Berchuck A, Barrett JC: PTEN/MMAC1 mutations in endometrial cancers. Cancer Res 1997;57: 4736-4738.

185. Tashiro H, Blazes MS, Wu R, et al: Mutations in PTEN are frequent in endometrial carcinoma but rare in other common gynecological malignancies. Cancer Res 1997;57:3935-3940.

186. Risinger JI, Hayes K, Maxwell GL, et al: PTEN mutation in endometrial cancers is associated with favorable clinical and pathologic characteristics. Clin Cancer Res 1998;4:3005-3010.

187. Mutter GL, Lin MC, Fitzgerald JT, et al: Altered PTEN expression as a diagnostic marker for the earliest endometrial precancers. J Natl Cancer Inst 2000;92:924-930.

188. Stambolic V, Tsao MS, Macpherson D, et al: High incidence of breast and endometrial neoplasia resembling human Cowden syndrome in pten+/− mice. Cancer Res 2000;60:3605-3611.

189. Mutter GL, Ince TA, Baak JP, et al: Molecular identification of latent precancers in histologically normal endometrium. Cancer Res 2001;61:4311-4314.

190. Mutter GL, Nogales L, Kurman R, et al: Endometrial Cancer. In:Tavassoli FA, Stratton MR, eds. WHO Classification of Tumors: Pathology and Genetics: Tumors of the Breast and Female Genital Organs. Lyon, France: IARC Press, 2002.

191. Mutter GL, Lin MC, Fitzgerald JT, et al: Changes in endometrial PTEN expression throughout the human menstrual cycle. J Clin Endocrinol Metab 2000;85:2334-2338.

192. Sherman ME, Bur ME, Kurman RJ: P53 in endometrial cancer and its putative precursors: Evidence for diverse pathways of tumorigenesis. Hum Pathol 1995;26:1268-1274.

193. Sherman ME. Theories of endometrial carcinogenesis: A multidisciplinary approach. Mod Pathol 2000;13:295-308.

194. Mutter GL, Baak JP, Fitzgerald JT, et al: Global expression changes of constitutive and hormonally regulated genes during endometrial neoplastic transformation. Gynecol Oncol 2001;83:177-185.

195. Baak JP, Kurver PH, Overdiep SH, et al: Quantitative, microscopical, computer-aided diagnosis of endometrial hyperplasia or carcinoma in individual patients. Histopathology 1981; 5:689-695.

196. Colgan TJ, Norris HJ, Foster W, et al: Predicting the outcome of endometrial hyperplasia by quantitative analysis of nuclear features using a linear discriminant function. Int J Gynecol Pathol 1983;1:347-352.

197. Baak JP, Nauta JJ, Wisse-Brekelmans EC, Bezemer PD: Architectural and nuclear morphometrical features together are more important prognosticators in endometrial hyperplasias than nuclear morphometrical features alone. J Pathol 1988;154:335-341.

198. Baak JP, Wisse-Brekelmans EC, Fleege JC, et al: Assessment of the risk on endometrial cancer in hyperplasia, by means of morphological and morphometrical features. Pathol Res Pract 1992;188:856-859.

199. Dunton CJ, Baak JP, Palazzo JP, et al: Use of computerized morphometric analyses of endometrial hyperplasias in the prediction of coexistent cancer. Am J Obstet Gynecol 1996;174: 1518-1521.

200. Bartels PH, Garcia FA, Davis J, et al: Progression curves for endometrial lesions. Anal Quant Cytol Histol 2001;23:1-8.

201. Garcia FA, Davis JR, Alberts DS, et al: Nuclear chromatin patterns in normal, hyperplastic and atypical endometrium. Anal Quant Cytol Histol 2001;23:144-150.

202. Barakat RR, Grigsby PW, Sabbatini P, Zaino RJ: Corpus: Epithelial Tumors. In Hoskins WJ, Perez CA, Young RC (Eds.): Principles and Practice of Gynecologic Oncology. Philadelphia: Lippincott-Raven, 2000.

203. Kurman RJ, Norris HJ: Evaluation of criteria for distinguishing atypical endometrial hyperplasia from well-differentiated carcinoma. Cancer 1982;49:2547-2559.

204. Randall TC, Kurman RJ: Progestin treatment of atypical hyperplasia and well-differentiated carcinoma of the endometrium in women under age 40. Obstet Gynecol 1997;90:434-440.

205. Hunter JE, Tritz DE, Howell MG, et al: The prognostic and therapeutic implications of cytologic atypia in patients with endometrial hyperplasia. Gynecol Oncol 1994;55:66-71.

206. Janicek MF, Rosenshein NB: Invasive endometrial cancer in uteri resected for atypical endometrial hyperplasia. Gynecol Oncol 1994;52:373-378.

207. Moukhtar M, Aleem FA, Hung HC, et al: The reversible behavior of locally invasive endometrial carcinoma in a chromosomally mosaic (45,X/46,Xr(X)) young woman treated with Clomid. Cancer 1977;40:2957-2966.

208. Kim YB, Holschneider CH, Ghosh K, et al: Progestin alone as primary treatment of endometrial carcinoma in premenopausal women: Report of seven cases and review of the literature. Cancer 1997;79:320-327.

209. Perez-Medina T, Bajo J, Folgueira G, et al: Atypical endometrial hyperplasia treatment with progestogens and gonadotropin-releasing hormone analogues: long-term follow-up. Gynecol Oncol 1999;73:299-304.

210. Bokhman JV, Chepick OF, Volkova AT, Vishnevsky AS: Can primary endometrial carcinoma stage I be cured without surgery and radiation therapy? Gynecol Oncol 1985;20:139-155.

211. Eichner E, Abellera M: Endometrial hyperplasia treated by progestins. Obstet Gynecol 1971;38:739-742.

212. Wentz WB: Progestin therapy in lesions of the endometrium. Semin Oncol 1985;12(1 Suppl 1):23-27.

213. Jasonni VM, Franceschetti F, Ciotti P, et al: Treatment of endometrial hyperplasia with cyproterone acetate histological and hormonal aspects. Acta Obstet Gynecol Scand 1986;65:685-687.

214. Ferenczy A, Gelfand M: The biologic significance of cytologic atypia in progestogen-treated endometrial hyperplasia. Am J Obstet Gynecol 1989;160:126-131.

215. Soh E, Sato K: Clinical effects of danazol on endometrial hyperplasia in menopausal and postmenopausal women. Cancer 1990;66:983-988.

216. Mariani L, Sedati A, Giovinazzi R, et al: Postmenopausal endometrial hyperplasia: Role of danazol therapy. Int J Gynecol Obstet 1994;44:155-159.

217. Abulafia O, Triest WE, Adcock JT, Sherer DM: The effect of medroxyprogesterone acetate on angiogenesis in complex endometrial hyperplasia. Gynecol Oncol 1999;72:193-198.

218. Amezcua CA, Lu JJ, Felix JC, et al: Apoptosis may be an early event of progestin therapy for endometrial hyperplasia. Gynecol Oncol 2000;79:169-176.

219. Amezcua CA, Zheng W, Muderspach LI, Felix JC: Down-regulation of bcl-2 is a potential marker of the efficacy of progestin therapy in the treatment of endometrial hyperplasia. Gynecol Oncol 1999;73:126-136.

220. Rose PG: Hyperglycemia secondary to megestrol acetate for endometrial neoplasia. Gynecol Oncol 1996;61:139-141.

221. Gal D, Edman CD, Vellios F, Forney JP: Long-term effect of megestrol acetate in the treatment of endometrial hyperplasia. Am J Obstet Gynecol 1983;146:316-322.

222. Lindahl B, Alm P, Ferno M, Norgren A: Endometrial hyperplasia: a prospective randomized study of histopathology, tissue steroid receptors and plasma steroids after abrasio, with or without high dose gestagen treatment. Anticancer Res 1990;10:725-730.

223. Masuzawa H, Badokhon NH, Nakayama K, et al: Failure of down-regulation of estrogen receptors and progesterone receptors after medroxyprogesterone acetate administration for endometrial hyperplasia. Cancer 1994;74:2321-2328.

224. Trimble CL, Kauderer J, Silverberg S, et al: Concurrent endometrial carcinoma in women with biopsy diagnosis of atypical endometrial hyperplasia: A Gynecologic Oncology Group (GOG) Study. SGO, 2004 Annual Meeting on Women's Cancer, February 8, 2004.

225. Barnholtz-Sloan JS, Tainsky MA, Abrams J, et al: Ethnic differences in survival among women with ovarian carcinoma. Cancer 2002;94:1886-1893.

226. Fathalla MF: Factors in the causation and incidence of ovarian cancer. Obstet Gynecol Surv 1972;27:751-768.

227. Bingham C, Roberts D, Hamilton TC: The role of molecular biology in understanding ovarian cancer initiation and progression. Int J Gynecol Cancer 2001;11(Suppl 1):7-11.

228. Boyd J: Molecular genetics of hereditary ovarian cancer. Oncology (Hunting) 1998;12:399-406; discussion, 409-410, 413.

229. Hamilton TC, Berek JS, Kaye SB: Basic research: How much do we know, and what are we likely to learn about ovarian cancer in the near future? Ann Oncol 1999;10(Suppl 1):69-73.

230. Orsulic S, Li Y, Soslow RA, et al: Induction of ovarian cancer by defined multiple genetic changes in a mouse model system. Cancer Cell 2002;1:53-62.

231. Hellstrom I, Goodman G, Pullman J, et al: Overexpression of HER-2 in ovarian carcinomas. Cancer Res 2001;61:2420-2423.

232. Gallion HH, Pieretti M, DePriest PD, van Nagell JR Jr: The molecular basis of ovarian cancer. Cancer 1995;76: (10 Suppl):1992-1997.

233. Kohler MF, Marks JR, Wiseman RW, et al: Spectrum of mutation and frequency of allelic deletion of the p53 gene in ovarian cancer. J Natl Cancer Inst 1993;85:1513-1519.

234. Abdollahi A, Bao R, Hamilton TC: LOT1 is a growth suppressor gene down-regulated by the epidermal growth factor receptor ligands and encodes a nuclear zinc-finger protein. Oncogene 1999;18:6477-6487.

235. Alper O, Bergmann-Leitner ES, Bennett TA, et al: Epidermal growth factor receptor signaling and the invasive phenotype of ovarian carcinoma cells. J Natl Cancer Inst 2001;93: 1375-1384.

236. Epe B: Role of endogenous oxidative DNA damage in carcinogenesis: What can we learn from repair-deficient mice? Biol Chem 2002;383:467-475.

237. Goodman MT, McDuffie K, Kolonel LN, et al: Case-control study of ovarian cancer and polymorphisms in genes involved in catecholestrogen formation and metabolism. Cancer Epidemiol Biomarkers Prev 2001;10:209-216.

238. Kawanishi S, Hiraku Y, Oikawa S: Mechanism of guanine-specific DNA damage by oxidative stress and its role in carcinogenesis and aging. Mutat Res 2001;488:65-76.

239. Ness RB, Cottreau C: Possible role of ovarian epithelial inflammation in ovarian cancer. J Natl Cancer Inst 1999;91:1459-1467.

240. Ness RB, Grisso JA, Cottreau C, et al: Factors related to inflammation of the ovarian epithelium and risk of ovarian cancer. Epidemiology 2000;11:111-117.

241. Persson I: Estrogens in the causation of breast, endometrial and ovarian cancers: Evidence and hypotheses from epidemiological findings. J Steroid Biochem Mol Biol 2000;74:357-364.

242. Narod SA, Sun P, Ghadirian P, et al: Tubal ligation and risk of ovarian cancer in carriers of BRCA1 or BRCA2 mutations: A case-control study. Lancet 2001;357:1467-1470.

243. Kerlikowske K, Brown JS, Grady DG: Should women with familial ovarian cancer undergo prophylactic oophorectomy? Obstet Gynecol 1992;80:700-707.

244. Schildkraut JM, Thompson WD: Familial ovarian cancer: A population-based case-control study. Am J Epidemiol 1988;128:456-466.

245. Prevalence and penetrance of BRCA1 and BRCA2 mutations in a population-based series of breast cancer cases. Anglian Breast Cancer Study Group. Br J Cancer 2000;83:1301-1308.

246. Risch HA, McLaughlin JR, Cole DE, et al: Prevalence and penetrance of germline BRCA1 and BRCA2 mutations in a population series of 649 women with ovarian cancer. Am J Hum Genet 2001;68:700-710.

247. Stratton JF, Thompson D, Bobrow L, et al: The genetic epidemiology of early-onset epithelial ovarian cancer: A population-based study. Am J Hum Genet 1999;65:1725-1732.

248. Foulkes WD: BRCA1 and BRCA2: Penetrating the clinical arena. Lancet 1998;352:1325-1326.

249. Arver B, Borg A, Lindblom A: First BRCA1 and BRCA2 gene testing implemented in the health care system of Stockholm. Genet Test 2001;5:1-8.

250. Narod SA: Modifiers of risk and hereditary breast and ovarian cancer. Nat Rev Cancer 2002;2:113-123.

251. Bansal A, Critchfield GC, Frank TS, et al: The predictive value of BRCA1 and BRCA2 mutation testing. Genet Test 2000;4:45-48.

252. Mogren I, Stenlund H, Hogberg U: Long-term impact of reproductive factors on the risk of cervical, endometrial, ovarian and breast cancer. Acta Oncol 2001;40:849-854.

253. Riman T, Dickman PW, Nilsson S, et al: Risk factors for epithelial borderline ovarian tumors: Results of a Swedish case-control study. Gynecol Oncol 2001;83:575-585.

254. Modugno F, Ness RB, Wheeler JE: Reproductive risk factors for epithelial ovarian cancer according to histologic type and invasiveness. Ann Epidemiol 2001;11:568-574.

255. Chiaffarino F, Pelucchi C, Parazzini F, et al: Reproductive and hormonal factors and ovarian cancer. Ann Oncol 2001;12:337-341.

256. Purdie D, Green A, Bain C, et al: Reproductive and other factors and risk of epithelial ovarian cancer: An Australian case-control study. Survey of Women's Health Study Group. Int J Cancer 1995;62:678-684.

257. Vachon CM, Mink PJ, Janney CA, et al: Association of parity and ovarian cancer risk by family history of breast or ovarian cancer in a population-based study of postmenopausal women. Epidemiology 2002;13:66-71.

258. Ness RB, Grisso JA, Vergona R, et al: Oral contraceptives, other methods of contraception, and risk reduction for ovarian cancer. Epidemiology 2001;12:307-312.

259. Balen A: Polycystic ovary syndrome and cancer. Hum Reprod Update 2001;7:522-525.

260. Schildkraut JM, Schwingl PJ, Bastos E, et al: Epithelial ovarian cancer risk among women with polycystic ovary syndrome. Obstet Gynecol 1996;88:554-559.

261. Solomon CG: The epidemiology of polycystic ovary syndrome: Prevalence and associated disease risks. Endocrinol Metab Clin North Am 1999;28:247-263.

262. Purdie DM, Bain CJ, Webb PM, et al: Body size and ovarian cancer: Case-control study and systematic review (Australia). Cancer Causes Control 2001;12:855-863.

263. Verkasalo PK, Kaprio J, Koskenvuo M, Pukkala E: Genetic predisposition, environment and cancer incidence: A nationwide twin study in Finland, 1976-1995. Int J Cancer 1999;83: 743-749.

264. Bosetti C, Altieri A, La Vecchia C: Diet and environmental carcinogenesis in breast/gynecological cancers. Curr Opin Obstet Gynecol 2002;14:13-18.

265. McCann SE, Moysich KB, Mettlin C: Intakes of selected nutrients and food groups and risk of ovarian cancer. Nutr Cancer 2001;39:19-28.

266. Huncharek M, Klassen H, Kupelnick B: Dietary beta-carotene intake and the risk of epithelial ovarian cancer: A meta-analysis of 3,782 subjects from five observational studies. In Vivo 2001; 15:339-343.

267. Bertone ER, Hankinson SE, Newcomb PA, et al: A population-based case-control study of carotenoid and vitamin A intake and ovarian cancer (United States). Cancer Causes Control 2001;12:83-90.

268. Tavani A, Gallus S, La Vecchia C, et al: Physical activity and risk of ovarian cancer: An Italian case-control study. Int J Cancer 2001;91:407-411.

269. Cottreau CM, Ness RB, Kriska AM: Physical activity and reduced risk of ovarian cancer. Obstet Gynecol 2000;96:609-614.

270. Bertone ER, Willett WC, Rosner BA, et al: Prospective study of recreational physical activity and ovarian cancer. J Natl Cancer Inst 2001;93:942-948.

271. Mink PJ, Folsom AR, Sellers TA, Kushi LH: Physical activity, waist-to-hip ratio, and other risk factors for ovarian cancer: A follow-up study of older women. Epidemiology 1996;7:38-45.

272. Green A, Purdie D, Bain C, et al: Cigarette smoking and risk of epithelial ovarian cancer (Australia). Cancer Causes Control 2001;12:713-719.

273. Marchbanks PA, Wilson H, Bastos E, et al: Cigarette smoking and epithelial ovarian cancer by histologic type. Obstet Gynecol 2000;95:255-260.

274. Kuper H, Titus-Ernstoff L, Harlow BL, Cramer DW: Population based study of coffee, alcohol and tobacco use and risk of ovarian cancer. Int J Cancer 2000;88:313-318.

275. Moysich KB, Mettlin C, Piver MS, et al: Regular use of analgesic drugs and ovarian cancer risk. Cancer Epidemiol Biomarkers Prev 2001;10:903-906.

276. Tavani A, Gallus S, La Vecchia C, et al: Aspirin and ovarian cancer: An Italian case-control study. Ann Oncol 2000;11:1171-1173.

277. Rodriguez-Burford C, Barnes MN, Oelschlager DK, et al: Effects of nonsteroidal anti-inflammatory agents (NSAIDs) on ovarian carcinoma cell lines: Preclinical evaluation of NSAIDs as chemopreventive agents. Clin Cancer Res 2002;8:202-209.

278. Hankinson SE, Colditz GA, Hunter DJ, et al: A prospective study of reproductive factors and risk of epithelial ovarian cancer. Cancer 1995;76:284-290.

279. Schildkraut JM, Calingaert B, Marchbanks PA, et al: Impact of progestin and estrogen potency in oral contraceptives on ovarian cancer risk. J Natl Cancer Inst 2002;94:32-38.

280. Ness RB, Grisso JA, Klapper J, et al: Risk of ovarian cancer in relation to estrogen and progestin dose and use characteristics of oral contraceptives. SHARE Study Group. Steroid Hormones and Reproductions. Am J Epidemiol 2000;152:233-241.

281. Riman T, Dickman PW, Nilsson S, et al: Hormone replacement therapy and the risk of invasive epithelial ovarian cancer in Swedish women. J Natl Cancer Inst 2002;94:497-504.

282. Rodriguez C, Patel AV, Calle EE, et al: Estrogen replacement therapy and ovarian cancer mortality in a large prospective study of US women. JAMA 2001;285:1460-1465.

283. La Vecchia C, Brinton LA, McTiernan A: Menopause, hormone replacement therapy and cancer. Maturitas 2001;39:97-115.

284. Lacey JV Jr, Mink PJ, Lubin JH, et al: Menopausal hormone replacement therapy and risk of ovarian cancer. JAMA 2002;288:334-341.

285. Hardiman P, Nieto JJ, MacLean AB: Infertility and ovarian cancer. Gynecol Oncol 2000;76:1-2.

286. Whittemore AS, Harris R, Itnyre J: Characteristics relating to ovarian cancer risk: Collaborative analysis of 12 US case-control studies. II. Invasive epithelial ovarian cancers in white women. Collaborative Ovarian Cancer Group. Am J Epidemiol 1992;136:1184-1203.

287. Ness RB, Cramer DW, Goodman MT, et al: Infertility, fertility drugs, and ovarian cancer: A pooled analysis of case-control studies. Am J Epidemiol 2002;155:217-224.

288. Rossing MA, Daling JR, Weiss NS, et al: Ovarian tumors in a cohort of infertile women. N Engl J Med 1994;331:771-776.

289. Nieto JJ, Rolfe KJ, MacLean AB, Hardiman P: Ovarian cancer and infertility: A genetic link? Lancet 1999;354:649.

290. Rossing MA, Weiss NS: Fertility drugs and breast and ovarian cancer [letter; comment]. Lancet 1995;346:1627-1628.

291. Miki Y, Swensen J, Shattuck-Eidens D, et al: A strong candidate for the breast and ovarian cancer susceptibility gene BRCA1. Science 1994;266:66-71.

292. Plaxe SC, Braly PS, Freddo JL, et al: Profiles of women age 30-39 and age less than 30 with epithelial ovarian cancer. Obstet Gynecol 1993;81:651-654.

293. Kramer BS, Gohagan J, Prorok PC: NIH Consensus 1994: Screening. Gynecol Oncol 1994;55:S20-S21.

294. Van Nagell JR Jr, DePriest PD, Puls LE, et al: Ovarian cancer screening in asymptomatic postmenopausal women by transvaginal sonography. Cancer 1991;68:458-462.

295. Karlan BY, Platt LD: The current status of ultrasound and color Doppler imaging in screening for ovarian cancer. Gynecol Oncol 1994;55:S28-S33.

296. Muto MG, Cramer DW, Brown DL, et al: Screening for ovarian cancer: The preliminary experience of a familial ovarian cancer center. Gynecol Oncol 1993;51:12-20.

297. Karlan BY: The status of ultrasound and color Doppler imaging for the early detection of ovarian carcinoma. Cancer Invest 1997;15:265-269.

298. Canis M, Pouly JL, Wattiez A, et al: Laparoscopic management of adnexal masses suspicious at ultrasound. Obstet Gynecol 1997;89:679-683.

299. van Nagell JR Jr, DePriest PD, Reedy MB, et al: The efficacy of transvaginal sonographic screening in asymptomatic women at risk for ovarian cancer. Gynecol Oncol 2000;77:350-356.

300. Berek JS, Bast RC Jr: Ovarian cancer screening: The use of serial complementary tumor markers to improve sensitivity and specificity for early detection. Cancer 1995;76(10 Suppl):2092-2096.

301. Bast RC Jr, Xu FJ, Yu YH, et al: CA 125: The past and the future. Int J Biol Markers 1998;13:179-187.

302. Brewer M, Utzinger U, Silva E, et al: Fluorescence spectroscopy for in vivo characterization of ovarian tissue. Lasers Surg Med 2001;29:128-135.

303. Petricoin EF, Ardekani AM, Hitt BA, et al: Use of proteomic patterns in serum to identify ovarian cancer. Lancet 2002;359:572-577.

304. Risch HA, Marrett LD, Howe GR: Parity, contraception, infertility, and the risk of epithelial ovarian cancer. Am J Epidemiol 1994;140:585-597.

305. Mosgaard BJ, Lidegaard O, Andersen AN: The impact of parity, infertility and treatment with fertility drugs on the risk of ovarian cancer: A survey. Acta Obstet Gynecol Scand 1997;76:89-95.

306. Mori M, Harabuchi I, Miyake H, et al: Reproductive, genetic, and dietary risk factors for ovarian cancer. Am J Epidemiol 1988;128:771-777.

307. Whiteman DC, Murphy MF, Cook LS, et al: Multiple births and risk of epithelial ovarian cancer. J Natl Cancer Inst 2000;92:1172-1177.

308. Rosenblatt KA, Thomas DB: Lactation and the risk of epithelial ovarian cancer. The WHO Collaborative Study of Neoplasia and Steroid Contraceptives. Int J Epidemiol 1993;22:192-197.

309. Piver MS, Jishi MF, Tsukada Y, Nava G: Primary peritoneal carcinoma after prophylactic oophorectomy in women with a family history of ovarian cancer. A report of the Gilda Radner Familial Ovarian Cancer Registry. Cancer 1993;71:2751-2755.

310. Speroff T, Dawson NV, Speroff L, Haber RJ: A risk-benefit analysis of elective bilateral oophorectomy: Effect of changes in compliance with estrogen therapy on outcome. Am J Obstet Gynecol 1991;164:165-174.

311. Brewer MA, Mitchell MF, Bast RC: Prevention of ovarian cancer. In Vivo 1999;13:99-106.

312. Guruswamy S, Lightfoot S, Gold MA, et al: Effects of retinoids on cancerous phenotype and apoptosis in organotypic cultures of ovarian carcinoma. JNCI 2001; 93:516-525.

313. De Palo G, Veronesi U, Camerini T, et al: Can fenretinide protect women against ovarian cancer? J Natl Cancer Inst 1995;87:146-147.

314. De Palo G, Mariani L, Camerini T, et al: Effect of fenretinide on ovarian carcinoma occurrence. Gynecol Oncol 2002;86:24-27.

315. Campbell MJ, Park S, Uskokovic MR, et al: Expression of retinoic acid receptor-beta sensitizes prostate cancer cells to growth inhibition mediated by combinations of retinoids and a 19-nor hexafluoride vitamin D3 analog. Endocrinology 1998;139:1972-1980.

316. Studzinski GP, Moore DC: Sunlight: Can it prevent as well as cause cancer? Cancer Res 1995;55:4014-4022.

317. Lefkowitz ES, Garland CF: Sunlight, vitamin D, and ovarian cancer mortality rates in US women. Int J Epidemiol 1994;23:1133-1136.

318. The reduction in risk of ovarian cancer associated with oral-contraceptive use. The Cancer and Steroid Hormone Study of the Centers for Disease Control and the National Institute of Child Health and Human Development. N Engl J Med 1987;316:650-655.

319. Risch HA: Hormonal etiology of epithelial ovarian cancer, with a hypothesis concerning the role of androgens and progesterone. J Natl Cancer Inst 1998;90:1774-1786.

320. Narod SA, Risch H, Moslehi R, et al: Oral contraceptives and the risk of hereditary ovarian cancer. Hereditary Ovarian Cancer Clinical Study Group. N Engl J Med 1998;339:424-428.

321. Walker GR, Schlesselman JJ, Ness RB: Family history of cancer, oral contraceptive use, and ovarian cancer risk. Am J Obstet Gynecol 2002;186:8-14.

322. Modan B, Hartge P, Hirsh-Yechezkel G, et al: Parity, oral contraceptives, and the risk of ovarian cancer among carriers and noncarriers of a BRCA1 or BRCA2 mutation. N Engl J Med 2001;345:235-240.

323. Depot-medroxyprogesterone acetate (DMPA) and risk of epithelial ovarian cancer: The WHO Collaborative Study of Neoplasia and Steroid Contraceptives. Int J Cancer 1991;49:191-195.

324. Rodriguez GC, Walmer DK, Cline M, et al: Effect of progestin on the ovarian epithelium of macaques: Cancer prevention through apoptosis? J Soc Gynecol Investig 1998;5:271-276.

325. Rodriguez GC, Nagarsheth NP, Lee KL, et al: Progestin-induced apoptosis in the Macaque ovarian epithelium: Differential regulation of transforming growth factor-beta. J Natl Cancer Inst 2002;94:50-60.

326. Cramer DW, Harlow BL, Titus-Ernstoff L, et al: Over-the-counter analgesics and risk of ovarian cancer. Lancet 1998;351:104-107.

327. Rosenberg L, Palmer JR, Rao RS, et al: A case-control study of analgesic use and ovarian cancer. Cancer Epidemiol Biomarkers Prev 2000;9:933-937.

328. Akhmedkhanov A, Toniolo P, Zeleniuch-Jacquotte A, et al: Aspirin and epithelial ovarian cancer. Prev Med 2001;33:682-687.

329. Goodwin JS: Prostaglandins and host defense in cancer. Med Clin North Am 1981;65:829-844.

330. Marnett LJ: Aspirin and related nonsteroidal anti-inflammatory drugs as chemopreventive agents against colon cancer. Prev Med 1995;24:103-106.

331. Ferrandina G, Ranelletti FO, Lauriola L, et al: Cyclooxygenase-2 (COX-2), epidermal growth factor receptor (EGFR), and Her-2/neu expression in ovarian cancer. Gynecol Oncol 2002;85:305-310.

332. Denkert C, Kobel M, Pest S, et al: Expression of cyclooxygenase 2 is an independent prognostic factor in human ovarian carcinoma. Am J Pathol 2002;160:893-903.

333. Masferrer JL, Leahy KM, Koki AT, et al: Antiangiogenic and antitumor activities of cyclooxygenase-2 inhibitors. Cancer Res 2000;60:1306-1311.

334. Trimble CL, Hildesheim A, Brinton LA, et al: Heterogeneous etiology of squamous carcinoma of the vulva. Obstet Gynecol 1996;87:59-64.

335. Gastrell FH, McConnell DT: Human papillomavirus and vulval intra-epithelial neoplasia. Best Pract Res Clin Obstet Gynecol 2001;15:769-782.

336. Joura EA: Epidemiology, diagnosis and treatment of vulvar intraepithelial neoplasia. Curr Opin Obstet Gynecol 2002;14:39-43.

337. Stern PL, Brown M, Stacey SN, et al: Natural HPV immunity and vaccination strategies. J Clin Virol 2000;19:57-66.

338. Flowers LC, Wistuba J II, Scurry CY, et al: Genetic changes during the multistage pathogenesis of human papillomavirus positive and negative vulvar carcinomas. J Soc Gynecol Investig 1999;6:213-221.

339. Rosenthal AN, Ryan A, Hopster D, et al: High frequency of loss of heterozygosity in vulval intraepithelial neoplasia (VIN) is associated with invasive vulval squamous cell carcinoma (VSCC). Int J Cancer 2001;94:896-900.

340. Jee KJ, Kim YT, Kim KR, et al: Loss in 3p and 4p and gain of 3q are concomitant aberrations in squamous cell carcinoma of the vulva. Mod Pathol 2001;14:377-381.

341. Pinto AP, Lin MC, Sheets EE, et al: Allelic imbalance in lichen sclerosus, hyperplasia, and intraepithelial neoplasia of the vulva. Gynecol Oncol 2000;77:171-176.

342. Rolfe KJ, Crow JC, Benjamin E, et al: Cyclin D1 and retinoblastoma protein in vulvar cancer and adjacent lesions. Int J Gynecol Cancer 2001;11:381-386.

343. Sauter ER, Nesbit M, Litwin S, et al: Antisense cyclin D1 induces apoptosis and tumor shrinkage in human squamous carcinomas. Cancer Res 1999;59:4876-4881.

344. Zamparelli A, Masciullo V, Bovicelli A, et al: Expression of cell-cycle-associated proteins pRB2/p130 and p27kip in vulvar squamous cell carcinomas. Hum Pathol 2001;32:4-9.

345. Ben-Hur H, Ashkenazi M, Huszar M, et al: Lymphoid elements and apoptosis-related proteins (Fas, Fas ligand, p53 and bcl-2) in lichen sclerosus and carcinoma of the vulva. Eur J Gynecol Oncol 2001;22:104-109.

346. Carlson JA, Amin S, Malfetano J, et al: Concordant p53 and mdm-2 protein expression in vulvar squamous cell carcinoma and adjacent lichen sclerosus. Appl Immunohistochem Mol Morphol 2001;9:150-163.

347. Kagie MJ, Kenter GG, Tollenaar RA, et al: P53 protein overexpression is common and independent of human papillomavirus infection in squamous cell carcinoma of the vulva. Cancer 1997;80:1228-1233.

348. Kagie MJ, Kenter GG, Tollenaar RA, et al: P53 protein overexpression, a frequent observation in squamous cell carcinoma of the vulva and in various synchronous vulvar epithelia, has no value as a prognostic parameter. Int J Gynecol Pathol 1997;16:124-130.

349. Tervahauta AI, Syrjanen SM, Vayrynen M, et al: Expression of p53 protein related to the presence of human papillomavirus (HPV) DNA in genital carcinomas and precancer lesions. Anticancer Res 1993;13:1107-1111.

350. Hietanen SH, Kurvinen K, Syrjanen K, et al: Mutation of tumor suppressor gene p53 is frequently found in vulvar carcinoma cells. Am J Obstet Gynecol 1995;173:1477-1482.

351. Kim YT, Thomas NF, Kessis TD, et al: P53 mutations and clonality in vulvar carcinomas and squamous hyperplasias: Evidence suggesting that squamous hyperplasias do not serve as direct precursors of human papillomavirus-negative vulvar carcinomas. Hum Pathol 1996;27:389-395.

352. Lee YY, Wilczynski SP, Chumakov A, et al: Carcinoma of the vulva: HPV and p53 mutations. Oncogene 1994;9:1655-1659.

353. Milde-Langosch K, Albrecht K, Joram S, et al: Presence and persistence of HPV infection and p53 mutation in cancer of the cervix uteri and the vulva. Int J Cancer 1995;63:639-645.

354. Pilotti S, D'Amato L, Della Torre G, et al: Papillomavirus, p53 alteration, and primary carcinoma of the vulva. Diagn Mol Pathol 1995;4:239-248.

355. Sliutz G, Schmidt W, Tempfer C, et al: Detection of p53 point mutations in primary human vulvar cancer by PCR and temperature gradient gel electrophoresis. Gynecol Oncol 1997;64:93-98.

356. Kohlberger P, Kainz C, Breitenecker G, et al: Prognostic value of immunohistochemically detected p53 expression in vulvar carcinoma. Cancer 1995;76:1786-1789.

357. Salmaso R, Zen T, Zannol M, et al: Prognostic value of protein p53 and ki-67 in invasive vulvar squamous cell carcinoma. Eur J Gynecol Oncol 2000;21:479-483.

358. Hantschmann P, Lampe B, Beysiegel S, Kurzl R: Tumor proliferation in squamous cell carcinoma of the vulva. Int J Gynecol Pathol 2000;19:361-368.

359. Hendricks JB, Wilkinson EJ, Kubilis P, et al: Ki-67 expression in vulvar carcinoma. Int J Gynecol Pathol 1994;13:205-210.

360. Scurry J, Beshay V, Cohen C, Allen D: Ki67 expression in lichen sclerosus of vulva in patients with and without associated squamous cell carcinoma. Histopathology 1998;32:399-404.

361. van Hoeven KH, Kovatich AJ: Immunohistochemical staining for proliferating cell nuclear antigen, BCL2, and Ki-67 in vulvar tissues. Int J Gynecol Pathol 1996;15:10-16.

362. Wu X, Xin Y, Yao J, et al: Expression of epithelial growth factor receptor and its two ligands, transforming growth factor-alpha and epithelial growth factor, in normal and neoplastic squamous cells in the vulva: An immunohistochemical study. Med Electron Microsc 2001;34:179-184.

363. Johnson GA, Mannel R, Khalifa M, et al: Epidermal growth factor receptor in vulvar malignancies and its relationship to metastasis and patient survival. Gynecol Oncol 1997;65:425-429.

364. Sirotnak FM, Zakowski MF, Miller VA, et al: Efficacy of cytotoxic agents against human tumor xenografts is markedly enhanced by coadministration of ZD1839 (Iressa), an inhibitor of EGFR tyrosine kinase. Clin Cancer Res 2000;6:4885-4892.

365. MacLean AB, Reid WM, Rolfe KJ, et al: Role of angiogenesis in benign, premalignant and malignant vulvar lesions. J Reprod Med 2000;45:609-612.

366. Hefler L, Tempfer C, Obermair A, et al: Serum concentrations of vascular endothelial growth factor in vulvar cancer. Clin Cancer Res 1999;5:2806-2809.

367. Lopez-Ocejo O, Viloria-Petit A, Bequet-Romero M, et al: Oncogenes and tumor angiogenesis: The HPV-16 E6 oncoprotein activates the vascular endothelial growth factor (VEGF) gene promoter in a p53 independent manner. Oncogene 2000;19:4611-4620.

368. Bancher-Todesca D, Obermair A, Bilgi S, et al: Angiogenesis in vulvar intraepithelial neoplasia. Gynecol Oncol 1997;64: 496-500.

369. Obermair A, Kohlberger P, Bancher-Todesca D, et al: Influence of microvessel density and vascular permeability factor/vascular endothelial growth factor expression on prognosis in vulvar cancer. Gynecol Oncol 1996;63:204-209.

370. Davis G, Wentworth J, Richard J: Self-administered topical imiquimod treatment of vulvar intraepithelial neoplasia: A report of four cases. J Reprod Med 2000;45:619-623.

371. Joura EA, Losch A, Haider-Angler MG, et al: Trends in vulvar neoplasia. Increasing incidence of vulvar intraepithelial neoplasia and squamous cell carcinoma of the vulva in young women. J Reprod Med 2000;45:613-615.

372. Sturgeon SR, Brinton LA, Devesa SS, et al: In situ and invasive vulvar cancer incidence trends (1973 to 1987). Am J Obstet Gynecol 1992;166:1482-1485.

373. Bergstrom R, Sparen P, Adami HO: Trends in cancer of the cervix uteri in Sweden following cytological screening. Br J Cancer 1999;81:159-166.

374. Liu S, Semenciw R, Probert A, Mao Y: Cervical cancer in Canada: Changing patterns in incidence and mortality. Int J Gynecol Cancer 2001;11:24-31.

375. Hildesheim A, Han CL, Brinton LA, et al: Human papillomavirus type 16 and risk of preinvasive and invasive vulvar cancer: Results from a seroepidemiological case-control study. Obstet Gynecol 1997;90:748-754.

376. Sellors JW, Lorincz AT, Mahony JB, et al: Comparison of self-collected vaginal, vulvar and urine samples with physician-collected cervical samples for human papillomavirus testing to detect high-grade squamous intraepithelial lesions. CMAJ 2000;163:513-518.

377. Stefanon B, De Palo G: Is vulvoscopy a reliable diagnostic technique for high grade vulvar intraepithelial neoplasia? Eur J Gynecol Oncol 1997;18:211.

378. Joura EA, Zeisler H, Losch A, et al: Differentiating vulvar intraepithelial neoplasia from nonneoplastic epithelial disorders. The toluidine blue test. J Reprod Med 1998;43: 71-674.

379. Hording U, Daugaard S, Junge J, Lundvall F: Human papillomaviruses and multifocal genital neoplasia. Int J Gynecol Pathol 1996;15:230-234.

380. Al-Ghamdi A, Freedman D, Miller D, et al: Vulvar squamous cell carcinoma in young women: A clinicopathologic study of 21 cases. Gynecol Oncol 2002;84:94-101.

381. Muderspach L, Wilczynski S, Roman L, et al: A phase I trial of a human papillomavirus (HPV) peptide vaccine for women with high-grade cervical and vulvar intraepithelial neoplasia who are HPV 16 positive. Clin Cancer Res 2000;6: 3406-3416.

382. Hopkins MP, Nemunaitis-Keller J: Carcinoma of the vulva. Obstet Gynecol Clin North Am 2001;28:791-804.

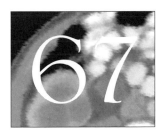

GYNECOLOGIC CANCER IN PREGNANCY

Afshin Bahador, M. Patrick Lowe, Joan Cheng, and Lynda D. Roman

---

 MAJOR CONTROVERSIES

- Are tumor markers useful in pregnant patients with an adnexal mass?
- What is the role of radiographic imaging in the pregnant patient with a pelvic mass?
- When is surgical intervention indicated in the pregnant patient with a pelvic mass?
- What route of surgery is best?
- What is the appropriate surgery for ovarian cancer diagnosed in pregnancy?
- Which chemotherapeutic agents should be used in treating ovarian cancer during pregnancy?
- When and how should cone biopsy in pregnancy be performed?
- What is the appropriate treatment for microinvasive cervical carcinoma in pregnancy?
- What is the role of radiologic imaging in pregnant women with cervical cancer?
- Is delay in treatment acceptable in early-stage disease?
- What is the optimal mode of delivery for women with cervical cancer?
- How should women with advanced lesions diagnosed in pregnancy be treated?
- What is the role of chemotherapy in the treatment of cervical cancer in pregnancy?

Although the diagnosis of cancer is always devastating, it is especially so in pregnancy. The welfare of both the mother and the fetus must be taken into account, and, frequently, optimal treatment of the cancer poses significant risk to the fetus. This is especially true in the case of gynecologic cancer complicating pregnancy, because definitive treatment usually requires direct manipulation of the very organs that are essential for fetal growth and well-being. The conflicting goals of aggressively treating the mother and protecting the fetus from harm can place enormous emotional stress on the patient and her family as well as her physician.

Of the gynecologic cancers, the one that is most common in pregnancy is cervical cancer, which affects 1.2 to 10.6 of every 10,000 pregnancies.[1-3] Ovarian cancer in pregnancy, which complicates 2 to 5 of every 100,000 deliveries,[4,5] is substantially less common. Endometrial and vulvar cancer in association with

pregnancy are extremely rare. The diagnosis of any of these cancers in the pregnant women poses its own set of dilemmas. Prospective trials of treatment of cancer during pregnancy are lacking (and will probably never be done), so the existing data are retrospective or anecdotal. As a result, controversy exists as to the optimal treatment of gynecologic cancer occurring in pregnancy. This chapter focuses on the controversies that surround the management of cervical and ovarian cancer in pregnancy, including the roles of imaging and serum markers, the timing of surgery and delivery, and the use of chemotherapy.

ADNEXAL MASSES IN PREGNANCY

The use of advanced ultrasonic technology has become commonplace in obstetric care and has led to an increased incidence of diagnosis of an adnexal mass during pregnancy. Historically, the incidence reported in the literature ranged from 1 in 81 to 1 in 8000 pregnancies.[6-8] This wide range resulted from variations in methods of detection and the criteria for diagnosis. Three publications from the late 1990s placed the incidence between 1in 800 and 1 in 1400 pregnancies.[9-11] The combined cohort included more than 256,000 live births, and 215 adnexal masses were detected during pregnancy.

The majority of adnexal masses in pregnancy are benign and do not represent an underlying ovarian malignancy. The incidence of malignancy in ovarian tumors complicating pregnancy is between 2% and 5%.[10,11] The most common ovarian tumors detected during pregnancy are functional cysts such as corpora lutea or follicular cysts. The majority of these do not persist into the second trimester and therefore pose no further risk. Dermoid cysts and cystadenomas have been reported to comprise up to 60% of adnexal masses removed in pregnancy.[10-12] The two most common ovarian malignancies diagnosed in pregnancy are germ cell tumors and epithelial ovarian cancers.[13] Germ cell tumors are known to be the most common ovarian malignancies in women of reproductive age. Epithelial ovarian cancers are most common in postmenopausal women, but the large majority of these associated with pregnancy are tumors of low malignant potential.[13]

Symptoms of adnexal masses in pregnancy range from none to the acute onset of pelvic pain. Methods of detection include clinical pelvic examination, routine obstetric ultrasonography, and size greater than date measurements. Reports in the literature indicate that one third to one half of adnexal masses in pregnancy are detected on routine prenatal examination. Whitecar and colleagues[11] diagnosed 47% of adnexal masses in their series by pelvic examination, and an additional 15% were diagnosed on routine obstetric ultrasound studies.[11] The acute onset of pelvic pain in these patients is primarily attributed to torsion, rupture, or hemorrhage into the cyst. This leads to unplanned surgery during pregnancy. The incidence of laparotomy for emergency conditions ranged from 1% to 27% in recently published series.[9-11] It is obviously preferable to approach surgery in the pregnant patient under a controlled environment, because studies show that emergency surgery in pregnancy carries a higher risk of unfavorable outcomes such as miscarriage, preterm labor, and preterm delivery.[10] Three important issues to address in the evaluation of an adnexal mass in pregnancy are the usefulness of tumor markers, the role of radiologic imaging in pregnancy, and the timing of surgical intervention.

Are tumor markers useful in pregnant patients with an adnexal mass?

The measurement of tumor markers such as CA 125, lactate dehydrogenase (LDH), α-fetoprotein (AFP), and human chorionic gonadotropin (HCG) in pregnancy poses a dilemma, because these values are elevated in normal pregnancy and their clinically utility in pregnancy is therefore debatable.

Serum CA 125 levels typically peak in the first trimester at 10 weeks with levels on the order of 1250 U/mL. These levels then decline and remain below 35 U/mL until the time of delivery. At delivery there is a transient increase and subsequent decrease to normal levels.[14] The use of CA 125 is therefore not advised in the first trimester, but it may be useful in the second or third trimester, especially if very elevated. LDH values change little in pregnancy (with the exception of preeclampsia and its variant, the HELLP syndrome). This hormone is used as a marker for dysgerminomas and has been used to monitor two patients with dysgerminomas during pregnancy.[15] AFP levels are elevated during pregnancy, and is the predominant serum protein; it is therefore difficult to use AFP to diagnose an endodermal sinus tumor in pregnancy. Similarly, HCG, which can serve as a valuable marker in the diagnosis of ovarian embryonal carcinomas, is not a reliable marker in pregnancy because of the physiologic elevation in HCG that normally occurs during this time.

What is the role of radiographic imaging in the pregnant patient with a pelvic mass?

When an adnexal mass has been diagnosed in pregnancy, questions arise as to the safety of radiologic imaging. The most common forms of radiation used today are ionizing and nonionizing. Ionizing radiation should be avoided in the first trimester because of its deleterious effects on the developing embryo. The preimplantation period (days 0 through 9 after conception) and the period of organogenesis (days 15 through 50 after conception) are the most sensitive times. Effects of ionizing radiation given in the first trimester include central nervous system malformations, radiation-induced abortion, mental retardation, congenital anomalies, and childhood cancers. It appears that, during the preimplantation period, an all-or-none effect is observed at a threshold of 5 to 10 rads. No malformations or growth restrictions are observed during this period, presumably because the cells are extraembryonic and no differentiation has occurred. Diagnostic imaging modalities that use ionizing radiation include x-radiography and computed tomography (CT). Chest radiography is the most common form of ionizing radiation used in pregnancy. Preferably avoided in the first trimester, chest radiography can be performed, if clinically warranted, with the use of an abdominal shielding to decrease the radiation exposure to the fetus. CT should be avoided in the first trimester.[16-18]

The best modality to evaluate an adnexal mass in the first trimester is transvaginal ultrasonography. This modality incorporates nonionizing radiation to create an image. No published reports have documented a deleterious effect of standard diagnostic ultrasound use in pregnancy. Ultrasonography provides important information that can be used in planning and management, including the architectural characteristics of the mass, the presence of ascites, and color Doppler flow data. Benign and malignant lesions demonstrate different characteristics, which can be used to categorize a lesion as benign appearing or suspicious for a malignancy.

Magnetic resonance imaging (MRI) is an additional nonionizing modality, but it is not recommended for use in the first trimester because of theoretical concerns about magnetic fields and heat generated from the study. These concerns stem from the possible effects at the cellular level of the high static magnetic fields that are used to generate an image. There are no reports that demonstrate adverse congenital or behavioral outcomes in a fetus exposed to MRI during pregnancy. Recent guidelines from the American College of Radiology state that there are no known risks to the fetus from a MRI examination.[19] However, the American College of Obstetrics and Gynecology recommends against its use in the first trimester of pregnancy.[20] In later trimesters, MRI may be useful for determining the nature of a mass, especially if there is suspicion that the mass may represent a fibroid.

MRI uses nonionizing radiation and provides multiplanar images with superior contrast resolution compared with CT and ultrasound. A report of 3-year follow-up data on women exposed to MRI while pregnant reported no adverse outcomes.[21] With a proven safety profile, no exposure to ionizing radiation, and published safety data, MRI should be performed preferentially in the second or third trimester instead of CT.

When is surgical intervention indicated in the pregnant patient with a pelvic mass?

The management of an asymptomatic adnexal mass in the first trimester of pregnancy is typically expectant. The majority of adnexal masses diagnosed at this time are physiologic cysts that resolve spontaneously by the second trimester. An initial transvaginal ultrasound examination is indicated to characterize the mass, and this is repeated at 12 to 14 weeks of gestation. If no lesion is present at that time, it is unlikely that a new mass will appear, and no further evaluation is necessary for the remainder of the pregnancy.

A persistent adnexal mass requires further evaluation, with importance focused on characterization of the lesion. Has it increased in size? Is the lesion cystic, solid, or complex? Are there internal septations or a thick cyst wall? Is there evidence of ascites or internal papillary projections? Options for management of a persistent adnexal mass in pregnancy are conservative or surgical in nature. Simple cysts smaller than 5 cm in diameter that persist into the second trimester warrant expectant management, because there is little chance

of an underlying malignancy and the risks associated with surgery are avoided.[16] A report by Platek and colleagues[9] described an algorithm for the conservative management of persistent simple adnexal masses in pregnancy. All masses including simple cysts greater than 10 cm and persistent complex adnexal masses warrant surgical intervention in the second trimester, which is best performed at 16 to 18 weeks of gestation to establish a tissue diagnosis and avoid surgical emergencies such as ovarian torsion or cyst rupture, which are associated with an increased risk of unfavorable pregnancy outcome. The risk of ovarian torsion, cyst rupture, or hemorrhage can be as high as 10% to 15%.[10] By this time, the majority of physiologic cysts have resolved, and the risk of spontaneous miscarriage and preterm labor is minimal.

Some controversy exists about the management of simple cysts measuring 5 to 9 cm in diameter. Thornton and Wells[22] suggested conservative management; however, in their report, 21% of simple cysts larger than 5 cm electively removed were tumors of low malignant potential. There were no reports of emergency surgery for torsion or cyst rupture in their series, but other reports demonstrate an incidence of up to 27% for emergency surgery for adnexal masses in pregnancy. Until other data become available, simple cysts between 5 and 9 cm in diameter should be electively removed in the second trimester.

An asymptomatic complex adnexal mass diagnosed in the third trimester can also be managed conservatively until after delivery, because only 2% to 5% of these lesions prove to be malignant.[10,11] The risk of preterm labor and delivery, with its sequelae, as a result of abdominal surgery in the early third trimester outweighs the possible benefits of surgery. If the lesion remains stable, surgical evaluation can be performed after delivery or through a combined cesarean section–ovarian cystectomy or oophorectomy followed by staging if necessary at term. If the patient is acutely symptomatic, surgical exploration may become necessary, with appropriate consultation with maternal-fetal medicine specialists.

What route of surgery is best?

Traditionally, adnexal masses in pregnancy have been surgically approached by laparotomy. The choice of incision is typically either midline or low transverse, usually based on the characteristics of the lesion and the preference of the surgeon. Surgical management consists of laparotomy, peritoneal washings, and cystectomy or unilateral salpingo-oophorectomy with frozen section examination intraoperatively. Early invasive epithelial lesions necessitate additional staging procedures (omentectomy, lymph node dissection, peritoneal and diaphragmatic biopsies) with or without removal of the remaining ovary.

The use of laparoscopy in pregnancy was very uncommon until recently because of concerns about trocar damage to the uterus, fetal risks during general anesthesia, and a lack of published experience with the technique. The majority of laparoscopic experience in pregnancy comes from laparoscopic cholecystectomy using the open-laparoscopy technique.[23] Few reports of laparoscopic management of adnexal masses in pregnancy exist in the literature, and these studies report only a small number of cases. In these series, laparoscopy is suggested as an alternative approach up until 14 to 16 weeks of gestation. Parker and colleagues[24] reported on the removal of 12 benign cystic teratomas from pregnant women. Gestational age ranged from 9 to 17 weeks. Intraoperative cyst rupture occurred in 93% of the women. Chemical peritonitis was not reported, and there were no major maternal or fetal complications. The extremely high rate of unintentional cyst rupture demonstrates the difficulty involved in performing laparoscopy in the second trimester. In another small series, Morice and coworkers[25] reported on the successful management of ovarian torsion during pregnancy in six patients. No maternal or fetal complications were reported. Similarly, Moore and Smith[26] reported on 14 women who underwent laparoscopic removal of an adnexal mass in the second trimester of pregnancy. No malignancies were found, and there was one instance of "mild peritonitis" that resolved without incidence. The rate of cyst rupture was not given.

There are some concerns regarding the safety of laparoscopy and the carbon dioxide pneumoperitoneum on the developing fetus. Questions concerning decreased uterine blood flow and possible fetal acidosis from the carbon dioxide pneumoperitoneum are still debated.[23] Cyst rupture is more likely to occur with laparoscopy than with laparotomy, increasing the risk of peritonitis. As with any surgical procedure, the benefit of the proposed procedure should outweigh the risk. The laparoscopic approach appears to be reasonable for women who are in the early second trimester of pregnancy, who have adnexal masses that appear to be benign and are limited in size, and in whom the procedure can be accomplished without a high likelihood of rupture. Until further data become available, the safest approach in most pregnant women with adnexal masses appears to be laparotomy.

OVARIAN CANCER IN PREGNANCY

Ovarian cancer in pregnancy is an uncommon phenomenon, with reported incidences ranging from 1 in 12,000 to 1 in 50,000 pregnancies. Ovarian malignancies in pregnancy typically are asymptomatic or produce symptoms that could be attributed to the pregnancy, such as abdominal distention, abdominal pain, and nausea and vomiting.[27] The diagnosis is usually made in the first or second trimester during routine prenatal physical examination or prenatal ultrasound examination. However, an ovarian malignancy can remain undiagnosed until the time of caesarian section.[28] Most patients reported in the literature have had early-stage disease. Rahman and associates[28] found that seven of their nine pregnant

patients with ovarian cancer had stage I disease. Carcinomas of germ cell and epithelial origin predominate. Not all malignant pelvic masses in pregnancy are of ovarian origin. Recurrent fallopian tube carcinoma[29] and retroperitoneal neuroblastoma[30] have also been reported.

What is the appropriate surgery for ovarian cancer diagnosed in pregnancy?

There is little controversy regarding surgical management of ovarian cancer during pregnancy. In most cases, the same basic principles applied to the management of ovarian cancer in a nonpregnant patient may be implemented. Although the level of suspicion may be high preoperatively, the diagnosis of a malignancy in an adnexal mass is made intraoperatively, and therefore knowledge and experience regarding the appropriate surgical management are essential. Most pregnant patients taken to the operating room for an adnexal mass are in their second trimester and have stage I disease, so that pelvic washings, unilateral oophorectomy, omentectomy, peritoneal biopsies, and ipsilateral pelvic and aortic lymphadenectomy can be performed without any significant harm to the gravid uterus. Management of more advanced disease should be individualized based on the following factors: gestational age, extent of disease, the expertise of the surgeon, and the wishes of the patient. Modification of the standard surgical staging procedure for invasive ovarian cancer may be required. If intraperitoneal dissemination is discovered intraoperatively and the patient is desirous of continuing the pregnancy, conservative cytoreduction (with the goal of avoiding a prolonged and traumatic procedure that could result in harm to the fetus) followed by adjuvant chemotherapy is appropriate. Hysterectomy and more extensive cytoreduction can be performed at the time of caesarian section, or in the immediate postpartum stage if the patient desires vaginal delivery.

Chemotherapy in pregnancy

The teratogenic potential of chemotherapeutic agents has been clearly demonstrated in animals.[31] Based on the U. S. Food and Drug Administration's assignment of risk categories to drugs in pregnancy, most chemotherapeutic agents are assigned as category C or D.[32] Category X (drugs that are contraindicated in pregnancy) is not usually assigned to chemotherapeutic agents because their use in pregnancy may be life-preserving for the mother.

The majority of the experience with the use of chemotherapy in pregnancy is in patients with leukemia or lymphoma.[33-35] It has been reported that there is a high incidence of congenital malformations when antineoplastic agents are administered during the first trimester, presumably because this period of organogenesis carries the highest risk.[36] Although there is a lack of prospective data showing its safety, a large collection of retrospective and anecdotal data demonstrate that chemotherapy, if indicated, can be given in the second and third trimesters without significant fetal sequelae. Reynoso and colleagues[35] reviewed more than 50 cases and concluded that the incidence of congenital malformations, at least in the second and third trimesters, is not significantly higher than that in uncomplicated pregnancies. Exposure during the second and third trimesters could, however, result in pregnancy-related complications such as intrauterine fetal demise, premature labor, and low birth weight. In addition, there have been reports of fetal or neonatal myelosuppression.[37]

It is of extreme importance that the patient makes an informed decision to undergo chemotherapy during her pregnancy. A multidisciplinary team of physicians comprising the oncologist, perinatologist, and neonatologist can aid the patient and her family by discussing the potential risks and benefits of the planned treatment. In addition, the patient and fetus should undergo close surveillance during the pregnancy.

Which chemotherapeutic agents should be used in treating ovarian cancer during pregnancy?

The reports in the literature consist mainly of case reports and small case series. Germ cell malignancies are treated with the same combination drug regimens as are used in nonpregnant women. These multidrug regimens include etoposide and cisplatin,[38] cisplatin/vinblastin/bleomycin,[39,40] cisplatin/ etoposide/ bleomycin,[41,42] and vincristin/adriamycin/ cyclophosphamide.[43-46]

There are only seven case reports in the literature describing the use of chemotherapy in epithelial ovarian carcinoma during pregnancy. King,[47] Malfetano,[48] and Bayhan[49] and their colleagues presented three patients who received a total of 14 cycles of a combination regimen of cisplatin and cyclophosphamide with excellent maternal results and no neonatal sequelae. Henderson and associates[50] reported using two cycles of cisplatin/cyclophosphamide in a patient with ovarian serous cystadenocarcinoma starting at 20 weeks of gestation. Because of ototoxicity, the cisplatin was changed to carboplatin for one more cycle before delivery. This patient also was disease free with a normally developed infant at the time of their report. Otton and coworkers[51] reported the use of single-agent cisplatin in a woman with unstaged papillary-serous adenocarcinoma with clear-cell features diagnosed at 16 weeks' gestation. The patient received 100 mg/m^2 cisplatin with the first cycle; however, this dose was reduced to 75 mg/m^2 because of ototoxicity. At 32 weeks' gestation, cesarean delivery was followed by total hysterectomy, bilateral salpingo-oophorectomy, omentectomy, and nodal staging with no evidence of residual disease. There were no neonatal sequelae. The patient received two cycles of carboplatin and taxol after delivery.

Koc and colleauges[52] reported treating a woman with ovarian cancer with three cycles of carboplatin in the antepartum period, followed by the delivery of a normal-term neonate. Information regarding maternal disease status was not provided.

As with other chemotherapeutic agents, paclitaxel has been shown to be teratogenic. When it was administered to rats in early pregnancy, significant fetal anomalies were noted.[53] However, when it was administered in advanced pregnancy, no short-term or long-term effects were observed.[54]

There have been only two reports on the use of taxanes in human pregnancies. The first case report presented a patient with recurrent advanced breast cancer who received three cycles of docetaxel and had a planned delivery at 32 weeks' gestation via a cesarean section. The neonate weighed 1620 g with Apgar scores of 8 and 9. The infant had a normal development at 20 months.[55] Sood and associates[56] reported the first published case of paclitaxel use in pregnancy. The patient had a diagnosis of optimally reduced stage IIIc papillary serous ovarian carcinoma. She then underwent three cycles of paclitaxel and cisplatin starting at 27 weeks of gestation. The authors stated that cisplatin was chosen over carboplatin to minimize the risk of thrombocytopenia during pregnancy. The patient had a caesarean delivery at 37 weeks, in addition to hysterectomy, contralateral salpingo-oophorectomy, and cytoreduction. The tumor recurred 6 weeks after completion of six cycles of chemotherapy, and the patient died at 29 months after diagnosis. The infant had a normal growth and development at 30 months of age.

Ever since the results of Gynecologic Oncology Group (GOG) 111 study were published in 1995, the combination of paclitaxel and platinum (cisplatin) has been considered standard first-line treatment of ovarian cancer in the adjuvant setting.[57] Although the experience with taxanes in pregnancy is based on only two case reports, the lack of significant adverse fetal outcomes reported by these authors sets the stage for further considerations in using a combination regimen that may have superiority over other combination regimens in terms of disease response and overall survival.

CERVICAL CANCER IN PREGNANCY

Approximately 1% to 3% of all women with cervical cancer are pregnant at the time of diagnosis.[58] The most common presenting symptom is vaginal bleeding, which occurs in 43% to 54% of patients.[59] In the remainder, the diagnosis usually is made after evaluation of abnormal cytology.[2,60,61] Because proper function of the cervix is essential to maintaining a viable pregnancy, definitive treatment of the cancer results in either loss of the pregnancy or severe fetal morbidity as a result of prematurity at all times other than in the last trimester. Issues that have been a source of controversy include how best to treat microinvasive cancers in the pregnant patient; whether it is safe to delay treatment of the cervical cancer and, if so, for how long; and how best to treat women with advanced disease, especially those wishing not to interrupt their pregnancy prematurely.

Microinvasive Cervical Cancer

Most women diagnosed with microinvasive cervical cancer in pregnancy present with abnormal cytology, which then leads to colposcopic biopsy. The diagnosis of microinvasive cervical cancer (carcinoma invading 3 mm or less into the stroma and the absence of lymph/vascular space invasion) on colposcopic biopsy is one of the few indications for cone biopsy in pregnancy.[62,63] The cone biopsy is both diagnostic (given the significant likelihood of frankly invasive disease when microinvasive cancer is present on punch biopsy) and potentially therapeutic, if the cone can clear a microinvasive lesion. The information gained is necessary for appropriate counseling of the patient regarding prognosis, treatment options, and mode of delivery.

When and how should cone biopsy in pregnancy be performed?

The optimal time to perform conization is somewhat controversial, as is the optimal surgical technique. Averette and colleagues[64] reported that 8 (24%) of 33 women undergoing cone biopsy in the first trimester had a fetal loss that was probably or possibly related to the cone (many of the losses were a result of delayed chorioamnionitis). In contrast, Hannigan and associates[65] reported no spontaneous abortions among 13 women undergoing cone biopsy in the first trimester. Both groups found that the rate of the fetal loss as a result of cone biopsy done in the second trimester was less than 10%, and that most patients undergoing cone biopsy in the third trimester delivered viable infants. In both reports, the estimated blood loss associated with the cone biopsy was highest in the third trimester, although transfusion was relatively uncommon. In 1991, Goldberg and coworkers[66] reported on 17 women undergoing cone biopsy at 10 to 32 weeks' gestational age. They used intracervical vasopressin, lateral sutures, and a McDonald cerclage placed at the time of the cone. None of the women had significant hemorrhage, and there were no second-trimester losses.

There are few data available on the utility of the loop electrosurgical excision procedure (LEEP) in pregnancy. In 1997, Robinson and colleagues[67] published a pilot study on the use of LEEP in pregnancy. Twenty pregnant women, most in the first trimester, underwent LEEP because of a clinical suspicion of cancer. Although no invasive cancers were found in the LEEP specimens, three women (15%) had preterm deliveries (one at 1 week and two at 8 weeks after LEEP); two women (10%), both of whom underwent LEEP in the third trimester, required blood transfusions for blood losses of 800 and 1000 mL; and there was one intrauterine fetal death occurring at 36 weeks (4 weeks after LEEP). The autopsy revealed chorioamnionitis and an umbilical cord thrombus.

Pregnant women who have microinvasive cancer diagnosed on colposcopic biopsy should be counseled about the need for cone biopsy. The cone biopsy is best avoided both during the period of organogenesis, when exposure to anesthesia is potentially harmful and the underlying spontaneous abortion rate is highest, and during the late second and early third trimesters, when the fetus is viable but so premature that delivery is associated with significant morbidity. Cone biopsies in the third trimester are associated with higher blood loss, but with the use of vasopressin and hemostatic sutures transfusions are not likely to be necessary. The routine performance of cerclage at the time of cone biopsy has not been well studied. It is certainly reasonable to perform cerclage when the cone biopsy is large enough to significantly affect the size of the cervix. The role of LEEP as an alternative to cold knife conization in the pregnant woman has also not been extensively studied. It is our preference to opt for cold knife conization rather than LEEP in the pregnant patient, because it is easier to control the size of the cone with a scalpel and also because of potential difficulty in passing the loop through the edematous pregnant cervix.

What is the appropriate treatment for microinvasive cervical carcinoma in pregnancy?

If the cone biopsy confirms microinvasive squamous carcinoma and the lesion is cleared, the patient can be monitored in pregnancy with Papanicolaou smears every 3 months and allowed to deliver at term. If future childbearing is not desired, simple hysterectomy is an option because it prevents recurrent disease in the cervix. Hysterectomy can be performed either in concert with elective caesarean section or in a delayed fashion at least 6 weeks after vaginal delivery. If the internal margins of the cone are involved, there is a risk that a more significant cancer is present in the residual cervix, especially if the margins are involved with microinvasive cancer as opposed to dysplasia. Such patients should be counseled similarly to patients with frankly invasive carcinoma (see later discussion), taking into account that the risk of delay in treatment is probably less, given the fact that many of these women do not harbor frankly invasive disease.

Whether microinvasive adenocarcinoma in pregnancy should be managed similarly to microinvasive squamous carcinoma is controversial. Although there have been numerous reports suggesting that microinvasive adenocarcinomas behave similarly to microinvasive squamous carcinomas,[68,69] the number of reports of women with microinvasive adenocarcinoma treated conservatively is far less than the comparable number with squamous carcinoma. Also, there is virtually no published experience of women with microinvasive adenocarcinoma in pregnancy. At this point, it would be most prudent to manage microinvasive adenocarcinomas similarly to women with stage Ib1 cancers.

Frankly Invasive Cervical Cancer

What is the role of radiologic imaging in pregnant women with cervical cancer? Radiologic imaging plays two major roles in the management of cervical cancer: the determination of stage based on ureteral status and the determination of extent of disease (particularly nodal status) to assist with optimal treatment planning. In pregnant women, MRI is the preferred mode of imaging because it avoids exposure to ionizing radiation (see Adnexal Masses in Pregnancy). MRI has utility in determining nodal status and ureteral status and in approximating tumor size.[70] Pregnant women with early-stage disease are at low risk for metastases, so abdominopelvic imaging is generally not warranted. An exception may be the patient with a stage Ib lesion diagnosed in the first or second trimester who is considering an appreciable treatment delay. If MRI suggests nodal metastases, this strategy should be reconsidered. All women with more advanced lesions should undergo either MRI or CT (with the latter being appropriate if the fetus is not viable) for assessment of extent of disease.

Is delay in treatment acceptable in early-stage disease?

Early reports of cervical cancer in pregnancy generally described immediate treatment of the cancer, which usually led to death of the fetus. Occasionally, when the diagnosis was made in the third trimester, a few weeks' delay was allowed to achieve fetal viability.[71-73] In 1989, Greer and colleagues[74] reported on five women, all diagnosed with cervical cancer in the second trimester, who delayed treatment for 6 to 17 weeks. All five remained without evidence of disease, with the exception of one patient with glass cell carcinoma who died from her cancer. The authors questioned the practice of immediate treatment of cervical cancer diagnosed in pregnancy, arguing that a delay of several weeks between diagnosis and treatment is common in general practice and that advancements in the field of neonatology have allowed fetal viability at earlier gestational ages. They recommended offering the possibility of delay in treatment to selected women.

Over the next several years, numerous studies were published detailing the experience with delay in treatment in women with cervical cancer diagnosed in pregnancy (Table 67-1). The majority of women reported had stage I disease and underwent radical hysterectomy when fetal maturity was established. The outcome using such an approach has been excellent. Progression of the cancer during pregnancy was uncommon, and the majority of women who delayed treatment were able to undergo radical hysterectomy successfully in the third trimester. The rate of reported nodal positivity was low. The few women who died from their disease had cancers with features associated with a poor prognosis. Based on this experience, it has become accepted practice to counsel women who are diagnosed with early cervical cancer at or after 20 weeks of gestation about the possibility of delay in treatment.

Whether allowing longer delays as an option, which would be necessary if the diagnosis were made in the first or early second trimester, is controversial. Only 9 of the 50 women described in Table 67-1 were diagnosed before 20 weeks' gestation, and only 4 were diagnosed in the first trimester. Eight of these nine women had an excellent outcome; details on the sole patient who died from her disease (after a 24-week delay) were not given, and it is unclear whether she was monitored closely during the pregnancy.

Women diagnosed with small cervical cancers early in pregnancy who are desirous of delay in therapy to allow a viable fetus should be counseled that the number of reported cases are small, especially if the diagnosis is made in the first trimester. Although the outcome appears to be favorable, the actual risk cannot be quantitated given the small denominator. Logistically, the size of the cancer and the histology of the lesion are important determinants in considering the feasibility of a prolonged delay.

Table 67–1. Cervical Cancer in Pregnancy: Results of Treatment Delay

Study and Year	N	Stage	Delay (wk)	No. Positive Lymph Notes	Outcome
Prem et al.[72] (1966)	9	I	6-17	?	All NED
Lee et al.[73] (1988)	8	Ib-II	1-12	?	All NED
Nisker and Shubat[75] (1983)	1	Ib	24	?	DOD
Greer et al.[74] (1989)	5	Ib	6,10,11,14,17	1 (20%)	1 DOD*
Monk and Montz[76] (1992)	1	Ia2	25	0	NED
Monk and Montz[75] (1992)	3	Ib	10-16 (mean, 13)	0	All NED
Duggan et al.[1] (1993)	5	Ib	7.5,12,19, 21,24	0	All NED
Sorosky et al.[77] (1996)	7	Ib	4-28 (mean, 14)	0	1 DOD†
Sood et al.[78] (1996)	11	Ia‡/Ib	3-32 wk (mean, 16)	?	All NED

DOD, dead of disease; NED, no evidence of disease.
*A glassy cell carcinoma.
†A 6-cm adenocarcinoma.
‡Three were stage Ia1.

What is the optimal mode of delivery for women with cervical cancer?

Some controversy exists as to whether women with cervical cancer should be allowed to deliver vaginally, particularly when gross tumor is present. Prospective studies comparing vaginal delivery with caesarean section in pregnant women with cervical cancer do not exist (and probably never will). Retrospective reports[72,76] have generally not shown a worse oncologic outcome in women with cervical cancer who underwent vaginal delivery. Jones and colleagues[79] reported a 75% survival rate, compared with 55% for women delivering vaginally; however, a statistical comparison was not performed.

One uncommon complication associated with vaginal delivery is episiotomy site recurrence. More than 10 such recurrences have been reported in the literature.[80-85] Of the nine women with isolated episiotomy recurrences, four died from their disease.[54] Although incisional site recurrences have also been reported in women undergoing caesarean delivery,[3,86,87] this particular complication appears to be more common in women with gross cervical tumors who undergo vaginal delivery.

Caesarean delivery has numerous logistic advantages over vaginal delivery. Trauma to the lesion is prevented, minimizing the risk of hemorrhage and obstructed labor. Concurrent radical hysterectomy can be performed, hastening the treatment of the cancer. Radical caesarean hysterectomy has previously been associated with greater blood loss, compared with radical hysterectomy[3,74,78]; however, the rate of blood transfusion usually has not been found to be significantly higher in the more recent studies.[3,78]

Caesarean section is the method of choice for pregnant women who are expected to deliver viable infants. Women with microinvasive cancers, in whom obstetric complications from the cancer are unlikely and in whom there is minimal risk to delaying definitive treatment further, can be offered vaginal delivery.

How should women with advanced lesions diagnosed in pregnancy be treated?

In women with large cervical lesions, radiation therapy is the mainstay of treatment. Traditionally, if the diagnosis is made in the late second or third trimester, a short delay is allowed to try to optimize fetal outcome. Thereafter, caesarean section is performed and pelvic radiation is started within 2 to 3 weeks after delivery.[72,73,88] Nodal status can be assessed at the time of caesarean section. If the diagnosis is made prior to fetal viability, pelvic irradiation is started with the fetus in situ. Most authors have reported that spontaneous abortion occurs at the dose of 40 Gy.[5,72,73] If the patient would benefit from pretreatment aortic nodal sampling, this can be performed via either a laparoscopic or a retroperitoneal technique, with the fetus in situ.

What is the role of chemotherapy in the treatment of cervical cancer in pregnancy?

Theoretically, neoadjuvant chemotherapy could play an important role in the treatment of pregnant women with advanced cervical cancer. Unlike radiation and hysterectomy, chemotherapy can be given without interruption of the pregnancy, thus allowing a vital interval of time to pass to achieve fetal viability. Such therapy is especially attractive when the diagnosis is made in the middle trimester, when the fetus is potentially viable but is likely to suffer severe morbidity as a result of premature delivery.

Tewari and colleagues[89] reported on two pregnant patients who underwent platinum-based neoadjuvant chemotherapy for locally advanced cervical carcinoma. The first patient was diagnosed with stage IIa cervical cancer at 20 weeks' gestation, and she elected to defer definitive treatment until the fetus was viable. She was given three cycles of vincristine and cisplatin, followed by three cycles of cisplatin alone, and attained a partial response. At 34 weeks' gestation, she delivered a healthy female infant via cesarean section and then underwent a radical hysterectomy with bilateral pelvic lymphadenectomy. Unfortunately, the disease recurred 5 months later.

The second patient was diagnosed with stage Ib2 (7cm) cervical cancer at 21 weeks' gestation. She also declined immediate cancer therapy and was treated with four courses of vincristine ($50 mg/m^2$) and cisplatin ($50 mg/m^2$). She underwent a surgical delivery followed by radical hysterectomy with pelvic lymphadenectomy. Two years later, both the patient and her child remained healthy.

In addition, a third pregnant patient with stage Ib1 squamous carcinoma of the cervix diagnosed in the second trimester was treated with weekly cisplatin ($40 mg/m^2$) starting in the second trimester at my own institution. Her tumor had been noted to progress in size during the pregnancy. Chemotherapy was given because the patient very much desired to delay delivery. The patient attained a partial response, and an additional delay of 8 critical weeks was gained before definitive surgical therapy without any apparent adverse fetal or maternal outcomes noted at 3-year follow-up.

Studies of neoadjuvant chemotherapy (most of which incorporated some combination of cisplatin and vincristine) in nonpregnant women with bulky cervical lesions have found that the majority of tumors respond to chemotherapy and that the incidence of nodal positivity at the time of radical hysterectomy is lower than what would be expected had chemotherapy not been given.[90-92] Randomized trials comparing neoadjuvant chemotherapy with radical hysterectomy and with irradiation are ongoing. Clearly, the data on the use of neoadjuvant chemotherapy in gravid patients with cervical carcinoma are limited, and this cannot be considered standard therapy. Based on the existing information, neoadjuvant chemotherapy is a treatment option for pregnant women who are highly motivated to continue their pregnancy to attain fetal viability.

REFERENCES

1. Duggan B, Muderspach LI, Roman LD, et al: Cervical cancer in pregnancy: Reporting on planned delay in therapy. Obstet Gynecol 1993;82:598-602.
2. Hacker NF, Berek JS, Lagasse LD, et al: Carcinoma of the cervix associated with pregnancy. Obstet Gynecol 1982;59:735-746.
3. Sivanesaratnam, V, Jayalakshmi P, Loo C: Surgical management of early invasive cancer of the cervix associated with pregnancy. Gynecol Oncol 1993;48:68-75.
4. Beischer NA, Buttery BW, Fortune DW, Macafee CAJ: Growth and malignancy of ovarian tumours in pregnancy. Aust N Z J Obstet Gynaecol 1971;11:208-220.
5. Creasman WT, Rutledge F, Smith JP: Carcinoma of the ovary associated with pregnancy. Obstet Gynecol 1971;38:111-116.
6. Tawa K: Ovarian tumors in pregnancy. Am J Obstet Gynecol 1964;90:511.
7. Graber EA: Ovarian tumors in pregnancy. In Barber HRK, Graber EA (eds): Surgical Disease in Pregnancy. Philadelphia, WB Saunders, 1974, pp 428-439.
8. Grimes WH, Bartholomew RA, Colvin ED, et al: Ovarian cyst complicating pregnancy. Am J Obstet Gynecol 1954;68:594-605.
9. Platek DN, Henderson CE, Goldberg GL: The management of a persistent adnexal mass in pregnancy. Am J Obstet Gynecol 1995;173:1236-1240.
10. Hess LW, Peaceman A, O`Brien WF, et al: Adnexal mass occurring with intrauterine pregnancy: Report of fifty-four patients requiring laparotomy for definitive management. Am J Obstet Gynecol 1988;158:1029-1034.
11. Whitecar P, Turner S, Higby K: Adnexal masses in pregnancy: A review of 130 cases undergoing surgical management. Am J Obstet Gynecol 1999;181:19-24.
12. Struyk APHB, Treffers PE: Ovarian tumors in pregnancy. Acta Obstet Gynecol Scand 1984;63:421-424.
13. Zanotti KM, Belinson JL, Kennedy AW: Treatment of gynecologic cancers in pregnancy. Semin Oncol 2000;27:686-698.
14. Kobayashi F, Sagawa N, Nakamura K, et al: Mechanism and clinical significance of elevated CA-125 levels in the sera of pregnant women. Am J Obstet Gynecol 1989;160:563-566.
15. Buller RE, Darrow V, Manetta A, et al: Conservative management of dysgerminoma concomitant with pregnancy. Obstet Gynecol 1992;79:887-890.
16. Steenvoorde P, Paumels E, Harding L, et al: Diagnostic nuclear medicine and risk for the fetus. Eur J Nucl Med 1998;25:195-199.
17. Brent RC: The effects of embryonic and fetal exposure to x-rays, microwaves, and ultrasound. Clin Perinatol 1986;13:615-648.
18. Stovall M, Blackwell CR, Cundiff J, et al: Total dose from radiotherapy with photon beams: Report of AAPM radiation therapy task group. No. 36. Med Phys 1995;22:63-82.
19. Thomas SR: Bioeffects of non-ionizing radiation. In American College of Radiology (ed): Radiation Bank: A Primer. Reston, VA: American College of Radiology, 1996, pp 45-50.
20. American College of Obstetricians and Gynecologists committee opinion. Guidelines for diagnostic imaging in pregnancy. Number 158, 1995.
21. Baker PN, Johnson IR, Harvey PR, et al: A three-year follow-up of children imaged in utero with echo-planar magnetic resonance. Am J Obstet Gynecol 1994;170:32-33.
22. Thornton JG, Wells M: Ovarian cysts in pregnancy: Does ultrasound make traditional management appropriate? Obstet Gynecol 1987;69:717-720.
23. Sharp HT: The acute abdomen in pregnancy. Clin Obstet Gynecol 2002;45:405-413.
24. Parker WH, Childers JM, Canis M, et al: Laparoscopic management of benign cystic teratomas during pregnancy. Am J Obstet Gynecol 1996;174:1499-1501.
25. Morice P, Louis-Silvestre C, Chapron C, Dubisson JB: Laparoscopy for adnexal torsion in pregnant women. J Reprod Med. 1998;43:160-161.
26. Moore RD, Smith WG: Laparoscopic management of adnexal masses in pregnant women. J Reprod Med 1990;44:97-100.
27. Creaseman WT, Rutledge F, Smith JP: Carcinoma of the ovary associated with pregnancy. Obstet Gynecol 1971;38:111-116.
28. Rahman MS, Al-Sibai MH, Rahman J, et al: Ovarian carcinoma associated with pregnancy: A review of 9 cases. Acta Obstet Gynecol Scand 2002;81:260-264.
29. Adolph A, Le T, Khan K, Biem S: Recurrent metastatic fallopian tube carcinoma in pregnancy. Gynecol Oncol 2001;81:110-112.
30. Arango HA, Kalter CS, Decesare SL, et al: Management of chemotherapy in a pregnancy complicated by a large neuroblastoma. Obstet Gynecol 1994;84:665-667.
31. Doll DC, Ringenberg S, Yarbo JW: Antineoplastid agents and pregnancy. Semin Oncol 1989;16:337-346.
32. FDA Drug Bulletin 1979;9:23-24.
33. Aviles A, Diaz-Maqueo J, Talavera A, et al: Growth and development of children of mothers treated with chemotherapy during pregnancy: Current status of 43 children. Am J Hematol 1991;36:243-248.
34. Blatt J, Mulvihill J, Ziegler J, et al: Pregnancy outcome following cancer chemotherapy. Am J Med 1980;69:828-832.
35. Reynoso E, Sheperd F, Messner H, et al: Acute leukemia during pregnancy: The Toronto leukemia study group experience with long-term follow-up of children exposed in utero to chemotherapeutic agents. J Clin Oncol 1987;5:1098-1106.
36. Doll D, Ringenberg S, Yarbro D: Management of cancer during pregnancy. Arch Intern Med. 1988;148:2058-2064.
37. Garcia, L, Valcacel M, Santiago-Borrero PJ: Chemotherapy during pregnancy and its effects on the fetus-neonatal myelosuppression: Two case reports. J Perinatol 1999;19:230-233.
38. Buller RE, Darrow V, Manetta A, et al: Conservative surgical management of dysgerminoma concomitant with pregnancy. Obstet Gynecol 1992;79:887-890.
39. Christman JE, Teng NNH, Lebovic GS, Sikic BI: Delivery of a normal infant following cisplatin, vinblastine, and bleomycin (PVB) chemotherapy for malignant teratoma of the ovary during pregnancy. Gynecol Oncol 1990;37:292-295.
40. Malone JM, Gershenson DM, Creasy RK, et al: Endodermal sinus tumor of the ovary associated with pregnancy. Obstet Gynecol 1986:68(Suppl):86S-89S.
41. Horbelt D, Delmore J, Meisel R, et al: Mixed germ cell malignancy of the ovary concurrent with pregnancy. Obstet Gynecol 1994;84:662-664.
42. Elit L, Bocking MD, Kenyon C, Natale R: An endodermal sinus tumor diagnosed in pregnancy: Case report and review of literature. Gynecol Oncol 1999;72:123-127.
43. Frederiksen MC, Casanova L, Schink JC: An elevated maternal serum alpha-fetoprotein leading to the diagnosis of an immature teratoma. Int J Gynecol Obstet 1991;35:343.
44. Kim DS, Park MI: Maternal and fetal survival following surgery and chemotherapy of an endodermal sinus tumor of the ovary during pregnancy: A case report. Obstet Gynecol 1989;73:503.
45. Metz SA, Day TG, Pursell SH: Adjuvant chemotherapy in a pregnant patient with endodermal sinus tumor of the ovary. Gynecol Oncol 1989;32:371.
46. Montz FJ, Horenstein J, Platt LD, et al: The diagnosis of immature teratoma by maternal serum alpha-fetoprotein screening. Obstet Gynecol 1989;73:522.
47. King LA, Nevin PC, Williams PP, Carson LF: Treatment of advanced epithelial ovarian carcinoma in pregnancy with cisplatin-based chemotherapy. Gynecol Oncol 1991;41:78-80.
48. Malfetano JH, Goldkrand JW: Cis-platinum combination chemotherapy during pregnancy for advanced epithelial ovarian carcinoma. Obstet Gynecol 1990;75:545-547.
49. Bayhan G, Aban M, Yayla M, et al: Cis-platinum combination chemotherapy during pregnancy for mucinous cystadenocarcinoma of the ovary: Case reprot. Eur J Gynaeccol Oncol 1999;20:231-232.
50. Henderson CE, Giovanni E, Garfinkel D, et al: Platinum chemotherapy during pregnancy for serous cystadenocarcinoma of the ovary. Gynecol Oncol 1993;49:92-93.
51. Otton G, Higgins S, Phillips KA, Quinn M: A case of early-stage epithelial ovarian cancer in pregnancy. Int J Gynecol Cancer 2001;11:413-417.
52. Koc ON, McFee M, Reed E, Gerson SL: Detection of plainum-DNA adducts in cord blood lymphocytes following in utero platinum exposure. Eur J Cancer 1994;30A:716-717.
53. Scialli AR, Waterhouse TB, Desesso JM, et al: Protective effect of liposome encapsulation on paclitaxel developmental toxicity in the rat. Teratology 1997;56:305-310.
54. Kai S, Kohmura H, Hiraiwa E, et al: Reproductive and developmental toxicity studies of paclitaxel: Intravenous administration

to rats during the prenatal and lactation periods. J Toxocol Sci 1994;19:93-111.

55. De Santis M, Lucchese A, De Carolis S, et al: Metatstatic breast cancer in pregnancy: First case of chemotherapy with docetaxel. Eur J Cancer Care 2000;9:235-237.

56. Sood A, Shahin M, Sorosky JI: Paclitaxel and platinum chemotherapy for ovarian carcinoma during pregnancy. Gynecol Oncol 2001;83:599-600.

57. McGuire WP, Hoskins WJ, Brady MF, et al: Cyclophosphamide and cisplatin compared with paclitaxel and cisplatin in patients with stage III and stage IV ovarian cancer. N Engl J Med 1996; 334:1-6.

58. Donegan WL: Cancer and pregnancy. CA Cancer J Clin 1983;33: 194-214.

59. Method MW, Brost BC: Management of cervical cancer in pregnancy. Semin Surg Oncol 1999;16:251-2560.

60. Creasman WT, Rutledge F, Fletcher G: Carcinoma of the cervix associated with pregnancy. Obstet Gynecol 1970;36:495-501.

61. Norstrom A, Jansson I, Andersson H: Carcinoma of the uterine cervix in pregnancy: A study of the incidence and treatment in the western region of Sweden 1973 to 1992. Acta Obstet Gynecol Scand 1997;76:583-589.

62. Nguyen C, Montz FJ, Bristow RE: Management of stage I cervical cancer in pregnancy. Obstet Gynecol Surv 2000;55:633-643.

63. Benedet JL, Selke PA, Nickerson KG: Colposcopic evaluation of abnormal Papanicolaou smear in pregnancy. Am J Obstet Gynecol 1987;157:932-937.

64. Averette HE, Nasser N, Yankow SL, Little WA: Cervical conization in pregnancy. Am J Obstet Gynecol 1970;106:543-549.

65. Hannigan EV, Whitehouse HH, Atkinson WD, Becker SN: Cone biopsy during pregnancy. Obstet Gynecol 1982;60:450-455.

66. Goldberg GL, Altaras MM, Bloch B: Cone cerclage in pregnancy. Obstet Gynecol 1991;77:315-317.

67. Robinson WR, Webb S, Tirpack J, et al: Management of cervical intraepithelial neoplasia during pregnancy with LOOP excision. Gynecol Oncol 1997;64:153-155.

68. Ostor A, Rome R, Quinn M: Microinvasive adenocarcinoma of the cervix: A clinical study of 77 women. Obstet Gynecol 1997; 89:88-93.

69. Schorge JO, Lee KR, Flynn CE, et al: Stage IA1 cervical adenocarcinoma: Definitoin and treatment. Obstet Gynecol 1999;93: 219-222.

70. Mayr NA, Magnotta VA, Ehrhardt JC, et al: Usefulness of tumor volumetry by magnetic resonance imaging in assessing response to radiation therapy in carcinoma of the uterine cervix. Int J Radiol Oncol Biol Phys 1996;35:915-924.

71. Hopkins MP, Morley GW: The prognosis and management of cervical cancer associated with pregnancy. Obstet Gynecol 1992;80:9-12.

72. Prem KA, Makowsky EL, McKelvey JL: Carcinoma of the cervix associated with pregnancy. Am J Obstet Gynecol 1966;95:99-108.

73. Lee RB, Neglia W, Park RC: Cervical carcinoma in pregnancy. Obstet Gynecol 1981;58:584-589.

74. Greer BE, Easterling TR, McLennan DA, et al: Fetal and maternal considerations in the management of stage IB cervical cancer during pregnancy. Gynecol Oncol 1989;34:61-65.

75. Nisker JA, Shubat M: Stage IB cervical carcinoma and pregnancy: Report of 49 cases. Am J Obstet Gynecol 1983;145: 203-206.

76. Monk BJ, Montz FJ: Invasive cervical cancer complicating intrauterine pregnancy: Treatment with radical hysterectomy. Obstet Gynecol 1992;80:199-203.

77. Sorosky JI, Cherouny PH. Podczaski ES, Hackett TE: Stage Ib cervical carcinoma in pregnancy: Awaiting fetal maturity. J Gynecol Techniques 1996;2:155-158.

78. Sood AK, Sorosky JI, Krogman S, et al: Surgical management of cervical cancer complicating pregnancy: A case-control study. Gynecol Oncol 1996;63:294-298.

79. Jones WB, Shingleton HM, Russell A, et al: Cervical carcinoma and pregnancy: A national patterns of care study of the American College of Surgeons. Cancer 1996;77:1479-1488.

80. Burgess SP, Waymont B: Implantation of a cervical carcinoma in an episiotomy site: Case report. Br J Obstet Gynaecol 1987;94: 598-599.

81. Copeland LJ, Saul PB, Sneige N: Cervical adenocarcinoma: Tumor implantation in the episiotomy sites of two patients. Gynecol Oncol 1987;28:230-235.

82. Gordon AN, Jensen R, Jones HW III: Squamous carcinoma of the cervical complicating pregnancy: Recurrence in episiotomy after vaginal delivery. Obstet Gynecol 1989;73:850-852.

83. Cliby WA, Dodson MK, Podratz KC: Cervical cancer complicated by pregnancy: Episiotomy site recurrences following vaginal delivery. Obstet Gynecol 1994;84:179-182.

84. Khalil AM, Khatib RA, Mufarrij AA, et al. Squamous cell carcinoma of the cervix implanting in the episiotomy site [review]. Gynecol Oncol 1993;51:408-410.

85. Van Dam PA, Irvine L, Lowe DG, et al: Carcinoma in episiotomy scars. Gynecol Oncol 1992;44:96-100.

86. Greenlee RM, Chervenak FA, Tovell HM: Incisional recurrence of cervical carcinoma: Report of a case. JAMA 1981; 246:69-70.

87. Stenson R, Jacobs AJ, Janney CG, Schmidt DA: Incisional recurrence of squamous cell cervical carcinoma following operative staging. Gynecol Oncol 1990;39:232-235.

88. Sood AK, Sorosky JI: Invasive cervical cancer complicating pregnancy: How to manage the dilemma. Obstet Gynecol Clin North Am 1998;25:343-352.

89. Tewari K, Cappuccini F, Gambino A, et al: Neoadjuvant chemotherapy in the treatment of locally advanced cervical carcinoma in pregnancy. Cancer 1998;82:1529-1534.

90. Pancini PB, Scambia G, Baiocchi G, et al: Neoadjuvant chemotherapy and radical surgery in locally advanced cervical cancer. Cancer 1991;67:372-379.

91. Dottino PR, Plaxe SC, Beddoe AM, et al: Induction chemotherapy followed by radical surgery in cervical cancer. Gynecol Oncol 1991;40:7-11.

92. Kim DS, Moon H, Kim KT, et al: Two-year survival: preoperative adjuvant chemotherapy in the treatment of cervical cancer stages Ib and II with bulky tumor. Gynecol Oncol 1989;33: 225-230.

CHAPTER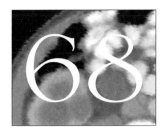

MELANOMA OF THE FEMALE GENITAL TRACT

Edward L. Trimble, Carol Kosary, Margaret Mooney, and Scott Saxman

---

 MAJOR CONTROVERSIES

- **Do melanomas of the female genital tract differ from cutaneous melanomas in biology and epidemiology?**
- **Should FIGO staging or AJCC melanoma staging be used to stage gynecologic melanomas?**
- **Do melanomas of the female genital tract differ from cutaneous melanomas in clinical behavior?**
- **What margins of resection are necessary in the primary surgical management of melanomas of the female genital tract?**
- **What is the role of sentinel lymph node biopsy in the management of gynecologic melanomas?**
- **What is the role of regional lymphadenectomy in the management of gynecologic melanomas?**
- **How should cervical and ovarian melanomas be treated?**
- **What is the role of adjuvant therapy after primary surgery for gynecologic melanoma?**
- **Are there reliable prognostic markers for women with vulvar melanoma?**
- **What is the recommended therapy for recurrent, metastatic disease?**
- **Is there a role for a prospective, multi-institutional effort to study gynecologic melanomas?**

Melanomas have been reported in a variety of locations within the female genital tract, including the vulva, vagina, cervix, and ovary. Vulvar melanomas may represent 5% to 10% of all vulvar cancers; the vast majority of vulvar cancers are squamous carcinomas. In the Surveillance, Epidemiology, and End Results (SEER) database of the National Cancer Institute (NCI), vulvar melanomas comprised 6% of all vulvar malignancies diagnosed between 1988 and 1999. Vaginal melanomas are less common. Cervical melanomas and ovarian melanomas arising in teratomas are sufficiently rare to be considered for case reports. The rarity of gynecologic melanomas renders the published literature scanty, clinical trials difficult to impossible, and clinical controversies hard to resolve. For guidance in many of these issues, we must fall back on the larger clinical experience with cutaneous melanomas, which may or may not be applicable.

Do melanomas of the female genital tract differ from cutaneous melanomas in biology and epidemiology?

Biostatistics. There are two population-based reports on the incidence of gynecologic melanoma, one from the SEER program and one from Sweden. Weinstock[1] reported on the incidence of vulvar and vaginal melanomas among women in the SEER database, collated from cancer registries that cover about 14% of the U. S. population. In their analysis, which included cancers diagnosed between 1973 and 1987, there were 203 cases of vulvar melanoma and 51 cases of vaginal melanoma. These represented 1.3% and 0.3% respectively, of all melanomas among women. The authors calculated an annual incidence rate of 0.108 per 100,000 women for vulvar melanoma and 0.026 per 100,000 women for vaginal melanoma. Ragnarsson-Olding and colleagues[2] calculated the incidence of vulvar melanoma in Sweden between 1960 and 1984, using data from the Swedish National Cancer Registry. The annual incidence of vulvar melanoma fell from 0.27 per 100,000 women in 1960-1964 to 0.14 per 100,000 women in 1980-1984. During the same period, the incidence of cutaneous melanoma among women in Sweden rose by 6% per year between 1960 and 1984. Based on this discrepancy, the authors hypothesized that cutaneous and vulvar melanomas have different etiologies.

Demographics. Vulvar melanoma appears to be less common among African-American and Asian-American women than among women of northern European descent. In the SEER data reported by Weinstock,[1] white women had an increased relative risk for development of vulvar melanoma of 2.6, compared with black women. There was no difference between white and black women in the risk for development of vaginal melanoma. Creasman and colleagues,[3] who reviewed 569 cases of vulvar melanoma reported to the American College of Surgeons Commission on Cancer National Cancer Database (NCDB) between 1985 and 1994, noted that more than 90% of patients were Caucasian.

The mean age at diagnosis for cutaneous melanoma is between 30 to 40 years. Vulvar melanomas tend to occur at later ages. In Weinstock's report, the median age at diagnosis was 66 years for vulvar melanoma and 70 years for vaginal melanoma.[1] In Creasman's report, the median age was 66 years for all patients (range, 7 to 97 years).[3] In the Swedish series, the mean age at diagnosis was 67.7 years for vulvar melanoma and 66.3 years for vaginal melanoma.[2]

Other risk factors. Cutaneous melanomas are related to sun exposure. Most gynecologic sites are rarely exposed to sun, and the etiologic factors associated with gynecologic melanomas are less well understood. Neither parity nor hormones, whether endogenous or exogenous, appear to play a role in the development of gynecologic melanomas.

Anatomy. Melanomas arise from melanocytes, cells that were originally part of the neural crest, which are present in the basal layer of the epidermis. Melanomas may also occur in the mucosa or in any other site to which neural crest cells migrate. In the skin, melanomas may arise from junctional nevi or compound nevi or de novo from epidermal melanocytes.

The most comprehensive anatomic study of gynecologic melanomas was performed by Ragnarsson-Olding and associates,[4] using 198 cases of vulvar melanoma diagnosed in Sweden between 1960 and 1984. This series represented 90% of all vulvar melanomas diagnosed during that period. The authors were able to distinguish between melanomas arising in hair-bearing skin and melanomas arising in mucosal or glabrous skin. In their series, the incidence of vulvar melanoma in hair-bearing skin was consistent with that of melanomas elsewhere in the skin. However, the glabrous or mucosal vulva, which covers only 0.7% of the body surface, bore 2% of all female melanomas.[4] In this study, 30% of all melanomas arose in the periclitoral area, 27% in the labia

majora, 19% in the labia minora, 11% in the periurethral area, and 4% in the vaginal introitus. The authors noted that 45% of the melanomas arose in the glabrous skin, 35% in the junction between hairy skin and glabrous skin, and only 12% in hairy skin. They also found pre-existing nevi associated with some melanomas arising in hairy skin but not in glabrous skin.

Pathology. The histologic subtypes reported for vulvar melanomas include superficial spreading melanoma, nodular, and lentiginous malignant melanoma. In the Swedish study, 57% of vulvar melanomas were lentiginous, 22% nodular, and only 4% superficial spreading.[4] The differential diagnosis includes Paget's disease, vulvar intraepithelial neoplasia, and dysplastic nevi. The gynecologic pathologist may need to use a panel of immunohistochemical stains to classify a lesion accurately. Consultation with a dermatologic pathologist, who sees melanoma more frequently, may also be helpful.

Screening. Health care providers should encourage women to perform routine surveillance of all skin surfaces, including the vulva. A handheld mirror may help with examination of the vulva.

Symptoms. At the earlier stages, patients report the presence of a lump or mass, or itching. Pain, bleeding, or discharge may accompany more advanced disease. Most vulvar melanomas are brown or black in pigmentation, and flat or nodular in shape. Up to 25% of melanomas occurring in the glabrous skin, however, may be amelanotic.[4]

Primary evaluation. Clinicians should promptly evaluate all vulvar lesions, including pigmented lesions that raise the possibility of vulvar melanoma. Small lesions may be resected in toto with the underlying subcutaneous tissue so that the full thickness of the lesion can be determined. Larger lesions should be evaluated with a full-thickness biopsy.

Should FIGO staging or AJCC melanoma staging be used to stage gynecologic melanomas?

Staging. Two different staging systems are commonly used. The International Federation of Gynaecologists and Obstetricians (FIGO) staging system for cancers of the vulva and vagina, developed for squamous carcinoma, is also applied to vulvar and vaginal melanomas. In addition, the American Joint Committee on Cancer (AJCC) staging for cutaneous melanomas is often used.[5] In one of the few prospective trials for women with vulvar melanoma ever conducted, the Gynecologic Oncology Group (GOG) found that AJCC staging (1992) had better correlation with survival than did FIGO staging (1969).[6] The authors concluded that AJCC staging should be used for patients with vulvar melanomas for the determination of prognosis and selection of therapies. Podratz and associates,[7] who conducted a retrospective study of 48 patients treated at the Mayo Clinic between 1950 and 1980, found

FIGO staging to be of little value in predicting outcome. The most recent FIGO and AJCC staging systems are shown in Table 68-1. The latest AJCC staging system includes microstaging of the primary melanoma lesion.[5,8] It is subdivided into clinical staging (after excision of the primary melanoma and clinical assessment of regional and distant metastases) and pathologic staging (after partial or complete regional lymphadenectomy has been performed). Although the AJCC staging system is far more complicated than FIGO staging, the AJCC system was based on clinicopathologic factors and outcome in 17,600 patients with cutaneous melanoma.[9] Such numbers clearly dwarf the limited series published on gynecologic melanomas. Nonetheless, the new AJCC system is based on data derived mostly from patients with nodular and superficial spreading melanomas, whereas the majority of gynecologic melanomas are lentiginous.

Microstaging of vulvar melanomas, using the anatomic level of local invasion[10] (Clark) or the vertical thickness of the lesion[11] (Breslow), has also been commonly performed.[10,11] Chung and coworkers proposed a modification of the Clark microstaging system specific to vulvar anatomy, in which the reticular dermis level may not be well developed. Beller and associates[13] proposed a microstaging system based on tumor volume. In general, thicker tumors and tumors with greater depth of invasion have a worse prognosis than thinner, shallower lesions. Differences among the four microstaging systems are shown in Table 68-2.

Staging has not been addressed prospectively in women with vaginal melanoma. Reid and coleagues[14] compiled data on 115 women with vaginal melanoma reported retrospectively from many different institutions. FIGO staging, reported for 42 of these patients, did not correlate with survival or time to recurrence. Tumor size appeared to be the key prognostic factor: women with lesions smaller than 3 cm in diameter had significantly better survival than those with larger lesions. Tumor thickness, which was reported for 31 patients, correlated with disease-free interval but not with survival.

Do melanomas of the female genital tract differ from cutaneous melanomas in clinical behavior?

Survival. As noted earlier, most of the data on vulvar and vaginal melanomas is derived from small retrospective case series, whereas outcome in cutaneous melanoma is derived from registry studies of large numbers of patients. We calculated the 5-year relative survival rates for 123 patients with vulvar melanoma recorded in the SEER registry between 1988 and 1999. and compared them, according to AJCC stage, with those of 31,482 patients with cutaneous melanoma recorded in the National Cancer Data Base between 1985 and 1989 is shown in Table 68-3.[15] Patients with vulvar melanoma appear to have worse relative survival than those with cutaneous melanoma.

What margins of resection are necessary in the primary surgical management of melanomas of the female genital tract?

Extent of primary surgery. There are no prospective data from randomized clinical trials evaluating the extent of surgical margins in patients with gynecologic melanomas. Among individuals with cutaneous melanomas, several trials have suggested that 3 cm or less is adequate. Balch and associates[16] conducted a trial of 468 patients with cutaneous melanomas 1 to 4 mm thick who were randomly assigned to resection with either 2- or 4-cm surgical margins. They found no difference in local recurrence or survival after a median follow-up period of 10 years. Patients who underwent resection with 2-cm margins were more likely to have successful primary wound closure, had shorter hospital stays, and were less likely to require skin grafts than those patients who underwent resection with 4-cm margins. Veronesi and Cascinelli also reported 8-year follow-up data on 612 patients with melanomas less than 2 mm in thickness who were randomly assigned to resection with either 1- or 3-cm margins. They found no difference between the two treatment arms in terms of disease-free survival or overall survival.

In a prospective GOG study, 37 patients underwent radical vulvectomy and 31 were treated with radical hemivulvectomy.[6] The GOG investigators were unable to make any definitive conclusions about the extent of surgery to be recommended for women with vulvar melanoma.

Numerous retrospective case series found similar survival rates associated with radical local excisions and with radical vulvectomy among women with vulvar melanoma.[18-25] Traditionalists have been known to recommend the standard radical vulvectomy with bilateral inguinal lymphadenectomy for any and all vulvar cancers, including melanoma. The most common practice today, however, is to perform a radical local excision, preserving as much normal tissue and function as possible. Based on the randomized phase III trials of patients with cutaneous melanoma, 1-cm margins should be adequate for melanomas less than 1 mm thick, and 2-cm margins should be adequate for melanomas 1 to 4 mm thick. In all cases, however, the margin should be at least 1 cm deep, extending through the subcutaneous fat to the muscular fascia.[26]

As noted earlier, there are limited retrospective data regarding the surgical management of women with vaginal melanoma. Two different sets of authors have analyzed the published reports in the literature. Reid and coworkers[14] added 15 patients from their institutions to 115 patients reported in the literature. In their analysis, there was no difference in survival between those women who underwent conservative surgery and those who underwent radical surgery. Van Nostrand and associates[27] added 8 patients from their institution to 111 reported in the literature. In their analysis, after 2 years of follow-up, survival was significantly better for women who underwent radical surgery than for those treated with conservative surgery. Tjalma and colleagues,[28] who added another 9 cases to the

Table 68–1. International Federation of Gynaecologists and Obstetricians (FIGO) and American Joint Committee on Cancer (AJCC) Staging Systems

FIGO Staging for Vulvar Cancer

Stage 0: Carcinoma in situ; intraepithelial neoplasia grade III
Stage I: Lesions ≤2 cm confined to the vulva or perineum, no nodal metastasis
Stage Ia: Stromal invasion <1.0 mm
Stage Ib: Stromal invasion >1.0 mm
Stage II: Lesions >2 cm confined to the vulva or perineum, no nodal metastasis
Stage III: Tumor of any size with adjacent spread to the lower urethra and/or vagina, or the anus, and/or unilateral regional lymph node metastasis
Stage IVa: Tumor invading any of the following: upper urethra, bladder mucosa, rectal mucosa, pelvic bone, and/or bilateral regional lymph node metastasis
Stage IVb: Any distant metastasis including pelvic lymph nodes

FIGO Staging for Vaginal Cancer

Stage 0: Carcinoma in situ; intraepithelial neoplasia grade III
Stage I: Carcinoma limited to the vaginal wall
Stage II: Carcinoma involving the subvaginal tissue but has not extending to the pelvic wall
Stage III: The carcinoma extending to the pelvic wall
Stage IVa: Tumor invading bladder and/or rectal mucosa and/or direct extension beyond the true pelvis
Stage IVb: Spread to distant organs

AJCC Staging for Cutaneous Melanoma (6th Edition)

Primary Tumor (T)

TX	Primary tumor cannot be assessed
T0	No evidence of primary tumor
Tis	Melanoma in situ
T1	Melanoma ≤1.0 mm in thickness with or without ulceration
T1a	Melanoma ≤1.0 mm in thickness and level II or III, no ulceration
T1b	Melanoma ≤1.0 mm in thickness and level IV or IV or with ulceration
T2	Melanoma 1.01-2 mm in thickness with or without ulceration
T2a	Melanoma 1.01-2 mm in thickness, no ulceration
T2b	Melanoma 1.01-2 mm in thickness, with ulceration
T3	Melanoma 2.01-4 mm in thickness with or without ulceration
T3a	Melanoma 2.01-4 mm in thickness, no ulceration
T3b	Melanoma 2.01-4 mm in thickness, with ulceration
T4	Melanoma >4.0 mm in thickness with or without ulceration
T4a	Melanoma >4.0 mm in thickness, no ulceration
T4b	Melanoma >4.0 mm in thickness, with ulceration

Regional Lymph Nodes (N)

Nx	Regional lymph nodes cannot be assessed
N0	No regional lymph node metastasis
N1	Metastasis in one lymph node
N1a	Clinically occult (microscopic) metastasis
N1b	Clinically apparent (macroscopic) metastasis
N2	Metastasis in two to three regional nodes or intralymphatic regional metastasis without nodal metastasis
N2a	Clinically occult (microscopic) metastasis
N2b	Clinically apparent (macroscopic) metastasis
N2c	Satellite or in-transit metastasis without nodal metastasis
N3	Metastasis in four or more regional lymph nodes, or matted metastatic nodes, or in-transit metastasis, or satellite(s) with metastasis in regional node (s)

Distant Metastasis (M)

Mx	Distant metastasis cannot be assessed
M0	No distant metastasis
M1	Distant metastasis
M1a	Distant metastasis to skin, subcutaneous tissues, or distant lymph nodes
M1b	Metastasis to lung
M1c	Metastasis to all other visceral sites or distant metastasis at any site associated with an elevated serum lactic dehydrogenase

Clinical Stage Grouping

Stage	T	N	M
Stage 0	Tis	N0	M0
Stage Ia	T1a	N0	M0
Stage Ib	T1b	N0	M0
	T2a	N0	M0
Stage IIa	T2b	N0	M0
	T3a	N0	M0
Stage IIb	T3b	N0	M0
Stage IIc	T4b	N0	M0

Table 68–1. International Federation of Gynaecologists and Obstetricians (FIGO) and American Joint Committee on Cancer (AJCC) Staging Systems—cont'd

Stage III	Any T	N1	M0
	Any T	N2	M0
	Any T	N3	M0
Stage IV	Any T	Any N	M1

Pathologic Stage Grouping

Stage 0	Tis	N0	M0
Stage Ia	T1a	N0	M0
Stage Ib	T1b	N0	M0
	T2a	N0	M0
Stage IIa	T2b	N0	M0
	T3a	N0	M0
Stage IIb	T3b	N0	M0
	T4a	N0	M0
Stage IIc	T4b	N0	M0
Stage IIIa	T1-4a	N1a	M0
	T1-4a	N2a	M0
Stage IIIb	T1-4b	N1a	M0
	T1-4b	N2a	M0
	T1-4a	N1b	M0
	T1-4a	N2b	M0
	T1-4a/b	N2c	M0
Stage IIIc	T1-4b	N1b	M0
	T1-4b	N2b	M0
	Any T	N3	M0
Stage IV	Any T	Any N	M1

From Pecorelli S, Benedet JL, Creasman WT, et al: FIGO annual report on the results of treatment in gynaecological cancer, Vol. 23. J Epidemiol Biostat 1998;3:103,111; American Joint Committee on Cancer. AJCC Cancer Staging Manual, 6th ed. New York, Springer, 2002.

literature and analyzed 5-year survival rates among 22 previously reported patients with long-term survival, found that the type of surgery (radical versus conservative) had no impact on survival. In the absence of prospective data, it seems reasonable to treat women with vaginal melanoma with the same surgical approach used for those with cutaneous melanoma.

What is role of sentinel lymph node biopsy in the management of gynecologic melanomas?

Sentinel lymph node biopsy. Among patients with cutaneous melanomas, the incidence of occult lymph node metastases is less than 5% for individuals with thin melanomas (<1 mm) and greater than 70% for individuals with thick melanomas (>4.0 mm). It is reasonable, therefore, to consider sentinel node biopsy

for those patients with tumor thicknesses between 1 and 4 mm. Dessureault and colleagues[29] analyzed the data from 14,914 patients in the AJCC Melanoma Staging Database and found a statistically significant survival advantage associated with sentinel lymph node biopsy among patients with melanomas thicker than 1 mm, compared with those patients whose regional lymph nodes were evaluated only by clinical examination. They concluded that lymphatic mapping and sentinel lymph node biopsy would provide the most accurate staging with least morbidity.

The role of sentinel lymph node biopsy in the management of gynecologic melanomas is unclear. In theory, those patients found to have disease in the sentinel lymph node could be advised to undergo regional lymphadenectomy, and those without such a finding could be spared this surgery. Such an algorithm, however, presupposes that regional lymphadenectomy prolongs survival, or that effective

Table 68-2. Microstaging Systems for Vulvar Melanoma

Level	Invasion (Clark[10])	Lesion Thickness, mm (Breslow[11])	Invasion (Chung[12])	Tumor Volume, mm³ (Beller[13])
I	Intraepithelial	<0.75	Intraepithelial	—
II	Extension to papillary dermis	0.76-1.5	<1 mm Invasion into dermis or lamina propria	<100
III	Filling dermal papillae	1.5-2.5	1.0-2.0 mm Invasion into subepithelial tissue	100-500
IV	Invasion of collagen in reticular dermis	2.26-3.0	>2 mm Invasion to fibrous tissue	>500
V	Subcutaneous fat	>3.0	Subcutaneous fat	

Table 68–3. Relative Survival Rates for 123 Women with Vulvar Melanoma and for 31,879 Patients with Cutaneous Melanoma, by American Joint Committee on Cancer (AJCC) Stage (Fifth Edition)

Stage	No. Patients	5-yr Survival Rate (%)
I		
Cutaneous	21,979	90
Vulvar	31	83
II		
Cutaneous	4,570	77
Vulvar	33	52
III		
Cutaneous	3,341	50
Vulvar	50	39
IV		
Cutaneous	1,592	37
Vulvar	9	14

Data for cutaneous melanoma modified from American Joint Committee on Cancer: AJCC Cancer Staging Manual, 5th ed. Philadelphia, Lippincott-Raven, 1977, p 165 (Figure 24.1). Data for vulvar melanoma from Surveillance, Epidemiology, and End Results (SEER) database, National Cancer Institute (http://www.cancer.gov/statistics/).

adjuvant therapy that reduces the risk of recurrent disease has been identified. There are no prospective clinical trials for women with gynecologic melanomas. Levenback and associates,[30] who were the first to report sentinel lymph node assessment in vulvar carcinoma, included two patients with vulvar melanoma in their published series of nine patients who underwent this procedure. De Hullu and coworkers[31] reported their experience in sentinel lymph node biopsy in nine women with vulvar melanoma. They used both preoperative lymphoscintigraphy with radioactive technetium-labeled colloid and blue dye and intraoperative identification of the sentinel lymph nodes with a handheld probe and dissection of blue-stained lymph channels. Two of the nine women, both of whom had thick primary tumors (5.9 and 8 mm), later developed in-transit metastases.

In the absence of any prospective data among women with vulvar melanoma, it is reasonable to recommend sentinel lymph node biopsy for women with melanomas greater than 1 mm and less than 4 mm in thickness, as with cutaneous melanoma. Should metastatic disease be found in the regional lymph nodes, then consideration of regional lymphadenectomy may again be reasonable.

What is the role of regional lymphadenectomy in the management of gynecologic melanomas?

Regional lymphadenectomy. Regional lymphadenectomy in cutaneous melanoma has been recommended both to remove metastatic disease and to identify patients who might benefit from adjuvant systemic therapy. To date, randomized phase III clinical trials for patients with cutaneous melanoma have failed to

show a survival advantage associated with regional lymphadenectomy for patients with thin tumors (<0.76 mm) or for those with thicker tumors (>4 mm). Balch and colleagues[32] did find a 6% absolute reduction in the 10-year survival rate associated with elective lymph node dissection among patients with tumor thickness of 1.0 to 2.0 mm. This benefit was found only in subgroup analysis. For the entire population of individuals with melanoma, elective lymph node dissection did not improve survival. In the retrospective analysis of AJCC data reported by Dessureault and associates,[29] however, patients who underwent sentinel lymph node biopsy survived better than those who underwent elective lymph node dissection. The authors concluded that sentinel lymph node assessment provided more accurate staging than did routine elective lymph node dissection.

The therapeutic benefit of sentinel lymph node assessment and "selective" complete lymph node dissection (SCLND) of regional lymph nodes (i.e., complete dissection based on evidence of metastatic disease in the sentinel lymph node) for patients with cutaneous melanoma is not known. The Multicenter Selective Lymphadenectomy Trial (MSLT), a clinical trial sponsored by the NCI and headed by Donald L. Morton of the John Wayne Cancer Institute, was initiated in 1994 to evaluate this benefit in patients with primary cutaneous melanoma (Breslow thickness ≥1 mm with Clark level III, or Clark level IV or greater regardless of Breslow thickness) with no evidence of regional nodal disease.[33] The primary aim of this trial is to assess whether there is a difference in overall survival for wide excision alone compared with sentinel lymph node assessment and SCLND. This trial randomized patients in a 60:40 distribution to wide excision alone versus wide excision plus sentinel lymph node assessment with SCLND. The trial closed at the end of 2001 after reaching its accrual goal of more than 1800 patients. The results of this trial will provide important information as to whether regional lymphadenectomy provides any survival advantage for patients with cutaneous melanoma.

The role of regional lymphadenectomy in the management of gynecologic melanomas has not yet been determined. There are no prospective clinical trials. In Creasman's report of the NCDB data, approximately half of women with vulvar melanoma underwent regional lymphadenectomy as part of primary surgical therapy. Based on the data from cutaneous melanoma, it may be reasonable to recommend a regional lymphadenectomy for women found to have metastatic disease in sentinel lymph nodes; however, investigators are awaiting the results of the Multicenter Selective Lymphadenectomy Trial to see whether any direct therapeutic benefit is associated with regional lymphadenectomy based on evidence of metastatic disease in sentinel lymph nodes for patients with cutaneous melanoma.

In the prospective GOG trial, capillary lymphatic space involvement and Breslow's depth of invasion correlated significantly with the risk of positive groin nodes.[6] In multiple regression analysis, independent predictors of lymph node metastasis were a central primary tumor and capillary lymphatic space involvement.

How should cervical and ovarian melanomas be treated?

Treatment of primary cervical melanomas. As noted previously, primary cervical melanomas are so rare that we have few published data on which to make recommendations.[34] It would seem reasonable to treat a melanoma confined to the cervix with primary radical hysterectomy. Radical surgery may also help control local symptoms in a woman with a primary cervical melanoma extending into the vagina, parametrium, uterine corpus, or other pelvic tissues. If the disease is inoperable or the patient has widespread metastatic disease, then primary radiotherapy may help control local disease.

Treatment of ovarian melanomas. Rarely, melanomas arise in ovarian teratomas.[35] Like cervical melanomas, these are so rare that there are few published data on which to base recommendations. Women found to

have a melanoma confined to the ovary should undergo primary resection. Recommendations regarding adjuvant therapy should be based on those for cutaneous melanoma.

What is the role of adjuvant therapy after primary surgery for gynecologic melanoma?

Adjuvant therapy. In two randomized trials involving patients with cutaneous melanomas, high-dose adjuvant interferon was shown to increase both progression-free and overall survival after surgical resection. The control arm of one trial was observation[36]; in the other, it was vaccine therapy.[37] However, the latter study was reported with a short median follow-up time. A subsequent review[38] of nine randomized controlled trials of adjuvant interferon found that wide clinical heterogeneity precluded meta-analysis and that a large randomized clinical trial would be necessary to determine whether adjuvant interferon is of benefit in individuals with cutaneous melanoma. Tolerability of the interferon regimen, however, has remained a barrier to patient acceptance. No improvement in

---

█ Table 68-4. Prognostic Factors for Women with Vulvar Melanoma

Survival

Demographics
Race
Weinstock[1]
Advanced Age at Diagnosis
Podratz et al.[7]
Rose et al.[4]
Bradgate et al.[19]
Trimble et al.[20]
Ragnarsson-Olding et al.[23]
Family History of Melanoma
Verschraegen et al.[39]

Anatomy
Presence of Groin Metastases
Scheistroen et al.[18]
Phillips et al.[6]
Trimble et al.[20]
Raber et al.[21]
Tumor Location (Central versus Lateral)
Scheistroen et al.[18]
Podratz et al.[7]

Tumor Characteristics
Angioinvasion
Scheistroen et al.[18]
DNA Ploidy
Scheistroen et al.[18]
High Mitotic Rate
Bradgate et al.[19]
Ragnarsson-Olding et al.[23]
Histologic Type
Podratz et al.[7]
Ragnarsson-Olding et al.[23]
Macroscopic Amelanosis
Ragnarsson-Olding et al.[23]
Tumor Thickness
Scheistroen et al.[18]

Verschraegen et al.[39]
Ragnarsson-Olding et al.[23]
DeMatos et al.[22]
Ulceration
Tasseron et al.[25]
Bradgate et al.[19]
Ragnarsson-Olding et al.[23]
DeMatos et al.[22]

Risk of Lymph Node Metastasis

Demographics
Advanced Age at Diagnosis
Scheistroen et al.[18]
Verschraegen et al.[39]

Anatomy
Tumor Location (Central versus Lateral)
Phillips et al.[6]

Tumor Characteristics
Angioinvasion
Scheistroen et al.[18]
Capillary Lymphatic Space Invasion
Phillips et al.[6]
DNA Ploidy
Scheistroen et al.[18]
Tumor Thickness
Scheistroen et al.[18]
Ulceration
Scheistroen et al.[18]

Risk of Recurrence

Demographics
Advanced Age at Diagnosis
Phillips et al.[6]

Anatomy
Tumor Location (Central versus Lateral)
Phillips et al.[6]

progression-free or overall survival has been documented with adjuvant radiation or chemotherapy. Vaccine therapy remains experimental.

There are only retrospective data on adjuvant therapy in women with vulvar and vaginal melanoma. Verschraegen and colleagues,[39] who reported a retrospective series of 51 women with vulvar melanoma treated at the University of Texas M.D. Anderson Cancer Center between 1970 and 1997, did find a statistically significant survival advantage associated with adjuvant therapy, which included a variety of regimens. Two recent small series, totaling 21 patients, documented long-term survival in women who had vaginal melanoma treated with wide local excision followed by adjuvant radiotherapy or primary radiotherapy.[40,41] In the absence of prospective data in patients with gynecologic melanomas, it is reasonable to extrapolate from the data on cutaneous melanomas and consider adjuvant high-dose interferon for patients who are at high risk of recurrence.

Are there reliable prognostic markers for women with vulvar melanoma?

Prognostic markers. Prognostic markers for cutaneous melanoma have largely been integrated into the latest AJCC staging system. Increased age at diagnosis also emerged as an adverse prognostic factor.[9] Prognostic markers that have been identified among women with vulvar melanoma in a number of different reports are shown in Table 68-4. These include demographics (race, advanced age), tumor location (central versus lateral), presence of groin node metastases, and various tumor characteristics (thickness, ulceration, mitotic rate, histologic type, DNA ploidy, angioinvasion, and macroscopic amelanosis). As Table 68-5 demonstrates, however, the majority of these studies were small and retrospective; the GOG cohort study was the only prospective study. The population-based retrospective Swedish series combined a relatively large data set with detailed clinical data and central pathologic review. Among patients with vaginal melanoma, tumor size appears to be the principal prognostic marker predicting survival.[14,28]

What is the recommended therapy for recurrent, metastatic disease?

Melanomas can spread by local extension through lymphatic channels and/or by hematogenous routes to distant sites. Any organ may be involved by metastases; lungs and liver are common sites. The risk of relapse decreases with time, but late relapses are not uncommon.

Interferon, interleukin-2, and dacarbazine have modest activity against metastatic or recurrent melanoma. Women with metastatic melanomas originally arising in the gynecologic tract should be considered for phase I to phase III trials of new anticancer regimens.

Table 68–5. Characteristics of Recent Reported Studies of Women with Vulvar and Vaginal Melanomas

Study	Site or Institution	N
Vulvar Melanoma		
Prospective Cohort Studies		
Phillips et al.[6]	Gynecologic Oncology Group	71
Population-Based Retrospective Series		
Bradgate et al.[19]	West Midlands, UK	50
Ragnarsson-Olding et al.[23]	Sweden	198
Weinstock[1]	14% of United States	203
Institutional-Based Retrospective Series		
DeMatos et al.[22]	1 cancer center	30
Podratz et al.[7]	1 cancer center	48
Raber et al.[21]	5 hospitals	89
Rose et al.[24]	1 cancer center	26
Scheistroen et al.[18]	1 cancer center	75
Tasseron et al.[25]	1 cancer center	30
Trimble et al.[20]	1 cancer center	80
Verschraegen et al.[39]	1 cancer center	51
Vaginal Melanoma		
Institutional-Based Retrospective Series		
DeMatos et al.[22]	1 cancer center	9
Irvin et al.[40]	1 cancer center	7
Petru et al.[41]	3 hospitals	14
Reid et al.[14]	2 cancer centers	15
Tjalma et al.[28]	1 cancer center	9
Van Nostrand et al.[27]	1 cancer center	8

Is there a role for a prospective multi-institutional effort to study gynecologic melanomas?

As the most recent data from SEER suggest, gynecologic melanomas are sufficiently rare as to make clinical trials very difficult to complete. Phase III trials may be impossible to perform; the only prospective study, reported by Phillips and colleagues,[6] was a cohort study. Phase II trials might be feasible in the context of an existing clinical trials cooperative group with an established track record of accruing patients with gynecologic malignancies.

The survival data from SEER suggest that women with gynecologic melanoma may face a worse prognosis than those with cutaneous melanoma of the same stage. It may be inappropriate, therefore, to consider the expansion of trials for individuals with cutaneous melanoma to include individuals with mucosal or glabrous melanomas such as those involving the vulva and vagina.

REFERENCES

1. Weinstock MA: Malignant melanoma of the vulva and vagina in the United States: Patterns of incidence and population-based estimated of survival. Am J Obstet Gynecol 1994;171: 1225-1230.
2. Ragnarsson-Olding B, Johansson H, Rutqvist L-E, et al: Malignant melanoma of the vulva and vagina: Trends in incidence, age distribution, and long-term survival among 245 consecutive cases in Sweden 1960-1984. Cancer 1993;71:1893-1897.

3. Creasman WT, Phillips JL, Menck HR: A survey of hospital management practices for vulvar melanoma. J Am Coll Surg 1999; 188:670-675.

4. Ragnarsson-Olding BK, Kanter-Lewensohn LR, Lagerlog B, et al: Malignant melanoma of the vulva in a nationwide, 25-year study of 219 Swedish females: Clinical observations and histopathologic features. Cancer 1999;86;1273-1284.

5. American Joint Committee on Cancer: Melanoma of the skin. In AJCC Cancer Staging Manual, 6th ed. New York, Springer, 2002, pp 209-217.

6. Phillips GL, Bundy BN, Okagaki T, et al: Malignant melanoma of the vulva treated by radical hemivulvectomy: A prospective study of the Gynecologic Oncology Group. Cancer 1994;73: 2626-2632.

7. Podratz KC, Gaffey TA, Symmonds RE, et al: Melanoma of the vulva: An update. Gynecol Oncol 1983;16:153-168.

8. Balch CM, Buzaid AC, Soong S-J, et al: Final version of the American Joint Committee on Cancer staging system for cutaneous melanoma. J Clin Oncol 2001;19:3635-3648.

9. Balch CM, Soong S-J, Gershenwald JE, et al: Prognostic factors analysis of 17,600 melanoma patients: Validation of the American Joint Committee on Cancer melanoma staging system. J Clin Oncol 2001;19:3622-3634.

10. Clark WH, From L, Bernadino EA, et al: The histogenesis and biologic behavior of primary human malignant melanoma of the skin. Cancer Res 1969;29:705-726.

11. Breslow A: Thickness, cross-sectional areas, and depth of invasion in the prognosis of cutaneous melanomas. Ann Surg 1970;172:902-908.

12. Chung AF, Woodruff JM, Lewis JL: Malignant melanoma of the vulva: A report of 44 cases. Obstet Gynecol 1975;45:638-646.

13. Beller U, Demopoulos RI, Beckman EM: Vulvovaginal melanoma: A clinicopathologic study. J Reprod Med 1986;31: 315-319.

14. Reid GC, Schmidt RW, Roberts JA, et al: Primary melanoma of the vagina: A clinicopathologic analysis. Obstet Gynecol 1989; 74:190-199.

15. Fleming ID, Cooper JS, Henson DE, et al. Malignant melanoma of the skin. In AJCC Cancer Staging Manual, 5th ed. Philadelphia, Lippincott-Raven, 1997, pp 163-167.

16. Balch CM, Soong SJ, Smith T, et al: Long-term results of a prospective surgical trial comparing 2 cm versus 4 cm excision margins for 740 patients with 1-4 mm melanomas. Ann Surg Oncol 2001;8:101-108.

17. Veronesi UU, Cascinelli N: Narrow excision (1 cm margin): A safe procedure for thin cutaneous melanoma. Arch Surg 1991; 126:438-441.

18. Scheistroen M, Trope C, Kaern J, et al: Malignant melanoma of the vulvar FIGO stage I: Evaluation of prognostic markers in 75 patients with emphasis on DNA ploidy and surgical treatment. Cancer 1995;75:72-80.

19. Bradgate MG, Rollason TP, McConkey CC, et al: Malignant melanoma of the vulva: A clinico-pathological study of 50 women. Br J Obstet Gynaecol 1990;97:124-133.

20. Trimble EL, Lewis JL Jr, Williams LL, et al: Management of vulvar melanoma. Gynecol Oncol 1992;45:254-258.

21. Raber G, Mempel V, Jackisch C, et al: Malignant melanoma of the vulva: Report of 89 patients. Cancer 1996;78:2353-2358.

22. DeMatos P, Tyler D, Seigler HF: Mucosal melanoma of the female genitalia: A clinicopathologic study of 43 cases at Duke University Medical Center. Surgery 1998;124:38-48.

23. Ragnarsson-Olding BK, Nilsson BR, Kaner-Lewensohn LR, et al: Malignant melanoma of the vulvar in a nationwide, 25-year

24. Rose PG, Piver MS, Tsukada Y, et al: Conservative therapy for melanoma of the vulva. Am J Obstet Gynecol 1988;159:520-525.

25. Tasseron EWK, van der Esch EP, Hart AAM, et al: A clinicopathological study of 30 melanomas of the vulva. Gynecol Oncol 1992;46:170-175.

26. Irwin WP, Legallo RL, Stoler MH, et al: Vulvar melanoma: A retrospective analysis and literature review. Gynecol Oncol 2001;83:457-465.

27. Van Nostrand KM, Lucci JA, Schell M, et al: Primary vaginal melanoma: Improved survival with radical pelvic surgery. Gynecol Oncol 1994;55:234-237.

28. Tjalma WA, Monaghan JM, de Barros Lopes A, et al: Primay vaginal melanoma and long-term survivors. Eur J Gynaecol Oncol 2001;22:20-22.

29. Dessureault S, Soong S-J, Ross MI, et al: Imporved staging of node-negative patients with intermediate to thick melanomas (> 1 mm) with the use of lymphatic mapping and sentinel lymph node biopsy. Ann Surg Oncol 2001;8:766-770.

30. Levenback C, Burge TW, Gershenson DM, et al: Intraoperative mapping for vulvar cancer. Obstet Gynecol 1994;84:163-167.

31. de Hullu JA, Hollema H, Hoekstra HJ, et al: Vulvar melanoma: Is there a role for sentinel lymph node biopsy? Cancer 2002; 94:486-491.

32. Balch CM, Soong S, Ross MI, et al: Long-term results of a multi-institutional randomized trial comparing prognostic factors and surgical results for intermediate thickness melanomas (1.0 to 4.0 mm). Intergroup Melanoma Surgical Trial. Ann Surg Oncol 2000;7:75-76.

33. Morton DL, Thompson JF, Essner R, et al: Validation of the accuracy of intraoperative lymphatic mapping and sentinel lymphadenectomy for early-stage melanoma: A multicenter trial. Multicenter Selective Lymphadenectomy Trial Group. Ann Surg 1999;230:453-463.

34. Clark KC, Butz WR, Hapke MR: Primary malignant melanoma of the uterine cervix: Case report with world literature review. Int J Gynecol Pathol 1999;18:265-273.

35. Vimla N, Kumar L, Thulkar S, et al: Primary malignant melanoma in ovarian cystic teratoma. Gynecol Oncol 2001;82: 380-383.

36. Kirkwood JM, Ibrahim JG, Sosman JA, et al: High-dose interferon alfa-2b significantly prolongs relapse-free and overall survival compared with the GM2-KLH/QS-21 vaccine in patients with resected stage IiB-III melanoma: Results of Intergroup Trial E1694/S9512/C509801. J Clin Oncol 2001;19:2370-2380.

37. Kirkwood JM, Ibrahim J, Lawson DH, et al: High-dose interferon alfa-2b does not diminish antibody response to GM2 vaccination in patients with resected melanoma: Results of the multicenter eastern cooperative oncology group phase II trial E2696. J Clin Oncol 2001;19:1430-1436.

38. Lens MB, Dawes M: Interferon alfa therapy for malignant melanoma: A systemic review of randomized controlled trials. J Clin Oncol 2002;20:1818-1825.

39. Verschraegen CF, Benjapibal M, Supakarapongkul W, et al: Vulvar melanoma at the MD Anderson Cancer Center: 25 Years later. Int J Gynecol Cancer 2001;11:359-364.

40. Irvin WP, Bliss SA, Rice LW, et al: Malignant melanoma of the vagina and locoregional control: Radical surgery revisited. Gynecol Oncol 1998;71:476-480.

41. Petru E, Nagele F, Czerwenka K, et al: Primary malignant melanoma of the vagina: Long-term remission following radiation therapy. Gynecol Oncol 1998;70:23-26.

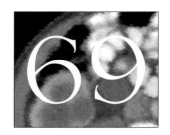

INTERVENTIONAL RADIOLOGY IN THE MANAGEMENT OF GYNECOLOGIC CANCER

Michael J. Wallace

 MAJOR CONTROVERSIES

- **What is an interventional radiologist?**
- **What is the utility of image-guided biopsy?**
- **What is the role of drainage procedures?**
- **What are arterial interventions and how do they affect patients with gynecologic neoplasms?**
- **What are venous interventions and how do they affect patients with gynecologic neoplasms?**

What is an interventional radiologist?

The interventional radiologist uses the standard imaging techniques that best define the target organ or lesion to guide minimally invasive vascular and non-vascular procedures. These procedures are adapted from standard surgical procedures to establish a diagnosis, initiate therapeutic management, or provide palliative care for patients with cancer. Minimally invasive approaches are often safer, less traumatic, and less painful but equally therapeutic and more cost effective for the patient and the health care provider when compared with the surgical alternative. Procedures used in the management of patients with gynecologic neoplasms include imaging-guided biopsy and drainage (gastrostomy, nephrostomy), arterial interventions (infusion, embolization, chemoembolization, balloon angioplasty, stent/stent-graft placement), and venous interventions (insertion and repositioning of long-term central venous access devices, stents, inferior vena caval filters, foreign body retrieval, thrombolysis), among others. State-of-the-art imaging modalities including fluoroscopy, ultrasonography, computed tomography (CT), and magnetic resonance imaging (MRI) are used to guide the placement of needles, catheters, and devices directly to the target site

deep within the body through a small skin incision. These procedures often are performed under local anesthesia with intravenous sedation and typically do not require general anesthesia.

NONVASCULAR INTERVENTIONS

What is the utility of image-guided biopsy?

Percutaneous image-guided biopsy has been one of the most cost effective contributions to the diagnosis and treatment of patients with cancer. Almost all tissues are accessible to the percutaneous biopsy approach. Needles ranging in size from 11 to 25 gauge typically are used to obtain core biopsy and fine-needle aspiration biopsy (FNAB) samples from the desired target lesion or organ. Special biopsy forceps and transvenous biopsy needles are available to acquire tissue samples via the vascular approach (endomyocardial biopsy, transvenous liver biopsy). Superficial palpable masses are usually biopsied by the cytopathologist, whereas masses requiring imaging techniques are biopsied by the radiologist. Depending on the size and location of the lesion to be sampled, CT, sonography, fluoroscopy, or MRI is used to guide the procedure.

The vast majority of these biopsies can be performed electively on an outpatient basis under intravenous sedation and local anesthesia. The preprocedure prothrombin time and platelet count are measured routinely, and any coagulopathy is corrected. Postprocedure observation time ranges from 1 to 3 hours depending on the lesion or organ sampled. A negative biopsy result does not exclude malignancy and may merely reflect an error in sampling.

The vast majority of gynecologic lesions that require biopsy can be accessed by image guidance with either CT or sonography. Sonography offers several advantages, including real-time visualization of the needle, shorter procedure time, lack of ionizing radiation exposure, and lower procedure cost, which make it the modality of choice in many situations.[1-4] Sonography plays a less important role when lesions are deep or situated behind bowel or bone, where the ultrasound waves do not adequately penetrate to provide a clear image to guide the biopsy. Unlike sonography, CT has the ability to provide precise localization of the lesion and adjacent structures regardless of their depth and proximity to bone or bowel. These advantages allow CT to fill the void when ultrasound falls short.

Abdomen-pelvis-retroperitoneum. CT is often the preferred imaging modality when small lesions or lymph nodes deep within the abdomen and pelvis or adjacent to the aorta (Fig. 69-1), inferior vena cava, or other vital structures are to be sampled.[5-7] Transvaginal ultrasound approaches have been effective for biopsies of lesions deep within the pelvis that are surrounded by bowel, bladder, or bone and for which a safe percutaneous route cannot be identified on CT.[8,9] Overall, image-guided abdominal biopsy can provide a high degree of accuracy with a low risk of complications.

Welch and colleagues,[7] in a prospective series of 1000 CT-guided abdominal biopsies, reported sensitivity and specificity of 91.8% and 98.9%, with positive and negative predictive values of 99.7% and 73.3%, respectively. In a small series of 29 patients with gynecologic malignancy, Kohler and associates[5] successfully used CT-guided FNAB of retroperitoneal lymph nodes. The biopsy success rate, defined by the adequacy of specimen cellularity, was 90%, with malignancy identified in 83% of the cytologic specimens. A review of our experience at the University of Texas M. D. Anderson Cancer Center with CT-guided biopsies of the abdomen, pelvis, and retroperitoneum for lesions smaller than 3 cm in diameter showed that adequate diagnostic material was obtained in 95% of samples from a subset of 41 patients with primary gynecologic malignancy. High rates of success, ranging from 85% to 97%, have been reported for sonographically guided biopsy of abdominal, pelvic, and retroperitoneal adenopathy.[4,10-12] The overall complication rate for image-guided biopsy is 1% or less,[7,13] with a potential for seeding of malignant cells along the needle tract in 0.05% of patients.

Thorax. Fluoroscopy and CT are typically used to guide biopsies of the lung and mediastinum. Because of the air within the lung, sonography is not feasible except for larger lesions that abut the pleura. Transthoracic image-guided percutaneous FNAB has been a reliable means of differentiating benign and malignant pulmonary lesions. Success rates have been well documented, with diagnostic accuracy rates in excess of 93%[14-16] and sensitivity rates in excess of 95%.[16-18] Aside from pneumothorax (16% to 44.6%) and chest tube insertion, reported complications are uncommon for image-guided FNAB.[16,17,19-22] Successful

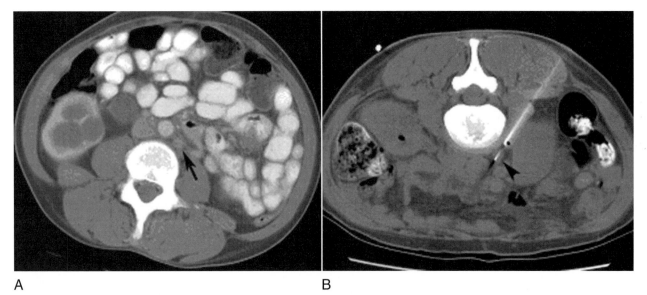

A   B

Figure 69-1. A, Contrast-enhanced computed tomogram of the abdomen in a patient (supine position) with cervical cancer, demonstrating a 1.1-cm paraaortic lymph node (arrow). **B,** Non-contrast computed tomogram in the same patient (prone position) during fine-needle aspiration of the para-aortic lymph node (arrowhead).

biopsy of lesions as small as 3 mm in diameter has been reported.[16,20] At M. D. Anderson, our review of 61 patients with pulmonary lesions equal to or less than 1 cm in diameter revealed an overall sensitivity of 82.1%, specificity of 100%, and diagnostic accuracy of 87.7% based on 57 evaluable patients. The results for lesions 0.8 to 1.0 cm in diameter (*n* = 47) were considerably better (sensitivity, 87.9%; accuracy, 91.5%) than for lesions 0.5 to 0.7 cm in diameter (*n* = 10; sensitivity, 50%; accuracy, 70%).

What is the role of drainage procedures?

Percutaneous catheter drainage is an additional major contribution of interventional radiology to the care of patients with malignancy. Catheters are placed into obstructed genitourinary, biliary, and gastrointestinal tracts as well as abnormal fluid collections such as abscesses, empyemas, bilomas, urinomas, seromas, and lymphocysts under radiologic guidance using the Seldinger technique, which makes use of a needle, guidewire, and catheter.

Percutaneous abscess drainage. The febrile patient is a common situation in the oncology setting. An intra-abdominal abscess can be life-threatening and is usually caused by perforation of a hollow viscus, either by a neoplasm or as a postoperative complication. A septic episode is often accompanied by renal, pulmonary, or cardiovascular failure and when untreated has a mortality rate of almost 100%. Thirty-six percent of intra-abdominal abscesses are located within the peritoneal cavity, 38% within the retroperitoneum, and 26% within the viscera.[23] In the past 15 to 20 years, percutaneous abscess drainage (PAD) has all but replaced surgical drainage as the treatment of choice for abscesses and other abnormal fluid collections (e.g., biloma, urinoma).[24] PAD is less invasive than surgical drainage, better maintains the integrity of surrounding structures and overlying skin, and can be done at the time of initial diagnosis, saving time and expense. CT and ultrasonography are used both to diagnose abscesses and guide their drainage. These cross-sectional techniques are used to determine the depth of the abscess, the cutaneous entry site, and the angle through which the collection is best approached so as to avoid adjacent vital structures such as bowel, organs, or major vessels. PAD also makes nursing care easier, because drainage systems are closed, with no extensive surgical wound that requires frequent dressing changes.

PAD is most successful when the fluid collection is well defined, unilocular, and free flowing, characteristics found in more than 90% of intra-abdominal collections. PAD may also be helpful in less favorable situations (e.g., multilocular collection, necrotic debris), particularly if the patient presents a high surgical risk. In these less optimal circumstances, PAD may improve the patient's condition so that a more definitive surgical drainage can be performed at a later time. The only absolute contraindication to PAD is the lack of a safe access route. This rarely is a problem when CT guidance is used. In very selected cases in which a fluid collection lies deep within the pelvis, transrectal or transvaginal routes may be used, with endocavitary ultrasound probes providing guidance.[25]

The most important step in PAD procedures is planning the access route. This is done after review of all pertinent imaging studies. In general, the shortest, straightest tract is the best approach. Care must be taken to avoid adjacent bowel, pleura, and major blood vessels. Diagnostic aspiration can be performed initially with an 18- to 22-gauge needle. The position of the needle is confirmed with ultrasound or CT, and the fluid is aspirated for culture and other diagnostic studies. If a decision is made to drain the fluid, a 10F to 20F catheter can be inserted into the collection using the Seldinger technique. The size of the drainage catheter depends on the type and viscosity of fluid obtained on the initial aspiration.

PAD compares favorably with surgical treatment in overall success, duration of drainage, and recurrence rate. The success of percutaneous management depends on the complexity of the collection. Unilocular and discrete collections can be effectively cured in 90% of cases. For collections that are more complex (e.g., abscess communication with bowel), the cure rate falls to between 80% and 90%. Pancreatic collections and tumors with abscess or phlegmon formation intermixed with necrosis are examples of situations in which PAD is much less effective, with cure rates falling as low as 30% to 50%.[26]

The overall complication rate for PAD in most series is 5% or less.[26] Minor complications include transient bacteremia, skin infection, and minor bleeding. Major complications include hemorrhage requiring transfusion, sepsis, and bowel perforation. The recurrence rate after PAD is approximately 5%. PAD compares favorably with surgical alternatives, for which the mortality rate is 10% to 20% and the recurrence rate is 15% to 30%.

Percutaneous nephrostomy. In cancer patients, urinary tract obstruction usually develops as a result of compression or direct extension of primary or metastatic neoplasms in the pelvis or retroperitoneum. Less frequently, obstruction is caused by benign iatrogenic strictures from surgical intervention or radiation therapy (or both) or from urinary calculi. Percutaneous nephrostomy (PCN) tube placement is an established intervention for urinary diversion in patients with supravesical urinary tract obstruction, urinary fistulas and leaks, or hemorrhagic cystitis. Percutaneous renal access is also the initial maneuver for more complex urologic interventions that include percutaneous nephrolithotomy and other endourologic procedures.

Urinary obstruction may become evident because of azotemia or urinary sepsis, or it may be diagnosed incidentally after ultrasound or CT examination of the abdomen for other reasons. The diagnosis of an obstructed collecting system can be confirmed by any number of imaging modalities. Ultrasonography is a good first-choice examination, especially if the patient's serum creatinine level is elevated and an obstructive uropathy is suspected.

Patients with pyonephrosis or infected hydronephrosis are at high risk for gram-negative sepsis. It is under these circumstances that urinary diversion must be performed as an emergency procedure. Patients often present with fever, flank pain, and evidence of urinary tract obstruction on cross-sectional imaging.

Percutaneous drainage has become the treatment of choice for initial decompression of an infected collecting system regardless of the underlying cause. In the presence of obstruction without infection, urinary diversion can be used to preserve renal function. It is particularly important for patients whose therapy regimens will include agents that depend on renal excretion and are potentially nephrotoxic. In patients with urinary leakage or fistulas, PCN tube placement can be used to divert an adequate amount of urine to allow healing to occur. If the leak or fistula is too large and simple diversion is inadequate, adjunctive embolization of the ureters (Fig. 69-2) above the fistula or leak can provide relief,[27] although the patient will then require lifelong percutaneous drainage. Similarly, percutaneous urinary diversion is one method of therapy for patients with hemorrhagic cystitis when more traditional local therapies have failed.[28] The decision

to perform a nephrostomy takes into consideration the patient's life expectancy and the available therapeutic options.

Overall success rates in excess of 98% have been reported for PCN tube placement.[29] Success rates are often lower in patients with nondilated collecting systems and in patients with complex stone disease. Complications occur in approximately 10% of patients when both major and minor complications are considered together.[29] Major hemorrhagic complications occur in approximately 2.5% of cases.[30,31] Other potential complications include septic shock and bowel transgression. Thoracic complications (pneumothorax, hydrothorax, hemothorax, and empyema) can occur if renal access is above the 12th rib.

Ureteric stenting. Ureteric stenting is a common alternative approach to PCN for internal urinary tract diversion in the management of benign or malignant causes of obstruction. Internal stents can be placed either from the retrograde approach via the bladder by cystoscopy or from the antegrade approach after PCN access. Like PCN tubes, ureteral stents can be used to maintain ureteral patency or to treat urine leakage to allow healing of the urothelium. Internal stenting is better tolerated by most patients because it does not require an external drainage bag or daily catheter care, as does PCN drainage.

The two basic types of ureteral stents are those made of plastic material and those constructed of metal. Most commonly used is the plastic catheter type of stent, which typically has a double-pigtail design ("double-J" stent). One end is situated in the renal pelvis and the other in the bladder. Proximal and distal sideholes in both pigtail portions allow drainage through the lumen, across the obstruction, and into the bladder. The "J" portion serves as a retention mechanism to prevent migration. In patients with malignant obstruction, the technical success of ureteric stenting ranges from 83% to 95%.[32] The longest recommended interval that these stents can remain in place without change is 6 months.[33] This compares favorably with nephrostomy tubes, which typically require exchange at roughly 3-month intervals.

Experience with conventional metal stents has demonstrated high rates of initial technical success but dismal short- and long-term patency, with a primary 12-month patency rate of 31%.[34] These devices are permanent implants that cannot be removed or exchanged. Newer stents with a biocompatible covering (stent grafts) may improve patency rates of metal stents.

Percutaneous gastrostomy. Percutaneous gastrostomy drainage can be used in patients who have chronic intestinal obstruction caused by unresectable neoplasm, and in those who have multiple enteric strictures secondary to irradiation, as a means of intestinal decompression. Percutaneous gastrostomy also offers a useful route for nutritional support in patients with esophageal or head and neck neoplasms that compromise swallowing function. Although it was previously

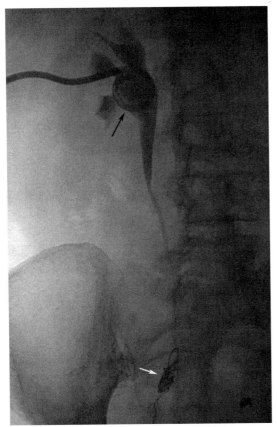

Figure 69-2. Antegrade nephrostogram obtained via a nephrostomy tube *(black arrow)* after coil embolization *(white arrow)* of the distal ureter in the treatment of a patient with vesicovaginal fistula.

considered a surgical procedure, placement of gastrostomy tubes can be performed by a percutaneous approach with fluoroscopic or endoscopic guidance in most cases.[35-37]

Overall, the percutaneous fluoroscopic technique that is used to insert gastrostomy tubes is efficient and safe, with success rates of 98% or greater, minor complication rates ranging from 1% to 12%, and major complications from 1% to 6%.[37-40] In a review of 92 consecutive outpatient gastrostomy tube insertions at M. D. Anderson over a 6-month period,[37] the success rate was 98%, with a major complication rate of 1% and a minor complication rate of 8%. Tube malfunctions were encountered in 13% of these patients.

Colonic stenting. Metallic stents have been used to manage vascular, gastrointestinal, biliary, and tracheobronchial stenoses. The use of these metallic stents within the gastrointestinal system is palliative, for nonsurgical management of esophageal, duodenal, and colonic obstruction. When resection is not feasible, stents can be used to palliate an obstruction for the remainder of the patient's life. Additionally, stents are being used to temporize an acute obstruction to allow adequate preoperative preparation before definitive surgical intervention. Acute left-sided malignant colonic obstruction is a frequently encountered surgical emergency. Colonic stenting offers a minimally invasive means of intestinal decompression that can quickly relieve an acute obstruction in these acutely ill patients. Once the patient's medical condition has improved, a definitive and often less complex surgical procedure can be performed at one session. Technical success in crossing the obstruction and deploying the device ranges from 80% to 100%, with clinical success (i.e., relief of obstruction) reported in 80% to 92%.[41]

Complications of colonic stenting included perforation, stent migration, and restenosis. Perforation has been reported in 0% to 16% of cases. Balloon dilation of the stent has been implicated as the cause of higher rates of perforation, and it is not recommended at the time of stent deployment. Without balloon dilation, the perforation rate may fall below 5%. Stent migration has been reported in as many as 40% of cases, and restenosis in 25%. The latter occurrence is often secondary to tumor ingrowth.[41]

VASCULAR INTERVENTIONS

What are arterial interventions and how do they affect patients with gynecologic neoplasms?

Over the past two decades, the role of the interventional radiologist has shifted from diagnosis to therapy in the care of patients with cancer. Although direct percutaneous therapeutic options have attracted recent interest, the transcatheter approach continues to play a significant role in the treatment of these

challenging cases. Techniques have traditionally included intra-arterial infusion, embolization, and chemoembolization. The delivery of therapeutic agents via the arterial system requires selective vascular catheterization, which is accomplished by tailoring the catheter configuration to the vascular anatomy. With improvements in catheter technology, coaxial microcatheter systems that range from 2F to 3F in outer diameter can be delivered through 4F to 5F standard angiographic catheters to facilitate the technical challenges involved in small-vessel catheterization. An additional advantage of these microcatheter systems is their potential for reducing arterial injuries (e.g. dissection, perforation) that can occur with larger catheters.

Although these transarterial infusions and embolizations are employed most commonly in the treatment of hepatic malignancy, they are also helpful means of reducing tumor burden preoperatively, as well as intraoperative blood loss. Nonhepatic embolizations have also been used for pain palliation in patients who are not candidates for surgical resection. Neoplastic, iatrogenic, and treatment-related hemorrhage can be effectively controlled with embolization techniques. Intra-arterial treatment of patients with malignancy requires close collaboration among the interventional radiologist, surgeon, oncologist, and radiotherapist to ensure the maximum potential benefit from these minimally invasive therapeutic options.

Intra-arterial infusion therapy. The goal of intra-arterial chemotherapy is to deliver high doses of chemotherapeutic agents into the artery supplying the neoplasm. Several experimental and clinical studies have shown that intra-arterial therapy can achieve a 20% to 30% higher response rate than can conventional systemic therapy. However, benefits such as prolonged survival and improved quality of life have not been demonstrated consistently, and patients are rarely cured.[42] These techniques have not gained enthusiastic support and have not been used as first-line therapy in many tumors; rather, they are employed after failure of other treatments and to test new drug regimens.

Embolization. Embolization involves the deliberate occlusion of the arterial supply to the tumor to create ischemia and tumor necrosis and to arrest tumor growth by intra-arterial delivery of particulate materials, sclerosing solutions, and substances introduced in a liquid state that eventually solidify or precipitate. Agents that allow peripheral (small-vessel) embolization are preferred over materials used to occlude the larger central vessels.

A central (proximal) occlusion of a vessel near its origin has an effect similar to a surgical ligation, with immediate formation of collateral circulation. The more proximal the occlusion, the more abundant is the development of collateral circulation. Proximal embolizations are not, however, the best approach for intra-arterial therapy to treat neoplasms directly, because this approach ultimately restricts the ability to re-treat the neoplasm from the same artery and requires pursuit of the technically challenging collaterals for further therapy. For the treatment of patients with bleeding (e.g., ulcer, diverticulum, trauma), the central embolic approach is desirable to sufficiently reduce the arterial pressure at the bleeding site until hemostasis can be achieved. The development of collateral arterial supply subsequent to the embolization is an added benefit in this particular application. The use of peripheral embolic agents would increase the risk of undesired tissue necrosis. Proximal embolizations can also be used to redistribute flow from one vessel to another, as described in the previous section.

The more peripheral the embolization is to the tumor, the less the opportunity for collateral circulation and the greater the likelihood of tumor necrosis. Although tumor necrosis is a desired effect, necrosis of adjacent nontarget tissue is not. Microcatheter coaxial systems allow subselective embolizations to access tumor vessels and avoid embolization of nontarget tissues. Peripheral embolization produces small-vessel occlusion without sacrificing the main arteries, allowing future re-embolization when necessary.

At the M. D. Anderson, peripheral embolization is usually achieved by introducing absorbable gelatin sponge particles (Gelfoam powder) or polyvinyl alcohol foam (Ivalon). Ivalon is an inert material with particles that range from 100 to 1000 µm in diameter and can be injected through 2F or 3F coaxial micro-catheter systems. The particles physically occlude the vessel and produce an inflammatory response, with fibroblast invasion and thrombus formation. Recanalization of the occluded vessel can occur with time. Ivalon is supplied in a dry form and requires suspension with dilute contrast material. Frequent agitation via a three-way stopcock and two syringes is needed before delivery to avoid clumping and premature catheter occlusion.

Gelfoam is an absorbable gelatin sponge that is available in sheet or powder form. Gelfoam powder particles range from 40 to 60 µm in diameter and produce embolization at the capillary level. Gelfoam sheet can be cut into cubes or "torpedoes" and used for embolization of larger vessels. Gelfoam embolization is temporary, with maximum local reaction within the first 2 weeks and recanalization in 1 to 2 months. Central occlusions are accomplished by delivering large absorbable gelatin sponge segments or stainless steel coils.

The indications for transcatheter embolization of neoplasms are (1) to control hemorrhage; (2) pre-operatively, to facilitate surgical resection by decreasing blood loss and operating time; (3) to inhibit tumor growth; and (4) to relieve pain by decreasing tumor bulk.

The complications that arise from embolization can be related to the catheterization (e.g., pseudoaneurysm, arteriovenous fistula, dissection, thrombosis, perforation) or to occlusion effects on tumor or nontarget arterial supply (e.g., pain, ischemia/infarction, abscess). In a series by Hemingway and Allison[43] representing a 10-year experience with 284 patients undergoing 410 embolizations, minor complications occurred in 16% of patients, serious complications in 6.6%, and death in 2%. The postembolization syndrome (i.e., fever, elevated white blood cell count, and discomfort) was encountered after 42.7% of the procedures. The underlying abnormality and its location usually determined the nature and risk of complications.

Carcinoma of the uterine cervix. The vast majority of transarterial interventions in women with uterine pathology relate to leiomyomata of the uterus. Pelvic malignancy accounts for only a fraction of all transarterial interventions, the majority involving embolization for hemorrhage.

At M. D. Anderson, patients with stage III or IV disease were treated with bilateral intra-arterial infusion of mitomycin C (10 mg/m^2 over 24 hours every other course) and bleomycin (20 to 40 mg/m^2 over 24 hours) and cisplasin (100 mg/m^2 over 2 hours every course) in the internal iliac arteries, while vincristine (2-mg bolus) was given intravenously. After three cycles spaced 3 to 4 weeks apart, the patients were evaluated for further definitive radiation therapy. Of the 44 patients who had received no prior therapy before intra-arterial chemotherapy was initiated, 35 (76%) responded to the regimen; 24 (52%) had a partial response, and 11 (24%) had a complete response. The 5-year survival rate for the study group was 30%, with a median survival duration of 18 months.

Nagata and coworkers[44] reported on 68 patients with stage I through IV carcinoma of the uterine cervix who received infusion of both internal iliac arteries with cisplatin (60 to 70 mg/m^2), doxorubicin (30 to 40 mg/m^2), mitomycin C (15 mg/m^2) and 5-fluorouracil (500 mg) at 2 to 3 mL/sec over 15 to 20 minutes. Fifty-eight (85%) of the 68 patients underwent subsequent radical hysterectomy, and 32 of these 58 patients received postoperative radiotherapy. Complete responses were noted in 10 (28%) of 36 patients with squamous cell carcinoma and in 1 of 22 patients with adenocarcinoma. The overall 5-year survival rates for stages I, II, and III were 92.3%, 62.2%, and 71%, respectively; the rates for those who underwent surgery were 100%, 66.3%, and 71.5%, respectively. Complications included leukopenia (75%), thrombocytopenia (79%), and ileus.[44]

Yamada and colleagues[45] reported their experience with unilateral continuous infusion of cisplatin (12.5 mg/day) via an implanted vascular access device. The infusion catheter was placed in the side of tumor dominance in 16 of 22 patients. The superior and inferior gluteal arteries as well as the contralateral uterine artery were also embolized to maximize the concentration of cisplatin at the target lesion. Scintigraphy was performed through the access device after implantation to assess the distribution of chemotherapy. The overall objective response rate of 22 patients was 73%.

Onishi and associates[46] evaluated 33 patients who underwent intra-arterial cisplatin infusion therapy and radiation therapy ($n = 18$) or radiation therapy alone ($n = 15$). They also compared different methods of cisplatin delivery. Eight patients received two one-shot infusions of cisplatin (100 mg/m²) at intervals of 2 to 3 weeks. Four patients received weekly infusions of carboplatin (100 mg/m² × 5 to 6 weeks) and daily injections of cisplatin (10 mg × 21 days) delivered via an implanted reservoir. The local complete response rates were 94% for the group receiving intra-arterial chemotherapy and radiation therapy and 67% for the radiation-only group. No significant differences in local response were detected for the three different delivery systems used. The 2- and 5-year overall survival rates did not differ significantly between the two groups: 54.5% and 44.4% for those receiving chemotherapy and radiation therapy versus 74.5% and 50% for those receiving radiation therapy only. Complications were more severe in the former group, contributing to the poorer performance status and poorer prognosis.[46]

Uterine leiomyomata. Selective transcatheter bilateral uterine artery embolization (UAE) has emerged as a viable nonoperative alternative to myomectomy and hysterectomy for the treatment of uterine leiomyomata (fibroids). Uterine leiomyoma is the most common benign tumor of the female genital tract, with a prevalence ranging from 20% to 77% of premenopausal women.[47] Factors associated with an increased frequency of fibroids include ethnicity (African and African-American women), family history of fibroids, nulliparity, and obesity.[47] Presenting symptoms can include menorrhagia, frequency of urination, problems with defecation, sexual dysfunction, or pain. Embolization produces infarction of the fibroids with subsequent hyaline degeneration, resulting in reduction in tumor size as well as decreased menstrual blood flow and relief of bulk-related symptoms. Bilateral embolization is important, because unilateral therapy is inadequate.[48,49]

UAE procedures are typically performed from a single femoral access site using 4F to 5F angiographic catheters. Bilateral femoral arterial access or coaxial 3F microcatheter techniques can be used in difficult circumstances. Polyvinyl alcohol particles ranging from 300 to 700 μm in diameter is the most commonly used embolic agent. The average procedure time ranges between 40 and 120 minutes, and patients typically develop pain subsequent to embolization that often requires narcotic analgesia. The postembolization hospital stay varies from several hours (for outpatient regimens) to 48 hours.

The reported technical procedural success rates with bilateral UAE exceed 96%.[48,50,51] Objective measures of response include shrinkage of fibroids and reduction in overall uterine volume, which can be assessed by physical examination, ultrasonography, or MRI. The average fibroid shrinkage or decrease in uterine volume has ranged from 40% to 69%.[49,52,53] Failure to achieve these responses has been noted in the presence of adenomyosis[54] or sarcomatous change. Improvement of symptoms associated with bleeding has been reported in more than 89% of patients.[50-52]

Complications of UAE can include (1) procedural complications involving the groin or pelvic/uterine arteries, (2) fibroid expulsion, (3) pain, (4) amenorrhea and ovarian compromise, and (5) sepsis. Spontaneous expulsion occurs in 4% to 10% of patients and is most often associated with submucosal or pedunculated intracavitary fibroids.[53,55-57] Shedding of a large fibroid can result in significant pain and may not be complete, requiring surgical intervention. Pain after embolization is variable and occurs subsequent to occlusion of the second uterine artery. Intra-arterial lidocaine has been used to reduce postprocedure pain without convincing benefit.[58] Regimens for pain management can include nonsteroidal anti-inflammatory medications or narcotics in addition to antiemetics to control the associated nausea. Reported rates of postembolization amenorrhea range from 3.5% to 7.4%.[59] Low-grade fever and nausea are common in the early postprocedure period. Pyrexia greater than 38.5° C, abdominal pain, or purulent discharge warrants readmission and antibiotic treatment. Sepsis is exceedingly rare: one death has been reported within 2 weeks after the procedure.[60] In a review by Lund and associates,[61] three patients (1%) required emergency hysterectomy secondary to ischemic necrosis and sepsis. The use of prophylactic antibiotics varies but has not yet been shown to add any significant benefit.

Vulvar cancer. In the United States, vulvar cancer accounts for 4% of cancers in the female reproductive organs and 0.6% of all cancers in women. The American Cancer Society estimated that in the year 2002, about 3800 cancers of the vulva would be diagnosed in the United States and about 800 deaths due to vulvar cancer would occur.

More than 90% of the cancers of the vulva are squamous cell cancers. This type of cancer usually forms slowly over many years and is usually preceded by precancerous changes that may last for several years. If vulvar cancer is detected early, it is highly curable. The overall 5-year survival rate if the lymph nodes are not involved is 90%; the rate declines to 20% to 55% if the cancer has metastasized to the lymph nodes. The second most common type of vulvar cancer (about 4%) is melanoma. About 5% to 8% of melanomas in women occur on the vulva, usually on the labia minora and clitoris. Adenocarcinomas, Paget's disease, and sarcoma are most unusual but do occur in the vulva.

At M. D. Anderson, our experience with percutaneous intra-arterial transcatheter chemotherapy in patients with recurrent carcinoma of the vulva and penis is limited. Therapy was usually delivered through the internal pudendal branch of the internal iliac artery, the external pudendal branch of the external iliac artery, or the external pudendal branch of the deep femoral artery. The chemotherapy regimen consisted of mitomycin C (10 mg/m² over 24 hours), bleomycin (20 to 40 mg/m² over 24 hours), and cisplatin (100 mg/m² over 2 hours). Although the number of patients treated with this regimen is too small for analysis, dramatic responses were observed in several patients.

Genitourinary hemorrhage. Hemorrhage from genitourinary neoplasms has been treated successfully in patients with neoplasms of the bladder, uterine cervix, and corpus, as has bleeding caused by irradiation cystitis.[62] Pelage and colleagues[63] reported the distribution of uterine pathology in 197 women who underwent embolization: leiomyoma (67.5%), primary and secondary postpartum hemorrhage (25%), postabortion hemorrhage (2.5%), postoperative hemorrhage (1%), adenomyosis (1.5%), uterine malformation (0.5%), and pelvic malignancy (2%).[63]

Chronic low-grade bleeding from a neoplasm may be managed by intra-arterial infusion of chemotherapy directly to the tumor. Embolization can be beneficial in the treatment of gynecologic neoplasms, but its effect may be only temporary (Fig. 69-3). In a series of 13 patients, Kramer and colleagues[64] reported their experience with embolization for hemorrhage in advanced cervical carcinoma. In 9 (69%) of 13 patients, the bleeding was controlled immediately with a single bilateral embolization treatment. One patient (7.7%) died during therapy secondary to uncontrolled bleeding. The remaining three patients (23%) showed slight persistent or recurrent bleeding that was controlled on follow-up intervention.

Iatrogenic bleeding within the pelvis can also be managed by endovascular techniques. Severe hemorrhagic cystitis is estimated to occur in fewer than 5% of patients after radiotherapy to the pelvis. Bilateral internal iliac embolization,[62] in addition to simple bladder irrigation; cystodiathermy; oral, parenteral, and intravesical agents; hyperbaric oxygen therapy; hydrodistention; urinary diversion; and cystectomy have been employed to control hemorrhage.[65] Bleeding secondary to a ureteroarterial fistula (Fig. 69-4) can occur in the presence of long-term ureterostomy diversion if the catheters erode into the adjacent iliac artery.[66-68] Percutaneous management originally involved embolization of the affected iliac artery to control bleeding, followed by extra-anatomic arterial bypass.[66,68] More recently, covered stents have been used to exclude the fistula while maintaining patency of the involved iliac artery.[67]

What are venous interventions and how do they affect patients with gynecologic neoplasms?

Before 1982, venous procedures predominantly involved ascending lower-extremity venography for the diagnosis of deep venous thrombosis (DVT) and pulmonary angiography for the diagnosis of pulmonary embolism. Since then, color flow Doppler imaging has supplanted diagnostic venography in the workup for DVT. Aside from the placement of central venous catheters, the current most common venous intervention is insertion of an inferior vena cava (IVC) filter for the prevention of new or recurrent pulmonary emboli. The majority of venous interventions use techniques that have been adapted from interventions in the arterial system. Venous thrombolysis, angioplasty, and stent placement are now used to treat stenoses and occlusions found in superior vena cava syndrome, Budd-Chiari syndrome, and hemodialysis access failure. Transjugular intrahepatic portosystemic shunt (TIPS) placement is a more recent venous intervention that involves creation of a percutaneous portosystemic shunt between the portal vein and the hepatic vein through the parenchyma of the liver to treat the complications of portal hypertension. Embolization techniques have also been applied in the venous system to occlude gastroesophageal varices as an adjunct to TIPS and to treat gonadal varicosities in the management of infertility in men and pelvic congestion syndrome in women.

Vena cava filters. Venous thromboembolic disease is a substantial health problem in the United States; the most lethal form, pulmonary embolus, is diagnosed in 355,000 patients per year.[69] Patients with malignancy are at greater risk for thromboembolic events than the general population. Anticoagulation remains the therapy of choice, with an expected risk for major hemorrhage of less than 5% in patients with no underlying sources of known active or potential bleeding.[70] In this subset of patients, IVC filters are an effective method of reducing the risk of life-threatening pulmonary embolus in those with a contraindication to anticoagulation and those who experience pulmonary embolism despite adequate anticoagulation. Other common indications for filter placement are listed in Box 69-1.

The majority of IVC filters are placed by an interventional radiologist under fluoroscopic guidance. Since development of the Greenfield filter in 1972, nine filters have been approved by the U.S. Food and Drug Administration and are available for use in the United States (Table 69-1). The delivery system of the initial version of the Greenfield filter was 29.5F in outer diameter; newer versions are delivered through a 14F system. Many of the delivery systems of the more recent filters range in outer diameter from 8F to 14F and can be placed from a femoral, jugular, or antecubital vein approach. The majority of the available filters are constructed of nonferromagnetic material and are considered safe for MRI imaging. Only the stainless steel Greenfield filter and the Bird's Nest filter are constructed of stainless steel and produce substantial MRI artifact. MRI can be performed safely in patients with these types of filters, but a delay of up to 6 weeks from implantation to imaging has been recommended by the manufacturer of the Bird's Nest filter.

In ex vivo tests, Katsamouris and associates[71] demonstrated that the Bird's Nest filter and the Simon Nitinol filter were the most efficient. Hammer and colleagues[72] concluded that the Bird's Nest filter had the highest clot-trapping capacity. The reported rates

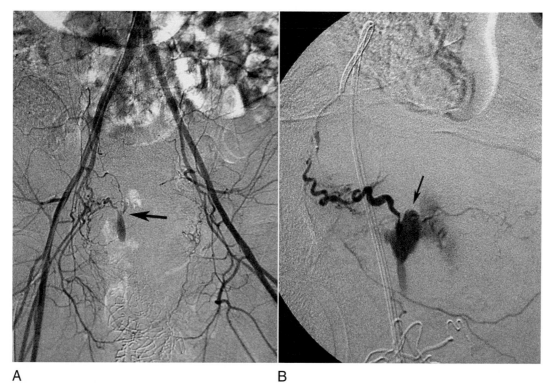

A

B

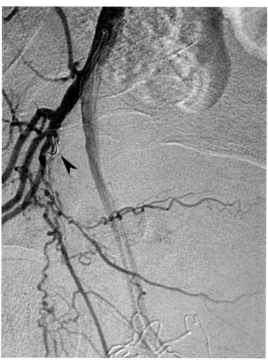

C

Figure 69–3. A, Digital subtraction pelvic angiogram demonstrating contrast extravasation *(arrow)* consistent with hemorrhage in a patient with cervical cancer and uncontrolled vaginal bleeding. **B,** A selective right uterine artery angiogram better demonstrates the site of hemorrhage *(arrow).* **C,** Right internal iliac angiogram after coil embolization *(arrowhead)* of the right uterine artery demonstrates no further angiographic evidence of hemorrhage.

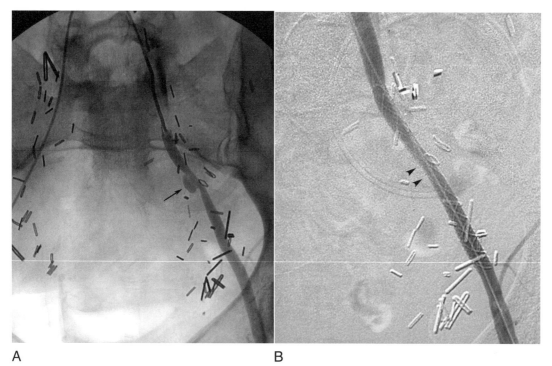

A   B

Figure 69–4. A, Pelvic angiogram of a patient with cervical cancer who had a history of surgery and radiation and presented with gross hematuria. Note the left iliac artery pseudoaneurysm *(arrow)* at the site of a fistula between the iliac artery and the left ureter. **B,** Angiogram taken after insertion of a covered stent reveals complete exclusion of the pseudoaneurysm *(arrowheads)* with the integrity of the iliac artery maintained.

Box 69–1

1. Absolute contraindication to anticoagulation
   A. Known recent hemorrhage: central nervous system, gastrointestinal, pulmonary, retroperitoneal
   B. Central nervous system neoplasm, aneurysm, or vascular malformation
   C. Heparin-associated thrombocythemia thrombosis syndrome
   D. Thrombocytopenia (<50,000/μL)
   E. Recent major trauma or surgery
2. Bleeding complication on anticoagulation
3. Failure of adequate anticoagulation

of clinically relevant postfilter pulmonary embolism range from 3.3% to 5.6%,[73-75] and almost and up to 2.5% of patients with filters overall are fatal.[73,74] To date, no randomized clinical trials have stratified patients with associated risk factors and those receiving concomitant anticoagulation therapy to adequately compare the various filter designs with respect to recurrence of pulmonary embolus and other complications such as caval or access site thrombosis. IVC thrombosis can be caused by thrombus formation on the filter itself, but it is more likely to be the result of an entrapped thrombus that has embolized from the pelvis or lower extremities. The rate of caval thrombosis varies dramatically depending on the diligence of the follow-up and the definition. In several large series using multiple filter designs, the thrombosis rate ranged from 2.7% to 19%.[73,74]

Table 69–1. Inferior Vena Cava Filters Approved by the U. S. Food and Drug Administration

Filter	Manufacturer	Year Approved
Stainless Steel Greenfield—Original	Boston Scientific—Medi Tech	1973
Titanium Greenfield	Boston Scientific—Medi Tech	1989
Stainless Steel Greenfield—Low Profile	Boston Scientific—Medi Tech	1995
Bird's Nest	Cook	1983
Simon Nitinol	Bard	1988
Vena Tech	B Braun	1989
Vena Tech—Low Profile	B Braun	2001
Trapease	Cordis	2000
Gunther Tulip	Cook	2001

REFERENCES

1. al-Mofleh IA: Ultrasound-guided fine needle aspiration of retroperitoneal, abdominal and pelvic lymph nodes: Diagnostic reliability. Acta Cytol 1992;36:413-415.
2. Buscarini L, Cavanna L: Ultrasound and ultrasonically guided biopsy in oncohematology. Haematologica 1991;76:53-64.
3. Nagano T, Nakai Y, Taniguchi F, et al: Diagnosis of paraaortic and pelvic lymph node metastasis of gynecologic malignant tumors by ultrasound-guided percutaneous fine-needle aspiration biopsy. Cancer 1991;68:2571-2574.
4. Tikkakoski T, Siniluoto T, Ollikainen A, et al: Ultrasound-guided aspiration cytology of enlarged lymph nodes. Acta Radiol 1991;32:53-56.
5. Kohler MF, Berchuck A, Baker ME, et al: Computed tomography-guided fine-needle aspiration of retroperitoneal lymph nodes in gynecologic oncology. Obstet Gynecol 1990;76:612-616.
6. Van Poppel H, Ameye F, Oyen R, et al: Accuracy of combined computerized tomography and fine needle aspiration cytology in lymph node staging of localized prostatic carcinoma. J Urol 1994;151:1310-1314.
7. Welch TJ, Sheedy PF 2nd, Johnson CD, et al: CT-guided biopsy: Prospective analysis of 1,000 procedures. Radiology 1989; 171:493-496.
8. O'Neill MJ, Rafferty EA, Lee SI, et al: Transvaginal interventional procedures: Aspiration, biopsy, and catheter drainage. Radiographics 2001;21:657-672.
9. Zanetta G, Brenna A, Pittelli M, et al: Transvaginal ultrasound-guided fine needle sampling of deep cancer recurrences in the pelvis: Usefulness and limitations. Gynecol Oncol 1994;54:59-63.
10. Memel DS, Dodd GD 3rd, Esola CC: Efficacy of sonography as a guidance technique for biopsy of abdominal, pelvic, and retroperitoneal lymph nodes. AJR Am J Roentgenol 1996;167: 957-962.
11. Fisher AJ, Paulson EK, Sheafor DH, et al: Small lymph nodes of the abdomen, pelvis, and retroperitoneum: Usefulness of sonographically guided biopsy. Radiology 1997;205:185-190.
12. Gupta S, Rajak CL, Sood BP, et al: Sonographically guided fine needle aspiration biopsy of abdominal lymph nodes: Experience in 102 patients. J Ultrasound Med 1999;18:135-139.
13. Nolsoe C, Nielsen L, Torp-Pedersen S, Holm HH: Major complications and deaths due to interventional ultrasonography: A review of 8000 cases. J Clin Ultrasound 1990;18:179-184.
14. de Gregorio Ariza MA, Alfonso Aguiran ER, et al: Transthoracic aspiration biopsy of pulmonary and mediastinal lesions. Eur J Radiol 1991;12:98-103.
15. Westcott JL: Direct percutaneous needle aspiration of localized pulmonary lesions: Result in 422 patients. Radiology 1980;137: 31-35.
16. Swischuk JL, Castaneda F, Patel JC, et al: Percutaneous transthoracic needle biopsy of the lung: Review of 612 lesions. J Vasc Interv Radiol 1998;9:347-352.
17. Laurent F, Latrabe V, Vergier B, et al: CT-guided transthoracic needle biopsy of pulmonary nodules smaller than 20 mm: Results with an automated 20-gauge coaxial cutting needle. Clin Radiol 2000;55:281-287.
18. Klein JS, Salomon G, Stewart EA: Transthoracic needle biopsy with a coaxially placed 20-gauge automated cutting needle: Results in 122 patients. Radiology 1996;198:715-720.
19. Tsukada H, Satou T, Iwashima A, Souma T: Diagnostic accuracy of CT-guided automated needle biopsy of lung nodules. AJR Am J Roentgenol 2000;175:239-243.
20. vanSonnenberg E, Casola G, Ho M, et al: Difficult thoracic lesions: CT-guided biopsy experience in 150 cases. Radiology 1988;167:457-461.
21. Tomiyama N, Mihara N, Maeda M, et al: CT-guided needle biopsy of small pulmonary nodules: Value of respiratory gating. Radiology 2000;217:907-910.
22. Yankelevitz DF, Henschke CI, Koizumi JH, et al: CT-guided transthoracic needle biopsy of small solitary pulmonary nodules. Clin Imaging 1997;21:107-110.
23. Altemeier WA, Culbertson WR, Fullen WD, Shook CD: Intra-abdominal abscesses. Am J Surg 1973;125:70-79.
24. vanSonnenberg E, Mueller PR, Ferrucci JT Jr: Percutaneous drainage of 250 abdominal abscesses and fluid collections.

Part I. Results, failures, and complications. Radiology 1984;151: 337-341.
25. Hovsepian DM: Transrectal and transvaginal abscess drainage. J Vasc Interv Radiol 1997;8:501-515.
26. vanSonnenberg E, Wittich GR, Goodacre BW, et al: Percutaneous abscess drainage: Update. World J Surg 2001;25:362-369, discussion 370-372.
27. Farrell TA, Wallace M, Hicks ME: Long-term results of transrenal ureteral occlusion with use of Gianturco coils and gelatin sponge pledgets. J Vasc Interv Radiol 1997;8:449-452.
28. Zagoria RJ, Hodge RG, Dyer RB, Routh WD: Percutaneous nephrostomy for treatment of intractable hemorrhagic cystitis. J Urol 1993;149:1449-1451.
29. Ramchandani P, Cardella JF, Grassi CJ, et al: Quality improvement guidelines for percutaneous nephrostomy. J Vasc Interv Radiol 2001;12:1247-1251.
30. Farrell TA, Hicks ME: A review of radiologically guided percutaneous nephrostomies in 303 patients. J Vasc Interv Radiol 1997;8:769-774.
31. Lee WJ, Patel U, Patel S, Pillari GP: Emergency percutaneous nephrostomy: Results and complications. J Vasc Interv Radiol 1994;5:135-139.
32. Seymour H, Patel U: Ureteric stenting: Current status. Semin Interv Radiol 2000;17:351-365.
33. Cardella JF, Castaneda-Zuniga WR, Hunter DW, et al: Urine-compatible polymer for long-term ureteral stenting. Radiology 1986;161:313-318.
34. Lugmayr HF, Pauer W: Wallstents for the treatment of extrinsic malignant ureteral obstruction: Midterm results. Radiology 1996;198:105-108.
35. Ponsky JL, Gauderer MW, Stellato TA: Percutaneous endoscopic gastrostomy: Review of 150 cases. Arch Surg 1983;118:913-914.
36. Preshaw RM: A percutaneous method for inserting a feeding gastrostomy tube. Surg Gynecol Obstet 1981;152:658-660.
37. Beaver ME, Myers JN, Griffenberg L, Waugh K: Percutaneous fluoroscopic gastrostomy tube placement in patients with head and neck cancer. Arch Otolaryngol Head Neck Surg 1998;124: 1141-1144.
38. Hicks ME, Surratt RS, Picus D, et al: Fluoroscopically guided percutaneous gastrostomy and gastroenterostomy: Analysis of 158 consecutive cases. AJR Am J Roentgenol 1990;154:725-728.
39. Ho CS, Gray RR, Goldfinger M, et al: Percutaneous gastrostomy for enteral feeding. Radiology 1985;156:349-351.
40. Wills JS, Oglesby JT: Percutaneous gastrostomy. Radiology 1983;149:449-453.
41. Mauro MA, Koehler RE, Baron TH: Advances in gastrointestinal intervention: The treatment of gastroduodenal and colorectal obstructions with metallic stents. Radiology 2000;215:659-669.
42. Charnsangavej C, Wallace S: Interventional radiologic techniques in the diagnosis and treatment of hepatobiliary malignancy. In Wanebo H (ed): Surgery for Gastrointestinal Cancer: A Multidiciplinary Approach. Philadelphia, Lippincott-Raven, 1997, pp 597-606.
43. Hemingway AP, Allison DJ: Complications of embolization: Analysis of 410 procedures. Radiology 1988;166:669-672.
44. Nagata Y, Okajima K, Kokubo M, et al: Clinical results of transcatheter arterial infusion for uterine cervical cancer. Am J Clin Oncol 1999;22:97-102.
45. Yamada T, Ohsugi F, Irie T, et al: Extended intraarterial cisplatin infusion for treatment of gynecologic cancer after alteration of intrapelvic blood flow and implantation of a vascular access device. Cardiovasc Intervent Radiol 1996;19:139-145.
46. Onishi H, Yamaguchi M, Kuriyama K, et al: Effect of concurrent intra-arterial infusion of platinum drugs for patients with stage III or IV uterine cervical cancer treated with radical radiation therapy. Cancer J Sci Am 2000;6:40-45.
47. Vollenhoven B: Introduction: The epidemiology of uterine leiomyomas. Baillieres Clin Obstet Gynaecol 1998;12:169-176.
48. Worthington-Kirsch RL, Popky GL, Hutchins FL Jr: Uterine arterial embolization for the management of leiomyomas: Quality-of-life assessment and clinical response. Radiology 1998;208:625-629.
49. Goodwin SC, Vedantham S, McLucas B, et al: Preliminary experience with uterine artery embolization for uterine fibroids. J Vasc Interv Radiol 1997;8:517-526.

50. Spies JB, Scialli AR, Jha RC, et al: Initial results from uterine fibroid embolization for symptomatic leiomyomata. J Vasc Interv Radiol 1999;10:1149-1157.

51. Goodwin SC, McLucas B, Lee M, et al: Uterine artery embolization for the treatment of uterine leiomyomata midterm results. J Vasc Interv Radiol 1999;10:1159-1165.

52. Ravina JH, Bouret JM, Ciraru-Vigneron N, et al: [Recourse to particular arterial embolization in the treatment of some uterine leiomyoma]. Bull Acad Natl Med 1997;181:233-243, discussion 244-246.

53. Bradley EA, Reidy JF, Forman RG, et al: Transcatheter uterine artery embolisation to treat large uterine fibroids. Br J Obstet Gynaecol 1998;105:235-240.

54. Smith SJ, Sewall LE, Handelsman A: A clinical failure of uterine fibroid embolization due to adenomyosis. J Vasc Interv Radiol 1999;10:1171-1174.

55. Berkowitz RP, Hutchins FL Jr, Worthington-Kirsch RL: Vaginal expulsion of submucosal fibroids after uterine artery embolization: A report of three cases. J Reprod Med 1999;44:373-376.

56. Worthington-Kirsch RL: Flow redistribution during uterine artery embolization for the management of symptomatic fibroids. J Vasc Interv Radiol 1999;10:237-238.

57. Worthington-Kirsch RL, Hutchins FL Jr, Berkowitz RP: Regarding sloughing of fibroids after uterine artery embolization. J Vasc Interv Radiol 1999;10:1135.

58. Goodwin SC, Walker WJ: Uterine artery embolization for the treatment of uterine fibroids. Curr Opin Obstet Gynecol 1998; 10:315-320.

59. Braude P, Reidy J, Nott V, et al: Embolization of uterine leiomyomata: Current concepts in management. Hum Reprod Update 2000;6:603-608.

60. Vashisht A, Studd J, Carey A, Burn P: Fatal septicaemia after fibroid embolisation. Lancet 1999;354:307-308.

61. Lund N, Justesen P, Elle B, et al: Fibroids treated by uterine artery embolization: A review. Acta Obstet Gynecol Scand 2000; 79:905-910.

62. Schwartz PE, Goldstein HM, Wallace S, Rutledge FN: Control of arterial hemorrhage using percutaneous arterial catheter techniques in patients with gynecologic malignancies. Gynecol Oncol 1975;3:276-288.

63. Pelage JP, Le Dref O, Soyer P, et al: Arterial anatomy of the female genital tract: Variations and relevance to transcatheter embolization of the uterus. AJR Am J Roentgenol 1999;172: 989-994.

64. Kramer SC, Gorich J, Rilinger N, et al: [Interventional treatment of hemorrhages in advanced cervical carcinoma]. Radiologe 1999;39:795-798.

65. Crew JP, Jephcott CR, Reynard JM: Radiation-induced haemorrhagic cystitis. Eur Urol 2001;40:111-123.

66. Quillin SP, Darcy MD, Picus D: Angiographic evaluation and therapy of ureteroarterial fistulas. AJR Am J Roentgenol 1994;162:873-878.

67. Feuer DS, Ciocca RG, Nackman GB, et al: Endovascular management of ureteroarterial fistula. J Vasc Surg 1999;30:1146-1149.

68. Gheiler EL, Tefilli MV, Tiguert R, et al: Angiographic arterial occlusion and extra-anatomical vascular bypass for the management of a ureteral-iliac fistula: Case report and review of the literature. Urol Int 1998;61:62-66.

69. Bick RL: Hereditary and acquired thrombophilia. Part I. Preface. Semin Thromb Hemost 1999;25:251-253.

70. Levine MN, Raskob G, Landefeld S, Kearon C: Hemorrhagic complications of anticoagulant treatment. Chest 1998; 114(5 Suppl):511S-523S.

71. Katsamouris AA, Waltman AC, Delichatsios MA, Athanasoulis CA: Inferior vena cava filters: In vitro comparison of clot trapping and flow dynamics. Radiology 1988;166:361-366.

72. Hammer FD, Rousseau HP, Joffre FG, et al: In vitro evaluation of vena cava filters. J Vasc Interv Radiol 1994;5:869-876.

73. Athanasoulis CA, Kaufman JA, Halpern EF, et al: Inferior vena caval filters: Review of a 26-year single-center clinical experience. Radiology 2000;216:54-66.

74. Ferris EJ, McCowan TC, Carver DK, McFarland DR: Percutaneous inferior vena caval filters: Follow-up of seven designs in 320 patients. Radiology 1993;188:851-856.

75. Greenfield LJ, Proctor MC: Twenty-year clinical experience with the Greenfield filter. Cardiovasc Surg 1995;3:199-205.

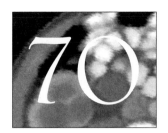
BIOLOGIC THERAPY
FOR GYNECOLOGIC
MALIGNANCIES

Samir N. Khleif

 MAJOR CONTROVERSIES

- **What is the best therapeutic strategy?**
- **What is the best trial design to test these strategies?**
- **What is the best population on which to test these biotherapy strategies?**
- **When may these strategies be taken into definitive phase III trials?**

Biologic therapy is considered the fourth modality of cancer treatment. It is a therapy that is geared toward the use of the patient's own biologic system or of natural biologic reagents to generate a rejection response against the malignant phenotype. This is a new area of cancer treatment, and it is gaining a large momentum because of the accelerated discoveries in both molecular biology and immunology of cancer.

There is no standard classification of biologic therapy. The term may be applied to many types of therapies that, in principle, affect the relationship between the biologic system of the patient and the malignant cell. These include, among others, bone marrow–enhancing reagents, hormone therapy, agents that affect tumor vascularization, and immunotherapy. The term immunotherapy is used interchangeably with biotherapy, and in this chapter the terms biotherapy and biologic therapy are used to describe immunotherapy for cancer.

This book has focused on controversies in standard therapy for gynecologic malignancies, including surgery, radiation therapy, and chemotherapy. The advances that have been made in these areas are noticeable, and the impact that they have exerted over the past decade has been significant. In contrast, biologic therapy for gynecologic malignancies is still in early development. Most of the approaches discussed

in this chapter are still in the investigational stage, and therefore the controversies presented are mainly controversies in the developmental process of this therapy.

The chapter reviews the basic principles of biologic therapy, the advances of the therapy in gynecologic malignancies, and current controversies in the development of such therapy. The controversies are presented as part of the discussion of each section, and they are summarized for the whole field at the end of the chapter.

The Immune System

The principal role of the immune system is to distinguish "self" from "foreign," providing the body with a defense mechanism against foreign antigens and harmful pathogen invaders. The ability to distinguish between self and foreign molecules is a learned process that leads in part to the development of tolerance to self-molecules and the generation of a specific immune response against foreign antigens.

There are two types of immunologic responses, both of which are employed by lymphocytes: (1) the humoral immune response, which is a B cell–dependent response, and (2) the cellular immune response, which is a T cell–dependent response.

Humoral immune response is antibody-dependent. Antibodies are released by B lymphocytes and are able to recognize extracellular domains of proteins that are expressed on the intact cell surface and antigens that reside in the extracellular space. The immunity mediated by antibodies is known as humoral immunity in reference to "humor" or body fluid, because antibodies are usually found in the body fluid components of the body. Among the various pathways by which antibodies exert their protective immune response against pathogens are neutralization and opsonization. Neutralization is the mechanism by which antibodies bind the pathogens, preventing their entrance into the target cells. This process is effective against organisms such as viral pathogens. Opsonization is the binding of antibodies to pathogens (e.g., bacteria) to make them recognizable by phagocytes for uptake and destruction. Other pathways that are relevant to tumor immunity are discussed separately with the specific antibodies.

Cell-mediated immune response is the function of T lymphocytes. This immune response recognizes antigens that are expressed intracellularly and are inaccessible to antibodies. The antigens that are recognized by the cell-mediated immune response are either foreign proteins that originate from intracellular organisms such as viruses, parasites, and some bacteria or altered native proteins. Lymphocytes are able to recognize antigens with a specific receptor on their surface, the T-cell receptor (TCR). TCR recognizes antigens that are presented on the surface of the target cells by the major histocompatibility complex (MHC).* The antigens are small peptides that are the result of endogenous protein processing (see later discussion). There are two types of T lymphocytes: CD4-positive T helper lymphocytes and CD8-positive cytotoxic T lymphocytes (CTLs). They are named according to the cluster determinant that they carry on their surface (4 and 8, respectively). The CD4+ cells are able to recognize peptide antigens that are presented in the context of MHC class II (MHC II), and CD8+ cells are programmed to recognize antigens displayed on MHC class I (MHC I). MHC I molecules are expressed on all nucleated cells, whereas MHC II molecules are expressed on professional antigen-presenting cells (APCs): dendritic cells (DCs), B cells, and macrophages. When activated, T-helper cells secrete cytokines, which can stimulate the growth and differentiation of B lymphocytes, activate macrophages, and induce the generation of CTLs. CTLs release mediators that can lyse or kill the target cells.

Antigen processing and presentation and T-Cell interaction. Antigens in nucleated cells are expressed on the cell surface for T cell recognition by a mechanism called antigen processing and presentation.[1] By this process, the proteins are converted into small peptides through a degradative mechanism that is ubiquitin-proteasome dependent. These peptides are then transferred to the cell surface in association with the MHC molecules.[2,3] With this process, intracellular antigens are presented at the surface of nucleated cells and become available to T lymphocytes.[4,5] This is an essential step for the interaction of the antigen with the TCR and further generation of immunologic response.[6]

Each of the two classes of MHC molecules is encoded by three genes that are all located on chromosome 6.[7] The three genes of MHC I are human leukocyte antigen (HLA) A, B, and C; the three genes of MHC II are HLA-DR, -DQ, and -DP. Both of these classes of molecules have a similar structure. This three-dimensional tertiary structure consists of two subunits that form a groove on their surface into which specific peptides can rest and be presented for recognition by a T cell.[8-11] The class I molecules are responsible for presenting peptides to CD8+ CTLs; they present antigens in the form of 8- to 12-amino-acid peptides. In general, these peptides are derived from endogenous native proteins that outlived their half-lives, proteins that originated from intracellular organisms such as viruses, or mutant or abnormally expressed proteins.[8,10] On the other hand, class II molecules, which are found on the surface of professional APCs, present antigens in the form of 12- to 25-amino-acid peptides. These antigens are derived from either proteins that originate from extracellular organisms or soluble proteins released from dying cells. The main role of these MHC II molecules is to display antigens to the CD4+ T-helper cells. When TCR binds to the peptides–MHC II complex, it activates the CD4+ cell, leading to the production of interleukin-2 (IL-2) and the activation of the IL-2 receptor gene. This, in turn, results in the activation of antigen-specific CTLs.[9,10,12,13]

The immunology of Cancer

The immune system is known to play a role in determining the natural history of cancer. This is evident from many anecdotal and systematic observations, including the following: (1) patients who are immune-suppressed after transplantation exhibit an increased incidence of malignancy[14-18]; (2) tumors are known to regress spontaneously[19-21]; and (3) biologic agents that work on modifying the immune response have been shown to be effective in treating tumors.[22-25] These observations indicate that tumors are potentially amenable for immune recognition; therefore, they are able to present antigens that are recognized by the immune cells. These antigens are called tumor-associated antigens (TAAs).

TTAs were described as early as the 1940s in studies which showed that mice could reject the transfer of live tumor cells that were induced by a specific carcinogen if they were immunized with the same syngeneic killed tumor.[26] These studies and others clearly indicated that tumors carry antigens that can generate a specific immune response which is capable of exerting protection against the growth of a tumor. These TAA usually reflect the new characteristics

---

*Historically, the term "MHC" has referred to the nomenclature of the mouse complexes, whereas the human counterpart has been referred to as human leukocyte antigens (HLA); however, the term "human MHC" is now acceptable as a general label.

acquired by the malignant cells, whether genetic or resultant phenotype. These new characteristics result from the accumulation of multiple genetic changes that are either spontaneous or acquired through oncogenic pathogens. These genetic events result in altered molecules or the acquisition of new molecules in cancer cells, which are processed and presented as outlined previously. These genetic events make the transformed cells express a novel antigenic profile, which is potentially perceived by the immune system as novel.[27,28] Classes of identified TAAs are discussed in the next segment.

Tumor-associated antigens. The TAAs are at the center of the development of biotherapy. In recent years, many human TAAs have been identified. This has led to the development of more specific and targeted cancer therapies, some of which are discussed later in this chapter.

TAA are grouped into two separate classes, which reflect their origin. The first class of TAA is called "self-antigens." This is composed of a group of antigens that have been generated from native molecules and maintain their native amino acid sequence. The second class of TAA is "non–self-antigens." This group includes antigens that are acquired by the tumor cells from exogenous sources, such as oncogenic viruses or parasites, or from native proteins that underwent molecular alterations leading to the production of novel amino acid sequences.

Self-antigens. Self-antigens are the product of alterations in tumor cells that contributed to or resulted from the transformation process while maintaining the original sequence of the protein. Alterations include activation of a silent gene or overexpression of a gene. Activation of a silent gene leads to the production of a protein in tumor cells that may not have been previously recognized as self and therefore could be antigenic for the naive immune system. An example of such an antigen is MAGE1 in melanoma.[29] Also in this category is the activation of genes that encode oncofetal antigens. Carcinoembryonic antigen (CEA) is the best characterized of this type of antigen.[30] Gene overexpression leads to higher expression of certain proteins in the tumor cell. This higher expression could overcome immune tolerance produced by a low level of protein expression in normal tissue. Antigens that result from this mechanism may be oncogenic (e.g., HER2/NEU) or non-oncogenic (e.g., the melanoma antigens MART1, gp100, and tyrosinase[31]).

Non–self-antigens. The first group of non–self-antigens are the products of organisms such as tumor viruses.[32-34] These microorganisms are RNA and DNA viruses implicated in the development of some human cancers. These viruses usually integrate their DNA into the genome of human cells, resulting in the expression of foreign proteins that form potential TAAs. The human papillomavirus (HPV), Epstein-Barr virus (EBV), hepatitis B virus (HBV), and hepatitis C virus (HCV) are known examples of the oncogenic viruses.

The second group of non–self-antigens are the products of genetic mutations that have led to the development of altered novel peptides, thereby acting as tumor antigens. This may occur as the result of a point mutation or translocation. Examples of such mutated genes include the oncogene *RAS* and the tumor suppressor gene *TP53*, both of which can acquire point mutations in human cancers (20% and 50%, respectively, for all solid tumors). T-cell responses specific for mutated *RAS* proteins and P53 proteins have been demonstrated both in mice and humans.[35-37] Bcr/Abl is an example of translocation that results in a TAA.[38-40]

TYPES OF BIOLOGIC THERAPIES

Biologic therapy for cancer can be divided into two types: humoral-based biotherapy, which is based on the active administration of specific antibodies, and cellular-based biotherapy, which is dependent on the generation of a cellular immune response against tumor targets. Each of these types of therapies can be either a defined-antigen–directed or a non–defined-antigen–directed therapy.

Defined-antigen–directed therapy is designed to specifically target a known antigen. Such therapies include monoclonal antibodies, defined-antigen–directed vaccines (DAV), and specific-antigen–activated lymphocytes. Non–defined-antigen–directed therapy is designed to enhance the immune response against a cluster of unidentified antigens, or nonspecifically against the tumor. Such therapies include non–defined-antigen–directed vaccines (NDAV), adoptive nonspecific immunotherapy, and cytokine therapy.

For the purpose of simplicity and because this chapter discusses biologic therapy for gynecologic malignancies, the discussion is limited to biotherapies that have been developed or are in the process of development for gynecologic malignancies, namely monoclonal antibodies (MoAb), vaccines, and cytokine therapy.

Monoclonal Antibodies

MoAb are biologic agents that are designed to target the extracellular domain of specific molecules expressed on the cell membrane or molecules that reside in the extracellular space. MoAb exert their antitumor effect through many mechanisms, including (1) blocking the targeted receptor and preventing its function in transmitting proliferative signals to the nucleus, (2) activating antibody-dependent cellular cytotoxicity (ADCC), and (3) internalizing the receptor and hence delivering toxic agents into the cells. MoAb technology has been very much improved in the past decade through the "humanization" of these biologic agents. Substituting the Fc murine portion of the molecule for the human equivalent leads to a significant decrease in the ability to generate human anti-mouse antibody (HAMA). This processing has made these biologic agents more usable to treat cancer patients. In general, MoAb are used either directly as therapeutic agents or as a delivery system for cellular toxins, radionuclides, or chemotherapeutic agents.

Cytokine Therapy

Cytokines are soluble proteins that have a hormone-like action and exhibit their effect on the immune system through regulation of other cells. They are glycoproteins with molecular weights that range between 15 and 40 kd. They are produced either by lymphocytes (lymphokines) or by monocytes (monokines). Currently, cytokines include interleukins ("between leukocytes"), of which there are 18 types (IL-1 through IL-18); interferons (IFN-α, IFN-β, and IFN-γ); tumor necrosis factor (TNF); and growth factors.[41] For a review, see *Principles and Practice of Biologic Therapy of Cancer*, edited by S. A. Rosenberg.

Cancer Vaccines

Cancer vaccinations aim to actively stimulate the immune system to generate a specific response against antigens that are expressed by malignant or premalignant cells. Cancer vaccines are used either as therapeutic agents in patients with established disease or as preventive therapy with the intent to prevent or eliminate an infection with a tumor-inducing pathogen, prevent the progression of a precancerous lesion to an invasive tumor, or prevent the recurrence of a completely regressed tumor.[42]

Vaccines can be designed to induce either humoral or cellular responses. Vaccines that produce humoral immune responses are usually most effective against extracellular organisms and pathogens and are more often used as cancer prevention vaccines. Vaccines that produce a cellular response generate specific T lymphocytes that are capable of recognizing cell-surface antigens produced by either intracellular pathogens or endogenous altered genes. These vaccines could be used for either preventive or therapeutic purposes.[42] Some investigators are developing humoral vaccines with therapeutic intent; these vaccines are directed against antigens such as Lewis y protein in ovarian cancer.[43,44]

Types of cancer vaccines. Cancer vaccines can use identified TAAs to generate the desired specific immune responses against cancer. However, the majority of antigens that are expressed on cancer cells have not yet been identified. Strategies have been developed to direct vaccination against specific TAAs and also against other collective antigens that are carried by tumor cells, which have not been identified. Therefore, vaccines can be classified into two groups: DAV and NDAV.

Defined-antigen–directed vaccines. DAV are specifically directed against known TAAs. They are administered either as a recombinant form that expresses the targeted antigen (or antigens) or as a synthetic form of the antigen. These defined antigens can be either a single antigen (peptide) or multiple antigens (polypeptides or full proteins). Recombinant vaccines may use live virus or naked DNA vectors. The specific gene-encoding sequence is introduced into a nonpathogenic or attenuated virus, or into a DNA plasmid, which is used for vaccination to express the desired antigen. The live virus technique has been used most commonly with vaccinia virus, although other viral vectors, such as fowl pox and adenovirus, are currently being tested in clinical trials. The nucleic acid/naked DNA vector vaccine is a simple and inexpensive method that is already being tested in clinical trials for advanced cancer.[45-48] Synthetic antigen vaccines may include a full known antigenic protein or synthetic peptide fragments.

Non–defined-antigen–directed vaccines. Tumor cells carry many potential TAAs that have not yet been identified but are able to activate the immune system if they are delivered under altered conditions that favor lymphocyte activation. NDAV do not target a specific antigen; rather, they use a collection of potential antigens derived from cancer cells that for the most part have not been identified. Methods include whole-cell vaccines and whole-cell lysate. Whole-cell vaccine technology uses whole tumor cells that have been treated to make them inactive. These cells are usually manipulated so that they present antigens to the host in a better fashion than the original tumor (e.g., over-expressing costimulatory molecules). Clinical protocols using this method have proved largely unsuccessful in advanced disease.[49,50] However, Vermorken and colleagues[51] showed that vaccinating patients who had stage II colon cancer with autologous irradiated tumor cells led to a longer recurrence-free survival time. Currently, new whole-cell tumor vaccine protocols are using modification techniques to render tumor cells more immunogenic. These modifications include introducing specific helpers (e.g., cytokine genes) into the tumor cell to make conditions more favorable for antigenic recognition.[52] Lysate of whole tumor cells can also be used as a source of TAA. The lysate contains all possible antigens that can be extracted by the lyses method. Many trials have been conducted to test this strategy in cancer patients and have shown promising results.[53-56]

Vaccination with any of these methods can be accomplished either by direct administration of the vaccine reagent through any of the known routes or by administration of the antigens using DCs as the delivery method. DCs are professional APCs that express all needed molecules for antigen presentation and proper interaction with lymphocytes. Transduction of DCs with genes expressing specific antigens can accomplish expression of the antigens on DCs, with the antigen expressed by viral vectors; loading the synthetic antigens on the DCs; or fusing tumor cells with DCs. DCs have been shown to be a powerful tool for generating specific cytotoxic immune response[57,58] and inducing total animal protection.[59,60] DCs are currently used in vaccination in two different ways. The first is the generation of DCs ex vivo with the use of appropriate cytokines such as IL-4 and granulocyte-macrophage colony-stimulating factor (GM-CSF). These cells then are made to express the antigen by one of the methods outlined. The second method is the activation of DCs directly in vivo with the use of cytokines such as GM-CSF.[61]

BIOLOGIC THERAPY FOR OVARIAN CANCER

Many advances have taken place in the past decade that have led to the identification of ovarian cancer as an immunogenic tumor. Many ovarian tumor antigens have been identified, leading to the development of biologic therapies against ovarian cancer. Therapies using MoAb, vaccines, and cytokines have been and are still being tested in ovarian cancer. The advances and controversies that are emerging from such therapies are discussed in the following sections.

Ovarian Cancer Tumor-Associated Antigens

As outlined earlier, it is to be expected that the accumulated genetic alteration in ovarian cancer and the resultant phenotype are the main contributors to the array of potential tumor antigens that are or will be identified in ovarian cancer. A few ovarian tumor antigens have been identified, including HER2/NEU, folate binding protein (FBP), P53, sialyl-Tn (STn), and MUC1. The following paragraphs give an overview of such antigens and the therapeutic approaches that are being undertaken to target them.[62]

HER2/NEU. The HER2/NEU transmembrane protein is a member of the epidermal growth factor receptor family. The protein consists of three domains: a cysteine-rich extracellular domain, a transmembrane domain, and an intracellular domain.[63,64] HER2/NEU gene amplification is seen in many cancers, including 20% to 30% of ovarian cancers.[65,66] Because of the biologic characteristics of the protein and the reasonable frequency of overexpression in ovarian cancer, HER2/NEU forms an attractive target for the development of biologic therapy for both humoral- and cellular-based approaches. In mice, protective immunity against the HER2/NEU-expressing tumor challenge can be achieved by vaccination with the full-length HER2/NEU antigen or a subunit[67] and can generate a CD8+ specific T-cell response.[68] Furthermore, Disis and others[29] have shown that HER2/NEU is an immunogenic protein; immunodominant epitopes are identified and are capable of generating a specific immune response.

Folate-binding protein. FBP is a membrane protein that functions as a transmembrane transporter for folate. It is highly expressed in the majority of ovarian cancers, with more than 80 times the normal expression.[70,71]

This makes FBP an attractive target for development of immune biologic therapy. Furthermore, it has been shown that FBP is an immunogenic protein. Peoples and associates[70] identified FBP HLA-A2 immunodominant peptides which are capable of generating specific T cells. These T lymphocytes can lyse tumor cells that overexpress the FBP.[70] Kim and colleagues[72] found that tumor-associated lymphocytes isolated from malignant ascites against FBP showed cytotoxic activity that was MHC I restricted.[72]

MUC1. MUC1 is a high-molecular-weight glycoprotein that is rich in serine and threonine residues, which are O-glycosylated. It is expressed on the membranes of many glandular epithelial cancer cells, including breast, ovary, and gastrointestinal epithelial carcinomas. The increase in the level of expression of MUC1 is usually accompanied by changes in the profile of glycosyl transferases involved in the synthesis of the O-glycans attached to the MUC1 core protein. This leads to aberrant glycosylation of the protein, which in turn makes cancer-associated mucin structurally different from the normal mucin. Accordingly, novel B and T cell epitopes get exposed for recognition by the immune system.[73,74] Specific MUC1 T-cell immune responses (CD8+ and CD4+) have been found in patients with ovarian and other types of cancers.[75-77] Vaccination of mice with the MUC1 antigen also elicited specific immune responses to mucin.[78] Furthermore, adoptive transfer of immune cells from wild-type mice primed in vivo with tumor cells and expressing the MUC1 protein into transgenic mice that express the MUC1 gene (MUC1.Tg) resulted in significant increases in the survival of MUC1.Tg recipients compared with unmanipulated control MUC.Tg mice challenged with B16.MUC1 tumor cells.[79] In humans, HLA-A2 epitopes have been identified in MUC1. These epitopes were found to generate specific T-cell responses in vitro that were capable of lysing tumor cells expressing MUC1 protein.[80]

Carcinoembryonic antigen. CEA is a glycoprotein with a molecular weight of 180 kd that is normally expressed on the cell surface of fetal colonic mucosa. Normal colonic mucosa has been found to have some expression of this antigen; however, CEA is usually overexpressed on the cell surface of many adenocarcinomas, including breast, colon, lung, and ovary. Many studies have shown that CEA is overexpressed in more than half of ovarian mucinous carcinomas and, to a much lesser degree (approximately 15%), in other types of ovarian cancer.[81]

P53. TP53 is a tumor suppressor gene that is commonly mutated in human cancers. TP53 is mutated in more 30% to 50% of ovarian cancers.[82] Mutations of the TP53 gene lead to an increase in the half-life and hence intracellular overexpression of the protein.[83] Therefore, this protein could function as an antigen through one of two different mechanisms: as a mutant "foreign" protein or as an overexpressed self-protein. CTL derived by mutant P53 peptide vaccination of mice can kill tumor cell targets endogenously expressing the corresponding mutant P53.[36] These CTLs are able to protect mice from challenge with tumors expressing mutant P53.[60,84] These responses are specific for tumor cells expressing the mutant sequence corresponding to the vaccinating peptide and not for tumors expressing other mutant P53 proteins. It has also been found that specific CTLs can be generated by in vitro stimulation of the primed T cells of the vaccinated mouse with the specific mutated peptides.[36,85] Wild-type P53 epitopes are also recognized by CTLs on murine tumor cells.[86] Mice were found to be protected by wild-type P53 peptide vaccination against challenge with tumors expressing the P53 protein.[60] Roth and associates[84] showed that vaccination of mice with recombinant wild-type P53 leads to a protective effect against challenge with tumors expressing high levels of mutant P53. In contrast, tumors with downregulated P53 escape immunologic rejection.

Multiple HLA-A2 P53 epitopes have been identified.[87-91] The P53 264-272 has been shown, by many investigators, to have high affinity for HLA-A2.[87-91] It is naturally processed and endogenously presented by HLA-A2 in different types of tumor cell lines.[92,93] P53 264-272 peptide-specific CD8+ T cells generated from HLA-A2 donors were able to lyse tumor cells overexpressing wild-type or mutant P53 protein.[92,93] On the other hand, these specific lymphocytes failed to lyse autologous cells derived from normal tissues.[92] In addition, CTLs generated against wild-type human P53 epitope 264-272, or against the murine P53 homologous peptide 261-269 in HLA-A2-transgenic mice, were found to recognize and lyse human and murine tumor cell lines expressing the P53 protein and failed to lyse nontransformed normal cells expressing normal levels of P53.[94,95]

Sialyl-Tn. STn is a disaccharide antigen that is expressed on the core region of aberrant underglycosylated mucin of many cancers.[96] The immunogenicity of STn is exhibited because of overexpression of the protein in ovarian tumors, which has been reported to be as high as 100%.[97-99] The expression of STn in ovarian cancer is more prominent in mucinous rather than serous carcinoma, which is a factor that needs to be taken into consideration in developing biotherapy based on this antigenic target.[100]

Many studies in animals have shown that vaccination with the carbohydrate antigen STn can generate a specific immune response and lead to meaningful tumor response with increased survival.[101,102]

Monoclonal Antibodies

Monoclonal Antibodies as Therapeutic Agents

Anti-HER2/NEU antibody trastuzumab. As outlined earlier, overexpression of HER2/NEU has been reported in up to 30% of ovarian cancer,[66] which makes it an attractive target for ovarian cancer treatment.[66] Antibodies against HER2/NEU have been developed and were shown to be effective in breast canrcinomas.[103] Trastuzumab was approved in 1998 by the U. S. Food and Drug administration for use in women with metastatic breast disease that overexpresses HER2/NEU as a single agent in second-line therapy or as first-line therapy in combination with Taxol.[104] In ovarian cancer, Cuello and coworkers[105] showed that HER2/NEU antibodies can downregulate the expression of the receptor in tumor cell lines. A phase II clinical trial testing the efficacy of Trastuzumab in ovarian cancer showed that it has limited clinical value as a single agent, with an overall response rate of less than 10% in a heavily pretreated population.[106] Based on the breast cancer data, the combination of Trastuzumab with chemotherapy may have a better chance of providing a meaningful result in patients with ovarian cancer. This strategy is currently being tested.

Anti–CA 125 antibody MoAb B43.14. Another antibody that has been developed and used in ovarian cancer is a MoAb against CA 125 antigen. CA 125 is overexpressed in ovarian cancer cells. Furthermore, this antigen in secreted into the bloodstream of ovarian cancer patients in more than 97% of cases of advanced disease.[107] MoAb B43.14 (OvaRex) is a murine MoAb that is generated against CA 125. This antibody binds to the circulating antigen and forms a complex that is recognized as "foreign." This leads to the development of human anti-mouse antibody (HAMA) and anti-idiotype antibody responses; in addition, it is able to generate a cellular immune response against the CA 125 protein. In a study conducted by Noujaim and colleagues,[108] investigators found that patients receiving MoAb B43.14 generated humoral and cellular anti–CA125 responses, including both B- and T-cell types of the latter. In addition, it was shown that the generation of CA 125–specific responses after MoAb-B43.14 injection correlated with improved survival.[108] Clinical trials are currently being conducted to further explore the role of MoAb B43.14.

Bispecific antibodies. Bispecific antibodies (BsAb) have also been developed against ovarian cancer targets. These reagents work by binding to an antigen on one end and to a receptor on an immune effector cell on the other end. This generates an effector cell-mediated lytic activity.[109] BsAb against HER2/NEU (MDX-210) were tested in a phase I trial in patients with tumors that overexpressed HER2/NEU. MDX-210 is a BsAb that recognizes FcγRI on monocytes and macrophages and the cell-surface product of the HER2/NEU oncogene. This trial, which included patients with ovarian and breast cancer, showed that MDX-210 is both immunologically and clinically active. It was able to generate monocyte/macrophage activation, and it did effectively localize tumors carrying the antigen, with some clinical response in one patient.[110,111] Other BsAb were also generated against other ovarian cancer antigens, such as folate receptor and CA 125. OCTR is a BsAb that is directed to the cluster determinant CD3 on T lymphocytes and to the folate receptor on ovarian carcinoma cells. In a phase II study with intraperitoneal administration of the antibody in 28 patients with limited intraperitoneal disease after first-line therapy, 27% of patients had a complete or partial intraperitoneal response with strict surgicopathologic evaluation.[112]

Radioimmunoconjugates. MoAb are also used as radionuclide β-emitter conjugates and have been tested in ovarian cancer. MoAb human milk fat globule (HMFG1), which binds specifically to polymorphic epithelial mucine (PEM), an antigen expressed in more than 90% of ovarian cancers, conjugated to yttrium 90 isotope, has been used in a phase I/II trial in ovarian cancer. Fifty-two ovarian cancer patients were treated with the conjugate antibody as a consolidated therapy after primary chemotherapy.

Immunotoxins. Antibodies can also be linked to chemotoxins to allow more specific targeting of these toxins to malignant cells. These toxin-conjugated antibodies require internalization to be able to exert their effect on the target cells. Immunotoxins have been tried in many cancers, including lymphomas, and have shown promising results.[113] In ovarian cancer, there have been few trials testing antibodies that can recognize ovarian antigens linked to toxins. One of these trials was conducted by Pai and colleagues,[114] using OVB3-PE, which is MoAb that recognizes human ovarian cancer linked to Pseudomonas exotoxin. This phase I trial demonstrated no activity when the immunotoxin was administered intraperitoneally. Immunotoxins are currently being developed against other known ovarian cancer antigens, such as HER2/NEU[115,116] or misothillin (a surface antigen that is predominantly expressed in ovarian cancer[117,118]) with promising preclinical results and may hold some promise in clinical trials.

Vaccines

With the discovery of the ovarian TAAs, vaccine development became a natural outcome in the effort to develop ovarian cancer–targeted therapy. Some of these antigens have been or are being tested in clinical trials. Several of the strategies outlined earlier are currently being tested in preclinical models or in clinical trials in ovarian cancers. Relatively few vaccine studies have been performed in patients with ovarian cancer. The following sections discuss the overall experience in the effort of vaccine development for ovarian cancer.

Defined-antigen–directed vaccines. HER2/NEU and MUC1 are the most studied TAAs and have the most accumulated experience in clinical trials in patients with ovarian cancers. Disis and colleagues[119,120] identified immunodominant epitopes derived from the HER2/NEU protein extracellular and intracellular domains and administered these 15- to 18-amino-acid peptides intradermally, along with GM-CSF, to ovarian

cancer patients with minimal disease. The patients were able to generate a specific immune response against the peptides, and this immune response was able to lyse tumor cells that overexpressed the HER2/NEU protein. Brossart and associates,[121] on the other hand, vaccinated patients who had bulky ovarian tumors with HER2/NEU and MUC1 peptides that were pulsed on DCs. They were able to demonstrate that advanced ovarian cancer patients can generate an immune response that is capable of lysing HLA-matched tumor cells in vitro. They also showed some data indicating that there is a potential clinical benefit with such treatment.

Another antigen that has been used in ovarian cancer clinical trials is STn. Many clinical trials have been conducted using this antigen.[122,123] Holmberg and coworkers[96] found that vaccinating breast and ovarian cancer patients with the STn antigen could protect these patients from relapse after high-dose chemotherapy and autologous stem cell rescue. In this trial, patients who had undergone autologous transplantation were immunized with sialyl-Tn–keyhole limpet hemocyanin (STn-KLH) vaccine (Theratope), which incorporates a synthetic STn antigen that mimics the unique tumor-associated STn carbohydrate. These patients were able to generate an effective CTL immune response to STn vaccine therapy. This therapy could potentially be useful in conjunction with high-dose chemotherapy regimens.[81]

Non–defined-antigen–directed vaccines. NDAV have also been tested in ovarian cancer, with tumor cell lysate used as a method of vaccination aimed at generating immune response to as many potential ovarian cancer antigens as possible. Zhao and coworkers[124] demonstrated that CTL generated against DC pulsed with ovarian cancer lysate can show significant killing activity against autologous tumor cells. In another study, Santin and colleagues[125] showed that eluted peptides from ovarian cancer cells generate specific CD8+ cells against autologous tumors. Clinical data using this method demonstrated some promise in a small trial conducted by Hernando and associates.[53] Immunization of ovarian cancer patients with autologous DC pulsed with tumor lysates and keyhole limpet hemocyanin as a helper antigen produced an immune response in two of six patients. Two of eight patients demonstrated immune response that coincided with stabilization of the disease.[53]

Vaccine development for ovarian cancer is a very active area of research. Therapeutic vaccination for ovarian cancer would most likely combine some of the strategies and methods that have been outlined in this chapter.

Cytokines

Few cytokines have been preclinically developed and clinically tested in the treatment of ovarian cancer. IFN-α and IFN-γ have shown some activity both in vitro and in vivo against ovarian cancer.[126,127]

In humans, IFN-α has been administered mainly by the intraperitoneal administration route. In a few studies, the use of IFN-α in patients with surgically documented minimal residual disease resulted in a response rate of 30% to 50%.[128-132] Studies have also used a combination of intraperitoneal IFN-α and chemotherapy. In two of these studies testing the efficacy of the intraperitoneal combination of IFN-α and carboplatin, clinical and pathologic complete responses were reported.[133,134] In the trial conducted by Frasci and associates,[133] patients with stage III minimal disease received IFN-α-2b, which was administered intraperitoneally along with carboplatin. Clinicopathologic response was as high as 91% in patients with residual disease of less than 5 mm and approximately 45% in patients with more than 5 mm disease.[133] However, the combination of IFN-α with chemotherapy has not been shown to have any advantage over IFN-α alone.[129-131] In one study, among 111 patients with small-volume residual disease, there was no difference between treatment with intraperitoneal carboplatin plus IFN-α versus carboplatin alone.[135] The use of IFN-α is an area that has not been fully settled in the development of ovarian cancer treatments, and further investigations are needed to determine the efficacy and the best strategy.

IFN-γ has also been used intraperitoneally, with results comparable to those of IFN-α in ovarian cancer patients (30% to 50% surgically confirmed response).[126,136-139] In a phase III trial conducted by Windbichler and colleagues,[140] IFN-γ was used subcutaneously in women with stages Ic-IIIc ovarian cancer that were treated with first-line cis-platinum. The addition of IFN-γ improved the response rate (68% versus 56%) and the disease-free survival rate (66% versus 53%).[140] Therefore, unlike IFN-α, IFN-γ has some advantages when combined with chemotherapy. This is another area in which further investigation is needed.

IL-2 is another cytokine that is used for the treatment of ovarian cancer. A phase II trial in which IL-2 was administered intraperitoneally to patients with taxane/platinum-refractory disease showed extended survival.[141] IL-2 has also been tested in combination with other cytokines in ovarian cancer. IFN-γ was combined with IL-2 and administered intraperitoneally in two of the trials, without any major clinical benefit.[142,143]

Recombinant human interleukin-12 (rhIL-12) was also tested in escalating doses to estimate its antitumor activity and toxicity in patients with recurrent or refractory epithelial ovarian cancer. As a single agent, rhIL-12 was found to be tolerable in advanced ovarian cancer, with a low response rate.[144] No further exploration of IL-12 is planned for the treatment of this disease with direct therapeutic intent.

In general, cytokines have not been shown to be of great benefit in ovarian cancer when used alone, and it is unlikely that such therapy would have a wide application in the treatment of this disease.[145] However, the combination of cytokines with other therapies, such as chemotherapy or vaccination, may have wider and more useful applications.

BIOLOGIC THERAPY FOR CERVICAL CANCER

Cervical cancer is one of the few malignancies in humans that is linked to a specific etiologic agent.[146-148] More than 99% of cervical cancers are caused by HPV, providing an excellent model for the development molecular targeted therapy. Therapeutic strategies against HPV-induced malignancies are designed for either prevention or treatment of the disease. HPVs are divided into low-risk and high-risk types, based on the type of clinical lesion with which they are associated. Low risk HPVs (e.g., HPV-6, HPV-11) are generally associated with benign lesions such as condyloma acuminata, and they usually maintain their DNA in cells as extrachromosomal circular episomes. High-risk types (e.g., HPV-16, HPV-18) are found in cervical intraepithelial neoplasia (CIN) II and III lesions and in invasive cervical cancers.[149] The genomes of high-risk types are integrated into the cellular DNA in most high-grade lesions and cervical carcinomas. The protein products of the early genes E6 and E7 in high-risk HPV types have been implicated in the oncogenic capability of the viruses. The continued expression of these proteins in cervical cells appears to be a critical event in the progression and maintenance of cervical neoplasia.[150] Therefore, the products of these two genes form very strong candidates as targets for biologic therapy.[151]

Cervical Cancer Antigens

There is strong evidence that the immune system plays a role in the natural outcome of the HPV infection and in cervical cancer. First, most lesions that are HPV induced regress spontaneously. Second, the incidence of malignancies induced by HPV increases in patients who are immune-suppressed, such as those with human immunodeficiency virus (HIV) infection, transplant recipients, and patients receiving immune suppressive therapy.[152-156] Third, the presence of lymphoproliferative responses in patients with CIN lesions is associated with higher likelihood for clearance of the infection and spontaneous resolution of the lesions.[157] Fourth, there is a higher tendency toward spontaneous clearance of warts that exhibit large infiltrates of lymphocytes.[158-160] Therefore, it is clear that the cervical cancer cell presents TAAs that are recognized by the immune system and that these antigens represent good targets for biologic therapeutic approach.

The HPV E6 and E7 are found to form TAAs in cervical cancer. These antigens are capable of inducing CTLs that can recognize and lyse tumor cells harboring HPV genome.[161,162] Vaccination of mice with HPV-16 E7 antigen was found to generate a specific immune response that was protective against transplanted tumors expressing the HPV-16 E7 antigen. This protection was found to be mediated by CD8+ lymphocytes.[163,164] Furthermore, HPV E6 and E7 epitope-specific CTLs are generated from cervical cancer patients with HPV-positive tumors.[162]

The identification of specific TAAs for cervical cancer has led to a new phase of therapeutic development for this disease. Currently, the largest effort in the development of biologic therapy is being directed toward HPV vaccines. However, other biologic therapies are also being developed for cervical cancer, including cytokine treatment. The following paragraphs discuss the latest developments of these strategies and the controversies relevant to the development process.

Cytokines

Evidence for a beneficial effect of cytokines in cervical cancer has not been very promising. IFN was found to have no tangible effect in patients with advanced disease in a multi-institutional phase II trial conducted by the Eastern Cooperative Oncology Group.[165] IFN-IFN-α has been used in combination with other agents such as retinoic acid. Veerasam and colleagues[166] used the combination of IFN-α and retinoic acid in patients with locally advanced disease concomitant with standard radiotherapy, demonstrating some enhancement in local control. In general, this treatment modality is not being further developed with the current known cytokines as therapeutic agents. However, cytokines are being explored in cervical cancer, mainly as immune enhancers for vaccine therapy (see later discussion).

Vaccines

Two types of vaccines are being developed in cervical cancer—a prophylactic vaccine and a therapeutic one.

Prophylactic vaccines. The principal goal of prophylactic vaccines is to prevent infection by the etiologic cause of cancer; accordingly, they are based on inducing a humoral immune response to generate neutralizing antibodies against the infectious agent. The traditional prophylactic use of viral vaccines has been with live, attenuated, or formalin-inactivated viral strains. Therefore, in general, development of a prophylactic vaccine against viruses requires the availability of a viral culture. Because it has been difficult to propagate HPV in a tissue culture system, prophylactic vaccines against HPV had lagged behind in development.

Recently, it was found that the HPV virion, which is composed of two late proteins, L1 and L2, is highly immunogenic and can generate humoral immune responses with high neutralizing titers.[167-169] This discovery provided a method for development of a vaccine that is potentially prophylactic against HPV infection. Many investigators have shown that L1 and L2, when expressed in nonmammalian cells, can self-assemble into HPV virus-like particles (VLP) that resemble the native viron[170-172] and exhibit the same immunogenicity as the authentic viron.[167,173] When used in animals, these VLP have the ability to fully protect against natural HPV infection.[174-176] This finding has paved the way to the beginning of clinical trials for the purpose of preventing cervical cancer through the prevention of HPV infection. Pastrana and colleagues[177] administered HPV-16 VLP to young women in a controlled trial and reported the induction of specific humoral immune response against the virus.[177] These VLP were shown by other investigators to reduce the incidence of HPV-16 infection and related CIN in volunteers.[178] These have been encouraging results, paving the way for the development of prophylactic HPV vaccines that may substantially decrease the incidence of cervical cancer worldwide.[151]

Another strategy of prophylactic vaccine development has been to prevent infection of HPV at the site of entry. Because HPV initiates infection at the mucosal surface, vaccines that are capable of inducing a mucosal immunity at the site of viral entry could potentially prevent such an infection. Vaccination in animal models through a mucosal route generates a neutralizing immunoglobulin A humoral immune response. This may have a reasonable impact on HPV infection incidence in high-risk populations.

Therapeutic vaccines. As outlined previously, E6 and E7 are the two antigens that have been shown to be potential targets for therapeutic vaccine development against cervical cancer. Various forms of vaccination have been developed and tested against these two antigens, including full-length protein, peptides, recombinant viruses, and naked DNA. E6- and E7-derived peptides that form human CTL epitopes have been identified,[179,180] and several clinical trials have been conducted testing this peptide-vaccine in patients with advanced cervical disease or high-grade CIN. Some trials using HLA-A2 peptides resulted in induction of specific immune response against the HPV antigens and cervical cancer–derived cells; others did not. Ressing and associates[181] performed a peptide-based phase I/II vaccination trial in patients with recurrent or persistent cervical carcinoma. Patients received two HLA-A2 peptides that were linked to a helper epitope and administered in an adjuvant agent. No CTL responses against the HPV-16 E7 peptides were detected. On the other hand, Wojtowicz and colleagues[182] demonstrated that vaccinating patients with advanced cervical disease with at least one of these HLA-A2–restricted peptides can induce a strong specific immune response.[182] Although these trials treated similar cohorts of patients and used the same antigens, the difference was the method of administering the peptide. Ressing[181] administered the peptide subcutaneously along with adjuvant, whereas Wojtowicz[182] administered the peptide pulsed on APCs intravenously. Muderspach and associates[183] also used the same peptides, with the same subcutaneous route of administration as in Ressing's trial, but to patients with CIN rather than advanced disease. They found that such patients can generate a strong immune response with some meaningful clinical response.

Full-length HPV E7 protein has also been used in clinical trials in cervical cancer and premalignant disease. As outlined previously, this strategy eliminates the need for identification of specific CTL epitopes, allowing the treatment of a wider cohort of patients by overcoming the need for HLA restriction. In addition, it provides a wider span of amino acid sequences that contain potential multiple peptide-antigens throughout the length of the protein. Full-length HPV-16 E7 has been fused to the heat shock protein Hsp65 to enhance antigen processing and presentation.[184] This construct was shown to have reasonable clinical effect when used in the treatment of patients with anal dysplasia,[185,186] and currently it is being tested in clinical trials of both cervical dysplasia and cervical carcinoma. Other reagents are also being developed that exploit the potential role of the full-length E6 and E7 proteins.[187]

Manipulation of the immune system against HPV as cervical cancer–specific therapy appears to be one of the most promising strategies that can be used to prevent progression of premalignant lesions and to treat invasive cervical cancers.

HPV antigens, whether in the form of proteins or peptides, can also be administered as naked DNA or recombinant viral vectors. This technology provides many advantages (see earlier discussion), but concern exists about the use of oncogenic proteins such as E6 and E7 under these circumstances. For this reason, mutated, functionally defective versions of the protein are used. Minigenes that consist of chains of identified CTL epitopes can be expressed from these vectors. Recombinant viruses such as vaccinia, adenovirus, and adenoassociated virus have been used to express HPV proteins.[33,57,61,188,189] However, viral infections may need to be used with care in patients with advanced disease who are immunocompromised. Naked DNA vectors cannot be delivered as efficiently as viral vectors, but they do not have the same risks and are stable and easy to produce. DNA vaccines that express a fusion protein targeting E7 proteins at the lysosomal/endosomal compartment enhanced the potency of the vaccine and increased tumor prevention and regression in mice.[190]

CONTROVERSIES

Biologic therapy for cancer is one of the most diverse treatments in medicine, because of the many different ways of manipulating the biologic system, the many antigens that are discovered or will be discovered, the various strategies for targeting those antigens, and the possible combinations of such strategies. This diversity generates a tremendous amount of debate and questions, including the controversies reviewed in this section. The majority of these questions have been addressed in relevance to each specific treatment discussed throughout the chapter; here, they are addressed for the field of biotherapy in a global fashion.

What is the best therapeutic strategy?

A wide range of agents, including antigen-vaccines, antibodies, toxins, and cytokines, are available or will be available with future discoveries to treat malignancies such as gynecologic cancers. In no other biotherapy can this be more obvious than vaccine therapy; therefore, for simplicity, the discussion of these questions is limited to vaccines as used in gynecologic malignancies. As outlined previously, vaccine therapy is a "basket" of agents that can be administered in various ways through various routes with various combinations of immune modulators. There are many factors that need to be determined when designing immunotherapy, and currently these remain areas of debate.

Type of antigen. As outlined earlier, many antigens have been identified in both ovarian and cervical cancers. The question of which is the best antigen to target for biotherapy is a major issue. The answer may not be any of the antigens described given separately, because targeting a single epitope invariably leads to loss of antigen expression.[191,192] The question may not be answerable, because many of these antigens work to some degree. The use of a multitude of antigens may present an advantage for few reasons, including the generation of multiple tumor-specific T-cell clones and the possibility of overcoming antigen loss. In addition, the potential antigenic heterogeneity of cancers may require use of multiple antigenic targets rather than targeting of a single molecule. This may be accomplished by using multiple DAV, such as multiple epitopes from the same antigen or a combination of epitopes from different antigens (as in some clinical trials of HPV multivariate vaccines) or by using NDAV.

Form of antigen. Antigen-vaccines can be used in many different forms. Antigens are used for vaccination either directly or on APCs as a vehicle for administration. These forms of antigens, particularly as used in gynecologic malignancies, were discussed in detail earlier in this chapter. Determining which form or combination of forms of antigen should be used is an active area of research and will continue to be a dynamic area because of the improved and enhanced technologies that are being developed in this field. Each form and strategies carries advantages and disadvantages. Peptide-antigens have the advantage of being specific vaccines, and they are easy to make and formulate, but they are HLA restricted and therefore limit the selection of patients. Most of the trials in cervical and ovarian cancer outlined earlier tested this method.[181-183,193] Full proteins possess a greater selection of antigenic epitopes, which helps in generating larger numbers of antigen-specific T-cell clones and which overcomes the HLA restriction in patient selection. However, this technology is challenging because it is difficult to produce these agents, maintain their stability, and process them suitably for human use.[184] DNA vaccines/vectors are easy to make and relatively inexpensive, can be produced on a large scale, are highly stable, and can be used repeatedly since no antivector immune response will be expected to occur. Concerns regarding such technology are mainly related to efficiency in expression and to the oncogenic potentials of some of these vectors, such as the HPV antigens and some of the antigenic oncogens of ovarian cancer (HER2/NEU, P53, and others), which can potentially integrate into the human genome and express oncoproteins. This concern may be of less importance in the case of viral vectors, which do not integrate into the human genome. However, viral vectors may pose other sets of disadvantages, including the production of neutralizing antibodies and the inherent safety concerns associated with these vectors.

Route of administration. Route of administration is another area of active debate in biotherapy. In MoAb, the route of administration has long been debated. In ovarian cancer, MoAb has been administered both intravenously and intraperitoneally, with the latter demonstrating a potential advantage over other routes in targeting intraperitoneal lesions.[194] On the other hand, distant metastases and larger intraperitoneal implantations may be better targeted with intravenous administration of MoAb, especially with the latest success of MoAb therapy in diseases like breast cancers.[195] The route of administration in vaccine therapy is also a highly debated area of research. Vaccines can be administered through any of the known routes, either as naked antigen or as part of APC-presenting antigen. Many trials are currently being conducted to try to answer this question.[193] In cervical cancer, HPV peptides have been administered intradermally, subcutaneously, or intravenously. These methods were discussed in detail in the section of vaccine therapy for HPV. No specific route has been identified to be better than others, and further research is needed in this area.

Immune-enhancing strategies. Many immune-enhancing strategies are used in vaccine development, including (1) immune adjuvants, such as emulsifying agents and polynucleotides; (2) cytokines, such as GM-CSF, IL-2,[196] and IL-12; (3) costimulatory molecules, such as B7.1, LFA, and intercellular adhesion molecule (ICAM)[197]; (4) helper molecules, such as Hsp65[184,186]; and (5) variant peptides.[198] As outlined earlier in the chapter, many trials are being conducted to test these methods, especially in combination, in either HPV vaccines or ovarian cancer vaccines. Further investigations are going to be crucial to determine the best type of vaccine and route of administration that would lead to the best immunologic response.

What is the best trial design to test these strategies?

Although early clinical trial development designs in chemotherapy apply to cytokine clinical development, it substantially differs from the clinical development of cancer vaccines or antibody therapy.[199] Because

vaccine therapy has been shown to be inert in causing toxicities, phase I escalating design trials are not needed in the development of such therapy. Furthermore, because biologic therapy often uses combinations of the multitude of agents that are available, and each of these regimens requires optimization for best response, trial designs that allow rapid screening of various strategies are needed for speedy development of effective therapies. Many designs have been suggested and are currently being applied in clinical trials (including phase II randomized designs[199]) to allow fast comparison of variations and a speedy way of adding and modifying these variations to reach the needed immune enhancement for better clinical response.

What is the best population on which to test these biotherapy strategies?

Another area of debate is the question of what patient population and disease stage should be used for biotherapy testing. All known ethical rules in clinical research dictate that early clinical development (i.e., phase I and most phase II studies) should be conducted in patients with advanced disease. In biotherapy, however, patients with advanced disease may be the least suitable group for such testing, for the following reasons: (1) patients with advanced disease are heavily pretreated with both chemotherapy and radiation therapy, which lead to suppression of T-cell function; (2) tumors secrete cytokines that suppress the immune system; and (3) the immune response obtained from biotherapy would not be sufficient to lead to tumor regression.[200] In conclusion, because the immune system does not react as efficiently in patients with bulky tumor as in normal people, evaluation of both toxicity and clinical response, both of which are dependent on immune response, is difficult in this population. Therefore, biotherapy may be better tested in patients with minimal disease. Patients with CIN or ovarian cancer who have no evidence of disease form an optimal cohort for testing nontoxic immunotherapy strategies, in particular vaccines, since most forms of vaccines are benign and nontoxic. The goal in these patients would be to elicit significant immunologic memory, capable of generating a sufficient magnitude of immune response to cross the threshold needed to provide meaningful clinical response. Toxic immunotherapies such as cytokines, antibodies, or vaccines administered with new untested viral vectors, still require phase I dose escalation studies[199] and need to be conducted in patients with advanced disease.

When may these strategies be taken into definitive phase III trials?

This issue is a hotly debated matter in the biotherapy field. With all the different possible combinations that could potentially be used to develop an effective biotherapy for cancer, the question usually arises of whether it is time for a phase III definitive trial. There are two schools of thought in this matter. The first advocates the continuation of "fast-track," randomized, phase II trials until a "best combination" is reached before starting phase III definitive studies. Because the "best combination" is always a debatable term, however, the other school of thought advocates taking any vaccine combination that demonstrates clinical activity into further development. Other factors do play a role in such a decision. Corporate financial issues with agents developed by biotechnology companies may be a consideration. Phase III trials are now being conducted in patients with CIN and in patients with ovarian cancer. Some biologic agents have no further development strategy, and testing of these agents may be needed in phase III trials.

In conclusion, biotherapy is a very promising field in the treatment of gynecologic malignancies. However, there are many issues in biotherapy that are highly debated, and further preclinical and clinical development will take this field in the coming few years into the mainstream of cancer therapy.

REFERENCES

1. Wilkinson KD: Ubiquitination and deubiquitination: Targeting of proteins for degradation by the proteasome. Semin Cell Dev Biol 2000;11:141-148.
2. Rock KL, Rothstein L, Benacerraf B: Analysis of the association of peptides of optimal length to class I molecules on the surface of cells. Proc Natl Acad Sci U S A 1992;89:8918-8922.
3. Brodsky FM, Lem L, Bresnahan PA: Antigen processing and presentation [see comments]. Tissue Antigens 1996;47:464-471.
4. Lurquin C, Van Pel A, Mariame B, et al: Structure of the gene of tum-transplantation antigen P91A: The mutated exon encodes a peptide recognized with Ld by cytolytic T cells. Cell 1989;58:293-303.
5. De Plaen E, Lurquin C, Van PA, et al: Immunogenic (tum-) variants of mouse tumor P815: Cloning of the gene of tum-antigen P91A and identification of the tum-mutation. Proc Natl Acad Sci U S A 1988;85:2274-2278.
6. Davis MM, Chien Y: Topology and affinity of T-cell receptor mediated recognition of peptide-MHC complexes. Curr Opin Immunol 1993;5:45-49.
7. Robinson MA, Kindt TJ: Major histo-compatibility complex antigens and genes. In Paul WE (ed): Fundamental Immunology. New York, Raven Press, 1989, p 489.
8. Solheim JC: Class I MHC molecules: Assembly and antigen presentation. Immunol Rev 1999;172:11-19.
9. Hanau D, Saudrais C, Haegel-Kronenberger H, et al: Fate of MHC class II molecules in human dendritic cells. Eur J Dermatol 1999;9:7-12.
10. Batalia MA, Collins EJ: Peptide binding by class I and class II MHC molecules. Biopolymers 1997;43:281-302.
11. Corradin G, Demotz S: Peptide-MHC complexes assembled following multiple pathways: An opportunity for the design of vaccines and therapeutic molecules. Hum Immunol 1997;54:137-147.
12. Wubbolts R, Neefjes J: Intracellular transport and peptide loading of MHC class II molecules: Regulation by chaperones and motors. Immunol Rev 1999;172:189-208.
13. Pareja E, Tobes R, Martin J, Nieto A: The tetramer model: A new view of class II MHC molecules in antigenic presentation to T cells. Tissue Antigens 1997;50:421-428.
14. Otley CC, Pittelkow MR: Skin cancer in liver transplant recipients. Liver Transpl 2000;6:253-262.
15. Penn I: Overview of the problem of cancer in organ transplant recipients. Ann Transplant 1997;2:5-6.
16. Konety BR, Tewari A, Howard RJ, et al: Prostate cancer in the post-transplant population. Urologic Society for Transplantation and Vascular Surgery. Urology 1998;52:428-432.
17. Flattery MP: Incidence and treatment of cancer in transplant recipients. J Transplant Coord 1998;8:105-110; quiz, 111-112.
18. Sheil AG: Cancer in immune-suppressed organ transplant recipients: Aetiology and evolution. Transplant Proc 1998;30:2055-2057.
19. Uenishi T, Hirohashi K, Tanaka H, et al: Spontaneous regression of a large hepatocellular carcinoma with portal vein tumor thrombi: Report of a case. Surg Today 2000;30:82-85.
20. Hachiya T, Koizumi T, Hayasaka M, et al: Spontaneous regression of primary mediastinal germ cell tumor. Jpn J Clin Oncol 1998;28:281-283.
21. Markowska J, Markowska A. [Spontaneous tumor regression]. Ginekol Pol 1998;69:39-44.
22. Royal RE, Steinberg SM, Krouse RS, et al: Correlates of response to IL-2 therapy in patients treated for metastatic renal cancer and melanoma cancer. J Sci Am 1996;2:91.
23. Bourantas KL, Hatzimichael EC, Makis AC, et al: Prolonged interferon-alpha-2b treatment of hairy cell leukemia patients [letter]. Eur J Haematol 2000;64:350-351.
24. Parkinson DR, Sznol M: High dose interleukin-2 in the therapy of metastatic renal cell carcinoma. Semon Oncol 1995;22:61-66.
25. Stadler WM, Vogelzang NJ: Low dose interleukin-2 in the treatment of metaststic renal call carcinoma. Semin Oncol 1995;22:67-73.
26. Landsteiner K, Chase MW: Experiments on transfer of cutaneous sensitivity to simple compounds. Proc Soc Exp Biol Med 1942;49:688.
27. Tsomides TJ, Eisen HN: T-cell antigens in cancer. Proc Natl Acad Sci U S A 1994;91:3487-3489.
28. Pardoll DM: Tumour antigens: A new look for the 1990s [news; comment]. Nature 1994;369:357.
29. van der Bruggen P, Traversari C, Chomez P, et al: A gene encoding an antigen recognized by cytolytic T lymphocytes on a human melanoma. Science 1991;254:1643-1647.
30. Bei R, Kantor J, Kashmiri SV, et al: Enhanced immune responses and anti-tumor activity by baculovirus recombinant carcinoembryonic antigen (CEA) in mice primed with the recombinant vaccinia CEA. J Immunother Emphasis Tumor Immunol 1994;16:275-282.
31. Kawakami Y, Nishimura MI, Restifo NP, et al: T-cell recognition of human melanoma antigens. J Immunother 1993;14:88-93.
32. Nevins JR: Cell cycle targets of the DNA tumor viruses. Curr Opin Genet Dev 1994;4:130-134.
33. Levine AJ: The origins of the small DNA tumor viruses. Adv Cancer Res 1994;65:141-168.
34. Rapp F, Cory JM: Viral oncogenesis and the immune system. Cancer Detect Prev 1990;14:437-444.
35. Peace DJ, Chen W, Nelson H, Cheever MA: T cell recognition of transforming proteins encoded by mutated ras proto-oncogenes. J Immunol 1991;146:2059-2065.
36. Yanuck M, Carbone DP, Pendleton DC, et al: A mutant p53 or ras tumor suppressor protein is a target for peptide-induced CD8+ cytotoxic T cells. Cancer Res 1993;53:3257-3261.
37. Khleif SN, Abrams SI, Hamilton JM, et al: A phase I vaccine trial with peptides reflecting ras oncogene mutations of solid tumors. J Immunother 1999;22:155-165.
38. Chen W, Peace DJ, Rovira DK, et al: T-cell immunity to the joining region of p210BCR-ABL protein. Proc Natl Acad Sci U S A 1992;89:1468-1472.
39. Cheever MA, Chen W, Disis ML, et al: T-cell immunity to oncogenic proteins including mutated ras and chimeric bcr-abl. Ann N Y Acad Sci 1993;690:101-112.
40. Bosch GJ, Joosten AM, Kessler JH, et al: Recognition of BCR-ABL positive leukemic blasts by human CD4+ T cells elicited by primary in vitro immunization with a BCR-ABL breakpoint peptide. Blood 1996;88:3522-3527.
41. Rosenberg SA: Principles of cancer management: Biologic therapy. In DeVita VT, Hellman S, Rosenberg SA (eds): Prnciples and Practice of Oncology. Philadelphia, Lippincott Williams & Wilkins, 2002, pp 307-332.
42. Khleif SN, Frederickson H: The role of vaccines in cancer prevention. Cancer Treat Res 2001;106:283-306.

43. Chapman PB, Morrissey DM, Panageas KS, et al: Induction of antibodies against GM2 ganglioside by immunizing melanoma patients using GM2-keyhole limpet hemocyanin + QS21 vaccine: A dose-response study. Clin Cancer Res 2000;6:874-879.

44. Sabbatini PJ, Kudryashov V, Ragupathi G, et al: Immunization of ovarian cancer patients with a synthetic Lewis(y)-protein conjugate vaccine: A phase 1 trial. Int J Cancer 2000;87:79-85.

45. Arvin AM, Mallory S, Moffat JF: Development of recombinant varicella-zoster virus vaccines. Contrib Microbiol 1999;3: 193-200.

46. Liljeqvist S, Stahl S: Production of recombinant subunit vaccines: Protein immunogens, live delivery systems and nucleic acid vaccines. J Biotechnol 1999;73:1-33.

47. Restifo NP, Rosenberg SA: Developing recombinant and synthetic vaccines for the treatment of melanoma. Curr Opin Oncol 1999;11:50-57.

48. Rolph MS, Ramshaw IA: Recombinant viruses as vaccines and immunological tools [see comments]. Curr Opin Immunol 1997;9:517-524.

49. Mitchell MS, Harel W, Kempf RA, et al: Active-specific immunotherapy for melanoma. J Clin Oncol 1990;8:856-869.

50. McCune CS, Schapira DV, Henshaw EC: Specific immunotherapy of advanced renal carcinoma: Evidence for the polyclonality of metastases. Cancer 1981;47:1984-1987.

51. Vermorken JB, Claessen AM, van Tinteren H, et al: Active specific immunotherapy for stage II and stage III human colon cancer: A randomised trial [see comments]. Lancet 1999;353: 345-350.

52. Chang EY, Chen CH, Ji H, et al: Antigen-specific cancer immunotherapy using a GM-CSF secreting allogeneic tumor cell-based vaccine. Int J Cancer 2000;86:725-730.

53. Hernando JJ, Park TW, Kubler K, et al: Vaccination with autologous tumour antigen-pulsed dendritic cells in advanced gynaecological malignancies: Clinical and immunological evaluation of a phase I trial. Cancer Immunol Immunother 2002;51: 45-52.

54. Sosman JA, Sondak VK: Melacine: An allogeneic melanoma tumor cell lysate vaccine. Expert Rev Vaccines 2003;2:353-368.

55. Zhou Y, McEarchern JA, Howard E, et al: Dendritic cells efficiently acquire and present antigen derived from lung cancer cells and induce antigen-specific T-cell responses. Cancer Immunol Immunother 2003;52:413-422.

56. Repmann R, Goldschmidt AJ, Richter A: Adjuvant therapy of renal cell carcinoma patients with an autologous tumor cell lysate vaccine: A 5-year follow-up analysis. Anticancer Res 2003;23:969-974.

57. Steinman RM: The dendritic cell system and its role in immunogenicity. Annu Rev Immunol 1991;9:271-296.

58. Takahashi H, Nakagawa Y, Yokomuro K, et al: Induction of CD8+ CTL by immunization with syngeneic irradiated HIV-1 envelope derived peptide-pulsed dendritic cells. Int Immunol 1993;5:849-857.

59. Celluzzi CM, Mayordomo JI, Storkus WJ, et al: Peptide-pulsed dendritic cells induce antigen-specific CTL-mediated protective tumor immunity [see comments]. J Exp Med 1996;183: 283-287.

60. Mayordomo JI, Loftus DJ, Sakamoto H, et al: Therapy of murine tumors with p53 wild-type and mutant sequence peptide-based vaccines. J Exp Med 1996;183:1357-1365.

61. Ahlers JD, Dunlop N, Alling DW, et al: Cytokine-in-adjuvant steering of the immune response phenotype to HIV-1 vaccine constructs: Granulocyte-macrophage colony-stimulating factor and TNF-alpha synergize with IL-12 to enhance induction of cytotoxic T lymphocytes. J Immunol 1997;158:3947-3958.

62. Knutson KL, Curiel TJ, Salazar L, Disis ML: Immunologic principles and immunotherapeutic approaches in ovarian cancer. Hematol Oncol Clin North Am 2003;17:1051-1073.

63. Samanta A, LeVea CM, Dougall WC, et al: Ligand and p185c-neu density govern receptor interactions and tyrosine kinase activation. Proc Natl Acad Sci U S A 1994;91:1711-1715.

64. Olayioye MA, Neve RM, Lane HA, Hynes NE: The ErbB signaling network: receptor heterodimerization in development and cancer. EMBO J 2000;19:3159-3167.

65. Press MF, Jones LA, Godolphin W, et al: HER-2/neu oncogene amplification and expression in breast and ovarian cancers. Prog Clin Biol Res 1990;354A:209-221.

66. Slamon DJ, Godolphin W, Jones LA, et al: Studies of the HER-2/neu proto-oncogene in human breast and ovarian cancer. Science 1989;244:707-712.

67. Foy TM, Bannink J, Sutherland RA, et al: Vaccination with Her-2/neu DNA or protein subunits protects against growth of a Her-2/neu-expressing murine tumor. Vaccine 2001;19:2598-2606.

68. Ikuta Y, Okugawa T, Furugen R, et al: A HER2/NEU-derived peptide, a K(d)-restricted murine tumor rejection antigen, induces HER2-specific HLA-A2402-restricted CD8(+) cytotoxic T lymphocytes. Int J Cancer 2000;87:553-558.

69. Disis ML, Calenoff E, McLaughlin G, et al: Existent T-cell and antibody immunity to HER-2/neu protein in patients with breast cancer. Cancer Res 1994;54:16-20.

70. Peoples GE, Anderson BW, Lee TV, et al: Vaccine implications of folate binding protein, a novel cytotoxic T lymphocyte-recognized antigen system in epithelial cancers. Clin Cancer Res 1999;5:4214-4223.

71. Li PY, Del Vecchio S, Fonti R, et al: Local concentration of folate binding protein GP38 in sections of human ovarian carcinoma by in vitro quantitative autoradiography. J Nucl Med 1996; 37:665-572.

72. Kim DK, Lee TV, Castilleja A, et al: Folate binding protein peptide 191-199 presented on dendritic cells can stimulate CTL from ovarian and breast cancer patients. Anticancer Res 1999; 19:2907-2916.

73. Gendler SJ, Spicer AP: Epithelial mucin genes. Annu Rev Physiol 1995;57:607-634.

74. Taylor-Papadimitriou J, Burchell J, Miles DW, Dalziel M: MUC1 and cancer. Biochim Biophys Acta 1999;1455:301-313.

75. Brossart P, Schneider A, Dill P, et al: The epithelial tumor antigen MUC1 is expressed in hematological malignancies and is recognized by MUC1-specific cytotoxic T-lymphocytes. Cancer Res 2001;61:6846-6850.

76. Agrawal B, Krantz MJ, Reddish MA, Longenecker BM: Rapid induction of primary human CD4+ and CD8+ T cell responses against cancer-associated MUC1 peptide epitopes. Int Immunol 1998;10:1907-1916.

77. Agrawal B, Krantz MJ, Parker J, Longenecker BM: Expression of MUC1 mucin on activated human T cells: Implications for a role of MUC1 in normal immune regulation. Cancer Res 1998;58: 4079-4081.

78. Pecher G, Finn OJ: Induction of cellular immunity in chimpanzees to human tumor-associated antigen mucin by vaccination with MUC-1 cDNA-transfected Epstein-Barr virus-immortalized autologous B cells. Proc Natl Acad Sci U S A 1996;93:1699-1704.

79. Tempero RM, VanLith ML, Morikane K, et al: CD4+ lymphocytes provide MUC1-specific tumor immunity in vivo that is undetectable in vitro and is absent in MUC1 transgenic mice. J Immunol 1998;161:5500-5506.

80. Brossart P, Heinrich KS, Stuhler G, et al: Identification of HLA-A2-restricted T-cell epitopes derived from the MUC1 tumor antigen for broadly applicable vaccine therapies. Blood 1999;93:4309-4317.

81. Hodge JW, Tsang KY, Poole DJ, Schlom J: General keynote: Vaccine strategies for the therapy of ovarian cancer. Gynecol Oncol 2003;88:S97-S104; discussion, S110-S113.

82. Berchuck A, Kohler MF, Marks JR, et al: The p53 tumor suppressor gene frequently is altered in gynecologic cancers. Am J Obstet Gynecol 1994;170:246-252.

83. Oren M, Maltzman W, Levine AJ: Post-translational regulation of the 54K cellular tumor antigen in normal and transformed cells. Mol Cell Biol 1981;1:101-110.

84. Roth J, Dittmer D, Rea D, et al: P53 as a target for cancer vaccines: Recombinant canarypox virus vectors expressing p53 protect mice against lethal tumor cell challenge. Proc Natl Acad Sci U S A 1996;93:4781-4786.

85. Skipper J, Stauss HJ: Identification of two cytotoxic T lymphocyte-recognized epitopes in the ras protein. J Exp Med 1993; 177:1493-1498.

86. Lacabanne V, Viguier M, Guillet JG, Choppin J: A wild-type p53 cytotoxic T cell epitope is presented by mouse hepatocarcinoma cells. Eur J Immunol 1996;26:2635-2639.

87. Zeh H Jr, Leder GH, Lotze MT, et al: Flow-cytometric determination of peptide-class I complex formation: Identification of p53 peptides that bind to HLA-A2. Hum Immunol 1994; 39:79-86.

88. Stuber G, Leder GH, Storkus WT, et al: Identification of wild-type and mutant p53 peptides binding to HLA-A2 assessed by a peptide loading-deficient cell line assay and a novel major histocompatibility complex class I peptide binding assay. Eur J Immunol 1994;24:765-768.

89. Houbiers JG, Nijman HW, van der Burg SH, et al: In vitro induction of human cytotoxic T lymphocyte responses against peptides of mutant and wild-type p53. Eur J Immunol 1993;23:2072-2077.

90. Nijman HW, Houbiers JG, van der Burg SH, et al: Characterization of cytotoxic T lymphocyte epitopes of a self-protein, p53, and a non-self-protein, influenza matrix: Relationship between major histocompatibility complex peptide binding affinity and immune responsiveness to peptides. J Immunother 1993;14:121-126.

91. Gnjatic S, Bressac-de Paillerets B, Guillet JG, Choppin J: Mapping and ranking of potential cytotoxic T epitopes in the p53 protein: Effect of mutations and polymorphism on peptide binding to purified and refolded HLA molecules. Eur J Immunol 1995;25:1638-1642.

92. Ropke M, Hald J, Guldberg P, et al: Spontaneous human squamous cell carcinomas are killed by a human cytotoxic T lymphocyte clone recognizing a wild-type p53-derived peptide. Proc Natl Acad Sci U S A 1996;93:14704-14707.

93. Gnjatic S, Cai Z, Viguier M, et al: Accumulation of the p53 protein allows recognition by human CTL of a wild-type p53 epitope presented by breast carcinomas and melanomas. J Immunol 1998;160:328-333.

94. Theobald M, Biggs J, Hernandez J, et al: Tolerance to p53 by A2.1-restricted cytotoxic T lymphocytes. J Exp Med 1997;185:833-841.

95. Theobald M, Biggs J, Dittmer D, et al: Targeting p53 as a general tumor antigen. Proc Natl Acad Sci U S A 1995;92:11993-11997.

96. Holmberg LA, Sandmaier BM: Theratope vaccine (STn-KLH). Expert Opin Biol Ther 2001;1:881-891.

97. Kobayashi H, Terao T, Kawashima Y: [Circulating serum STN antigen as a prognostic marker in epithelial ovarian cancer]. Gan To Kagaku Ryoho 1991;18:1651-1655.

98. Kobayashi H, Terao T, Kawashima Y: Sialyl Tn as a prognostic marker in epithelial ovarian cancer. Br J Cancer 1992;66:984-985.

99. Kobayashi M, Fitz L, Ryan M, et al: Identification and purification of natural killer cell stimulatory factor (NKSF), a cytokine with multiple biologic effects on human lymphocytes. J Exp Med 1989;170:827-845.

100. Federici MF, Kudryashov V, Saigo PE, et al: Selection of carbohydrate antigens in human epithelial ovarian cancers as targets for immunotherapy: Serous and mucinous tumors exhibit distinctive patterns of expression. Int J Cancer 1999;81:193-198.

101. Singhal A, Fohn M, Hakomori S: Induction of alpha-N-acetylgalactosamine-O-serine/threonine (Tn) antigen-mediated cellular immune response for active immunotherapy in mice. Cancer Res 1991;51:1406-1411.

102. Fung PY, Madej M, Koganty RR, Longenecker BM: Active specific immunotherapy of a murine mammary adenocarcinoma using a synthetic tumor-associated glycoconjugate. Cancer Res 1990;50:4308-4314.

103. Slamon DJ, Leyland-Jones B, Shak S, et al: Use of chemotherapy plus a monoclonal antibody against HER2 for metastatic breast cancer that overexpresses HER2. N Engl J Med 2001;344:783-792.

104. Baselga J: Clinical trials of Herceptin (trastuzumab). Eur J Cancer 2001;37(Suppl 1):S18-S24.

105. Cuello M, Ettenberg SA, Clark AS, et al: Down-regulation of the erbB-2 receptor by trastuzumab (Herceptin) enhances tumor necrosis factor-related apoptosis-inducing ligand-mediated apoptosis in breast and ovarian cancer cell lines that overexpress erbB-2. Cancer Res 2001;61:4892-4900.

106. Bookman MA, Darcy KM, Clarke-Pearson D, et al: Evaluation of monoclonal humanized anti-HER2 antibody, trastuzumab, in patients with recurrent or refractory ovarian or primary peritoneal carcinoma with overexpression of HER2: A phase II trial of the Gynecologic Oncology Group. J Clin Oncol 2003;21:283-290.

107. Eagle K, Ledermann JA: Tumor markers in ovarian malignancies. Oncologist 1997;2:324-329.

108. Noujaim AA, Schultes BC, Baum RP, Madiyalakan R: Induction of CA125-specific B and T cell responses in patients injected with MAb-B43.13: Evidence for antibody-mediated antigen-processing and presentation of CA125 in vivo. Cancer Biother Radiopharm 2001;16:187-203.

109. Kirby TO, Huh W, Alvarez R: Immunotherapy of ovarian cancer. Expert Opin Biol Ther 2002;2:409-417.

110. Valone FH, Kaufman PA, Guyre PM, et al: Clinical trials of bispecific antibody MDX-210 in women with advanced breast or ovarian cancer that overexpresses HER-2/neu. J Hematother 1995;4:471-475.

111. Valone FH, Kaufman PA, Guyre PM, et al: Phase Ia/Ib trial of bispecific antibody MDX-210 in patients with advanced breast or ovarian cancer that overexpresses the proto-oncogene HER-2/neu. J Clin Oncol 1995;13:2281-2292.

112. Canevari S, Mezzanzanica D, Mazzoni A, et al: Bispecific antibody targeted T cell therapy of ovarian cancer: Clinical results and future directions. J Hematother 1995;4:423-427.

113. Longo DL, Duffey PL, Gribben JG, et al: Combination chemotherapy followed by an immunotoxin (anti-B4-blocked ricin) in patients with indolent lymphoma: Results of a phase II study. Cancer J 2000;6:146-150.

114. Pai LH, Bookman MA, Ozols RF, et al: Clinical evaluation of intraperitoneal *Pseudomonas* exotoxin immunoconjugate OVB3-PE in patients with ovarian cancer. J Clin Oncol 1991;9:2095-2103.

115. Xu F, Leadon SA, Yu Y, et al: Synergistic interaction between anti-p185HER-2 ricin A chain immunotoxins and radionuclide conjugates for inhibiting growth of ovarian and breast cancer cells that overexpress HER-2. Clin Cancer Res 2000;6:3334-3341.

116. Schmidt M, McWatters A, White RA, et al: Synergistic interaction between an anti-p185HER-2 pseudomonas exotoxin fusion protein [scFv(FRP5)-ETA] and ionizing radiation for inhibiting growth of ovarian cancer cells that overexpress HER-2. Gynecol Oncol 2001;80:145-155.

117. Bera TK, Williams-Gould J, Beers R, et al: Bivalent disulfide-stabilized fragment variable immunotoxin directed against mesotheliomas and ovarian cancer. Mol Cancer Ther 2001;1:79-84.

118. Hassan R, Viner JL, Wang QC, et al: Anti-tumor activity of K1-LysPE38QQR, an immunotoxin targeting mesothelin, a cell-surface antigen overexpressed in ovarian cancer and malignant mesothelioma. J Immunother 2000;23:473-479.

119. Disis ML, Grabstein KH, Sleath PR, Cheever MA: Generation of immunity to the HER-2/neu oncogenic protein in patients with breast and ovarian cancer using a peptide-based vaccine. Clin Cancer Res 1999;5:1289-1297.

120. Knutson KL, Schiffman K, Disis ML: Immunization with a HER-2/neu helper peptide vaccine generates HER-2/neu CD8 T-cell immunity in cancer patients. J Clin Invest 2001;107:477-484.

121. Brossart P, Wirths S, Stuhler G, et al: Induction of cytotoxic T-lymphocyte responses in vivo after vaccinations with peptide-pulsed dendritic cells. Blood 2000;96:3102-3108.

122. Yacyshyn MB, Poppema S, Berg A, et al: CD69+ and HLA-DR+ activation antigens on peripheral blood lymphocyte populations in metastatic breast and ovarian cancer patients: Correlations with survival following active specific immunotherapy. Int J Cancer 1995;61:470-474.

123. Reddish MA, MacLean GD, Poppema S, et al: Pre-immunotherapy serum CA27.29 (MUC-1) mucin level and CD69+ lymphocytes correlate with effects of Theratope sialyl-Tn-KLH cancer vaccine in active specific immunotherapy. Cancer Immunol Immunother 1996;42:303-309.

124. Zhao X, Wei YQ, Peng ZL: Induction of T cell responses against autologous ovarian tumors with whole tumor cell lysate-pulsed dendritic cells. Immunol Invest 2001;30:33-45.

125. Santin AD, Bellone S, Ravaggi A, et al: Induction of ovarian tumor-specific CD8+ cytotoxic T lymphocytes by acid-eluted peptide-pulsed autologous dendritic cells. Obstet Gynecol 2000;96:422-430.

126. Allavena P, Peccatori F, Maggioni D, et al: Intraperitoneal recombinant gamma-interferon in patients with recurrent

ascitic ovarian carcinoma: modulation of cytotoxicity and cytokine production in tumor-associated effectors and of major histocompatibility antigen expression on tumor cells. Cancer Res 1990;50:7318-7323.

127. Nehme A, Julia AM, Jozan S, et al: Modulation of cisplatin cytotoxicity by human recombinant interferon-gamma in human ovarian cancer cell lines. Eur J Cancer 1994;30A: 520-525.

128. Nardi M, Cognetti F, Pollera CF, et al: Intraperitoneal recombinant alpha-2-interferon alternating with cisplatin as salvage therapy for minimal residual-disease ovarian cancer: A phase II study. J Clin Oncol 1990;8:1036-1041.

129. Berek JS, Markman M, Stonebraker B, et al: Intraperitoneal interferon-alpha in residual ovarian carcinoma: A phase II gynecologic oncology group study. Gynecol Oncol 1999;75: 10-14.

130. Berek JS, Markman M, Blessing JA, et al: Intraperitoneal alpha-interferon alternating with cisplatin in residual ovarian carcinoma: A phase II Gynecologic Oncology Group study. Gynecol Oncol 1999;74:48-52.

131. Berek JS, Welander C, Schink JC, et al: A phase I-II trial of intraperitoneal cisplatin and alpha-interferon in patients with persistent epithelial ovarian cancer. Gynecol Oncol 1991;40: 237-243.

132. Feun LG, Blessing JA, Major FJ, et al: A phase II study of intraperitoneal cisplatin and thiotepa in residual ovarian carcinoma: A Gynecologic Oncology Group study. Gynecol Oncol 1998;71:410-415.

133. Frasci G, Tortoriello A, Facchini G, et al: Carboplatin and alpha-2b interferon intraperitoneal combination as first-line treatment of minimal residual ovarian cancer: A pilot study. Eur J Cancer 1994;30A:946-950.

134. Ferrari E, Maffeo DA, Graziano R, et al: Intraperitoneal chemotherapy with carboplatin and recombinant interferon alpha in ovarian cancer. Eur J Gynaecol Oncol 1994;15:437-442.

135. Bruzzone M, Rubagotti A, Gadducci A, et al: Intraperitoneal carboplatin with or without interferon-alpha in advanced ovarian cancer patients with minimal residual disease at second look: A prospective randomized trial of 111 patients. G.O.N.O. Gruppo Oncologic Nord Ovest. Gynecol Oncol 1997;65: 499-505.

136. Colombo N, Peccatori F, Paganin C, et al: Anti-tumor and immunomodulatory activity of intraperitoneal IFN-gamma in ovarian carcinoma patients with minimal residual tumor after chemotherapy. Int J Cancer 1992;51:42-46.

137. Guastalla JP, Pujade-Lauraine E, Colombo N, et al: [Intraperitoneal recombinant gamma interferon (RU 42369) efficacy in ovarian carcinomas. European BRM Study Group]. Pathol Biol (Paris) 1992;39:831-832.

138. Pujade-Lauraine E, Guastalla JP, Colombo N, et al: Intraperitoneal recombinant interferon gamma in ovarian cancer patients with residual disease at second-look laparotomy. J Clin Oncol 1996;14:343-350.

139. D'Acquisto R, Markman M, Hakes T, et al: A phase I trial of intraperitoneal recombinant gamma-interferon in advanced ovarian carcinoma. J Clin Oncol 1988;6:689-695.

140. Windbichler GH, Hausmaninger H, Stummvoll W, et al: Interferon-gamma in the first-line therapy of ovarian cancer: a randomized phase III trial. Br J Cancer 2000;82:1138-1144.

141. Edwards RP, Gooding G, D'Angelo G, et al: A phase II trial of intraperitoneal interleukin-2 demonstrates extended survival in taxane platinum refractory ovarian cancer. Proc ASCO 2003;22.

142. Freedman RS, Kudelka AP, Kavanagh JJ, et al: Clinical and biological effects of intraperitoneal injections of recombinant interferon-gamma and recombinant interleukin 2 with or without tumor-infiltrating lymphocytes in patients with ovarian or peritoneal carcinoma. Clin Cancer Res 2000;6:2268-2278.

143. Han X, Wilbanks GD, Devaja O, et al: IL-2 enhances standard IFNgamma/LPS activation of macrophage cytotoxicity to human ovarian carcinoma in vitro: A potential for adoptive cellular immunotherapy. Gynecol Oncol 1999;75:198-210.

144. Hurteau JA, Blessing JA, DeCesare SL, Creasman WT: Evaluation of recombinant human interleukin-12 in patients with recurrent or refractory ovarian cancer: A Gynecologic Oncology Group study. Gynecol Oncol 2001;82:7-10.

145. Berek JS: Interferon plus chemotherapy for primary treatment of ovarian cancer. Lancet 2000;356:6-7.

146. Munoz N, Bosch FX: The causal link between HPV and cervical cancer and its implications for prevention of cervical cancer. Bull Pan Am Health Organ 1996;30:362-377.

147. Zunzunegui MV, King MC, Coria CF, Charlet J: Male influences on cervical cancer risk. Am J Epidemiol 1986;123:302-307.

148. Arends MJ, Donaldson YK, Duvall E, et al: HPV in full thickness cervical biopsies: High prevalence in CIN 2 and CIN 3 detected by a sensitive PCR method. J Pathol 1991;165:301-309.

149. Schiffman MH, Bauer HM, Hoover RN, et al: Epidemiologic evidence showing that human papilloma virus infection causes most cervical intraepithelial neoplasia. J Natl Cancer Inst 1993;85:958-964.

150. Nindl I, Rindfleisch K, Lotz B, et al: Uniform distribution of HPV 16 E6 and E7 variants in patients with normal histology, cervical intra-epithelial neoplasia and cervical cancer. Int J Cancer 1999;82:203-207.

151. Khleif SN: Human papillomavirus therapy for the prevention and treatment of cervical cancer. Curr Treat Options Oncol 2003;4:111-119.

152. Lee AK, Eisinger M: Cell-mediated immunity (CMI) to human wart virus and wart-associated tissue antigens. Clin Exp Immunol 1976;26:419-424.

153. Chretien JH, Esswein JG, Garagusi VF: Decreased T cell levels in patients with warts. Arch Dermatol 1978;114:213-215.

154. Schneider V, Kay S, Lee HM: Immunosuppression as a high-risk factor in the development of condyloma acuminatum and squamous neoplasia of the cervix. Acta Cytol 1983;27:220-224.

155. Halpert R, Fruchter RG, Sedlis A, et al: Human papillomavirus and lower genital neoplasia in renal transplant patients. Obstet Gynecol 1986;68:251-258.

156. Laga M, Icenogle JP, Marsella R, et al: Genital papillomavirus infection and cervical dysplasia: Opportunistic complications of HIV infection. Int J Cancer 1992;50:45-48.

157. Kadish AS, Ho GY, Burk RD, et al: Lymphoproliferative responses to human papillomavirus (HPV) type 16 proteins E6 and E7: Outcome of HPV infection and associated neoplasia. J Natl Cancer Inst 1997;89:1285-1293.

158. Coleman N, Birley HD, Renton AM, et al: Immunological events in regressing genital warts. Am J Clin Pathol 1994; 102:768-774.

159. Okabayashi M, Angell MG, Christensen ND, Kreider JW: Morphometric analysis and identification of infiltrating leucocytes in regressing and progressing Shope rabbit papillomas. Int J Cancer 1991;49:919-923.

160. Vardy DA, Baadsgaard O, Hansen ER, et al: The cellular immune response to human papillomavirus infection. Int J Dermatol 1990;29:603-610.

161. Evans EM, Man S, Evans AS, Borysiewicz LK: Infiltration of cervical cancer tissue with human papillomavirus-specific cytotoxic T-lymphocytes. Cancer Res 1997;57:2943-2950.

162. Alexander M, Salgaller ML, Celis E, et al: Generation of tumor-specific cytolytic T lymphocytes from peripheral blood of cervical cancer patients by in vitro stimulation with a synthetic human papillomavirus type 16 E7 epitope. Am J Obstet Gynecol 1996;175:1586-1593.

163. Chen L, Thomas EK, Hu SL, et al: Human papillomavirus type 16 nucleoprotein E7 is a tumor rejection antigen. Proc Natl Acad Sci U S A 1991;88:110-114.

164. Feltkamp MG, Smits HL, Vierboom MP, et al: Vaccination with cytotoxic T lymphocyte epitope containing peptide protects against a tumor induced by human papillomavirus type 16-transformed cells. Eur J Immunol 1993;23:2242-2249.

165. Wadler S, Burk RD, Neuberg D, et al: Lack of efficacy of interferon-alpha therapy in recurrent, advanced cervical cancer. J Interferon Cytokine Res 1995;15:1011-1016.

166. Veerasarn V, Sritongchai C, Tepmongkol P, Senapad S: Randomized trial radiotherapy with and without concomitant 13-cis-retinoic acid plus interferon-alpha for locally advanced cervical cancer: A preliminary report. J Med Assoc Thai 1996;79:439-447.

167. Kirnbauer R, Booy F, Cheng N, et al: Papillomavirus L1 major capsid protein self-assembles into virus-like particles that are highly immunogenic. Proc Natl Acad Sci U S A 1992;89: 12180-12184.

168. Dvoretzky I, Shober R, Chattopadhyay SK, Lowy DR: A quantitative in vitro focus assay for bovine papilloma virus. Virology 1980;103:369-375.

169. Lowy DR, Schiller JT: Papillomaviruses: Prophylactic vaccine prospects. Biochim Biophys Acta 1999;1423:M1-M8.

170. Volpers C, Schirmacher P, Streeck RE, Sapp M: Assembly of the major and the minor capsid protein of human papillomavirus type 33 into virus-like particles and tubular structures in insect cells. Virology 1994;200:504-512.

171. Roden RB, Hubbert NL, Kirnbauer R, et al: Assessment of the serological relatedness of genital human papillomaviruses by hemagglutination inhibition. J Virol 1996;70:3298-3301.

172. Kirnbauer R, Taub J, Greenstone H, et al: Efficient self-assembly of human papillomavirus type 16 L1 and L1-L2 into virus-like particles. J Virol 1993;67:6929-6936.

173. Roden RB, Greenstone HL, Kirnbauer R, et al: In vitro generation and type-specific neutralization of a human papillomavirus type 16 virion pseudotype. J Virol 1996;70:5875-5883.

174. Suzich JA, Ghim SJ, Palmer-Hill FJ, et al: Systemic immunization with papillomavirus L1 protein completely prevents the development of viral mucosal papillomas. Proc Natl Acad Sci U S A 1995;92:11553-11557.

175. Jansen KU, Rosolowsky M, Schultz LD, et al: Vaccination with yeast-expressed cottontail rabbit papillomavirus (CRPV) virus-like particles protects rabbits from CRPV-induced papilloma formation. Vaccine 1995;13:1509-1514.

176. Breitburd F, Kirnbauer R, Hubbert NL, et al: Immunization with viruslike particles from cottontail rabbit papillomavirus (CRPV) can protect against experimental CRPV infection. J Virol 1995;69:3959-3963.

177. Pastrana DV, Vass WC, Lowy DR, Schiller JT: NHPV16 VLP vaccine induces human antibodies that neutralize divergent variants of HPV16. Virology 2001;279:361-369.

178. Koutsky LA, Ault KA, Wheeler CM, et al: A controlled trial of a human papillomavirus type 16 vaccine. N Engl J Med 2002;347:1645-1651.

179. Kast WM, Brandt RM, Sidney J, et al: Role of HLA-A motifs in identification of potential CTL epitopes in human papillomavirus type 16 E6 and E7 proteins. J Immunol 1994;152:3904-3912.

180. Kast WM, Brant RM, Drijfhout JW, et al: Human leukocyte antigen-A2.1 restricted candidate cytotoxic T lymphocyte epitopes of human papillomavirus type 16 E6 and E7 proteins identified by using the processing-defective human cell line T2. Immunotherapy 1993;14:115-120.

181. Ressing ME, van Driel WJ, Brandt RM, et al: Detection of T helper responses, but not of human papillomavirus-specific cytotoxic T lymphocyte responses, after peptide vaccination of patients with cervical carcinoma. J Immunother 2000;23:255-266.

182. Wojtowicz M, Hamilton JM, Khong H, et al: Vaccination of Cervical Cancer Patients with Papilloma Virus Type 16 E6 and E7 Peptides. Atlanta, GA, American Society of Clinical Oncology, 1999.

183. Muderspach L, Wilczynski S, Roman L, et al: A phase I trial of a human papillomavirus (HPV) peptide vaccine for women with high-grade cervical and vulvar intraepithelial neoplasia who are HPV 16 positive. Clin Cancer Res 2000;6:3406-3416.

184. Hunt S: Technology evaluation: HspE7, StressGen Biotechnologies Corp. Curr Opin Mol Ther 2001;3:413-417.

185. Palefsky JM, Goldstone LS, Boux LJ, Neefe JR: Pathological Response to Treatment with HspE7 in Anal Dysplasia of Multiple HPV types. New York, Cabcer Vaccine 2000, 2000.

186. Goldstone SE, Palefsky JM, Winnett MT, Neefe JR: Activity of HspE7, a novel immunotherapy, in patients with anogenital warts. Dis Colon Rectum 2002;45:502-507.

187. Murakami M, Gurski KJ, Marincola FM, et al: Induction of specific CD8+ T-lymphocyte responses using a human papillomavirus-16 E6/E7 fusion protein and autologous dendritic cells. Cancer Res 1999;59:1184-1187.

188. Borysiewicz LK, Fiander A, Nimako M, et al: A recombinant vaccinia virus encoding human papillomavirus types 16 and 18, E6 and E7 proteins as immunotherapy for cervical cancer [see comments]. Lancet 1996;347:1523-1527.

189. He Z, Wlazlo AP, Kowalczyk DW, et al: Viral recombinant vaccines to the E6 and E7 antigens of HPV-16. Virology 2000;270:146-161.

190. Koutsky LA, Ault KA, Wheeler CM, et al: A controlled trial of a human papillomavirus type 16 vaccine. N Engl J Med 2002;347:1645-1651.

191. Ringhoffer M, Schmitt M, Karbach J, et al: Quantitative assessment of the expression of melanoma-associated antigens by non-competitive reverse transcription polymerase chain reaction. Int J Oncol 2001;19:983-989.

192. Jager E, Ringhoffer M, Altmannsberger M, et al: Immunoselection in vivo: Independent loss of MHC class I and melanocyte differentiation antigen expression in metastatic melanoma. Int J Cancer 1997;71:142-147.

193. Herrin VE, Behrens RJ, Achtar MS, et al: Wild-type p53 peptide vaccine can generate a specific immune response in low burden ovarian adenocarcioma. American Society of Clinical Oncology Annual Meeting, Chicago, Illinois, 2003.

194. Colcher D, Esteban J, Carrasquillo JA, et al: Complementation of intracavitary and intravenous administration of a monoclonal antibody (B72.3) in patients with carcinoma. Cancer Res 1987;47:4218-4224.

195. Cobleigh MA, Vogel CL, Tripathy D, et al: Multinational study of the efficacy and safety of humanized anti-HER2 monoclonal antibody in women who have HER2-overexpressing metastatic breast cancer that has progressed after chemotherapy for metastatic disease. J Clin Oncol 1999;17:2639-2648.

196. Achtar MS, Behrens RJ, Herrin VE, et al: Mutant ras vaccine in advanced cancers. American Society of Clinical Oncolgy Annual Meeting, Chicago, Illinois, 2003.

197. Schlom J, Sabzevari H, Grosenbach DW, Hodge JW: A triad of costimulatory molecules synergize to amplify T-cell activation in both vector-based and vector-infected dendritic cell vaccines. Artif Cells Blood Substit Immobil Biotechnol 2003;31:193-228.

198. Steller MA, Gurski KJ, Murakami M, et al: Cell-mediated immunological responses in cervical and vaginal cancer patients immunized with a lipidated epitope of human papillomavirus type 16 E7. Clin Cancer Res 1998;4:2103-2109.

199. Simon RM, Steinberg SM, Hamilton M, et al: Clinical trial designs for the early clinical development of therapeutic cancer vaccines. J Clin Oncol 2001;19:1848-1854.

200. Cheever MA, Chen W:. Therapy with cultured T cells: Principles revisited. Immunol Rev 1997;157:177-194.

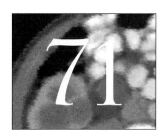

IMAGING OF GYNECOLOGIC MALIGNANCIES

Hedvig Hricak and Svetlana Mironov

 MAJOR CONTROVERSIES

- **Why imaging?**
- **What do we expect from imaging?**
- **Which imaging modality should be used?**
- **Is imaging cost-effective?**

Imaging has become an important adjunct to the clinical assessment of gynecologic cancer. It aids in tumor detection, characterization, staging, treatment planning, and follow-up. Imaging, integrated with clinical findings, can optimize cancer care and assist in the development of a treatment plan specific for the individual patient and extent of disease. The pretreatment evaluation of uterine (endometrial and cervical) and ovarian cancer has traditionally consisted of clinical evaluation, laboratory tests, and conventional radiographic studies (e.g., barium enema, intravenous pyelogram). Cross-sectional imaging is increasingly considered a necessary complement to other methods of tumor evaluation by either clinical or surgical assessment. Over the last two decades, advances in cross-sectional imaging—ultrasonography (US), computed tomography (CT), magnetic resonance imaging (MRI), and positron emission tomography (PET)—have yielded new insights into the evaluation of morphologic and metabolic tumor prognostic factors. As a tool in the evaluation of tumor location, volume, and extent, imaging can contribute to planning of the surgical approach, subspecialty referral, and alternative treatment management in patients with surgically nonresectable disease. Imaging continually evolves in response to changes in clinical practice and technologic improvement. The choice of imaging modality depends not only on the cancer site but also on local gynecology practice, radiology expertise, and equipment availability. An imaging study should never be ordered routinely but should be tailored to specific clinical questions that can be answered by the appropriate imaging test. Although the efficacy of diagnostic imaging in gynecologic oncology has been documented, imaging has not been incorporated into widespread gynecologic oncology practice. This chapter reviews controversies in the use of imaging for cancer of the endometrium, cervix, and ovary. For each cancer site, the potential value of imaging is examined in light of controversies and added value to patient management.

IMAGING MODALITIES USED IN GYNECOLOGIC ONCOLOGY

Modern Cross-Sectional Imaging

US, CT, MRI, and PET/CT are the main imaging modalities used in modern gynecologic oncologic imaging.

US is often the preferred initial imaging study in the evaluation of the female pelvis. In the evaluation of benign uterine masses or detection and characterization of an adnexal mass, US can be regarded as an extension of the physical examination. A combination of transabdominal and transvaginal US is 80% to 90% accurate in detecting adnexal masses.[1] The transvaginal approach improves the efficacy of US in the evaluation of pelvic pathology. Transvaginal US uses high-frequency probes placed into the vagina and allows high-resolution assessment of all pelvic organs (uterus and ovaries), peritoneal pouch, lower urinary tract, and pelvic side-wall without interference from bowel.

CT is used primarily for the preoperative staging and treatment planning of ovarian cancer, for the evaluation of advanced cancer of the endometrium and cervix, and for the detection of recurrent gynecologic malignancy.[2] In the evaluation of gynecologic disease, both oral and intravenous contrast administration are necessary. The advantages of CT are rapid acquisition time, lack of bowel motion artifact, and the ability to image organs during the peak of vascular enhancement, thus allowing differentiation between blood vessels and lymph nodes. The limitations of CT are difficulties in direct tumor visualization and differentiation between the tumor and normal uterine or cervical tissue. Assessment of early parametrial invasion in cervical cancer is limited. Advances in CT technology (e.g., multidetector scanners) are improving the ability of CT to detect and characterize primary gynecologic tumors. Multidetector CT uses thinner-section collimation and higher table speed per rotation, allowing better spatial and contrast resolution compared with single-detector helical CT. This improves detection of small lesions (<1.0 cm).

MRI is used in gynecologic malignancy for pretreatment evaluation of cervical and endometrial carcinoma and as an adjunct to US in the characterization of ovarian masses. The two types of coils most commonly used in pelvic imaging are the standard gradient body coil and the phased-array surface coil. Compared with body coils, phased-array coils provide better spatial resolution by improving the signal-to-noise ratio and contributing to field homogeneity. The use of either endoluminal coil (transvaginal or transrectal) improves visualization of small tumors of the uterine cervix; however, endoluminal coils did not significantly improve the accuracy of assessment of parametrial invasion.[3]

PET/CT imaging is an effective adjunct to CT and MRI for detecting distant metastases and evaluating treatment response.[4-6] Most PET/CT studies performed today are diagnostic fluorodeoxyglucose (FDG) scans, based on the elevated rate of glucose metabolism by cancer cells. The magnitude of elevated FDG uptake and accumulation within tumors is expressed by the standardized uptake value (SUV). An SUV value 2.5 times greater than normal suggest a malignant rather than a benign lesion. The ability to disinguish viable from necrotic tissue is an important application of PET. However, the difficulty of separating viable tumor from post-therapy inflammation reduces the reliability of FDG as a quantitative index of response. New, cancer-specific tracers under clinical investigation and in development are a promising tool for PET studies in tumor biology. Carbon 11 (^{11}C)-methionine is a radiotracer that differentiates tumor from normal tissue based on elevated protein synthesis in the tumor cell.[6,7] Radiolabeled fluorine 18 (^{18}F)-difluoroestradiol is another potential PET scanning agent under investigation as a noninvasive method to quantify hormone receptors. The selection of radiotracers for tumor diagnosis and follow-up depends on the organ site.

The continuing developments in radiotracer technology promise significant advances in gynecologic cancer care.

Conventional Radiologic Studies

Chest radiography is performed as a staging procedure to identify pleural effusion or pulmonary metastases, which occur in the late stages of gynecologic malignancies. Chest CT is superior to radiography for both of these indications and is becoming the mainstay for the radiologic evaluation of the thorax.

Intravenous urography (IVU) has been widely used for evaluation of suspected ureteral obstruction or iatrogenic injury during surgical procedures. However, cross-sectional techniques specifically CT, can demonstrate urinary obstruction or injury with better detail. The use of IVU is declining, and the new technique CT urography (CTU) is gaining acceptance. CTU demonstrates intrinsic and extrinsic causes of ureteral obstruction or injury, differentiating lymphadenopathy from solid-organ metastases, and in addition it demonstrates the degree of obstruction and its effect on the renal parenchyma.

Barium enema is also becoming an uncommon method in the radiologic assessment of gynecologic cancer. It is primarily reserved for patients in whom bowel resection is being considered and patients with equivocal findings on CT or MRI. Barium enema can be easily replaced by modern CT with coronal and sagittal reformatting of the volumetric CT data.

Hysterosalpingography has no role in the evaluation of a patient with pelvic malignancy. The test is indicated primarily in the assessment of infertility.

CANCER OF THE ENDOMETRIUM

Why imaging?

The International Federation of Gynaecologists and Obstetricians (FIGO) surgical staging system has been recommended for all patients with endometrial cancer since 1988. Whereas 80% of patients with endometrial cancer have stage I disease at the time of diagnosis and therefore are candidates for routine surgical treatment (simple hysterectomy and bilateral salpingo-oophorectomy), the remaining 20% either require more extensive surgery or are not surgical candidates. Even in patients with stage I disease, in addition to tumor grade, the decision to perform lymph node sampling or lymph node dissection depends on the depth of myometrial invasion, a finding that is difficult to determine from clinical data. The introduction of new treatments, such as hormone treatment for low-grade stage I tumor, poses new demands on pretreatment staging.[8] Imaging can assist in the evaluation of tumor location and extent, and it therefore can contribute to planning of the treatment approach and subspecialty referral. Preoperative identification of patients who could benefit from hormone therapy or from appropriate surgical expertise, if extensive surgery is required, is an all important challenge.

In the community setting, preoperative identification of deep myometrial invasion or spread beyond the uterus should assist in the decision of whether to refer the patient to a gynecologic oncologist.[9] In a tertiary center, detection of deep myometrial invasion indicates the need for lymph node dissection, and cancer extension to the cervix or beyond the corpus indicates the need for a more extensive surgical approach. Because not every patient is a candidate for surgery, findings from cross-sectional imaging can facilitate stratification of patients into surgical and nonsurgical (radiation and/or chemotherapy) treatment groups.

What do we expect from imaging?

The main role of imaging in the evaluation of endometrial cancer is the assessment of morphologic prognostic factors. The three main prognostic factors for endometrial cancer factors are depth of myometrial invasion, endocervical tumor extension, and lymph node status. The depth of myometrial invasion is probably the single most important morphologic prognostic factor, because it correlates with tumor grade, isthmus/cervix extension, and the incidence of nodal metastasis. It ultimately determines the surgical approach and patient survival.[10] Preoperative imaging in the evaluation of deep myometrial invasion, isthmus-cervix extension, and lymphadenopathy, as well as other extrauterine disease, is feasible and should be utilized as indicated.

Which imaging modality should be used?

Of the four modern cross-sectional imaging modalities, transabdominal US is not recommended in the staging of endometrial cancer. Reports on the use of endovaginal sonography (EVUS) in the evaluation of myometrial invasion have shown promise, but the disparity in the range of reported accuracy limits its widespread use (Fig. 71-1).[11] Furthermore, EVUS is not applicable for the assessment of cervical extension, lymph node status, or overall staging. Soft tissue contrast resolution is suboptimal because of similar echogenicity of tumor and the normal myometrium, cervical stroma, or coexisting benign pathology (e.g., uterine leiomyomata). Assessment of a large tumor is often precluded by the relatively small field of view. Furthermore, patients with endometrial carcinoma are often obese and of short stature, a physique that is well recognized as a limitation for the widespread use of US in this disease.

CT, including multidetector CT, has been preferred by the gynecologic community in the evaluation of endometrial carcinoma. The reported accuracy of CT in the assessment of myometrial invasion markedly varies and is generally poor.[12] The main limitation of CT has been in the assessment of cervical extension and overall staging. CT assessment of lymph node status is similar to that of MRI, with both modalities unable to differentiate enlarged metastatic from

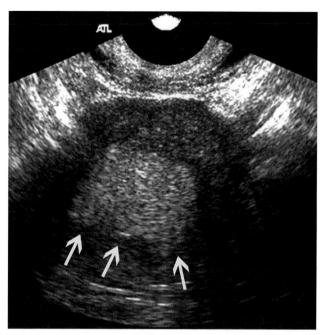

Figure 71-1. A 65-year-old woman with moderately differentiated endometrial carcinoma (endometriod type), stage FIGO Ib (T1b). Transverse endovaginal ultrasonographic image of the uterus demonstrates a hyperechoic mass with irregular tumor-myometrial interface *(arrows)*, consistent with superficial myometrial invasion.

hyperplastic nodes or to detect nodal disease in normal-sized nodes (Fig. 71-2).[13] There are no reports on the efficacy of multidetector CT in the evaluation of endometrial cancer.

A meta-analysis review showed that MRI provides the most accurate and consistent pretreatment evaluation of patients with endometrial cancer.[14,15] It is essential that the use of MRI include contrast enhancement. Intravenous contrast injection significantly improves the detection of endometrial abnormalities; the sensitivity of contrast-enhanced MRI is 88%, compared

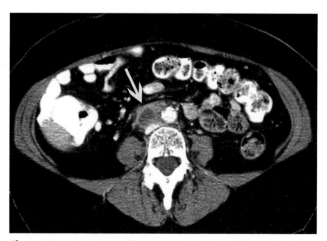

Figure 71-2. A 67-year-old woman with poorly differentiated endometrial carcinoma (endometrioid type), stage FIGO IIb (T2bN1). Contrast-enhanced computed tomographic scan demonstrates enlarged necrotic nodes in the aortocaval location *(arrow)*.

with 71% for nonenhanced MRI).[16] Assessment of the depth of myometrial invasion is also improved by the use of contrast media (Fig. 71-3). The positive predictive value for assessing deep myometrial invasion increases from 75% for noncontrast-enhanced scans to 95% for contrast-enhanced scans.[14,17-20] In the evaluation of myometrial invasion, review of the literature demonstrates that MRI is better than US or CT (accuracy of 92%, 40%, and 64%, respectively).

Tumor extension into the cervix is also better demonstrated by MRI than by either US or CT (see Fig. 71-3). A meta-analysis of the use of MRI for extent of tumor to the endocervix showed a sensitivity of 86% (range, 66% to 100%) and a specificity of 97% (range, 92% to 100%).[21] In the evaluation of lymph node metastases, CT and MRI have similar efficacies. Both modalities rely on an anatomic finding of nodal size (≥7 mm in short axis) and the number of detectable nodes. According to published reports, the detection of more than three nodes (located in the regional and juxtaregional sites), regardless of their size, correlates significantly with nodal involvement by tumor.[15]

Is imaging cost-effective?

Preoperative imaging has cost implications. No studies address the cost-effectiveness of the various imaging methods in endometrial cancer. However, net cost savings of MRI over frozen-section analysis have been

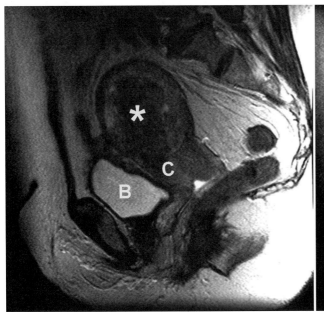

A

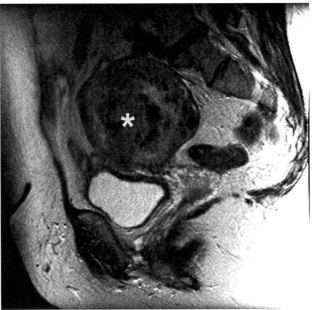

B

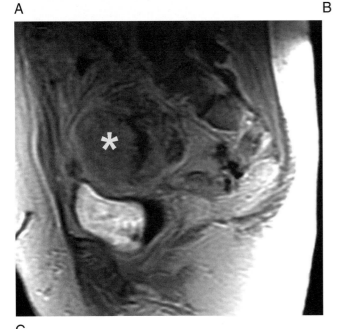

C

Figure 71-3. A 67-year-old woman with poorly differentiated endometrial carcinoma (endometrioid type), stage FIGO IIb (T2b). **A,** T2-weighted sagittal magnetic resonance image demonstrates a large endometrial tumor *(asterisk)* extending into the cervix (C). The urinary bladder (B) is not invaded. Corresponding sagittal plane T2-weighted **(B)** and gadolinium-enhanced T1-weighted **(C)** images demonstrate a large endometrial cancer *(asterisk)* with deep myometrial invasion anteriorly.

shown in the evaluation of myometrial invasion.[22] The use of MRI resulted in shorter operating room time and in an earlier forewarning of probable findings oncologic gynecologist.

Suggested Imaging Guidelines for Endometrial Cancer

In the staging (pretreatment) workup of endometrial cancer, imaging studies are requested only after a histologic diagnosis has been established. Based on the review of the literature, the following imaging guidelines are suggested:

1. The choice of the primary imaging modality should consider
   - The patient's pretest probability for myometrial invasion, cervical extension, or lymph node disease
   - The patient's body habitus
   - The local expertise of the physician in care of imaging
2. For patients with a low pretest probability of deep myometrial invasion (tumor grade 1)
   - No routine imaging is required if the uterus is normal size on physical examination unless non surgical treatment is contemplated (i.e., the diagnosis of stage Ia disease needs to be confirmed)
   - US (combined transabdominal and endovaginal approach) can be used for lower-grade tumors
   - MRI is suggested if US scans are technically inadequate or if US raises the suspicion of deep myometrial or endocervical extension
   - CT should be reserved for patients with contraindications to the use of MRI or in whom US demonstrates advanced disease
3. For patients with a high pretest probability of deep myometrial invasion (grade 2 or 3 tumor, papillary or clear cell tumor type), suggested cervical extension (bulky cervix or positive endocervical curettage), or lymph node metastases (high-grade tumor, papillary or clear cell tumor):
   - MRI offers a versatile single scan procedure for the evaluation of all prognostic factors
4. In patients for whom preoperative imaging is not used:
   - Intraoperative evaluation of the depth of myometrial invasion in the uterine specimen should be performed by gross visual inspection or frozen-section diagnosis
   - Appropriate surgical personnel should be available if deep myometrial invasion is encountered and lymph node sampling is required

▌ CANCER OF THE CERVIX

Why imaging?

Staging of cervical cancer is still based on clinical FIGO criteria. This includes findings by physical examination, colposcopy, lesion biopsy, and radiologic and endoscopic studies (chest radiography, cystoscopy, sigmoidoscopy, IVU, and barium enema).[23,24] FIGO clinical staging, compared with surgical staging, results in errors in 17% to 32% of cases in stage Ib disease and in up to 65% to 90% in stage III and IV disease.[25] The greatest difficulties in the clinical evaluation of patients with cervical cancer are the assessment of parametrial and pelvic sidewall invasion, the estimation of tumor size (especially if the tumor is primarily endocervical in location), and the evaluation of lymph node metastases. Pretreatment evaluation of these prognostic factors facilitates patient triage (surgery versus radiation therapy) in early disease.

What do we expect from imaging?

The assessment of cervical cancer prognostic parameters is critical to staging and appropriate treatment decisions. Critical prognostic factors in the treatment decision are tumor size, parametrial invasion, and lymph node status.[26] As in the case of endometrial cancer, a body of literature exists to show the efficacy of imaging in the evaluation of morphologic cervical cancer prognostic factors.

The official FIGO guidelines do not incorporate modern imaging findings (neither CT nor MRI) into the staging of invasive cervical cancer. However, as knowledge of cancer risk factors and the value of cross-sectional imaging have been disseminated, extended clinical staging systems have developed that include imaging findings. CT and MRI have gained acceptance in treatment planning, and the use of conventional radiologic examinations (IVU, barium enema, and lymphangiography) has decreased.[27] Examination under anesthesia as a staging test is also less frequently used, because the reported errors in staging of cervical cancer (18% to 25%) detract from its value.

Which imaging modality should be used?

Neither transabdominal US nor EVUS is recommended for the evaluation of cervical cancer. CT is recommended for suspected advanced disease, mostly for the evaluation of lymph node metastasis. MRI is the single best modality for the evaluation of cervical cancer prognostic factors (Fig. 71-4). A comparison of MRI and CT in the evaluation of parametrial invasion yielded the following data: accuracy, 85% to 93% versus 70% to 80%, respectively; sensitivity, 71% to 100% versus 50%; specificity, 46% to 87% versus 73% to 75%; positive predictive value, 28% to 77% versus 31% to 33%; and negative predictive value, 94% to 100% versus 67%.[30] The presence of a low-signal-intensity stripe of cervical stroma on T2-weighted MRI scans is 88% accurate in assessing parametrial invasion (Figs. 71-5 and 71-6).[28] In comparison with contrast-enhanced T1-weighted imaging, nonenhanced T2-weighted MRI demonstrates a higher accuracy in assessing the degree of invasion in the early stage of

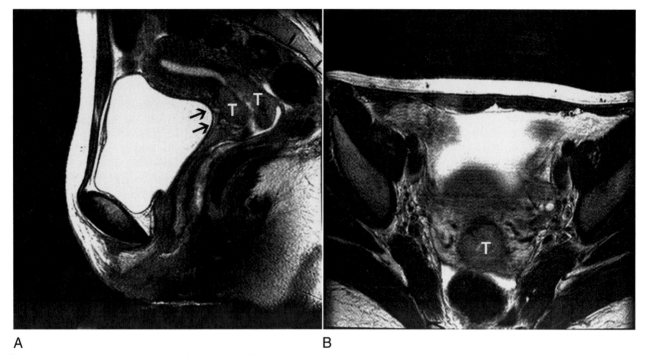

A   B

Figure 71-4. A 31-year-old woman with stage FIGO Ib (T1b) invasive adenocarcinoma of the cervix, mucinous type. **A,** Sagittal T2-weighted magnetic resonance image demonstrates large infiltrating cervical tumor (T) extending from the external to the internal os of the cervix. The tumor demonstrates full-thickness stromal invasion. The urinary bladder is not invaded, because the low-signal-intensity bladder wall is intact *(arrows)*. **B,** Axial T2-weighted image shows no evidence of parametrial invasion. T, tumor.

cervical cancer (57% versus 85%).[28,29] The high predictive value of MRI in determining the absence of parametrial invasion is valuable in identifying lesions that could be surgically resected (Fig. 71-7). MRI also demonstrates high accuracy in the detection of urinary bladder invasion by cervical carcinoma (sensitivity,

83%; specificity, 100%; accuracy, 99%), although bladder invasion is a very uncommon finding (Fig. 71-8).[30]

Compared with surgical staging, MRI is significantly better than CT (80% versus 63%, respectively).[31] Although the performance of MRI versus CT in the detection of nodal metastasis is considered to be

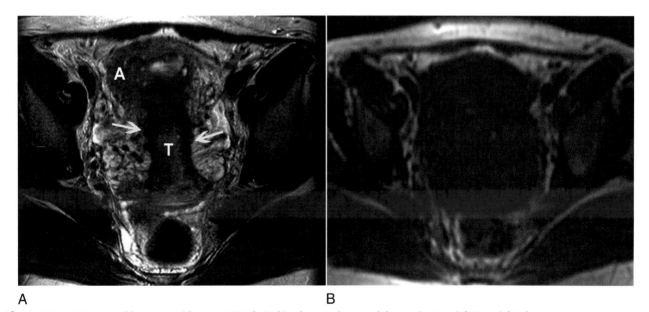

A   B

Figure 71-5. A 43-year-old woman with stage FIGO Ib (T1b) adenocarcinoma of the cervix. **A,** Axial T2-weighted magnetic resonance image shows a large tumor (T) in the endocervical canal. The low signal intensity of the cervical stroma on the right and left sides *(arrows)* is intact, indicating no parametrial invasion. Of note is widening of the junctional zone with high-signal-intensity foci within it, consistent with adenomyosis (A). **B,** T1-weighted image is inadequate for direct tumor visualization or evaluation of parametrial tumor extension.

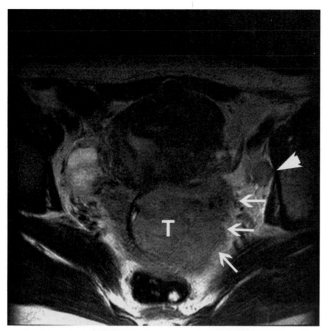

Figure 71-6. A 48-year-old woman with moderately differentiated squamous cell carcinoma of the cervix, stage FIGO IIb (T2bN1). Axial T2-weighted magnetic resonance image shows a large cervical tumor (T) with left-sided parametrial invasion *(arrows)* and enlarged obturator lymph node *(arrowhead)*.

similar,[30,33,34] significantly higher accuracy was shown for MRI (88%, versus 83% for CT; $P < .01$) in a single-institution report of 99 patients with cervical cancer.[35] This superiority was attributed to the higher contrast resolution and the ease of differentiating nodes, vascular

structures, and ovaries with MRI. Both MRI and CT rely on size criteria (nodal enlargement ≥7 mm) to diagnose lymphatic metastases, because of the inability of either modality to detect metastases in normal-size nodes. Furthermore, both techniques have a limited ability to differentiate between tumor and hyperplasia.[36] PET is being used increasingly in the initial evaluation of cervical cancer (mainly in the assessment of nodal disease). It's use has been reported for the evaluation of recurrent disease (Fig. 71-9).[4,7,37]

In addition to presurgical evaluation, imaging of the cervical cancer is used before treatment planning. Anatomic information from helical scanners yields consistent, high-quality images devoid of motion artifact; this is even more true for multidetector CT. MRI provides improved soft tissue contrast, relative to CT. In the evaluation of cervical cancer, MRI demonstrates the zonal anatomy of the cervix as well as tumor location, size, and local extent. However, MRI by itself may not be sufficient for treatment planning, because it does not provide anatomic information in terms of electron density, as needed for dose calculations. The combination of x-ray attenuation data from CT and tissue contrast from MRI provides a powerful planning tool when the images from the two modalities are spatially registered. Furthermore, information on tumor vascularity based on contrast-enhanced MRI has been used as a prognostic factor in the treatment of cervical cancer.

Another modality that has been used in cervical cancer treatment planning is FDG PET. Initial data are very encouraging but prospective, multi-institutional studies, wide availability of technology, and further

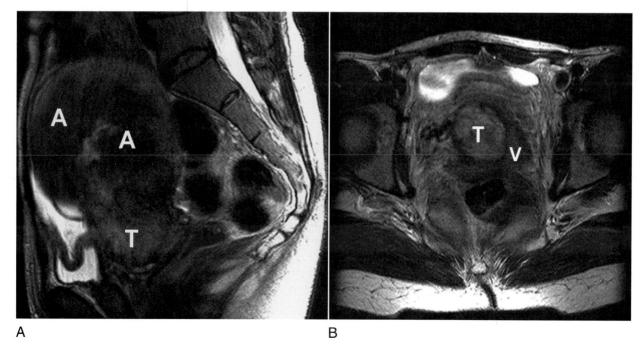

A   B

Figure 71-7. Adenomyosis and cervical adenocarcinoma with squamous differentiation, stage FIGO Ib (T1b), in a 47-year-old woman with a history of exposure to diethylstilbestrol (DES). On clinical examination, the uterus was markedly enlarged. **A,** Sagittal T2-weighted magnetic resonance image shows enlarged uterus with diffuse widening of the junctional zone, consistent with diffuse adenomyosis (A). Cervical tumor (T) measures 3 cm in the transverse diameter. **B,** Axial T2-weighted image demonstrates mass within the cervix (T); the outer cervical stroma is intact and demonstrates low signal intensity. There is no parametrial invasion. V, posterior fornix of the vagina.

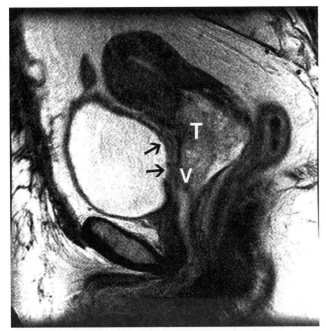

Figure 71-8. A 56-year-old woman with invasive, well-differentiated cervical adenocarcinoma, stage FIGO IVa (T4a) adenocarcinoma. Sagittal T2-weighted magnetic resonance image demonstrates large cervical tumor (T) with full-depth stromal invasion and tumor extension to the anterior fornix of the vagina (V) and urinary bladder (arrows).

technical improvements (e.g., ability to use respiratory gating so that tumor volume measurements can be used) are needed before PET scanning can be widely recommended.[38]

Is imaging of cervical cancer cost-effective?

Cost analysis of the diagnostic tests recommended by FIGO for clinical stage Ib disease demonstrated that the routine use of cystoscopy, proctoscopy, barium enema, or IVU is not justified.[39] All these studies can be replaced by a single cross-sectional imaging examination such as MRI.

By avoiding additional testing such as examination under anesthesia, IVU, cystoscopy, and proctoscopy, the initial use of MRI results in fewer tests and invasive procedures.[39] The judicious use of MRI, despite its relatively high cost, results in cost minimization and net cost savings, compared with the conventional diagnostic workup recommended by FIGO.[39]

Suggested Imaging Guidelines for Cervical Cancer

In formulating diagnostic guidelines, we have considered test efficacy defined by accuracy, sensitivity and specificity, and incremental change from pretest to post-test probabilities for the specific clinical question.

1. For extended clinical staging, CT and MRI are not recommended routinely. The decision as to whether

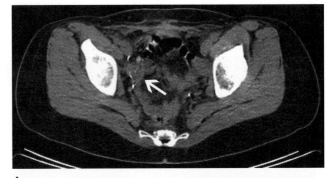

A

B

Figure 71-9. A 34-year-old woman with stage FIGO Ia (T1a) adenocarcinoma of the cervix, treated with total abdominal hysterectomy and pelvic/retroperitoneal lymph node dissection. Positron emission tomography (PET) with computed tomography (CT) demonstrates the utility of this modality for detection of recurrent tumors. **A,** CT part of the PET/CT examination shows a 2-cm mass (arrow) adjacent to the surgical clips on the right. **B,** This mass (arrow) demonstrates increased uptake of fluorodeoxyglucose (FDG) on FDG-PET part of the study, indicating tumor recurrence.

to use imaging is based on tumor size and the pretest probability of parametrial or nodal disease.
2. For the assessment of tumor size, MRI is the recommended imaging approach because it allows direct tumor visualization.
3. For a tumor size smaller than 2 cm, the data suggest that neither CT nor MRI is justified.

4. MRI is recommended as the initial examination of choice for clinical stage Ib disease with a tumor diameter greater than 2 cm, or for an endocervical tumor location.

5. In most patients, MRI alone provides sufficient information for initial patient management.[39] If the MRI findings are equivocal for urinary bladder or rectal invasion, endoscopic studies should be performed. CT-guided biopsy is warranted if enlarged lymph nodes are detected by MRI and a histologic diagnosis is essential for treatment decision-making.

The value of imaging increases with larger tumor size and more advanced stage, for which an accurate definition of the disease optimizes treatment planning. MRI is significantly better than CT in identifying operable candidates. Furthermore, MRI provides valuable data on concomitant pelvic masses and is suitable for the evaluation of pregnant patients, because it poses no known radiation risk to the fetus. If preoperative imaging is considered, MRI is preferred to CT. The use of "expensive" high technology imaging upfront achieves better patient care at a lower cost.

OVARIAN CANCER

Why imaging?

The imaging findings that are critical for the management of ovarian cancer may be divided into those related to characterization of the primary tumor, identification of metastatic disease to decrease understaging, identification of disease that may be an indication for neoadjuvant chemotherapy, detection of cancer recurrence, and evaluation of the feasibility for secondary cytoreduction. In each category, there are a number of clinical challenges for which imaging information can be used as an adjunct to clinical and laboratory evaluation.

If an adnexal lesion is detected, lesion characterization (benign versus malignant) assists in treatment planning and subspecialty referral. A benign lesion can be resected by a general gynecologist, but malignant lesions require surgical staging and referral to a gynecologic oncologist.

Approximately 30% of ovarian cancers are understaged during primary surgery.[39] The main reasons for understaging are the assumption that the lesion is benign, the presence of a much greater disease extent than initially expected, and the failure to perform a selective retroperitoneal lymphadenectomy.[23,24,39,40] Identification of ovarian metastases by imaging helps prevent understaging, guides subspecialist referral, and assists surgical planning.

Modern management of ovarian cancer is related to the stage and extent of disease and includes surgery and neoadjuvant chemotherapy (in patients with nonresectable disease) or primary chemotherapy (in patients with stage IV disease).[23,24,40-46] The standard of care for FIGO stage Ia through IIIb ovarian cancer is comprehensive staging laparotomy. The standard of care for resectable FIGO stage IIIc ovarian cancer is

primary surgical cytoreduction (i.e., debulking), followed by the adjuvant combination chemotherapy with a platinum compound and paclitaxel. Optimal debulking refers to the reduction of all tumor sites to a maximal diameter of less than 1 cm. The management of FIGO stage IV disease is primary chemocytoreduction.[23,24,40-46]

In considering the various management options, the importance of imaging lies in distinguishing between FIGO stage IIIc and stage IV disease.[47] In making this distinction, there are two important issues in imaging. First, the most common finding indicative of stage IV disease is a malignant pleural effusion. However, the radiologic detection of a pleural effusion is not in itself sufficient to constitute stage IV disease; the effusion must be demonstrated to be malignant. CT rarely contributes to the determination of whether an effusion is benign or malignant, except when pleural thickening or nodules are identified (Fig. 71-10). Another important distinction is the differentiation of liver surface implants (peritoneal spread—stage III) from true intraparenchymal liver metastases (hematogenous spread—stage IV). Surface implants are usually well defined, biconvex, and peripheral, and they indent the liver rather than replace liver parenchyma (Fig. 71-11). True intraparenchymal metastases are often ill-defined, circular, and partially or completely surrounded by liver tissue (Fig. 71-12).

In the category of FIGO stage IIIc disease, the importance of imaging is in establishing the presence of nonresectable disease.[47-51] In practice, the percentage of advanced ovarian cancers that are successfully (i.e., optimally) debulked varies from 17% to 87%.[52] This wide variation most likely reflects differences in surgical expertise, but it indicates that even in tertiary centers a significant fraction of patients have inoperable disease

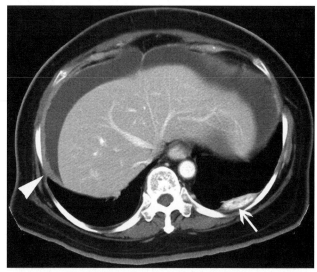

Figure 71-10. A 63-year-old woman with ovarian cancer who presented with left pleural effusion. Computed tomographic scan after thoracic synthesis demonstrates enhancing left pleural mass (*arrow*), indicating FIGO stage IV disease. Also demonstrated is irregular nodular peritoneal thickening (*arrowhead*) and ascites.

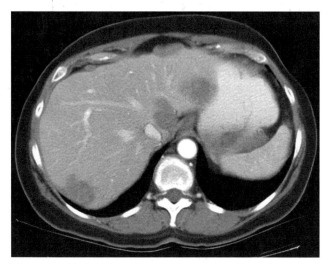

Figure 71-11. A 56-year-old woman with stage IIIc ovarian carcinoma. Contrast-enhanced computed tomogram shows extensive liver surface and subcapsular liver implants.

and gain no benefit from primary cytoreduction.[41] The optimal management of ovarian cancer that is considered inoperable is not established, but a review of the clinical and radiologic literature suggests that neoadjuvant (i.e., preoperative) chemotherapy with interval (or delayed) cytoreductive surgery after tumor shrinkage is a viable management option meriting a randomized controlled trial[44,45] and that cross-sectional imaging can help treatment planning by identifying, with a high degree of accuracy, patients with probable inoperable disease.[50,51] There is no agreement on the established surgical criteria that indicate inoperable disease. Some institutions consider radical surgery appropriate to achieve optimal debulking, even if it

includes resection of the liver, spleen, or kidneys.[42] Therefore, the role of imaging is not to describe disease as resectable or unresectable, but rather to describe the findings that are important for surgical management, so as to alert the surgeon to extensive disease that indicates complex surgery or the indications neoadjuvant chemotherapy. Findings that are important for surgical planning and the decision for probable inoperable disease are invasion of the pelvic sidewall and, in the abdomen, tumor deposits greater than 1 to 2 cm in the gastrosplenic ligament, gastrohepatic ligament, lesser sac, fissure for the ligamentum teres, porta hepatis, subphrenic space, small bowel mesentery, or retroperitoneum above the renal hila (Fig. 71-13).[46,50,51] These imaging findings directly influence clinical management, and therefore imaging plays a key role in optimizing patient-specific care.

Which imaging modality should be used?

Characterization of adnexal lesions. In patients with a known or suspected adnexal mass, US is highly accurate in the assessment of tumor location (e.g., differentiation of uterine from adnexal masses) and in distinguishing between a benign and a malignant adnexal lesion (Fig. 71-14). The optimal use of US requires the analysis of morphologic features and Doppler findings.[53-55] Despite recent advances in US technology, there are still a number of adnexal lesions classified as equivocal or indeterminate, particularly in cases of endometrioma and cystic teratoma. In the setting of sonographically indeterminate adnexal masses, MRI is recommended for further evaluation.[56-59] In both a prospective study and a meta-analysis review, the efficacy of MRI was shown to be superior to that of either US or CT in the characterization of

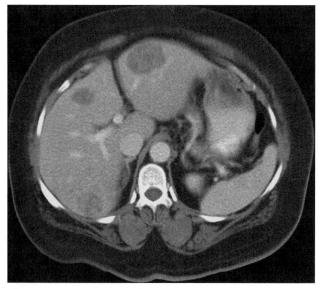

Figure 71-12. A 67-year-old woman with stage IV ovarian carcinoma. Contrast-enhanced computed tomogram demonstrates intraparenchymal liver metastasis.

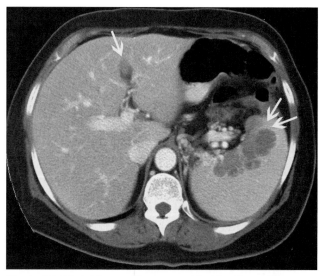

Figure 71-13. A 66-year-old woman with stage IIIc papillary serous carcinoma. Contrast-enhanced computed tomogram shows disease present in the fissure of the ligamentum teres *(arrow)*, in the gastrosplenic ligament, and in the splenic hilum *(arrows)*.

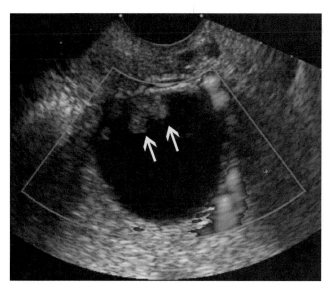

Figure 71-14. A 56-year-old woman with a clinically palpable left adnexal mass. Ultrasound study shows a cystic lesion with papillary projections *(arrows)*; Doppler imaging demonstrated flow within the papillary projection. The findings indicate a malignant lesion.

adnexal masses.[53,60,61] When MRI is used, the performance is considerably better if gadolinium contrast material is administered (Fig. 71-15).[58] The use of contrast media allows a better characterization of solid nodules within a cystic lesion or demonstration of the presence of necrosis within a solid lesion. In the characterization of adnexal masses, MRI also shows high interobserver and intraobserver agreement.

Although CT has not traditionally been used in the characterization of an adnexal mass, studies have shown that the utility of CT is equivalent to that of US. CT characterization of adnexal masses (similar to US and MRI) relies on the depiction of morphologic features with mural nodularity or heterogeneity and necrosis within the solid lesion. The presence of ancillary findings such as ascites or peritoneal implants is a strong indicator of malignant etiology of an adnexal mass by either US, CT, or MRI (Fig. 71-16).

The use of PET imaging with current radiotracers (FDG) can be applied to the characterization of adnexal masses, but its efficacy is not contributory after US and MRI findings are evaluated.[62] However, new tracers such as ^{11}C-methionine (cell membrane proliferation tracer), used for the assessment of tumor aggressiveness, may be of use in the future.

Ovarian cancer staging. Ovarian cancer spreads primarily by local continuity to the opposite ovary (6% to 13%), to the uterus (5% to 25%), and to the adjacent structures such as the sigmoid colon, urinary bladder, and pelvic sidewall.

Peritoneal dissemination is the most common route of ovarian cancer spread. The presence of nodal metastases in ovarian cancer is an important feature. The frequency of nodal metastases in a patient with T1 or T2

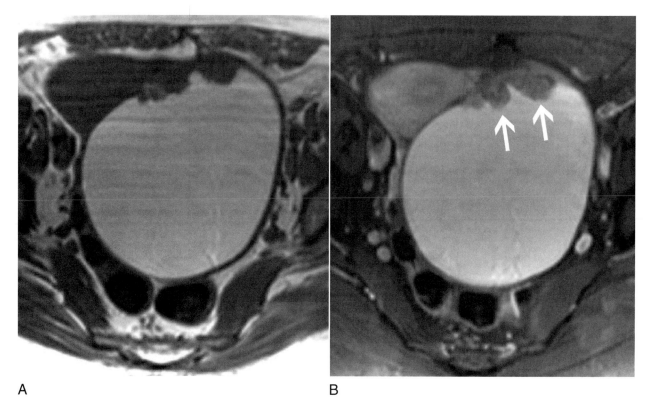

A   B

Figure 71-15. A 66-year-old woman with sonographically indeterminate left adnexal mass. Axial T1-weighted magnetic resonance image **(A)** and contrast-enhanced, fat-suppressed T1-weighted image **(B)** demonstrate a hemorrhagic lesion with enhancing papillary projections *(arrows)*. The findings indicate that the lesion is malignant. At surgery, it was found to be a clear cell carcinoma present within an endometrioma.

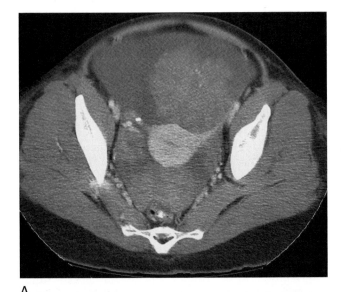

A

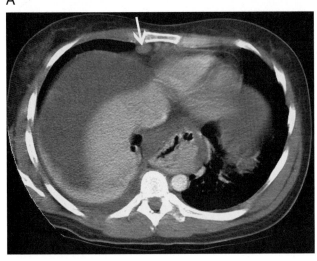

B

Figure 71-16. Contrast-enhanced computed tomograms of a 31-year-old woman with immature ovarian teratoma. **A,** Image though the pelvis demonstrates bilateral irregular adnexal masses with calcifications and malignant ascites. **B,** Image of the upper abdomen demonstrates supra- diaphragmatic adenopathy *(arrow),* indicating unresectable disease and a grave prognosis.

disease is 15% to 17%; it rises to 64% in those with M1 disease. In ovarian cancer patients, the use of a size threshold of 1 cm or greater in the short axis to define malignant adenopathy by CT showed a disappointingly low sensitivity of only 50%. However, the specificity with that threshold was as high as 95%.[48,63]

Stage M1 disease refers to the presence of metastases outside the peritoneal cavity, including hematogenous spread (most commonly liver and lung), and lymph node disease beyond the regional nodal spread. Among those with distant nodal disease, supra-diaphragmatic adenopathy is detected in approximately 15% to 28% of patients with advanced ovarian cancer (see Fig. 71-16).[64]

Although M1 disease at the time of diagnosis is rare, the common sites of distant metastasis at autopsy include liver (45% to 48%), lung (34% to 39%), pleura

(25%), adrenal gland (21%), and spleen (20%); bone and brain metastases are found in fewer than 10% of these cases.[65] The knowledge of the frequency of distant metastases in ovarian cancer guides the imaging algorithm for patient surveillance.

In ovarian cancer site-specific metastatic disease, CT is superior to MRI in the evaluation of peritoneal metastases (Fig. 71-17).[48,66] Nonhelical CT in the diagnosis of peritoneal metastases in ovarian cancer has a sensitivity of 63% to 79% and a specificity of 100%. The use of helical CT improves the CT performance, demonstrating a sensitivity of 85% to 93% and a specificity of 78% to 96%.[49,66] This increased accuracy probably reflects the increasing use of thinner sections and the absence of slice misregistration artifact on helical CT, which aids the detection of small implants and helps in distinguishing unopacified bowel from tumor implants (Fig. 71-18). However, implants measuring 1 cm or less remain difficult to detect, and for these lesions the CT sensitivity decreases to less than 50%.[66]

In the evaluation of nodal disease, using a size threshold of 1 cm in the short axis, the sensitivity (50%) and specificity (95%) of preoperative CT are similar to those of MRI. Although enlarged nodes are likely to be metastatic, CT and MRI are unable to exclude disease in nonenlarged nodes.

In the evaluation of liver parenchymal metastases, the performance of CT and that of MRI are similar. In the setting of preexisting liver disease, MRI may be superior to CT.

In summary, the value of imaging is in integration of the radiologic findings with the clinical presentation, so as to optimize patient care and develop a tailored, patient-specific management plan. Although CT is the primary modality for the staging of ovarian cancer, the Radiologic Diagnostic Oncology Group (RDOG) study showed that MRI may be equally or even more accurate than CT.[63] However, the use of MRI is currently limited by expense, lack of availability, prolonged scanning time, and the relative shortage of physicians with adequate reading experience.

Is imaging cost-effective?

In the characterization of an ovarian lesion, both a cost-benefit study and a net cost analysis showed that the use of MRI in the evaluation of sonographically indeterminate adnexal lesions resulted in fewer surgical procedures, better patient triage, and net cost savings.[64,65] There are no data on the cost benefit of imaging in staging or treatment follow-up.

Ovarian Cancer Treatment Follow-Up

The role of imaging in the evaluation of ovarian cancer after the initial treatment has not been thoroughly investigated. The use of imaging to monitor treatment has not reached a consensus. CT is considered to be the primary imaging modality in ovarian cancer treatment

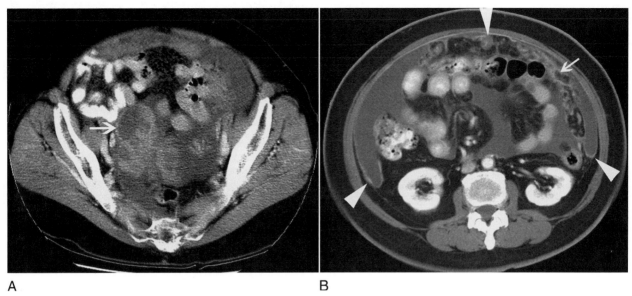

A   B

Figure 71-17. Contrast-enhanced computed tomograms of a 67-year-old woman with high-grade ovarian adenocarcinoma, endometrioid type, demonstrating bilateral irregular adnexal masses. **A,** The presence of solid components within a cystic lesion *(arrow)* is strongly suggestive of the malignant nature of these lesions. **B,** In the abdomen, the presence of ancillary findings such as nodular enhancement of peritoneum *(arrowhead)*, ascites, and omental nodules *(arrow)* are consistent with FIGO stage III disease.

follow-up.[67,68] The practice of obtaining a baseline CT scan after completion of the initial treatment is gaining acceptance. Currently, a combination of physical examination findings, CA-125 levels, and findings on CT scan of the abdomen and pelvis are considered to be an effective method to follow up patients with ovarian cancer. Chest CT should be eliminated from the routine follow up, because chest CT has been shown to be valuable only in patients who have elevated serum tumor markers but no evidence of abdominal or pelvic disease.[69,70,74] PET/CT is rapidly gaining acceptance. The initial data show an outstanding performance in the detection of recurrent disease.

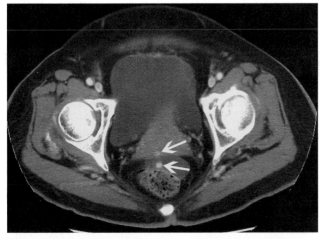

Figure 71-18. A 63-year-old woman with ovarian carcinoma. Contrast-enhanced computed tomogram shows enhancing nodules in cul-de-sac *(arrows)*, outlined by small amount of ascites.

Suggested Imaging Guidelines in Ovarian Cancer Treatment Follow-Up

1. The role of imaging in persistent disease and platinum-resistant disease is limited unless the patient develops acute clinical symptoms (e.g., bowel or urinary obstruction).

2. In refractory, unresponsive, or progressive tumors, imaging is rarely used unless clinical symptoms develop (e.g., bowel or urinary obstruction). However, in this patient cohort imaging can be used to document disease progression and can potentially assist in the development of new treatment regimens.

3. In recurrent ovarian cancer, the treatment depends on tumor bulk and extent and may include surgical debulking, chemotherapy or palliation, to medical therapy.[71-73,75] In this patient group, survival benefit is seen only if cytoreduction is optimal. Therefore, pretreatment identification of unresectable recurrent cancer is clinically relevant, assisting in management and outcome. Survival rates after attempted secondary cytoreduction vary from 17% to 62%.[23] To spare the patient unnecessary surgery, an attempt should be to predict resectability preoperatively.[76] As in primary ovarian cancer, bulky upper-abdominal disease, such as disease in the gastrohepatic ligament, gastrosplenic ligament, gallbladder fossa, or perisplenic location, precludes optimal surgical debulking. If the upper-abdominal disease is deemed resectable (Fig. 71-19) and the bulk of the tumor burden is in the pelvis, some patients are selected for secondary cytoreduction. A study evaluating the role of helical CT in patients undergoing secondary cytoreduction showed that the significant indicators of tumor nonresectability in recurrent disease of the pelvis are the presence of hydronephrosis

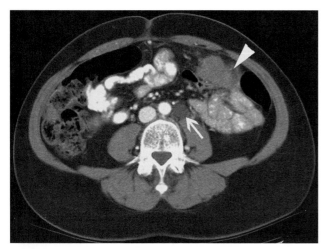

Figure 71-19. A 56-year-old woman with recurrent ovarian cancer. Contrast-enhanced computed tomogram demonstrates retroperitoneal adenopathy *(arrow)* and mesenteric implant adjacent to bowel loops *(arrowhead)*, indicating the need for bowel resection.

and pelvic sidewall invasion (Fig. 71-20).[72] The size of a pelvic mass is not an indicator of tumor nonresectability.[72] However, extension of a mass into the pelvic sidewall is indicative of surgical outcome. The presence of large-bowel obstruction is a strong indication of tumor nonresectability. In fact, in the presence of large-bowel obstruction, a second cytoreductive surgery is usually replaced by palliative approaches.[72]

In summary, in patients with recurrent ovarian cancer considered for secondary cytoreductive surgery, preoperative CT identifies the presence and extent of disease. Furthermore, it points out indicators of tumor nonresectability that affect management, tailor the surgical approach, and consequently have an impact on patient survival.

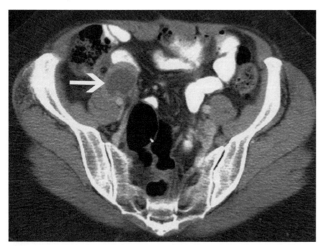

Figure 71-20. A 66-year-old woman with recurrent papillary serous adenocarcinoma. Computed tomogram demonstrates recurrent tumor *(arrow)* inseparable from the psoas muscle and the common iliac vessels.

REFERENCES

1. Kurtz AB, Tsimikas JV, Tempany CM, et al: Diagnosis and staging of ovarian cancer: Comparative values of Doppler and conventional US, CT, and MR imaging correlated with surgery and histopathologic analysis. Report of the Radiology Diagnostic Oncology Group. Radiology 1999;212:19-27.
2. Yu KK, Hricak H, Subak LL, et al: Preoperative staging of cervical carcinoma: Phased array coil fast spin-echo versus body coil spin-echo T2-weighted MR imaging. AJR Am J Roentgenol 1998;171:707-711.
3. Kim MJ, Chung JJ, Lee YH, et al: Comparison of the use of the transrectal surface coil and the pelvic phased-array coil in MR imaging for preoperative evaluation of uterine cervical carcinoma. AJR Am J Roentgenol 1997;168:1215-1221.
4. Umesaki N, Tanaka T, Miyama M, et al: The role of 18F-fluoro-2-deoxy-D-glucose positron emission tomography (18F-FDG-PET) in the diagnosis of recurrence and lymph node metastasis of cervical cancer. Oncol Rep 2000;7:1261-1264.
5. Makhija S, Howden N, Edwards R, et al: Positron emission tomography/computed tomography imaging for the detection of recurrent ovarian and fallopian tube carcinoma: A retrospective review. Gynecol Oncol 2002;85:53-58.
6. Suguwara Y, Eisbruch A, Kosuda S, et al: Evaluation of FDG PET in patients with cervical cancer. J Nucl Med 1999;40:1125-1131.
7. Lapela M, Leskinen-Kallio S, Varpula M, et al: Imaging of uterine carcinoma by carbon-11-methionine and PET. J Nucl Med 1994;35:1618-1623.
8. Montz FJ, Bristow RE, Bovicelli A, et al: Intrauterine progesterone treatment of early endometrial cancer. Am J Obstet Gynecol 2002;186:651-657.
9. Frei KA, Kinkel K, Bonel HM, et al: Prediction of deep myometrial invasion in patients with endometrial cancer: Clinical utility of contrast-enhanced MR imaging. A meta-analysis and Bayesian analysis. Radiology 2000;216:444-449.
10. Atsukawa H, Sasaki H, Tada S: A multivariate analysis of assessment of myometrial invasion of endometrial carcinoma by magnetic resonance imaging. Gynecol Oncol 1994;54:298-306.
11. Artner A, Bosze P, Gonda G: The value of ultrasound in preoperative assessment of the myometrial and cervical invasion in endometrial carcinoma. Gynecol Oncol 1994;54:147-151.
12. Hardesty LA, Sumkin JH, Hakim C, et al: The ability of helical CT to preoperatively stage endometrial carcinoma. AJR Am J Roentgenol 2001;176:603-606.
13. Connor JP, Andrews JI, Anderson B, Buller RE: Computed tomography in endometrial carcinoma. Obstet Gynecol 2000;95:692-696.
14. Kinkel K, Kaji Y, Yu KK, et al: Radiologic staging in patients with endometrial cancer: A meta-analysis. Radiology 1999;212:711-718.
15. Hricak H, Rubinstein LV, Gherman GM, Karstaedt N: MR imaging evaluation of endometrial carcinoma: Results of an NCI cooperative study. Radiology 1991;179:829-832.
16. Sironi S, Colombo E, Villa G, et al: Myometrial invasion by endometrial carcinoma: Assessment with plain and gadolinium-enhanced MR imaging. Radiology 1992;185:207-212.
17. Kim SH, Kim HD, Song YS, et al: Detection of deep myometrial invasion in endometrial carcinoma: Comparison of transvaginal ultrasound, CT, and MRI. J Comput Assist Tomogr 1995;19:766-772.
18. Seki H, Kimura M, Sakai K: Myometrial invasion of endometrial carcinoma: Assessment with dynamic MR and contrast-enhanced T1-weighted images. Clin Radiol 1997;52:18-23.
19. Hricak H, Hamm B, Semelka RC, et al: Carcinoma of the uterus: Use of gadopentetate dimeglumine in MR imaging. Radiology 1991;181:95-106.
20. Ito K, Matsumoto T, Nakada T, et al: Assessing myometrial invasion by endometrial carcinoma with dynamic MRI. J Comput Assist Tomogr 1994;18:77-86.
21. Seki H, Takano T, Sakai K: Value of dynamic MR imaging in assessing endometrial carcinoma involvement of the cervix. AJR Am J Roentgenol 2000;175:171-176.
22. Hardesty LA, Sumkin JH, Nath ME, et al: Use of preoperative MR imaging in the management of endometrial carcinoma: Cost analysis. Radiology 2000;215:45-49.

23. Nicolet V, Carignan L, Bourdon F, Prosmanne O: MR imaging of cervical carcinoma: A practical staging approach. Radiographics 2000;20:1539-1549.
24. Young RC, Perez CA, Hoskins WJ: Cancer of the ovary. In DeVita VT Jr, Hellman S, Rosenberg SA (eds): Cancer: Principles and Practice of Oncology, 4th ed. Philadelphia, JB Lippincott, 1993, pp 1226-1261.
25. Pannu H, Corl F, Fishman E: CT evaluation of cervical cancer: Spectrum of disease. Radiographics 2001;21:1155-1168.
26. Kamura T, Tsukamoto N, Tsuruchi N, et al: Multivariate analysis of the histopathologic prognostic factors of cervical cancer in patients undergoing radical hysterectomy. Cancer 1992;69: 181-186.
27. Montana GS, Hanlon AL, Brickner TJ, et al: Carcinoma of the cervix: Patterns of care studies—Review of 1978, 1983, and 1988-1989 surveys. Int J Radiat Oncol Biol Phys 1995;32:1481-1486.
28. Okuno K, Joja I, Miyagi Y, et al: Cervical carcinoma with full-thickness stromal invasion: Relationship between tumor size on T2-weighted images and parametrial involvement. J Comput Assist Tomogr 2002;26:119-125.
29. Lien HH, Blomlie V, Iversen T, et al: Clinical stage I carcinoma of the cervix: Value of MR imaging in determining invasion into the parametrium. Acta Radiol 1993;34:130-132.
30. Subak LL, Hricak H, Powell CB, et al: Cervical carcinoma: Computed tomography and magnetic resonance imaging for preoperative staging. Obstet Gynecol 1995;86:43-50.
31. Kim SH, Han MC: Invasion of the urinary bladder by uterine cervical carcinoma: Evaluation with MR imaging. AJR Am J Roentgenol 1997;168:393-397.
32. Cobby M, Browning J, Jones A, et al: Magnetic resonance imaging, computed tomography and endosonography in the local staging of carcinoma of the cervix. Br J Radiol 1990;63:673-679.
33. Scheidler J, Hricak H, Yu KK, et al: Radiological evaluation of lymph node metastases in patients with cervical cancer: A meta-analysis. JAMA 1997;278:1096-1101.
34. Yang WT, Lam WW, Yu MY, et al: Comparison of dynamic helical CT and dynamic MR imaging in the evaluation of pelvic lymph nodes in cervical carcinoma. AJR Am J Roentgenol 2000;175: 759-766.
35. Kim SH, Choi BI, Han JK, et al: Preoperative staging of uterine cervical carcinoma: Comparison of CT and MRI in 99 patients. J Comput Assist Tomogr 1993;17:633-640.
36. Roy C, Le Bras Y, Mangold L, et al: Small pelvic lymph node metastases: Evaluation with MR imaging. Clin Radiol 1997;52: 437-440.
37. Grigsby PW, Siegel BA, Dehdashti F: Lymph node staging by positron emission tomography in patients with carcinoma of the cervix. J Clin Oncol 2001;19:3745-3749.
38. Malyapa RS, Mutic S, Low DA, et al: Physiologic FDG-PET three-dimensional brachytherapy treatment planning for cervical cancer. Int J Radiat Oncol Biol Phys 2002;54:1140-1146.
39. Hricak H, Powell CB, Yu KK, et al: Invasive cervical carcinoma: Role of MR imaging in pretreatment work-up-cost minimization and diagnostic efficacy analysis. Radiology 1996;198: 403-409.
40. McGowan L, Lesher LP, Norris HJ, et al: Missstaging of ovarian cancer. Obstet Gynecol 1985;65:568-572.
41. Munoz KA, Harlan LC, Trimble EL: Patterns of care for women with ovarian cancer in the United States. J Clin Oncol 1997; 15:3408-3415.
42. Barakat RR, Hricak H: What do we expect from imaging? [review]. Radiol Clin North Am 2002;40:521-526, vii.
43. Hoskins WJ: Surgical staging and cytoreductive surgery of epithelial ovarian cancer. Cancer 1993;71:1534-1540.
44. Curtin JP, Malik R, Venkatraman ES, et al: Stage IV ovarian cancer: Impact of surgical debulking. Gynecol Oncol 1997;64:9-12.
45. International Federation of Obstetrics and Gynecology: Annual report on the results of treatment in gynecological cancer. Int J Gynecol Obstet 1989;28:189-190.
46. Schwartz PE, Rutherford TJ, Chambers JT, et al: Neoadjuvant chemotherapy for advanced ovarian cancer: Long-term survival. Gynecol Oncol 1999;72:93-99.
47. Vergote I, De Wever I, Tjalma W, et al: Neoadjuvant chemotherapy or primary debulking surgery in advanced ovarian carcinoma: a retrospective analysis of 285 patients. Gynecol Oncol 1998;71:431-436.
48. Heintz APM, Hacker NF, Berek JS, et al: Cytoreductive surgery in ovarian carcinoma: Feasibility and morbidity. Obstet Gynecol 1986;67:783-788.
49. Coakley FV: Staging ovarian cancer: Role of imaging [review]. Radiol Clin North Am 2002;40:609-636.
50. Fostner R, Hricak H, Occhipinti KA, et al: Ovarian cancer: Staging with CT and MR Imaging. Radiology 1995;197: 619-626.
51. Byrom J, Widjaja E, Redman CW, et al: Can pre-operative computed tomography predict resectability of ovarian carcinoma at primary laparotomy? Br J Obstet Gynecol 2002;109:369-375.
52. Nelson BE, Rosenfield AT, Schwartz PE: Preoperative abdominopelvic computed tomographic prediction of optimal cytoreduction in epithelial ovarian carcinoma. J Clin Oncol 1993;11:166-172.
53. Meyer JI, Kennedy AW, Friedman R, et al: Ovarian carcinoma: Value of CT in predicting success of debulking surgery. AJR Am J Roentgenol 1995;165:875-878.
54. Boente MP, Chi DS, Hoskins WJ: The role of surgery in the management of ovarian cancer: Primary and interval cytoreductive surgery. Semin Oncol 1998;25:326-334.
55. Kinkel K, Hricak H, Ying Lu, et al: US characterization of ovarian masses: A meta-analysis. Radiology 2000;217:803-811.
56. Cohen LS, Escobar PF, Scharm C, et al: Three-dimensional power Doppler ultrasound improves the diagnostic accuracy for ovarian cancer prediction. Gynecol Oncol 2001;82:40-48.
57. Kurjak A, Kupesic S, Anic T, Kosuta D: Three-dimensional ultrasound and power Doppler improve the diagnosis of ovarian lesions. Gynecol Oncol 2000;76:28-32.
58. Yamashita Y, Torashima M, Hatanaka Y, et al: Adnexal masses: Accuracy of characterization with transvaginal US and precontrast and postcontrast MR imaging. Radiology 1995;194:557-565.
59. Rieber A, Nussie K, Stohr I, et al: Preoperative diagnosis of ovarian tumors with MR imaging: Comparison with transvaginal sonography, positron emission tomography, and histologic findings. AJR Am J Roentgenol 2001;177:123-129.
60. Hricak H, Chen M, Coakley FV, et al: Complex adnexal masses: Detection and characterization by MR imaging- multivariate analysis. Radiology 2000;214:39-46.
61. Brown DL, Zou KH, Tempany CM, et al: Primary versus secondary ovarian malignancy: Imaging findings of adnexal masses in the Radiology Diagnostic Oncology Group Study. Radiology 2001;219:213-218.
62. Huber S, Medl M, Baumann L, Czembirek H: Value of ultrasound and magnetic resonance imaging in the preoperative evaluation of suspected ovarian masses. Anticancer Res 2002; 22:2501-2507.
63. Stevens SK, Hricak H, Stern JL: Ovarian lesions: Detection and characterization with gadolinium-enhanced MR imaging at 1.5 T. Radiology 1991;181:481-488.
64. Altman CF, Travis AFB, Feller JF: MR imaging of sonographically indeterminate adnexal masses. Radiology 1995;197:354.
65. Schwartz LB, Panageas E, Lange R, et al: Female pelvis: Impact of MR imaging on treatment decisions and net cost analysis. Radiology 1994;192:55-60.
66. Fenchel S, Grab D, Nuessle K, et al: Asymptomatic adnexal masses: Correlation of FDG PET and histopathologic findings. Radiology 2002;223:780-788.
67. Tempany CM, Zou KH, Silverman SG, et al: Staging of advanced ovarian cancer: Comparison of imaging modalities. Report from the Radiological Diagnostic Oncology Group. Radiology 2000; 215:761-767.
68. Holloway BJ, Gore ME, A'Hern RP, Parsons C: The significance of paracardiac lymph node enlargement in ovarian cancer. Clin Radiol 1997;52:692-697.
69. Dvoretsky PM, Richards KA, Angel C, et al: Distribution of disease at autopsy in 100 women with ovarian cancer. Hum Pathol 1988;19:57-63.
70. Coakley FV, Choi PH, Gougoutas CA, et al: Peritoneal metastases: Detection with spiral CT in patients with ovarian cancer. Radiology 2002;223:495-499.
71. Prayer L, Kainz C, Kramer J, et al: CT and MR accuracy in the detection of tumor recurrence in patients treated for ovarian cancer. J Comput Assist Tomogr 1993;17:626-632.
72. Funt S, Hricak H, Ruustum N, et al: Recurrent ovarian cancer: Role of CT scan in patient management. AJR (in press).

73. Sella T, Rosenbaum E, Edelmann DZ, et al: Value of chest CT scans in routine ovarian carcinoma follow-up. AJR Am J Roentgenol 2001;177:857-859.

74. Dachman AH, Visweswaran A, Battula R, et al: Role of chest CT in the follow-up of ovarian adenocarcinoma. AJR Am J Roentgenol 2001;176:701-705.

75. Rose PG: Surgery for recurrent ovarian cancer. Semin Oncol 2000;27(3 Suppl 7):17-23.

76. Chi DS, Liao JB, Leon LF, et al: Identification of prognostic factors in advanced epithelial ovarian carcinoma. Gynecol Oncol 2001;82:532-537.

77. Eisenkop SM, Friedman RL, Wang HJ: Complete cytoreductive surgery is feasible and maximizes survival in patients with advanced epithelial ovarian carcinoma: A retrospective study. Gynecol Oncol 1998;69:103-108.

INDEX

Note: Page numbers followed by f refer to figures; page numbers followed by t refer to tables.